SKILLS FOR PROFESSIONAL NURSING PRACTICE

BARBARA A. NORTON, B.S., M.P.H, R.N.
Associate Professor
Indiana University School of Nursing
Indianapolis, Indiana

ANNA M. MILLER, B.S.N., M.S.N., R.N.
Assistant Professor
DePauw University School of Nursing
Greencastle, Indiana

SKILLS FOR PROFESSIONAL NURSING PRACTICE

COMMUNICATION, PHYSICAL APPRAISAL, AND CLINICAL TECHNIQUES

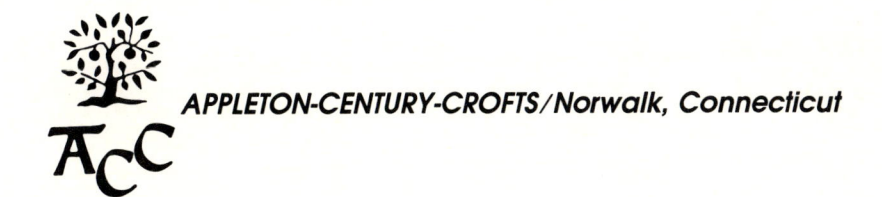

APPLETON-CENTURY-CROFTS/Norwalk, Connecticut

0-8385-8565-5

Notice: Our knowledge in clinical sciences is constantly changing. As new information becomes available, changes in treatment and in the use of drugs become necessary. The authors and the publisher of this volume have taken care to make certain that the doses of drugs and schedules of treatment are correct and compatible with the standards generally accepted at the time of publication. The reader is advised to consult carefully the instruction and information material included in the package insert of each drug or therapeutic agent before administration. This advice is especially important when using new or infrequently used drugs.

Copyright © 1986 by Appleton-Century-Crofts
A Publishing Division of Prentice-Hall, Inc.

All rights reserved. This book, or any parts thereof, may not be used or reproduced in any manner without written permission except for all Performance Checklists and Table 6–1, "Guide for Observing Nonverbal Behaviors." For information, address Appleton-Century-Crofts, 25 Van Zant Street, East Norwalk, Connecticut 06855.

86 87 88 89 / 10 9 8 7 6 5 4 3 2 1

Prentice-Hall of Australia, Pty. Ltd., Sydney
Prentice-Hall Canada, Inc.
Prentice-Hall Hispanoamericana, S.A., Mexico
Prentice-Hall of India Private Limited, New Delhi
Prentice-Hall International (UK) Limited, London
Prentice-Hall of Japan, Inc., Tokyo
Prentice-Hall of Southeast Asia (Pte.) Ltd., Singapore
Whitehall Books Ltd., Wellington, New Zealand
Editora Prentice-Hall do Brasil Ltda., Rio de Janeiro

Library of Congress Cataloging-in-Publication Data
Norton, Barbara A.
   Skills for professional nursing practice.

   Includes index.
   1. Nurse and client. 2. Interpersonal relations.
3. Medicine, Clinical.   I. Miller, Anna M. II. Title.
[DNLM: 1. Communication. 2. Nurse-Patient Relations.
3. Nursing Process. WY 100 N882s]
RT86.3.N67   1986   610.73′0699   85-26808

ISBN 0-8385-8565-5

Design: Jean M. Sabato-Morley

PRINTED IN THE UNITED STATES OF AMERICA

CONTENTS

Preface / ix

Acknowledgments / xi

General Organization of the Text / xvii

How to Use This Book / xix

PART ONE Professional Communication Skills / 1

☐ CHAPTER 1
Awareness of Self in the Helping Relationship　　　　　7

Skill 1 The Helping Relationship / 8
　　　 2 Knowing Ourselves / 17
　　　 3 Needs Identification / 24
　　　 4 Values Identification / 30
　　　 5 Self-Disclosure / 36

☐ CHAPTER 2
Communication Through Nonverbal Channels　　　　　45

Skill 6 Understanding Nonverbal Behavior / 46
　　　 7 Time and Silence / 55
　　　 8 Space and Touch / 60

☐ CHAPTER 3
Facilitative Communication Skills　　　　　69

Skill 9 Attending Behavior / 70
　　　10 Attentive Listening / 74
　　　11 Reflection of Content / 79
　　　12 Reflection of Feelings / 85
　　　13 Questioning / 91
　　　14 Offering Assistance / 97

CHAPTER 4
Structured Nurse-Client Interactions 107

Skill **15** Interviewing / 108
　　　16 Teaching-Learning / 126

CHAPTER 5
Written Communication 141

Skill **17** Using the Health Record / 141
　　　18 Nursing Records / 148

PART TWO *Professional Clinical Nursing Skills* / 165

CHAPTER 6
Physical Appraisal Skills 169

Skill **19** Inspection / 169
　　　20 Palpation / 171
　　　21 Percussion / 173
　　　22 Auscultation / 177

CHAPTER 7
Common Techniques for Measuring Health Status 181

Skill **23** Temperature Appraisal / 182
　　　24 Pulse Appraisal / 194
　　　25 Respiration Appraisal / 205
　　　26 Blood Pressure Appraisal / 210
　　　27 Height and Weight Appraisal / 223

CHAPTER 8
Medical Asepsis 239

Skill **28** Handwashing / 241
　　　29 Isolation Techniques / 248

CHAPTER 9
Surgical Asepsis 267

Skill **30** Sterile Supplies / 268
　　　31 Donning Sterile Gloves / 286
　　　32 Dressings and Wound Care / 292
　　　33 Suture Removal / 311
　　　34 Wound Culture Specimen Collection / 318
　　　35 Wound Drains and Irrigations / 328
　　　36 Wet Sterile Dressings / 343
　　　37 Wet-to-Dry Dressings / 351

CHAPTER 10
Personal Hygiene 357

Skill 38 Skin Care / 358
   39 Perineal Care / 372
   40 Oral Care / 383
   41 Hair Care / 397
   42 Nail Care / 406
   43 Vaginal Irrigation / 411
   44 Breast Examination / 417
   45 Care of the Corpse / 425

CHAPTER 11
Supportive and Protective Treatments 433

Skill 46 Thermal Applications / 433
   47 Massage / 446
   48 Applying Bandages and Binders / 453
   49 Mechanical Restraints / 464
   50 Cast Care / 473

CHAPTER 12
Nutritional Care 481

Skill 51 Monitoring Fluid Balance / 482
   52 Nutritional Assessment and the Serving of Food / 499
   53 Assistance with Eating / 515
   54 Enteral Nutritional Support / 527
   55 Total Parenteral Nutrition / 546

CHAPTER 13
Elimination Assistance 561

Skill 56 Insertion and Care of Gastrointestinal Tubes / 562
   57 Bedpans and Urinals / 588
   58 Bowel Elimination Procedures / 605
   59 Urinary Incontinence Care / 620
   60 Urinary Catheterization / 629
   61 Ostomy Care / 658

CHAPTER 14
Mobility Assistance 685

Skill 62 Assistance with Ambulation / 691
   63 Maintenance of Range of Motion / 704
   64 Turning, Moving, and Positioning / 717
   65 Transfer Activities / 744
   66 Bed Making Procedures / 757

CHAPTER 15
Respiratory Care 773

Skill 67 Chest Therapy Exercises / 774
   68 Oxygen Therapy / 785

69 Tracheostomy Care / *799*
70 Suctioning the Airway / *815*

☐ CHAPTER 16
Medication Administration   **827**

Skill **71** Oral Medication Administration / *847*
       72 Topical Medication Administration / *865*
       73 Injectable Medication Administration / *890*
       74 Intravenous Fluid and Medication Administration / *928*

☐ CHAPTER 17
Emergency Techniques   **969**

Skill **75** Cardiopulmonary Resuscitation / *971*
       76 Removal of Airway Obstruction / *988*

Appendix I Keys to Chapter Entry Tests / *999*

Appendix II Keys to Learning Activities / *1013*

Index / *1017*

PREFACE

This book is written for students and graduate nurses who are committed to the practice of nursing as professional persons. The book evolved from the authors' work in baccalaureate curriculum development, interactions with academic peers and colleagues on clinical units, and from teaching students in the classroom, laboratory, and clinical units. These experiences provide the basis for our belief that clinical practice must incorporate findings from nursing research and other disciplines in addition to using principles from the biologic and social sciences.

Communication and psychomotor skills are combined in this text to represent a blending of technology with holism and caring. All of the skills in this book are developed within the context of client care, rather than as separate tasks to be implemented. Skills in professional nursing practice are implemented as part of an overall goal for the client; they are executed and evaluated as an integral part of the therapeutic regime in relation to the goals established with the client, not as a separate entity. The format of the book reflects the value of psychomotor skills as an integral and significant portion of nursing practice. Psychomotor skills are valued by the consumer and often serve as the context in which assessment and communication skills are used. The inclusion of interpersonal and recording skills in a basic book reflects the authors' belief that those skills are equally important to psychomotor skills.

Physical appraisal skills are presented within the context of clinical practice rather than as skills reserved for an expanded nurse role since these skills are now accepted as an integral part of nursing practice. The data base for each psychomotor skill identifies subjective and objective data that would be gathered from multiple sources using various techniques for both skill preparation and implementation. These data serve as the basis for making accurate nursing assessments and developing relevant evaluation criteria.

The design used in this text was conceived by the authors to meet students' demonstrated need to have a knowledge base for developing clinical practice skills that meet professional standards and facilitate their application of the nursing process. Professional standards require that the nurse possess knowledge and understanding of why, when, and how each skill is performed. The nurse as a student or as a graduate is accountable and responsible for his or her own actions. To learn and use these skills appropriately in nursing practice, a nurse must know the available scientific evidence that supports the practices and techniques which are an integral part of the skill and its execution. If professional standards of nursing practice are to be met, the rational basis for nursing activities must be continually and critically examined and modified to be consistent with research findings.

Rote learning and the development of habitual behaviors are of limited value if a nurse's practice is to meet the expectations of an informed society for quality nursing care. To be usable, skill learning must be established to the point where it functions as needed. The automaticity of a skill increases its efficiency but decreases its effectiveness if the performer is unable to adapt the skill appropriately to different and varying complex situations. Adaptation requires an increase in thought and judgment. Learning a skill and being capable of adapting any skill to meet varying situations moves the automatic skill to a conceptual skill. This is the ultimate goal of a professional person. Skills are part of the self; how they are learned and how they are applied in practice relates to how the self is perceived as a therapeutic agent. A person approaches a skill as an integrated being and skill learning requires that the learner engage in thinking, feeling, and moving behaviors. Each type of skill in this book requires different combinations of these behaviors. As the student progresses through the various nursing skills, he or she will become aware of the interplay of these behaviors and their significance to the learning process.

ACKNOWLEDGMENTS

There is no senior author for this book, both authors have collaborated on its development, reviewed and critiqued all of the work in this book. Thus, this book represents the joint commitment of two persons to a common goal.

The authors wish to express their sincere appreciation to all of those persons, agencies, and manufacturers of health-care products who made significant contributions in making this book a reality.

☐ CONTRIBUTORS

Nancy Hess Bishop, B.S.N., R.N., CCRN
  Venice Hospital, Venice, Florida
  Author of the cardiopulmonary resuscitation and removal of airway obstruction skills.

Melissa R. Ganza, B.S.N., M.S.N., R.N.
  Assistant Professor, Indiana Central University, Indianapolis
  Author of the intravenous fluid and medication administration skill.

CONSULTANTS AND MANUSCRIPT REVIEWERS

Cheryl Boucher, O.T.R.
  Occupational therapist, Staff Builders Home Health Care, Indianapolis

Mary A. Carder, R.D., M.S.
  Program Director, Dietetic Internship, Methodist Hospital of Indiana, Inc., Indianapolis, and part-time Instructor, DePauw University, Greencastle and Indianapolis

Carole A. Gartner, B.S.N., M.S.N., R.N.
  Former Nutritional Support Clinical Specialist, Methodist Hospital of Indiana, Inc., Indianapolis

Richard F. Graffis, M.D.
  General Surgeon, Indianapolis

Pamela J. Houchens, E.T., R.N.
  Supervisor, Enterostomal Therapy Department, Methodist Hospital of Indiana, Inc., Indianapolis

Virginia Kummer, B.S.N., R.N., R.P.T.
  Former physical therapist with Merrill A. Ritter, M.D., Orthopedic surgeon, Indianapolis

Douglas L. Miller, B.S.
  Computer scientist, Naval Avionics Center, Indianapolis

James N. Miller, M.S.W., ACSW
  President, Family Service Association, Indianapolis

Rebecca D. Neal, B.S.N., R.N.
   Staff nurse, Methodist Hospital of Indiana, Inc., Indianapolis
Evelyn Oldsen, B.A., M.S.
   Associate Professor of Dental Auxillary Education and Director of Dental Hygiene Program, Indiana University, School of Dentistry, Indianapolis
M. Jean Steiner, R.N.
   Director, Infection Control, Wishard Memorial Hospital, Indianapolis
Anne E. Ward, E.T., R.N.
   Former Supervisor, Enterostomal Therapy Department, Methodist Hospital of Indiana, Inc., Indianapolis
Barbara J. Wilder, B.A.
   Former Infection Control Coordinator, Methodist Hospital of Indiana, Inc., Indianapolis

MANUSCRIPT REVIEWERS

The authors are particularly indebted to

Ruth Harboe, M.S., R.N.
   University of Colorado School of Nursing who reviewed almost the entire manuscript and made numerous valuable suggestions.

Other reviewers who provided helpful critiques for portions of the manuscript include:

Marcia E. Blicharz, M.S.N., R.N.
   Trenton State University, Trenton, New Jersey
Jean Bradley, Ph.D.
   University of Illinois, Chicago
Marguerite Casey, M.S.N., R.N.
   Assistant Professor, Indiana University School of Nursing, Indianapolis
William Gillette, D.D.S.
   Assistant Chief of Dental Services, Richard L. Roudebush Veterans Administration Hospital, Indianapolis
Susan Gottschalk, B.S., R.N.
   Former Manager of Infection Control, St. Vincent Hospital and Health Care Center, Indianapolis
Carl Graves, Jr., Ph.D., R.N.
   University of Texas, Houston
Mary Louise Haben
   St. Johns Hospital, Detroit, Michigan
Teresa J. Hudspeth, B.S.N., R.N.
   Patient Care Manager, Methodist Hospital of Indiana, Inc., Indianapolis
Jean Hutten, M.S.N.Ed., R.N.
   Associate Professor, Indiana University School of Nursing, Indianapolis
Carol Kammer, M.S.N., Ed.D., R.N.
   Associate Professor, Indiana University School of Nursing, Indianapolis
Leigh Kasyk, M.S.N., R.N.
   Nurse Specialist, Penrose Cancer Hospital, Colorado Springs, Colorado
Theresa A. Kessler, B.S., M.S.N., R.N.
   Assistant Professor, DePauw University School of Nursing, Greencastle and Indianapolis
Barbara A. Killila, B.S.N., R.N.
   Former Patient Care Manager, Methodist Hospital of Indiana, Inc., Indianapolis
Gayle Lawrence, B.S.N., M.S.N., R.N.
   Unit Director Indiana University Hospitals, Indianapolis
Flora Meiseheimer
   California State University, Long Beach, California
John S. Mikesell, M.T.
   I.V. Team Supervisor, Methodist Hospital of Indiana, Inc., Indianapolis

Carol Montoya, M.Ed., R.N.
 Staff Development Coordinator, Medical Nursing, Indiana University Hospitals, Indianapolis
Peter J. Parashoes, Pharm.D.
 Clinical Pharmacist, Oncology/Nutritional Support, Methodist Hospital of Indiana, Inc., Indianapolis
Barbara Resler, M.S.N., R.N.
 Former Assistant Professor, Indiana University School of Nursing, Indianapolis
Beverly Ross, M.S., R.N.
 Assistant Professor, Indiana University School of Nursing, Indianapolis
Mary Ann Scharf, M.S.N., Ph.D
 Seton Hall, Seton Hall University, South Orange, New Jersey
Richard Smith, D.D.S.
 Chief of Dental Services, Richard L. Roudebush Veterans Administration Hospital, Indianapolis
Sherry Smith, B.S.N., M.S.N., Ed.D., R.N.
 Director, DePauw University School of Nursing, Greencastle and Indianapolis
Teresa Smith, M.S.N., R.N.
 Assistant Professor, Indiana University School of Nursing, Indianapolis
Davis R. Steup, R.Ph.
 Indianapolis
Ann Talley, B.S.N.
 Unit Director, Indiana University Hospitals, Indianapolis
Doris Toney, R.N.
 Former Patient Care Coordinator, Winona Memorial Hospital, Indianapolis
Kathleen Vorholt, M.S.N., R.N.
 Former Assistant Professor, Indiana University School of Nursing, Indianapolis

In addition the authors wish to recognize the following for their support and contributions:

DePauw University for released time and financial aid.
Ann Marriner, Ph.D., R.N.
 Former Associate Dean, Baccalaureate Program, Indiana University School of Nursing, Indianapolis
Stanley D. Miller
 Student Journalist, Indiana University, Indianapolis
Lana C. Phillips, B.S.
 Department Head, Supply, Processing and Distribution, Methodist Hospital of Indiana, Inc., Indianapolis, for assistance in finding information about equipment and supplies.
Staff, supervisors, and **administrators** of Indiana University Hospitals, Methodist Hospital of Indiana, Inc., and Winona Memorial Hospital, Indianapolis, for their support and assistance.
Students, faculty, and **graduates** of DePauw University School of Nursing for their support and for serving as photography subjects.
Ann Van Camp, M.L.S.
 Director of Information and Online Services, Indiana University School of Medicine Library, Indianapolis, for numerous computer searches for literature and audiovisual resources.

We also wish to express our appreciation to

Charles Bowers for illustrations
James Haines for photography
Carol Hash, Marla Riggan, and **Deborah Thompson** for their fast and accurate typing

In addition we wish to recognize the following persons from Appleton-Century-Crofts who have worked closely with us in various capacities during the duration of this project.

John Allison, former Executive Editor
Karen Emilson, former Editor
Marion Kalstein-Welch, Executive Editor, Nursing
Robin Millay, Associate Managing Editor
Lisa Pinto, Developmental Editor
Terry Sternberg, former Developmental Editor

*In appreciation and with love to our husbands,
Kenneth Hamilton and Jim Miller.*

GENERAL ORGANIZATION OF THE TEXT

This text is divided into two parts, an introduction sets the tone for each part. Both parts follow the general organization described here. Differences between the organization of Part One and Part Two are described below.

Part One is devoted to the cognitive and affective aspects of verbal, non-verbal, and written communication skills. Part Two concentrates on psychomotor skills which are often referred to as clinical techniques. Each chapter of the text begins with an *Introduction* which includes basic concepts and background information relevant to all of the skills included in each chapter and concludes with the titles of all of the skills. The general model for each skill included in the text is designed with major sections presented in the following sequence: *Student Objectives* provide a focus for the student's study; an *Introduction* addresses the purpose of the skill; *Preparation* contains content that enables the student to make appropriate nursing judgments about skill implementation; *Execution* addresses some specific aspects of the skill implementation; *Critical Points Summary* highlights the major points the student should learn; *Learning Activities* provide the student with experiential learning; *Review Questions* based on objectives permit the self-evaluation on the content; *References* are those cited within the skill; *Bibliography* includes supplementary material used by the authors; *Suggested Readings* are those a student may find particularly helpful; and *Audiovisual Resources* demonstrate either specific aspects of the skill or the entire skill.

☐ PART ONE

The skills in Chapters 1 through 4 focus on elements inherent to the helping relationship and the use of basic communication skills. Skills in these chapters are designed to be used in the sequence in which they are presented because the skills build upon one another. In this part the learning activities are interspersed throughout each skill. It is important that the student engage in each learning activity before progressing on to the next aspect of the skill. Performance checklists for evaluation of skill achievement are included in selected skills. Chapter 5, which focuses on written communication, may be used at any time deemed appropriate by the instructor.

☐ PART TWO

The chapter introductions in Part Two, "Professional Clinical Nursing Skills," differ from those in Part One in that each introduction concludes with an entry level test on prerequisite knowledge from the biologic sciences that the student is expected to know as a minimal basis for learning each skill. A key is provided in the appendices for the student to validate his or her responses. The information contained in each of the keys is intended to serve as a resource to help the student recall previously learned content; it is not intended to be a substitute for all of the content included in the prerequisite biologic sciences courses a student is required to take in a nursing education program. The student may find it beneficial to use additional texts to enlarge his or her basic knowledge.

Each skill in Part Two begins with a list of prerequisite skills for which the student is expected to demonstrate competency before beginning that particular skill. In a few skills these prerequisite learnings include content from a specific chapter introduction. The Preparation section is modified to include additional subsections. *Data Base* identifies subjective and objective data that the student needs to obtain as a basis for deciding whether or not to execute the skill and for evaluating the outcome of the implemented skill. The pertinent data are identified and categorized according to the sources from which they are obtained. These subsections include *Client History and Recorded Data* and *Physical Appraisal Skills.* An additional subsection, *Equipment,* describes the types of equipment and supply items needed to implement the skill. In the Execution section, *Skill Sequences* provide a step by step procedure for the skill implementation and include an accompanying rationale for each step which is drawn from the content presented previously. The last section included in the Execution section is *Recording;* this subsection presents two methods of recording, the problem oriented recording and the narrative recording method. The same examples are used for each method to provide models for recording in both systems. Learning activities are grouped together near the conclusion of each skill.

TO THE STUDENT: HOW TO USE THIS BOOK

This book is designed to help you learn the following three types of professional nursing practice skills:

1. Communication: basic communication skills, interviewing, client teaching, and recording;
2. Physical appraisal skills: inspection, palpation, percussion and auscultation as entities themselves and as they are used within the context of other clinical techniques;
3. Traditional clinical nursing techniques.

Within the context of learning all of these skills you will be engaging your total person, that is to say, you will be using your intellectual abilities (cognitive), your emotional responses (affective), and your fine and gross motor (psychomotor) abilities. The content, sequence, and method of presentation have been selected to permit you to assume a great deal of responsibility for your own learning, which is an expectation of a professional person.

Learning the proper technique used for any skill takes time, practice, and patience to acquire a minimum level of competence that you need to be able to use the skills. As is true for all skill development, spaced and consistent practice is essential for anyone learning a skill. When learning a skill, it is important to validate your performance with more experienced nurse practitioners. Frequent practice and validation help to develop good technique which gives you a sense of confidence in your performance.

The authors believe that skill and comfort with the ability to communicate clearly and efficiently is an essential part of any helping person's professional practice. We suggest that you begin your course of study with Part One, Chapters 1 through 4, learning the skills in the sequence presented.

Upon completion of Part One, we suggest that you concentrate on learning and demonstrating competence in handwashing, Skill 28. This skill is used consistently before and after any contact with a client so it is wise to develop competence in it before attempting to progress to other skills. Next, we suggest that you concentrate on the skills in Chapter 6 because they also are an integral part of all subsequent skills. All other skills may be approached in whatever sequence is appropriate.

TO USE THIS BOOK WE SUGGEST THAT YOU

1. Carefully read the chapter introduction, answer the entry test questions and then validate your responses with the key provided in the Appendix One. Seek out additional resources according to your own needs.

2. Review the prerequisite skills listed for the skill you are going to study. In the event that you have not demonstrated competency in the prerequisite skills, proceed to do so before attempting to learn the skill you had intended to study.
3. Study the objectives so that you have a good sense of what you are expected to achieve by the end of the skill.
4. Concentrate on the content included in the skill, progressing through all of it in the sequence in which it is presented.
5. Carefully examine the illustrations pertinent to the content.
6. Participate in each of the learning activities as directed in each skill. Practice the skill sequences using available manikins and peers in a simulated setting such as a learning laboratory.
7. Use the critical points summary to reinforce your learning.
8. Answer the review questions on a separate sheet of paper. Compare your responses with peers and then validate your responses with your instructor. Review and study those areas in which you demonstrate a weakness.
9. Have a peer use the performance checklist to evaluate your skill performance. If necessary modify your skill execution to meet the performance criteria.
10. Use available consultants such as the course or laboratory instructor to clarify content areas and improve your technique.

NOTE:

Permission is granted to the user of this text to copy the following: all performance checklists and Table 6-1, "Guide for Observing Nonverbal Behaviors."

SKILLS FOR PROFESSIONAL NURSING PRACTICE

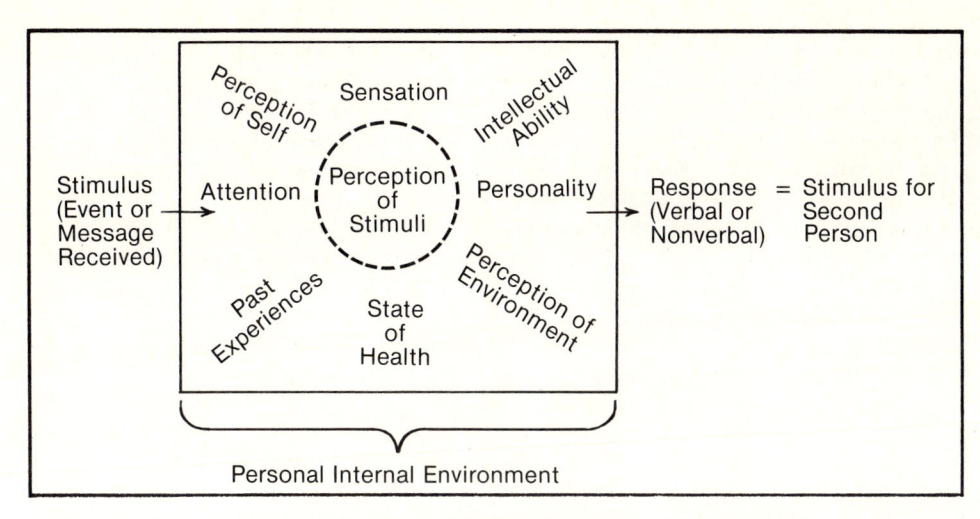

Figure 1. Intrapersonal and interpersonal communications model. The response of one person becomes the stimulus for the second person. (Adapted from Pluckhan ML: Human Communication: The Matrix of Nursing. New York, McGraw-Hill, 1978, with permission.)

person needs to pay attention to it. A person's past experiences, personality, perceptions of self and environment, intellectual ability, and state of health—all have an impact on how that person perceives this stimulus. A person's response flows from this perception and in turn becomes a stimulus for the person with whom he or she is communicating. The second person responds on the basis of his or her own unique combination of internal factors; therefore, the communications model becomes *inter*personal.

According to Satir (1967), communication occurs at both the denotative and metacommunication levels. Denotative communication refers to the literal verbal content of a message, while metacommunication refers to messages *about* that verbal message. Metacommunication occurs through the context in which something is said and through the nonverbal behaviors that always accompany the spoken message. Metacommunication also can be verbal when the speaker comments on or explains the verbal message, such as by saying "I was only trying to make you laugh," or "I thought you were angry with me and I wanted to explain what I meant." When communication is clear, this metacommunication is congruent with, or fits, the literal verbal content of the message.

In any interpersonal relationship, stimuli are given and perceived at both the denotative and metacommunication levels. Developing effective communication skills involves learning to recognize both of these levels in our own and others' responses to stimuli. It also means learning to increase the helpful nature of our own responses to those with whom we interact.

LEARNING COMMUNICATION SKILLS

Pluckhan (1978) indicates that communication skills are best learned experientially, and that effective communication cannot be learned except through interactions with others. She reports a study involving senior student nurses who studied a series of 10 lessons in interpersonal relationships, working in dyads and interacting in pairs. Retention testing 11 weeks after the sessions ended revealed a 92 percent retention, much greater than from conventional didactic methods.

While it takes a lot of time, thought, energy, and a fair degree of insight to develop effective communication skills, once these skills are learned, they will always be part of the nurse's repertoire of skills (Blondis and Jackson, 1977). Communication skills involved in working with people on a one-to-one basis are useful in all areas of human service and are particularly relevant for the development and maintenance of the helping relationship that characterizes nurse–client interactions. The learning activities for many of the skills in Part

One are highly interactional and experiential, with no right and wrong answers. Since effective learning requires knowledge of the outcome of the learning activity (Combs et al., 1971), it is important that the student receive a reaction (feedback) from someone else about his or her use of the learning activities. Receiving feedback helps a person evaluate his or her own behavior from someone else's viewpoint, and makes it possible to modify ineffective behavior or reinforce effective behavior. Giving feedback to someone else helps a person learn to observe, listen, evaluate behaviors, and contribute to someone else's growth and learning—all of which are parts of a helping relationship.

Feedback is helpful when given in a way that the receiver both understands and is able to accept. It has been found to be more effective if given soon after the incident or exchange has occurred (Brammer, 1979; Clift, 1981; Combs et al., 1971; Finley et al., 1979). Feedback is best when given in concise, nontechnical language, in small amounts, and when it includes only observed behaviors. Helpful feedback does not include bringing up past behaviors or unfinished emotional business. Leveling responses and I-messages (as discussed in Skill 5) are important skills in giving feedback, because they focus on specific and observable behaviors and are nonthreatening and impersonal in nature. Feedback is nonhelpful and counterproductive when it focuses on personality, character, and physical traits or when it contains value judgments and moralizations.

During practice sessions and simulated sessions presented in the following skills, the student is often asked to validate his or her experiences or communication responses with other students. This validation is a form of feedback in which a person compares perceptions and experiences with others, checks the accuracy of his or her communication, or verifies that the skill has been used correctly.

Because of the experiential nature of the learning activities in Part One, it is important for the student to participate fully in the activities in an open and honest manner. It also is important to respect the individuality, integrity, and personality of other students so that each student's self-worth is enhanced and growth is permitted to take place. The skills and learning activities are designed so that students can use them independently or with the direction of a teacher. Depending on the needs of the class, the teacher may want to focus selectively on some aspects of a learning activity in preference to others.

Videotaping is a helpful way to obtain feedback about communication skills and has been found to be useful in mastering interpersonal skills (Finley et al., 1979; Talento and McKeever, 1983). If it is available, videotaping is recommended for the learning activities in Chapter 3, and in Chapter 4, Skill 15. When using videotaping for learning communication skills, the student will find it helpful to practice working with the equipment in advance of taping the suggested interactions. Initially, it is quite common for students to be concerned with how they look, sound, and act; however, repeated videotaping experiences tend to increase comfort with the activity.

Students are encouraged to play back and review their interactions with a teacher immediately after taping. Helpful teacher feedback is direct and nonambiguous, focused on specific behaviors and learning objectives, and preferably is used for learning rather than evaluation purposes.

Although the communication skills are presented separately, it is important to remember that no one skill is appropriate to use under all circumstances. The student is expected to integrate these skills into his or her own unique way of communicating with others. As a helping person, the nurse develops a range of communication skills to use intentionally and deliberately in order to achieve a specific purpose within the nurse–client interaction.

☐ OVERVIEW OF PART ONE

Helping skills can be learned and helping characteristics can be developed, either initially or as added expertise to a helper's existing skills (D'Augelli et al.,

1980; Martin and Carkhuff, 1968; Truax and Carkhuff, 1976). To do this requires a knowledge of the helping relationship, knowledge of one's self, one's needs, and one's values, and the ability to disclose that self to another in a way that facilitates the other's growth. These skills are developed in Chapter 1.

There are other less personal factors that enter into a person's ability to establish and maintain a helping relationship. They are focused more directly on the client and the environment, rather than on the helper, and include observation of nonverbal behavior and the use of time, silence, space, and touch. These skills are presented in Chapter 2.

Chapter 3 presents six specific components of communication to be learned and practiced separately and then integrated later. This approach is similar to the "microskills training" methods of teaching communication skills that are used and described by Brammer (1979), D'Augelli et al. (1980), Ivey (1977), and Marson (1979). The method also is comparable to skills training in sports such as golf and tennis, where the fundamentals of grip, stance, and swing are learned separately and then combined into a single performance, using each component as needed. These facilitative skill components include attending behavior, attentive listening, reflection of content, reflection of feelings, questioning, and offering assistance.

Chapter 4 provides the framework for integrating and using facilitative communication skills in a purposeful way through interviewing and teaching.

In addition to communicating with clients, nurses also communicate with other health-care professionals about the care of those clients. Chapter 5 describes the use of written health records.

REFERENCES

Bernstein L, Bernstein RS: Interviewing: A Guide for Health Professionals, ed 3. New York, Appleton-Century-Crofts, 1980.

Blondis MN, Jackson BE: Nonverbal Communication with Patients: Back to the Human Touch. New York, John Wiley & Sons, 1977.

Brammer, LM: The Helping Relationship, ed 2. Englewood Cliffs, NJ, Prentice-Hall, 1979.

Clift JC, Imrie BW: Assessing Students, Appraising Teaching. New York, Halsted Press, 1981.

Combs AW, Avila DL, Purkey WW: Helping Relationships: Basic Concepts for the Helping Professions. Boston, Allyn & Bacon, 1971.

D'Augelli AR, Danish SJ, et al: Helping Skills: A Basic Training Program (Leader's Manual), ed 2. New York, Human Sciences Press, 1980.

Finley B, Kim KK, Mynatt S: Maximizing videotaped learning of interpersonal skills. Journal of Nursing Education 18(1):33–41, 1979.

Freemon BL, Korsch BM, et al: How do nurses expand their roles in well child care? American Journal of Nursing 72(10):1866–1871, 1972.

Gerrard BA, Boniface WJ, Love BH: Interpersonal Skills for Health Professionals. Reston, VA, Reston, 1980.

Gluck M, Carter R: Personal qualities of nurses implying need for continuing education to increase interpersonal and leadership effectiveness. The Journal of Continuing Education in Nursing 11(4):29–36, 1980.

Ivey AE: Microcounseling: Interviewing Skills Manual, ed 2. Springfield, IL, Charles C Thomas, 1977.

Jourard SM: The Transparent Self, rev ed. New York, D. Van Nostrand, 1971.

Marson SN: Nursing, a helping relationship? Nursing Times 75(12):541–544, 1979.

Martin J, Carkhuff RR: Changes in personality of counselors-in-training. Journal of Clinical Psychology 24(1):109–110, 1968.

Peitchinis JA: Therapeutic effectiveness of counseling by nursing personnel: Review of the literature. Nursing Research 21(2):138–147, 1972.

Pluckhan ML: Human Communication: The Matrix of Nursing. New York, McGraw-Hill, 1978.

Satir V: Conjoint Family Therapy, rev ed. Palo Alto, CA, Science & Behavior Books, 1967.

Skipper JK: Communication and the hospitalized patient. In Skipper JK, Leonard RC, (eds): Social Interaction and Patient Care. Philadelphia, JB Lippincott, 1965.

Smith D: A clinical nursing tool. American Journal of Nursing 68(11):2384–2388, 1968.

Talento B, McKeever LC: Improving interviewing techniques. Nursing Outlook 31(4):234–235, 1983.

Travelbee J: Interpersonal Aspects of Nursing. Philadelphia, FA Davis, 1971.

Truax C, Altmann H, Millis WA: Therapeutic relationships provided by various professionals. Journal of Community Psychology 2(1):33–36, 1974.

Truax C, Carkhuff RR: Toward Effective Counseling and Psychotherapy. Chicago, Aldine Publications, 1976.

BIBLIOGRAPHY

Brockhaus JPD, Woods M, Brockhaus RH: Structured experiential learning exercises: A facilitation to more effective learning in clinical settings. Journal of Psychosocial Nursing and Mental Health Services 19(10):27–32, 1981.

Goldsborough J: Involvement. American Journal of Nursing 69(1):66–68, 1969.

AUDIOVISUAL RESOURCE

The Meaning of Communication
 Film (16mm). (1971, B & W, 30 min.)
 Available through:
  Instructional Media Center
  University of Nebraska
  3835 Holdrege Street
  Lincoln, NE 68583

1 Awareness of Self in the Helping Relationship

☐ INTRODUCTION

A primary goal of professional nursing is to implement nursing care in a way that is helpful for the client. This means that nursing care increases clients' sense of self-worth, facilitates their communication with health-care professionals, and assists them to participate in their own recovery. Whether this goal is achieved depends on the nature of the relationship that develops between the nurse and the client. When the nurse–client relationship has the characteristics of a helping relationship, clients are more likely to perceive their needs as being met and to view the nurse as a helpful, caring person who is interested in them as individuals.

To develop and maintain a helping relationship with clients requires the person of the nurse to become involved with the person of the client. For this involvement to be growth-producing and helpful for the client, the nurse consciously and deliberately acts in the client's best interests rather than acting for the primary purpose of meeting his or her own needs. To do this requires that the nurse know who he or she is, both as a person and as a nurse.

Learning to know ourselves requires conscious effort, time, and a fair degree of introspection. It involves a willingness to risk looking at ourselves and sharing that self with others. This is not always an easy process, because knowing ourselves increases our recognition of both pleasant and unpleasant aspects of the inner self. That recognition, however, helps bring our actions under more conscious and deliberate control.

Self-awareness involves understanding what we experience in everyday situations, that is, what is happening, how we feel about it, what we think and do about it, and what our motives are in our interactions with others.

Self-concept comprises our own beliefs and perceptions of what we are like and what we perceive others think of us. *Self-understanding* involves knowing something about the factors in our background and psychosocial development that contribute to being the kind of people we are at this time.

Behaviors are actions, both verbal and nonverbal. Behaviors are how we function in everyday situations and respond to them. *Feelings* are emotions that occur in response to what we experience and often provide a motivating force for further behaviors.

Needs are motivating forces for behavior in that we act in ways that meet our perceived needs. Needs are basic, universal, and common to all people, and they are specific to each individual. Our *values* are whatever has worth or value for us. Values are motivating forces for behavior, because in general, we act on the basis of what we believe to be important.

Self-disclosure is the process of sharing ourselves with another person. It involves revealing our thoughts, feelings, and purposes to someone for the purpose of promoting that person's growth and health.

The skills in this chapter are focused on increasing an awareness of oneself as a person and as a nurse who is learning to function within a helping relationship with clients who seek or need help. These skills present abstract concepts that are essential for developing a helping nurse–client relationship. Within each skill there are experiential learning activities to help the student understand those concepts and incorporate them into both personal and professional relationships. For maximum benefit, each of the learning activities should be used carefully and thoughtfully before going on to the next skill. Once the skills in this chapter are completed, the student will have developed a sound basis for moving on to more client-focused aspects of professional communication skills.

This chapter presents "The Helping Relationship" and how it applies to nursing (Skill 1), "Knowing Ourselves" (Skill 2), "Needs Identification" (Skill 3), "Values Identification" (Skill 4), and "Self-Disclosure" (Skill 5).

SKILL 1 The Helping Relationship

The two keys to the helping process are the helper as a person and his or her skills.
—Brammer, p. vii

☐ STUDENT OBJECTIVES

1. Describe the characteristics of a helping relationship.
2. Describe the characteristics of an effective helper.
3. Explain the significance of the helping relationship to the practice of nursing.
4. Describe the characteristics of the concepts of acceptance, trust, empathy, and caring.
5. Explain the correlation of acceptance, trust, empathy, and caring with the development of a helping relationship.
6. Recognize your own ability to accept, trust, empathize with, and care for another person.
7. Recognize your own experiences of accepting and trusting another person, receiving empathy, and being cared for.
8. Illustrate the value of acceptance, trust, empathy, and caring in a nursing framework.

☐ INTRODUCTION

The helping relationship is an interaction between two persons wherein at least one of the persons has the intent of actively seeking the good of the other (Benjamin, 1981; Brammer, 1979). According to Rogers (1958, p. 6), it is a deliberate, intentional process directed toward "promoting the growth, development, maturity, improved functioning, improved coping with life of the other [person]". This helping relationship is a necessary component in interactions between health care and social service professionals and their clients, and it is sometimes called a *therapeutic relationship* because of its healing nature. Within the context of providing nursing care, it is often called the *nurse–client relationship* or the *nurse–patient relationship*.

The characteristics of a helping relationship have grown out of the work of observant and perceptive counselors and therapists and have been validated experientially by clients and by therapists, nurses, and others involved in helping professions. Other research has explored the characteristics of the helping relationship. In their observations of effective counselors and therapists, Truax and Carkhuff (1967) found that accurate empathy, nonpossessive warmth, and genuineness occurred consistently. Research at the University of Florida found that dealing with people in purely objective terms was correlated with ineffectiveness on the part of counselors (Combs, 1969; Combs et al., 1971).

When asked what they value most in a nurse, clients generally emphasize the nurse's interpersonal skills. In a study where the clients were asked what was ideally expected from a nurse, 81 percent stressed the importance of both personalized care and empathic attitudes, while 45 percent expected prompt and efficient services, and only 29 percent mentioned knowledge and technical skills. Most clients admitted that they were reluctant to reveal their apprehensions, fears, and dissatisfactions to the nurse, and that they regarded demands for physical care rather than demands for emotional support as being legitimate (Sundeen et al., 1981).

Rogers (1961) indicates that the attitudes and feelings of a helper are more important than the technique or methods used in helping. Stetler's research indicates that verbal behaviors of the nurse are not the most important factors in the client's perception of empathy (1977). A study of 3596 cases in 266 family service agencies showed that the quality of the counselor–client relationship had a statistically significant association with positive client change, and had the strongest association with positive client outcomes of any client or service characteristic analyzed in that study (Beck and Jones, 1975).

Most important, it is the client's perception of the helper's attitudes and feelings that is crucial. When the client perceives that he or she is accepted as an individual, a helping relationship becomes possible. When the helper is a trustworthy person, the client can more readily trust the helper; when the helper is able to communicate to clients an empathic understanding of what they are experiencing, those clients perceive the helper as a caring person who values them as individuals. This skill presents the concepts of acceptance, trust, empathy, and caring within the context of the helping relationship that is nursing.

☐ PREPARATION

THE HELPING RELATIONSHIP

There are common characteristics of the helping relationship that can be described, studied, and learned. The helping relationship is a caring relationship between the helper and the client, characterized by mutual respect, genuineness, and congruence, through which nonpossessive warmth, accurate empathy, and acceptance (sometimes called unconditional positive regard) are conveyed to another person (Biestek, 1957; Jourard, 1971; Rogers, 1961; Travelbee, 1971). It is an *individualized* relationship where the client is treated as a person rather than as a case or number, and it also is a *confidential* relationship in which the client can share needed information without it becoming public knowledge. Through the helping relationship the client is given the opportunity to express both negative and positive feelings and to involve those feelings in the problem-solving process.

The helping relationship is *purposeful;* its purpose is to establish a relationship between two human beings that can be a means for promoting problem solving and personal growth. In nursing it also includes providing nursing care and meeting the client's nursing needs. The responsibility for developing and maintaining the helping relationship lies primarily with the professional helper, although the relationship generally is satisfying and rewarding for both parties.

Characteristics of a Helper

Characteristics of an effective helper have been described through the same observational process as for the helping relationship itself, and they are considered prerequisite skills for developing a helping relationship. These characteristics include:

- A knowledge of human behavior
- An awareness of biases and prejudices
- The ability to listen and observe what is said and not said
- The ability to empathize
- The capability of being involved with the other person and yet remain separate

An effective helper also is able to express himself or herself clearly; he or she is perceived as trustworthy, dependable, and consistent; and is able to experience caring, warmth, liking, respect, and interest and is able to convey those characteristics to the other person.

If as helpers we are warm, caring, accepting, and able to enter into someone else's feelings and experiences, then our clients will feel loved, accepted, and understood. When people experience these feelings they tend to be more receptive to the process of being helped than when they feel threatened or rejected. To feel threatened is to feel unsafe, and growth and change are difficult when we feel unsafe. When we feel threatened we tend to become angry and resistive to change. In the nurse-client relationship the need for change may relate to coping with physical problems, such as learning to live with a low-sodium diet for reducing hypertension, attempting to alter life style to decrease the risks of coronary artery disease, learning to adapt colostomy care to the home setting, or accepting the needed short-term dependency associated with surgery. The need for change also may be of an interpersonal nature, such as when working with a teenage mother whose inadequate mothering skills are causing behavior problems in her children, a family that is suspected of abusing aging relatives, or adolescents who come to a health clinic for venereal disease care and information.

The words *genuine, authentic,* and *congruent* have been used to describe an effective helper. They describe a person who is open and honest both with himself or herself and with others, one who does not need to play a role in relationships with others. The words, actions, and feelings of an authentic person are in harmony (congruent) with each other—there are no games or hidden agendas. Combs et al. (1971) note that such persons have a tremendous advantage in that they can forget themselves and give more freely to the task at hand in a straightforward and uncomplicated way.

The Nurse-Client Relationship

The nurse-client relationship is a helping relationship that often develops between nurse and client during the process of providing nursing care, although it is possible to provide nursing care without the development of this type of relationship. Some interactions between nurses and clients are too brief for a helping relationship to develop, and sometimes neither nurse nor client is ready for this type of relationship. However, the nurse who consistently possesses the characteristics of an effective helper can relate to clients in such a way that a helping relationship is possible.

Looking at several descriptions of the nurse-client relationship clarifies its similarity to the helping relationship. Peplau (1952) described the nurse-client relationship as a supportive one in which nurse and client know and respect each other and work together cooperatively to face the client's problems. According to Orlando (1961), "What a nurse says or does is the exclusive mode through which she serves the patient" (p. 6). Orlando views a helpful nurse-client interaction as a deliberate, validating approach in which the client's perception of the situation is identified, and the nurse then helps the client avoid or alleviate the distress that occurs from unmet needs.

Travelbee (1971) describes the nurse-client relationship as a "human-to-human relationship," because a relationship is possible only between persons who see each other as human beings rather than as roles or stereotypes. She states:

The human-to-human relationship in nursing situations is the means through which the purpose of nursing is accomplished, namely to assist an individual (or family) to prevent, or cope with, the experience of illness and suffering, and to help him (or his family) to find meaning in these experiences. (p. 119)

The goal of the relationship is to know the client as a human being and thus to be able to determine and meet the client's (or family's) nursing needs.

Sundeen et al. (1981) also view the nurse-client interpersonal interrelationship as the vehicle through which nursing is accomplished and the nursing process is implemented. They state that achievement of nursing-care goals is often directly related to the nature of the nurse-client relationship.

In any helping relationship the primary focus is

on the client's needs and responses, rather than on the helper's needs. In nearly every interaction the nurse has with clients, and regardless of how task-oriented the interaction may be, the kind of person the nurse is and how the nurse responds to and treats the client affects how that person feels about the nurse, about himself or herself, and about the current situation. When clients function better and feel better about themselves as the result of a nurse's interaction, that nurse has used himself or herself in a therapeutic manner (sometimes called the therapeutic use of self), and some degree of a helping relationship has been established.

The helping relationship promotes increased self-care ability for the client and collaboration between nurse and client as they determine nursing care goals, plan interventions, and evaluate the effectiveness of those interventions. However, during the course of the relationship the nurse also recognizes the client's right of self-determination, that is, the client's right and need to make decisions and choices about his or her own life, even when those choices differ from the nurse's own choices.

One deterrent to the development of a helpful nurse–client relationship is for the nurse to substitute the external authority of roles or rules for his or her own personal authority of experience and knowledge. When nurses feel insecure or inexperienced, they sometimes assume a nurse *role* and interact on the basis of nurse and client in a rather authoritarian way. Or they may use the authority of the physician or of rules and policies to bolster their own position.

For example, consider the types of authority used by nurses in making the following statements: "You will need to get out of bed today" (nurse role); "All patients on this unit get out of bed their first day post-op" (rules and policies); "Your doctor says you must get out of bed today" (physician); "People usually get along better if they get out of bed soon after surgery" (knowledge). The last statement is nonauthoritarian and begins to involve the client in acting on his or her own behalf.

Cultural Variables in Helping
The concept of helping has individual meanings for each of us and also culturally determined meanings. Brammer (1979) indicates that helping, in the sense of counseling, largely is an American white middle-class phenomenon. In most other cultures, these helping functions are performed within the family. As indicated earlier, the helping relationship between nurses and clients involves interpersonal interactions, physical care, and health-promotion activities. In order to make helping acceptable to the recipient (client), the nurse considers the special meanings that various racial, ethnic, and religious groups place on helping and being helped. The nurse can draw from social science and humanities courses and from personal and vicarious experiences with persons from other cultures. The nurse can remain sensitive and open to cues from clients by questioning and validating perceptions rather than assuming that the nurse's norms are the same as the client's norms. A genuine concern for a client's well-being motivates the nurse to act positively toward persons from another culture.

Mead (1956) indicates that if nurses are aware that a client's behavior may be culturally determined, they will be more accepting of persons from cultures other than their own. Leininger (1978) proposes that those professional caring behaviors (including, among others, compassion, empathy, helping behaviors, and nurturance)

... which are congruent with the social structure and values of a particular culture will show greater client satisfactions and acceptance than those caring behaviors which show incongruencies with the values and social structure of a given culture. (p. 37)

KEY COMPONENTS OF THE HELPING RELATIONSHIP

Four key components of the helping relationship are acceptance, trust, empathy, and caring.

Acceptance
Acceptance is a major requirement for creating an atmosphere that promotes a helpful relationship with a client (Biestek, 1957; Combs et al., 1971). Acceptance has been defined as a

... principle of action wherein the helper perceives and deals with the client as he really is, including his strengths and weaknesses, his congenial and uncongenial qualities, his positive and negative feelings, his constructive and destructive attitudes and behavior, maintaining all the while a sense of the client's innate dignity and personal worth. (Biestek, 1957, p. 72)

Acceptance is nonjudgmental in that it recognizes and accepts what exists without exercising good or bad value judgments.

An accepting, nonjudgmental attitude grows out of the inner conviction that judging clients denies them their basic right to individuality and therefore is therapeutically harmful. Acceptance is therapeutic in that it assists the helper in understanding clients as they really are, which in turn helps clients feel safe in disclosing information about themselves and helps them look at what they are doing. This enables clients to deal with their problems and themselves.

The experience of being accepted by others brings a release from the negative feelings associated with threats or judgments. When we do not feel as though our feelings and actions are condemned as wrong or inappropriate, we feel less risk in acknowledging and talking about them. For example, when a nurse's attitude conveys disapproval to a mother who has failed to keep several clinic appointments, the mother is neither likely to share spontaneously her reasons for not coming (perhaps a lack of transportation, money, or child care, or negative experiences at the clinic) nor be apt to follow the advice of a nurse whom she perceives as judgmental and noncaring.

Biestek (1957) emphasizes that a nonjudgmental attitude is perceived by the client only if the helper feels it; it is not something that can be feigned. A nonjudgmental attitude can be developed as the helper becomes aware of his or her own feelings about being judged by others. This self-awareness increases the helper's sensitivity to clients' feelings about being judged. Biestek also indicates that "self-awareness leads to the acceptance of self and ultimately to the acceptance of others" (1957, p. 80), and Hein writes that "acceptance of others begins with self-acceptance because we cannot accept imperfections and qualities in others until we have admitted to similar characteristics in ourselves" (1980, p. 123).

A helper can become more accepting by being observant of and open to others and by attempting to understand his or her own experiences with people. Perlman (1969) suggests that the capacity to accept may grow with widened experiences. She indicates that there is probably little acceptance of what is unknown or strange, and that we accept what we understand. Hein (1980) indicates that while we may not totally understand someone else's reactions, way of thinking, or way of communicating, such understanding is less important than recognizing who that person is right now as a unique individual.

A nonaccepting, judgmental attitude can be conveyed through both verbal and nonverbal behaviors. Voice tone, facial expressions, gestures, and words can be condemning and judgmental. Judgment also can be conveyed by making unfavorable comparisons to others, by jumping to conclusions, and by too quickly giving assurances that the helper understands—before hearing all of what the client is saying. The following activity is designed to examine feelings associated with personal acceptance.

Activity 1-A:
The Experiencing of Acceptance

1. Recall an incident in which you felt judged, scolded, or criticized by another person for doing something that was either misunderstood or inappropriate—from their perspective. First describe the nonverbal behaviors that communicated these messages to you and then describe your feelings and reactions to this experience.
2. Recall an incident in which you felt loved and accepted, even though you may have done something inappropriate or foolish. Describe the nonverbal behaviors that communicated these messages to you and then describe your feelings and reactions to this experience.

Trust

Trust can be defined as a firm reliance on or confident belief in another person (Webster, 1976). In the context of the helping relationship, trust is described by Travelbee as "the assured belief that other individuals are capable of assisting in times of distress and will probably do so" (1971, p. 80). Placing trust in someone involves a confident belief that the other person will act in our own best interests, or will at least do us no harm.

Trust grows out of positive, trusting experiences with trustworthy persons. Some people find it easier to trust than others. One of the earliest stages of psychosocial development described by Erickson is the development of trust versus mistrust, which is related to Maslow's basic need for safety and security (Maier, 1969; Maslow, 1954). (These concepts are discussed in Skill 3.) When this developmental stage is positively resolved, the infant or young child experiences the world as a trustworthy place and learns to feel safe and secure. People with these early experiences find it fairly easy to trust others and feel safe in their environment. Adults who had less positive experiences in this developmental stage may find it more difficult to trust others.

Some people approach a relationship in a trusting way, while others reserve that trust until they find the other person to be a *trustworthy person*, that is, someone who can be trusted safely. A trustworthy person relates to other people in *reliable, dependable, honest,* and *consistent* ways, as evidenced to others through both nonverbal and verbal behaviors. In fact, a helper's nonverbal behavior and manner appear to have a greater impact on the perceived trustworthiness of the helper than words (Brammer, 1979). The following activity is designed to focus on the experience of placing trust in someone else and depending on that person for physical and emotional safety.

Activity 1-B:
Experiencing Trust

Work in pairs for this activity.

1. Partner A closes his or her eyes or is blindfolded and allows Partner B to guide him or her on a walk lasting at least 5 minutes. The walk should involve minor obstructions or problems such as stairs, elevators, streets, sitting in a chair, or getting a drink. *All* communication is to be *nonverbal.*
2. As the blindfolded partner, describe how you felt initially, as the walk progressed, and at the end of the walk. Let your partner know what helped you feel safe or unsafe (for example, "I felt safe when you . . . ," or "When you . . . , I felt unsafe").
3. Exchange roles and repeat the activity.

To foster the development of a helping relationship and to be perceived by clients as trustworthy, the nurse demonstrates trustworthiness behaviorally. The nurse is perceived as reliable and dependable when he or she pays attention to clients' requests, whether the requests are for ice water, pain medication, diet changes, or information about the waiting time to see the physician at a well-child clinic. To illustrate, an elderly woman at an older adult clinic asked the nurse when her next appointment was scheduled at the eye clinic. While checking on the appointment, the nurse became involved in discussing staffing problems with a co-worker and then saw several other clients. The woman waited for over an hour, missed her bus, and became quite weary and discouraged. She thought, "No one really cares what happens to an old woman like me."

Whatever trust might have been established could be severely strained. From the client's perspective, in the often unfamiliar and unpredictable world of health-care delivery systems, responses to requests that may seem insignificant to the nurse often indicate to the client how well he or she can expect to be cared for. When the nurse forgets small things, it raises the question of how available the nurse would be if the client "really needed" something.

Honesty is essential for the development of trust in a nurse–client relationship. If a nurse does not have the information the client wants or does not know the answer to a question, it is best to acknowledge this. For instance, it is better to say, "I don't know very much about that question, but I will find out and get back to you," than to give a vague or incorrect response. When something happens to delay responding to a request, an honest explanation or acknowledgement is helpful: "I haven't yet been able to find out . . . , but before I leave today, I will check that out for you." Or, "The doctor will be at least an hour late because of an emergency. Are you able to wait, or would you like to make an appointment for another day?" Both of these comments communicate caring and help the nurse to be perceived as a trustworthy person.

The client will perceive the nurse as dependable and trustworthy when the nurse has consistent expectations and gives clear, consistent explanations of what is expected. For example, if the nurse is teaching someone how to give insulin and yesterday emphasized a point that today he or she says is unimportant (without valid reason for the change), the person may well begin to question the accuracy of other parts of the nurse's teaching and his or her credibility and competence in general. A client should be able to trust, or confidently believe, that the nurse will look out for the client's best interests even when the client is unable to do so unaided. The client should be able to believe that the nurse can be counted on to alleviate pain, decrease anxiety, promote comfort and safety, and even sustain life for the client, if necessary.

Some clients and families may have had little contact with the health-care professions and no previous basis for trust; others may have had negative or traumatic experiences; and still others have had positive, trusting encounters. Although some trust grows out of previous positive experiences with trustworthy persons, trust must be newly developed in each new situation, between each nurse and client or nurse and family. The client often tests this trust, especially if there have been previous experiences with nurses regarded as untrustworthy. This testing may take the form of questioning the nurse's judgment, making numerous requests for help, or making negative remarks about the nurses or the agency in general. With this testing, the client is asking, "Can I really count on this nurse, or will he or she reject me if I complain, ask for too many things?" The nurse's response to testing will influence the client's perception of the nurse's trustworthiness.

Empathy

The ability to empathize is considered to be a major part of a helping relationship and a characteristic of an effective helper (Carkhuff, 1969; Combs et al., 1971; Rogers, 1958; Travelbee, 1971). Rogers (1958) has observed that even a minimal amount of empathic understanding is helpful for a client.

Empathy has been described as the "ability to enter into the life of another person, to accurately perceive his current feelings and their meanings" (Kalisch, 1973, p. 1548). It is the ability to enter into someone's current intrapersonal experiences to "get inside him (or her)" or "walk a mile in his (or her) shoes," to enter his or her internal frame of reference or perceive his or her private world—and it is the ability to communicate this understanding to that person (Biestek, 1957; Brammer, 1979; Travelbee, 1971; Zderad, 1969). Empathy is an

. . . almost instantaneous process characterized by the ability to comprehend the meaning and relevance of the thoughts and feelings of the individual concerned. . . . To empathize is to form a bond with another and experience closeness without being submerged by the involvement. (Travelbee, 1971, p. 136)

Empathy implies a perception of another's nonverbalized feelings and moods. It is a conscious process in which each person is aware that something meaningful has occurred during the interaction. It is not necessarily dependent on liking the other person.

Empathy is characterized by both sharing and separateness. Although the empathic helper shares in the thinking and feelings of the other person, the helper remains separate and apart, retaining a sense of objectivity and detachment. Empathy occurs in response to subtle, almost unconscious cues from the other person, and it involves a sensation of being "with" that person. Zderad (1969) describes the process of developing empathy as first a conscious perception of how the situation appears to the client, followed by an inner-feeling response (more unconscious than conscious) that is harmonious with the client's feelings, and, finally, a return to an objectivity in which the empathizer becomes aware of the client's experience as it compares to his or her own.

Brammer (1979) suggests that helpers can enter the client's internal frame of reference by listening attentively to the client and asking themselves several questions: "*What* is the person *feeling* right now? *How* does he view this *problem*? *What* does she see in her *world*?" (p. 37).

In his research on empathy, Carkhuff (1969) has developed and used a scale for measuring the degree of empathic understanding achieved in an interpersonal interaction. The scale ranges from verbal and nonverbal responses that indicate no awareness of the other person's expression of feelings and meaning (Level 1) to responses that indicate an accurate awareness of the other person's deep and surface feelings and meanings (Level 5). Responses in Levels 1 and 2 produce nonhelpful, neutral, or even negative effects on interpersonal relationships. Level 3 is considered the minimal level for facilitative interpersonal interactions. Responses in Levels 4 and 5 are more highly empathic in that they reflect more than a superficial recognition of what the other person is actually experiencing.

- *Level 1.* The listener's responses either *do not attend to* or *detract significantly from* the other person's verbal and nonverbal expressions. Responses ignore the other person or communicate significantly less of the meaning and feelings that the other person communicated. There is no indication that the listener is aware of even the most obvious expressed feelings.
- *Level 2.* The listener responds to expressed feelings and meanings in a way that decreases the feeling level and distorts the meaning of the other person's communication. Responses are incongruent with what the other person is expressing.
- *Level 3.* The listener responds to expressed feelings in a way that accurately reflects the surface feelings and meanings of the other person. Responses do not respond to deeper feelings or may misinterpret them.
- *Level 4.* The listener's responses express feelings and meanings a level deeper than the other person was able to express for himself or herself. Responses add noticeably to the other person's expression and communicate an understanding that is a level deeper than the expressed surface level.
- *Level 5.* The listener's responses add significantly to the feeling and meaning expressed by the other person. Responses either (1) accurately express both surface and the deepest feelings and meanings, below what the other person may be able to express; or (2) reflect an awareness and understanding of the other person's deep feelings and meanings.

Carkhuff's research also identified that respect, genuineness, and self-disclosure vary with the level of empathy. *Level of respect* for the other person ranges from lack of respect at Level 1 to deep respect at Level 5; *genuineness* ranges from a discrepancy between the listener's verbal and nonverbal experience at Level 1 to a completely open, nonexploitive relationship at Level 5; and *self-disclosure* ranges from detachment in Level 1 to fairly intimate self-disclosure at Level 5.

There are many factors that affect a person's ability to empathize with another person. Travelbee (1971) believes that a *desire* to comprehend or understand another person is a prerequisite for developing empathy, regardless of whether that be a desire to help, to exploit, or even to satisfy one's curiosity. Similarity of experience between the two persons is also a significant factor in the ability to develop empathy, as is the ability to be perceptive of and open to unconsciously perceived cues from others. An empathic person is able to be spontaneous and flexible, is mentally healthy, and has the ability to observe himself or herself and to know that self well. Behaviors such as selective inattention and absentmindedness, and characteristics such as aggression, hostility, competitiveness, and authoritarianism decrease the ability to empathize. Any factor that causes a person to focus on self rather than on the other person also decreases the ability to empathize; examples are fear, anxiety, personal problems, or even unmet physical needs such as hunger or lack of sleep.

It is not possible to have had experiences similar to those of each person the nurse cares for. Travelbee (1971) proposes that student nurses with a limited exposure to persons of a wide variety of ages, cultures, and backgrounds can increase their ability to empathize in several ways: They can learn from human experiences as recorded in nursing literature, the behavioral sciences, and the humanities; they can be purposefully assigned to care for clients with varying backgrounds; and they can be helped by nurse educators to recognize similarities and dissimilarities between their own experiences and the experiences of their clients.

Prejudice, bias, and stereotyping make an empathic helping relationship difficult to achieve. Any one of these causes us at least initially to relate to a person as a type; thus we see "an elderly person," "a black," "a WASP," or "a welfare recipient," rather than an individual. Prejudice interferes with the nurse's ability to give individualized care, decreases communication between nurse and client, and produces decreased feelings of self-worth and loss of trust for the client. An empathic nurse recognizes stereotypes and generalizations for what they are, and avoids basing responses and nursing interventions on those inaccurate perceptions. This kind of nurse also cares enough to become knowledgeable about a particular client's culture and life style. Biestek (1957) even points out that it is not enough to treat a person as a human being, but as *this* human being with all of his or her personal uniqueness.

Few people, including helping professionals, are totally free from bias and prejudice. Becoming aware of his or her own biases and prejudices helps the nurse develop the ability to set aside those attitudes and feelings within a professional setting in order to provide quality nursing care. For example, a nurse who is aware that he or she feels that gross obesity is disgusting can make a conscious effort not to let those feelings interfere with the amount and kind of care provided. When biases and prejudices are not acknowledged to oneself, they often are communicated verbally or nonverbally to others. The following activity is designed to focus on giving and receiving empathy.

Activity 1-C: Experiencing Empathy

Work in groups of three, with two partners and one observer.

1. Partner A: Select a meaningful or interesting experience you have had and discuss it with partner B.
2. Partner B: In your responses to partner A, try to use responses characteristic of the various levels of empathy.
3. Observer: Make written notes about partner B's responses as they illustrate each level, and about partner A's verbal and nonverbal reactions.
4. When the exchange is completed, observer and partner B validate with each other the kinds of responses used. Partner A validates his or her reactions with those responses.
5. Exchange roles and repeat the activity until each person has been both partner A and partner B.

Caring

Caring is an integral part of helping, since the helping relationship is a caring relationship in which one person seeks to help another person grow. Leininger (1977) contends that "there can be *no* curing *without* the elements and processes of caring" (p. 2). A person who feels cared for as an individual also feels secure and has greater ability to trust. A caring nurse is a trustworthy person whose care provides an empathic experience that helps the client perceive that he or she is being understood.

To care means to show genuine concern for the welfare of another (Brammer, 1979). Caring is a "feeling of concern, regard, respect that one human being may have for another" (Sobel, 1969, p. 2612). It is primarily nonverbal and is conveyed through the *manner* in which things are said or done—or left unsaid or undone—rather than *what* is done or said. As Wisser (1978) so aptly states, "Caring is a state of mind, not additional work" (p. 1017). Travelbee (1971) describes the concept of caring as a "process wherein an individual is able to comprehend the distress of another, be moved or touched by another's distress, and desires to alleviate the cause" (p. 142). It is a sharing of feelings and an experience of compassion.

To care about someone implies a commitment to that person. It also calls for an emotional closeness and involvement, as well as the ability to translate those attitudes into helpful behaviors. When we are sensitive to others' circumstances, are aware of their needs, offer help, and in any way reach out to them, we show caring behavior. To care is to respect the other person as having worth, regardless of age, sex, socioeconomic status, or cultural background. Caring is a genuine attitude that cannot be feigned; it is more than courtesy or kindness, although it includes both. It is more than intuition or treating someone else the way you would like to be treated. Caring conveys warmth and compassion from one human to another. The following activity is designed to help recognize components of caring through personal life experiences.

Activity 1-D: Experiencing Caring

Work in small groups with people you know reasonably well.

1. Recall and describe incidents or experiences in which you have felt cared about. Try to analyze what gave you that feeling, that is, what actions, words, and feelings were communicated to you. Are there any common elements in your experiences?
2. Recall and describe incidents in which you knew or felt that people around you did not care for or about you. Again, try to analyze what caused you to feel that way and look for common elements in your experiences.
3. Describe how you behave (what you do, say, or feel) when you care about someone as compared with how you behave when you do not care about someone.
4. Describe how you behave when those around you care for or about you as compared with how you behave when they do not.

In a caring relationship, the nurse does become emotionally involved with the client but does not become blinded or incapacitated by that involvement. Generally speaking, the nurse is over-involved emotionally when he or she is unable to see a situation from any perspective other than the client's own. This over-involvement is not productive for either party, because neither the nurse's goal of helping nor the client's goal of being helped can be reached. On the other hand, a lack of emotional involvement with clients easily can result in a depersonalized manner on the part of the nurse and in a feeling that no one cares on the part of the client.

Caring causes the nurse to be vulnerable to experiencing pain, since as humans we share the pain of someone we care about. Caring also places the nurse in a position that is vulnerable to rejection or lack of appreciation, because the nature of the nurse–client relationship leaves the nurse open for the potential experience of caring for someone who does not reciprocate. In a professional relationship, caring is not reciprocal in the same way it is with friends. The nurse is important to the client primarily as an instrument for becoming or remaining well. Thus, the nurse may feel rejected and unappreciated if he or she is not aware of the difference between caring in a professional relationship and caring in a personal relationship. The nurse who uses work to meet all or most needs for love and affection is also vulnerable to feeling rejected. Since feelings affect behavior, the nurse's feelings of rejection or lack of being appreciated are quite likely to make it difficult for the nurse to relate to clients who do not express appreciation in some way.

Caring actions can be both verbal and nonverbal, and include touching, talking, listening, or perhaps being firm and setting limits (Fig. 1-1). Rohweder (1969) indicates that caring actions need to be based on a wide knowledge of human behavior in general, on how and why people respond as they do in a wide variety of situations and events. However, it is essential to refrain from assuming that each individual fits that general pattern, to avoid acting out personal motivations and needs in the guise of caring, and to assume that personal experiences are not a completely adequate guide for determining how caring is implemented.

At one agency, the nursing staff has developed standards for person-centered caring that are used as both process and outcome criteria (defined in Skill 18). The standards include caring behaviors such as introducing self to the client and family, calling the client by the name the client wishes, maintaining the client's privacy, respecting the client's values and life style, providing adequate information to the client and family, inquiring how illness and health status affects the client's work, laughing with the client and treating him or her like a human being (Paulen and Rapp, 1981). Information about those behaviors is gathered through interviews with clients, families, and nurses, and then used to evaluate and improve the personal quality of nursing care.

Caring is complementary to the systematic problem-solving approach of providing nursing care known as the nursing process. (Similar to the scientific process, the nursing process is further described in the introduction to Chapter 3.) However, neither caring nor nursing process alone is adequate to provide quality nursing care. By itself, the nursing process readily can become a technical and mechanical activity. When nursing is only rational and scientific, the health and illness needs of clients may be met adequately, but in an impersonal manner that causes clients to feel dehumanized and unsatisfied. By itself, caring can be an intuitive, kind, and compassionate activity. This kind of caring can be quite beneficial to clients, because they usually perceive the nurse's intent and feel that the nurse is a kind person who really wants to help. However, this intuitive caring may also be quite unhelpful, especially when it is used primarily to meet the nurse's own needs for love and affection.

When caring, knowledge, and rational thought are combined, the process of meeting human needs becomes a personal human interaction; knowledge and rational thought help determine the behaviors used to express caring to individuals. Through this combination of a caring and systematic approach to nursing care, clients are more adequately served and nurses receive more personal satisfaction and fulfillment from their work.

☐ EXECUTION

A helping relationship between helper and the recipient of help develops as a process. The process presented here is described by Mitchell and Loustau (1981) as the *movement* that occurs within a helping relationship in the nursing context. It proceeds from a superficial level to a personally involved level.

At the earliest, most *superficial level* the nurse and client are strangers and perceive each other in their stereotyped roles. Together they begin to gather information and clarify the needs of the client and the kind of help the nurse is able to provide. As the relationship continues to the *identity level,* the person of the nurse and the person of the client begin to emerge. The two begin to respond to each other in terms of their actual roles, as *this* client and *this* nurse. The client begins both to trust and test the nurse, and the nurse develops empathy for the client. At the *involvement level,* nurse and client no longer assume roles, but work together as persons and partners. At this level, Mitchell believes empathy leads to compassion (caring), and testing gives way to trust. This level is similar to Travelbee's development of rapport (1971).

The nurse–client relationship may end at the superficial, identity, or involvement level. The client may refuse help and leave; the nurse may be reassigned and leave the agency; or one or both may be unable to move to a higher level within the relationship.

Either the nurse or the client may initiate termination of a relationship. If the nurse initiates termination, the client should be prepared for this. Preferably, this preparation begins at the outset of the relationship, when the nurse explains his or her role in the relationship. An unannounced termination by the

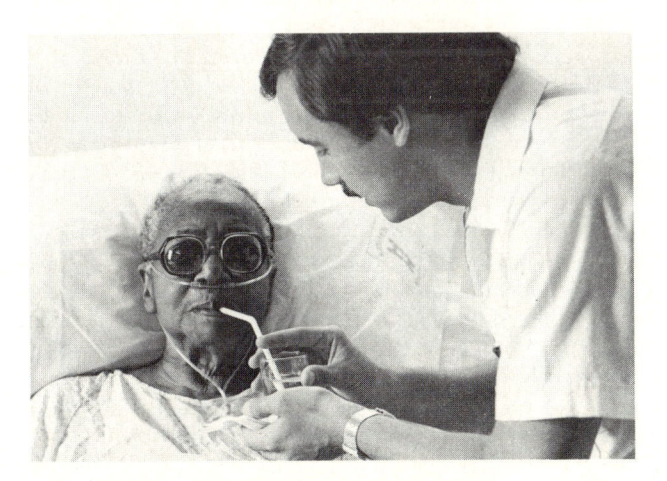

Figure 1-1. *Caring can be conveyed both verbally and nonverbally. (Photo by James Haines.)*

nurse, especially in a higher-level relationship, leaves both client and nurse emotionally vulnerable and may make it difficult for that client to develop trust in the next nurse. Termination and feelings about it need to be discussed openly. It is helpful if the nurse periodically reminds the client that termination is near. Although not actually a termination but an interruption, nurses also generally tell their clients when they have days off or a vacation, so the client does not feel abandoned or forgotten.

Establishing a helping relationship with clients requires presenting oneself as a trustworthy person who is able to receive others' trust and who is able and willing to accept, empathize with, and care for those clients. As with all of the skills in this chapter, developing these characteristics takes time, energy, and some introspection. There are different ways to facilitate their development: First, it is possible to observe our own verbal and nonverbal behaviors and make some judgment about personal trustworthiness, empathic abilities, and caring attitudes. Second, using the self-awareness wheel in Skill 2 helps us look at our own level of trust, empathy, and caring in our everyday lives. Since others do not always see us in the same ways we see ourselves, it is also helpful to solicit observations from a friend or teacher whose judgment and honesty can be trusted. This feedback can provide additional information about the way we present ourselves to others and help us modify personal behaviors we may dislike.

☐ CRITICAL POINTS SUMMARY

1. A helping relationship is accepting, nonjudgmental, individualized, confidential, and respectful.
2. The client's *perception* of the feelings and attitudes of the helper is the most crucial part of a helping relationship.
3. A skillful helper is empathic yet objective, reasonably free from bias, able to listen and observe, and able to work at a client's own pace.
4. Acceptance, trust, empathy, and caring are essential components of any helping relationship.
5. Acceptance is a nonjudgmental attitude on the part of the helper that helps the client feel safe in disclosing feelings and information.
6. A trustworthy person is one whom others perceive as reliable and dependable, honest and consistent.
7. Empathy is the ability to understand the meaning of another person's experience and to communicate that understanding to the other person.
8. Caring is a genuine concern for another person's welfare that conveys warmth, interest, and respect.

☐ REVIEW QUESTIONS

1. In what way or ways do you see the characteristics of a helping relationship as being different from a social or business relationship?
2. How would you describe an effective helper?
3. What does this statement mean to you? "The nurse–client relationship is a specific kind of helping relationship."
4. From the perspective of the person receiving help, what are the most significant characteristics of both the helper and the helping relationship?
5. In your own words, define acceptance, trust, empathy, and caring.
6. What role does helper acceptance play in developing a helping relationship?
7. How does being a trustworthy person help promote the development of a helping relationship?
8. In what way would lack of empathic ability make it difficult to develop a helping relationship with a client?
9. What factors make it easier for a client to trust a nurse? more difficult?
10. For what reasons is caring important in a helping relationship?
11. What personal situations can you identify in which you have accepted or trusted someone else? in which someone has empathized with you?
12. What personal situations can you identify in which you have felt accepted or trusted by someone else? in which you have empathized with someone else?

REFERENCES

Beck DF, Jones MA: Progress on Family Problems: A Nationwide Study of Clients' and Counselors' Views on Family Agency Services. New York, Family Service Association of America, 1975.

Benjamin A: The Helping Interview, ed 3. Boston, Houghton Mifflin, 1981.

Biestek FP: The Casework Relationship. Chicago, Loyola University Press, 1957.

Brammer LM: The Helping Relationship, ed 2. Englewood Cliffs, NJ, Prentice-Hall, 1979.

Carkhuff RR: Helping and Human Relations: A Primer for Lay and Professional Helpers, 2 vols. New York, Holt, Rinehart, and Winston, 1969.

Combs AW: Florida Studies in the Helping Professions, part 3. Gainesville, FL, University of Florida Press, 1969.

Combs AW, Avila DL, Purkey WW: Helping Relationships: Basic Concepts for the Helping Professions. Boston, Allyn & Bacon, 1971.

Hein EC: Communication in Nursing Practice, ed 2. Boston, Little, Brown, 1980.

Jourard SM: The Transparent Self, rev ed. New York, D Van Nostrand, 1971.

Kalisch BJ: What is empathy? American Journal of Nursing 73(9):1548–1552, 1973.

Leininger M: The phenomenon of caring, part V. Nursing Research Report 21(1):2, 14, 1977.

Leininger M: Transcultural Nursing: Concepts, Theories, and Practices. New York, John Wiley & Sons, 1978.

Maier HW: Three Theories of Child Development, rev ed. New York, Harper & Row, 1969.

Maslow AH: Motivation and Personality. New York, Harper & Row, 1954.

Mead M: Understanding cultural patterns. Nursing Outlook 4(5):260–262, 1956.

Mitchell PH, Loustau A: Concepts Basic to Nursing, ed 3. New York, McGraw-Hill, 1981.

Orlando IJ: The Dynamic Nurse–Patient Relationship. New York, GP Putnam's Sons, 1961.

Paulen A, Rapp C: Person-centered caring. Nursing Management 12(9):17–21, 1981.

Peplau HE: Interpersonal Relations in Nursing: A Conceptual Frame of Reference for Psychodynamic Nursing. New York, Putnam, 1952.

Perlman HH (ed): Helping: Charlotte Towle on Social Work and Social Casework. Chicago, University of Chicago Press, 1969.

Pluckhan ML: Human Communication: The Matrix of Nursing. New York, McGraw-Hill, 1978.

Rogers CR: Characteristics of a helping relationship. Personnel Guidance Journal 37(1):6–16, 1958.

Rogers CR: On Becoming a Person. Boston, Houghton Mifflin, 1961.

Rohweder AW: Can love, compassion, and involvement be scientific? Nursing Clinics of North America 4(4):701–707, 1969.

Sobel D: Love and pain. American Journal of Nursing 69(12):2612–2613, 1969.

Stetler CB: Relationship of perceived empathy to nurses' communication. Nursing Research 26(6):432–438, 1977.

Sundeen SJ, Stuart GW, et al: Nurse–Client Interaction: Implementing the Nursing Process. St Louis, MO, CV Mosby, 1981.

Travelbee J: Interpersonal Aspects of Nursing. Philadelphia, FA Davis, 1971.

Truax CB, Carkhuff RR: Toward Effective Counseling and Psychotherapy. Chicago, Aldine Publishing, 1967.

Webster GC (ed): Third New International Dictionary, Unabridged. Springfield, MA, Merriam, 1976.

Wisser SH: When the walls listened. American Journal of Nursing 78(6):1016–1017, 1978.

Zderad LT: Empathic nursing: Realization of a human capacity. Nursing Clinics of North America 4(4):655–662, 1969.

BIBLIOGRAPHY

Avila DL, Combs AW, Purkey WW: The Helping Relationship Sourcebook, ed 2. Boston, Allyn & Bacon, 1977.

Fromm E: The Art of Loving. New York, Harper & Row, 1956.

Group Child Care Consultant Services: The Child Care Worker: Separation; Instructor Manual III. Chapel Hill, NC, School of Social Work, University of North Carolina, 1977 (DHEW Contract 105-75-1122).

Haspedis BL: Creating a caring climate. Nursing Clinics of North America 4(4):683–690, 1969.

Johnson DW: Reaching Out: Interpersonal Effectiveness and Self-actualization. Englewood Cliffs, NJ, Prentice-Hall, 1972.

Kalisch BJ: An experiment in the development of empathy in nursing students. Nursing Research 20(3):202–211, 1971.

Kauffman M: On developing empathy: Sharing the patient's experience. American Journal of Nursing 78(5):860–861, 1978.

McGoran S: On developing empathy: Teaching students self-awareness. American Journal of Nursing 78(5):859–861, 1978.

Naugle EH: The difference caring makes. American Journal of Nursing 73:1890, 1973.

Peplau HE: Talking with patients. American Journal of Nursing 60(7):962–966, 1960.

Skipper JK: Communication and the hospitalized patient. In Skipper JK, Leonard RC (eds): Social Interaction and Patient Care. Philadelphia, JB Lippincott, 1965.

Triplett JL: Empathy is . . . . Nursing Clinics of North America 4(4):673–681, 1969.

AUDIOVISUAL RESOURCES

Communication Processes in Nursing
  Videocassette. (1971, B & W, 30 min.)

The Meaning of Communication
  Film (16 mm). (1971, B & W, 30 min.)
  Available through:
    Instructional Media Center
    University of Nebraska
    3835 Holdrege Street
    Lincoln, NE 68583

The Nurse–Patient Relationship
  Videocassette. Includes techniques of acceptance, establishment of trust. (1981, Color, series of 8, 4 hr.)
  Available through:
    Health Sciences Consortium
    103 Laurel Avenue
    Carrboro, NC 27510

SKILL 2 Knowing Ourselves

One of the essentials of helping others is understanding and facing ourselves.
— Hamilton, p. 296

☐ STUDENT OBJECTIVES

1. Explain the contributions of self-awareness, self-concept, and self-understanding to self-knowledge.
2. Explain the relationship of self-knowledge to the ability to help others.
3. Describe the influence of self-worth on a person's concept of self.
4. Distinguish between feelings and behaviors.
5. Describe the relationship of basic-need satisfaction and level of psychosocial growth and development to feelings and behaviors.
6. Increase your own awareness of how you function in everyday situations.

INTRODUCTION

Knowing ourselves involves being able to recognize what we are like and how we function interpersonally; it involves understanding the effect those characteristics have on the nature and quality of our interpersonal relationships. Knowing ourselves is requisite to our ability to help others because it is essential for productive communication that is therapeutic for the client and based on mutual respect between nurse and client.

When we know ourselves we also tend to become more comfortable with and accepting of ourselves. Therefore, the ability to develop a helping relationship with another person depends on how well we have learned to know, understand, and accept ourselves. Acceptance of self is a positive recognition of our own worth and value, coupled with a knowledge of our strengths and weaknesses and how they affect our relationships with others, as opposed to having a self-centered or complacent attitude about what we are like. Sundeen et al. (1981) state that a positive concept of self is directly related to good mental health and has been found to be correlated with good interpersonal communications. Jourard (1971) believes that a nurse who is afraid or unaware of his or her own self is likely to be threatened by a client's genuine self-expressions.

Knowing ourselves helps us to take care of ourselves and meet our own needs, yet it precludes a primary or exclusive focus on self while working with clients. This makes it possible to set aside our own needs in preference to the client's needs when that becomes necessary. (See Skill 3.)

To provide quality total client care, a nurse treats each person as a unique and worthwhile individual. This is possible only when the nurse first knows and accepts himself or herself as a unique and worthwhile person. Learning to know ourselves takes time, effort, and thoughtful introspection, but it is possible.

There is a reciprocal relationship between what we do and say (our behavior) and our basic needs, level of psychosocial development, self-concept, and the feedback we receive about ourselves from others (Group Child Care Consultant Services, 1977). This relationship is illustrated in Figure 2-1. These concepts are developed as part of the following discussion of self-awareness, self-concept, and self-understanding.

PREPARATION

Whatever makes us distinctively *us* is our *self*. To know that self involves an awareness of how we feel and respond in everyday situations (self-awareness), a comprehension of how we perceive and feel about ourselves (self-concept), and some sense of who we are (self-understanding).

SELF-AWARENESS

Feelings and Behaviors

An important part of knowing ourselves is to become consciously aware of our own feelings and behaviors. Feelings are emotions that simply occur; they are not necessarily associated with rational, logical thought. All of us have feelings in response to our experiences, whether or not we are aware of them or are comfortable expressing them. Our bodies give us cues about our feelings: heart rate, respirations, perspiration, warm or cold sensations, skin color, and muscle tension or relaxation—all reflect varying kinds and degrees of emotions. The following activity is designed to help identify personal feelings.

Activity 2-A: Feelings Identification

Listed in Activity Figure 2-A are feelings most people have in different situations. Indicate how often you are aware of experiencing each emotion: never, seldom, sometimes, or frequently. There are no right or wrong answers, because each of us is different. Try to be honest with yourself about the feelings that are a part of you.

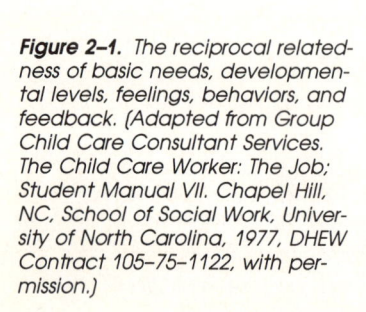

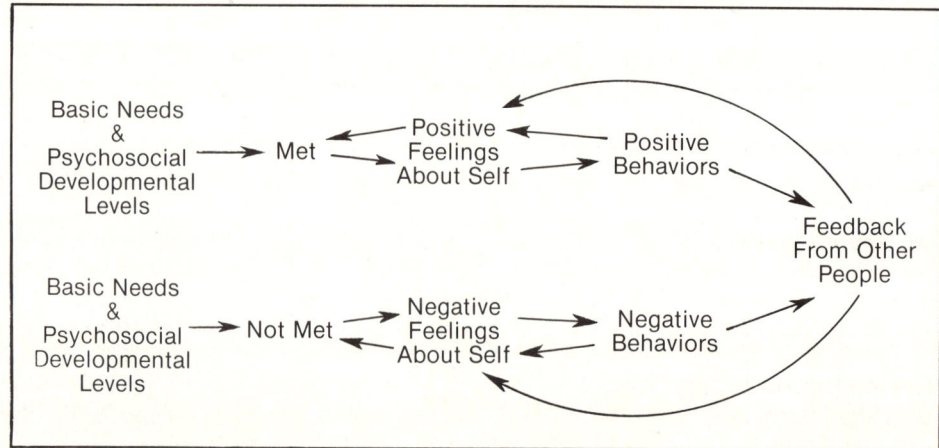

Figure 2-1. The reciprocal relatedness of basic needs, developmental levels, feelings, behaviors, and feedback. (Adapted from Group Child Care Consultant Services. The Child Care Worker: The Job; Student Manual VII. Chapel Hill, NC, School of Social Work, University of North Carolina, 1977, DHEW Contract 105-75-1122, with permission.)

Feelings	Never	Seldom	Sometimes	Frequently	Feelings	Never	Seldom	Sometimes	Frequently
stubborn					contented				
loving					sad				
angry					excited				
jealous					fearful				
disappointed					bored				
grateful					proud				
embarrassed					depressed				
cautious					shy				
daring					lonely				
confused					tender				
anxious					pleased				
sexy					guilty				
frustrated					appreciative				
surprised					happy				

Activity Figure 2–A. (From Miller S, Nunnally EW, Wackman DB: Couple Communication: Talking Together. Minneapolis, Interpersonal Communication Programs, 1979, p. 52.)

Behaviors are actions, both verbal and nonverbal; they are how we respond to and function in situations. All behavior consciously or unconsciously is meaningful to an individual and serves as a means of coping with or responding to circumstances. The result of many factors, behavior can be an expression of our feelings about past or present experiences, our reaction to our environment, or our current state of physical or emotional health.

We express our feelings through both constructive and destructive behaviors, whether or not we have a conscious awareness of this process. Because behavior is meaningful, it can be interpreted, although it is important to note that a given behavior may reflect more than one feeling. For instance, crying may represent sadness or the very opposite feeling of joy.

The relationship between feelings and behavior is reciprocal and reinforcing: feelings result in behavior, we have feelings about that behavior, and those feelings result in further behavior. For example, suppose a young woman is very angry at someone and really "tells off" the offender. When it is all over, she may feel embarrassed at her outburst, she may be pleased that she finally stood up for herself, or she may have ambivalent feelings of regret and satisfaction. How she feels about her outburst will help determine her future behavior around the other person.

Becoming aware of our own feelings and how they influence our behavior can enable us to change behavior patterns that interfere with our ability to reach out to others. For example, suppose a nurse has strong feelings of disgust and anger toward grossly obese people and prefers to avoid them. If the nurse is aware of these negative feelings, it will be easier to focus on that individual as a person and monitor verbal and nonverbal interactions than if the nurse did not acknowledge those feelings.

Developing Self-Awareness
Self-awareness involves knowing what we are experiencing at the time it is happening. This knowledge is enhanced by an understanding of how we process information. The self-awareness wheel (Fig. 2–2) is a tool that can help us do that (Miller et al., 1980). The five dimensions of the wheel (sensations, interpretations, feelings, intentions, and actions) are interrelated components in every situation we experience. The degree to which we are conscious of each component reflects our level of self-awareness.

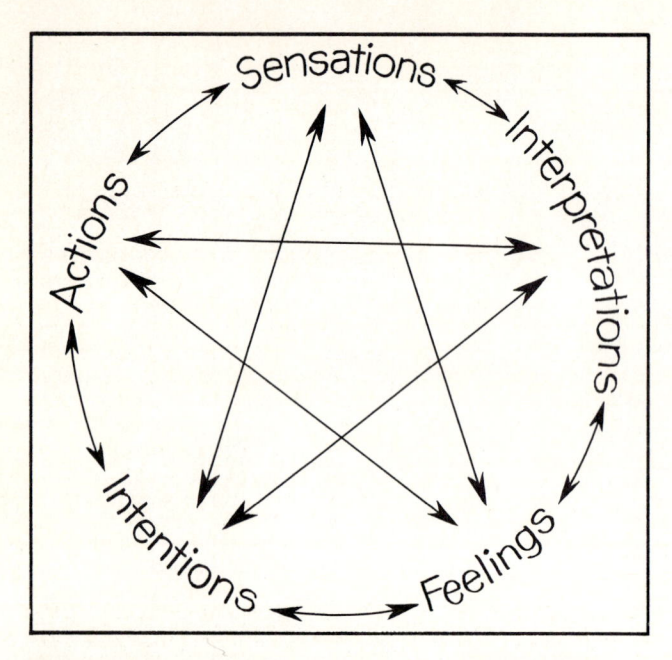

Figure 2-2. The self-awareness wheel. (From Miller S, Nunnally EW, Wackman DB: Couple Communication: Talking Together. Minneapolis, Interpersonal Communication Programs, 1979, p. 26, with permission.)

Sensations are the raw data provided by our senses: what we see, hear, touch, taste, and smell. *Interpretation* is the process of making meaning out of sensory data: what we think is happening. How we interpret data depends on our previous experiences, assumptions, expectations, and what we are aware of in that particular situation. *Feelings* are spontaneous emotional responses to our expectations and interpretations of a situation, as well as to the anticipated and actual outcome. If the outcome is better than we anticipated, good feelings usually occur; but if the outcome is not what we had hoped for, as happens when our expectations are greater than what is realistic for the situation, troublesome feelings usually occur. *Intentions* are what we want to be or do, or what we would like to have happen. Intentions are like purposes or goals (long-range intentions) and objectives (short-range intentions). In a given situation intentions may range from persuading, clarifying, and being friendly to ignoring, hurting, or demanding. Sometimes intentions are difficult to identify, and they sometimes are conflicting. For example, a student might want to help a classmate with his or her studies but at the same time might not want that classmate to get the better grade on the next exam. If we are aware of our intentions in situations, we have the option of choosing which ones we will act upon. *Actions* are verbal and nonverbal expressions of what we intend to do. Becoming aware of our actions can give us information about how we respond in situations. We can then use this information to change our behavior, if we so choose.

Initially, we become aware of what we are experiencing at any given point on the self-awareness wheel (Fig. 2-2) and then become aware of at least some of the other components. The point of initial awareness varies with the individual. For example, some people do or say something (act) before becoming aware of what they are feeling or intending; others may respond less quickly but may have become aware of what they were feeling, thinking, or intending before they took any action.

It is important to recognize that having an initial awareness at any one point is not necessarily better than having an initial awareness at any other point. However, to become more completely aware of what we are experiencing, it is necessary to be able to move from that one point of awareness to the others.

In our reactions to situations, we often bypass some of the components of the self-awareness wheel, and this can result in behavior that we or others may regard as inappropriate. Practiced use of each component of the wheel can increase our awareness of what is being experienced and how we respond in various situations. The following activity is designed to increase awareness of reactions to a specific experience.

Activity 2-B: Using the Self-awareness Wheel

Think about something that happened recently: something interesting, pleasant, difficult, or troublesome. Ask yourself these questions about the situation and write the responses on a separate sheet of paper. (Writing them down helps you to be more specific.)

- What happened? (Sensations)
- What did you think about the experience? (Interpretations)
- What emotions did you experience? (Feelings)
- What did you want to have happen? (Intentions)
- What did you do, verbally and nonverbally? (Actions)
- Which one of these were you most readily able to identify?
- Which was the most difficult?
- Is this pattern a usual one for you?

The self-awareness wheel can be used regularly to examine daily experiences in retrospect. To do this, take the time to determine the point on the wheel where awareness of a situation first occurred and move from there. For example, in a new and unfamiliar work setting some people find that they feel quite anxious, without having taken the time to think about what the new situation requires and how they might best function. Actions based only on those anxious feelings may be quite inappropriate, incongruent, or out of proportion to the actual situation. However, we can act more appropriately if we take the time first to become aware of our feelings and then to identify what is happening, what the situation means for us, and what we hope will be the outcome. On the other hand, some people respond first by thinking about and

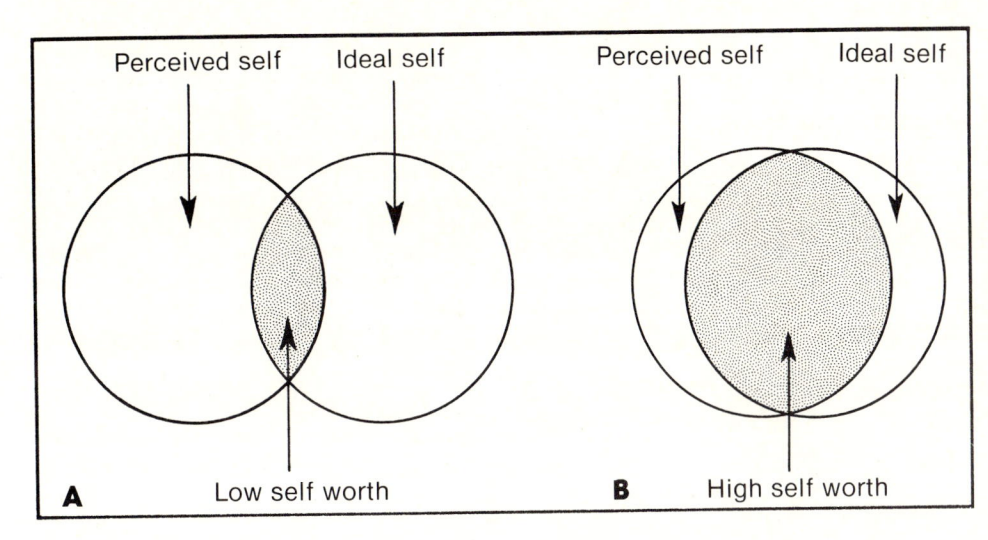

Figure 2–3. *The relationship of perceived self and ideal self to self-worth.* **A.** *Represents a person with a low level of self-worth resulting from a large discrepancy between perceived self and ideal self.* **B.** *Represents a person with a high level of self-worth resulting from greater conformity of perceived self and ideal self. (From Sundeen SJ, Stuart GW, et al: Nurse–Client Interaction: Implementing the Nursing Process (ed 2). St Louis, MO, CV Mosby, 1981, p. 62, with permission.)*

analyzing a situation before they become aware of their feelings, and only later are aware of the feelings they experienced. Although each of us processes information in different ways and at different levels, it is possible to increase our capacity to understand what is happening around us. One way is to develop an awareness of how we are responding initially to any situation, and then make a conscious and deliberate identification of the other response components before taking any action.

Conscious and deliberate focus on identification of sensations, interpretations, feelings, intentions, and actions in various situations increases our level of self-awareness and generally results in less interpersonal conflict caused by misunderstandings. It also helps us to meet our own needs in positive ways and to respond more sensitively to the needs and concerns of other people. Becoming more aware of what is happening and what we are thinking, feeling, intending, and doing increases our awareness and understanding of what our clients may be experiencing, thinking, feeling, intending, and doing.

SELF-CONCEPT

Self-concept is a subjective belief system about oneself. Our concept of self includes our own beliefs, values, and feelings, as well as our perceptions of our own experiences, abilities, and appearance. It also includes our own perceptions of what we are like and how we believe others see us. Self-concept serves as a frame of reference from which we view the world and as a filter through which we screen all information. Self-concept is not genetically determined or present at birth; rather, it is learned and developed throughout one's lifetime.

Our self-concept is influenced by *feelings of self-worth*. Self-worth, or self-esteem, is the value we place on ourselves. Satir (1972) says that a crucial factor in what happens inside each person and between people relates to each person's own concept of his or her self-worth. How we feel about ourselves depends, in a large part, on how others have felt about us. If others have felt positively toward us, loved us, and cared for us, we generally feel good about ourselves. Basically, self-worth is learned in the family during childhood and reinforced through daily experiences during an entire lifetime. It is partly determined by how we perceive ourselves in comparison with others, and by the expectations we have of ourselves and that others have of us. If we meet those expectations, we tend to feel that we have worth; if we do not, we tend to feel less than good about ourselves. Although it requires a conscious effort and a lot of time, it is possible for adults to develop a more positive sense of self-worth.

Each of us has a perceived self and an ideal self. The perceived self is what we believe ourselves to be like. This perception of self is based on our belief about what other people think of us. That belief is a subjective judgment and may or may not be accurate, which can create misunderstandings. The ideal self is the self we wish we were or the self we wish others would see us as. When the perceived and ideal selves are relatively congruent, we experience a high degree of self-worth and, as Rogers expresses it, "feelings of comfort and freedom from tension" (1947, p. 364). As the discrepancy between our perceived and ideal selves increases, our sense of self-worth decreases and our feelings of tension and discomfort increase. Figure 2–3 illustrates this relationship of perceived self and ideal self to self-worth (Sundeen et al., 1981). The following activity focuses on feelings of self-worth in personal experiences.

Activity 2–C: Looking at Self-worth*

1. Think of a recent situation in which you felt good about yourself and your spirits were high. Perhaps it had to do with a new and attractive

---

* *(Based on Satir V: Peoplemaking. Palo Alto, CA, Science & Behavior Books, 1972, pp. 22–24.)*

outfit, a well-earned high grade, or a new job. Try to feel those same feelings again. Such feelings are associated with adequate self-worth.
2. Think of a time when you really goofed, were scolded, or felt helpless and frustrated. Recall those feelings, even though painful. Such feelings are associated with low self-worth.
3. Relax. Note your state of self-worth today.

Self-concept also is influenced by a person's *level of growth and development* and the extent to which all previous developmental tasks were completed in a satisfactory manner. For example, someone who completed satisfactorily the developmental task of autonomy versus shame and doubt as a child, generally is able to accept reasonable limits and respond to necessary external controls and constraints without hostility. Someone who did not resolve this developmental task satisfactorily may continue to struggle with the authority issue into adulthood, demonstrating this by being habitually late and having others wait for him or her. This behavior frequently becomes irritating to other people and results in negative feedback from them. Since self-concept is so dependent on others' perspectives, this feedback can produce negative feelings and more negative behavior.

The level and nature of *basic-need satisfaction* also influences self-concept. Unmet basic needs may result in negative feelings about self and in behaviors that are perceived negatively by others. People are not always fully aware of what their basic needs are and therefore may be expending their energy on behavior that does not meet either their real or perceived needs, which generally results in negative feedback from other people. For example, adults who perceived themselves to have been loved and accepted as children usually are able to give freely of themselves to others, to accept and enjoy others as they are, and to find their world to be generally safe and satisfying. Adults who did not perceive themselves to have been loved and accepted as children often have a strong need for approval. Seeking approval within adult relationships may cause others to respond negatively, and receiving these negative responses further decreases positive feelings about self.

To illustrate the relationship between basic-need satisfaction and self-concept, consider Mary, a college junior. Mary treated her new roommates to a movie or hamburgers at least once a week, even though she needed to work part-time to put herself through college. At first her roommates enjoyed the treats, but eventually they felt guilty and angry. They told Mary it seemed she was trying to bribe them into liking her. Mary was hurt because she thought she was being generous and kind. She was only vaguely aware that what she found to be most satisfying was her roommates' gratitude, not the sharing of her resources—but she was keenly aware that she felt unloved and unwanted. As time went by, Mary assumed that her roommates did not like her and became convinced they put up with her only because they had to, although she did not validate these perceptions with them. She became moody and tearful, and when her roommates asked her to join them for pizza she responded, "Sure, I'll go—if you *really* want me along!" The roommates felt irritated at Mary's indirect request for their approval but responded, "Of course we want you!" Mary sensed their irritation, and so the destructive interpersonal cycle continued. While it is not possible to explain or describe precisely one's own self-concept, the following exercise is designed to look at self-perception and self-identity.

Activity 2-D: Looking at Self-identity

On a separate sheet of paper, write ten spontaneous answers to each of these questions:

1. Who are you?
2. What are you like?

Write down whatever comes to your mind without deliberation. Answers to the first question will usually be nouns and answers to the second question will usually be descriptive adjectives.

> Examples: "Who are you?" "I am a woman (man, student)."
> "What are you like?" "I am attractive (healthy, energetic)."

Look at the words you have used to describe yourself. What do they tell you about your perceptions of yourself? Are they task-oriented? role-oriented? person-oriented? Are they positive? negative?

SELF-UNDERSTANDING

Self-understanding is the awareness of factors in our own background and development that have contributed to the kind of persons we have become. Understanding ourselves helps us to recognize how we are similar and yet unique from other people. This can help our awareness of what we are like as nurses. For example, some of us may have grown up in homes and communities where male and female roles were defined very clearly and traditionally. Males might not have been expected to do their own laundry, to prepare food, or to clean up after themselves. Females might not have been expected to be independent, to manage money, or to plan their own social life. In addition to the family, there were relatives or neighbors who gave advice and helped make decisions, or who gave support in crises. When young people with such a background attend school or live away from home for the first time they may feel overwhelmed by the experience of being completely in charge of their own lives. They may feel a great need for support and togetherness from a roommate or friend. Others of us may have grown up with different expectations, and looking after ourselves may be a well-established pattern with which we are very comfortable. Discussing these kinds of past experiences and expectations with other persons can increase our understanding of our own expectations and behaviors.

Self-understanding is more than a cognitive recognition of background factors. It also involves looking at how those factors affect our present relationships with others. Understanding ourselves can help us to identify conflicts from our past in order to deal with them in the present. For example, a nurse may be able to recognize a relationship between anger at a client who does not follow instructions and childhood experiences of being severely scolded and punished for disobedience or mistakes. Being aware of this relationship can help the nurse to be more creative and less punitive in working with this client, and the client will generally respond by following instructions more carefully!

As with self-concept, self-understanding is achieved gradually and with a degree of introspection. The following activity is designed to look at your own background and how it might be related to your behavior.

Activity 2-E: Past Experiences and Behavior

1. Recall how men and women, parents and children, and teenagers and adults related to each other in your family and community. Compare these relationships with those experienced by several friends.
2. Observe situations in which people respond to each other in ways that seem strange and inappropriate to you. Consider how someone in your own family would have reacted.
3. Observe your own interactions with other people, or ask for feedback from someone whose judgment and objectivity you trust. Ask yourself these questions: How do you respond to directions or requests for help from other people? Do you have frequent arguments with people? Are you often critical of other people's behavior?

☐ EXECUTION

None of us can ever know our inner self completely or be fully known by someone else. We can, however, increase our level of understanding and awareness of ourselves. The Johari window (Fig. 2-4) illustrates this idea (Luft, 1984). The four quadrants represent the total self as it is known or unknown to self and others. A change in the size of any one quadrant affects the sizes of other quadrants.

Quadrant 1, the *public self*, is an *open area* that includes behaviors and motivations known to ourselves and to others. Quadrant 2, the *semipublic self*, is a *blind area* because it includes those things others perceive in us, of which we are unaware. Quadrant 3, the *private self*, is a *hidden area* that contains things we know about ourselves, but which are not revealed to others. Quadrant 4, the *inner self*, is an *unknown area* that contains aspects of the self of which neither we nor others are aware.

When quadrant 1 is large, levels of communication and interpersonal relationships are generally high and productive. When quadrant 1 is small, the reverse is true. Learning about self, its relationship to behaviors, and how that affects others increases the size of the first quadrant, making one or more of the other quadrants correspondingly smaller (Fig. 2-4). This increased knowledge of self provides a person with more internal freedom and an increased ability to interact spontaneously and honestly with others (Haber et al., 1982; Jourard, 1971; Luft, 1984).

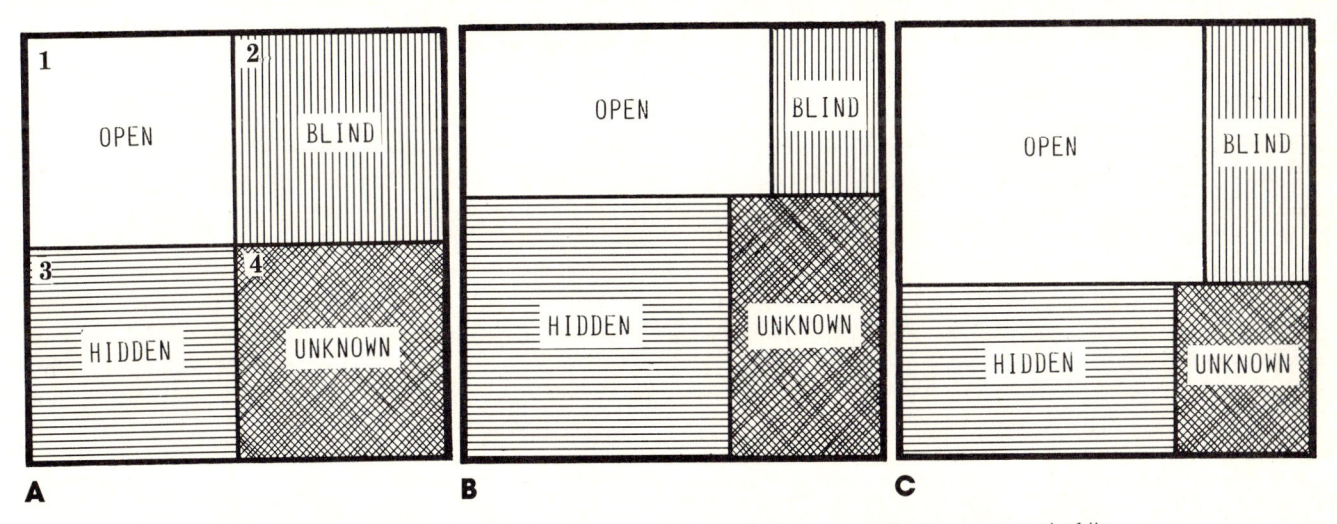

Figure 2-4. The Johari window. **A.** Each quadrant, or windowpane, reflects one aspect of the self. The relative sizes of the quadrants reflect varying degrees of self-awareness. **B.** Represents a person with little self-awareness and openness. **C.** Represents a person with great self-awareness and openness. (From Luft J: Group Processes: An Introduction to Group Dynamics. With permission, Mayfield Publishing Company, Palo Alto, CA. Copyright © 1984, 1970, 1963 by Joseph Luft.)

Learning about self requires that we be able to observe ourselves and be honest with ourselves. It requires that we be sensitive and open to ourselves and to other people, and that we be willing to look at what we and others do and are. Developing an increased understanding of ourselves takes time, energy, and thoughtful introspection. It takes a willingness to risk learning some things about ourselves that might be uncomfortable or even painful. The process of knowing ourselves can also be facilitated by asking for and receiving feedback from people who care about us and want to help us grow.

☐ CRITICAL POINTS SUMMARY

1. Self-knowledge is necessary for effective helping.
2. Self-awareness, self-concept, and self-understanding are integral to knowing oneself.
3. Self-worth derives from our experiences with others, the expectations they have of us, the degree of congruence between our perceived and ideal selves, our developmental level, and the degree to which our basic needs are satisfied.
4. Self-awareness involves being conscious of our sensations, interpretations, feelings, intentions, and actions in situations we experience.
5. Being aware of what we experience and how we respond increases our awareness of what a client is experiencing and helps us respond to his or her needs rather than our own.
6. The ability to understand and accept ourselves increases our ability to understand, accept, and help others.

☐ REVIEW QUESTIONS

1. What is the major difference between self-understanding and self-awareness?
2. What is the difference between self-concept and self-worth?
3. What three factors influence our sense of self-worth?
4. How do self-worth, developmental level, and basic-need satisfaction affect our self-concept?
5. How is behavior related to self-worth, basic-need satisfaction, and developmental level?
6. In what ways are the five components of the self-awareness wheel interrelated?
7. How can using the self-awareness wheel influence our own level of self-awareness?
8. What is the relationship between self-understanding and self-awareness, and the ability to help other people?

REFERENCES

Group Child Care Counsultant Services. The Child Care Worker: The Job; Student Manual VII. Chapel Hill, NC, School of Social Work, University of North Carolina, 1977 (DHEW Contract 105-75-1122).

Haber J, Leach AM, et al: Comprehensive Psychiatric Nursing, ed 2. New York, McGraw-Hill, 1982.

Hamilton G: Helping people—The growth of a profession. Journal of Social Casework 29(8):296, 1948.

Jourard SM: The Transparent Self, rev ed. New York, D Van Nostrand, 1971.

Luft J: Of Human Interaction. Palo Alto, CA, National Press Books, 1984.

Miller S, Nunnally EW, Wackman DB: Couple Communication: Talking Together. Minneapolis, Interpersonal Communication Programs, 1980.

Rogers CR: Some observations on the organization of personality. American Psychologist 2:358–368, 1947.

Satir V: Peoplemaking. Palo Alto, CA, Science and Behavior Books, 1972.

Sundeen SJ, Stuart GW, et al: Nurse–Client Interaction: Implementing the Nursing Process, ed 2. St Louis, MO, CV Mosby, 1981.

SKILL 3 Needs Identification

The human being is motivated by a number of basic needs which are species-wide, apparently unchanging, and genetic or instinctual in origin.
—Goble, p. 38

☐ STUDENT OBJECTIVES

1. Describe the relationship of basic need satisfaction to a positive or negative self-concept.
2. Explain the hierarchic nature of basic needs.
3. Describe the relationship between needs and behavior.
4. Describe the relationship between needs and values.
5. Examine the relationship between basic needs and self-concept.
6. Explain how illness affects the ability to satisfy basic needs.
7. Identify your own met and unmet physical and psychological needs.
8. Recognize ways that you meet your own needs.
9. Identify ways of resolving conflicting nurse and client needs.

INTRODUCTION

Basic needs are internal motivating forces for human behavior. According to psychologist Abraham Maslow, these needs are species-wide, apparently unchanging, and genetic or instinctual in origin. They are both physiological and psychological in nature and are described as deficiency needs because they are necessary for health. Their absence breeds illness, their presence prevents illness, their restoration cures illness, and their level is low in the healthy person (Goble, 1970; Maslow, 1968).

Understanding the connection between basic needs and behaviors can help us understand both our own behaviors and the behaviors of others. Recognition of causes for behavior helps us to become less judgmental and better able to relate to clients and peers who exhibit wide ranges of behavior. For example, soon after being admitted to the clinical unit, an elderly woman put her call light on every few minutes for what seemed to the nurses to be minor requests, such as for adjusting the pillows, adding a blanket, removing the blanket, or asking for the bedpan or a drink. Although she was unable to identify her real need, the woman's primary concern was that she was feeling quite unsafe in her new environment. The nurses were irritated until they recognized their client's unmet need and planned ways to increase her feelings of safety and security. They made sure her light was answered promptly, they anticipated what she might need and offered it before she asked, they told her when they would return (and returned regularly), and they asked her what she might need. Before long the call light was on only infrequently, the nurses were able to plan their time more effectively, and everyone felt better.

Awareness of our own needs helps us to choose positive ways of meeting those needs rather than meeting them at the expense of others. To illustrate, a nurse who is unaware of her unsatisfied needs for love and belonging often keeps clients dependent on her much longer than is helpful to them, or does things for them that they would benefit from doing unaided. For this nurse, feelings of being needed and the client's gratitude and appreciation provide such a deep sense of reward that she may be unable to put them aside in order to promote self-care and independence in the client. If the nurse were aware of those unmet needs for love, affection, and belonging when working with clients, she could consciously observe and evaluate whose need is being met and then could look for ways to meet her own unmet needs in ways other than through work.

PREPARATION

THE CONCEPT OF BASIC NEEDS

Maslow describes a hierarchy of basic needs. *Physiological needs for survival* include air, food and water, shelter, sleep, activity, and reproduction. After the physiological survival needs are met, the need to feel safe and secure within one's world and relationships emerge. Safety has both physical and psychological connotations for Maslow. When physiological needs and safety needs are met, *needs for love, affection, and belonging* emerge. For Maslow, love involves both giving and receiving, and belonging has to do with attaining a place within the group and a sense of belonging somewhere. After these needs are satisfied, the need for esteem emerges. This need includes both self-esteem (feelings of competence, independence, achievement) and esteem from others (such as respect, recognition, and appreciation) (Goble, 1970).

When the basic needs of love and esteem are reasonably satisfied, the need for self-actualization emerges. This innate need for growth, development, and utilization of potential is described by Maslow as "the desire to become more and more what one is, to become everything that one is capable of becoming" (Maslow, 1954, p. 92).

Beyond the basic needs, Maslow later identified what he termed nonhierarchic *growth needs* or *being-values,* which are also essential for human beings. Some of the growth needs or being-values he described are wholeness, individuality, justice, playfulness, completeness, and goodness (Goble, 1970).

Basic needs generally emerge in the order presented here. Gratification very early in life, especially in the first 2 years, of the needs for safety, love, and esteem is very important for developing a healthy personality, according to Maslow. If basic needs are met adequately within the first 2 years of life, a person can withstand a later loss or frustration of these needs and still remain a secure and strong person. The following activity is designed to look at ways your basic needs are met. It is for personal information only and need not be shared unless desired.

Activity 3-A: Looking at Basic Needs

1. In the first column of Activity Figure 3-A the basic needs described by Maslow are listed. In the second column write ways you are currently meeting those needs and in the third column indicate the degree to which you perceive the needs are being met, using the following scale:

   1 = very little   4 = above average
   2 = less than average 5 = very well
   3 = average

   In the last column indicate whether you perceive your needs as being met in a positive or negative way.

2. Look at your responses. Take note of the needs that you have indicated are being met at a less than average level or in a negative way. What could you do to raise the level of meeting these needs or how could you develop more positive ways of meeting them?

Basic Need	How Need Is Being Met	Degree to Which Need Is Being Met	Positive/Negative
Air			
Food and Water			
Shelter			
Sleep and Activity			
Reproduction (sex)			
Safety (physical/psychological)			
Love and Belonging			
Esteem from Self and Others			
Growth (list several that are relevant for you)			

Activity Figure 3–A

Basic Needs and Developmental Levels

There are some relationships between Maslow's basic need theory and Erikson's theory of psychosocial human development that may help explain the hierarchic and developmental nature of basic needs. The basic needs of safety and security identified by Maslow are met through satisfactory resolution of the developmental task of *trust versus mistrust* identified by Erikson (Maier, 1969). In this phase, the development of trust brings with it a sense of being loved and cared for. The need for esteem from self and others is met through resolving the issues of *autonomy and initiative*. Resolution of these issues as well as the next higher developmental issues of *identity and intimacy* also increases one's sense of belonging. Finally, self-actualization is strived for during the years identified by Erikson as being concerned with *generativity and integrity*. This is also the time during which one is concerned with the nonhierarchical growth needs described by Maslow.

Basic needs are general ways of looking at human needs and can be translated into specific needs for individuals in specific situations. For example, the elderly woman with the unmet general need for safety had specific needs for reassurance, information, and consistency. Meeting these specific needs helped meet the woman's greater need for safety and security in an unfamiliar setting. This concept is congruent with Orlando's (1961) definition of a need as "a requirement of a [person] which, if supplied, relieves or diminishes his immediate distress or improves his immediate sense of adequacy or well-being" (p. 5).

BASIC-NEED SATISFACTION

In our society some people have their basic survival needs well met, while others struggle to meet those needs at subsistence levels. This is especially true for many elderly persons, for the unemployed, and for the urban and rural poor. It is difficult to be concerned about meeting higher needs when lower ones remain unmet.

Beyond the physical survival needs, it is primarily a subjective judgment whether or not one's basic needs are met adequately. If a person does not feel that his or her needs are met, then for that person they are not met, regardless of others' perceptions. A person may have a good job, loving family, and friends, and may appear to be successful, and yet may feel quite inadequate. When basic needs are satisfied adequately as they emerge, they remain at a low level of deficiency throughout life. When basic needs are satisfied inadequately as they emerge or even remain unmet, the resulting higher level of deficiency produces strong behavioral motivation forces as the person continues to strive to meet those needs throughout life. As Maslow indicates, "I am motivated when I feel desire or want or yearning or wish or lack" (1968, p. 22). When basic needs are satisfied inadequately, they become sources of problems throughout life. For example, a child who does not experience a reliable, consistent, and predictable world in which he or she feels safe becomes anxious and insecure. As an adult, he or she may avoid the strange and unexpected and may have a compulsive need to make order out of his or her environment. He or she behaves as if some danger were always imminent.

Needs may be met in healthy ways, such as becoming highly successful in one's profession as a way of meeting a need for esteem from self and others. Behaviors that satisfy needs are healthy if they meet those needs successfully, are nondamaging to others, and are legally and socially approved by one's own culture. Needs may be met in unhealthy ways, such as satisfying a need for esteem from others through exerting power and control over them. Behaviors that satisfy needs are unhealthy when they are exploitive and manipulative of others, disregard others' needs, or are unacceptable legally and socially.

SELF-CONCEPT AND NEED SATISFACTION

A person's sense of self-worth affects both the ability to meet basic needs and the perception of whether or not those needs are met. A person who chooses the most healthy available ways of meeting basic needs will generally feel accepted, loved, worthwhile, and successful. Positive responses from other people reinforce these feelings. When basic needs are met in unhealthy ways, the person will tend to feel unaccepted, unloved, worthless, and unsuccessful, and negative responses from others will reinforce these negative feelings. When we feel good about ourselves, we are able to form open, comfortable, and mutually satisfying relationships with other people, without having a need to make excessive demands on others as a way of bolstering our own self-concept and sense of self-worth. People with a low self-concept often see themselves as lacking esteem from both self and others, and as being inadequately loved and accepted. Because of this, they may put themselves down, hoping that someone will contradict them and tell them that they are good, competent, or attractive. This approach to meeting basic needs tends to make others feel manipulated and uncomfortable.

To illustrate the relationship of self-concept and basic needs, consider Sally, who always puts herself down by making statements like: "You always look so much nicer than I do when we go out together"; "You'd better get someone else to do that for you—you know I always mess things up"; or "You really want to go on a trip with a loser like me?" Although Sally's friends feel uncomfortable about Sally's unspoken bids for compliments and reassurance, they tend to respond: "Nonsense—you always look good!" or "Now Sally, you know you're not a loser!" Sally's need for esteem is valid, but the way she unconsciously meets that need does not invite positive feelings from others.

VALUES AND NEED SATISFACTION

One way of identifying individual needs is to look at what a person regards as important, that is, what he or she values. Values can be regarded as the opposite side of human needs (Hall, 1976). Whatever we value highly becomes essential for our feelings of well-being and is thus something we perceive we need. For example, a person who values order and neatness can become quite uncomfortable and irritable when his or her surroundings are disorganized or untidy. For this person order and neatness are psychological needs. If the person is not aware that his or her discomfort is related to a need for and a value of order and neatness, he or she may lash out at the roommate or co-worker who caused the disorder. When the person becomes aware of the value and need for order, he or she can make a deliberate choice as to how to meet that need, such as choosing to ignore the disorder, to take care of it personally, or to convey the discomfort to the person (or persons) responsible. Regardless of the alternative chosen, making a conscious decision is a freeing process in that it produces a higher level of self-responsibility, which results in increased feelings of self-worth and self-confidence. The following activity is designed to help identify needs and values as they relate to personal behaviors and to other people.

Activity 3-B: Needs and Behavior in Conflict

1. Recall a recent situation in which you were in conflict, either within yourself or with someone else. Briefly describe the situation to yourself or to someone else.
2. Using the self-awareness wheel from Figure 2–2 (Skill 2) ask yourself:
   - What happened? What was I experiencing through my *senses?*
   - How did I interpret or *think* about what happened?
   - What were my *feelings* about the situation?
   - What did I *intend* or wish to have happen?
   - What did I *do* in the situation, both verbally and nonverbally?
3. Try to identify what your need was in the situation and what you were attempting to do to satisfy it. Name the need. For example, "In this situation I had a need for _____"; or "I had a need to _____."
4. State the need as a *value*. For example, "I valued _____"; or "_____ was quite important to me in this situation."
5. Identify how you are *acting* on that value. For example, "Since I valued _____, I _____."
6. Was your need met positively and productively for yourself? For others? If not, what might you have done to meet that need more productively?

Example: After examining a situation with the self-awareness wheel concept, you might determine that your need was independence: to be in charge of your own life and destiny. Often this need is demonstrated by managing or controlling other people and the situation. So for you, being in charge and controlling the outcome or the other persons involved was important. Your responses to the above questions might be: "I had a need to be independent." "I valued self-sufficiency." "Since I valued self-sufficiency, I attempted to control what others did so that I would be in charge."

Attempting to control others probably made them irritated with you and resulted in your feeling miserable. Therefore, your need for independence was not met productively. To meet that need in a more positive manner, you could consider controlling your own behavior and responses (rather than those of others), as that generally results in greater degree of self-sufficiency, a higher level of independence, and more positive feedback from others.

ILLNESS AND NEED SATISFACTION

Illness often interferes with a person's ability to meet basic needs. For example, having abdominal surgery interferes with meeting the survival needs for food and water; fear of anesthesia may create problems with one's sense of safety; and becoming a dependent "patient" does not meet esteem needs as adequately as functioning in an independent role such as that of a homemaker, carpenter, or business executive. Under the stress of illness, a person's need for *receiving* becomes intense, and the need to have a helper becomes important. For example, a person who is having surgery that has an uncertain outcome may feel very unsafe. He or she may express this through demanding behavior, through many questions, or through withdrawal—all of which say "I need you to help me feel more safe."

Whenever we are ill, most of us experience some degree of regression to earlier levels of need satisfaction. It feels good to be taken care of, to forget about our responsibilities, and to have no obligations. If we're not feeling too badly, we even enjoy the extra attention. Once we feel better we are ready to resume our usual roles and responsibilities. These are normal, healthy dependency reactions to illness. Some people find the dependency and rewards of being sick (secondary gains from illness) more personally satisfying than being well and assuming usual responsibilities. They may manipulate the nurse into doing more for them than is necessary or even helpful physically, and often find ways to prolong a hospital stay or delay a return to work.

The following example tells us something about secondary gains from illness. The discharge planning nurse arranged for a community health nurse to visit Mr. King, a 48-year-old man returning home after abdominal surgery. Although the physician had instructed Mr. King to increase his activities gradually, the community health nurse found him in a hospital bed at home, with his wife providing almost complete care. Mr. King said he just didn't feel very good but had no specific complaints. Besides, he said his wife enjoyed looking after him. He also was planning to ask for an extension of his sick leave from his job. In this example, Mr. King's need to be taken care of is stronger than his need for independence. It is hoped that by giving Mr. King adequate acceptance and support, by exploring his perceptions of his illness, and by explaining his recovery needs, the community health nurse can help him to return to his usual roles without excessive delays.

The nature of the nurse–client relationship can facilitate growth and movement toward self-actualization, particularly when the nurse is able to assist clients to understand what they are experiencing, to feel good about themselves, to maintain their self-respect, and to achieve some sense of control over their destiny or come to terms with the inevitable. Travelbee (1971) proposes that illness can become a time of personal growth and self-actualization if the person is able to find meaning in the experience. She proposes that nurses can find as much satisfaction in helping people find meaning in illness as in assisting them toward recovery.

☐ EXECUTION

Like self-knowledge (Skill 2), becoming aware of our own needs takes time, energy, conscious thought, and some degree of introspection. One benefit from becoming aware of our own needs is that we can then make conscious and deliberate choices about how we will meet those needs from the options available to us.

While basic needs are general and common to all, the way they are met is unique to each individual. Recognizing the relationship between our own needs and behaviors can help us to recognize need-satisfaction behaviors in others. This recognition of the commonality and individuality of need satisfaction can help us to be less judgmental about ourselves and about others. The following activity is designed to increase awareness of basic and individual needs in specific situations through the use of the self-awareness wheel (Fig. 2–2) from Skill 2.

Activity 3–C:
Needs and Behavior in Success

1. Recall a situation in which things went well for you: a successful happening at work, school, or with your friends or family.
2. Using the self-awareness wheel from Figure 2–2, think about the experience. Ask yourself:
   - What happened? What was I experiencing through my *senses?*
   - How did I interpret or *think* about what happened?
   - What were my *feelings* about the situation?
   - What did I *intend* or wish to have happen?
   - What did I *do* in the situation, both verbally and nonverbally?
3. What basic and individual needs were being satisfied through this experience?
4. Now recall a situation in which things did not go well for you.
5. Ask yourself the same questions as in 2.
6. What basic and individual needs were not being satisfied very well through this experience, or which ones were you trying to meet unsuccessfully?

7. How could you have met your needs more productively?

Sometimes a nurse needs to set aside or modify his or her own need satisfaction for the purpose of meeting a client's needs. For example, Sandra Jones, a community health nurse, had several important home visits planned for the morning and a personal appointment to keep during her lunch break. She was also scheduled to be at a clinic in the afternoon. Sandra's second visit of the morning is with a mother of a premature infant whom she had visited 2 weeks ago when the infant had been home only a few days. At that time the mother had a number of questions about the infant's care. She initially seemed somewhat anxious but eagerly listened to and apparently understood Sandra's instructions. The mother was visibly relaxed and seemed confident when the nurse left. Today, however, the mother is anxious, looks tired, and appears disheveled in contrast to her previous well-groomed appearance. The baby is fretful and looks slightly dehydrated. The mother tells Sandra that the baby has been wakeful for 3 or 4 days and nights, cries a lot, does not take as much formula as he had earlier, and wants to be held all the time. She is in tears and says, "I just don't know what to do! My husband has to sleep at night so he can go to work, so I try to keep the baby quiet as much as I can. He says I must not be a very good mother or the baby wouldn't cry so much!" The nurse also learns that the mother's neighbor has told her she will spoil the baby by holding him so much and that the reason he cries so much is because he needs cereal and other baby foods. So the mother has begun feeding the baby cereal, fruit, and egg yolk, although both the clinic doctor and Sandra had recommended waiting until later to begin solid food.

Sandra recognizes that the mother is not coping adequately with the additional demands the baby is making, that she needs much support and encouragement right now, and that she needs help in solving the problem. However, Sandra also feels some irritation that the mother is not following instructions. Sandra knows that the family she is scheduled to visit next has no telephone so she cannot call and change the appointment she made last week. She is also concerned about keeping her personal appointment at lunchtime.

In this situation, the nurse needs to decide how to respond to the mother's obvious need for help, the baby's need for more adequate care, and her own needs for being on time, keeping the next client's trust, and tending to personal needs. To meet what seem to be conflicting needs, the nurse first identifies which needs have the highest priority so that a process of negotiation can begin. It is hoped that some needs can be met for all three individuals. For example, Sandra might say to the mother, "It sounds as though a lot of things aren't going very well for you right now! The family I'm scheduled to visit when I leave here doesn't have a telephone, so I can't call and change that appointment and I need to be at the clinic after that. I do have about a half hour right now, so we could work on whatever is giving you the most difficulty and then I could come back again tomorrow afternoon. How does that sound to you?" On another day when Sandra had no lunchtime commitments, she might very well have decided to spend more time with the young mother, be late for the next appointment, and eat a quick sandwich in the car enroute to the clinic.

A crucial part of being a professional helper involves the ability to reorder priorities or set aside one's own needs temporarily and in preference to the needs of someone seeking help. This does not mean that the nurse negates his or her own needs. What it does mean is that the nurse develops an awareness of when and how it is necessary to give priority to clients' needs in order to promote their growth and health.

☐ CRITICAL POINTS SUMMARY

1. Basic human needs are universal and hierarchic in nature.
2. Basic human needs are a controlling factor of behavior.
3. Successfully meeting basic needs contributes to a positive self-concept.
4. Unsuccessfully meeting basic needs contributes to a negative self-concept.
5. Basic needs can be translated into specific needs for individual situations.
6. Illness interferes with or modifies the ability to meet one's basic needs.
7. Values often reflect a person's needs.
8. Recognizing one's own needs helps to keep those needs from interfering with personal and professional relationships.

☐ REVIEW QUESTIONS

1. List the basic physiological and psychological needs.
2. Why are basic needs sometimes called deficiency needs?
3. Discuss the meaning of the following statements: "Basic needs are hierarchic in nature." "Basic needs are met through satisfactory resolution of developmental tasks."
4. Give two examples of individual needs that could be associated with (a) the need for safety and security, (b) the need for love and belonging, and (c) the need for esteem.
5. How is self-concept related to basic-need satisfaction?
6. In what way do our values help us to understand what our needs are?
7. Give one example each of how illness can interfere with meeting physiological and psychological basic needs.

8. What relationship exists between basic-need satisfaction and the ability to be helpful to others?
9. How does recognition of one's own basic needs increase the ability to help?
10. What examples can you give from your experience of positive and negative ways of meeting basic needs?

REFERENCES

Goble FG: The Third Force. New York, Pocket Books, 1970.

Hall BP: The Development of a Confluent Theory of Values. New York, Paulist Press, 1976.

Maier HW: Three Theories of Child Development. New York, Harper & Row, 1969.

Maslow AH: Motivation and Personality. New York, Harper & Row, 1954.

Maslow AH: Toward a Psychology of Being, ed 2. New York, Van Nostrand Reinhold, 1968.

Orlando IJ: The Dynamic Nurse–Patient Relationship. New York, GP Putnam's Sons, 1961.

Travelbee J: Interpersonal Aspects of Nursing. Philadelphia, FA Davis, 1971.

SKILL 4 Values Identification

If a man does not keep pace with his companions, perhaps it is because he hears a different drummer. Let him step to the music he hears, however measured or far away.
—Henry David Thoreau

□ STUDENT OBJECTIVES

1. Distinguish among values, valuing, and value system.
2. Explain how one's perception of the world influences the development of one's values.
3. Distinguish between internal and external value sources.
4. Explain the relationship of feelings, behaviors, needs, and vision to values.
5. Explain the five aspects of a valuing process.
6. Relate professional codes and standards to values associated with client care.
7. Discuss the significance of values identification for positive personal and professional relationships.
8. Recognize behavioral expressions of your own values.
9. Become aware of your own values and value conflicts.

□ INTRODUCTION

A *value* is something that has worth or merit; it is what we believe and accept to be worthwhile. Hall (1976) defines a value as "any person, relationship, or object which when freely chosen and acted upon contributes to the self's meaning and enhances its growth" (p. 24). Values arise from our beliefs and feelings and are demonstrated through our behavior; that is, we act on the basis of what we believe or feel to be worthwhile. Thus, values are motivating forces for behavior and give direction to our lives. For example, our values influence many decisions in life such as the job we choose, whether we marry or have children, or how we spend time and money.

A person may or may not be aware of the values he or she holds and may or may not recognize how those values are expressed behaviorally. Because our behavior reflects our values, other people may be more aware of the values we hold than we ourselves are.

Recognizing our own values and looking at how they affect our behavior increases our understanding of ourselves. It also helps us to recognize the values other people hold and how those values affect others' behavior and choices. Identifying our own values increases our ability to make choices about value-laden issues that are congruent with those values. In the health-care field there are many ethical dilemmas that involve a nurse, such as prolongation of life, abortion, research involving human subjects, and priorities for community services offered. As with recognizing our own needs, recognizing our own values makes it possible to choose our response in a given situation and act in a client's best interest, rather than responding automatically out of an unclear value base. Leininger (1978), a nurse-anthropologist, has written about values that many nurses have, such as cleanliness, time, and optimal good health. These and other more personal values affect the way nurses relate to the people with whom they work.

The practice of professional nursing requires that nurses respect the values of the patients they care for. For example, the Code for Nurses, revised by the American Nurses' Association in 1976, states that

The nurse provides services with respect for human dignity and the uniqueness of the client unrestricted by considerations of social or economic status, nationality, race, personal attributes, or the nature of health problems. (American Nurses' Association, 1976, p. 3)

Similarly, included in the International Council of Nurses' 1973 Code for Nurses are these statements:

Inherent in nursing is respect for life, dignity and rights of man. . . . The nurse, in providing care, respects the beliefs, values and customs of the individual. (Davis and Aroskar, 1983, p. 12)

☐ PREPARATION

VALUES AND BASIC NEEDS

Basic needs are considered to be *shared values* because the needs for survival, security, esteem from self and others, love and belonging, and self-actualization are valued by all people regardless of age, sex, ethnic group, or religious background. However, many other values held by individuals are not shared values, and so personal values and value systems vary greatly from one person to another. Values serve as motivators for basic-need satisfaction. For example, as the basic need for esteem from self and others emerges during a person's growth and development, a person's choices about how to meet that need are guided by values such as friendship, being liked and appreciated, feeling competent, and becoming successful. (The relationship between needs and values is discussed at greater length in Skill 3.)

DEVELOPMENT OF VALUES

Many of our values are inculcated in us when we are young through the influence of family and significant others and before we have a conscious awareness of the process. This means that initially our source of values is external rather than internal. When a value is primarily external in origin, it may be held without a full understanding of its basis or rationale. If our source of values remains external into adulthood, we tend to feel insecure and easily threatened when confronted with values different from our own. When we do not understand those external values clearly, we hold onto them rather rigidly, inconsistently, or irrationally. For example, a nurse who places a high value on justice, without having examined and owned that value, tends to treat all clients exactly alike (fairly and equitably) whether or not that is in the clients' best interests. In a clinic setting, this nurse would follow protocols exactly, would require all clients to wait their turn, and would make no exceptions for handicaps, child-care or transportation problems, or age. To other nurses in the clinic this nurse may seem very rigid. When values are internalized and understood, we are able to be more flexible and rational, making appropriate allowances for varying circumstances.

Rather than being static, values tend to change over time. New experiences, exposure to different life styles, and ideas other than our own cause us to become aware of the values we now hold and to reexamine values we held without question when we were younger. When we have consciously identified and examined a value we hold, we can then choose to own it as valid for ourselves, modify it, or reject it.

The process of identifying and owning a value is known as *internalizing* and is sometimes called *values development* or *valuing*. Kirschenbaum (1973) has described the components of the valuing process as feeling, thinking, communicating, choosing, and acting.

In the process of recognizing and owning our values, it is necessary both to be aware of and to accept our *feelings*, whether they are positive or negative. Kirschenbaum (1973) states that without feelings the other parts of the valuing process become distorted. Awareness of feelings has to do with being open to and aware of our inner experiences, as discussed in Skill 2. Critical, logical, and creative *thinking* bring clarity and rationality to the process of valuing.

The ability to *communicate* verbally and nonverbally—to send clear messages, to listen, to validate, to give and receive feedback, and to resolve conflict—helps us to identify our values and share them with someone else. Kirschenbaum (1973) further suggests that "appropriate sharing" of values with peers and friends helps us to understand and accept ourselves. This self-disclosure helps to clarify our values as we hear ourselves communicate and listen to others' reactions.

To become internalized, a value must be *chosen* freely from among alternatives. This choice needs to be based on thoughtful consideration of the consequences and possible outcomes of the alternatives available. Kirschenbaum (1973, p. 98) states that by "an ongoing process of identifying and sorting through our feelings" we can continue to arrive at choices we can prize and cherish.

For a value actually to become internalized it must serve as a guide for *action*, because what we do is an indicator of what we value. The more we act on a value and integrate it into our life style, the more consistent our behavior becomes. When our values finally become internalized through this process of valuing, they are our own values rather than externally imposed values from others.

In addition to being derived from our personal thinking and feeling experiences, values arise from our view of the larger world—our consciousness of what is happening in our community, our nation, and the world. Values also develop from our sense of vision of what could be rather than simply what is (Hall, 1976). The following activity is designed to look at ideals and vision about the systems in which we function and how they relate to the values we hold.

Activity 4–A: Values and Ideals

1. Think of a social system such as your family, church, community, or nation.
2. What would make it an ideal system, from your point of view? List these characteristics in writ-

ing. Your list may include items such as harmony, caring, and productivity.
3. Study your list. Do the items represent characteristics you value?
4. Within the social system you selected, how could you act on those values? The idea is not to attempt to change the entire system but to act within that system in ways that are possible and congruent with your values.

VALUES AND BEHAVIOR

Rogers (1973) indicates that to the extent a person can freely be in touch with the valuing process within himself or herself, that person will behave in ways which are self-enhancing.

Behaviors may be called value indicators because they reflect our values. Therefore, behaviors help us to identify what our own values are and what others' values may be. A value indicator includes actions and choices along with their emotional content. The following activity is designed to look at value indicators; that is, what we do and how highly we prize those activities.

Activity 4-B: "Things I Love to Do"*

1. In the first column of Activity Figure 4-B list 15 things you love to do (Abramowitz and Macari, 1973).
2. Characterize each activity in your list by checking the other appropriate column or columns. In the last column write down when you last actually did each activity.
3. Examine your list and the characteristics you have checked.
   a. Look for patterns. These can give you some idea of what kind of values you hold. For example, many check marks in the "alone" col-

*Abramowitz MW, Macari C: Values clarification in Junior High School. In Kirschenbaum H, Simon SB (comps): Reading in Values Clarification. Minneapolis, Winston Press, 1973.

Things I Love to Do	Alone	With people	Costs $5 or more	Mental	Physical	Competitive	Aesthetic	Skilled	Creative	Risk—mental or physical	Last time done
1.											
2.											
3.											
4.											
5.											
6.											
7.											
8.											
9.											
10.											
11.											
12.											
13.											
14.											
15.											

Activity Figure 4-B

umn may indicate that you value independence or solitude. Many check marks in the "physical" column may indicate that you value strength and endurance.

b. Think about the frequency with which you engage in these activities. Are there things you love to do (value) but seldom actually do? If so, what are the reasons for this? There could be many reasons, such as time, money, and higher priorities.

Another way to examine the values we hold is to identify things we believe are important to us and then look at our behaviors to see if we are acting on those values. The following activity is designed to look at whether our actions support our stated values.

Activity 4–C:
Values and Actions

1. List five personal values that you hold, five things that are important to you. Example: friendship, family, order, leisure, and comfort. Make them uniquely yours.
2. For each value in your list write five things you do that indicate this is a value for you. Example: If friendship is a value for you, some action indicators might be: "I spend an hour each day visiting with friends"; "I include my friends in my plans for leisure activities"; and "I am willing to listen and help out when my friends need me."

VALUES AND FEELINGS

As indicated earlier, feelings are involved in value choices. The following activity is designed to assess how feelings and behaviors in conflict situations relate to values.

Activity 4–D:
Values and Feelings in Interactions

1. Recall a conflict situation that you recently experienced and resolved; describe it briefly to yourself or to someone else.
2. Diagram the major participants in the situation as follows: Draw a rectangle for the location. Draw circles for the persons in the situation. Draw these in proportionate sizes on the basis of how you perceived yourself and the others *at that time*. Label the circles and the rectangle as in the sample diagram (Activity Fig. 4–D).
3. Ask yourself the following questions:
   - What were my negative and positive feelings during this conflict?
   - What was the overt or covert issue?
   - What value might this relate to?
4. Now add dotted lines to your diagram to indicate your perception of yourself and of the others as the situation was resolved.

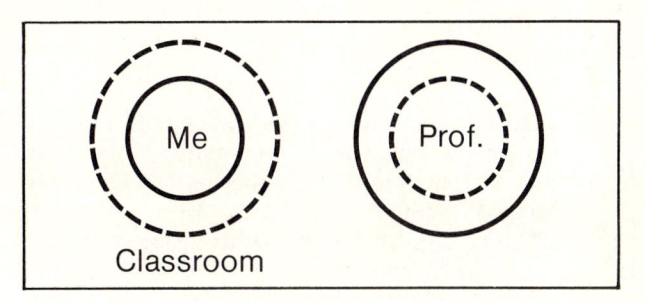

Activity Figure 4–D. (Adapted from Abramowitz MW, Macari C: Values Clarification in Junior High School. In Kirschenbaum H, Simon SB (comps): Readings in Values Clarification. Minneapolis, Winston Press, 1973, p. 301, with permission.)

Sample Situation: Classroom exchange between student and teacher about controversial subject.

Negative feelings: "I felt embarrassed and angry because he (she) was trying to make me feel and look stupid and ignorant."

Positive feelings: "I was proud I held my own ground, even though I knew he (she) was right and I was wrong."

Possible issues: Who was right?
Who would win?

Possible values: Being competent
Being right
Winning

Your situation may have more than two participants. It may be resolved with all circles the same size, rather than as illustrated in Activity Figure 4–D.

When something is important to us, its misuse or expropriation by other people arouses strong feelings within us. On the other hand, unimportant things generally do not have the same power to irritate us. For example, if time is important to a nurse, he or she may experience feelings of irritation, annoyance, or anger with people who are chronically late or who waste time. If daily showers, perfume, and deodorants are important, the nurse may find that unwashed bodies, natural body odors, bad breath, or alcohol odors arouse feelings of disgust and dislike. If, however, the nurse is aware of the connection between his or her feelings and values, that nurse can *choose* how to respond, rather than responding automatically and probably unproductively. This does not change the nurse's basic values, but simply the way he or she expresses them. When we act on the basis of conscious thought, we experience the freedom and self-affirmation that comes from being in charge of our own behavior. The following activity is designed to look at things and behaviors that irritate and annoy us, as well as the values that may correspond with those irritants.

Activity 4-E: Values and Irritants

1. Look at the following list. Choose the five you find most irritating. Now rank order your choices from 1 to 5, with 1 being the most irritating.
   - I become quite irritated with people who:
     - ___ are always late.
     - ___ are always right.
     - ___ never say what *they* want to do but make someone else decide.
     - ___ can't always be counted on to tell the truth.
     - ___ cheat on income tax.
     - ___ butter up professors or bosses.
     - ___ are quick to point out others' faults.
     - ___ always take charge.
     - ___ are lazy.
     - ___ are on welfare.
   - I get irritated or annoyed with situations such as:
     - ___ messy, cluttered rooms.
     - ___ "Keep off the grass" signs.
     - ___ dirty floors, windows, or bathrooms.
     - ___ unplanned, nonstructured committee meetings.
     - ___ disorganized planning or execution of a plan.
     - ___ immaculate, orderly surroundings.
2. Translate the five irritants you chose into a value. For example, if you chose "are always late," a corresponding value might be "time." Or, for "always take charge," corresponding values might be "control" or "independence."
3. Are the values you have named true for you? Do they "fit" internally?
4. Translate the other characteristics and situations into values.

VALUE CONFLICTS

Personal values vary with the individual and may lead to conflict with other people. For example, someone who values pacifism may have a conflict with a neighbor who is a career military person; or a nurse who values communication skills equally with technical skills may have conflict with a task-oriented supervisor.

Sometimes we experience *conflicting values within ourselves,* such as the conflict between a value of success (high grades on the final exam) and a value of honesty (not using the copies of last year's exams that are for sale from another student).

Value conflicts also occur between the individual and the systems in which he or she functions, such as one's profession, one's employing institution, or the social structure in which one lives. An example of a *conflict with an institution's values* occurred when a public health maternal–child clinic officially offered contraceptive devices and information. Several staff nurses who were opposed to birth control of any kind did not mention the service to the women with whom they worked. The institution's policy reflected a value of offering complete health care for women of varying value stances, and the nurses' actions reflected their personal values. Both the personal values of the nurses and the institutional values of the agency were valid, but some reconciliation of conflicting values was needed in order to serve clients adequately and meet professional accountability. In this situation, this might require that the nurses remove themselves from a position of needing to provide that service, perhaps by arranging for other nurses to discuss contraception with women who come to the clinic, or by asking for transfer to a pediatric or older adult clinic where contraceptive information is not offered.

Nurses may experience *personal and professional conflicts* over issues such as abortion, euthanasia, human research, or transplants. *Societal conflicts* may involve issues such as equal rights and right-to-life amendments, capital punishment, registration for the draft, or funding for neighborhood health centers. In a society as complex and diverse as ours, it is quite likely that there will be discrepancies and conflict between the value structure within which a person operates and the value process within the person's self.

Trade-offs in our values may be necessary from time to time. That is, at a particular time we may decide that one value has priority over something else that we also value. For example, a full-time student with a family to care for probably will need to modify the value placed on a clean house and homemade foods, or at least set it aside for a while. This does not mean that the student does not value those things, only that a decision has been made to act on a different value at this time.

☐ EXECUTION

Once our values have been examined and reaffirmed or altered, they become our own values rather than being externally imposed. Or we may decide to surrender them. The following illustration involves surrendering a value: A clinic nurse who placed a high value on physician and nurse time always scheduled clinic appointments close together so that there was a continual backlog of clients waiting to be seen. When someone pointed out to the nurse that the waiting room was highly congested with much noise and confusion and that clients were frustrated because they had to wait for long periods of time, the nurse was able to reexamine her value of time. She subsequently surrendered her high value of physician and nurse time and changed the scheduling so that clients' time was given more value than previously.

As with other skills of self-awareness (developing helping characteristics, knowing ourselves, identifying our own needs, and learning self-disclosure), the process of identifying and examining our own values takes time, energy, and introspection. It may also be disturbing and uncomfortable, because our values are such a basic part of ourselves. The outcome, however, is a greater internal comfort and congruence, which can result in less internal conflict and increased levels of self-respect and self-confidence.

Being aware of our own values helps to keep them from interfering with our professional and personal relationships. Understanding both our own values and how values affect people's behavior helps us be more open to clients' value systems. Professional helpers have a responsibility to provide care that is individualized, nonjudgmental, and which does not impose the helpers' own values on the people for whom they provide care. To illustrate, Juan Perez has been assigned to care for a woman who had an elective abortion. Juan's values include abortion only in very specific extenuating circumstances. If Juan's feelings are strong enough to interfere with his ability to relate to the woman and Juan finds himself unable to provide adequate care, he may want to ask for a change in assignment. If there is no other option (for example, if Juan is the only night nurse), his awareness both of his own strong value stance and of his commitment to quality care regardless of individual differences can help him to provide the needed care without expressing disapproval and nonacceptance either verbally or nonverbally.

When helping clients and families explore value-laden issues such as prolongation of life with life-support systems, organ donation, or abortion, it may or may not be appropriate for the nurse to share his or her own values with them. The nurse ensures that personal values are not used to control and manipulate others' decisions about these issues, but instead that they are used to facilitate the process of making choices. This is achieved through helping clients and families explore their own thoughts and feelings about the issues. When asked about his or her personal value stance, the nurse responds with a brief explanation of the value he or she holds, followed by comments that identify and recognize the validity of other options. For example, in response to a question about the nurse's opinion about signing a permit for organ donation, the nurse might say: "I personally think it's a good idea to donate a kidney to help people who are waiting for a transplant, but I also recognize that for many people the idea of removing something from a loved one is quite disturbing and so I believe the decision must be an individual one." This response avoids giving a message about what the nurse thinks the family should do; rather, it allows them to make a decision that is congruent with their values and with which they are comfortable.

☐ CRITICAL POINTS SUMMARY

1. Values are products of our own experiences, view of the world, and sense of vision.
2. Values are developmental in nature and change over time.
3. Values direct our actions and shape our life style.
4. Feelings, behaviors, and needs help us to identify our values.
5. When a value is chosen, prized, and acted on, it becomes our own.
6. Identification of our own values can help us decide to keep, modify, or surrender those values.
7. Internalized values provide for a wider choice of action than external value sources.
8. Recognition of the value base for our behavior helps make it possible for us to choose our behavior.
9. A professional nurse avoids imposing personal values on others.
10. A professional nurse provides nonjudgmental care that is congruent with professional standards and codes.

☐ REVIEW QUESTIONS

1. What is a value?
2. How do values influence choices and behaviors?
3. What benefits can be derived from identifying your own values?
4. How does recognition of values and their role influence the ability to be a helper?
5. In what way is an internalized value different from a value with an external source?
6. What does it mean to choose, prize, and act on a value?
7. How are basic needs related to the values people hold at different psychosocial developmental levels?
8. In what way do your values reflect how you view your surroundings and life experiences?
9. What does it mean to "not impose your values on someone else"?
10. What are some ways in which a nurse's values might influence client care?

REFERENCES

Abramowitz MW, Macari C: Values Clarification in Junior High School. In Kirschenbaum H, Simon SB (comps): Readings in Values Clarification. Minneapolis, Winston Press, 1973.

American Nurses' Association. Code for Nurses with Interpretive Statements (ANA Publication Code No. 656 25M,

9/76). Kansas City, MO, American Nurses' Association, 1976.

Davis AJ, Aroskar MA: Ethical Dilemmas and Nursing Practice, ed 2. Norwalk, CT, Appleton-Century-Crofts, 1983.

Hall BP: The Development of a Confluent Theory of Values. New York, Paulist Press, 1976.

Kirschenbaum H: Beyond values clarification. In Kirschenbaum H, Simon SB (comps): Readings in Values Clarification. Minneapolis, Winston Press, 1973.

Leininger M: Transcultural Nursing: Concepts, Theories, and Practices. New York, John Wiley & Sons, 1978.

Rogers C: Toward a modern approach to values: The valuing process in the mature person. In Kirschenbaum H, Simon SB (comps): Readings in Values Clarification. Minneapolis, Winston Press, 1973.

BIBLIOGRAPHY

Harmin M, Simon SB: Values. In Kirschenbaum H, Simon SB (comps): Readings in Values Clarification. Minneapolis, Winston Press, 1973.

Partridge KB: Nursing values in a changing society. Nursing Outlook 26(6):356–360, 1978.

Simon SB, Howe LW, Kirschenbaum H: Values Clarification: A Handbook of Practical Strategies for Teachers and Students. New York, Hart Publishing, 1972.

Smith M: A Practical Guide to Value Clarification. LaJolla, CA, University Associates, 1977.

Steele SM, Harmon VM: Values Clarification in Nursing. New York, Appleton-Century-Crofts, 1979.

Steiner E: The teaching of values and moral education. Presented at the Symposium on Philosophy of Education, State University of New York at Fredonia, 1977.

SKILL 5 Self-Disclosure

Make thyself known, and thou shalt then know thyself.
—*Jourard, p. 7*

☐ STUDENT OBJECTIVES

1. Discuss the relationship of self-disclosure to self-understanding.
2. Explain the relationship between openness and development of positive helping relationships.
3. Distinguish between productive and nonproductive professional self-disclosure.
4. Distinguish between productive and nonproductive personal self-disclosure.
5. Discuss the need to disclose within a nurse–client interaction.
6. Describe ways of disclosing within nurse–client interactions.
7. Assess your own ability to self-disclose.
8. Practice disclosing thoughts, intentions, and feelings in direct, open ways.

☐ INTRODUCTION

Self-disclosure is the process or act of revealing thoughts, intentions, and feelings to another person so that the other person can understand those perceptions. Jourard (1971) believes self-disclosure is a means of becoming a mentally healthy person and that the ability to self-disclose indicates mental health.

There is evidence that the ability to self-disclose varies among individuals and with age, sex, education, and cultural background. M. Johnson (1980) cites studies which indicate that in general: Self-disclosure is highest among young adults and lower in older persons; women self-disclose at higher levels than men; people with higher educational levels self-disclose at higher levels than their counterparts; whites self-disclose at higher levels than blacks; and blacks self-disclose at higher levels than Mexican-Americans. Jourard (1971) indicates that people who are able to self-disclose more easily are likely to be competent, flexible, adaptive, and somewhat socially extroverted. In addition, the ability to self-disclose increases the ability to establish close communication with others. For example, Jourard (1971) found that nursing students who had a higher level of self-disclosure with their parents and peers were better able to establish close communicative relationships with their patients than did nursing students with low levels of self-disclosure.

While self-disclosure and personal growth generally are productive for anyone, they are especially necessary for persons entering a helping profession, where a special kind of self-disclosure is needed. Self-disclosure by a helper is an intentional or deliberate action, a sharing of oneself for the purposes of establishing a human to human relationship and fostering self-disclosure on the part of the person receiving help. Whereas self-disclosure for personal growth focuses on the discloser and primarily serves his or her own needs, self-disclosure for helping purposes is directed toward meeting the client's needs and promoting that person's growth.

As discussed in the other skills in this chapter, the ability to know and to accept one's self is regarded as essential for a helping professional. Jourard (1971) proposes that it is only through self-disclosure that a person can fully understand and accept himself or herself. A person who understands and accepts himself or herself is generally comfortable with that self and is likely to be perceived by others as genuine, open, honest, accepting, and caring. These characteristics are necessary for involvement in the kind of helping relationship where mutual respect exists between helper and client.

☐ PREPARATION

Self-disclosure may be intentional or unintentional. Intentional self-disclosure is a deliberate disclosure to another person. It involves revealing to someone else how we react to or perceive the present situation, and may include giving the other person relevant information about our past (D. Johnson, 1981). Recall that communication is the exchange of meaning, not simply information, and intentional self-disclosure is one way of including meaning in our communication with others. Intentional self-disclosure is personally beneficial, particularly when it is reciprocal; the shared intimacy of self-disclosure can raise one's sense of self-worth, can increase trust in others, is a self-affirming process, and in general helps a person feel good.

Self-disclosure is unintentional in that we disclose something of ourselves to others continually, through both our verbal and nonverbal interactions. During the socialization process of growing up, most of us learn to monitor and screen what we disclose during everyday circumstances, but under stress we sometimes remove our concealing masks and disclose a great deal about ourselves inadvertently.

PERSONAL SELF-DISCLOSURE

Intentional self-disclosure helps us to understand and accept ourselves in several ways. First, as social beings our self-concept is developed largely through interactions with other people and from their feedback to the behaviors, thoughts, and feelings we disclose to them. As we share our inner experiences, we learn to receive acceptance from others or to cope with the rejection that we encounter. This process helps us to accept ourselves or forces us to deal with those parts of self that we find unacceptable. Second, self-disclosure has a clarifying effect. Thoughts, feelings, and intentions become clearer to us as they are expressed and then perhaps explained and clarified to another person. Third, self-disclosure is therapeutic in and of itself, since expression of feelings and thoughts can be a beneficial, cathartic experience, resulting in feelings of relief and freedom from tension.

Self-disclosure is reciprocal in nature, in that self-disclosure on the part of one person fosters self-disclosure on the part of the other person. As Jourard (1971) expresses it, ". . . behavior begets its own kind. Manipulation begets counter-manipulation. Self-disclosure begets self-disclosure" (p. 142).

Self-disclosure involves risk because there is no way of knowing for certain how the other person will respond. In disclosing ourselves we may feel that we are at the other person's mercy or that our disclosed thoughts, feelings, and intentions will cause other people to think less well of us. We also may fear that our own sense of self-worth may be threatened or that an existing relationship may be damaged.

Willingness to self-disclose is partly related to our self-concept. People with low self-worth who have experienced repeated or continuous negative feedback from other people are less likely to take the risks involved in self-disclosure. People who have experienced more positive feedback from significant others in the past are less likely to be threatened by the possibility of a new rejection, and thus are more likely to take the risks involved in self-disclosure.

The degree of self-disclosure that we permit ourselves depends on the level of trust we have in the person to whom we are disclosing. Usually we disclose ourselves to family or close friends, but sometimes a professional counselor is the most helpful person for self-disclosure. Highly personal things are usually harder to disclose, even to those persons whom we know well. Sometimes people choose to disclose all kinds of personal things to a total stranger, such as when riding a bus, plane, or train, or in a waiting room. Sharing with a total stranger usually involves little risk, because a stranger is safe and anonymous; he or she will not be around as a reminder of what or how much was disclosed. The following activity is designed to look at the nature and extent of our openness to other people and our past experiences in self-disclosure.

Activity 5–A: Self-Disclosure

In the space provided in Activity Figure 5–A, indicate the degree to which you have shared thoughts and feelings about various subjects. Place the appropriate rating scale number in each of the columns that represent various people with whom you interact. Be candid with yourself; it is for your information and use only.

Rating Scale:
0 = have not shared myself
1 = have shared myself in general terms
2 = have shared myself in full detail
3 = have lied about myself

Person Code:
M = Mother
F = Father
MF = Male friend
FF = Female friend
SP = Spouse
A = Associates (work or school)

SUBJECT AREA	PERSON						SUBJECT AREA	PERSON					
ATTITUDES/OPINIONS	M	F	MF	FF	SP	A	MONEY	M	F	MF	FF	SP	A
my religion							how much I make						
other religious groups							how much I owe						
communism							who I owe						
present government							amount of savings						
racial integration							amount others owe me						
drinking							my gambling habits						
sexual morality							my total income						
desirable qualities in a man							my financial worth						
desirable qualities in a woman							my greatest need for money now						
how parents should raise children							how I budget my money						
TASTES AND INTERESTS	M	F	MF	FF	SP	A	WORK OR STUDIES	M	F	MF	FF	SP	A
food preferences							pressures & strains of work						
beverage preferences							most boring aspects						
music preferences							most enjoyable part						
reading preferences							my shortcomings						
movies I like							my qualifications						
taste in clothes							how I am or am not appreciated						
houses & furnishings I like							my ambitions						
social gathering preferences							my feelings about salary						
ways I like to spend spare time							my feelings about career						
presents I would like							my feelings about co-workers						
PERSONALITY	M	F	MF	FF	SP	A	BODY	M	F	MF	FF	SP	A
parts of me I dislike							my feelings about my face						
feelings I have trouble expressing and controlling							how I wish I look						
facts of my sex life							feelings about different parts of my body						
feelings of attractiveness							worries about my appearance						
things I feel ashamed about							health problems I have						
things that make me furious							long-range concerns about health						
things that make me depressed							past illnesses						
things that worry me							my efforts to stay fit, healthy, attractive						
how my feelings get hurt							my present physical measurements						
things I am proud of							my adequacy and style in sexual behavior						

Activity Figure 5–A. *(Adapted from Jourard SM: The Transparent Self. New York, D Van Nostrand, 1971, pp. 213–217, with permission.)*

SELF-DISCLOSURE AND THE NURSE–CLIENT RELATIONSHIP

One of the goals of the early phases of the nurse–client helping relationship is to encourage clients to communicate freely with the nurse; to disclose their concerns, thoughts, questions, and feelings. It is quite useful for the nurse to foster this self-disclosure in clients, because client self-disclosure helps the nurse to understand the meanings and interpretations a client attaches to his or her circumstances and provides the nurse with valuable information about the client's state of health or illness. Through self-disclosure, clients also reveal their level of anxiety. However, a high level of anxiety makes it difficult for some people to disclose themselves to others. When clients are anxious, the nurse assesses the level of that anxiety and intervenes, if necessary, to lower the anxiety to a manageable level.

Within the nurse–client relationship, the nurse can foster client self-disclosure simply by encouraging the client to talk about himself or herself. This helps the client become known as a person to the nurse, which can be particularly helpful when the client is

BUSINESS REPLY MAIL
FIRST CLASS PERMIT NO. 150 E. NORWALK, CT

POSTAGE WILL BE PAID BY ADDRESSEE

APPLETON-CENTURY-CROFTS
MEDICAL/NURSING PUBLISHERS

DEPARTMENT B
25 VAN ZANT STREET
EAST NORWALK, CT 06855

NO POSTAGE
NECESSARY
IF MAILED
IN THE
UNITED STATES

☐ Yes, I want the #1 authority!

GOVONI & HAYES
Drugs and Nursing Implications

5TH EDITION

A1788-7, $29.95
flexibound

☐ **Please send me _____ copies of the 5th Edition on 30-day approval.**
☐ **Payment enclosed.** (Publisher pays postage and handling). Please include appropriate state sales tax.
☐ **Bill me later.**

Name _____
Address _____
City _____
State _____ Zip _____

Please bill my credit card as follows:
☐ VISA   ☐ MasterCard

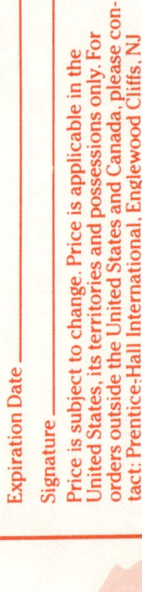

Account # _____
Expiration Date _____
Signature _____

Price is subject to change. Price is applicable in the United States, its territories and possessions only. For orders outside the United States and Canada, please contact: Prentice-Hall International, Englewood Cliffs, NJ 07632 USA

APPLETON-CENTURY-CROFTS
Medical/Nursing Publishers, Dept B
25 Van Zant St. East Norwalk, CT 06855

ACC454-9

from a cultural, economic, or ethnic background quite dissimilar to that of the nurse.

Since *self-disclosure is reciprocal in nature,* client self-disclosure is fostered through appropriate self-disclosure by the nurse. The nurse might choose to share past experiences that are relevant to the client's current experience. Or the nurse might choose to share (disclose) his or her observations of client behaviors. This disclosure can elicit valid information, such as information about the congruence between the client's verbal and nonverbal disclosures. An example would be a nurse who observes a young woman alternately staring off into space and crying. In response to the nurse's query, she says "I'm fine—don't worry, I'll be OK!" The nurse can help the young woman bring her verbal and nonverbal behaviors into congruence by sharing the nurse's perception of what is happening, perhaps by saying, "Your words tell me you're fine, but your eyes tell me something else." As the nurse shares those perceptions, the young woman is likely to feel safe enough to disclose her concerns. Or the nurse might have observed that the young woman's pulse, respirations, and blood pressure were higher than usual, with no obvious physical reasons. In this instance, the nurse could foster the client's self-disclosure by saying, "You say you're feeling fine today, but I notice your pulse and blood pressure are a little higher than usual this morning. I don't see anything specific that might be causing it." Again, this self-disclosure on the part of the nurse may foster the disclosure of something that is disturbing to the young woman.

It is important that self-disclosure be *authentic* or real, the opposite of fake or contrived. A self-disclosing nurse tries not to hide behind a professional role or facade, but to respond to client comments and questions with appropriate and authentic responses. Rogers (1961) and others describe self-disclosure in the helping relationship as *genuineness,* meaning that a helper's words are consistent with his or her own nonverbal behavior. For example, if a nurse says, "I'm glad to see you today," his or her voice quality and body language hopefully will reflect a welcome.

Another term used in this context is *congruence* (Rogers, 1961). Congruence refers to a harmony between a helper's words and basic attitudes. When a helper is perceived as a congruent person, the client's responses are more likely to be congruent with his or her own internal experiences and behaviors. However, when a helper's words are inconsistent with his or her basic feelings, this discrepancy is apparent to the client and results in loss of confidence or annoyance at the helper's pretended interest.

The following situation illustrates authentic and genuine self-disclosure from a congruent nurse that in turn fostered a reciprocal self-disclosure in the client: A community health nurse was making a home visit to a newly referred family with an elderly parent in failing health who lived alone across town. On the first visit the nurse introduced himself, shook hands with the husband and wife, and said, "Hello, I'm Steven Brown from the Public Health Department. I'm the nurse who is assigned to this part of town. I understand you called our office and asked to talk to someone about your mother, who is still living alone. I believe you have some concerns for her safety."

After this open, honest introduction of himself and his reason for coming, the family responded by beginning to tell Steven about their concerns. They perceived him as being genuinely interested in what they were worried about. As they talked, Steven commented, "I have some appreciation for what you are struggling with because I remember when my parents were facing a similar decision with my grandfather, and I know how hard it was for them to decide at what point to intervene." If that event were not a part of his own experiences, Steven might have said, "I know something about the difficult decision you face. When I was a student and worked in a nursing home, some of the elderly people there would talk about how difficult it had been to leave their homes, while others were glad to have come to the nursing home."

In either response, Steven would have shared (disclosed) in an open, honest way his own experiences and some of his feelings and reactions to the situation the family was facing. This openness fostered openness on the part of the family, who readily shared their worries and questions about various kinds of protective care. Although they had never met Steven Brown before, his ability to share himself made this first encounter a profitable one for the family and a satisfactory one for Steven. If Steven had been cool and impersonal, or if he had said all of the right words but looked at his watch frequently or sounded superficial, the lack of genuineness and congruence on his part would have been quite apparent and the outcome would have been very different.

While self-disclosure in a professional nurse–client relationship does foster personal growth for the nurse, the primary purpose of self-disclosure is to benefit the client. Sometimes the nurse may choose to disclose fairly personal thoughts and feelings to the client. However, he or she always exercises judgment in such self-disclosures, and discloses only what is necessary in that particular helping relationship. The nurse determines the purpose to be served by any given self-disclosure within a nurse–client interaction, and then chooses to disclose or not to disclose on the basis of the client's need rather than the nurse's own needs.

Too much self-disclosure can cause confusion about who is the helper and who is being helped. Thus the helper's need to self-disclose never takes precedence over the need to facilitate the desired level of disclosure in the person being helped. If Steven had gone into great detail about his own experiences with elderly persons and their adjustment to leaving home, the family might have felt a need to give him support in his own concerns and they certainly would have felt he was more interested in what he had done than in what they needed.

Reciprocal self-disclosure in a professional relationship does not mean "I'll tell you my troubles if you'll tell me yours." Some kinds of self-disclosure are inappropriate in a professional helping relationship even though the disclosure might add to the helper's own personal growth. For example, if the client happens to be a banker, it is inappropriate to disclose financial difficulties; if the client is a counselor, it is inappropriate to disclose marriage or family problems and seek advice; or if the client is a physician, it is inappropriate to ask for medical advice or a consultation.

HINDRANCES TO SELF-DISCLOSURE

Sometimes nurses are unwilling to become involved with clients enough either to self-disclose or to foster self-disclosure. This may arise from various sources: from the nurse's concern about having too much work to do and too little time simply to talk and listen; from the nurse's uncertainty about himself or herself and how to react to or cope with what the client might self-disclose; or from the nurse's attitude that it is unprofessional to become involved with the client to such an extent.

Sometimes nurses are unwilling to share a client's self-disclosure with other professionals, even though it may be necessary for providing quality client care. Jourard (1971) indicates that nurses are sometimes reluctant to report or record what they have observed, felt, guessed, or thought in connection with a client for fear of being criticized or laughed at. He proposes that in addition to fostering self-disclosure, nurses ought to record those self-disclosures regularly and use the data in a systematic way to assess progress or to help guide therapy.

The following illustration points out both the value of fostering client self-disclosure and the need to share this information with other professionals: A student nurse working in a community health setting had developed a trusting relationship with an older woman who had a nonhealing leg ulcer. During one visit the woman confided, "I put tobacco juice on my ulcer when I change the dressing, because that's what we use where I come from—but don't tell the nurse what I'm doing! She'd get mad at me!" The student nurse considered the issues of both confidentiality and safety, and decided to share the disclosure with her teacher and her staff nurse. However, by discussing with the woman her decision to share this information before she actually shared it, the student nurse was able to meet both the need for privacy and the need for quality care.

COMMUNICATION AND SELF-DISCLOSURE

The way we choose to disclose to others, both for personal growth and as a part of the nurse–client relationship, can either enhance growth in ourselves and others, or hinder it; can either draw us closer to other people, or cause alienation; can either alleviate someone else's distress, or contribute to it; and can either help heal sick bodies and minds and promote wellness, or delay the healing process.

As a result of her many years of counseling experience, Satir (1972) identified five universal patterns of communication: placating, blaming, computing, distracting, and leveling. Of these five, only leveling responses result in productive self-disclosure. The other four patterns are ways we respond to stress when our self-esteem is threatened. Although we may be unable to identify this threat directly, we use these response patterns to divert the threat of rejection from others. Satir (1972) describes these responses as double-level messages, because the words used convey one message while the body language and voice tone convey another. Double-level messages do not convey an accurate disclosure of what we are feeling or thinking.

Placating is agreeing and going along with everything so that the other person does not get mad. People who placate feel worthless, talk in an ingratiating manner, always try to please, and never disagree. *Blaming* is disagreeing and finding fault so that the other person perceives you as being strong. People who blame act superior, dictate to others, and cut others down, but actually they feel lonely and unsuccessful. *Computing* is being very correct and ultrareasonable, with no emotions visible. Nothing bothers people who compute. They are always calm, cool, and collected, even though inwardly they usually feel very vulnerable. *Distracting* is doing or saying things that are totally irrelevant to what anyone else is saying or doing. People who distract never respond to the point at hand. They feel that no one cares for them and that they do not belong anywhere.

Placating, blaming, computing, and distracting are uncomfortable communication patterns that are reflected in body tension and increased blood pressure, and are usually accompanied by common aches and pains such as headache, backache, and digestive difficulties. Satir (1972) suggests that whenever our self-esteem is in doubt, our bodies know it.

A *leveling* response is a productive kind of communication pattern. It is direct and honest, and it conveys what the person is thinking and feeling at the time; it is a total response of the whole person. Unlike the other responses, it is a single-level response, where words are congruent with body language and voice tone. With leveling responses, relationships are easy, free, and honest, and people are able to disclose thoughts and feelings with little threat to self-esteem. Leveling responses can heal differences between people, break impasses, build bridges between people, and also help bodies to become or remain well.

The following activity is designed to help experience different ways of responding to others' communications.

Activity 5-B:
Self-Disclosure Through Communication Patterns

Work individually, within small groups.

1. Respond to the following comments by writing a placating, blaming, computing, distracting, and leveling response for each:
2. Comments:
   - "Let's go to Canada for vacation this summer."
   - "I accidentally made a hole in the sweater I borrowed from you."
   - "Dad and Mom—Bob and I want to get married next month!"
   - "I've just found out I'm pregnant!"
3. Read each of your responses aloud to your group. Check each other's response patterns for validity. What feelings are generated by the different types of responses? Which do you prefer?

Example:
Comment: "Let's go see that space movie again tonight!"
Placating Response: "Whatever movie you want to see is fine with me, dear."
Blaming Response: "You know we can't afford that! Besides, I don't have time for such foolishness."
Computing Response: "Well, let's sit down and figure out our priorities on time and money."
Distracting Response: "Just a minute—I just have to tell you about . . ."
Leveling Response: "I'd like to go with you to a movie, but I don't feel like seeing the space movie tonight"; or "I'd love to do that! What time shall I be ready?"

The concepts of I-messages and You-messages described by Ginott (1965) are similar to Satir's communication patterns. An I-message gives the listener information about the effect of the listener's behavior on the speaker. It reports both the behavior itself and the feelings generated in the speaker. Because I-messages focus on the behavior, they do not attack the listener's self, character, or personality.

An example of an I-message (direct response) would be, "When I find the TV room in such a mess, I really get irritated and wonder why I bothered to clean it." By contrast, a You-message (indirect response) would focus on the listener, often to blame and attack. For example, "You've made such a mess in the TV room again—how come you're always so sloppy?"

The following activity is designed to help experience giving both I-messages and You-messages to someone else.

Activity 5-C:
Self-Disclosure Through I-messages and You-messages

Work individually, within small groups.

1. Respond to the following situations by writing first a You-message and then an I-message for each:
   - Your best friend borrowed your favorite shirt and returned it with a large grease spot—without telling you. What will you say the next time you see him or her?
   - Your roommate left the bathroom in a terrible mess again. What will you say when he or she returns?
   - A friend is late for the umpteenth time, and you will both be late to your destination. What will you say when he or she finally arrives?
   - You are a parent responding to information that your son or daughter had an accident with the family car, that he or she is failing chemistry, or is dropping out of school.
   - Your family leaves the kitchen without helping clean up. How will you let them know your feelings about this?
2. Read each of your responses aloud to your group. Check each other's responses for validity. What feelings are generated by the two types of responses? Which do you prefer?

Both leveling responses and I-messages disclose what a person is experiencing and thinking at the time, in ways that promote honest and open communication. They respond to the issue at hand and avoid blaming and dredging up old interpersonal garbage, such as "You always . . ." or "That's just like you to . . . ."

As we learn to use positive and direct ways to disclose our own thoughts, feelings, and intentions, we will experience personal growth and improved interpersonal relationships. We will also find that self-disclosure promotes client health, growth, and well-being, and that it fosters healthy and productive work relationships with other health-care professionals.

☐ EXECUTION

When we have learned to use self-disclosure with peers and friends for personal growth, we become more accepting of ourselves and others. In a nurse–client relationship, this acceptance encourages the client to self-disclose to the nurse, knowing that what he or she discloses will be accepted by the nurse without judgment. In order to self-disclose deliberately to another person, we must have the ability to verbalize our own ideas, beliefs, and feelings and a willingness to take the risks involved in sharing ourselves. Since self-disclosure generally is a reciprocal process, it also requires a willingness to place our trust in another person as well as the ability to be trusted with someone else's self-disclosure. In addition, self-disclosure requires that the nurse be aware of what is happening in the situation and what he or she is experiencing and feeling, as discussed in Skill 2.

The following activity is designed to increase the ability to self-disclose to others in productive ways.

Activity 5–D: Self-Disclosure to Others

1. Look back at the situations you recalled in Skills 2, 3, and 4. Select one to disclose to a partner whom you know fairly well.
2. Describe your thoughts, feelings, and intentions in that situation to your partner.
3. Answer these questions:
   a. Which were easiest for you to describe: thoughts, feelings, or intentions? Which were hardest?
   b. Does your partner agree with you?
   c. In what ways did your partner facilitate your self-disclosing?
4. Reverse roles and allow your partner to share an experience with you.
5. Answer these questions:
   a. Which were easiest for my partner to describe: thoughts, feelings, or intentions? Which were hardest?
   b. How did you facilitate or hinder your partner's self-disclosure?

Specific communication techniques presented in subsequent skills will help develop self-disclosure skills such as the abilities to validate perceptions, to listen, and to reflect content and feelings. Practiced use of the direct I-messages and leveling responses presented in this skill also promote accurate and productive self-disclosure. When giving these messages and responses, it is important to avoid labeling, sarcasm, accusations, and judgments.

In addition to sharing experiences and feelings, nurses can disclose themselves to clients in other ways. For example, a nurse might disclose his or her *own identity* and the *purpose* of a specific nurse–client interaction. This provides clients with the *information* they need in order to cope with a procedure or to participate knowledgeably in an interview. A nurse might disclose his or her identity and intent in this way: "Hello Ms. Johnson. I'm Sally Smith, the evening charge nurse. I'm making rounds and talking to everyone. Is there anything you need or want to ask me about?"; or "I'm Steven Brown and I understand you've been having some problems with your diet. In what way can I be of help to you?"

The nurse discloses *competence* to the client by the way procedures and techniques are done, by knowing how to operate equipment, by the way direct physical care is given, by skillful interviewing, by knowing policies and procedures, and by being able to make knowledgeable referrals.

The nurse also discloses a *caring and accepting attitude* to the client through words, actions, and technical competence. Technical competence can convey caring, in that the nurse cares enough to have become competent (although technical competence does not necessarily equate with caring). When the nurse discloses himself or herself as an accepting and caring human being, clients are more likely to perceive themselves as persons of individual worth and dignity. Caring is disclosed through the nurse's verbal and nonverbal behaviors and attitudes, and clients generally perceive this message clearly. The concept of caring was discussed in Skill 1.

☐ CRITICAL POINTS SUMMARY

1. Self-disclosure helps us to understand and accept ourselves.
2. Self-disclosure helps clarify our thoughts, feelings, intentions, and beliefs, and is therapeutic in itself.
3. Self-disclosure involves the risks of rejection and loss of self-esteem.
4. People with a high degree of self-esteem are more willing to risk self-disclosure than are people with lower levels of self-esteem.
5. Leveling responses and I-messages are direct and productive ways of disclosing thoughts, feelings, and intentions to clients, peers, and co-workers.
6. In nurse–client interactions, the nurse discloses information, intent, competence, and caring.
7. Self-disclosure in a helper fosters self-disclosure in the one seeking or receiving help.

☐ REVIEW QUESTIONS

1. What does it mean to self-disclose?
2. What positive results occur from self-disclosure?
3. In what way is self-disclosure risky?
4. On what variables does the ability to self-disclose depend?
5. In what ways can the nurse use self-disclosure both personally and professionally?
6. What do the terms congruence, authenticity, and genuineness mean in the context of self-disclosure?
7. What are some benefits to both nurse and client when client self-disclosure is fostered?
8. How would you distinguish leveling responses from the nonproductive responses of placating, blaming, computing, and distracting?
9. What are the benefits of open, direct, and leveling self-disclosure?
10. How does the focus and effect of an I-message differ from the focus and effect of a You-message?

REFERENCES

Ginott HG: Between Parent and Child. New York, Macmillan, 1965.

Johnson DW: Reaching Out: Interpersonal Effectiveness and Self-Actualization, ed 2. Englewood Cliffs, NJ, Prentice-Hall, 1981.

Johnson MN: Self-disclosure: A variable in the nurse–client relationship. Journal of Psychiatric Nursing and Mental Health Services 18(1):17–20, 1980.

Jourard SM: The Transparent Self. Princeton, NY: D Van Nostrand, 1971.

Rogers CR: On Becoming a Person. Boston, Houghton Mifflin, 1961.

Satir V: Peoplemaking. Palo Alto, CA, Science & Behavior Books, 1972.

BIBLIOGRAPHY

Tubesing DA, Tubesing NL: Tune In: Empathy Training Workshop, Participant Workbook. Duluth, MN, Listening Group, 1973.

2 Communication Through Nonverbal Channels

Communication between people occurs with and without words. Nonverbal communication is the transmission of messages without the use of words (Travelbee, 1971) and "includes any intentional or unintentional nonverbal behavior which affects the interaction between two people" (Smith and Bass, 1979, p. 80). It is continuously present in all interactions. It occurs either alone or in conjunction with verbal messages and must be considered when interpreting the meaning of any interaction. It is estimated that from 55 percent (Sweeney, 1977) to 70 percent (Birdwhistle, 1970) of all communication is through nonverbal avenues. Some authors place the percentage as high as 90 percent to 93 percent (Kron, 1972; Tubesing and Tubesing, 1973).

Nonverbal communication includes the ways we use our bodies, voice, eyes, appearance, and surroundings to transmit messages to others or to disclose our thoughts, feelings, and perceptions of ourselves to others. Morain describes communication through nonverbal behaviors as an "elaborate and secret code that is written nowhere, known by none, and understood by all" ("all" meaning members of the same culture) (1978, p. 19). The manner in which nonverbal modes of expression are used and interpreted is often dictated by cultural-ethnic and individual differences. If these differences are not understood, both nurse and client may unintentionally make invalid assumptions about the real meaning or perceived intent of a message. For example, Stern (1981) reports that the practice of beckoning to a person with the hand (such as might occur in a clinic or office) instead of saying the person's name is considered disrespectful by Filipino persons.

We also communicate with others and reveal ourselves through the ways we use time, silence, space, and touch. Since these modes of expression either enhance verbal communication or serve as the exclusive medium of communication, the way a nurse uses them can add to or detract from the relationship that develops between nurse and client. The nurse can also use nonverbal methods of communication to create an interpersonal environment in which nursing procedures will have the greatest therapeutic benefit.

As individuals we have varying degrees of ability to observe and attend to our own and others' nonverbal communication. The skills presented in this chapter are designed to sensitize the student to the significance of nonverbal communication, to help evaluate how each of the modes of nonverbal communication is used, and to increase the ability to use each mode in a manner that enhances the helping relationship. Throughout each of the skills are activities that help increase the ability to observe nonverbal behaviors and provide opportunities to experience the use of time, silence, space, and touch. The experiential learning that results from these activities help the student to understand the relevance of each of the skills to nonverbal communication and also to know the feelings that are generated when time, silence, space, and touch are used intentionally and purposefully in nurse–client relationships.

This chapter presents "Understanding Nonverbal Behavior" (Skill 6), "Time and Silence" (Skill 7), and "Space and Touch" (Skill 8).

REFERENCES

Birdwhistle RL: Kinesics and Context: Essays on Body Motion Communication. Philadelphia, University of Pennsylvania Press, 1970.

Kron T: Communication in Nursing. Philadelphia, WB Saunders, 1972.

Morain GG: Kinesics and cross-cultural understanding, ERIC Document Reproduction Service No. 7. Arlington, VA, Center for Applied Linguistics, 1978.

Smith VM, Bass TA: Communication for Health Professionals. New York, JB Lippincott, 1979.

Stern PN: Solving problems of cross-cultural health teaching: The Filipino childbearing family. Image 13(2):47–50, 1981.

Sweeney MA: Evaluating the nonverbal communication skills of nursing students. Journal of Nursing Education 16(3):5–11, 1977.

Travelbee J: Interpersonal Aspects of Nursing. Philadelphia, FA Davis, 1971.

Tubesing DA, Tubesing NL: Tune In: Empathy Training Workshop, Participant Workbook. Duluth, MN, Listening Group, 1973.

SKILL 6 Understanding Nonverbal Behavior

The real value of body language, however, still remains in a blending of all levels of communication.
— Fast, p. 173

☐ STUDENT OBJECTIVES

1. Describe the significance of nonverbal communication.
2. Explain how the meaning of nonverbal behaviors can be determined.
3. Give examples of nonverbal communication as demonstrated through eyes, facial expressions, body language, voice, and environment.
4. Practice giving and receiving feedback on your own nonverbal communication and that of others.
5. Identify congruence or noncongruence between your own verbal and nonverbal behaviors and those of your peers in both simulated and real settings.
6. Become aware of your own nonverbal messages to other people.
7. Practice consciously modifying your own nonverbal responses.

☐ INTRODUCTION

Nonverbal behaviors are an integral part of the way we communicate verbally with other people. We use our eyes, facial expressions, body language, voice, and environment to clarify, modify, or enhance our verbal expressions. For example, when we are introduced to someone we evaluate their reaction through more than simply the words they say. A "hello" accompanied by a warm voice tone, a smile, and a firm handshake gives an entirely different message than a "hello" accompanied by an aloof voice tone, a look of indifference, and a limp handshake.

Through nonverbal behaviors we also reveal to others what we are experiencing, thinking, and feeling or what we think of ourselves, even when we are not engaged in an encounter with another person. We reveal something about ourselves through our general appearance: by how we stand and walk, by how we hold and carry our bodies, by where we place ourselves in relationship to others, by the kind of clothes we wear, and the type of environment we provide for ourselves when we have the opportunity. For example, if a man walks with his head erect, has a confident and relaxed gait, and glances easily at people he meets, we usually understand his nonverbal behavior to tell us that he feels safe in his environment, feels good about himself, and knows where he is going. By contrast, if a man walks uncertainly or unsteadily and glances around furtively he gives far different messages about himself.

Nonverbal behavior also serves a metacommunication function in that it gives the listener a message about the verbal message. That is, the speaker's nonverbal behavior gives the listener information about how to interpret the literal verbal message (Satir, 1967). (The concept of metacommunication was discussed in the introduction to Part One.)

A relatively new approach to observation and interpretation of nonverbal behavior is neurolinguistic programming (NLP), developed by Grinder and Bandler (1976). According to these authors, people access (take in) and process (make sense out of) information through three basic sensory modalities called representational systems: auditory, visual, and kinesthetic.

A person's representational system is reflected in the words and phrases that person uses. For example, depending on his or her representational system a person would likely say, "I see what you are saying to me" (a visual person); "I hear what you are telling me" (an auditory person); or, "What you are saying feels right to me" (a kinesthetic person). Other cues to a person's representational system include eye movements and the direction in which that person looks while talking (Brockopp, 1983; Grinder and Bandler, 1976; King et al., 1983; Knowles, 1983). (This skill uses a more general approach to identifying and interpreting nonverbal behavior; students will find additional information about NLP from the sources listed in the references.)

☐ PREPARATION

Much nonverbal behavior is the result of a lack of conscious thought. We begin to communicate nonverbally as infants, before cognitive thought processes have developed. Infants and preverbal children are skillful in communicating their needs and wants nonverbally, particularly when that nonverbal behavior is

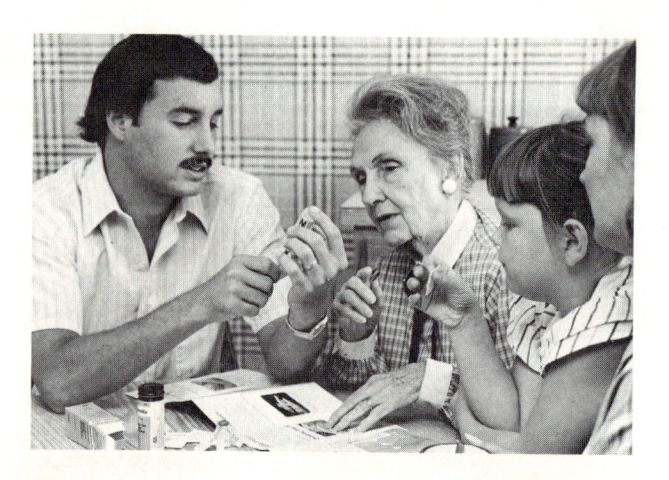

Figure 6–1. Nonverbal communication often speaks more clearly than words. (Photo by James Haines.)

being observed and interpreted by a sensitive, caring adult. As children we learn nonverbal behavior by imitating those who are important to us, such as parents, teachers, and peers. We also acquire nonverbal behavior patterns from our cultural background, racial and ethnic heritage, educational experiences, and geographic location. In addition, each of us has a unique pattern of combining learned nonverbal behavior that makes us distinctively ourselves, sets us apart from others, and helps others to recognize who we are.

Nonverbal behavior is usually closely allied with both verbal behavior and feelings (Fig. 6-1). We often communicate feelings, preferences, and intentions through nonverbal behavior, which either reinforces or contradicts our verbal expressions. When there is a contradiction between verbal and nonverbal behavior, the nonverbal is generallly considered to be more accurate, as it is likely to be harder to fake, particularly when feelings are being communicated (Haber et al., 1982; D. Johnson, 1972; Pluckhan, 1978). The following activity focuses on nonverbal behavior without any accompanying verbal behavior.

Activity 6-A: Nonverbal Communication

1. Using nonverbal communication *only*, communicate to another person where you would like to go for dinner and what you would like to eat. How successful were you? What kinds of feelings did you experience?
2. Observe a preverbal child for 30 minutes or more. How does the child make his or her needs known? What specific behaviors does the child use to show affection, joy, fear, anger, and other emotions?
3. Compare the skill level and the complexity of the messages in 1 and 2. Consider what may contribute to any observed differences.

MODES OF NONVERBAL COMMUNICATION

General Appearance

The general appearance we present conveys many messages about who we are and what we are like. When observing another person's general appearance, we take note of their approximate height and weight, skin color, personal hygiene, clothing, and affect. General appearance can tell us about a person's physical, mental, or emotional health. Pale-colored skin may indicate fear or physical illness, while a flushed face may indicate embarrassment, anger, or elevated temperature. Perspiration may result from anxiety or simply from being hot. Disheveled clothing and poor grooming may indicate an inability to care for oneself, inadequate facilities for personal care, or depression.

Clothing can tell us something about a person's personality, socioeconomic status, or the value he or she places on clothing as a status symbol. Clothing can be used to enhance or conceal physical characteristics, such as with maternity clothes, tight sweaters, or long sleeves on a drug addict. Clothing such as that worn by some priests and nuns or the Amish indicates a religious persuasion. In many hospital settings, hospital clothing designates people as patients.

We disclose our emotional status through what is known as affect. *Affect* is a person's nonverbal expression of feelings, mood, or frame of mind through a total combination of all modes of nonverbal communication and the person's general appearance (Haber, 1982). A person's affect may be described in terms such as flat (expressionless and nonresponsive), dull (lifeless and dreary), warm (vibrant and alive), or elated (joyful and exuberant). (The concept of feeling tones, as discussed in Skill 10, is similar to the concept of affect.)

Appearance also conveys a variety of messages. Clean uniforms, clothing, and shoes, and good grooming convey a sense of respect and caring for self, client, and employer. Excessive use of makeup, jewelry, and perfume, and inappropriate clothing and shoes can convey aloofness and social distance or can be distracting and offensive.

Eye Communication

The messages sent with the eyes are quite varied. For example, a glance can be warm, cold, curious, questioning, loving, or hateful. When wide open, eyes may speak of fear or amazement. When narrowed, they may speak of skepticism. A person's eyes can appear open and alert, and we know we are being seen and heard; or they can appear closed or blank, and we feel we are being shut out or ignored.

Eye contact is the ability to look directly into someone's eyes while interacting with him or her. The nature of eye contact can communicate the level of interest in a current interaction or the level of involvement with it. Having good eye contact consists of looking at another person in a spontaneous, easy, and natural way when talking with that person. Poor eye contact consists of never looking at the other person, looking away as soon as the person looks at you, or staring intently and relentlessly.

The nature of eye contact is often psychologically, socially, and culturally determined. Some Spanish-Americans look down when talking with a Caucasian. Mexican-American children may avoid eye contact when an adult discusses their behavior or reprimands them. This is considered an act of deference, not disrespect or indifference (Anthony-Tkach, 1981). Culturally determined patterns of respect rather than furtive avoidance cause Puerto Rican and rural Appalachian children to avoid looking at a middle-class American adult who is speaking to them (Morain, 1978). Direct eye contact is considered disrespectful for many American Indian tribes (Primeaux, 1977). People who perceive themselves as powerless often hesitate to have eye contact with those whom they perceive as powerful.

Morain (1978, pp. 24-25) indicates that the role of

eye contact in a conversational exchange between Americans is clearly, but unconsciously, defined. That is, the speaker initially makes brief eye contact with the listener and then glances away as he or she continues to talk. The speaker reestablishes eye contact every few minutes to see if the listener is still attentive and then glances away again. Listeners, however, keep their eyes attentively on the speaker and only occasionally glance away. They may nod and murmur "mmhmm" to indicate they are listening. By contrast, according to British custom, both speaker and listener focus attentively on each other, with the listener remaining silent. Germans tend to maintain a steady gaze toward the listener, and Arabs and some South Americans consider a lack of eye contact to be rude and insulting. It has also been observed that members of poor black families look at each other less often when talking than do middle-class white families, and may even reverse the speaker–listener pattern of eye contact.

Avoiding eye contact may serve other purposes. In embarrassing or personal situations, avoiding eye contact helps preserve the ego. When someone comes too close physically, we often close or turn our eyes, since those actions help us to become less aware of the actual proximity involved. For example, when in the dentist's chair, we tend to feel uncomfortable if our gaze meets the dentist's at close proximity. If we avert or close our eyes, we feel as though the dentist is farther away, although the distance may remain unchanged. A similar phenomenon occurs in the confined space of an elevator.

Facial Expressions

Facial expressions are considered a major source of nonverbal messages (Haber et al., 1982). They include a wide variety of movements, such as frowns, smiles, wrinkled brows, raised eyebrows, or clenched jaws, and express a myriad of feelings that range from indifference and aloofness to love and excitement. Or, if a person is trying to conceal feelings, his or her face may be flat and expressionless. Facial expressions carry messages about feelings and responses to other people and circumstances; it is true that feelings can be written all over one's face. However, facial expressions, like other nonverbal behavior, can be difficult to interpret and must be considered in context. For example, a frown may mean anger, puzzlement, or disgust.

Nurses find it helpful to be aware of the messages they give through their facial expressions and to learn how to control those expressions in situations where unmonitored expressions may interfere with caregiving, client functioning, or communication. For instance, facial expressions of revulsion, disgust, or pity help neither the nurse nor the client to cope with bedpans, colostomies, roaches, or terminal illness. It is important to realize that people who are in need of physical, economic, or emotional assistance usually become very sensitive to the attitudes of those who are providing that help. These attitudes are often communicated to clients through facial expressions. Conversely, a nurse's observations of clients' facial expressions can give clues about reactions to the nurse's interaction, as well as provide some index to their physical comfort level or inner feelings.

Body Language

The study of communication through body movements is known as *kinesics* (Birdwhistle, 1970) and includes posture, gait, and gestures.

Posture and gait are the way we hold and use our bodies. Posture can be relaxed, tense, slouched, or upright; gait can be shuffling, even, wide-based, confident, or ataxic. Both posture and gait tell us something about physical, mental, and emotional status. A nurse's posture and gait as he or she approaches a client can convey confidence, calmness, anxiety, fear, dominance, coolness, or warmth. Both posture and gait can reflect physiological problems. For example, a person who has had a slight stroke is likely to walk somewhat slouched and with a shuffling gait. For someone else, these same signs may indicate depression. Arms crossed over the chest may indicate defensiveness and closed-mindedness to another's communication; hands on the hips may mean rejection or judgment; and arms relaxed and apart may indicate openness and receptivity.

Change in body position when two people are talking may mean a change in emotional state. Movement toward the other person may mean acceptance and trust, while movement away may mean hesitancy or uncertainty. During an interview, discomfort with the subject under discussion may be indicated by shifting uncomfortably, stiffening visibly, or turning away. However, it is important to be careful of unvalidated assumptions; crossed arms may mean being chilled, and shifting position may mean tired muscles.

Gestures are movements of the hands, arms, legs, feet, head, and entire body. They may be used to emphasize a verbal message, or they may convey a variety of feelings such as indifference, relaxation, anxiety, and impatience. Gestures tend to reveal our degree of emotional comfort or level of anxiety. Fidgeting, tapping feet, biting nails, drumming fingers, and cracking knuckles are usually considered signs of tension or uneasiness. However, as with all nonverbal behavior, gestures may mean any one of several emotions. For example, fidgeting may also result from sleepiness or boredom.

Voice

The words we speak are verbal communication, but the way we speak them is part of nonverbal communication. This *paralinguistic* behavior also includes nonlanguage verbalizations such as sobbing, laughing, and grunting. Words may convey a given message, but unless the voice tone is congruent with the words, the verbal message is not believable. Vocal cues to consider include rate, pitch, volume, intonation, quality, inflection, fluency, and vocal patterns.

Rate is the speed with which we speak, including pauses. *Pitch* refers to the highness or lowness of the voice, while *volume* is loudness, measured in decibels. Both pitch and volume relate to the frequency and intensity of sound waves. Changes in rate, pitch, and volume can reflect emotions; for example, a sudden change to a higher pitch with a faster rate may reflect excitement or fear. *Intonation* or modulation represents the melody pattern our speech follows, how we use rate, pitch, and volume, or how we stress our phrases. Voice *quality* or *tone* can be described as resonant, nasal, breathy, or strident. *Inflection* is an alteration in vocal pitch or tone. *Fluency* relates to the ease with which we speak. A fluent person has few pauses, repetitions, or hesitations in his or her speaking. The level of fluency usually decreases when under stress. *Vocal patterns* refer to the ways we combine words, phrases, and inflections, and to our regional patterns or dialects.

Usually, we perceive all of these vocal cues fairly simultaneously and use them to evaluate the verbal messages being given. Vocal cues also give us general messages about an individual's personality. For example, someone who speaks rapidly, fairly loudly, and with a great deal of inflection is often regarded as outgoing, and someone who speaks more quietly and slowly may be regarded as reserved or shy.

Environment

When we have a choice we surround ourselves with items that reflect our personality and provide comfort, pleasure, and a sense of security. The items people bring to a health-care institution often reflect their own interests, family, or occupation.

In the home setting, *furnishings* (or lack of them) often represent the owner's current socioeconomic status, personality, interests, occupation, or the value placed on possessions. A retirement apartment usually reflects the owner's past life, family, and current interests. A community nurse may be asked to assess a home setting for suitability for home care of an ill person, an elderly or handicapped family member, or a premature infant. She or he would note nonverbal indicators of the family's preparation for accommodating the client's needs, such as rearranged furniture, added ramps or elevators, and the general state of cleanliness and ventilation. It is important to be able to distinguish between the clutter and disarray of family living and nonhygienic conditions.

Odors are another aspect of environment that convey messages about ourselves and give clues about a client's environment and state of health. There are many odors associated with sickness that are usually considered unpleasant, such as odors of vomitus, excreta, and unwashed bodies. Some physical illnesses have specific odors associated with them, such as the acetone odor of ketoacidosis or the foul smell of purulent drainage. Body odors may represent personal habits, such as poor hygiene or the use of alcohol, tobacco, or marijuana. Nurses who work in the community encounter odors in public buildings, apartments, homes, and on the streets and sidewalks. These odors may represent a particular culture, such as ethnic foods or incense. They may also indicate neighborhood conditions, such as decay, dampness, presence of rodents, or fresh paint. Nurses find it helpful to be able to identify many odors and to learn to tolerate unpleasant ones. The ability to tolerate unpleasant odors can be increased by concentrating on the verbal interaction or focusing on the task at hand. Breathing shallowly or through the mouth also helps, because prolonged odors fatigue the olfactory receptors and, therefore, eventually decrease the perception of an odor.

Many Americans spend much time, energy, and money masking or removing natural body odors. Media advertising often conveys the message that natural odors are offensive or undesirable. However, this cultural value is not necessarily held by all ethnic groups or all individuals.

NONVERBAL BEHAVIOR AND THE NURSE–CLIENT RELATIONSHIP

The nonverbal behavior of both nurse and client affects the development of a helping nurse–client relationship. Sometimes clients' nonverbal cues are difficult to identify because they may be subtle or almost nonexistent. Therefore, it is possible for such cues to be picked up only by a sensitive observer with repeated contacts over time. This may be especially true when a nurse works with clients from a cultural-ethnic background with which the nurse is unfamiliar. Sometimes clients withhold nonverbal cues from the nurse until they feel able to trust the nurse with those messages about themselves. Sometimes people intentionally control or modify their nonverbal expression in order to convey a desired image to others, such as being stoical or invulnerable. In addition, there is some thought that because of physiological differences in facial musculature, not all people are physiologically capable of showing the same degree of emotion through their facial expressions.

Recipients of help usually are aware of their dependence on the helper and, therefore, may be extrasensitive to nonverbal cues of acceptance, support, disgust, or anger. Some recipients of help are able to ignore negative nonverbal cues, either out of a sense of entitlement to services or because their own sense of self-worth enables them to look beyond the negative messages. John McDonald's experience illustrates the negative effect a nurse's nonverbal behavior can have: John, a community health nurse, made a visit to a large family who lived in a very untidy home. He sat gingerly on the edge of an overstuffed chair and held himself quite erect, as his nose involuntarily wrinkled at the unfamiliar, unpleasant sights and smells. His nonverbal behavior clearly communicated discomfort and disapproval, and the client found it difficult to respond positively to him.

Understanding and interpreting nonverbal communication is dependent on observing the behavior of others. While some people are naturally more keen observers, it is possible to become more skillful in this. Practice in making and reporting observations of others can help identify how accurately and carefully we observe and can give some indication of the need for growth in this area. The following activities focus on observing general appearances of others and on personal patterns of nonverbal behavior.

Activity 6-B:
Making and Reporting Observations

Work in pairs for this activity.

1. Sit facing each other in a comfortable and relaxed position. Look intently at each other for a full minute, noting as many characteristics as possible. Create a mental picture of the other person.
2. Turn away from each other and take turns describing what you saw. Be specific, giving color of hair, eyes, skin, kind and color of clothing, jewelry, or makeup.
3. After each person has described the other, you may check your observations by turning around looking at each other. (NOTE: As an alternative, observations may be written and then checked for accuracy.)

Activity 6-C:
Personal Modes of Nonverbal Behavior

1. Make an audiotape of your own voice as you read something aloud or have a conversation with a friend. Play it back and write a description of the rate, pitch, volume, intonation, quality, inflection, fluency, and vocal patterns of your voice. Have a friend describe the same characteristics of your voice and compare the descriptions.
2. Videotape a conversation between yourself and a friend. Play it back, watching and listening for nonverbal behavior rather than content.

INTERPRETING NONVERBAL BEHAVIOR

Consciously or unconsciously, behavior is meaningful for the person expressing it and can be observed and interpreted by other people. Observation and interpretation are made almost simultaneously. Perceptions of the meaning of nonverbal behavior have a significant effect on the way people respond to each other. For example, if someone is perceived to be angry or afraid in an interaction, others will respond in that interaction as if that person really is angry. If someone is perceived as accepting and caring, people will respond accordingly.

Interpretation of nonverbal behavior is often difficult. This is because nonverbal messages are often ambiguous, and it is not possible to say that any one nonverbal behavior always has the same meaning. A given nonverbal behavior can arise from a variety of feelings; for example, blushing may indicate pleasure, embarrassment, or even hostility. On the other hand, a given feeling may be exhibited in several ways; anger can be expressed through agitated movements, angry voice tones, or immobilization.

Perceptions and interpretations of nonverbal behavior are influenced by a number of factors, such as previous experiences with the other person's behavioral responses, past experiences with similar behaviors exhibited by other persons, or the nature of the present situation. In addition, the self-concept, values, and cultural-ethnic background of the observer influence perceptions of nonverbal behavior. People with low self-concept often expect to be devalued and may interpret nonverbal messages as negative, even though someone else may perceive the same behaviors as positive or neutral. Values and cultural-ethnic background influence perceptions of nonverbal behavior in that those factors help determine what people regard as acceptable and unacceptable behavior in others, often on the basis of what is personally regarded as acceptable.

Generalizations about nonverbal behavior are just that, and the specific meanings of any nonverbal behavior must be interpreted from the perspective of the individual's cultural-ethnic background. In a mobile and multicultural society, it is important for nurses to remember that the meaning of a specific nonverbal behavior for a given individual is influenced not only by his or her cultural-ethnic group, but also by that person as an individual within that group. Therefore, interpretations of nonverbal behavior are to be made cautiously and sensitively. Anthropologist Margaret Mead (1956) proposed that a conscious recognition of the possibility that behaviors are culturally based can help the nurse to avoid making inappropriate or stereotyped interpretations of nonverbal behavior and also to avoid becoming judgmental about behaviors different from the nurse's own norms.

Birdwhistle (1970) believes that no body motions or gestures have an identical meaning in all societies, while Eible-Eibesfeldt (Morain, 1978) points out that deaf-blind children exhibit typical facial expressions of smiling with pleasure, crying, fear, and surprise, although they cannot acquire those expressions from other people. Ekman et al. (1972) indicate that primary emotions (happiness, anger, sadness, fear, surprise, and disgust) are identical and agreed upon in varied cultures such as in the United States, Japan, and Brazil. However, the rules that govern when it is appropriate to exhibit or conceal the expression of these emotions vary with the culture.

Two examples: A reticent Swedish-American client was able to talk about his fears only after a nurse began to join him in a regular Swedish social break of juice and homemade cookies; sharing food was culturally important to this man. A Vietnamese immigrant family mourned the death of a small child with loud wailing and crying. The emergency room nurse and physician were able to recognize the cultural nature of this activity and provided the family with the needed time for it (Leininger, 1970; Shubin, 1980).

Nurses also find it helpful to know and understand the cultural norms of the people with whom they work and to interpret their behaviors from that perspective. For example, Taylor (1979) writes about how rural and mountain people usually express themselves to outsiders in short phrases, single words, and long pauses, and how this can be incorrectly interpreted as depression by a verbally oriented nurse. She gives the example of an adolescent who was hospitalized outside of his community. He did not talk or respond verbally to anyone and was put through many diagnostic tests to find out what was wrong. A few weeks later his family visited, and the nurses observed the boy talking freely with his family. When the surprised staff asked the family about his talking, the older brother replied, "Wouldn't, not couldn't. Doesn't like strangers." The father said "Should have asked the boy!" (p. 143).

Verbal-Nonverbal Congruence
When the perceived nonverbal meaning corresponds to the verbal message being communicated, the two communication modes are said to be congruent with each other. Generally, congruence or lack of congruence between verbal and nonverbal messages is evident to an observer. However, when noncongruence exists, the reasons for that discrepancy are not always clear and are subject to misinterpretation by the receiver of the message, and therefore can be a source of misunderstandings between individuals. Noncongruent messages are confusing because the receiver is not quite sure which message to believe. Since actions do speak louder than words, people usually believe what they deduce from our nonverbal behavior.

Blondis and Jackson (1977) indicate that when a nurse's words and actions are not congruent, clients may perceive those words as having been learned by rote and delivered much the same as medications are administered, rather than as a genuine involvement in an interaction with another human being. Congruence is an important factor in the helping relationship since it affects the way clients perceive and react to the nurse. For example, a nurse who glances frequently at the clock during a conversation gives a clear message that he or she either is in a hurry or is not interested—regardless of what that nurse may be saying. The following activity focuses on various interpretations that may be attached to nonverbal behaviors.

Activity 6-D: Interpreting Nonverbal Behavior

Work in pairs or small groups for this activity.

1. Watch a 15-minute segment of a television show with the sound turned off or with earphones on to eliminate the sound. Have your partner watch the same show with the sound turned on. Compare what you thought happened on the show with what your partner heard happen. How are your versions alike? How are they different?
2. View a short film such as *Do You Know Dr. Jones?* (1970) first without sound and then with sound. After the first viewing, describe what you thought was happening between the nurse and the client and compare with others who may be viewing the film. Identify the major nonverbal messages being communicated by each and the specific behaviors that conveyed those messages. After the second viewing, compare what actually happened with what you thought happened. How were your versions alike? How were they different? In what ways did the verbal communication alter your understanding of the nonverbal communication?
3. View the film *The Eye of the Beholder* (1958), which portrays the variable perceptions of an individual who observed one episode in the life of a young artist and a model. Compare those perceptions and for each individual identify factors that influenced his or her perceptions.

VALIDATING PERCEPTIONS OF NONVERBAL BEHAVIOR

Validation of the perceived meaning of client behaviors helps the nurse to avoid misinterpretation of nonverbal behavior. It can also facilitate the client's ability to express his or her feelings and perceptions more clearly. Validation is particularly important when the client is from a culture that is different from the nurse's own culture or the dominant culture in which the nurse usually functions. Validation is also important when the nurse becomes aware of a lack of congruence between verbal and nonverbal behavior, or when the meaning of the client's behavior is unclear.

Verbal validation of noncongruent behavior is illustrated by a nurse who found that a hospitalized woman had eaten only a small amount of lunch. In response to the nurse's comment "You didn't eat very much lunch today," the woman replied, "The food wasn't any good." However, her face was expressionless and her voice was flat. At this point, the observant nurse identified a discrepancy between the verbal and nonverbal messages, and validated her observations with the woman by responding, "You say the food wasn't any good, but you sound quite discouraged—would you like to talk about it?"

Whenever the nurse is uncertain about the meaning of a client's nonverbal behavior, it is generally appropriate and safe to report those observations to the client and find out what that behavior may mean to him or her. For example, a nurse might say to a hospitalized client who is awake at 2:00 A.M.: "I see that you are not sleeping tonight—what seems to be the matter?" Another way to validate nonverbal behavior is for the nurse to act on his or her observations and see whether the other person's response to those actions confirms or denies the accuracy of the observations. For example, when a nurse perceives someone to be angry, he or she may choose to become conciliatory; or if the person is perceived as fearful, the nurse can give more information about the present or anticipated circumstances. If the nurse's perceptions of the nonverbal behavior are correct, the other person's level of anger or fear tends to decrease, thus giving validity to the nurse's observations and approach.

Other ways to validate nonverbal messages are to universalize or personalize perceived observations. *Universalizing* involves articulating how many people would feel or behave in similar circumstances and inquiring if that is true for this person. A universalizing comment would be, "A lot of people having this experience act as if they are scared." *Personalizing* involves articulating how you might feel or behave in similar circumstances and inquiring if that is true for this person. A personalizing comment would be, "When I'm faced with something I don't understand, I feel rather anxious." Both universalizing and personalizing give the other person an opportunity to name his or her feelings and behaviors and to see them as usual and acceptable. They also communicate that the nurse understands their experiences. (Additional communication skills presented in Chapter 3 provide more tools for validating perceptions of nonverbal behavior.)

☐ EXECUTION

Observation of nonverbal behavior begins with the ability to observe both our own behaviors and the reactions of other people to those behaviors. Once we become aware of the nonverbal messages we actually give to others, we can begin to avoid giving negative messages that interfere with clients' responsiveness. For example, a nurse may be unaware that his or her voice tone, eyes, and posture convey control and rigidity. But when this nurse becomes aware of how those nonverbal behaviors are perceived, change is possible. In addition, observations and interpretations of others' behavior helps us begin to monitor our own nonverbal behavior, achieve more control over ourselves, and begin to function more effectively (Fast, 1970).

OBSERVATION OF CLIENTS

Observation of nonverbal behavior provides significant data about clients' physical and emotional health and helps identify nursing or medical needs. Nonverbal data may be the only direct information available from a client who is unable to verbalize, or it may serve to complement and validate a client's verbal comments and the nurse's observations.

People who are ill often have a decreased ability to communicate verbally for reasons such as impaired speech or perceptual difficulties, oral surgery, tubes in the throat, overwhelming fatigue, or pain. Clients in home settings and in the hospital sometimes report their needs inaccurately or unclearly, perhaps because they do not want to bother the nurse or because they do not understand what to communicate to the nurse in order to receive the care they need. For example, Mr. Jacobson received no pain medication the day after his abdominal surgery because each time the nurses asked him how he was and if he had much pain, he said "I'm OK, and the pain is not too bad." The night nurse found him wakeful with elevated vital signs. She noticed that he gritted his teeth as he slowly turned on his side. The night nurse told him what she observed and how that differed from what she had been told about his pain. Mr. Jacobson acknowledged that he was quite uncomfortable but said that he was afraid of getting addicted to pain medication. He said he knew he could stand more pain than this if he had to, and, besides, the nurses were always in a hurry when they came into his room—so he knew other patients needed their help more than he did. After giving him a much-needed injection for pain, the nurse recorded both his nonverbal and verbal behavior in the record and reported the incident to the nurses on the next shift.

Nonverbal behavior from clients also provides feedback about the nurse's own nonverbal behavior. For example, in the previously cited example with John McDonald, the mother avoided eye contact, answered questions very briefly or remained silent, volunteered no information, and frequently turned to scold the children playing nearby. Her nonverbal behavior gave John the message that she was uncomfortable, but he did not recognize that her behavior was most likely a response to *his nonverbal messages* rather than to what he was talking about. Later, as he discussed his experience with his supervisor, John began to understand how his nonverbal behavior had a negative effect on the mother's responsiveness. Clients sometimes give verbal feedback about the nurse's verbal and nonverbal congruence. In the example of the nurse who glanced frequently at the clock, the client, Mrs. Childers, stopped talking and said "I'm sorry, I know you're in a hurry and too busy. I won't bother you anymore." The nurse, Sandra James, believed that her own need to leave the room and attend to other things was known only to herself and that she was responding appropriately to Mrs. Childers' conversation. However, her nonverbal glances clearly conveyed another message, which the client interpreted as lack of interest. If Sandra were to have used a direct and leveling response as discussed in Skill 5, she might have said something like, "Mrs. Childers, I'd love to hear more about your grandchildren, but I have several urgent medications to give. Later in the day, I'll try to stop by to see their pictures." Had the nurse done this, both she and Mrs. Childers would have felt more comfortable and satisfied.

To be a keen observer and careful reporter of nonverbal information requires a mental attitude of

TABLE 6-1. Guide for Observing Nonverbal Behavior

Name: _____
Guide completed by: _____
Self _____ Observer _____

BEHAVIOR OBSERVED	BRIEF DESCRIPTION	
	Sender Behaviors	Receiver Behaviors

1. General appearance
   a. Height and weight
   b. Skin color
   c. Personal hygiene
   d. Clothing
   e. Affect
   f. Body position in relation to others		

2. Eye communication
   a. Eye messages
   b. Eye contact		

3. Facial Expressions		

4. Body language
   a. Posture
   b. Gait
   c. Gestures
   d. Distracting behaviors		

5. Voice
   a. Rate
   b. Pitch
   c. Volume
   d. Intonation
   e. Quality
   f. Inflection
   g. Fluency
   h. Vocal patterns		

6. Environment
7. Summary of verbal content
8. Verbal and nonverbal congruent?
   a. Examples of congruency
   b. Examples of noncongruency
	Yes___ No___
	
	Sometimes___
		Yes___ No___
		
		Sometimes___

alertness and attentiveness to self, others, and the surroundings; a receptivity to others' nonverbal communication; an awareness of one's own nonverbal effect on others; and the mental ability to integrate verbal and nonverbal messages. The nurse also makes observations sensitively, without violating the client's sense of self-worth; remembers what is observed; and has an adequate vocabulary to describe and record those observations. As with any data gathering, it is helpful to make observations about clients' nonverbal behavior in a systematic way. Table 6-1 may be used to increase skill in observation of nonverbal behavior or to guide the gathering of nonverbal information about clients.

When describing nonverbal behavior it is important to be objective and specific, rather than evaluative, subjective, or general. For example, describing a person as confused or uncooperative is evaluative, subjective, and general. Objective reporting of observations in this case means describing the specific behaviors that caused the observer to use the label confused or uncooperative. Record nonverbal observations in the health record with the same sense of commitment that verbal data, diagnostic and therapeutic measures, and physical signs and symptoms are recorded.

DEVELOPING OBSERVATIONAL SKILLS

The ability to observe nonverbal behavior can be increased through practice. The following activity focuses on making systematic observations of nonverbal behaviors during verbal interactions with peers.

Activity 6-E:
Observing Nonverbal Behavior: Simulated Settings

Work in groups of four; each group has a sender, a receiver, and observers 1 and 2. Each participant should have two copies of Table 6-1. A video camera may be used to supplement the observation.

1. Each participant recalls an interesting, discouraging, sad, or pleasant event, or selects a topic about which he or she feels strongly.
2. The sender talks about his or her event or topic to the receiver for 2 or 3 minutes. The receiver listens, responding enough to keep the conversation going but not enough to take over.
3. During the exchange, observer 1 takes written notes on the sender's nonverbal behavior, while observer 2 takes notes on the receiver. Both use Table 6-1.
4. When the exchange is finished, the sender and the receiver make written notes on the nonverbal behaviors they were aware of in themselves, again using Table 6-1.
5. The sender and the receiver compare and validate observations and perceptions with their observers.
6. Exchange roles and repeat the exercise until each person has been a sender, a receiver, and an observer.
(*NOTE:* At the conclusion of the activity, each person should have two tables, one completed by himself or herself while in the sender and receiver roles and the other completed by the observers.)

The following activity is designed to be completed *before proceeding to the next skill*. It provides a structure for practicing nonverbal observational skills in everyday situations. Three copies of Table 6-1 are needed for this activity.

Activity 6-F: Observing Nonverbal Behavior: Real-Life Settings

1. Use Table 6-1 to record remembered observations about yourself after two conversations: (a) when you were talking about a subject that is important to you, and (b) when you were listening to someone else tell about something important to him or her. How do the results of this observation compare with the simulated ones you did in Activity 6-E?
2. Find a place to sit comfortably and unobtrusively where people gather together, such as a restaurant, park, or waiting room.
    a. Observe an exchange between two or three people from a distance close enough to observe nonverbal behavior and hear voice sounds, but not close enough to eavesdrop on the conversation.
    b. Complete Table 6-1 again, observing both the sender and the receiver. In item 7 indicate what you *think* they were talking about. In item 8, indicate if body language and voice tones are congruent.
3. Repeat the activity in another location with two other people.

☐ CRITICAL POINTS SUMMARY

1. Nonverbal and verbal communication usually complement and validate each other.
2. Nonverbal behaviors are communicated through general appearance, eye communication, facial expressions, body language, voice, and environment.
3. Nonverbal behaviors need to be considered within the context of the present situation.
4. When verbal–nonverbal noncongruence exists, the nonverbal message is generally considered to be more accurate.
5. Interpretations of nonverbal behavior should be validated verbally to avoid misunderstandings.
6. Nurses convey much information about themselves and their attitudes toward others through nonverbal behaviors.
7. Nurses' own nonverbal behavior and the congruence between their verbal and nonverbal behavior impact directly on clients.
8. Professional nurses develop the ability to observe both their own nonverbal behaviors and those of their clients while giving physical care or interacting with clients.
9. Observations of nonverbal behavior form a basis for responding to clients in helpful, appropriate ways.

☐ REVIEW QUESTIONS

1. Why is nonverbal behavior by itself an inadequate indicator of what is happening?
2. To have some understanding of nonverbal behavior, what needs to be considered in addition to the behavior itself?
3. What benefits occur when nurses validate their perceptions of the meaning of nonverbal behavior?
4. What nonverbal components are included in observations of general appearance?
5. What is the difference between good and poor eye contact?
6. What is meant by vocal rate, pitch, volume, intonation, quality, inflection, fluency, and patterns?
7. How do clothing, home furnishings, and possessions contribute information to nonverbal observations about clients?
8. What nonverbal messages could a client receive if you:
    a. Speak indistinctly? hurriedly? hesitantly?
    b. Enter or leave a room abruptly?
    c. Are always smiling regardless of the situation?
9. What nonverbal messages could a nurse send through:
    a. Standing with hands on hips while talking?
    b. Walking briskly when entering a room?
10. What nonverbal messages could a client send through:
    a. Avoiding eye contact?
    b. Lying in bed with the covers over his or her head?
    c. Sitting and staring blankly out of the window?
    d. Lying curled up in bed?

11. How might you validate the meaning of the behaviors listed in question 10?

REFERENCES

Anthony-Tkach C: Care of the Mexican-American patient. Nursing and Health Care 2(8):424–427, 432, 1981.

Birdwhistle RL: Kinesics and Context: Essays on Body Motion Communication. Philadelphia, University of Pennsylvania Press, 1970.

Blondis MM, Jackson BE: Nonverbal Communication with Patients: Back to the Human Touch. New York, John Wiley & Sons, 1977.

Brockopp DY: What is NLP? American Journal of Nursing 83(7):1012–1014, 1983.

Ekman P, Wallace VF, Ellsworth P: Emotion in the Human Face: Guidelines for Research and an Integration of Findings. New York, Pergamon Press, 1972.

Fast J: Body Language. New York, M Evans, distributed in association with JB Lippincott, 1970.

Grinder J, Bandler R: The Structure of Magic, vol II. Palo Alto, CA, Science & Behavior Books, 1976.

Haber J, Leach AM, et al: Comprehensive Psychiatric Nursing, ed 2. New York, McGraw-Hill, 1982.

Johnson DW: Reaching Out: Interpersonal Effectiveness and Self-Actualization. Englewood Cliffs, NJ, Prentice-Hall, 1972.

King M, Novik L, Citrenbaum C: Irresistible Communication; Creative Skills for the Health Professional. Philadelphia, WB Saunders, 1983.

Knowles RD: Building rapport through neuro-linguistic programming. American Journal of Nursing 83(7):1011–1014, 1983.

Leininger M: Nursing and Anthropology: Two Worlds to Blend. New York, John Wiley & Sons, 1970.

Mead M: Understanding cultural patterns. Nursing Outlook 4(5):260–262, 1956.

Morain GG: Kinesics and Cross-Cultural Understanding, ERIC Document Reproduction Service No. 7. Arlington, VA, Center for Applied Linguistics, 1978.

Pluckhan ML: Human Communication: The Matrix of Nursing. New York, McGraw-Hill, 1978.

Primeaux M: Caring for the American Indian patient. American Journal of Nursing 77(1):91–94, 1977.

Satir V: Conjoint Family Therapy, rev. ed. Palo Alto, CA, Science & Behavior Books, 1967.

Shubin S: Nursing patients from different cultures. Nursing80 10(6):78–81, 1980.

Taylor C: Cultural Barriers: An Anthropological Perspective. In Hymovich DP, Barnard MU (eds): Family Health Care, vol 1, ed 2. New York, McGraw-Hill, 1979.

BIBLIOGRAPHY

Cooper J: Actions really *do* speak louder than words. Nursing79 9(4):113–116, 118, 1979.

Milner J: Clothes maketh a patient. Nursing Mirror 154(11):30–31, 1982.

Sundeen SJ, Stuart GW, et al: Nurse–Client Interaction: Implementing the Nursing Process, ed 2. St Louis, MO, CV Mosby, 1981.

Sweeney MA: Evaluating the nonverbal communication skills of nursing students. Journal of Nursing Education 16(3):5–11, 1977.

AUDIOVISUAL RESOURCES

Do You Know Dr. Jones?
Film. Illustrates good and poor listening and attending behaviors, with hospitalized client in preoperative setting. Effective both with and without soundtrack. (1970, B & W)
Available through:
McGraw-Hill Book Company
1221 Avenue of the Americas
New York, NY 10020

The Eye of the Beholder
Film. Illustrates perceptual differences of six people for the same situation. (1958, B & W, 25 min.)
Available through:
Stuart Reynolds Productions
9465 Wilshire Boulevard
Beverly Hills, CA 90212

Kinesics: The Study of Body Language
Filmstrip with audiocassette. (1975, Color, 20 min.)

The Silent Vocabulary
Filmstrip with audiocassette. (1975, Color, 16 min.)
Both available through:
Concept Media
P.O. Box 19542
Irvine, CA 92714

SKILL 7 Time and Silence

For everything there is a season, and a time for every purpose under heaven . . . a time to keep silence, and a time to speak.
—*The Preacher in Ecclesiastes 3:1–7*

☐ STUDENT OBJECTIVES

1. Describe various messages conveyed through the nurse's use of time.
2. Identify the value and meaning time may have to the nurse and to the client.
3. Assess your own valuing of and use of time.
4. Discuss possible meanings of silence for the nurse and client.
5. Describe ways silence may be used in interviews and interactions.
6. Describe problems associated with the use of silence.

7. Identify your own use of silence in interpersonal interactions.

☐ INTRODUCTION

Time is a silent language in the sense that our use of time conveys nonverbal messages about our regard and respect for others. For example, when we value and respect others, we tend to be on time for our commitments to them, we voluntarily spend time with them, we avoid interrupting them, and we are careful not to control them through our own use of time. The passage of time can be experienced and measured quantitatively, but the value and use of time varies with the individual. Some people are very time-conscious; they make lists, use every moment efficiently, and worry if they get behind time, while others treat time more casually, even though they may be just as aware of its passage.

Nurses tend to be time-oriented, as are many of their work settings. Hospitals are time-structured, with shift schedules and rotations, many tasks to do for many clients at specific time intervals, and often too much to do in a given period of time. Time demands can make a hospital nurse feel fragmented and frustrated. Nurses in community settings often relate to only one client or family at a given time, but they experience the pressure of having many places to go, each of which may have an unpredictable time element.

Silence is a specific use of time; a period of time during which there is no verbal exchange. Verbal communication is highly valued in our society, and many people find 2 or 3 minutes of silence in a conversation to be an intolerably long time. When a silence occurs, we tend to think we have not been heard or understood, so we rephrase, repeat, or change the subject. Hein (1980) points out that nursing is an activity-oriented profession and that talking is an activity. She also indicates that effective use of silence in a helping relationship is one of the most difficult communication skills to develop. In an interview situation, the nurse conducting the interview is more likely to break periods of silence than is the person being interviewed (Bloch, 1970). This would tend to indicate that the nurse rather than the client determines how silence is used and whether that use is effective (Hein, 1980).

Both time and silence can be used in therapeutic and nontherapeutic ways in the nurse–client relationship. For example, spending time with a client or remaining silent can convey acceptance and caring, while either continuous talking or being too busy to talk and listen can convey opposite feelings. The nurse's perception of time and the value placed on time influences his or her management of time-structured situations and helps determine the amount and character of time actually spent with clients. The nurse's comfort level with silence determines the extent to which he or she uses silence as a communication tool. When used selectively and consciously, the nonverbal skills of time and silence can be an effective complement to the nurse's verbal communication skills.

☐ PREPARATION

USE OF TIME

The issue of *control* is central to the concept of time as communication (Hein, 1980). We plan and protect our time, but also find ourselves controlling others' time. When we are late and cause others to wait, we control them and their use of time. We view time as a commodity that belongs to someone (my time, your time) and that can be spent, bought, given, saved, or wasted.

Waiting refers to a perception of the passage of time before an anticipated event actually occurs. Power, dominance, and control are implied in waiting, since the person who is being waited for generally has control over the length of time the other person waits. Health-care professionals tend to keep clients waiting for routine services, sometimes for long periods of time. Often a client does not understand the reasons for lengthy waiting and may perceive the waiting as deliberate, because health-care professionals are viewed as having power and management capability within the health-care setting and as being able to avoid making people wait if they so choose.

Waiting often arouses anxiety, helplessness, and anger. For an ill person, it can also mean prolonged discomfort, feelings of decreased self-worth, a sense of abandonment, or even fear of intolerable pain or dying (Hein, 1980). Nurses frequently say "I'll be back in a minute," or "The doctor will be here right away," although usually neither materializes in such a short time span. A nurse may make these unrealistic promises out of a sincere desire for the client to have prompt service, out of habit, or as an excuse to leave for an indeterminate length of time. Regardless of the reason, the nurse's credibility is suspect when these unfulfilled promises are made.

In most health-care settings, waiting is a one-way process. The client is expected to be on time, or even early. A professional person rarely waits for a client but assumes it is all right for the client to wait for the professional. Some delays inevitably occur because of the unpredictable nature of illness and health care, but at least two studies indicated that the basic causes for client waiting were physician lateness and poor design of the appointment system (Johnson and Rosenfield, 1968).

Interruptions are another way we use time to control others. An interruption is anything verbal or nonverbal that distracts the client's thinking prematurely or interrupts the readiness to continue with an interaction or interview (Hein, 1980). An interruption forces a change in the speaker's use of time and often substitutes the listener's use and value of time for that of the speaker. It is important to recognize that nonverbal interruptions such as glancing at a watch or getting up to leave change the flow of a conversation as surely as verbal interruptions do. A person who has been interrupted tends to feel that his or her time has been usurped, and that the other person either is disrespectful or disinterested. There are circumstances when time and work-load constraints necessitate interruptions, but in such cases the untoward effects of interruptions can be minimized by explanation and apology. If interruptions are anticipated (such as returned phone calls), giving clients that information in advance helps them more readily accept an interruption of the nurse's time. Other interruptions can be avoided by attending to the client's indications of being finished with a subject, such as by the finality of his or her ending comments or by nonverbal cues that indicate readiness to proceed with another subject.

Time is used consciously or unconsciously to *convey feelings* toward others or to *express personal needs*. When possible, most of us spend time with those whom we enjoy and avoid those whom we dislike. Letters to those with whom we are uncomfortable may go unanswered for a long time. Nurses often are reluctant to answer a call light from dying or demanding clients, and any necessary care is given quickly (Kastenbaum and Aisenberg, 1972). Unwillingness to give time to those clients may reflect discomfort with death or an attempt to avoid receiving criticism. A nurse who works in a community setting may limit the time he or she has available for a home visit with a difficult family by scheduling the visit a short time before he or she is due at a clinic.

Clients often use time to express their needs to the nurse. For example, clients may be indirectly asking the nurse to spend time with them when they make repeated requests for items and services or are slow in completing procedures with which the nurse is assisting. From the nurse's perspective, this time may be given grudgingly because of the pressure from other demands.

To understand how you can use time in nurse–client relationships, it is helpful to look at your usual patterns of time use. Awareness of how you generally use time and react to others' use of time can help you to avoid having those patterns interfere with productive interpersonal relationships with peers, coworkers, and clients.

Activity 7-A: Personal Use of Time

Respond to the following questions in writing. Ask a friend or relative who knows you well to do the same for you. Then compare your responses. How are they alike and different?

1. Which of these descriptors best fits you?
   a. Clock-watcher
   b. Procrastinator
   c. On time
   d. Late
2. For whom or what are you usually on time? Who or what do you usually make wait for you?
3. How do you react to people who are late? How do you respond when you have to wait? (What are your behavioral, emotional, and physiological reactions?) What do you do to pass the time while waiting?
4. How do you react when you make people wait for you? If you are late, do you expect others to wait for you?
5. Do you feel differently about waiting or being waited for if the waiting time is 10 minutes or an hour?

USE OF SILENCE

Silence is a significant way to use time, both personally and professionally. Silence is not passivity or an absence of overt activity, but is a covert activity in and of itself. Silence may be complete or it may include sounds such as "mmm" and "mmhmm," since this minimal verbal encouragement does not interrupt or make demands on the speaker. In the context of the nurse–client relationship, silence is defined as a period of time during which the nurse waits without interruption for the client to begin or resume talking (Hall, 1969).

Silence on the part of the nurse serves a number of functions in the nurse–client relationship. It communicates acceptance and caring (Skill 1), facilitates self-disclosure (Skill 5), and is a necessary component of productive attending behavior (Skill 9), and attentive listening (Skill 10). Silence can be helpful when words are inadequate or superfluous. Sometimes simply being with someone who is in grief, pain, or fear eases the feelings of aloneness. Silence combined with touch when appropriate can be more eloquent and convey more caring than dozens of words.

For both client and nurse, silence can be used to clarify one's own thoughts and ideas, as well as to formulate questions and responses. For the client, silence can provide rest and relaxation and freedom from demands to be sociable. It can provide time to gather inner strength and to reestablish stressed coping mechanisms.

For the nurse, silence provides an opportunity to observe how the client reacts to what is being discussed; to note both the nurse's own level of anxiety and that of the client; to observe the client's use of silence and patterns of pauses in the conversation; and to determine the client's readiness to move on to another subject. Silence is not a time for daydreaming or turning one's attention to the next task.

The nurse's silence also invites a response of some sort from the client. It is important for the nurse to remember to allow enough time for clients to formulate responses, since some people respond verbally to questions and comments more readily than others. Some people take time to consider and think through their responses, while others respond quickly. Older people, people with limited intellectual capability, and people who are sick or in mental or physical distress often need more time to respond.

Nurses have varied natural comfort levels with silence. A nurse who is naturally uncomfortable with silence will at least initially have difficulty using it at all, let alone using it effectively or therapeutically. Excessive talking on the part of the nurse makes it difficult for clients to talk about their concerns. Clients may perceive a talkative nurse as too busy with his or her own agenda to attend to their concerns. Talkative nurses sometimes unwittingly interrupt clients' thought processes and expressions. A too-talkative nurse can also tire clients who are fatigued or in distress and do not have the energy to listen and respond.

Nurses who are naturally quiet, shy, and comfortable with silence can be therapeutic and comforting. However, their silence may be as much a liability as excessive talking, because excessively silent nurses sometimes have difficulty gathering data, conducting interviews, or using verbal communication skills. Clients may perceive a too-silent nurse as being disinterested in them, preoccupied with personal concerns, cool and aloof, bored, or noncaring. This is especially true if the nurse remains silent and does not respond to clients' verbal and nonverbal communications.

Prolonged silences can occur when the nurse is uncomfortable with silence and does not know how to end it and move on to something else, or when the nurse misinterprets the client's signals of being finished with a subject. Generally speaking, a silence has become too long when both persons are noticeably uncomfortable. Since silence is an unfamiliar skill for many people, it is helpful to experience silence and identify our own feelings about and comfort level with silence. This is the focus of the following activity.

Activity 7-B: Experiencing Silence

Work independently or in small groups.

1. Sit quietly in a comfortable chair in an upright position. Note the time of day.
2. Close your eyes and quietly be aware of your environment, both internal and external. Try not to respond to environmental stimuli but simply be aware of them.
3. When you feel comfortable with the silence and after what seems to be at least 5 to 10 minutes, open your eyes. Note the time. Did the silence seem longer or shorter than the actual time? What kind of feelings did you experience while silent?
4. Compare your experiences with another person.

Looking at ways other people use silence in communication can also help us to understand its function and actual use in interpersonal interactions. This in turn helps us to use silence more comfortably and knowledgeably.

Activity 7-C: Observing Silence in Others

1. Situate yourself inconspicuously in a place where people gather together, such as a restaurant, lounge, or waiting room.
2. From enough distance so as not to eavesdrop, observe two people talking with each other. Record the number of times there are silent pauses of 5 to 10 seconds or more. Note who initiated the silences and who broke them. Was silence overused or underused? What messages seemed to be conveyed through silence?
3. Repeat the observations in at least one other location.

Increased awareness of our present use of time and silence makes it possible to modify our use of those activities in ways that promote client growth.

☐ EXECUTION

TIME

Nurses often become very time-conscious because there are so many aspects of their work that are time-related, such as medications, treatments, tests, and clinic schedules. It is helpful to learn to plan one's time, but with the goal of remaining flexible when the unexpected happens. Agendas and lists can help in planning, and written notes of what happens make it easier to recall and record appropriate information. Mentally attending to the task at hand rather than thinking of what comes next helps in using time more efficiently—and certainly is more effective interpersonally.

Nurses often occupy positions of control over waiting in hospitals, clinics, and home settings. There are several ways to reduce client waiting time: One is to avoid making unrealistic time commitments for oneself and others. Another is to keep clients as informed as possible about times for tests, treatments, nursing care, and appointments. When clients do have to wait, the nurse can check back, keep them informed, and help them to use the time constructively. Waiting periods can be a good time for assessment interviewing. In clinic or office settings it is helpful to analyze the appointment system and make necessary changes to minimize client waiting. Feedback to chronically late health-care personnel about the effect their lateness has on others can also be constructive.

Many hospitalized clients need to be kept oriented to the passage of time. Clocks and calendars are often helpful to children, the elderly, or the chronically ill whose usual time indicators are absent or changed during hospitalization. A distorted sense of time can occur with narcotics, some stimulants, anesthesia, serious illness, or isolation. A nurse who tries to view time from the client's perspective is likely to remember to keep the client informed about waiting times, to provide orientation to time as needed, to schedule clinic or home visits with the client's needs in mind, and to gain some appreciation for the time demands and constraints placed on clients by the healthcare system.

To develop the ability to use time constructively with clients, it is helpful to become aware of how we usually use time. Some of us are habitually late, others are always early. Some people frequently interrupt others or finish sentences for them, and others never do. Becoming aware of how others react to our use of time and being sensitive to others' nonverbal behavior helps us to determine whether we wish to modify our use of time.

SILENCE

Some nurses are uncomfortable being silent and spend more time talking than listening, while other nurses prefer to say little. Both the overly silent and the overly talkative nurse will find it helpful to evaluate the effect those behaviors have on clients. If either nurse or client seems uncomfortable when the nurse is providing care silently or if the nurse tends to gather less data than other nurses, he or she may be too silent and may want to consider doing more talking. It is also possible for a talkative nurse to gather inadequate data if he or she is not using enough silence to allow clients time to respond. A balance between silence and talking is needed. An old proverb says, "We were given two ears and one mouth and we ought to use them in that proportion."

If we find ourselves uncomfortable using silence, we can try to identify the source of our discomfort. We may feel the constraint of thinking we really ought to be saying something instead of being silent; that being silent is a waste of valuable time; or that we are inept as interviewers if silences occur. If silence is more comfortable than client interactions, it is again important to try to identify the reasons: We may have a quiet personality that causes us to be naturally comfortable with silence; we may feel some reticence about exploring issues with other people and feel that we are prying into their personal business; or we may not feel a need to fill time with words.

The first step in determining whether our use of silence facilitates or hampers client interactions is to become aware of how we use silence and how clients react to our use or nonuse of this skill. Observing ourselves and soliciting feedback from peers and clients will help us to determine whether modification of our use of silence would increase our professional competence. Planned or practiced use of silence can help us learn to use silence more appropriately and increase our comfort level in using it. The following activity provides a structured situation in which to use silence and observe its effect on others and self.

Activity 7-D: Using Silence in Interactions

Work in groups of three: partners A and B, and an observer. A video camera may be used to supplement the observer's activities.

1. Partner A: Select a topic of special concern to you and interview partner B about his or her views on the subject.
   Partner B: Respond in a natural manner, but at some appropriate time in the interview become silent. The interview should last 4 to 5 minutes, with at least a 45- to 60-second silence.
   Observer: Observe and take notes on the basis of the following questions:
   a. How long was the silence (*actual* time elapsed)?
   b. What was being discussed before the silence? After the silence?
   c. Who broke the silence?
   d. What nonverbal or verbal indicators of comfort or discomfort were evident in partner A? In partner B?
   e. What feelings were being communicated by partner A? By partner B?
2. Partners A and B: Examine your exchange, using feedback from the observer or videotape and the following questions as a guide:
   a. How long did the silence *seem* to each of you?
   b. What feelings did each of you experience during the silence?
   c. How would you rate your partner's comfort or discomfort level during the silence? Your own? Use a scale of 0 to 5, with 5 being a high level of discomfort.
3. Exchange roles and repeat the activity.

☐ CRITICAL POINTS SUMMARY

1. Time can be used to dominate and control other people.
2. The way time is used in providing care can communicate the provider's feelings to the client.
3. Waiting implies that power and dominance are with the one being waited for.
4. Nurses can act to decrease waiting time and to minimize its effects on clients.
5. Silence can be a purposeful nonverbal activity used alone or interspersed with verbal communication.
6. To use time and silence effectively, be aware of usual patterns of time and silence and how they affect the messages communicated to clients.

☐ REVIEW QUESTIONS

1. What does this statement mean to you? "The issue of control is central to the concept of time as communication."

2. How can a nurse minimize the negative effects of client waiting?
3. What are some helpful and unhelpful ways silence can be used?
4. What problems with the planned use of silence does a naturally talkative person have? The naturally shy, quiet person?
5. How can a nurse help clients maintain a perspective of the passage of time when the usual time indicators have been removed?

REFERENCES

Bloch DW: Privacy. In Carlson CE, (coordinator), Behavioral Concepts and Nursing Interventions. Philadelphia, JB Lippincott, 1970.
Hall ET: The Hidden Dimension. Garden City, NY, Doubleday, 1969.
Hein EC: Communication in Nursing Practice, ed 2. Boston, Little, Brown, 1980.
Johnson WL, Rosenfield LS: Factors affecting waiting time in ambulatory care services. Health Services Research 286–295, Winter 1968.

Kastenbaum R, Aisenberg R: The Psychology of Death. New York, Springer Publishing, 1972.

BIBLIOGRAPHY

Bradley JC, Edinburg MA: Communication in the Nursing Context. New York, Appleton-Century-Crofts, 1982.
Edwards BJ, Brillhart JK: Communication in Nursing Practice. St Louis, MO, CV Mosby, 1981.
Pluckhan ML: Human Communication: The Matrix of Nursing. New York, McGraw-Hill, 1978.
Sundeen SJ, Stuart GW, et al: Nurse–Client Interaction: Implementing the Nursing Process. St Louis, MO, CV Mosby, 1981.

AUDIOVISUAL RESOURCE

Proxemics: Space and Human Experience
Filmstrip. (1975, Color, 20 min.)
Available from:
  Concept Media
  P.O. Box 19542
  Irvine, CA 92714

SKILL 8 Space and Touch

Where people sit and stand in relation to each other reflects how they feel about one another.
— Stillman, p. 1671

Only when someone listens, only when someone touches, can the body and spirit be restored.
— Naugle, p. 1891

☐ STUDENT OBJECTIVES

1. Distinguish among intimate, personal, social, and public distance zones.
2. Describe ways of modifying the impact of entering clients' intimate and personal distance zones while providing nursing care.
3. Identify appropriate distance zones for various nursing activities.
4. Explain the concept of territoriality as it relates to nursing activities.
5. Distinguish between procedural and nonprocedural or caring touch.
6. Describe the various meanings and uses of touch.
7. Describe nonverbal messages that may be conveyed through specific uses of space and touch.
8. Recognize your own patterns in the use of space and touch.
9. Assess your own feelings when others enter your intimate or personal distance zone.
10. Assess your own feelings about entering the intimate or personal distance zone of other persons.
11. Identify your own feelings about touching and being touched.

☐ INTRODUCTION

Space is an invisible area that surrounds us and sets us apart from others; it is room in which to move about and a place for our bodies to be in (Pluckhan, 1978a). Personal space is the area immediately around the individual; it has invisible boundaries that move about with the individual and expand and contract under different situations (Little, 1965). Lyman and Scott (1967) describe the space occupied by the human body as body territory. Territoriality involves a spatial relationship with people and things. It is a dimension of space that refers to the desire (or instinct) to control the occupancy and use of the space we define as our own (Edwards and Brilhart, 1981). Hall defines territoriality as "the behavior by which an organism characteristically lays claim to an area and defends it against members of his own species" (1966, p. 7).

Touch involves personal space and action. Through the action of physical contact with another person, we enter his or her personal space. Touch is regarded as the most profound and primitive of all our senses (Hall, 1966) and the most elemental medium of communication between people (Barnett, 1972b).

Touch may be procedural or nonprocedural (Goodykoontz, 1979). *Procedural touch* is the touching that is an essential part of nearly all nursing activities, while *nonprocedural touch* is the spontaneous touching that is used to convey feelings and attitudes. When it conveys empathy and concern, nonprocedural touch can be described as *caring touch* and is perceived by clients as a therapeutic gesture (Bradley and Edinberg, 1982).

Barnett (1972b) indicates that the act of touch is an integral part of nursing intervention and is to be used judiciously between nurse and client as a basis for establishing communication and as a fundamental mechanism of communicating emotions and ideas. One study has shown that the response to treatment was significantly better in seriously ill clients who were touched during verbal interactions as compared with seriously ill clients who were not touched (McCorkel, 1974). The effectiveness of nonprocedural touch depends on the comfort level of both the nurse who initiates the touch and the client who receives the touch.

Hospitalized clients experience a great deal of intrusion into their personal space because of the lack of privacy in hospitals, the nature of diagnostic and therapeutic procedures, and the physical (often personal and intimate) care involved in nursing care activities. When nurses enter someone else's personal space and use procedural or nonprocedural touch, they communicate nonverbally their own level of comfort with those kinds of touch. In general, nurses seem to be more comfortable with procedural touch than with nonprocedural touch, and their use of touch is quite variable. A study of utilization of nonprocedural touch involving 900 health-team personnel and 540 hospitalized clients in two general hospitals had some interesting results. In this study, registered nurses touched clients more frequently than other health-team personnel and twice as often as junior nursing students. Senior nursing students and medical interns used no touch. Younger personnel, aged 18 to 25, used touch the most frequently; women touched more frequently than men; the hands, forehead, and shoulders were the most frequent body areas touched; newborns and infants of one year or less and adults between ages 26 and 33 were touched most frequently; and the most frequent use of touch occurred in the pediatric units, labor and delivery rooms, and intensive care areas (Barnett, 1972a).

☐ PREPARATION

SPACE

As with the use of time in Skill 7, the basic issue in communication through the use of space is *control*. We seek to protect and control our own space, and in turn seek to exert control over others' space. We send messages about our feelings for others through the distance we place between us and them.

In his study of *proxemics*—theories of observations about territorial zones and their use—Hall (1966) defines the functional use of space in terms of four distance zones. Each of the zones differs in sensory input and has a near and a far phase. *Intimate distance* is from 0 to 18 inches. Usually this zone is reserved for contact with people with whom we are close and of whom we are fond. Intimate distance is used for comforting, protecting, and lovemaking. This closeness allows for body contact and perceptions of breath and odor, and produces visual distortion. Vocal communication is usually soft, even whispered. *Personal distance* is from 1½ to 4 feet and is considered an extension of the self. This is the zone where private conversation is conducted. At these distances, voice volume is moderate, body odors are not usually apparent, and visual distortion is absent. *Social distance,* 4 to 12 feet, is reserved for impersonal business transactions or social conversation at a party. At these distances, the perceptual information we receive about the other person is much less detailed. *Public distance,* beyond 12 feet, is an impersonal distance in which the voice must be projected and subtle facial expressions are lost to us.

Acceptable and comfortable distances between persons are culturally and socially defined and vary with the individual. For example, Hall (1966) reports that middle-class Americans of northern European descent tend to determine interpersonal space visually and maintain a greater conversational distance than do Arabs, who generally involve both the visual and olfactory senses and stand close enough to smell each other's breath. Americans usually find this conversational closeness uncomfortable.

Children tend to use space more freely than adults. As we grow older, we learn the socially accepted spatial norms for our own cultural-ethnic group, such as to respect the space reserved by a coat draped over an empty seat or to know how close to stand when talking with someone. When we talk with someone from too far away we feel a need to move closer, but if he or she moves too close we feel uncomfortable and may even retreat. Allekian (1973) cites several studies demonstrating that close approach within the personal space causes physiological responses and embarrassment. In a crowded elevator or bus, most of us feel that our own space is being intruded on and that we are intruding into others' space. In an effort to achieve some distancing and to protect our psychologic self, we tend to hold ourselves erect, not relaxing against others, to avoid eye contact, and even to avoid conversation. However, when an elevator or bus breaks down the shared emergency tends to decrease the social barriers, and strangers relate to each other more intimately.

Territoriality and Personal Space

In our daily lives we regard our community, street, home, room, or closet as our own territory: a place that is ours to control or in which to act as we choose. A sense of having our own space helps us feel secure, especially in new and unfamiliar surroundings. Our body territory is regarded as the most inviolable of all the territories to which we lay claim.

Personal space extends about an arm's length away from the body, although its size varies with the individual and does not extend equally in all directions. We usually can tolerate having a person stand closer to our sides than in front and facing us, and allow some people to come closer than others. Sometimes this personal space and extension of ourselves is described as a life-space bubble that we carry with us at all times and reinforce in various ways, such as with an aloof manner or by wearing heavy perfume to help maintain the boundaries of that bubble. The concept of life space also can expand to include the topics an individual considers private and personal. For example, a person may consider job, income, religion, sexual activities, or elimination habits as private information and therefore send clear nonverbal and verbal messages that these are part of his or her personal space.

The following activity focuses on the effect that variable distances between people have on comfort level and the ability to communicate.

Activity 8–A: Communication Distances and Comfort

Work in pairs for this activity.

1. Position yourself about 15 feet away from your partner and tell him or her about an experience you had recently. While you are talking, your partner moves toward you at a pace of about 1 foot each 15 seconds and continues moving forward until one of you calls a halt. Each of you notes the distance at which you first became uncomfortable and at which you could not tolerate the closeness—if that occurred.
2. Describe your feelings about having someone approach and enter your life-space bubble. Have your partner describe the feelings he or she experienced about entering someone's life-space bubble uninvited.
3. At what distances did you find it easy to talk to your partner? At what distances was it difficult?
4. Exchange roles and repeat the activity.

Whether we allow someone to enter our personal space depends on the person and the situation. Through nonverbal cues, we give some people permission to come close and even to enter into our personal life space and we keep other people at a greater distance. It is similar to inviting someone into your house versus keeping him or her on the porch while you talk. When we go to a physician's office or to a hospital, we expect to have our personal space entered, and health-care providers expect to enter that personal space (Fig. 8–1). While this does lend objectivity to intrusions and touch that would ordinarily be unaccept-

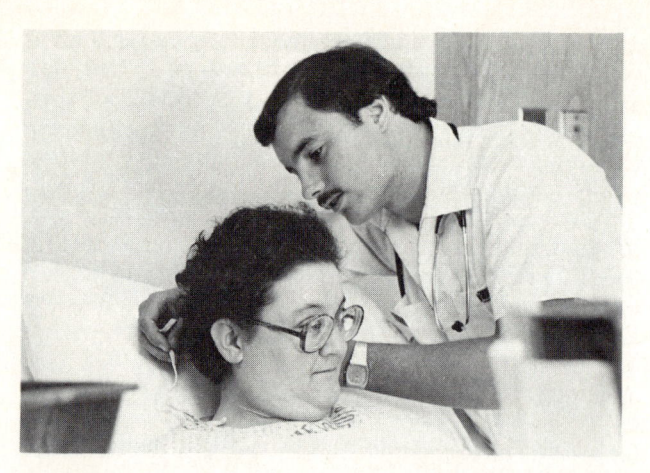

Figure 8–1. Most nursing care is provided within the life-space bubble. (Photo by James Haines.)

able, the health-care provider is usually far more comfortable with this intrusion than is the client. Unfortunately, the health-care provider's comfort level sometimes translates into nonchalant haste or an assumed right to perform intimate procedures without explanation or permission and is regarded by the client as highly depersonalizing and intrusive.

The Use of Space in Nursing

When hospitalized, a client enters unfamiliar surroundings, which usually are considered to be nurses' territory because of their 24-hour presence there. Minckley (1968) suggests that this places the client in the role of transgressor into the nurses' territory, with some resultant guilt and tension.

Although the hospital room, bed, bedside stand, and closet are considered the client's temporary territory, a virtual parade of people intrude into this space, often without knocking and without introductions and explanations. Personal possessions frequently are rearranged and moved to create space for treatments; and a nurse often rearranges bedside table items, thus intruding into the client's territory. A nurse may intrude into the client's personal space by leaning across the bed or the client to reach a nurse-call signal or other object (Pluckhan, 1968).

In a study of anxiety and intrusions of territorial and personal space involving 76 clients, Allekian (1973) found that territorial intrusions by hospital personnel produced more anxiety than did intrusions into personal space (including body territory). No personal space intrusions were regarded favorably, and the greatest client anxiety was elicited by feeling the nurse's breath against the client's face. Allekian found that clients had greater anxiety levels when they perceived the personnel's actions to be inconsistent with the client's best interests, comfort and well-being. In addition, there seemed to be less territoriality associated with objects that were somewhat unrelated to the client's sense of identity; for example, one client reacted with more annoyance when "his" bedside stand was moved than when "the chair in his room" was removed. Allekian suggests that this reaction may occur because people may anticipate personal space intrusions when they enter the hospital, but are unprepared for territorial intrusions which may be perceived as reducing their personal control and identity.

Although entering a hospital usually means loss of territory and space, for some people it may mean the opposite. Stillman reports that homeless transients who were hospitalized for frostbite, malnutrition, or alcoholism often welcomed having a bed, a chair, and space of their own, and frequent intrusions from personnel were seen as opportunities for interactions (Stillman, 1978).

Nurses use space to communicate with clients by the way they place themselves physically in relationship to those clients. For example, when a nurse stands in the doorway to talk with a client rather than entering the room, the client tends to feel that the nurse is hurried or disinterested. If the nurse interviews a client while standing at the foot of the bed, the client is likely to perceive dominance, control, and lack of time on the part of the nurse and to experience a sense of depersonalization. This physical relationship requires the client to look up while the nurse looks down, a clear status indicator. An interview is generally more successful when the nurse is seated near the client, with the physical indicators of status difference minimized.

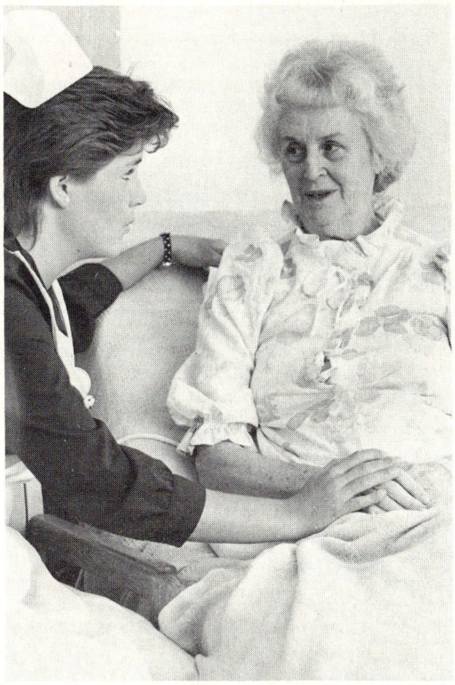

TOUCH

Touch serves many functions. For the blind, it is one of the two primary senses that provide input about their world. Touch can be used to get someone's attention or to give a greeting; for example, a tap on the shoulder or a handshake. It can convey pleasure, reassurance, or comfort. Touch can also provide a contact with reality for the severely ill, withdrawn, or disturbed person, and can convey a sense of caring to the person in grief or pain. As the "last stage in reducing the distance between people" (Jourard, 1968, p. 136), touch reduces our sense of aloneness and separateness from others. Research indicates that the use of touch helps to establish rapport quickly with seriously ill clients and indicates to them that the nurse does care about them (McCorkle, 1974).

Touch is an almost universally understood nonverbal way of conveying feelings and attitudes. Although often combined with words, touch is a tactile language that by itself can express human concern more powerfully and expressively than words. For example, a 32-year-old father of three died from a cerebral aneurysm, despite heroic medical efforts for 3 days. His wife had been there constantly, visiting him whenever visiting hours permitted. It was the duty of the night intensive care nurse to tell the wife her husband had died. The nurse found the wife in the waiting room and said simply "I'm sorry," embracing her for a few moments, as they both cried softly. The wife understood the message and felt sustained and strengthened from the nurse's caring touch.

Figure 8–2. Touch conveys the quality and intent of a message. (Photo by James Haines.)

As with all nonverbal communication, touch conveys primarily the quality and intent of a message, rather than its content, and the recipient often responds largely to those aspects (Fig. 8–2). People readily perceive whether the intent of touch is to help or to hurt. Although not always evident to an observer, in most instances the recipient of touch is also aware of the nonverbal message conveyed. For example, when one person greets another with a hug, bystanders may see only cordiality and affection, while the recipient readily knows whether the hug is warm and caring or perfunctory and cool, and will respond on the basis of that perception.

As with personal space, the amount of touching with which people feel comfortable varies. In North America it is not unusual for people to apologize when they accidentally touch someone else. People raised in families where physical affection was easily expressed may feel more comfortable with touching others as adults. In some families the members, men and women alike, hug and kiss as both a welcome and a farewell. In other families only a handshake or pat on the back is used, even when a son or daughter is leaving for college or overseas. Some families continue to display physical affection to children through adolescence, while others stop when the child leaves infancy, enters school, or begins puberty. For boys, this discontinuation of physical display of affection often comes earlier than for girls.

The following activity focuses on familial and cultural patterns of space and touch use.

Activity 8-B:
Personal Patterns of Space and Touch Use

1. Compare your familial and cultural patterns of touching and physical closeness with at least four other persons, preferably both male and female, and of different ages and ethnic groups. Consider these factors:
   a. Who touches whom and under what circumstance
   b. Any gender, age, or relational prohibitions or requirements for touching
   c. Parental expression of physical affection to each other and to children
2. How are your own patterns like or different from the patterns of the persons with whom you compared? What could contribute to the similarities or differences?

The Use of Touch in Nursing

Nurturing activities such as bathing, giving back rubs, and cuddling of children and infants are regarded as acceptable touching activities by both nurse and client. Nurses generally have unspoken "professional permission" from themselves and clients to touch people in ways and places considered unacceptable in other circumstances. However, the degree to which this is accepted varies with individuals and cultural groups. For example, Shubin (1980) reports a recent study revealing that Israeli clients generally do not like a lot of touching when ill. According to Shubin, an Hispanic psychiatrist indicates that Puerto Rican adults feel much the same way.

When touching norms are violated, the person being touched may become quite uncomfortable. In fact, Jourard indicates that to actually touch a person who does not wish to be touched "is often to invite violence or panic" (1968, p. 137).

On the basis of their studies of the role of body contact in American society, Jourard and Rubin (1968) indicate that for most people, touching has conscious or unconscious sexual connotations. Sometimes hospitalized male clients who are seeking reinforcement for their sense of masculinity may pinch, pat, or attempt to kiss a female nurse. The beginning nurse may be alarmed by this behavior and may become angry with the client. When this happens, the nurse can do several things: She can consider the possible meaning of the client's behavior. She can confront the client with his behavior and disclose her own feelings to him, using an I-message (see Skill 5) such as, "I become uncomfortable when you do that, and I am asking you not to touch me like that anymore." She can also look at her own behavior to see if she may have given permission for the client's approach through a too-familiar social relationship rather than a professional one.

The way a nurse uses touch conveys important nonverbal messages to clients and their families about how the nurse feels about them, their circumstances, and their problems. When personal care is given gently but firmly, carefully, and with provision for privacy, nurses communicate caring, respect for the individual, and confidence in themselves. When personal care is given roughly or hastily, touching conveys disinterest, depersonalization, or even dislike. When personal care is given tentatively and hesitantly, touch can convey fear, anxiety, or insecurity.

When a person is critically ill and in an intensive care unit, the monitoring and life-sustaining devices often seem to demand more attention from the nurse than the client. In these circumstances it is not uncommon, and is sometimes necessary, for a nurse to do a complete assessment of the client's status with minimal touching and handling of the client. Some touching does seem to be necessary, however. For example, Roberts (1976) indicates that clients experience an emotional deprivation when the nurse's touching is limited to handling the equipment.

Giving a back rub is a special type of touching that can be used creatively. In addition to stimulating circulation and preventing skin breakdown, back rubs relieve tension and stiff muscles and promote relaxation and sleep, as discussed in Skill 47.

Although all touch used in a caring manner is therapeutic in that it conveys warmth and concern, touch can be used in specific ways as a distinct therapy. Research over the past several years suggests that healing energy can pass from or through one person to another, providing relief of pain and discomfort, decreasing anxiety, and promoting relaxation and healing. The nurse-healer learns to sense areas where the client is experiencing difficulty by placing his or her hands on or near different parts of the client's body. The nurse-healer then either rearranges the client's energy fields through an energy exchange or serves as a channel for other more universal healing energies to flow through the nurse-healer to the client. With either method, the nurse-healer enters a centered meditative state of consciousness prior to beginning the therapeutic touch treatment (Boguslawski, 1979; Heidt, 1980; Krieger, 1975, 1979; Krieger et al., 1979; Macrae, 1979; Miller, 1979; Quinn, 1979).

□ EXECUTION

SPACE AND TOUCH IN NURSING CARE

The use of space and touch in nursing needs to be a knowledgeable, deliberate, and judicious part of all nursing activities, not simply an intuitive activity. On the basis of Hall's (1966) analysis of distance zones, Levine (1973) suggests that nurses can use territory and distance to contribute positively to clients' well-being and comfort. Raising or lowering the volume of the voice has the psychological effect of altering the perception of distance zones. For example, when giving nursing care within the intimate distance zone of 0 to 18 inches, nurses can psychologically increase both their own perception and the client's perception of the distance involved by using a voice and tone appropriate for personal distance, rather than using the whisper associated with intimate distance. This approach lessens the client's anxiety about having someone so close and increases the nurse's comfort about being so close.

Eye contact can also be used to alter the perception of distance between people. Maintaining eye contact when talking to a client from across the room reduces the feeling of distance. On the other hand, using intermittent eye contact when very close to a client or when performing intimate care increases the feeling of distance, providing psychological relief from intrusion into the client's life-space bubble. As much as possible, avoid leaning or reaching directly over a client, especially over the face. It usually takes only a little extra time and energy to walk around the bed or chair to obtain or adjust equipment.

The space between client and nurse should be appropriate for the activity being performed, and the voice volume and tone generally consistent with what is usual for that distance. This means that the nurse moves into the personal distance zone of 1½ to 4 feet and uses a moderate voice volume when discussing personal matters with clients. Standing at a greater distance and using a loud tone to discuss personal matters (such as bowel and eating habits or use of contraceptives) psychologically moves the interaction into the impersonal social distance zone and is perceived by clients and bystanders as highly invasive, intrusive, embarrassing, and depersonalizing. A similar effect would occur if the nurse physically remained within a personal distance but raised his or her voice volume to that used in social distance. For the exception of a client who has impaired hearing, increasing the voice volume and lowering the pitch is usually more effective and is perceived as less intrusive.

Interviews are best conducted when the nurse is seated within the far personal distance zone, defined as 2½ to 4 feet, which is the usual range for conversation. This distance allows both nurse and client to drop the voice volume and tone to a more personal level for more intimate subjects and still be heard clearly. It also allows the nurse to reach out and communicate nonverbally through touch.

When entering the intimate distance zone for giving personal care, it is important to take care not to be intrusive or abrupt. Giving prior explanations, avoiding haste, protecting privacy, and being gentle all communicate respect and caring for the client and his or her personal integrity. When consciously using touch for comfort, reassurance, orientation, or other purposes, sensitivity to the client's mood and response to such an approach is needed. For example, if a client withdraws his or her hand when it is touched or moves away, touch is probably not appropriate at that time. However, if the client stiffens when touched, it might be beneficial to continue the touch for a short time to see if relaxation occurs. Whether or not the client then relaxes and accepts the touch will indicate if the touch is appropriate. It is important to recognize that a client who rejects being touched at one time may or may not reject it later or under other circumstances. For example, people are more likely to be receptive to our touch when there is privacy, when they have learned to know and trust us, and when they perceive us as warm and caring.

PERSONAL COMFORT LEVEL WITH TOUCH

Since much of nursing involves entering the intimate and personal distance zones of others, it is important to develop the ability to function comfortably within those zones and still convey respect for privacy and personal space. There are several ways to increase our comfort level in using both procedural and nonprocedural touch. The first is to become aware of our own patterns of touching and being touched and the degree of comfort we experience when we enter someone's intimate and personal distance zones, or when someone enters ours. To do this, begin by observing the circumstances, frequency, and ways in which we touch and allow ourselves to be touched by persons of the same and opposite sex.

The following activity focuses on identifying body areas where you are comfortable touching and being touched. This activity is primarily for your own use but may be shared if desired.

Activity 8-C: Personal Comfort with Touch

1. Look at the "good friend" picture, Activity Figure 8-C. Using a pencil, shade in the body areas you would feel comfortable *touching* when with a good friend of either sex in public or in private.

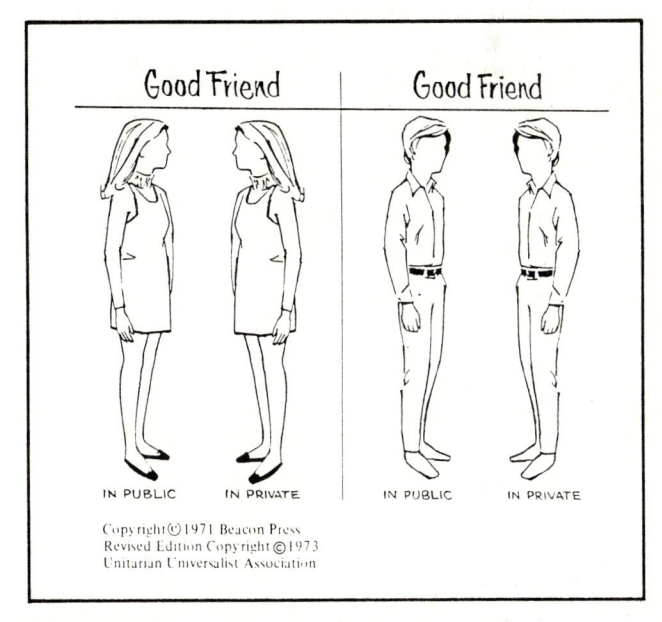

Activity Figure 8–C. (From About Your Sexuality by Deryck Calderwood, a multi-media curriculum published by the Unitarian Universalist Association. Used with permission. Revised edition copyright © 1973 by the Unitarian Universalist Association.)

2. Now shade in the areas you are comfortable *being touched,* using a different color pencil.
3. Note any differences in touching versus being touched, public versus private, and male versus female.
4. Identify the situations and circumstances in which you would touch the body areas you have identified (or in which you would permit others to touch you).
5. As additional information for your own use, you may want to validate your perceptions of your own use of touch with someone you know and trust.
6. On the basis of your assessment, you may want to modify your usual use of space and touch. For example, if you rarely touch anyone or usually touch only impersonal areas such as the hands, you may want to consciously increase your use of touch to convey caring and helpfulness.

As indicated earlier in this skill, for many people in our society touching has sexual overtones. For this reason, many of us experience minimal or brief touching contact with people outside our own families. When we are not accustomed to touching someone else deliberately and purposefully, we may not be aware of the relaxation and warmth that can be communicated through caring touch. Becoming aware of the feelings clients experience through caring touch can help us to feel more comfortable using that touch.

The following activity focuses on experiencing feelings of pleasure, relaxation, and rest through being touched, as well as the experience of touching someone else.

Activity 8-D: Touching and Being Touched

Work in pairs and groups of three for this activity, preferably with mixed male and female partners. Switch partners for each exercise.

For each of the following exercises, respond to these questions:

- How did you feel when you were the receiver? The giver? What sensations were you aware of?
- With which role did you feel more comfortable?
- How do the different persons in the group vary in their use of touch?
- With which activity did you feel most comfortable? Least comfortable?
- How do your experiences compare with the others within your small group? (Remember that there are no norms for this experience, as each of you is unique.)

1. Give and receive a "body rub." Work in groups of three, taking turns being the recipient.
    Recipient: Stand in a comfortable, relaxed position, with feet slightly apart and arms hanging at sides.
    Partners: Stand on either side, facing the recipient. Using both hands, begin patting the recipient's shoulder nearest to you, checking with the recipient to see if your patting is too light or too harsh. Working simultaneously and fairly quickly but not hastily, begin to pat the recipient, using this sequence:
    a. Down the outside of the arms
    b. Up the inside of the arms and onto the shoulders
    c. Down the back
    d. Single firm pat on the posterior
    e. Down the outside of the legs
    f. Up the inside of the legs
    g. Up the back and neck
    Now, "walk" your fingers over the recipient's head, especially the temporal areas, and down the back of the neck to the shoulders. Give three firm, quick "good-bye" pats on the shoulders.
2. Exchange roles and repeat until each has given and received a "body rub."
3. Describe your feelings about receiving and giving a full "body rub." Compare with your partners and with your friends.
4. Give and receive a foot massage, using either lotion on bare skin or dry hands over feet with socks. Work in pairs.
    Recipient: Sit in a relaxed position on a chair, a couch, or the floor.
    Partner: Position yourself comfortably in front of the recipient. Using a firm, smooth rubbing and kneading stroke, gently massage the entire foot and ankle areas. Spend at least 3 minutes massaging first the right foot and then the left, ending with smooth rubbing strokes on both feet simultaneously.
    (*NOTE:* You may extend a stroking movement up to the calf of the leg if you wish, but avoid rubbing or kneading the calves because of the potential that exists for deep vein thrombosis in some persons.)
5. Reverse roles and repeat.
6. Describe your feelings about receiving and giving a foot rub. Compare with your partner.

☐ CRITICAL POINTS SUMMARY

1. Use and perceptions of space and touch are culturally and socially influenced.
2. The nurse's use of space and touch communicates his or her feelings about clients' concerns.
3. The nurse's use of space and touch reflects respect for clients' territorial needs and life-space bubble.
4. The nurse's intent to be helpful and caring is conveyed through both procedural and nonprocedural caring touch.
5. Space and touch can be deliberately used for specific therapeutic purposes.

6. Perception of space can be psychologically altered by modifying voice volume and eye contact.
7. Client integrity and privacy must be maintained when performing nursing activities within the intimate and personal distance zones.
8. The nurse can learn to observe his or her own use of space and touch and how it affects clients, and can find ways to modify it to enhance the nurse–client relationship.

☐ REVIEW QUESTIONS

1. What does this statement mean to you? "The basic issue in communication through space is control."
2. What does the concept of life space comprise?
3. When a person's life-space bubble is entered, what meanings may that have for him or her?
4. What is the range (in feet) for each of Hall's four distance zones?
5. What professional or personal activities might occur in each distance zone?
6. Give examples of how you can minimize the intrusiveness of giving personal care in the intimate distance zone.
7. As a nurse, how might you respect the territorial needs of clients?
8. Give several examples of procedural and nonprocedural touch.
9. Why is nonprocedural touch also called caring touch?
10. What are at least six purposes for which touch can be used?
11. What messages can the nurse convey to the client through use of touch?
12. In what way is therapeutic touch different from caring touch?

REFERENCES

Allekian CI: Intrusions of territory and personal space: An anxiety-inducing factor for hospitalized persons—An exploratory study. Nursing Research 22(3):236–241, 1973.

Barnett K: A survey of the current utilization of touch by health team personnel with hospitalized patients. International Journal of Nursing Studies 9:195–208, 1972a.

Barnett K: A theoretical construct of the concepts of touch as they relate to nursing. Nursing Research 21(2):102–110, 1972b.

Boguslawski M: The use of therapeutic touch in nursing. Journal of Continuing Education in Nursing 10(4):9–14, 1979.

Bradley JC, Edinberg MA: Communication in the Nursing Context. New York, Appleton-Century-Crofts, 1982.

Calderwood D: About Your Sexuality (Student Activity Packet). Rev. ed. Boston, Unitarian Universalist Association, 1973.

Edwards BJ, Brilhart JK: Communication in Nursing Practice. St Louis, MO, CV Mosby, 1981.

Goodykoontz L: Touch: Attitudes and practice. Nursing Forum 18(1):4–17, 1979.

Hall ET: The Hidden Dimension. Garden City, NY, Doubleday, 1966.

Heidt P: Effect of therapeutic touch on anxiety level of hospitalized patients. Nursing Research 30(1):32–37, 1980.

Jourard, S: Disclosing Man to Himself. New York, D. Van Nostrand Co., 1968.

Jourard S, Rubin JE: Self-disclosure and touching: A study of two modes of interpersonal encounter and their interrelation. Journal of Humanistic Psychology 8(1):39–48, 1968.

Krieger D: Therapeutic touch: The imprimatur of nursing. American Journal of Nursing 75(5):784–787, 1975.

Krieger D: The Therapeutic Touch. Englewood Cliffs, NJ, Prentice-Hall, 1979.

Krieger D, Peper E, Ancoli S: Therapeutic touch: Searching for evidence of physiological changes. American Journal of Nursing 79(4):660–662, 1979.

Levine ME: Introduction to Clinical Nursing. Philadelphia, FA Davis, 1973.

Little KB: Personal space. Journal of Experimental Social Psychology 1(3):237–247, 1965.

Lyman SM, Scott MB: Territoriality: A neglected sociological dimension. Social Problems 15(2):236–249, 1967.

Macrae J: Therapeutic touch in practice. American Journal of Nursing 79(4):664–665, 1979.

McCorkle R: Effects of touch on seriously ill patients. Nursing Research 23(2):125–132, 1974.

Miller LA: An explanation of therapeutic touch. Nursing Forum 18(3)278–287, 1979.

Minckley B: Space and place in nursing care. American Journal of Nursing 68(3):510–516, 1968.

Naugle EH: The difference caring makes. American Journal of Nursing 73(11):1890–1891, 1973.

Pluckhan ML: Human Communication: The Matrix of Nursing. New York, McGraw-Hill, 1978.

Pluckhan ML: Space: The silent language . . . . Nursing Forum 7(4):386–397, 1968.

Quinn J: One nurse's evolution as a healer. American Journal of Nursing 79(4):664–665, 1979.

Roberts S: Behavioral Concepts and the Critically Ill Patient. Englewood Cliffs, NJ, Prentice-Hall, 1976.

Shubin S: Nursing patients from different cultures. Nursing80 10(6):78–81, 1980.

Stillman MJ: Territoriality and personal space. American Journal of Nursing 78(10):1670–1672, 1978.

BIBLIOGRAPHY

Sundeen SJ, Stuart GW, et al: Nurse–Client Interaction: Implementing the Nursing Process. St Louis, MO, CV Mosby, 1981.

Ujhely GB: Touch: Reflections and perceptions. Nursing Forum 18(1):18–32, 1979.

Weiss SJ: The language of touch. Nursing Research 28(2):76–80, 1979.

3 Facilitative Communication Skills

☐ INTRODUCTION

Facilitative communication skills are skills that assist the process of sending and receiving messages. The use of these skills makes it easier to establish a caring relationship with clients in which help can be requested, offered, or received without depersonalization or excessive dependency. Facilitative communication skills help the nurse to gather more relevant and accurate information and also enable clients to express themselves and their concerns more freely to the nurse. Perhaps more importantly, during the process of using facilitative communication skills the client gradually becomes a real person to the nurse: It is difficult to listen actively and attentively to someone's messages and to reflect accurately the content, feelings, and meaning of those messages without seeing that person as a unique individual—and without beginning to care.

Since most nursing care delivery occurs within the health-care system with the client requesting services, the nurse is perceived as the provider of care and services. However, the term facilitative communication skills implies that the client is being helped to do something for himself or herself rather than having it done by someone else. Nursing at its best is a collaborative relationship between nurse and client, where each contributes from his or her own area of strength. The nurse can contribute knowledge of health and illness as well as technical, interpersonal, and problem-solving skills. The client can contribute knowledge of personal goals, strengths, and resources.

This chapter presents six components of communication as separate skills, which are then combined in Chapter 4 through Skill 15, "Interviewing," and Skill 16, "Teaching–Learning."

Attending behavior refers to the ways in which we pay attention to what someone is saying to us. Attending behavior is productive when it communicates respect, interest, and understanding.

Listening is a process of hearing and perceiving messages. *Attentive listening* requires the listener's attention to and involvement in what is being said.

Reflection of content and feelings is possible when the listener has heard with understanding. Reflection of content is a restatement of the main thought or meaning in a person's message. Reflection of feelings is an empathic response that communicates understanding of the emotional experience of another person.

Questioning refers to the use of inquiries when determining client status and response.

Offering assistance involves providing direct physical help with basic needs and activities of daily living, providing appropriate reassurance, and helping to identify and resolve problems.

The process of learning a specific communication skill first involves reading theory about that skill in order to understand the ideas on which it is based. Interspersed throughout the theory are learning activities to help the student understand and internalize the concepts being discussed. The student then views models of appropriate and inappropriate use of the particular skill. This is followed by practice in using the skill in both an effective and ineffective manner. Through evaluation by self and peers, the student receives feedback about his or her ability to use the skill in these simulated settings and then practices using that skill in real-life situations before progressing to the next skill.

Research indicates that practicing specific communication skills and seeing models (examples) of those skills provide better learning than simple discussion, and that individuals learn well through contrasting experiences (Brammer, 1979; D'Augelli et al., 1980). Seeing models of ineffective, nonhelpful, and inappropriate communication skills and then experiencing them helps the student to distinguish and learn effective, helpful, and appropriate skills more readily. At times the use of ineffective skills may seem exaggerated and silly, but it is important for the student to experience them *before* practicing the effective skills.

Because of the more specific nature of the facilitative communication skills in this chapter, each skill includes a performance checklist. Audiovisual resources for the facilitative communication skills are listed here rather than in each separate skill because of the overlapping and interrelated nature of the content.

This chapter presents the facilitative skills of "Attending Behavior" (Skill 9), "Attentive Listening" (Skill 10), "Reflection of Content" (Skill 11), "Reflection of Feelings" (Skill 12), "Questioning" (Skill 13), and "Offering Assistance" (Skill 14).

REFERENCES

Brammer LM: The Helping Relationship: Process and Skills, ed 2. Englewood Cliffs, NJ, Prentice-Hall, 1979.

D'Augelli AR, Danish SJ, et al: Helping Skills: A Basic Training Program (Leader's Manual), ed 2. New York, Human Sciences Press, 1980.

AUDIOVISUAL RESOURCES

Art of Helping Training Videotapes: Attending Skills Module
  Videorecording. (30 min.) By discussing and demonstrating the specific skills of physical posturing, observing, and listening, this videorecording promotes trainees' ability to set the stage for effectiveness.

Art of Helping Training Videotapes: Responding Skills Module
  Videorecording. (30 min.) Responding to content, feeling, and meaning.

Life Skills Model Videotapes: Helping Model Module
  Videorecording. (1 hr.) Introduces attending, responding, personalizing, and initiating behaviors.
  Available for purchase from:
  Human Resource Development Press
  Box 863
  Amherst, MA 01002

Communication: Concepts and Complexities
  Film or videocassette. (1979, Color, 30 min.)

Creative Listening
  Film or videocassette. (1981, Color, 42 min.)

Therapeutic Silence
  Film or videocassette. (1981, Color, 30 min.)
  Available through:
  American Journal of Nursing Company
  Educational Services Division
  555 West 57th St.
  New York, NY 10019

Communication Processes in Nursing, Lesson 4
  Videorecording. (1971, B & W, 30 min.)

Utilizing Effective Communication
  Film (16 mm). (1971, B & W, 30 min.)
  Available through:
  Instructional Media Center
  University of Nebraska
  3835 Holdrege Street
  Lincoln, NE 68583

Do You Know Dr. Jones?
  Film. (1970, B & W) Illustrates good and poor listening and attending behaviors, with hospitalized client in preoperative setting. Effective both with soundtrack and without.
  Available through:
  McGraw-Hill Book Company
  1221 Avenue of the Americas
  New York, NY 10020

Interpretation of Patient Responses
  Filmstrip (76 slides with cassette and guide). (1979, Color, 12 min.)

Report on Assertiveness: Verbal Assertiveness
  Filmstrip with cassette and script. (1979, Color, 19 min.)
  Available through:
  Medcom, Inc.
  P.O. Box 116
  Garden Grove, CA 92642

Step-by-Step
  Videorecording. (1975) Series of isolated vignettes illustrating the facilitative skills of attending, open questions, closed questions, reflection of content, and reflection of feelings; the action-oriented skills of helper expression of content, expression of feelings, and interpretation of client situation.
  Available through:
  Human Resource Center
  Graduate School of Social Work
  University of Texas at Arlington
  Arlington, TX 76019

Techniques of Therapeutic Communication
  Filmstrip. (1970, Color, 20 min.)
  Available through:
  Concept Media
  P.O. Box 19542
  Irvine, CA 92714

Therapeutic vs. Non-Therapeutic Communication
  Videocassette. (1978, Color, 20 min.)
  Available through:
  Health Sciences Consortium
  103 Laurel Avenue
  Carrboro, NC 27510

Verbal Questioning Techniques: Verbal Questioning in Clinical and Classroom Teaching
  Videorecording. (1977, Color, 30 min.)
  Available through:
  AudioVisual Concepts
  1525 East 53rd Street
  Chicago, IL 60615

SKILL 9 Attending Behavior

Good attending behavior demonstrates . . . that you respect him as a person, and . . . are interested in what he has to say.
—Ivey, 1971, p. 149

☐ STUDENT OBJECTIVES

1. Describe the components of productive and counterproductive attending behaviors.

2. Discuss the relationship between attending behavior and the helping principle of acceptance.
3. Illustrate the experience of being accepted and accepting others.
4. Recognize the nature of one's own and others' attending behavior.
5. Identify your own counterproductive attending behavior.
6. Demonstrate the ability to use productive attending behavior in simulated and real settings.

☐ INTRODUCTION

Attending behavior refers to the way we pay attention or do not pay attention to someone who is talking to us. It involves nonverbal posture, gestures, and eye contact, plus verbal encouragement (Ivey, 1971, 1977). Attending behavior may be either productive or counterproductive.

Productive attending behavior grows out of an attitude of acceptance on the part of the helper. When the helper is nonjudgmental and accepts the client as he or she really is, that attitude is readily conveyed nonverbally to the client through the helper's attending behavior.

With productive attending behavior a helper uses gestures, eye contact, posture, and verbal encouragement in ways that convey to clients that the helper is interested in, has respect for, and wants to understand them (Brammer, 1979; Ivey, 1971, 1977). In using productive attending behavior, the helper indicates that he or she is giving full attention to the speaker's story through use of appropriate verbal and nonverbal responses. Productive attending behavior encourages people to express themselves freely without fear of criticism or rejection. For example, when we tell someone about a personal problem, we feel that we are being heard, listened to, and understood without being judged if our listener sits or stands quietly, maintains fairly steady eye contact, and occasionally gives appropriate brief comments.

With *counterproductive attending behavior* a helper's gestures, eye contact, posture, and verbal responses are used in ways that convey disinterest or being in a hurry to get on to something the helper considers more important. The client may feel that the helper is being judgmental and does not care for him or her as an individual. In the previous example, if our listener fidgets, glances away, or interrupts, we usually feel that he or she is not interested in us or does not care enough to listen to our concerns.

Productive attending behavior fosters the development and maintenance of a helping relationship in that it communicates caring and empathy to the client, promotes trust, and conveys an attitude that is perceived by the client as warm and accepting. Counterproductive attending behavior, on the other hand, has a negative impact on the helping relationship. Since the client's perception of the helper is a significant factor in the helping relationship, it is crucial that helpers become aware of their own attending behaviors and how those behaviors affect others. Furthermore, it is beneficial if they learn to modify counterproductive behavior and develop the skill of attending to others' communications in a productive way.

As with all aspects of communication, it is important to recognize that attending behavior varies within different cultural frameworks and with individuals within a culture. Attending behavior is presented in this skill primarily from the perspective of the North American middle class. When working with clients from other cultures, nurses find it helpful to inquire about or observe the norms for attending behavior that are held by those clients. If nurses are aware of these norms, they can avoid making incorrect assumptions about the meaning of a client's behavior; or they may decide to adapt their own attending behavior to fit the client's cultural norms.

☐ PREPARATION

COMPONENTS OF ATTENDING BEHAVIOR

As just discussed, attending behavior includes the use of posture, gestures, eye contact, and verbal encouragement. The productive and counterproductive aspects of each of these are described in the following sections.

Posture

Productive attending posture is comfortable and relaxed, yet alert. It is neither so stiff and straight that the helper appears anxious or rigid, nor so slouched and reclined that he or she appears bored, sleepy, or disinterested. With productive attending posture, the helper faces the client and is on the same level; that is, if the client is seated or in bed, the helper is seated. This position allows for maximum nonverbal communication to occur and helps to avoid talking down to the client.

In North American culture, a distance of 3 or 4 feet (far personal distance zone) is considered appropriate for helping conversations (Hall, 1966). Morain (1978) indicates that, in general, Arab, Latin American, Greek, and Turkish people usually stand close to each other. Therefore, it is possible that a somewhat closer distance would be appropriate when interacting with these people.

Leaning slightly forward toward the client helps to convey concern and interest. A helper with a relaxed manner fosters relaxation in the client, making it easier for the client to talk. Tenseness in the helper fosters tenseness in the client and tends to shift the focus of the exchange from client to helper. However, an overly relaxed manner, such as slouching or leaning backward in a chair with arms crossed behind one's head is counterproductive, since it tends to be too casual and socially oriented to be helpful professionally.

Gestures

Relaxed and open arms with hands that are placed on one's lap, the desk, or the arm of a chair convey a message of receptivity to the client. Arms crossed over the chest tend to give closed and negative messages, and the client often perceives disapproval, rejection, and a feeling of being shut out. Other counterproductive gestures include fidgeting with pencils, jewelry, or hair. Keeping one's hands in one's pockets would certainly be relaxed but would be too casual and uninvolved to be considered helpful professionally.

Eye Contact

Direct eye contact generally conveys interest in what the client is saying, and gives a message that the helper is attentive and caring. Eye contact is helpful when it is spontaneous, fairly steady, yet varied by occasional disengagement. Too intense and persistent eye contact is intimidating and artificial, while complete avoidance of eye contact communicates discomfort, embarrassment, or disinterest in the client or topic of discussion. These guidelines may need to be modified when the helper is talking with clients from cultures that use either minimal eye contact, such as some Puerto Ricans, rural Appalachians, or poor blacks; or more intense eye contact, such as some South Americans, British, or Germans (Morain, 1978).

Simply maintaining periodic eye contact does not ensure that productive attending behavior is occurring. Direct eye contact can also communicate boredom, disinterest, or skepticism; and there are times when nonverbal messages are not exchanged even though direct eye contact occurs. For example, it is possible to use blank looks deliberately to avoid conveying a message with the eyes.

Verbal Encouragement

Minimal but purposeful verbal responses can be used to convey interest and encouragement to clients and can help them to continue talking about their concerns. Minimal verbal encouragement is an active mental process during which the helper stays engaged with the client's story and uses minimal verbal responses in a way that indicates he or she is paying attention to what is being said. These minimal responses must relate directly to what the client has said and should not introduce new ideas or change the subject.

Minimal verbal encouragement may be used nondirectively or directively. Nondirective responses simply encourage the client to continue telling his or her story in whatever direction the client chooses. Examples of nondirective minimal responses include words and phrases such as "yes," "mmhmm," "go on," "and then." Or, a key word or words used by the client may be restated by the helper as a question or statement, such as "Your father . . . ," or "You hurt your back?" Gestures such as nods of the head often accompany and reinforce the message conveyed by these minimal verbal responses.

In the more directive approach, the helper comments selectively on aspects of the client's story that the helper believes need to be focused on, expanded, or explained. Examples of directive minimal responses include questions and phrases such as "What happened next?"; "Could you give me an example?"; "What does that mean to you?"; or "I'm not sure I understand when you say that. . . . "

The helper's use of minimal but purposeful verbal encouragement does not include counterproductive behaviors such as talking about oneself, interrupting, and finishing sentences for the client, because these behaviors make it difficult for the client to continue (McHugh, 1978). Sighing, yawning, and a bored, disinterested tone of voice are other verbal attending behaviors that are counterproductive in a helping relationship.

The following activity focuses on observing attending behavior used by others.

Activity 9-A: Observing Attending Behavior of Others

Work in pairs for this activity.

1. Both partners observe a 15-minute segment of the same televised interview show, either alone or together. Independently, write down the specific attending behaviors used by both the interviewer and the person being interviewed, as well as the nonverbal messages being communicated through these behaviors. Note which verbal and nonverbal attending behaviors you consider to be productive and which you consider to be nonproductive.
2. Discuss and compare your observations with your partner.

☐ EXECUTION

To use productive attending behavior within a helping relationship requires that, as helpers, we are able to (1) observe our own verbal and nonverbal behavior, (2) observe others' responses to our behavior, (3) observe others' verbal and nonverbal behavior, (4) have an open, accepting attitude toward others.

Productive attending behavior focuses on the client and involves a basic attitude of acceptance and an understanding of the client's self and circumstances as they are, not necessarily as they ought to be. This requires that, as much as possible, the helper sets aside value judgments and makes a deliberate, conscious effort to avoid evaluating the client's words and actions.

We can expand our ability to use productive attending behavior by observing how others attend to us when we talk to them and noting which behaviors help us to feel heard and understood. It is helpful to be aware of the attending behaviors we usually use and to ask for feedback about them from someone we trust. We then can decide what modifications would be most beneficial to our interpersonal relationships.

The following activities focus on observing and experiencing productive and counterproductive attending behaviors and the messages they communicate.

Activity 9-B: Simulations of Attending Behavior

In a group setting, observe simulated live or videotaped examples first of counterproductive behavior and then of productive behavior. Discuss the simulations among yourselves, focusing on these questions: What specific nonverbal and verbal attending behaviors cause the examples to be either counterproductive or productive? What behavioral responses and feelings are communicated by the person who is being attended to in counterproductive and productive ways? What feelings did you experience as you observed the two kinds of attending behavior?

Activity 9-C: Experiencing and Using Attending Behavior

Work in groups of three, with two partners and one observer. A video camera may be used to supplement the observer. Use the Performance Checklist, p. 74, to evaluate productive attending behavior.

1. *Counterproductive attending behavior*
   a. Partner A: Talk to partner B for 3 minutes on a recent event or a topic of interest to you.
   b. Partner B: Use counterproductive attending behavior as you listen to partner A.
   c. Observer: Write down the specific attending behaviors used by both partners and the feelings communicated.
   d. Observer and partner A: Give feedback to partner B about his or her attending behavior. Review the videotape if available.
   e. Exchange roles and repeat the exercise until each person has assumed each role.
2. *Productive attending behavior*
   a. Partner A: Talk to partner B for 3 minutes on a recent event or a topic of interest to you.
   b. Partner B: Use productive attending behavior in a way that is natural for you.
   c. Observer: Write down the specific attending behaviors used by both partners and the feelings communicated.
   d. Evaluate partner B's attending skills by using the Performance Checklist, p. 74, the observer's notes, and the videotape if available.
   e. Exchange roles and repeat the exercise until each person has assumed each role.

3. Discuss the experience of using and receiving both nonproductive and productive attending behaviors. In your discussion, focus on what you observed or experienced that would cause you to value either productive or nonproductive attending behavior. What aspects of attending behavior would you want to avoid in your interpersonal interactions?

BEFORE THE NEXT SKILL

Before progressing to the next skill, spend some time observing the attending behavior of others, because this will help to increase your awareness of the role that attending behavior plays in interpersonal interactions. At a distance that precludes eavesdropping, observe at least three interactions between persons in a public setting. Use the Performance Checklist, p. 74, as a guide for your observations. Make a list of each person's specific use of posture, gestures, eye contact, and verbal encouragement. Identify the nonverbal feelings or messages each person is communicating through his or her attending behavior, and rate that behavior in general as excellent, fair, or poor.

After you have finished these observations, observe at least three interactions between persons you know well enough to listen to without being intrusive, such as persons in your dormitory, classroom, or home. Again, make a list of each person's specific use of posture, gestures, eye contact, and verbal encouragement. Identify the nonverbal feelings or messages each person is communicating through his or her attending behavior, and rate that behavior in general as excellent, fair, or poor.

☐ CRITICAL POINTS SUMMARY

1. Productive attending behavior communicates interest, caring, respect, and acceptance, and encourages client expression.
2. Productive attending posture is alert, comfortable, and relaxed.
3. Relaxed attending gestures are open and receptive.
4. Spontaneous and fairly steady eye contact conveys interest and attentiveness.
5. Verbal encouragement through use of minimal but purposeful responses allows the client to be the focus of the interaction.

☐ REVIEW QUESTIONS

1. What purposes does productive attending behavior serve in the helping relationship?
2. How does the ability to accept the client affect the helper's use of productive attending behavior?
3. What type of attending posture tends to result in productive and counterproductive behaviors?

4. How are gestures used in productive and counter-productive behaviors?
5. What kind of eye contact constitutes productive attending behaviors? counterproductive?
6. What is meant by minimal but purposeful verbal encouragement?
7. Give examples of ways that minimal verbal encouragement can be used in nurse–client interactions.

☐ PERFORMANCE CHECKLIST

OBJECTIVE: To demonstrate the ability to communicate productive attending behavior.

EVALUATION OF SELF[a]		BEHAVIORS	EVALUATION BY PARTNER B[a]		EVALUATION BY OBSERVER[a]	
S	U		S	U	S	U
		1. Uses alert, attentive body posture.				
		2. Faces the speaker.				
		3. Uses fairly steady, spontaneous eye contact.				
		4. Uses head nods appropriately.				
		5. Uses relaxed, appropriate gestures.				
		6. Uses nondirective minimal verbal encouragement (give examples).				
		7. Uses directive minimal responses (give examples).				
		8. Communicates acceptance verbally and nonverbally.				
		9. Needs strengthening in certain areas (specify).				

[a] S = Satisfactory; U = Unsatisfactory.

REFERENCES

Brammer LM: The Helping Relationship: Process and Skills, ed 2. Englewood Cliffs, NJ, Prentice-Hall, 1979.
Hall ET: The Hidden Dimension. Garden City, NY, Doubleday, 1966.
Ivey AE: Microcounseling: Innovations in Interview Training. Springfield, IL, Charles C Thomas, 1971.
Ivey AE: Microcounseling: Interviewing Skills Manual, ed 2. Springfield, IL, Charles C Thomas, 1977.
McHugh C: The Helping Relationship. Springfield, IL, Lincolnland Community College, 1978 (course handouts, mimeo).
Morain GG: Kinesics and Cross-Cultural Understanding, ERIC Document Reproductive Service No. 7. Arlington, VA, Center for Applied Linguistics, 1978.

BIBLIOGRAPHY

Anthony WA, Carkhuff RR: The Art of Health Care: A Handbook of Psychological First Aid Skills. Amherst, MA, Human Resource Development Press, 1976.
Carkhuff RR: Helping and Human Relations: A Primer for Lay and Professional Helpers, 2 vols. New York, Holt, Rinehart, & Winston, 1969.
Gerrard BA, Boniface WJ, Love BH: Interpersonal Skills for Health Professionals. Reston, VA, Reston, 1980.

SKILL 10 Attentive Listening

And in the naked light I saw ten thousand people, maybe more. People talking without speaking, people hearing without listening ...
—Paul Simon, 1964

☐ STUDENT OBJECTIVES

1. Distinguish between hearing and listening.
2. Describe therapeutic functions of active listening.
3. Identify factors that interfere with listening.
4. Compare effective and ineffective listening habits.
5. Describe attitudinal characteristics of a good listener.
6. Describe ways of becoming a more active listener.
7. Identify your own listening habits.

☐ INTRODUCTION

Listening is defined by Webster (1976) as applying oneself to hearing something, or paying attention.

Hearing is simply becoming aware of sounds, which happens automatically when sound waves stimulate functional auditory nerves. Hearing is a passive act; listening is an active process requiring attention and participation.

The purpose of listening is to receive and understand messages from another person. Listening is regarded by some as the most effective therapeutic communication tool available. Hollis states:

When a person knows that he has a good listener to talk to, he'll share his thoughts more fully, which in turn, makes it easier . . . to help him with his problems. And, moreover, as he talks, the person needing help often finds a good solution to his problem himself. (Borman et al., 1969, p. 178)

Illness, loss, and personal problems tend to make us more self-focused and ready to talk to someone who is willing to listen. Therefore, in a helping relationship, listening often is more important than talking. Listening to clients helps them to verbalize their feelings and experiences as they attempt to cope with many of the difficult events happening to them, such as pain, loss of function, or impending death.

It is through listening that the helper can gain information about the client and become aware of client needs. The information the nurse gains about the client's physical, emotional, spiritual, and social status is important for the following reasons:

1. Information from the client is a crucial aspect of the data base needed for appropriate problem identification and effective planning and intervention.
2. Teaching and information-giving are effective when related to what the client already knows.
3. The client's present status is the starting point for personal growth.

It is possible to intervene, teach, and promote growth appropriately only when the nurse has listened with enough comprehension to know what that individual client needs and can use.

☐ *PREPARATION*

Listening is closely allied with attending behavior in that productive attending behavior accompanies active listening, and counterproductive attending behavior accompanies ineffective listening.

EFFECTIVE LISTENING BEHAVIOR

An effective helper is an effective listener. The client has the right and the need to be listened to in a competent manner, and active listening on the part of the helper conveys respect and caring for that client and his or her concerns. Active listening involves careful observation of the person who is speaking. It is an active mental process of hearing words and silences and perceiving their meanings. Active listening requires thought about the other person's message, method of presentation, and intent, as well as comprehension of the message itself. "Comprehension involves the attempt to understand and grasp the true idea or meaning of what is heard" (Lewis, 1973, p. 37). Comprehension is crucial in the helping relationship because the helper must be certain that his or her perception of the client's message is accurate. The helper can validate those perceptions through "Reflection of Content" (Skill 11), "Reflection of Feelings" (Skill 12), and "Understanding Nonverbal Behavior" (Skill 6).

Active listening also includes some *response* by the helper to the message heard. This verbal or nonverbal response may include validation of what was heard, encouragement to continue, or an attempt to clarify what was heard.

An active listener *attends* to what is said and what is not said through both verbal and nonverbal communication. Many times the most vital concerns are expressed indirectly and subtly, in an offhand manner or a soft voice—and can be missed by an inattentive listener. However, an effective listener knows to listen for these cues.

Listening for *key words or themes* in the conversation helps in understanding the client's message, because often the client will repeat what is important to him or her. The helper may hear specific words, phrases, or names that come up with regularity during a conversation. These words may describe feelings such as hopefulness or anger; symptoms such as pain or constipation; or the names or titles of persons who currently are important, such as a spouse, child, parent, friend, or physician. Conversation may also be characterized by recurrent themes such as those described by Hein (1980): self-effacement, "me-focus," loss, loneliness, wellness, poverty, and humor.

In addition to listening for the primary verbal message being communicated, the effective helper also listens to what Hein describes as "underlying secondary information transmitted through the feelings the patient experiences at the time" (1980, p. 232). These *secondary messages,* called feeling tones, can assist the helper in identifying emotional states the client may be experiencing, such as anger, fear, happiness, satisfaction, or sadness. It also is helpful to note whether the feeling tones are congruent with the client's primary verbal message. All of this information can be validated with the client in the same ways that meaning is validated.

The importance of *silence* in listening may seem obvious but cannot be overestimated. Barbara (1958) indicates that an effective listener is one who *uses* silence with as much eagerness as talking. In the helping relationship, silence provides time for the listener to hear and consider the meaning and verbal–nonverbal congruence of the client's message, to note mentally any repeated themes or unspoken messages, and to think about how to respond to the client's message. For the client, silence provides time for organizing thoughts and ideas, identifying feelings, and observing the helper's response to his or her comments. Comfort level with silence varies with the individual; some nurses as well as some clients are uncomfortable with silence.

The following activities focus on developing an increased sensitivity to what is heard and understood.

Activity 10-A:
Learning to Listen

Work in groups of three or four.

1. Close your eyes and sit or stand quietly for several minutes. Listen to all of the different sounds you can hear.
2. Open your eyes and write down all of the sounds you can remember.
3. Compare your list of sounds with the lists of other persons in your group. How many were alike? How many different sounds were heard by only one person? Did anyone have different names for the same sounds?

Activity 10-B:
Listening for Meaning

Work in pairs or small groups.

1. Watch a television commercial with your partner or group.
   a. Summarize in writing the message you receive from this commercial and then compare summaries. You may find that you hear very different messages!
   b. Repeat this exercise with four or five more commercials until it becomes relatively easy to identify messages.
2. Watch a segment of the evening news with your partner or group.
   a. Summarize its content in writing and then compare summaries.
   b. Repeat this exercise with several more news segments until it becomes relatively easy to summarize complex messages.

INEFFECTIVE LISTENING BEHAVIOR

While attentive listening is therapeutic, *poor listening* is a barrier to effective communication and helping because it conveys disinterest, boredom, haste, or self-centeredness. Many people are not good listeners, for a variety of reasons. *A physiological reason* is that humans have the capacity to hear and understand at a rate much faster than they can talk. Most people can speak at a rate of about 125 words per minute but can think and comprehend about four times that fast. "It is what we do with this extra time that makes us either good or poor listeners" (Barbara, 1958, p. 4).

There are also *physical characteristics* that make it more difficult to be an effective listener. Some people have a hearing loss without knowing it, especially with increasing age. Health problems can be a deterrent to good listening; when a person is tired, in pain, or worried, it is difficult for him or her to pay full attention to what someone else is saying. This undoubtedly applies to clients as well as helpers, and may be the reason why clients do not hear all that nurses tell them.

Personal factors may interfere with the ability to listen. Crisis events such as placing a parent in a nursing home, breaking up a significant relationship, or a child having an automobile accident can distract a person's thoughts and divert energies from active listening. Arguments with co-workers or family members or being reprimanded by a supervisor or parent can produce guilt or anger, which takes the focus of the helper's attention away from what the client is saying. The frustration of having too heavy a work load or having work assigned inequitably can make it difficult to take time and energy to listen.

Distracting behaviors on the part of the helper convey the impression of being a poor listener and thus interfere with the client's perception of being listened to. When the helper doodles, twists a pen or ring, or looks out the window or at his or her fingers or shoes, he or she appears to be preoccupied mentally with something other than what the client is saying.

Environmental factors contribute to poor listening. Excessive noise levels, uncomfortably high or low temperatures, inadequate ventilation, or a room design that allows for no privacy interfere with the ability to listen.

Listening habits also affect a person's ability to listen attentively. Kron (1972) describes four poor listening habits that detract from a person's ability to listen: failure to concentrate, selective inattention, self-interest, and prejudice. *Failure to concentrate* can result from the listener's failure to expend sufficient mental effort. It is common not to concentrate as a parent, supervisor, or nurse gives a standard pep talk or uses familiar clichés. It also is possible to be preoccupied with one's next task, tomorrow's test, or tonight's date and only listen superficially. *Selective inattention* refers to the ability to hear only part of a message and then stop listening. This often occurs when the listener expects certain responses, has predetermined ideas about what information is important, or wants to avoid hearing something that is uncomfortable or unfamiliar or difficult to cope with readily. Some people are more *interested in themselves* than in other people and always are ready to break into a conversation at the slightest evidence of a pause. Or they may interrupt with statements such as, "That reminds me of when I. . . ." *Prejudices* also can cause people to listen poorly. When a person uses words or expressions that are not acceptable to the listener's beliefs and values, it is common for the listener to stop listening and either discount what the speaker is saying or gather mental arguments to refute the speaker's position. Sometimes a listener discounts what is being said simply because of who the other person is or because of previous experiences with that person.

Sometimes people give the appearance of listening when they really are not. They may appear interested, nod, smile, and even occasionally answer, yet be thinking of something entirely different and ignoring what the other person is saying. Adler and Towne (1981) describe this kind of behavior as "pseudolistening" and regard it as counterfeit communication.

☐ EXECUTION

To be an effective listener in a helping relationship requires that helpers have (1) a sincere interest in other people, (2) a real desire to hear what the other person has to say, (3) a belief that what the other person has to say is important, (4) a genuine acceptance of the other person's feelings and concerns, (5) a feeling of trust in the other person's capacity to explore and help resolve his or her own circumstances.

Helpful active listening is oriented toward the other person and includes using productive attending behaviors to convey that concern for the other person. This means that the helper faces the client and leans forward slightly, uses appropriate gestures, maintains spontaneous and fairly direct eye contact, and uses minimal verbal encouragement. All of these actions help the client know that the helper is listening as well as hearing.

The ability to listen effectively can be enhanced by becoming aware of your own listening habits and by practicing being a good listener. Observe yourself while listening to someone. Are you a doodler? Do you find that your mind often wanders and that you often have to ask people to repeat what they have said? Do you argue mentally with or criticize the speaker, frequently interrupt, or finish sentences and supply words during pauses? Consider whether you tend to feel that people are not very interesting or that what they say is unimportant (Kron, 1972). Since it is difficult to be objective about oneself, you will find it helpful to ask these same questions of someone who knows you fairly well. This person could also give you feedback about whether you look interested when someone is talking to you, and whether you tend to hear all or part of what people say to you. After you have examined your listening habits, decide what modifications would be most beneficial to your personal and professional interpersonal relationships. As you practice being a good listener, you will find that it is helpful to stop talking and avoid interrupting, to listen with all your senses to verbal and nonverbal messages, and to concentrate on what is being said. The following activities focus on using effective and ineffective listening skills in simulated settings.

Activity 10-C:
Simulations of Listening Behavior

In a group setting, observe simulated live or videotaped examples first of ineffective listening behavior and then of effective listening behaviors. Discuss the simulation among yourselves, considering these questions: What specific behaviors cause the examples to be ineffective or effective? What effects do the two kinds of listening have on the person doing the talking? Describe your reactions as you watch someone being listened to in ineffective and effective ways.

Activity 10-D:
Experiencing and Using Listening Behavior

Work in groups of three, with two partners and one observer. A video camera may be used to supplement the observer. Use the Performance Checklist, p. 78, to evaluate the high-level listening behaviors.

1. *Ineffective listening behavior*
   a. Partner A: Talk to partner B for 3 to 5 minutes on a subject or event that is interesting or important to you.
   b. Partner B: Respond to partner A with very ineffective listening skills, poor listening habits, etc.
   c. Observer: Note in writing the negative listening behaviors used by partner B as well as partner A's reactions.
   d. Observer and partner A: Give feedback to partner B about his or her listening behaviors. Review the videotape, if available.
   e. Exchange roles and repeat the exercise until each person has assumed each role.
2. *Effective listening behavior*
   a. Partner A: Talk to partner B for 3 to 5 minutes on a subject or event that is interesting or important to you.
   b. Partner B: Use effective listening skills in a way that is natural for you.
   c. Observer: Note in writing the specific listening skills used and the feelings communicated by both partners.
   d. Evaluate partner B's listening skills by using the Performance Checklist, p. 78, the observer's notes, and the videotape if available.
   e. Exchange roles and repeat the exercise until each person has assumed each role.
3. Discuss the experience of listening and being listened to in both ineffective and effective ways. In your discussion, focus on which way you would prefer to be listened to, and for what reasons. What listening behaviors did you find gave you negative reactions?

BEFORE THE NEXT SKILL

Before progressing to the next skill, spend some time identifying effective and ineffective listening behaviors in others. At a distance that precludes eavesdropping, observe people talking to each other in three situations, such as at a party, restaurant, or lounge. Use the Performance Checklist, p. 78, as a guide for your observations. Make a list of each person's use of effective and ineffective listening behaviors. What environmental and physical factors contributed to the two kinds of listening? What percentage of the persons you observed practiced effective listening behaviors? In casual conversations with others, try to observe yourself for effective and ineffective listening behaviors.

Other helpful activities that can increase your listening abilities are to contract with a friend to give each other feedback about listening behavior and to continue the practice of mentally summarizing the content of news broadcasts, lectures, and conversations.

CRITICAL POINTS SUMMARY

1. Active listening is receiving and understanding the obvious and hidden meanings of messages from another person.
2. Active listening is therapeutic in itself.
3. Ill persons generally have an increased need to talk about themselves and to have someone listen to them.
4. Active listening is necessary for the development and maintenance of a helping relationship.
5. Active listening is needed to gather relevant data and to plan nursing care.
6. Listening behavior communicates the helper's feelings about the client to that individual.

REVIEW QUESTIONS

1. How is listening different from hearing?
2. Why does a nurse need to be able to listen actively and effectively?
3. How is listening therapeutic in itself?
4. How does active listening promote the development and maintenance of a helping relationship?
5. What factors contribute to ineffective listening? How does each of these factors affect the quality of listening?
6. How do a helper's mental attitudes affect listening?
7. What specific things can you do to improve your ability to listen?

PERFORMANCE CHECKLIST

OBJECTIVE: To demonstrate the ability to listen attentively.

EVALUATION OF SELF[a]		BEHAVIORS	EVALUATION BY PARTNER B[a]		EVALUATION BY OBSERVER[a]	
S	U		S	U	S	U
		1. Listens more than talks.				
		2. Appears to be concentrating on speaker.				
		3. Responds appropriately to both feelings and content.				
		4. Uses productive attending behaviors: 　Posture 　Gestures 　Eye contact 　Verbal encouragement				
		5. Uses other effective listening behaviors (give examples).				
		6. Avoids ineffective listening habits: 　Distracting behaviors (specify) 　Lack of concentration 　Inattention 　Disinterest 　Others (be specific)				
		7. Communicates interest and acceptance nonverbally.				
		8. Needs strengthening in certain areas (specify).				

[a] S = Satisfactory; U = Unsatisfactory.

REFERENCES

Adler RB, Towne N: Looking Out—Looking In, ed 3. New York, Holt, Rinehart, & Winston, 1981.

Barbara DA: The Art of Listening. Springfield, IL, Charles C Thomas, 1958.

Borman EG, Howell WS, et al: Interpersonal Communication in the Modern Organization. Englewood Cliffs, NJ, Prentice-Hall, 1969.

Hein EC: Communication in Nursing Practice, ed 2. Boston, Little, Brown, 1980.

Kron T: Communication in Nursing, ed 2. Philadelphia, WB Saunders, 1972.

Lewis GK: Nurse–Patient Communication. Dubuque, IA, WC Brown, 1973.

Simon P: The Sounds of Silence. NY, Paul Simon, 1964, 1965.

Webster GC: Third New International Dictionary, Unabridged. Springfield, MA, G & C Merriam, 1976.

BIBLIOGRAPHY

Bernstein L, Bernstein RS, Dana RH: Interviewing: A Guide for Health Professionals, ed 3. New York, Appleton-Century-Crofts, 1980.

Brammer LM: The Helping Relationship, ed 2. Englewood Cliffs, NJ, Prentice-Hall, 1979.

Egan G: The Skilled Helper: A Model for Systematic Helping and Interpersonal Relating. Monterey, CA, Brooks/Cole, 1975.

Freund H: Listening with any ear at all. American Journal of Nursing 69(8):1949–1953, 1969.

Johnson DW: Reaching Out: Interpersonal Effectiveness and Self-Actualization. Englewood Cliffs, NJ, Prentice-Hall, 1972.

Perlman HH (ed): Helping: Charlotte Towle on Social Work and Social Casework. Chicago, University of Chicago Press, 1969.

Raudsepp E: 7 ways to cure communication breakdowns. NursingLife 4(1):51–53, 1984.

Sundeen SJ, Stuart GW, et al: Nurse–Client Interaction: Implementing the Nursing Process. St Louis, MO, CV Mosby, 1981.

Travelbee J: Interpersonal Aspects of Nursing. Philadelphia, FA Davis, 1971.

SKILL 11 Reflection of Content

I know you believe that you understand what you think I said, but I am not sure you realize that what you heard is not what I meant.
—*Anonymous*

☐ STUDENT OBJECTIVES

1. Describe the purpose, uses, and misuses of reflection of content.
2. Describe the relationship of effective reflection of content to attentive listening and productive attending behaviors.
3. Discuss the significance of accurate reflection of content in a helping relationship.
4. Reflect the content of statements back to the speaker accurately.
5. Recognize when your own and others' statements have been reflected accurately.
6. Use content reflecting skills consistently in interpersonal interactions.

☐ INTRODUCTION

Reflection of content is the listener's restatement of another person's message as the listener understands it. Sometimes called paraphrasing, it is a reflection of the main thought, idea, or meaning of the speaker's message and grows out of that message. Sometimes the listener might use the same words as the speaker (verbatim reflection); usually the listener's reflection is a shorter and more concise distillation of the speaker's message.

A major function of reflection of content is to validate and clarify information being given and messages being exchanged. Reflection of content helps both parties understand each other and minimizes the potential for incorrect assumptions and misunderstandings in any relationship. When people fail to validate or clarify, they risk making inappropriate recommendations or decisions on the basis of incorrect assumptions.

Validating the meaning of clients' messages through reflection of content helps the nurse provide quality nursing care. When clients' messages are not understood or are interpreted incorrectly, it is possible that data gathering will be incomplete or inaccurate and that inappropriate plans will be made and implemented. In one medical study project involving the application of interview techniques in a pediatric setting, it was found that the amount and scope of data gathered was increased when physicians indicated verbally that they understood what the mother was communicating. This validation also resulted in greater cooperation with the treatment regime and more satisfying professional–patient relationships (Korsch, 1956).

A nursing research study by Bochnak et al. (1962) found that when nurses did not explore and validate the meaning of clients' complaints of pain, they made hasty, inaccurate judgments and often gave unnecessary medications. It is not uncommon for a hospitalized client to ask for sleeping medication when pain is keeping him or her awake. Usually, however, the sedative will neither ease the pain nor produce sleep when pain is present. The nurse who has not validated the client's message verbally may give a noneffective or unnecessary medication.

In human communications, content and feelings cannot be separated; in this text they are presented separately for learning purposes. This skill focuses on reflecting the meaning of the content, while Skill 12 focuses on reflecting the feeling (affective) component of an interaction.

☐ PREPARATION

Content reflection or paraphrasing seems simple and has powerful effects, but it often is very difficult to put into practice. Most people entering a helping profession have little or no experience in using content reflection and may have difficulty seeing its significance (D'Augelli et al., 1980; Johnson, 1972).

All individuals see themselves as the center of their own universe and as the frame of reference from which everything is observed and comprehended. According to Combs et al. (1971), many of us assume that others' perceptions are the same as our own and that people with different perceptions are stupid, stubborn, or prejudiced. We also assume that what we *understand* from a statement is what the other person intended. It is an interesting paradox that most of us expect to validate a name or phone number given to us verbally, but assume that we understand more complex communications and therefore will agree or disagree with the speaker without validation!

EFFECTIVE REFLECTION OF CONTENT

In their psychological studies, Truax and Carkhuff (1967) have gathered considerable evidence to indicate that a sensitive understanding of the client and his or her situation is an essential characteristic of therapeutic counseling. Reflection of content is one way the helper can validate that understanding with the client. A helper who does not understand correctly what the client is telling or asking may fail to reach out in a caring way to someone in need. According to Johnson,

If you paraphase a message, that act tends to reduce the sender's fears about revealing himself to you and decreases the sender's defensiveness about what he is communicating. It facilitates psychological health and growth. (1972, p. 75)

In the helping relationship, reflection of content serves a number of purposes. As an *empathic response,* reflection of content lets the client know that he or she is being listened to. It conveys the message that the helper is a caring person who respects the client, is interested in the client, and is attempting to understand what the client is saying. Being misunderstood is a frustrating experience that tends to lower a person's sense of self-worth. *Validating* the helper's perception of the client's message is useful when that message is unclear to the helper or seems to have double meanings. It also is useful when the helper believes a client may be unclear about the meaning of his or her own message. People usually understand their own ideas, circumstances, or values more clearly when they hear them reflected or restated by someone else. In addition, reflection of content can give the helper *time to think* about the client's message before exploring it further; or the helper may use reflection of content to help the client expand on what he or she is talking about.

Since reflection of content helps us to understand what someone else is saying, it also is a useful tool in conflict situations and negotiations. In *conflict situations* it can help avoid the assumptions and misunderstandings that escalate conflict. In *negotiations,* where it is crucial that both sides understand what the other is saying, it helps clarify the positions of the involved parties and promotes settlement of issues.

The tone of voice and nonverbal manner used when reflecting content should convey interest and should be fairly neutral or in harmony with the original message. It is important to avoid conveying approval, disapproval, or blame through voice and manner, as this affects the meaning of the restatement.

The following are some suggested initial phrases that are useful when the listener believes that his or her perceptions of the speaker's message are accurate, and that the speaker will be receptive to the listener's response:

- "From your point of view . . ."
- "As you see it . . ."
- "It seems to you that . . ."
- "What I hear you saying . . ."
- "You believe . . ."
- "In other words . . ."
- "If I understand you correctly . . ."
- "It seems to me that . . ."

These additional phrases are useful when the listener is unsure of his or her perceptions of the speaker's message or believes that the speaker might not be very receptive to the listener's response:

- "I'm not sure if I'm with you, but . . ."
- "Correct me if I'm wrong, but . . ."
- "This is what I think I hear you saying . . ."
- "As I hear it, you . . ."
- ". . . Is that what you mean? . . . Is that the way it is?"
- "Let me see if I understand; you . . ."

Examples of Effective Reflection of Content

Client: "The days get awfully long here with nothing to do. I've been here ever since I broke my hip a month ago. My family is from Georgetown, over 100 miles away, so they don't get over here very often. I don't get much other company, either."

Helper's response: "In other words, you're quite alone here in the big city."

Client: "Yes, I really am. The nurses are real nice, but..."

Speaker: "I could just die! You know that neat guy in Soc. class? Well, he's asked me for a date Saturday night! And guess what! I already had a date with that creep from downstairs! Guess that's just too bad for him!"

Listener's response: "I'm not sure I understand; are you telling me you just accepted a second date for Saturday night?"

Speaker: "Well, yes and no. Since I really don't care for that other guy, it wasn't really a date—just going out somewhere."

The following activity focuses on accurate reflection of the content and meaning contained in structured situations.

Activity 11-A: Reflecting Content Statements

Work in groups of three. A video camera may be used to provide additional feedback.

1. *Reflecting prepared statements*
   a. Read the following statements individually. Restate the *content* in writing, each person using his or her own words. Be concise and specific.
      (1) "Did you count the pages we have to read for next week? And all for one class! They must think their class is the only one we have to study for!"
      (2) "I don't know how I'm going to tell my parents. They'll really be disappointed with me! I just can't have an abortion—and I'm sure not ready to get married yet! What'll I say to them?"
      (3) "If they would just bring me my briefcase so I could finish that project, then I'd relax! How am I supposed to 'take it easy' when things have to get done and there is no one else to do them? 'Just lie quietly and rest!' That's like telling the wind to stop blowing!"
   b. Compare your written statements with those of the other persons in your group to validate the accuracy of your responses.
2. *Making relevant responses*
   Designate one person as partner A, one as partner B, and one as observer.
   a. Partner A: Make a statement to partner B about yourself, about partner B, or about something meaningful to both of you. Avoid bland, trite, or meaningless statements.
   b. Partner B: Reflect the content of the statement to partner A.
   c. Partner A and observer: Validate the accuracy of the reflected message.
   d. Repeat the exercise using a different statement from partner A.
   e. Exchange roles and repeat the exercise until each person has assumed each role.
3. *Negotiating for meaning*
   Use the same partners as in the previous exercise.
   a. Partner A: Make a more detailed statement about yourself, about partner B, or about something meaningful to both of you, as in number 2a of this activity.
   b. Partner B: Respond to partner A, beginning with "What I think you mean is..."
   c. Partners A and B: Negotiate and restate the original message and content until partner A is able to say, "Yes, that is exactly what I mean."
   d. Observer: Follow this negotiation and confirm that agreement has been reached.
   e. Exchange roles and repeat the exercise until each person has assumed each role.
4. After completing these exercises, ask yourselves the following questions:
   a. How accurately was the content reflected by yourself and by others?
   b. What problems in reflection of content were noted?

INEFFECTIVE REFLECTION OF CONTENT

Since accurate reflection of content is dependent on attentive listening, people with ineffective or inadequate listening skills have difficulty reflecting the content of messages. They may not even hear what is being said to them and may therefore make no response. In a nurse–client situation, this nonresponse leaves the client in limbo, not knowing if the nurse simply did not hear or is choosing not to respond.

Some approaches to reflection of content are nonhelpful in the nurse–client relationship because they make it difficult for the client to continue telling his or her story and cause the client to feel devalued. A listener may *respond to one part of what is being said* and thereby change the discussion to something more interesting to himself or herself. Johnson (1972) refers to this as an asyndetic response, and calls it a polite way to introduce one's own ideas into the conversation.

Sometimes beginning helpers try to *reflect too much content* at one time, and this tends to become cumbersome and sound artificial. Or, they may pay attention to details and miss the main message. Using *verbatim reflection* or simply *rearranging words* can be helpful when employed selectively or for special emphasis; but when it is overused or is the only approach a listener uses, it tends to sound like mimicking, and both listener and speaker feel uncomfortable. Other problems with reflection of content occur when the listener either does not hear all that was said and *omits important aspects*, or when the listener *adds content* to the original message. Both of these approaches tend to cause the speaker to feel as if the listener is not paying careful attention and is making an interpretation of the message that is different from what the speaker intended.

The nonverbal manner in which content is reflected can change the meaning of the response. Instead of being simply reflection of content, nonverbal behavior can *evaluate* that content. Johnson (1972) indicates that giving evaluative responses is a common tendency in all conversations. Especially when deep feelings and emotions are involved, the two parties tend to evaluate each other's statements from their own points of view. This evaluation may be verbal, such as "I think you're wrong (or right) when you say . . ."; or the evaluation may be internal and mental. For the most part, approval and disapproval can be conveyed nonverbally as clearly as verbally, and disapproval tends to alienate the speaker from the listener. As Combs et al. indicate, the "beliefs of helpers are conveyed to clients despite the words they use" (1971, p. 252).

A limitation to the usefulness of reflection of content is that it can easily be overdone. In either casual conversation or nurse–client interaction, communications can be slow and frustrating if everything must be restated and validated before a response can be made. A constant replay of messages is distracting and can interfere with communication rather than facilitate it.

Examples of Ineffective Reflection of Content
A 12-year-old girl is being interviewed during her first visit to a family planning clinic.

Client: "My best friends are taking pills because their mothers don't want them to have a baby. They told me I should get some pills here like they did."

Helper's response: "You are too young to be having sex and taking birth control pills."

Client: "I'm the same age as my friends and they got pills here."

Speaker: "Do I need to get a signed permission from each child's parents in addition to the director of day care before I can test hearing at the day care center?"

Listener's response: "The director at the day care center really likes to work with student nurses and have them test hearing; she'll give her permission. Last year some students tested all of the children and found two cases of significant hearing loss. The day care teacher had suspected that those children had hearing problems because they did not respond normally and had impaired speech. The students really had a great time and enjoyed working with the children."

The following activity focuses on accurate reflection of content through the contrast of ineffective reflection of content.

Activity 11–B: Ineffective Reflection of Content

Work in groups of three or four, using an audio recorder or video camera if available.

1. *Ignoring messages and giving irrelevant responses*
    a. Within the group, talk with each other for 5 minutes about an agreed-upon topic of interest or concern to the group, such as classes, professors, clinical experiences, or communications exercises. All comments must be about the agreed-upon topic, but no one should respond directly to someone else's comments. Rather, responses should be characterized by using silence or avoidance (ignoring) or by being irrelevant in nature. Each person should both make and respond to statements.
2. *Changing the subject*
    a. Talk with each other for 5 minutes, beginning with a topic such as suggested in number 1 of this activity. Listen to what each of the others says, but only as a springboard for changing the subject to one you prefer. The other persons' messages must be partially acknowledged, but only as a polite means of introducing your own ideas. Each person should both make and respond to statements.
3. Discuss your experience with each other and listen to the audiotape or view the videotape if available. What was your reaction to having others ignore your comments, respond in an irrelevant manner, or change the subject to their own ideas? What was your reaction to doing those things to others?

☐ EXECUTION

To reflect content in an accurate and appropriate manner requires that the helper possess the ability to (1) understand and speak the client's language, (2) attend to the client's message, (3) listen attentively, and (4) use an adequate vocabulary to restate messages.

The process of reflection of content begins with attentive listening to the themes and ideas being conveyed by the client. The helper mentally processes the message and restates the message as he or she hears it.

After this response is made, the helper observes for responses or cues from the client that confirm or deny the accuracy of the reflection of content, such as nonverbal facial expressions and gestures and verbal comments. If no response is heard or observed, the helper may want to ask for validation. It is sometimes helpful to validate verbally one's interpretation of nonverbal cues, especially if the cues lend noncongruence to the client's message. The following situation illustrates validation of response to content reflection: A 28-year-old mother of three children had just finished describing to Sally Jackson, a home-care nurse, a difficult family situation involving physical abuse. Sally reflected what she heard: "As I understand it, your husband has struck you before—about twice a month for several years." The mother was silent and expressionless. After a few moments of silence, Sally asked gently, "That is what I heard you saying, is it not?" The mother glanced quickly at Sally and nodded only slightly. Another woman might have burst into tears and nodded affirmatively in response to Sally's first comment. With either response, Sally's reflection has been validated as correct.

There are endless ways to paraphrase or reflect content. Each person and each exchange are unique, and require individualized responses. When learning to reflect content, it is helpful to begin with ways that feel natural and then experiment with others. Using only a few standard cliché phrases is limiting, stilted, and can convey uninterest in the other person. The ability to reflect content can be expanded through increasing listening and attending skills, observing others' ability to reflect content, and consciously practicing accurate reflection of content in social and professional situations.

The following activities focus on observing and experiencing effective and ineffective reflection of content and the messages those behaviors communicate.

Activity 11-C: Simulations of Reflection of Content

In a group setting, observe simulated live or videotaped examples first of ineffective reflection of content and then of effective reflection of content.

As you discuss the simulations, identify the specific characteristics that cause the examples to be ineffective or effective. In what ways do you react differently to the two ways of reflecting the content of what someone says? What feelings were communicated by the persons involved in the simulations?

Activity 11-D: Experiencing and Using Reflection of Content

Work in groups of three with two partners and one observer. Use an audio tape recorder or video camera if available.

1. *Ineffective reflection of content*
   a. Partner A: Talk to partner B for 3 to 5 minutes on a subject of interest to you.
   b. Partner B: Respond to partner A with a variety of very ineffective content reflection behaviors.
   c. Observer: Note in writing the specific negative and ineffective reflecting behaviors used by partner B, as well as partner A's reactions to partner B's responses.
   d. Observer and partner A: Give feedback to partner B about the kinds of negative reflecting behaviors observed. View the videotape if available.
   e. Exchange roles and repeat the exercise until each person has assumed each role.
2. *Effective reflection of content*
   Each person chooses a subject he or she feels strongly about, such as nuclear power, euthanasia, or abortion.
   a. Partner A: Comment on your chosen subject.
   b. Partner B: *Before* responding with your own views, you *must* restate the content of partner A's comments to the satisfaction of both partner A and the observer. Use effective methods of reflection of content, and continue this exchange for 5 minutes.
   c. Complete the Performance Checklist, p. 84. Give feedback to partner B about the reflecting behaviors you observed. Review any available audiotapes or videotapes.
   d. Exchange roles and repeat the exercise until each person has assumed each role.
3. Discuss the experiences of reflecting someone else's messages and of having your own messages reflected in both effective and ineffective ways. In your discussion, focus on (1) whether content was accurately reflected, (2) which approaches to reflection of content have the most positive effect on the speaker (and for what reasons), and (3) which approaches have negative effects (and for what reasons). What approaches do you believe you will find personally helpful in interacting with others?

BEFORE THE NEXT SKILL

Before progressing to the next skill, practice accurate reflection of content at least four different times during your usual interpersonal interactions. Summarize the situations in writing, indicating what effect the use of reflection of content did or did not have, and how you felt about reflecting content in those particular situations. Observe how other persons reflect content and examine your own reaction to different ways of reflecting content.

You will find it helpful to plan and implement a simulation exercise involving one or two other persons and yourself. Audiotape or videotape a series of exchanges or a conversation in which you reflected content several times. For self-learning, listen to and evaluate the taped responses, using the criteria in the Performance Checklist as a guide. For additional critique and learning, bring the tape to class for peer and faculty feedback.

☐ CRITICAL POINTS SUMMARY

1. Reflection of content is a restatement of the message being communicated.
2. Accurate reflection of content is based on effective listening.
3. Reflection of content provides validation of messages and inappropriate and ineffective actions.
4. To reflect accurately the content of a message:
   a. *Listen* to what is being said.
   b. *Restate* the basic message, or content, concisely in your *own* words.
   c. *Observe* for a cue or ask the client for a response that indicates whether the reflection is accurate.
5. Ineffective reflection of content makes it difficult for the client to communicate his or her message to the helper.
6. Using a variety of ways to reflect content avoids a routine approach.

☐ REVIEW QUESTIONS

1. How is reflection of content different from verbal encouragement?
2. How does effective listening contribute to the ability to reflect content accurately?
3. How would accurate reflection of content help the nurse to collect more adequate and relevant data from a client?
4. What kind of nonverbal cues might indicate that reflection of content is accurate?
5. For what reasons are verbatim reflection and rearranging of words not considered the most generally helpful ways to reflect content?
6. What messages are conveyed to the client when the helper ignores messages, responds to only part of a message, adds content to a message, or evaluates a message both verbally and nonverbally?

☐ PERFORMANCE CHECKLIST

OBJECTIVE: To demonstrate the ability to reflect the content of a message in an effective manner.

EVALUATION OF SELF[a]		BEHAVIORS	EVALUATION BY PARTNER B[a]		EVALUATION BY OBSERVER[a]	
S	U		S	U	S	U
		1. Restates content in own words, avoiding mimicking or rearranging of words.				
		2. Avoids evaluating, blaming, giving of advice, approval/disapproval.				
		3. Prefaces remarks with a phrase that indicates perception of the communication (give examples).				
		4. Uses nonverbal behavior that is interested and neutral or congruent with the original communication.				
		5. Identifies when own statements were correctly reflected.				
		6. Needs strengthening in certain areas (specify).				

[a] S = Satisfactory; U = Unsatisfactory.

REFERENCES

Bochnak MA, Rhymes JP, Leonard RC: Comparison of two types of nursing activity on the relief of pain. In Innovations in Nurse–Patient Relationships: Automatic or Reasoned Nurse Actions (Clinical Papers No. 6). New York, American Nurses' Association, 1962.

Combs AW, Avila DL, Purkey WW: Helping Relationships: Basic Concepts for the Helping Professions. Boston, Allyn & Bacon, 1971.

D'Augelli AR, Danish SJ, et al: Helping Skills: A Basic Training Program (Leader's Manual), ed 2. New York, Human Sciences Press, 1980.

Johnson DW: Reaching Out: Interpersonal Effectiveness and Self-Actualization. Englewood Cliffs, NJ, Prentice-Hall, 1972.

Korsch BM: Practical techniques of observing, interviewing, and advising parents in pediatric practice as demonstrated in an attitude study project. Pediatrics 18(3):467–490, 1956.

Truax CB, Carkhuff RR: Toward Effective Counseling and Psychotherapy. Chicago, Aldine Publishing, 1967.

BIBLIOGRAPHY

Benjamin A: The Helping Interview, ed 3. Boston, Houghton Mifflin, 1981.

Bernstein L, Bernstein RS, Dana RH: Interviewing: A Guide for Health Professionals, ed 2. New York, Appleton-Century-Crofts, 1974.

Brammer LM: The Helping Relationship: Process and Skills, ed 2. Englewood Cliffs, NJ, Prentice-Hall, 1979.

Carkhuff RR: Helping and Human Relations: A Primer for Lay and Professional Helpers, 2 vols. New York, Holt, Rinehart, & Winston, 1969.

Hein EC: Communication in Nursing Practice, ed 2. Boston, Little, Brown, 1980.

SKILL 12 Reflection of Feelings

There can be no feeling except about something, and no knowing without some personal reference.
—*Combs et al., p. 100*

☐ STUDENT OBJECTIVES

1. Describe the relationship of productive attending behavior and attentive listening to the ability to reflect feelings.
2. Explain the relationship between the client's need to express feelings and the helper's ability to reflect feelings.
3. Describe ways the helper can identify another person's feelings.
4. Describe effective and ineffective ways to reflect the feeling content of a message.
5. Develop the ability to identify different kinds and intensities of feelings.
6. Reflect the feeling content of messages in simulated and practice settings.
7. Increase your vocabulary of words that describe feelings.

☐ INTRODUCTION

Reflection of feelings is a way of responding to the emotions another person experiences. It is an identification and verbalization of the feelings that the listener perceives are being communicated through the other person's words, nonverbal behaviors, or feeling tones. It may also include an identification and reflection of the reasons for those feelings. Reflection of feelings builds on reflection of content in that reflection of content clarifies the meaning of a situation and reflection of feelings acknowledges the other person's emotional response to that situation.

Reflecting the feeling aspect of a message lets a person know that he or she has been heard and understood. As an empathic response, it is helpful in conversations with friends or family and is especially useful in nurse–client interactions. As with reflection of content, reflection of feelings can help a person recognize or clarify his or her own feelings through hearing them reflected accurately. Reflecting a client's feelings can also help the client regard those feelings as legitimate.

For example, if a nurse recognizes that a hospitalized client is anxious about an anticipated surgery and responds by reflecting that anxiety in a nonjudgmental way, the client will most likely feel that it is acceptable or even expected for him or her to feel that way. The client also will feel that it is all right to talk about those feelings and that the nurse understands and accepts those feelings as real and valid. This kind of experience is very reassuring.

Like other helpers, nurses often deal with persons who are in the midst of crises and are experiencing the emotions that accompany crisis situations. Identifying and responding to those emotions in a productive way increases the nurse's ability to be a caring and empathic professional. Furthermore, it increases the level of trust and respect in the nurse–client relationship.

☐ PREPARATION

A feeling is a description of an emotional experience. Although all people have feelings, our awareness of our own feelings and our ability to identify those feelings varies. "Feelings are aroused by what we do and what is done to us; they are reflected in what we subsequently do and think; they condition how we act toward others and how we treat ourselves" (Carkhuff and Anthony, 1979, p. 75).

Feelings are real for the person who is experiencing them. Feelings simply exist; they cannot be argued with, denied, or told to go away, and it is not helpful to tell someone that he or she ought or ought not to have certain feelings. Feelings find expression through the way people move their bodies, the energy level in their voices, their voice tone, and the content of what they say.

A helper can learn to recognize feelings through the use of careful observation, productive attending behavior, and attentive listening. In addition, the helper can try to see the situation from the client's frame of reference and ask mentally, "If I were that person and had to cope with what he or she is facing, how might I feel?" If the nurse has some idea of what the client is facing, it can be helpful to share these perceptions with the client. Two ways to do this are through *universalizing* and *personalizing* (discussed in Skill 6). An example of a universalizing comment about a client's feelings would be, "I don't know if this is your experience or not, but a lot of people seem to feel . . . when this kind of thing happens to them. Is this true for you?" An example of a personalizing comment would be, "If I were in circumstances similar to yours, I might feel . . . . Is that true for you?" Both of these approaches suggest feelings the client may be experiencing, but they do not impose the helper's feelings or assume that those feelings are the same as the client's; the client is free to accept or reject the suggestion.

Once the helper is fairly certain that he or she understands the client's feelings, the helper can verbalize those feelings to the client. If the helper's perceptions and reflections of the client's feelings are accurate, the client will recognize them as such. This usually is a clarifying and empathic experience for the client and validates the accuracy of the helper's perceptions (Anthony and Carkhuff, 1976).

Feelings occur in response to something; that is, they have causes. As with awareness of feelings, the ability of individuals to recognize the causes or sources of their feelings varies. Carkhuff and Anthony (1979) believe that the helper needs to listen for the cause of what the client is feeling as well as for the feeling itself, and to reflect that cause to the client—again from the helper's perspective. The client's recognition of the reflected cause as being true for his or her own experience again serves to validate the helper's perceptions.

EFFECTIVE REFLECTION OF FEELINGS

The helper's ability to reflect his or her perception of the feelings a client is experiencing can help the client with purposeful expression of his or her own feelings, which is one of the client's needs in a helping relationship. When people are in some kind of difficulty, the need to express feelings is felt more keenly. Biestek (1957) believes that to deny the client the opportunity to express feelings is the same as not dealing with the whole person. Purposeful expression of feelings on the part of the client can relieve some of his or her pressures and tensions, and is a form of psychological support. It also can help the client to see and understand his or her own problems more clearly and objectively.

Many people are not accustomed to recognizing and expressing their own feelings, let alone having those feelings recognized and expressed by someone else. In the helping situation, expression of feelings comes fairly naturally and easily for the client when (1) the helper has established a helping relationship through the use of productive attending behavior and attentive listening, and (2) when the client has developed some degree of trust and confidence in the helper as an empathic person.

In addition to recognition and expression of the feeling itself, the intensity associated with the feeling needs to be identified and reflected. A response becomes "interchangeable in feeling with the patient's own statement" when both the same feeling and the same intensity are reflected and the client recognizes them as his or her own (Carkhuff and Anthony, 1979, p. 81). Anthony and Carkhuff (1976) have designed a model based on seven kinds or categories of feelings: happy, sad, angry, scared, confused, weak, and strong (Activity Figure 12-A). Each of these feeling categories has three possible levels of intensity: strong, mild, or weak. The authors propose that a helper can use these categories and intensity levels to choose a response that is congruent with and reflects the client's feelings accurately.

To reflect feelings back to a client accurately requires an adequate vocabulary of words that describe feelings. The ability to use specific feeling words helps the nurse reflect others' feelings in a caring and individualized way. For example, before surgery clients generally experience some degree of anxiety or fear. They may simply feel uneasy, uncertain, or slightly apprehensive; or they may feel afraid, scared, terrified, or panic-stricken, depending on the person or situation. In this and many other circumstances, the helper needs to know how to use a wide variety of words to reflect accurately a particular person's specific feelings.

Rankin (1981) indicates that it often is difficult for students to identify clients' feelings when practicing interview skills, and Doona (1979) points out that a common cause of this difficulty is lack of practice. Rankin also states that "in order to increase their awareness of the role that feelings play in maintaining emotional health, students must first become more cognizant of different kinds of feelings" (1981, p. 37). She describes an instructional game designed to provide practice in identifying specific feelings.

The following activity focuses on identifying a variety of kinds and intensities of feelings.

Activity 12-A: Identifying Feelings

Work in small groups.

1. Activity Figure 12-A gives examples of seven kinds and three intensity levels of words that describe feelings. Add at least two words of your own choice to each intensity level of each feeling. Use a thesaurus if necessary.
2. Select seven words from your completed chart, one from each of the categories of feelings. Include words from each intensity level in your selection. Recall a situation or personal experience in which each of those words would be an accurate reflection of the feelings you experienced. Write one or two sentences describing the feeling and the situation. For example, "I was really upset when I failed that test"; "I felt so proud because I had really done a good job." Compare your sentences with others.
3. Select four additional words from your completed chart. Take turns conveying the feelings you selected to the others in your group. You

LEVELS OF INTENSITY	CATEGORY						
	Happy	Sad	Angry	Confused	Scared	Weak	Strong
Strong	Excited Great Overjoyed	Hopeless Lost Crushed	Furious Disgusted Enraged	Numb Trapped Panicky	Terrified Afraid Fearful	Ashamed Vulnerable Exhausted	Powerful Potent Aggressive
Mild	Alive Proud Up	Lonely Hurt Upset	Frustrated Irritated Sore	Doubtful Mixed up Uncomfortable	Shaky Worried Anxious	Embarrassed Helpless Powerless	Tough Confident Brave
Weak	Calm Glad Pleased	Down Bad Dull	Annoyed Mad Uptight	Unsure Surprised Foggy	Nervous Shy Uneasy	Tired Shaky Worn out	Healthy Firm Able

Activity Figure 12-A. (Adapted with permission of the publisher from Anthony WA, Carkhuff RR: *The Art of Health Care*, pp. 28–29, © 1976, Human Resource Development Press, 22 Amherst Road, Amherst, Massachusetts. All rights reserved.)

may use any nonverbal behaviors, but the only word you may say is the name of someone in the group. Use inflection and voice tone that match the feeling. The other persons in the group are to write down the feeling they perceive you are conveying and to show the words to you for validation.
4. How well are you able to convey feelings to others, and how readily can you identify others' feelings?

Examples of Reflection of Feelings

Since we cannot know for certain what someone else is feeling, it is best to introduce the reflection tentatively. Some examples of introductory phrases are:

- "It sounds as though you are feeling . . . (sad, happy, elated)"
- "You look . . . (furious, fearful, joyful)"
- "You seem . . . (troubled, nervous, satisfied)"

When the feelings seem evident, a more direct response may be appropriate, such as:

- "You feel . . . (pleased, hurt)"
- "You are feeling . . . (excited, angry)"

The following statements were used in Skill 11 as examples of reflection of content. They are used again here to illustrate reflection of feelings and to help clarify the distinctions between the two types of reflection. The first example contains only a reflection of the feeling itself, while the second includes the cause.

Client: "The days get awfully long here with nothing to do. I've been here ever since I broke my hip a month ago. My family is from Georgetown, over 100 miles away, so they don't get over here very often. I don't get much other company, either."

Helper's response: "It sounds as if you're feeling rather lonely."
Client: "Yes, I guess I am! Everyone here has been really good to me, but it's not quite the same as family!"

Speaker: "I could just die! You know that neat guy in Soc. class? Well, he's asked me for a date Saturday night! And guess what! I already had a date with that creep from downstairs! Guess that's just too bad for him!"
Listener's response: "You look a little doubtful about what you have done."
Speaker: "Well, I guess I am! It's really kind of a mean thing to do, even to a creep!"

The following activity focuses on accurate reflection of feelings in simulated situations.

**Activity 12-B:
Reflecting Feelings**

Work in small groups.

1. Respond to the following prepared situations in writing. Focus only on the feeling being communicated. You will note that these statements are the same as the ones you used for preparing written content responses in Skill 11. After you have finished, compare your written statements with those of the other persons in your group to validate the accuracy of your responses.
    a. "Did you count the pages we have to read for next week? And all for one class! They must think their class is the only one we have to study for!"

b. "I don't know how I'm going to tell my parents. They'll really be disappointed with me! I just can't have an abortion—and I'm sure not ready to get married yet! What'll I say to them?"

c. "If they would just bring me my briefcase so I could finish that project, then I'd relax! How am I supposed to 'take it easy' when things have to get done and there is no one else to do them? 'Just lie quietly and rest!' That's like telling the wind to stop blowing!"

2. Using the same situations as in number 1 of this activity, write another response to each situation, this time including what you perceive as the cause of the feeling. Compare your responses with those of the other persons in your group.

3. Respond to statements made by another person in the group. Designate one person as partner A, one as partner B, and one as observer.
   a. Partner A: Make a statement to partner B on something about which you feel strongly.
   b. Partner B: Reflect the feelings expressed in what partner A is saying, matching the intensity of the words you choose with the intensity of the feeling expressed by partner A. Use voice tone and manner that are either neutral or congruent with partner A's nonverbal behavior.
   c. Partner A and observer: Validate the accuracy of the reflected message.
   d. Repeat the exercise using a different statement from partner A.
   e. Exchange roles and repeat the exercise until each person has assumed each role.

4. After completing these exercises, ask yourselves the following questions:
   a. How accurately were feelings reflected?
   b. What problems in reflection of feelings were noted?
   c. What was your reaction to reflecting the feelings you understood someone to be communicating to you?
   d. How did it feel to have your own feelings reflected by someone else?

INEFFECTIVE REFLECTION OF FEELINGS

As with reflection of content, reflection of feelings is dependent on attentive listening; therefore, people with poorly developed listening skills have difficulty identifying and reflecting the feelings connected with a client's messages. It also is difficult to recognize and reflect another person's feelings if the listener has a low level of awareness of his or her own feelings and emotional reactions to situations; or if the listener does not view the other person as an individual but sees him or her as simply another client. In addition, a listener who is uncomfortable with the expression either of his or her own feelings or of others' feelings will find it more difficult to encourage expression of feelings through reflection of observed feelings.

Occasionally beginning helpers are so anxious about their own functioning that they are unable to recognize that clients even *have* feelings about their circumstances, let alone *respond* to those feelings. When this happens, the beginning helper's level of anxiety must be dealt with and brought to manageable levels before responding behaviors can be developed.

There are several approaches to reflection of feelings that are nonhelpful in a helping relationship. These sidetrack a client from telling his or her own story, and discount the value of the client's feelings, as well as the value of the client as an individual. Consciously or unconsciously, the listener may choose to *disregard the feelings* that are being communicated and respond only to the content. Occasionally, a skilled and experienced helper may have appropriate reasons for doing this; however, it usually is not helpful to ignore the feeling content in a client's message. Another way of disregarding a client's feelings is to assume that we understand exactly how the client feels. While similar experiences can give us some idea of how others may feel, it is not possible to be someone else and experience his or her feelings. A statement such as, "I know how you feel," ignores the individuality of the person's feelings and tends to focus the attention of the exchange on the helper rather than the client. This does not help the client to feel heard. Sometimes beginning helpers use their own feelings about a situation as a *substitute* for the client's feelings, rather than as a guide for determining the client's frame of reference. They tend to think that the way they would feel in a given situation is exactly how someone else would feel; that is, they assume that their perspective is the norm for others.

As with reflection of content, *approval, disapproval, or blame* can be conveyed through the way feelings are reflected. The words and tone of voice used to describe the observed feeling can convey the message that the feelings are appropriate and valid or inappropriate, wrong, or stupid. For example, Steven O'Brien, R.N., is teaching Jack McAllister, a newly diagnosed diabetic, to give his own insulin. Jack's words and nonverbal manner have indicated to Steven that he is quite fearful of doing this. Steven could say to Jack, "You're kind of scared about giving insulin to yourself, aren't you?" in a way that is empathic, warm, and nonjudgmental; or he could use the same words in a surprised or disapproving manner that might cause Jack to become defensive or discouraged.

Examples of Ineffective Reflection of Feelings

A 68-year-old man is slowly dying from terminal cancer. The man's son says to the nurse who is caring for his father, "I'll be so glad when it's all over!" The nurse responds, "How can you say that about your father! As long as there is life there is hope!" Had she responded to the son's feelings of grief over the suffering his father was experiencing, the nurse might have said, "You're feeling really sad to see your dad suffer so much," and the son would most likely have felt heard and understood.

A hospitalized middle-aged woman is scheduled for an abdominal hysterectomy in the morning. At 10:00 P.M. when the nurse responds to her call light, the woman has an anxious look on her face and says in a questioning voice, "I'm not sure I really want to go through with this surgery tomorrow!" The nurse may respond by (1) disregarding the feelings conveyed: "It's fairly usual to feel that way. I brought the sleeping pill the doctor ordered for you. It will help you get a good sleep"; (2) substituting the nurse's own feelings: "The same anesthesiologist who did my surgery last year is scheduled to do yours tomorrow. I really felt safe in his hands and didn't worry at all"; or (3) with a disapproving value judgment: "You're not sure you want to go through with it? You've already had your lab work and prep and everything is planned and ready for tomorrow morning!" However, if the nurse responds to the feelings the woman is communicating, the nurse might say, "You seem rather worried about the surgery." The woman might then feel free to describe her concerns.

☐ EXECUTION

Responding to the feelings contained in a client's message requires that the helper be able to (1) use an adequate vocabulary and adequate verbal skills, (2) listen attentively, (3) use productive attending behavior, and (4) experience a genuine caring for other persons.

The process of reflecting feelings begins with listening to the verbal and nonverbal messages being communicated by the client, making a mental note of the congruence of those messages, and identifying the feelings being communicated. Sometimes intuition or hunches can help identify what the client is experiencing. After identifying the feelings that are present, the helper selects words that describe both the kind (category) and intensity of those feelings and states his or her perceptions of those feelings. Next the helper observes for responses or cues from the client that confirm or deny the accuracy of the reflected feelings, such as nonverbal facial expressions and gestures or verbal comments. If no response is heard or observed, the helper may want to ask the client for validation. Sometimes verbal validation of the helper's interpretation of nonverbal cues is helpful, particularly if the cues lend noncongruence to the client's message. Consider the illustration from Skill 11, with the 28-year-old mother of three who has just finished describing a difficult family situation involving physical abuse. Depending on the situation, the nurse, Sally, might decide to respond to the mother's feelings rather than the content, and reflect, "You sound confused about what has been happening." If Sally's perceptions of the mother's feelings are correct, the mother may give Sally a glance of appreciation and respond, "You're right! I know he loves me, but when he beats me, I just want to leave and never come back!" And so the nurse's perceptions are validated as correct.

The ability to reflect feelings can be expanded through increasing our listening and attending skills, increasing our vocabulary of words that describe feelings, identifying feelings we are experiencing and that we observe others to be experiencing, and practicing a conscious reflection of feelings in social and professional situations.

The following activities focus on observing and experiencing effective and ineffective reflection of feelings and noting the messages those behaviors communicate.

Activity 12-C:
Simulations of Reflection of Feeling

In a group setting, observe simulated live or videotaped examples first of ineffective reflection of feelings and then of effective reflection of feelings. Discuss the simulations among yourselves, focusing on these questions: What specific characteristics cause the examples to be ineffective or effective reflection of feelings? What were your reactions to observing both kinds of reflection? What kinds of feelings were communicated by the participants?

Activity 12-D:
Experiencing and Using Reflection of Feeling

Work in groups of three, with two partners and one observer. Use a video camera or an audio recorder if available.

1. *Ineffective reflection of feelings*
   a. Partner A: Talk to partner B for 3 to 5 minutes on a subject or event of personal interest or importance.
   b. Partner B: Respond to partner A with a variety of very ineffective reflections of feelings.
   c. Observer: Note in writing the specific negative and ineffective ways partner B reflected the feelings contained in partner A's message, as well as partner A's reactions to partner B's reflections.
   d. Observer and partner A: Give feedback to partner B about the kinds of negative reflections observed. Review the audiotape or videotape if available.
   e. Exchange roles and repeat the activity until each person has assumed each role.
2. *Effective reflection of feelings*
   Each person chooses a subject he or she feels strongly about or recalls an experience about which he or she has strong feelings.
   a. Partner A: Describe your experience or subject to partner B.

b. Partner B: Use effective methods of reflecting feelings to respond to partner A. Reflect the specific feelings, their intensity, and associated nonverbal behaviors as accurately as possible.
c. Observer: Take written notes on partner B's listening skills, including the words and nonverbal behaviors used to reflect feelings.
d. Complete the Performance Checklist, p. 91. Give feedback to partner B about the reflecting behaviors you observed. Review the audiotape or videotape if available.
e. Exchange roles and repeat the activity until each person has assumed each role.
3. Discuss the experience of reflecting someone else's feelings and having your own feelings reflected in both effective and ineffective ways. In your discussion, focus on whether the feelings were reflected accurately; which approaches to reflecting feelings seem most appropriate to you as a speaker and as a listener, and for what reasons; and the positive and negative results from each approach. What learning can you apply to other interpersonal situations?

BEFORE THE NEXT SKILL

Several times in the next few days, reread your chart of words that describe feelings (Table 12–1). Observe your own feelings in interpersonal situations and give them a specific descriptive label. Observe other people's reactions in everyday situations and give a specific descriptive label to the feelings you believe they are experiencing. After you have practiced identifying and labeling feelings, begin to reflect those feelings back to the other person. Take note of the validation you receive, both verbally and nonverbally.

It will be helpful to plan and implement a simulation exercise involving one or two other persons and yourself. Audiotape or videotape a series of exchanges or a conversation in which you reflected someone's feelings several times. For self-learning, listen to and evaluate the taped responses, using the criteria in the Performance Checklist, p. 91, as a guide. For additional critique and learning, bring the tape to class for peer and faculty feedback.

☐ CRITICAL POINTS SUMMARY

1. All people have feelings that are expressed both verbally and nonverbally.
2. A helper becomes aware of a client's feelings through active listening, productive attending behavior, and careful observation.
3. Effective reflection of feelings helps the client to recognize, clarify, and express his or her own feelings.
4. An adequate vocabulary of words that describe feelings is needed for accurate reflection of feelings.
5. To reflect accurately the feelings in a message:
   a. *Listen* to what is being said.
   b. *Observe* nonverbal behavior.
   c. *State* the kind and intensity of feelings, using specific descriptive words.
   d. *Observe* for a cue or ask for a response from the client that indicates the accuracy of the reflection.
6. Ineffective reflection of feelings makes it difficult for the client to communicate his or her message to the helper.

☐ REVIEW QUESTIONS

1. In what ways is accurate reflection of feelings helpful, with both friends and clients?
2. Why is reflection of feelings a necessary part of a helping relationship?
3. How do attentive listening and productive attending behavior contribute to accurate reflection of feelings?
4. What messages are conveyed to the client when the helper disregards feelings, assumes he or she understands what the client is feeling, substitutes his or her own feelings for the client's, or gives value judgments about feelings?
5. What does it mean for the client to recognize a reflected feeling as his or her own?

REFERENCES

Anthony WA, Carkhuff RR: The Art of Health Care: A Handbook of Psychological First Aid Skills. Amherst, MA, Human Resource Development Press, 1976.

Biestek FP: The Casework Relationship. Chicago, Loyola University Press, 1957.

Carkhuff RR, Anthony WA: The Skills of Helping: An Introduction to Counseling. Amherst, MA, Human Resource Development Press, 1979.

Combs AW, Avila DL, Purkey WW: Helping Relationships: Basic Concepts for the Helping Professions. Boston, Allyn & Bacon, 1971.

Doona M: Travelbee's Intervention in Psychiatric Nursing, ed 2. Philadelphia, FA Davis, 1979.

Rankin NM: Name that feeling! An innovative teaching tool. Journal of Psychosocial Nursing and Mental Health Services 19(12):37–39, 1981.

BIBLIOGRAPHY

Benjamin A: The Helping Interview, ed 3. Boston, Houghton Mifflin, 1981.

Bernstein L, Bernstein RS, Dana RH: Interviewing: A Guide for Health Professionals, ed 3. New York, Appleton-Century-Crofts, 1980.

Brammer LM: The Helping Relationship, ed 2. Englewood Cliffs, NJ, Prentice-Hall, 1979.

Johnson DW: Reaching Out: Interpersonal Effectiveness and Self-actualization. Englewood Cliffs, NJ, Prentice-Hall, 1972.

☐ PERFORMANCE CHECKLIST

OBJECTIVE: To demonstrate the ability to reflect the feeling content of a message in an effective manner.							
EVALUATION OF SELF[a]			EVALUATION BY PARTNER B[a]		EVALUATION BY OBSERVER[a]	
S	U	BEHAVIORS	S	U	S	U
		1. Uses productive attending behavior.				
		2. Uses attentive listening skills.				
		3. Attends to verbal and nonverbal messages.				
		4. Reflects type of feeling congruent with the message.				
		5. Reflects intensity level congruent with the message.				
		6. Uses appropriate words to describe feelings (give examples).				
		7. Needs strengthening in certain areas (specify).				

[a] S = Satisfactory; U = Unsatisfactory.

SKILL 13 Questioning

Perhaps the central method of interviewing is the fine art of questioning.
—Garrett, p. 37

☐ STUDENT OBJECTIVES

1. Explain the functions of questions in the helping relationship.
2. Describe the influence of a helper's manner on the client's response to questions.
3. Distinguish between open and closed questions.
4. Illustrate appropriate use and benefits of both open and closed questions.
5. Compare the messages conveyed to clients through the use of open and closed questions.
6. Describe problems associated with the use of questions.
7. Demonstrate your own ability to use open and closed questions appropriately in simulated and real settings.

☐ INTRODUCTION

A question is "an expression of inquiry that invites or calls for a response" (Webster, 1976). Questions are part of nearly all casual or routine nurse–client interactions, as well as being a significant aspect of the more formalized context of a structured interview setting.

Questions serve a number of functions in the nurse–client relationship. They may be used to gather information, to validate and clarify the content and feeling of a client's messages, to explore a client's situation or thinking, or to help a client explore his or her own circumstances and values. Questions may also be used to offer assistance, as discussed in Skill 14.

In her classic text on interviewing, Garrett (1972) indicates that the fine art of questioning most likely is the central method used in interviewing. Hein says that the "information received by a nurse is as pertinent and relevant as the question asked" (1980, p. 42). However, Benjamin (1981) advises caution concerning the use of questions, because although questions are necessary and helpful, it is possible (1) to ask too many meaningless questions that either interrupt or confuse the client, (2) to ask questions that the client cannot answer, or (3) to use questions to obtain information that is not needed. Benjamin also states that using questions and answers as the primary format for an interview produces an expectation in both helper and client that the helper has the answers to the client's problem. As opposed to working together to resolve problems, this approach sets up the helper as the authority and expert and the client as the one who supplies specific information only when he or she is asked for it. The question–answer format is considered an impersonal approach that

... does not create an atmosphere in which a warm, positive relationship can develop; in which the client may find a valuable experience; in which he may discover more about himself, his strengths and weaknesses; in which he has the opportunity to grow. (Benjamin, 1981, p. 72)

The two major kinds of questions discussed in this skill are open and closed questions. Acquiring the skill of asking appropriate questions in effective ways and for specific purposes enhances a nurse's ability to develop therapeutic relationships with clients and become an effective helper.

☐ *PREPARATION*

When asking questions during interactions with clients, nurses are mindful both of their reason for asking a question and of the kind of information they are seeking. It is not valid to ask questions for no particular reason; this does not contribute to the development of a positive nurse–client relationship.

The vocabulary used to ask questions should be appropriate for the particular client's educational and occupational background, level of comprehension, and past experiences. Some nurses talk down to clients in a patronizing manner and use excessively simple language, while others use highly technical terminology and professional jargon without considering whether the client understands what is being talked about. For example, a committee for a community health center consisting of both professional and lay members was considering the addition of a nurse practitioner with expertise in obstetrics and gynecology to the clinic staff. Some of the medically oriented board members often used the terms OB-Gyn and prenatal during the discussion without considering the other members' lack of understanding of these terms. Finally, one local resident board member who had a high degree of self-confidence said, "Wait a minute! What *is* OB-Gyn?"

Questions can convey messages other than those contained in the actual content. Depending on how they are spoken, the same words can convey suspicion, accusation, sarcasm, or friendliness. For example, consider the different meanings that can result simply from emphasizing a different word in the following sentence:

- "Are *you* leaving early for the holidays?"
- "Are you *leaving* early for the holidays?"
- "Are you leaving *early* for the holidays?"
- "Are you leaving early for the *holidays?*"

Additional meanings can be added to this sentence by using nonverbal expressions and voice tones that convey surprise, pleasure, sarcasm, or disgust. If a nurse asks a question in a hostile or sarcastic manner, the client will tend to respond in a hostile fashion. If the tone is accusatory, the client may become defensive and angry. If the tone is friendly, the nurse has a better chance of receiving the information he or she seeks, although not everyone will automatically respond in a friendly way.

OPEN AND CLOSED QUESTIONS

In most nurse–client interactions, open questions are considered more effective than closed questions. Open questions involve client participation in care, generally provide more complete information, and invite clients to express their own perceptions. However, closed questions can be useful and appropriate for specific purposes.

Open Questions

Open questions are broad queries that allow the client to determine the direction and extent of the answer and encourage the client to describe and elaborate on what is being disclosed. Open questions neither restrict the client to limited choices or responses nor convey expectations of specific kinds of responses. Rather, they allow the client to verbalize in his or her own way without forcing disclosure, yet at the same time increase the client's willingness to disclose. Open questions convey acceptance of and caring for the individual as a person rather than as just another client and do not impose values, judgments, or certain expectations of behavior.

Open questions are particularly valuable for validation, clarification, exploration, and giving advice. Since responses to open questions tend to be longer than responses to closed questions, the nurse using open questions has a greater opportunity to observe the client's nonverbal behavior and vocabulary and gain an understanding of the client's values and perception of his or her situation.

An open question can be made even more open by stating it indirectly. In contrast to direct questions, which are clear, straight queries, indirect questions inquire without seeming to do so. Although they do not sound like questions, indirect questions clearly pose a question and seek an answer. For example, the open question, "How is the new diet working out for you?" can be made more open if stated as the indirect question, "I would like to hear how the new diet is working out for you."

Examples of Open Questions

These open questions are of the type that seek fairly specific information:

- "What plans have you made for help when you first go home?"
- "What do you think is keeping you awake?"
- "How is it working out for you to give your own insulin?"
- "I would like to hear how it is working for you to be giving your own insulin."

The following open questions are of the type that explore and encourage elaboration:

- "What happened then?"
- "What was your reaction to . . .?"
- "Could you tell me more about . . .?"
- "What are you hoping this hospitalization will do for you?"
- "I'm wondering what you are hoping this hospitalization will do for you."

Closed Questions

Closed questions are narrow in scope and consciously or unconsciously are designed to elicit a specific response. Closed questions focus on specific factual information rather than on an exploration of the client's circumstances. The most common closed questions are those that can be answered "yes" or "no." Other closed questions require brief, several-word answers. With closed questions, the helper, rather than the client, sets the parameters of the response to the question, and the client usually does not elaborate beyond what is asked specifically.

Hein (1980) points out that nurses tend to use more closed questions than open questions during initial interviews, when under stress, or when feeling ill at ease around clients. Some nurses use closed questions because they can obtain information quickly and sound knowledgeable about their clients. Some nurses who are unable or unwilling to communicate freely and flexibly with clients will use primarily closed questions that are directed toward factual information.

Although limited in scope, closed questions can be useful in some circumstances. Closed questions are more efficient when brief factual information is needed, such as demographic data when admitting a client to a health-care facility. Closed questions are appropriate when minimal client involvement is required, such as when asking about menu selections, determining whether personal care or exercise programs have been carried out, or checking on readiness for an x-ray procedure.

Closed questions may be used to probe for further information, such as when trying to identify the source and nature of discomfort or pain, or to determine exactly what happened in an incident needing investigation. For example, when investigating the nature and extent of pain, the nurse might ask a series of closed questions: "Does it hurt when you take a deep breath? When you move? Would you describe it as an aching, sharp, or dull pain? When did the pain begin?"

Closed questions are useful when circumstances limit a client's choices. Sometimes the diagnostic or therapeutic regime requires activities that the client might not freely choose, such as getting out of bed for exercise even when tired or uncomfortable, receiving injections, or having blood drawn for tests. When choices are limited, the nurse can use closed questions to maximize the choices that are possible, giving the client some sense of control over his or her own situation. For example, when a client needs an injection, the nurse can offer a limited but viable choice through a closed question such as: "Would you like your shot in your left or right hip?" Not all closed questions would offer this clear-cut choice. For example, the closed question "Would you like your shot now?" is likely to elicit a specific response: "No!" If medication is a necessary part of a treatment plan, the choice of having or not having the injection is not a viable choice, and this is obviously not what the nurse would intend to be asking. On the other hand, an open question can also be unproductive. If the nurse asks, "Where would you like your shot?" a client might answer "In my left hip"; but the depressed or indecisive client may not be able to cope with that choice; the frightened child may begin to cry; or the joker may respond "Nowhere!" or "In *your* hip!"

Examples of Closed Questions

These closed questions can be answered with yes or no:

- "Are you having pain?"
- "Are you allergic to penicillin?"
- "Is this your first time at this clinic?"

The following closed questions appropriately seek brief, factual material:

- "How many people are in your family?"
- "Where do you usually go for medical care?"
- "When did you have your last menstrual period?"

The following closed questions are used to probe after an open question:

Open question:	"Could you tell me about your pain?"
Closed, probing questions:	"Exactly where does it hurt?"
	"Does it hurt when you move?"
	"When you cough or sneeze?"
	"Does it go away when you rest?"
	"On a scale of one to ten, with ten being the most pain you could possibly tolerate, how would you rate your pain?"

The following activity focuses on the use of open and closed questions in structured situations.

Activity 13-A: Using Open and Closed Questions

Work individually and as partners within a small group.

1. *Responding to prepared statements*
   a. Respond in writing to each of the following client statements with both an open and a closed question. Validate your written questions with other group members before doing number 2 of this activity.
   "I just can't get to sleep tonight."
   "I have been so constipated lately."
   "I don't think my diet is helping me lose weight."
   "The food here is terrible."
   b. For each of the open and closed questions you wrote in number 1a, write what you think would be a probable client response.
   c. Within your group, compare written responses for both open and closed questions, noting general characteristics, similarities, and differences.

2. *Asking closed questions*
    Divide your group into pairs, partners A and B, pairing people who do *not* know each other well.
    a. Partner A: Introduce yourself to partner B, indicating that you would like to get acquainted. Using only closed questions, spend 3 or 4 minutes finding out about partner B.
    b. Reverse roles and repeat number 2a.
    c. How well do you feel you know each other? Compare your reactions to asking and responding only to closed questions.
3. *Asking open questions*
    Select a different partner for this exercise.
    a. Partner A: Introduce yourself to partner B, indicating that you would like to get acquainted. Using only open questions, spend 3 or 4 minutes finding out about partner B.
    b. Reverse roles and repeat number 3a.
    c. How well do you feel you know each other? Compare your reactions to asking and responding only to open questions.
4. Compare the nature and volume of the information you gained through using closed versus open questions.

PROBLEMS WITH QUESTIONS

Both open and closed questions can be abused and misused in ways that are nonproductive in the helping relationship and are ineffective in gathering data and exploring a client's circumstances.

Using open questions to gather specific factual information can be unnecessarily time-consuming. If open questions are too broad, are too vague, or lack direction, the client is likely to be confused and not know what information is being requested.

Value judgments can be implied in closed questions, such as when a question is phrased in such a way that the client is able to determine the answer the helper would approve. This was illustrated in Korsch's (1956) study of mothers in an outpatient pediatric setting. This study found that when asked, "Do you hold the baby in your lap when you feed him?" most mothers answered positively because they inferred that this was the approved answer. When the question was rephrased as, "How many times are you able to hold the baby when you feed him, and how often do you have to let him take the bottle in the crib?" nearly all of the mothers acknowledged that they were propping some of the bottles each day and often for very legitimate reasons (pp. 478–479).

Value judgments also can be conveyed through questions that place the client on the defensive or question his or her judgment. For example, a young nurse asked a 24-year-old mother of three children who was recovering from voluntary sterilization surgery, "Don't you think you are a little young to have had this kind of surgery?" Any response to such a question places the client in the defensive posture of having to justify why she made the decision.

Sometimes a helper asks many closed questions in rapid succession, following his or her own agenda and waiting only for the information he or she wants and expects. With this approach, the client likely will feel bombarded and not really heard or understood. When the client is not given some freedom to respond from his or her own ideas, thought processes, or concerns, an interaction can deteriorate into an interrogation.

Some questions contain two questions at one time. These double questions confuse both client and helper. For example, consider this question: "Are you moving around more easily today, and is your dressing staying in place?" The client must choose which question to answer—or ignore both and respond with something irrelevant. Although people often respond to the first part of a double question, the helper cannot really know which question the client is answering without further clarification.

A misuse of closed questions occurs when the questions indicate what the client's response ought to be. Benjamin (1981) considers these kinds of questions to be even more closed than closed questions, because the question contains the answer and assumes that the predetermined or expected answer is the one the client would give if he or she actually was asked. The only option the client has other than agreeing with the predetermined answer is to contradict the helper directly. This is difficult for most clients to do, particularly since a value judgment tends to be implied in the question. The following are examples of questions that contain an expected answer:

- "Of course you wouldn't hurt your children because you love them, don't you?"
- "You really didn't mean to hit them, did you? It was just because you were tired and upset, wasn't it?"

Prefacing a question with *why* is inappropriate and nonhelpful in nearly all circumstances. An individual may not understand why he or she did something or may not want to share the reasons, and so becomes defensive about his or her behavior. Consider the difference in these two questions:

- "Why did you miss your last clinic appointment?"
- "What happened with your last clinic appointment?"

The first question focuses the responsibility for not coming to the clinic on the client and has an accusatory tone; the client probably will feel a need to make excuses or defend himself or herself. The second question focuses on the issue and inquires about the circumstances of not coming to the clinic; the client is asked to explain, probably will not feel accused, and has less need to become defensive.

☐ EXECUTION

To use questions in a productive way requires that the helper be (1) sensitive to others' needs, (2) able to listen attentively, using productive attending behaviors, (3) able to follow the flow of a conversation, (4) conscious of the purpose in asking questions.

It also is important to use a vocabulary that is appropriate to the client's educational level, occupation, background, and level of comprehension; convey a sense of respect for the client as a worthwhile individual; avoid including value judgments in the questions; ask one question at a time; use open questions whenever feasible; and allow the client time to respond to the questions being asked.

Productive questioning begins with attentive listening, which includes productive attending behavior. As the client talks, the helper pays attention to and considers the messages he or she is receiving from the client. The helper then can clarify, explore, or seek more information about what the client is saying. To do this, the helper asks relevant questions in a way that will achieve his or her purposes. There is no single kind of question that is most appropriate for a given purpose or situation. Having learned productive and nonproductive ways to ask questions, a helper's sensitivity, attentiveness, and listening skills will provide guidance in formulating questions.

The way the helper asks questions influences the response a client may give. This can be illustrated with the example of a clinic nurse, Mrs. Andrews, who is talking with a client, Mr. Wilson, about his new medication regime for his recently diagnosed hypertension. The amount and kind of information Mrs. Andrews receives about Mr. Wilson's adaptation to his changed circumstances will vary according to how she asks the question. If Mrs. Andrews asks the closed question, "Are you having any problems with your new medications?" Mr. Wilson might answer, "No." At that point, Mrs. Andrews would not know if his interpretation of "problems" is the same as hers or if more exploration is needed. If he were to answer "Yes," she would need to ask more questions to learn the nature of those problems.

If Mrs. Andrews asks the closed question, "You're not having any problems with your new medications, are you?" she clearly indicates that she expects him *not* to have any problems, which makes it difficult for Mr. Wilson to disclose any problems he might have. On the other hand, Mrs. Andrews might ask the open question, "What kind of problems are you having with your medications?" This may be an appropriate question if problems with these medications are an expected part of therapy, but it does assume that he *is* having problems. The open question, "How are you managing with your new medications?" leaves it more open for Mr. Wilson to respond that all is well, that he feels better (or worse), that some problems exist—in short, he can respond with his own experience and ideas rather than respond to Mrs. Andrews' preconceived ideas.

While the way a question is worded influences the client's response, learning the so-called correct way to phrase questions will not necessarily ensure that the helper's goals are met. Garrett (1972) believes that although the words are important, the helper's manner and voice tone are more important. She indicates that a helper needs to use a "method of friendliness" when asking questions, that is, to use an empathic and encouraging manner to ask questions and have an intent to understand and assist the client (Garrett, 1972, p. 37). As discussed in earlier skills, helper attitudes are perceived by the client, who often responds more to the manner than to the words spoken.

Asking questions in an effective manner is enhanced by becoming aware of the distinctions between open, closed, effective, and ineffective questions; by observing and experiencing the different responses each kind elicits; and by noting the relationship between the intent of an inquiry and the questioning approach that seems to be the most productive. It is also helpful to pay conscious attention to the ways in which we usually ask questions in both social and professional settings and then decide what modifications in asking questions would be most beneficial to our personal and professional interpersonal relationships.

The following activities focus on observing and experiencing the productive and nonproductive use of questions.

Activity 13-B: Simulations of Questioning

In a group setting, observe simulated live or videotaped examples of open and closed questions used first in ineffective ways and then in effective ways. Discuss the simulations among yourselves, focusing on these questions: What specific characteristics caused the questions to be open or closed, ineffective or effective? What feelings seem to be conveyed by the person asking different kinds of questions? How does the other person's response vary with the type of question asked? Which kinds of questions do you believe will be most helpful to you in nurse–client interactions?

Activity 13-C: Questioning and Being Questioned

Work in groups of three, with two partners and one observer. Use a video camera or an audio recorder if available.

1. *Nonproductive use of questions*
   Select a topic that is controversial or about which you or your partner have strong feelings, or plan to role-play an employment interview situation.
   a. Partner A: Interview partner B, using only nonproductive questions, such as closed questions with yes and no or brief answers, questions with implied answers, questions that

contain value judgments, bombarding questions, and broad, vague, open questions.
  b. Partner B: Respond to the questions in a way that is natural for you.
  c. Observer: Take written notes on the kinds of nonproductive questions used by partner A, the ability of partner B to respond, and the feelings you perceive partner B to be experiencing.
  d. Observer and partner B: Give feedback to partner A about the kinds of nonproductive questions you observed. Review the audiotape or videotape if available.
  e. Exchange roles and repeat the exercise until each person has assumed each role.
2. *Productive use of questions*
  a. Partner A: Interview partner B in a similar way as in number 1a. Ask only productive kinds of direct and indirect, open and closed questions.
  b. Partner B: Respond to the questions in a way that is natural for you.
  c. Observer: Take written notes on the kinds of productive questions used by partner A, the ability of partner B to respond, and the feelings you perceive partner B to be experiencing.
  d. Complete the Performance Checklist for partner A. Observer and partner B: Give feedback to partner A about the productive kinds of questions you observed. Review the audiotape or videotape if available.
  e. Exchange roles and repeat the activity until each person has assumed each role.
3. Discuss the experience of asking and receiving open and closed questions in effective and ineffective ways. In your discussion, consider the following questions: Which kinds of questions do you prefer to answer and for what reasons? Which kinds of questions do you dislike responding to, and for what reasons? Was there a difference in the nonverbal messages that accompanied the open and closed questions? In future nurse–client interactions, what uses do you expect to make of both open and closed questions?

BEFORE THE NEXT SKILL

Before progressing to the next skill, listen to others' use of questions in everyday conversations. Mentally label the questions as open or closed and observe the responses that are given to those questions. Listen to the questions other people ask you and observe your own response and level of comfort with various kinds of questions. Practice using both open and closed questions intentionally in everyday conversations and note any differences in the way people respond to the different kinds of questions.

☐ CRITICAL POINTS SUMMARY

1. Open questions encourage description, elaboration, and exploration.
2. The client determines the direction and parameters of the response to an open question.
3. Closed questions elicit specific information.
4. The helper determines the direction and parameters of the response to a closed question.
5. Both open and closed questions have valid uses in nurse–client interactions but both can be misused.
6. Both the words and the nonverbal manner used with questions influence the effectiveness of the question.
7. Nonproductive questions contain value judgments, double questions, and predetermined answers; ask why; or interrogate the client.
8. Knowing the intent or purpose of a question increases the helper's ability to ask appropriate questions.

☐ REVIEW QUESTIONS

1. Explain the differences between open and closed questions.
2. In what ways do both the phrasing of a question and the helper's manner influence the client's response?
3. In each of these situations, indicate whether open (O) or closed questions (C) would be preferable for *most* of the questions asked:
  ___ a. Admitting clerk filling out admission forms
  ___ b. Hospital nurse admitting a client to clinical unit
  ___ c. Community health nurse encouraging a mother to immunize her children
  ___ d. Pediatric nurse caring for a child with a tonsillectomy
  ___ e. Student conducting an assessment interview
  ___ f. Staff nurse working with a confused elderly person
4. What benefits might result from using both open and closed questions in an interaction?
5. What helps determine whether open or closed questions are asked?
6. How can a closed question be helpful in giving a client limited choices of action?
7. What problems can arise when questions convey an expectation of the "correct" answer?
8. What problems are associated with asking "why?"
9. What kinds of questions contain value judgments?

☐ PERFORMANCE CHECKLIST

OBJECTIVE: To demonstrate the ability to use questions in a productive manner.						
EVALUATION OF SELF[a]		BEHAVIORS	EVALUATION BY PARTNER B[a]		EVALUATION BY OBSERVER[a]	
S	U		S	U	S	U
		1. Creates appropriate simulated open questions.				
		2. Creates appropriate simulated closed questions.				
		3. Listens attentively.				
		4. Recognizes own use of open and closed questions.				
		5. Chooses open or closed questions as relevant to the situation.				
		6. Uses attentive listening and productive attending behavior.				
		7. Needs strengthening in certain areas (specify).				

[a] S = Satisfactory; U = Unsatisfactory.

REFERENCES

Benjamin A: The Helping Interview, ed 3. Boston, Houghton Mifflin, 1981.

Garrett A: Interviewing: Its Principles and Methods, ed 2. New York, Family Service Association of America, 1972.

Hein EC: Communication in Nursing Practice, ed 2. Boston, Little, Brown, 1980.

Korsch BM: Practical techniques of observing, interviewing, and advising parents in pediatric practice as demonstrated in an attitude study project. Pediatrics 18(3):467–490, 1956.

Webster GC: Third New International Dictionary, Unabridged. Springfield, MA, G & C Merriam, 1976.

BIBLIOGRAPHY

Bernstein L, Bernstein RS, Dana RH: Interviewing: A Guide for Health Professionals, ed 3. New York, Appleton-Century-Crofts, 1980.

Brammer LM: The Helping Relationship: Process and Skills, ed 2. Englewood Cliffs, NJ, Prentice-Hall, 1979.

Carkhuff RR, Anthony WA: The Skills of Helping: An Introduction to Counseling. Amherst, MA, Human Resource Development Press, 1979.

Gerrard BA, Boniface WJ, Love BH: Interpersonal Skills for Health Professionals. Reston, VA, Reston, 1980.

Peplau HE: Talking with patients. American Journal of Nursing 60(7):962–966, 1960.

SKILL 14 Offering Assistance

Not what we give, but what we share, for the gift without the giver is bare.
—*James Russell Lowell, 1848*

☐ STUDENT OBJECTIVES

1. Distinguish between offering help to someone and doing for someone.
2. Illustrate individual and family needs for direct physical help, reassurance, and assistance with decision making.
3. Compare false and genuine reassurance.
4. Identify nursing behaviors that provide genuine reassurance.
5. Compare productive and nonproductive ways to give advice and help others make decisions.
6. Illustrate appropriate ways to offer direct physical help, reassurance, and assistance with decision making.
7. Identify your own patterns of offering assistance to others.
8. Develop the ability to offer direct physical help, reassurance, and assistance with decision making in appropriate and helpful ways.

☐ INTRODUCTION

To offer assistance is to offer help or aid to someone (Webster, 1976). A need for assistance of some sort is implied when a person assumes the role of client. Although Lewis (1978) indicates that few nurses ask questions that offer comfort and assistance, such as,

"May I help you?" or, "Can I help you?" the willingness and ability to offer assistance is implied when a person assumes the role of helper.

Offering assistance includes three components: direct physical help, reassurance, and assistance with decision making. *Direct physical help* is a common part of nursing care, because illness alters a person's ability to meet his or her own basic needs and carry out activities of daily living. *Reassurance* helps people gather their own inner resources to cope with their circumstances. Unfamiliar, uncomfortable, or painful experiences often occur in health-care institutions, and even the act of entering a hospital is threatening to an individual's self-concept and his or her feelings of physical and psychological safety. *Providing assistance with decision making* helps people resolve problems through exploring alternative courses of action, providing information, or making recommendations that are in their own best interests.

When offering assistance of any kind, the nurse first assesses the client's need for assistance and then determines the kind of assistance that would be of the greatest benefit and best used by that individual. There is a fine line between assistance that promotes independence and self-care and assistance that promotes excessive dependency. Giving assistance in ways that are productive for the individual helps the nurse develop and maintain a therapeutic nurse–client relationship and promotes client growth and independence.

☐ **PREPARATION**

PROVIDING DIRECT PHYSICAL HELP

Direct physical help refers to providing physical comfort and safety measures, helping meet basic physiological needs, and helping carry out activities of daily living. Much of a nurse's energy in a direct-care setting is focused on providing this kind of help. When nurses offer and provide help with basic needs and activities of daily living, they communicate to the client that they care enough both to notice and to help with personal needs. In addition, providing direct physical help promotes psychological comfort and safety.

The nurse often must make a judgment as to whether a client receives the most benefit from having the nurse provide direct physical help, being required to assist with the activity, or performing the activity independently. There are a number of circumstances in which it is appropriate to offer and provide direct physical help:

1. When the client is unable to do necessary activities for himself or herself, such as reaching for a drink, combing hair, navigating stairs, or using the bathroom
2. When doing the activity independently would cause the client to expend energies that should be reserved for more important activities; for example, a client should not bathe himself or herself if that activity causes him or her to be too tired for needed physical therapy
3. When the client is uncomfortable physically, for example, a client who is lying crumpled up in a wrinkled bed and is unable to reposition himself or herself
4. When the client is experiencing emotional distress and the energy for meeting basic needs is being diverted
5. When it is a simple act of kindness or courtesy, for example, pouring coffee at lunch or getting fresh water.

Direct physical help tends not to be appropriate if the goal is for the client to gain increased confidence, strength, and independence by performing the activity for himself or herself. For example, a client who has only partial use of one or both arms, as may occur after a stroke, will gain more benefit from self-feeding than from being fed. The process may be slow and messy, and the nurse probably would need to give some preparatory help and assist when fatigue develops.

Some people find it difficult to ask for or accept needed physical help, perhaps because of a strong sense of independence and self-sufficiency. These people tend to feel that they have failed themselves or others if they cannot take care of themselves independently. People who feel inadequate and have a low concept of self-worth may feel that they are not worthwhile enough for a nurse to want to help them. Other people may have difficulty accepting the invasion of their personal space and privacy that often accompanies direct physical help.

When a client requests help with an activity that he or she seems capable of performing unassisted, this is a cue for the nurse to consider what circumstances might be prompting that request. For example, there may be a new health problem causing increased fatigue or pain, an emotional upset may have reduced the client's ability to function, or the client may simply want someone near for comfort and reassurance. The request may be a manipulative attempt to control the nurse and the situation, so as to continue secondary gains from the illness or maintain nonproductive dependency levels. It also may mean that the client assumes that a given level of services is the norm for that agency. A careful assessment of the total situation will help the nurse determine whether meeting or refusing the present request for assistance has the most long-term benefit.

Offering Direct Physical Help
Direct physical help can be offered in ways that support and enhance a client's self-worth and independence, or in ways that are belittling and promote dependence. A client's self-worth is generally enhanced

when the nurse's offer of direct physical assistance is combined with the observation of that need for assistance, as in the following examples:

- "It looks as if it is difficult for you to get those shoes on—let me give you a hand."
- "You look uncomfortable—what could I do that would make you more comfortable?"
- "It looks like your pain is coming back—would you like some medication before it gets too severe?"

Sometimes the client only needs to have someone available if help is necessary. In this case the nurse could say something like, "I believe you'll be able to get out of bed alone today, but I will stay near and give you a hand if you need it."

When a client is temporarily dependent on nurses for physical care and would prefer not to be, it can be helpful to acknowledge those feelings along with the offer to help; for example, "I know you would rather be able to bathe yourself, but until you are stronger, I will help you." If the nurse's judgment indicates that the client needs physical assistance, it is preferable to offer help directly rather than asking if the client wants or needs help, since some people have great difficulty either in acknowledging the need for help or asking for it. Statements like, "Let me help you . . . ," "In what way can I help you with . . . ," or, "I will help you with . . . and you can take care of . . . " tend to be easy to accept and to promote self-worth, control, and decision making. On the other hand, statements like, "Do you want any help with . . . " or, "If you want me to . . . I will be glad to do it" require clients to ask for help directly, tend to force them into a dependent relationship, and may cause them to feel less good about themselves.

PROVIDING APPROPRIATE REASSURANCE

To reassure means to restore confidence and promote feelings of ease and comfort (Webster, 1976). Reassurance essentially is a subjective experience the client has in response to a helper's actions or statements. Although "give reassurance" is listed in care plans as a nursing intervention by both beginning and experienced nurses, reassurance cannot be *given* to someone else. Hein (1980) describes reassurance as a restorative concept—a provision of external sources of influence, confidence, and belief when clients are unable to provide these things for and within themselves.

The need for reassurance arises in a variety of situations, such as when clients

1. Need to talk (often indicated by frequent requests for services or through a direct request for the nurse to come and talk)
2. Need information the nurse can provide
3. Need services and information beyond what the nurse is able to provide
4. Are dependent on the nurse for taking care of their basic physical needs
5. Have experiences during which being alone intensifies feelings of pain, grief, or fear
6. Have experiences that are new or unfamiliar for the individual

Bernstein et al. (1980) and Garrett (1972) distinguish between *genuine reassurance* and *false reassurance*. They indicate that genuine reassurance conveys respect to clients as individuals, and helps them feel understood and more comfortable and safe in their situations. According to Gregg, clients feel reassured "when they are helped to use their own skills to work with problems that seem overwhelming at the outset. [Clients] probably feel reassured when someone is willing to listen and value them as persons, accepting what they say without condemning them for expressing what they feel" (1955, p. 173). Clients also feel reassured when they understand what is happening and are able to cope with their circumstances.

Genuine Reassurance

Genuine reassurance can be communicated in a variety of ways. Active listening and reflection of content and feelings are reassuring in that a person feels he or she has been heard. Correct information and explanations given at the time they are needed and by someone in whom the individual has confidence help a person feel he or she is being cared for or helped by knowledgeable persons.

Explanations are helpful and reassuring because the unknown generally is a greater source of anxiety than the known. Information about what is happening or is going to happen gives clients more control over themselves and the situation, and helps them to cope with whatever happens. In one study, the most critical aspect of medical care was poor explanations, while clear and adequate explanations decreased anxiety, put clients at ease, and indicated to them that the physician understood their illness and was able to help (Skipper, 1965).

Adequate information is less likely to result in the fantasy of expecting the worst. Out of a desire to avoid causing anxiety, health-care personnel sometimes minimize or omit information about the amount of pain or discomfort a specific procedure or test will cause. Nichols (1976) points out that this practice may increase anxiety, as people tend to feel more safe and secure (one of Maslow's basic needs) when they know what to anticipate and can psychologically prepare themselves. Similarly, when a nurse expects a client to do something or report observations, the instructions need to be clear and specific. For example, it is preferable for the nurse to say, "Call me if your arm should get sore or puffy where the IV needle is placed," rather than, "Call me if anything goes wrong with your IV."

When explanations about treatments or procedures are given in great detail or too far in advance of the actual event, the client may become more anxious. Assessment of a client's knowledge level and previous experiences should precede giving explanations, so that the explanation is appropriate for that person. For example, the nurse may ask, "What have you been told about preparation for this test?" or, "Have you ever had this test done before?" Or the nurse may inquire as to what the client would like to know about a situation; for example, "You are having a glucose tolerance test done today. Is there anything you would like for me to explain about that test?" Sometimes people ask for information the nurse does not have. When this happens, it is best to be honest and say, "I don't know, but I will find out," or, "I don't know very much about that, but Ms. Jones is quite knowledgeable about that. I will ask her to come talk with you."

Technical competence in using equipment and skill in performing nursing care are reassuring for an ill person, since this conveys the message that the person is in safe hands. The actual *presence of the nurse* can be very reassuring in difficult or unfamiliar experiences, such as during labor, preoperative waiting time, or examinations done by a physician or another nurse. Sometimes simply staying with the client is helpful. For example, a newly diagnosed diabetic found it reassuring to have someone sit with her while experiencing her first insulin reaction as she waited for the laboratory to draw a blood specimen to determine her blood sugar level before she drank the orange juice to relieve her symptoms.

Setting limits, that is, defining parameters of activity and behavior, can be reassuring. This can range from establishing activity levels for a client with a recent heart attack to maintaining a nurse–client relationship at a professional level rather than allowing it to become a social one.

Helping clients mobilize their own resources and strengths increases the ability to manage their own affairs and cope with their own situation and thus is reassuring. The nurse needs to be alert to whatever strengths clients already possess, such as a supportive family, a determination to get well, or the ability to handle difficult situations. Family, friends, or church groups can help clients gain their inner coping strengths. Self-help groups such as Recovery, Inc., Alcoholics Anonymous, Reach for Recovery, and Parents Without Partners provide support and help develop the ability to cope with specific problems.

Appropriate referrals to other agencies or to persons with special training and knowledge can be quite reassuring to a client, as this indicates that the nurse knows his or her own capabilities and limits, and also knows how to augment his or her skills by using appropriate resources. For example, the community health nurse cannot provide food stamps, welfare, or rehabilitation services, but he or she does know community resources well enough to make helpful referrals.

False Reassurance

Bernstein et al. (1980) indicate that much of what health-care professionals do in the name of reassurance actually is false reassurance, and serves to protect and reassure the professional rather than the client. Hein (1980) indicates that false reassurance denies the existence of a client's capabilities, feelings, and problems, as well as his or her right to overcome those problems. She also describes false reassurance as an undeliverable promise and guarantee initiated by and for the benefit of the nurse. Health-care professionals tend to be uncomfortable with clients' anxiety and attempt to keep that anxiety under control by using false and superficial statements such as, "Let us do the worrying—you just lie there and get well!" Statements like this do not provide reassurance; rather, they deny the reality and urgency of the client's concerns and help the nurse avoid dealing with his or her own discomfort or with the client's concerns. Some health-care professionals use false and superficial reassurance to avoid arousing concern. However, it is a safe assumption that when a client brings up a subject or raises questions, he or she already is concerned and wants and needs information.

False reassurance is communicated in a variety of ways. Health-care professionals sometimes avoid dealing with the reality of a situation through *misrepresentation* or outright false statements, supposedly to gain cooperation or avoid causing worry. For example, children sometimes are told that an injection will not hurt, when obviously it will and does. This betrayal by supposedly trustworthy adults results in suspicion, lack of trust, and unwillingness to cooperate during future encounters with a physician or nurse. Sometimes when a hospitalized client dies, others on the unit are told that he or she was transferred. If the lie is discovered, the nurse's credibility is damaged.

Nurses sometimes avoid dealing with the anxiety or concerns of both clients and families by denying the reality of those concerns and responding with *trite platitudes and clichés,* such as, "I am sure everything will be all right"; "Your doctor knows what is best for you"; or "Don't cross your bridges before you come to them." Responses such as these indicate superficial recognition and minimal understanding of the situation and offer empty consolation.

Another way to avoid dealing with clients' concerns and give false reassurance is to *change the subject* rather than discussing something that is uncomfortable for the nurse. For example, sex and death are subjects with which nurses are most often uncomfortable (Bernstein et al., 1980). However, talking about and dealing with painful subjects usually alleviates anxiety and increases coping ability. Changing the subject delays this process and prolongs the anxiety. An example of changing the subject occurred when a middle-aged woman asked the nurse, "What is wrong with me? Do I have cancer?" The nurse hesitated and replied, "Let me fix your pillows for you so you will be more comfortable."

Some statements that are meant to be reassuring actually *belittle the feelings* a client is expressing. These statements equate or associate a given feeling with the feelings of other people and substitute being told how to feel for an acknowledgment of what is felt.

Examples of these kinds of statements include, "You don't need to feel anxious about . . ."; "Everyone feels like that"; and "You should be grateful it is not more serious."

A major problem with false reassurance is the denial it involves. By not dealing directly with client concerns, the health-care professional behaves as if the problem does not exist and also ignores the client's feelings about the problem. False reassurance may give the message that a subject is taboo or trivial, or that the client is incapable of understanding or coping with the situation. When clients experience such lack of responsiveness from the health-care professional, their anxiety levels are raised and they begin to wonder, "Why won't anyone answer me? What is wrong with me?"

False reassurance has a negative impact on clients and nurses alike. It usually causes the client to doubt that the nurse really understands the situation or is able to help; and it does not change the situation, the client's perception of it, or the client's ability to cope with it. False reassurance neither reassures the client nor gives the nurse the satisfaction that comes with giving genuine reassurance. Both persons are cheated out of meaningful human to human interactions. The following situation is an example of denying reality and avoiding dealing with it: Three members of a family were injured seriously in an automobile accident and were admitted to an intensive care unit. The father and teenage son did not survive, and the mother remained in the hospital for a long time. Because of her injuries, the staff did not tell her that her husband and son had died. Rather, they answered questions and requests to see the husband and son with comments such as, "Don't worry about them right now—just concentrate on getting well" and, "They can't come see you now." Although the nurses alternately charted "cheerful" and "crying" and reported that she was "holding up well under the circumstances," no one would talk openly with the woman about her concerns because they did not want to upset her. Through the nurses' denial and avoidance, the woman was deprived of human comfort and caring, and the nurses were deprived of the experience of providing that comfort and caring.

The following activity focuses on identifying the characteristics of genuine and false reassurance.

Activity 14-A: Genuine and False Reassurance

Work independently, within small groups.

1. *Receiving reassurance*
    a. Recall a situation in which you received reassurance that you recognized as genuine. What actions, statements, or circumstances helped you to know that the reassurance was genuine?
    b. Recall a situation in which you received reassurance that you perceived to be false, either then or later. What actions, statements, or circumstances helped you to decide that the reassurance was false?
    c. Compare experiences of receiving genuine and false reassurance with others in your group.
2. *Giving reassurance*
    a. Recall a situation in which you gave genuine reassurance. What helped you to know or believe that the reassurance you gave was genuine?
    b. Recall a situation in which you gave reassurance that you either knew or later determined to be false. What helped you to become aware that the reassurance was false?
    c. Compare experiences of giving genuine and false reassurance with others in your group.

ASSISTING WITH DECISION MAKING

Because of their knowledge and role, nurses frequently are placed in a position of helping people make decisions or resolve problems about physical and psychosocial health-care problems. People sometimes approach the nurse directly and ask for help, or a physician may request that the nurse provide this kind of assistance. At other times, the nurse's professional judgment may prompt him or her to approach a person about making a decision that is in the best interests of that person's physical and psychosocial health, even though the person may or may not initially perceive the situation as a problem needing resolution.

Assistance with decision making may take the form of a problem-solving approach, providing information, disclosing one's own practices or beliefs, making referrals, or giving direct advice. It is important that the decision-making process promote the client's independence, self-reliance, and self-confidence, since this will increase the probability of a successful resolution that is acceptable to the client. Therefore, the nurse avoids being judgmental and imposing a resolution that is based on the nurse's own values, life style, or circumstances.

Problem Solving

A problem-solving approach to decision making involves both nurse and client working together, combining their knowledge and skills. The nurse provides the expertise of knowledge about health care and health promotion, and the client provides the expertise of his or her own health-care knowledge base, past experiences, capabilities, and motivation. A problem-solving approach to decision making begins with a thorough assessment of the individual's problem and his or her perception of that problem, plus some judgment about the individual's ability and willingness to assume responsibility for doing something about the problem. A thorough assessment helps the nurse avoid the risks of making suggestions too quickly without adequate information or suggesting something that the client has already found unsuccessful or that would be unacceptable.

One problem-solving approach is to *explore possible alternative solutions* to the problem. After determining the client's perception of the problem, the nurse next investigates what the client has already done in an attempt to resolve the situation, such as by asking, "What have you done so far to try to work this out?" or, "Have you found anything that worked before in this kind of situation?" Third, the nurse explores other ideas the client has thought of but has not tried, such as by asking, "What else had you thought of doing?" Fourth, the nurse clarifies his or her own perception of the client's intent or purpose in the situation, such as by asking, "As I understand it, what you hope to do is. . . . Is that correct?" *Now* the nurse may be ready to suggest additional alternatives, such as, "Had you thought of trying . . .?" "What would you think of . . .?" or, "Some people have found that. . . ." Or, the nurse may want to reinforce the client's own ideas, such as, "It sounds like that would be a workable plan for you. Let me know how it turns out." Very often the client expresses the same solution the helper intended to suggest, but if it is the client's own idea, it is more likely to be implemented successfully.

Another problem-solving approach involves *discussing available options and the probable outcomes* of each, leaving the client free to make the choice from those options. For example, an elderly man may be trying to decide whether to continue living at home, move to a retirement home, or go live with a relative. The nurse's role in this situation is to help him look at the likely results of each of the options open to him so that he can make the choice that is best for him. The nurse may want to role-play the proposed solution with the client as a way of exploring various outcomes and providing a simulated learning experience.

Providing Information

People often solicit information and recommendations from nurses and other health-care professionals about matters ranging from birth control, diet, child rearing, and nursing homes, to laxatives, vitamins, and suntan lotions. Specific information can sometimes help a person reach a goal he or she wishes to achieve. For example, a person may have a goal of losing weight and wants to do this by learning to eat balanced meals. The nurse can provide specific information about nutritional requirements, the four food groups, and nutritional content of foods that can help the person reach his or her goal.

Another way to give information that may influence decision making is to let individuals know the known risks and outcomes of what they are doing. In this situation, the nurse would first determine whether the individuals are aware of those risks and outcomes. If not, the nurse is responsible for providing that information. If the individuals already are aware of the risks and outcomes and choose not to act on that information, remember that the ultimate choice belongs to them, and accept and respect that choice. For example, when working with a client who has a positive family history for heart disease, eats and smokes excessively, and exercises inadequately, the nurse is responsible for pointing out the increased risk of developing heart disease. However, the *client* is responsible for choosing whether to change his or her life style; the nurse cannot make or enforce that decision for another person.

It is important to remember that a request for specific information may or may not reflect the total problem situation the client is facing, and it might not be the most important question he or she wants to ask. For example, the nurse would want to explore the nature and extent of the person's gastrointestinal disturbance before responding to the question about "the best laxative." If this is not done, the nurse might give inappropriate and unsafe information and recommendations that ignore the possibility of serious factors that contribute to constipation, such as cancer of the large bowel. In addition, the client's most urgent yet unspoken question might be, "Do I have cancer?" Therefore, although giving information can be quite helpful in making decisions, information always is preceded by and based on an assessment of the client's presenting problem, present situation, and past experiences.

Self-Disclosure

Another way to assist people in making decisions is through *self-disclosure,* that is, by sharing one's own and others' experiences and observations. For example: "I have found that regular meals with no snacking helps me keep from gaining weight"; "I have observed that when some people have this kind of discomfort, they find relaxation exercises are helpful"; or, "Some people report that a salt substitute tastes better if it is used during cooking rather than added afterward."

Referrals

Sometimes the best way to help resolve a problem or make a decision is to make a referral to a person or agency that has more expertise and resources in a particular area than does the nurse. For example, a nurse may suggest that a client discuss dietary problems with a dietitian; financial problems with a financial counselor; personal and emotional concerns with a social worker, psychiatrist, or psychologist; or spiritual concerns with a minister, priest, or rabbi. Clients should be consulted before making a referral to another person or agency. This consultation not only involves clients in decision making, but also demonstrates respect for their privacy and right of self-determination.

Follow-up on Decision Making

As much as possible, successful assistance with decision making includes a follow-up to determine the outcome for the client and to identify whether more assistance is needed. This follow-up and evaluation conveys caring and a continuing interest in the client. It also indicates that the nurse is willing to be flexible, adaptable, and helpful. Follow-up may be done on the next contact the nurse has with the client, such as when providing care the following day, on a return visit to a clinic, through a home visit, or by a telephone call. For example, a clinic nurse might say, "The last time we talked together, you were planning to.... How has that worked for you?" A referral to a home-care agency can provide needed follow-up to determine the outcome of the client's decision and actions.

Sometimes people make choices that have negative results, such as a person who continues to smoke and eventually develops emphysema and respiratory problems. In these circumstances, it is more helpful for the nurse to continue to be supportive in helping the person deal with his or her current situation than it is to blame and criticize for not having made other choices.

Giving Advice
There are times when the nurse offers direct advice, makes specific recommendations, or gives instructions about a course of action that the nurse knows are in the best interests of the client's health status.

Direct advice is used to make recommendations to someone; it focuses on what the person can or should do or not do. For example, a nurse gives direct advice when instructing clients about how to take medications or under what circumstances to call the physician or nurse. Clients will require more specific and direct advice about health-care activities when they are not highly motivated to act in their own best interests or when they are unable to make appropriate judgments.

Nurses may offer direct yet unsolicited advice and recommendations when they believe their experiences or expertise would help the client meet his or her needs. For example, the nurse may determine that a client has a need for certain information, is doing something harmful to self or others, or needs help in making decisions and following through on a course of action. However, even when the nurse gives direct advice, the ultimate decision about a course of action should be left to the client, since advice ought not be coercive or take charge of the decision-making process. Taking over decision making for another person generally is appropriate only for people who are too old, too young, or too sick (emotionally or physically) to make decisions.

According to Sundeen et al. (1981) giving advice frequently becomes a judgmental technique and implies that the recipient has an inferior status and is unable to direct himself or herself. Advice becomes dictatorial when it conveys the message that the giver of the advice has the only possible solution. Although it is particularly tempting to give direct advice when people openly seek that advice, the nurse will want to be cautious about assuming responsibility for other people's decisions. Some people consciously or unconsciously prefer to avoid responsibility for their own actions, choosing instead to have someone else make decisions or tell them what to do. This allows them to place the responsibility for the outcome of the advice on the person who gave the advice, rather than assuming that responsibility themselves.

Nonproductive ways to give advice often include "should," "ought," or "you have to," and reflect the values, beliefs, and biases of the advice-giver. These admonitions tend to be dictatorial because they are external sources of direction for the person rather than internal messages of self-direction. Self-directed decisions are more productive because they tend to be acted upon more reliably and consistently than decisions proposed or imposed by others.

Brammer (1979) suggests that the most productive way to respond to a request for advice is first to reflect and clarify the feelings involved in the request and then to decide how to respond to the request itself. Sometimes the best advice in a situation is to take no new or additional action, but simply to wait and allow time to help resolve the problem. For example, sometimes people expect to be back to normal within a few weeks after surgery and become impatient and discouraged when they are not. Or, a widow may not expect the symptoms of grief to last beyond a few months. In actuality, a complete physiological and psychological healing process takes much longer, and a return to health may take up to a year. These people need to be reminded to be more patient with themselves and allow more time to regain their usual strength and energy.

The following activity focuses on the experience of giving and receiving advice, both solicited and unsolicited.

Activity 14-B: Experiences with Giving Advice

Work in small groups.

1. Recall situations in which you have received both solicited and unsolicited advice. Write down the specific statements that were made and recall the nonverbal behaviors that accompanied the advice. What reactions to the advice do you recall having?
2. Recall situations in which you gave both solicited and unsolicited advice. Write down the specific statements you used. Was your advice followed? If it was followed, did you receive either credit or blame? If it was not followed, what were the reasons?
3. Compare your experiences of giving and receiving advice with the others in your group.

☐ EXECUTION

Giving assistance in helpful ways requires that the helper possess the ability to (1) be sensitive to others' needs, (2) observe others' verbal and nonverbal behaviors, and (3) use productive communication skills.

There are many circumstances in which nurses are expected to give assistance as part of their professional role. The way this is done can enhance the client's self-confidence and self-worth, promote independence, and contribute to the development of a positive nurse–client relationship. However, the reverse is also true, and assistance can have a negative impact on the client.

We can increase our ability to provide reassurance and assist in making decisions through observing how others do these things and by paying attention to our own reactions to the reassurance and decision-making assistance others give to us. As we observe others offering and providing direct physical help, we can note the ways clients respond to the different approaches of various health-care personnel. After making these observations, we can decide whether we want to modify our own approaches to offering and providing direct physical help, providing reassurance, and assisting with decision making.

The following activities focus on the experiences of reassurance and assisting with decision making.

Activity 14-C:
Simulation of Reassurance and Assisting with Decision Making

In a group setting, observe simulated live or videotaped examples of first nonproductive and then productive ways of providing reassurance and helping others to make decisions. Discuss the characteristics that distinguished the two approaches. Which statements or actions would you most likely find reassuring, and for what reasons? If you were the person receiving the help in decision making, which approach or advice would you be most likely to follow, and for what reasons? What feelings were communicated by the participants in these simulations?

Activity 14-D:
Experiencing Reassurance and Assistance with Decision Making

Work in pairs.
1. *Nonproductive reassurance and help with decision making*
   a. Role-play two situations: one that requires providing reassurance and one that requires help with decision making. Partner A offers nonproductive reassurance and advice to partner B, using situations such as those listed in b and c.
   b. Suggested situations for giving reassurance:
      - A student who is anxious about passing tomorrow's examination
      - A student who may not have enough money to return to school next year
      - A friend whose mother has just been diagnosed as having breast cancer
      - A friend who has just broken up with a boyfriend or girlfriend
   c. Suggested situations for helping with decision making or giving advice:
      - A school counselor recommending a course of study or career choice
      - A mother advising her teenage daughter on clothing and hairstyles
   d. Partner B: Did you feel reassured? Why or why not? Did you feel like accepting the suggestions partner A gave you? Why or why not?
   e. Reverse roles and repeat the exercise.
2. *Productive reassurance and help with decision making*
   a. Role-play two more situations with partner B providing productive reassurance and advice to partner A.
   b. Partner A: Did you feel reassured? Why or why not? Did you feel like accepting the suggestions partner B gave you? Why or why not?
   c. Use the relevant sections of the Performance Checklist, p. 105, to evaluate your skill in providing reassurance and helping others make decisions.
   d. Reverse roles and repeat the exercise.
3. Compare your reactions with your partner's reactions to providing and receiving productive and nonproductive reassurance and decision-making help.

BEFORE THE NEXT SKILL

In everyday situations, practice intentionally using approaches that provide genuine rather than false reassurance, helpful rather than nonhelpful assistance with decision making, and (if relevant) direct physical care that increases self-worth and coping ability. When involved in direct nurse–client interactions, use the Performance Checklist, p. 105, to evaluate the characteristics of the direct physical help, reassurance, and assistance with decision making that you provide for clients in any setting.

☐ CRITICAL POINTS SUMMARY

1. Direct physical assistance is offered in response to observed need or requests for help in carrying out activities of daily living or meeting basic needs.
2. The nurse distinguishes when direct physical help should be offered, not offered, or refused.
3. Feelings about receiving help need to be recognized and acknowledged.
4. Genuine reassurance promotes physical and psychological safety, comfort, understanding of the situation, and increased sense of self-worth and ability to cope.

5. Genuine reassurance is conveyed through attentive listening, reflection of content and feeling, providing correct information, technical competence, physical presence of the nurse, setting limits, and by helping people mobilize their own resources.
6. False reassurance essentially is a denial of the existence of a problem or any feelings associated with it.
7. False reassurance is conveyed through misrepresentation, using clichés, changing the subject, belittling, and avoidance.
8. Assistance with decision making includes solving problems, providing information, self-disclosure, making referrals, and giving direct advice.
9. Follow-up on decision making conveys caring and serves to evaluate the outcome.
10. Giving advice carries the risks of being too hasty, being inappropriate, promoting dependency, being judgmental, and assuming responsibility for someone else's behavior.
11. Assisting with decision making and giving advice should be preceded by learning about the situation, investigating what has been done, and determining what ideas the person may have.

☐ REVIEW QUESTIONS

1. On what basis would the nurse decide to offer, not offer, or refuse to provide direct physical help?
2. How can the nurse use direct physical help to enhance a client's self-esteem?
3. How might the nurse diminish an individual's sense of self-worth when offering direct physical help?
4. What is your understanding of the differences between genuine and false reassurance?
5. Under what circumstances have you known or observed false reassurance to occur?
6. How is reassurance related to basic psychological needs?
7. What does this statement mean to you? "Reassurance is much more a subjective experience of the client than activities performed by the nurse."
8. What problems are associated with false reassurance?
9. In what ways might the nurse provide reassurance for these persons:
    A man waiting for a diagnostic x-ray
    A family whose child is ill
    A critically injured teenager
    A demanding, worried middle-aged woman
    An elderly woman who lives alone
    A child receiving an unwanted injection
10. In what way is problem solving with someone else a productive way to help make decisions?
11. What can the nurse do to decrease the probability of giving inappropriate or hasty advice, and help with decision making?
12. How is productive assistance with decision making different from giving advice that promotes dependency?

☐ PERFORMANCE CHECKLIST

OBJECTIVE: To demonstrate the ability to offer assistance by offering and providing direct physical help, reassurance, and assistance with decision making.			
CHARACTERISTIC	RANGE OF ACCEPTABILITY	SATISFACTORY	UNSATISFACTORY
1. Recognizes need to offer direct physical help.	No deviation		
2. Offers direct physical help in a way that promotes the client's self-worth and ability to cope.	No deviation		
3. Acknowledges client's feelings about receiving help.	No deviation		
4. Recognizes client's need for reassurance.	No deviation		
5. Communicates genuine reassurance verbally and nonverbally.	No deviation		
6. Recognizes situations where assistance with decision making or advice is needed (give specific illustrative examples).	No deviation		
7. Provides helpful, productive decision-making assistance or advice that supports and utilizes client strengths and resources.	No deviation		

REFERENCES

Bernstein L, Bernstein RS, Dana RH: Interviewing: A Guide for Health Professionals, ed 3. New York, Appleton-Century-Crofts, 1980.

Brammer LM: The Helping Relationship, ed 2. Englewood Cliffs, NJ, Prentice-Hall, 1979.

Garrett A: Interviewing: Its Principles and Methods, ed 2. New York, Family Service Association of America, 1972.

Gregg D: Reassurance. American Journal of Nursing 55(2):171–174, 1955.

Hein EC: Communication in Nursing Practice, ed 2. Boston, Little, Brown, 1980.

Lewis GK: Nurse–Patient Communication. Dubuque, IA, WC Brown, 1978.

Nichols KA: Talking point: A reason to worry. Nursing Times 72(51):1990–1991, 1976.

Skipper JK: Communication and the hospitalized patient. In Skipper JK, Leonard RC (eds): Social Interaction and Patient Care. Philadelphia, JB Lippincott, 1965.

Sundeen SJ, Stuart GW, et al: Nurse–Client Interaction: Implementing the Nursing Process, ed 2. St Louis, MO, CV Mosby, 1981.

Webster GC: Third New International Dictionary, Unabridged. Springfield, MA, G & C Merriam, 1976.

4 Structured Nurse–Client Interactions

☐ **INTRODUCTION**

In this chapter, the student has the opportunity to integrate and apply all of the previously learned communication skills within the context of interviewing and teaching–learning. The interview is an important method of collecting subjective data for the assessment phase of the nursing process, and the teaching–learning process has many similarities to the nursing process. Both activities require the use of quite complex and well-developed communication skills.

The nursing process is a problem-solving method that is similar to the scientific method and is used to provide a systematic framework for nursing practice. It is a cyclical process of assessment, planning, intervention, and evaluation. The *assessment* phase usually includes collection of subjective and objective data as well as identification of a nursing diagnosis or nursing problem statement based on those data. Subjective data refer to information provided by the client about himself or herself. Objective data are information derived from the health record and from appraisal of the client's status. *Planning* includes determination of long-term goals and short-term objectives and identification of interventions that have the potential for meeting those goals and objectives and resolving the nursing problem. *Interventions* should be specific and selected for the individual client. In the intervention phase, the nurse actually carries out the planned activities.

Evaluation involves determining whether the interventions were successful in meeting the goals and objectives and resolving the problem. After comparing present data with the original data, the nurse determines whether the desired result has been achieved, if alternate interventions would be appropriate, or if more data need to be gathered, a different diagnosis made, or the goals reconsidered. As much as possible, each phase of the nursing process is a joint and collaborative effort between the nurse and the client, since client participation has a positive effect on the relevance and success of the intervention.

Careful assessment is a crucial aspect of the nursing process, since incomplete or inaccurate assessment can lead the nurse to an incorrect nursing diagnosis and result in inappropriate goals and interventions. The *assessment interview* is a systematic method of gathering desired data about the client, often based on an assessment guide. Because the initial contact between the client and the nurse most commonly is focused on assessment, the skill of interviewing as presented here is directed primarily toward assessment. Because of the exploratory nature of an assessment interview, *problem identification and clarification* is often an integral aspect of this interview process. The interviewing principles and guidelines presented here are not restricted to assessment interviews but may be applied to any type of interview setting or purpose. Whether the primary focus of the interview is assessment or intervention, the nurse's interviewing skills have a distinctly therapeutic or nontherapeutic effect on the nurse–client relationship.

Teaching–learning activities may be directed toward both individuals and groups and may be formal or informal in nature. A teaching–learning plan often is developed to meet the client's needs and concerns that have been identified through the assessment interview. The medical diagnosis, plan of care, and client's function also may determine the nature and scope of planned teaching. Regardless of the reason teaching is initiated, the teaching–learning process (client education) is an integral aspect of all nursing, medical, and health care. The nurse's role in client education may be that of actual teaching or it may be that of coordinating the teaching activities of various members of the health-care team. In an institutional setting, some nurses may focus primarily on client education, whereas others provide direct care or supervision; *both* teaching and direct care, however, are essential aspects of total client care and are not separate entities.

Skills used in interviewing are essential for the teaching–learning process, because they enable the nurse to assess a client's learning needs and they also serve as guidelines for the nurse during the actual nurse–client exchanges involved in teaching and responding to client comments and concerns.

As nurses assume more independent functions and greater responsibilities in a wide variety of settings, the ability to interview and teach successfully becomes more crucial. The professionally accountable nurse knows how to gather and use data for planning, implementing, and evaluating the care provided to any client. The professional nurse also is expected to be able to use interviewing and teaching skills as therapeutic interventions to promote client growth and change.

This chapter discusses the skills of "Interviewing" (Skill 15) and "Teaching–Learning" (Skill 16).

SKILL 15 Interviewing

Interviewing is an art, a skilled technique that . . . might be called professional conversation.
—Garrett, p. 5

☐ STUDENT OBJECTIVES

1. Explain the purposes and uses of interviewing in a health-care setting.
2. Describe the preparation needed for conducting the interview.
3. Identify guidelines for conducting an interview.
4. Discuss the relationship of communication skills to interviewing.
5. Identify factors that hinder or promote successful interviewing.
6. Identify ways of dealing with recurrent themes, contradictions, and distress during an interview.
7. Identify guidelines for using printed forms and taking notes in interviews.
8. Develop the ability to gather needed information through interviewing.
9. Integrate previously learned communication skills into the process of interviewing.
10. Demonstrate the ability to prepare for and conduct an assessment interview in a simulated setting.
11. Apply guidelines for interviewing during simulated and real interviews.
12. Examine your own techniques of interviewing and interactions with clients.

☐ INTRODUCTION

An interview is a purposeful and structured interaction between two or more persons, with each party actively and intentionally involved in the process. It is an art that is based on sound principles and combines a knowledge of human behavior with warmth, understanding, and caring. More than an exchange of questions and answers, interviewing is a skilled communication technique that is sometimes called professional conversation (Garrett, 1972). Bernstein and Bernstein (1980, p. 24), regard the interview as "the major vehicle for conducting the relationship between the health professional and the client."

Every nurse–client interaction has some aspects of an interview, but not all interactions are interviews. A nurse is most likely to use an interview for assessment and problem-identification purposes, that is, to gather information as a basis for nursing interventions and to assist the client in identifying and clarifying problems. The nurse may also use the interview as a framework for helping clients resolve problems or to offer assistance. Interviews may be initiated either by the client seeking help or by the nurse seeking information, offering assistance, or both. Many agencies require that each newly admitted client be interviewed to determine his or her usual ways of meeting basic needs, managing activities of daily living, strengths, and actual or potential problem areas. Some agencies have specific forms for recording this assessment data and identified problems, such as the Admitting Nursing Assessment form shown in Figure 15-1. This form was developed for the above purposes by nurses in one hospital. The forms are completed by a registered nurse within 48 hours of admission, are used as a basis for planning nursing care, and become a part of the permanent record. An additional assessment form (not shown here) completed by the nursing assistant contains information about vital signs, possessions brought to the hospital, allergies, and routine admission data.

This skill focuses on interviewing for assessment and problem-identification purposes. It is not intended to prepare the nurse for using what is known as a therapeutic interview for resolving interpersonal or mental health problems, since that type of inter-

FOR USE IN PLANNING NURSING CARE. NOT INTENDED TO REPLACE MEDICAL HISTORY AND PHYSICAL.

A. NURSING ADMITTING HISTORY
1. Reason for hospitalization __Blood in urine__
2. Chief complaint __Blood in urine__
3. General observations: Alert ✓ Stuporous___ Drowsy___ Coma___ Other___
4. Past medical history:
   a. Medical __Good health – arthritis__
   b. Surgical __Prostatectomy, Supra-pubic 25 years ago. Cataract surgery__
   c. Past education or instruction: Diabetes___ Cardiac Rehab.___ Ostomy___ Pulmonary Rehab.___ Other ✓
   d. Activities of normal daily living: Check appropriate level.
      I - Independent   A - Assistance Needed   C - Complete dependence
      Bathing _I_ Hygiene _I_ Eating _I_ Mouth Care _I_ Dressing _I_ Locomotion _I_
   e. Allergies or sensitivities: Include type of reaction.
      (1) Medications __Codeine__
      (2) Food __None__
      (3) Allergy band on: Yes ✓
   f. Medications (Include anticoagulants, hormones, thyroid and hypoglycemics): Those taken at home __Thorazine 50 mg. h.s. daily__
5. Family history: Diabetes - Hypertension - Cancer - Heart - T.B. - Anemia - Sickle cell disease/Trait - Other __Cancer – mother and sister__
6. Habits:
   Smokes: Yes___ No ✓ How much ___
   Alcoholic drinks: Yes___ No ✓ How much ___
   Exercise: Yes ✓ No___ How much __Plays Golf 2X week__
   Sleep: # Hours _8_ Normal bedtime _10 P_ Sleep aids (meds, radio, etc.) __Thorazine 50 mg.__
   Dietary: Special diet __Regular Diet__ Likes __Most foods__
   Dislikes ___ Daily fluid intake __2 quarts__
7. Psycho-social history:
   a. Expectation of this hospitalization __Have cysto exam and go to Florida.__
   b. Behavior indicative of mental/emotional status:
      Alert ✓   Cooperative ✓   Flat affect ___   Sad ___
      Anxious ✓   Demanding ___   Guarded ___   Talkative ✓
      Apprehensive ✓ Depressed ___   Hyperactive ___   Trustful ___
      Calm ___   Distrustful ___   Mentally slow ___   Withdrawn ___
      Other ___
   c. Occupation: Present ___ Past __Dentist__ Working Hours __Retired__
   d. Special interests and hobbies ___
8. Safety factors:
   Over 65 ✓   Hx of falls ___   Nocturia ___
   Language barrier ___ Obese ✓   Incontinent ___
   Senile ___   Smokes ___   X-ray prep. ___
   Confused ___   Dec. sensation ___   Sleeping pills ___
   Mentally retarded ___ Loss of balance ___ Anticoagulants/Cuts ___
   Emotional instability ✓ Seizures ___   Allergy ✓
   Overly independent ___ (Vision)/hearing prob. ✓ Hypotension ___
9. Discharge planning:
   a. # of children _2_ Age range _45 – 49_ Role in family __Husband__ # in household _2_
   b. Plan for discharge (Independent)/need assistance). If assistance needed, send social service consult (date ___)
   Date __1-2-81__ Time __2:15 p.m.__ Signature __L. Brown R.N.__
Informant if other than patient ___

Winona Memorial Hospital
3232 North Meridian Street
Indianapolis, Indiana 46208
07-03390-7

JACOB SCHLONEGAR   406-W
592-00-8130   59890
ANDREW MC CLARENDEN, M.D.
FREDERICK JONES, M.D.
9/11/18   06/30/84

17-K

ADMITTING NURSING ASSESSMENT

Figure 15–1. Admitting Nursing Assessment. **A.** Nursing Admitting History. (Courtesy of Winona Memorial Hospital, Indianapolis, IN.)

view requires more complex skills and theoretical knowledge about psychiatric–mental health problems and is beyond the scope of this text. Nevertheless, any interaction or interview can have either a positive or negative impact on the client insofar as it engages or disengages that client in the relationship with the nurse. In that sense, any interview can be therapeutic or nontherapeutic, and the way the nurse gathers information helps or hinders the development and maintenance of the helping relationship.

B. NURSING HISTORY
(Circle = + response)

1. INTEGUMENTARY
(Do you have or have you had problems with?)
1. Eczema
2. Psoriasis
3. Dry - Oily skin

Comments: Pt denies any problems

NURSING OBSERVATION/ASSESSMENT
1. General hygiene: good
2. Problems: None noted
3. Hydration: Good
Skin turgor firm
Mucous membranes pink
Comments: Intact skin

2. SENSORY
(Do you have or have you had problems with?)
1. Ears: (Hard of hearing) (R/L)
Dizziness, ringing in ears
2. Eyes: (Vision) (R/L)
Blurring, spots, double vision
3. Nose: Bleeding, post-nasal drip, obstruction

OBSERVATION/ASSESSMENT
1. Ears Bilateral Hearing Aids
2. Eyes Bilateral Cataract soft lenses and glasses
3. Nose Deviated septum
Comments:

3. CARDIOVASCULAR - RESPIRATORY
(Do you have or have you had?)
1. Heart disease No
2. Chest pain (describe) No
3. Hypertension, Phlebitis
4. S.O.B. (exert/non-exert) #Pillows
5. Lung disease
6. Colds - frequent (infrequent)
7. Chronic cough Yes (No)
If yes, describe

Comments:

OBSERVATION/ASSESSMENT
1. Pulse - Radial rate 84 Regularity Reg. Quality Strong
Other
2. Extremities - Edema None
Color Rosy - Pink Warm/Cold W
Comments: No cardiac symptoms
3. Respirations - Rate 16 Depth deep Pattern Regular
If abnormalities in above, assess breath sounds & describe.
Comments: No resp. problems noted.

4. GASTROINTESTINAL
(Do you have or have you had?)
1. Problems with: Swallowing, heartburn/indigestion, Hiatal hernia, N&V, gas, abd. pain, recent wt. gain/loss, constipation, diarrhea, abnormal stool color, rectal pain/bleeding, distention

Comments: Denies any problems

OBSERVATION/ASSESSMENT
1. If problems, describe: None
2. Bowel habits: Last B.M. today Normal freq. q.d.
Time of day a.m. Aids (laxatives, fluids, etc.) none

5. GENITOURINARY
(Do you have or have you had?)
1. Problems with frequency (day x____, night X___)
Urgency, pain, burning, difficulty starting stream, incontinence, (retention) (bloody urine) infection, prostate problems
2. Breasts - Lumps R/L, Drainage, pain, tenderness
Breasts: Self exam Yes/No
Do you desire instruction? Yes/No
3. Menses: L.M.P. NA Interval NA

Comments:
Last pap test NA
Vaginal discharge, itching

OBSERVATION/ASSESSMENT
1. If problems, describe:
Cysto 1/30/81
Had supra-pubic prostatectomy 25 years ago

6. MUSCULOSKELETAL - NEUROLOGICAL
(Do you have or have you had?)
1. Problems with: (Joint pain) or swelling, aches, muscle cramps, (numbness) tremors, seizures, weakness, paralysis, fractures, amputations.
Dizziness/Loss of balance. Fainting/Blackout spells.

Comments:

OBSERVATION/ASSESSMENT
1. If problems, describe: arthritis
2. (R)/L handed
3. Gait: Not observed, (normal) abnormal. Describe:
normal for age

Date 1/29/81 Time 2 45 p Signature L. Brown, R.N.

Informant if other than patient

07-03390-7

Figure 15–1. ***B.*** *Nursing History. (Courtesy of Winona Memorial Hospital, Indianapolis, IN.)*

□ PREPARATION

Most people have been interviewed at some time, such as when applying for a job or to enroll in school, and most have also sought information from other people in either structured or unstructured ways. Looking at those experiences can help identify factors that contribute to successful or unsuccessful interviewing.

The following activity examines past experiences with interviewing and being interviewed.

Activity 15-A:
Experiences with Interviewing

Recall situations in which you were being interviewed, such as for a job, school, or a scholarship. Mentally reconstruct the physical environment in which the interview took place. Recall the placement of the interviewer in relation to yourself. Describe the interviewer's manner and approach to you. In what ways did the interviewer contribute to your feeling either at ease or uncomfortable before, during, and after the interview? How similar were your expectations of the interview with those of the interviewer?

What helpful and nonhelpful interview techniques and principles did your interviewer use? What aspects of your experience with interviewing have relevance for interviewing clients in a health-care setting?

A basic purpose of most interviews is to collect data for the initial phase of the nursing process. The focus of the interview may be broad or narrow, depending on how recently the client has entered the health-care system and on the type of data being collected. If the purpose of the interview is to make an initial assessment, it will be more intensive and comprehensive than if the purpose is to explore a specific problem or the functioning of a given body organ system. A complete initial assessment interview or nursing history is usually conducted by the staff nurse soon after the client is admitted, by the visiting nurse on an initial visit to a client's home, or by the clinic nurse on a client's first clinical appointment. This initial assessment interview usually includes past and current health status, daily living habits and activities, functional status of the various body organ systems, and the client's perception of his or her health problems. If the client is in acute distress, either emotionally or physically, the initial interview must be much shorter, focusing on the immediate problem and gathering enough minimal data for providing safe initial care. After the crisis situation has been addressed, the nurse can conduct a more extensive interview.

Interviews are often modified and focused selectively on a specific health or illness problem, body organ system, or client population. For example, the initial assessment interview for obstetric clients will of necessity be different than that done for adult medical-surgical clients. Similarly, clients with heart disease will need to be interviewed in more depth about their cardiovascular system's function than about their motor ability. In a pediatric unit, an assessment interview will include gathering data about the child's developmental level as well as physical status.

During the process of gathering data in an assessment interview, the nurse frequently identifies problems that need to be explored more completely. By using communication skills such as listening, questioning, reflecting, and validating, the nurse can clarify the nature of the problem as a natural part of the assessment interview. Throughout the interview, the focus may shift back and forth between data gathering and problem clarification. For example, while the nurse is gathering data about the gastrointestinal system during an initial assessment interview, the client may indicate that he or she has problems with constipation. Rather than simply making a note of that fact and continuing to gather other information, the nurse would take the time to elicit additional data about that specific problem. These data might include food and fluid consumption, activity, life style, or use of laxatives. Exploration and clarification of a problem area helps the nurse make an initial nursing diagnosis and at a later time discuss with the client what might contribute to constipation and what the client might do to alleviate it.

Rather than simply making casual observations during direct care, it is important to learn how to gather data about a client's functional status in a systematic manner and also how to judge what type of data to gather. A sound theoretical basis from medical, nursing, behavioral, and social sciences helps the nurse determine this. A variety of guides and frameworks are used to structure and organize collection of these data. One framework is presented in Figure 15-2. It was developed by P. H. Mitchell and based on earlier authors' works (McCain, 1965; McPhetridge, 1968; D. Smith, 1968) and her own clinical experiences (Mitchell and Loustau, 1981). The assessment guide is divided into 13 areas for assessment of the client's ability to function. The first three areas for assessment focus on the client's psychosocial, mental, emotional, and environmental health status. The remaining ten areas serve as guides for assessing a client's physiological health status.

When the nurse is beginning to learn how to assess a client's functional abilities, he or she needs to collect complete information about each area of functional status. This helps the nurse to become familiar with the scope of data that can be gathered about any given functional area. Once the nurse is competent in eliciting the broad scope of data that are pertinent to each functional area, he or she can then become selective in the interview process and focus only on those functional areas that have the highest priority at the moment.

PREPARATION FOR THE INTERVIEW

Whenever possible, it is helpful to do some preparation before interviewing, regardless of who initiates the interview.

First, *become familiar with what is known about the client.* When the nurse knows something about the client—especially something as basic as the client's name—it helps build a relationship. It is frustrating to

Data Which May Be Collected in Each Assessment Area*

I. *Psychosocial Status.* This area deals with the person's roles in relationship to others—family, work group, health professionals. If the nurse is attempting to diagnose the problems of a group of persons, this area would include the social relationships within that group—patterns of leadership, methods of resolving conflict. However, beginning practice generally deals primarily with individuals, and the outline of data needed will focus only on that needed for an individual.
  A. General Social Status
    1. Ethnic background
    2. Occupation—status or position in that occupation
    3. Economic status
    4. Religious practices
       a. Religious affiliation
       b. Practices or beliefs which might affect reaction to health care (proscriptions against immunization or blood transfusion, dietary laws, beliefs about the cause of disease)
       c. Concept of deity
       d. Sources of hope
    5. Type of housing accommodation
    6. Contacts or previous referrals to social agencies
  B. Family or Peer Group Social Status
    1. Position in the family (father, mother, etc.)
    2. Others in family
    3. With whom the person lives; whom he or she considers close if he or she lives alone
    4. Marital Status
    5. Role in family (e.g., source of support during crisis, "black sheep," etc.)
    6. Perceptions of social support available
  C. Social Developmental Status
    1. Age
    2. Sex
    3. Marital status
    4. Degree of dependence and independence (prior to and during health deviation)
    5. Diversional and recreational interests

II. *Mental and Emotional Status.* These are considered as one category since one's intellectual growth bears on reactions to self and others, and vice versa. There is overlap between the psychosocial area and the mental-emotional area, but the student need not waste energy trying to fit an item of data precisely into one category. The important thing is to note the information *somewhere*.
  A. Mental Status
    1. Level of consciousness (response to verbal stimuli, response to noise and light, response to touch and painful stimuli, spontaneous activity)
    2. Orientation to time, place, and person
    3. Intellectual development relative to age
    4. Mental skills (level of education, ability to read and write, vocabulary, ability to comprehend and follow directions, attention span, memory span, ability to understand abstraction)
    5. Perception and understanding of health problems and goals of medical and nursing therapy
    6. Beliefs and attitudes about disease
    7. Previous experience with and reaction to illness and hospitalization
  B. Emotional Status
    1. Affect (general mood and emotional response)
    2. Reactions to stressful situations (includes kinds of situations person considers stressful)
    3. Patterns of relating to others
    4. Special concerns or fears
    5. Concept of self—self-esteem (prior to and in relation to current health problem; body image)
    6. Substances taken to alter emotional response (includes prescribed medications—tranquilizers, sedatives, mood-elevating drugs; alcohol; mind-expanding drugs; amphetamines)

III. *Sexuality Status.* This area evaluates sexual function, sexual roles and the person's perceptions of sexuality in relation to health and illness. It combines data regarding both physiological and psychosocial functioning.
  A. Gender
  B. Level of Sexual Development
  C. Attitudes toward Own Sexuality
  D. Reproductive Data (male and female)
    1. Number of children, number of pregnancies, number of live births (self, spouse, or significant sexual partner)
    2. Attitudes toward contraception, contraceptive methods used
    3. Difficulties related to menopause or male climacterium
  E. Reproductive Organs
    1. Appearance of genitalia, presence or absence or absence of lesions, abnormal innervation
    2. Unusual genital discharge
    3. Menstrual pattern, age of menarche
    4. History of disease, or surgery affecting reproductive organs
  F. Effects of State of Health on Sexuality
    1. Changes in sexual function necessitated by illness, disability
    2. Changes in sexual role
    3. Changes in sexual self-concept

IV. *Environmental Status.* Factors in the patient-client's home, work, or institutional environment are assessed in several other areas. However, some factors, related to safety, control of infection, and environmental effects upon illness, need to be assessed in their own right.
  A. Safety Factors
    1. Age
    2. State of mobility
    3. Arrangement of objects in physical environment; other potential safety hazards
    4. Sensory deficits
    5. Orientation-disorientation to environment
    6. Use of restraining devices—bed rails, restraints
    7. Use of prosthetic and other supportive devices—crutches, artificial limbs, mechanical lifting devices
  B. Infection Control
    1. Presence of infectious disease or infected wounds in patient, family, or others in proximity
    2. Barriers to cross-infection (isolation techniques, handwashing facilities, distance from infected persons or infectible persons)
    3. Patient and family understanding and beliefs about transfer of pathogens
    4. Equipment potentially harboring pathogens (isolettes, humidifiers, pulmonary therapy equipment)
  C. Environmental Effects on Illness
    1. Patterns of activity, light, noise, color (varied, steady, excessive, absent)
    2. Arrangement of environment in relation to functional abilities or disabilities (Are pictures and reading material placed where bedfast person can see them? Are implements placed where handicapped person can reach them?)

---

* The outline is meant to serve as a guide to data collection, not as an exhaustive outline. The guide was developed from those published by R. Faye McCain and associates (1965), L. Mac McPhetridge (1968), and Dorothy Smith (1968), and modified by this author's own clinical experience.

Figure 15–2. Assessment Guide, with data that may be collected in each assessment area. (From Mitchell PH, Loustau A, Concepts Basic to Nursing, ed 3. New York, McGraw-Hill, 1981 used with permission.)

112

V. *Sensory Status.*† This area refers to the state of the perceiving senses—vision, hearing, smell, taste, touch. Language perception and formation are categorized here although they are dependent upon both sensory and motor function.
   A. Visual Status
      1. Visual acuity (ability to distinguish objects at a specified distance), pupillary responses
      2. Field of vision (lateral, horizontal, vertical), extraocular movements
      3. Known deficits (myopia, presbyopia, astigmatism, color blindness, blindness)
      4. Corrective or prosthetic devices (glasses, contact lenses, artificial eye)
      5. Unusual sensations (rainbows around lights, blind spots, flashing lights)
   B. Auditory Status
      1. Ability to distinguish voice (distance, loudness)
      2. Known deficits (extent—i.e., one ear, both ears, complete, partial)
      3. Corrective devices
      4. Unusual sensations (ringing, buzzing, dizziness)
   C. Olfactory Status
      1. Ability to discriminate odors
      2. Unusual sensations (lack of smell, heightened sensitivity to smell, smelling odors with no stimulus present)
   D. Gustatory Status
      1. Ability to discriminate sweet, sour, salt, bitter
      2. Unusual sensations (lack of taste, aftertaste, substances taste alike)
   E. Tactile Status
      1. Ability to discriminate sharp and dull, light and firm touch; head and extremities
      2. Ability to perceive heat, cold, and pain in proportion to stimulus
      3. Ability to differentiate common objects by touch (stereognosis)
      4. Intactness of body image
      5. Aberrant sensation (lack of pain, touch, heat, cold sensation; increased or decreased pain in proportion to stimulus; diffuse burning, pricking, or pain)
   F. Language Perception and Formation
      1. Intactness of speech organs (mouth, teeth, tongue, palate, larynx)
      2. Deficits in phonation (stammering, lisping, repetition, jargon, mutism, staccato speech)
      3. Ability to understand, initiate, and imitate speech
      4. Ability to read, write, and copy figures
   G. Sensory Environment
      1. Intensity
      2. Pattern
      3. Variety
      4. Appropriateness to developmental level
VI. *Motor Status.*† This area evaluates the ability of the person's nervous system to initiate action in response to stimuli perceived by the sensory organs. Many of the data center around the state of the structural organs of movement—the muscles and the bones.
   A. Medical Restrictions on Activity (physician's prescription for bed rest; bed rest with bathroom privileges, restraints)
   B. Musculoskeletal Status
      1. General movement (coordination, ease, stability)
      2. Movement of head and neck structures (eyes, facial muscles, tongue, mouth, jaw, neck, shoulders)
      3. Muscle strength, tone, and mass (all extremities, trunk and abdomen; symmetry; prior to and during health problem)
      4. Range of joint motion (all joints, active and passive motion)
      5. Posture
      6. Handedness
      7. Deformities (intactness of extremities, prosthetic devices)
      8. Abnormal innervation to muscles (paralysis, weakness)
   C. Mobility
      1. Method of ambulation (unassisted, with supportive aids such as cane, crutch, wheelchair)
      2. Gait (mode of walking, coordination, stability)
      3. Endurance (amount of activity tolerated)
VII. *Nutritional Status.* This area deals not only with obvious data about intake of foods but also with attitudes toward eating and toward special diets.
   A. Dietary Habits
      1. Usual eating habits (number and timing of meals, inclusion of "basic four" categories of food, preferred foods, excesses)
      2. Appetite
      3. Changes related to health problem (appetite changes, special diet prescribed by physician or by patient-client)
      4. Person responsible for preparing food at home
   B. Adequacy of Diet
      1. Height, weight; gain-loss pattern
      2. General appearance (obese, normal, thin; appearance of skin, hair, nails)
   C. Attitudes toward Eating
      1. Importance of food to feeling of well-being
      2. Religious dietary restrictions
      3. Symbolic meaning of food—reward, love, punishment
   D. Factors in Food Ingestion
      1. State of teeth (dentulous, partially or completely edentulous; disease of teeth and gums; oral hygiene habits)
      2. State of mouth (intactness of mucous membranes; disorders of salivary glands; moistness; odor; presence of debris)
      3. State of consciousness
      4. Ability to swallow
      5. Gastrointestinal motility, bowel sounds
   E. Digestion
      1. Ease of digestion
      2. Nausea, vomiting, retching
      3. Eructation (belching)
      4. Medications affecting digestion and metabolism of foods
   F. Nonoral Means of Feeding
      1. Parenteral fluids, hyperalimentation
      2. Nasogastric tube, gastrostomy
VIII. *Elimination Status.* This category includes elimination via the urinary and gastrointestinal tracts.
   A. Normal Patterns (frequency, amount, color, consistency of stool)
   B. Aids to Elimination Normally Used (beverages, laxatives, position)
   C. Changes Due to Health Problem
      1. Character of urine (color, odor, specific gravity, unusual constituents)
      2. Character of stool (color, odor, consistency, presence of unusual constituents)
   D. Method of Eliminating (toilet, commode, bedpan)
      1. Artificial orifices (ileal conduit—urine; colostomy, ileostomy—bowel)
      2. Method of care for excretions from artificial orifices

---

† Areas V and VI, which deal with sensory-motor status, evaluate the individual's ability to perceive the world and to act on those perceptions. Functions in these areas are mediated by the central nervous system, and their status is one clue to the intactness of motor and sensory nerves and tracts. Deficits in one modality often correspond to deficits in the other. For example, the person who is hemiplegic (paralyzed on one side) often has decreased sensation to touch on the paralyzed side. For this reason, the two areas should be assessed in relation to each other, although a systematic evaluation is made of each.

Figure 15–2. (Continued)

E. Special Problems
1. Incontinence (urine, stool; ways of coping)
2. Urinary retention
3. Constipation
4. Diarrhea
5. Abnormal bowel sounds

IX. *Fluid and Electrolyte Status.* Maintenance of a balance of body fluids and electrolytes is essential to homeostasis and to life. Although the physician has primary responsibility in restoring this balance, nurses' observations often provide key data for the medical management. In addition, the nurse may play an important role in helping to maintain this balance.
A. Normal Patterns of Fluid Intake and Output
1. Ingestion of food and fluids (amounts in 24 h, types preferred)
2. Output (urine, stool, perspiration)
B. Changes Due to Health Problem (increase or decrease in intake or output)
C. Measurements
1. Oral and parenteral intake (includes type of solid foods)
2. Output (urine, liquid stool, number of formed stools, drainage from wounds, occasionally perspiration and respiratory loss)
D. Indirect Data
1. State of fluid balance
a. Weight
b. Thirst
c. Skin turgor, dryness
d. Condition of mouth, mucous membranes (dry, moist, coated, presence of crusts)
e. Edema
f. Blood pressure, lying and standing
2. Venous state (distended, flattened, filling time)
3. Level of consciousness
4. Depression or elevation of fontanels in infants
5. Neuromuscular flaccidity or irritability
6. Laboratory values of electrolytes, pH
7. Medical therapy (drugs, parenteral fluids, blood)

X. *Circulatory Status.* These observations give indirect data about the state of the heart and blood vessels.
A. Pulse
1. Rate
2. Quality (thready, weak, bounding, strong)
3. Rhythm (regular, irregular, paired beats)
4. Apical-radial differences
5. Response to activity, emotional stress
6. Medications which alter heart rate or rhythm
B. Heart Sounds
C. Blood Pressure
1. Systolic, diastolic
2. Lying and standing
3. Discrepancies between arms
4. Factors altering accuracy of reading (obesity, cuff size)
D. General Appearance
1. Color (skin, lips, nails)
2. Evidence of volume depletion or edema
3. Urine output, fluid intake
4. Warmth and color of extremities
5. Undue fatigue after exertion
6. Pains in legs after walking
7. Chest or epigastric pain, precipitating factors
E. Special Observations. If the patient has acute cardiac disease and his or her condition is being specially monitored, the list may also include data from monitoring devices such as the character of the electrocardiogram, central venous pressure, arterial pressure, laboratory values

XI. *Respiratory Status.* The state of the respiratory function may be assessed both directly and indirectly. The indirect measurements give some clues to the state of cellular respiration.

A. Direct Measurements
1. Patency of the airway
2. Respirations
a. Rate, rhythm, depth, ease, use of accessory muscles
b. Factors altering character (position, emotion, cough, humidity, air pollution)
c. Breath sounds
3. Cough
a. Patterns (upon arising, continuous, random, after smoking)
b. Productive of sputum
c. Character of sputum (color, viscosity, odor, hemoptysis)
B. Indirect Measurements
1. Smoking history
2. Medications affecting respiratory rate, patency of bronchial tree
3. Color (skin, lips, nails)
4. Clubbing of nails
5. Posture, skeletal defects such as kyphosis
6. Level of consciousness (increase or decrease)
7. Anxiety or apprehension (diffuse or specific regarding breathing)
8. Laboratory values (Pa_{O_2}, Pa_{CO_2}, pH)
C. Supportive Devices
1. Nebulizers, aerosols (patterns of use, effectiveness)
2. Positive-pressure breathing
3. Tracheostomy
4. Assisted or controlled ventilation with respirator

XII. *Temperature Status*
A. Subjective Feeling of Warmth and Cold
B. Usual Measures for Temperature Comfort
C. Body Temperature
1. Oral
2. Rectal
3. Axillary
D. Perspiration
1. Presence or absence
2. Pattern (night, day, intermittent)
E. Environmental Temperature and Humidity
F. Methods of Altering Temperature
1. Convection, conduction, radiation, evaporation
2. Special equipment (hypo-hyperthermia blanket)

XIII. *Integumentary Status.* This area refers to the condition of the skin and underlying tissues, nails, and hair.
A. Skin Condition and Mucous Membranes
1. Color, turgor, elasticity, wetness, dryness
2. Intactness (presence of wounds, incisions, ulcers, pressure sores, diaper rash)
3. Character of any lesions present (dry, draining, infected)
4. Areas of ischemia
5. Factors predisposing to skin breakdown (prolonged pressure, lack of position change, unprotected bony prominences, incontinence, age, hyperactivity, self-destructive tendencies)
B. Condition of Nails and Hair
C. Habits of Personal Hygiene
D. Odors and Excretions (oily, perspiration, abnormal)

XIV. *Comfort and Rest Status*
A. Sleep
1. Normal sleep pattern (numbers of hours, time, feeling of being rested)
2. Alterations due to health problem
3. Aids used for sleep (beverages, warm bath, medications)
B. Comfort
1. Presence of pain or discomfort (location, duration, degree, extent, character, precipitating factors)
2. Use of aids to relieve pain or discomfort (prior to and during current health problem)
3. Changes in pain or discomfort with current health problem
4. Cultural expressions of comfort, discomfort, pain

Figure 15–2. *(Continued)*

a client to be asked to report the same information again and again to various health-care workers, and tends to make the client feel that no one listened the first time. If health-care workers communicate among themselves and document their communication through adequate record systems, this needless repetition—and its attendant frustration—can be minimized. Each health-care worker should assume responsibility for finding out what others have recorded.

If the client is newly admitted to the health-care agency, there may be only minimal information available, such as biographic data and the client's reason for coming to the agency. Records for newly admitted hospitalized persons usually contain physician's admitting orders and possibly a problem list and a brief past history. Before beginning the interview, the nurse briefly reviews the medical diagnostic and treatment plans, test results, and other records that are available. This gives some idea of the person's medical condition, progress, and prognosis. The nurse also reviews nursing orders and problems already identified. If the client's diagnosis or records indicate that the client is too ill, unresponsive, or has lost the ability to speak, family members may need to be interviewed instead of the client.

Some caution is needed when preparing for an interview. Overpreparation with accumulation of large amounts of detailed information is not always helpful. The goal of preparation is to obtain enough information to personalize the interview, avoid needless repetition of data gathering, and have a framework in which to conduct the interview.

Second, *know what specific areas need investigating during the interview.* If the interview is for assessment purposes, the interviewer needs to be thoroughly familiar with the assessment categories. The interviewer may find it helpful to jot down those categories in a notebook or on paper and use them to refresh the memory. If this memory help is needed, a simple, honest statement should be made, such as, "Let me check if there are other areas I need information about." If the interview is to explore a specific problem, the interviewer needs to have enough background information and experience with the problem to know what to explore. For example, it would be difficult to explore a problem of constipation if the interviewer does not know what factors contribute to or relieve constipation, or to interview a family where child abuse is suspected if the interviewer has no knowledge of the dynamics and indicators of child abuse.

Third, *assess the client's level of comfort and ability to participate in the interview.* Discomfort—pain, an uncomfortable position, the need to defecate or urinate—makes it difficult for the client to concentrate on an interview. As much as possible, alleviate the client's discomfort before beginning the interview. If the client is too ill or uncomfortable to participate, it is best to delay the interview. If this is not possible because the information is necessary for care, the nurse can acknowledge that he or she is aware of the client's condition and explain the reason for needing to have the information at that particular time. For example, the nurse could say, "I know you're quite uncomfortable, but there is some information I need to have from you so that we can work together to help you be more comfortable." This approach generally will increase the client's willingness to participate in the interview, and the interview then should be as brief as possible.

It is best to avoid scheduling interviews during times when the client may have other commitments—for example, during visiting hours, mealtimes, or a favorite television show, when tests are scheduled, or just after strenuous activities such as physical therapy or some diagnostic procedures. Before beginning an interview it is common courtesy for the nurse to ask the client if it is an appropriate time and explain approximately how much time is needed. For example, the nurse may say, "I need to have some information about.... This is the best time for me to talk with you today and I would need about 20 to 30 minutes. Would that be all right for you?"; or, "I will be free right after lunch and would like to talk with you then about.... Would that be a good time for you?" However, if the suggested time is the only time the nurse has or is the preferred time, that should be stated along with the request, rather than offering a choice that does not exist.

Fourth, *prepare the environment.* Although the physical plan of many health-care agencies does not promote privacy, do whatever is possible to provide privacy during the interview. If available, a separate room may be used, or the door to an office or room may be closed, or others asked to leave the room for the duration of the interview. Pulling the curtain around the bed in a ward or semiprivate room provides some privacy. When the environment cannot be adapted to provide privacy, a client's psychological perception of privacy is enhanced if the interviewer sits near the client (2 to 3 feet) and keeps his or her voice volume low.

Distractions in the environment can be reduced, such as by turning off the television or radio or closing the door. In a clinic or outpatient department, ask the receptionist to hold other phone calls and request other staff to avoid interruptions. The client has the right to expect the interviewer's undivided attention. If interruptions or delays are unavoidable, it is helpful to explain the situation briefly and let the client know what to expect—for example, "I am expecting a phone call from Dr. Jones about another patient. I will need to answer the call but will be as brief as possible and then come back to finish our conversation."

Fifth, *consider clients' special needs.* Additional planning is needed for clients who are hard of hearing, deaf, have difficulty speaking or are unable to speak, have distorted thought processes, or who speak a different language from the nurse.

For a hearing-impaired person, check to make sure the hearing aid (if one is used) is functional, turned on, and has good batteries. Face the client to facilitate lipreading and speak slowly and clearly without exaggerated slowness or yelling. When clients have impaired verbal ability—for example, persons with strokes or laryngectomies—use short-answer or yes-and-no questions, or perhaps a magic slate or paper and pencil.

Arrange for an interpreter if the interview is with a person who speaks another language or a hearing-impaired person who uses sign language. Since literal word-for-word translations seldom convey accurate meanings, the interpreter must be reasonably fluent in both languages, not someone with simply a year of high school language study. If a client has some use of the nurse's major language, or vice versa, written communication may be helpful, since people sometimes have a better written than verbal grasp of their second language.

Some people have disordered thought processes due to conditions such as organic brain syndrome, cerebrovascular insufficiency, senility, depression, or paranoia. In general, these persons tend to respond more readily and clearly to short-answer questions, but a more specific understanding of a given client's thought process will help the nurse adapt the interview process successfully.

GUIDELINES FOR INTERVIEWING

There is no set formula for interviewing because every interview is a unique exchange between two individuals. There are, however, some helpful guidelines to keep in mind during the interview.

Establish the Purpose
It is important that the nurse state his or her intent to conduct an interview. Although much relevant information is obtained during casual nurse–client interactions, it is inappropriate to "see how much you can find out by just talking" without ever disclosing to the client that an assessment interview or nursing history is taking place. In addition, it is important to communicate to the client the purpose of the interview, why the information is being sought, and how that information will be used. In addition, the client has the right to know who the nurse is, what position he or she has in the agency, and who will have access to the information. This establishes the nurse's credibility with the client. The nurse does not have the right to gather information for its own sake or simply out of curiosity.

Begin with the Client's Concerns
Before pursuing his or her own agenda, the nurse first inquires about any concerns or questions the client may have. This communicates to the client that those concerns are important. When the nurse focuses on his or her own purposes first, the client receives the message that his or her own concerns are less important than those of the nurse or the agency. Listening to a client's concerns helps establish rapport with the nurse and engages the two in meaningful conversation and is a way of individualizing the interview. Additionally, a client is more able to attend to content areas the nurse wishes to discuss if his or her own concerns have already been dealt with. In a study of doctor–patient communications, Korsch et al. (1971) found that if the client's expectations in an interchange are not met, the client is likely to be preoccupied with his or her own concerns and unable to respond to the health-care professional's questions or advice.

At the outset of an interview, it is possible to establish the purpose for the interview and attend to the client's concerns. For example, the nurse may say, "Mr. Jackson, my name is Sally Smith. I'm the nurse who will be taking care of you most of the time during your hospital stay. I'm here to get some information from you that will help us to provide proper care. There are some specific things I need to know, such as your usual habits of eating, sleeping, and going to the bathroom. Before I begin, is there anything you want to ask me? . . ."

The interviewer will want to pay close attention to his or her initial impressions of the client, the situation, and the client's opening remarks. Opening words may convey the client's feelings about the interview and the interviewer, and initial impressions often have validity. The way in which a client states his or her concerns may reflect their meaning and significance to the client.

Individualize the Interview
Individualization consists of both an internal process and external activities on the part of the interviewer. Internal individualization involves the nurse's attitude toward the client and the client's perception of that attitude. To be able to regard clients as individuals, the nurse needs to be able to recognize and set aside his or her own biases, prejudices, and stereotypes about people. The nurse also needs to understand human behavior, have the ability to listen and observe, and be able to empathize with someone else's feelings while maintaining a separate perspective. Other ways to individualize an interview are to begin with the client's concerns, help the client be comfortable, and avoid hurrying the client or forcing him or her to talk about something he or she does not want to, unless it is absolutely necessary. When the nurse regards the client as an individual, the client is likely to respond favorably; if the client perceives that the nurse does not regard him or her as an individual, however, he or she tends to "react by giving the bare objective facts . . . rather than his subjective feelings which are often the most important items" (Garrett, 1972, p. 27).

Individualization is conveyed externally in many different ways, such as by using the client's name, considering the client's obligations and time when scheduling interviews, providing privacy, and acting to increase the client's comfort level. Knowing and using the client's name is an essential feature of individualizing an interview. With the exception of children and teenagers, it is considered more appropriate to use a title and last name for initial contacts, for example, Mr. Jones, Mrs. Smith, or Ms. Johnson. When interviews and relationships continue over a period of time, first names may become appropriate. A client may indicate a preference for the name he or she chooses to use. The nurse may consider the client's culture or inquire about the name the client prefers. Use of terms like "Gramps," "Pop," "Honey," and "Hon," tend to dehumanize and stereotype and should be avoided as one's name is a significant part of one's individuality.

Use Learned Communications Skills

The professional nurse incorporates learned communication skills into his or her own way of relating to people and develops the ability to use any one or a combination of these skills in a selective and intentional manner (Fig. 15–3). Sometimes the novice interviewer finds a comment or a response that "really worked" with a given client and attempts to repeat it in the same fashion with another client, only to find it does not work nearly as well the next time. It is important for the nurse to develop a style that is natural and comfortable, professional, and yet adaptable to the individual client. There is no prescribed way to combine and use communication skills in an interview, nor is there a given approach that works with every client or situation. There is also no standard approach for groups of people, such as the "right" way to interview old people, young people, pregnant women, blacks, Hispanics, and so forth.

The most productive approach to interviewing is to focus on the person being interviewed rather than on the techniques and phrases being used. In a sense this means being able to forget one's own self while still being able to use that self in a deliberate way to promote someone else's well-being.

Terminate the Interview Appropriately

It is best to terminate the interview at the agreed-upon time. In one study reported by Pluckhan (1978), the average length of an assessment interview in an ambulatory care clinic was 45 minutes. Garrett (1972) believes it seldom is beneficial to have an interview last more than 1 hour. Long interviews exhaust both the client and the nurse. A prearranged time frame helps the nurse direct the interview more efficiently and helps the client organize and plan what he or she wants to say.

As the end of the time allotted for the interview approaches, begin to reflect on what has been discussed and to summarize what has occurred during the interview. This summarization might include general content areas discussed and the problems and concerns that have been identified and resolved as well as those requiring continuing exploration. Point out that the time allotted for the interview is nearly over and also determine with the client when and where the next interview (if any) will take place.

Summarization also includes informing the client of what he or she is expected to do for follow-up before the next interview, such as practicing a psychomotor or psychosocial skill, reading some material, or thinking about something. This is particularly true if the interview focused on problem solving or if teaching needs were identified. The client also is told what the interviewer will do prior to the next interview, such as research some information, find materials, or make a referral. These semicontractual agreements help involve the client in a continuing relationship and avoid having an interview be an isolated experience. If this interview is to be the only contact the nurse has with this particular client, the client needs to be informed of that fact and be told who will follow up on the interview, when, and in what way.

If the interviewer has initiated the interview with a request for information, he or she concludes the interview session with an acknowledgment of appreciation for the client's time, energy, information, or participation. For example, "I appreciate your taking the time to talk with me about these things today. The information will help me and the other nurses to provide the kind of care you want and need." Words of encouragement, such as for progress being made or effort expended, also help maintain nurse–client involvement between interview sessions. The conclusion of an interview also can include a client's summary of what the interview meant or what he or she intends to do next.

New material is not introduced near the end of the interview, as this can either cause a delay in termination or leave both parties with an unfinished feeling. The interviewer also avoids offering platitudes or clichés as a closing statement, such as, "I'm sure everything will be fine" or, "Keep a stiff upper lip."

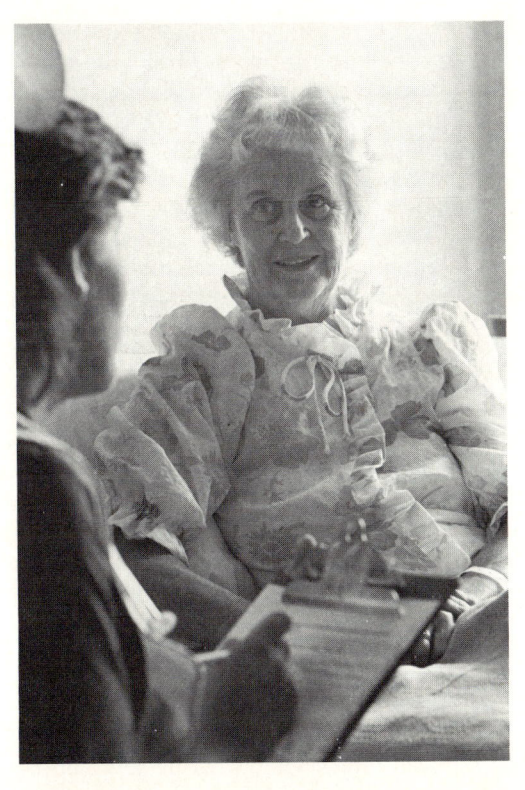

Figure 15–3. Attentive listening facilitates data gathering during an interview. (Photo by James Haines.)

SPECIAL SKILLS FOR INTERVIEWING

Recording Information During the Interview

The nurse must decide in advance how to manage all the information that is obtained during the interview. There is some disagreement about whether an interviewer should take notes during an interview. Those opposing the taking of notes believe it is distracting and rude to the client. Unfortunately, some interviewers try to resolve this issue by attempting to take notes surreptitiously, without explaining what they are doing. Most of us cannot remember large amounts of information accurately and do need notes. If the nurse decides to take notes, it should be explained to the client; "I usually take notes when I interview someone, because I have difficulty keeping everything in my head. Will that cause a problem for you?"

Note-taking should not be a continuous activity, as it might be during a class, for example, as it eliminates or drastically reduces eye contact and observation of nonverbal behaviors (see p. 122). Complete sentences are unnecessary; brief phrases or single words can serve as reminders for later recording.

During the interview, the nurse records information and facts. Share all notes with the client, if requested. There are unsettled issues over the extent of a client's access to personal information contained in agency records. (See Skill 17 for a further discussion of this issue.) The safest policy is to avoid recording, either in interview notes or the health record, any information that the nurse would be unwilling to share with the client. If the nurse retains the notes written during the interview for his or her own personal study, care must be taken to ensure the client's privacy. For example, full client names are not included in a student's interview notes or in nursing histories and care plans that are used primarily for learning purposes. Nor should client affairs be discussed in the cafeteria, elevator, lounge, or dormitory.

Listening for Meaning and Contradictions

In addition to listening carefully to factual information and observing the related nonverbal behavior, the nurse needs to listen for recurrent themes, concealed meanings, contradictions, and inconsistencies. When a client returns frequently to a given subject during an interview, that subject may be of particular importance to the client, or the client may be reluctant to go on to something else. Recurrent themes must be listened to and discussed with the client. For example, the nurse may say, "I've noticed that you've referred to that subject several times. Do you want to say more about that?" Or, "That's come up several times. Maybe we should take the time to talk about it."

An interviewer needs to learn to listen to what the client means as well as what he or she says. A sensitive listener "reads between the lines" and picks up on unspoken cues that guide his or her responses to the client. A client often makes a quite casual remark or a passing reference to something that has a great deal of meaning for him or her. The nurse is alert to these cues and responds to them by either requesting more information or reflecting upon the feelings that seem to be present. To illustrate: A student nurse was interviewing a woman who recently had a radical mastectomy. During the interview the woman related that the surgeon had asked her if he could use her as a case for "rounds." The student asked if she was planning to do this and the woman replied, "Yes, if it will help someone else to avoid making the same mistake I did." When the student explored what she meant by "mistake," the woman revealed that she had found the lump over a year before seeing the physician. The student allowed her to verbalize her guilt and anger at herself and arranged a counseling referral. Had the student not clarified the meaning of "mistake," the woman might not have received the help she needed desperately.

Sometimes the client presents contradictions and inconsistencies that result in unclear messages. For example, verbal and nonverbal messages may be contradictory, such as when a person who is obviously in pain reports that he or she feels fine, or when the distraught, crying person says that nothing is wrong. Or the client may also offer conflicting versions of the same episode and facts at different times or to different persons, such as the man who shouts angrily at a nurse's aide about the way she took his temperature but pleasantly assures the charge nurse that there has been no problem between him and the aide. Sometimes stated facts conflict with other information already given or with the nurse's own observations; for example, the client may say this is a new health problem and yet there is a referral letter for the same problem in the health record. Or a client says she is taking no medications, but the physician's admitting notes list several current medications. Clients also may omit some information or be reluctant to discuss something such as sexual problems, the reason for leaving a job, or changing physicians, or they may talk about all family members except one. Inconsistencies and gaps can be due to ordinary memory lapses, confusion, senility, or can represent real problem areas. Single episodes tend not to be significant, but cumulative and repeated episodes usually warrant attention.

When aware of contradictions, inconsistencies, or gaps in what the client reports or does, it is necessary to confront the client with that information. This confrontation focuses on the situation and identifies the observed contradictions. For example, "To me you look like you're in a great deal of pain, but you tell me you feel fine. I'm getting two messages and am wondering which one is correct." Or, "I don't understand; Miss Jones said you were quite angry about the way she took your temperature, but you tell me nothing happened between you and her. I'd like to hear from you what happened, so we can work at resolving it." Or, "Can you clear something up for me? Earlier you said this was a new problem for you, but I have here a letter from Dr. Smith that says he saw you for this same problem last month."

The purpose of identifying inconsistencies is to

clarify, not psychoanalyze, the client's messages. The purpose in confrontation is to give or receive information, not accuse, blame, or "catch" the other person. After receiving the information, clients should be left free to make their own use of the information, modifying their behavior as they choose.

Anthony and Carkhuff (1976) emphasize that before the health-care professional confronts a client, he or she must first listen to, reflect upon, and clarify the client's message. When this is not done, confrontation may cause the client to feel defensive. In the previous example regarding temperature taking, a nonhelpful confrontation might go like this: The nurse enters the room and says, "I understand you were angry about the way Miss Jones took your temperature." The client answers, "No, I wasn't angry." Without exploring the situation, the nurse responds, "She said you were angry and you say you weren't. That doesn't fit!"

During the interview, the interviewer often formulates interpretations of client behaviors that help the interviewer's understanding of the situation. Sharing these interpretations with the client is generally considered inadvisable (Garrett, 1972, p. 48). For example, the nurse may hypothesize that an overweight client is a compulsive eater. Rather than reporting this interpretation to the client, the nurse tests out the assumption through his or her own or others' observations of the client's eating behaviors.

Dealing with Distress
During the interview process, the nurse generally tries to avoid creating unnecessary distress and often acts to relieve distress. There are times, however, when an interview or interaction causes—rather than relieves—distress for either the nurse or the client, or both. Because they view themselves primarily as helpers and healers, nurses are often uncomfortable when what they do or say causes increased pain or discomfort. Because of the intensely personal nature of nursing, however, many things a nurse deals with *are* uncomfortable or painful. It is painful to work with a woman who has been raped, a family where child abuse is suspected, or a person who has recently discovered he or she has cancer. It is threatening and uncomfortable to deal with promiscuity, threats of suicide, homosexuality, death, depression, or intractable pain. The temptation is to avoid discussing these and other uncomfortable, painful, or threatening situations because it causes pain, both for the client to talk about it and for the nurse to listen. But because these are things the client is experiencing—and often it is the client who initiates direct or indirect communication about them—the nurse must not back away or try to avoid painful situations. Although the client may need more help than the nurse is able to offer, the nurse can explore the situation enough to know the nature of the problem and make a knowledgeable referral.

Nurses may avoid uncomfortable situations in a variety of ways. For example, a depressed person may say that life just is not worthwhile anymore, and the nurse responds, "Oh, but you have so many things to be grateful for! Count your blessings!" Or a person with intractable pain may say that he does not know how much longer he can go on like this and the nurse replies, "Maybe tomorrow will be a better day." Or the parents in a suspected child-abuse situation insist the injuries resulted from an accident and the nurse says, "You really need to watch that child more carefully." In uncomfortable situations such as these, the nurse can focus on reflecting the content and feelings in the client's message and communicating acceptance, caring, and empathy. Another way of avoiding dealing with uncomfortable issues is through stereotyping, such as the nurse who explains her attitude toward a client by saying, "He's gay. I can always tell by looking!"

Changes in health status often necessitate other life changes, which can produce distress for the client. An assessment interview can help determine whether the client is cooperative and amenable to change or is resistant to change. A client who volunteers information and participates readily in the interview is usually receptive to change, whereas a client who avoids eye contact, rejects all suggestions, or complains about previous health care frequently is resistant to change.

The process of growth and change may bring resistance and pain. A sincere desire to alleviate pain may cause the nurse to overreassure and avoid conflict, anger, resistance, or discomfort. If the nurse always backs away from discomfort, he or she tends to reinforce the client's status quo rather than promote growth and change. Obviously, the nurse never makes a client uncomfortable just for the sake of doing so. There is much discomfort that is not related to growth. People can change without growing, but it is not possible to grow without changing—and change tends to be uncomfortable.

Using Printed Forms
Sometimes the information needed by the nurse is determined in advance by a printed form or guide such as the admitting nursing assessment guide shown in Figure 15-1.

When using guides and forms, it is essential to be thoroughly familiar with the questions and understand the purposes and significance of each item. Otherwise, the questions tend to be asked in a perfunctory manner that minimizes their importance. Furthermore, an interviewer is more inclined to accept superficial and incomplete answers to questions if he or she does not understand the reason for the question. For example, a nurse is gathering information about usual diet and activity from a man who has congestive heart failure. If the nurse understands the relationship between heart failure and diet, fluid intake, edema, urinary output, and respiratory problems, he or she is more likely to gather specific information about those factors than is someone who has no understanding of heart failure and simply fills out the form, indicating number of meals per day, likes and dislikes, and amount of exercise.

When the nurse understands the intent of the question, he or she can rephrase it successfully or translate it into terms appropriate for the individual client. An assessment interview is a structured rather than free-flowing interview, but the information can and usually should be gathered in a nonstructured way, using a combination of open and closed questions.

AFTER THE INTERVIEW

Following an assessment interview, the information obtained is recorded on the appropriate forms. A nursing note is written that indicates where the interview was conducted, who conducted it, and something about the client's status, general appearance, and response to being interviewed. The nurse also records relevant information not placed on other agency forms, any problems identified during the interview, and initial plans for dealing with these problems.

INTERVIEW ANALYSIS

A systematic examination of the interview process can enhance the nurse's understanding of the client's situation and increase his or her interviewing skills. Table 15-1 presents a method of looking at the total interview itself.

PROCESS RECORDING

A process recording is a verbatim record of the verbal comments of the nurse and the client, associated nonverbal behaviors of each, and the nurse's impressions about what was happening in the interaction (Pluckhan, 1978; Schweer and Gebbie, 1976; L. Smith, 1979). A process recording can be used to examine the nurse–client interactions within an interview for the purpose of identifying strengths and weaknesses in the nurse's approach and to look for the client's themes and messages. Table 15-2 gives a format for recording data and impressions, and Table 15-3 presents a process recording written by a student nurse.

It is important to record verbatim exchanges very soon after the interaction or interview, using notes taken during the interaction as a guide. With the passage of time, details of the interview are forgotten, especially in areas that are sensitive or uncomfortable for either the nurse or the client.

Nonverbal behaviors are also recorded, as they may shed additional light on verbal responses. Nonverbal behavior may be incongruent with the verbal comments and need further validation, or it may be congruent and lend validity to the verbal comments.

The interpretation of nurse and client behaviors in the third column of Tables 15-2 and 15-3 includes an examination of the nurse's feelings during the in-

---

TABLE 15-1. Interview Analysis Guide

A. General descriptions
  1. Client: age, appearance, state of health, etc.
  2. Environment, both physical and psychological
  3. Nurse and client positions relative to each other
  4. General purpose of interview
B. Opening of interview
  1. Verbatim quotes of any of the following as applicable:
     Opening remarks of nurse, with client response
     Opening remarks of client, with nurse response
     Nurse's statement of intent of interview, with client response
     Client statement of problem, with nurse response
  2. Client affect at outset of interview
  3. Nurse's feeling at outset of interview
C. Body of interview
  1. Summarize the general direction or content of the interview
  2. Note problems or concerns identified
  3. Look at use of learned communication skills:
     Productive attending behavior
     Active listening
     Reflection of content
     Reflection of feelings
     Open-ended questions
     Closed questions
     Offering assistance appropriately (direct physical help, genuine reassurance, helpful advice)
     Touch
     Silence
     Caring
     Self-awareness
     Self-disclosure
  4. Note any blocks to communication:
     Environmental
     Client characteristics
     Interviewer attitudes and behaviors
  5. Note any contradictions, recurrent themes, etc.
D. Termination of interview
  1. Length of interview
  2. Reason for termination
  3. Verbatim terminating statements of nurse, with client's response
  4. Plan made with client for next interview, use of information, expectations of nurse and client
  5. Client affect at termination of interview
  6. Nurse's feelings at termination of interview

---

teraction; the intent or purpose in the nurse's comments; the possible meaning of the client's response; and any observations that might be helpful at a later time. It also is worthwhile to record whether the nurse's response was helpful or if a different approach might have been more productive.

After recording data and impressions, a summary paragraph is usually written, in which the interviewer's overall views of the interaction are given. This may include a brief description of the client situation; whether or not the approach used was helpful or if an alternate approach might have been more helpful; the benefits the client may have received; or learning that occurred on the part of the interviewer.

Schweer and Gebbie (1976) indicate that process recordings are best examined jointly by the student and a more experienced person such as a teacher or preceptor who understands the dynamics of human behavior. This analysis gives the student an opportu-

TABLE 15-2. Process Recording Guide

FORMAT

Nurse	Client	Analysis of Interaction
Verbal response + (Nonverbal communication behaviors)	Verbal response + (Nonverbal communication behaviors)	Interpretation of nurse and client behaviors, nurse–client interactions

INSTRUCTIONS

1. Record a verbatim, sequential 5-minute conversation between the nurse and the client, using notes, recall, or a tape recorder, depending on agency policies.
2. Record nurse and client verbal comments and responses under Nurse (column 1) and Client (column 2), respectively. Include related nonverbal behaviors, in parentheses. Indicate any silences and their estimated length, as well as accompanying nonverbal behavior.
3. Consider the possible meaning of the responses in columns 1 and 2 and record them under Analysis of Interaction (column 3). Complete sentences are not necessary. Identify:
   a. Congruency/noncongruency between verbal and nonverbal behaviors
   b. Use of specific communication skills
   c. Communication blocks
   d. Intent or purpose of responses
   e. Client and nurse coping mechanisms
   f. Helpful/appropriate or nonhelpful/inappropriate responses, explaining why the response was helpful or nonhelpful, and what might have been a more appropriate response
   g. Nurse responses regarded as planned interventions and their success
4. Write a summary paragraph that includes any recurrent themes, general patterns noted in the interaction, outcome or general effect of the interaction, and plans for follow-up interactions.

(Adapted from Coghill M, Smith L: Process Recording Guide. Indianapolis, IN, Indiana University School of Nursing, 1980.)

---

nity to explore cause-and-effect relationships of given responses, providing a basis for modifying future exchanges. Process recordings also serve as a data source for planning interventions.

☐ EXECUTION

Successful interviewing skills include the ability to (1) relate to others as individuals, (2) use learned communication skills, (3) be sensitive to others' needs and concerns, (4) observe the client's response, (5) use flexible and adaptable methods, (6) follow the flow of an interview process, and (7) organize and analyze information.

An interview is best conducted within the far personal distance zone, 2½ to 4 feet, which is the area used for conversation. Less distance may be perceived as intrusive or inviting inappropriate intimacy, and greater distance as being aloof. The nurse and the client are seated in the same horizontal plane so as to minimize status differential based on role. The interviewer is responsible for providing direction and focus to the interview, maintaining its momentum, and bringing it to a successful termination.

Nurses who are learning to interview are generally fearful about several things. "Will the person talk?" "Will I say the right things to draw him or her out?" "Will I say the wrong thing?" "Will I damage the person by what I say?"

Generally, a client will talk and the nurse will know what to say if the nurse concentrates on getting to know the client rather than on worrying, "How will I do?" When a client does not talk, try closed questions with yes or no or brief answers, and then intersperse open-ended questions. This gives the client an opportunity to begin to talk if he or she feels like it. If the client continues to avoid talking, acknowledge verbally that the client does not feel like talking now and plan with the client to return later, if at all possible. It is important not to become angry with the client for not talking.

Although the beginning interviewer probably will say inappropriate things or make mistakes, it is likely that most of these will not be damaging—as long as the interviewer is caring. Caring can usually be perceived by the client, and when caring exists, both the client and the healing process are quite forgiving. On the other hand, if the nurse becomes judgmental, authoritarian, and noncaring, even the best techniques will not lead to successful interviewing.

During the interview, be observant, alert, and attend simultaneously to both verbal and nonverbal behaviors as well as process the meaning of the interaction while it is happening. This is not an easy task and it requires effort and concentration as well as complete attention to that particular interaction with that particular client.

The following activities provide practice in interviewing, using an assessment guide, and evaluating the interview.

TABLE 15-3. Sample Process Recording

NURSE	CLIENT	ANALYSIS OF INTERACTION
Verbal response + (Nonverbal communication behaviors)	Verbal response + (Nonverbal communication behaviors)	Interpretation of nurse and client behaviors, nurse–client interactions

This process recording is my second visit to the M. family. Mrs. M. is a 27-year-old, obese, pregnant woman with three children. The children are, John, Jr. (Johnny), age 6, Julie, age 4, and Jimmy, age 3. The family lives in a rented four-room home. Their home is located at the end of a dirt road, and is rather isolated from the other homes on the road.

NURSE	CLIENT	ANALYSIS OF INTERACTION
"How have you been getting along since your last visit to the prenatal clinic?" (Nurse sitting on davenport.)	"Oh fine." (Smiles and puts hand to mouth.) "I have been gaining weight so fast. I bet I gained five pounds last week. With the other pregnancies I gained very little weight. Afterwards though, I gained weight fast." (Mother on straight chair across room, about 6 feet away.)	I should have found a way to sit closer to her—that's too far away for social conversation!
"But you're gaining weight earlier with this pregnancy?" (Questioning expression, leaning forward.)	"I sure am! I try to watch what I eat. I have a calorie sheet and I try to stick to 1000 calories per day."	Good question—a validating response! Mother is aware and a little disturbed about her obesity and brings up weight gain before nurse has a chance to.
"Is that what the clinic doctor suggested?"	"So far he hasn't said anything about it." (Smiles and shrugs shoulders.)	Needs teaching about diet during pregnancy and in general. She and children have dental problems.
	"I had some water tablets that the doctor gave me 6 months ago. I started to take them, but since I am pregnant, I was afraid to."	Seems to use good judgment in this situation.
"It is best that you do not take these pills anytime. Medicine sometimes changes when it has been lying around for a long time and it could be harmful. Old medicine should be poured down the drain or flushed down the toilet since you have small children around. Since you are pregnant, it is best that you take only what the doctor in the prenatal clinic prescribes."		Mother seems receptive to teaching. However, I sounded like I was preaching. Should have verified what she has done with them first.
(Recognizes Julie's gesture and smiles at her.)	(Four-year-old Julie is now tired of blowing bubbles. She comes near nurse and sits down beside her on davenport and starts playing with the handles on nurse's bag. Julie sits there for a minute or two, then she takes off for the bedroom again.)	Starts to relate to nurse but is still cautious. Sizes situation up. Decides this is close enough for now and takes off. Children at this age are very energetic and have short attention spans.
"Mrs. M., what did you have for breakfast?" "And lunch?" "And supper?"	"Coffee..." (Pause) "Usually I eat a sandwich." (Pause) "Usually meat like chicken or pork chops."	Abrupt change of subject. Could have gone back to the weight gain and tied it into diet. Mother is hesitant; having trouble remembering. Is probably aware that she is not eating a proper diet.
"What about vegetables?"	(Pause) "The children like peas, beans, and corn. We have these quite often."	My value judgments are showing! I should have said, "What do you usually fix to go along with the meat?"
"Does Johnny eat breakfast before he goes to school?" "What do they usually eat?"	"Oh yes. He and Jimmy get up and eat breakfast at the same time." "Usually cereal and milk. Sometimes cookies or crackers, if we're out of milk for the cereal."	No fruit or juice mentioned. Teaching regarding proper diet for mother and possibly children, too, is indicated. Will, however, concentrate on mother for present.
"Since you are pregnant, it is very important that you eat a well-balanced diet that is high in protein, minerals, and vitamins."		Does she know what a "balanced diet" is? Maybe I should have been more specific.

(continued)

NURSE	CLIENT	ANALYSIS OF INTERACTION
Verbal response + (Nonverbal communication behaviors)	Verbal response + (Nonverbal communication behaviors)	Interpretation of nurse and client behaviors, nurse-client interactions
"Have you tried to sit down and eat breakfast with the children in the morning?"	"I have never been able to eat breakfast. It makes me sluggish all day and I am not able to get anything done. I also get sick if I have anything besides coffee for breakfast."	
"Do you eat between meals or after you put the children to bed at night?"	"No, I do not eat between meals. I drink plenty of milk and sometimes I may have a cookie or two before I go to bed. Occasionally, the children have candy but I try to give them crackers and fresh fruit instead of too much sweet food. I eat graham crackers sometimes."	Is probably eating more between meals than she realizes but will not come right out and say this. Tried a "strategy."
"About how many graham crackers do you eat a day?"	"About two."	
"That shouldn't make that much difference in your weight."		I see now that I asked too many closed questions—even though she answered. Also think she may be giving me the answers she thinks I want to hear. Have to watch my implied answers!
"I do not have anything with me. I will see what is available at the office and will bring you something on this subject on my next visit. You can also see what the doctor in the prenatal clinic recommends."	"Do you have any books on dieting? The other nurses gave me a book but when I moved, I lost it."	Realizes that something will have to be done and very soon. Seems concerned and interested and is taking initiative in requesting help. However, also thinks just a diet book will help. She'll need support in using it and planning meals.
	"I would appreciate any help because I know that I am gaining weight too fast and that it will be hard to lose it after the baby is born."	
"How about writing down everything you eat between now and next Tuesday? I will come back next Wednesday afternoon if it is all right with you— and with the list of food that you have eaten and a book on diet during pregnancy, we'll see if we can plan a diet that will be adequate yet low in fat and carbohydrate."	"That will be fine because I know that I am gaining weight too fast."	Receptive of teaching; seeking help. Seems motivated and ready to learn.

Activity 15-B: Conducting an Assessment Interview

Work in groups of three, partners A and B and an observer, using an audio or video tape recorder for later analysis and feedback.

1. Using one of the assessment guides presented in this skill, partner A conducts an assessment interview that incorporates several assessment categories and lasts approximately 10 to 15 minutes.
2. Based on the interviewer's (partner A) and observer's notes, use the Performance Checklist, p. 125, to evaluate the interview. Compare and discuss the three evaluation columns of self, partner B, and observer.
3. Reverse roles and repeat exercise until each person has assumed each role. Each person should use a different section of the assessment guide as a basis for the interview.
4. Discuss your reactions to asking for and giving personal information. Do your reactions vary according to different subject areas in the assessment guide? If so, in what areas and for what reasons?

Activity 15-C: Evaluating the Interview

Review the taped role play from Activity 15-B with a preceptor or teacher, using the Interview Analysis Guide (Table 15-1), and the Performance Checklist, p. 125. You may want to identify illustrative examples of each checklist item. The interviewee and other students may be included in the review process, if acceptable to the interviewer.

With which aspects of interviewing do you feel competent? Which aspects give you the most difficulty? How similar are your own and others' evaluation of your interviewing capabilities?

(NOTE: If taping equipment is unavailable, the activity may be modified by having the preceptor or teacher present during the interview, taking notes.)

The ability to interview effectively and efficiently comes with time, practice, and an examination of your interviewing and interactional skills. The Interview Analysis Guide (Table 15-1) and the Performance Checklist, p. 125, can be used to evaluate your ability to interview, and the Process Recording Guide (Table 15-2) is useful for examining your one-to-one interactions with clients. You may wish to have a teacher or preceptor evaluate your ability to interview, since the added objectivity and expertise of either one can be beneficial. At intervals during your career, you will find it helpful to use similar techniques to reevaluate your ability to interview.

The following activities provide practice in conducting and analyzing an interview in a clinical setting, and in analyzing the interaction between yourself and a client.

Activity 15-D: Client Interviews

1. Select a client in any health-care setting. Negotiate and conduct an assessment interview with that client, taking notes as needed.
2. Examine the interview, using the Interview Analysis Guide (Table 15-1) and the Performance Checklist, p. 125.
3. Review your interview and analysis with a teacher or preceptor. Identify your own strengths and areas needing improvement.

(NOTE: You may want to use a 5- or 10-minute segment of this interview to examine specific interactional responses, as in Activity 15-E.)

Activity 15-E: Analyzing Interactions

Select a 5- to 10-minute segment of a client interview. Using the format of the Process Recording Guide (Table 15-2), record and examine the verbatim verbal exchanges between yourself and the client. Include nonverbal behaviors and interpretations as indicated. Review and discuss this process recording with a skilled teacher or preceptor.

As a way of continuing to increase your interactional skills, repeat this evaluation at regular intervals during your ongoing nurse–client interactions.

☐ CRITICAL POINTS SUMMARY

1. The assessment interview is used to gather data for the assessment phase of the nursing process.
2. Interviews are useful in identifying and clarifying problems.
3. An interview or interaction has either a positive or negative therapeutic impact on the client.
4. Before interviewing, determine what is known about the client, the specific information that is to be obtained, and the client's level of comfort; prepare the environment; and consider any special client needs.
5. During an interview, establish the purpose; begin with the client's concerns; individualize the interview; use learned communication skills; and terminate appropriately.
6. During the interview, note any recurrent themes, hidden meanings, contradictions, and inconsistencies.
7. Deal with client distress rather than avoiding it.
8. Learned communication skills are incorporated into an interview in the interviewer's own unique manner.
9. Successful interviewing requires a warm, caring attitude combined with knowledge of human behavior, communication skills, and interview guidelines.
10. Skill in interviewing is enhanced through practice and through critical analysis of both the interview and specific interactions.

☐ REVIEW QUESTIONS

1. What purpose does an assessment interview serve?
2. What general content areas are included in an assessment interview?
3. How can an interview be used to identify and clarify problems?
4. What is your understanding of the following statement? "Any interaction or interview has either a positive or negative impact."
5. What can a nurse do to reduce distractions and provide privacy during an interview?
6. Cite three guidelines for note-taking during an interview.
7. What benefits occur when the nurse begins an interview by inquiring about the client's concerns?
8. What type of information needs to be shared with the client as part of establishing the purpose in an interview?
9. Why is individualization an important aspect of interviewing?
10. In an interview, how is individualization conveyed internally and externally?
11. What is the purpose in confronting contradictions and inconsistencies?
12. What does the nurse do with his or her interpretations of client behaviors?
13. What is the purpose of a process recording?
14. What is to be accomplished in an interview analysis?
15. How can the nurse individualize gathering information for a printed form?
16. In an interview setting, what factors are most likely to contribute to ease in talking for both the nurse and the client?
17. How should the nurse respond to the client who does not talk during an interview?

☐ PERFORMANCE CHECKLIST

OBJECTIVE: To use principles of interviewing to conduct an assessment interview.						
EVALUATION OF SELF[a]			EVALUATION BY PARTNER B[a]		EVALUATION BY OBSERVER[a]	
S	U	BEHAVIORS	S	U	S	U
		1. Attends to physical and psychological environment.				
		2. Uses appropriate opening statements.				
		3. States intent of interview clearly.				
		4. Begins with the other person's concerns.				
		5. Individualizes the interview.				
		6. Promotes a warm, trusting relationship.				
		7. Avoids creating barriers in the interview process.				
		8. Uses learned communication skills to respond to verbal and nonverbal messages.				
		9. Assumes responsibility for direction and movement of interview.				
		10. Responds to recurrent themes and contradictions, and responds to discomfort and conflict.				
		11. Uses appropriate terminating statements.				
		12. Plans for next interview, use of information, or for intended activities of client and nurse.				
		13. Records and reports information as appropriate.				
		14. Areas of strength:				
		15. Needs strengthening in certain areas (specify).				

[a] S = Satisfactory; U = Unsatisfactory.

REFERENCES

Anthony WA, Carkhuff RR: The Art of Health Care: A Handbook of Psychological First Aid Skills. Amherst, MA, Human Resources Development Press, 1976.

Bernstein L, Bernstein RS: Interviewing: A Guide for Health Professionals, ed 3. New York, Appleton-Century-Crofts, 1980.

Garrett A: Interviewing: Its Principles and Methods, ed 2. New York, Family Service of America, 1972.

Korsch BM, Freemon B, Negrete VF: Practical implications of doctor–patient interaction analysis for pediatric practice. American Journal of the Disabled Child 121(2):110-114, 1971.

McCain RF: Nursing by assessment—Not intuition. American Journal of Nursing 65(4):82-84, 1965.

McPhetridge LM: Nursing history: One means to personalize care. American Journal of Nursing 68(1):68-75, 1968.

Mitchell PH, Loustau A: Concepts Basic to Nursing, ed 3. New York, McGraw-Hill, 1981.

Pluckhan ML: Human Communication: The Matrix of Nursing. New York, McGraw-Hill, 1978.

Schweer JE, Gebbie KM: Creative Teaching in Clinical Nursing. St Louis, CV Mosby, 1976.

Smith D: A clinical nursing tool. American Journal of Nursing 68(11):2384-2388, 1968.

Smith L: Communication skills. Nursing Times 75(2): 926-929, 1979.

BIBLIOGRAPHY

Freeman BL, Korsch BN, et al: How well do nurses expand their roles in well child care? American Journal of Nursing 72(10):1866-1871, 1972.

SUGGESTED READING

Devillers L: What to do when you just can't communicate. NursingLife 2(2):34-39, 1982.

Mengel A: Getting the most from patient interviews. Nursing82 (Horsham) 12(11):46-49, 1982.

Richardson B: A tool for assessing the real world of diabetic noncompliance. Nursing82 (Horsham) 12(1):68-73, 1982.

AUDIOVISUAL RESOURCES

Nursing History: Guidelines for Accuracy
  Slides, filmstrip, videocassette, film. (1978, Color, 16 min.)

Nursing History: Interviewing Techniques
  Slides, filmstrip, videocassette, film. (1978, Color, 15 min.)

Process Recording Guide
  Audio-Tape Cassette. (1975, 20 min.)
  Available through:
    Medcom, Inc.
    P.O. Box 116
    Garden Grove, CA 92642

SKILL 16 Teaching–Learning

He that complies against his will is of the same opinion still.
—Samuel Butler

☐ STUDENT OBJECTIVES

1. Discuss the nurse's obligation to teach clients.
2. Distinguish between teaching and learning.
3. Compare incidental and planned teaching.
4. Describe various approaches to identifying learning needs.
5. Describe factors that influence client readiness to learn.
6. Discuss ways the nurse can enhance the client's readiness for learning.
7. Describe readiness factors that contribute to client learning.
8. Compare the nursing process and the teaching–learning process.
9. Develop the ability to create realistic goals and objectives when teaching clients.
10. Use a task analysis to determine the content, objectives, and instructional methods of teaching–learning tasks.
11. Recommend valid ways to determine effectiveness of the teaching–learning process.
12. Describe the characteristics of a productive nurse-teacher.

☐ INTRODUCTION

Teaching and learning are two elements of a single process in which both the teacher and the learner are actively involved.

Teaching can be defined as the process of facilitating learning. It is a "deliberate, intentional action . . . undertaken to help another person learn to do something he presently cannot do" (Narrow, 1979, p. 3).

Learning means that a person "becomes capable of doing something he could not do before and actually carries this out" (Narrow, 1979, p. 5). This learning may be intellectual or cognitive, social, behavioral, or psychomotor in nature.

Teaching has been within the scope of nursing practice for many years. In the 19th century, nursing leaders emphasized the need to teach families about sanitation, cleanliness, and the care of the sick. As early as 1918, National League for Nursing statements included a concern about teaching as a function of nursing (Redman, 1980). For many years public health nurses have considered teaching a major part of their role.

Teaching is an essential nursing intervention, not an optional activity. The American Nurses' Association Standards of Practice developed in 1976 include teaching as a nursing function (American Nurses' Association, 1976). The Nurse Practice Acts of many different states specify teaching as one of the functions that are within the legal scope of nursing practice. Increasingly, the nurse is being held accountable for teaching clients and may be held liable for failure to do so.

There are many reasons for an increased emphasis on teaching as a nursing function, and over the years the nature of what needs to be taught has changed. Since World War II there has been an increase in long-term illnesses and disabilities, where both the client and family need to achieve a thorough understanding of the illness and its treatment. Changes in longevity, the nature of medical care, increased lifesaving technology, and new procedures expand the need for teaching, as well as its scope. A trend toward consumerism, self-care, and holistic health indicates people wish to be knowledgeable about health promotion, illness, and illness prevention. Efforts at reducing hospital and medical costs depend directly on the existence of well-informed health-care consumers. Hospital stays are likely to be shortened, readmission rates reduced, and visits to medical facilities decreased if clients understand illness prevention, early diagnosis, and home care of illness.

This increased need for teaching has generated a new career for some nurses who enjoy teaching. To fill a void, some nurses are engaging in private practices and contracting with physicians to provide health teaching for those physicians' clients. The role of health educator or teaching specialist is becoming more common in hospital, clinic, and home-care settings.

Several authors (Redman, 1980; Rosenberg, 1976)

have reported accumulating evidence to suggest health teaching is effective in reducing health-care system use and expense. In one study, a continuing education program for clients with congestive heart failure resulted in improved adherence to the therapeutic plan, higher levels of functioning, and a reduction in hospital readmissions (Rosenberg, 1976). In another study, hospitalized clients who had pre- and postoperative instruction about pain requested less postoperative pain medication and were discharged an average of 2.7 days earlier than clients who were not instructed (Redman, 1980, p. 7). Substantial economic savings through decreased hospital and outpatient costs occurred as a result of a self-treatment project for hemophiliac patients (Rosenberg, 1976). Hypertensive patients who agreed to accept home visits for teaching and follow-up from a nurse exhibited a higher degree of adherence to therapeutic regimens and had lower blood pressures than those who refused home visits (Haynes, 1976b).

With their traditional concern for the whole person and for clients' ability to function optimally, it is logical for nurses to assume an active role in teaching. Yet some studies indicate that many nurses neither teach nor perceive teaching to be part of their job (Redman, 1980). Redman (1980, pp. 15–17) discusses numerous reasons for this, ranging from confusion about the nurse's role in teaching to lack of time and lack of preparation for the teaching role. Rosenberg (1976, p. 93) proposes that in most acute-care institutions, "patient and family education, if provided, is usually on an incidental, accidental, and ad hoc basis."

☐ PREPARATION

Teaching and learning are familiar activities; everyone has been involved in planned formal teaching–learning situations and most people regularly encounter situations in which they are required to learn something new or explain something to another person. Looking at those experiences can help identify factors that promote or inhibit learning and produce effective or ineffective learning. The following activity examines past experiences with teaching and learning.

Activity 16-A: Experiences with Teaching and Learning

Work individually within small groups.

1. Recall and examine personal situations in which you were expected to learn something but did not. Identify reasons why you did not learn. Group those reasons into three categories: factors related to yourself, your teacher, and the teaching–learning situation. What was needed in this situation to make it possible for you to learn? Discuss and compare your situation with others in the group.

2. Compare two learning experiences you have had—one in which you were actively involved in doing something and another in which you were a passive observer. Which one provided the best learning experience for you? For what reasons? Discuss and compare with others in your group.

3. Recall and examine teaching experiences you have had, such as teaching swimming at summer camp, teaching a sibling to ride a bicycle, or teaching a child to tie shoelaces. Give reasons why your teaching did or did not result in learning. Discuss and compare with others in your group.

Teaching in a health-care setting may be incidental (informal) or planned (formal). *Incidental teaching* occurs when clients ask about things that are important to them or attempt to validate previous information or perceptions. The nurse who values client teaching is alert for teaching needs and opportunities that are expressed both directly and indirectly. A client may say, "I need help in learning about this new salt-free diet!" or, "Leave my menus in my drawer so I'll know what to eat when I get home." The first is a direct request for information; the second an indirect way of communicating the same request. Incidental teaching also occurs in the process of giving direct care to clients. Many spontaneous opportunities for informal teaching can be utilized during this time if nurses are alert and sensitive to their own observations of client verbal, nonverbal, or psychomotor behaviors that indicate a need for client teaching. For example, the nurse may comment on the correct way to apply and position support stockings while helping the client reapply them after bathing. If the nurse discusses the importance of correct placement of the stockings in the context of both comfort and prevention of complications, the client is more likely to learn and practice the correct technique.

Planned teaching is necessary for patients with special needs. For example, clients with diabetes, hypertension, heart disease, new babies, or a handicapped relative often need extensive information and practice to help them cope adequately with their circumstances. Planned teaching may be done on either an individual or group basis.

ASSESSMENT OF THE LEARNER

Background Information

To assess the learning needs of clients, there are three categories of information to be gathered: data *about the client's medical and nursing diagnoses;* data *about the client;* and *data from the client.*

Information *about the medical and nursing diagnoses* and therapeutic regime determines what the client and family need to know in order to manage the client's medical condition. These data will be found in the client's health record, nursing-care kardex, or computer care plan.

Data about the client can be obtained from a variety of sources such as direct observation of the client, client records or referral forms, and the client's family. It is crucial, however, that written data be verified with the client to avoid operating on assumptions that may not be correct.

Data from the client provides insight into the client's ability to function and his or her readiness to learn. The effectiveness with which information is gathered from the client is directly related to the nurse's ability to use communications skills. Assessment interviews combined with direct observations enable the nurse to determine how the client is functioning in terms of the ability to care for self, accomplish the activities of daily living, and meet basic needs. For example, if a client has problems with ambulation, the nurse would assess the alterations from normal that are present, the client's potential ability to ambulate, the kind and degree of assistance needed, and what the client needs to know to ambulate at his or her optimal level. This particular client's teaching–learning need may involve learning to use a walker, crutches, cane, or a prosthesis or it might involve reeducation about more effective ways to use crutches. It is crucial to involve the client in the process of assessing his or her own learning abilities, needs, readiness, and attitude because the process of learning is enhanced when the client is interested in learning, wants to learn, and is actively involved in both the planning and implementation of teaching–learning activities.

Readiness for Learning

Readiness is a "state or condition of being both willing and able to make use of instruction. The degree of readiness to learn depends upon the degrees of willingness and ability; therefore, a high level of readiness presumes that the student is eager and fully able to respond to instruction. On the other hand, if either willingness or ability is diminished, readiness to learn is also decreased" (Narrow, 1979, p. 79). Without readiness, learning tends to be limited, but with readiness, Narrow indicates that even less than mediocre instruction (activities of teaching) can be profitable.

Client readiness is difficult to assess accurately. Health and illness problems alter a person's usual ability to learn, and in most agencies, the time available for both assessment of learning needs and teaching may be quite brief. In a health-care setting there are four factors that Narrow believes influence client readiness—motivation to learn, client comfort, client energy levels, and client capabilities.

Client Motivation. Motivation refers to an incentive or stimulation for action (Webster, 1976) and is described by Redman (1980) as "emotional readiness." Motivation may be either external or internal in nature. Internal, self-directed motivation is generally considered to be far more effective in achieving learning than when motivation is only external. In the latter case, the motivation often disappears as soon as the external motivating source is withdrawn. An example of primarily external motivation is the diabetic client who remains on a prescribed diet only as long as someone else is monitoring his or her food intake, and when left alone, goes on eating binges.

Motivation to learn is highly individualized. A variety of *desires or needs* may motivate clients' learning: to get well; to understand their illness; to please others; to be able to return to work; to be a "good patient"; to be self-sufficient; to protect themselves from the mistakes of health-care workers; to feel better; or to avoid complications of illness and criticism from others (Narrow, 1979).

Personal relevance of material to be learned affects motivation, since people are more able to focus on and learn material they perceive to be personally relevant (Combs et al., 1971). This perception of relevance is highly personal and may or may not coincide with someone else's perceptions. For example, a family may perceive that it is important for the father to quit smoking and follow a weight reduction diet, but until the father perceives these things as important to *him*, no amount of information, bribing, or nagging will motivate him to change his behaviors.

The *attitude of the health-care worker* can affect clients' motivation. There is some indication that a supportive, nonjudgmental, and accepting nurse can increase a client's willingness to learn new health behaviors. In her study of diabetic client learning, Casey (1979) found that clients initially carried out desired activities such as diet and insulin regimes because of their relationship with the health-care worker and then gradually developed internal motivation to continue these activities for their own reasons. A supportive family may provide a similar initial motivation (Haynes, 1976a).

Challenge can sometimes motivate a person to learn. However, the same learning situation may be viewed by different people as either challenging or threatening, depending on the individual's perceived ability to cope with the situation. When people encounter a situation they are interested in and feel reasonably able to handle, they usually feel challenged and are motivated to master the situation. However, when people see themselves as inadequate to handle something, they tend to feel threatened and may withdraw from the situation or function quite inappropriately and inadequately.

There is good evidence to indicate that threats from the health-care worker seldom enhance motivation or learning (Combs et al., 1971; Combs and Taylor, 1952). When a person feels threatened, his or her perceptual field becomes narrowed, thus decreasing the ability to process information. Additionally, a person who feels threatened perceives a need to defend his or her own practices and beliefs. This is obviously not conducive to change. As discussed in earlier skills, it is important to remember that if the individual *feels* threatened, for all intents and purposes, he or she *is* threatened in that situation, regardless of anyone else's perceptions.

Some degree of *anxiety* can produce motivation to learn, but high levels tend to decrease perceptual awareness and hamper learning. A study reported by Bernstein et al. (1974) indicated a positive correlation between memory and moderate anxiety, with both high and low anxiety levels producing less recall than moderate levels of anxiety.

Assessment of Motivation. Motivation can be assessed through observation of behavior and by listening to what the client says. When clients are motivated to learn, they usually ask questions, take notes on what is being discussed, ask for additional explanations, request books and pamphlets, or exhibit other behaviors that indicate interest. Clients may not be fully aware of their own motivation to learn; they may not choose to share it with the nurse, and it may be different from what the nurse thinks it should be. Narrow (1979) suggests that any motivation to learn is valid. As a professional person, the nurse learns to accept and respect the client's current motivation, recognizing that it may change over time. For example, an overweight executive with hypertension may initially adopt an exercise and diet program simply because of orders from the company physician, while the nurse may think the client should be concerned about avoiding complications, not just obeying orders. Eventually the client may find that he or she feels better on the new regime or may decide that hypertension and excess weight are detrimental to good health, and begin to follow the new regime for those reasons.

Client Comfort. Both physical and psychological comfort affect learning. Learning is generally decreased when a person is physically uncomfortable and weary, or emotionally drained by unsettling events. Some common sources of *physical discomfort* for a hospitalized individual are pain, nausea, dizziness, itching, fatigue or weakness, hunger or thirst, or the need to urinate or defecate. Emotions such as fear, anxiety, worry, grief, anger, and guilt can cause *psychological discomfort* for a client in any setting. Actually, any intense emotion interferes with learning, including positive ones like elation. Nearly everyone has had the experience of being too excited to study when anticipating a special event. Interruptions, lack of privacy, and excessive noise levels also cause psychological discomfort. There is a reciprocal relationship between physical discomfort and psychological discomfort, in that either can initiate or intensify the other, and intervention to reduce either has a beneficial effect on both.

Assessment of Comfort Level. Comfort levels can be assessed through direct observations by the nurse and validated with subjective data from the client. If a client is experiencing physical or psychological discomfort, the nurse intervenes to relieve or decrease that discomfort before continuing with planned teaching activities. This might mean rescheduling the teaching for a later time or date. If this is not possible, specific teaching activities should be directed toward reducing the client's anxiety, such as by giving explanations and information, or by helping the client cope with the discomfort, such as through teaching relaxation methods.

Client Energy Levels. Energy levels affect the ability to concentrate and attend to a learning task. They vary with time of day, state of health, mental attitude, medications, and motivation. Because of body rhythms, some people learn more readily in the morning and others learn more easily in the late afternoon. Since learning requires the active involvement of the learner, the fatigue associated with illness often makes learning difficult, and when large amounts of physical or psychic energy are being expended to cope with crisis and illness, there may be very little energy left for learning. Some medications dull the client's perception of his or her surroundings. This dulling effect may be very helpful for relief of pain, but it diminishes the client's capacity to learn.

Assessment of Energy Level. Energy levels can be assessed by observing the client's general appearance state of health and illness, and by paying attention to the client's comments. When at all possible, teaching should be planned for times when a client's energy is at a maximum level.

Client Capabilities. Capability refers to the ability to learn something or implement a psychomotor skill. It is a more objective aspect of readiness than are motivation, comfort, and energy. Redman (1980) describes capabilities as "experiential readiness." Capability may be assessed by considering physical capability, intellectual capability, past learning, and previous experiences (Narrow, 1979). *Physical capabilities* include strength, size, coordination, dexterity, and the ability to see, hear, smell, taste, and feel. *Intellectual capability* refers to clients' ability to read, perform basic mathematics, comprehend instructions, problem solve, and communicate verbally. *Past learning and experiences* affect clients' present level of knowledge, their attitudes toward what is being taught, and their current level of related skills. For example, a pregnant woman may not attend a clinic regularly or follow advice about caring for herself because she has had no previous experience with the benefits of regular health care and has not yet learned to value that care.

Assessment of Capability. To determine whether a client is capable of learning something or performing a psychomotor skill, the nurse identifies the capabilities required to learn the skill and then determines whether the client possesses those capabilities. For example, a client with very limited eyesight will have difficulty learning to self-administer insulin because of the visual acuity required by that task. In addition, a client's perception of his or her own capability affects the capacity to learn and perform. For example, two people may seem to have the same degree of physical handicap, but because of attitude, philosophy, and personality, one may be able to use his or her capabilities more completely and accomplish much more than the other.

THE TEACHING-LEARNING PROCESS

The process of teaching–learning is very similar to the nursing process. In the teaching–learning process, learner needs and learner readiness are identified from subjective and objective data, comparable to assessment with its nursing diagnosis. This learning need can also be considered to be the teaching–learning task, for which goals, objectives, content, teaching strategies, and evaluative criteria can be developed, similar to the way the nursing process is implemented.

Setting Goals and Objectives

Long-term goals generally relate to the desired outcome or resolution of the learning need. Short-term objectives are more narrow and specific, with more immediate outcomes, and can be termed instructional objectives. They are directly related to the teaching-learning task. To illustrate the concepts of long-term goals and short-term objectives, consider a newly diagnosed insulin-dependent diabetic. For this client, a long-term teaching-learning goal could be, "To be able to assume self-care and management of diabetes." A short-term instructional objective could then be "To give my own insulin correctly and safely."

Goals and objectives are best created jointly with the client, since it is the client who must work to achieve them. A goal or objective that seems completely appropriate to the nurse may be totally unacceptable to the client, the client's family, or both. For example, the nurse's goal may be to have the diabetic client achieve total self-care, including administration of insulin. Because of the interpersonal relationships among the family members, the client and spouse may have quite different goals, and either one or both may assume that the wife manages the care for the husband, or vice versa. Some degree of agreement on goals and objectives obviously is necessary if any successful teaching is to take place.

When creating goals or objectives with clients, Narrow (1979, p. 110) suggests coupling the desired behavior with the client's reason for wanting to learn it, that is, "to learn . . . in order to . . ." For example, "To learn how to plan my diet in order to avoid insulin reactions." The client's stated reason may alert the nurse to additional teaching needs. In this example, the additional need might be discussing reasons for insulin reactions other than imbalances in the dietary program.

Some educational authorities propose that all educational or instructional objectives ought to be measurable and specific, indicating the behavior to be achieved, the criteria (how well the behavior is to be done), and the conditions (circumstances under which the behavior is to be carried out). Although it may not always be necessary to specify each of these components when creating objectives with the client, the nurse considers them in the teaching plan. For example, if a diabetic is going to self-administer insulin (the behavior) at home with a reusable glass syringe (the conditions), the nurse alters the teaching plan to incorporate glass syringe care in order to meet the crite-

TABLE 16-1. Sample Task Analysis

MAJOR SKILL	LONG-TERM GOAL
Insulin self-administration	Involve self in the care of diabetes
	Learner's Objective
	Give own insulin correctly and safely
Subskills	**Instructional Objectives**

1. Handle sterile equipment.
   a. Differentiate among clean, sterile, and nonsterile equipment.
   b. Wash hands.
   c. Open disposable syringe and needle package without contamination.
   d. Sterilize reusable equipment.[a]
      i. Rinse syringe and needle with cold water after each use.
      ii. Boil unassembled syringe for 20 minutes, covered with water.
      iii. Reassemble syringe and attach needle, touching only the barrel, plunger head, and needle hub.
2. Withdraw correct dosage of insulin.
3. Select appropriate injection site.
4. Inject insulin in a safe manner.
	1. Describe the differences among clean, sterile, and nonsterile.
	
	2. Demonstrate the ability to use a sterile syringe and needle without contamination.
	3. Demonstrate the ability to clean and resterilize reusable equipment.[a]
	
	4. Obtain correct amount of insulin for prescribed dosage.
	5. Locate available sites for insulin injection.
	6. Plan a rotation process for insulin injection.
	7. Inject insulin correctly.

[a] Appropriate when using glass syringes or reusable needles.

ria of giving the insulin in the correct manner without contamination of the syringe.

It is important to remember that unplanned, unexpected learning often occurs, and its relevance frequently surpasses what could be planned or predicted (Styles, 1975). These serendipitous learning experiences can often be the most meaningful ones and may involve attitudinal changes, integration of information, or a new, better way to do something.

Analyzing the Teaching-Learning Task
After the teaching-learning task has been identified, Dick and Carey (1978) advise analyzing the task to determine necessary content before identifying instructional objectives. They suggest asking two questions: "What steps are necessary to achieve this task or learn this material?" and, "What knowledge is necessary for each step?" This process identifies the necessary skills and subskills and the supporting information that comprise the total teaching-learning task, including the content to be learned. According to Dick and Carey, the next step is to create short-term instructional objectives that are directly related to these skills and their subskills. When the skill to be learned has been broken into subskills, the nurse then considers what information and experiences the client requires in order to accomplish each subskill.

Returning to the example of the diabetic client, where the long-term goal is, "To be able to assume self-care and management of diabetes," an instructional objective might be, "To give my own insulin correctly and safely." In order to accomplish the skill of insulin self-administration, the client will need to learn the subskills of handling sterile equipment, withdrawing correct dosages of insulin, selecting the appropriate injection site, and injecting the insulin in a safe manner. To make this possible, the nurse will instruct the client in sterile technique, site selection and rotation, and withdrawal and injection of the insulin. The client then must practice each subskill. Table 16-1 presents an illustration of how this task analysis and development of objectives might be done, again using diabetes as an example. Subskill 1 is defined in detail as an example of the task analysis process.

Although this process sounds lengthy and complicated, it ensures that important material is not omitted, promotes organized presentation of the learning materials, and avoids last-minute hasty inclusion of information and searching for equipment or teaching aids.

The following activity provides practice in analyzing a teaching-learning task by analyzing a familiar activity for its component skills and objectives.

Activity 16-B: Examining a Learning Situation

This activity is to be done in writing; work alone or with a partner.

1. Recall an activity, task, or subject you have learned in the past year, such as yoga, skiing, baking bread, or learning French.
2. State in writing your own original objective for the activity. Example: "To learn to bake bread."
3. Sequentially identify the basic subskills necessary to reach this goal.

   Examples: Read and follow the recipe correctly.
   Measure ingredients accurately.
   Knead the dough adequately.
   Provide optimum rising conditions.
   Shape dough into loaves.
   Provide proper baking environment.

   Each of these could be subdivided into more subskills, such as how to measure dry versus liquid ingredients. There is some basic knowledge that is needed to be able to perform most of these tasks, such as knowing the proper temperature for bread to rise properly. Each of these subskills can also be stated as an objective, for example, "To develop the ability to read and follow a recipe accurately."

4. Describe the activities in which you engaged to help you carry out these subskills or meet the objectives.

   Example: Objective: "To develop the ability to read and follow a recipe correctly."
   Activities: Read entire recipe; research or ask about unclear terms or measurement units.

5. Compare your learning sequence, goals, subtasks, objectives, and activities with other students.

Teaching-Learning Content

Selecting Content. Select content that is *relevant* for the learning task and the learner, meets the client's perceived needs, and also provides information the nurse knows the client needs to have. A knowledge of health and illness, medical and nursing diagnoses and therapies, anatomy and physiology, and the social sciences helps the nurse determine what the client needs to know. Communication skills help the nurse assess what the client already knows, wants to know, and his or her level of readiness. If there is any question about the nature and depth of the content, or of its compatibility with the medical plan of care, planned teaching is validated with the nursing supervisor, the client's physician, or both.

Content needs to be sufficiently specific and clear so that the client will understand what he or she is expected to learn to do. The type of content being presented will influence the organization of the material and the instructional methods used. For example, when teaching diabetic clients to self-administer insulin, theory content about diabetes and insulin usually precedes instruction about injecting insulin, and essential instructional methods include demonstrations, practice, and return demonstrations.

Establishing Priorities. The constraints of time and sometimes limited client contact do not always permit the amount of teaching the nurse believes is necessary. There are several ways to determine priorities for the content and sequence of planned teaching. One approach is to divide content between basic and advanced levels and present advanced content at a later time. For example, when teaching a client about angina, symptoms and treatment could be considered basic content, whereas the action of nitroglycerin and the distinction between angina and a heart attack could be considered more advanced content. Another approach is to determine what is essential information and then add helpful or interesting material as time permits. For example, it is essential for a diabetic to know how to maintain sterility during self-administration of insulin. It is helpful to understand the concept of sterility, and interesting to know the meaning of U-100 and labels such as protamine zinc. If assessment of learning needs has identified significant misconceptions or omissions in the client's existing knowledge or skill, the first priority for teaching is to remedy those gaps and errors. For example, if a client believes insulin will cure diabetes, the teaching content would first focus on the nature and management of diabetes as a chronic condition.

Organization of Content. Planned content should be presented in an organized manner because organization promotes retention and application of learning (Pohl, 1978). Content is best divided into manageable segments, based on the amount of time available, the nature of the subject matter, and the capabilities of the individual or group. Although no single organizational pattern fits all material or individuals, it is worth noting the research reported by Bernstein and Bernstein (1980). They indicate that material that is presented first is remembered more clearly than material presented second, and that the rate of recall drops as the amount of information presented increases.

The most appropriate length for a teaching–learning session is no more than 1 hour, and preferably less than that. Learning is generally increased when content is presented in shorter successive segments, thus allowing review, practice, and reinforcement between sessions.

Instructional Methods and Activities

When the nurse and client together have created written or verbal objectives that identify the focus of learning and the nurse has analyzed the task for content and sequential steps, the nurse then develops a written teaching plan. This plan includes the goals and objectives, teaching–learning tasks, a time schedule for presenting the material, and the activities to be used. Activities used to implement teaching plans are known as instructional methods or activities. They may include discussions, lectures, printed materials, audiovisual aids, demonstrations, and return demonstrations. Variety in instructional methods is helpful, but too much variety is confusing and fatiguing. It is best to be selective, choosing methods appropriate to the objectives, the material being taught, and the client involved. When the client has been given reading materials, the nurse should follow up with a discussion or provide time for questions and clarification.

When one or two persons have the primary responsibility for the actual teaching, it is possible to provide greater continuity and increased levels of client involvement. However, when the plan is available for all staff involved with the client, all staff can reinforce teaching and have consistent expectations.

Learner Involvement

The teaching–learning process is an active process and requires involvement and participation on the part of the learner in order to achieve long-term benefits (Combs et al., 1978; DuGas, 1977). However, regarding the client as a participant does not mean trying to find ways to manipulate him or her into doing what the nurse wants. To be a participant implies the active involvement of a client and includes decision-making power and actual choices for that client. Sometimes the choices may not be what the nurse would prefer, but if the client truly is a participant, those choices are to be respected. A compromise acceptable to both nurse and client can usually be reached.

There are many ways to involve the client learner. As described earlier, goals and objectives are more realistic and achievable when determined jointly by the nurse and the client, and often the family. In addition, teaching activities are most effective when planned in consultation with the client and his or her family. It has been found that teaching is more effective when families as well as clients are involved. A study of weight reduction in cardiac patients indicated that patients whose spouses were involved in the teaching plan lost more weight than those whose spouses were not involved (Casey, 1979). The client's life style and home environment also need to be known and considered when developing the teaching plan. It does no good to teach a diabetic client about meat exchanges if he or she is a vegetarian, or to teach a person with a stroke how to move from a wheelchair to a toilet if the bathroom door in the home is too narrow for the wheelchair.

Effective teaching is a give-and-take process, with the nurse giving information or demonstrating a skill, the client asking questions, and the nurse validating the client's understanding of what is being taught. The nurse can get some idea of the client's involvement in the teaching–learning process by observing whether the client seems interested, follows what is being said, and asks questions. Negative reactions on the part of the client can alert the nurse to the need

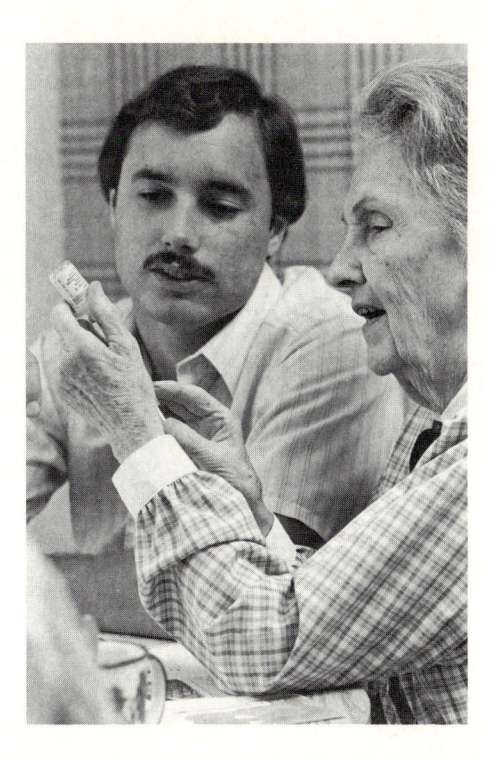

Figure 16–1. Supervised practice facilitates learning. (Photo by James Haines.)

for exploring the client's attitudes and perceptions about what is being taught. For example, if a client grimaces while preparing insulin for self-injection, the outcome of the teaching will be more successful if the nurse identifies the nonverbal reaction and validates its meaning with the client before continuing to teach the manual skill.

Whenever manual skills are taught, involve the client in that learning by having him or her give a return demonstration, practice independently, and then again demonstrate the skill to the nurse for validation of accuracy as shown in Figure 16-1. It is best if practice occurs soon after the initial teaching has taken place because learning is retained longer when it is put to immediate use than when its application is delayed (DuGas, 1977).

Reinforcement
Reinforcement is essential for learning. It can take the form of repetition, praise for a task well done, positive feedback from the nurse and the family, recognition within the group, or even concrete rewards such as tokens or candy, which might be used with disturbed or retarded persons. During the teaching–learning process, it is important to give clients *feedback* about their learning, since effective learning requires knowledge of the results (Combs et al., 1971). The client is given feedback about what he or she is doing successfully, as well as what requires more work or could be improved. This feedback focuses on the learning task, rather than on the client's personality or character.

Positive feedback reinforces a person's self-concept, which enhances learning. For two reasons, it is helpful to give positive feedback about successes prior to feedback about problem areas. People tend to focus on failures rather than successes, and also remember best what they hear first (Bernstein and Bernstein, 1980). The "sandwich" approach of inserting the criticism between positive comments tends to diminish the effectiveness of the criticism. For more discussion of feedback, see the Introduction to Part One.

Repetition strengthens learning (Talarico, 1978). Periodic reviews of what already has been learned can help the client see the progress already made as well as provide reinforcement for the learning. These reviews might take place before and after a teaching–learning session, perhaps on a daily or weekly basis. The frequency depends on the newness and nature of the material, the characteristics of the learner, and the setting.

Follow-up is an essential element of the teaching–learning process. Follow-up helps reinforce learning and demonstrates the health-care professional's concern for the client. It can be used to determine a client's long-term learning of manual skills, knowledge, or attitudes, as well as to identify needed modifications of the teaching plan and any additional learning needs. Follow-up can be accomplished in a number of ways. Clinic or private clients can be asked to return for follow-up visits. A clinic or hospital client can be referred to a public health or home-care agency. A community or public health nurse can plan regular follow-up visits or telephone calls. Clients can be encouraged to telephone the health educator, the clinic, physician's office, or the community health nurse when questions or problems occur during or after a teaching program.

Some nurses have found written contracts to be a helpful way to facilitate and reinforce learning. The contract is jointly created by the nurse and the client and clearly identifies what each will do and what each one can expect from the other. One study indicated that when nurses used written contracts with diabetic clients, more than twice as many clients were able to meet at least half of their learning objectives (Bell and Bell, 1980).

Evaluation of Learning
As in the nursing process, teaching–learning includes examining the results of the teaching–learning process in an effort to determine whether or not objectives were met, goals were reached, and teaching activities were successful. When goals and objectives are clearly stated at the outset of teaching activities, they can serve as the criteria by which to evaluate learning. Probably the best way to determine whether or not learning has occurred, however, is to observe for changes in the client's health-care behavior. Research cited by Haynes (1976a) tends to suggest that although a change in behavior is usually thought to indicate a change in attitude, it is also possible for health-care behaviors to change before a change in be-

liefs and attitude has occurred. Other research indicates that health beliefs and attitudes change as compliance develops and as the client follows the recommended course of treatment and experiences its benefits (Becker et al., 1979). This is true of the client who initially practices the change in behavior for someone else, and later for himself or herself.

Compliance has been defined as "the extent to which a person's behavior . . . coincides with medical or health advice" (Haynes, 1979, pp. 1–2). The term adherence can be used interchangeably with compliance; both are intended to be nonjudgmental and to imply an active willingness to participate on the part of the client (Haynes, 1979; Rosenberg, 1976). The acquisition of knowledge by itself is known to have a low correlation with compliance or adherence behavior (Haynes, 1976a,b). Knowledge accompanied by a change in attitude results in a much higher level of adherence to the desired health-care behavior.

Similar to all other aspects of the teaching–learning process, evaluation is a joint effort of the nurse and the client and includes examining the process itself, the teaching program, and the client benefits. By looking objectively at behaviors and discussing feelings and concerns, the nurse and the client can determine whether or not the teaching plan has been successful and what alterations or additions might need to be included. Evaluation is best done as an ongoing activity—during as well as after the teaching-learning process. During the interaction, the nurse watches for nonverbal feedback that would indicate understanding or lack of understanding on the client's part; and asks for verbal feedback at intervals. For example, the nurse can ask questions such as "Is there anything else you may be wondering about?" or "Is any part of what we've talked about not clear for you?"

ASSESSING ONESELF AS A TEACHER

"The effectiveness of teaching depends largely upon what the nurse brings to the situation" (Narrow, 1979, p. 92). When assessing oneself as a teacher, the nurse must consider his or her own attitudes both toward the client and toward the material to be taught. If teaching–learning is to be successful, the nurse must demonstrate an accepting, open attitude and have the ability to develop a supportive rapport with the client rather than make the client feel stupid or inadequate because of either not knowing something or having incorrect information. Veninga (1978) indicates that interpersonal communication may be the most crucial variable in determining whether or not learning occurs. As a teacher, the nurse uses learned communication skills discussed earlier in this text, is aware of personal and client values and beliefs, and makes a genuine attempt to avoid stereotyping and prejudging those with differing values and beliefs.

Some nurses are unable to teach material with which they are not comfortable, such as sex or pain; other nurses may be uncomfortable when working with people from some religious and ethnic groups, the very rich, or the very poor. It is important that nurses be aware of their own limits and either learn to avoid having their own values interfere with client care or learn when to arrange for someone else to do teaching with which they are uncomfortable.

It is important for the nurse to be aware of his or her own energy, knowledge, and skill levels. Teaching requires energy in the form of alertness to the meaning of nurse–client interactions, attention to direct and indirect requests for information, and a commitment to the importance of teaching. If nurses find their knowledge in given areas is less than adequate to meet client needs, it is their responsibility either to upgrade those skills and knowledge or to request relocation to an area in which they are more competent.

Nurses sometimes find it easier to teach individuals before attempting to teach groups of clients. Teaching individuals alerts the nurse to the types of concerns, issues, and questions that clients with specific learning needs tend to raise. This helps the nurse to be better prepared to answer questions from a group or to raise issues and questions that have been relevant to other individuals with similar learning needs. It also helps the nurse to become familiar with available resources within the agency and community and to learn how to find answers to client concerns.

THE TEACHING-LEARNING SITUATION

Health-care agencies vary in their commitment to client education and the amount of resources and staff allocated to teaching. The *degree of commitment* can contribute to or detract from teaching–learning. For client teaching to be included in the expected functions of the nursing staff, there must be an administrative commitment to client education from both the agency and nursing administration. This commitment translates into adequate staffing levels that permit teaching to occur, adequate salaries to retain competent staff, and in-service programs to increase the staff's teaching skills. For client teaching to be implemented successfully, it is important for both staff nurses and nursing management to value teaching, for physicians and nurses alike to recognize the collaborative role each has in planning and providing client teaching, and for families and clients to value the nurse's teaching function. To illustrate these concepts, consider the difficulty encountered by a nurse who values client teaching if (1) administration fails to budget enough staff to permit teaching time, (2) supervisors are task oriented and regard "just talking" to clients as wasted time, (3) physicians have a proprietary attitude toward patients and believe that no one other than themselves should teach their patients, (4) fellow nurses do not value or practice teaching, or (5) clients or families believe nurses should do everything for the client and refuse to assume responsibility for any aspects of their own care.

Availability of resources also affects the process of teaching–learning. Space, time, staffing, and audiovisual materials all have budgetary implications but are necessary parts of planned teaching, particularly for groups of clients. For informal, individual teaching, time and even a limited amount of space are the primary resources needed.

When planning group teaching, care must be taken to see that the *physical environment* is comfortable, attractive, well-lighted, and well-ventilated and has furniture and visual aids appropriate to the age and physical status of the participants. It is recommended that group education be conducted at the eighth-grade level. Equipment and materials used in teaching should be comparable to what clients will use in their homes, for example, home dialysis equipment, reusable insulin syringes, dressing supplies, or blood pressure equipment.

DOCUMENTATION OF TEACHING–LEARNING

Teaching activities and any identified client learning must be documented in the health record. Having this information in the client's record fulfills nurse accountability and provides for continuity of care. The Joint Commission for Accreditation of Hospitals (JCAH) includes documentation of teaching in their standards for nursing service and looks for this documentation during the process of reaccreditation (Joint Commission, 1984). Documentation of teaching can be a part of the regular narrative nurses' notes or be entered on a special teaching documentation form that becomes a part of the client's permanent health record.

Specially created forms or guides can be useful when a number of clients have similar teaching–learning needs or specific content needs to be communicated to many clients. These guides provide an efficient way of documenting teaching and learning and serve as a reference point for the nurses who are doing the teaching. Guides are especially useful when several different nurses participate in teaching the same client over the course of several shifts or days. Teaching–learning guides are usually developed by nurses for their own particular setting or client population and often include both general items applicable to many clients and items that can be adapted to meet individual needs (McConnell, 1980).

The use of teaching–learning guides provides some standardization of teaching content, but the focus is on documentation rather than on developing a standardized approach to teaching. The Diabetic Therapy and Education Sheet in Figure 16–2 provides space for documentation of nurse teaching and client learning focused on self-care on a long-term basis. This guide is used to document specific, measurable behavioral outcomes. The sequence of teaching activities is staff demonstration, explanation, or both, followed by a return demonstration, explanation, or both, from the client or a family member or friend. The review column helps the nurse identify new teaching goals and activities. The second and third pages of a three-page form are shown here; the first page (which appears in Fig. 18–3) provides space for recording tests and therapies. Results of diagnostic tests such as urine glucose may indicate additional teaching needs or represent progress in learning. Other guides, such as preoperative checklists, are used to document that the client was prepared adequately for a diagnostic or therapeutic procedure.

☐ EXECUTION

A nurse who is able to teach successfully and enable others to learn is one who is able to (1) care about other people, (2) develop empathic relationships, (3) use effective communication skills, (4) accept others' values and motivation, (5) work collaboratively with clients, (6) help clients become motivated for learning, (7) assess, plan, and evaluate, and (8) create realistic goals and objectives. This nurse also has a commitment to developing teaching skills, an adequate vocabulary for explaining diverse subjects, and competence within the content area being taught.

Some client teaching must be done by nurses with specialized training for specific areas, for example, home dialysis or neurologic rehabilitation. However, most teaching can be done by nurses who are comfortable with the content and willing to acquire the necessary knowledge, develop teaching skills, and explore the meaning of the client's condition or situation for him or her and the family (Narrow, 1979).

Teaching plans, like discharge plans, are best begun at the time the client is first admitted to the health-care facility. When physicians and nurses coordinate and communicate their plans for teaching, enough time for teaching and learning usually is available. It is most unfortunate when this kind of physician order is written: "Instruct patient about low-sodium diet and discharge in A.M." This allows insufficient time for the teaching–learning process to occur and certainly provides less than quality care. The client benefits when all health-care personnel are alert to client teaching needs and each one considers teaching as his or her business.

Sometimes nurses will want to create opportunities for teaching, using their knowledge of the client's medical and nursing diagnoses, treatment plan, and family situation. For example, Miss Smith-Jones is an elderly wealthy woman who lives alone in a fashionable condominium. She has always been independent, loves to travel, entertain, dine out, and socialize. Recently she has been identified as being severely hypertensive and is now on a very-low-salt weight reduction diet and antihypertensive medications. She has commented several times that she will be able to manage

DIABETES EDUCATION CHECKLIST

	STAFF DEMO &/OR EXPLAINED	PT./OTHER DEMO. &/OR EXPLAINED	NEEDS REVIEW
I. DEFINITION, DIAGNOSIS, TREATMENT PATIENT/OTHER VERBALIZES: 1. BASIC DEFINITION OF DIABETES MELLITUS	3/16 CC	3/17 CC	
2. NORMAL BLOOD SUGAR VALUES	3/16 CC	3/17 CC	
3. DIET, EXERCISE, AND MEDICATION (IF NEEDED) ARE PART OF THE PROGRAM FOR DIABETIC CONTROL	3/16 CC	3/17 CC	
II. URINE TESTING PATIENT/OTHER VERBALIZES: 1. IMPORTANCE OF URINE TESTING AS A MEANS OF ASSESSING DIABETIC CONTROL	3/17 CC	3/18 CC	
2. WHEN TO TEST FOR GLYCOSURIA	3/17 CC	3/18 CC	
3. UNDERSTANDING OF RESULTS OF URINE TEST	3/17 CC	3/18 CC	
4. WHY KETONES ARE PRODUCED AND WHEN TO TEST FOR THEM	3/17 CC	3/18 CC	✓
5. NEED TO TEST URINE BEFORE EACH MEAL DURING TIMES OF ILLNESS	3/17 CC	3/18 KD	✓
PATIENT/OTHER DEMONSTRATES: 6. COLLECTION OF DOUBLE-VOIDED SPECIMENS AT RECOMMENDED TIMES	3/17 CC	3/18 KD	✓
7. ACCURATE TIMING AND COLOR MATCHING FOR URINE TEST USED (CIRCLE): DIASTIX (KETODIASTIX) OTHER:	3/17 CC	3/18 KD	✓
8. RECORDING OF RESULTS	3/17 CC	3/18 CC	
III. FOOT CARE PATIENT/OTHER VERBALIZES: 1. FOOT CARE IS AN IMPORTANT ASPECT OF THE DAILY DIABETIC REGIMEN	3/17 CC	3/18 CC	✓
2. SPECIAL PRECAUTIONS FOR LEGS AND FEET	3/17 CC	3/18 CC	✓
PATIENT/OTHER DEMONSTRATES: 3. PROPER DAILY FOOT CARE	3/17 CC		
IV. MISCELLANEOUS 1. PATIENT HAS BEEN GIVEN OR WEARS SOME FORM OF DIABETIC IDENTIFICATION		3/18 CC	
2. REFERRED TO O.T. PROGRAM (CIRCLE) YES NO (EXERCISE PROGRAM) / (MEAL PREPARATION)	3/16 BJ	3/20 BJ	
PATIENT/OTHER DEMONSTRATES: 3. PLANNING AND PREPARATION OF MEAL ACCORDING TO DIET IN O.T. DEPARTMENT	3/17 BJ	3/17 BJ	
PATIENT/OTHER VERBALIZES: 4. ACTIVITY/EXERCISE LOWERS THE BLOOD SUGAR	3/16 BJ	3/18 BJ	
5. PHYSICAL OR EMOTIONAL STRESS CAN ELEVATE THE BLOOD SUGAR	3/16 CC	3/17 CC	
6. FEELINGS REGARDING COPING WITH DIABETES AFTER DISCHARGE	3/16 CC	3/18 CC	
7. AT LEAST TWO SYMPTOMS OF HYPERGLYCEMIA			
8. THE HEART, EYES, EXTREMITIES, SKIN, NERVE SENSATIONS, AND HEALING ABILITY CAN BE AFFECTED BY DIABETES			
9. THE NEED FOR ONGOING PHYSICIAN, NURSING, AND DIETITIAN SUPERVISOR AND/OR COMMUNICATIONS			
10. SOME COMMUNITY RESOURCES & PUBLICATIONS AVAILABLE FOR CONTINUING EDUCATION			

Winona Memorial Hospital
3232 North Meridian Street
Indianapolis, Indiana 46208
0703359-6

Figure 16–2. Diabetic Therapy and Education Sheet. (Courtesy of Winona Memorial Hospital, Indianapolis, IN.)

perfectly well when she gets home and does not want to attend diet classes. From this minimal information and her own knowledge base, the nurse knows that dietary management is a major part of treatment, that this woman will need to know how to select low-salt foods in a variety of eating circumstances, and that she is unaccustomed to asking for or receiving help. To create an opportunity either to discuss diet or arouse interest in discussing diet modifications, the nurse could plan to serve the woman's lunch tray, and ask if she minds if the nurse joins her for a cup of coffee while she eats. Since this woman is socially outgoing, this probably would be an acceptable invitation. The nurse can listen actively with productive attending behavior, observe for nonverbal and verbal comments about the food, reflect feelings and content in a sensitive way—and perhaps be able to determine what might motivate this woman to learn how dietary information could have personal meaning for her.

The following activity provides practice in determining client teaching–learning needs in a simulated client-care situation.

V. DIET PATIENT/OTHER VERBALIZES: 1. TYPE OF DIET AND NUMBER OF CALORIES	3/16 NH	3/17 NH	
2. IMPORTANCE OF A WELL-BALANCED DIET	3/16 NH	3/20 NH	
3. DEFINITION OF AN EXCHANGE	3/16 NH	3/17 NH	✓
4. IMPORTANCE OF FOOD INTAKE AND ENERGY EXPENDITURE IN WEIGHT REGULATION AND MANAGEMENT OF DIABETES	3/18 NH	3/20 NH	
5. RATIONALE FOR AVOIDING CONCENTRATED SWEETS	3/18 NH	3/20 NH	
6. CONSISTENCY IN EATING PATTERN IS IMPORTANT ON A DAILY BASIS	3/16 NH	3/20 NH	
7. ALTERATION OF MEAL PLAN FOR SICK DAYS	3/18 NH	3/20 NH	✓
PATIENT/OTHER DEMONSTRATES: 8. USE OF SCALES, MEASURING CUPS, SPOONS, ETC.	3/17 NH	3/20 NH	
9. ABILITY TO UTILIZE DIFFERENT UNITS OF MEASUREMENT	3/17 NH	3/20 NH	✓
10. HOW TO READ AND USE A NUTRITION CONTENT LABEL	3/19 NH	3/20 NH	
11. HOW THE MEAL PLAN CAN BE INDIVIDUALIZED BY WRITING A DAY'S MENU FOR HOME USE	3/17 NH	3/18 NH	✓
12. UNDERSTANDING OF MEAL PLAN BY DAILY FOOD SELECTION FROM HOSPITAL MENU	3/16 NH	Daily	
VI. INSULIN/ORAL HYPOGLYCEMIC AGENTS PATIENT/OTHER VERBALIZES: 1. BASIC ACTION OF INSULIN AND ORAL AGENTS	3/18 CC		
2. NAME, DOSAGE, AND TIME MEDICINE SHOULD BE TAKEN *Lente Insulin*	3/18 CC		
3. ONSET, PEAK, AND DURATION OF INSULIN ACTION	3/18 CC		
4. DIABETIC PILLS ARE NOT INSULIN BY MOUTH	3/18 CC		
5. IMPORTANCE OF FOOD INTAKE EVERY 4-5 HOURS TO BALANCE WITH DIABETIC MEDICINE TAKEN	3/18 CC		
6. INSULIN THERAPY SHOULD CONTINUE ON SICK DAYS			✓
PATIENT/OTHER DEMONSTRATES: 7. MEASUREMENT OF INSULIN(S) DOSE WITHIN PLUS OR MINUS 2 UNITS OF ACCURACY	3/16 CC	3/18 LB	✓
8. INJECTION OF INSULIN USING PROPER TECHNIQUE AT LEAST TWICE	3/16 CC	3/18 LB	
9. ROTATION OF INJECTION SITES	3/18 CC	3/18 LB	
VII. INSULIN REACTION PATIENT/OTHER VERBALIZES: 1. AT LEAST TWO CAUSES OF INSULIN REACTION			
2. AT LEAST TWO SYMPTOMS OF INSULIN REACTION			
3. PROPER TREATMENT OF INSULIN REACTION			

INITIALS	SIGNATURE		
L.B.	Linda Bailey, R.N.	NH	Nancy Hester, R.D.
		CC	Cheri Casey, R.N.
K.D.	Kathy Doak, R.N.	BJ	Brenda Johnson, O.T.R.

Figure 16-2. *(Continued)*

Activity 16-C:
Analyzing a Client-Care Situation

Work individually, within a small group.

1. Read the following situation:

    A nurse is caring for a hospitalized elderly woman who has had a hip pinning for a hip that was fractured 2 weeks ago. Objective assessment indicates dry mouth and lips, decreased skin turgor, dark brown urine, and intake and output below recommended levels. The woman receives a stool softener daily, has had several enemas and laxatives, and receives a selective diet based on her choices. Subjectively, the woman indicates she does not like to bother the nurses for the bedpan and so she does not drink very much water or eat much food.

2. Based only on the information provided, analyze the situation in writing:
   a. State a probable learning need.
   b. State a long-term goal for teaching.
   c. Identify the subskills of the teaching goal and state them as short-term objectives.
   d. Describe the learning activities and instructional activities you would use to help reach the teaching goal and objectives.
3. Compare your analysis with the others in your group.

Time, practice, and careful examination of your teaching skills will increase your ability to teach clients in ways that foster learning. The Performance Checklist, p. 139, can be used to evaluate your ability to teach clients. You may also wish to have a teacher or preceptor evaluate your teaching skills, since their added objectivity and expertise can be beneficial. At intervals during your career, it can also be helpful to reevaluate your teaching skills in a similar manner.

The following activity requires implementation of teaching-learning principles in an actual client-care situation and provides an opportunity to evaluate your own teaching-learning skills.

Activity 16-D: Evaluation of Teaching-Learning Skills

In a direct-care setting, select a client with a particular learning need. Plan and implement teaching activities, using the principles and methods discussed in this skill. Use the Performance Checklist, p. 139, to evaluate your own ability to provide for teaching and learning. If possible, validate your plans and activities with a faculty or staff preceptor before implementing the teaching activities.

☐ CRITICAL POINTS SUMMARY

1. Teaching has occurred when learning is demonstrated by a change in behavior.
2. Learning can occur when client readiness exists and appropriate instructional activities are provided.
3. Learner readiness can be evaluated through assessment of motivation, comfort and energy levels, and client capabilities.
4. Motivation is enhanced when the learning task is perceived as personally relevant, internally directed, challenging, produces a moderate level of anxiety, and when family and nurses are supportive.
5. Learning is increased when the client and family are active participants in all phases of the teaching-learning process.
6. Learning effectiveness is increased through feedback, reinforcement, repetition, practice, and follow-up by a health-care professional.

☐ REVIEW QUESTIONS

1. Name several teaching-learning situations where the nurse can take advantage of incidental teaching opportunities.
2. In your own words, state the relationship between the teaching-learning process and the nursing process.
3. What assessment data would you want to have about a client before beginning a planned, formal teaching session or series of classes?
4. What factors influence a person's readiness to learn? How can they be assessed?
5. In what ways can a nurse have a negative or positive effect on a client's ability to learn?
6. How do basic needs relate to the identification of learning needs and readiness to learn?
7. How do threats, challenge, and anxiety affect the ability to learn?
8. In what ways do motivation, comfort levels, energy levels, and capabilities influence the ability to learn? How does the nurse assess for each of these factors?
9. How do goals and objectives relate to each other and to the skill and subskills to be learned?
10. What factors might influence the choice of content and instructional activities when planning client teaching sessions?
11. In which specific parts of the teaching-learning process is the client most actively involved? Which parts are primarily the nurse's responsibility?
12. How do feedback, repetition, and follow-up reinforce and enhance learning?
13. In what ways do staffing, finances, and agency administration affect teaching-learning outcomes?
14. What methods can be used to determine the effectiveness of the teaching-learning process?
15. What personal and professional attributes increase a nurse's effectiveness as a teacher?
16. How could a nurse manage his or her personal discomfort with teaching-learning situations?

☐ PERFORMANCE CHECKLIST

OBJECTIVE: To use appropriate principles in implementing a teaching-learning plan.

EVALUATION OF SELF[a]		Behaviors	EVALUATION BY PRECEPTOR[a]	
S	U		S	U

		1. Gathers needed data:
		   a. About the medical and nursing diagnoses
		   b. About the client
		   c. From the client		

		2. Assesses learner readiness:
		   a. Determines client motivation for learning
		   b. Identifies client comfort level
		   c. Identifies client energy level
		   d. Identifies client capabilities		

		3. Negotiates appropriate and feasible goals and objectives with the client.		
		4. Determines specific content components and subskills.		
		5. Identifies specific instructional objectives for subskills.		

		6. Plans instructional materials and approaches appropriate for:
		   a. the client
		   b. the content
		   c. the situation		

		7. Includes the client in each phase of the teaching-learning process.		
		8. Gives feedback to client about learning.		
		9. Provides opportunities for use and practice of learned materials.		
		10. Makes follow-up plans or referrals.		
		11. Identifies ways to determine if learning has occurred.		
		12. Identifies own strengths, abilities, and weaknesses in teaching situations (specify).		

		13. Recognizes and uses available support systems and resources:
		   a. Staff
		   b. Space
		   c. Materials
		   d. Other		

		14. Records teaching activities.		
		15. Needs strengthening in certain areas (specify).		

[a]S = Satisfactory; U = Unsatisfactory.

REFERENCES

American Nurses Association: Code for Nurses with Interpretive Statements. (ANA Publication Code No. G56 25 M, 9/76.) Kansas City, MO, American Nurses Association, 1976.

Becker MH: Sociobehavioral determinants of compliance. In Sackett DL, Haynes RB (eds): Compliance with Therapeutic Regimens. Baltimore, The Johns Hopkins University Press, 1976.

Becker MH, Maiman LA, et al: Patient perceptions and compliance: Recent studies of the health belief model. In Haynes RB, Taylor DW, Sackett DL (eds): Compliance in Health Care. Baltimore, The Johns Hopkins University Press, 1979.

Bell DF, Bell DL: The effect of contracting on patient compliance. Diabetes 29(5)(Suppl 2); Abstract No. 21, 1980.

Bernstein L, Bernstein RS, Dana RH: Interviewing: A Guide for Health Professionals, ed 2. New York, Appleton-Century-Crofts, 1974.

Bernstein L, Bernstein RS: Interviewing: A Guide for Health Professionals, ed 3. New York, Appleton-Century-Crofts, 1980.

Casey CL: Comparison of health beliefs and behaviors among compliant and noncompliant diabetic patients. Diabetes 28(5)(Suppl 3); Abstract No. 98, 1979.

Combs AW, Avila DL, Purkey WW: Helping Relationships: Basic Concepts for the Helping Professions. Boston, Allyn & Bacon, 1971.

Combs AW, Taylor C: The effect of perception and mild degrees of threat on performance. Journal of Abnormal and Social Psychology 47(2):420–424, 1952.

Dick W, Carey L: The Systematic Design of Instruction. Glenview, IL, Scott, Foresman, 1978.

DuGas B: Introduction to Patient Care, ed 3. Philadelphia, WB Saunders, 1977.

Haynes RB: A critical review of the "determinants" of patient compliance with therapeutic regimens. In Sackett DL, Haynes RB (eds): Compliance with Therapeutic Regimens. Baltimore, The Johns Hopkins University Press, 1976a.

Haynes RB: Strategies for improving compliance: A methodologic analysis and review. In Sackett DL, Haynes RB (eds): Compliance with Therapeutic Regimens. Baltimore, The Johns Hopkins University Press, 1976b.

Haynes RB: Introduction. In Haynes RB, Taylor DW, Sackett DL (eds): Compliance in Health Care. Baltimore, The Johns Hopkins University Press, 1979.

Joint Commission on Accreditation of Hospitals: Accreditation Manual for Hospitals. Chicago, JCAH, 1984.

McConnell EA: Preop teaching helps. Nursing80 10(3):90, 1980.

Narrow BW: Patient Teaching in Nursing Practice: A Patient and Family Centered Approach. New York, John Wiley & Sons, 1979.

Pohl ML: The Teaching Function of the Nursing Practitioner, ed 4. Dubuque, IA, William C. Brown, 1981.

Redman BK: The Process of Patient Teaching in Nursing, ed 4. St Louis, CV Mosby, 1980.

Rosenberg SG: Patient education: An educator's view. In Sackett DL, Haynes RB (eds): Compliance with Therapeutic Regimens. Baltimore, The Johns Hopkins University Press, 1976.

Styles MM: Serendipity and objectivity. Nursing Outlook 23(5):311–313, 1975.

Taylor P: Patient teaching: Keys to more success more often. NursingLife 2(6):25–32, 1982.

Talarico D: Four basic steps to successful patient teaching. Canadian Nurse 74(5):22–24, 1978.

Veninga R: Are you a successful communicator? Canadian Nurse 74(10):34–37, 1978.

Webster GC: Third New International Dictionary, Unabridged. Springfield, MA, G & C Merriam, 1976.

BIBLIOGRAPHY

Adom D, Wright AS: Dissonance in nurse and patient evaluations of a patient-teaching program. Nursing Outlook 30(2): 132–136, 1982.

Herje PA: Hows and whys of contracting. Nurse Educator 5(1):30–34, 1980.

Langford T: Establishing a nursing contract. Nursing Outlook 26(6):386–388, 1978.

Squyres WD (ed): Patient Education: An Inquiry into the State of the Art. New York, Springer, 1980.

SUGGESTED READING

Grosser LR: Health belief model aids understanding of patient behavior. AORN Journal 35(6):1056–1059, 1982.

Taylor P: Patient teaching: Keys to more success more often. NursingLife 2(6):25–32, 1982.

AUDIOVISUAL RESOURCES

The Nurse is a Teacher: The Nurse's Role in Teaching
Slides, filmstrip, videocassette, film. (1978, Color, 13 min.)

The Nurse is a Teacher: Principles of Learning
Slides, filmstrip, videocassette, film. (1978, Color, 13 min.)

The Nurse is a Teacher: Principles of Teaching
Slides, filmstrip, videocassette, film. (1978, Color, 13 min.)

The Nurse is a Teacher: Teaching and the Nursing Process
Slides, filmstrip, videocassette, film. (1978, Color, 16 min.)

The Nurse is a Teacher: Teaching Methods
Slides, filmstrip, videocassette, film. (1978, Color, 16 min.)
Available through:
Medcom, Inc.
P.O. Box 116
Garden Grove, CA 92642

5 Written Communication

☐ INTRODUCTION

Health records have many functions. Within an agency, records are used as a communication tool among professionals, for documentation of medical and nursing care, and for education of staff and students. The information contained in health records is often used as data for retrospective and concurrent clinical research. An agency's utilization review committee uses the health record to determine "certification of need," that is, to evaluate the client's need for admission to the agency and for continued care from that agency. Records are audited (examined and evaluated) regularly by an agency audit committee; the committee examines randomly selected records of discharged clients, using predetermined criteria for evaluating the completeness and quality of the documentation contained in the record. The audit process has a built-in feedback mechanism through which agency staff are given information about record strengths and deficits, along with a plan for correcting deficits.

Although designed primarily for intraagency use, health records also contain information with broad community and societal functions. Health records are legal records of an agency's business with the public. Records may serve as a basis for employment, disability and unemployment claims, life and health insurance decisions, and judgments about private and governmental third-party payments; they may also provide evidence in a court of law. Epidemiologic and vital statistical data are gathered from health agency records and sent to the appropriate local, state, or federal governmental agency for compilation. These and other client statistics become part of planning data for both the individual agency and for state, local, and regional planning bodies.

The nurse is *responsible* for maintaining accurate nursing records; that is, the nurse has an obligation to do so. In addition, the nurse can be held professionally and legally *accountable* (answerable) for the kind of records he or she prepares. The nurse fulfills this professional and legal responsibility by recording relevant, current data about the client's health status and the care the client receives.

This chapter presents the health record as two separate skills: "Using the Health Record" (Skill 17) and "Nursing Records" (Skill 18). The two skills include a brief history of health and nursing records, a discussion of two types of record systems, legality issues, and guidelines for creating quality nursing records. The intent of this chapter is to help the student use existing health records, appreciate the need for adequate written communication of care, and produce the kind of record that improves as well as proves client care.

SKILL 17 Using the Health Record

At the very heart of all health care is the information that describes or symbolically represents that care.
—Waters and Murphy, p. 33

☐ STUDENT OBJECTIVES

1. Discuss the purposes of a health record and its various parts.
2. Describe the legal status of the health record and its contents.
3. Describe the components of the Problem-Oriented Medical Record (POMR) system.
4. Compare problem-oriented and traditional, source-oriented records.
5. Cite several advantages of the POMR system.
6. Give examples of record modification for health agencies in varied settings.
7. Locate data in sample client health records.

□ INTRODUCTION

A health record, often called a medical record or chart, is a written accounting of a client's health status and the care given while receiving services from any health agency. Health records are used to document the client's condition, the actual medical and nursing care given, and the client's response to that care. These records vary in form and content, depending on whether the setting is a hospital, physician's office, outpatient department, or public health or home-care agency.

The nurse uses health records to gather objective data for the independent function of planning and implementing nursing care and for the dependent function of carrying out the medical plan while the client is under the agency's care.

Medical records apparently have been in existence as long as medical care has been given, and as medical care has become more varied, sophisticated, and complex, so have its records. As long ago as 450 B.C., Hippocrates kept detailed clinical records of sick persons. In London, England, St. Bartholomew's Hospital still has some patient records that date from its medieval beginnings in 1137 A.D. In the United States, handwritten medical records still exist from the founding of Pennsylvania Hospital in 1752 and New York Hospital in 1793 (Huffman, 1972).

Since the early 1900s, medical records have gradually become more standardized, complete, and systematic. The Joint Commission on Accreditation of Hospitals (JCAH) has specific requirements for the contents and completeness of records kept by its accredited agencies (Joint, 1984). In many health-care settings, professionally trained medical record librarians are responsible for knowing the detailed requirements of the JCAH and communicating them to agency personnel. Trained medical record librarians are members of the American Medical Records Association (AMRA), and use the letters RRA (Registered Records Administrator) to indicate their professional status (Waters and Murphy, 1979). They are in charge of record storage and retrieval systems and review records of discharged clients for completeness. If the record is incomplete, the medical record librarian returns it to the physician or nurse for completion. Health records are available through the medical record librarian for retrieval when a client is readmitted or for professional education purposes.

Health agencies often have microfilm records on file for easier storage. Storage space and agency policy, rather than law, usually control the length of time records are kept, except for records of minors. Although laws vary, it generally is accepted that juvenile records should be kept until the age of majority (age 21 in most states) (Waters and Murphy, 1979).

The most recent development in medical records is the increasing use of automated informational systems, or computers. There are four general kinds of automated informational systems—medical, communications, ancillary, and transactional. A *medical informational system* computerizes the recording of nursing and medical care, allowing for input and retrieval of all information generated for the medical record by the client, physicians, nurses, social workers, or other health-care professionals. *Communications systems* transmit data among personnel and departments, replacing printed requisition forms and manual dispatch systems for ordering medications, diagnostic tests, or therapeutic procedures. *Ancillary support systems* are used for activities of a specific unit, such as a pharmacy or laboratory. *Transactional systems* deal with finances, billing, and the use of goods and services (Hurst and Walker, 1972). An agency may choose to use one or more of these systems either to supplement its manual record-keeping system or as the primary mode of generating, transmitting, storing, and retrieving information.

In some agencies, nurses learn how to access and input information into computerized systems; in other agencies, unit managers or secretaries perform these functions. Agencies that use computerized record-keeping systems provide all new employees with extensive orientation to the particular system in use at that agency. When medical informational systems are used, many agencies continue to maintain handwritten nursing-care plans for each client, usually in a kardex form, as described in Skill 18. Nursing-care plans that are kept on kardexes tend to be more easily accessible than those that are kept on a computer system, since computer terminal space may be limited, the terminal occupied, or the system "down."

□ PREPARATION

Institutions may satisfy JCAH record-keeping requirements by using either a problem-oriented or a traditional, source-oriented medical record system.

PROBLEM-ORIENTED MEDICAL RECORD (POMR) SYSTEM

The POMR system focuses on client needs or problems. It was initiated by Lawrence Weed in 1968 while attempting to teach and evaluate clinical decision making to medical students and hospital staff. There are three parts in the POMR system: the problem-oriented record (POR); the audit process; and the correction of deficiencies. Figure 17-1 illustrates the interrelationship of these three components. The audit process uses established criteria for care as a basis for systematically examining the completeness and clarity of reporting and recording medical and nursing care provided to clients. Agencies may create their own criteria, incorporating professional standards of care from various professional organizations, or they may use existing published criteria, such as those developed by Phaneuf (1976). Based on information gath-

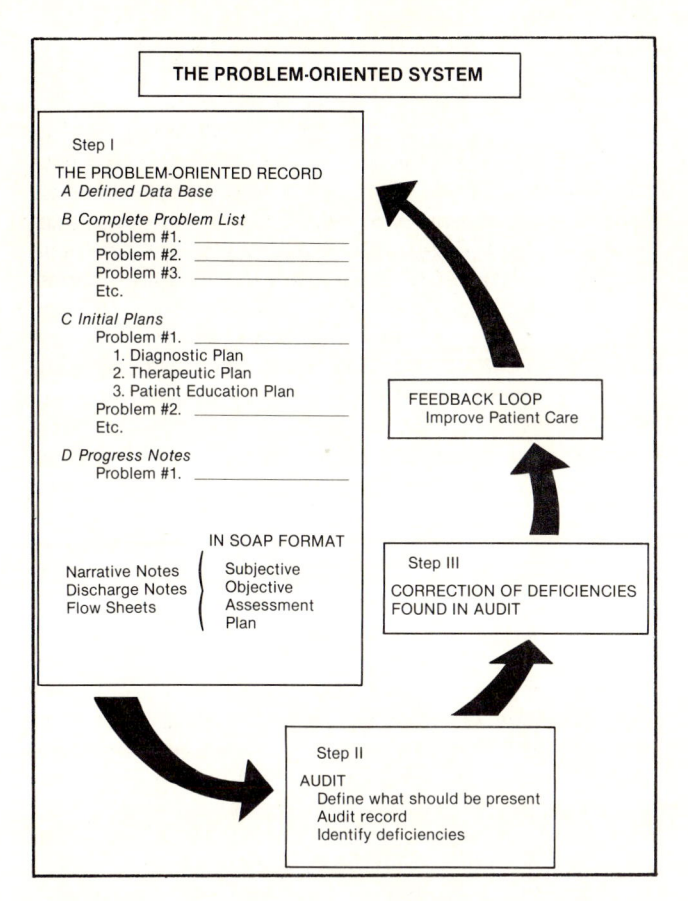

Figure 17-1. *The problem-oriented system. The record is the tool used to chart [client] care, to audit that care and the performance of the care-givers, and thus to improve the quality of [client] care. (Figure and legend from the American Journal of Nursing 73(7):1169, 1973, with permission.)*

ered in the audit process, changes can be made in nursing and medical care policies and practices that will correct deficiencies identified in the audit process. This creates a feedback loop that results in improvement of client care (Woody and Mallison, 1973). The individual nurse is most directly involved in the creation and use of the POR itself. A detailed discussion of the audit process and correction of deficiencies involves the total institution and is beyond the scope of this text.

Problem-Oriented Record (POR)

The POR has four major components: (1) a data base; (2) a problem list; (3) initial plans with interdisciplinary orders; and (4) progress notes. A variety of forms may be used to record data in each of these components. All health-care professionals may contribute information to the forms in any of these components, so that the resultant record is an interdisciplinary product.

Data Base. The data base consists of data known or determined at the time of a client's entry into the health-care agency—for example, demographic data, initial observations and assessments, and data specific to the kind of agency or service unit to which the client is being admitted. The data base is developed by an interdisciplinary group of health-care providers and includes an admitting form, reports of the physician's history and physical examination, nursing history and assessment, laboratory data, and assessments by other professionals, such as social workers, clinical specialists, and various therapists. Data on these record forms may be in narrative style, checklists, or summaries.

Problem List. The *problem list* summarizes the known problems and serves as a numbered "index" to the POR. This master problem list is placed at the front of the record. Ideally it includes medical, physical, functional, and psychosocial problems and is created jointly by professionals from several disciplines. Tentative or temporary problems are usually entered on a separate sheet.

Initial Plans. *Initial plans* are titled and numbered to correspond with the problem list and include diagnostic, therapeutic, and educational plans, along with specific orders for implementation. This approach provides a rationale for these orders and serves as a baseline for measuring future progress.

Progress Notes. *Progress notes* are used to record progress and changes in identified problems, list new problems, or indicate resolution of identified problems. They include narrative notes, a variety of flow sheets, and several summaries.

Narrative Notes. These notes are sequential, dated notations describing client status and the care provided by the staff; they are numbered and titled to correspond with the master problem list. In the POMR system, narrative notes are written in a format that is called "SOAP": "S" for *subjective* data, "O" for *objective* data, "A" for *assessment* or analysis, and "P" for *plan* of care. (Narrative notes and the SOAP format are described further in Skill 18.) In the POMR system, all health-care professionals providing client care use this format to record their contributions in the one progress notes section (Weed, 1970; Berni and Readey, 1974). Weed (1970) indicates that progress notes need to be written only when the client's condition has changed. However, most acute-care institutions require at least one progress note in SOAP format every 24 hours. When flow sheets are completed properly, they can substitute for narrative documentation of routine care, thus saving time and avoiding unnecessary duplication of recording.

Flow Sheets. These forms are concise records of various kinds of repetitive, serial, or quantifiable data such as vital signs measurement, urine and blood tests, or basic nursing tasks. Flow sheets are used in both a problem-oriented record and the traditional, source-oriented record described below. Flow sheets are discussed further in Skill 18.

Summaries. Transfer and discharge summaries are written when a client is transferred from one clinical area to another or is discharged from the agency itself, thus providing data needed for continuity of care. In the POMR system, these summaries present a brief review of each problem at its current level of resolution.

Advocates of the POMR system perceive many advantages from its use (Berni and Readey, 1974; Walker and Hurst, 1972). They maintain that it promotes learning a core of behavior, that is, it promotes the development of problem-solving skills rather than memorization of a core of knowledge. They also believe that this process fosters professional growth more advantageously than traditional, source-oriented or memory-dependent systems. Another advantage of the POMR system is that it is focused on the *client* rather than on the delivery of medical services, nursing care, social work services, and other professional care. If the POMR system is used properly, data are well documented and tied to an existing framework of numbered problems rather than recorded as isolated, sequential facts and are retrieved more easily for professional education and audit purposes. In addition, there generally is a more clear documentation of client education and the process of planning care than in the more traditional record.

Hurst and Walker (1972) state that the POMR format facilitates computerization of client care and that computerization augments POMR's medical capabilities. Computerization makes it "possible to retrieve all data on one problem sequence" and for "data to be organized separate from its source in the record." Their experience with this kind of computerization indicates that it facilitates assessment of client problems (Hurst and Walker, 1972, pp. 203, 249).

Some difficulties with the POMR system relate to staff uncertainty about learning to use a new recording format and hesitancy in writing an "assessment" that involves putting one's analysis of a situation in writing for others to read. Using a problem-oriented approach requires the ability to think analytically; therefore, deficiencies in information and assessment are quite visible, which is often threatening to the nursing staff. In addition, during the initial stages of learning to use the SOAP format, more charting time (record-keeping time) is often required. It should also be noted, as Mitchell (1973, p. 205) has pointed out, that adopting the POMR system does not guarantee improved care, for "sloppy thinking documented is still sloppy thinking," regardless of the format.

TRADITIONAL, SOURCE-ORIENTED, MEDICAL RECORD SYSTEMS

Although the POMR system is gaining rapid acceptance and is increasingly used throughout the country, many institutions prefer the traditional approach to record keeping, which has been called a source-oriented system. These records are organized around the care given by the various health-care disciplines, that is, according to the kind of health-care professional who made the observations and recorded the information—those persons who are the *source* of the data. A traditional, source-oriented record has the following discrete sections or components, arranged in a variable sequence: admission data sheet, consent forms, physicians' order sheets, history and physical examination sheets, physicians' progress notes, flow sheets for vital signs and other basic data, nurses' notes, nursing assessment or nursing history forms, medication records, admission and discharge forms, laboratory reports, x-ray reports, and other miscellaneous records (such as diagnostic procedures, specialized tests or treatment reports, operative procedures, therapy and social services records, and discharge or continuity of care summaries).

In the source-oriented system, persons from each discipline record their information only on forms designated for their own use; therefore, information about a specific problem a client is having will be found in a variety of places within the record. For example, when providing care to a client with a stroke, a staff nurse would use the nurses' notes to record information about the client's ability to move, speak, and carry out the activities of daily living; the physical therapist would use the physical therapy record to record information about the client's progress in learning exercises to increase his or her functional level; the physician would use the physician's progress record to record current status of the recovery from the stroke; the social worker or chaplain would record psychological, spiritual, and home-care concerns in the social services record; and so on.

Similar record forms may be used in both the POMR and traditional systems; the difference between the two systems lies in who records information on the various forms, as indicated earlier. For example, the flow sheets described in Skill 18 can be used in either system; nurses' notes and progress notes can be written in SOAP or paragraph style regardless of the system; and some data always are recorded on source-specific forms in both the POMR and traditional systems, such as laboratory, x-ray, and surgery reports.

Traditional, source-oriented records are easy for the individual professional to use, as each discipline can locate the section for his or her own entry of factual information quite readily. However, the process of gathering data from a traditional record can sometimes be quite time-consuming and difficult. This is particularly true if the record is very large and the reader wants to determine the overall status of the client or trace the progress of a particular client problem, since it is left to the reader to sort out and analyze the data mentally.

It is important to recognize that the quality of record keeping is not as dependent on the nature of the record-keeping system as it is on the persons who contribute to the record. It is possible to record observations and document nursing care well or poorly in either system, and nurses' notes in a traditional record can reflect an analytical thought process as well as those that are made using the SOAP format of the

POMR system. For example, the paragraph narrative notes of the traditional system can include all the components of the SOAP format even though the structure itself is not used.

HEALTH RECORD FORMATS

All health-care agencies use some form of record keeping for basic client information and for identification and resolution of client problems. Records in acute-care settings are generally detailed and lengthy because of the short-term and urgent nature of the care given. In chronic, long-term, or custodial institutions such as some nursing homes, the records are similar to those used in acute-care settings, but data entries are less frequent.

In an inpatient setting, health records are kept in a three-ring notebook or a spring-loaded clipboard style holder as shown in Figure 17–2. They are divided into sections by colored or numbered dividers for easy access and stored in some kind of stationary or portable rack in the nurses' station area or in the client's room.

In outpatient areas, clinics, health centers, and physicians' offices, records may be kept in manila folders. These folders contain basic data sheets, history and physical examination sheets, and ongoing records of care provided on a dated visit basis. In home-care or public health agencies, basic client information may be written on the record folder itself, with recurrent visits noted on additional inserted pages. These records are often smaller in size than institutional records, so they can be taken on home visits more conveniently. Any of these records may be written in either the POMR or the traditional format.

LEGAL STATUS OF RECORDS

By law, any corporation dealing with the public is required to keep official records of those transactions. As a record made in the regular course of business, the medical record is considered the property of the health-care agency. The issue of ownership of the health record as distinct from ownership of the information it contains has not yet been resolved. Case law indicates that although the agency has a property right to the *record* itself, the client has a property right to the *information* contained in it and cannot be denied access to that information (Annas, 1975; Rocereto and Maleski, 1982). In actual practice, in most health-care institutions everyone except the client has somewhat casual access to the record, including transportation and clerical persons as well as direct caregivers.

There is no uniform policy about clients' access to their own records, and policies and practices vary from one state or agency to another. Some institutions limit the record sections to which the client may have access, some limit the total number of pages that may be copied, some charge substantial fees for each copied page, some require the physician's permission, and in some states, clients must resort to court procedures in order to have access to their own records. The American Hospital Association's 1975 Patient's Bill of

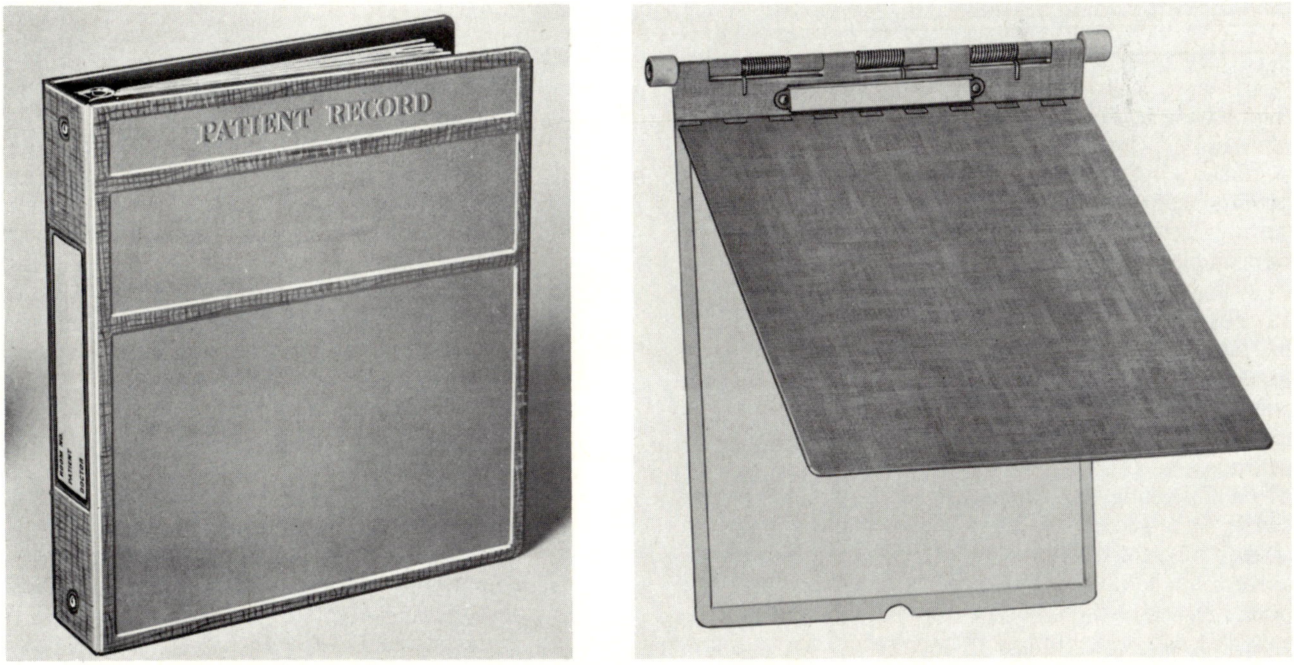

A

B

Figure 17–2. **A.** *Side-opening ring binder chart holder.* **B.** *Top-opening springloaded clipboard style chart holder. (Courtesy Carstens Health Industries, Chicago, IL.)*

Rights does not speak specifically to the issue of record access (Waters and Murphy, 1979). In their 1978 position paper, the American Medical Record Association (AMRA) indicated that the concept of self-care must be broadened to include client knowledge of the record, its contents, and its uses. They recommend that, upon written request with reasonable notice and subject to specific contraindications by the attending physician and to any legal constraints such as those governing minors or mentally incompetent persons, clients have access to their own records for review. Photocopies should also be provided on written request and payment of a reasonable fee (American Medical Record Association, 1978).

Many states are in the process of developing bills of rights for clients in health-care settings. These documents usually include the standards indicated in the Privacy Act of 1974 that govern record use and access in federal agencies. This act allows individuals to have access to their records, have a copy made, and amend or correct the records (Waters and Murphy, 1979).

Some physicians oppose giving clients access to their records, as they fear clients will misunderstand the contents. Some hospitals fear that they may receive unreasonable demands for changing record data. However, Weed (1970) and others believe a person should have only one health record that can accompany him or her to any physician or health-care agency in any location. Initial studies in Vermont indicate that when clients were routinely given a complete copy of their medical records, cooperation was stimulated, anxiety was decreased, and no adverse effects were noted. Annas (1975) and Steiner (1978) cite studies that indicate positive effects of sharing written medical information with clients.

☐ EXECUTION

A nurse who prepares and uses health records in a professional manner is one who is able to (1) read carefully, (2) think critically, (3) describe observations in writing clearly, and (4) write legibly. In addition, it is crucial that the professional nurse respect and protect the client's privacy by maintaining the record and its information as confidential. Much private personal information comes to a nurse's attention, both through the health record and during interpersonal interactions. The client has the right to keep this personal information private. Therefore, it is important to avoid discussing this kind of information in nonprofessional settings such as the elevator, cafeteria, or the nurse's place of residence. In addition, a health record is returned to its rack after use rather than being left open and visible on a countertop or table.

The age of computers makes maintenance of privacy more difficult because of the large numbers of persons who have legitimate access to a computer system from any available terminal in the agency. When working with a computer system, the professional nurse restricts the use of a personal computer access code to professional purposes and neither shares it with others nor uses it to gather information for purposes other than legitimate care-giving or educational purposes. It is important to remember that divulging private client information is a breach of professional conduct and can expose the nurse to a suit for invasion of privacy.

When working in an agency with actual client records, it is necessary to become familiar with that agency's record systems and to know the policies and practices regarding record keeping and retrieval. As a professional person, the nurse has an obligation to help create accurate records and use the information they contain to provide quality nursing care.

Thorough and careful examination of representative records increase the student's ability to use records effectively when he or she is in an actual nursing-care situation. The following activity is designed to help the student become familiar with the two general styles of health records. The records that are used are actual client records and contain confidential information about a person. The use of these records is for professional learning purposes only.

Activity 17-A:
Health Record Examination

Work in pairs.
   Use the following guide to examine an actual health/medical record for either a current or discharged patient. If possible examine both a problem-oriented and a traditional, source-oriented record from both an acute-care and community-agency setting.

1. Identify the location, identification, and placement of health records from both current and previous admissions. Who has access to these records, and what happens to them when the client is discharged?
2. Glance through the record, noting its various sections, their paging sequence, method of client identification, dividers, color or number coding, arrangement, and legibility. Locate the record sections or information listed below. Some sections are found in both problem-oriented and traditional, source-oriented records, whereas others are found in only one or the other. Indicate the type of record in which you find each section with a "P" for problem-oriented, "T" for traditional, and "B" for both.
    a. *Face sheet or admitting room sheet:* Identify the types of information found on this sheet, who would obtain it, and what might have significance to you as a nurse. (____)
    b. *Numbered problem list:* Identify which problems are focused on disease entities, functional status, or psychosocial problems. Note any additional categories of problems. (____)

c. *Problem-oriented initial impressions and interdisciplinary orders:* Look for indications of diagnostic, therapeutic, and educational impressions and the corresponding orders. Determine which health professionals have written these orders. (___)
d. *Consent sheet (may be part of admitting room record):* In your own words, tell *what* has been consented to when the sheet was signed, *when* the consent was given, who *gave* the consent, and who *witnessed* the consent. Is there a release of information paragraph? (___)
e. *Physician's order sheet:* Locate verbal, written, and telephone orders, noting similarities and differences. If more than one doctor has written orders, see if you can determine why. What process is involved in conveying the orders to the appropriate persons and departments? (___)
f. *History and physical sheets:* Read an admission note, a client history, or a physical exam with findings, conclusions, or diagnoses. Interpret in your own words. (___)
g. *Progress record:* Identify the health team members who use this sheet, the frequency with which comments are written, and the general purpose and function of these comments. (___)
h. *Nursing history or nursing assessment record:* Generalize about the kind of information given on this record. Identify the writer's position on the health team and discuss the clarity and completeness of the information recorded. (___)
i. *Nurses' notes:* Identify the health team members who use this sheet. Read an admission note, and note the description of the client (physical, mental, emotional condition, medical problem, and subjective and objective symptoms). Identify the kind of information that is recorded most consistently, recurrent phrases, and the health team personnel who recorded the data. Pick a 1-day period of time and describe the physical and emotional status and activities of the client for that day. Trace the progress of the client from admission to discharge or present status. (___)
j. *Clinical records, graphic sheet, or TPR sheet:* List the information recorded on these flow sheets, the frequency with which it is recorded, and the time span covered by each page. Note any indications of personal accountability for recorded information. (___)
k. *Other flow sheets:* List the various flow sheets in the record. State the purpose of each in your own words. Make some generalizations about the nature or purpose of the flow sheets. (___)
l. *Laboratory reports:* Note the difference in this section as compared with all previous sections. Find out how the reports are placed on the chart. Note color coding of lab reports. Find a report about blood values—preferably a hematology or complete blood cell count (CBC) report. Using your knowledge of anatomy and physiology, determine if the values are within normal limits. Using another lab report, compare stated norms with actual values. Refer back to the physician's order sheet to determine when a test was ordered, and compare that date with the date the test was performed. X-ray and ECG reports may be in this section or in separate ones. Read one of these reports and give the results in your own words. (___)
m. *Other records:* There may be many other record forms in the health record, such as a surgery report, anesthesia record, pathology report, recovery room record, blood pressure graphs, diabetic or anticoagulant records, coronary care or intensive care records, emergency room records, property records, and so on. Examine some of these and state in your own words what is being communicated. (___)

☐ CRITICAL POINTS SUMMARY

1. The health record is a legal document, containing confidential information.
2. Client access to health record information varies with the state and the agency.
3. Problem-oriented records are interdisciplinary in nature and contain a data base, problem list, initial plans, and progress notes.
4. Traditional, source-oriented records provide a separate section for each professional group to record its information about the client.
5. Health records are modified to fit the agency situation.
6. The nurse has a responsibility to maintain the client's privacy when using health records.
7. The nurse needs to know record systems used within an agency and be able to use them correctly.

☐ REVIEW QUESTIONS

1. What is the current status of the issue of client access to health record information?
2. What does the following statement mean to you? "The agency has a property right in the record, and the client has a property right in the information."
3. What are three intraagency and three societal or community functions for health records?
4. In the POMR system, how are the audit process and the problem-oriented record related?
5. What would you expect to find in each of the four components of the problem-oriented record?

6. In what ways are problem-oriented and traditional, source-oriented records alike? Different?
7. How does the use of the POMR system benefit professionals, clients, and agencies?
8. How does a home-care agency record differ from an acute-care agency record? A chronic, long-term inpatient record from an acute-care record?
9. As an individual and a professional nurse, how do adequate health records benefit you?

REFERENCES

American Medical Record Association: Confidentiality of patient health information: A position statement of the American Medical Record Association. Medical Record News 49(2):8–25, 1978.

American Nurses' Association: Standards of Nursing Practice. Kansas City, MO, ANA, 1973.

Annas GJ: The Rights of Hospital Patients: The Basic ACLU Guide to a Hospital Patient's Rights. New York, Avon Discus Books, 1975.

Berni R, Readey H: Problem Oriented Medical Record Implementation: Allied Health Peer Review. St Louis, CV Mosby, 1974.

Huffman EK: Medical Record Management, ed 6. Revised by the American Medical Association, Price EA (ed). Berwyn, IL, Physicians' Record Company, 1972.

Hurst WH, Walker HK (eds): The Problem-Oriented System. New York, Medcom Press, 1972.

Joint Commission on Accreditation of Hospitals. Accreditation Manual for Hospitals. Chicago, JCAH, 1984.

Mitchell PH: A systematic nursing progress record: The problem-oriented approach. Nursing Forum 12(2):187–210, 1973.

Phaneuf M: The Nursing Audit: Self-Regulation in Nursing Practice, ed 2. New York, Appleton-Century-Crofts, 1976.

Rocereto LaV R, Maleski CM: The Legal Dimensions of Nursing Practice. New York, Springer, 1982.

Waters KA, Murphy GF: Medical Records in Health Information. Germantown, MD, Aspen Systems, 1979.

Weed LL: Medical Records, Medical Education, and Patient Care. Cleveland, OH, Case Western University Press, 1970.

Woody M, Mallison M: The problem-oriented system for patient-centered care. American Journal of Nursing 73(7):1168–1175, 1973.

BIBLIOGRAPHY

Barnett GO, Zielstorff RD: Data systems can enhance or hinder medical, nursing activities. Hospitals 51(20):157–161, 1977.

Bloom JT, Dressler J, et al: Problem-oriented charting. American Journal of Nursing 71(11):2144–2148, 1971.

Blount M, Green SS, et al: Documenting with the problemoriented record system. American Journal of Nursing, 78(9):1539–1542, 1978.

Colton, MR: A note on professional record keeping. Supervisor Nurse 9(8):56–58, 1978.

Creighton HC: Law Every Nurse Should Know, ed 4. Philadelphia, WB Saunders, 1981.

Documenting Patient Care Responsibly. Horsham, PA, Intermed Communications (Nursing Skillbook series), 1978.

Hemelt MD, Mackert ME: Dynamics of Law in Nursing and Health Care. Reston, VA, Reston Publishing, 1978.

Mitchell PH, Atwood J: Problem-oriented recording as a teaching–learning tool. Nursing Research 24(2):99–103, 1975.

Schell PL, Campbell AT: POMR—not just another way to chart. Nursing Outlook 20(8):510–514, 1972.

Spaulding EK, Notter LE: Professional Nursing: Foundations, Perspectives, and Relationships. Philadelphia, JB Lippincott, 1976.

Steiner P: Patient access to the medical record: A study of physicians' attitudes. Medical Record News 49(4):77–78, 1978.

The Problem-Oriented System—A Multidisciplinary Approach. New York, National League for Nursing Publ. No. 20-1546, 1974.

Ware WH: Old patterns in a new age endanger information privacy. Hospitals 151:133–140, 1977.

AUDIOVISUAL RESOURCES

Medical Records: A Legal Tool; Legal Aspects of Charting
   Filmstrip. (1979, Color, 19 min.)
   Available through:
     St. Paul Fire and Marine Insurance Co.
     385 Washington St.
     St. Paul, MN 55102

Problem Oriented Medical Record
   Film or videocassette. (1975, Color, 25 min.)
   Available through:
     American Journal of Nursing Company
     Educational Services Division
     555 West 57th St.
     New York, NY 10019

SKILL 18   Nursing Records

Charting means telling the needed story, and telling it every day.

—E. T. Eggland

PREREQUISITE SKILL

Skill 17, "Using the Health Record"

☐ STUDENT OBJECTIVES

1. Describe the purposes of nursing records.
2. Discuss the legal status of nursing records.
3. Describe the nurse's responsibilities for maintaining the record as a legal document.

4. Describe each component of the SOAP format for narrative notes.
5. Discuss the nursing implementation of the POMR system.
6. Compare nursing narrative notes for problem-oriented and for traditional, source-oriented records.
7. Accurately interpret objective data on flow sheets.
8. Using appropriate terminology and abbreviations, record a sample client situation in both problem-oriented and traditional-style narrative nurses' notes.
9. Appreciate the role of the nurse in creating worthwhile health records.

☐ INTRODUCTION

Nursing records are the written reporting of dependent and independent nursing functions involved in providing or supervising nursing care. They are legal and professional documentation of actual medical and nursing care given and the client's response to that care. They serve as a communication tool among nurses, physicians, and other health-care workers and provide a source for subjective and objective health data about the client.

Although nurses are responsible for knowing about and using other sections of the health record, nursing records are the part for which they are most directly responsible. It is through these records that nurses discharge their professional and legal responsibilities.

Records of medical care have been common since the time of Hippocrates, but nursing records apparently began in the 19th century, along with the trained nurse movement. Florence Nightingale expected her nurses to keep accurate and detailed mental records of their patients' condition and believed written notes were an unnecessary crutch. In 1859, she wrote, "If you find it helps you to note down such things on a bit of paper in pencil, by all means do so. I think it more often lames than strengthens the memory and observation" (Nightingale, 1946, p. 63). For patients who are ill for months or a year, she recommended that there is a "necessity of recording in words from time to time, for the information of the nurse, who will not otherwise see, that he cannot do this or that, which he could do a month or a year ago" (Nightingale, 1946, p. 66). One wonders what she would think of today's emphasis on written records!

Nursing records, often called nurses' notes, are thought to have begun in 1874 with Linda Richards, known as America's first trained nurse (Bullough and Bullough, 1978, p. 115). In her first year at Bellevue Hospital in New York City, she began writing notes to other nurses on patient progress and care instead of relying completely on verbal reports. These written notes found immediate approval and acceptance with supervisors and physicians alike (Bellevue, 1923).

Nurses' notes have often been maligned as worthless and meaningless. In some states, they are not considered a part of the permanent record and are destroyed or stored elsewhere after the client has been discharged from the hospital (Annas, 1974; Huffman, 1972). In their university medical center study of nurses' notes, Walker and Selmanoff (1965) found that nurses' notes were rarely used by medical center physicians and had little significance to either the medical or nursing staff. Studies reported by Healy (1968) support the impression that nurses' notes are considered repetitive and incomplete and are characterized by statements of procedure rather than observation of response to care. More recently, nurses' notes have been described as something that have to be done—like paying taxes—and are put off until the last minute (Kunkel, 1983); it also has been found that nurses often have difficulty giving high priority to the documentation of client care (Barbiasz et al., 1981).

Nurses can no longer be content with creating inadequate, incomplete nursing notes. Adequate and accurate nurses' notes are essential since this is the part of the health record where documentation of actual care provided is recorded most visibly and on a regular basis. It is the responsibility of each individual nurse to create high quality, meaningful nurses' notes that *will* be read and used. Additionally, nurses must begin to look critically at the recording systems used and make recommendations for improvements where needed.

Social and professional forces have been pushing strongly for improved nurse recording of client care, observation, and judgments. For example, in many settings, nurses are seeking greater professional autonomy and visibility with increased responsibility and accountability for direct client care. This requires adequate, accurate record keeping that documents the care given, provides for continuity of care, serves as a useful source for writing reports and referrals, and can be used for third-party payment purposes. Health-care consumers are increasingly aware of and involved in their own health care and in its documentation. Documentation of care is also essential for the legal protection of the nurse, the client, and the agency.

More professional emphasis is being placed on *nursing audit* of nursing records as a method of evaluating and improving the nature and quality of care provided. Phaneuf (1976) describes a nursing audit as "a method for evaluating quality of care through appraisal of the nursing process as it is reflected in the patient care records." Nursing audits are either retrospective or concurrent examinations of nursing records, using process or outcome criteria as guidelines. *Process criteria* are desired nursing actions for a given client situation. *Outcome criteria* refer to desired client function or ability. Through this evaluation process, deficiencies either in nursing practice or in its documentation can be identified. Isler (1974) reported that nursing audits resulted in increased independent nursing actions, increased attention to total client-care needs, and a decreased level of dependence on physicians' orders for the care provided. Nurses at a major medical center hospital discovered that corrective action based on an audit process resulted in greater standardization of documentation of nursing care and a substantial increase in the total amount of documentation (Hoffman, 1980). Some agencies use a charting format that incorporates client outcomes, thus providing a basis for outcome audits (Gamberg et al., 1981).

Bernhardt (1978) reminds us that recording is a *service* rendered to clients by nurses. In one state, an estimated 5 to 10 percent of rejected Medicare claims would have been accepted had nurses documented specific items such as the need for pain medication or physical assistance, rather than vague generalities such as "offered no complaints." Specific documentation of care would have indicated to claims analysts that inpatient care was both needed and given (Austin, 1978).

☐ PREPARATION

The content and format of nursing records vary according to whether the POMR system or a source-oriented record system is used. Records also vary with the agency itself, since each agency develops forms to suit its own needs. Orientation to an agency always includes the use of records.

There is some indication that using a problem-oriented record (POR) increases the quantity and quality of documentation in nursing records. For example, problem-oriented notes are reported to improve nursing care (Bloom et al., 1971) and increase the amount of documentation of care provided (Blount et al., 1978). When compared with students who used traditional, source-oriented records, students who were taught and used a POR method identified more nursing-focused problems, integrated the recording of nursing procedures into the context of the client's problems rather than recording them as isolated tasks, and were able to document more clearly their ability to plan and problem solve (Mitchell and Atwood, 1975).

In a POMR system, the nurse is responsible for contributing information to the clearly defined *data base*. Using interview and physical appraisal skills, the nurse collects information about the client's functional abilities, activities of daily living, assets and liabilities, and psychosocial status. Many agencies have a specific format for this information, known as a nursing assessment, nursing history, admission history, or a client profile. With this system, the nurse is also expected to contribute nursing problems or nursing diagnoses to the multidisciplinary problem list and record observations and judgments about client problems and status in the progress notes along with the notes of other professionals. The nurse also records repetitive and routine data on a variety of flow sheets and contributes to a problem-oriented discharge summary.

Sometimes nurses implement problem-oriented recording on their own initiative, without physician staff involvement. In this circumstance, the numbered problem list is exclusively a nursing problem list, usually kept at the front of the record. Progress notes in SOAP format are written on nurses' notes or general purpose sheets, and any needed flow sheets are developed.

Nursing records can be divided into three basic types—narrative notes, flow sheets, and kardex care plans.

NARRATIVE NOTES

Narrative notes are sequential notations written by the nursing staff to document the client's status and the nursing care that has been implemented. Each notation is dated, a time of day given, and the nurse's signature and title are added at the conclusion of each entry. Narrative notes are written in a SOAP format in a problem-oriented record and in paragraph style in a traditional, source-oriented record.

POMR System

In a problem-oriented record used in the POMR system, narrative notes are written in the following SOAP format:

- S—Subjective data
- O—Objective data
- A—Assessment
- P—Plan (diagnostic, therapeutic, and client education)

Subjective data refer to the information provided by the client. When the client is unable to provide information because of age, impaired health status, or inadequate developmental level, a relative or friend may supply these data. If at all possible, this nonquantifiable type of data is written as direct quotes. Subjective data do *not* include the *nurse's* subjective perspective of the client.

Objective data refer to quantifiable information, such as direct observations about skin color, nonverbal behavior, or physical signs such as blood pressure, laboratory tests, and intake–output levels. Objective data may also include any therapy or interventions that were carried out prior to or during the time the subjective and objective observations were gathered.

Assessment refers to the interpretation and conclusion the observer makes after analyzing the subjective and objective data. "The nurse describes what she thinks is happening to the patient and why, the effects of treatment and the responses of the patient to a particular approach; she may also indicate her perceptions of the patient's progress on a particular problem" (National League for Nursing, 1974, p. 40). Most nurses find the assessment section the most difficult one to write, since "putting this kind of judgment in writing takes courage, but once the nurse has done it, and particularly once she has received a positive response from others on the health team, it becomes a more and more comfortable process, reflecting her thinking about the patient care she is giving and the

TABLE 18-1. Sample POR Format

PROBLEM	INITIAL PLANS	PROGRESS NOTE

GI bleeding	Goal: Stop bleeding
	Plan of Care:
	  Diagnostic: Monitor VS q2h
	    Note ↑ pulse or ↓ BP
	    Hematest stools
	  Therapeutic: Iced water lavage q2h, Maalox q1h c̄ NG tube clamped. NPO c̄ ice chips. O₂ 5 L until Hct ↑
	  Education: Explain treatment; teach about bland diet when bleeding stops
		S — c/o slight nausea when NG tube is clamped. "I feel so tired! Am I going to be alright? I'm so thirsty—may I have more ice?"
		O — P98, BP 98/68. Color pale. No blood noted in NG returns for past 2 hours. BM hematested positive.
		A — No current gastric bleeding; is anxious about condition.
		P — (Diag.) Continue monitoring as planned.
		    (Ther.) Give oral and nasal care q2–4h. Obtain physician order for throat lozenges.
		    (Educ.) Reinforce teaching about ice chips and NG tube.

observations she is making. It is the assessment that demonstrates to others the nurse's thinking and her analyses of observations and reactions" (National League for Nursing, 1974, p. 40).

Plan refers to immediate and long-term actions and solutions for the identified problem. Plans involve the same three aspects as the initial plan component in a problem-oriented record: diagnostic, therapeutic, and client education aspects. The *diagnostic* aspect identifies additional data that need to be collected about the situation; the *therapeutic* aspect indicates the interventions that will be used in an effort to resolve the situation or alleviate the client's problem; and the *client education* aspect includes the information the client needs to receive. Interventions that were performed in response to the assessment the nurse made are recorded primarily in flow sheets and do not need to be duplicated in the SOAP format. Interventions are also incorporated into the objective data portion of the next SOAP note in the form of observations of the success of the planned interventions, that is, as an evaluation of interventions. Berni and Readey (1978, pp. 50–51) indicate that interventions ("what you do for the patient") can be included in the plan or in the objective data component, and that the patient's reaction to the treatment can be included either in the therapeutic or client education aspect of the plan.

SOAP notes are more meaningful when they are tied to the problems on the master problem list, to the initial plans made when the client was admitted to the agency, or to a revision of those plans. Like the nursing process, SOAP notes are cyclical; that is, implementation of the plan provides additional data to be incorporated into successive SOAP notes. Not all SOAP components need to be written at each entry; only the information that is relevant and available is required (Berni and Readey, 1978; Weed, 1970; Woody and Mallison, 1973).

Implementation of the SOAP format varies somewhat within the literature and in actual practice. The decision about where a given type of information is located within the SOAP format is less important than having an agency policy about how SOAP is to be used and then having that policy implemented consistently.

Table 18-1 presents a sample SOAP narrative note based on a defined health problem from a master problem list and initial plans and goals. The plan component of the SOAP entry includes diagnostic, therapeutic, and client education aspects.

Traditional, Source-Oriented Systems

Narrative notes are written in paragraph style in a traditional, source-oriented record. They are dated, timed, and signed in the same way as SOAP format notes. Although not structured to emphasize the problem-solving process as is a SOAP format, problem solving and analytical thinking are possible within this paragraph format since the content of a narrative note depends as much on the nurse as it does on the system being used. The subjective and objective data, assessment, and planning included in a SOAP note can be written in paragraph narrative style; however, at times, relevant subjective data, objective data, and interventions are recorded without an assessment or plan.

FLOW SHEETS

Flow sheets are record forms designed for recording a variety of data related to client care. These data may be measurable and recorded numerically or they may describe signs and symptoms specific to a client's particular health problem. Flow sheets provide a concise, easily read record that can be evaluated over time. Each agency designs its own flow sheets to meet the specific needs of its client population, agency purpose, and staff. In a POR, flow sheets are organized according to the problems on the master problem list. Flow sheets may also be created for a specific client care area, such as an intensive care unit, or for specific purposes, such as to monitor vital signs.

Some flow sheets have specified time periods when observations are to be made, such as the graphic

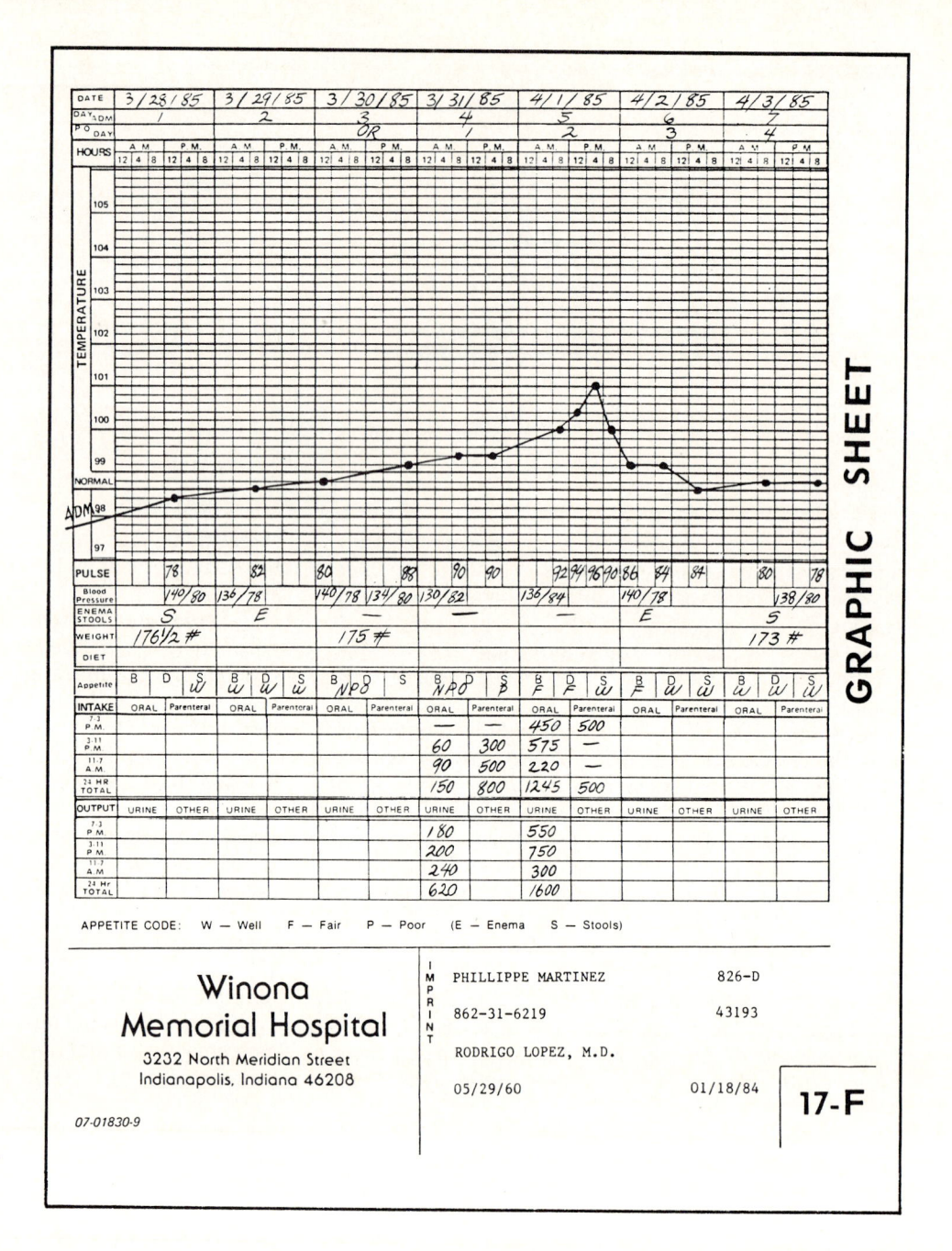

Figure 18-1. Flow Sheet: Graphic Sheet. (Courtesy of Winona Memorial Hospital, Indianapolis, IN.)

sheet shown in Figure 18-1. This record contains vital signs, nutrition and elimination data, and fluid intake and output values for a 1-week time span. Other flow sheets are more general and allow the nurse to determine the frequency of observations necessary for a specific client-care situation, such as the vital sign record (Fig. 26-11). The specified time intervals may be as frequent as every 15 minutes to 1 hour in an intensive care unit; other flow sheets may be designed for observations four times a day or daily in acute-care settings, or weekly and monthly in long-term and home-care settings.

Some flow sheets are preprinted with the aspects of care that need to be monitored, such as the basic care sheet shown in Figure 18-2 and the diabetic therapy sheet shown in Figure 18-3. The basic care sheet is kept at the bedside and used by the direct caregiver. The diabetic therapy sheet is the first page of a 3-page, 5-day form for recording urine tests, blood sugars, insulin and hypoglycemic agent administration, and any special related data. Pages 2 and 3 of the form focus on diabetic teaching and are shown in Figure 16-2.

Other flow sheets have blank spaces for nurses to designate the observations needed for a particular client. For example, a person with a cardiac problem who has peripheral edema and is experiencing shortness of breath would be monitored for data such as intake and output measurements, weight, degree of edema present, and rate and character of respirations. On the other hand, a person with a cardiac problem who is experiencing chest pain would be monitored for data

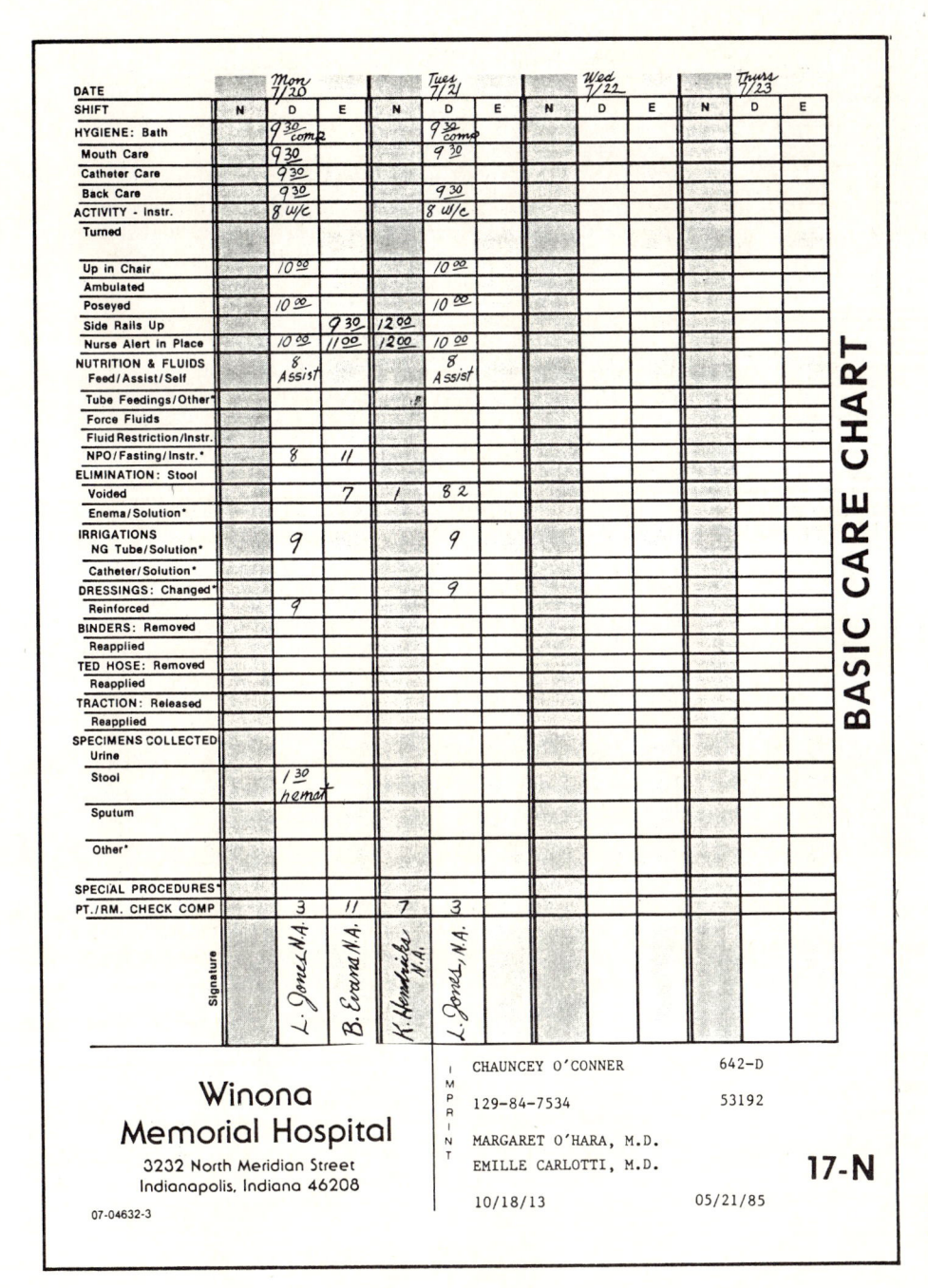

Figure 18-2A. Flow Sheet: Basic Care Chart, front. (Courtesy of Winona Memorial Hospital, Indianapolis, IN.)

such as color, skin temperature, blood pressure, and cardiac rate and rhythm.

Weed (1970) suggests using general flow sheets, where the desired observations can be filled in as needed, and he proposes that flow sheets may be the only progress notes needed on some occasions. One reliability study of nursing flow sheets reported statistically significant interrater reliability among flow sheets completed independently by different nurses for the same client situation (Cohn, 1975).

KARDEX SYSTEMS

A kardex system usually accompanies either a problem-oriented record or a traditional, source-oriented record in both acute and long-term hospital settings. The kardex is a series of index cards in a portable flip-style file as shown in Figure 18-4. Significant current client data and nursing-care plans are placed on these cards for quick, easy reference by various health-team members. These nursing-care plans may be newly handwritten for each client; they may include either algorithms (behavioral steps in basic nursing care for given nursing diagnoses) or prototype plans of care for clients with a particular medical diagnosis. Sometimes computer printouts of the medical and nursing care plans are kept in a kardex file. The kardex normally is used as a reference during hospital intershift reports. Sometimes a separate kardex system is used for medication administration.

In most agencies, the kardex is not considered

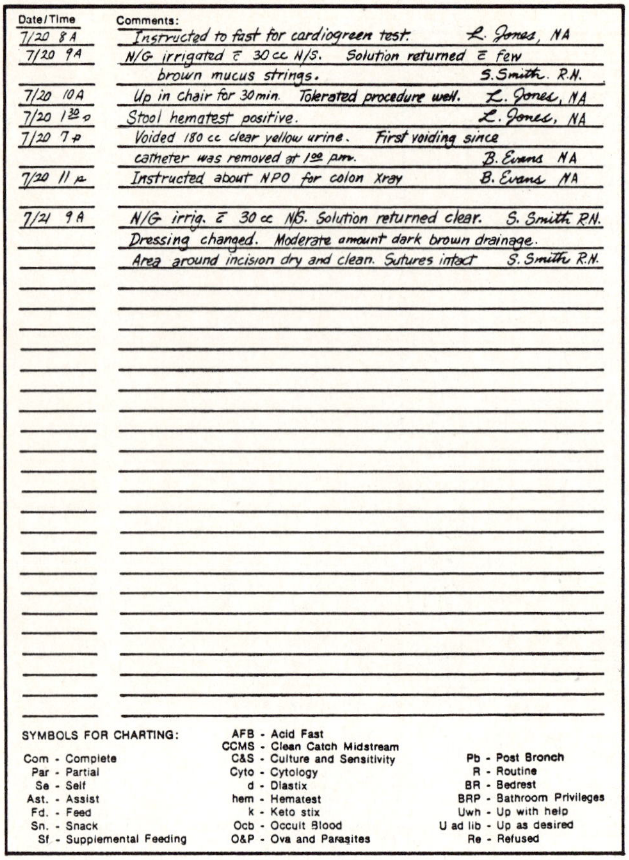

Date/Time	Comments:
7/20 8 A	Instructed to fast for cardiogreen test. L. Jones, NA
7/20 9A	N/G irrigated c̄ 30 cc N/S. Solution returned c̄ few
	brown mucus strings. S. Smith. R.N.
7/20 10A	Up in chair for 30 min. Tolerated procedure well. L. Jones, NA
7/20 1³⁰ p	Stool hematest positive. L. Jones, NA
7/20 7 p	Voided 180 cc clear yellow urine. First voiding since
	catheter was removed at 1⁰⁰ pm. B. Evans NA
7/20 11 p	Instructed about NPO for colon Xray B. Evans NA
7/21 9 A	N/G irrig. c̄ 30 cc N/S. Solution returned clear. S. Smith R.N.
	Dressing changed. Moderate amount dark brown drainage.
	Area around incision dry and clean. Sutures intact S. Smith R.N.

SYMBOLS FOR CHARTING:

	AFB - Acid Fast	
	CCMS - Clean Catch Midstream	
Com - Complete	C&S - Culture and Sensitivity	Pb - Post Bronch
Par - Partial	Cyto - Cytology	R - Routine
Se - Self	d - Diastix	BR - Bedrest
Ast. - Assist	hem - Hematest	BRP - Bathroom Privileges
Fd. - Feed	k - Keto stix	Uwh - Up with help
Sn. - Snack	Ocb - Occult Blood	U ad lib - Up as desired
Sf - Supplemental Feeding	O&P - Ova and Parasites	Re - Refused

Figure 18–2B. *Flow Sheet: Basic Care Chart, back. (Courtesy of Winona Memorial Hospital, Indianapolis, IN.)*

part of the permanent legal record; often it is written in pencil and erased and updated as needed. Unfortunately, if nursing-care problems and plans are noted only in the kardex, they cannot be retrieved for nursing education and audits. Figure 18–5 shows a 3-page kardex in use at one hospital. These large ($8\frac{1}{2} \times 11$ in) cards provide a format for using nursing diagnosis and nursing process in clinical practice, as well as a place to record basic data about the client's medical problems, functional status, diagnostic tests, and therapeutic procedures. These data provide a framework for both independent and dependent nursing practice.

REPORTING OBSERVATIONS

A large amount of verbal communication accompanies both the POMR and the traditional, source-oriented record systems. For example, students and other nursing-team members usually report significant happenings verbally to team leaders; decisions are discussed with head nurses, other team members, or both; and reports of client status, plans, and necessary tasks are communicated verbally between shifts in acute-care agencies. Intershift reports may be tape recorded or given orally. One four-state survey reported that nurses in specialty areas preferred an oral report to a taped report because it allowed them to communicate more information about critical patients. On general-care units, the taped report remained increasingly popular, as it seemed to save time for nurses on both shifts (Mitchell, 1976).

Oral reports, like written recordings, should be clear, concise, and relevant. Depending on the situation, these reports reflect nursing observations, judgments, plans, evaluations, or the client's response to care given.

Legal Status of Nursing Records

Nursing records are part of the legal health record. Creighton (1981) reminds us that the nurse is an employee of the agency, not the client, and is responsible for keeping adequate records that protect the agency. Failure to keep adequate records is considered *negligence*. Negligence for a professional nurse is failure "to apply that degree of skill and learning in treating and nursing a patient which is customarily applied in . . . the same community" (Spaulding and Notter, 1976, p. 116). Inadequate records may be the basis for a tort liability claim against a nurse. (A tort is a wrongful act for which a civil suit can be brought, such as for redress of injury or neglect.)

Nursing records are considered a prime source of evidence in malpractice or bodily injury lawsuits. An investigator for a hospital malpractice insurance firm says the leading causes of claims against nurses are the failure to chart; failure to notify physicians of changes; failure to identify patients for medications and treatments; and paying insufficient attention to patients (Mumme, 1977). In her excellent discussion on nurses' notes, Kerr (1975) says trial lawyers in malpractice or bodily injury cases are intensely interested in nurses' notes because that is where much of their evidence comes from, as nurses' notes are dated, written frequently, and provide detailed information about daily care and events. Kerr suggests that as the nurse charts, he or she should consider the questions that might be asked about what is being charted. Other authors also provide guidelines for the creation of nursing records that meet professional and legal standards (Creighton, 1980; Kunkel, 1983; Lee and Fraser, 1981; Schaefer, 1981).

☐ *EXECUTION*

Records are an integral part of every nursing work setting. The nurse has a professional obligation to help produce an accurate and complete record of client care. Preparing that kind of record requires that the professional nurse use correct terminology and grammar, become familiar with agency record forms and systems, use interpersonal and observational skills to collect needed data, and be able to record observations and interventions in an accurate and concise manner.

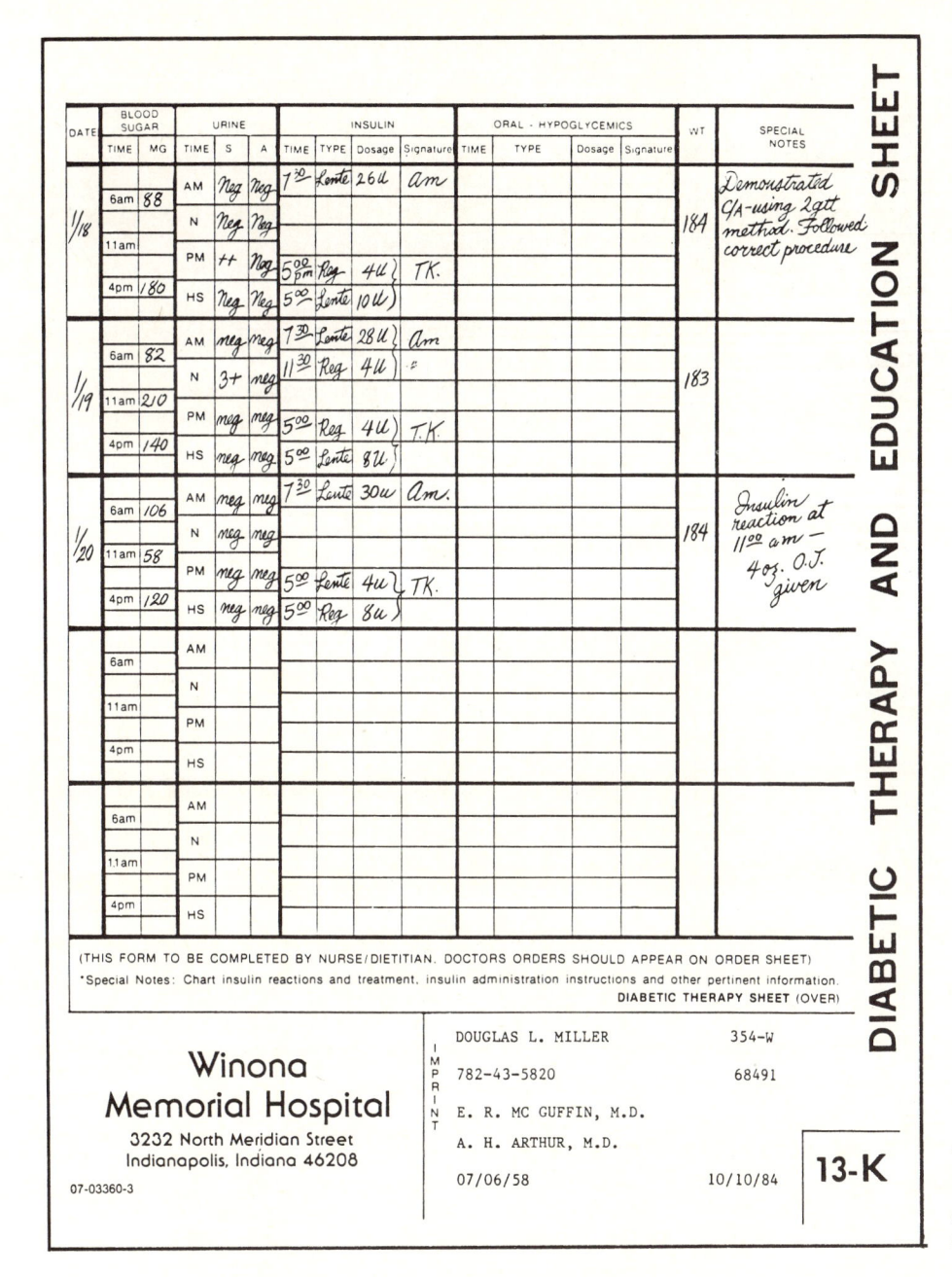

Figure 18-3. Flow Sheet: Diabetic Therapy and Education Sheet, page 1 of a 3-page form. (Courtesy of Winona Memorial Hospital, Indianapolis, IN.)

GUIDELINES FOR LEGALLY ACCEPTABLE NURSING RECORDS

Although the format, structure, and complexity of the record varies with the setting, the following guidelines will help you produce nursing records that meet accepted legal standards for both traditional and SOAP format recordings.

1. *Write or print legibly, in black ink.*
2. *Record date and time, and sign all entries.* Signature includes first initial, last name, and title; for example, M. Johnston, S. N. (student nurse); or M. Johnston, R. N. (registered nurse).
3. *Leave no blank spaces in the record.* Use the entire line, including the signature line. Draw a line through any lines or parts of lines inadvertently left blank and date and sign the blank space.
4. *Make no erasures or obliterations.* Both arouse strong suspicion in lawyers as to what and why something was deleted. When an error occurs, simply circle it or draw a line through the error, write "error," date, and sign the notation. In addition, nurse–lawyer Greenlaw (1982) states that "... removing, discarding, and writing an entire new page is not a sound practice as someone may have acted in reliance on the information before it was discovered to be erroneous. It is preferable that the chart shows the error instead of someone discovering, at a later time, the attempt to conceal it" (p. 173).

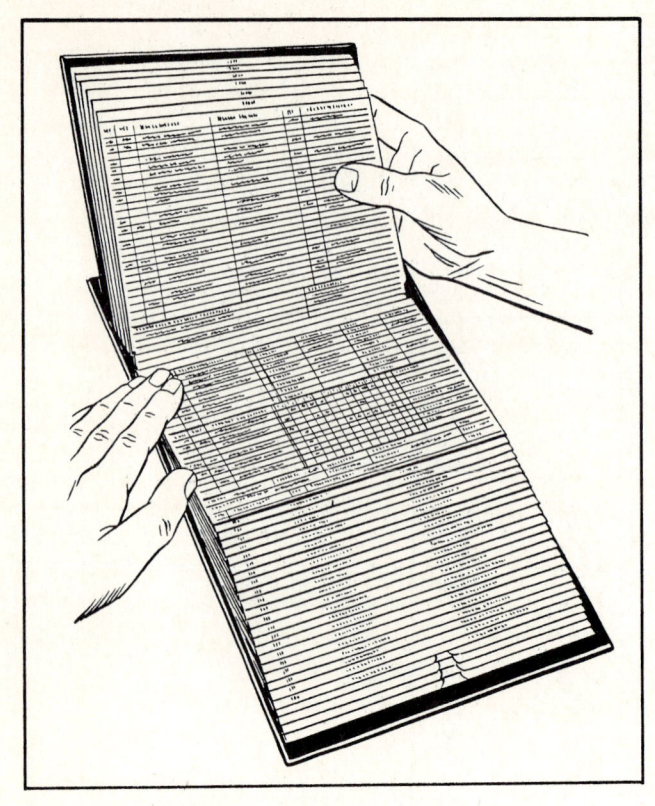

Figure 18–4. Portable kardex holder.

5. *Do not insert or add material later.* In a survey by Nursing74, 48 percent of the nurses reported that they had charted on blank lines or between lines to insert information (Kerr, 1975). A nurse may be held legally accountable for falsification of records if disputes arise and he or she is shown to have added data after a time lapse, or if the insertion looks as if it is meant to cover up an error. Sophisticated ink analyses can determine if the same pen was used for an insertion as for the original note. A malpractice commission report indicates that 24 percent of attorneys surveyed felt that altered records raise questions in jurors' minds about the credibility of the entire record (Hershey and Lawrence, 1976).

6. *Record significant data accurately.* Give exact times and events, especially for medication administration and during emergencies. Record factual information, rather than subjective terms and generalities. For example, Murchison and Nichols (1970, p. 45) state that "probably the most common error made by nurses in entering their notes—and one that decreases the value of the record when offered to court—is to report value judgments, opinions, and conclusions instead of factual information." Examples of these types of comments include "she is drinking *well*"; "reports *good* relief from pain"; "ambulating *well*."

Figure 18–5. The large cards in this three-card kardex contain nursing-care plans and summary data about the client in a readily available form. (Script writing indicates pencilled notations; printing indicates information written in ink.) (Courtesy of Winona Memorial Hospital, Indianapolis, IN.)

Date	Nursing Dx/Problem	Nursing Order	Inl.	EVALUATION/OUTCOME
1-29	1. Anxiety related to fear of cancer	1. Allow ventilation of feelings 2. Reassure 3. Promote calm environment 4. Promote environment conducive to asking questions 5. Explain all procedures + tests	K.T.	Decrease anxiety Promote understanding of tests and procedures
1-29	2. Possibility of alteration in urinary elimination related to hematuria and urinary retention	1. Strict I & O 2. Force fluids 3. Note amount, color, consistency of urine 4. Note bladder distention (related to retention)	K.T.	Promote "normal" urinary elimination, which is "normal" for patient.
1-29	3. Sensory deprivation related to cataract extraction and being hard of hearing	1. Assist with ambulation (related to poor vision) 2. Set up tray and assist with meals 3. Assist with a.m. care 4. Speak distinctly to patient (face patient when talking) 5. Speak slowly. 6. Keep necessary items within reach of patient	K.T.	Promote safety.
1-29	4. Alteration in thought process related to age.	1. Re-orient to time, place, and person everytime you are in patients' presence 2. Provide calendar to assist in orientation to time. 3. Side rails in place at all times.	K.T.	Maintain optimal mental functioning

Discharge Objectives/Long Term Goals
1-29 Discharge:
1- Able to perform own ADL's with minimal assistance
2- Without hematuria, voiding without difficulty.

PRIMARY NURSE:
L. Brown, R.N.
K. Thompson R.N.

Date	INL	PRN TREATMENTS	CK	RISK	ACTION	RISK	ACTION
1-29	AM	CATHETERIZE Q 12° p.r.n. FOR 3 DAYS IF UNABLE TO VOID		(Over 65) Language Barrier (Senile) (Confused) Mentally Retarded Alcoholic (Emotional Instability) Overly Independent Hx of falls (Obese) Smokes	ASSIST SIDERAILS REORIENT, USE CALENDAR REASSURE, EXPLAIN	Dec. Sensation Loss of Balance Seizures (Vision)(hearing) prob. Nocturia Incontinent X-ray prep. (Sleeping pills) Anticoagulants/cuts (Allergy) Hypotension	 ASSIST - SPEAK CLEARLY SIDERAILS @ H.S. SHRIMP-ALLERGY BAND on.

Date	Initials	STANDARD TREATMENTS	8/9	10/11	12/1	2/3	4/5	6/7	8/9	10/11	12/1	2/3	4/5	6/7	24hr CK	DC Date	
1-29	AM	V.S. DAILY					4										Bladder Function
1-29	AM	HEMATEST ALL URINE															Bowel Function
1-29	AM	I & O (N.M.)				2				10				6			INDEPENDENT Q.A.M.

Special Medications
THORAZINE 50 MG. H.S. DAILY.

Intravenous (Yes) No
Meds at Bedside Yes (No)
Meds in Locked Drawer Yes (No)
Valuables in Safe Yes (No)

Bath: Self (Assist)
Complete   Shower
Partial at B.S.   Tub
Partial in B.R.

Activity: Self (Assist)
Bedrest   (BRP) c̄ HELP
Dangle   Amb.
Commode 1/29 (Up) c̄ HELP
Chair

Allergies CODEINE	Adm. Date 1-29-81	Religion Sacr. of Sick PROT.	Condition Classification Satisfactory	Cons. MD
Prominent Med. Problems/Conditions ARTHRITIS			Surgery	Ref. M.D.
Room No. 209	Name JOHN JONES	Age 80	Diagnosis HEMATURIA	Adm. M.D. A.J. WOODS

Figure 18–5. (continued)

7. *Use only abbreviations and symbols that are common* to the employing agency. Personal shorthand styles often mean something different to another person and can be the source of error.
8. *Use correct spelling and punctuation* to avoid misunderstanding. For example, when written carelessly, perineal and peritoneal look alike although they have entirely different meanings.
9. *Record movement of clients to other departments.* For example, document the time a client leaves the nursing-care area for specialized services, such as the operating room, laboratory, or physical therapy department, and record the time the client returns to the unit.
10. *Record visits from physicians, other health-team members, and family.*
11. *Do not omit information, even if it reflects on yourself or someone else in a negative manner.* A Nursing76 survey indicated that nearly one out of ten respondents had at some time omitted information because they thought it might make them look bad. These same nurses were also ones who tended to record inaccurate information and add to or later alter the data (Kerr, 1975). Creighton (1978) reports that a surgeon and a supervisor nurse who concealed nonrecorded information were found guilty of falsifying business records in the first degree. Legality aside, professional accountability dictates that a nurse be truthful and accurate in reporting.
12. *Record instructions given to clients and any refusal to follow those instructions.* An injury that occurs after a client refuses to follow instructions often is regarded by courts as contributory negligence on the part of the client; thus, the nurse is not held liable.
13. *You are accountable for what precedes your signature.* Be accurate in what you write and leave no space for others to insert something prior to your signature. Professional nurses often need to record results of procedures performed by nurse aides or assistants without having personally seen the client or the test results. Nurses may be asked to countersign record entries made by licensed practical nurses, students, or aides. In situations like these, the nurse's signature attests to the authenticity of events of which he or she has no firsthand knowledge. Hemelt and Mackert (1978, p. 134) remind us that countersigning means to "place one's signature to a writing already signed by another to attest to the authenticity of that writing." They suggest that the facts be recorded carefully, and in such a way that the source of data and the nurse's role in recording and signing or countersigning is clarified. For example, the nurse can record, "Enemas given by L. Jones, L.P.N., who reports patient expelled large amounts of flatus, highly colored solution, and 'large amount' of stool. Also reports patient states he feels better."

GUIDELINES FOR PROFESSIONAL ACCOUNTABILITY IN NURSING RECORDS

Both the Joint Commission on Accreditation of Hospitals (JCAH) and the American Nurses Association (ANA) in their standards of care state that nursing records of care given should reflect the use of the nursing process (American, 1973; Joint, 1981). That is, records are to include subjective and objective data; nursing problem identification; and planning, implementation, and evaluation of care given. Nursing records need to reflect the dependent function of implementing physicians' orders and the independent functions of reporting observations about client status and judgments about medical and nursing interventions, as well as indicating the actual care given.

The following guidelines will help you produce professional nurses' notes in either SOAP or paragraph style:

1. *Record objective data*—what you *see, hear, feel,* and *smell* through direct and instrumental observation.
2. *Record subjective data.* Use direct quotes from the client or family whenever possible.
3. *Indicate relationships* among observed data, plans of care, and actual care given. For example, administration of pain medication should be accompanied by a documentation of the client's pain, followed later by documentation of the effectiveness of the medication.
4. *Document the care actually given.* Record nursing and medical interventions that were ordered by the physician, independent nursing actions based on nursing judgments, observations about actions based on nursing judgments, and observations about results and effectiveness of care given.
5. *Record baseline data.* That is, record current client status or initial observations as a basis for comparison with the client's status at a later time and to help evaluate changes in condition.
6. *Record presence or absence of significant data.* That is, include data that are relevant to the medical or nursing diagnoses or both, because this also helps develop a data base for assessment and evaluation of client status.
7. *Use specific and meaningful terminology.*
   a. Avoid general, nonspecific, and nondescriptive terms, such as "good condition," "better day," or "good night."
   b. Measure whenever possible, such as the circumference of a distended abdomen or swollen ankle.
   c. Use metric measurements such as milliliter (ml) and centimeter (cm) rather than ounces, cups, or inches. Learn to estimate fairly accurately. Minimize the use of imprecise terms like small, moderate, and large.
   d. Describe the exact nature and location of symptoms. Use drawings, if that will make the recording more clear.

TABLE 18-2. Common Abbreviations

ABBREVIATION	MEANING	ABBREVIATION	MEANING
A.M.	morning; after midnight, before noon	KDS	ketodiastix
A-R	apical-radial pulse rate	LLQ	left lower quadrant of abdomen
abd	abdomen	LUQ	left upper quadrant of abdomen
AMA	against medical advice	NPO	nothing by mouth
amt	amount	N.S.	normal saline
approx	approximately	OD	right eye
BM	bowel movement	OS	left eye
BP	blood pressure	OU	both eyes
BRP	bathroom privileges	OT	occupational therapy
c̄	with	p.o.	telephone order
CCU	coronary care unit	PT	physical therapy
CBC	complete blood count	per	by way of
CCMS	clean-catch midstream urine specimen	pt	patient
C & S	culture and sensitivity	q	every
c/o	complains of; complaint	q.s.	a sufficient quantity
DC	discontinue	q.o.d.	every other day
DOA	dead on arrival	RLQ	right lower quadrant of abdomen
DTV	due to void	RUQ	right upper quadrant of abdomen
D/W	distilled water	ROM	range of motion
D_5W	dextrose, 5% in water	s̄	without
ECG, EKG	electrocardiogram	S/A	sugar and acetone
EEG	electroencephalogram	SSE	soap suds enema
EMG	electromyogram	t.o.	telephone order
FF	force fluids	TCDB	turn, cough, deep breathe
GB	gallbladder	RHC	respirations have ceased
GI	gastrointestinal	TPR	temperature, pulse, respirations
GU	genitourinary	U/A	urinalysis
h.s.	hour of sleep, bedtime	wt.	weight
H_2O	water	w/c	wheelchair
I & O	intake and output	WNL	within normal limits
IPPB	intermittent positive pressure breathing	via	by way of
IV	intravenous	v.o.	verbal order

e. Use accepted abbreviations only. Table 18-2 lists abbreviations in common use.

8. *Sentences need not be grammatically complete.* Since all information in the record refers to the client, comments need not begin with, "Client says" or, "Client went." For example, write: "To x-ray per w/c for chest x-ray," rather than "The client went to the x-ray department in a wheelchair for a chest x-ray." Be sure punctuation provides a correct meaning. Begin each comment with a capital letter and end with a period.

9. *Make precise and accurate notations on flow sheets.* Draw lines to connect dots or circles on graphic sheets. This provides a visual picture of data such as temperature, pulse, or blood pressure.

10. *Be brief and concise.* However, include sufficient detail to reflect in an accurate way the client's status and the care given.

Bernhardt (1978) poses several questions for evaluating one's own record keeping: Based on your written account, could your nursing care be duplicated? Would your care be considered appropriate by your peers? Would *you* pay for nursing care you recorded as being given? If you were in court, would your written record reflect the nursing care you gave, or would you want to change or add something?

Thorough and careful examination of representative nursing records will increase your ability to use those records effectively when you are in actual nursing-care situations. The following activities are designed to help you become familiar with the primary types of nursing records: narrative notes, flow sheets, and kardex forms.

Activity 18-A: Writing Nurses' Notes

1. Read the following sample client-care situation and the sample SOAP and paragraph charting notes.

Client Situation A: Mrs. Smith is a newly diagnosed diabetic who is in the hospital for regulation of her diabetes. At 4 A.M., the night nurse finds Mrs. Smith sitting on the side of the bed, holding her abdomen and reporting that she has just vomited for the second time in a half hour. The nurse notes that the young woman is pale and her skin is cool and damp.

Nurse: "Do you feel as if you might be having an insulin reaction, Mrs. Smith?"

Mrs. Smith: "I don't know—I've never had one!"

Nurse: "Well, that's what I suspect is happening right now. I notice that you're sweating and your skin is quite cool, and you look rather pale."

Mrs. Smith: "I hadn't really noticed—I guess because of my stomach."

Nurse: "Everyone feels a little different when they have a reaction, but it's quite common to be nauseated, to sweat, and be pale and cool when having a reaction. I am going to do the things for you that we usually do when someone has a reaction, and if it turns out to be a reaction, then you'll have learned something else about your diabetes—how *you* feel when having a reaction! If it doesn't, then we'll do something else about your nausea. The first thing I'm going to do is call the lab and have them draw a stat blood sugar, which they'll do in less than 10 minutes. After that, I'll bring you some orange juice and crackers, and I suspect you'll soon feel much better. I'll also send someone to stay with you for a while."

The nurse asks the student nurse to stay with the client, monitor her condition, provide moral support, and discuss diabetes as the young woman might be interested and the student able to do so. After leaving the room, the nurse calls the lab for the stat blood sugar.

SOAP Format Charting Note

4 A.M. S—"I feel so sick! I just vomited twice in the last half hour. I've never had an insulin reaction, so I don't know if I'm having one or not."

O—Sitting on edge of bed, holding abdomen. Skin pale, cool, and clammy, with moderate diaphoresis.

A—Experiencing hypoglycemic reaction.

P—(Therapeutic) Have someone stay with Mrs. Smith for safety, monitoring, and reassurance. (Diagnostic) Explore understanding of hypoglycemic reaction. (Education) Reinforce teaching about symptoms, cause, and Rx of reactions.

Traditional Charting Note

4 A.M. Found sitting @ bedside. Says she has just vomited for the second time in a half hour & is quite nauseated. Color pale, skin cool and clammy; holding abdomen with arms. Says has never had insulin reaction and doesn't know how it would feel. Believe she is having hypoglycemic reaction. Briefly explained reaction symptoms. Nursing student/aide staying with Mrs. Smith. Called lab for stat BS.

2. Read the following sample client-care situation. Write two nurses' notes entries, one in a SOAP format for a problem-oriented record, and the other in a paragraph style for a traditional, source-oriented record. Validate your notes with peers or faculty.

Client Situation B: Mr. Jones, 73 years old, had surgery 5 days earlier for an abdominal aneurysm. He is currently receiving a liquid diet and is to be up walking as much as possible, which he is reluctant to do. A student nurse is assisting him with his breakfast because his appetite has been rather poor. After drinking 80 ml of juice, 30 ml of hot cereal with milk, and a few sips of tea, Mr. Jones says that is all he wants.

Student: "Are there any other liquids you might like better than these?"

Mr. Jones: "No, these foods are OK—I just don't want any more."

Student: "You've not eaten a very large breakfast—are you not feeling well?"

Mr. Jones: "Yes. I'm fine. I'm just stuffed. I keep eating all this food and can't move my bowels—I'm so bloated."

Student: "I see; not sick or nauseated, just bloated. Are you passing any gas?"

Mr. Jones: "I don't think so—but I feel like I should!"

Student: "Let me listen to your abdomen for bowel sounds and see if they are active.... (Listens with stethoscope in several places) .... There are good bowel sounds all across there ... (Gestures to midabdominal area, and then proceeds to palpate Mr. Jones' abdomen gently, being careful not to cause incisional pain).... Your abdomen feels rather firm, too, so I suspect you do feel 'bloated.' As you move around more in bed and walk more, that gas will begin to move on and out. Some warm water or tea with lemon juice might help, too. Would you want to try some more tea now? In about an hour I would have time to go with you for a walk in the hallway. I'll come back then."

Activity 18-B:
Using Flow Sheets

Locate the following data on the sample flow sheet in Figure 18-1.

1. Blood pressure: on admission _____ March 31 _____
2. Pulse: day of surgery _____ February 1 _____
3. Respirations: second postoperative day _____ March 29 _____
4. Temperature: first postoperative day _____ March 31 _____
5. Diet received: second postoperative day _____ April 1 _____
6. Appetite: lunch, March 28 _____, third postoperative day _____
7. Oral fluid intake: day of surgery, 3-11 shift _____ 24-hour intake, first postoperative day _____
8. Bowel activity: March 28 _____ April 1 _____
9. Urinary output: March 30, 7-3 shift _____ 24 hours _____
10. Activity: March 28 _____ day of surgery _____

Activity 18-C:
Using a Kardex System

Use the following guide to examine an actual kardex card, computer nursing-care plan, or the sample kardex cards shown in Figure 18-5.

1. Locate client identification data (name, age, sex, room number, admission date).
2. Compare the types of information written in pencil with those in ink.
3. Determine the method of accountability for information placed on the kardex.
4. Identify any information you would consider confidential.
5. Locate the following:
   - Medical diagnoses
   - Nursing diagnoses
   - Attending physician(s)
   - Nursing plan of care
   - Nursing orders
   - Medical orders
   - Surgery performed and the date
   - Special tests or procedures
   - Laboratory tests ordered
   - Therapist or specialist services
   - Diet and fluids
   - Activities
   - Allergies
   - Medications

☐ CRITICAL POINTS SUMMARY

1. Write or print legibly, in black ink.
2. Date, time, and sign all entries.
3. Leave no blank spaces.
4. Make no erasures or obliterations.
5. Do not insert or add material later.
6. Be truthful and accurate.
7. Create complete, accurate, and precise flow sheets.
8. Record objective and subjective data, nursing observations, judgments, and evaluations.
9. Document current and changed client status and the actual medical and nursing care given.
10. Record both independent and dependent nursing functions.
11. Use specific, meaningful, and descriptive terminology.
12. Use accepted abbreviations, symbols, and terminology.
13. Well-written nurses' notes are significant and worthwhile legal and professional documents.

☐ REVIEW QUESTIONS

1. Describe legal and professional functions of nursing records.
2. What obligation does the nurse have to the client for preparing and keeping adequate records? to the agency?
3. In what way does the nurse indicate legal accountability when charting?
4. What implications for accountability do signing and countersigning carry?
5. How can nurses' charting provide legal protection for themselves and their agency?
6. List five guidelines for preparing legally correct records.
7. In what ways are source-oriented and problem-oriented nurses' notes similar and different?
8. What does the acronym SOAP represent?
9. List five guidelines that help produce more concise recording.
10. What categories of information are included in narrative notes?
11. What functions are served by flow sheets?
12. How does a kardex system facilitate giving nursing care?
13. Of what professional value are well-written nursing records?

REFERENCES

American Nurses' Association: Standards of Nursing Practice. Kansas City, MO, ANA, 1973.

Annas GJ: The Rights of Hospital Patients: The Basic ACLU Guide to a Hospital Patient's Rights. New York, Avon Discus Books, 1974.

Austin E: How your nursing notes can rob your patients of benefits. RN 41(9):58, 1978.

Barbiasz JE, Hunt V, Lowenstein A: Nursing documentation: A format not a form. Journal of Nursing Administration XI(6):22-26, 1981.

Bellevue Hospital: Training School for Nurses: 1873-1923. Fiftieth Anniversary, Bellevue Training School for Nurses. New York, NY, Bellevue Hospital, 1923.

Bernhardt JH: Record keeping—Key to professional accountability. Occupational Health Nursing (NY) 26(8):22-28, 1978.

Berni R, Readey H: Problem Oriented Medical Record Implementation: Allied Health Peer Review, ed 2. St Louis, CV Mosby, 1978.

Bloom JT, Dressler J, et al: Problem-oriented charting. American Journal of Nursing 71(11):2114-2148, 1971.

Blount M, Green SS, et al: Documenting with the problem-oriented record system. American Journal of Nursing 78(9):1539-1542, 1978.

Bullough V, Bullough B: The Care of the Sick: The Emergence of Modern Nursing. New York, NY, Prodist, 1978.

Cohn S, Fulcher A, Gastafson N: Reliability study of a nursing flow sheet. Journal of Nursing Administration 5(9):30-33, 1975.

Creighton H: Liability for falsifying records. Supervisor Nurse 9:16-17, 1978.

Creighton H: Nurse's charting—Part II. Supervisor Nurse 11(6):61-62, 1980.

Creighton H: Law Every Nurse Should Know, ed 4. Philadelphia, WB Saunders, 1981.

Gamberg D, Hushower G, Smith N: Outcome charting. Nursing Management 12(10):36-38, 1981.

Greenlaw JG: Documentation of patient care: An often underestimated responsibility. Law, Medicine, & Health Care 10(4):172-174, 1982.

Healy KM: Does preoperative instruction make a difference? American Journal of Nursing 68(1):68-71, 1968.

Hemelt MD, Mackert ME: Dynamics of Law in Nursing and Health Care. Reston, VA, Reston Publishing, 1978.

Hershey N, Lawrence R: The influence of charting upon liability determinations. Journal of Nursing Administration 6(3):35-37, 1976.

Hoffman J: Personal Communication, Feb. 21, 1980. Indiana University Hospital, Indianapolis, IN.

Huffman EK: Medical Record Management, ed 6. Revised by the American Medical Association, Price EA (ed). Berwyn, IL, Physicians' Record Company, 1972.

Isler C: Nursing audit: New yardstick for patient care. RN 37(12):31-35, 1974.

Joint Commission on Accreditation of Hospitals: Accreditation Manual for Hospitals. Chicago, JCAH, 1984.

Kerr AH: Nurses' notes: That's where the goodies are! Nursing75 5(2):34-41, 1975.

Kunkel JA: Charting: Some pointers for doing it better. NursingLife 3(2):57-64, 1983.

Lee G, Fraser SS: ED nursing SOAP notes. Journal of Emergency Nursing 7(5):216-218, 1981.

Mitchell M: Intershift reports—To tape or not to tape. Supervisor Nurse 7(10):38-39, 1976.

Mitchell PH, Atwood J: Problem-oriented recording as a teaching-learning tool. Nursing Research 24(2):99-103, 1975.

Mumme JL: Seven surefire ways to lose a malpractice case. RN 40(11):60-64, 1977.

Murchison IA, Nichols TS: Legal Foundations of Nursing Practice. New York, Macmillan, 1970.

National League for Nursing: The Problem-Oriented System—A Multidisciplinary Approach. New York, National League for Nursing (Publ. No. 20-1546), 1974.

Nightingale F: Notes on Nursing: What It Is and What It Is Not, ed 2. New York, Dover, 1946.

Phaneuf M: The Nursing Audit: Self-Regulation in Nursing Practice, ed 2. New York, Appleton-Century-Crofts, 1976.

Schaefer MS: To avoid a lawsuit, keep the record straight. RN 44(11):81-82, 1981.

Spaulding EK, Notter LE: Professional Nursing: Foundations, Perspectives, and Relationships. Philadelphia, JB Lippincott, 1976.

Walker BH, Selmanoff ED: A study of the nature and use of nurses' notes. Nursing Research 13(2):113-121, 1964.

Weed LL: Medical Records, Medical Education, and Patient Care. Cleveland, Case Western University Press, 1970.

Woody M, Mallison M: The problem-oriented system for patient-centered care. American Journal of Nursing 73(7):1168-1175, 1973.

BIBLIOGRAPHY

Allen RS: Proper charting is important. Nursing76 6(2):72, 75, 1976.

Bergerson SR: Charting with a jury in mind. NursingLife 2(4):30-33, 1982.

Documenting Patient Care Responsibly. Horsham, PA, Intermed Communications (Nursing Skillbook Series), 1978.

Eggland ET: Charting: How and why to document your care daily—and fully. Nursing80 10(2):38-43, 1980.

Katz BF: Reporting and review of patient care: The nurse's responsibility. Law, Medicine & Health Care 11(2):76-79, 1983.

Kozier B, Erb GL: Fundamentals of Nursing: Concepts and Procedures, ed 2. Reading, MA, Addison-Wesley, 1983.

Mancini M: Documenting clinical records. American Journal of Nursing 78(9):1556, 1561, 1978.

McIntosh JB: Record keeping—A boon or a bind? No. 1. Record content. Nursing Mirror 147(1):43-44, 1978.

McIntosh JB: Record keeping—a boon or a bind? No. 3. The way forward. Nursing Mirror 147(3):36-37, 1978.

Moore K: Closing the audit cycle. Nursing Management 12(10):32-34, 1981.

Richards L: Reminiscences of Linda Richards. Boston, M Barrows, 1911.

Rocereto LaV R, Maleski CM: The Legal Dimensions of Nursing Practice. New York, Springer, 1982.

Rosenberg M, Carriker D: Automating nurses' notes. American Journal of Nursing 66(5):1021–1023, 1966.

Veazie S, Dankmyer T: HISs, MISs, DBMSs: Sorting out the letters. Hospitals 51(20):80–84, 1977.

Walker M, Geller D: Ambulatory pediatric assessment: A computerized system for nurses. Pediatric Nursing 3(5):37–41, 1977.

Watson A, Mayers M: Evaluating the quality of patient care through retrospective chart review. Journal of Nursing Administration 6(3):17–21, 1976.

Zielstorff RD (ed): Computers in Nursing. Rockville, MD, Aspen Systems Corporation, 1980.

SUGGESTED READING

Kerr AM: Nurses' notes: That's where the goodies are! Nursing75 5(2):34–41, 1975.

Kunkel JA: Charting: Some pointers for doing it better. NursingLife 3(2):57–64, 1983.

Lee G, Fraser SS: ED nursing SOAP notes. Journal of Emergency Nursing 7(5):216–218, 1981.

AUDIOVISUAL RESOURCES

The Nursing History: Foundation for Total Patient Care (13 min.)

The Nursing History: Guidelines for Accuracy (16 min.)

The Nursing History: Interviewing Techniques (15 min.)
  Each available as filmstrip, slides, cartridge, videotape. (Color, 1979)
  Available through:
  Medcom, Inc.
  P.O. Box 116
  Garden Grove, CA 92642

PART TWO
PROFESSIONAL CLINICAL NURSING SKILLS

☐ INTRODUCTION

The scope of professional nursing practice includes provision of direct nursing care for clients in acute-care, extended-care, and home settings. The skills used to provide this care are often called basic nursing skills, technical skills, psychomotor skills, or sometimes simply, skills. It is these skills with which the public is most familiar, and which are most often associated with the concept of "nurse." Public expectations, as well as professional standards, demand that a high level of skill competency be demonstrated at all times. It is essential that these expectations and standards be met because of the importance of promoting client safety, preventing injury, and avoiding the negative consequences that may result from improper skill execution.

Clinical nursing skills are not used in isolation from the communication skills presented in Part One. Verbal and nonverbal communication skills enable the nurse to develop rapport with the client, help the client to establish trust in the nurse, and facilitate the data collection that is vitally important for safe and effective implementation of clinical nursing skills. Written communication skills enable the nurse to communicate to other members of the health-care team the relevant data gathered during the process of skill implementation.

Recent efforts to control the high costs of health care include changes in federal and private insurance reimbursement practices, resulting in decreased lengths of stay in acute-care hospitals and an accelerated demand for home or extended-care services for increasingly complex types of care. In addition, increased numbers of elderly and chronically ill persons produce an escalating demand for home health-care services (Spradley, 1985). In the past, home-care services consisted primarily of basic care to assist with personal hygiene, nutrition, elimination, mobility, and wound care. In addition to meeting these traditional needs, home-care services now include enterostomal therapy, intravenous therapy, chemotherapy, and antibiotic therapy as well as special programs for the psychiatric, diabetic, and cardiac client (Weinstein, 1984). To meet this demand, the total number of home-care agencies has grown phenomenally. Therefore, increased numbers of nurses are practicing in settings that require them to function much more independently than in the immediate past, without the strong support usually experienced while working amid larger numbers of professional peers.

LEARNING CLINICAL NURSING SKILLS

Learning the clinical nursing skills presented in Part Two requires that the student combine behaviors from the cognitive, affective, and psychomotor domains of learning. The cognitive domain is concerned with intellectual behaviors; adequate functioning in the cognitive domain is demonstrated by the ability to acquire and use the knowledge base required for safe implementation of each skill. The affective domain addresses the feeling, emotional, and value aspects of self, client, and family; adequate functioning in this domain is demonstrated by integrating these aspects into the process of skill learning and implementation. The psychomotor domain combines the mental and physical actions required to perform a given task; adequate functioning in the psychomotor domain is demonstrated by using intellectual processes simultaneously with the physical movements required for actual performance of the skill.

Since standards for professional nursing practice require that a nurse's actions are based on a current, sound knowledge base and that individualized care be provided within the nursing process framework, it is essential that the student assume responsibility for integrating each of these domains of learning into the process of skill learning. If possible, it is recommended that each skill be practiced within a simulated laboratory setting with models and peers before implementing the skill with clients in the clinical setting.

OVERVIEW OF PART TWO

Professional implementation of psychomotor skills requires that a nurse gather an adequate data base prior to execution of a skill and be able to identify and evaluate changes in the client's status during and after the process of implementing the skill. In the same way that communication skills are basic to gathering adequate subjective data about the client's psychosocial and functional status through the interview process, physical appraisal techniques are basic to gathering objective data through direct observation of the client's physical status. As with communication skills, physical appraisal techniques are learned as distinct components and then integrated into the process of data gathering.

Chapter 6 provides an opportunity to learn the physical appraisal skills of inspection, palpation, percussion, and auscultation in a nonclinical setting, focusing on the *techniques* themselves. Physical appraisal skills are now accepted as an essential component of professional clinical nursing skills (Sana and Judge, 1982), although in the relatively recent past they were considered to be a part of only the physician's repertoire of skills. Competence in physical appraisal skills enables the nurse to exercise more sophisticated clinical judgments because their use makes it possible to obtain a more accurate and complete data base and to evaluate more fully the effectiveness of nursing interventions. In succeeding chapters, these skills are integrated appropriately within the context of each additional skill presented.

In Chapter 7, these physical appraisal techniques are applied to the skills of gathering basic data about a client's vital signs. This chapter includes the skills of measuring and appraising temperature, pulse, respirations, blood pressure, and height and weight.

Safe implementation of all psychomotor skills requires use of either medical or surgical aseptic techniques, or a combination of both, as well as the ability to determine when each is necessary. The concept of medical asepsis is presented in Chapter 8, along with the skills of handwashing and isolation techniques. Chapter 9 presents concepts of surgical asepsis, along with the skills of handling sterile supplies, donning sterile gloves, providing wound care and applying wound dressings, removing sutures, obtaining wound culture specimens, caring for and irrigating wounds, and applying wet sterile dressings and wet-to-dry dressings.

Chapter 10 presents the basic skills of assisting clients with personal hygiene needs which are an integral aspect of direct client care in any setting. This chapter includes care of the skin, perineum, mouth, hair, and nails, as well as vaginal irrigation, breast examination, and care of the corpse.

The skills in Chapter 11 are used to provide functional support for and protection of clients in a variety of circumstances. These skills include thermal applications, massage, application of bandages and binders, use of mechanical restraints, and care of casts.

Chapters 12 and 13 present skills related to providing assistance with the basic life functions of nutrition and elimination. Nutritional care is presented in Chapter 12, and includes monitoring fluid balance, assessment of nutritional status and serving food to clients, assisting clients to eat, and providing nutritional support through both the enteral and parenteral routes. Chapter 13 presents skills related to assisting with elimination, and includes insertion and care of gastrointestinal tubes, use of bedpans and urinals, bowel elimination procedures, urinary incontinence care, urinary catheterization, and care of an ostomy.

Chapter 14 presents the principles of safe and effective body mechanics for both the nurse and the client and integrates these principles into the skills of assisting the client with maintenance of functional mobility. These mobility-related skills include assistance with ambulation, maintenance of range of motion, transferring and positioning clients, and making a bed.

Skills related to assisting with maintenance of the basic life function of respiration are presented in Chapter 15. These skills include chest therapy exercises, oxygen therapy, tracheostomy care, and airway suctioning.

Medication administration is presented in Chapter 16. This chapter includes basic concepts of medication administration and dosage calculations, as well as the skills of administering oral, topical, injectable, and intravenous medications.

Chapter 17 presents two emergency techniques that may be needed in life-threatening situations in acute, nonacute, home, or community settings. These skills are cardiopulmonary resuscitation and removal of an obstruction in the airway.

REFERENCES

Sana JM, Judge RD (eds): Physical Appraisal Methods in Nursing Practice, ed 2. Boston, Little, Brown, 1982.

Spradley BW: Community Health Nursing: Concepts and Practice, ed 2. Boston, Little, Brown, 1985.

Weinstein SM: Specialty teams in home care. American Journal of Nursing 85(3):342–345, 1985.

6 Physical Appraisal Skills

☐ INTRODUCTION

Inspection, palpation, percussion, and auscultation are important skills in the professional nurse's repertoire. They are used either singly or in combination to collect data and to evaluate nursing activities. For example, a skin appraisal requires the use of inspection and palpation. Measuring blood pressure involves inspection, palpation, and auscultation. Improper execution of any one of the skills will produce erroneous measurements.

Proper execution of the physical appraisal skills requires the application of knowledge and the use of particular motor activities. The fine and gross motor movements necessary for some of the skills require adaptations of normal body movements.

The student is first expected to master the skills of "Inspection" (Skill 19), "Palpation" (Skill 20), "Percussion" (Skill 21), and "Auscultation" (Skill 22). Then he or she will learn to apply these skills in more complex procedures.

SKILL 19 Inspection

☐ STUDENT OBJECTIVES

1. Describe the purpose of general and specific inspection.
2. Explain the factors that affect accuracy of the findings obtained by inspection.
3. Apply the skill of inspection to collect data about the general and specific characteristics of a specific object.
4. Record the data in a clear and concise report.

☐ INTRODUCTION

Inspection is careful, detailed visual investigation. It is a process that requires unhurried and concentrated attention. The act of inspection is intended to provide data about the presence or absence of any landmarks that may be usual or unusual. It involves notation of location, position, color, texture, size, and temperature. The symmetry, type, and movement of body parts are appraised by comparison with the opposite side. Inspection includes investigation of both the general appearance and the specific characteristics of an entity. It is always conducted before as well as in conjunction with the other physical appraisal skills.

In this text, the term inspection is also applied to many other aspects of a nurse's responsibilities that are concerned with ensuring the safety of clients. For example, the skill of inspection is used to evaluate the integrity and proper function of all equipment used either by the client or by the nurse during the course of care, and it is used to detect hazards in the client's environment.

The use of inspection in nursing practice follows a tradition that dates back to Hippocrates, who developed it as a scientific method to study the physical signs of his patients.

☐ PREPARATION

Anders describes inspection as "the act of looking intelligently and attentively" (1907, p. 28). It is important for the student to be aware of any uncorrected personal visual deficiencies that may interfere with perception. Color blindness and loss of acuity and depth perception will prevent the appraiser from obtaining complete and accurate data. Because preconceived notions of what will be seen have a significant influence on what is seen, it is also important for the student to be aware of how knowledge and past experiences can distort perception. Judge and Zuidema (1982) explain that the mind may subconsciously use past experiences to fill in gaps with false information. This invented subjective data becomes incorporated with objective data and results in false findings. For example, when a nurse expects a client's temperature to be normal, on the basis of previous measurements, he or she may read a thermometer as normal when it is not, or wait so long to record it that the correct measurement is actually forgotten. In either situation, the nurse's mind can conjure up a mental substitution so that something can be placed on the client's health record as a temperature measurement. We can reduce this natural tendency by concentrating on one thing at a time, repeating the appraisal to validate the original findings, and making notes of the findings immediately. Inspection provides the most valuable and reliable information when the appraiser concentrates on the task at hand and proceeds systematically.

☐ EXECUTION

Unnecessary distraction during inspection can occur when the appraiser or the client is physically or psychologically uncomfortable. The nurse can help to put the client at ease by being courteous, protecting his or her privacy, and explaining what is to occur.

Proper body position for the nurse and the client and sufficient exposure of the area to be inspected in adequate natural or artificial light are essential. It is best to begin inspection by focusing upon the general characteristics of the area before concentrating on specific details.

☐ CRITICAL POINTS SUMMARY

1. Use a systematic approach.
2. Concentrate on the task at hand.
3. Position yourself and the client properly.
4. Expose the area to be examined.
5. Ensure adequate light.
6. Begin inspection with general characteristics.
7. Repeat inspection to verify findings.
8. Record findings immediately while they are fresh in your mind.

☐ LEARNING ACTIVITIES

1. Place a fruit or vegetable on a table under a good light. Concentrate your attention on noting the general characteristics of the object. Describe the size (in centimeters and inches), shape, color, tone, landmarks, and texture. When describing shape, include irregularities in contour. Record your findings clearly and concisely.
2. Select an irregularity present on the object and describe its distance from other landmarks. Describe the specific details of the irregularity.
3. Change the distance between the object and your eyes and then repeat activities 1 and 2.
4. Discuss and validate your findings from each activity with a peer. Do your descriptions agree? Consider what changes in your recording would improve communicating the findings of your inspections.

☐ REVIEW QUESTIONS

1. What are five examples of the types of information obtained by inspection?
2. Name two causes of inaccurate findings.
3. How can the factors creating errors in the findings be corrected?

REFERENCES

Anders HS: Physical Diagnosis. New York, D Appleton, 1907.

Judge RD, Zuidema GD (eds): Physical Diagnosis: A Physiological Approach to the Clinical Evaluation, ed 2. Boston, Little, Brown, 1973.

BIBLIOGRAPHY

Buckingham WB: A Primer of Clinical Diagnosis, ed 2. Hagerstown, MD, Harper & Row, 1979.

Malasanos L, Barkauskas V, et al: Health Assessment. St Louis, MO, CV Mosby, 1981.

AUDIOVISUAL RESOURCES

Physical Examination Techniques
   Videotape (3/4 in). (1976, Color, 9 min.)
   Available through:
      Medical Electronic Educational Services
      954 West Grant
      Tucson, AZ 85705

Physical Appraisal of the Adult in Nursing Practice: General Techniques
   Videotape (3/4 in). (1976, Color, 25 min.)
   Available through:
      University of Michigan, School of Nursing
      Medical Media Center
      Ann Arbor, MI 48109

PORTLAND COMMUNITY COLLEGE
Nursing Department

Student _____ Date _____

Skill _____ Pass: Yes ___ Evaluator _____
                              No ___

Advisor _____
****

Assessment:

****

Evaluation Comments:

I have met the criteria for successful demonstration of this procedure and feel competent to perform with patients.

Student Signature: _____

3/88

Time	PROGRESS NOTES

PORTLAND COMMUNITY COLLEGE
Nursing Department

Student _____ Date _____

Skill _____ Pass: Yes ___ Evaluator _____
                                No ___

Advisor _____
****

Assessment:

****

Evaluation Comments:

I have met the criteria for successful demonstration of this procedure and feel competent to perform with patients.

Student Signature: _____

3/88

Time | PROGRESS NOTES

SKILL 20 Palpation

PREREQUISITE SKILLS

Skill 19, "Inspection"
Skill 28, "Handwashing"

☐ STUDENT OBJECTIVES

1. Describe palpation.
2. Differentiate between the types of palpation.
3. Select the type of palpation appropriate for specific appraisals.
4. Become aware of what is perceived through the sense of touch.

☐ INTRODUCTION

Palpation is the use of touch to examine body parts to determine the characteristics of tissues or organs. Some data obtained by inspection may be confirmed by palpation. An examination of the parts of the body accessible by palpation provides information about the presence or absence of masses, pulsations, enlargement of organs, pain or tenderness, swelling, muscle spasm or rigidity, elasticity, and differences in texture. Temperature, moisture, movement, consistency, and form can also be determined by palpation.

The simplicity of palpation belies the experience necessary to use the skill well; consequently, it is frequently neglected by beginners. The manual operations of palpation must be combined with the ability to discriminate and interpret what is being felt, if valid information is to be obtained for use in clinical judgments.

☐ PREPARATION

Palpation is performed slowly and gently with warm, clean hands. Different parts and movements of the hands are used for various purposes. Because of their extreme sensitivity, the tips of the fingers are used for fine discriminations such as determining the texture of the skin or the size of a small lymph node. The dorsum of the hand is used to estimate temperature differences, because the skin is thinner and more sensitive there than on the palmar surface. The palmar aspects of the metacarpophalangeal joints are particularly sensitive to vibration. A grasping action of the fingers is used because the fingers can be curved to fit around an organ or mass. The quality and quantity of data collected depends on the selection of the proper aspect of the hand and on the development of a systematic and symmetrical pattern of appraisal.

☐ EXECUTION

The appropriate position of the appraiser and the client depends on the body area to be palpated and the purpose of the palpation. For example, the chest may be palpated with the client in a sitting or supine position. Specific positions are described within each skill that requires palpation. Since palpation is used to appraise many body areas that are normally considered private, it is essential that the student consider the client's need for modesty. Towels, sheets, or clothing should be draped to expose only the area to be appraised.

Light palpation is preferred for most appraisals because the sensitivity of the hand can be dulled by heavy and continuous pressure. The fingertips are used for light palpation. Fingertips on one or both hands may be used simultaneously depending on the purpose of the appraisal. After placing the hand over the area to be palpated, pressure on the fingers is increased slowly from a point of merely laying the hand on the part to gradually exerting more pressure until the desired finding is perceived or the purpose of the appraisal is attained. Firm pressure applied too rapidly may obscure the findings and cause the client discomfort. The amount of pressure needed for light palpation varies with the size of the client and the area being palpated. For example, palpating the pulse of a client with a heavy layer of fat or muscle over the artery may require more pressure than is normally necessary in order to detect the pulse. On the other hand, the same amount of pressure applied over the pulse of a thin person whose vessels are close to the skin could obliterate the pulse. When changing the location of the hand, lift rather than drag it across the skin to the next site. Figure 20–1 depicts light palpation.

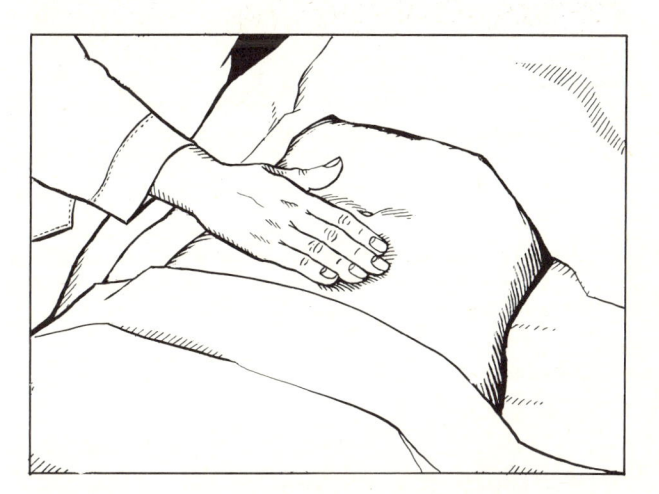

Figure 20–1. Light palpation. The hand indents the skin slightly as pressure is applied to the fingertips.

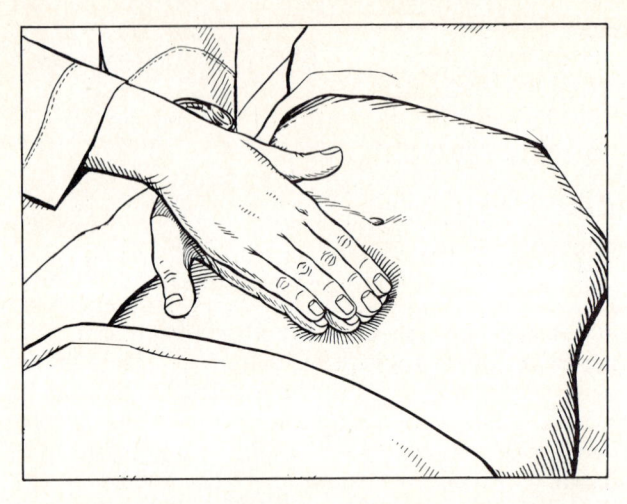

Figure 20-2. Deep palpation. The distal interphalangeal joints of the sensing hand receive pressure from the superimposed hand. Increased pressure results in more indentation than in light palpation.

Deep palpation is necessary to feel the contents of the abdomen. Deep palpation is usually performed with two hands and therefore is called bimanual. One hand, the sensing hand, is placed on the area to be examined and held in a relaxed position while the fingers of the second hand are placed immediately over the first set of fingers. Pressure is applied by the top hand to the distal interphalangeal joints of the sensing hand, forcing it deep into the tissue. The pressure is gradually released before removing the hands in order to avoid discomfort to the client, unless the purpose of the palpation is to determine the presence of tenderness. If an area of tenderness is suspected, it should be examined last to allow the client to remain relaxed as long as possible. When the intent is to identify an area of tenderness, the hands are removed abruptly and the facial expression is observed for reaction. As in light palpation, the hands are lifted from the skin prior to relocation for repeated palpation. Figure 20-2 depicts deep palpation.

Palpation may be difficult to perform on a client who is anxious, in discomfort, in pain, or even ticklish. These problems may be dealt with by explaining what is to be done and by having the client place his or her hand under the examiner's hand during the initial movements of the appraisal. After the client relaxes somewhat, his or her hand is removed. Muscular tension may interfere with the effective use of palpation and distort the findings, so it is important that the client be relaxed and in a comfortable position whenever possible. Relaxation may be promoted by having the client concentrate on deep breathing or by bending the knees, which also serves to relieve stress on the abdominal muscles.

☐ CRITICAL POINTS SUMMARY

1. Wash and warm hands.
2. Explain to the client what is to be done.
3. Position yourself and the client appropriately.
4. Facilitate client relaxation.
5. Expose the area to be examined.
6. Protect the client's modesty with appropriate draping.
7. Use proper aspect of the hand for the appropriate appraisal.
8. Apply and release pressure gradually.
9. Lift the hand (or hands) when changing position.
10. Reserve suspected areas of tenderness for last.

☐ LEARNING ACTIVITIES

1. Select two objects of different textures such as fabric, raw wood, fruit, or vegetables that have rough and smooth textures. Lightly stroke the objects first with the palmar aspects of the fingers and then with the tips of the fingers to note the difference in perception of textures. Describe your findings in a clear and concise written report.
2. Select two objects of different temperatures: one from a refrigerator and the other at room temperature. Compare the difference in temperature of each object by first using the palmar aspect of the hand and then the dorsal aspect.
3. Turn on the radio or television with the sound at a low volume. Place the palm of your hand lightly against the surface of the cabinet, noting the vibratory sensations. Remove and relocate your hand so that the palmar aspects of the fingers are in contact with the cabinet in a hyperextended position, that is, so that the metacarpophalangeal joints are the primary points of contact with the case. Compare the difference in vibrations with the first experience. Increase the volume of the appliance as necessary for each comparison until you are sure that you can detect the differences.
4. In a learning laboratory with a peer simulating a client, practice palpating the dorsal chest and abdomen; exchange roles. Have the client put on a hospital gown or a shirt so that the opening is in the back. Wash and warm your hands. Draw the cubicle curtain to provide privacy.
   a. While sitting in a low-back chair, have the client lean forward so you can place both of your hands flat against the upper back of the chest on each side of the spinal column. Ask the client to begin speaking softly, gradually increasing in loudness as you concentrate on feeling changes in the vibrations created in the chest by the voice sounds.
   b. Have the client remove clothing from the lower part of the body and lie flat in the bed. Use a sheet or large towel to cover the pubic area and then instruct the client to place both feet against the bed and bend the knees to reduce tension in the abdomen. Perform light palpation by placing one hand lightly on the abdomen as shown in Figure 20-1, gradually increasing pressure on the fingers. Note the amount and type of

resistance present in the abdomen and try to determine whether you are palpating muscle or adipose tissue. Remove your hand to a different location, then perform deep palpation as shown in Figure 20-2. Compare the difference in the findings from both palpations.

☐ REVIEW QUESTIONS

1. What data are obtained by palpation?
2. What is the difference between the methods of light and deep palpation?
3. Which method of palpation should be used to obtain data about each of the following: pulse, temperature, organ position, skin texture, chest sounds.

BIBLIOGRAPHY

Buckingham WB: A Primer of Clinical Diagnosis, ed 2. Hagerstown, MD, Harper & Row, 1979.

Judge RD, Zuidema GD (eds): Physical Diagnosis: A Physiological Approach to the Clinical Evaluation, ed 2. Boston, Little, Brown, 1973.

Judge RD, Zuidema GD, Fitzgerald FT (eds): Physical Diagnosis: A Physiological Approach to the Clinical Evaluation, ed 4. Boston, Little, Brown, 1982.

Malasanos L, Barkauskas, V, et al: Health Assessment, ed 2. St Louis, MO, CV Mosby, 1981.

Sana JM, Judge RD: Physical Assessment Skills for Nursing Practice, ed 2. Boston, Little, Brown, 1982.

AUDIOVISUAL RESOURCES

Physical Examination Techniques
  Videorecording (3/4 in). (1976, Color, 9 min.)
  Available through:
    Medical Electronic Educational Services
    954 West Grant
    Tucson, AZ 85705

Physical Appraisal of the Adult in Nursing Practice: General Techniques
  Videotape (3/4 in). (1976, Color, 25 min.)
  Available through:
    University of Michigan, School of Nursing
    Medical Media Center
    Ann Arbor, MI 48109

SKILL 21 Percussion

PREREQUISITE SKILLS

Skill 19, "Inspection"
Skill 28, "Handwashing"

☐ STUDENT OBJECTIVES

1. Explain percussion.
2. Differentiate between the different qualities of percussion sound.
3. Associate each type of sound with its particular characteristics and location.
4. Practice the technique of mediate percussion.
5. Use mediate percussion to elicit each of the four percussion sounds.
6. Record the findings obtained from each of the percussive appraisals clearly and concisely.

☐ INTRODUCTION

Percussion is the act of striking or tapping a surface of the body such as the chest or abdomen in order to produce a sound or to determine the resistance of tissue. The disturbance produced by a percussive blow results in sounds that can be heard with or without a stethoscope and vibrations that can be felt. The density of the underlying structure determines the quality of sound. Percussion is valuable in identifying the normal or abnormal presence of air, fluid, or tissue in an organ or cavity.

Auenbrugger, a Viennese physician who was concerned with finding objective evidence of disease, invented and first described percussion in 1761. He found that judging the character of sounds elicited from a blow required an appreciation of anatomy in order to infer the nature of an internal abnormality. Auenbrugger's technique, known as direct or immediate percussion, consisted of a direct blow to the body by the tips of the fingers of one hand.

A second method, known as indirect or mediate percussion, was devised in 1826. In this method, a small metal plate (later rubber) called a *pleximeter* was held against the patient's body, and either the fingers or a small hammer (*plexor*) was used to strike a blow. Indirect percussion produced a more definite note than that obtained by the direct method.

Both types of percussion are in use today. The value of the findings depends on the appraiser's understanding of anatomy and physiological processes, as well as correct execution of the technique and accurate interpretation of the sounds and vibrations elicited. It is important for the student to be aware of any hearing deficiencies that may interfere with the accurate perception of percussed sounds.

☐ PREPARATION

Percussion combines the techniques of palpation and auscultation. A percussive blow generates vibrations that produce audible sound waves. Sound is characterized by loudness, pitch, and quality. While there are objective measurements for each of these characteristics, the more important consideration is how each of these is interpreted by the nurse. Because equipment to measure the characteristics of sound is not used in physical appraisal, the accurate assessment of sounds is entirely dependent on the nurse's perception of those sounds.

CHARACTERISTICS OF SOUND WAVES

Loudness is the subjective auditory perception of the intensity of sound waves. Sound is measured in amplitude; the intensity is determined by the amount of energy imparted to the vibrating structure as it is moved from its position of rest. Volume controls on radios or television sets regulate the loudness of sound waves. Because assessment of sound is a subjective matter, what is perceived as a loud sound for one person may be scarcely noticed by another.

Pitch is the subjective auditory perception of the frequency of sound waves. Objectively, frequency refers to the number of vibrations per second and is recorded in cycles per second (cps) or hertz (Hz). As the frequency of a sound wave increases, it is perceived as increasingly higher tones; as the frequency decreases, it is perceived as lower tones. The human ear is capable of hearing sounds in the frequency range of 20 to 20,000 cps, but the maximum sensitivity for hearing lies within the speech range of about 1000 to 2000 cps. Because the human ear does not respond equally to different pitches, tones of the same intensity but of different frequencies produce different subjective perceptions of loudness.

Age and noise pollution reduce normal hearing sensitivity for high-pitched sounds. For example, a person over the age of 60 usually cannot hear sounds above 8000 cps, and a person who works in a noisy environment or who frequently listens to very loud music generally loses the ability to hear higher-pitched sounds. Low-pitched tones are more difficult to hear at a low volume because they are masked by higher-pitched tones and overtones. Increasing the volume increases the person's ability to hear low tones; hence, a hi-fi buff will turn up the volume to hear the lower tones better.

Quality of sound is determined by the presence of overtones added to the pitch of a given fundamental or pure tone. A pure tone is produced by a single frequency. However, most natural sounds are composed of overtones that are superimposed on the basic frequency. A vibrating object simultaneously vibrates as a whole and as parts. Overtones are produced by the vibrations of the parts and are higher pitched than the fundamental tone. The quality of a sound is determined by the presence and relative intensity of the various overtones. A richer and more complex tone is produced when overtones are added to pure tones. Overtones help the listener to distinguish between different sounds of the same pitch and same loudness. For example, the same note sounds different when played on a violin, piano, and trumpet because of the different overtones produced by each instrument.

Although this is not one of the basic characteristics of sound, *duration* is a factor that has significance for sound perception in physical appraisal. Duration is the length of time a sound lasts and is determined by how long the vibrating structure is in motion. As the energy originally imparted to the vibrating structure is dissipated in the form of heat from friction, the vibrations tend to die out. If the resistance from the friction is increased, the vibratory motion lasts for a shorter time period because the amplitude is decreased. This is known as *damping*. Vibrations of internal body structures are damped by surrounding soft tissues (Rushmer, 1976).

PERCEPTION OF SOUND

Perception of sound is affected by factors other than loudness, pitch, quality, and duration. A person's hearing acuity, amount of earwax, and state of ear hygiene all influence the perception of sound. Sound perception is also influenced by the ability to listen selectively to specific sounds or components of sounds. A person can intentionally focus on a single type of sound or a specific tone while ignoring others that are present in the environment. For example, when listening to an orchestra, a person can choose to attend only to the string section or even only to the violins. Sound patterns and selective sounds can be stored by the brain for future use. A mother can distinguish her own child's voice in a crowd because she has learned to attend selectively to that sound and recall it. In the same way, nurses can learn to attend selectively to the sounds of body tissues and can increase their ability to hear and distinguish them through repeated practice and validation from more experienced persons.

PERCUSSION SOUNDS IN PHYSICAL APPRAISAL

The sounds emanating from a correctly executed blow are classified according to the acoustic characteristics of their tones. Different types of tissue produce different sounds, because the sounds are dependent on the density of the tissues underlying the area percussed and the nature of the vibrations produced by the tissue. Although the terms used to describe the perceived

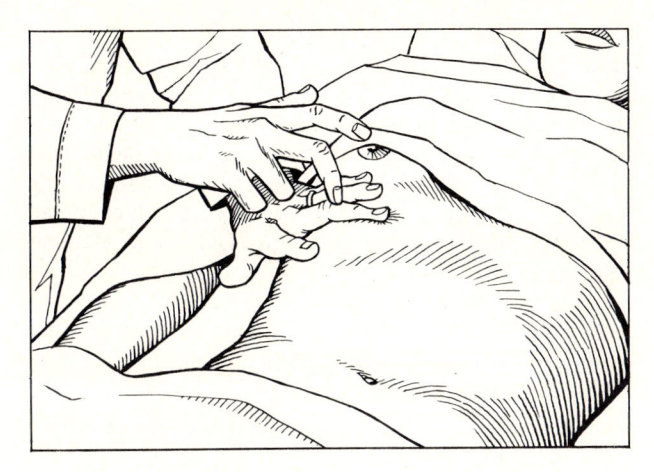

Figure 21-1. Percussion over the intercostal space below the right breast to elicit resonance.

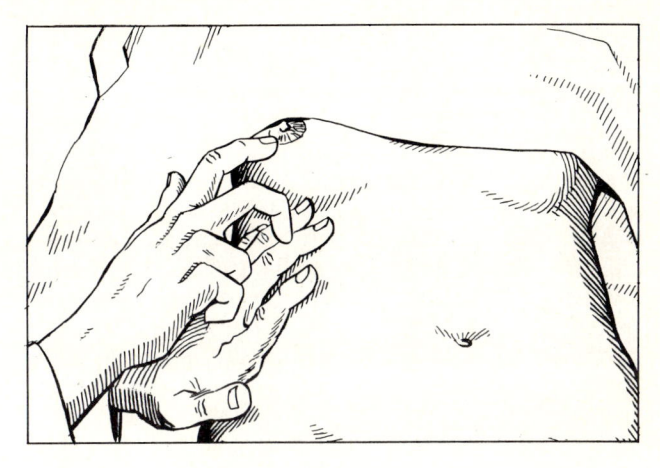

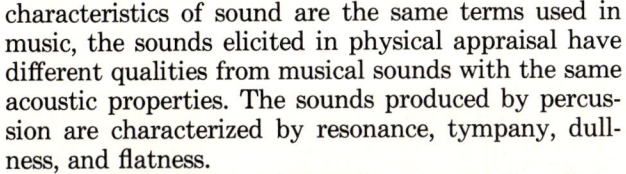

Figure 21-3. Percussion of the right chest just above the rib margin to elicit dullness.

characteristics of sound are the same terms used in music, the sounds elicited in physical appraisal have different qualities from musical sounds with the same acoustic properties. The sounds produced by percussion are characterized by resonance, tympany, dullness, and flatness.

A *resonant* sound is heard on percussion of the right chest over the rib cage below the breast. It occurs because of air in the lung tissue, which is under the area being percussed. A resonant sound has a clear, hollow note that is not loud but easily heard. It is nonmusical, of moderate pitch, and well-sustained. Figure 21-1 depicts percussion to elicit resonance.

A *tympanic* sound is heard on percussion of the left chest just above the rib margin. It occurs because of air in the stomach or colon, which is under the area being percussed. A tympanic sound is higher pitched than a resonant sound because percussion causes increased vibrations when air is trapped in a closed chamber with elastic walls, such as the stomach or colon. A tympanic sound is a somewhat high-pitched, loud musical sound with rich overtones. It is clear and hollow and well sustained, like the sound of a kettle drum. Figure 21-2 depicts percussion to elicit tympany.

A *dull* sound is heard on percussion of the right chest below the breast, just above the rib margin. It occurs because of the dense organ tissue of the liver, which is under the area being percussed. A dull sound is high-pitched, nonmusical, and short. It sometimes is described as a soft thud. Figure 21-3 depicts percussion to elicit dullness.

A *flat* sound is heard on percussion of solid tissues such as the muscles of the thigh or arm. It occurs because there is little air trapped in these tissues. A flat sound is high-pitched, very short, and nonmusical. Figure 21-4 depicts percussion to elicit flatness.

Using a systematic method that elicits resonant sounds before dull sounds facilitates hearing percussed tones. Resonant sounds are clear, of moderate pitch, and well sustained, while dull sounds are high-pitched and of short duration. Any organ or mass more than 4 to 5 centimeters below the surface will not produce vibrations from percussion.

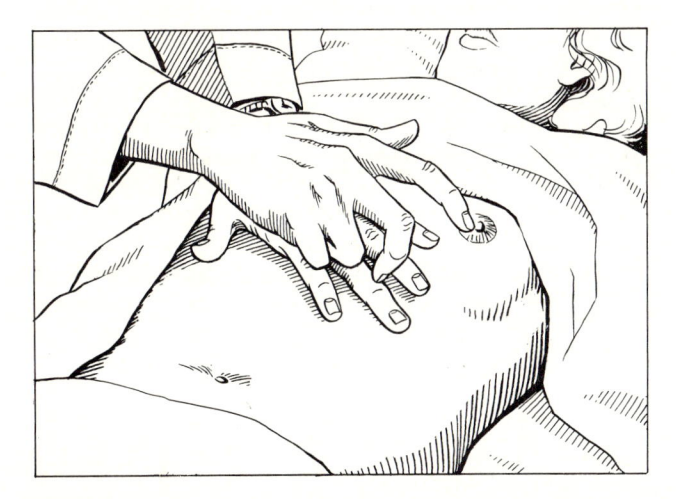

Figure 21-2. Percussion of the left chest just above the rib margin to elicit tympany.

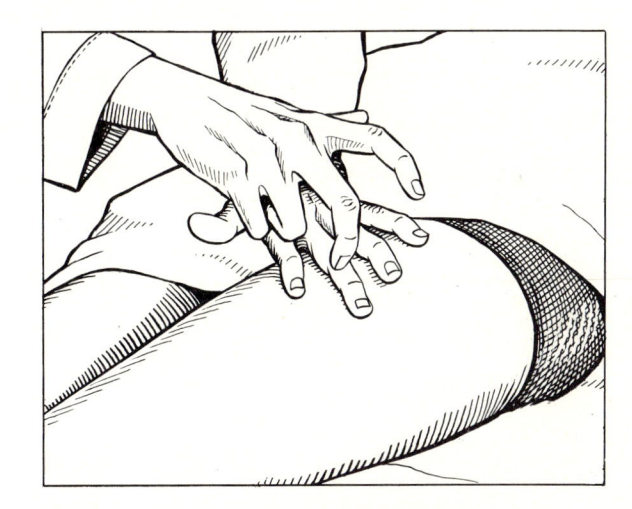

Figure 21-4. Percussion of the thigh muscle to elicit flatness.

☐ EXECUTION

Mediate or indirect percussion is the most commonly used technique and is the method included in the appropriate skills in subsequent chapters. As shown in Figure 21-5, it is performed by placing the middle finger of the nondominant hand, serving as the pleximeter, flat and firmly against the body surface to be examined. The palm and remaining fingers are held away from the skin to prevent interference with the percussed sound. The tip of the middle finger of the dominant hand is used as a plexor to strike a brisk, short blow to the distal joint. This is the area most sensitive to the vibrations arising from the underlying tissues. The plexor is curved and extended downward and held in a stationary position. The index finger is adducted (extended away), and the third and fourth fingers are curled toward the palm. The blow of the plexor is struck by holding the forearm stationary and flexing the wrist in a snapping action to transmit the speed and force of the blow. The wrist is the only moving part in this action. The plexor is removed immediately to prevent interference with the vibrations.

The blow must be brisk and short to produce a crisp, sharp note. The plexor fingernail should be short, or else the tip of the finger cannot be used and a poor quality sound will result. The amount of force and the speed of each blow should be uniform to prevent distortion of sound and to permit comparison of each percussed note. The ideal blow is the lightest blow that will produce a sound which can be heard. The best results are obtained by striking one blow and noting the sound and vibrations before striking a second blow.

The appropriate position of the appraiser and the client depends on the body area to be percussed and the purpose of the percussion. The chest is usually percussed with the client in the sitting position, if this is possible, and the appraiser stationed in a position of comfort and convenience so that the appropriate wrist and hand actions can be properly executed. Percussion of the abdomen is performed with the client in the supine position and the appraiser standing at the side of the bed or examining table so that he or she is over the body area to be percussed.

As in palpation, the appraiser should begin percussion with warm, clean hands. Percussion of the chest and abdomen requires that the client be properly draped to avoid unnecessary exposure of the private parts of the body.

☐ CRITICAL POINTS SUMMARY

1. Wash and warm hands.
2. Keep plexor fingernail trimmed short.
3. Position yourself and the client appropriately.
4. Place pleximeter flat and firmly against the body surface to be percussed.
5. Prevent contact of the palm and other fingers with the body surface.
6. Use only the tip of the plexor to strike a single uniform blow.
7. Hold the forearm stationary while snapping the wrist to transmit a brisk blow.
8. Strike the percussive blow against the distal joint of the pleximeter.
9. Use the lightest blow that will produce sound.
10. Elicit resonant sounds before dull sounds.

☐ LEARNING ACTIVITIES

1. Holding your forearm stationary, practice flexing and snapping the wrist and hand downward and upward in a rapid but smooth manner.
2. Curve and extend the plexor of the percussing hand downward, so that the tip of the finger is vertical to the horizontal plane. Hold the plexor in a stationary position and the index finger adducted (extended away), while the third and fourth fingers are curled toward the palm. Add the flexing, snapping action of the wrist and try to strike the same spot on a designated target, such as a tabletop, with a deliberate, sharp single blow. Note the sound and vibratory sensation elicited from each single blow.
3. Place the pleximeter of the nondominant hand flatly and firmly against a table surface. Hold the palm and remaining fingers away from the table surface. Use the plexor to strike the pleximeter on the distal joint or the area immediately distal to the joint. Attempt to strike the pleximeter at the same point each time. Note the sound and vibratory sensation elicited from each blow. Rapid and successive blows obscure the sound quality; be patient and strike one blow at a time.
4. Practice mediate percussion with a partner in a quiet environment that will permit concentration on the technique, sounds, and vibrations. The partner should be lying down for these exercises.

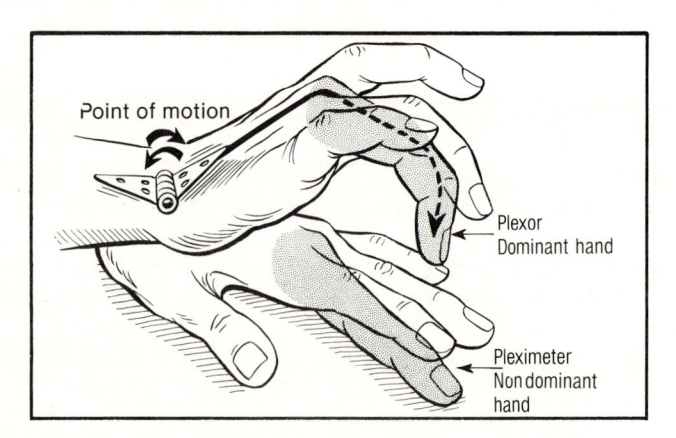

Figure 21–5. Method of percussion. The only point of motion is the wrist. The middle finger of the dominant hand serves as the plexor, and the middle finger of the nondominant hand serves as the pleximeter. The palm and remaining fingers are held away to prevent interference with the action and the sound.

a. Percuss the right chest above the rib cage margin but below the breast. Place the pleximeter flat and firmly against and parallel to the intercostal space. Percuss and listen for the resonant sound elicited from the air-filled lung. Percuss at the same level on the chest but near the surface of the bed; note the difference in sound quality resulting from the interference of the bed.
b. Percuss the left chest just above the rib cage margin in the same manner as in activity 4a to elicit tympany.
c. Use the same method to percuss the right chest immediately above the rib cage margin to elicit the dull sound over the liver.
d. Percuss the muscles of an arm or thigh to elicit a flat sound.

☐ REVIEW QUESTIONS

1. Why is percussion a useful technique?
2. How would you describe each of the percussion sounds with respect to their loudness, pitch, quality, and duration?
3. What is the percussion sound that would be normally heard over the lung tissue, the liver, the stomach, the biceps, and the colon?
4. What is the advantage of mediate over immediate percussion?
5. What is the proper sequence for each of the steps used to execute mediate percussion correctly?

REFERENCE

Rushmer RF: Cardiovascular Dynamics, ed 4. Philadelphia, WB Saunders, 1976.

BIBLIOGRAPHY

Bennet CE: Physics without Mathematics. New York, Barnes & Noble, 1970.
Buckingham WB: A Primer of Clinical Diagnosis, ed 2. Hagerstown, MD, Harper & Row, 1979.
Emerson CP: Physical Diagnosis, ed 2. Philadelphia, JB Lippincott, 1929.
Judge RD, Zuidema GD (eds): Physical Diagnosis: A Physiological Approach to the Clinical Evaluation, ed 2. Boston, Little, Brown, 1973.
Judge RD, Zuidema GD, Fitzgerald FT (eds): Physical Diagnosis: A Physiological Approach to the Clinical Evaluation, ed 4. Boston, Little, Brown, 1982.
Malasanos L, Barkauskas V, et al: Health Assessment, ed 2. St Louis, MO, CV Mosby, 1981.
Performing Percussion. Nursing83 (Horsham) 13(2):63-64, 1983.
Sana JM, Judge RD: Physical Assessment Skills for Nursing Practice, ed 2. Boston, Little, Brown, 1982.

AUDIOVISUAL RESOURCES

Physical Examination Techniques
 Videorecording (3/4 in). (1976, Color, 9 min.)
 Available through:
  Medical Electronic Educational Services
  954 West Grant
  Tucson, AZ 85705

Physical Appraisal of the Adult in Nursing Practice: General Techniques
 Videotape (3/4 in). (1976, Color, 25 min.)
 Available through:
  University of Michigan, School of Nursing
  Medical Media Center
  Ann Arbor, MI 48109

SKILL 22 Auscultation

PREREQUISITE SKILLS

Skill 19, "Inspection"
Skill 20, "Palpation"
Skill 28, "Handwashing"

☐ STUDENT OBJECTIVES

1. Describe auscultation.
2. Describe the parts of the stethoscope.
3. Explain the purpose of cleaning the stethoscope.
4. Select a properly fitting stethoscope.
5. Practice auscultation of the chest and abdomen.
6. Identify single sound or sounds emanating from the heart and blood vessels.

☐ INTRODUCTION

Auscultation is the act of listening to sounds arising from the organs within the body such as the heart, blood vessels, lungs, and abdomen. Auscultation is performed to determine the normal or abnormal status or the degree of change in important sounds arising from specific areas. It can be performed by directly applying the ear to the body or by using a stethoscope.

Immediate or direct auscultation was practiced by Hippocrates. Mediate or indirect auscultation was introduced in 1816 by René Laennec, a French surgeon, as a hygienic device to avoid placing his ear directly on the chest of dirty patients. He invented the first stethoscope, which was a rolled up piece of paper in the shape of a tube with one end placed against the patient's chest and the other end to the ear. The improvement in sound conduction stimulated Laennec to improve on the design. By the 1890s, the monaural model had been replaced by the acoustically superior binaural stethoscope.

☐ PREPARATION

As in percussion, it is important for the student to be aware of any hearing deficits that may interfere with accurate perception of the auscultated sounds. Special stethoscopes are available for persons who have diminished hearing acuity. It is becoming more common for nurses to purchase their own instruments. Figure 22–1 shows one type of stethoscope.

EQUIPMENT

The stethoscope provides a closed acoustic system for conducting sounds from the body to the listener's ear. The mechanical or acoustic stethoscope is the most common type of instrument used in clinical practice. The stethoscope is composed of a chestpiece, flexible tubing, and a headset which includes earpieces and ear tips.

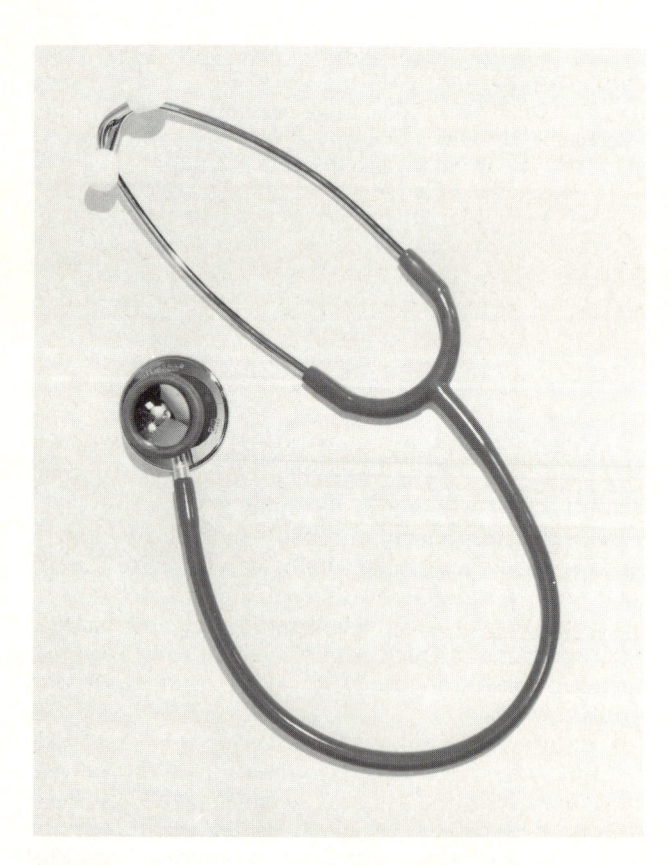

Figure 22–1. Stethoscope with bell and diaphragm chestpieces and plastic ear tips. (Courtesy 3M Medical Products, St Paul, MN 55133.)

Components of the Stethoscope

The *chestpiece* is a head that picks up sounds. There are two types of chestpieces: the open bell, which is a short cone or funnel-shaped head, and the Bowles or closed diaphragm. The open bell conducts sound with very little distortion of pitch or quality. It is used to listen to low-frequency sounds such as those produced by the third and fourth heart sounds or by heart murmurs. Since the diameter of the bell is usually 1 inch or less, the volume of sound it can pick up is more limited than for the closed diaphragm. The size and shape of the bell permit better contact with the skin on small or bony chests than the closed diaphragm, so that sound leaks are avoided. A rubber or plastic sleeve around the lip of the bell avoids chilling the client and also decreases air leaks. Air leaks interfere with the transmission of sound and permit environmental sounds to enter the chestpiece. When the bell is used to detect low-pitched sounds, it is lightly placed against the chest wall. When increased pressure is applied to the bell, the sounds become higher pitched because the skin beneath the bell serves as a diaphragm which in itself has a higher natural frequency. This higher natural frequency attenuates the lower-frequency components of the organ sounds listened to and emphasizes the higher-frequency components, thus distorting the original low-pitched organ sounds. Skill in the use of the bell is beyond the scope of this text.

The Bowles or closed diaphragm is larger than the bell and therefore picks up more sound. The diaphragm is made of material, usually plastic, that has a natural frequency in the desired range for listening to high-pitched sounds and suppresses the lower-frequency sounds. *All of the auscultations presented in this text presume the use of this type of chestpiece.*

Some stethoscopes have a dual, reversible chestpiece with both a bell and a diaphragm. The listener can select the desired chestpiece by either changing a valve or rotating the chestpiece.

The *flexible tubing* serves as a link between the chestpiece and the earpieces. Sound is transmitted through the closed column of air within the tubing. The plastic or rubber tubing used is rigid enough not to vibrate and create extraneous sounds, so that sounds picked up by the chestpiece are not distorted. The length of the tubing should be as short as can be conveniently used, with the optimal length being 10 to 12 inches. The inside of the tubing should be 1/8th inch in diameter. Stethoscope tubing may be single or double. Although double tubing is believed to conduct sound better, the two tubes can produce distracting sounds when they touch during use. They also add to the weight and bulk of the instrument. An internal or external Y brace between the tubing and the earpieces serves to keep the tubing rigid and prevents obstruction of sound. The brace also serves as a tension spring to hold the headset snugly in place.

The *headset* on some models has a front and a back position. On these models, the *earpieces* incline anteriorly to conform to the normal contour of the ear canals. Other models have straight earpieces. Hard plastic or soft pliant rubber *ear tips* are attached to the ends of the earpieces. A snug fit of the ear tips in the central opening of the ear canal is of paramount importance to prevent room noise from interfering with the auscultated sounds. Soft rubber ear tips are available in at least two sizes and hard plastic tips in four sizes. Use of the largest possible size that can be comfortably placed in the external auditory canal is suggested. Plastic and rubber ear tips should be tried in varying sizes to find the best individual fit. However, even with a well-fitting set of ear tips, sound leaks may be created by movement of the head or jaw during use. Consequently, the wearer should become aware of the sounds created by these movements so they are not confused with organ sounds.

Maintenance of the Stethoscope

The acoustic effectiveness of the stethoscope may be significantly reduced if the stethoscope is not maintained properly. Since the stethoscope is a closed system that conducts sound from the body area to the listener's ears, the parts must be kept intact. The nurse periodically inspects the instrument for the following defects: cracked or loose ear tips, stretched or broken Y brace, dried and cracked tubing (particularly at the junction with the metal parts at the headset or chestpiece), cracked or torn diaphragm, and chipped or cracked open bell. Each defective part is replaced with new parts from the manufacturer, because makeshift replacements are not adequate to maintain the acoustic quality of the instrument. There is no rule of thumb regarding when a stethoscope should be replaced. It is a matter of personal preference or of the availability of replaceable parts from the manufacturer. Most companies will tune up their instruments for a reasonable service charge.

Cleaning the Stethoscope. The ear tips may become occluded with earwax and debris-like lint, or shreds of tobacco may accumulate on the diaphragm or on the inside of the tubing. Because such debris will interfere with sound conduction or even generate extraneous sounds, the parts that can be disassembled for cleaning should be frequently checked and cleaned.

The stethoscope may also serve as an instrument of cross-infection between users of a common instrument or between user and client. Quadrucci (1977) conducted a nursing study to determine if the ear tips are unhygienic. She found that 75 percent of the nurses studied who had been in practice for more than 1 year had complaints of at least one type of ear condition. At least one ear condition was also reported by 35.7 percent of nurses in practice less than 1 year. Only 10 percent of the nurses in the study reported cleaning the ear tips before and after every use. The nurses who had suffered the ear conditions considered the use of the stethoscope to be linked to their conditions. Routine cleaning of the ear tips was recommended by 90.9 percent of the nurses who had experienced an ear condition.

The stethoscope as a source of infection between clients was the focus of a study by Mangi and Andriole (1972). Bacterial cultures taken from the chestpieces of 50 stethoscopes obtained from equal numbers of medical interns, residents, and clinical fellows, faculty engaged in client care, and nurses assigned to intensive care and medical units revealed a total of 125 different organisms. Fifteen of these organisms were classified as potential pathogens. Physicians and nurses using stethoscopes contaminated with pathogenic organisms expose each client they examine to these organisms. Ten additional stethoscopes belonging to medical interns and residents were swabbed with 70 percent alcohol before the bacterial culture was taken. These yielded only three different nonpathogenic bacteria. Of the 60 study participants, only three had ever cleaned their stethoscopes and then not routinely before and after each use.

The potential for stethoscopes to serve as vehicles for cross-infection between users and between clients indicates a need for preventive action by proper cleansing with alcohol before and after every use. The stethoscope should not be immersed in any liquid. If the stethoscope must be sterilized because of contamination by organisms not destroyed by 70 percent alcohol, gas sterilization with a cold cycle in a Steri-Vac Gas Sterilizer should be used. After sterilization, the instrument must be aerated either in a Steri-Vac cabinet for 8 hours or at room temperature for 5 days.

☐ EXECUTION

Use of the stethoscope for the specific appraisal of particular organs or body areas is dealt with in the context of individual procedures presented in subsequent chapters. As in the other physical appraisal skills, it is important for the appraiser to be conscientious about having clean hands and providing for the client's modesty with appropriate draping.

☐ CRITICAL POINTS SUMMARY

1. Select appropriate-sized ear tips for snug fit.
2. Inspect all of the component parts for defects and insecure connections.
3. Remove earwax from the ear tips and debris from inside the tubing.
4. Cleanse the chestpiece, earpieces, and exterior tubing with 70 percent alcohol.
5. Identify the front of the headset before inserting ear tips.
6. Place the ear tips securely in the central opening of the ear canal.
7. Select the appropriate chestpiece for the tones to be auscultated.

☐ LEARNING ACTIVITIES

1. Inspect the stethoscope to make sure all of the component parts are intact, properly attached, and secure.
2. Remove the ear tips from the ear tubes and remove any wax by using swabs and 70 percent ethylene alcohol. Replace the ear tips. Use the same agent to clean the chestpiece.
3. Identify the front of the stethoscope and rotate the chestpiece or change the position of the valve which controls the patency of the channel to the diaphragm.
4. Place the ear tips in the central opening of the ear canal, adjusting their position for comfort and occlusion.
5. Firmly place the diaphragm flat against a convenient location on your own chest. The left breast is usually within easy reach for most stethoscope lengths and permits listening without moving your head or body. Standing in front of a mirror is helpful for self-observation.
6. Concentrate on listening carefully to the sounds. If the room noise is louder than the auscultated sounds, check the ear tips to make sure that they are snug and in the proper place.
7. Identify a single sound such as the heartbeat and focus on it, ignoring the breath sounds.
8. Listen to a partner in a similar way. Note the similarities and differences in the auscultated sounds.

☐ REVIEW QUESTIONS

1. What is auscultation?
2. What are the functions of each part of a stethoscope?
3. Before using a stethoscope, how would you inspect it to determine its condition?
4. How would you clean a stethoscope? Give the reasons for each action.
5. What problems and what solutions would you consider if you were unable to hear auscultated sounds clearly?

REFERENCES

Mangi RJ, Andriole VT: Contaminated Stethoscopes: A Potential Source of Nosocomial Infections. Yale Journal of Biology and Medicine 45(12):600-604, 1972.

Quadrucci J: The Hygiene of Stethoscopes. Nursing Times 73(6):193-195, 1977.

BIBLIOGRAPHY

Bennet CE: Physics without Mathematics. New York, Barnes & Noble Books, 1970.

Buckingham WB: A Primer of Clinical Diagnosis, ed 2. Hagerstown, MD, Harper & Row, 1979.

Judge RD, Zuidema GD, Fitzgerald FT (eds): Physical Diagnosis: A Physiological Approach to the Clinical Evaluation, ed 4. Boston, Little, Brown, 1982.

Lehmann J, Sr: Auscultation of heart sounds. American Journal of Nursing 72(7):1242-1246, 1972.

Littman D: Stethoscopes and auscultation. American Journal of Nursing 72(7):1239-1241, 1972.

Malasanos L, Barkauskas V, et al: Health Assessment, ed 2. St Louis, MO, CV Mosby, 1981.

Performing Percussion. Nursing83 (Horsham) 13(2):63-64, 1983.

Raiser S: The medical influence of the stethoscope. Scientific American 240(2):148-154, 1979.

Rapport MB, Sprague HB: Physiologic and physical laws that govern auscultation and their clinical application. The American Heart Journal 21(3):257-318, 1941.

Sana JM, Judge RD: Physical Assessment Skills for Nursing Practice, ed 2. Boston, Little, Brown, 1982.

Straight P, Saukaup M, Sr: How to hear it right: Evaluating and choosing a stethoscope. American Journal of Nursing 77(9):1477, 1977.

AUDIOVISUAL RESOURCES

Physical Appraisal of the Adult in Nursing Practice: General Techniques
Videotape (3/4 in). (1976, Color, 25 min.)
Available through:
  University of Michigan, School of Nursing
  Medical Media Center
  Ann Arbor, MI 48109

Physical Examination Techniques
Videorecording (3/4 in). (1976, Color, 9 min.)
Available through:
  Medical Electronic Educational Services
  954 West Grant
  Tucson, AZ 85705

7 Common Techniques for Measuring Health Status

☐ INTRODUCTION

Temperature, pulse, respiration, blood pressure, and height and weight are measurements that provide information about a person's current health status. They are used to monitor the way in which an individual's state of balance is maintained by physiological and psychological adjustments to internal and external forces. Temperature, pulse, respiration, and blood pressure are often referred to as *vital signs* because of the important information they reveal about the state of health. Collectively these measurements are obtained in health-screening programs to identify real and potential health problems, upon admission to health-care programs and agencies, and then periodically thereafter as part of the data base used to plot the progress of health, illness, and recovery from illness.

Since decisions about the appropriate courses of action are based on the data provided by these measurements, it is important that they be accurately obtained and correctly recorded. Although a single measurement may be significant, it is usually more valuable to look at a pattern of serial measurements, evaluate it in light of the expected course of events for the particular situation or problem, and be alert for deviations from this course. Obtaining accurate and safe measurements requires skill and knowledge; interpreting them requires knowledge and clinical judgment.

All of these measurements are obtained by professional health workers, auxiliary personnel, the client and his or her family, as well as members of the general public in a variety of settings. When auxiliary personnel obtain the measurements, the nurse is responsible for teaching them accurate and safe methods and supervising them during the execution. The nurse is also accountable for the accuracy of the measurements; if there is a doubt about the results obtained, he or she has them checked again.

The nurse is also in a position to teach clients and their families how to obtain and understand the meaning of each of these measurements as part of a therapeutic regime. Currently, the general public has an increased interest in preventive health-care practices and a desire to assume a more active role in managing their own health needs. This interest provides numerous opportunities for the nurse to become involved in teaching people how to obtain the measurements correctly, how to use the equipment accurately, and what implications changes in the measurements have for modification of life-style behaviors that affect health status.

The skills in this chapter include "Temperature Appraisal" (Skill 23), "Pulse Appraisal" (Skill 24), "Respiration Appraisal" (Skill 25), "Blood Pressure Appraisal" (Skill 26), and "Height and Weight Appraisal" (Skill 27).

☐ ENTRY TEST

1. How is body temperature controlled?
2. What are seven factors that affect body temperature?
3. How does the body produce heat?
4. How is heat lost from the body?
5. Name the major structures that make up the cardiovascular system.
6. Compare the structure and function of the arteries and veins and capillaries.
7. Describe the circulation of the blood from the right side of the heart to the left. Name the major arteries and veins, heart chambers and valves.
8. Describe the basic functions of the circulatory system.
9. Identify the mechanisms that control heart rate.
10. Identify the circulatory factors that influence arterial blood pressure.
11. Name three circulatory reflexes that influence arterial blood pressure regulation.
12. What role does the kidney play in arterial blood pressure regulation?
13. What are the anatomic structures of the respiratory tract that are involved in breathing?

14. At which level of the respiratory tract does gas exchange occur?
15. What gases are exchanged during respiration?
16. Where is the respiratory center located?
17. What are three important stimuli for respiration?
18. What are the major muscles used in normal inspiration and expiration?
19. What is a kilocalorie?
20. How many kilocalories are in 1 gram of protein, carbohydrate, and fat?
21. What purpose do protein, carbohydrate, and fat have in the diet?
22. What determines the daily caloric and nutrient requirements of an individual?
23. What is metabolism?

SKILL 23 Temperature Appraisal

PREREQUISITE SKILLS

Skill 19, "Inspection"
Skill 20, "Palpation"
Skill 28, "Handwashing"

□ STUDENT OBJECTIVES

1. Explain the purpose of measuring body temperature.
2. Convert between Celsius and Fahrenheit scales.
3. Describe the types of thermometers used to measure temperature.
4. Explain how to maintain thermometers in an aseptic condition.
5. Describe the sites used to monitor temperature.
6. Indicate the precautions to be observed with each site.
7. Summarize the factors that create errors.
8. Use the appropriate method to measure body temperature accurately.
9. Record the temperature measurement accurately.

□ INTRODUCTION

The term *temperature* usually is used to refer to the interior or core temperature of the body. The core temperature, which reflects about two-thirds of the body mass, represents the balance of heat generated by the tissues in metabolic activity and heat loss to the environment. A clinical measurement of body temperature is an estimation of the heat of arterial blood.

Body temperature is measured to determine the presence of a deviation from the person's normal range of temperature. Damage to body tissue can occur with deviations beyond the normal homeostatic range. Early detection of marked deviations permits intervention to prevent tissue damage. Temperature is also monitored to determine when normal involuntary physiological responses such as ovulation occur.

Concern about the body temperature as an important indicator of health status is documented in writings by Hippocrates, who estimated temperature by palpation. Measurement of temperature was made possible by Santorius's development in 1625 of the first thermometer used to measure a fever (Beck and St. Cyr, 1974).

□ PREPARATION

The thermoregulatory system of the body maintains a relatively constant core temperature in the healthy individual, with variation of less than 0.6°C (1°F). Individuals manifest highest and lowest core temperatures in circadian rhythms. For most persons who operate on a regular day work and night sleep pattern, the highest temperature occurs between 4 P.M. and 8 P.M. and the lowest between 12 A.M. and 6 A.M. However, there are exceptions whereby persons in this same population will have their highest temperature in the morning. Knowledge of a person's normal pattern is important if a temperature measurement is to be interpreted correctly. Environmental changes can also shift the times for the peak high and low temperatures (Felton, 1970).

The normal range of body temperature measured orally is from 36°C (97°F) to beyond 37.2°C (99°F) depending on the time of day, the environmental temperature, the person's emotional state, and the amount of physical energy expended in work or exercise. The average normal temperature is considered to be 37°C (98.6°F).

The scale used to measure temperature may be either Celsius (centigrade) or Fahrenheit. On the *Celsius* scale, which is being used increasingly, water freezes at 0° and boils at 100°. On the *Fahrenheit* scale, water freezes at 32° and boils at 212°. To convert from Celsius to Fahrenheit, multiply by 9/5 and add 32. For example, the following formula would be used to change a Celsius temperature of 37° to Fahrenheit:

$$C \times 9/5 + 32 = F$$
$$37 \times 9/5 = 66.6$$
$$66.6 + 32 = 98.6$$

To convert Fahrenheit to Celsius, subtract 32 and multiply by 5/9. For example, a Fahrenheit temperature of 98.6° is changed to Celsius by use of the following formula:

$$F - 32 \times 5/9 = C$$
$$98.6 - 32 = 66.6$$
$$66.6 \times 5/9 = 37.0$$

MEASUREMENT SITES

Body temperature can be measured by placing the thermometer (mercury glass, electronic, or chemical dot) in either the mouth, rectum, or axilla. Once a pattern of taking temperature by one route has been established, it is not wise to change. Because different sites in the same person may produce different readings, data collected in this way might lead to inappropriate therapeutic intervention. The following studies suggest the range of readings that different sites might produce: In Kintzel's study (1967), the difference between the majority of oral and rectal temperatures ranged from .6° to .84°C (1° to 1.4°F); however, individual differences revealed a broader range of 0° to 1.4°F. Nichols et al. (1966) revealed a range of 0° to 2.8°F difference for oral versus rectal temperatures and from 0° to 4.2°F difference for oral versus axillary temperatures.

Although agency policy or a physician's order may indicate the site to be used, the nurse's clinical judgment ultimately determines the appropriate site for each measurement on a given individual. The data on which the nurse forms a clinical judgment on the site selection include the client's age, state of mental alertness, and ability to cooperate; the type and extent of external influences on the client; the presence of injury or inflammation at any given site; the closeness of major arteries to the site; and the convenience of the site as dictated by the particular setting. For example, if there is an order for an oral thermometer, but the client seems confused and might bite the thermometer, the nurse would use the axillary or rectal site.

The temperatures measured at any site can be adversely affected by *hot baths,* which can elevate the reading as much as .5° to 1°C (.83° to 1.6°F), and the effect can last as long as 45 minutes. Strenuous *exercise* such as physical therapy can also elevate the temperature .6°C (1°F). When a person moves from one *environmental temperature* to another and significant differences are present, time should be allotted for the person to adjust to the new climate before the temperature is measured. Otherwise, an inaccurate reading will result.

Oral

This site is most commonly used unless contraindicated because of age (less than 5 years), injury or inflammation of the mouth, inability to keep the mouth closed, or a state of mental confusion or unconsciousness (Blainey, 1974). Direct measurement of core temperatures taken from the esophagus, external auditory meatus, and the tympanic membrane correlate well with the sublingual temperature (Erickson, 1976).

The accuracy of the oral measurement is claimed to be superior to the accuracy of measurements taken at the rectal and axillary sites, since the core temperature of the head and trunk remains relatively constant because of the arterial circulation. A branch of the external carotid artery forks into branches of the lingual artery at the posterior base of the tongue. A heat pocket between the base of the posterior aspect of the tongue near the molars serves as an ideal location to measure body temperature. Figure 23–1 shows the location of the heat pockets. All types of oral thermometers should be placed in the heat pocket. The temperature in the heat pocket is most stable in people who have their own teeth; the presence of dentures can lower the temperature as much as .3°C (0.5°F) (Beck and Campbell, 1975). The temperature in other parts of the mouth beneath the frenum can be .7°C (1.2°F) lower than the heat pocket.

Although it is still commonly believed that the mercury glass oral thermometer should be left in place for 3 minutes, nursing studies by Nichols and Ruskin et al. (1966), Nichols and Verhonick (1967), Nichols (1968), Nichols and Fielding (1969), and Nichols and Kucha (1972) indicate that 9 to 11 minutes are required for an individual's maximum temperature to register on a mercury thermometer. *Maximum temperature* as defined by Nichols and Verhonick (1967) is the highest reading of a thermometer. The client's age and the room temperature affect the amount of time required. Only 13 percent of the sample population reached maximum temperature in 3 minutes (Nichols and Verhonick, 1967).

Regardless of the type of instrument used to measure oral temperature, consideration must be given to client activities that affect the accuracy of the mea-

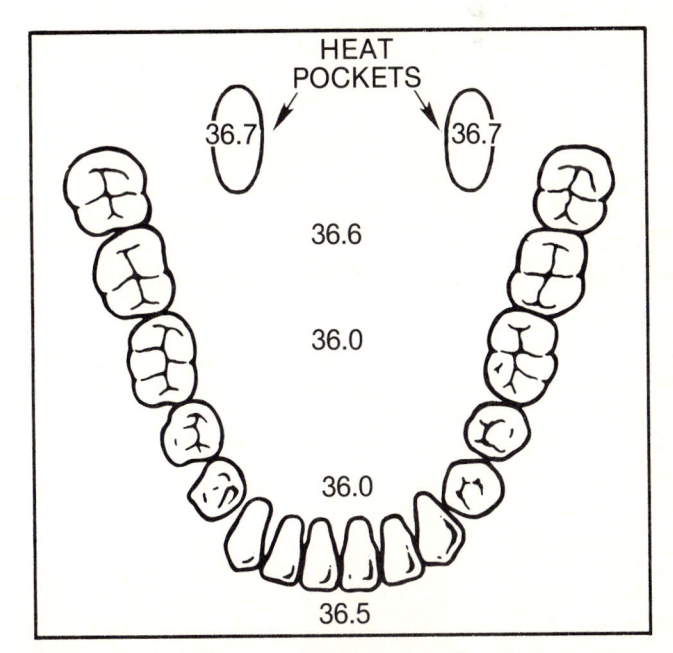

Figure 23–1. Heat pockets. The highest reading occurs when the thermometer is placed in the heat pocket. Lower readings are obtained at other locations in the mouth.

surement. For example, *iced liquids* can lower the temperature from .12° to .96°C (0.2° to 1.6°F) if measurement occurs immediately after ingestion. Fifteen minutes after ingestion, the reading may still be .12°C (.20°F) lower than the base (Woodman et al., 1967). One study, which used electronic thermometers, showed a drop of 3.3°C (5.5°F) after ingestion of iced liquids, and the effect lasted for 15 minutes (Forster et al., 1970). *Hot liquids* can elevate the temperature 1.2° to 1.8°C (2° to 3°F), and it takes 30 minutes for the temperature to return to .14°C (.24°F) above the base reading (Larkin, 1974). *Smoking* prior to measurement produces an increase of only .3°C (.5°F); however, vigorous puffing while the thermometer is in place can raise the temperature to 38.8°C (102°F) (Lee and Atkins, 1972). *Gum chewing* generates heat in the mouth because of the muscular activity and also serves to elevate the temperature. Temperature returns to normal after 3 minutes without chewing (Blainey, 1974). There has been some question about the accuracy of an oral temperature when *oxygen* is administered. However, findings by Graas (1974), Kintzel (1967), and Dressler et al. (1983) do not support changing the site from oral to rectal for a client being given oxygen. The presence of a *tracheostomy* does not require a change from the oral site (Biskey, 1973); however, the thermometer must be placed accurately.

Rectal

The use of the rectal site poses its own problems. Rectal measurements are consistently higher than measurements by oral or axillary route for yet undetermined reasons. It is known that rectal measurements do not respond as readily to changes in the arterial blood temperature as do sublingual measurements. The presence of stool in the rectum may prevent proper placement of the thermometer. Accurate comparisons of serial readings are possible only if the thermometer is placed at the same depth and in the same place for all readings.

There continues to be a controversy as to whether anal stimulation from insertion and presence of the thermometer provokes the vagus nerve to cause bradycardia (slowed heart rate), which could be detrimental to clients with certain heart conditions. An increased heart rate may result from the embarrassment some clients experience from having their temperatures taken rectally. Other hazards of using this site include causing discomfort if the client has hemorrhoids, and possibly perforating the rectum or causing ulcerations of the mucous membranes, particularly in infants (Blainey, 1974).

The time required for maximum temperature to register with a mercury glass thermometer in adults is 2 to 4 minutes according to Nichols' (1972) findings. For infants, the time required is 3 minutes.

When the rectal site is used, whether for adults or for children, the thermometer must be held in place while the temperature is being measured. Water soluble lubricant is applied to the bulb end, which is extended up to a maximum of 1/2 inch for infants and up to 3 inches for adults. The client's upper buttock is

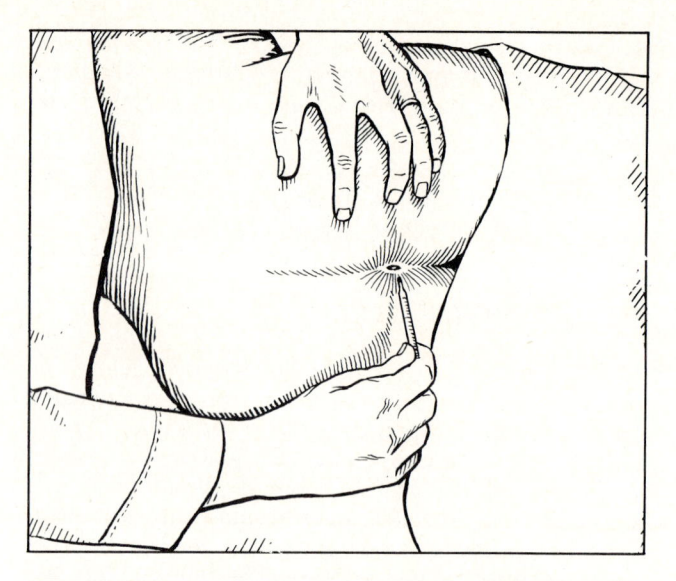

Figure 23-2. Insertion of rectal thermometer. Water soluble lubricant is applied to the bulb end, which is extended up to a maximum of 1/2 inch for infants and up to 3 inches for adults. The upper buttock is raised to expose the anus. The thermometer is inserted anteriorly (toward the front of the client).

raised to expose the anus. The rectal sphincter is gently touched to stimulate relaxation before the thermometer is inserted forward and upward toward the client's navel. Figure 23-2 illustrates the technique used for rectal insertion.

Axillary

The axilla provides a safe and convenient site for temperature measurement. The axillary route is indicated for infants as well as for adults whose other sites cannot be used because of injury, surgery, or potential trauma for the thermometer. The axilla is also used when the client cannot cooperate during oral or rectal measurements.

Sims-Williams (1976) advocates using the same axilla each time the temperature is taken, because the left side provides a slightly higher reading. The axillary site is best used when environmental temperature is carefully controlled (Blainey, 1974). However, it may be difficult for some clients to stay in one position for the 9 to 11 minutes required for the temperature to register. Figure 23-3 illustrates the proper way to insert the axillary thermometer and hold it in place.

DATA BASE

Client History and Recorded Data

Monitoring body temperature at times other than those scheduled or more frequently than directed by agency policy may be indicated by the clinical judgments made by the nurse. These judgments may be based on objective data obtained from inspection and palpation, the graphic pattern of previously recorded temperature, or subjective reports from clients such as feeling cold or hot, sweating or shivering, or com-

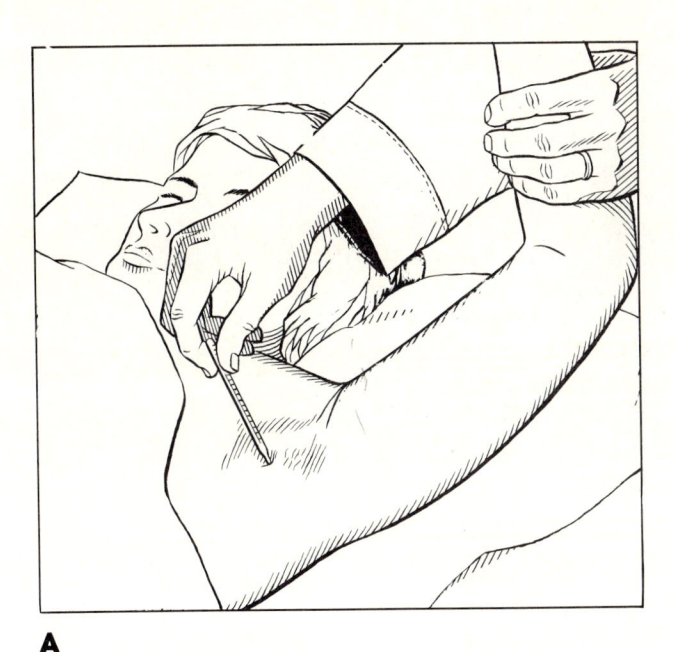

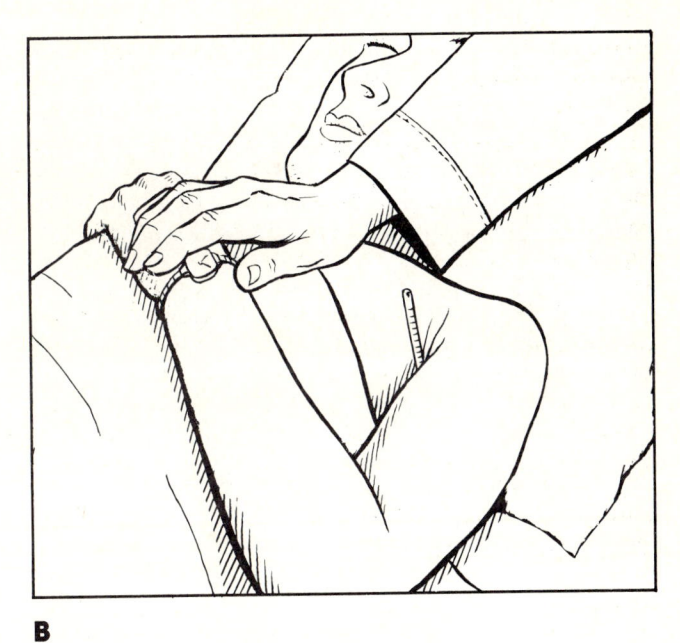

Figure 23-3. **A.** *Inserting an axillary thermometer. After the axilla has been dried, the bulb end of the thermometer is pointed toward the top of the shoulder in the axillary pocket. The elbow is lowered to the side of the body while the thermometer is held in place.* **B.** *Keep the axillary thermometer in place by holding arm close to body.*

plaints of thirst. Since changes in temperature correspond with changes in pulse and respiratory rate, these signs may also indicate a need for temperature measurement.

Physical Appraisal Skills
The decision to take a temperature may evolve from an analysis of objective data obtained by the use of inspection and palpation.

Inspection. *Inspection* may reveal that the client's skin is pale or flushed; that perspiration or goose flesh is present, or that the client is experiencing shivers. Inspection is also used for proper placement and reading of the thermometer.

Palpation. *Palpation* is used to determine if the skin is warm, hot, or cool.

EQUIPMENT

There are three types of thermometers used widely: the mercury glass thermometer, the electronic thermometer, and the chemical probe thermometer. The following sections contain the information that the nurse must have to use each type effectively.

Mercury Glass Thermometer
In most clinical settings, the mercury glass thermometer is used to measure body temperature. It consists of a glass bulb containing mercury and a hollow stem, which permits the mercury to expand and contract. A Celsius thermometer usually has gradations from a low of 34° to a high of 43°. Fahrenheit thermometers are usually calibrated from a low of 94° to a high of 110°. The site used for temperature measurement dictates the shape of the bulb. The stubby tip and pear-shaped bulb are used for rectal and axillary sites as well as for oral sites. The long tip bulb is used only for the oral site because it can cause discomfort in the axilla or perforate the internal tissues of the rectum. The United States Department of Commerce sets standards for the accuracy of measurement, acceptable ranges of deviation, range of calibration, and specifications for the construction of the stem and bulb. Figure 23-4 illustrates three types of mercury glass thermometers.

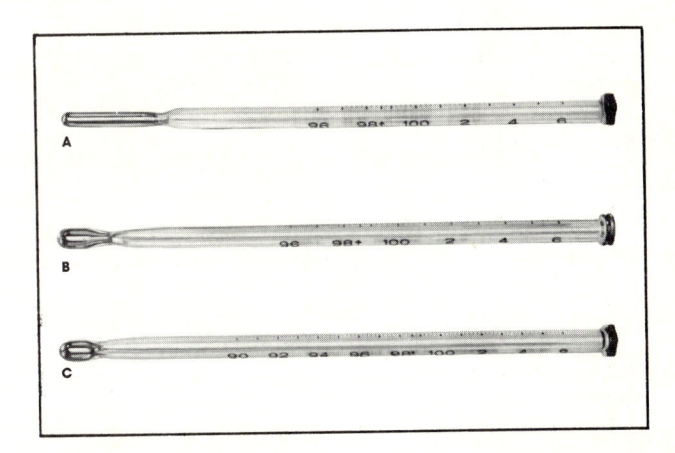

Figure 23-4. *Mercury glass thermometers.* **A.** *long tip, used for oral measurements;* **B.** *and* **C.** *pearshaped and stubby tip used for axillary or rectal measurements. Each type is available in Celsius or Fahrenheit scale. (Courtesy of Becton Dickinson and Company, Rutherford, NJ 07070.)*

Before using a mercury glass thermometer, the nurse inspects it for defects according to the following standards:

1. The scale range should be at least 35° to 41°C (96° to 106°F); the marking should be legible, and the glass should have no fire cracks (cracks in the glass resulting from stress of heat during manufacturing).
2. Gas bubbles should not be present in the bulb, and the mercury column should not have breaks in it above the bulb constriction.
3. Shaking the mercury column down below 35.5°C (96°F) should not be excessively difficult (Beck and St. Cyr, 1974).

Determining the accuracy of a thermometer's measurements is not feasible in the clinical setting. This test requires a water bath with a constant temperature and another thermometer of known accuracy. If there is reason to doubt the accuracy of an instrument, the client's temperature should be measured again with particular attention given to the correct procedure. Doubts about the second reading indicate a need for a third measurement using a new thermometer.

Numerous research studies have documented that mercury glass thermometers do not register accurately. Beck and St. Cyr (1974) found 28 percent of the thermometers evaluated to be inaccurate at 98.6°F. Purintum and Bishop (1969) detected that 48 percent of their sample thermometers measured beyond the acceptable range of deviation. The accuracy tests of Nichols et al. (1966) revealed that 10 percent of the oral thermometers and 6 percent of the rectal thermometers in their sample provided correct readings at six different points ranging from 35.2° to 41°C (95.4° to 105.8°F).

Hazards. The most obvious hazard is broken glass if the thermometer breaks while in the client's mouth or rectum. Mercury poisoning is a frequently mentioned possibility if ingestion occurs; however, this is not a real hazard because mercury oxidizes too slowly in the intestinal tract to permit absorption. Swallowed glass presents the greatest danger. Spilled mercury is a hazard because mercury vaporizes in the presence of heat and can then be absorbed into the lungs. Careless handling and disposal of mercury in sink or toilet drains and open waste receptacles provides opportunities for mercury to vaporize into the environment (Mitchell, 1977; Sims-Williams, 1976).

Cleaning. Keeping the glass thermometer free from microorganisms begins with handwashing before and after each individual measurement (Skill 28). Touching a client's mouth, axillary skin, or rectal area contaminates the hands and provides an opportunity for the transfer of bacteria to the thermometer and to other clients.

There are essentially three different systems used in health-care facilities for storing mercury glass thermometers. Litsky (1976) describes these systems in a study of microbiologic evaluations of each system. A *recycle system* is one in which the central service department of the agency cleans and repackages thermometers after each use. Positive microbial colony counts occurred in about 60 percent of the thermometers taken from this system. *Escherichia coli, Proteus vulgaris, Staphylococcus albus,* alpha streptococci, *Bacillus subtilis,* fungi, and *Neisseria* were among the organisms cultured. Recontamination of the "clean" thermometers resulted from processing the thermometers with nonsterile materials such as a tap water rinse after disinfection and the use of ungloved, nonsterile hands and towels. The *wet kit system* consists of a thermometer in a holder containing a liquid disinfectant, which is provided for the client at the time of admission. Over 80 percent of these thermometers had positive microbial cultures and more than 75 percent of the cultures revealed organisms such as *Neisseria catarrhalis, Proteus vulgaris, Diplococcus pneumoniae,* and *Klebsiella pneumoniae*. The third system described by Litsky is a *dry kit system*. Each client is issued a thermometer and holder upon admission; no liquid disinfectant is used in the holder. After the thermometer is used, it is wiped with a tissue and replaced in the holder. Cultures taken on these thermometers after 3 days of use produced positive colony counts with an average of 11,900 colonies per thermometer. After 5 days of use, the average colony count per thermometer rose to 16,350. The microorganisms cultured from the thermometers from each system are found on the hands, in the mouth, and in feces. They result from human contamination and cause cross-infection.

The Communicable Disease Center Nosocomial Infections Study Report (1976) recommends the following procedures for aseptic handling of thermometers: Each client should be provided with his or her own thermometer. Before and after each use, the thermometer should be washed with soap, rinsed with cool water, and dried with a paper towel at the sink in the client's room, or disinfected after washing and drying with 70 to 90 percent ethyl or isopropyl alcohol. If a wet kit system is used, the disinfectant recommended is 70 to 90 percent ethyl or isopropyl alcohol with 0.2 percent iodine. This solution should be discarded and replaced at least every 3 days. After each use, the thermometer should be washed and dried with a tissue before being returned to the solution holder. The holder should have a warning label attached, because the alcohol solution poses a fire hazard and is harmful if ingested.

Electronic Thermometer

Electronic thermometers use a thermistor in the tip of the probe as a temperature sensing element. A thermistor is composed of a material that changes its electrical resistance in response to a change in temperature.

Two types of electronic thermometers are available for measuring body temperature. The *temperature monitor* type is a direct-reading thermometer, which displays the actual temperature sensed by the probe. It is primarily used for continuous monitoring of body temperature during special procedures and is frequently one component of physiological monitoring systems used with critically ill clients. The second *intermittent-reading* type is used in much the same way a mercury thermometer is used periodically to measure temperature at a single point in time. Intermittent-reading thermometers can be either steady state or predictive. Steady state thermometers operate in a direct-reading mode, while predictive thermometers operate by measuring the temperature at two or more different points in time before the probe reaches thermal equilibrium. This measurement of the rate of temperature rise is used to compute the final temperature reading (Mercury, 1972).

The electronic thermometer consists of two separate parts, the thermometer unit and a charger/storage base. The small portable unit houses a readout panel that displays the temperature in digits; a red light appears when the optimum temperature has been reached. The readout panel also has a charge light indicator that stays on when the unit is recharging on its base. Other components of the thermometer unit include a storage area for the probe covers, a receptacle well for the probe, and a probe that attaches to the unit by a connector. A carrying strap attached to the unit enables the user to keep his or her hands free. When the unit is not in use, it rests on a charger/storage base that automatically recharges the unit batteries when the base is plugged into a proper power source. To prevent transferring organisms from client to client, the base should not be carried to the client's bedside.

Most models use the single disposable probe cover to prevent contamination of the probe and the client. Oral probe covers are translucent whereas rectal probe covers are red. The probe cover should be easy to apply and remove to facilitate aseptic handling. It should also be resistant to tearing and puncturing. Different probes are used for oral and rectal temperatures. The temperature appears on the display panel in Celsius or Fahrenheit scales or both.

The accuracy of the direct-reading thermometer can be checked by use of a constant-temperature water bath. Some of the predictive models cannot be checked because of the difference in the thermal characteristics of water and the mucous membrane surfaces of the mouth and rectum (Mercury, 1972).

The electronic thermometer registers the optimum temperature in 20 to 30 seconds. *Optimum temperature* is the maximum temperature minus 0.2°F (Nichols and Verhonick, 1967).

Chemical Probe Thermometer

This single-use disposable thermometer (Fig. 23-5) consists of many colored dots, each of which changes color at intervals of 0.2°F according to its chemical makeup. For example, the first dot changes color at 96.2°F, the second dot changes color at 96.4°F, and so forth until the thermometer registers optimum temperature. The chemical probe thermometer registers temperatures from 96.0° to 104.8°F. A Celsius version is scaled from 35.5° to 40.4°C. The correct temperature is determined by the last dot to change color. In a study comparing the accuracy of the chemical probe thermometer with the mercury glass thermometer conducted by St. Cyr and Beck (1973), the overall accuracy of the chemical probe thermometer was found to be 94.4 percent, while the accuracy of the mercury glass thermometer was 92.1 percent. The deviation in accuracy in the case of the mercury glass thermometer seemed to be due to the instrument and in the case of the chemical probe thermometer, to the lack of proper placement.

The chemical probe thermometer registers oral temperature in 45 seconds, rectal temperature in 90 seconds, and axillary temperature in 2 minutes. The merits of the chemical probe thermometer are its accuracy, sterility, disposability, sturdiness, short measurement time, and ease of reading.

Kirkpatrick and Stanley (1976) conducted a study to evaluate the merits of a single-use thermometer as compared with the more traditional glass mercury thermometer. They found the single-use thermometer quick and easy to read, accurate when correctly placed, and well accepted by clients. Some clients were relieved because they did not have to worry about glass breaking or about contracting an infection from the last client to use the instrument.

☐ EXECUTION

A routine schedule of taking temperatures at 8 A.M. and 4 P.M. may be mandated by agency policy. This schedule is usually selected because these measurements will reflect the body's temperature between the expected physiological low and high temperatures. Thus, an elevation of temperature at 8 A.M. could be clinically significant. However, unit personnel frequently take temperatures at any time between 5 A.M. and 7 A.M. and between 2 P.M. and 4 P.M. because these times are convenient. They thus miss the times when the clients' temperatures are most apt to be clinically significant.

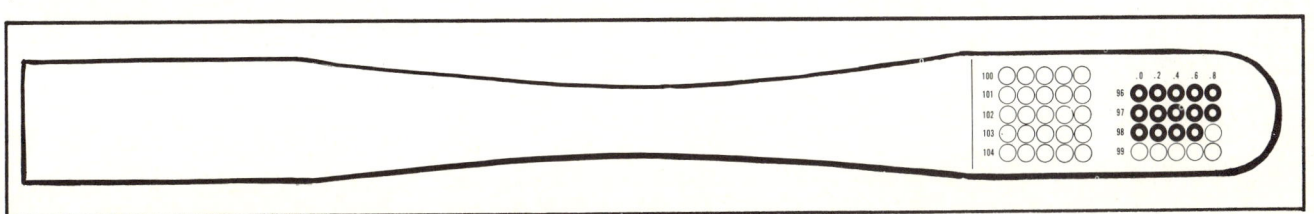

Figure 23-5. Tempa-DOT single-use thermometer. (Used with permission of Organon Hospital Products, Organon, Inc., West Orange, NJ 07052.)

☐ SKILL SEQUENCES

ORAL TEMPERATURE WITH A MERCURY GLASS THERMOMETER

Step	Rationale
1. Wash hands.	Prevents contamination of thermometer.
2. Obtain oral thermometer.	
3. Explain procedure to client.	Allays client's anxiety.
4. Inspect thermometer for fire cracks, loss of color from calibrations, separation of mercury in column.	Prevents inaccurate measurement.
5. Note calibration: °C or °F.	
6. Hold at end distal to bulb.	Prevents contamination of hands.
7. Wash with soap and rinse under cool running water if holder has disinfectant solution. (If dry kit is used, disinfect thermometer with 70 to 90 percent alcohol. The recycle system provides a sterile thermometer that does not require cleansing before use.)	Removes disinfectant solution or retained oral mucus. Hot water causes mercury to expand, could break thermometer.
8. Dry with paper towel, wiping from fingers toward bulb. (Omit this step with recycle system.)	Wipe from part least contaminated toward part most contaminated to maintain asepsis of least contaminated end.
9. Wipe with disinfectant solution of 70 to 90 percent ethyl or isopropyl alcohol. (Omit this step with recycle system.)	Removes residual microorganisms.
10. Hold thermometer horizontal at eye level in right hand.	Holding in left hand makes reading scale more difficult.
11. Rotate thermometer slowly until mercury line is clearly visible.	
12. Read measurement to closest calibration: 1/10th for Celsius and 2/10ths for Fahrenheit.	
13. If mercury above 35°C (96°F), prepare to shake down the mercury.	For accurate reading, mercury must be below 35°C (96°F).
14. Move away from walls, furniture, and equipment.	Prevents breaking thermometer.
15. Hold thermometer tightly at end distal to bulb.	
16. Keep wrist loose and snap hand vigorously up and down.	
17. Reread to make sure mercury is below 35°C (96°F).	
18. Have client moisten lips if able, or wet them with cool water.	Prevents tissue damage from thermometer adhering to mucous membranes.
19. Have client open mouth and raise tongue slightly.	Permits location of site for placement.
20. Gently slide thermometer under tongue until bulb is in place in heat pocket.	Temperature measured in other sites yields lower reading.
21. Tell client not to bite down, merely close lips.	Prevents breaking thermometer.
22. Leave thermometer in place 9 to 11 minutes. Remain with client.	Client should not open mouth. If mouth opens start timing again from the beginning. Use time to perform other nursing actions.
23. Hold end of thermometer and have client open mouth.	Prevents thermometer from falling when mouth opens.
24. Remove thermometer carefully, wipe with tissue using friction in turning motion from least contaminated end to bulb.	Enables more accurate reading; removes saliva.
25. Hold thermometer at eye level; rotate until mercury line and calibrations are visible.	Permits accurate reading.
26. Read thermometer as in step 12.	
27. Record reading immediately.	Prevents forgetting reading.
28. Wash thermometer with soap, rinse with cool water, dry with paper towel. (If the agency uses a recycle system, omit steps 28 to 30. Return thermometer to receptacle provided by central service department.)	Removes remaining saliva. Prevents dilution of disinfectant.
29. Wipe with disinfectant as in step 9.	Removes bacteria, which would multiply on thermometer while in holder.
30. Shake down mercury as in steps 14 to 16.	
31. Return thermometer to holder or recycle system container.	
32. Wash hands.	Prevents cross-infection to next client.

RECTAL TEMPERATURE WITH A MERCURY GLASS THERMOMETER

Step	Rationale
1. Follow steps 1 to 17, "Oral Temperatures," using rectal thermometer.	
2. Close room door; pull cubicle curtains.	Ensures privacy.
3. Have client turn on side, assisting as necessary. Flex client's upper leg if possible. Can also have client lie on abdomen if side not possible.	Allows better visualization of anal sphincter.
4. Apply water soluble lubricant to thermometer bulb end, extending up for 1/2 inch for infant and up to 3 inches for adult. Obtain tissue.	Facilitates insertion. Oil-based lubricant interferes with bowel function of water absorption of stool and may also interfere with accurate transfer of heat to bulb.
5. Raise client's upper buttock to expose anus. Client may be asked to bear down to improve exposure of anus.	Permits visualization of anus and sphincter.
6. Gently touch anal sphincter with bulb tip.	Spontaneous involuntary reaction is to tighten anus. Gentle touch stimulates this response, then anus relaxes so that easy insertion is possible.
7. Gently insert thermometer bulb tip into anal opening, directing thermometer anteriorly and inward (toward client's navel), sliding thermometer along wall of rectum to a maximum depth of 1/2 inch for infant, and up to 3 inches for adult.	Follows normal shape of rectum, prevents damage to rectum.
8. Hold in place 2 to 4 minutes. May monitor pulse and respirations during this time.	Ensures accurate measurement by keeping thermometer in place.
9. Remove thermometer in reverse direction of insertion.	
10. Use tissue to wipe from fingers to bulb end; use friction and turning motion.	Protects hand and stem from contamination and removes lubricant and fecal matter.
11. Discard tissue.	
12. Cleanse anal area with tissue.	Removes lubricant and fecal matter.
13. Assist client into a comfortable position; replace covers.	
14. Read thermometer as in "Oral Temperature."	
15. Record temperature immediately. Write "R" for rectal.	
16. Complete procedure as in "Oral Temperature," steps 28 to 32.	

AXILLARY TEMPERATURE WITH A MERCURY GLASS THERMOMETER

Step	Rationale
1. Repeat steps 1 to 17, "Oral Temperature," using axillary thermometer.	
2. Have client lying down in bed.	Prevents thermometer from falling out of place.
3. Remove sleeve of client's gown, assisting as necessary.	Exposes axilla.
4. Have client raise elbow to expose axilla, assisting as necessary.	
5. Use tissue to dry axilla gently.	Skin is cooled by moisture.
6. Place thermometer bulb end pointed directly toward top of shoulder in axillary pocket. Lower client's elbow to side of body. Hold in place with other hand. Always hold for infant or child.	Holds thermometer in axilla over artery.
7. Leave in place 10 minutes for all age groups. If thermometer is disturbed from location, restart time count.	Ensures accurate measurement.
8. Hold thermometer and raise client's elbow; remove thermometer.	
9. Use tissue to wipe thermometer with twisting motion moving from stem end toward bulb.	Wipe from least contaminated to most contaminated portion.
10. Replace client's gown and covers.	
11. Read thermometer as in "Oral Temperature," p. 194.	
12. Record temperature immediately. Write "A" for axillary.	
13. Complete procedure as in "Oral Temperature" steps 28 to 32.	

ELECTRONIC THERMOMETER

To use an electronic thermometer such as the IVAC (see Figure 23-6). For rectal measurements apply a red probe cover. Insert the thermometer in the same manner as the mercury glass thermometer. Axillary temperatures can be obtained with the oral probe using the same technique and time (9 to 11 minutes) required for a mercury glass thermometer.

CHEMICAL PROBE THERMOMETER

To use the chemical probe thermometer such as the Tempa-Dot:

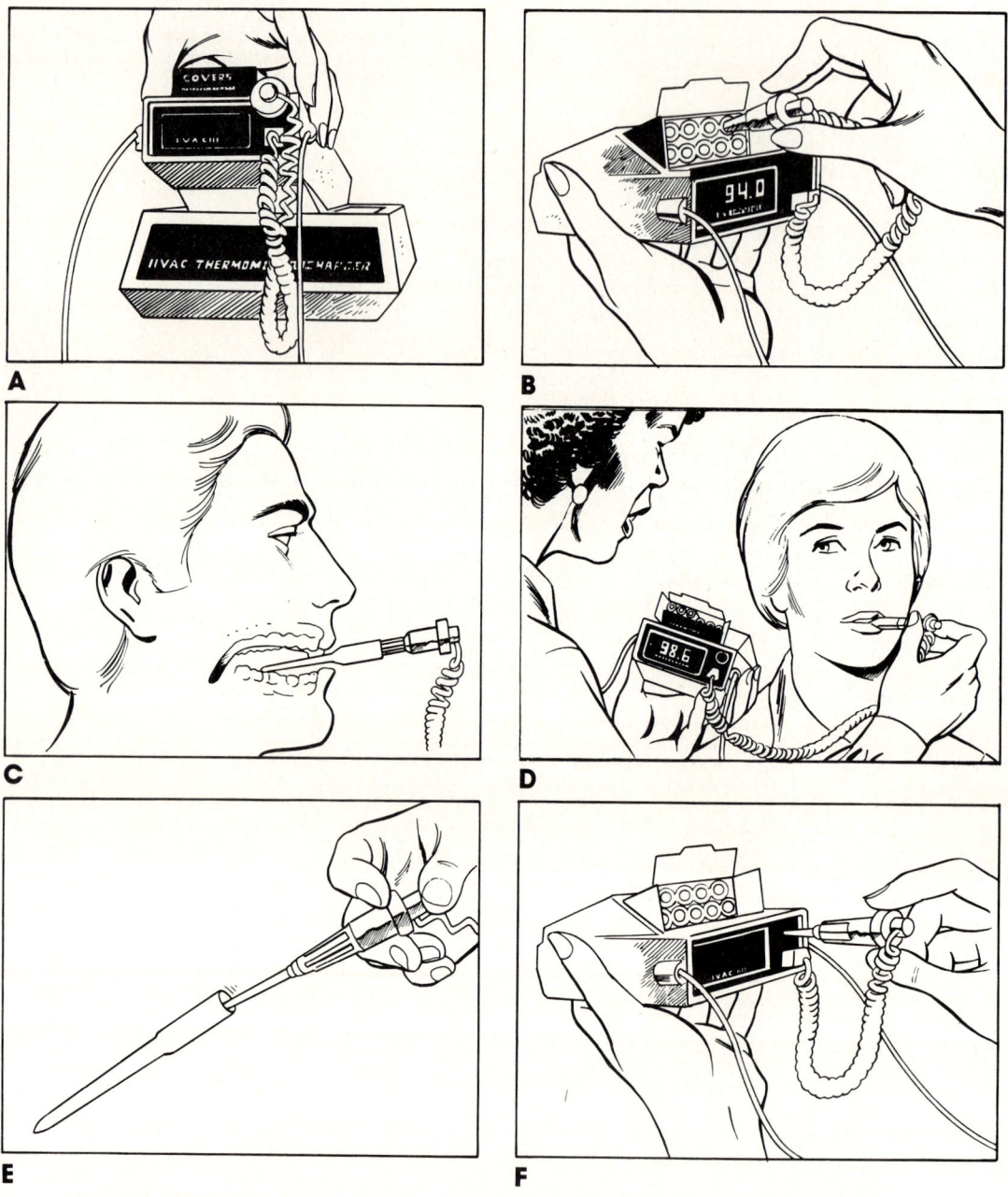

Figure 23–6. Technique for using the IVAC electronic thermometer. **A.** Remove the thermometer from the charger base and place the carrying strap around the neck. **B.** Grasp the probe by the large ring at the top and insert the probe into a disposable cover. Do not push the top of the probe; it is the ejection button. **C.** For an oral measurement, slowly slide the probe under the front of the tongue along the gum line, back to the sublingual pocket at the posterior base of the tongue. **D.** Hold the probe in place. Do not watch the digital display but watch the position of the probe in the client until an audible signal tells when the client's temperature is reached and displayed. **E.** Remove the probe from the client's mouth; push the ejection button with the thumb to remove the cover. **F.** Read the temperature from the display and record it before returning the probe to its storage well. Return the thermometer to the charger base when finished. (Adapted with permission from IVAC® Corporation, San Diego, CA 92121.)

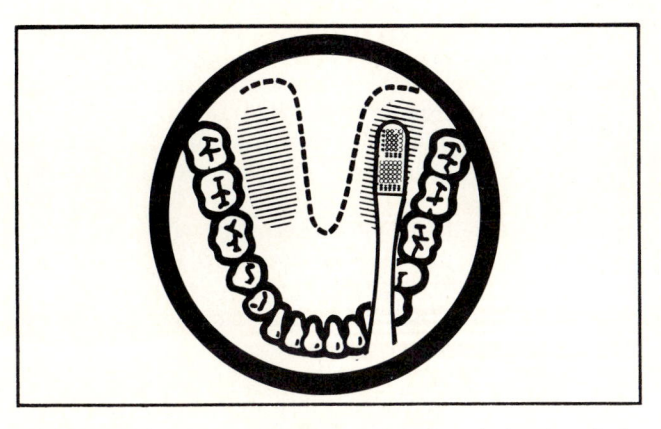

Figure 23-7. Tempa-DOT thermometer in place in heat pocket. (Used with permission of Organon Hospital Products, Organon Inc., West Orange, NJ 07052.)

1. Remove the thermometer from the paper wrapper by peeling it back to expose the handle end. Do not touch the sterile indicator dots or the shaft.
2. For an oral temperature have the client open his or her mouth and insert the thermometer as far back as possible into the sublingual heat pocket. (Figure 23-7 illustrates the proper oral position of the chemical probe thermometer.)
3. Have the client press his or her tongue down on the thermometer, then close and keep mouth shut.
4. Remove the thermometer after a minimum of 45 seconds. Read and record the temperature, which is indicated by the last dot that has changed color.

For an axillary temperature, place the sensor tip deep into the axillary pocket with the matrix against the body and the instrument parallel to the length of the body. Hold the thermometer in place for 2 minutes.

For a rectal temperature, attach a rectal adaptor and insert the thermometer as in the mercury glass thermometer procedure. Hold the thermometer in place for at least 90 seconds.

RECORDING

After reading the thermometer accurately, write the measurement down immediately, exactly as it was read. If the site used is other than oral, note this by using "R" for rectal and "A" for axillary. Record the time of the measurement. Transfer of the reading to the client record is usually done at the nurse's desk, or the reading may be placed on a record kept at the client's bedside. Figure 23-8 illustrates the graphic recording of body temperature.

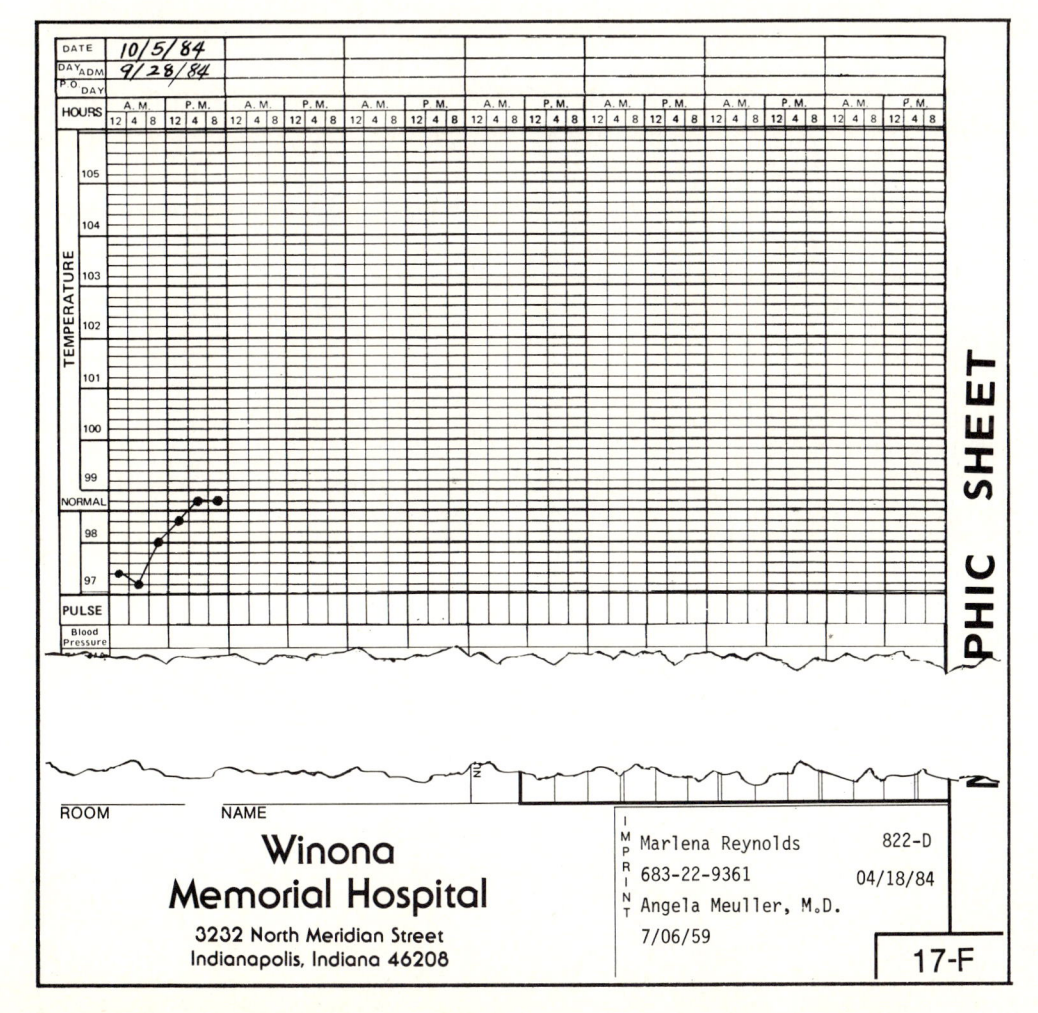

Figure 23-8. Graphic recording of body temperature. (Used with permission of Winona Memorial Hospital, Indianapolis, IN 46208.)

Walker and Selmanoff (1965) found serious discrepancies between measured and recorded temperatures. Only 37 percent of all temperatures taken and recorded by nursing personnel were the same as those taken by the investigators. Sixty-one percent of clients whose temperatures were subnormal had higher measurements recorded, and 66 percent of those with normal or elevated temperatures had temperatures recorded that were too low. The investigators speculate that nursing personnel had preconceived notions of what the client's temperature should be. When their expectation was not met, they attributed the discrepancy to a fault in their technique and so changed the recording to meet their expectation.

If body temperature measurements are to be used as indicators of health and illness status upon which decisions about treatment are made, then measurement and recording must be accurate. A variety of designs for vital-sign data records are used in healthcare agencies. The agency policies must be followed for recording.

□ CRITICAL POINTS SUMMARY

1. Determine the appropriate site for temperature measurement.
2. Use the same site for successive measurements.
3. Select the correct thermometer for the measurement site.
4. Inspect the thermometer for defects: mercury column broken above bulb, scale not readable, gas bubbles in the mercury.
5. Consider factors that affect the accuracy of measurement: ingestion of hot or cold liquids, smoking, gum chewing, and exercise.
6. Disinfect the thermometer.
7. Shake down the mercury to below 35°C (96°F).
8. Place the thermometer in proper site correctly.
9. Leave thermometer in for required period of time.
10. For mercury glass thermometers, wipe with tissue after removal.
11. Read and record measurement correctly.
12. Disinfect thermometer and replace in appropriate receptacle.

□ LEARNING ACTIVITIES

1. Inspect oral, rectal, and axillary thermometers to note the difference in the bulb design.
2. Practice snapping your wrist while holding a pencil, as if to shake down a thermometer before actually using it.
3. Select a mercury glass thermometer.
    a. Clean it according to the aseptic procedure previously described.
    b. Obtain a base oral temperature on yourself or a friend, leaving the thermometer in for 10 minutes.
    c. Drink 8 ounces of a hot or cold beverage in a brief period of time, such as 2 to 3 minutes, and take your temperature immediately.
    d. Obtain a third measurement 15 minutes after the drink was consumed. Note the differences in the three measurements.
4. Use the sample graphic form (Fig. 23–8) to record the following temperatures in the proper time slot:
    8 A.M.—98.6°F; 12 noon—99.4°; 4 P.M.—100.2°;
    8 P.M.—101°; 12 midnight—97.2°; 4 A.M.—97.6°.

□ REVIEW QUESTIONS

1. Why is body temperature measured?
2. What types of instruments are available to measure body temperature?
3. How does the mercury glass thermometer bulb differ in models designed for use in the mouth, rectum, and axilla?
4. What calculations are used to change a Fahrenheit reading to a Celsius (Centigrade) reading?
5. How do you maintain the asepsis of a thermometer in a wet kit system? In a dry kit system?
6. How would you explain to someone the correct placement of a thermometer in each of the sites?
7. What precautions, if any, should be observed with each site?
8. Why can serial measurements not be compared when the measurement site is changed?
9. What sources of error in temperature measurement can be attributed to the equipment, the nurse, or the client?
10. What data should be included in a temperature recording?

□ PERFORMANCE CHECKLIST

OBJECTIVE: To use the appropriate method to measure body temperature accurately.

CHARACTERISTIC	RANGE OF ACCEPTABILITY	SATISFACTORY	UNSATISFACTORY
1. Washes hands.	No deviation		
2. Determines correct site for measurement.	No deviation		
3. Selects correct thermometer for site.	No deviation		
4. Explains procedure to client.	No deviation		

(continued)

CHARACTERISTIC	RANGE OF ACCEPTABILITY	SATISFACTORY	UNSATISFACTORY
5. Inspects thermometer for defects.	No deviation		
6. Holds securely, rinses under cool water.	No deviation		
7. Dries with paper towel.	No deviation		
8. Wipes with disinfectant.	No deviation		
9. Reads mercury level.	No deviation		
10. Shakes down to 95°F (35°C).	No deviation		
11. Places thermometer in proper site.	No deviation		
12. Leaves in for required time.	No deviation		
13. Removes thermometer safely.	No deviation		
14. Cleans thermometer with proper technique.	No deviation		
15. Reads thermometer accurately.	0.1°C or 0.2°F		
16. Disinfects thermometer before replacing in receptacle.	No deviation		
17. Washes hands.	No deviation		
18. Records temperature accurately.	No deviation		

REFERENCES

Aseptic handling of thermometers and other equipment for measuring patient temperatures. Communicable Disease Center Nosocomial Infections Study Report Annual Summary, 1976. Hospital Infections Branch, Bacterial Diseases Division, Bureau of Epidemiology, April, 1978. Unpublished report from the Special Investigations Section, Hepatitis Laboratories Division, Bureau of Epidemiology, Centers for Disease Control. Mimeograph.

Beck WC, Campbell R: Clinical thermometry. Guthrie Bulletin 44(4):82–90, 1975.

Beck WC, St. Cyr B: Oral thermometry. Guthrie Bulletin 43(4):170–185, 1974.

Biskey V: Oral Temperatures and Their Validity in Patients with Tracheostomies. Unpublished manuscript. Indianapolis, Indiana University, 1973.

Blainey CG: Site selection in taking body temperature. American Journal of Nursing 74(10):1859–1861, 1974.

Dressler DK, Smejkal C, Ruffolo ML: A comparison of oral and rectal temperature measurement on patients receiving oxygen by mask. Nursing Research 32(6):373–375, 1983.

Erickson R: Thermometer placement for oral temperature measurement in febrile adults. International Journal of Nursing Studies 13(4):199–208, 1976.

Felton G: Effect of time cycle change on blood pressure and temperature in young women. Nursing Research 19(1):56–57, 1970.

Forster B, Adler DC, Davis M: Duration of effects of drinking iced water on oral temperature. Nursing Research 19(2):169–170, 1970.

Graas S: Thermometer sites and oxygen. American Journal of Nursing 74(10):1862–1863, 1974.

Kintzel KC: A comparative study of oral and rectal temperatures in patients receiving two forms of oxygen therapy. In American Nurses Association Clinical Sessions, paper presented at the American Nurses' Association Convention, San Francisco, 1966. New York, Appleton-Century-Crofts, 1967.

Kirkpatrick M, Stanley SM: Evaluation of a new single-use thermometer. Occupational Health Nursing 24(12):9–18, 1976.

Larkin J: Effects of Ingestion of Hot and Cold Fluids on Oral Temperatures of Afebrile Adults. Unpublished manuscript. Indianapolis, Indiana University, 1974.

Lee R, Atkins E: Spurious fever. American Journal of Nursing 72(6):1094–1095, 1972.

Litsky BY: A study of temperature taking systems. Supervisor Nurse 7(5):48–53, 1976.

Mercury vs. electronic thermometers. Health Devices 2(1):3–20, 1972.

Mitchell P: Concepts Basic to Nursing, ed 2. New York, McGraw-Hill, 1977.

Nichols G: Placement times for oral thermometers: A nursing study replication. Nursing Research 17(2):159–161, 1968.

Nichols G: Taking adult temperatures: Rectal measurements. American Journal of Nursing 72(6):192–193, 1972.

Nichols G, Fielding JT, et al: Taking oral temperatures of febrile patients. Nursing Research 18(5):448–450, 1969.

Nichols G, Kucha D: Oral measurements. American Journal of Nursing 72(6):191–193, 1972.

Nichols G, Ruskin M, et al: Oral, axillary and rectal temperature determinations and relationships. Nursing Research 15(4):307–310, 1966.

Nichols G, Verhonick P: Time and temperature. American Journal of Nursing 67(11):2304–2306, 1967.

Purintum L, Bishop B: How accurate are clinical glass thermometers? American Journal of Nursing 69(1):99–100, 1969.

St. Cyr G, Beck W: A new disposable thermometer in clinical use. Guthrie Bulletin 42(4):94–104, 1973.

Sims-Williams AJ: Temperature taking with glass thermometers: A review. Journal of Advanced Nursing 1(6):481–493, 1976.

Walker V, Selmanoff ED: A note on the accuracy of temperature, pulse and respiration procedure. Nursing Research 14(1):72–76, 1965.

Woodman E, Parry S, Simms L: Sources of unreliability in oral temperatures. Nursing Research 16(3):276-279, 1967.

BIBLIOGRAPHY

Baker NC, Cerone SB, et al: The effect of type of thermometer and length of time inserted on oral temperature measurements of afebrile subjects. Nursing Research 33(2):109-111, 1984.

Campbell K: Taking temperatures. Nursing Times 79(32):63-65, 1983.

Eaff MJ, Meier RS, Miller C: Temperature measurement in infants. Nursing Research 23(6):457-460, 1974.

Evaluation: Clinical electronic thermometers. Health Devices 2(1):13-20, 1972.

Hasler ME, Cohen JA: The effect of oxygen administration on oral temperature assessment. Nursing Research 31(5):265-268, 1982.

Higgins P: Can 98.6 degrees be a fever in disguise? Geriatric Nurse 4(2):101-102, 1983.

AUDIOVISUAL RESOURCES

Body Temperature
  18 slides. (1974, Color)
  Available through:
    Robert J. Brady Company
    Route 197
    Bowie, MD 20715

How to Take Your Patient's Temperature
  Filmstrip and cassette. (1975, Color, 40 min.)
  Available through:
    Techniques Learning Council
    921 East Green Street
    Pasadena, CA 91106

Measuring Vital Signs/Temperature
  Videocassette (½ in, ¾ in). (1979, Color, 14 min.)
  Available through:
    Indiana University, School of Nursing
    NICER Department
    1100 West Michigan Street
    Indianapolis, IN 46223

Temperature, Pulse, and Respiration
  Filmstrip and cassette. (1974, Color, 15 min.)
  Available through:
    Medcom, Inc.
    P.O. Box 116
    Garden Grove, CA 92642

SKILL 24 Pulse Appraisal

PREREQUISITE SKILLS

Skill 19, "Inspection"
Skill 20, "Palpation"
Skill 22, "Auscultation"
Skill 28, "Handwashing"

☐ **STUDENT OBJECTIVES**

1. Explain the purpose of appraising the pulse.
2. Describe the terms used for the characteristics of the pulse.
3. Describe the location of each pulse site.
4. Differentiate the pulse sites usually used to determine rate, rhythm, and quality from those used to determine only presence and quality.
5. Identify the pulse sites appropriate for different situations.
6. Summarize the factors that create errors in pulse appraisal.
7. Use the correct method to appraise peripheral pulses, the apical pulse, and an apical–radial pulse.
8. Record the characteristics of the pulse accurately in graphic and narrative form.

☐ **INTRODUCTION**

Each heartbeat forces blood from the left ventricle into the arterial circulation, creating a pulse wave that may be palpated in several superficial arteries of the body. There are some pulse waves, such as the carotid, that may be visible. The pulse reflects the physical and emotional state of a person. It is an important indicator of the heart's ability to respond to the physiological demands of metabolism, exercise, fever, fluid, blood loss or gain, and tissue damage in the heart.

The pulse also provides information about the condition of the blood vessels and the adequacy of the circulation to the extremities. With age, disease, or both, the blood vessels become less resilient, the inner diameter is reduced, and the vessel may even become occluded, thereby blocking the flow of blood. When an inadequate amount of blood flows to an extremity, the tissues do not get the proper amount of nutrition and oxygen and the waste products are not removed adequately. These changes in tissue perfusion can be detected by appraising the pulse and the skin of the extremities. The color of the skin may become pale or bluish, and the temperature is cooler to palpation than other body areas.

Pulse monitoring dates back to 1500 B.C. to Ebers Papyrus, who noted the synchrony of the pulse with the heartbeat, and palpated it in many parts of the body. The rate and rhythm of the pulse has been used as a guide for medical therapy since the middle of the 18th century.

Monitoring of the pulse is a very common but deceptively simple procedure. In one study, 28 percent of the recorded pulse rates counted by nursing personnel differed by a minimum of 12 beats when compared with those taken by the investigators (Walker and Selmanoff, 1965). Another study identified some problems encountered in pulse appraisal (Jones, 1970). Both student and graduate nurses had problems in finding the pulse site and holding it for the time required for counting. Some students applied so much pressure while palpating that their finger pads left imprints on the person's skin. Other errors noted were counting the movement of the second hand of the clock instead of the pulse beat and counting before and after the time interval specified for measurement.

☐ PREPARATION

CHARACTERISTICS OF THE PULSE

The pulse has three characteristics that are appraised each time the pulse is monitored: rate, rhythm, and quality. All three characteristics change in relation to metabolic needs, exercise, body temperature, and fluid or blood volume changes.

Rate

The *rate* is the number of pulse waves that occur in 1 minute. It is normally counted by palpation or auscultation. An electrocardiograph can also be used to count the pulse rate, but it is usually not used by the nurse in ordinary situations. The rate is used to gauge a person's response to normal activity and to stresses encountered during illness. The normal pulse rate varies with age and sex. An infant has a rate from 120 to 140 beats per minute. A decrease occurs as the child grows, so that by age 3 the rate is about 110 beats per minute, and by age 12 a boy's pulse ranges between 65 and 105 beats per minute and a girl's is slightly faster at 70 to 110 beats per minute. The adult rate is usually established by age 18. For males it ranges between 50 and 80, and for females it ranges between 55 and 95.

Pulsus bigeminus, or bigeminy, is a double-beat pulse. A strong pulse wave caused by a regular sinus beat is coupled with a weak pulse wave caused by a premature contraction of the ventricle before it is completely filled with blood (Fig 24-1; Davis and Nelson, 1978). The interval between successive beats differs and results in an irregular rhythm. Bigeminy is

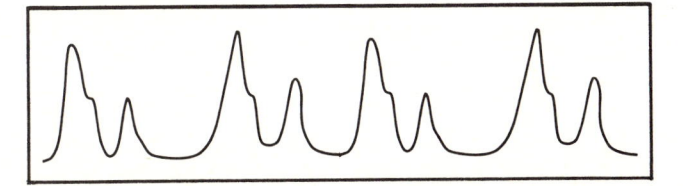

Figure 24-1. Pulsus bigeminus, or bigeminy, a double-beat pulse. Normal pulse wave and premature ventricular contraction. (From Understanding Cardiology © 1978. By Hywel Davies and William P. Nelson, Butterworth Publishers, Inc., 19 Cummings Park, Woburn, MA 01801. With permission.)

most commonly caused by digitalis intoxication. It may not be identified by palpation; if the weak beat is too faint to be palpated, the pulse may appear to be bradycardia. It may be necessary to use a stethoscope to listen over the apex of the heart to count the pulse rate accurately. (The method for obtaining an apical pulse rate is described later in this skill.)

Quality

Quality or volume is the third characteristic of a pulse. It is a reflection of the strength of the ventricular contraction, the amount of blood ejected with each contraction, and the quality of the perfusion of blood to the peripheral vessels in the body. While palpating the pulse, the nurse feels the strength of the pulse wave bouncing against the finger pads. A normal pulse is usually felt without difficulty. However, layers of large muscles or adipose tissue over a superficial artery can make it difficult to appraise pulse volume accurately.

A *weak pulse* has less force because of a low stroke volume and an increase in vascular resistance. This type of pulse is referred to as weak and thready because it is often found in conjunction with an increased rate. The observer may mistakenly count his or her own pulse if the pulse in one's own fingers is stronger than the client's pulse; using the pads of the fingers instead of the flat palmar surface of the fingers reduces this possibility.

The terms used to describe slow and fast pulse rates are bradycardia and tachycardia. *Bradycardia* is the term used for a pulse rate below 60 beats per minute. A rate this slow may be the result of physical conditioning of the cardiovascular system, such as in the case of athletes or persons engaged in regular strenuous exercise. In others, it may be caused by cardiotonic medications, partial or complete block of the impulses conducted through the heart, or increased intracranial pressure. Some people can deliberately and consciously decrease their heart rate.

Tachycardia is the term used for a pulse rate over 100 beats per minute. The increased rate may be a normal physiological response to exercise, anger, anxiety, or fear. It may also be caused by some pathological conditions of the heart or other disease problems.

Rhythm

Rhythm, the second characteristic of pulse waves, is usually synchronous with the heartbeat in a normal person. It may be altered by a change in heart function, electrolyte imbalance, or the effect of drugs. Two common irregular patterns of pulse are *atrial fibrillation* and *pulsus bigeminus.*

Atrial fibrillation is an irregular heart rhythm. It occurs when the sinus node no longer controls the rhythm. The atria do not contract in coordination, and there is a complete irregularity of the ventricular beats. This creates an irregular pattern of pulse waves that do not have any pattern within the irregularity.

A *bounding pulse* has strong force because of increased stroke volume and decreased vascular resistance. It is a normal response to exercise, fear, anxiety, or fever, and occurs in some women during a normal pregnancy. It is also present in abnormal conditions such as anemia, complete heart block, and liver failure.

The quality of a pulse is particularly important when there is a pathological condition present in the cardiovascular system. Scales are used to quantify the pulse volume so that a more precise record of changes can be maintained. The gradations of the scale vary among institutions; some use a four- and others a five-point scale. The four-point scale usually includes the following: 3+, bounding pulse; 2+, normal pulse; 1+, weak pulse; and 0, absent pulse. The five-point scale provides an additional point for levels of weakness. It is necessary to be aware of the system used in the setting in which one is practicing, so that there will be consistency in documenting the pulse quality. The judgment required in using the scale is subjective, but with the experience of validating one's findings with competent practitioners, learners develop confidence in their judgments.

Pulsus paradoxus and *pulsus alternans* are two types of pulses that have a combination of weak and strong beats. *Pulsus paradoxus,* also referred to as paradoxical pulse, refers to an exaggerated weakening of the pulse wave during inspiration. Some imperceptible waning of the pulse volume occurs during inspiration because of a normal pressure change in the thorax as the diaphragm is lowered. This happens because more blood is trapped in the lungs with a decreased amount returned to the left ventricle to be ejected into the systemic circulation. A paradoxical pulse occurs when the blood pressure falls 10 mm Hg during inspiration, which is more than normal. Pulmonary diseases such as asthma, emphysema, and airway obstruction as well as congestive heart failure and cardiac tamponade are conditions in which paradoxical pulse may occur. Since its rhythm is regular, the presence of a paradoxical pulse may be difficult to confirm by palpation. Although the pulse is weakened, the intensity of the heart sounds remains constant. Paradoxical pulse may be confirmed by inflating a blood pressure cuff on the upper arm until no sounds can be heard with the stethoscope bell over the brachial artery. As the cuff pressure is reduced, the first sounds will be heard only during expiration (Fig. 24-2; Fowler, 1972; Kinnebrew, 1981).

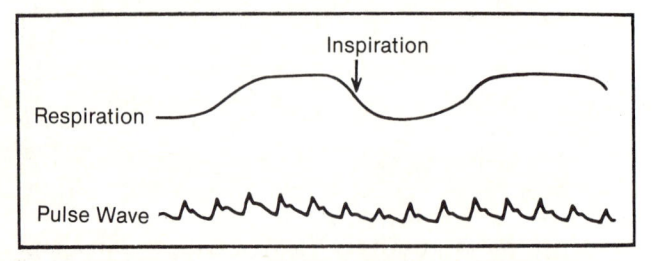

Figure 24-2. Pulsus paradoxus. The relationship between a weak pulse wave and inspiration; strong waves occur during expiration in a client with pulmonary emphysema. (Adapted from Inspection and Palpation of Venous and Arterial Pulses by Noble O. Fowler, M.D. Part II of Examination of the Heart series. American Heart Association, 1972. With permission.)

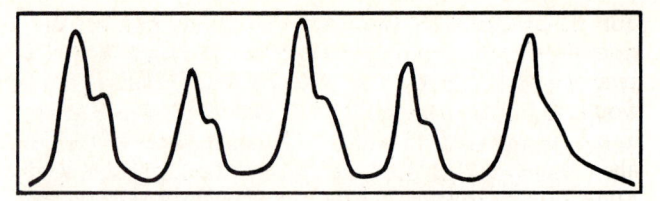

Figure 24-3. Pulsus alternans. The strength of the beats alternates but the rhythm is regular. (From Understanding Cardiology © 1978. By Hywel Davies and William P. Nelson, Butterworth Publishers, Inc., 19 Cummings Park, Woburn, MA 01801. With permission.)

Pulsus alternans, or alternating pulse, refers to a pulse that results from ventricular contractions that alternate in strength. Weak contractions produce weak beats and strong contractions produce strong beats. The weak beats may be only slightly weaker than the strong beats (Fig 24-3). The rhythm is regular but on rare occasions it may appear to be irregular on palpation, because the sensation perceived by palpation may be slightly delayed. Davis and Nelson (1978) recommend that when pulsus alternans is suspected, it may be detected by using one finger to apply pressure over the radial artery to eliminate the weak beats, and a second finger distal to the first to sense the stronger beats. This technique reduces the pulse rate by half (Fig. 24-4).

A blood pressure cuff may also be inflated to a pressure that eliminates the weaker beats and permits palpation or auscultation of only the stronger beats. Pulsus alternans is an important sign of left ventricular failure.

SITES FOR PULSE APPRAISAL

The site selected for pulse appraisal depends on the specific purpose for which the pulse is to be obtained and the presence of any constraints on a given site.

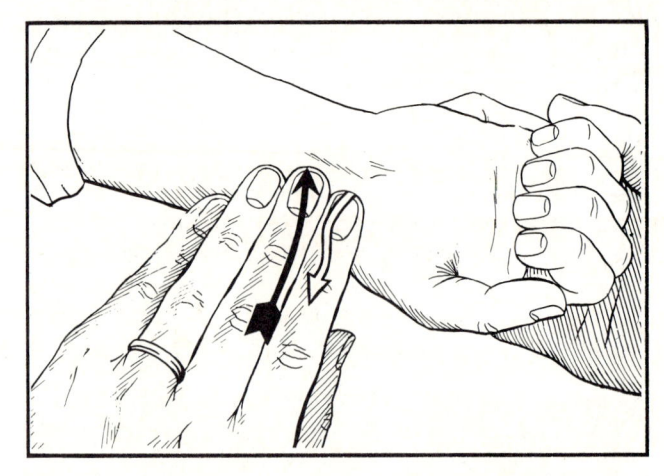

Figure 24-4. Palpation technique to detect pulsus alternans. Pressure on the radial artery with the proximal finger eliminates the weak beats; the distal finger senses the strong beats. The rate is reduced by half. (From Understanding Cardiology © 1978. By Hywel Davies and William P. Nelson, Butterworth Publishers, Inc., 19 Cummings Park, Woburn, MA 01801. With permission.)

For example, the radial pulse is normally used for routine vital signs, but if both arms are injured and swathed in dressings or plaster casts, another site would be used. It is important to develop competence in using all of the pulse sites, so that accurate appraisals may be obtained regardless of the circumstances. Figure 24-5 shows the location and position used to palpate each pulse site.

The *temporal* artery is frequently used in children and infants. It lies just above the zygomatic bone between the lateral aspect of the eye and the hairline. Use gentle palpatory pressure.

The *facial* artery is found along the lower mandible, approximately in line with the outer aspect of the eye. It may be used when other pulses on the head or neck are not available. Use gentle palpatory pressure.

The *carotid* artery occurs below the angle of the jaw medial to the sternocleidomastoid muscle. It is a strong pulse and is used when the radial artery is not available; for example, in emergency situations. To palpate the carotid artery, turn the client's head slightly toward the side being palpated so that the sternocleidomastoid muscle is relaxed. Use gentle pressure and examine only one side at a time. In normal healthy persons, massage or compression of the carotid sinus which lies above the bifurcation of the common carotid artery often causes temporary slowing of the heart rate and a mild drop in blood pressure. Singly or in combination, these responses can seriously compromise the circulation and result in syncope or loss of consciousness in healthy persons. In elderly persons who may have heart disease, the effects may be dramatic and cause serious problems.

The *radial* artery is the most commonly used site in most appraisals because of its accessibility. It lies on the inner aspect of the wrist along the radial bone near the base of the thumb.

The *brachial* artery is most commonly used for measuring blood pressure but is also used for pulse appraisal when the radial artery cannot be used. It is found above the elbow on the anterior surface of the arm slightly above the cubital space and along the medial side of the biceps and lateral side of the triceps.

The *femoral* artery lies deep in the groin between the anterior iliac spine and the symphysis pubis. It is used most often to determine the adequacy of circulation to the extremity. It may be used for pulse appraisal when other sites are not available.

The *popliteal* artery, an extension of the femoral artery, is located deep in the tissues in the back of the knee, along the lateral (outer) side of the medial tendon. It is a difficult artery to palpate. The knee must be slightly flexed regardless of whether the person is lying on his or her back (supine) or abdomen (prone). This pulse site is used to measure blood pressure on the thigh and also to check circulation in the extremity.

The *dorsalis pedis* artery is a superficial artery on the dorsum of the foot. It lies lateral to the extensor tendon of the great toe. One or both of these arteries may be absent in about 10 percent of the population. The foot must be held in a dorsiflexed position at an angle of about 90 degrees to reduce the tension on the artery before palpation. Palpation must be light or the pulse will be obliterated. This pulse is also used to check circulation in the extremity.

The *posterior tibialis* artery is located behind the inner ankle bone, the medial malleolus. The foot must be held in a dorsiflexed position to palpate this artery also. This site is used to check circulation to the foot.

The *apical* site refers to the apex of the heart. The location of the apical pulse is found by using the fingers to palpate, identify, and count the intercostal spaces. In adults, it is used when a radial pulse is abnormal, when cardiotonic medications are administered, and when heart sounds are appraised. The use of this site requires inspection, palpation, and auscultation. In adults and children over age 4, the pulse site is usually located medial to the midclavicular line (it may be on or to the left of the line) at the fifth intercostal space, usually below the nipple. In children under age 4, it is found in the fourth intercostal space and lateral to the midclavicular line. Figure 24-6 depicts the anatomic landmarks of the chest wall. The palm and the fingers are used as shown in Figure 24-7A to palpate the general area in search of the small 2-centimeter diameter spot where the apical pulse is found. The pads of the fingers are then placed on the specific pulse site where the stethoscope diaphragm will be placed. This is shown in Figure 24-7B. The apical site is used in infants and children under 2 to 3 years old for routine appraisal of the pulse.

COMPARISON OF PULSES

The pulses in the arms, legs, and feet (the *peripheral pulses*) are palpated to determine their *presence* and *quality* in a physical examination as part of the evaluation of the cardiovascular system. Nurses are expected to compare the presence and quality of a pulse on one side of the body with its counterpart on the other side. This is particularly important when there is concern about the adequacy of blood flow to a part of the body. Pulses on both sides of the body are appraised and compared when casts or restrictive dressings are in place, after major surgery on the vascular system, and in clients who have arteriovascular diseases or diseases that have arteriovascular complications, such as diabetes mellitus. Monitoring the change in the quality of pulses may be necessary as often as every hour in some situations. The use of the rating scale is valuable in documenting changes in the pulse volume. In events that require appraisal of peripheral pulses for evaluation of blood flow, the color and temperature of the skin near and distal to the pulse site are also appraised. Inadequate blood circulation results in changes in the skin with increased paleness and decreased temperature.

The nurse may also need to compare a peripheral pulse with the apical pulse to determine if a pulse deficit is present. A *pulse deficit* occurs when a ventricular contraction is not strong enough to produce a palpable peripheral pulse. A deficit is present when the number

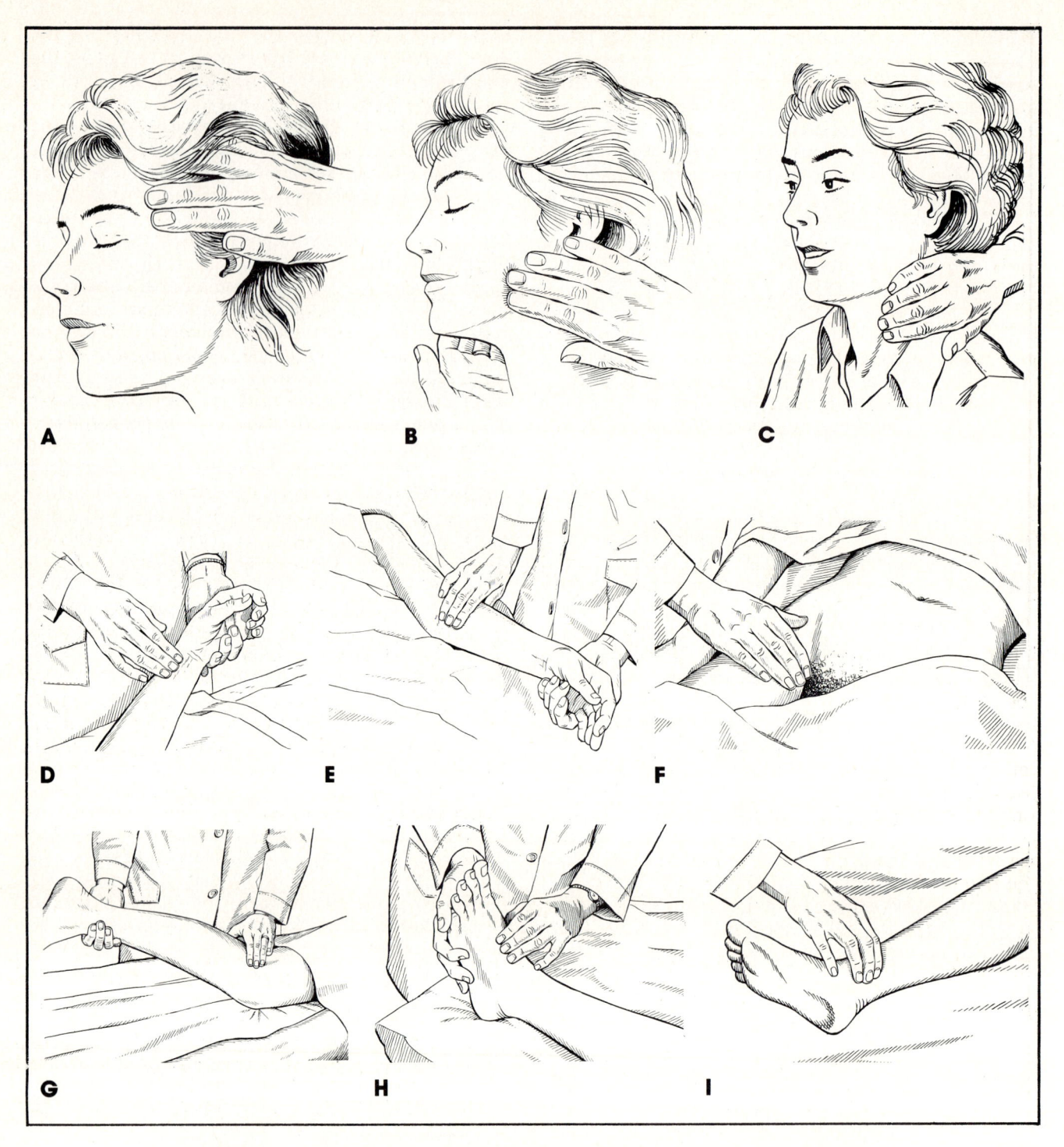

Figure 24–5. Pulse sites. **A.** Temporal artery. Gentle palpation of the temporal artery above the zygomatic bone between the lateral aspect of the eye and the hairline. **B.** Facial artery. Gentle palpation of the facial artery along the lower mandible, approximately in line with the outer aspect of the eye. **C.** Carotid artery. Gentle palpation of the carotid artery below the angle of the jaw medial to the sternocleidomastoid muscle. The head is turned slightly toward the side being palpated to relax the sternocleidomastoid muscle. Only one side is palpated at a time to avoid reducing the pulse rate. **D.** Radial artery. Palpation of the radial artery on the inner aspect of the wrist along the radial bone near the base of the thumb. **E.** Brachial artery. Palpation of the brachial artery above the elbow on the anterior surface of the arm slightly above the cubital space and along the medial side of the biceps and lateral side of the triceps. **F.** Femoral artery. Palpation of the femoral artery deep in the groin between the anterior iliac spine and the symphysis pubis. **G.** Popliteal artery. Palpation of the popliteal artery deep in the tissues in the back of the knee, along the lateral side of the medial tendon. The prone position is demonstrated. **H.** Dorsalis pedis. Palpation of the dorsalis pedis artery on the dorsum of the foot, lateral to the extensor tendon of the great toe. **I.** Posterior tibialis. Palpation of the posterior tibialis artery behind the medial malleolus.

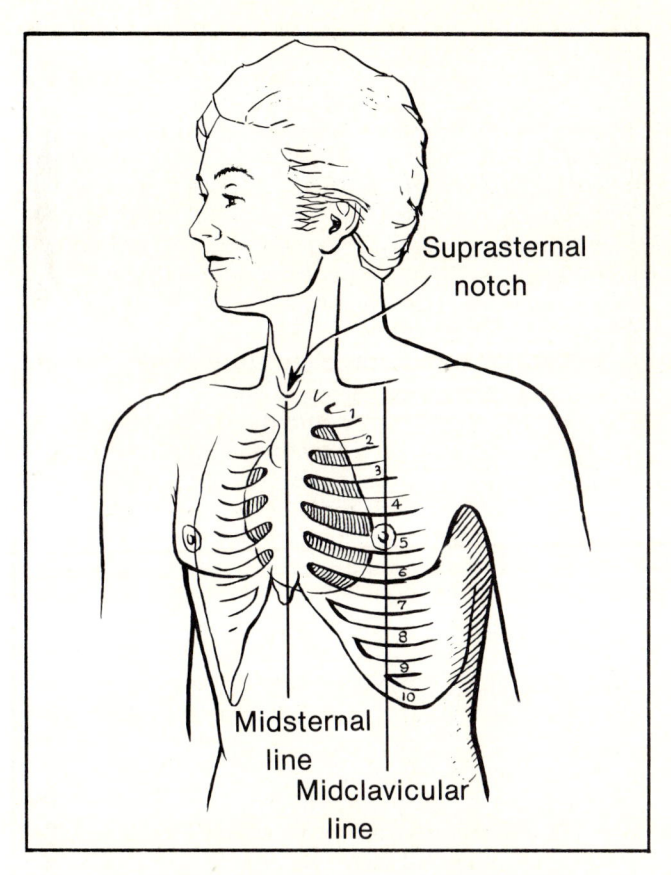

Figure 24-6. The anatomic landmarks of the chest wall.

of counted apical and peripheral pulsations is not the same. Pulse deficits may occur when a client has premature ventricular contractions or atrial fibrillation.

A pulse deficit is detected by simultaneously counting the apical and radial pulse beats. This requires two persons, one listening to and counting the apical pulse while the other simultaneously palpates and counts the radial pulse. If only one nurse is available to take the pulse, then he or she listens to and counts the apical beats while simultaneously palpating the radial pulse to determine if both beats are in synchrony and have approximately the same rate. It is not possible for one nurse to count both pulses accurately at the same time.

DATA BASE

The pulse is normally monitored with other vital signs. A change in temperature, respiration, or blood pressure may indicate a need for more frequent monitoring, even as often as every 5 minutes in certain situations. The relationship among them is such that marked increases or decreases of one sign affect another.

Client History and Recorded Data

In any incident where an unexpected or undesired response to a medication or treatment occurs, and when there is evidence of fluid or blood loss, the pulse is frequently the first vital sign to be taken. The pulse is always taken before a cardiotonic medication is administered. Knowledge of the client's pattern of previous pulse rates, rhythms, and volume permits a more intelligent understanding of what changes in any pulse characteristic mean for that particular individual. Objective data obtained from the health record and the use of physical appraisal skills combined with subjective information from the client, provide a rational basis for monitoring the pulse and making clinical judgments. Verbal and nonverbal expressions of weakness, difficulty in breathing, and chest pain are a few of the indicators that mark a need for pulse appraisal.

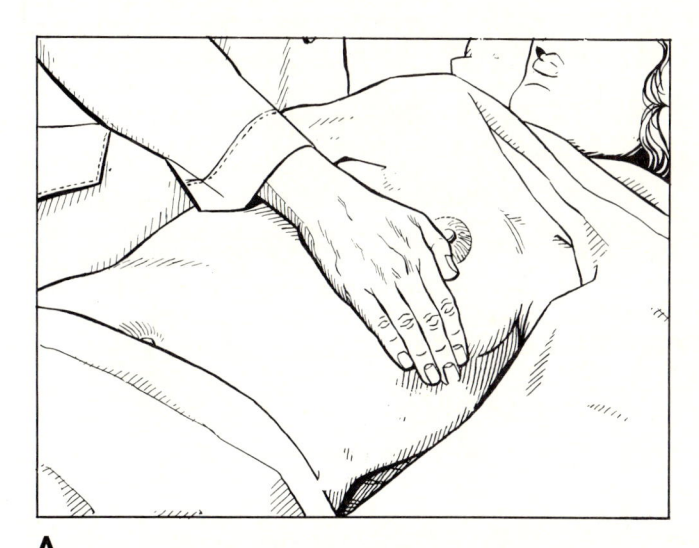

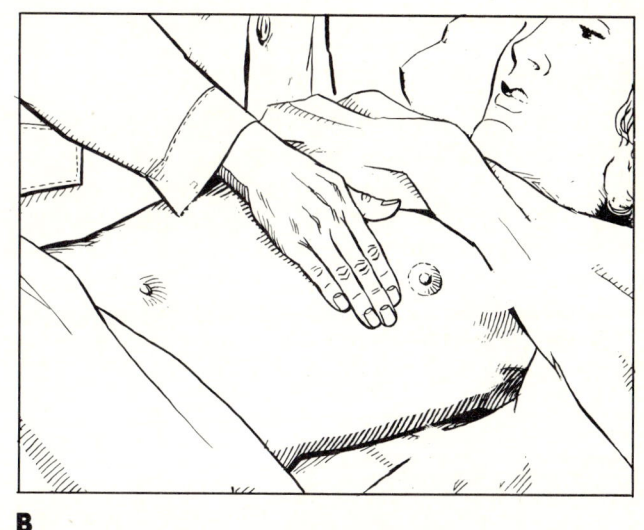

Figure 24-7. Palpation of the apical pulse site. **A.** The palm and fingers are placed over the chest wall at the midclavicular line at the fifth intercostal space to locate the pulse site. **B.** Apical site. The pads of the fingers are placed over the exact location of the apical pulse.

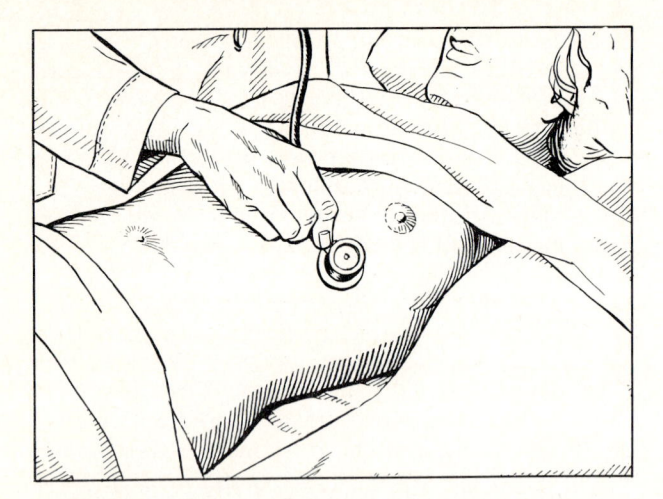

Figure 24-8. The stethoscope diaphragm in place over the apical pulse site for auscultation to count the rate.

Physical Appraisal Skills

Inspection. Inspection is used to identify the appropriate landmarks for the specific site selected before attempting to locate the arterial pulsation by palpation.

Palpation. Palpation is used to find the strongest pulsation of the artery and to detect the rhythm and quality of the pulse. When sensitively executed, it is also possible to identify any vibrations that may be present. The finger pads are placed flat and lightly against the pulse site to prevent obliterating the pulse. Gradual pressure is applied once the pulse is detected and until the pulse is obliterated, and then the pressure is released until the strongest pulse is perceived. Too little pressure or too much pressure obscures the real quality of the pulse and can also alter the rhythm.

Auscultation. Auscultation is necessary to hear the sounds of the apical heartbeat. Figure 24-8 shows how the stethoscope diaphragm is placed over the apical pulse site.

EQUIPMENT

There is no special equipment used to appraise the pulse in most routine situations, other than the palpating fingers. A stethoscope is used to obtain an apical pulse. The hands and the instrument need to be clean.

☐ EXECUTION

The length of time during which the pulse rate should be counted is a matter of considerable disagreement. There is no hard and fast rule that can be applied. The guiding principle to be observed in making a decision is to know the purpose for which the pulse is being monitored and to determine the rhythm of the pulse and its quality before selecting a 15-, 30-, or 60-second time interval. In a study by Jones (1970), the 15-second time period resulted in the most accurate counts for pulses with normal rhythms. Pulse rates over 120 beats per minute, as determined by electrocardiographs, were least accurate when counted for 30 seconds by graduate nurses. Jones suggests the use of a method other than palpation for rapid rates. The auscultatory method with the apical beat provides another option to improve accuracy.

Regardless of the time period used to count the pulse rate, the count should be started with zero, not one. This is because it is necessary to count the beats that occur during the interval. The first pulse beat that occurs at the beginning of the time interval is counted as zero, the second beat as one, the third beat as two, and so on, until the time interval is complete. Only the beats that occur within the time interval are counted, not those before or after. The error in a count started with one will be at least four beats in a 60-second interval when the number of beats is counted for 15 seconds and multiplied by four to obtain the rate for 1 minute. Larger errors result when beats occurring before or after the time interval are also counted (Hargest, 1974).

There are also factors in the environment that may alter the pulse rate and interfere with obtaining an accurate pulse appraisal. It is important for the nurse to recognize when this occurs. For example, a roommate, noise, confusion, visitors, or health-care personnel may cause stress for the client and result in a change in the pulse rate, volume, or even rhythm. In such situations, the pulse should be monitored again when the client is relaxed, so that a more accurate data base is established. It is important to know how a client responds to stress and the extent to which the pulse reflects a change in emotional state.

A quiet and nondistracting environment enables the nurse to concentrate on the task of accurately monitoring the pulse.

☐ SKILL SEQUENCES

RADIAL PULSE

Step	Rationale
1. Wash hands.	Prevents cross-infection.
2. Have client in comfortable position with arm relaxed, wrist extended, and palm down. Placing client's arm over abdomen or chest facilitates counting the respirations later.	Promotes comfort of client and observer; decreases distractions from skill.

(continued)

Step	Rationale
3. Place pads of your first three fingers flat against client's skin along the radial artery at base of thumb where pulse is expected.	Pads are more sensitive; weak pulse in this area.
4. Apply light pressure; press artery against radius, keeping your fingers in same spot for about 10 seconds to feel pulse if present. If pulse is not present, move fingers slightly to right or left until found.	Pulsation is felt better when artery is pressed against bone.
5. Once pulse is felt at strongest point, apply pressure until pulse disappears; release pressure until pulse is strong again.	Too little pressure prevents feeling pulse; too much pressure obliterates pulse; need to find correct pressure.
6. Palpate pulse, noting rhythm and quality.	Identify pattern of pulse; if irregular or weak, may not feel all beats and may need to take apical pulse. Determine time interval for rate count.
7. Use second hand on watch or clock to count beat. Start count with zero; include only those beats that occur within the interval.	Inaccurate count occurs when first beat is counted as one; error is increased by counting beats before and after time interval.
8. Record pulse characteristics immediately.	

APICAL PULSE

Step	Rationale
1. Wash hands.	Prevents transfer of microorganisms.
2. Explain procedure to client.	
3. Close room door, draw cubicle curtains.	Provides privacy.
4. Clean stethoscope ear tips and diaphragm with alcohol.	Prevents transfer of microorganisms from stethoscope between observer and clients.
5. Position client in supine or sitting position.	Provides full access to chest for palpation and auscultation.
6. Remove client's gown and bed covers to expose left chest.	Permits identification of landmarks.
7. Drape covers and gown over shoulders and right chest.	Preserves modesty and prevents client from chilling.
8. Identify midclavicular line.	First landmark for pulse site.
9. Palpate and count intercostal spaces to the fifth intercostal space.	Second landmark.
10. Place your palm and fingers flat against client's skin over apical area; move hand until pulse is found. If unable to locate apical beat, have client turn on left side; resume palpation to find site. Pulse may be appraised in this position.	Provides better coverage of precordium to find exact pulse site. Moves heart closer to chest wall.
11. Remove your hand and place pads of fingers over exact spot of pulse. Note site.	Identifies site for stethoscope diaphragm placement.
12. Warm chestpiece by rubbing it against the palm of your hand.	Cold diaphragm can cause discomfort and increase pulse rate.
13. Place ear tips in ears properly.	
14. Place diaphragm on apical site, holding it firmly in place.	Diaphragm is used to hear high-pitched heart sounds.
15. Listen for lub-dub sounds of heartbeat; ignore breath and other sounds.	Two sounds of heartbeat for each contraction.
16. Note rhythm and quality of heartbeat.	
17. Count rate as in radial pulse for 1 full minute.	Rapid and abnormal pulse rates are counted accurately during a 60-second time interval.
18. Replace gown and bed covers; reposition client if necessary.	
19. Record findings.	
20. Clean stethoscope as in step 4.	

BRACHIAL PULSE

Step	Rationale
1. Wash hands.	Prevents transfer of microorganisms.
2. Have client in comfortable position, with arm relaxed and fully extended or slightly flexed with anterior surface up.	Provides access to pulse site.
3. Place pads of your fingers against skin in space above client's elbow, between biceps and triceps.	Locate pulse site.
4. Follow steps 4 to 8, "Radial Pulse."	

APICAL–RADIAL PULSE

Step	Rationale
1. Select a second nurse.	Two people needed to take both pulses simultaneously.
2. Determine who will take which pulse.	Nurse taking apical pulse is in charge.
3. Explain procedure to client.	
4. Each nurse locates own site.	
5. Position watch so both nurses can accurately view second hand.	Use of single timepiece ensures more accurate count.
6. Command nurse signals time to start count when both are ready.	Each notes characteristics of pulse.
7. Command nurse calls "time" at end of interval.	
8. Compare results discretely.	Differences of more than one or two beats are considered real; may need to repeat count if reason to believe it is not accurate.
9. Complete procedure as in "Apical Pulse."	

FEMORAL PULSE

Step	Rationale
1. Wash hands.	Prevents transfer of microorganisms.
2. Close door, draw cubicle curtains.	Provides privacy for client.
3. Explain procedure to client.	Site near genital area may be embarrassing to client.
4. Have client in supine position. Expose groin area on one side, drape sheet.	Protects client's modesty.
5. Use pads of your fingers to locate pulsation; relocate fingers as necessary to find pulse.	Prevents perception of own pulse.
6. Apply pressure to obliterate pulse; release until pulse is strong.	Ensures palpation of femoral artery pulse.
7. Note rhythm and quality; quantify volume using rating scale.	Use as base for comparison with other side and other previous appraisals.
8. Obtain pulse on other side.	Compare rhythm and quality.
9. Replace bed covers.	
10. Record findings.	
11. (NOTE: Both pulses can be palpated simultaneously.) Drape client's genital area.	Facilitates comparison of quality. Protects client's modesty.

POPLITEAL PULSE

Step	Rationale
1. Follow steps 1 to 3, "Femoral Pulse."	
2. Have client in supine or prone position.	
3. Flex client's knee slightly.	Reduces tension on tendons.
4. Press fingertips deep into popliteal fossa, slightly lateral to midline.	Pulse deep and not as clearly defined as at other sites.
5. If unable to feel pulse, have client assume alternate position.	Shift of body position may facilitate finding pulse site.
6. Follow steps 6 to 11, "Femoral Pulse."	

DORSALIS PEDIS PULSE

Step	Rationale
1. Wash hands.	Prevents transfer of microorganisms.
2. Explain procedure.	
3. Have client in supine or sitting position. Remove bed covers, hosiery to expose foot.	Exposes foot.
4. Place client's foot in dorsiflexed position, about 90 degrees.	Releases tension on artery.
5. Place pads of your fingers lightly on extensor of great toe.	Landmark to find pulse site.
6. Move fingers lateral to the tendon to locate pulse.	
7. Use only light pressure to palpate pulse once found.	Pulse normally not strong; too much pressure will occlude it.
8. Note presence or absence of pulse, quality.	Pulse absent in 10 percent of normal population.
9. Inspect foot for pallor, temperature, presence of skin lesions.	Changes may be result of decreased or absent blood flow.
10. Obtain pulse data on other side.	Compare quality.
11. Replace bed covers.	
12. Record findings.	
13. (NOTE: Both pulses can be palpated simultaneously.)	

POSTERIOR TIBIALIS PULSE

Step	Rationale
1. Follow steps 1 to 4, "Dorsalis Pedis Pulse."	
2. Place pads of your first fingers behind medial malleolus.	Landmark to find pulse site.
3. Start with light pressure and gradually increase pressure until pulse is found.	Pulse normally not strong; too much pressure will occlude it.
4. Relocate fingers until pulse is found.	
5. Follow steps 8 to 13, "Dorsalis Pedis Pulse."	

RECORDING

Pulse rates are usually recorded on a graph. Some flow sheets provide space for a numerical entry. Other characteristics of the pulse are written in narrative form using the standardized terms previously described in the text. It is customary to record only abnormal characteristics when monitoring heart function. When appraising the quality of perfusion in the extremities, however, it is important to describe normal and abnormal qualities. The rating scale is frequently used in combination with a stick figure (drawing) to indicate the pulse volume at each peripheral site, as shown in Figure 24–9.

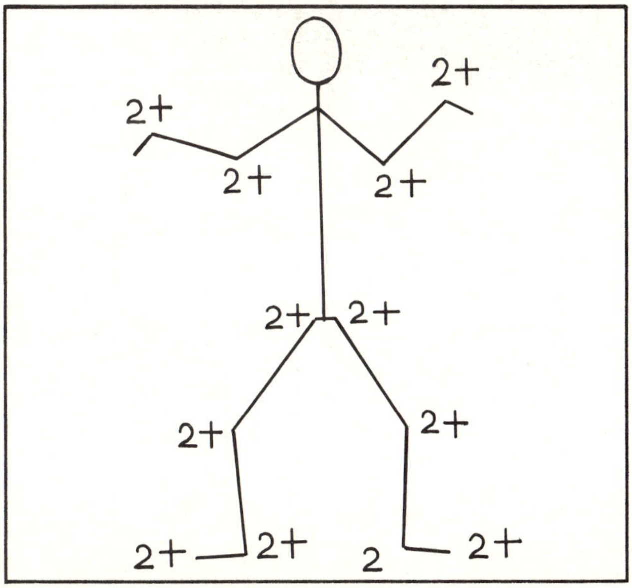

When a stick figure is not used, each pulse site is listed and the right and left side is specified for each rating. Set up in column form, it is concise and easy to read. Table 24–1 presents an example of this method of recording peripheral pulses.

Figure 24–9. Stick figure to record the quantified volume of the peripheral pulses.

TABLE 24–1. Rating Scale for Peripheral Pulses[a]

PULSE SITE	R	L
Brachial	2+	2+
Radial	2+	2+
Femoral	2+	2+
Popliteal	2+	2+
Dorsalis pedis	2+	2+
Posterior tibialis	2+	2+

[a]Scale key: 3+ = bounding; 2+ = normal; 1+ = weak; 0 = absent.

Sample Narrative Recording
Radial pulse rate 65 and weak, apical rate 86, irregular without a pattern, some beats weak, majority are strong.

☐ CRITICAL POINTS SUMMARY

1. Wash hands.
2. Position client properly.
3. Identify landmarks for pulse site.
4. Use pads of fingers to palpate.
5. Use moderate amount of pressure in palpation.
6. Observe rhythm and quality before counting rate; note irregular rhythms.
7. Determine the time interval appropriate for the type of pulse.
8. Keep track of count.
9. Start count with zero.
10. Count only beats occurring within the time interval.
11. Count beats, not the second hand of the clock.
12. Count rate accurately.
13. Use alternate sites when indicated.
14. Recognize events that temporarily increase the pulse rate.
15. Record the characteristics and rate accurately.
16. Report the abnormal findings.

☐ LEARNING ACTIVITIES

Select a partner for the following exercises.

1. Palpate and describe your partner's pulse at each site while he or she is at rest and again after 2 to 3 minutes of vigorous exercise. Compare the difference in rate and quality. Record your findings in narrative form.
2. Locate and listen to the apical pulse beat.
3. Select a third person to serve as a subject for an apical–radial pulse appraisal.
4. Observe your own response to anxiety or fear by noting changes in your pulse rate.
5. Examine your own feelings about having an apical pulse and peripheral pulses taken. Consider the sense of privacy, modesty, and concern about whether the findings are normal.
6. Record these pulses on a graph:
   8ᴀᴍ 72   12ɴ 78   2ᴀᴍ 76   8ᴘᴍ 72   12ᴍ 68

☐ REVIEW QUESTIONS

1. Why are pulses appraised?
2. How does bradycardia differ from tachycardia?
3. What term is used for a pulse that has no discernible pattern?
4. What term is used for a pulse that has coupled beats, one strong and the other weak?
5. What mechanism is available to quantify a pulse volume when it is recorded?
6. Which pulse sites are usually used to obtain all of the pulse characteristics?
7. Which pulse sites are used to determine the adequacy of blood perfusion?
8. Describe the location of each pulse site.
9. What situations indicate a need to take an apical pulse? An apical–radial pulse?
10. How would you instruct someone to count a pulse rate?
11. What data are included in the recording of a pulse?

☐ PERFORMANCE CHECKLIST

OBJECTIVE: To use the appropriate method to monitor pulse accurately.			
CHARACTERISTIC	RANGE OF ACCEPTABILITY	SATISFACTORY	UNSATISFACTORY
1. Washes hands.	No deviation		
2. Positions client comfortably and properly for site.	No deviation		
3. Provides privacy when appropriate.	No deviation		
4. Uses landmarks to identify site.	No deviation		
5. Palpates lightly with finger pads to identify pulse.	No deviation		
6. Obliterates pulse, then releases pressure until strongest pulse is felt.	No deviation		
7. Notes rhythm and quality.	No deviation		
8. Selects appropriate time interval.	No deviation		
9. Counts pulse accurately.	No deviation		
10. Records pulse characteristics using standard terms.	No deviation		

REFERENCES

Davies H, Nelson WP: Understanding Cardiology. Woburn, MA, Butterworth Publishers, 1978.

Fowler NO: Inspection and Palpation of Venous and Arterial Pulses: II. Examination of the heart. Dallas, American Heart Association, 1972.

Hargest T: Start your count with zero. American Journal of Nursing 74(5):887, 1974.

Kinnebrew MN: Add paradoxical pulse to your assessment routine. RN 44(11):32–33, 1981.

Jones ML: Accuracy of pulse rates counted for fifteen, thirty, and sixty seconds. Military Medicine 135(12):1127–1135, 1970.

Walker V, Selmanoff E: A note on the accuracy of the temperature, pulse and respiration procedure. Nursing Research 14(1):72–76, 1965.

BIBLIOGRAPHY

Hurst J, Logue RB, et al: The Heart: Arteries and Veins, ed 3. New York, McGraw-Hill, 1974.

O'Dell ML: Vital signs of surgical patients on routine admission to the hospital and three and six hours past admission. Military Medicine 139(9):719–721, 1974.

Patient assessment: Pulses. American Journal of Nursing 79(1):115–132, 1979.

Sparks C: Peripheral pulses. American Journal of Nursing 75(7):1132–1133, 1975.

SUGGESTED READING

Kinnebrew MN: Add paradoxical pulse to your assessment routine. RN 44(11):32–33, 1981.

AUDIOVISUAL RESOURCES

How to Take Your Patient's Pulse and Respiration
Filmstrip and cassette. (1975, Color, 40 min.)
Available through:
Techniques Learning Council
921 East Green Street
Pasadena, CA 91106

Measuring Vital Signs/Pulse
Videocassette (½ in, ¾ in). (1977, Color, 14 min.)
Available through:
Indiana University, School of Nursing
NICER Department
1100 West Michigan Street
Indianapolis, IN 46223

SKILL 25   Respiration Appraisal

PREREQUISITE SKILLS

Skill 19, "Inspection"
Skill 20, "Palpation"
Skill 22, "Auscultation"
Skill 28, "Handwashing"

☐ STUDENT OBJECTIVES

1. Explain the purpose of appraising respiration.
2. Explain the terms used for the characteristics of respiration.
3. Explain the methods used to obtain basic information about respiratory status.
4. Use the correct method to appraise respiration.
5. Record correctly the data pertinent to respiration.

☐ INTRODUCTION

Respiration is the vital and complex process common to all living things taking in oxygen and eliminating carbon dioxide, water, and waste products of cell metabolism. One respiratory cycle is comprised of inspiration and expiration. An appraisal of the functional status of the respiratory system is usually conducted at the same time other vital signs such as temperature and pulse are monitored. A more in-depth appraisal of ventilation is presented in Chapter 15.

Traditionally, the only datum routinely recorded about the respiratory status of a client is the rate, and there is evidence from several research studies to indicate that this is seldom measured accurately. Walker and Selmanoff (1965) found that 43 percent of the measurements made by the nursing personnel varied by more than four respirations per minute from the investigators' counts. Kory (1957) also documented consistent discrepancies between the counts made by personnel and the counts made by investigators. Eisman (1970) found that while more than half of the nurses interviewed actually counted the rate, the others only estimated it.

The clinical value of measuring respiratory rate without appraising other characteristics of respiration is relatively low, and when the rate measurement is inaccurate it is of no value. In fact measurement of rate alone may be detrimental to the client because it provides incomplete data about the client's respiratory status. Kory (1957) suggests that a more efficient use of personnel's time would be to appraise and describe the character and rate of breathing only on clients who have a specific medical order for it to be done.

Many agencies now omit the routine respiration appraisal for clients with normal patterns. The nurse has a responsibility to be aware of the respiratory status of clients who do not have a specific medical order, so that changes will be detected. This monitoring is done by observing the respiratory characteristics to determine if there are changes that indicate some type of respiratory distress. This information is then used to decide if more frequent systematic appraisals of each of the characteristics should be done.

☐ PREPARATION

CHARACTERISTICS OF RESPIRATION

The process of respiration is described by the characteristics of rate, rhythm, depth, and pattern.

Rate

The *rate* of respirations is the number of cycles that occur in 1 minute. A cycle consists of one inspiration and one expiration. This can be counted by inspection or palpation. The normal rate, like that of the pulse, varies with age but there is no sex-related difference. The ratio of respiration to pulse is 1:4. An infant's respiratory rate ranges from 30 to 80 per minute and slows as the child matures. By age 2, it ranges from 25 to 35 per minute and continues to decrease as the efficiency of gas exchange increases. By the adult years, the normal range is from 14 to 20 per minute. According to the results of the study by Zikria et al. (1974), the normal rate per minute may actually be 14 plus or minus 4 for adults. As the metabolic rate decreases in older age, the respiratory rate also decreases. A respiratory rate of less than 10 per minute is called *bradypnea* and may be caused by opiates or a depressed respiratory center. *Tachypnea* is a rate that exceeds 24 per minute and is seen in pneumonia, respiratory insufficiency, and fever. For every degree of elevation above the normal temperature, the respiratory rate increases by four cycles.

Rhythm

The *rhythm* of normal respirations is even, with equal intervals between each cycle; the chest usually moves symmetrically. The rhythm is described as either regular or irregular. *Eupnea* means easy, effortless, quiet breathing and is used to describe normal respirations.

Depth

The *depth* of respiration refers to the volume of air inhaled and exhaled. Accurate measurement of this characteristic is possible only with special pulmonary equipment. Without such equipment, the depth can be grossly appraised by observing the amount of effort used in the act of breathing and the extent to which the accessory muscles of the neck and shoulder girdle are used during inspiration. When at rest, children and men normally use the diaphragm in breathing, and women tend to use the thorax or intercostal muscles. In addition to inspiration of the chest during respiration, the depth can be gauged by holding the back of the hand near the nose to feel the flow of air passing through the nostrils during expiration. Depth of respiration can be described as deep or shallow. *Hyperpnea* is the term used for an increase in depth of respiration.

Pattern

The *pattern* of respiration, sometimes referred to as the character, is described as an appraisal of the *rate, rhythm,* and *depth* characteristics found in normal and abnormal conditions. In a normal state, it is a pattern of fairly rapid inspiration, a pause, and then expiration, which is slightly longer than inspiration, followed by another prolonged pause before the next inspiration.

Hyperventilation is deep and rapid breathing in which more air is inspired but little or no change occurs in the amount of oxygen taken to the lungs. However, an increased amount of carbon dioxide eliminated through expiration causes a decrease in the blood level of carbon dioxide. This is seen in normal persons during moderate to extreme physical exertion, anxiety, fear, or fever and in clients with abnormal conditions such as damage to the midbrain, overdose of salicylates, and diabetic or hepatic coma. *Kussmaul respirations* are a type of hyperventilation presented by deep breathing with long sighing exhalations, which is seen in diabetic coma. *Hypoventilation* usually has an irregular or slow rate and shallow depth. It results in a decreased amount of oxygen and an increase in the amount of carbon dioxide retained. Bed rest, conscious splinting of the chest because of pain, drugs that depress the central nervous system, neurologic impairment, and diseases that decrease the surfaces of the alveoli are some of the causes of hypoventilation. The adequacy of the gas exchange in either hyperventilation or hypoventilation can only be determined by laboratory tests for blood gas levels.

Apnea means a cessation of respirations. It may be periodic or prolonged due to obstruction of the airway by a foreign body, mucous plug, or vomitus; damage to the respiratory center in the brain; drugs that depress the central nervous system; or insufficient carbon dioxide in the blood. There obviously is a limit on how long apnea can be present and life be sustained. *Cheyne-Stokes respiration* is a pattern consisting of cycles of increased rate and depth, followed by decreased rate and depth, then a period of apnea. It may be a variation of normal respiration seen in children or the aged during sleep, or it may be an abnormal respiration related to heart failure, drug overdose, meningitis, or increased intracranial pressure (Fig. 25–1).

Dyspnea is a term that is often used to describe two different types of client responses to respiratory difficulty. For objective data, dyspnea describes a condition in which several respiratory characteristics are

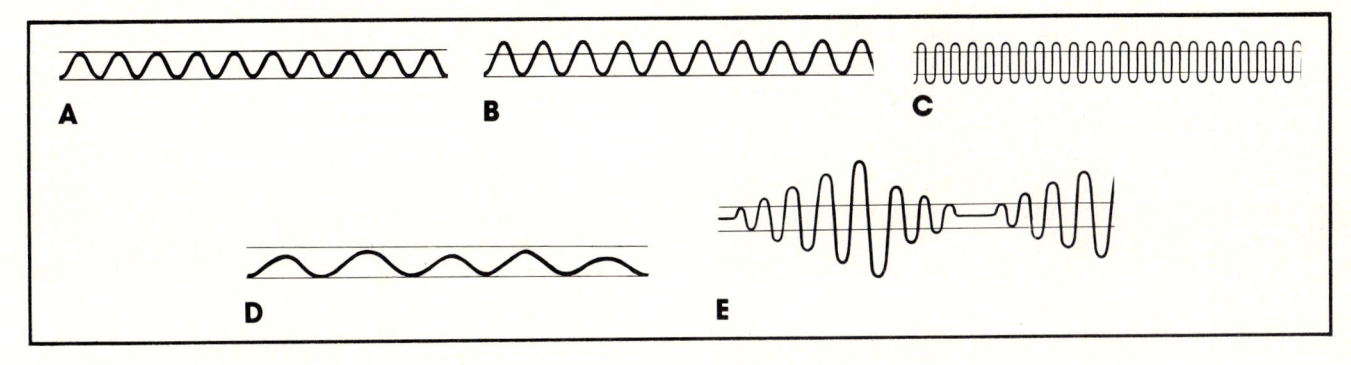

Figure 25–1. **A.** *Eupnea. Normal respirations. Even inspiration and expiration at a rate of 10 to 18 per minute for adults.* **B.** *Hyperpnea. Only the depth is increased. The rate is unchanged.* **C.** *Hyperventilation. The depth and rate of inspiration and expiration is increased.* **D.** *Hypoventilation. The rate is irregular or slow, and the depth is shallow.* **E.** *Cheyne-Stokes. The cycle consists of a gradual increase in the rate and depth, then a decrease in the rate and depth, followed by a period of apnea.*

combined into a specific pattern. A client is considered dyspneic when he or she has tachypnea, nasal flaring, tensing of the chest and neck muscles in an attempt to take in more air, and a facial expression of distress. The client may not be aware of the respiratory difficulty he or she is experiencing, and the nurse needs to be alert to the cues offered by these physical signs as well as to behavior changes. For example, the client may unconsciously pause in the middle of an activity for a rest to "catch some breath." It is important that the nurse be able to identify the degree of dyspnea the client is experiencing in relation to the amount of physical exertion, because this information may be indicative of the extent of heart or lung disease. The most severe degree of dyspnea is known as *orthopnea*. Orthopnea is present when the client must elevate the head and trunk in an upright position while at rest in order to breathe adequately (DeGowin and DeGowin, 1981).

For subjective data, dyspnea is used to describe what a client is experiencing when he or she is not getting enough air. The client may state that he or she is short of breath, smothering, or having a tightness in the chest. These sensations may or may not be accompanied by physical manifestations described earlier.

BREATH SOUNDS

Normal respiration is silent, so when sounds are heard without the use of a stethoscope, the nurse listens carefully in order to describe them accurately. *Sighing* is heard on prolonged expiration that follows deep inspiration. Occasional sighing is normal; however, frequent sighing is a sign of emotional tension. *Stertor* is a snoring respiration that occurs while awake as well as in sleep and results from secretions in the trachea or large bronchi of the upper airway. *Wheezing* occurs with expiration and is caused by air passing through a partially obstructed small bronchi and bronchioles. It is a high-pitched musical whistling sound often heard in persons who have asthma or emphysema. *Stridor* occurs on inspiration and is caused by an obstruction in the larynx or trachea. A harsh crowing sound is produced on inspiration or expiration when foreign bodies, laryngitis, or laryngeal spasm (as in croup) are present.

DATA BASE

Client History and Recorded Data
The client's previous pattern of respirations, medical diagnosis, and current health status make up the data base on which decisions are made regarding the frequency and scope of respiration appraisal. Abnormal respiratory characteristics are frequently found in clients who have cardiac disease such as congestive heart failure; pulmonary infections or diseases such as pneumonia, emphysema, or cancer; or neurologic disease such as amyotrophic lateral sclerosis. The nurse is also aware that anesthesia depresses respiratory function, and that the pain that accompanies surgical incisions and other wounds of the chest or abdomen affects the movements required by normal respiration. Clients with such pain often attempt to reduce the pain by breathing less deeply, thus reducing their respiratory function. There are also specific symptoms that indicate to the nurse a need for more frequent appraisals. These symptoms include shortness of breath, wheezing, dyspnea, orthopnea, and chest pain.

Physical Appraisal Skills
Respiration appraisal can be done either overtly (with the client's knowledge) or covertly (with the client unaware that an appraisal is being done). Since the character of respirations may be altered if the client is aware of being observed, covert appraisal is more common for routine monitoring. However, the amount of data the nurse is able to obtain is limited with a covert appraisal, because the position of the client and the presence of clothing may prevent good visualization of the chest movements.

Inspection. The rate of respiratory cycles per minute is determined by *inspection*. This is done by watching the rise and fall of the chest and the symmetry of the chest expansion during each cycle. Another method frequently used to count the respiratory rate is to place the client's arm over his or her chest or upper abdomen at the time the pulse is monitored and then to observe the rise and fall of the client's arm while it moves during the respiratory cycle. When undergoing either procedure, clients usually keep their clothing on, but if there is some question about a client's respiratory status, it is best to remove the clothing. The amount of effort used during respiration and the extent to which the pectoral, sternocleidomastoid, scalene, and intercostal and abdominal muscles are used as accessories for inspiration or expiration is noted. In some conditions, the nostrils may flare on inspiration. An anxious facial expression, the degree of mental alertness, and the color of the skin around the mouth, lips, nose, and earlobes are also noted for evidence of inadequate gas exchange during respiration. Inadequate gas exchange and perfusion is eventually reflected by a color change to a dusky blue hue (cyanosis).

The position the person chooses to assume during respiration is also important. Persons with respiratory problems often alter their posture by sitting upright with the shoulders hunched forward and arms elevated to permit more chest expansion.

Palpation. *Palpation* can be used to feel the rise and fall of the chest during respiration. This is done by placing the hand directly on the chest.

Auscultation. *Auscultation* without a stethoscope is used to listen for the quality of breath sounds during inspiration and expiration.

☐ EXECUTION

The rate, rhythm, depth, and pattern of respiration can be appraised with the client in any position that permits visualization of the chest movements. It is important that there be adequate light to permit inspection of the chest. When the characteristics of respiration are abnormal, it may be necessary to place the client in a sitting position so that the abnormal findings can be reappraised in a body position that facilitates respiratory function. Respirations are appraised with the client at rest. It is also necessary to determine respiratory changes that occur with physical activity when the client has a disease condition that affects respiratory function. This enables the nurse to plan aspects of nursing care within the activity tolerance of the client.

☐ SKILL SEQUENCE

RESPIRATION APPRAISAL

Step	Rationale
1. Wash hands.	Prevents transfer of microorganisms.
2. Explain procedure to client for overt appraisal only.	Prevents alteration of the respiratory pattern. Explanation is usually omitted so that client does not unconsciously alter respirations.
3. Remove client's gown if necessary to observe the chest movement. Close room door, draw cubicle curtains.	Clothing may prevent accurate appraisal of movements. Curtains provide privacy.
4. Place hand flat on chest and observe depth and symmetry of movement. Place client's arm across chest as if to monitor pulse.	Depth and symmetry may be difficult to visualize without using the hand. Covert method used to count rate, distracts client while chest is being observed.
5. Determine rhythm.	
6. Count rate of cycles for 30 seconds if regular, for 1 minute if irregular. If respirations have irregular rhythm, may need to count for more than 1 minute.	Accurate count of irregular respiratory cycles requires 1 minute.
7. Listen for breath sounds; note abnormal sounds.	Normal respiration is silent.
8. Record characteristics, using standard terms.	Documents findings for data base.

RECORDING

The form used for vital signs usually has a space for the rate of respirations. A description of the other characteristics is written in narrative form in the nurse's record.

Sample POR Recording
- S—NA
- O—Respirations shallow, irregular, and slow; chest movement symmetrical; color pale; rate 8.
- A—Hypoventilating.
- P—Placed in semi-Fowler's position, notified physician.

Sample Narrative Recording
Respirations shallow, irregular, and slow; chest movement symmetrical; color pale; rate 8. Physician notified.

4. Observe the respiratory pattern of a person with temporary or permanent respiratory problems. Note the facial expression, skin color, and use of accessory muscles. Listen for abnormal sounds.

☐ CRITICAL POINTS SUMMARY

1. Use the data base to determine the scope of the appraisal.
2. Determine rhythm, depth, and pattern before counting rate.
3. Listen for breath sounds.
4. Inspect each characteristic of respiration.
5. Count the true rate.

☐ LEARNING ACTIVITIES

Select a partner for the following exercises.

1. Note the rhythm, depth, pattern, rate, and sound of respirations at rest and again after 2 to 3 minutes of vigorous exercise. Compare the differences. Write a report of your findings.
2. Remove the clothing from the chest, use a drape for the sake of modesty, if necessary, and inspect the posterior or anterior chest for depth of movement and symmetry. Count the rate by inspection and then by palpation.
3. Observe the respiratory pattern of an infant, a child, a young adult, and an elderly person at rest and after activity. Compare the similarities and differences in each of the characteristics. Write a report of each appraisal.

☐ REVIEW QUESTIONS

1. Why are respirations appraised?
2. What characteristics of respirations are appraised?
3. How does bradypnea differ from tachypnea?
4. What does it mean when a person is described as having eupnea?
5. How would you determine the depth of a person's respiration?
6. Describe the process of normal respiration.
7. List the term or terms used to describe respirations that:
   a. are shallow and slow or irregular.
   b. have stopped for a period of time.
   c. are cycles of increased depth and rate alternated with shallow and slow respirations and periods of no breathing.
8. Name the breath sounds you would expect from someone who has:
   a. an obstruction in the larynx.
   b. partial obstruction of the small bronchi and bronchioles.
   c. secretions in the trachea.
9. What objective respiratory characteristics are obtained by inspection? By palpation? By auscultation?
10. What term is used to describe a person who says he or she is not getting enough air?
11. What information would you include in a narrative description of respirations?

☐ PERFORMANCE CHECKLIST

OBJECTIVE: To use the appropriate method to appraise respirations.			
CHARACTERISTIC	**RANGE OF ACCEPTABILITY**	**SATISFACTORY**	**UNSATISFACTORY**
1. Washes hands.	No deviation		
2. Explains procedure as appropriate to situation.	Omit when necessary.		
3. Observes for signs of abnormal respirations.	No deviation		
4. Removes gown if necessary; provides privacy.	Omit if not necessary.		
5. Places hand on chest or moves client's arm across chest.	No deviation		
6. Observes rhythm, depth, symmetry of chest movement.	No deviation		
7. Counts rate for required time interval.	No deviation		
8. Listens for breath sounds.	No deviation		
9. Accurately records characteristics of respiration using standard terms.	No deviation		

REFERENCES

DeGowin EL, DeGowin RL: Bedside diagnostic examination, ed 4. New York, Macmillan, 1981.

Eisman R: Criteria Registered Nurses Reportedly Use in Making Decisions Regarding the Observation of Respiratory Behavior of Patients. Unpublished master's thesis. Seattle, University of Washington, 1970.

Kory RC: Routine measurement of respiratory rate. Journal of the American Medical Association 165(5):448–450, 1957.

Walker V, Selmanoff E: A note on the accuracy of the temperature, pulse and respiration procedure. Nursing Research 14(1):72–76, 1965.

Zikria BA, Spencer JL, et al: Alterations in ventilatory function and breathing patterns following surgical trauma. Annals of Surgery 179(1):1–7, 1974.

BIBLIOGRAPHY

Basford P: Anatomy of respiration. Nursing Mirror 158(6):30–33, 1984.

Rochester DF: Respiratory muscle function in health. Heart and Lung 13(4):349–354, 1984.

Sorensen KC, Luckmann J: Basic Nursing: A Psychophysiologic Approach. Philadelphia, WB Saunders, 1979.

Sweetwood H: Bedside assessment of respirations. Nursing73 3(9): 50–51, 1973.

SUGGESTED READING

Sweetwood H: Bedside assessment of respirations. Nursing73 3(9): 50–51, 1973.

AUDIOVISUAL RESOURCES

Measuring Vital Signs/Respirations
Videocassette (½ in, ¾ in). (1977, Color, 10 min.)
Available through:
  Indiana University, School of Nursing
  NICER Department
  1100 West Michigan Street
  Indianapolis, IN 46223

Respirations
9 Slides. (1974, Color)
Available through:
  Robert J. Brady Company
  Route 197
  Bowie, MD 20715

SKILL 26 Blood Pressure Appraisal

PREREQUISITE SKILLS

Skill 19, "Inspection"
Skill 20, "Palpation"
Skill 22, "Auscultation"
Skill 28, "Handwashing"

STUDENT OBJECTIVES

1. Describe the purpose of measuring blood pressure.
2. Compare the methods used to measure blood pressure indirectly.
3. Explain the procedures used to measure arterial blood pressure indirectly.
4. Describe the Korotkoff sounds pertinent to each phase.
5. Explain what is meant by an auscultatory gap.
6. Summarize the factors that create errors in measurement.
7. Use the appropriate method to measure blood pressure accurately.
8. Record blood pressure accurately.

INTRODUCTION

Blood pressure is the pressure exerted by the blood against the arterial walls as it flows through the vessels. It is measured to determine the maximum pressure exerted against the arterial walls during left ventricular contraction (systole), and the lowest pressure maintained by the elastic recoil in the arterial walls during relaxation of the ventricle (diastole). Blood pressure reflects the circulating blood volume, the efficiency of the heart as a pump, the peripheral vascular resistance, the viscosity of the blood, and the elasticity of the arterial walls.

Blood pressure readings are expressed in millimeters of mercury (mm Hg). Normal readings increase gradually over the life span as each of the factors affecting blood pressure changes. For example, in the brachial artery a reading of 96 mm Hg systolic and 60 mm Hg diastolic blood pressure is normal for a 4 year old. An adult's normal blood pressure reading is 120 mm Hg systolic and less than 90 mm Hg diastolic. In the popliteal artery, systolic blood pressure may be as much as 10 to 40 mm Hg higher than in the radial artery; the diastolic blood pressure varies little from the measurement in the radial artery. During the middle and later years of life, more rapid increases may occur due to changes in vascular resistance and other physiological factors. Current recommendations from national task forces on blood pressure control and hypertension are that annual blood pressure measurements should begin at age 3 (National Heart, Lung, and Blood Institute, 1977). A baseline can thus be established as the individual grows. This enables early detection and evaluation of above-normal blood pressure measurements. A single blood pressure measurement is of little value in the detection of hypertension. Persons with one initial above-normal blood pressure reading need to have repeated measurements taken before medical evaluation is initiated.

The significance of blood pressure measurement as an indicator of health status has been attested to by numerous experimental and clinical studies. Blood pressure is a frequently measured indicator of health status obtained by nursing personnel. Combined with other data, it can be used as part of a health screening examination to determine the degree of illness or to indicate a need for change in medication or treatment.

☐ PREPARATION

Stephen Hales first measured blood pressure of animals directly through the wall of an artery in 1733. Clinically, however, the most practical method of obtaining blood pressure measurements is by the indirect method, that is, without direct contact with the blood. Indirect measurement is considered to be only an estimate of the true blood pressure; however, when it is done correctly the results correlate well with true blood pressure, which is obtained by direct measurements taken by a catheter placed into an artery. Unfortunately, there are some investigations which show that indirect measurements taken by nursing personnel are not always valid and reliable. In Wilcox's (1961) nursing research study, there was enough variation in the blood pressure readings taken by graduate nurses to raise serious questions regarding the nurses' knowledge, understanding, and interpretation of what they were measuring. Mitchell and Van Meter (1971) also found significant variations in the recorded measurements taken by four levels of nursing personnel in the clinical setting. The registered nurses' measurements varied the most. It is interesting to note that, like Glor et al. (1970), Mitchell and Van Meter found that the use of a standardized and controlled method of measuring blood pressure (as described in this skill) produced valid and reliable readings.

Indirect measurement of blood pressure dates back to 1855, when Karl Vierordt estimated the amount of counterpressure required to obliterate a peripheral arterial pulse. All of the methods by which indirect measurements can be obtained are based on the same principle: external pressure is applied to a superficial artery by means of a compression cuff so that blood pressure sounds can be detected from the artery as the pressure in the compression cuff is slowly released.

AUSCULTATORY METHOD OF MEASURING BLOOD PRESSURE

Auscultation is the most commonly used technique for measuring blood pressure in the clinical and community setting; thus, it is considered in detail throughout this skill. The equipment used includes a sphygmomanometer and a stethoscope. The sphygmomanometer includes an inflation system, through which external pressure is applied to a superficial artery, and a calibrated pressure manometer that indicates the pressure at which the blood pressure can be heard. The stethoscope is used to auscultate the blood pressure sounds. When the auscultatory method is properly executed, the measurements compare favorably with those obtained by direct arterial cannulation.

Korotkoff Sounds

Blood pressure sounds are named for a Russian surgeon, Nikolai Korotkoff, who discovered them in 1905. This led to the auscultatory method of blood pressure measurement. While the exact cause of these sounds has not yet been confirmed, it is believed that they are caused either by the vibratory motion of the arterial wall or by motion within the blood as the blood flow is reestablished with the release of the pressure in the compression cuff. There is no sound when the artery is compressed by external pressure greater than the systolic pressure, nor is there any sound when the external pressure is insufficient to collapse the artery.

As the pressure applied by the compression cuff is reduced, the sounds from the artery vary in character and pass through four phases until they disappear. The disappearance of the sounds marks the fifth phase. These phases have specific sound characteristics. The numerical points at which the specific Korotkoff sounds occur and disappear on the manometer scale must be noted to determine the systolic and diastolic blood pressure measurements.

Phase I is the systolic pressure. It is marked when two consecutive faint, clear taps have been heard. The tapping begins as soon as the pressure within the cuff has decreased enough to permit the first spurt of blood to flow through and distend the artery during ventricular contraction. The intensity of the sound seems to be related to the forcefulness of the stream of blood, which in turn depends on the speed of the rise of pressure in the artery and the volume of blood flowing. The systolic pressure measurement is read on the calibrated pressure manometer as the number at which the two clear taps are detected.

Phase II occurs when the tap changes to a murmur. This phase usually begins 10 to 15 mm Hg below the onset of phase I. The murmur is thought to be produced by the vibratory motion of the blood within the vessel wall as a result of the change in the size of the artery from narrow under the cuff to wider distal to the cuff.

Phase III begins with the disappearance of the murmur. The tapping remains and the sounds become crisper, increase in intensity, and become relatively loud and high pitched.

Phase IV is marked by sudden change as the tapping becomes lower pitched and less intense; it is described as a muffled sound that has a soft, blowing quality. The pressure reading for this phase is currently used as the diastolic reading for children. In the past, phase IV was considered the diastolic reading for adults also; therefore, some personnel may still be using this phase as the diastolic measurement for adults.

Phase V occurs when the muffled sound disappears. This phase is currently used as the diastolic reading for adults. The ability to hear the point at which the sounds disappear depends on the observer's hearing and concentration and the quality of the stethoscope (Report of the Joint National Committee on Detection, Evaluation, and Treatment of High Blood Pressure, 1978). Figure 26-1 is a pictorial representation of the sounds of Korotkoff (Ravin, 1972).

Valid comparisons of serial measurements of the systolic and diastolic blood pressure depend on the consistent use of the same point of reference for the diastolic reading by all observers. The American Heart Association recommends that the first, fourth, and fifth phases be recorded so that comparisons will be valid (Kirkendall et al., 1967). Mitchell and Van Meter (1971) found that some of the staff in their study used the fourth sound and others used the fifth sound for the diastolic pressure measurement.

Auscultatory Gap

In persons with abnormalities of the cardiovascular system, a period of silence may exist between the first and third phases. When there are no sounds in the second (murmur) phase, an auscultatory gap exists. The arterial pulse is palpable, but there are no sounds. The gap is important to recognize because it can cover a range of 40 mm Hg (Askey, 1974) and cause a significant underestimation of the systolic pressure or an overestimation of the diastolic pressure. Phase I may not be heard at all if the pressure cuff is not inflated beyond the second phase. This serious problem is eliminated by inflating the pressure cuff 30 mm Hg beyond the point at which the arterial pulse is no longer palpable. Figure 26-2 shows where the auscultatory gap occurs (Ravin, 1972).

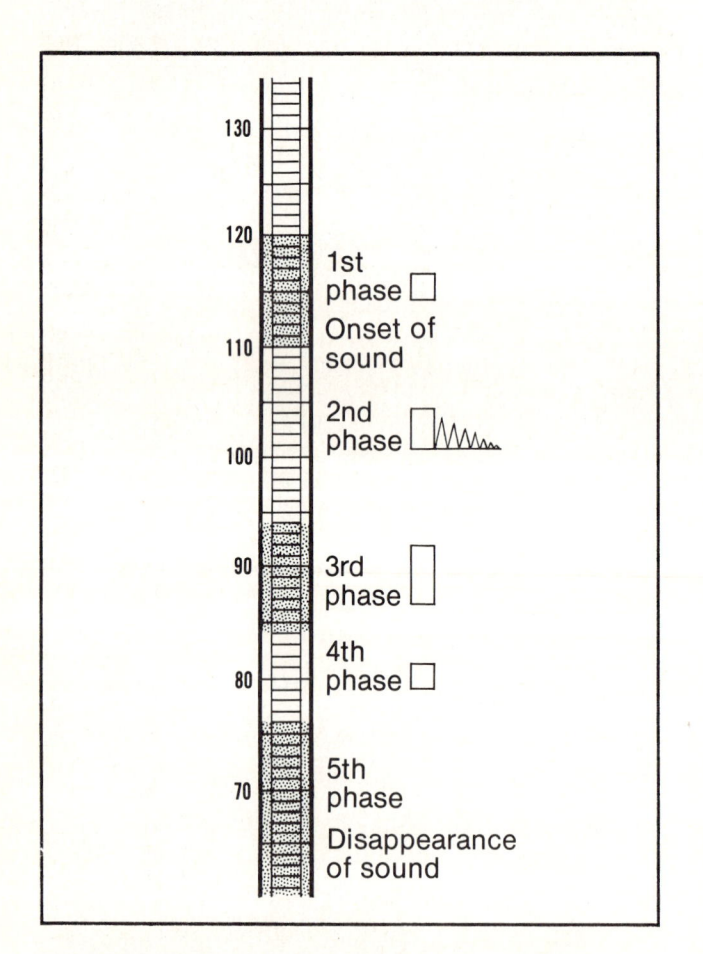

Figure 26–1. Normal blood pressure. The sounds of Korotkoff. (From Ravin A: The Clinical Significance of the Sounds of Korotkoff, audiovisual manual. West Point, PA, Merck, Sharp & Dohme, 1972, with permission.)

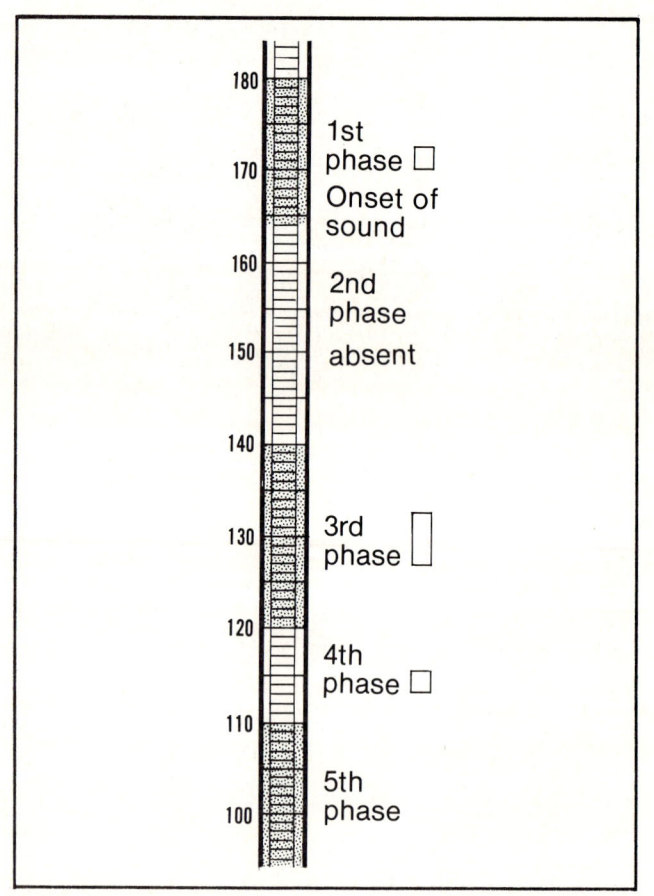

Figure 26–2. Blood pressure with an auscultatory gap; the second phase is absent. (From Ravin A: The Clinical Significance of the Sounds of Korotkoff, audiovisual manual. West Point, PA, Merck, Sharp & Dohme, 1972, with permission.)

Augmentation of Korotkoff Sounds

There are situations where the Korotkoff sounds are too faint to be heard adequately for accurate measurement. The sounds may be augmented by one of the following methods:

1. Rapid inflation of the compression cuff reduces the amount of blood in the forearm and thereby increases the difference in pressure between the upper and lower arm, resulting in louder sounds. Conversely, slow or hesitant cuff inflation decreases the sounds.
2. Elevation of the client's arm above heart level for several seconds drains out the venous blood. When the cuff is inflated with the arm raised, the sounds are louder.
3. Having the client open and close the fist several times after the cuff is inflated above the systolic level increases the capacity of the vessels in the hand and forearm to hold blood and increases the loudness of the tap and murmur.

If good technique, a quiet environment, accurate equipment, and these augmentation methods do not succeed in producing audible sounds, it may be necessary to use another method to obtain the measurement.

OTHER METHODS OF MEASURING BLOOD PRESSURE

The auscultatory method is by far the most common method of measuring blood pressure, and the equipment and procedures for auscultation of blood pressure are considered in depth later in this skill. However, alternate methods for measuring blood pressure are available when auscultation is not possible for various reasons.

Palpatory Method

This method may be used when the auscultatory method is not possible because the Korotkoff sounds are too faint to be heard and the electronic equipment necessary for other indirect methods is not available. In place of the stethoscope, some tactile sensing device, usually the fingers (or an electronic or mechanical apparatus), is used to detect the pulsations. Instead of listening for the sounds, the pulse is palpated as the compression cuff pressure is released at a rate of 2 to 3 mm Hg per heartbeat. The systolic pressure is recorded at the point when the pulse in the artery returns. As described by Enselberg (1961), the diastolic pressure is best detected with light to moderate palpatory pressure applied to the brachial artery. It is identified by a single whip-like vibration, which is felt in addition to the arterial pulsation and occurs at the point when the pressure in the cuff nears the diastolic blood pressure. The sensation quickly disappears when the cuff pressure is below the diastolic level. Its presence may be more marked in some persons than in others. Putt (1966) conducted a direct comparison study of auscultatory and palpatory readings, and concluded that measurements obtained by palpation of the brachial artery were within the acceptable range of error of plus or minus 8 mm Hg set by the American Heart Association, p. 308.

Flush Method

The flush method is used on infants when the Korotkoff sounds are too faint to permit using the auscultatory method and the electronic equipment necessary for measurement by other methods is not available. The measurement depends on a vascular flush. This is a skin color change in the extremity from pallor to redness when circulation resumes as the compression on the extremity is released.

The flush method must be done while the infant is quiet, because crying increases the blood pressure. Soothe the infant with a pacifier or bottle, and wrap an infant-size cuff (2.5 centimeters (1 in) wide) snugly around the extremity above the wrist or ankle. Then squeeze the extremity just below the cuff with a hand or a tightly wrapped elastic bandage. Simultaneously pump the manometer up to 120 to 140 mm Hg; this blanches the extremity below the cuff. The hand or bandage must be released at the same time the pressure is released at a rate of no faster than 5 mm Hg per second. This usually requires two persons to be involved in taking the measurement. The point at which the flushing occurs in the extremity is the mean diastolic pressure.

In a comparison study by Virnig and Reynolds (1974), the flush method results correlated well with the mean aortic pressures obtained in well and sick infants, particularly in the right arm. However, in a report issued by the Task Force on Blood Pressure Control in Children (National, 1977), this method is considered most useful in determining if there is a difference between the pressures in the upper and lower extremities. They consider use of the ultrasonic device to be preferable to use of the flush method, because the former records the systolic and diastolic pressures and can be executed by only one person, while the latter provides only a mean pressure.

DATA BASE

Client History and Recorded Data

Clients with medical diagnoses such as heart disease, hypertension, or intracranial pressure often require more frequent monitoring of their blood pressure. A medical order may specify that blood pressure measurements be taken on a regular basis; or, the nurse may take a measurement because the data available indicate the need for more frequent monitoring of blood pressure. Data that could signal a need for more frequent measurements include a change in pulse rate, rhythm, or quality; a change from the baseline blood pressures; a change in the client's temperature; or sudden changes in other aspects of the client's condition. Subjective data indicating a need to measure blood pressure could include a client's complaints of weakness or faintness, severe headache, chest pain, or difficulty in breathing.

Physical Appraisal Skills

Inspection. Inspection is used to confirm the correct position of the body and the physical condition and position of the extremity before taking a measurement. Blood pressure should not be measured on an extremity with surgical wounds, intravenous fluids, renal dialysis shunts, or paralysis. Clients who have had a radical mastectomy should not have the arm on the operative side used for measurements. Inspection is also used to select the appropriate pulse site for measurement.

Palpation. Palpation is used to identify the strongest impulse from the artery to be used for measurement. Slight adjustments of the palpatory pressure may be necessary in order to detect the strongest impulse. Too much pressure may obliterate the impulse; too little pressure may prevent finding the correct pulse pressure. There are cases in which a slight internal or external rotation of the forearm will change the position of the brachial artery and permit easier palpation and auscultation.

Auscultation. Auscultation is used to detect and discriminate among the different phases of sound over the blood pressure range. If the strongest impulse has not been identified properly, the observer may not be able to distinguish adequately among the four phases of the blood pressure sounds. The sounds may be obliterated or changed if too much pressure is applied over the arterial pulsation with the stethoscope chestpiece.

EQUIPMENT

The sphygmomanometer is the standard instrument used to measure blood pressure. There are two types of calibrated pressure manometers: mercury and aneroid. Since 1875, the mercury manometer has served as the standard for measurement; therefore, blood pressure readings are obtained in millimeters of mercury (mm Hg). Both types of manometers have an inflation system to compress the artery and a calibrated instrument from which the measurement is read. The component parts of the mercury and aneroid manometers and the inflation system are shown in Figure 26-3.

The Inflation System

The inflation system consists of a compression cuff with an inflatable rubber bladder and a rubber pressure bulb with a control valve used to inflate and deflate the cuff. It is connected to the manometer by rubber tubing.

The cuff fabric should be made of a nonstretch material, so that the pressure created by the inflatable

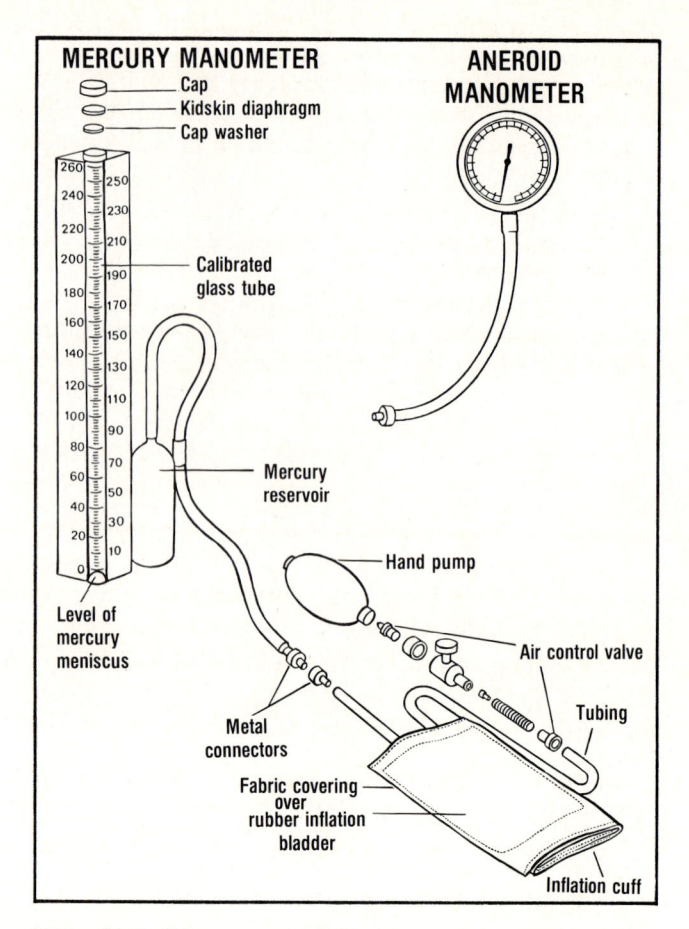

Figure 26-3. Sphygmomanometer. Mercury and aneroid manometers with the component parts of the inflation system. (Adapted from: Baumometer Service Manual. WA Baum Co, Inc, Copiague, NY 11726, 1975.)

bladder is distributed evenly over the extremity. The inflatable bladder must be 20 percent wider than the diameter of the extremity in order to compress an adequate length of the artery for valid measurements (Fig. 26-4). The bladder length should be adequate to encircle at least half of the extremity, and particular attention must be given to placing the bladder directly over the artery. These standards, recommended by the American Heart Association in 1967 (Kirkendall et al., 1967), are supported by studies conducted by Burch and Shewey (1973). King (1967, 1969) suggests that a more accurate estimation of the true arterial pressure is obtained with an inflatable bladder that encircles the entire extremity. Cuffs and bladders are available in different lengths and widths for use on both arms and thighs of infants, children, and obese persons. It is the size of the extremity that is important in selecting a cuff, not the age of the person.

When soiled, the fabric cuff is sponged clean with a damp cloth or hand washed with a detergent disinfectant after the inflation bag has been removed. After rinsing, the cuff is air dried. The exterior of the inflation system is cleaned by wiping it with 70 percent alcohol or a detergent disinfectant.

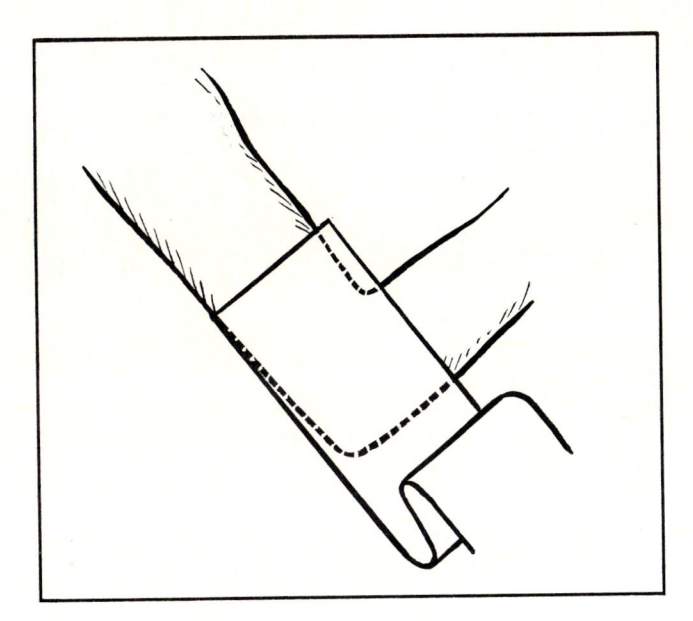

Figure 26-4. Measurement of the cuff with the extremity to ensure the appropriate size. The cuff must be 20 percent wider than the diameter of the extremity.

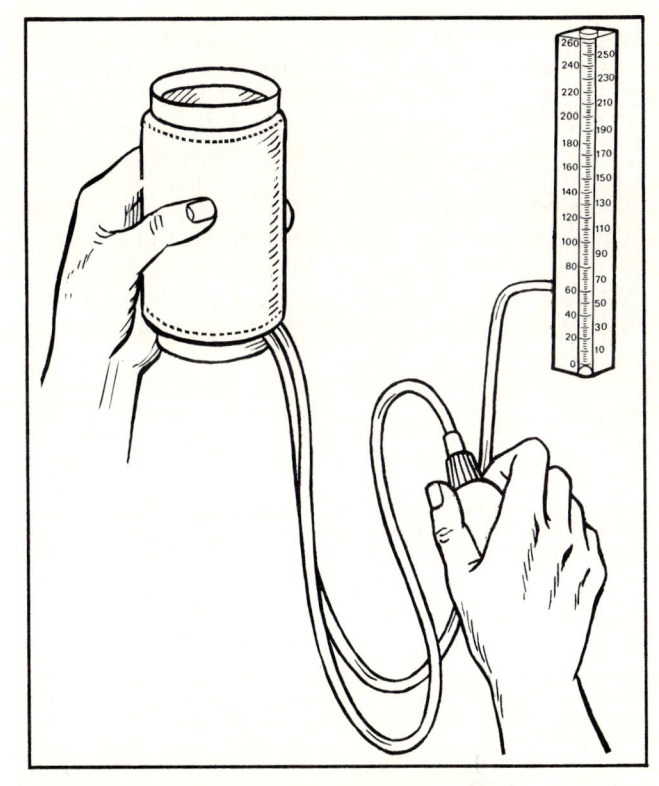

Figure 26-5. Testing the inflation system for air leaks. Close the control valve; then begin at the bladder end to roll the cuff tightly and hold it securely. Inflate the cuff to 250 mm Hg, release the control valve to reduce the pressure to 200 mm Hg, and then close the valve. Observe the manometer for a drop in pressure.

Faulty equipment may result in inaccurate blood pressure measurements. If the compression system does not seem to be properly responding to inflation and deflation of the manometer, it should be inspected to determine the problem. Although many institutions have persons available to service equipment, it falls to the nurse to identify faulty equipment and, in some cases, to make minor repairs.

To check the inflation system for leaks, inspect the outer fabric of the cuff to determine if there are any ripped seams that would permit the bladder to bulge during inflation, thereby reducing the pressure exerted against the artery. The tubing and hand pump should be inspected for cracks or punctures. Each metal connector in the rubber tubing must be tightened securely. If a leak is found at the end of a segment, short sections of the rubber tubing may be cut off. A faulty pressure bulb must be replaced.

Less obvious leaks can be identified as follows: Wrap the cuff tightly and secure it at the end. With the control valve closed, pump up the pressure to 250 mm Hg, open the valve slightly to reduce the pressure to 200 mm Hg, and reclose the valve (Fig. 26-5). Any drop in pressure on the manometer indicates a leak. To find the source of the leak, pinch off different segments of tubing at several points between the manometer and the cuff and the cuff and the control valve, checking each segment for a leak. Remove the leaking section if possible. Reinflate the manometer as often as necessary to complete the test.

If no leaks are found in a malfunctioning system, check the bulb, control valve, and tubing for debris. Conceicao et al. (1976) reported that almost half of the mercury manometers in a teaching hospital had sticky, leaky, or blocked control valves that interfered with accurate readings. Many of the instruments that functioned improperly had excessive air resistance because of dirty filters in the air control valve. This is resolved by separating the bulb and the valve from the tubing and squeezing the hand pump several times to dislodge the debris. In some models, the bulb can be removed from the valve to clean the filter.

The Mercury-Gravity Manometer

This instrument consists of a vertical glass column calibrated in units with a mercury reservoir at the bottom. The reservoir must have sufficient mercury to fill the vertical column to the level of zero on the scale before any pressure is applied to the mercury. The pressure contained in the cuff exerts force against the mercury in the manometer and thrusts it up the glass column. The mercury manometer does not have to be recalibrated and is considered more accurate than the aneroid manometer. However, it does need to be checked at least once a year to ensure accurate functioning.

The mercury manometer is available in portable, upright, and wall-mounted models. It must be placed on a level surface at a height that permits the observer to view the mercury meniscus at eye level. The meniscus shape at the zero point on the scale should have a smooth and well-defined curve. Dirt in the mercury or the glass tube will give an irregular shape to the meniscus, elevate the level above zero, and cause bubbles in the column during inflation.

If cleaning is needed, remove the mercury by unscrewing the cap at the top of the glass column, removing the diaphragm and the washer, and then tip the manometer back and forth to facilitate pouring out the mercury. Insert a paper cone with a pinhole in the apex into a clean, dry container, pour the mercury into the cone and let it drip through slowly. The dirt will float to the top. Discard the last drop.

To remove the glass tube from the manometer, place the manometer on its side with the reservoir below the tube. Pull the mechanism that releases the tube and lift or slide the tube out of place (Fig. 26–6). Wash the tube in water with detergent and rinse it with water; then use alcohol to dry it. Or, use pipe cleaners or cotton swabs to clean out debris. To force the dirt out of the reservoir, squeeze the hand pump a few times.

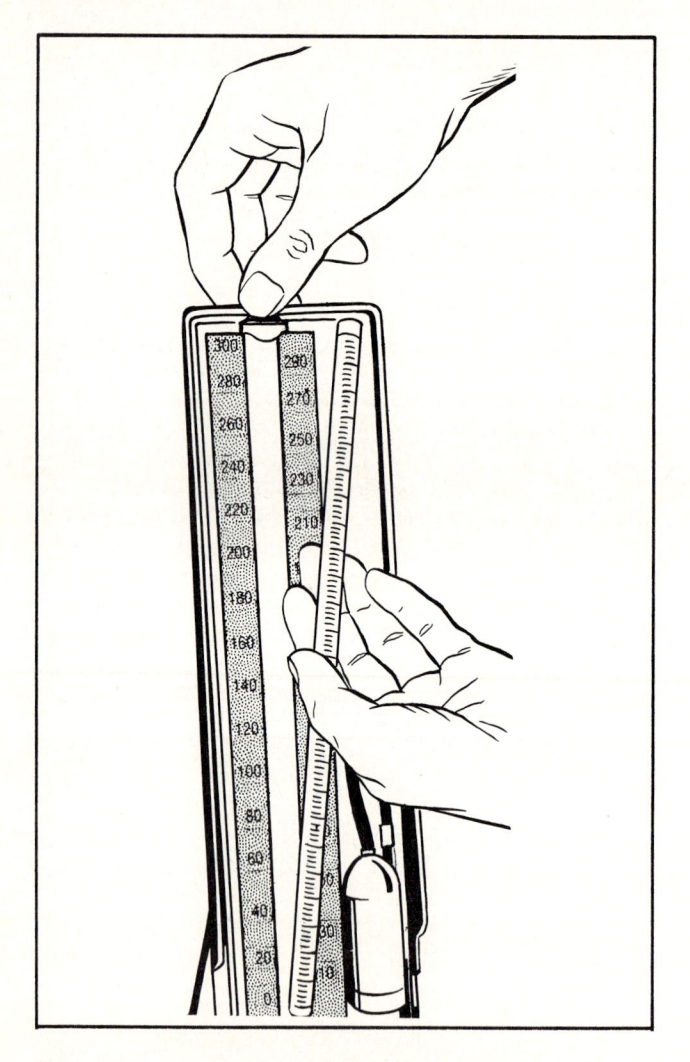

Figure 26–6. Removing the glass column for cleaning or replacement. (Adapted from Baumometer Service Manual. WA Baum Co, Inc, Copiague, NY 11726, 1975.)

Replace the glass tube and use a paper funnel to return the mercury to the glass tube. Once the mercury is replaced, check the level of the meniscus to make sure it is at zero. If it is below zero, add mercury a drop at a time with a medicine dropper. If it is above zero, slowly pour off the excess. Reassemble all the other components of the manometer.

Leaks of mercury around the top of the glass column may be caused by a loose top cap or a faulty washer. After tightening the top cap, the integrity of the washer can be checked by rolling the cuff tightly and securing it, then inflating the manometer to a pressure higher than the full calibration. A careful inspection around the top cap, the bottom of the glass tube, and the bottom of the reservoir will reveal drops of mercury if a leak is present. Faulty washers must be replaced.

A slow mercury response to inflation or deflation may be caused by a nonporous kidskin diaphragm, which is located at the top of the glass column under the top cap. If it has lost its pliancy, rolling it between the fingers will renew it temporarily until a replacement is available.

The Aneroid Manometer
This type of manometer functions by way of an internal metal bellows, which responds to pressure within the system by expanding and collapsing. A needle pivots over the calibrated dial as a result of gear rotation from the bellows movement. The aneroid manometer must be positioned so that the center of the dial face is viewed straight on.

The aneroid manometer can be cleaned by wiping with a cloth dampened with a detergent disinfectant or 70 percent alcohol. The metal parts are vulnerable to wear and abuse from frequent usage. The needle may not start or return to zero when the pressure is released and can thereby give erroneous readings. Some models are designed with a stop pin that prevents the needle from moving below the zero point; this design prevents the user from knowing when the manometer is obviously inaccurate.

To ensure the instrument's accurate functioning, the aneroid manometer should be checked against a mercury manometer of known accuracy at least once a year. If it is used frequently on a regular basis, it should be checked once a month. Perlman et al. (1970) found that almost one-third of the aneroid manometers used in seven hospitals had more than the acceptable deviation of plus or minus 3 mm Hg and 18 percent had a deviation of more than plus 7 mm Hg.

To check an aneroid manometer against a mercury manometer, connect the single end of a Y-connector to the control valve end of the pressure bulb; attach the tubing from the aneroid manometer to one branch of the Y-connector; and attach the tubing from the mercury manometer to the other branch (Fig. 26–7). Close the control valve and inflate the pressure to 250 mm Hg. Slowly release the pressure, stopping at at least five different points on the scale to

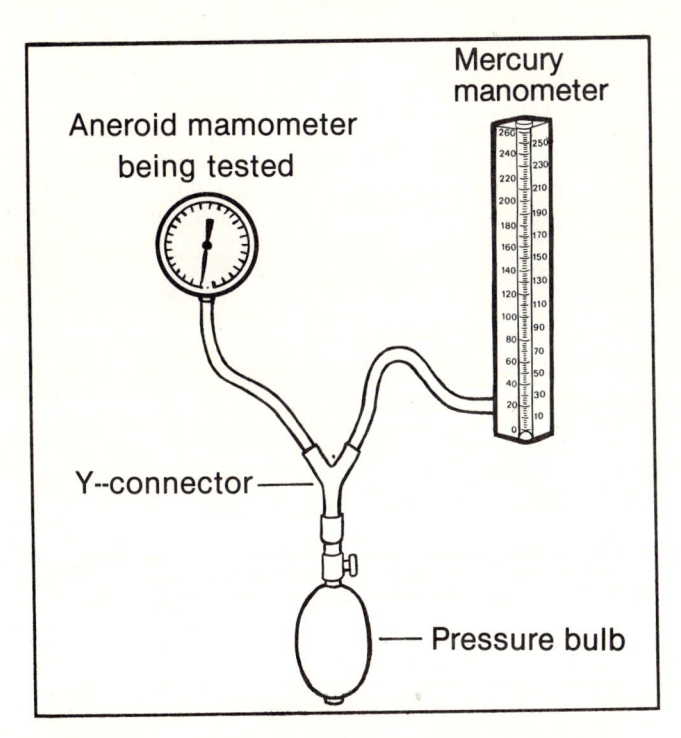

Figure 26–7. Checking an aneroid manometer against a mercury manometer for accuracy. (Adapted from Baumometer Service Manual. WA Baum Co, Inc, Copiague, NY 11726, 1975.)

note the consistency of the readings on the two manometers. Any difference greater than plus or minus 3 mm Hg over the entire range indicates a need for recalibration by the manufacturer.

☐ EXECUTION

Blood pressure measurement can be very anxiety-provoking to some persons, and anxiety affects blood pressure. An explanation of the purpose of and steps in the procedure and an unhurried approach reassure the client and elicit cooperation. Prior to the taking of a reading, have the client sit or lie supine for at least 5 minutes. Whenever possible, the client should have an empty bladder, should refrain from smoking, and should not be unusually hungry; all these factors alter the blood pressure measurement.

The observer can most effectively concentrate on the procedure and auscultate the sounds if the door to the room is closed, the radio and television are turned off, and the client is requested to not talk during the measurement. Others in the room may also be requested to be quiet while the measurement is obtained. Intrusion of environmental noise can prevent hearing the Korotkoff sounds adequately.

The *mental attitude* and set of the observer during the use of the physical appraisal skills to obtain a blood pressure measurement can affect the accuracy of the measurement and what is reported. A preference for specific digits may cause the observer to round a reading up or down, and a preconceived notion of what the reading should be instead of what it actually is can interfere with the accurate reporting of an accurately obtained measurement.

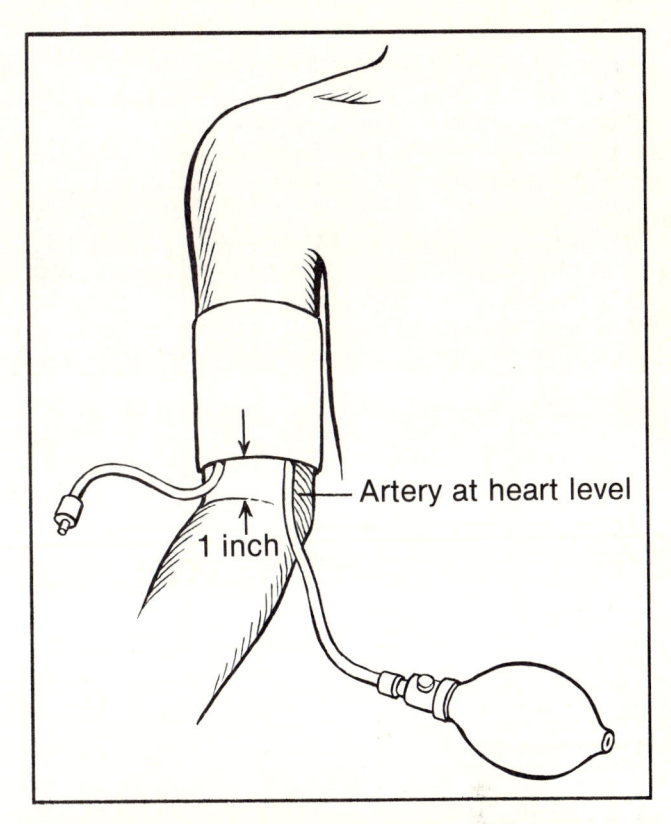

Figure 26–8. Cuff placement on the arm to compress an adequate length of the artery. The cuff is placed 2.5 cm (1 in) above the cubital space to permit auscultation of the pulse without interference of the cuff edge.

As previously mentioned, an accurate sphygmomanometer and a quality stethoscope are essential for accurate blood pressure measurements. Check out the equipment before using it. Select the appropriate size compression cuff for the circumference of the extremity to be used for the measurement. Wrap the cuff snugly around the extremity 2.5 cm (1 in) above the artery and position the extremity at heart level (Fig. 26–8). The client should not hold his or her own extremity extended without support. If necessary, use a pillow or over-bed table to hold it at heart level. Place the manometer at an angle that permits accurate readings. Palpate the artery pulsation while rapidly inflating the compression cuff until the manometer pressure is 30 mm Hg beyond the point at which the pulse disappears. Place the stethoscope chestpiece *lightly* over the location of the pulsation (Fig. 26–9). Release the compression cuff pressure at a rate of 2 to 3 mm Hg per heartbeat while simultaneously listening to the Korotkoff sounds and noting the point on the manometer at which each occurs.

The position of either the client or the arm has been implicated as a source of error. The systolic and diastolic pressures may show marked variations in cli-

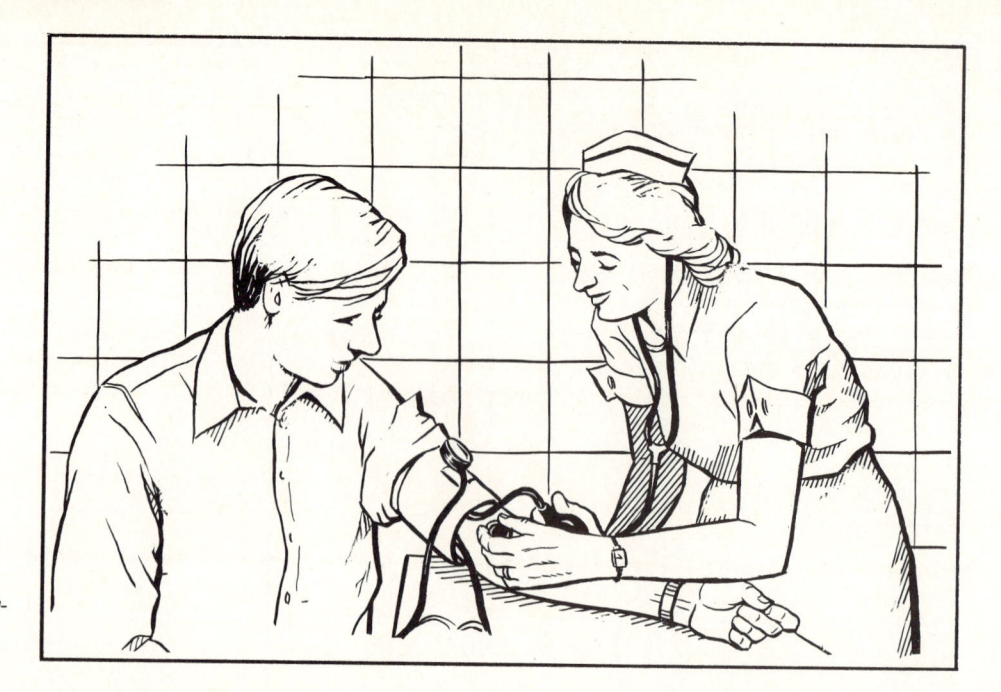

Figure 26–9. Arm properly positioned at heart level, manometer gauge placed at angle for accurate reading, and stethoscope diaphragm placed over the brachial pulse site.

ents lying in the lateral recumbent position. Foley (1971) reported the results of a nursing study that investigated normal subjects and recovery room clients, and revealed marked variations in blood pressure when they were lying in the right or left lateral recumbent position. Measurements taken in the uppermost arm showed a drop from the baseline measurements in both the systolic and the diastolic readings, and this drop was sustained for the whole time the position was maintained. Readings taken in the downward arm revealed a lesser drop in the systolic reading and an increase in the diastolic. All pressure readings rose when the client was turned over to the supine position.

A false rise in systolic and diastolic blood pressure may occur if the arm on which the measurement is being made is unsupported during the measurement. Thompson et al. (1977) report a medical study in which both the systolic and diastolic pressures became elevated when either the arm used for the measurement or the opposite arm was unsupported during the measurement. The isometric contractions in the arm cause increased heart rate and increased peripheral resistance. These increases are greater in clients who are hypertensive and even greater still in clients who are on beta-blocking drugs.

Another source of either a false high systolic reading or a false low diastolic reading can occur when a repeat measurement is taken immediately. The error occurs because of blood trapped in the forearm. To obtain an accurate measurement from subsequent attempts, completely deflate the cuff, wait about 30 seconds, and then raise the client's arm above heart level before inflating the cuff.

In observing nursing personnel measure blood pressure, Mitchell and Van Meter (1971) found that clients frequently were not required to be at rest for any period of time before the pressure was read, and that many clients changed position to assist the staff in the procedure. The staff often neglected to raise the arm being measured to heart level before inflating the compression cuff on clients who were sitting during the measurement.

In another nursing study, Hochberg and Westhoff (1970) found that in readings taken simultaneously on both arms, only 3 out of 100 subjects had the same blood pressure in both arms. The remaining subjects

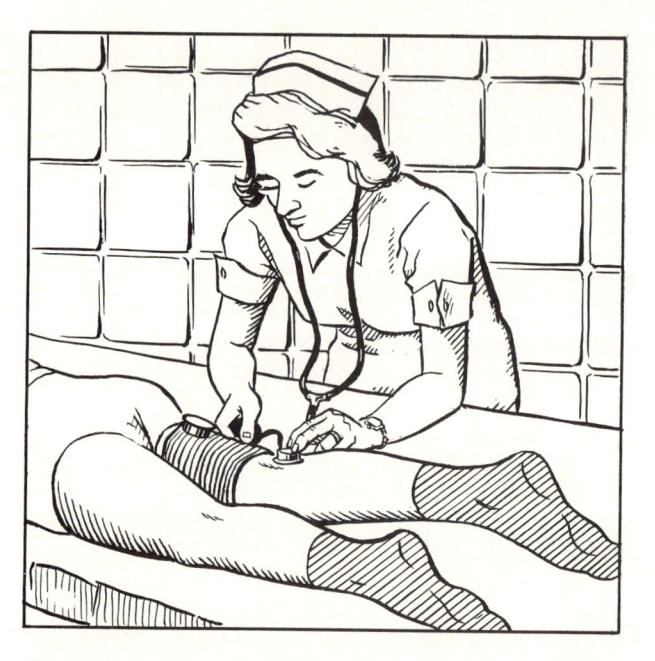

Figure 26–10. Measuring blood pressure in the thigh with the client in the prone position.

had differences in both systolic and diastolic readings. Although the majority did not have pressure differences that exceeded 10 mm Hg, the investigators recommend that baseline pressures be obtained on both arms and that the extremity used be noted when the pressure is recorded.

Thigh pressure may be taken if the arms are not available for measurement. For measurement of blood pressure in the thigh, the client must lie flat, either prone or supine. The cuff must be wider and longer than that used on the arm. The center of the cuff bladder is placed above the popliteal artery located behind the knee. A slight bend in the knee permits placement of the stethoscope over the artery, but the knee should not be elevated above heart level if the client is in the supine position. Figure 26–10 shows the measurement of blood pressure in a thigh. The procedural steps are the same as for obtaining a blood pressure on the arm.

The systolic pressure reading in the thighs may be as much as 10 to 40 mm Hg higher than in the arms, while the diastolic pressure is usually about the same. It is important to note on the recording that the thigh was used for measurement.

☐ SKILL SEQUENCE

AUSCULTATORY METHOD OF MEASURING BLOOD PRESSURE

Step	Rationale
1. Inspect equipment for defects.	Faulty equipment can cause errors.
2. Wash hands.	Prevents transfer of microorganisms.
3. Explain procedure to client.	Allays anxiety.
4. Place client in a sitting or supine position if possible. Permit client to rest in position for 5 minutes.	Lateral recumbent position can cause systolic and diastolic readings lower than supine position. Measurements taken immediately following activity are elevated above baseline measurements.
5. Position arm at heart level with palm up.	Arm above heart level gives a false low reading; arm below heart level gives a false high reading.
6. Measure cuff against arm to determine correct width and length.	Cuff too narrow does not compress adequate length of artery, results in false high pressure reading.
7. Apply deflated cuff bladder with the center (either arrow or rubber tubing) over brachial artery (located at medial aspect of anticubital fossa). Lower edge of the cuff is at least 2½ centimeters (1 inch) above site where maximum arterial pulse is palpated.	Bladder must be in position to compress artery. Space must be open for palpation of arterial pulse and placement of stethoscope without touching cuff.
8. Wrap cuff around arm snugly. Avoid contact with clothing. Support arm with own if necessary.	Loose cuff gives a false high reading; tight cuff gives a false low reading and is uncomfortable. Unsupported arm can cause false high systolic and diastolic readings.
9. Place self 3 feet or less from manometer. Aneroid type directly in front of vision; mercury type on level surface with meniscus level at eye level.	If scale numbers are too far away or not at eye level, errors in reading occur.
10. Palpate brachial artery, keeping fingers in place while inflating cuff rapidly to 30 mm Hg above point where pulse disappears.	Ensures hearing systolic phase; identifies auscultatory gap if present.
11. Place diaphragm of stethoscope over pulse site; hold securely with fingers without excess pressure.	Too much pressure can distort sounds and change reading.
12. Release cuff pressure 2 to 3 mm Hg per heartbeat.	Too slow release causes falsely elevated diastolic pressure. Too rapid release makes it difficult to read points on the scale accurately with the sounds.
13. Note the manometer numbers at which the first, fourth, and fifth Korotkoff sounds are heard.	These numbers are systolic and diastolic pressures.
14. Rapidly deflate cuff to zero when sounds have disappeared.	Relieves discomfort caused from tight cuff.
15. If the reading is to be repeated immediately, wait 30 seconds, elevate the arm above heart level to drain trapped blood from forearm, inflate cuff, lower arm, and repeat steps 9 to 12.	Venous congestion in forearm for a prolonged period of time causes false high systolic readings and false low diastolic readings.
16. If unable to hear sounds after applying methods to augment sounds, take reading by palpation as described in text.	
17. Remove cuff after reading is obtained.	
18. Place client in position of comfort.	
19. Record measurement in health record promptly.	Documents measurement.

RECORDING

The American Heart Association recommends that three points be recorded: phase I for the systolic pressure and phases IV and V for the diastolic pressure. To avoid confusion it is best to follow agency policy. When methods other than auscultatory are used, the method should be recorded. In a written recording, the date, time of day, and extremity used for the measurement are included with the measurement. For example: 1/5/80, 8 A.M., 120/94/90, r. arm. In the event that the fourth and fifth phases are the same, both figures are still recorded, for example: 120/94/94.

In plotting the measurement on a graphic recording, the date and time of day are entered in the appropriate column, the points are plotted in the same column, and the extremity used and the position of the client are also noted (Fig. 26–11). Some graphic recordings have other vital signs plotted on the same form; it is important that the recording is clear and legible and not confused with other data.

☐ CRITICAL POINTS SUMMARY

1. Inspect the equipment for defects.
2. Prepare and position the client and extremity correctly.

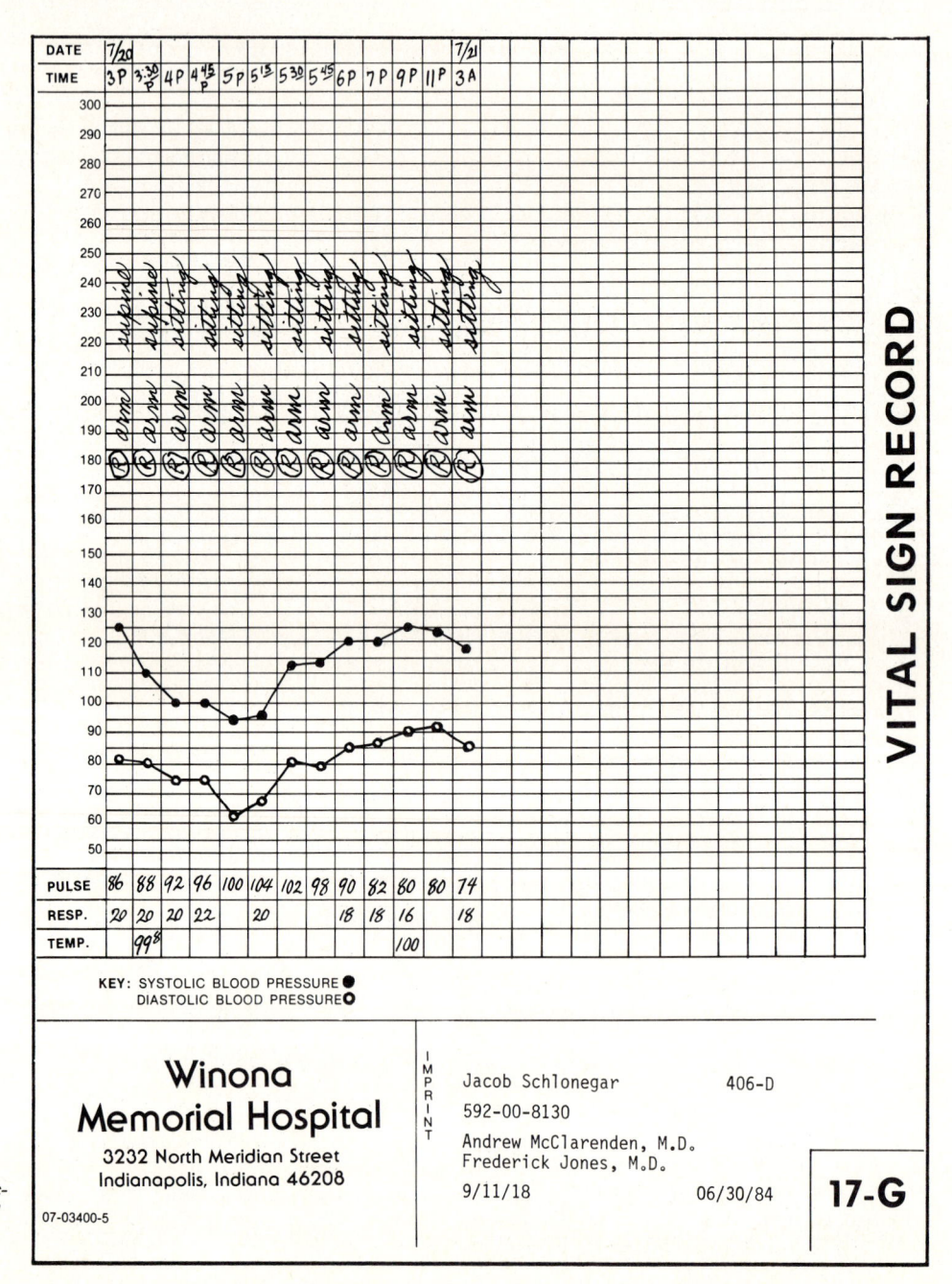

Figure 26–11. Graphic recording for blood pressure. (Vital signs record courtesy of Winona Memorial Hospital, Indianapolis, IN 46208, with permission.)

3. Select the correct size cuff for the extremity.
4. Apply the cuff centered and snugly 2½ centimeters (1 inch) above the antecubital or popliteal fossa.
5. Inflate the cuff 30 mm Hg beyond the point at which the palpated arterial pulse disappears.
6. Release the cuff pressure at a rate of 2 to 3 mm Hg per heartbeat.
7. Listen for all phases of Korotkoff sounds.
8. Apply techniques to augment the sounds if needed.
9. Record the measurement accurately.

IV. Have the sounds validated by someone else using a two-way stethoscope.

☐ REVIEW QUESTIONS

1. What are two reasons for measuring blood pressure?
2. Which components of the sphygmomanometer should be inspected before use?
3. How would you find a leak in the inflation system?
4. How would you check the accuracy of an aneroid manometer?
5. Under what circumstances would blood pressure be taken by the flush method?
6. How are inspection, palpation, and auscultation used in blood pressure measurement?
7. What are Korotkoff sounds? What do they represent? What does each phase sound like?
8. What are the ways to increase the loudness of the Korotkoff sounds?
9. How can you identify an auscultatory gap? Why is it important?
10. What should you consider about the selection and placement of the compression cuff?
11. What happens if the cuff pressure is reduced at a rate other than 2 to 3 mm Hg per heartbeat?
12. Why should the same extremity be used for serial measurements whenever possible?
13. What can be done to ensure an accurate repeat measurement?
14. What data should be recorded about a blood pressure reading?
15. What are the errors in measurement that can be attributed to the equipment, the observer, the person, and the environment?

☐ LEARNING ACTIVITIES

1. In your own words, explain blood pressure to someone who does not know about it.
2. Examine your own feelings when your blood pressure is taken by a physician or a nurse.
3. Explain how accurate blood pressure measurements serve to protect the client.
4. Examine each type of sphygmomanometer to identify all the component parts and locate any defects that may be present.
5. Determine the accuracy of an aneroid instrument by using a Y-connector to check it against a mercury manometer of known accuracy.
6. Compare blood pressure readings taken on the same person after resting for 5 minutes and then again after moderate exercise.
7. Compare blood pressure readings taken on the same person with the arm at heart level and again at levels above and below the heart.
8. Obtain blood pressure measurements on persons of different ages and compare any difference in the quality of Korotkoff sounds for each of phases I to

☐ PERFORMANCE CHECKLIST

OBJECTIVE: To use the correct technique to measure blood pressure by the auscultatory method accurately.

CHARACTERISTIC	RANGE OF ACCEPTABILITY	SATISFACTORY	UNSATISFACTORY
1. Washes hands.	No deviation		
2. Explains procedure to client.	No deviation		
3. Positions client and extremity correctly.	No deviation		
4. Selects appropriate cuff size.	No deviation		
5. Applies cuff snugly at 1 inch above the fossa.	No deviation		
6. Supports extremity.	No deviation		
7. Locates strongest impulse of artery.	No deviation		
8. Holds stethoscope lightly and flat over pulse site.	No deviation		
9. Inflates cuff rapidly to 30 mm Hg above pulse disappearance.	Deviation of 5 mm Hg permitted.		

(continued)

OBJECTIVE: To use the correct technique to measure blood pressure by the auscultatory method accurately (cont.).			
CHARACTERISTIC	RANGE OF ACCEPTABILITY	SATISFACTORY	UNSATISFACTORY
10. Releases cuff pressure at 2 to 3 mm Hg per heartbeat.	Deviation of 1 mm Hg permitted.		
11. Notes phase I, IV, and V Korotkoff sounds.	No deviation		
12. Deflates cuff completely and elevates extremity before next reading.	No deviation		
13. Validates reading of blood pressure.	Within 5 mm Hg of first reading.		
14. Records reading correctly.	No deviation		

REFERENCES

Askey JM: The auscultatory gap in sphygmomanometry. Annals of Internal Medicine 80(1):94-97, 1974.

Baum WA: Baumanometer service manual. Copiague, NY, WA Baum Co., Inc., 1975.

Burch GE, Shewey L: Sphygmomanometric cuff size and blood pressure recordings. Journal of the American Medical Association 225(10):1215-1218, 1973.

Conceicao S, Ward MK, Kerr DNS: Defects in sphygmomanometers: An important source of error in blood pressure recording. British Medical Journal 1(6014):886-888, 1976.

Enselberg CD: Measurement of diastolic blood pressure by palpation. New England Journal of Medicine 265(6):272-274, 1961.

Foley MF: Variations in blood pressure in the lateral recumbent position. Nursing Research 20(1):64-94, 1971.

Glor BAK, Sullivan EF, Estes ZE: Reproducibility of blood pressure measurements: A replication. Nursing Research 19(2):170-172, 1970.

Hochberg A, Westhoff ME: Simultaneous bilateral blood pressures. In ANA Clinical Conferences: Medical-Surgical Clinic Sessions, ANA 1969, Minneapolis/Atlanta. New York, Appleton-Century-Crofts, 1970.

King GE: Errors in clinical measurement of blood pressure in obesity. Clinical Science 32(4):223-237, 1967.

King GE: Taking the blood pressure. Journal of the American Medical Association 209(12):1902-1904, 1969.

Kirkendall W, Burton AC, et al: Recommendations for Human Blood Pressure Determination by Sphygmomanometers. New York, American Heart Association, 1967.

Mitchell P, Van Meter MJ: Reproducibility of blood pressures recorded on patients' records by nursing personnel. Nursing Research 20(4):348-352, 1971.

National Heart, Lung, & Blood Institute: Report of the task force on blood pressure control in children. Pediatrics 59(suppl, pt 2): 797-820, 1977.

Perlman LV, Chiang BN, et al: Accuracy of sphygmomanometers in hospital practice. Archives of Internal Medicine 6(125):1000-1003, 1970.

Putt AM: A comparison of blood pressure readings by auscultation and palpation. Nursing Research 15(4):311-316, 1966.

Ravin A: The Clinical Significance of the Sounds of Korotkoff, audiovisual manual. West Point, PA, Merck, Sharp & Dohme, 1972.

Report of the Joint National Committee on Detection, Evaluation, and Treatment of High Blood Pressure. US Dept of Health, Education, and Welfare publication No. (NIH) 78-1088. Bethesda, MD, National Institutes of Health, Public Health Service, 1978.

Thompson DG, Pease CT, Howard AJ: The unsupported arm: A cause of falsely raised blood pressure readings. British Medical Journal 2(6098):1331, 1977.

Virnig NL, Reynolds JW: Reliability of flush blood pressure measurements in the sick newborn. The Journal of Pediatrics 84(4): 594-598, 1974.

Wilcox J: Observer factors in the measurement of blood pressure. Nursing Research 10(1):16-17, 1961.

BIBLIOGRAPHY

American Journal of Nursing Editors: Correcting common errors in blood pressure measurement. American Journal of Nursing 65(10):133-164, 1965.

Beaumont E: Blood pressure equipment. Nursing75 5(1):56-62, 1975.

Burch GE, DePasquale NP: Primer of Clinical Blood Pressure. St Louis, MO, CV Mosby, 1962.

Corns RH: Maintenance of blood pressure equipment. American Journal of Nursing 67(5):776-777, 1976.

Cranwell PD: Blood pressure teaching and screening program for school children grades 5-8. Home Healthcare Nurse 2(3):42-44, 1984.

Evans MJ: Tips for taking a child's blood pressure quickly. Nursing83 (Horsham) 13(3):61, 1983.

Guyton AC: Textbook of Medical Physiology, ed 4. Philadelphia, Saunders, 1971.

Jarvis CM: Vital signs: How to take them more accurately and understand them more fully. Nursing76 6(4):31-37, 1976.

Kaplan N, Lieberman E: Clinical Hypertension, ed 2. Baltimore, Williams & Wilkins, 1978.

Keeping your sphygmomanometer accurate and in good repair. Patient Care 8(8):146, 1974.

Krausman DT: Methods and procedures for monitoring and recording blood pressure. American Psychologist 30(3):285-294, 1975.

Lancour J: How to avoid pitfalls in measuring blood pressure. American Journal of Nursing 67(5):773-775, 1976.

Lichti EL, Lyson JD, Terry BE: Use of Doppler ultrasonic flowmeter to monitor blood pressure during ileal loop bypass for extreme obesity. American Surgeon 40(7):398-399, 1974.

Warren FM: Blood pressure readings: Getting them quickly on an infant. Nursing75 5(4):13, 1975.

SUGGESTED READING

Correcting common errors in blood pressure measurements. *American Journal of Nursing* 65(10):133–164, 1965.

AUDIOVISUAL RESOURCES

Blood Pressure
   Videorecording (¾ in). (1976, Color, 20 min.)
   Available through:
      Comprenetics, Inc.
      5805 Uplander Way
      Culver City, CA 90230

How to Measure Your Patient's Blood Pressure
   Filmstrip and Cassette. (1975, Color, 80 min.)
   Available through:
      Techniques Learning Council
      921 East Green Street
      Pasadena, CA 91106

Measuring Vital Signs/Blood Pressure by Sphygmomanometer
   Videocassette (½ in, ¾ in). (1977, Color, 18 min.)
   Available through:
      Indiana University, School of Nursing
      NICER Department
      1100 West Michigan Street
      Indianapolis, IN 46223

The Clinical Significance of the Sounds of Korotkoff
   Audiocassette. (1972)
   Available through:
      Merck, Sharp & Dohme
      West Point, PA 19486

The Measurement of Blood Pressure
   Film (16 mm). (1971, Color, 10 min.)
   Available through:
      National Medical Audiovisual Center
      Washington, DC 20409

SKILL 27 Height and Weight Appraisal

PREREQUISITE SKILLS

Skill 19, "Inspection"
Skill 20, "Palpation"
Skill 28, "Handwashing"

☐ STUDENT OBJECTIVES

1. Explain the purposes in measuring body height and weight.
2. Describe how to balance a scale.
3. Differentiate between desired weight, underweight, overweight, and obesity.
4. Describe the conditions under which a person should be weighed.
5. Describe how to obtain the height of persons of varying ages and abilities.
6. Describe how to weigh a person on a bed scale safely.
7. Explain the methods used to determine the amount of body fat.
8. Summarize the factors involved in obtaining accurate height and weight measurements.
9. Record height and weight accurately.

☐ INTRODUCTION

Measurements of body height and weight are used as indicators of health status. Throughout infancy (to about age 2 years), serial measurements are made on length, weight, head circumference, and chest circumference. These data are compared with norms for the age and sex to evaluate the growth progress and normalcy of an individual child. After about age 2, only height and weight measurements are usually obtained unless there is reason to be concerned with a particular measurement or the general proportions of growth. The word *length* is commonly used for stature measurements until an infant is old enough to stand; then stature is referred to as height.

Weight is often considered to be the best indicator of nutritional status. Weight is usually viewed as either meeting or deviating from the ideal or desired weight for height. This is determined according to sex and frame size as cited on tables or charts that are based on data obtained from surveys of selected populations. Deviations from the desired standard of weight may require therapeutic intervention; diet therapy is indicated when nutrition is the cause of deviation.

Accurate weight measurement is also critical when monitoring fluid balance. Persons with disease conditions of the cardiovascular or renal systems can retain fluid and may require weighing as often as once per day. Copious loss of body fluids from diarrhea, vomiting, metabolic diseases, burns, or draining wounds can also cause significant changes in weight within a short period of time. In some situations, even surgical dressings must be weighed to quantify the amount of fluid loss, so that adequate amounts of fluid can be replaced. The frequency of weight measurements depends on a person's diagnosis and condition, and on the medical regimen. During the years of physical growth, height is measured to assess bone growth at regular time intervals. When adult stature is attained, height is usually measured only at the time of admission to a health-care service.

☐ PREPARATION

WEIGHT

Total body weight (gross weight) is composed of blood, water, bone, muscle, fat, and adipose tissue. However, gross weight does not identify the percent that each of these contributes to the total weight. Changes in weight may occur as a result of increases or decreases in any of the components. In healthy people after the growth years, most changes occur in muscle, bone, adipose tissue, and the amount of water.

Body Composition

Water. Water is a major constituent of body weight. The percentage of water in the healthy individual decreases over the life span. In the newborn, water makes up 77 percent of body weight, and by age 2 years it makes up 60 percent. In males, water content remains at this level until about age 40, when it decreases to 55 percent. In females, it decreases to 50 percent at about age 20 and changes little after that (Beland and Passos, 1981; Luckmann and Sorensen, 1980). Gains or losses of more than 1.1 pounds (0.5 kilograms) within 24 hours indicate a change in the amount of body fluid. Slower gains or losses are more apt to reflect changes in caloric intake, activity level, or both (Mitchell, 1977, p. 415).

Fat. About half of total body fat is found in layers of subcutaneous tissue called adipose tissue. Adipose tissue is composed of about 80 to 85 percent fat, 10 percent water, and 2 percent protein. The percent of total body weight composed of fat in adipose tissue varies among individuals, and it may change in the same individual at different ages. When the amount of adipose tissue is increased, the proportion of body fat increases slightly (Craddock, 1978).

It takes about five times as much fat as lean muscle mass to equal 1 pound of fat. The percentage of fat in persons who are in the upper weight range according to the standard tables should be no more than 22 to 25 percent for females and 16 to 19 percent for males. Females normally have 5 to 10 percent more fat than males, and the fat tends to be stored in different places. Males can store large amounts of fat in the greater omentum, with evidence of excess body weight revealed only by an expanding waistline. A certain amount of fat is beneficial because it provides a reserve of fuel for energy during exercise and rest. Adipose tissue has the important metabolic function of assimilating carbohydrates and lipids for fat synthesis and storage, so that the fat can be used as an energy reserve when and if the nutritional intake is inadequate to meet the body's needs (Craddock, 1978). Desired weight according to frame size for men and women age 25 and older is in Tables 27-1 and 27-2.

Nutrition and Weight

Undernutrition is present when an inadequate amount of nutrients is consumed, or when the diet is adequate in nutrients but the body is unable to utilize the food because of some disorder. Weight loss occurs when the

TABLE 27-1. Desired Weights for Men of Ages 25 and Older, According to Frame[a]

HEIGHT		FRAME		
Feet	Inches	Small	Medium	Large
5	2	128–134	131–141	138–150
5	3	130–136	133–143	140–153
5	4	132–138	135–145	142–156
5	5	134–140	137–148	144–160
5	6	136–142	139–151	146–164
5	7	138–145	142–154	149–168
5	8	140–148	145–157	152–172
5	9	142–151	148–160	155–176
5	10	144–154	151–163	158–180
5	11	146–157	154–166	161–184
6	0	149–160	157–170	164–188
6	1	152–164	160–174	168–192
6	2	155–168	164–178	172–197
6	3	158–172	167–182	176–202
6	4	162–176	171–187	181–207

[a]Weights at ages 25 to 59 based on lowest mortality. Weights in pounds according to frame (in indoor clothing weighing 5 pounds, shoes with 1-inch heels).
(Source: 1983 Metropolitan Height and Weight Tables. Courtesy of Metropolitan Life Insurance Company. Used with permission.)

TABLE 27-2. Desired Weights for Women of Ages 25 and Older, According to Frame[a]

HEIGHT		FRAME		
Feet	Inches	Small	Medium	Large
4	10	102–111	109–121	118–131
4	11	103–113	111–123	120–134
5	0	104–115	113–126	122–137
5	1	106–118	115–129	125–140
5	2	108–121	118–132	128–143
5	3	111–124	121–135	131–147
5	4	114–127	124–138	134–151
5	5	117–130	127–141	137–155
5	6	120–133	130–144	140–159
5	7	123–136	133–147	143–163
5	8	126–139	136–150	146–167
5	9	129–142	139–153	149–170
5	10	132–145	142–156	152–173
5	11	135–148	145–159	155–176
6	0	138–151	148–162	158–179

[a] Weights at ages 25 to 59 based on lowest mortality. Weights in pounds according to frame (in indoor clothing weighing 3 pounds, shoes with 1-inch heels).
(Source: 1983 Metropolitan Height and Weight Tables. Courtesy of Metropolitan Life Insurance Company. Used with permission.)

body draws on the tissues to meet its nutritive requirements (Wenke et al., 1980).

Overnutrition occurs when food intake exceeds the body's need. The excess calories are stored in the liver and adipose tissue. Overnutrition results in overweight, but the overweight person may not be adequately nourished if the diet is deficient in basic nutrients (Wenke et al., 1980).

Overweight is considered to exist when an individual's weight exceeds the maximum weight on the standard tables according to height and frame size. However, this definition presents some problems because there is no criterion for frame size. While not commonly done, frame size can be determined by anthropometrists using several body measurements of girth and diameter. The average adult 25 years or older gains 1 pound of additional weight per year, while bone and muscle mass decreases by about 0.25 to 0.5 pounds during each of these years. This makes a net gain in fat of about 1.25 to 1.5 pounds per year; thus, the sedentary middle-age person is heavier and fatter than the sedentary young person (Pollack et al., 1978). Even when weight stays the same through the adult years, fat can be added at the expense of muscle (Craddock, 1978).

Obesity, or overfatness, is defined as excess weight of anywhere from 10 to 20 percent beyond the desired weight for height. Females who have 30 to 35 percent of total body weight in fat and men who have 25 percent weight in fat are considered obese by some authorities (Pollack et al., 1978).

STANDARDS FOR MEASUREMENTS

Measurements of height and weight are usually evaluated against tables that list standards for such measurements. For children, there are charts that show expected growth patterns at various ages. Weight-for-height tables list normal weights for adults on the basis of sex, age, size, and height.

While such tables are used because they provide criteria against which to judge height and weight measurements, the nurse is aware of their limitations. For evaluating growth patterns in children, reliance on a growth chart alone may be deceiving. Each child must be evaluated in relation to the many factors that affect growth, not all of which may have been taken into account in creating a particular chart.

There are no tables against which to judge growth or weight for young adults. Maximum height is reached between ages 16½ and 18 for females and between 17½ and 20 for males; yet growth charts for adolescents stop at age 18, and tables for adults are based on populations of age 25 and over.

The weight-for-height tables used to evaluate weights of adults do not take into account desirable ratios of lean body mass (all body tissue except stored fat) to fat. Persons engaged in regular heavy exercise and athletes such as football players may seem to be overweight, but the weight is in lean body mass, not fat. Standard tables may indicate that such individuals are overweight, when in fact the proportion of lean body mass to fat in their bodies is within the normal range. This limitation of weight-for-height tables is now being decreased by the use of skinfold tests to determine the amount of body weight that is in fat.

DATA BASE

Weight and height measurements reflect body system function and, therefore, are an integral part of the overall data base by which clients are evaluated. Body weight is also used to calculate the correct dose of medications and diagnostic testing materials.

Measurements of height and weight are routine procedures on admission to health-care facilities and programs. The frequency of measurements thereafter may be directed by medical orders or agency policy, or may be left to the judgment of the nurse.

The nurse is alert for signs and symptoms of possible changes in height and weight, which would indicate the need for measurement. For example, there may be an observable increase or decrease in body proportions, particularly in the face, abdomen, hands, feet, and lower legs; or, clients may report that the fit of clothes, shoes, slippers, or rings has changed or that their personal appearance has changed enough to be noticeable to themselves or others.

Client History and Recorded Data

While initial measurements of weight and height are significant in themselves, they are of greater value when they can be compared with previous measurements. For a child, serial measurements of weight and height indicate whether the growth process is normal. For adults, changes in weight and height measurements over a period of time may indicate an abnormal condition. Factors in a client's history that might cause weight changes include recent surgery, medication such as diuretics and steroids, and diseases that cause fluid loss or accumulation. Height changes may be the result of atrophy of the intervertebral discs or changes in posture.

Physical Appraisal Skills

Inspection. *Inspection* is used to determine the accurate position of the individual for measurement of height and weight. It is also used to appraise the relative proportions of the body to estimate underweight or overweight before or after weighing. Accurate balance of the scale prior to use and correct positioning of the bed scale before weighing must also be observed if reliable measurements are to be made.

Palpation. *Palpation* is used to test the skinfold thickness to determine the amount of fat present.

EQUIPMENT

Height–Length Measure

A nonstretch tape measure or a yardstick may be used to measure height or length. The attachment on an upright scale is used to measure height. The system of measurement used in health-care facilities varies.

Weight Measure

Scales are used to measure body weight, and calipers are used to determine skinfold thickness.

Bathroom Scales. Bathroom scales found in many homes are spring scales, not balanced scales, and are not considered to be reliable. They tend to give inconsistent readings on successive weighings even with the same test weight (Consumer Research Magazine, 1978). Some models may weigh one quantity correctly but may be inaccurate for amounts above or below that quantity.

Balance-Beam Scales

Balance-beam scales used in health-care and other public settings are more accurate and dependable than bathroom scales. These scales are available in the avoirdupois system, the metric system, or both. In addition to the physician's stand-on model (Fig. 27-1), there are models that may be used for infants and for persons confined to wheelchairs or beds. Other models have built-in supports for the person unable to stand without assistance. The bedside balance-beam scale may be used for ambulatory or bed clients. When the

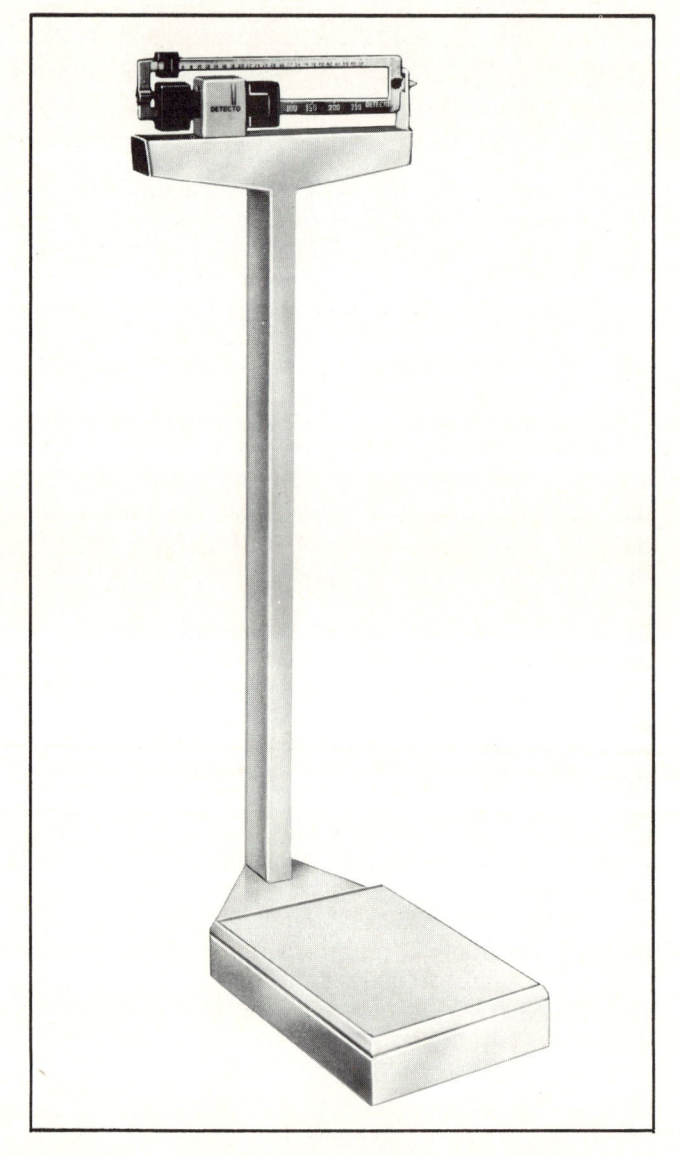

Figure 27-1. Physician's scale. This type of balance-beam scale has an adjustment screw to restore the beam balance to zero. It is located at the lower left of the beam. (Courtesy of Detecto Scales Company, Brooklyn, NY 11236.)

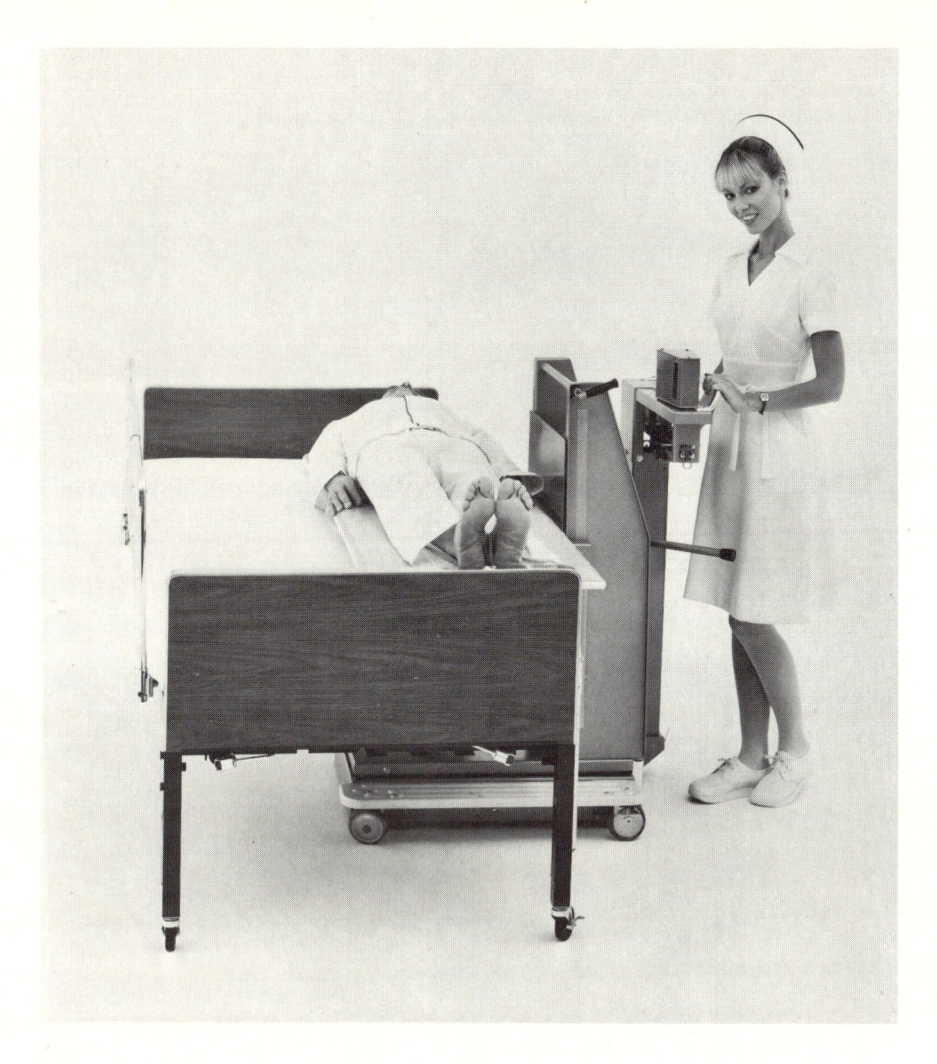

Figure 27-2. Bedside balance-beam scale. The client is positioned for weight measurement. (Courtesy of Acme Scale Company, San Leandro, CA 94577.)

bedside scale is used to weigh a bed client, the weighboard used to hold the client can be adjusted in height by the use of a hydraulic lift (Fig. 27-2). This facilitates transferring the client from the bed to the scale. Brakes on the scale prevent it from rolling and possibly causing injury to the client or the nurse.

When a balance-beam scale has two beams, such as the physician's stand-on model, each beam has a rider that can be moved separately to a balanced position that indicates the client's weight. The lower beam is calibrated in large increments, and the upper beam in small increments. Bedside scales may have one or two beams. A scale having only one beam operates with a combination of beam settings with a rider and ratio weights. A set of ratio weights consists of three or four weights, each corresponding to the value shown on the weight (50, 100, 200 pounds or 10, 20, 50, 100 kilograms). The ratio weights are individually added to a weight holder that is attached to the end of the main beam. They are added in increments to total the amount closest to but less than the client's weight. The rider is moved on the beam to provide additional weight required to balance the beam and obtain the client's weight. (Some bed scales also have a secondary beam that permits greater accuracy of measurement.) The client's weight is the sum total of the values of the ratio weights and the weight read on the beam (or beams) when the scale is in balance. The component parts of the bedside scale are shown in Figure 27-3.

Checking Scale Accuracy

The balance of a scale may be disturbed by moving the scale from place to place. Prior to each use, the balance should be checked. This can be done by placing the rider (riders) on the beam (beams) on zero and noting if the pointer on the side of the beam moves equally above and below the center marker on the right. If the beam rests at the top or bottom or floats unevenly, then an adjustment of it is necessary. On some scales the beam balance is restored by using a coin to turn the screw located at the far left of the beam. The screw moves a fixed back-balance weight on the beam. Usually a very slight turn is sufficient to restore the balance. When the beam float is low, the adjustment is made by turning clockwise; when it is high, the adjustment is counterclockwise. The balance of a bedside scale is checked after the scale is in place at the bedside with the ratio weight holder attached to the beam. Bedside scales have a special balance knob that does not require the use of a coin or tool.

Scales used frequently should be tested for accuracy at least every 6 months by applying various

228 PROFESSIONAL CLINICAL NURSING SKILLS

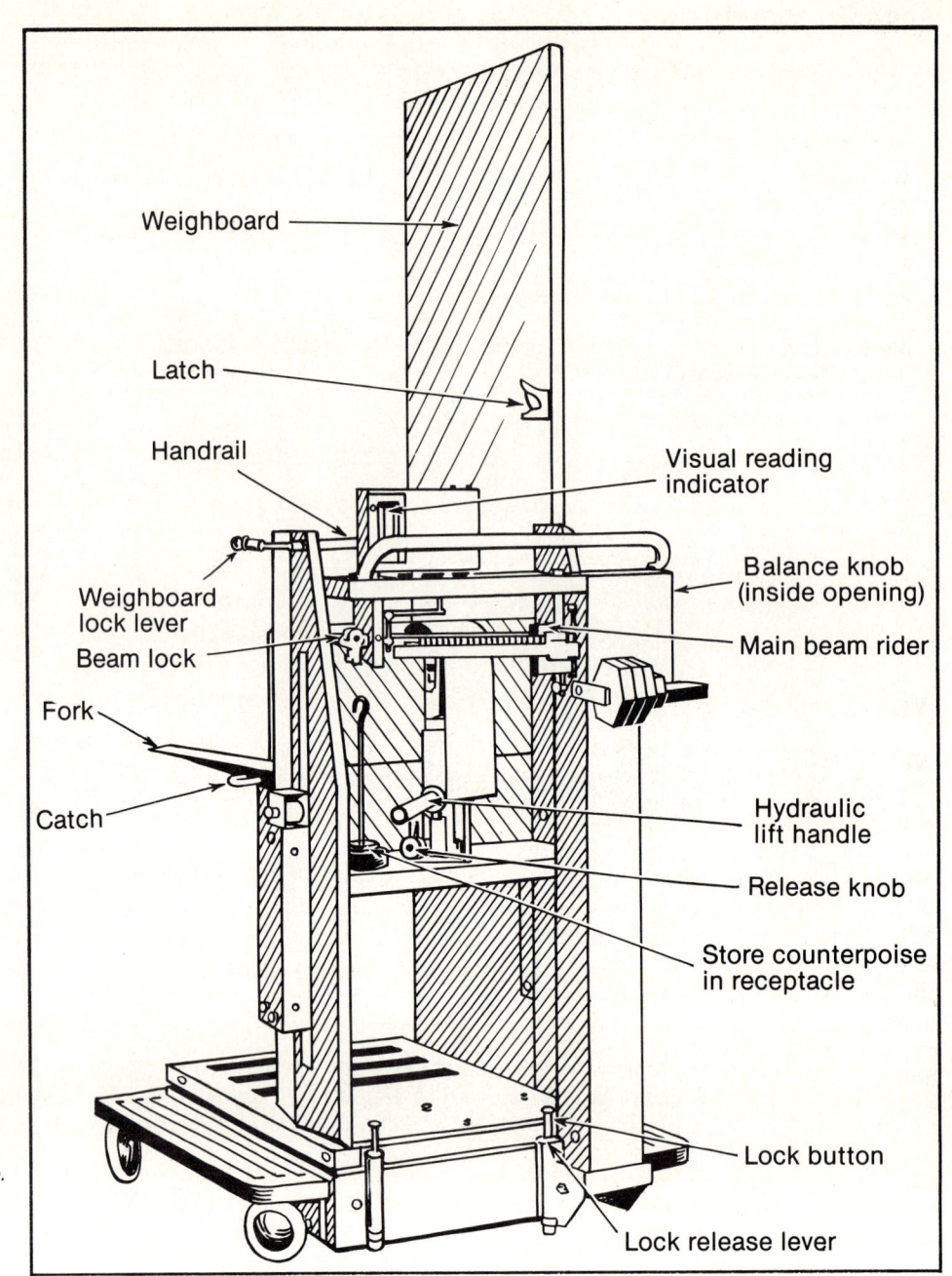

Figure 27-3. Component parts of the bedside balance-beam scale. (Adapted from the operating instruction manual, Acme Scale Company, San Leandro, CA 94577, with permission.)

known test weights up to the capacity of the scale. Since the calibration can be altered by a number of different factors, adjustments should be made by a skilled scale technician or trained maintenance personnel following the manufacturer's service manual.

Calipers

Calipers measure skinfold thickness in millimeters. Calipers used in medical and research settings are designed to exert a pressure on the caliper face of 10 grams per square millimeter. This ensures that the same amount of pressure is applied by the caliper to each skin fold, thus permitting valid comparison of reliable measurements.

☐ EXECUTION

HEIGHT DETERMINATION

Height or length can be measured with the person in the standing or supine position. When persons are capable of standing, it is important that they stand erect and in stocking feet. For the supine position, they should lie fully extended on a firm, flat surface without any bend in their knees.

Length or height can be obtained in centimeters (metric system) or in feet and inches (1 inch equals 2.54 centimeters).

☐ SKILL SEQUENCE

MEASURING HEIGHT–LENGTH

Step	Rationale
1. Wash hands.	Prevents transfer of microorganisms.
2. Select accurate nonstretch measuring device.	Stretchable measures give inconsistent data.
3. Have client in fully extended position if possible. Use flat, firm surface if supine. Clients able to stand should be erect.	Slouching or bending prevents accurate measurements.
4. Remove shoes; place paper towel on scale platform.	Shoes prevent accurate measurement. Paper towel protects client from possible contamination of the sole.
5. Measure a straight line from vertex (highest point) of head to sole of heel with foot in dorsiflexed position. When using the measuring device on a stand-on scale, raise the device above client's estimated height before helping client on the scale. Extend the arm attached to the measuring device and lower it until it rests level on vertex of head.	Simulates foot positions when standing. Otherwise, measurement would be greater or lesser than true length.
6. Read measure to nearest ¼ inch or nearest centimeter.	
7. Record measurement.	
8. Help client step off scale, or obtain client's weight if necessary.	

WEIGHT DETERMINATION

Weight Measurement

Weight is most accurately measured when the person is in a dry state, usually between 6:00 and 7:00 a.m., before breakfast and after the bowel and bladder have been emptied. The least possible amount of clothing should be worn by the person being weighed. A half-full bladder can contain 500 milliliters of urine, which weighs 1.1 pounds (0.5 kilograms). Body weight changes constantly throughout the day as intake is balanced by loss of urine, feces, and insensible perspiration at a rate of about 3.3 ounces (100 milliliters) per hour (Guyton, 1978, pp. 385–386). When a client wears more than minimal clothing during weighing, it is best to weigh the clothing separately at a later time and subtract clothing weight from gross weight to get a more accurate net weight. The frequency of weight measurement depends on the purpose. In clinical situations, weight is often closely observed in order to monitor fluid balance, nutritional deficiencies, or special weight-loss regimens for obesity. Accurate weights at the same time each day can produce a reliable data base.

Weight can be obtained in the avoirdupois system of pounds and ounces or in the metric system of kilograms and grams (2.2 pounds equals 1 kilogram; 0.3527 ounces equals 10 grams).

☐ SKILL SEQUENCES

MEASURING WEIGHT

Step	Rationale
1. Wash hands.	Prevents transfer of microorganisms.
2. Secure appropriate scale for client's age and physical ability.	
3. Check and adjust scale balance.	Ensures accurate measurement.
4. Have client remove as much clothing as feasible. Place paper towel on scale platform.	Provides greater consistency for serial weight measurements. Protects feet from possible contamination and soil.
5. Position client on center of scale.	Off-center position affects accuracy of weight.
6. Move weights on upper and lower arms to balance points.	
7. Read weight to nearest ¼ pound or 0.1 kilogram.	
8. Record weight on scratch pad.	Prevents forgetting weight value.
9. Help client move off scale.	
10. Return riders to zero.	Prepares scale for next user. Prevents possible embarrassment to client.
11. Record weight on client's record.	

MEASURING WEIGHT WITH BEDSIDE SCALE

Step	Rationale
1. Wash hands.	Prevents transfer of microorganisms.
2. Secure enough help to transfer and weigh client. At least two persons may be required if client is heavy or unable to help.	Prevents injury to staff or client.
3. Explain procedure to client.	Allays client's concern about being placed on scale.
4. Move scale parallel to bed and client. Carefully lower weighboard into its locked position.	Latch maintains weighboard in a safe, stable horizontal position during weighing.
5. Check beam balance at zero by: a. Setting rider (riders) at zero. b. Attaching ratio-weight holder to loop at tip of beam with hook facing away from scale. c. Releasing lock on beam to permit it to float freely up and down. d. Noting swing of beam for equal distance above and below center marker. Correct beam balance if necessary by turning screw or knob clockwise if beam is low or counterclockwise if it is high.	Ensures accurate balance of beam (beams). Low beam will give underweight readings and high beam will give overweight readings if uncorrected.
6. Turn release knob on hydraulic lift clockwise to close it; then pump lift handle to elevate weighboard to just above mattress surface.	Lift will not elevate if it is not closed. Elevated weighboard can be moved over mattress.
7. Turn client onto his or her side facing away from scale.	Places client in a position to be turned back onto scale.
8. Roll scale toward bed so that weighboard is over mattress and centered to client. Make sure no part of scale is touching bed.	Contact between bed and scale interferes with accurate weighing.
9. Lock brakes on each side of scale with sole of your shoe.	Prevents scale from moving and causing possible injury to client or staff.
10. Turn release knob on hydraulic lift slightly counterclockwise to lower weighboard slowly to bed surface.	
11. Position client so that he or she is aligned as straight as possible along edge of weighboard.	Facilitates transfer to weighboard.
12. Turn client onto his or her back on weighboard. If desired, a lift sheet can be used to transfer client. Make sure sheet is entirely on scale. Weigh sheet afterward and deduct sheet weight from gross weight of client.	Sheet hanging over scale will affect accurate weighing.
13. Turn release knob on lift in a clockwise direction to close it; then pump lift handle to elevate weighboard above mattress surface. Make sure board is clear of bed.	Contact between bed and scale interferes with accurate weighing.
14. Place appropriate ratio weights on weight holder one at a time until addition of one more would cause balance beam to fall. Then move rider on beam to right until scale balances. When available, use rider on secondary beam for more precise weights.	Provides for accurate weight measurement.
15. Read value to nearest small quantity: ½ ounce, ¼ pound, 10 grams, or 100 grams.	
16. Total value of ratio weights and rider (riders) on beam (beams) to obtain client's weight.	
17. Record weight on a scratch pad.	Prevents forgetting the weight.
18. Slowly release lift to lower client to bed.	Too much and too rapid a release of lift lowers weighboard with a load quickly; this can be hazardous and frightening to client.
19. Turn client back onto mattress.	
20. Close lift and elevate weighboard enough to clear mattress.	Facilitates removal of weighboard from mattress.

(continued)

Step	Rationale
21. Release brake on each side of scale with tip of sole of your shoe. Withdraw scale from bedside.	
22. Lower weighboard as low as possible and leave release knob slightly open.	Releases pressure from hydraulic system.
23. Release weighboard latch and return board to its vertical position. Lock it.	
24. Return ratio weights to their storage place on scale. Remove weight holder and place it in location provided.	Leaving ratio weights and weight holder on scale may affect beam balance. Weights may fall off during transport and cause damage or injury.
25. Return beam lock to secure beam.	Movement of scale without lock in place can damage weighing mechanism of scale.
26. Assist client into a comfortable position and adjust bed linen.	
27. Remove scale from room.	
28. Record weight on client's record.	Provides ongoing data base; fulfills nurse accountability.

Skinfold Measurement

The limitations of standard height and weight tables, the current interest in illness prevention and physical fitness, and an increase in the incidence of obesity have promoted the use of skinfold thickness to determine how much of body weight is fat. Skinfold thickness measurements are becoming a routine part of health-screening examinations at health fairs and physical fitness centers as well as in some traditional medical-care settings. Skinfold measurements are a practical and economical method of determining the amount of fat in body weight. More sophisticated methods such as calculating body density by chemical analysis or underwater weighing, soft-tissue x-rays, and multiple measurements of body girth and diameter are expensive and not feasible for general use.

The Pinch Test. Adipose tissue overlying the main point of the triceps is considered to be a representative site for body fat. The triceps measurement is taken at the midpoint of the back of the arm. To find this point, the arm is flexed at a 90 degree angle and the midpoint between the tip of the olecranon (elbow) and the tip of the acromion process (shoulder) is located with a tape measure and marked. The arm hangs straight and relaxed for measurement, which involves pinching at about ½ inch below the mark. The pinch test provides a gross estimation of body fat. To test this area, pinch up a vertical fold of skin and subcutaneous tissue with the left forefinger and thumb, pull it away from the underlying muscle, and hold it. There should be only skin and subcutaneous tissue in the skinfold. Use a nonstretch tape measure or ruler to determine the width of the thickness at the base of the fold. It should be less than ½-inch thick; a measurement of more than 1 inch indicates obesity. The pinch test of the triceps tends to be more reliable in women than in men.

Calipers. More precise measurement of skinfold thickness is achieved by using calipers. Measurements are taken with the person standing. The side of the body used for skinfold measurements is important. Measurements should be taken on the same side that has been used to establish the standards for estimating the percentage of body fat. (Some standards are established by measuring the right side and others the left; Powers, 1980.) Two sites are used for women: the triceps and the suprailiae (at the crest of the ilium in the middle of the side of the body immediately under the costal margin and close to the umbilicus). (See Fig. 27–4, A and B.) Men are also measured at two sites: the subscapula (the lower point of the shoulder blade) and the thigh (the anterior, midway between the hip and the knee joint). (See Fig. 27–4 C and D.) These locations for each sex are where fat is generally representative of total body fat. The skin folds are measured with the person standing. Each site is pinched vertically except for the subscapula, which is picked up at about a 45 degree angle that conforms to the natural skin fold (Getchell, 1979). The pinching technique is used. (The procedure for using calipers is presented in the Skill Sequence, "Skinfold Thickness Measurement.") If several attempts are required to pinch the skin and subcutaneous tissue away from the underlying muscle, move on to the next site and let the first site rest. Repeated pinching forces the water from the tissues and produces a false low reading. Return to the first site in a few minutes, after it has returned to normal.

The percentage of body fat can be derived by using the values of the skinfold thickness on sex-specific nomograms (as in Fig. 27–5), or by using tables that have skinfold thickness correlated with percent body fat for each sex (Brozek et al., 1963; Getchell, 1979; Sloan, 1967; Sloan et al., 1962). There are also formulas to calculate body density and percentage of body fat from skinfold measurements.

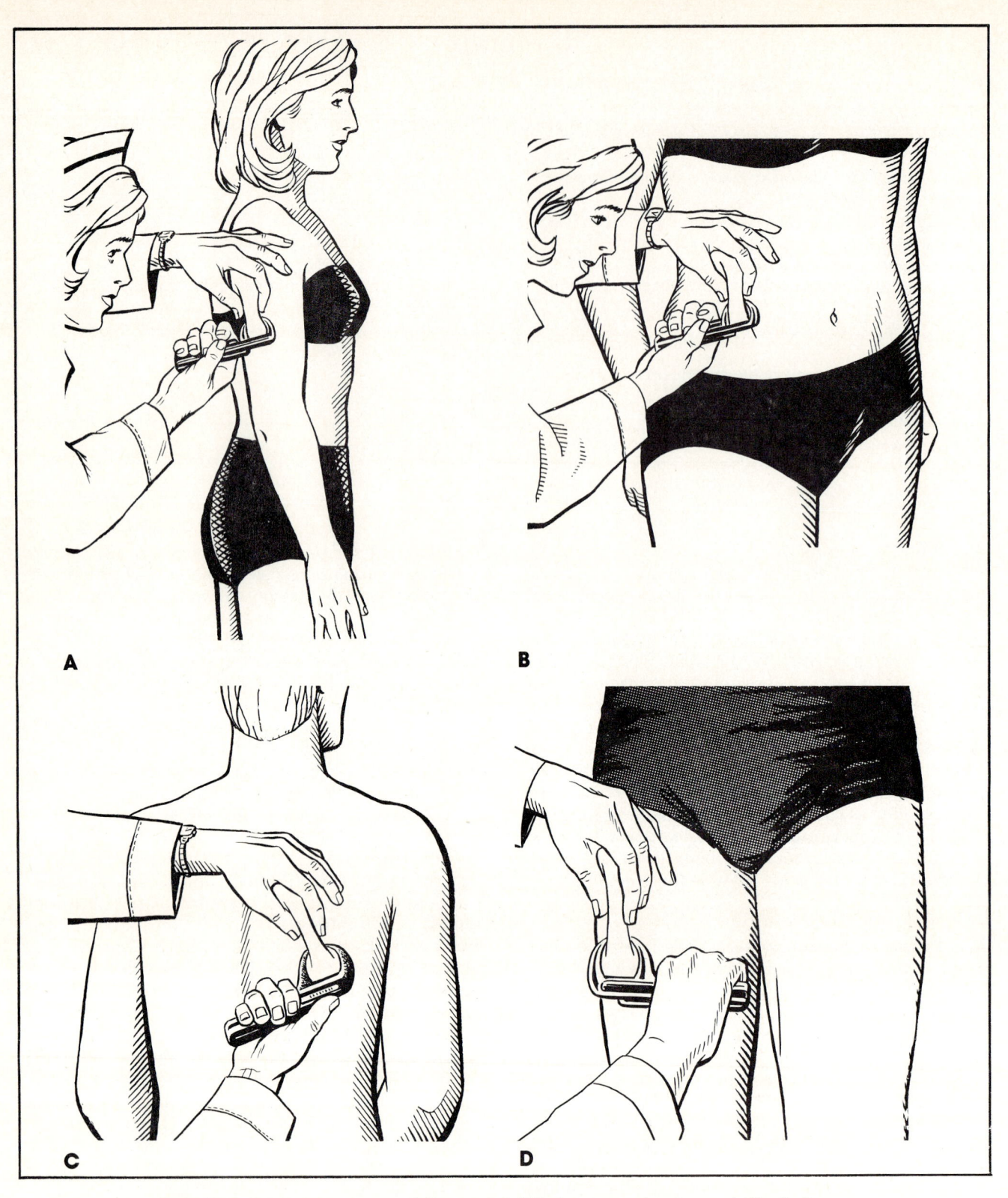

Figure 27-4. **A.** *Triceps measurement (for women).* With the person standing and after finding the midpoint of the arm, have the arm hanging freely at the side of the body. Pinch a vertical fold thickness of skin and subcutaneous tissue at the midpoint of the back of the arm. With the left forefinger and thumb, pull it away from the underlying muscle and hold it. Apply the calipers ½ inch (1.25 centimeters) below the fingers holding the skin fold. Place the calipers at a depth equal to the skinfold thickness. **B.** *Suprailiac measurement (for women).* With the person standing, use the same technique to pinch a vertical fold thickness of skin at the crest of the ilium (hip bone). Have the person lean slightly toward the side being measured; this helps to obtain this measurement. **C.** *Subscapular measurement (for men).* With the person standing, use the same technique to pinch a fold thickness of skin at the bottom point of the scapula at about a 45 degree angle from the vertical. **D.** *Thigh measurement (for men).* With the person standing, use the same technique to pinch a vertical fold thickness of skin midway on the anterior thigh between the hip and the knee joint.

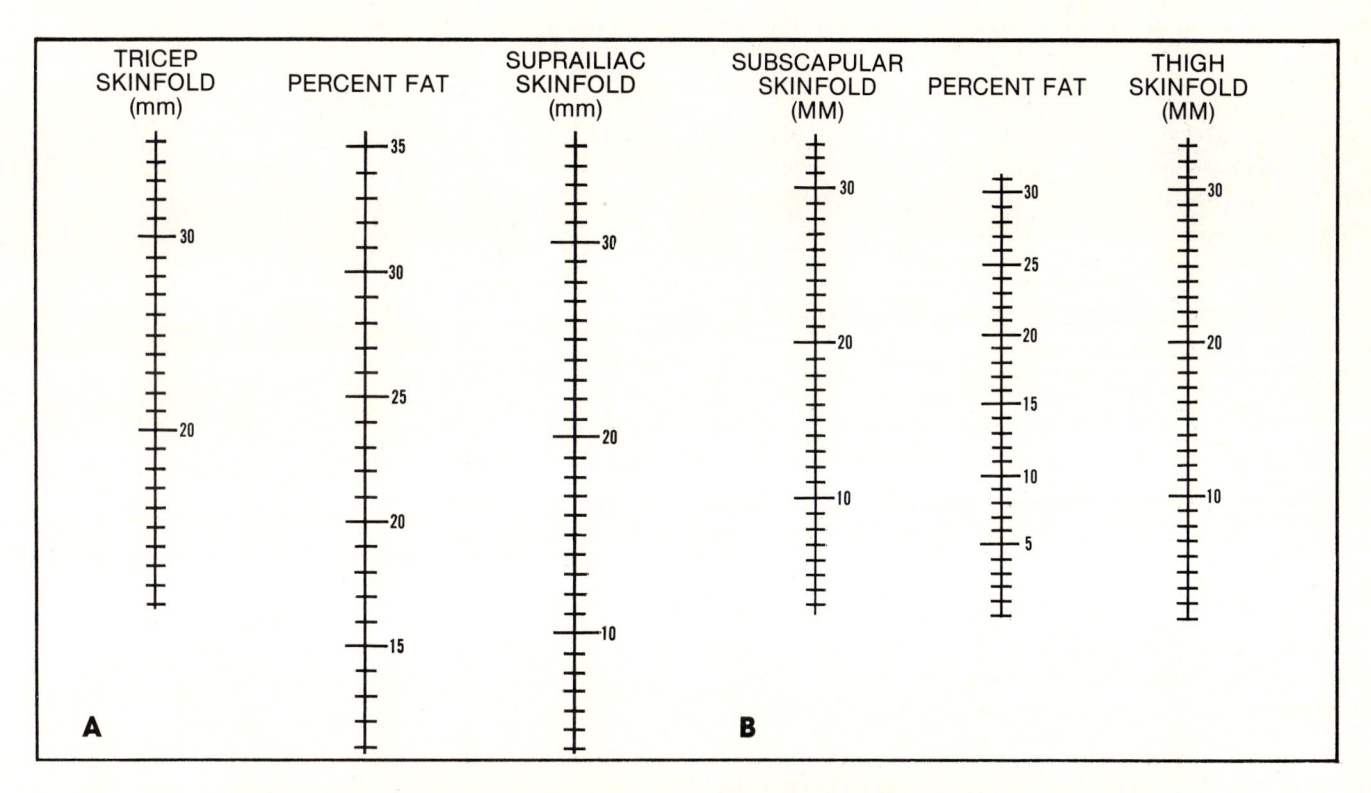

Figure 27–5. A. Nomogram for conversion of women's right-sided skinfold measurements to percent body fat. **B.** Nomogram for conversion of men's right-sided skinfold measurements to percent body fat. (From: Getchell B: Physical Fitness: A Way of Life, ed 2. New York, John Wiley & Sons, 1979, with permission. Nomogram based on formulas developed by: Sloan AW: Estimation of body fat in young men. Journal of Applied Physiology 23(3):311–315, 1967. Brozek J, Grande F, et al: Densitometric analysis of body composition: Revision of some quantitative assumptions. Annals of the New York Academy of Sciences 110:113–139, 1963.)

☐ SKILL SEQUENCE

SKINFOLD THICKNESS MEASUREMENT WITH CALIPERS

Step	Rationale
1. Wash hands.	Prevents transfer of microorganisms.
2. Clean tips of calipers with 70 to 90 percent ethyl or isopropyl alcohol.	Prevents spread of contaminants.
3. Have client standing, relaxed, with the arms at sides.	Facilitates even distribution of body tissue and more accurate measurement. All sites become accessible.
4. Depending on client's sex, select recommended site. Use side of body specified by standard that will be used to determine percent of body fat according to skinfold thickness measurements.	
5. Use left thumb and forefinger to grasp a thickness of skin and subcutaneous tissue, separating it from underlying muscle. (You may need to release and regrasp skinfold to get only skin and fat.) If a site requires several pinches to grasp skinfold, move to next site to let first rest. Hold tissues between finger and thumb.	Calipers must be held in right hand so that measurement scale is read right-side up. Repeated grasps force water from tissues and give false low reading.
6. Use right hand to squeeze calipers open.	Places scale on calipers right-side up.
7. Apply calipers about ½ inch (1.25 centimeters) below fingers holding skinfold; place them at depth equal to skinfold thickness.	Permits pressure on skinfold to be exerted by caliper tips, not fingers.

(continued)

SKINFOLD THICKNESS MEASUREMENT WITH CALIPERS (Cont.)	
Step	**Rationale**
8. Read millimeter value 2 to 3 seconds after caliper tips are placed on skinfold. Read value to nearest 0.5 millimeter.	Allows pressure on skinfold to stabilize and results in a more accurate measurement.
9. Open calipers and remove from skinfold. Release fingers.	
10. Record value.	
11. Repeat measurement at same site after letting skin rest a minute. If measured difference is greater than 0.5 millimeters, take a third reading. Use average of two closest readings as value for that site.	
12. Record final value.	
13. Measure second site.	
14. Use values to determine percentage of body fat. Use nomogram if it is appropriate for person's age. Otherwise, use method prescribed in your clinical settings.	

Nomogram. A nomogram is a series of scales arranged to permit calculations to be performed graphically. The nomograms presented in Figure 27–5 are based on right-sided measurements; they are used to convert skinfold measurements to percent body fat. To use a nomogram, place a point on the scale for each skinfold measurement and join the points with a straight line. The line will intersect the value for the percentage of fat. The percentage of fat can then be used to calculate desirable weight that is more individualized than that provided by the weight-for-height charts.

Body fat norms are available on charts drawn from different populations. Norms classified for college-age men and women are presented in Table 27–3 (Getchell, 1979). These are average ratings of the percentage of fat and not necessarily an ideal rating.

Desirable Weight Calculation

To find a young adult's desirable weight (Getchell, 1979), use the percentage of fat identified on the nomogram from the skinfold measurement. For example, say that you are a female of college age and that 25 percent of your weight of 130 pounds is fat. According to Table 27–3 this is above an average amount. Now the question becomes: How much would you weigh if

TABLE 27–3. Body Fat Norms for College-Age Adults

CLASSIFICATION	PERCENTAGE OF BODY FAT	
	Women	Men
Very low of fat: skinny	14.0–16.9	7.0–9.9
Low: trim	17.0–19.9	10.0–12.9
Average: normal	20.0–23.9	13.0–16.9
Above normal: plump	24.0–26.9	17.0–19.9
Very high: fat	27.0–29.9	20.0–24.9
Obese: overfat	30.0 and higher	25.0 and higher

(Source: Getchell B: Physical Fitness: A Way of Life, ed 2. New York, John Wiley & Sons, 1979. Used with permission.)

your body fat were only 20 percent, which is a low normal value? First, calculate how much of your present weight is in fat:

CALCULATION

$$\text{Fat weight} = \text{weight} \times \frac{\text{percentage of fat}}{100}$$

$$= 130 \times \frac{25}{100}$$

$$\text{Fat weight} = 32.5 \text{ pounds}$$

Next, determine your fat-free weight, that is, your lean body mass weight:

CALCULATION

$$\text{Fat-free weight} = \text{weight} - \text{fat weight}$$
$$= 130 - 32.5 = 97.5$$
$$\text{Fat-free weight} = 97.5 \text{ pounds}$$

Now, to get your desired weight, you need to know how much you would weigh if you had only 20 percent fat, that is, if your fat-free weight were 80 percent of your total weight:

CALCULATION

$$\text{Desired weight for 20 percent fat} = \frac{\text{fat-free weight}}{80 \text{ percent}}$$

$$= \frac{97.5}{.80}$$

$$\text{Desired weight for 20 percent fat} = 122 \text{ pounds}$$

So you would have to shed 8 of your 130 pounds to have only 20 percent of your weight in fat, instead of 25 percent.

RECORDING

Height and weight are usually recorded in numbers on the same form used for vital signs. When serial measurements are obtained during the growth years, they may be plotted on a graph for easier comparison with standard charts. Weights of adult clients with cardiac, renal, or metabolic disorders may also be plotted on graph forms. The same system of measurement should be used for all recordings so that changes can be easily identified.

CRITICAL POINTS SUMMARY

HEIGHT
1. Use a nonstretch measure.
2. Have client fully extended in standing or supine position.
3. Remove client's shoes.
4. Measure to nearest ¼ inch or to nearest centimeter.
5. Record accurately.

WEIGHT
1. Weigh at same time of day whenever possible.
2. Have client empty bowel and bladder before weighing.
3. Remove as much of client's clothing as possible.
4. Check and adjust scale balance before weighing.
5. Center client on scale platform.
6. Observe safety precautions.
7. Return riders on beams to zero after weight is obtained.
8. Record accurately.

LEARNING ACTIVITIES

1. Have a friend measure your height while you are slouching, wearing shoes with heels, then standing erect without shoes. Compare the measurements.
2. Weigh yourself on a spring-balance scale and a balance-beam scale in the same clothing and at the same time of day. Compare the measurements.
3. Weigh yourself on a balance-beam scale before and after emptying your bowel and bladder and before breakfast. Identify the reasons for any differences.
4. Have someone weigh you on a bed scale. Examine your feelings about safety during the entire procedure.
5. When in settings where people are in swim, gym, or running clothes, look critically at males and females of all ages to identify the general proportions of their bodies and the presence and location of fat and muscle development.
6. Have a friend do the pinch test on you to determine if you are overfat. If calipers are available, use them to measure the correct sites to obtain skinfold thicknesses. Use the values on the nomogram (Fig. 27–5A or B) to determine the percentage of fat and calculate your desired weight following the formulas from the text.

REVIEW QUESTIONS

1. What are some of the reasons height and weight measurements are obtained?
2. How does overweight differ from obesity?
3. Why could someone who is considered overweight according to standard table data actually be underweight?
4. Which type of scale is considered more reliable and why?
5. How can you check the balance of a scale? Why is this important?
6. When should a scale be cleaned?
7. How would you instruct someone to obtain accurately the height of a person who cannot stand up?
8. What steps would you use to weigh someone on an upright scale?
9. How can you determine if someone is fat?
10. What is the procedure for using skinfold calipers?

PERFORMANCE CHECKLISTS

OBJECTIVE: To use the correct method to measure body height or length.			
CHARACTERISTIC	RANGE OF ACCEPTABILITY	SATISFACTORY	UNSATISFACTORY
1. Washes hands.	No deviation		
2. Selects nonstretch measure.	No deviation		
3. Has client remove shoes if standing.	No deviation		
4. Has client fully extended or erect.	No deviation		
5. Measures from vertex of head to sole of heel in a straight line.	No deviation		
6. Reads measure to nearest ¼ inch or to nearest centimeter.	No deviation		
7. Records measurement.	No deviation		

236 PROFESSIONAL CLINICAL NURSING SKILLS

OBJECTIVE: To use the correct method to weigh a client accurately and safely.

CHARACTERISTIC	RANGE OF ACCEPTABILITY	SATISFACTORY	UNSATISFACTORY
1. Washes hands.	No deviation		
2. Secures appropriate scale for client's age and physical ability.	No deviation		
3. Checks and adjusts scale balance.	No deviation		
4. Has client remove all clothing feasible.	No deviation		
5. Positions client on center of scale.	No deviation		
6. Moves riders on lower and upper beams to balance points.	No deviation		
7. Reads weight to nearest 1/4 pound or 1/10 kilogram.	No deviation		
8. Helps client move from scale.	No deviation		
9. Returns riders to zero.	No deviation		
10. Records weight.	No deviation		

OBJECTIVE: To use the correct method to weigh a client on a bedside scale accurately and safely.

CHARACTERISTIC	RANGE OF ACCEPTABILITY	SATISFACTORY	UNSATISFACTORY
1. Washes hands.	No deviation		
2. Secures sufficient help to transfer client to scale safely.	No deviation		
3. Explains procedure to client. Moves scale parallel to bed and client; lowers weighboard.	No deviation		
4. Checks and adjusts balance.	No deviation		
5. Closes lift; elevates weighboard.	No deviation		
6. Turns client to side of bed facing away from scale.	No deviation		
7. Releases lift slowly to lower weighboard to mattress.	No deviation		
8. Sets brake securely.	No deviation		
9. Aligns client straight along edge of weighboard.	No deviation		
10. Turns client onto his or her back on the weighboard.	No deviation		
11. Closes lift and elevates weighboard above the mattress.	No deviation		
12. Places ratio weights on weight holder, moves rider (riders) on beam (beams) until beam balances; totals the value of the ratio weights and the riders on the beam.	No deviation		
13. Records weight on scratch pad.	No deviation		
14. Slowly releases lift to lower client to bed.	No deviation		
15. Turns client to bed.	No deviation		
16. Closes lift and elevates weighboard.	No deviation		
17. Releases brakes; withdraws scale from bedside.	No deviation		
18. Lowers weighboard; leaves lift release knob slightly open.	No deviation		

(continued)

CHARACTERISTIC	RANGE OF ACCEPTABILITY	SATISFACTORY	UNSATISFACTORY
19. Returns ratio weights and weight holder to storage place.	No deviation		
20. Secures beam lock.	No deviation		
21. Assists client to comfortable position.	No deviation		
22. Removes scale from room.	No deviation		
23. Records weight on client's record.	No deviation		

REFERENCES

Beland I, Passos JY: Clinical Nursing: Pathophysiology and Psychosocial Approaches, ed 4. New York, Macmillan, 1981.

Brozek J, Grande F, et al: Densitometric analysis of body composition: Revision of some quantitative assumptions. Annals of the New York Academy of Sciences 110:113–139, 1963.

Consumer Research Magazine 61(10):161, 1978.

Craddock D: Obesity and Its Management, ed 3. Edinburgh, Churchill Livingstone, 1978.

Getchell B: Physical Fitness: A Way of Life, ed 2. New York, John Wiley & Sons, 1979.

Guyton AC: Textbook of Medical Physiology, ed 6. Philadelphia, WB Saunders, 1981.

Luckmann J, Sorensen KC: Medical–Surgical Nursing: A Psychophysiologic Approach, ed 2. Philadelphia: WB Saunders, 1980.

Mitchell P: Concepts Basic to Nursing. NY, McGraw-Hill, 1977.

Pollack ML, Wilmore JH, Fox SM: Health and Fitness Through Physical Activity. New York, John Wiley & Sons, 1978.

Powers PS: Obesity: The Regulation of Weight. Baltimore, Williams & Wilkins, 1980.

Sloan AW: Estimation of body fat in young men. Journal of Applied Physiology 23(3):311–315, 1967.

Sloan AW, Burt JJ, Blyth CS: Estimation of body fat in young women. Journal of Applied Physiology 17(6):967–970, 1962.

Wenke DA, Baren M, Dewan SP: Nutrition: The Challenge of Being Well Nourished. Reston, VA, Reston, 1980.

BIBLIOGRAPHY

Gibbons A: Weighing the patient. Nursing Times 63(46):1550–1551, 1967.

Goodhart RS, Shils ME: Modern Nutrition in Health and Disease, ed 5. Philadelphia, Lea & Febiger, 1973.

Mayer J: Overweight. Englewood Cliffs, NJ, Prentice-Hall, 1968.

Vitale F: Individualized Fitness Programs. Englewood Cliffs, NJ, Prentice-Hall, 1973.

8 Medical Asepsis

☐ INTRODUCTION

Microorganisms capable of causing infections are present within and on all people and in all environments. *Asepsis* literally means "without infection." Aseptic techniques are those procedures used to prevent and control infection. There are two types of aseptic techniques: medical and surgical. *Medical asepsis*, or clean technique, is used to prevent patient contamination from the environment, by individuals and among individuals. The number and growth of pathogenic microorganisms are reduced by proper use of cleaning agents. *Surgical asepsis*, which is presented in Chapter 9, involves the use of objects or materials that have no living microorganisms, either pathogenic or nonpathogenic. The correct use of each type of aseptic technique for any given procedure is important in any setting where good health is valued.

Microorganisms to which the client is exposed in health-care facilities, especially in acute-care hospitals and long-term care facilities, are more likely to pose problems than those encountered in the home. The type and number of microorganisms in health-care facilities are frequently different from those to which a person is normally exposed in the community. The client is exposed to microorganisms through contact with the personnel and materials used for treatment. People are more vulnerable to infection when they are aged or have had surgery, debilitating illnesses, or medical treatments that weaken the body's normal defenses. Antibiotic-resistant strains of microorganisms, which are difficult to treat, are a particular problem for the debilitated client.

An infection may be classified as either *community acquired*, which means that the client entered the facility with it, or *nosocomial*, which means it was acquired after admission to the facility. Nosocomial infections pose a major health problem in today's health-care system, particularly in hospitals. Data from an ongoing national study of nosocomial infections by the Centers for Disease Control (CDC) reveal that nosocomial infections are diagnosed in 3 to 6 percent of all hospitalized patients. There also is an untold number of nosocomial infections that remain undiagnosed. The costs of nosocomial infections to the client are enormous; such infections can result in extended hospital stays, suffering, disability, and loss of life. It has been estimated by the CDC that up to $6 billion per year are spent because of nosocomial infections and that at least $1 billion per year could be saved by a significant reduction of infections that are frequently preventable (Reinarz, 1978).

A study by Freeman et al. (1979) indicates the cost of nosocomial infections. Clients who acquired one nosocomial infection had an average extended hospital stay of 13 days. Those with two nosocomial infections stayed an average of 35.4 days longer. The increased vulnerability of the elderly to nosocomial infections is illustrated by Brem and Torok's (1979) analysis of data from a community teaching hospital's nosocomial infection rate for 1 year. People under age 65 had an infection rate of 2.1 percent; those over age 65 had a rate of 10 percent, five times greater than their younger counterparts. Inhalation therapy and urinary catheterization were the two procedures most commonly associated with the infections.

Since the advent of antibiotics, the increase in nosocomial infections has been attributed in part to an increase in the number of resistant strains of pathogenic microorganisms. Some microorganisms that had been nonpathogenic are now causing infections because of an increase in client susceptibility. Recognition of the problem and the need to take positive action against nosocomial infections started in 1958. The American Hospital Association (AHA) and the Joint Commission on Accreditation of Hospitals (JCAH) recommended that every hospital have an infection control program. Such a program is now a requirement for hospital accreditation by the JCAH. The American Hospital Association publishes a manual of recommended procedures for an infection control program. The program includes a committee with members from the medical, nursing, and administrative staff and representatives from other hospital departments. The committee is charged with the responsibility for developing infection control policies and procedures for all departments and for surveillance activities for the institution. These activities include prevention and control of infections in health-care personnel, clients, and visitors. An infection control practitioner (ICP), freqently a nurse, and an epidemiologist, usually a physician, both provide services that are vital to the implementation of isolation policies and surveillance activities. The ICP trains the institution's personnel on the proper use of the isolation techniques and provides consultation to the nurses and other staff and serves as a resource for community agencies. The epidemiologist consults with the medical staff and supervises the proper isolation techniques.

Because infection control is a responsibility shared by all personnel in the facility, nurses can assume an active role in working with the infection control committee by critically examining the techniques used and determining their adequacy. Hardy (1973) suggests that the nurse make the effort to determine what percent of clients enter the hopsital with an infection and what percent acquire an infection. This information provides a basis for evaluating the effectiveness of aseptic practices. If the number of clients with nosocomial infections is seen to increase on the clinical unit, the nurse is then aware of the need for changes in procedures or more stringent implementation of existing procedures.

There also is a legal component to the problem of nosocomial infections. The hospital may be held legally liable for harm suffered by the client if he or she can establish that the harm from an infection resulted from negligence on the part of the hospital or its personnel, or that the hospital knowingly permitted the use of nonaseptic techniques (American Hospital Association, 1979).

The nurse has a responsibility, along with other health professionals, to provide an environment for clients, their families and visitors, other personnel, and themselves that is as free as possible from disease-causing microorganisms. The nurse serves as a role model for others through personal hygiene habits and appearance as well as in the use of appropriate aseptic techniques while providing nursing care. In practice, the nurse is responsible for all of the functions that are essential to the prevention, recognition, and management of infection regardless of the setting. He or she protects the clients from exposure to infection from their families, visitors, the hospital staff, other clients, and from the materials and equipment used during diagnostic and treatment procedures. The nurse also serves as a teacher and a supervisor for other members of the nursing team, clients, their families, and visitors. On occasion, it may be necessary to remind supervisors and physicians about appropriate techniques to prevent infection.

Frequent and intimate contacts with clients designate the nurse for a key role in the prevention and control of infection. The nurse must combine knowledge of microbes with an understanding of how infection occurs in order to prevent microorganisms from causing an infection and to control existing infections from spreading. The ability of any microorganism to cause an infection is related to its characteristics, the support provided for it to survive in the environment, and the strengths of the host's defenses.

The cycle of infection, frequently known as the infection chain, requires the presence of six elements. The absence or elimination of any one of them prevents an infectious process from occurring. When each of the elements is present, an infection may occur at any point in the cycle. The cycle includes:

1. An infectious agent present in numbers and virulence sufficient to cause an infection
2. A reservoir or place available for the microorganisms to grow and multiply
3. An available exit for the microorganisms to leave the reservoir
4. A means of transportation available for movement to another site
5. An available entrance at another site
6. A susceptible host available for the microorganisms to enter

The goal of providing a safe environment is attained by interrupting the cycle of events through the use of techniques that remove pathogens and potentially pathogenic microorganisms from the cycle or by limiting their ability to be transported. All nursing-care activities require the use of aseptic techniques to break the cycle of infection.

The skills presented in this chapter are in the category of medical asepsis. Handwashing (Skill 28) is considered to be the most important procedure used to prevent nosocomial infections. Even though handwashing is learned at an early age as part of personal hygiene practice, the handwashing techniques required for medical asepsis are more rigorous and complete in order to prevent the spread of microorganisms from oneself to others or to the materials used in clinical practice. To be effective, handwashing must be complete and used at the appropriate time.

Isolation techniques (Skill 29) are used to limit the contact an infected person has with others or the contact a susceptible client has with personnel and visitors. The techniques and procedures serve as barriers so that the transmission of microorganisms is controlled. The degree of the isolation depends on the site of the infection and how the microorganism causing the infection is transmitted.

☐ ENTRY TEST

1. What do the terms host, reservoir, carrier, fomite, vector, and contaminant mean?
2. What are the main routes by which microorganisms are transmitted?

3. How are each of these routes described?
4. What are the routes through which disease-causing microorganisms enter or leave the body?
5. What are the barriers of the human body that prevent microorganisms from entering?
6. Which microorganisms are normally found on the skin, conjunctiva of the eye, nose, throat, and mouth, the intestines, and genital tract?
7. Which body area has the greatest number of microorganisms?
8. How do antiseptics and disinfectants differ in their action on microorganisms?

REFERENCES

American Hospital Association: Infection Control in the Hospital, ed 4. Chicago, AHA, 1979.

Brem AM, Torok EM: Nosocomial infections in the elderly. Hospital Topics 57(6):10, 40–43, 1979.

Freeman J, Rosner BA, McGowan JE: Adverse effects of nosocomial infection. The Journal of Infectious Diseases 140(5):732–740, 1979.

Hardy CS: Infection control. Nursing73 3(8):18–21, 1973.

Reinarz JA: Nosocomial infections. Clinical Symposia 30(6):2–32, 1978.

SKILL 28 Handwashing

PREREQUISITE SKILLS

Skill 19, "Inspection"

STUDENT OBJECTIVES

1. Describe the purpose of handwashing.
2. Identify sources of hand contamination.
3. Identify activities that require handwashing.
4. Explain the steps in the handwashing procedure.
5. Wash hands correctly to remove transient and resident bacteria.

INTRODUCTION

Handwashing removes soil and invisible microorganisms from the skin and nails when all surfaces are thoroughly cleaned with running water, friction, and soap or detergent. It is the single most important technique used in nursing practice in all health-care settings and its value in preventing infections cannot be overemphasized.

Long before Louis Pasteur established the germ theory of disease and Joseph Lister discovered antiseptics, Ignaz Semmelweiss made the association between contaminated hands and infection in a maternity hospital in 1847. He found that the incidence of maternal infections and death decreased significantly when physicians and students rinsed their hands in a solution of chlorinated lime after leaving the autopsy room and before attending and examining the women in labor and delivery (Walker, 1955).

PREPARATION

Everyone has *resident* organisms on the skin and mucous membranes. Resident organisms are usually the same as the normal flora indigenous to the body. They tend to be stable in both numbers and variety according to the particular body area in which they reside. Resident organisms found on each person vary somewhat from person to person depending on age, physiology, skin type, activity, and the external environment. The normal bacteria in residence help to prevent harmful organisms from becoming established. But they are also capable of becoming parasites and causing an infection if the opportunity is available for increased numbers of them to enter different sites of the body, such as the blood or deeper tissues. For example, organisms found in the intestines can cause an infection when they are transferred to another body area such as the urinary tract or skin. Washing and scrubbing reduces the number of resident bacteria but it can never completely eliminate them because they lie in the deeper layers of the skin. Soon after removal, they rapidly reestablish themselves on the surface. The hair, face, axilla, and groin usually have more resident bacteria than the arms and hands. The area around and under the fingernails holds the greatest number of bacteria on the hands. Moist body areas such as the groin, perineum, and axilla harbor gram-negative bacteria whereas gram-positive bacteria are more common on other areas (Steere and Mallison, 1975).

Transient bacteria are those that do not normally survive on the skin longer than 24 hours; they are not firmly attached to the skin and can be easily washed away or may die because of inadequate support for their growth and multiplication. Some are destroyed by the normal resident bacteria. Transient bacteria are acquired through contacts with materials on which they are present. Depending on the person, some organisms may be transient or resident. Resident bacteria may also be acquired from transient bacteria either because of repeated exposure to the organisms or because of the loss of normal resident organisms that would prevent the prolonged life of the transient organisms. Bacteria that are resident on one area of the body become transient when transferred to another part.

A study on the quality and frequency of handwashing by Fox et al. (1974) revealed that the washing techniques used by registered nurses were poorer than those of other nursing personnel, although none of the subjects used a perfect technique. Handwashing was not done after performance of dirty activities in 93 percent of the incidents observed by the investigators. Taylor (1978) also found that nursing personnel washed more often after clean than dirty activities; however, the registered nurses' technique in washing was less deficient than that of the other nursing personnel. Both studies reflect a persistent lack of concern for and attention given to handwashing as an important preventive measure in cross-contamination.

The pervasiveness of pathogenic bacteria is illustrated by Flournoy's study (1979) on nosocomial infections from gram-negative bacteria. Sink drains throughout a hospital were found to be a source of antibiotic-resistant gram-negative bacteria contamination for hands. Even when sinks were disinfected regularly, the organisms recolonized when the disinfection was discontinued over the weekend. Bacteriological cultures revealed that the water was not the source of contamination but that the sink traps served as the reservoir. Prevention of the problem may be resolved by redesigning the sinks.

Paper towel dispensers near every sink are essential for handwashing to maintain medical asepsis.

HAND-CARE AGENTS

Soap in any form, if used properly, is effective in removing transient bacteria. A common bar of soap left at the sink has been considered a source of contamination, but there are no studies to support this. When bar soap is used, the bar should be small and changed frequently. It should rest on a draining rack and not be permitted to sit in a pool of water that would permit the growth of bacteria. Liquid soap dispensers may become contaminated and have been associated with outbreaks of nosocomial infections (Steere and Mallison, 1975). Simmons recommends that liquid soap dispensers be emptied at least once a month and the container cleaned, dried, and refilled with fresh solution. The use of disposable dispensers may be preferable to reusable ones (1981, p. 5).

Alcohol, one of the most effective antiseptics, can disinfect the skin in 15 to 30 seconds and reduce the bacterial count by an average of 92 percent when used for washing for 1 to 3 minutes. But alcohol dries the skin and evaporates quickly. It is also hazardous because of its flammability. When combined with other disinfectants, alcohol becomes even more effective in cleaning, and the addition of emollients reduces drying of skin.

Iodine in tincture form (with alcohol) is also an effective germicide, but it is not recommended for routine handwashing because of the possibility of tissue damage from chapping, burning, and allergic reactions. Water-soluble preparations of iodine and organic compounds, called *iodophors,* are also effective disinfectants, but their action appears to be limited because once they are rinsed from the skin, reduction of bacteria ceases. When used frequently, they are reported to be more drying to the skin than other antiseptic handwashing preparations (Steere and Mallison, 1975).

There are some significant disadvantages found with the use of *hexachlorophene* preparations as handwashing agents. Although they reduce the number of S. aureus able to survive on the skin when used at least once a day for 3 to 5 days, they have not been shown to be more effective than soap and water in reducing S. aureus infections in clients. Hexachlorophene preparations also disrupt the film left on the skin when alcohol is used, and have a minimal effect on gram-negative bacteria and fungi. They have also been shown to support the growth of *Pseudomonas aeruginosa, Serratia marcescens,* and *Alcaligenes faecalis,* which are all gram-negative organisms associated with nosocomial infections (Steere and Mallison, 1975). In addition, because hexachlorophene can be absorbed from the skin in large amounts it might have toxic effects on the central nervous system, particularly in premature infants (Simmons, 1981, p. 3).

Aqueous benzalkonium chloride products are quickly inactivated by contact with organic materials such as protein and cellulose fibers and are therefore rather ineffective antiseptics. Furthermore, *Pseudomonas* and *Enterobacter* organisms have been found growing in them (Steere and Mallison, 1975).

Antiseptic foams consisting of alcohol, with or without an additional antiseptic, have been found to be effective in killing transient bacteria, but they do not remove soil from the hands. This substitute for handwashing is easy to use and the dispenser may be carried about in the pocket or mounted on the wall for use in places where sinks are not available. Len and Deshmukh (1974) found an ethanol foam product to be superior to one that was combined with hexachlorophene when they compared cultures taken after routine clean activities, after routine handwashing, and after examining clients. Beck (1978) compared cultures before and after the use of ethanol and hexachlorophene foam and found it effective in killing transient bacteria.

The foam is massaged into the hands with the same technique used for traditional washing. The amount used must be adequate to keep the hands feeling moist for about 1 minute and it should be dispersed around and under the nails for complete cleaning. Nursing personnel who used the foam repeatedly reported that it was not drying to the skin.

Where sinks are available, soap and water are recommended for handwashing before all routine contacts with clients. Antiseptic preparations for handwashing are best reserved for situations where the risk of infection is the greatest, such as in surgical scrubs, and before procedures that invade the body, such as catheterization. Many antiseptics considered safe for the skin cause excessive dryness, cracking, and dermatitis. Personnel with dermatitis pose a greater risk to clients if they are reluctant to wash in order to avoid aggravating their skin condition. Antiseptics do not reduce bacteria counts on skin with dermatitis (Steere and Mallison, 1975).

The use of *hand creams* between washings is discouraged for individuals working in a clinical setting because hand creams are not sterile and have been found to be a source of pathogens that cause nosocomial infections. Hand cream containing hexachlorophene has been found to be contaminated with gram-negative bacteria and *Candida albicans* (France, 1968; Knights and Harvey, 1964). A septicemia outbreak in a medical intensive care unit was traced to a dispensing bottle of lanolin hand cream contaminated with *Klebsiella pneumoniae* (Morse et al., 1967). Of 26 brands of commercially available hand lotions cultured by Morse and Schonbeck (1968), 4 were found to be contaminated. In one nationally distributed brand, *S. marcescens* was found in 9 of the 13 previously unopened bottles cultured. Both new and used bottles of another brand that were distributed by a hospital to clients on admission were found to be contaminated with *Pseudomonas aeruginosa*. From all new and used samples cultured in a third brand also distributed by a hospital for use by clients and staff, *Escherichia intermedia, K. pneumoniae, Alcaligenes faecalis,* and *P. aeruginosa* were found. Samples of a fourth brand, manufactured by a hospital pharmacy, distributed throughout the institution and commercially available from the pharmacy, yielded *S. marsescens* and *A. faecalis* when cultured.

DATA BASE

Because microorganisms are invisible, the presence or absence of visible soil on the hands is an inadequate indication of the presence or absence of contamination. The nurse must make a conscious decision about when to wash the hands based on knowledge of sources of contamination. All nursing activities can be classified according to the probability of the presence of pathogenic organisms. Such a classification provides a useful guide for deciding if the hands should be washed before and after, only before, or only after engaging in a particular activity. The nurse must be able to evaluate each activity to determine if it is clean or dirty. Unnecessary handwashing can be eliminated in many instances by organizing work flow from clean to dirty tasks. For example, within a brief period of time the nurse may perform the following tasks for a single client: administer medications, assist the client with a meal, change bed linen, and measure urine output. When it is possible to sequence these activities from clean to contaminated tasks, as they are listed here, time and handwashing are saved, while contamination is prevented. Ranking of client-care activities provides a useful guide for knowing when the hands may be considered contaminated or clean (Fox et al., 1974).

Contaminated activities are those in which the nurse has direct or indirect contact with people, materials, or objects known or highly suspected to have pathogenic organisms present. These activities include personal events in which one may engage apart from client care. The hands should be washed after contact with each contaminated activity so that the organisms from each source are not transferred. The activities in the contaminated category are sequenced below from the *most* contaminated to the *least* contaminated contacts that may occur during client care. They include contact with:

1. Client body surfaces that are infected, such as abscesses or infected traumatic and surgical wounds.
2. Items or hands that have been in direct contact with blood, secretions or excretions from known infections (such as blood on needles or syringes), respiratory discharges on tissues or equipment, or dressings with wound drainage.
3. Fecal matter, which may be encountered while cleansing the anal area after defecation, during the process of fecal disimpaction, or while administering an enema.
4. Materials bearing fecal matter, such as bedpans, toilet seats, bed linen, and protective clothing.
5. Urine, which may be touched while obtaining urine specimens or while emptying bedpans or urinary drainage bags.
6. Materials contaminated with urine, such as clothing, linen, or protective pads.
7. A client who has direct contact with body area secretions, such as those from the genital organs, nose, mouth, and ears.
8. Items that have been in contact with or contain blood or secretions that are not known or expected to be contaminated, such as used needles and syringes and saliva on used tissues or napkins.

Clean activities are those in which the nurse has direct or indirect contact with people, materials, or objects that are *known* to be free of pathogenic organisms. The hands should be clean before engaging in clean activities to prevent the transfer of contaminants during the contacts. The activities in the clean category are sequenced below from the *least* clean to the *most* clean contacts that may occur during client care, and thus are on a continuum with the preceding activities. They include contact with:

9. Body surfaces of the client that do not have secretions or excretions present. Included in this group are brief contacts, such as obtaining a pulse or blood pressure, touching to reassure, and shaking hands.
10. Items that have been in intimate contact with clients but are not known to have contaminating secretions and excretions. Included here are relatively clean surfaces of bedside tables, used clothing, and linen.
11. Items that have had brief or infrequent contacts with clients or those on which a significant degree of contamination is not expected, including such things as blood pressure cuffs, meal trays, and scales.
12. Items that are separated from client contact and thus are not routinely cleaned. Supplies and equipment used by personnel in nonclient areas, such as the nursing station, medicine room, and clean storage areas, are included in this group.
13. Materials that are thoroughly washed or cleaned after direct or indirect contact with the client's environment, or his or her secretions or excretions. This cleaning process may include disinfection but not sterilization. Included here are such items as linen, clothing, instruments, equipment, and furniture.
14. Materials that are sterile. Such materials are enclosed in protective wrappers and then processed so that all pathogenic and nonpathogenic organisms are killed. The exterior wrapper prevents exposure to microorganisms after sterilization. The intact package may be handled with clean hands. The sterile materials remain sterile only if contacted by other sterile materials. Manual contact requires the use of sterile gloves, but clean hands may be used if the materials do not have to remain sterile.

Physical Appraisal Skills

Inspection. Inspection is used to note the presence of soil on one's hands and to monitor one's skin condition. Dryness, cracking, dermatitis, torn cuticles, and hangnails provide opportunities for bacterial invasion. The skin is an important natural barrier that should be kept intact. Early signs of problems with the skin must be attended to promptly. In some situations, it may be necessary to wear gloves while on duty to protect oneself and others from hands that cannot be thoroughly cleaned by routine handwashing. Medical treatment for dermatitis may be necessary.

EQUIPMENT

The availability of sinks for handwashing by personnel varies among institutions. The most convenient location for washing may be in the client's room or bathroom. However, there is an unresolved debate about personnel's use of sinks that are also used by clients. Some feel that the microorganisms deposited by clients may be a source of hand contamination. Others feel that if the client's sink is the only washing facility available within a short distance, it is better to allow personnel to use it, observing proper precautions against hand contamination, than to risk their not washing at all.

Short faucet handles require the use of the hands to turn them on and off, which can result in contamination of washed hands. Long wing tip blades can be operated with the arm. Foot pedal faucets are normally found in the nursery, labor, delivery, and operating room areas where surgical scrubs are necessary. They may also be available on sinks located on clincial units.

☐ EXECUTION

Rings, chipped nail polish, and long fingernails should be avoided; they provide places for transient bacteria to harbor and grow. (Some agencies permit the wearing of rings during clean activites; if rings are worn, they are moved up and down during the washing so that the area around and under them can be cleaned.) Watches are worn high on wrists to permit proper cleaning of the wrist. The water should be comfortably warm, because hot water enlarges the pores and more oil is lost from the skin, thus promoting dryness and cracking. Warm water also has a lower surface tension than hot water, which facilitates removal of bacteria. A moderate flow of water is left running during the washing and rinsing process to prevent hand contamination from occurring when touching the faucets (see Fig. 28-1). Too strong a flow splashes water onto clothing and the floor, which spreads bacteria and poses additional hazards. Friction from the running water also aids in the physical removal of bacteria.

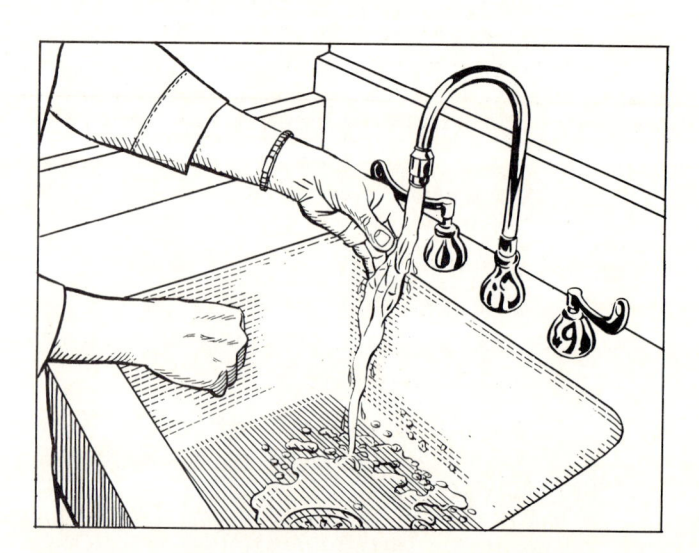

Figure 28-1. Position at sink, hands down, water running.

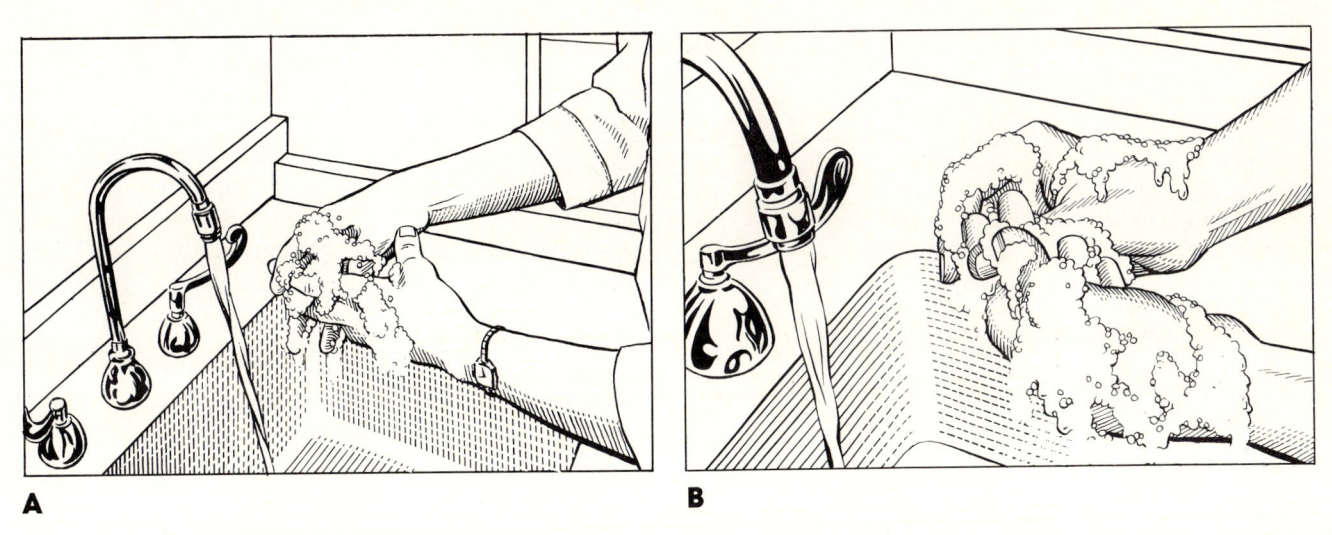

Figure 28–2. A. Vigorous massaging of areas between fingers. **B.** Vigorous massaging of areas around and under nails.

Rubbing the hands vigorously together creates a soap lather, and the friction removes bacteria. Attention is paid to massaging all skin areas, around and under the nails, the knuckles, the back, palmar surfaces, sides of the hands, and the areas between the fingers, as shown in Figure 28-2. The hands are rubbed together for a minimum of 15 seconds under running water before rinsing. They are held downward so that the water drains down from the fingertips into the sink. Paper towels are used to prevent contamination. Overly vigorous rubbing to dry the hands can also cause irritation, although the friction of the towels is thought to remove some of the bacteria that may be present after washing and rinsing. Use a clean paper towel to turn off water faucets in order to prevent recontamination of the hands (see Fig. 28-3).

There is no specific length of time for handwashing, although some authorities cite 2 to 3 minutes as optimum. The actual length of time depends on the nature and degree of contamination and the amount of soilage. Handling of grossly contaminated materials requires longer washing.

The hectic pace encountered in some clinical situations need not prevent personnel from washing. Sprunt et al. (1973) have shown that transient bacteria can be removed by a quick washing of about 30 seconds with running water and friction and drying with paper towels. This method is almost as effective as a longer wash using soap.

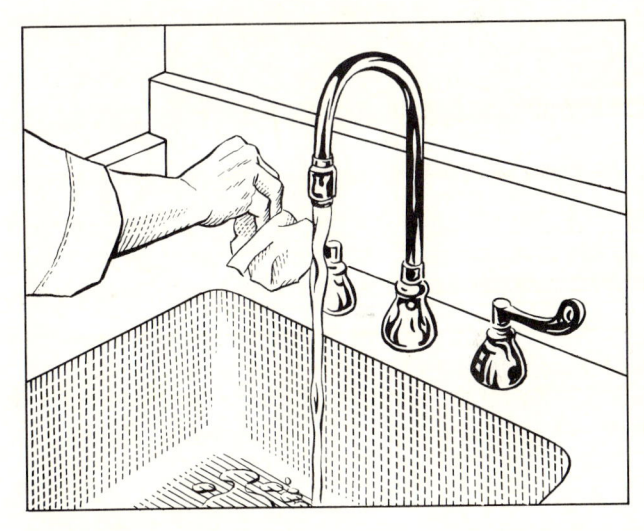

Figure 28–3. A dry paper towel is used to turn off the faucet to prevent recontamination of hands.

☐ SKILL SEQUENCE

HANDWASHING

Step	Rationale
1. Remove rings, push watch up above wrist.	Rings and watches may harbor microorganisms.
2. Turn faucet on and adjust moderate flow of water to warm temperature.	Too strong a water flow splashes clothing and floor, creating potential for contamination of self and making floor slippery. Warm water has lower surface tension, increases removal of microorganisms.

(continued)

HANDWASHING (Cont.)

Step	Rationale
3. Wet hands and wrists, holding hands down so that water drains from fingertips into sink. Avoid touching sides with hands.	More lather produced when hands are wet first. Sink and faucets are contaminated. If touched while washing, must restart washing.
4. Rinse bar soap under running water before and after lathering or obtain liquid soap from dispenser.	Rinses off contaminant present on soap.
5. Rub palms together to create visible lather.	Lather helps to remove microorganisms and soil.
6. Apply vigorous friction from one hand to thoroughly massage all hand and finger surfaces of other; flex fingers and thumb so skin creases at joints can be thoroughly cleaned. Massage wrist area with soap lather.	Friction is the most important step in removing bacteria.
7. Rub loosely interlocked fingers and thumbs together to wash spaces between them. (If ring is worn, move it up and down on fingers and wash under it.)	Areas where microorganisms hide.
8. Use fingernails of one hand to clean under nails of other hand. (Use brushes, nail files, and orange sticks if available.)	
9. Massage around nail beds.	Areas where microorganisms hide.
10. Rub hands together vigorously under running water to rinse, starting with the wrists to remove all soap. If hands are grossly contaminated, repeat steps 4 to 10.	Running water flushes soil and organisms away. Residual soap is drying to the skin. Prevents contaminating arms.
11. Use paper towels to dry hands with gentle rubbing or patting. Discard towels in waste basket.	Overzealous rubbing creates skin irritation, promotes chapping.
12. Use dry towels to turn off water.	Wet towels permit microorganisms to move through them from faucet to recontaminate hands.

☐ CRITICAL POINTS SUMMARY

1. Identify the activities that require handwashing before and after, before only, or after only.
2. Attend to your personal grooming practices to eliminate sources of contamination.
3. Prevent hands from becoming dry, chapped, or developing dermatitis. Treat dermatitis promptly.
4. Use correct handwashing technique.
   a. Remove rings, push watch above wrist.
   b. Use moderate stream of warm running water for handwashing.
   c. Avoid touching sink and faucets after handwashing has begun.
   d. Avoid wetting clothing and floor; hold hands down so water runs off fingertips.
   e. Create a visible soap lather.
   f. Use friction to massage all surfaces of hands and wrists vigorously. Clean area under and around nails.
   g. Rinse soap from all surfaces thoroughly under running water.
   h. Dry hands thoroughly and gently with paper towels.
   i. Turn off faucets with dry paper towel.

☐ LEARNING ACTIVITIES

1. List in sequence each item or body site you have touched since you last washed your hands.
   a. Place a "C" before the clean items and a "D" before the dirty (contaminated) items.
   b. Note the number of dirty contacts that were followed by a clean contact.
   c. Name the organisms that you are most apt to have transferred from the dirty to the clean site.
2. In a clinical setting, discreetly observe the aseptic practices of a physician, a nurse, and an aide while they perform their routine functions.
   a. Note when and how often each person proceeds from a dirty to a clean activity without handwashing.
   b. Observe each person's handwashing technique and note how complete each of them is. Note the key points included and omitted.
   c. Consider which persons you would or would not want to take care of you if you were a client. What are the reasons for your selection?
3. Interview a member of the housekeeping department to learn the frequency and method with which sinks are cleaned.
4. Tour a clinical unit and check each handwashing facility for general sanitation and complete supplies.
5. Compare the type of handwashing facilities available in different health-care settings.
6. Rank the following items from the most contaminated to the cleanest, designating the most contaminated as 1 and the cleanest as 6. Compare and discuss the reasons for your rankings with a peer.
   a. ____ solution returned from a cleansing enema
   b. ____ hosiery removed from a person's leg
   c. ____ a dressing removed from a draining wound
   d. ____ a used hypodermic needle
   e. ____ used bed linen
   f. ____ a nurse's uniform at the beginning of the day

7. Completely immerse both of your hands and wrists in flour or loose earth so that all surfaces are covered. Wash your hands according to the previously described procedure and note the areas that require the most effort to clean. Are these areas the same as those where microorganisms hide?

☐ REVIEW QUESTIONS

1. Why do hands need to be washed?
2. What type of organisms are removed during handwashing?
3. What are some sources of contamination that can occur from the equipment used in handwashing?
4. To what extent is washing without soap effective in cleaning the hands?
5. How is inspection used in relation to maintaining medically aseptic hands?
6. Why is it necessary to differentiate between contaminated and clean activities?
7. What factors determine whether an activity is contaminated or clean?
8. What are some of the objective and subjective data the nurse should know about clients so that cross-infection does not occur?
9. How can personal grooming and hygiene practices affect the safety of the client's environment?
10. On what areas of the hands are most transient bacteria found?
11. How would you teach someone handwashing to remove transient bacteria?

☐ PERFORMANCE CHECKLIST

OBJECTIVE: To use the appropriate washing technique to remove pathogenic microorganisms from the hands.			
CHARACTERISTIC	RANGE OF ACCEPTABILITY	SATISFACTORY	UNSATISFACTORY
1. Removes rings.	Wearing flat, even-surfaced wedding rings is permitted by some facilities.		
2. Pushes watch up on arm above wrist.	No deviation		
3. Turns faucet on and adjusts flow and temperature of water.	No deviation		
4. Wets hands and wrists with hands held down over sink.	No deviation		
5. Rinses bar soap or dispenses liquid soap.	No deviation		
6. Rubs palms together vigorously.	No deviation		
7. Creates visible lather.	No deviation		
8. Rinses bar soap, replaces on drain.	No deviation		
9. Uses friction and lather on all surfaces of hands, fingers, and under and around nails.	No deviation		
10. Rinses all hand surfaces, starting with wrists, under running water.	No deviation		
11. Holds hands down and over sink to rinse.	No deviation		
12. Dries all surfaces with paper towels.	No deviation		
13. Turns off faucet with dry paper towels.	No deviation		

REFERENCES

Beck WC: Handwashing substitute for degerming. The American Journal of Surgery 56(5):728, 1978.

Flournoy DJ, et al: Nosocomial infection linked to handwashing. Hospitals 53(15):105–107, 1979.

Fox MK, Langner SB, Wells RW: How good are handwashing practices? American Journal of Nursing 74(9):1676–1678, 1974.

France DR: Survival of *Candida albicans* in hand creams. New Zealand Medical Journal 67(432):552–554, 1968.

Knights HT, Harvey J: Hand creams containing hexochlorophene and cross infection with gram-negative bacteria. New Zealand Medical Journal 63(386):653–655, 1964.

Len JJ, Deshmukh NJ: Septisal antiseptic foam versus handwashing in patient care—An effective technique. The Guthrie Bulletin 44(1):19–24, 1974.

Morse L, Williams HL, et al: Septicemia due to *Klebsiella pneumoniae* originating from a hand cream dispenser. The New England Journal of Medicine 277(9):472–473, 1967.

Morse LJ, Schonbeck LE: Hand lotions—A potential nosocomial hazard. The New England Journal of Medicine 278(7):376–378, 1968.

Simmons BP: In consultation with Hooten TM, Mallison GF: Guideline for Hospital Environmental Control. From: Guidelines for the Precaution and Control of Nosocomial Infections. Atlanta, GA, U.S. Department of Health and Human Services, Public Health Service, Centers for Disease Control, 1981.

Sprunt K, Redman W, Leidy G: Antibacterial effectiveness of routine handwashing. Pediatrics 52(2):264-271, 1973.

Steere AC, Mallison GF: Handwashing practices for the prevention of nosocomial infections. Annals of Internal Medicine 83(5):683-690, 1975.

Taylor LJ: An evaluation of handwashing techniques—2. Nursing Times 74(3):108-110, 1978.

Walker K: The Story of Medicine. New York, Oxford University Press, 1955.

BIBLIOGRAPHY

American Hospital Association: Infection Control in the Hospital, ed 4. Chicago, AHA, 1979.

Breitung J: Are you fudging on handwashing routines? RN 40(6):71, 1971.

Brem AM, Torok EM: Nosocomial infections in the elderly. Hospital Topics 57(6):10, 40-43, 1979.

DeLaat ANC: Microbiology for the Allied Health Professions, ed 2. Philadelphia, Lea & Febiger, 1979.

Freeman J, Rosner BA, McGowan JE: Adverse effects of nosocomial infection. The Journal of Infectious Diseases 140(5):732-740, 1979.

Hardy CS: Infection control. Nursing73 3(8):18-21, 1973.

Litsky BY: Infection control and hospital design. Supervisor Nurse 3(2):23-25, 28-31, 1972.

Reinarz JA: Nosocomial infections. Clinical Symposia 30(6):2-32, 1978.

Speers R, et al: Contamination of nurses' uniforms with *Staphylococcus aureus*. The Lancet 2(7614):233-235, 1969.

Williams WW: CDC Guideline for infection control in hospital personnel. Infection Control (Suppl):4(4):326-347, 1983.

Wilson M, Mizer HE, Morello JA: Microbiology in Patient Care, ed 3. New York, Macmillan, 1979.

SUGGESTED READING

Current handwashing issues. Infection Control 5(1):15-17, 1984.

Fox MK, Langner SB, Wells RW: How good are handwashing practices? American Journal of Nursing 74(9):1676-1678, 1976.

Sedgewick J: Hand-washing in hospital wards. Nursing Times 80(20):64-67, 1984.

AUDIOVISUAL RESOURCES

Handwashing in Patient Care
  Film (16 mm). (1961, Color, 16 min.)
  Available through:
    U.S. Public Health Service
    National Audio-visual Center
    Order Section EQ
    Washington, DC 20409

Handwashing and Personal Hygiene
  Filmstrip and cassette. (1977, Color, 7 min.)
  Available through:
    Medcom, Inc.
    P.O. Box 116
    Garden Grove, CA 92642

SKILL 29 Isolation Techniques

PREREQUISITE SKILLS

Skill 19, "Inspection"
Skill 28, "Handwashing"

☐ STUDENT OBJECTIVES

1. State the purpose of isolation.
2. Identify the settings in which isolation is used.
3. Differentiate between the category- and disease-specific systems used for isolation precautions.
4. Explain the rationale for the isolation categories in the category-specific isolation system.
5. Give examples of the diseases and conditions for which each category of isolation is used.
6. Describe the supplies used by personnel to protect themselves against disease-producing microorganisms.
7. Explain the rationale for each item of equipment used to implement isolation technique.
8. Describe the points that should be included when teaching clients and families about isolation precautions in the hospital and home.
9. Summarize the factors that promote effective isolation technique.
10. Identify psychosocial implications of being placed on isolation precautions.
11. Demonstrate the ability to don and remove isolation garments correctly.
12. Describe safe handling of contaminated client-care equipment, body secretions and excretions, and personal belongings, and the safe transport of isolated clients.

INTRODUCTION

The word *isolate* means "to set apart." In health care, the term *isolation* or *isolation precautions* is used broadly to refer to practices that involve the use of mechanical barriers and special procedures and techniques to prevent the spread of pathogenic and potentially pathogenic organisms. These techniques include the wearing of protective gowns and masks and the special care of contaminated items and wounds. The type of organism, its transmission route, and its routes of entry and exit determine the specific practices necessary to prevent and control a given infection. Isolation precautions are designed to isolate the microorganisms, not the client. However, to prevent movement of microorganisms between individuals and between the environment and individuals, it is sometimes necessary to isolate the client.

Although the need for and use of isolation precautions is concentrated in hospitals, these techniques are also necessary in any setting where people may receive health-care services. Hospitals have infection control committees that are responsible for determining appropriate isolation techniques for that agency; this is usually not true for ambulatory- or extended-care facilities, health-care offices, or in the home. The 1983 Centers for Disease Control (CDC) guidelines and consultation from an infection control practitioner provide appropriate assistance for the nurse without an infection control committee (Garner and Simmons, 1983; Williams, 1983).

In hospitals, the need for isolation varies according to the population served and the type of clinical unit. It is important to be aware that this same variation may extend to other settings. Garner and Kaiser (1972) analyzed data from eight community hospitals included in the CDC's Comprehensive Hospital Infection Study and found that an average of 2 percent of the 6000 patients included in the study required some type of isolation. In community hospitals the average rate was 1.6 percent, compared with a rate of 4.6 percent for a city-county hospital. Within clinical units, the variation in the rate ranged from 10.8 percent for the pediatric service to 1 to 2 percent for the medical-surgical units; the lowest rate—less than 1 percent—was found in the obstetrics and psychiatric units.

The use of isolation adds to the already high cost of health care. In addition to the increased expense for extra equipment, supplies, and a private room, the staff work load is increased because of the special procedures and techniques required when providing client care. Additional staff are needed when several clients on a clinical unit require isolation precautions.

Although most hospitals have an infection control committee that is responsible for determining appropriate isolation techniques for that agency, this is not usually the case in ambulatory- or extended-care facilities, in health-care offices, or in the home. The procedures and techniques contained in this skill are based on information contained in the 1975 and 1983 CDC guidelines and are applicable in any setting (CDC, 1975; Garner and Simmons, 1983; Williams, 1983). Agency policy may dictate additional or alternate practices to those presented here. The nurse is advised to learn and follow those practices, as consistency in practice is crucial to effective control of infectious diseases.

PREPARATION

In addition to the use of isolation precautions to isolate disease-producing organisms, an important aspect of the control of infectious disease is the health and immunization status of the agency personnel who provide care and come in contact with clients. Hospitals are people-intensive work settings, and clients come in contact with a variety of employees during the course of a usual day. Any one of these employees or a visitor may be a potential host or transport vehicle for disease-producing organisms.

EMPLOYEE HEALTH AND INFECTION CONTROL

The CDC (Williams, 1983, pp. 329–330) suggests that the following personnel health services be part of a hospital's general program for infection control:

1. Placement evaluations for all personnel at the time of initial employment or reassignment to a different job or work area. One important component of these evaluations is a health inventory that includes immunization status and a history of any health conditions that may predispose the employee to the transmission or acquisition of infectious diseases. This inventory can help determine the need for a physical examination or laboratory tests.
2. Health and safety education for all personnel about the elements of the infection control program.
3. Immunization programs that maintain appropriate levels of immunity to protect the health of the employees and prevent transmission of infectious diseases to clients.
4. Screening for susceptibility to hepatitis B or rubella when the prevalence of either disease warrants it. Rubella immunization can be administered to both sexes without requiring serologic testing as long as females are known to be not pregnant.
5. Provision for prompt diagnosis and management of job-related illnesses and provision of preventive interventions for specific preventable infectious diseases to which personnel may be exposed.
6. Provision of access to health counseling about diseases that may be acquired from or transmitted to clients.

7. Coordination of the activities of personnel working in employee health service with the infection control program and with other departments in the hospital.

TECHNIQUES USED IN ISOLATION PRECAUTIONS

Specific practices used to eliminate or reduce each mode of microorganism transmission include handwashing, the use of physical barriers to prevent the microorganisms from coming in contact with other persons and materials, and the use of special procedures while handling the client and his or her secretions, excretions, and infective materials, as well as the equipment and supplies used in providing care. Not all of these practices are used with each type of isolation, but only those that are relevant for the particular type of isolation.

Handwashing

As indicated in Skill 28, handwashing is the single most important means of preventing the spread of microorganisms. Even when gloves are used, hands should be washed after caring for a client who is either infected or colonized with microorganisms that are of special clinical significance, after contact with clients' excretions or secretions, before performing invasive procedures, and before touching wounds or providing care to clients who are particularly vulnerable to infection. Handwashing between all client contacts in both the intensive care area and newborn nurseries is also essential. Despite the clear evidence supporting the importance of handwashing in preventing the spread of infection, studies continue to document the unacceptable handwashing practices of health-care personnel (Albert and Condie, 1981; Larson and Killen, 1982; Preston et al., 1981).

Physical Barriers

Physical barriers are used to prevent contact of the microorganism with other persons and materials. Barriers employed in isolation precautions include the use of a private room to confine the client, protective clothing worn by the personnel and client, and the bagging of items used in the care of infective clients.

A *private room* serves as a barrier by separating the infected or colonized client from other susceptible clients and thus reducing the opportunity for airborne transmission of microorganisms. An additional benefit of a private room is that it may reinforce the importance of handwashing before personnel leave the room to care for other clients. A private room is indicated for clients who are infected with organisms that are highly virulent or infectious, or it may be indicated for clients who are colonized with microorganisms that are of special clinical significance. Clients whose personal hygiene practices are poor may need to be placed in a private room even when the nature of their infection may not otherwise require it, for example, infants, children, and adults with altered mental status.

Private rooms used for isolation purposes need to have bathing, handwashing, and toilet facilities for the client, as well as separate handwashing facilities for the staff. Rooms specifically designed for isolation purposes have a connecting anteroom that provides storage for the necessary clean protective clothing and other supplies required for the particular type of isolation being used. When an anteroom is not available, a special cart containing the isolation supplies can be placed outside the client's room. It is recommended that room air have six exchanges per hour and either be ventilated to the outdoors or be filtered with a high-efficiency filter before being recirculated to other client rooms.

Generally, clients infected with the same organism may share the same room. However, infected clients should not share a room with a client who is likely to become infected or who is likely to suffer severe consequences from acquiring an infection. When a noninfected client shares a room with an infected client, both the personnel and the infected client need to use appropriate techniques to prevent the transfer of organisms and the spread of infection.

Protective clothing most often includes a mask, gown, and gloves. These items are worn by personnel when providing client care, or sometimes by the client when he or she is being transported to areas outside the room.

Masks are used to prevent the spread of infectious microorganisms through large and small droplets that are transmitted either by close contact or from being suspended in the surrounding air. It is also believed that masks help to prevent transmission of some infections that are spread by direct contact with mucous membranes because wearing masks may discourage personnel from touching their mouths, eyes, and nose until after the mask has been removed and their hands have been washed.

Gowns are used to prevent soiling the nurse's clothing with infective secretions or excretions while providing client care, such as when changing the bed of an incontinent client who has an infectious diarrhea or when changing a dressing on an infected wound. A gown may also be worn by all persons entering the room of a client who has an infectious disease that would result in serious illness if transmitted to other clients in the hospital. For example, chicken pox poses a risk for all clients in the hospital, not only those who are compromised because of immunosuppression.

Booties and caps are not currently used as part of the protective clothing worn for isolation precautions in most agencies. In the past they were worn in protective isolation to prevent the introduction of potentially pathogenic microorganisms from the care-giver's hair and shoes into the client's environment.

Special Procedures

Disposal of Contaminated Items. The method used to dispose of equipment and supplies used in client care depends on whether the item is contaminated with infective material and if the item is disposable or reusable. *Infective material* may include any one or a combination of the following substances when they contain infectious organisms: blood, body fluids, spinal fluid, body tissues, lesion secretions or drainage, secretions from infected sites, respiratory secretions, pus, purulent exudate, feces, urine, and genital and vaginal discharges.

When contaminated items are removed from the client's room, they are placed in a bag inside the room, and then removed using a method known as the "double-bag" technique. With this method, the person providing the care inside the client's room (the contaminated person) places the closed bag and its contents into a second bag held by the helper (the clean person) outside the room. The clean person folds the top end of the bag back over his or her hands to form a cuff that prevents the outside of the bag from becoming contaminated, as shown in Figure 29-1. The bag is then closed securely and labeled "Isolation" or "Contaminated," to alert all personnel to the nature of its contents. The purpose of double bagging is to prevent exposure of personnel to infectious material on the bagged items and to avoid contamination of the environment outside the client's room.

Disposable Items. The use of disposable equipment and supplies is considered to be the safest and most cost-effective method of achieving infection control (Kirkis, 1982). If contaminated items are discarded safely, they are much less likely to serve as fomites than are reusable items that must be cleaned and disinfected or resterilized. Items contaminated with infective material should be bagged, labeled, and disposed of according to agency policy for disposing of infective waste.

Reusable Items. Reusable equipment and supplies are bagged, labeled, and then returned to central service for decontamination, cleansing, and reprocessing by trained personnel. A single bag is sufficient to contain the item if the bag is not easily punctured, and if the item can be placed in the bag without contaminating the exterior of the bag. If this is not possible, use the double-bag technique. Dismantle large items of equipment that have easily removable parts before bagging them. Use a germicide-detergent solution to wipe the outside of the equipment that cannot be bagged and return it to central service for further decontamination and cleaning.

Care of Specific Items. Following is a description of the type of care required for a wide variety of equipment, supplies, items used in client care, clients' personal items, the room and visitors, as well as ways to protect hospital personnel and other clients when the isolated client must leave the room for special services in other areas of the hospital.

Needles and Syringes. All syringes and needles should be handled with caution, since it is not usually known which clients have blood that is contaminated with hepatitis virus or other pathogenic microorganisms. That is, the nurse should be careful to avoid needle punctures and direct contact with clients' blood, especially if there are breaks in the skin on the nurse's hands. Disposable needles and syringes are preferred, particularly when the client's blood is known to be infective. To avoid needle puncture injuries, the nurse does not recap used needles or bend and break them, but, rather, places them in a well-labeled, puncture-proof container and disposes of them according to agency policy. Reusable needles and syringes must be double bagged, labeled, and returned to central service for decontamination and reprocessing.

Sphygmomanometer and Stethoscope. Special handling of a sphygmomanometer and stethoscope are necessary only if they have become or are likely to become contaminated with infective material. If there is a potential for contamination, place a clean towel on the bed to protect the sphygmomanometer cuff and be sure the client's arm is clean and dry. If only the diaphragm of the stethoscope touches a client's clean dry skin, the stethoscope requires no more than routine cleaning. If these items become contaminated, they should be sent to central service for appropriate disinfection.

Thermometers. As with clients not on isolation precautions, every client should have his or her own thermometer. Prior to use by any other client, a thermometer is either sterilized or disinfected. Disinfection may be done on the clinical unit by cleansing the ther-

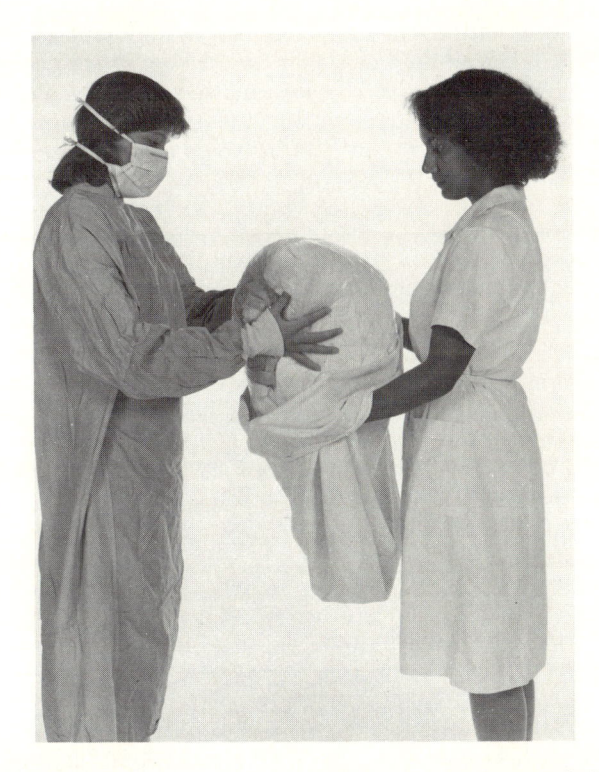

Figure 29-1. The double-bag technique. The clean nurse holds a clean impermeable bag with a folded cuff over the hands outside of the room as the contaminated nurse prepares to put the contaminated bag inside. The clean nurse then closes and labels the outside bag. (Photo by James Haines.)

mometer and then immersing it in 70 to 90 percent isopropyl alcohol for 30 minutes. Sterilization is done by the central service department. When using an electronic thermometer, discard the protective cover in the client's trash can inside the room.

Bed Linen. Handle both clean and soiled linen with a minimum of movement to reduce the dispersion of organisms into the environment. When in the client's room, the nurse places soiled linen in a water-soluble or washable linen bag that is color-coded or labeled to identify it as an isolation container. Linen bags are filled only two-thirds full because the linen will be washed for decontamination purposes before it is removed from the bag. Double bag all linen bags as they are removed from the client's room. The mattress and pillows used in an isolation room are encased in plastic covers to avoid contamination and to facilitate cleaning (CDC, 1975).

Dishes and Eating Utensils. If contamination of dishes and utensils is likely to occur, it is best to use disposable materials. Special precautions for reusable dishes and eating utensils are not necessary unless these items are grossly contaminated with infective material such as blood, drainage, or secretions. Contaminated reusable items are bagged and labeled before being returned to the kitchen. Food personnel should wear gloves while handling these items and then wash their hands before touching other dishes or food.

Tissues and Dressings. All used facial tissues and dressings that are soiled with infective material should be bagged, labeled, and disposed of as directed by hospital policy for infective waste disposal.

The *dressing technique* used to change a dressing depends upon the nature of the infected wound or lesion. Two techniques are recommended (CDC, 1975). A *special dressing technique* should be used for all wound or skin infections with excessive purulent drainage, regardless of the type of microorganism. In addition, wounds that are infected with microorganisms listed in the strict and contact isolation precaution categories should be dressed with the special dressing technique. The *standard dressing technique* should be used for all other types of infected wounds and lesions. Table 29-1 lists the specifications for each of these techniques. It should be noted that *two sets of gloves* are required to dress a wound using the special technique. This is essential to protect the nurse's hands from contact with microorganisms that may be present on the outside of a dressing.

Urine and Feces. Urine and feces are flushed down the toilet when a standard sewage system is available, as sewage systems provide adequate disposal of pathogens. A bedpan, urinal, or bedside commode should be emptied into the toilet and then cleaned, dried with paper towels, and replaced at the bedside. Drying helps to control microbial growth. Before they

TABLE 29-1. Dressing Techniques

	STANDARD	SPECIAL
Handwashing before and after	yes	yes
Gloves, two sets	no	yes
Gown[a]	no	yes
Mask	no	yes
Sterile equipment	yes	yes
Double-bag technique for soiled dressings and equipment	yes	yes
No-touch technique[b]	yes	yes

[a] Sterile only if advisable to prevent cross-infection of extensive wounds.
[b] Dressing or wound must not be touched by bare ungloved hands.
(Adapted from CDC Isolation Techniques for Use in Hospitals, 1975, p. 25.)

are used for another client, urinals and bedpans should be cleaned and either disinfected or sterilized.

Laboratory Specimens. A laboratory specimen container should have a secure lid to prevent leakage during transport. Avoid contamination of the outside of the container when obtaining the specimen. Whether the specimen container is bagged for removal from the client's room and for transport to the laboratory depends on the type of specimen and how it is collected, handled, and transported to the laboratory.

The Health Record. The client's health record should not be permitted to come in contact with infective material or items that may be contaminated. With strict isolation, the care-giver can write vital sign values and other data on paper that is kept in the client's room and transfer the information verbally to the helper outside the room. Documentation in the health record can be done outside the room after care is completed.

Visitors. Before entering a room or cubicle of a client who is on isolation precautions, visitors should talk with a nurse about the isolation requirements and be instructed in the appropriate use of gowns, masks, gloves, or any other techniques as necessary. Depending on the nature of the infectious disease or the purpose of the isolation precautions, visitors may be limited to the immediate family or to a specific number at a given time. Visitors are required to be free of infectious or communicable diseases that might be communicated to the client.

Transportation to Other Areas. When clients are taken to other areas of the hospital, both the client and the transport personnel should use appropriate garment barriers to prevent the transmission of infective material. Personnel in the area to which the client is being taken should be alerted as to the type of isolation precautions needed. In addition, clients should be taught how they can assist in preventing the transmission of their infectious microorganisms to others while in and out of their room. Clients who are infected with microorganisms that are either virulent or epidemiologically important because they are unusually resistant to antibiotics should leave the room only if it is absolutely essential.

Personal Clothing and Effects. If personal items are contaminated with infective material, they should be double bagged and sent to the client's home. The family must be instructed as follows in the method of handling and decontaminating the clothing. After removing the clothing from the bag and placing it in a washing machine or washing receptacle, the bag is then put inside another clean bag and placed in the trash or burned; the person doing the above should then thoroughly wash his or her hands. Fabrics that will tolerate hot water should be washed in a washing machine with laundry detergent and a cup of household chlorine bleach. Items to be washed by hand should be soaked at least 10 minutes in hot water with laundry detergent and 1 ounce of household bleach per gallon of water. To machine wash delicate fabrics requiring warm water, add 1 cup of 5 percent phenol disinfectant (such as Lysol) along with the laundry detergent. After the rinse cycle, wash the items without the phenol in a normal manner to remove the phenol residue. For handwashing delicate fabrics, add 1 ounce of 5 percent phenol per gallon of warm water and detergent. Rinse the items three times to remove phenol residue (CDC, 1975, p. 95).

Toys, Books, and Magazines. If these items become soiled with infective materials, they must be disinfected or destroyed. Otherwise, no special precautions are needed.

Room Cleaning. Routine cleaning of the room is referred to as *concurrent cleaning.* Concurrent cleaning of isolation rooms is the same as for other rooms. However, when a client has an infection that necessitates that he or she be placed in a private room, disinfect the cleaning equipment before it is used in other clients' rooms. Bag and label cleaning cloths and mop heads that are contaminated with infective material or blood before they are sent to the laundry.

Terminal cleaning refers to the cleaning that is done after isolation precautions have been discontinued. Unless the surfaces in the room are visibly contaminated, cleaning can be directed toward items that have been in direct contact with either the client or the client's infective material. Use a freshly prepared disinfectant–detergent solution. Housekeeping personnel should wear the same barrier garments that would be worn if the client were still infected. A mask may be omitted if it would have been worn only for direct or close contact with the client. Wash all surfaces that have been in contact with the client's infective material, horizontal surfaces of the furniture, and the mattress and pillow covers. Wash other surfaces only if visibly soiled with contaminated material. Reusable and disposable supplies and equipment are handled as described earlier. The procedures used to clean the room of a client who is suspected of having either smallpox or Lassa fever (or other hemorrhagic fever) should be determined by consulting experts at the State Board of Health or the Centers for Disease Control Hospital Infections Program. These serious illnesses are highly contagious and require additional terminal cleaning of the room.

Postmortem Care. After the death of a client, the same procedures are generally used to protect the personnel and environment as would be used if the client were still alive, except that masks are not generally needed. The body should be labeled to indicate the type of protective care needed later.

IMPLEMENTING ISOLATION PRECAUTIONS

The physician is responsible for ordering a client to be placed on isolation precautions. However, it is appropriate for the nurse to recommend to the physician that isolation precautions be initiated and to specify the type of isolation required. In some agencies, the infection control practitioner (ICP) or other member of the infection control committee may be assigned the authority to order a client isolated when the physician is not available or has neglected to do so. In this event, the physician must be notified of the decision to isolate. The nurse should ensure that the order is both written and signed or countersigned by the attending physician to ensure payment of the added costs by the client's insurance company.

Criteria for isolating a client are established by the infection control committee. The nurse in charge of a clinical unit must know these criteria, as he or she is usually the first person to become aware of the need to isolate a client. It is usually unwise to wait for laboratory confirmation before isolating a client because the organisms can spread to other clients or staff during the interval between a suspected and confirmed infectious condition.

The charge nurse is also responsible for informing other agency departments about the need to use isolation precautions for specific clients. It is also this nurse's responsibility to see that the necessary equipment and supplies are available for the staff to use in implementing the required procedures and techniques and to determine that unit personnel are executing the procedures correctly. The charge nurse or team leader can facilitate the staff's ability to maintain the integrity of the isolation procedures and techniques and assist them to provide safe and efficient care by assigning a helper to the care-giver who works with the isolated client. This helper must be available to obtain clean supplies for the care-giver in the isolation room and to assist with removing contaminated articles from the room by double bagging them. If there is no helper, the care-giver must spend additional time leaving and entering the isolation area, and breaks in isolation technique are more likely to occur. To isolate successfully, all personnel and visitors must follow the designated procedures. One break in the technique by one person is all that is necessary to defeat the purpose of isolation precautions.

In addition to teaching and supervising staff in the use of isolation precautions, the nurse must also teach the client, family, and other visitors how to perform the necessary procedures and techniques, as well as provide an accurate, brief explanation of the purpose for the isolation precautions. Without an understanding of the rationale, isolation procedures and techniques become meaningless rituals that may not be valued or implemented properly. Genvert et al. (1979) describe an information booklet about isolation that was developed to reinforce the teaching provided for clients and visitors. The use of the booklet has had very positive responses from both clients and their visitors.

When monitoring housekeeping staff's cleaning practices or when teaching families how to clean and disinfect infectious material, it is important to emphasize the need for scrubbing items with soap and water to remove all visible organic matter mechanically before using a disinfectant agent. This practice enables the disinfectant to come in direct contact with the surface of the item being disinfected. Regular household chlorine bleach and 5 percent phenol preparations (such as Lysol) are effective disinfectants when they are used with the mechanical action of scrubbing. The specific type of agent used will depend on the material to be disinfected. When in doubt, consult an expert resource such as an infection control practitioner at a hospital or public health department.

In addition to teaching the client and family prior to discharge from the hospital, the nurse is also responsible for conveying information about a client's infectious disease to any agencies involved in his or her care after discharge from the hospital, such as a home-care agency or extended-care facility. This information should include what the client and family have been taught about infection control. Shared information enables the next agency to provide more appropriate follow-up care without duplicating the referring nurse's efforts. In some agencies, this responsibility may be assumed by the infection control practitioner (ICP).

Although nurses are not responsible for cleaning clients' rooms, they should know about the procedures used by the housekeeping personnel to contain organisms.

Because the need for infection control through the use of isolation techniques extends beyond the hospital, nurses are often in a position to teach others how to prevent the spread of infection in the home. People need to know how to wash their hands properly (Skill 28), handle and dispose of wound dressings (Skill 32), and clean and disinfect contaminated articles, clothing, and furnishings when necessary. When clients with contaminated wounds or secretions are being cared for at home or are being discharged from the hospital, it is important that they and their families be taught how to provide adequate care for infected materials.

PSYCHOSOCIAL IMPACT OF ISOLATION

The client, family, or visitors may be apprehensive about the isolation procedures and techniques. This apprehension can cause inadequate use of the needed procedures, therefore resulting in ineffective infection control. Apprehension can also cause family and friends to avoid visiting out of fear of catching something from the client. They may also be concerned about their ability to carry out the prescribed procedures and techniques correctly. When this happens, the client is needlessly deprived of psychological support at a time when it is particularly important for his or her well-being.

Other factors contribute to a client experiencing a sense of psychological isolation and loneliness in addition to the experience of physical isolation. For example, the number of visitors may be limited to help decrease the potential spread of microorganisms; direct physical contact with visitors may be discouraged; limits may be set on the amount and type of recreational and personal items a client may have; and in some instances, facial features of all staff and visitors are almost completely hidden by a face mask, thus depriving the client of a significant amount of nonverbal communication. Agency staff also are likely to enter the isolated client's room less often, for reasons of efficiency in implementing isolation techniques. In addition, staff may be unrealistically fearful of their own probability of contracting the client's infection. Clients in isolation are usually quite appreciative when staff take the time and initiative to enter their room for non-task related purposes. If the particular type of isolation precaution does not require that the door of the room be closed, clients may appreciate having the door open so hallway activity can be observed and heard and so staff can chat from the doorway at more frequent intervals.

SPECIFICATIONS FOR ISOLATION PRECAUTIONS

The isolation procedures and techniques used to control any given infection are based on specifications and recommendations from the CDC. These guidelines have been established and published by the CDC since 1970. They are revised and updated periodically, based on new information about pathogenic organisms and their transmission and on information about the development of new infectious diseases. The fourth set of guidelines published in 1983 is based on either epidemiologic studies or on reasonable theoretical rationale (Garner and Simmons, 1983; Williams, 1983).

The new guidelines are significant in that they contain major changes from all previously published guidelines. All former guidelines were based on one system whereas now there are two systems—one based on disease categories and an alternative that is disease-specific. Many institutions are now studying the new guidelines, evaluating their own systems of isolation, and deciding whether to use an isolation system based on categories of disease or one based on specific diseases. The CDC recommends that a hospital choose one or the other system and not attempt to combine the two, as this would be extremely confusing for staff. An additional option is for the hospital to create a new system based on information provided in the CDC guidelines.

In the meantime, most hospitals continue to use their previously adopted system. For this reason it is important to know the categories in the old system: strict isolation, respiratory isolation, protective (reverse) isolation, enteric precautions, wound and skin precautions, discharge precautions, secretions (oral) precautions, and blood precautions. Under the new guidelines some of these categories have been combined, others eliminated, and some new ones created. For example, wound and skin precautions have been combined with discharge precautions and secretion (oral) precautions to create a new category labeled drainage/secretion precautions. Blood precautions have been expanded to include body fluids. Protective (reverse) isolation has been eliminated and two completely new categories have been created, one specifically for tuberculosis and a second for clients who have a highly transmissible disease but do not require strict isolation. The changes in the revised categories are intended to minimize unnecessary use of isolation equipment such as gowns and gloves. The disease-specific system is thought to avoid unnecessary over-isolation and to be more conserving of supplies.

The CDC has instruction cards for both isolation precaution systems. The front of each card specifies the major steps required for anyone entering the client's room, and the back of the card lists the disease(s) and condition(s) for which those isolation precautions are required, as shown in Figure 29-2. Institutions often design their own instruction cards to incorporate the modifications their own infection control committee believe are necessary. When a client is placed on isolation precautions, the appropriate card is placed

---

SAMPLE INSTRUCTION CARDS FOR CATEGORY-SPECIFIC ISOLATION PRECAUTIONS

(Front of Card)

Strict Isolation

Visitors—Report to Nurses' Station Before Entering Room

1. Masks are indicated for all persons entering room.
2. Gowns are indicated for all persons entering room.
3. Gloves are indicated for all persons entering room.
4. HANDS MUST BE WASHED AFTER TOUCHING THE PATIENT OR POTENTIALLY CONTAMINATED ARTICLES AND BEFORE TAKING CARE OF ANOTHER PATIENT.
5. Articles contaminated with infective material should be discarded or bagged and labeled before being sent for decontamination and reprocessing.

(Back of Card)

Diseases Requiring Strict Isolation*

Diphtheria, pharyngeal
Lassa fever and other viral hemorrhagic fevers, such as Marburg virus disease§
Plague, pneumonic
Smallpox§
Varicella (chickenpox)
Zoster, localized in immunocompromised patient, or disseminated

*A private room is indicated for Strict Isolation; in general, however, patients infected with the same organism may share a room.
See Guideline for Isolation Precautions in Hospitals for details and for how long to apply precautions.
§A private room with special ventilation is indicated.

Figure 29-2. The CDC's instruction card system for isolation. **A.** Category-specific isolation precautions.

Sample Instruction Card for Disease-Specific Isolation Precautions

(Front of Card)

Visitors—Report to Nurses' Station Before Entering Room

1. **Private room indicated?** _____ No
   _____ Yes
2. **Masks indicated?** _____ No
   _____ Yes for those close to patient
   _____ Yes for all persons entering room
3. **Gowns indicated?** _____ No
   _____ Yes if soiling is likely
   _____ Yes for all persons entering room
4. **Gloves indicated?** _____ No
   _____ Yes for touching infective material
   _____ Yes for all persons entering room
5. Special precautions _____ No
   indicated for handling blood? _____ Yes
6. **Hands must be washed after touching the patient or potentially contaminated articles and before taking care of another patient.**
7. Articles contaminated with _____ should be
                                       infective material(s)
   discarded or bagged and labeled before being sent for decontamination and reprocessing.

(Back of Card)

Instructions

1. On Table B, Disease-Specific Precautions, locate the disease for which isolation precautions are indicated.
2. Write disease in blank space here: _____
3. Determine if a private room is indicated. In general, patients infected with the same organism may share a room. For some diseases or conditions, a private room is indicated if patient hygiene is poor. A patient with poor hygiene does not wash hands after touching infective material (feces, purulent drainage, or secretions), contaminates the environment with infective material, or shares contaminated articles with other patients.
4. Place a check mark beside the indicated precautions on front of card.
5. Cross through precautions that are *not* indicated.
6. Write infective material in blank space in item 7 on front of card.

Figure 29–2. B. Disease-specific isolation precautions.

---

on the door of his or her room so that all staff and visitors are alerted to the isolation requirements. A color-coded sticker is usually placed on the front of the client's health record, thus providing information for the staff when planning care. When isolation precautions do not require the use of a private room, the isolation card may be attached to the client's bed or placed on the wall near the bed.

Category-Specific Isolation

Category-specific isolation precautions are identified as "System A" by the CDC. The seven categories in this system were derived by grouping together the most common infectious diseases found in the United States on the basis of the similarity of the barriers and techniques required to prevent their transmission. The advantages of the category-specific system are that it is familiar and easy to use and teach to personnel. Its disadvantage is that in each category there are diseases for which more isolation precautions are prescribed than are really necessary to prevent the transmission of that particular disease, thus resulting in overuse of isolation procedures. Overuse of isolation increases the amount of time required to provide nursing care, deprives the client of attention from staff and visitors, and increases the amount of supplies needed.

The seven categories in the new category-specific system are strict isolation, contact isolation, respiratory isolation, tuberculosis (AFB) isolation, enteric isolation precautions, drainage/secretions precautions, and blood/body fluids precautions. Table 29-2 summarizes the specifications for each category and identifies the diseases and conditions included in each category.

1. *Strict isolation* is intended to prevent the transmission of highly contagious or virulent infections that may be spread by both air and contact.
2. *Contact isolation* is intended to prevent the transmission of highly transmissible or epidemiologically important infections (or colonization) that do not warrant the use of strict isolation. All diseases in this category are spread primarily by close or direct contact.
3. *Respiratory isolation* is designed to prevent the transmission of infectious diseases over short dis-

TABLE 29-2. Category-Specific Isolation Precautions

		BARRIERS[a]			
DISEASE/CONDITION	CATEGORY	Private Room	Mask	Gown	Gloves
Diseases Requiring Strict Isolation Diphtheria, pharyngeal Lassa fever and other viral hemorrhagic fevers, such as Marburg virus disease Plague, pneumonic Smallpox Varicella (chickenpox) Zoster, localized in immunocompromised patient, or disseminated	Strict isolation	R	R	R	R
Diseases or Conditions Requiring Contact Isolation Acute respiratory infections in infants and young children, including croup, colds, bronchitis, and bronchiolitis caused by respiratory syncytial virus, adenovirus, coronavirus, influenza viruses, para-influenza viruses, and rhinovirus Conjunctivitis, gonococcal, in newborns Diphtheria, cutaneous Endometritis, group A Streptococcus Furunculosis, staphylococcal, in newborns Herpes simplex, disseminated, severe primary or neonatal Impetigo Influenza, in infants and young children Multiply-resistant bacteria, infection, or colonization (any site) with any of the following: 1. Gram-negative bacilli resistant to all aminoglycosides that are tested. (In general, such organisms should be resistant to gentamicin, tobramycin, and amikacin for these special precautions to be indicated.) 2. Staphylococcus aureus resistant to methicillin (or nafcillin or oxacillin if they are used instead of methicillin for testing). 3. Pneumococcus resistant to penicillin. 4. Haemophilus influenzae resistant to ampicillin (beta-lactamase positive) and chloramphenicol. 5. Other resistant bacteria may be included if they are judged by the infection control team to be of special clinical and epidemiologic significance. Pediculosis Pharyngitis, infectious, in infants and young children. Pneumonia, viral, in infants and young children. Pneumonia, S. aureus or Group A Streptococcus Rabies Rubella, congenital and other Scabies Scalded skin syndrome, staphylococcal (Ritter's disease) Skin, wound, or burn infection, major (draining and not covered by dressing or dressing does not adequately contain the purulent material) including those infected with S. aureus or group A Streptococcus Vaccinia (generalized and progressive eczema vaccinatum)	Contact isolation	R	CC	S	DC

Diseases Requiring Respiratory Isolation
Epiglottis, H. influenzae
Erythema infectiosum
Measles
Meningitis
  H. influenzae, known or suspected
  Meningococcal, known or suspected
Meningococcal pneumonia
Meningococcemia
Mumps
Pertussis (whooping cough)
Pneumonia, H. influenze, in children (any age)
	Respiratory isolation	R	CC	—	—

Tuberculosis, pulmonary or laryngeal	Tuberculosis isolation	R	DP	PC	—

(continued)

TABLE 29-2. (Cont.)

DISEASE/CONDITION	CATEGORY	Private Room	Mask	Gown	Gloves

Diseases Requiring Enteric Precautions
  Amebic dysentery
  Cholera
  Coxsackievirus disease
  Diarrhea, acute illness with suspected infectious etiology
  Echovirus disease
  Encephalitis (unless known not to be caused by enteroviruses)
  Enterocolitis caused by Clostridium difficile or S. aureus
  Enteroviral infection
  Gastroenteritis caused by
    Campylobacter species
    Cryptosporidium species
    Dientamoeba fragilis
    Escherichia coli (enterotoxic, enteropathogenic, or enteroinvasive)
    Giardia lamblia
    Salmonella species
    Shigella species
    Unknown etiology but presumed to be an infectious agent
    Vibrio parahaemolyticus
    Viruses—including Norwalk agent and ratovirus
    Yersinia enterocolitica
  Hand, foot, and mouth disease
  Hepatitis, viral, type A
  Herpangina
  Meningitis, viral (unless known not to be caused by enteroviruses)
  Necrotizing enterocolitis
  Pleurodynia
  Poliomyelitis
  Typhoid fever (Salmonella typhi)
  Viral pericarditis, myocarditis, or meningitis (unless known not to be caused by enteroviruses)
	Enteric precautions	DP	—	S	DC

Diseases Requiring Drainage/Secretion Precautions
  The following infections are examples of those included in this category provided they are not
    (a) caused by multiply-resistant microorganisms,
    (b) major (draining and not covered by a dressing or dressing does not adequately contain the drainage) skin, wound, or burn infections, including those caused by S. aureus or group A Streptococcus, or
    (c) gonococcal eye infections in newborns. (See Contact isolation if the infection falls into one of these categories.)
  Abscess, minor or limited
  Burn infection, minor or limited
  Conjunctivitis
  Decubitus ulcer, infected, minor or limited
  Skin infection, minor or limited
  Wound infection, minor or limited
	Drainage/Secretions	—	—	S	DC

Diseases Requiring Blood/Body Fluid Precautions
  Acquired immunodeficiency syndrome (AIDS)
  Arthropodborne viral fevers (for example, dengue, yellow fever, and Colorado tick fever)
  Babesiosis
  Creutzfeldt–Jakob disease
  Hepatitis B (including HBsAg antigen carrier)
  Hepatitis, non-A, non-B
  Leptospirosis
  Malaria
  Rat-bite fever
  Relapsing fever
  Syphilis, primary and secondary with skin and mucous membrane lesions
	Blood/Body Fluids	DP	—	S	DC

[a]R—recommended at all times, CC—close contact, S—if soiling likely, DC—direct contact, DP—depends upon patient ability to cooperate with requirements, PC—protect clothing.
(Adapted from Garner JS, Simmons BP: CDC guidelines for isolation precautions in hospitals. Infection Control 4(4):258–260, 1983.)

tances through droplets in the air. Some of the diseases listed in this category are also occasionally transmitted by direct and indirect contact.

4. *Tuberculosis isolation (AFB isolation)* is a category created for clients who have acid-fast bacilli (AFB) with pulmonary tuberculosis (TB), a positive sputum smear for AFB, and chest x-ray evidence of current infection (active) TB, or laryngeal TB. Infants and young children with pulmonary tuberculosis do not usually require this type of isolation because they seldom cough and their bronchial secretions have few AFB when compared with adults with pulmonary TB.

5. *Enteric precautions* are used when microorganisms in infected feces can be transmitted by direct or indirect contact with feces. A common illness included in this category is viral hepatitis type A (HAV), which is transmitted through the fecal–oral route. Although type B viral hepatitis (HBV) is not transmitted through that route, many institutions do not have the necessary laboratory capability to differentiate between types A and B. Under those circumstances, any client suspected of having either type of hepatitis must be placed on enteric precautions (Favero et al., 1979).

6. *Drainage/secretion precautions* are designed to prevent transmission of infections by direct or indirect contact with purulent material or drainage from an infected body site. If a disease that produces purulent drainage is also included in another isolation category with more rigid isolation requirements, it would be dealt with according to those requirements.

7. *Blood/body precautions* are designed to prevent transmission of infection by direct and indirect contact with infected blood or body fluids. If a disease that produces infected blood or body fluids is also included in another isolation category with more rigid isolation requirements, it would be dealt with according to those requirements. To avoid contamination from blood spills, clean them promptly with a solution of 5.25 percent sodium hypochlorite diluted 1:10 with water.

Disease-Specific Isolation

Disease-specific isolation precautions are identified as "System B" by the CDC. In this system, each individual infectious disease is considered separately, so that only those barriers and techniques that are necessary for interrupting the transmission of that particular disease are recommended. The diseases and infectious agents listed in the 1983 guidelines are those likely to be found in U.S. hospitals (Garner and Simmons, 1983). They are listed alphabetically by anatomic site or syndrome (such as cellulitis or abscess), etiologic agent (such as *Escherichia coli*), or a combination of these two factors. The recommendations for some diseases or conditions may be more stringent for children than for adults because the risk of transmission and the consequences of acquiring an infection are often greater for younger children.

The rationale for this system is that it saves on time and supplies because only those isolation practices actually needed for a particular condition are required, thus eliminating unnecessary use of gowns and masks. It is thought that personnel may comply more fully with isolation precautions when only those practices that are essential are used. The disease-specific system requires that the physician or nurse selecting the type of isolation precautions to be instituted for a given disease be knowledgeable about the mode of transmission of the microorganisms so that the appropriate procedures are adopted. An accurate medical diagnosis and a laboratory report indicating the causative microorganism are not always available at the time the client may need to be isolated. In such cases, isolation precautions are initiated on the basis of a presumptive diagnosis. This system allows the nurse to have flexibility to respond to these situations.

DATA BASE

Client History and Recorded Data

The decision to place a client in isolation and the selection of the type of isolation is determined by the client's condition, admitting diagnosis, and the criteria established by the infection control committee. At the time of admission, the nurse considers whether the client's condition warrants isolation and notes the presence of wounds, burns, lesions, discharges, excretions, and secretions. An elevated body temperature may be an indicator of the presence of infection. When clinical signs and symptoms of pathogenic microorganisms are confirmed by positive bacteriology reports and blood tests, the nurse initiates the use of isolation procedures by notifying the physician or the appropriate person designated within the institution with the authority to order isolation. The ICP can give valuable assistance in determining whether a positive bacteriology report indicates an actual infection, a colonization, or contamination. As mentioned previously, it is not always wise to wait for laboratory confirmation before isolating a client. The nurse must use the criteria established by the infection control committee or consult the ICP while waiting for bacteriology and blood test reports.

Physical Appraisal Skills

Inspection. Proper execution of isolation procedures and techniques requires that *inspection* be used to monitor the activities included in the isolation precautions. Inspection validates the extent to which the staff, the client, and visitors are adhering to the necessary practices. It is also used to inventory the equipment and supplies needed for the isolation procedures and techniques as well as for client-care activities. Inspection should ensure that no client is neglected because he or she is isolated.

In some situations gloves are not required to protect the hands from pathogenic organisms, but inspection of the hands may reveal breaks in the skin that indicate a need for wearing gloves. Inspection is also used to assess changes in wounds, the nature of wound drainage, and the containment of wound drainage by the surgical dressing.

EQUIPMENT

The supplies used to implement isolation procedures serve as barriers to prevent the spread of organisms from the client to the staff, other clients, and visitors and vice versa.

Gowns may be either washable or disposable. They must be full length to cover the clothing and have long sleeves with snug cuffs, a high neck, and ties at the neck and waist. The gown is worn once and then discarded before the user leaves the contaminated area. In the event that the gown becomes wet before client care is completed, it should be changed, because wet material does not provide a barrier to the transmission of organisms. Sterile gowns may be used in some agencies with clients who have extensive burns or wounds. An adequate supply of gowns must be available outside of the room on the isolation cart or in the anteroom.

Masks may be made of washable cotton or disposable material. The current trend in isolation procedures is to use only the high-efficiency disposable mask that is used in surgery because it has a smaller pore size. Masks serve as an air filter, and the size of the pores in the material is considered to be an important factor in preventing the passage of droplets from the wearer into the environment and from the client or the environment to the care-giver or visitor. It is generally believed that cotton or thin paper masks are ineffective in preventing aerosol particles from penetrating the mask. There is no substantial research to support either position at this time. A mask serves to redirect the flow of air from the mouth. Instead of flowing directly forward during respiration or normal speech, the air flow is deflected to the sides, thereby providing some protection to a wound from the direct fallout of microorganisms in droplets. The respiratory tract also receives the same type of protection. It is important to remember that droplets expelled during coughing, sneezing, or yelling can penetrate the mask and enter the environment. Regardless of the type of mask used, once it becomes damp it is ineffective and should be changed (Dechario, 1978).

In spite of the frequency with which one sees the mask lowered around the neck and then replaced back over the nose and mouth, this is not considered to be acceptable practice. Although there is no documented evidence to indicate the reasons why the practice is unacceptable, it might be surmised that part of the rationale is that the mask becomes contaminated when it is touched by the hands. Whenever the mask is removed from the mouth and nose it should be discarded, the hands should be washed, and a new mask put on. When client care extends beyond the time a mask remains dry, the mask will have to be changed. This requires that the care-giver wash his or her hands, remove the damp mask by touching only the strings, and obtain a new one from the supply on the isolation cart outside of the room. To eliminate the need for the care-giver to remove his or her gown to obtain a clean mask, an assistant outside the room can hand a fresh mask to the fully gowned care-giver.

Gloves may be either the surgical type or the looser-fitting vinyl or latex examination type. Use of sterile surgical gloves in isolation is unnecessarily costly and wasteful. When gloves are worn with a gown, the glove cuff should be long enough to extend up over the cuff of the gown. Gloves are worn once and then discarded. They must be changed when they have come into direct contact with contaminated secretions and excretions even if client care is not completed. Gloves may also be indicated in those situations where potentially infectious material could be left on the hands and not removed without special attention to additional cleaning under the fingernails and rings. In situations where more than one pair of gloves is needed to provide care, the clean gloves must be brought into the room in an unopened package or in a clean impermeable bag. Whether or not the gloves need to be sterile depends on their use. An adequate supply of additional gloves must be available outside of the room.

Caps used for isolation are usually made of a disposable material. Their design is similar to that of a shower cap, with an elastic band for a snug fit. Because they are worn for protective isolation, they should be large enough to cover all of the hair to prevent a fallout of microorganisms from the hair into the environment.

Booties or shoe covers should extend upward to cover the open ends of trousers or slacks.

Bags of different sizes and colors are required for the removal of all contaminated materials from the room and to protect clean items brought into the room. They must be large and strong enough to hold the contents without tearing. Small clear plastic bags are normally used to protect laboratory specimens. They are also needed to protect the nurse's watch from contamination when it cannot be worn because of the gown but is needed in the room for measuring the pulse and respirations. Tissue and dressing bags may be made of plastic or foil-lined paper. Large, color-coded linen bags made of heavy washable cotton or water-soluble plastic are kept inside the room in the laundry hamper. Clean bags of the same or greater size must be kept outside the room for the double-bag procedure. The second bag should be of a designated color (such as red) to alert personnel to the contaminated contents.

Germicidal detergents must be freshly prepared and diluted to the proper concentration for the specific use. For example, when it is necessary to use such a preparation for handwashing, the concentration will be less than when the same chemical is used for disinfection. Too strong a solution may be irritating to the skin and too weak a solution does not destroy pathogens, thus giving a false sense of protection. Thorough handwashing procedure is required to remove organisms picked up on the hands.

☐ EXECUTION

Proper execution of isolation procedures and techniques requires that the nurse be constantly aware of the purpose of isolation and how the specific infective organisms are transmitted. It is common to observe lax technique being implemented, and students should be wary of basing their techniques on those they may observe. A critical factor in using the correct technique is a basic understanding of what is and should be kept clean or sterile and what is considered contaminated. When a clean item touches a contaminated item, the clean item becomes contaminated also.

When a gown, mask, and gloves are worn, put them on in the following sequence. First put on the gown and secure the ties, next the mask, and lastly the gloves. This sequence provides the maximum amount of time to wear the mask while it is dry and serves as an effective filter; donning the gloves after the gown and mask makes it possible to draw the wrist portion of the glove up over the cuff of the gown; it is also easier to tie the mask in place without gloves on.

To minimize the amount of times handwashing is necessary while removing contaminated garments, use the following steps:

1. Untie the waist strings of the gown while the gloves are still on. The gloves and the waist strings are considered contaminated.
2. Remove the gloves.
3. Untie the neck strings of the gown, which are considered clean. Remove the gown.
4. Untie the mask strings and remove the mask.
5. Wash the hands.

In the event that one's hands become contaminated through contact with contaminated parts of the garments, they must be washed before moving on to the next item to prevent showering oneself with microorganisms.

☐ SKILL SEQUENCES

DONNING AND REMOVING A GOWN

Step	Rationale
1. Remove watch and rings. Place watch and rings in a clear plastic bag and place in pocket.	Prevents contamination of watch while in the room. Hands are better cleaned without rings.
2. Pull long hair away from face and secure at neck.	Handling hair while in isolation transfers microorganisms from nurse to client and vice versa.
3. Wash hands.	
4. Pick up folded clean gown by grasping it at neck or shoulders. Raise arms high enough to allow gown to open so that it does not touch the floor. The inside of gown faces uniform.	Gowns are folded to open when grasped at top. Prevents contaminating clean gown.
5. Open gown by spreading arms outward (Fig. 29–3A). Slip arms into sleeves and adjust gown by drawing it around body (Fig. 29–3B).	Facilitates putting gown on correctly.
6. Tie neck strings (Fig. 29–3C).	
7. Overlap outer back edge of gown over under side. Secure inside ties if available.	Gown must cover all of uniform.
8. Grasp waist strings and tie them (Fig. 29–3D).	Holds gown securely wrapped around body. Having strings in front makes it easier to untie them for removal.
9. To remove gown:	
a. Untie waist strings. (If gloves are worn, keep them on for this step and then remove them.)	The waist strings are considered contaminated.
b. Remove gloves if worn.	
c. Wash hands.	Removes resident bacteria and transient bacteria if gloves have been punctured.
d. Untie neck strings.	The neck strings are considered clean.
e. Grasp each side of neck band of gown with both hands and pull gown down over arms inside out. Do not touch outside of gown.	The neck band is considered clean. Places clean side of gown outside to prevent transfer of organisms to hands.
f. Pull gown away from body and hold it inside out.	Keeps contaminated outside of gown away from uniform.
g. Fold gown so that inside is folded outside. Roll it into a bundle with a minimum of movements and discard it in linen hamper or wastebasket.	Prevents scattering pathogenic microorganisms.
h. Wash hands.	

(continued)

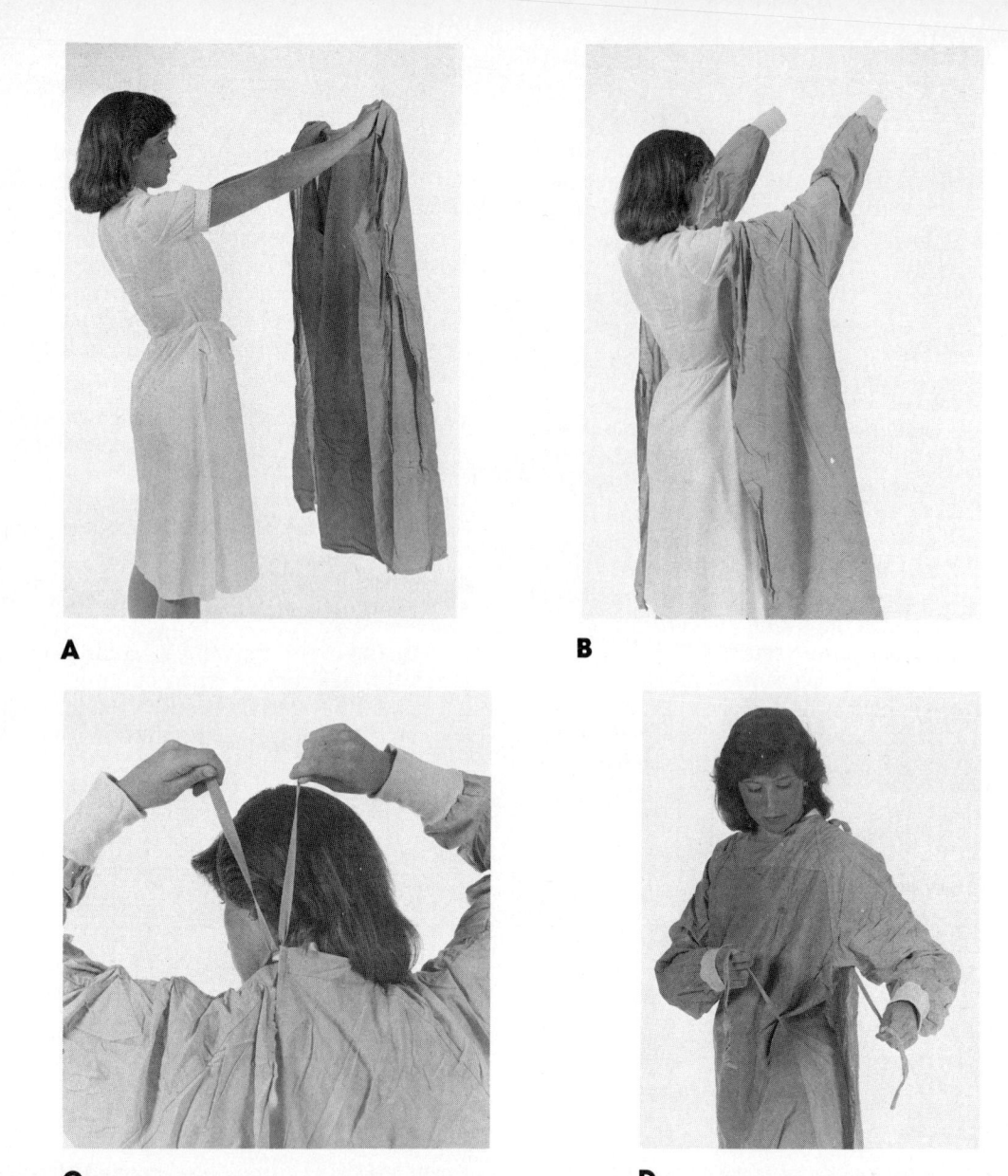

Figure 29–3. Technique for donning a gown. **A.** Hold the clean gown by the neck or shoulders, with the arms held high. Open the gown by spreading the arms outward. **B.** Slip the arms into sleeves and adjust the gown around the body. **C.** Tie the neck strings. **D.** Overlap the outer back edge of gown over the underside and tie the waist strings.

DONNING AND REMOVING A MASK

Step	Rationale
1. Wash hands.	Prevents contamination of mask.
2. Pick up clean mask and adjust it snugly over top of nose and mouth.	A used mask is an ineffective filter.
3. Use both hands to extend top strings over ears and around to back of head; tie them securely.	Holds mask in place on nose.
4. Extend lower strings below and around lower jaw and tie them at back of neck (Fig. 29–4A). Do not touch front of mask while it is being worn. Mask should never be lowered around neck and then reused.	Holds mask in place over mouth. Must fit snugly on face to be effective. The front of mask is considered contaminated once it is in place. Wearing mask around neck transfers microorganisms to oneself.
5. To remove mask when task is completed:	
a. Wash hands.	Prevents contaminating oneself.
b. Untie bottom strings first, then top ones, using both hands.	The strings are considered clean.
c. Touching only strings or mask corners, pull mask away from face.	
d. Hold mask by strings and discard reusable masks in linen bag and disposable masks in wastebasket (Fig. 29–4B).	Center of mask is assumed to be grossly contaminated.

SKILL 29: ISOLATION TECHNIQUES   **263**

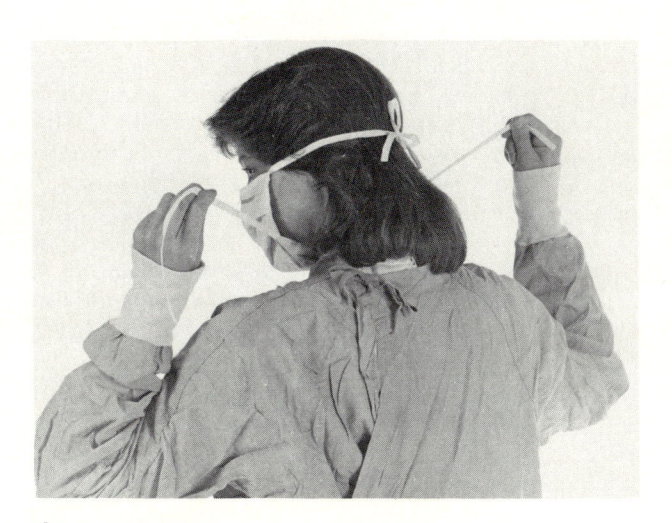

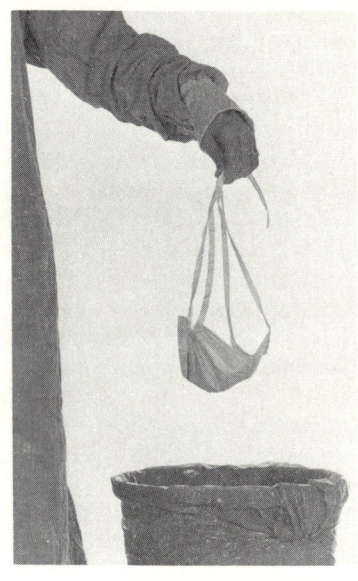

A   **B**

Figure 29–4. **A.** *Technique for donning a mask. Adjust the mask snugly over the nose, using both hands to extend and tie the strings around the back of the head and neck.* **B.** *Technique for discarding a mask. Hold the mask by the strings to discard it. (Photos by James Haines.)*

DONNING AND REMOVING GLOVES

Step	Rationale
1. Put on the gown as in "Donning and Removing a Gown."	Gown is donned before gloves so glove cuffs can be drawn up over gown cuffs.
2. If using surgical gloves, either sterile or unsterile, see Skill 31.	
3. Loose-fitting vinyl or latex gloves are put on like street gloves. Extend available glove cuff over gown cuff or wrist.	Provides protection for wrists and gown cuff.

4. To remove gloves after untying waist strings of gown:
  a. Grasp first glove below top edge of cuff and peel it off inside out and discard it in plastic-lined wastebasket.
  b. Place an ungloved finger inside upper edge of second glove; peel it off inside out and discard it as first glove.
	Gloved hand is contaminated, as is area grasped on cuff of other hand.
	Ungloved hand is considered clean so must not touch outside of gloved hand.

5. Wash hands.	Resident microorganisms multiply rapidly on hands while gloves are worn. Transient microorganisms from isolated client may have been acquired through a puncture in the gloves.

RECORDING

A note is entered on the client's record when any type of isolation precautions are ordered, implemented, and terminated.

Data relevant to the client's psychological status and ability to understand and cooperate with the necessary procedures and techniques, along with any teaching the nurse does of the client and family should also be entered on the health record.

Sample POR Recording
- S—NA
- O—Purulent drainage from ulcer on l. leg.
- A—Drainage may have pathogenic microorganisms.
- P—Consulted ICP about initiating isolation precautions to prevent cross-infection.

Sample Narrative Recording
Purulent drainage from ulcer on l. leg. ICP consulted about need for isolation precautions to prevent cross-infection of others.

☐ CRITICAL POINTS SUMMARY

1. Handwashing is an essential component of infection control.
2. The isolation precautions used must be appropriate for the route of organism transmission and the client's ability to cooperate with the procedures.
3. Consult with an infection control practitioner, the state or county board of health, or the CDC manual when unsure of the correct isolation category to implement.

4. A card system for isolation alerts all personnel and visitors of the necessary requirements.
5. Understand the purpose for the isolation precautions and the transmission route of the causative microorganism.
6. Be able to identify what is considered clean and what is considered contaminated.
7. Have a clean helper outside of the room to assist in obtaining needed supplies.
8. Contaminated items removed from the isolation unit must be double bagged and labeled.
9. Contaminated needles are not capped or bent.
10. Contaminated needles are placed in a puncture-proof container.
11. Client and visitor teaching is a vital part of effective infection control.
12. Housekeeping personnel must be knowledgeable about cleaning requirements for each category of isolation.
13. Germicidal detergents must be freshly prepared and properly diluted.
14. Isolation garments are used only once.
15. Even if the procedure does not require them, gloves are worn when there are breaks in the skin on the hands.

☐ LEARNING ACTIVITIES

1. Tour an isolation unit to observe the type of facilities available. Interview a member of the infection control committee to find out what types of issues the committee deals with in their meetings. Interview a member of the housekeeping staff to determine what training and staff development programs they attend.
2. Practice donning and removing the isolation garments. Have a peer critique your performance using the Performance Checklist.
3. Select two peers to simulate with you the use of different isolation techniques and procedures to give various types of nursing care. Have one act as the client, one the care-giver, and the third as observer. Simulate giving a bed bath, making a linen change, preparing contaminated items for return to central supply, and giving an injection. Reverse roles.
   a. Summarize the most common errors made by each member of the group.
   b. Describe how the isolation garments were used.
   c. Characterize the completeness of the preplanning before entering the isolation unit.
   d. Discuss ways to eliminate the errors.
4. Interview a client who is confined in any category of isolation. Find out how much he or she understands about the purpose of the various procedures and techniques used during his or her care.

☐ REVIEW QUESTIONS

1. What is the purpose of isolation?
2. What is the difference between the two alternative systems for isolation precautions?
3. Indicate how you would explain to a client the reasons for each of the different categories of isolation.
4. What are some of the diseases and conditions for which strict, contact, respiratory, and enteric isolation are used?
5. What are some of the diseases and conditions for which drainage/secretion and blood/body fluid precautions are used?
6. What types of data determine whether strict isolation or contact isolation precautions are used?
7. What are some of the factors that cause isolation to be ineffective?
8. When and why is it necessary to wear gowns? Gloves? Masks?
9. Why are gloves put on after the gown?
10. When and why is it necessary to use two pair of gloves to change a wound dressing?
11. How is the skill of inspection used in relation to isolation practices?
12. List the points you would include in a teaching plan for a client with a wound infection and his or her family while in the hospital and in preparation for discharge.

☐ PERFORMANCE CHECKLISTS

OBJECTIVE: To use the correct technique to don and remove an isolation gown.			
CHARACTERISTIC	RANGE OF ACCEPTABILITY	SATISFACTORY	UNSATISFACTORY
1. Removes watch and rings.	Watch may be worn if it is not to be used during client care.		
2. Pulls long hair away from face and secures at neck.	Not necessary if cap is worn for protective isolation		
3. Washes hands.	No deviation		
4. Picks up folded clean gown by neck or shoulders; keeps arms high.	No deviation No deviation		

(continued)

CHARACTERISTIC	RANGE OF ACCEPTABILITY	SATISFACTORY	UNSATISFACTORY
5. Opens gown with arms spread outward.	No deviation		
6. Slips arms into sleeves and adjusts gown around body.	No deviation		
7. Ties neck strings.	No deviation		
8. Overlaps the back of gown.	No deviation		
9. Ties waist strings in front.	No deviation		
10. Gown removal: Unties waist strings.	No deviation		
11. Washes hands.	No deviation		
12. Unties neck strings.	No deviation		
13. Grasps each side of neck band and pulls gown down inside out over arms without touching outside of contaminated gown.	No deviation		
14. Holds gown inside out and folds it so the contaminated outside is inside; rolls it in a bundle.	No deviation		
15. Discards gown in appropriate container.	No deviation		
16. Washes hands.	No deviation		

OBJECTIVE: To use the correct technique to don and remove a mask.

CHARACTERISTIC	RANGE OF ACCEPTABILITY	SATISFACTORY	UNSATISFACTORY
1. Washes hands.	No deviation		
2. Picks up clean mask and places it snugly over nose and mouth.	No deviation		
3. Uses both hands to draw tie top strings over ears and ties at back of head.	No deviation		
4. Uses both hands to draw lower strings around lower jaw and ties them at back of neck.	No deviation		
5. Avoids touching front of mask.	No deviation		
6. To remove mask: a. Washes hands.	No deviation		
b. Uses both hands to untie top, then lowers strings.	No deviation		
c. Pulls mask away from face.	No deviation		
d. Holds mask by strings to discard it in appropriate container.	No deviation		

OBJECTIVE: To use the correct technique to don and remove gloves.

CHARACTERISTIC	RANGE OF ACCEPTABILITY	SATISFACTORY	UNSATISFACTORY
1. Puts on each glove and extends cuff up over gown cuff or wrist.	No deviation		
2. a. To remove gloves, grasps the outside edge of one glove cuff and peels it off inside out and discards in plastic-lined wastebasket.	No deviation		
b. Grasps the inside edge of the other glove, peels it off inside out, and discards as the first.	No deviation		
3. Washes hands.	No deviation		

REFERENCES

Albert RK, Condie F: Handwashing patterns in medical intensive care units. New England Journal of Medicine 304(24):1465-1466, 1981.

Centers for Disease Control: Isolation Techniques for Use in Hospitals, ed 2. Atlanta, GA, U.S. Department of Health, Education, and Welfare, (CDC) 78-8314, 1975.

Dechario DC: Isolation. In Barrett-Connor E, Brandt SL, et al (eds): Epidemiology for the Infection Control Nurse. St. Louis, CV Mosby, 1978, chap. 6.

Favero MS, Maynard JE, et al: Guidelines for the care of patients hospitalized with viral hepatitis. Annals of Internal Medicine 91(6):872-876, 1979.

Garner JS, Kaiser AB: How often is isolation needed? American Journal of Nursing 72(4):733-737, 1972.

Garner JS, Simmons BP: CDC guidelines for isolation precautions in hospitals. Infection Control (Suppl): 4(4):245-325, 1983.

Genvert G, Theil J, et al: Isolation information booklet stimulates dialog, allays fears. Hospitals 53(3):72-75, 1979.

Kirkis EJ: Tactics to hold microbes at bay. RN 45(6):81, 1982.

Larson EL, Killen M: Factors influencing handwashing behavior of patient care personnel. American Journal of Infection Control 10(3):93-99, 1982.

Preston GA, Larson EL, Stamm WE: The effect of private isolation rooms on patient care practices, colonization, and infection in an intensive care unit. American Journal of Medicine 70(3):641-645, 1981.

Simmons BP: In consultation with Hooten TM, Mallison GF: Guideline for Hospital Environmental Control. From: Guidelines for the Precaution and Control of Nosocomial Infections. U.S. Department of Health and Human Services, Public Health Service, Centers for Disease Control, Atlanta, GA, 1981.

Williams WW: CDC guideline for infection control in hospital personnel. Infection Control (Suppl):4(4):326-347, 1983.

BIBLIOGRAPHY

Castle M: Isolation: Precise procedures for better protection. Nursing75 5(5)50-57, 1975.

Dubay EC: Infection: Prevention and control, ed 2. St. Louis, CV Mosby, 1978.

Garner JS, Brachman PS: Isolation policies and procedures. In Bennett JW, Brachman PS (eds): Hospital Infections. Boston, Little, Brown, 1979.

Golden W: Routine protective isolation: Worth the trouble in neutropenic patients? Journal of the American Medical Association 242(19):2045, 1979.

Rycoft P: Infection control in the community. Paper presented at the meeting of National League for Nursing, New York, March, 1975. Infection Control, New York, National League for Nursing 20-1582, 1975.

AUDIOVISUAL RESOURCES

Controlling Transmission of Infection
Videocassette (¾ in). (1984, Color 28 min.)
Available through:
American Journal of Nursing Company
Educational Services Division
555 West 57th Street
New York, NY 10019

Psychosocial Needs of the Patient in Isolation
Videocassette (¾ in). (1980, Color, 20 min.)
Available through:
Medical University of South Carolina
80 Barre Street
Charleston, SC 29401

Protective Isolation
Filmstrip and cassette. (1975, Color, 15 min.)
Available through:
Medcom, Inc.
P.O. Box 116
Garden Grove, CA 92642

Infection Control III
Program 1. Overview & Disease-specific Isolation (17 min).
Program 2. Precautionary Measures in Isolation (22 min).
Program 3. Category-specific Isolation, Part I (17 min).
Program 4. Category-specific Isolation, Part II (18 min).
Filmstrip and cassette. (1984, Color.)
Available through:
Concept Media
P.O. Box 19542
Irvine, CA 92713

9 Surgical Asepsis

☐ INTRODUCTION

As discussed in Chapter 8, microorganisms capable of causing infections are present within and on all people and in all environments. The use of surgical aseptic procedures decreases the potential for these microorganisms to cause infections when open wounds are present or when an object is introduced into sterile body cavities.

Sterilization is the process by which all living organisms are killed, both pathogenic and nonpathogenic. This includes all vegetative bacteria and fungi, spores, and viruses. *Asepsis,* which literally means "without infection," is commonly regarded as meaning the absence of disease-producing organisms. *Surgical asepsis* refers to the use of techniques designed to exclude *all* microorganisms, in contrast to medical asepsis, which is designed to exclude agents capable of causing infectious disease but not all other microorganisms. *Aseptic technique,* often equated with surgical asepsis, refers to those practices maintaining the sterility of objects and areas. *Contamination* is the introduction of microorganisms into a previously sterile area.

The skills presented in this chapter cannot be viewed in isolation from each other or from the concepts and practices of medical asepsis and correct handwashing techniques (Skill 28). To use sterile equipment for any sterile procedure, it is important to be able to discriminate between the concepts of *clean, sterile,* and *contaminated.* In the context of medical asepsis, "clean" involves the known or assumed absence of pathogens, and "contamination" refers to contact with items known or highly suspected to have pathogenic microorganisms present. By contrast, when something is sterile, it has no living microorganisms of any kind. In the context of using sterile items with aseptic technique, contamination refers to the introduction of *any* microorganisms, whether pathogenic or nonpathogenic, from any source into a previously sterile area. This may be unintentional and accidental during a procedure, or intentional, such as when a procedure is finished.

The differences among the concepts of clean, sterile, and contaminated are illustrated with bed linen use. Fresh bed linen is considered *clean,* but even with thorough laundry processes, it is not *sterile* or microorganism-free because laundry processes do not sterilize. If double-wrapped and autoclaved with steam under pressure for an appropriate time-to-temperature ratio, it is considered sterile as long as it remains wrapped and sealed. When the sterilized linen is unwrapped, it can be kept sterile only if handled with sterile gloves, forceps, or hemostats, or if placed on another sterile area. If handled with clean ungloved hands or placed on an unsterile but clean surface, it automatically becomes *contaminated* from the perspective of surgical asepsis, because it is no longer free from all microorganisms. From a medical aseptic perspective, it could still be considered clean and usable for client care.

Sterility is an all-or-nothing concept. It is not possible for something to be "almost sterile"—it either is or is not sterile. The term *surgically clean* is not to be confused with *sterile.* Surgically clean means that something has been thoroughly cleaned (mechanically, physically, or chemically) and perhaps given a terminal sterilization as an added precaution, such as when instruments are cleaned in the operating room. This results in a marked reduction of microorganisms and minimizes the disease-producing capability of the items, but does not render them sterile.

Beck (1977) opposes the concept of "abridged sterility" as being adequate for many surgical procedures. Abridged sterility refers to destruction of all microbial life except resistant spores. Beck's strong opposition to this practice is based on the premises that (1) pathogens not currently recognized as disease-producing could become so in the future and that (2) although there are no reliable ways to measure abridged sterility, there are methods to test sterility. He concludes that "we should accept no less than sterility for any human contact when skin or mucous membranes will be or probably could be broken" (Beck, 1977, p. 244). Others believe that instruments such as endoscopes, bronchoscopes, or laparoscopes can safely be used after careful cleaning and disinfection, rather than sterilization.

Sterility is an invisible attribute of an item or area, but breaks in aseptic technique are visible to the observant user or onlooker. The nurse must know when something is sterile, when it is not, how to keep sterile items sterile and separate from nonsterile items, and how to recognize immediately and act to correct breaks in aseptic technique. Close attention and careful movements are needed to avoid unintentional contamination during an aseptic procedure. When there is any question about whether contamination has occurred, the item or area is *always* considered contaminated. Gruendemann et al. (1977) advocate developing a "surgical conscience" that constantly monitors one's own and others' use of aseptic technique and acts to correct breaks and contamination. This surgical conscience is necessary because "human beings possess a tendency for covering up their own errors, for ignoring risks, and for letting embarrassing faults go uncorrected" (Gruendemann et al., 1977, p. 53).

The nurse is involved in supervising, monitoring, and setting standards for other health-care personnel, including nursing assistants, practical nurses, nursing and medical students, and physicians. The nurse often teaches aseptic procedures to clients and their families, such as for insulin administration, dressing changes, or self-catheterization. The nurse determines which sterile supplies are to be ordered and how they are stored. In small clinics, physicians' offices, and home settings, the nurse may be responsible for the actual sterilization of some equipment and supplies.

This chapter presents the methods of sterilization, storage, and handling of sterile supplies, "Sterile Supplies" (Skill 30); use of sterile gloves, "Donning Sterile Gloves" (Skill 31); "Dressings and Wound Care" (Skill 32); "Suture Removal" (Skill 33); "Wound Culture Specimen Collection" (Skill 34); "Wound Drains and Irrigation" (Skill 35); "Wet Sterile Dressings" (Skill 36); and "Wet-to-Dry Dressings" (Skill 37). This chapter does not present techniques used primarily or exclusively in the operating room or delivery room, which are usually specific to the institution and are well presented in current operating room textbooks (Brooks, 1975; Ginsberg, 1966; Gruendemann and Meeker, 1983; LeMaitre and Finnegan, 1980).

☐ ENTRY TEST

1. Respond to the questions in the Chapter 8 Entry Test, p. 240.
2. How do pathogenic and nonpathogenic bacteria differ?
3. What is the difference between medical and surgical asepsis?
4. What are the differences between facultative spore-forming and nonspore-forming bacteria?
5. How do the vegetative and spore forms of spore-forming bacteria differ?
6. How do aerobic bacteria differ from anaerobic bacteria?
7. What is meant by "facultative anaerobes?"

REFERENCES

Beck WC (guest ed): Abridged sterility: A level of disinfection. AORN Journal 26(2):242, 244, 1977.

Brooks SM: Fundamentals of Operating Room Nursing, ed 2. St Louis, MO, CV Mosby, 1979.

Ginsberg F: A Manual of Operating Room Technology. Philadelphia, JB Lippincott, 1966.

Gruendemann BJ, Casterton SB, et al.: The Surgical Patient: Behavioral Concepts for the Operating Room Nurse, ed 2. St Louis, MO, CV Mosby, 1977.

Gruendemann BJ, Meeker MH: Alexander's Care of the Patient in Surgery, ed 7. St Louis, MO, CV Mosby, 1983.

LeMaitre GD, Finnegan JA: The Patient in Surgery: A Guide for Nurses, ed 4. Philadelphia, WB Saunders, 1980.

SKILL 30 Sterile Supplies

PREREQUISITE SKILL

Skill 19, "Inspection"
Skill 28, "Handwashing"

☐ STUDENT OBJECTIVES

1. Explain the purposes for using sterile supplies and sterile fields.
2. Describe principles and uses of various methods of sterilization.
3. Discuss the nurse's role and responsibility to the client when preparing and implementing aseptic procedures.
4. Relate medical aseptic techniques to the use of sterile supplies.
5. Relate principles of microorganism transfer and aseptic technique to the use of sterile supplies.
6. Cite specific situations where various sterile supplies and sterile fields are required.
7. Describe various indicators of sterility for commercially and institutionally packaged sterile items.
8. Relate storage conditions and packaging materials to maintenance of sterility.

9. Using correct aseptic technique:
   a. Open sterile packages, both institutional and commercial.
   b. Prepare a sterile field.
   c. Add sterile items to a sterile field.
   d. Add sterile liquids to a sterile area.

□ INTRODUCTION

The term *sterile supplies* refers to any sterilized item or liquid that can be used in a client-care procedure requiring the use of aseptic technique. Some examples of sterile supplies are dressings, bandages, drapes, gowns, gloves, urinary catheters, surgical drains, basins, syringes, and sterile water or solutions for injection or irrigation. Some sterile items such as wrappers or basins may be used to create a sterile field, that is, an area on which to place other sterile items.

The many types of sterile supplies available are used in numerous diagnostic and therapeutic procedures and in nearly every kind of health-care setting. Knowledge of how to handle, use, and store sterile supplies is a prerequisite for correctly executing any aseptic procedure. Combined with correct handwashing techniques, conscientious implementation of correct aseptic technique when using sterile supplies is a basic method for preventing infections.

When sterile supplies have been opened and sterile areas created, the nurse needs to know how to maintain the area as sterile. Following are some principles of microorganism transfer that have implications for maintaining sterility.

PRINCIPLES OF MICROORGANISM TRANSFER

1. Microorganisms are unable to travel independently from one place to another but require a vector.
2. Skin and mucous membranes normally harbor microorganisms.
3. Shedding skin flakes carry thousands of usually nonpathogenic organisms, spread through air currents.
4. Gravity causes microorganisms to shed along with nonsterile skin flakes onto a sterile area.
5. Coughing, sneezing, or yelling spreads microorganisms for short distances through the air by way of moisture droplets. These microorganisms can fall on sterile areas.
6. Microorganisms can be transferred whenever a sterile item touches a nonsterile item, making the sterile item nonsterile.
7. Microorganisms cannot penetrate the surface of a double layer of *dry* sterile cotton fabric or nonwoven barrier fabric.
8. When a sterile nonwaterproof surface in contact with a nonsterile surface becomes wet, capillary attraction allows microorganisms to transfer upward from the nonsterile surface and contaminate the sterile surface.
9. Moisture facilitates growth and movement of microorganisms.

This skill presents basic principles and practices of sterilization, plus techniques for preparing a sterile field and opening and using sterile supplies. The use of some specific sterile items will be discussed in separate skills; for example, syringes and needles are discussed in Skill 73, intravenous equipment in Skill 74, and urinary catheters in Skill 59.

□ PREPARATION

Sterile supplies may be classified as either disposable or reusable. Most disposable sterile supplies are prepackaged and sterilized in small, ready-to-use units by the manufacturer. However, some disposable supplies, such as dressing rolls and gauze squares and sponges, are bought in bulk by the institution and then repackaged and sterilized in smaller units. Reusable sterile supplies may be sterile or nonsterile when received from the manufacturer and are cleaned, disinfected, and resterilized at the institution after each use, following agency policy.

There are differences of opinion about whether disposables are more effective in reducing costs and infections than are reusables. Increased cost of disposables must be weighed against increased worker time in cleaning, repairing, and resterilizing reusables, and Perkins (1969) indicates that hospital practices rather than the type of supplies used determine the incidence of infection. Ryan (1976) reports documented studies that support the use of reusable as well as disposable supplies. Mallison (1979b) recommends that in-hospital sterilization not be used for gloves, masks, sponges, and any syringes except the most sophisticated special-use ones, since dependable, high-quality disposable equipment is cheaper and safer than resterilizing these items.

Another aspect of the question of disposables versus reusables is the ecologic issue. It has been estimated that an average of 10 pounds of solid waste per person per day is generated in the average hospital (Wolff et al., 1979).

METHODS OF STERILIZATION

Modern sterilization had its beginning in 1865 when Joseph Lister began to use carbolic acid solution to disinfect instruments, hands, and wounds, and as an operating room spray. In the middle 1880s, boiling was introduced as another method of destroying bacteria. Around the year 1888, Ernst von Bergmann and his associates developed steam sterilization much as it is known today (Berry and Kohn, 1974).

Modern sterilization methods include steam, dry heat, ethylene oxide gas, ionizing radiation, and chemical sterilization. Boiling and ultraviolet radiation, although sometimes referred to as "sterilization," actually achieve only disinfection. They are discussed under sterilization, however, because these methods may be safely used in the home to destroy pathogens and prepare items for use or reuse, as an alternative to using disposable sterile supplies.

Adequate sterilization depends on a combination of factors. For example, the item must be free from dirt, tissue, or other debris; all surfaces to be sterilized must be in direct contact with the sterilizing agent; sufficient time must be allowed; and, in the case of steam sterilization, an adequate time-temperature-pressure combination is required.

All items being sterilized must be packaged in a wrapper or container suitable for the particular item. The packaging method must be appropriate for both the item and for the method of sterilization that item requires. Sterilized packages are handled and stored in a way that maintains their sterility, and they are opened in a manner that maintains the sterility of the contents. Sterility of package contents is evidenced by sterilizing indicators specific to the method of sterilization used.

Hospitals, nursing homes, surgicenters, large clinics, and other agencies have a central service area where sterile supplies are stored. Commonly called Central Supply, this department also assumes the responsibility for cleaning, repairing, and resterilizing reusable supplies. In smaller settings, nurses may be responsible for these functions.

Steam Sterilization
Saturated steam under pressure is the most widely used, safest, most reliable and economic method of sterilization used today (Gruendemann and Meeker, 1983; LeMaitre and Finnegan, 1980; Sorensen and Luckmann, 1979; Wilson et al., 1979).

Heat destroys microorganisms through denaturation and coagulation of the enzyme-protein within the cell. When moisture as well as heat is present, that is, steam, microorganisms are killed at lower temperatures than when dry heat is used. Free-flowing steam has a temperature of 100°C (212°F), but under pressure and in a vacuum, steam temperature rises considerably.

Steam sterilization usually is done in an autoclave, in which steam is under pressure within a vacuum. The steam flows around the items to be sterilized, permeating the wrappers.

When exposed to heat, microorganisms do not die all at once. Instead, they die in a logarithmic pattern. This means that with time, more and more bacteria die until eventually all cells are dead. Standard time and temperature requirements for steam sterilization at 15 to 17 pounds per square inch (1.1 to 1.2 kg per cm^2) are: 121°C (250°F) for 15 minutes, or 132°C (270°F) for 5 minutes (American Hospital Association, 1979; LeMaitre and Finnegan, 1980; Wilson et al., 1979). Mallison (1979b) advises that exposure to saturated steam at 121° to 123°C (250° to 253°F) for 15 to 45 minutes (depending on the size of the package being sterilized) dependably sterilizes most materials without excessively damaging them.

Items for institutional steam sterilization must be wrapped in materials that allow steam to penetrate the package freely and sterilize the contents, such as double muslin, paper, or nonwoven fabrics. Liquids are sterilized in large flasks with a self-sealing closure consisting of a collar and cap that allows for escape of air as the flask contents expand due to the rise in temperature and pressure during sterilization. As the internal flask pressure drops during cooling, the cap seals itself tightly against the collar, preserving the vacuum and sterility of the contents.

Although steam sterilization is used widely, there are some items that can be damaged by this heat, such as rubber goods, plastics, sensitive surgical instruments, cutting edges, and ground glass items.

In the home setting, steam sterilization can be achieved in a pressure cooker. The item is placed on the rack above the water level, and the pressure maintained at 15 pounds per square inch for 15 minutes, which is a recommended time, temperature, and pressure relationship. Ironing with steam at a medium to high setting provides some degree of disinfection appropriate for home use (Wolff et al., 1979).

Gas Sterilization
A gas known as ethylene oxide began to be used for sterilization purposes in the 1950s. It is used for heat-sensitive materials that would be damaged by other more efficient methods of sterilization. For example, plastic and rubber items, heart valves, lensed instruments, ground glass instruments such as glass syringes, books, papers, mattresses, and face masks can be sterilized safely with ethylene oxide. This gas is effective against all microorganisms, as it causes cell alkylation and inactivates cell reproduction. Ethylene oxide penetrates dry materials readily, does not require high temperatures or pressures, and is noncorrosive and nondamaging.

A disadvantage of ethylene oxide is that it is slower and more expensive than steam sterilization. It also is toxic; workers need protection from its fumes, and rubber goods often absorb the gas and retain it for up to 24 hours, resulting in skin burns if the items are used before the gas dissipates. Porous materials must be well aerated before they are allowed to contact any body tissue (Mallison, 1979b). Ethylene gas is recommended for use only when steam sterilization will damage the article.

It is difficult to obtain an even distribution of ethylene oxide during sterilization. Items intended for gas sterilization must be dried throughly and may be wrapped in muslin, paper, or thin plastic film, as these materials readily allow gas penetration. Gas cannot penetrate glass or aluminum foil wrappers.

Dry Heat Sterilization

Some substances that are impenetrable to steam can be sterilized with dry heat. These items include powders, waxes, oils, glycerin, petroleum jelly, or petrolatum gauze. Dry heat also is used for items such as glass tubes and syringes, needles, and cutting edge instruments. Dry heat does not cause corrosion of sharp instruments nor erode the ground glass surfaces of syringe plungers, as often happens with steam (Perkins, 1969).

Dry heat sterilization causes microorganism death by coagulation and oxidation of cell protein. Recommended temperatures for dry heat sterilization are 160° to 165°C (320° to 330°F) for 2 hours or 170° to 175°C (338° to 347°F) for 1 hour (Wilson et al., 1979). Laboratory studies indicate that dry spores of *Bacillus steatothermophilus* are destroyed by 160°C for 1 hour (Perkins, 1969). Disadvantages of dry sterilization include: (a) an increased length of time needed for sterilization as compared to steam sterilization; (b) destructiveness to fabrics (linens, dressings, and wrappers); and (c) overexposure to dry heat is more damaging than overexposure to moist heat.

Items to be sterilized with dry heat may be wrapped in muslin or foil, as permeability is not a requirement for a wrapping material used for dry heat sterilization. In the home setting, items can be sterilized by baking them in a 325° oven for 1 to 2 hours. To check the accuracy of the oven thermostat, use an oven thermometer.

Ionizing Radiation Sterilization

In sufficient dosage, some types of radiation are destructive to living microorganisms such as bacteria and viruses. The shorter and higher energy wavelengths from X-rays, high-speed electrons, and gamma or beta rays destroy the cell's ability to propagate.

Ionizing radiation can be used safely with heat-sensitive and delicate instruments, as there is virtually no thermal reaction involved. It also is used to sterilize tissues for transplant purposes. It is considered reliable and effective, easy to monitor sterility levels, and works well with liquids and solids. It is not considered practical for general institutional use, owing to the cost of building and operating the sophisticated equipment needed. The major disadvantages of ionizing radiation are: (a) some organisms are radio-resistant and are reduced but not completely destroyed; and (b) radiation can be mutagenic rather than lethal to some microorganisms (MacClelland, 1977; Wilson et al., 1979).

Liquid Chemical Sterilization

Liquid chemical sterilization, also called cold sterilization, can be achieved by soaking items in a solution of activated aqueous glutaraldehyde (Cidex) for 10 hours. If used properly, this solution is considered an effective sterilizing agent and is capable of destroying all microorganisms, including bacteria, fungi, spores, the tubercle bacillus, and viruses (Gruendemann and Meeker, 1983). It often is used to sterilize lensed instruments such as bronchoscopes and cystoscopes. Activated aqueous glutaraldehyde is noncorrosive, penetrates easily, rinses off readily, is not inactivated by organic matter, does not cause protein or blood to coagulate, and does not affect the sharpness of delicate instruments.

Only one other solution is capable of cold sterilization—aqueous formaldehyde. It is not commonly used because of its irritating, pungent odor (Gruendemann and Meeker, 1983; Perkins, 1969). Solutions such as 70 percent alcohol, povidone iodine (Betadine), or benzalkonium chloride (Zepharin) are capable of disinfection, but not sterilization.

Boiling Water Disinfection

Nonpressurized boiling water does *not* sterilize, as it does not destroy spores or reliably kill all viruses. *Disinfection*, rather than sterilization, is achieved by boiling. If there is no other method of sterilization available, sodium carbonate (sal soda or washing soda) may be added to the water to make a 2 percent solution (4 teaspoons per quart). Perkins (1969, p. 315) reports several studies that indicated bacterial spores which resisted destruction in boiling water for 10 hours were destroyed in 10 to 30 minutes in this 2 percent soda solution. This solution has been found to decrease the corrosive action on metal instruments and increase the disinfecting power of boiling water. However, it is not used for rubber goods or glassware because it is destructive to both.

Instruments must be covered with at least 1 inch of water above them. Moderate boiling is recommended, as simmering does not produce boiling temperatures and too vigorous boiling results in rapid depletion of the water level, necessitating adding more water.

The boiling temperature of water varies with elevation. At sea level, the boiling temperature of water is 100°C (212°F), and the recommended boiling time for disinfection is 30 minutes (Perkins, 1969). As the altitude rises and atmospheric pressure decreases, the boiling temperature drops. For example, in Denver, Colorado (altitude 1609 meters, or 5280 feet), water boils at 94.4°C (202.0°F), and in LaPaz, Bolivia (altitude 3900 meters, or 12,795 feet), water boils at 86.6°C (188.0°F). Because it is the temperature of the water rather than the actual boiling that accomplishes disinfection, boiling times must be lengthened at higher elevations to provide adequate disinfection. Perkins (1969) recommends lengthening the boiling time by 5 minutes for each 1000 feet of elevation. Based on this standard, Table 30-1 presents approximate boiling time recommended for disinfection at various elevations (Perkins, 1969; Todd, 1970).

In the home setting, boiling is considered adequate for items such as syringes, catheters, or instruments. People generally are more resistant to bacteria within their own environment, and the home lacks the major cross-contamination potential present in most

TABLE 30-1. Boiling Times for Disinfection at Various Altitudes

ALTITUDE[a]		BOILING POINT OF WATER		APPROXIMATE BOILING TIME
(meters)	(feet)	(C°)	(F°)	(minutes)
0	0	100.0	212.0	30
305	1000	99.0	210.2	35
610	2000	98.0	208.4	40
915	3000	96.9	206.5	45
1219	4000	95.9	204.7	50
1524	5000	94.9	202.9	55
2134	7000	92.9	199.2	65
2743	9000	90.9	195.6	75
3353	11000	88.8	191.9	85
3963	13000	86.8	188.2	95
4572	15000	85.0	185.0	105

[a]U.S. Standard Atmosphere is assumed.
(Adapted with permission from Todd DK (ed): The Water Encyclopedia: A Compendium of Useful Information on Water Resources. Syosset, NY, Water Information Center, Inc., 1970.)

health-care settings where many and varied bacteria are present. The problem of lime deposit buildup on items boiled frequently in hard water can be decreased somewhat by boiling the water for 10 minutes before adding the instruments. Some of the lime precipitates out during that interval (Perkins, 1969). Adding vinegar or water softener to the water also tends to decrease lime buildup.

Ultraviolet-Radiation Disinfection

Ultraviolet rays are short light rays from the invisible light spectrum, found naturally in sunlight and produced artificially with ultraviolet lamps. These lamps were often used to help prevent airborne infections in confined areas of public use (elevators or school rooms) or in critical areas of a hospital (operating rooms, nurseries, or infectious disease areas). The effectiveness of ultraviolet disinfection is limited to the surfaces of objects. Ultraviolet lights are not to be used where people are directly exposed because of the potential for retinal and skin burns. Ultraviolet lamps require frequent monitoring, as their effectiveness diminishes before they stop glowing.

When used as a home method of disinfection, articles must be exposed to bright, direct sunlight for several hours, so as not to obstruct the ultraviolet rays (Wilson et al., 1979; Wolff et al., 1979).

STERILIZING INDICATORS

It is important that items be exposed to the sterilizing agent for a sufficient time to render them sterile. Since sterility is not evident visibly, there are a number of methods used to determine sterility in institutionally prepared sterile supplies. One of these is a sealed glass tube containing pellets that melt when time and temperature conditions favorable to sterilization have been achieved. These tubes are placed in the center of an operating room linen pack or of a loaded autoclave. Other monitoring devices include chemical indicator cards or strips that can be inserted into surgical packs or procedure sets. When sufficiently exposed to steam or gas, the dye changes color.

Biologic control of sterility is considered the only accurate method of determining the effectiveness of steam sterilization. Commercially prepared spore strips or ampules containing a known population of *Bacillus steatothermophilus* spores are placed within the center of dense linen packs or in the middle of a loaded autoclave. This microorganism is highly heat-resistant and spore-forming, but is nonpathogenic. After sterilization, the ampules or strips are sent to the bacteriology lab, a commercial lab, or to the manufacturer for determination of microorganism destruction. Some newer spore tubes are designed to be read in the central supply area. The effectiveness of dry heat and ethylene oxide sterilizers usually is monitored with known populations of *Bacillus subtilis* spores.

All sterile packages prepared within an institution should be closed with sterilizing indicator tape. This tape has imprinted lines, squares, or words that change color when the sterilization method used has functioned properly. Usually the colors darken and become much more visible. Each time the nurse opens a sterile package, he or she must note the sterilizing indicators to determine if the sterilization process actually has occurred. Color change in sterilizing indicators does not actually guarantee sterility, only that the items have been through the sterilization process, and sterility is presumed to have occurred.

Institutionally prepared bottles of liquids often have a chemical indicator on a tag placed around the bottle neck. When using institutionally prepared bottles with large rubber caps, the sound of the vacuum seal being released indicates sterility.

Sterile packages are dated according to their shelf life, or the length of time they are considered sterile. The date represents the last date on which the item may be used as sterile. After that date, reusable items must be returned to central supply and resterilized. Commercially sterilized products generally have a fairly long shelf life if stored properly, but if outdated they may be used only as clean supplies. Regular checking of expiration dates and a habit of placing new supplies at the back of the shelf help prevent supplies from becoming outdated.

Commercially prepared sterile supplies are clearly labeled "Sterile," and often say "Patient-Ready" or "Sterility guaranteed unless package is damaged or opened." With commercial supplies, the manufacturer, rather than the institution, assumes the responsibility for sterility. The frequency of microbiologic contamination of commercially prepared sterile items is so low that routine microbiologic sampling and testing by health-care agencies is not recommended. Instead, it is recommended that if, in the monitoring of disease patterns, sterile products are suspected as the cause of a disease, all items with the same lot number should be quarantined and investigated by local, state, and federal agencies (Mallison, 1979b).

STORAGE AND HANDLING

Sterile packages must be stored in a clean, dry, well-ventilated but dustproof and verminproof area. There should be no sharp corners, and extremes of temperature and humidity are to be avoided. Temperatures between 18° and 25°C (64° and 77°F), and a relative humidity no lower than 30 percent or higher than 75 percent are recommended (Mallison, 1979a). Items sterilized in a double muslin wrapper or paper wrapper generally are considered to have a shelf life of 21 to 30 days, but according to Mallison and Standard (1974), this can be doubled if items are kept in a closed cabinet instead of on open shelves. A plastic dust cover placed over sterile packages increases their shelf life to 6 months or more. Plastic or plastic and paper combination wraps that are heat-sealed will remain sterile for 6 months to 1 year. Theoretically, commercially prepared disposable items that are heat-sealed in nonwoven envelopes inside plastic sealed wrappers are sterile indefinitely, if handled and stored carefully (Gruendemann and Meeker, 1983).

It is recommended that storage shelves for sterile items should be at least 12 inches from the floor, 18 inches from the ceiling, and 2 inches from outside walls. A sterile package is never placed on the floor (Mallison, 1979a; Mallison and Standard, 1974). Sterile packages that have been handled excessively or have been stored under uncertain conditions must be considered nonsterile and either discarded or resterilized.

DATA BASE

A wide variety of information enables the nurse both to use sterile supplies correctly and to provide necessary explanations to the client and family.

Client History and Recorded Data

Knowing the client's diagnosis and medical and nursing problems helps the nurse understand, explain, and implement the procedure within the context of the particular client's plan of care. As a basis for explanations and answering questions, the nurse assesses the client's level of knowledge about and previous experience with the procedure. The nurse also assesses the client's level of consciousness, mobility, and ability to cooperate and assist with the procedure as needed so that the integrity of the sterile supplies is not compromised by client actions.

Physical Appraisal Skills

Inspection. Although the skill of inspection generally is used as a method of gathering data by observing a client, it is necessary to use the same careful attention to details and to evaluate what is observed when examining a sterile package prior to its use. The nurse *inspects* sterile items for indicators of sterility, that is, intactness, dryness, expiration date, and the color and notations of sterilizing indicators. If any of these four factors is not absolute, the package must be considered contaminated and discarded if it is a single-use item, or returned to the central service area for resterilization if the item is reusable.

EQUIPMENT

A wide variety of supplies and equipment is sterilized for use in client-care situations. Before equipment and supplies can be sterilized, they must be clean and free from debris and gross contamination from blood, tissue, and body secretions. After they have been sterilized, all sterile supplies must have some method for protecting and maintaining their sterility. Various wrappers, containers, packaging techniques, and sterilizing indicators serve as methods for ensuring that a sterile item remains sterile until its use.

Sterile Wrappers and Containers

Sterile supplies are usually packaged in cloth, paper, or plastic wrappers, or some combination of these three. The wrapper provides protection against contact contamination during handling, protects against the entry of insects or vermin during storage, and serves as a dust filter.

Cloth. Two thicknesses of *dry muslin* of a good quality 140-thread count (per square inch) have been found to prevent migration of bacteria (Perkins, 1969). However, the American Hospital Association (1979) recommends using four layers of muslin, and indicates that newer nonwoven single-use fabrics may have some advantages over muslin. If a fabric is too thin or has holes in it, it provides inadequate protection against contamination, but if the fabric is too dense or woven too tightly (as are some single-use fabrics), steam penetration is seriously retarded and sterility compromised. Muslin wrappers must be sent to the laundry before being resterilized to avoid superheating and fiber damage (Ryan, 1976).

Paper. Disposable and reusable *paper wraps* of a variety of kinds may be used. Paper allows steam to pass freely, although not quite as rapidly as muslin. It provides a satisfactory dust filter and is relatively inexpensive, but it can be noisy and not very flexible. Paper packages are more likely to become punctured or torn, with resulting contamination, although newer laminated paper wraps are sturdier. If the paper is too dense, steam penetration is slower. Some institutions use double paper bags for packaging items such as cotton balls or dressings.

Plastic. Presterilized commercially prepared liquids for both external and internal use are often contained in *plastic bottles or bags. Plastic film* is also used as a packaging material and is especially useful with ethylene oxide gas sterilization. Since plastic is practically impermeable to air or steam, it cannot be used in a steam sterilizer. Plastics are pliable, transparent, impervious to dust, resist tearing more than paper, and are heat sealable. They are frequently used as an outer protective wrap over paper wraps, or as dust covers in storage areas.

Glass. Liquids are sterilized in *glass* containers. Fluids for intramuscular or intravenous injection should be commercially prepared (Mallison, 1979b). Institutionally prepared sterile fluids (for example, sterile water, distilled water, normal saline, acetic acid, boric acid, and magnesium sulfate solutions.) can be used for water, external or irrigating purposes.

Institutionally prepared solutions often are sterilized in reusable glass containers with large rubber caps. They must be clearly labeled with the contents and the expiration date. Commercially prepared solutions for external use are available in nonreusable glass or plastic containers that have a seal over the screw cap. They are labeled with the contents, a clear notation "Sterile" or "Sterile: Patient-Ready," the sterilization or expiration date, and whether they are for irrigation or for injection.

Packaging of Sterile Supplies

Institutionally prepared packages of either disposable or reusable items usually are wrapped envelope-style and closed with sterilizing indicator tape.

Commercially prepared disposable sterile packages may be wrapped in paper, plastic, or a combination of the two. Items may be envelope-wrapped in paper and placed in a heat-sealed plastic bag, or they may be placed inside a paper or plastic wrap with heat-sealed edges. A commercial package with heat-sealed edges has labeled flaps or tabs that can be pulled apart to open the package.

Some commercial packages contain all the items needed for a given procedure, such as a urinary catheterization. The items may be inside a cardboard or plastic box or tray, envelope-wrapped in paper, and inserted in a heat-sealed plastic bag. Or the plastic tray may have a heat-sealed paper top that can be pulled off without contamination. All commercially prepared sterile packages have a clear label on the outside or have the label visible through the plastic bag. Labeling includes the term "Sterile," the name of the product, the various items in the package, and directions for both opening the package and using its contents. Since all manufacturers have their own variations of package-opening procedures, it is advisable to take time to *read and follow* the directions on the package or bottle.

Transfer Forceps

Sterile transfer forceps (also called lifting forceps) may be used to add dressings, swabs, or instruments to an existing sterile field when sterile gloves are not being worn. They also may be used to arrange or handle sterile supplies when sterile gloves are not being worn.

In the past, transfer forceps frequently were used to remove sterile items from a common storage container, such as a jar of sterilized cotton balls. Currently, these forceps are considered undesirable for general institutional use since there is great potential for cross-contamination when used repeatedly by many people in a busy nursing-care unit (Wolff et al., 1979). If transfer forceps are used in an operating room, clinic, or a physician's office, they should be washed and resterilized daily and fresh disinfectant solution placed in their container. Seventy percent alcohol is often used for this purpose because it dries quickly and is noninjurious if it comes in contact with body tissues. A transfer forceps must be removed from and returned to the storage container with care, as both the top edges and the insides of the container above the liquid level are considered contaminated. The portion of the forceps located beneath the fluid level is considered sterile, while the handles and the portion above the fluid are considered unsterile. The Bard-Parker transfer forceps is designed with a spring-loaded inner cylinder which rises above the outer container edges when the forceps is removed. The forceps can then be returned to the cylinder without contamination. This transfer forceps is not used to pick up anything with an adhering base, such as petrolatum gauze, as this action introduces foreign bodies into the disinfectant solution. When used to add items to a sterile field, the forceps is not allowed to touch the field, as this provides a potential cross-contamination when later used with another sterile field.

Single-use transfer forceps usually are wrapped separately, sterilized, and used for only one procedure. This one-time use of dry transfer forceps is considered safer than keeping forceps in a solution, because there is no possible contamination prior to opening the wrapper. This type of forceps usually has ratchets (or catches) on the handles, so the forceps can be closed. This design helps keep the forcep tips from accidentally separating and possibly becoming contaminated.

When a single-use sterile transfer forceps is used with ungloved hands, the forceps tips are considered sterile and are kept well within the sterile area, while the handles are considered unsterile and are placed at the edge of or extending off the sterile field. When a single-use sterile transfer forceps is used with sterile gloves, the entire forceps is considered sterile and is placed completely within the sterile field.

When using transfer forceps stored in a solution, or when handling wet items with a single-use transfer forceps, the forceps tips *must* be kept pointed downward at all times. When forceps tips are turned upward, liquids can flow by gravity from the sterile tips to the contaminated handles, and then back to the sterile tips, thereby contaminating the forceps tips. When sterile gloves are used with a single-use sterile transfer forceps, this is not a problem, but it is considered safest to be in the habit of always holding forceps tips downward. When using forceps, keep the elbows abducted (away from the body), as this helps keep the forceps tips pointed downward. When removing items from a sterile package with forceps, the forceps tips must not touch the edges of the package, as the package edges may be contaminated.

Care of Used Sterile Equipment
When a sterile procedure is completed, single-use items are discarded. Glass items and needles are disposed of in specially designated containers separate from other debris because they are not burnable and have a potential for breakage with puncturing of trash bags and transfer of microorganisms.

Reusable items are placed in containers in designated areas for pick-up and transfer to the central supply area. Mallison (1979a) recommends that reusable supplies be returned to central supply without precleaning in the clinical area, because this precleaning can be unsafe, is inefficient, and is unnecessary with central processing. Common practice, however, often continues to include prewashing in the clinical area, because body proteins (blood and tissues) are more readily removed by rinsing with cool water before they become dried and hardened. This is especially true for forceps and hemostats with their corrugated tips and ratchet handles (See Skill 32 for illustrations of these items).

If items are known or suspected to be contaminated with infectious material, they are not rinsed, but are placed in impervious plastic bags and clearly labeled "contaminated" before sending them to central supply. Reusable surgical instruments are washed in a mechanical washer-sterilizer with a decontamination cycle or in an ultrasonic cleaner before being resterilized. Manual cleaning of used instruments is not recommended because it is difficult, time-consuming, and potentially unsafe, as it contributes to microorganism spread through droplets and aerosols during the washing. It also is quite difficult to remove manually all microorganism-harboring blood and tissue debris from hemostat and forceps joints, hinges, and ratchets.

Because smaller clinics and physicians' offices may do their own instrument cleaning and resterilization, some guidelines for manual instrument cleaning are included here, based on Perkins' (1969) recommendations:

1. Rinse in cool water immediately after use before blood and soil can harden in the instrument's crevices and serrations. Hot water causes coagulation of blood and tissue protein.
2. Soak in *warm* (52°C or 125°F) solution of a blood solvent or detergent such as Edisonite, Reliance, Solvent, or Haemosol. Avoid soap (produces a film) and abrasives (scratches surfaces).
3. Scrub all aspects of the instrument with a stiff-bristled, newly sterilized brush. All adhering debris, blood, and lime salts must be removed because they harbor microorganisms and cause difficulty in sterilization. Avoid splashing on clothing and surrounding work areas, as this contact spreads contaminants.
4. Rinse with *hot* water and dry thoroughly. Residual moisture can cause rusting.

Other reusable items for resterilization should be rinsed and washed using similar procedures. More detailed information is available from the Centers for Disease Control (CDC), U.S. Public Health Services, Atlanta, Georgia.

☐ EXECUTION

Before beginning an aseptic procedure, the nurse must know how to implement the procedure, what supplies are needed, and what the supplies will be used for. Sometimes the supplies are predetermined by the items within the package. Commercially prepared packages sometimes have directions for use of the contents. Before beginning a procedure, think through the procedural steps as they relate to the specific client, as this helps determine whether additional equipment or procedural modifications are necessary. As part of this assessment, identify the focal anatomic area on the client's body, the placement of sterile equipment, and the need for a sterile back-up supply area.

Before implementing a procedure using sterile supplies, the area around the client must be clean and tidy in order to decrease the potential for microorganism transfer. This means changing soiled bed linen or clothing, removing used linen and trash from the room, and, cleansing obvious soiling from the client's skin. When possible, implement sterile procedures after bathing the client, changing the linen, and allowing time for air currents and dust thus generated to subside.

Before implementing a sterile procedure, wash your hands thoroughly, using careful medical aseptic technique (See Skill 28).

In an operating or delivery room, a 3 to 10 minute surgical hand scrub is used prior to operative or delivery procedures. For this kind of handwashing, sterile scrub brushes, foot-controlled faucets, skin antiseptic solutions, and a specific washing methodology (known as a surgical scrub) are used.

The skin can never be sterilized, but it can be made surgically clean by reducing the number of microorganisms present. A full surgical scrub in the operating room has been found to reduce the microbial count to near zero, and some antiseptic soaps leave an antimicrobial residue on the skin for several hours (Gruendemann and Meeker, 1983). Each institution has specific guidelines for surgical scrubs and provides orientation for persons needing to use this procedure.

GUIDELINES FOR ASEPTIC TECHNIQUE

Based on the principles of microorganism transfer (see p. 269), the following guidelines enable you to use correct aseptic technique to maintain surgical asepsis.

1. Never assume sterility. Always check package intactness, sterilizing indicators for color changes, or package label "Sterile."
2. Sterile items become unsterile and contaminated when touched by unsterile items or when allowed to sit exposed to the air for prolonged periods of time.
3. Always keep sterile items clearly visible to the worker.
4. Keep sterile items above the waist or table.
5. Always face the sterile field. *Do not turn your back* toward a sterile field.
6. The outer 1 inch of a sterile field is generally considered contaminated.
7. Do not reach across a sterile field. Reach around the field, move yourself around the field, or turn the sterile field carefully by reaching underneath the wrapper or by touching only the wrapper edges.
8. Avoid speaking, coughing, sneezing, or laughing over a sterile field. Turn your head away from the sterile field if these actions are necessary, unless wearing a surgical mask.
9. Decrease contamination from air currents by closing doors, windows, or curtains; by moving slowly; and by minimizing the shaking of drapes and linens.
10. A sterile field is considered contaminated when it becomes damp if there is no sterile waterproof barrier underneath. Damp surfaces also attract contaminating microorganisms from the air.
11. Avoid splashing on the sterile field when adding liquids to a sterile receptacle. Pour liquids slowly.
12. Contamination does not generally change the appearance of a previously sterile item. Only the person who saw contamination occur knows it happened and can change it. *If sterility is questioned, assume the item is unsterile.*

OPENING STERILE PACKAGES

While the principles for opening different kinds of packages are similar, the actual technique used varies according to the unique features of each package style. If the package is enclosed in a plastic wrap, the plastic usually is torn open or pulled apart at a designated place. If a scissors must be used, exercise extreme care not to cut the inner package, which would result in contamination. The outer plastic bag may be folded back at the top edges and used as a container for disposing used supplies during the procedure being implemented. The inner package may either be envelope-wrapped or have heat-sealed edges.

Envelope Wrap

The following procedures are illustred in Figure 30–1. To open an *envelope-wrapped package,* first place the

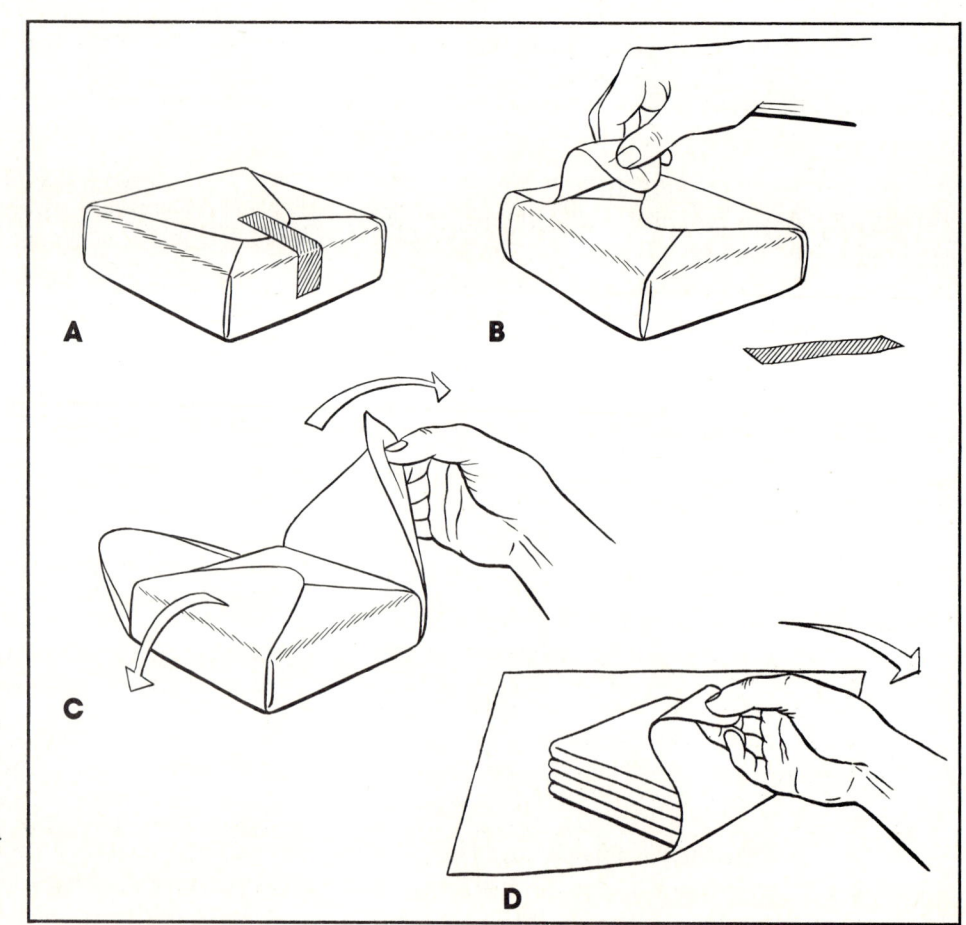

Figure 30–1. Opening an envelope-style wrapped sterile package. **A.** Place package with top flap facing self. Remove sterilizing indicator tape, if opening an institutionally sterilized package. **B.** Open flap farthest away from self, grasping outside of wrapper. Reach around, not over, the package. **C.** Open right flap (next visible flap) with right hand. Open left flap with left hand. **D.** Open last flap forward toward self.

package with the top flap pointing toward yourself (Fig. 30-1A). After checking and removing the sterilizing indicator tape, grasp the outer surface of the flap and unfold it away from yourself by reaching around rather than over the package (Fig. 30-1B). One at a time, grasp the two side flaps by the folded-back tips and unfold them completely (Fig. 30-1C). Last, grasp the folded-back tip of the flap directly in front of yourself (Fig. 30-1D), being careful to stand sufficiently far back from the sterile field so as not to contact and contaminate it with your clothing or uniform. If there are no folded-back tips, grasp the *outer* surface of the flap at least 1 inch from the corner. Do not reach across the sterile area, or handle the folded edges of the cuffed corner tips. This method avoids contamination if the wrap happens to reclose spontaneously, which sometimes happens with stiff, nonflexible paper wrappers.

After adding additional supplies or solution to an envelope-wrapped sterile package, the package may need to be reclosed temporarily, such as while carrying it to the client's room or during an unavoidable wait.

If you have unwrapped the package carefully and touched only the cuff tips, it is possible to reclose the package without contaminating the contents. Close the package in reverse sequence, beginning with the tip nearest yourself and avoiding reaching across the sterile field.

☐ SKILL SEQUENCE

OPENING ENVELOPE-WRAPPED STERILE PACKAGES

Step	Rationale
1. Wash hands thoroughly.	Decreases potential for cross-contamination from transient microorganisms.
2. Select proper package.	
3. Explain procedure to client.	Preserves client's right to know; promotes cooperation.
4. Place package on table or in center of work space with top wrapper corner facing self.	Facilitates opening package.
5. Examine sterilizing indicator tape for color or marking changes.	Color change or presence of dark lines or designs indicates sterility.
6. Remove tape and discard. Do not allow it to remain on wrapper.	Interferes with laundry processes.
7. Completely open top flap of package by grasping outside of flap and unfolding it away from your own body. Reach around, not across package.	Avoids contaminating inside of wrapper. Avoids reaching across sterile field.
8. Grasp topmost folded-back tip and completely unfold laterally. Repeat for other side. Do not touch inside of wrapper. If no folded-back tips are present, grasp outer surface of wrapper, rather than edge of tip.	Touching both sides of wrapper tip that has not been turned back contaminates inner surface of wrapper; this contaminates sterile contents or sterile field if wrapper is reclosed, either intentionally or inadvertently.
9. Stand at least 6 to 12 inches from package, completely unfold last flap toward self; grasp only folded-back tip or top surface of wrapper.	Avoids contamination of sterile field from uniform. Avoids contamination of inner surface of wrapper.
10. Complete procedure.	
11. Wash hands.	Removes any acquired transient bacteria.
12. Record results of procedure in client's record.	Documents nurse's accountability.

Heat-Sealed Packages

The following procedures are illustrated in Figure 30-2. To open a *heat-sealed package,* grasp the labeled unsealed flaps and pull them apart gently, firmly, and completely (Fig. 30-2A). Keep the inside of the wrapper sterile and do not touch it. When the package is completely opened, the area inside the heat-seal line is considered sterile. The sterile item may then be picked up with a gloved hand, forceps, or at the corners with an ungloved hand for a simple dressing. To open a sterile box with a heat-sealed top, grasp the labeled tab and remove the top completely. Remember to hold only the outside of the box, so as not to contaminate the contents (Fig. 30-2B).

Package contents also can be removed with a sterile forceps or a gloved hand while someone else holds the package partly open. To do this, the second person pulls the package flaps back far enough to expose the contents, and extends the package toward the person wearing the sterile gloves (Fig. 30-2C). Some styles of packages may need to have the package edges compressed, which causes the opening to separate. This makes it possible to grasp the contents with a forceps, or extend them toward a person wearing sterile gloves (Fig. 30-2D).

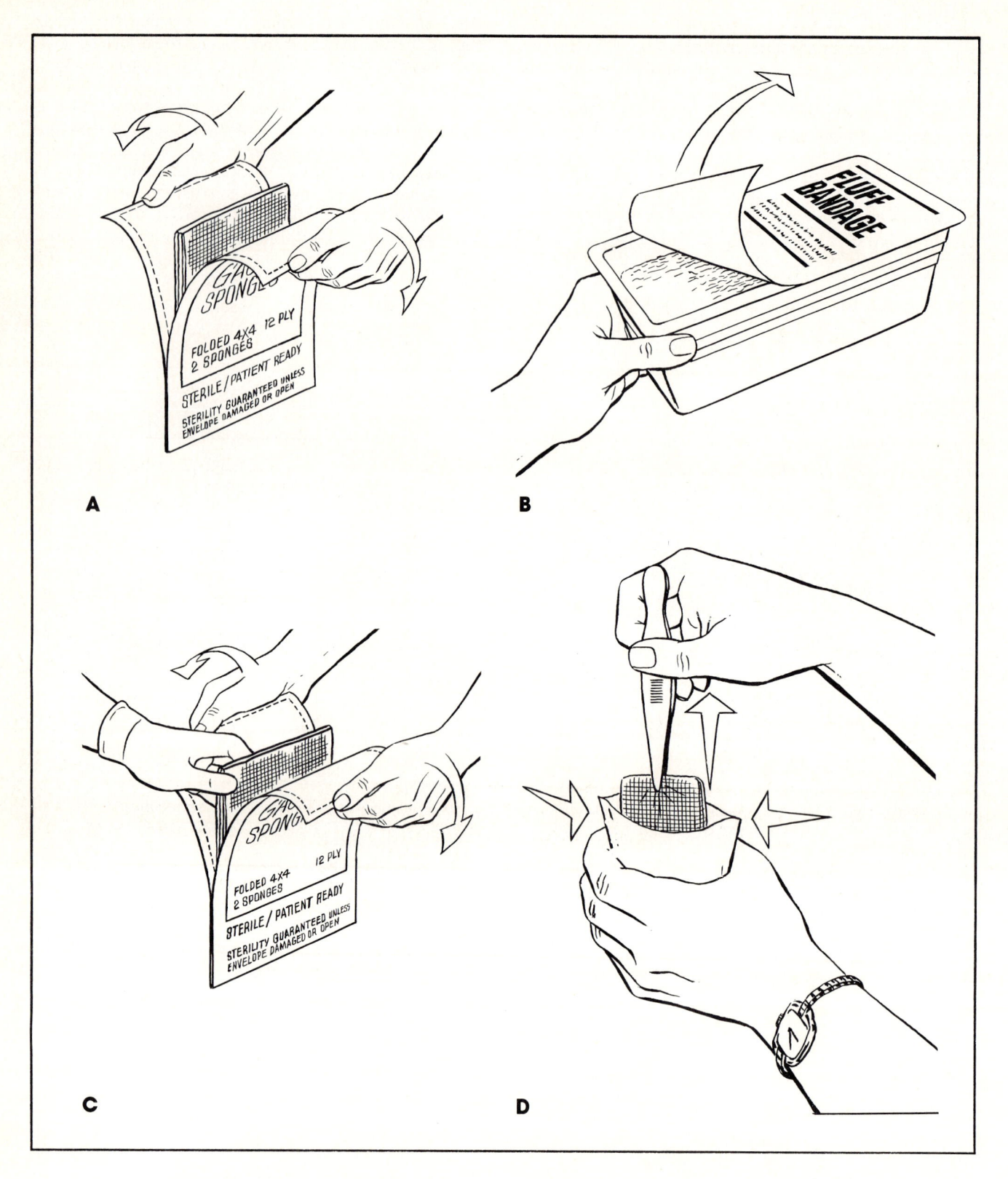

Figure 30–2. Opening heat-sealed sterile packages. **A.** Grasp the top flaps and pull apart. Area inside heat-seal line (indicated by dotted lines) is guaranteed sterile if opened properly.
B. Hold container securely. Grasp corner of the top marked "To Open—Peel Down" and peel off cover completely. If opened correctly, inside of container is guaranteed sterile.
C. Extending contents of a heat-sealed package to another person. **D.** Compress sides of package and remove contents with forceps.

☐ SKILL SEQUENCE

OPENING HEAT-SEALED STERILE PACKAGES

Step	Rationale
1. Wash hands thoroughly.	Decreases potential for cross-contamination from transient microorganisms.
2. Select appropriate package. Read contents and note intactness and indicators of sterility.	Helps determine whether choice is correct. Monitors safety of product used.
3. Explain procedure to client.	Preserves client's right to know; promotes cooperation.
4. Open package: a. Read directions. b. Grasp unsealed flaps or tabs as designated, and pull apart firmly and completely. c. Lay wrapper on work surface. Inside may be used as sterile field. Alternative: item may be added to another sterile field (Skill Sequences, "Adding Heat-sealed Items to a Sterile Field" and "Adding Envelope-wrapped Items to a Sterile Field," p. 281.).	Opening procedure varies with the manufacturer and type and size of package. Complete opening helps wrapper lie flat. Area within heat-seal line is considered sterile.

PREPARING STERILE FIELDS

A *sterile field* is a sterile area of any size that contains or will contain sterile items. A sterile field may be created at the anatomic site where the procedure is being done, such as an incision, laceration, or catheter insertion. This *sterile work* area or *field* keeps sterile equipment and gloves from becoming contaminated during the procedure. A sterile field also may be created to serve as a *sterile supply field*, providing a sterile area on which to place instruments, dressings, and other supplies before and during the procedure. Depending on the specific procedure, one or both of these types of sterile fields may be needed. For example, only a sterile supply field is required to change most dressings or remove sutures, while both a sterile supply field and a sterile work field are required to insert a urinary catheter. In the latter instance, the sterile work field would be around the urethral meatus.

The inside surface of a sterile package wrap often is used to provide a sterile field. A sterile field may also be created or enlarged by the use of *drapes,* which are made of fabric or disposable flexible paper. Drapes may be of any size, usually are rectangular or square, and may be arranged in any way that provides the best protection from contamination for the equipment to be used in any given procedure.

Large drapes are used in the operating room to provide a sterile operative work area; smaller drapes are used for procedures such as a spinal tap, bone marrow aspiration, or application of large dressings. Drapes may be specially designed for a given purpose, such as a drape with an oval or octagonal opening designed to fit over the perineum during urinary catheterization. Drapes with an opening in them are known as *fenestrated* drapes.

In the operating room and for any procedure involving blood or water, the drape must be moisture-resistant and thus provide a barrier to microorganisms. *Barrier drapes* may be made of chemically treated tightly woven cotton cloth or of a nonwoven disposable synthetic fiber. Muslin is not an effective barrier, as it does not retard moisture passage effectively. Perkins cites a study demonstrating that when sterile cloth becomes damp (even with sterile water), contamination of the exposed sterile surface occurs if the fabric is lying on an unsterile surface or is in contact with an unsterile item. Another study indicated that bacteria pass readily through two layers of wet cloth, but not through dry cloth (Perkins, 1969).

☐ SKILL SEQUENCE

PREPARING A STERILE FIELD

Step	Rationale
1. Wash hands thoroughly.	Decreases potential for cross-contamination from transient microorganisms.
2. Select appropriate size and type of packaged drapes.	Facilitates adequate draping.
3. Explain procedure to client.	Preserves client's right to know; increases self-care knowledge.
4. Open package, following Skill Sequence, "Opening Envelope-wrapped Sterile Packages," steps 4 to 9, p. 277.	Continues preparation for procedure.

(continued)

PREPARING A STERILE FIELD (Cont.)

Step	Rationale
5. Pick up a corner of drape with one hand. (If not wearing sterile gloves, touch only folded-back tip or outer surfaces of drape.)	Outside and outer 1 inch are considered unsterile.
6. Allow to open freely; do not shake vigorously. Grasp a parallel corner of drape with other hand to help open drape. (Stiff paper drapes may need gentle shaking or unfolding.)	Shaking drapes sets up air currents that cause microorganism transfer.
7. Hold drape within own visual field and away from clothing. Gently place drape in desired location. If one side of drape is plasticized, that surface should be placed on tabletop or bed, with fabric or paper side upward.	Avoids contamination. Fabric or paper surface absorbs small amounts of moisture while plasticized coating prevents contamination.
8. Place sterile supplies on sterile field as needed for procedure.	Provides sterile work area; maintains sterility of supplies.

Adding Sterile Items to a Sterile Field

The following procedures are illustrated in Figure 30–3. If a sterile item in a heat-sealed package is to be added to an existing sterile field, first pull the package partly open while holding it away from the sterile field. Then hold the package upside down over the sterile field, pull it apart completely and allow the item to drop on the sterile field from a height of about 15cm (6 in) (Fig. 30–3A). This is done from the side of the sterile field that provides the most ready access and the least reaching across the field. If the item drops less than 1 inch from the edge, it is considered contaminated and must be removed by grasping only the part of the item extending into the 1-inch area.

Small, lightweight envelope-wrapped items such as dressings, bowls, or instruments often are added to an existing sterile field or handed to someone wearing sterile gloves. These items can be held in one hand and opened with the other hand (Fig. 30–3B). To transfer these items to the sterile field or another person, grasp all the corners or edges of the wrap in one hand and hold them out of the way (usually back around the wrist) with the holding hand completely covered by the wrap (Fig. 30–3C). This action avoids contamination of the field or the other person's sterile garb from uncontrolled wrapper edges.

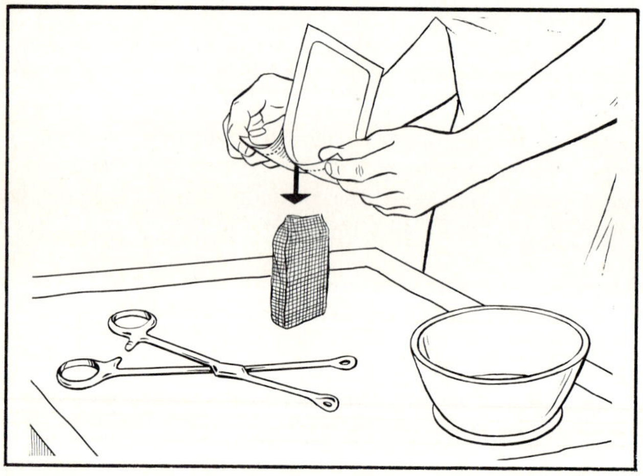

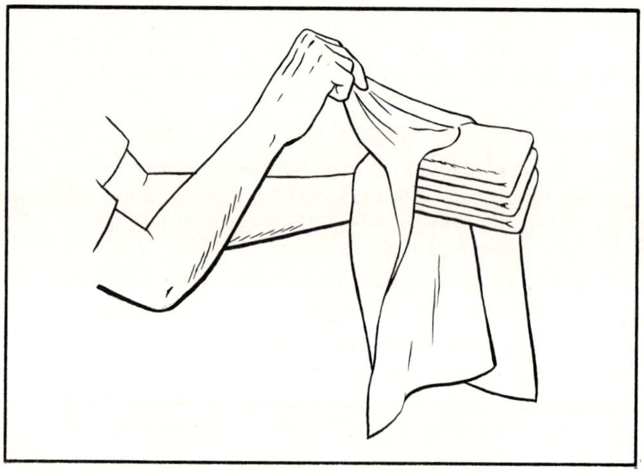

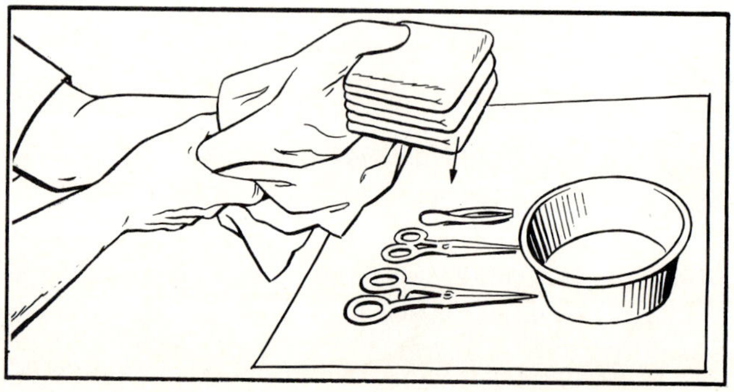

Figure 30–3. Adding sterile items to a sterile field. **A.** Heat-sealed packages: Pull package apart and allow contents to drop on near side of sterile field. Note transfer forceps with its serrated ring tips. **B.** Envelope wrap: Hold package in hand to unwrap. **C.** Gather ends of wrapper securely around wrist. Deposit contents on near side of sterile field or offer to another person wearing sterile gloves.

SKILL SEQUENCES

ADDING HEAT-SEALED ITEMS TO A STERILE FIELD

Step	Rationale
1. Prepare a sterile field, as in Skill Sequences, "Preparing a Sterile Field," pp. 279–280, or "Opening Envelope-wrapped Sterile Packages," p. 277.	Initial preparation for procedure.
2. Select appropriate package and inspect for intactness and sterility; read directions for opening.	Ensures use of correct and safe equipment.
3. Standing back from sterile field, grasp unsealed flaps and pull partially open. Completely remove pull-tab tops.	Decreases probability of microorganisms falling by gravity onto sterile field.
4. Reach over near side of sterile field, pull flaps completely apart, invert the package, and allow it to drop on sterile field from a height of about 15 cm (6 in), and more than 1 inch from edge of field. Remove hands from above field. OR: a. Extend partially opened package toward another worker who is wearing sterile gloves or holding a sterile forceps. b. Hold package edges firmly while other worker removes sterile item.	An item dropped closer than 1 inch from edge is considered contaminated and must be removed. Appropriate method for assisting another worker in a sterile procedure.
5. Dispose of wrapper, following agency policy.	Cloth wrappers are laundered and resterilized. Some paper wrappers are reusable.

ADDING ENVELOPE-WRAPPED ITEMS TO A STERILE FIELD

Step	Rationale
1. Prepare a sterile field, as in Skill Sequence, "Preparing a Sterile Field," pp. 279–280, or "Opening Envelope-wrapped Sterile Packages," p. 277.	Initial preparation for procedure.
2. Select appropriate package and inspect for intactness and sterility; read directions for opening.	Continues preparation for procedure.
3. Hold item on palm of nondominant hand or between thumb and fingers; grasp folded-back tip and unfold flap farthest from self, allowing it to drop freely. If wrap is of stiff paper, bend downward and backward.	Avoids reaching across partially opened package.
4. Unfold side flaps as in step 3.	Continues exposing sterile item.
5. Unfold flap nearest self. Grasp all corners of wrap with dominant hand, bring back toward wrist, covering hand and wrist.	Contains all edges of wrapper to avoid contamination.
6. Hold edges of wrapper firmly in dominant hand and drop sterile item directly onto sterile field from a height of about 10 cm (4 in), and more than 1 inch from edge of field. OR: Hold edges of wrapper firmly around wrist as in step 6 and extend opened sterile package toward another worker who is wearing sterile gloves or holding a sterile forceps.	Avoids contamination of sterile field. Items falling less than 1 inch from the edge are considered contaminated and must be removed. Appropriate method for assisting another worker in a sterile procedure.
7. Dispose of wrapper, following agency policy.	Cloth wrappers are laundered and resterilized. Some paper wrappers are reusable.

Pouring Sterile Solutions

Frequently it is necessary to add sterile water, antiseptics, or cleansing solutions to a dressing tray, to a diagnostic tray for a procedure such as a spinal tap, or to a sterile field for an operative procedure. Prepackaged special-use trays or sets often include premeasured amounts of solutions contained in plastic or foil packets and therefore it is not necessary to pour solutions from larger containers. Because of cost factors and increasing ecologic and environmental concerns about disposing of single-use items, not all agencies will use these kinds of trays. It is important, therefore, to know how to pour sterile liquids within a sterile field without contaminating that field.

Sterile liquids are most frequently poured from a larger stock or multiple-use container into a smaller basin, cup, or pan already placed on a sterile field. When opening and reclosing the bottle, touch only the outside of the bottle cap and either hold it between thumb and fingers or place it on a table with the top side down. The outside of the cap and bottle are considered clean but contaminated, and the insides of both are considered sterile. Always turn the bottle label away from the direction the fluid is being poured, as wet or stained labels are difficult to read (see Fig. 30–4).

Place sterile receiving containers near the edge of the sterile field for minimal reaching across the sterile field. Trays often are prepared with this action in mind, or you may use a forceps or reach under the sterile wrap to adjust the location of the receiving container. Some sources recommend pouring a small amount of solution into a sink or wastebasket to cleanse the bottle lip before pouring into the sterile receiving container. Hold large bottles 10 to 15 cm (4 to 6 in) above the receiving container and pour the liquid steadily, without splashing. Smaller bottles may be held lower, but at no time should the bottle touch the receiving container, as this would result in contamination from the outside of the bottle. When the desired amount of liquid has been poured, turn the bottle upright quickly and remove it from above the sterile field to avoid dripping on the field. Replace the bottle cap carefully, touching only the outside surface. Sterile solutions are considered sterile for 24 hours if the cap reseals the bottle. To avoid inadvertent use of outdated solutions, write the date and time on a reusable bottle after pouring from it. Place the bottle on the bedside table or in the client's supply area. Wipe stock bottles of solution with a germicidal solution and return them to the stock supply area.

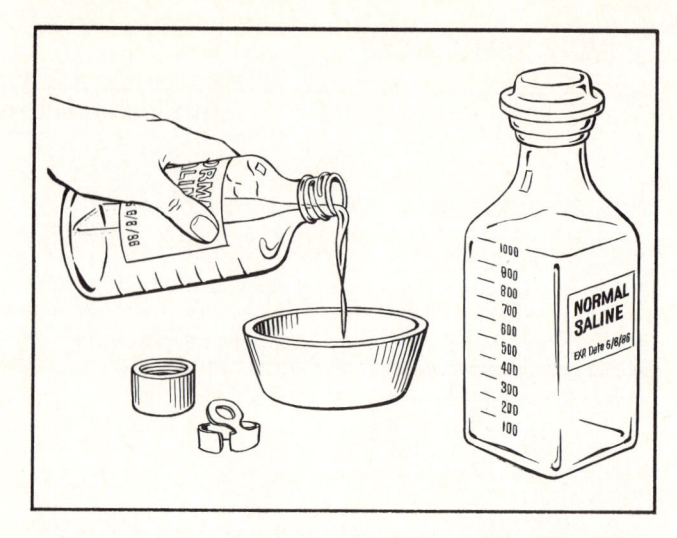

Figure 30–4. Pouring sterile solutions. Read label; Remove seal and cap. Place cap upright on table (or hold between thumb and fingers). With label facing palm and bottle 10 to 15 cm (4 to 6 in) above pan, pour steadily, without splashing.

☐ SKILL SEQUENCE

POURING STERILE SOLUTIONS

Step	Rationale
1. Prepare a sterile field, as in Skill Sequence, "Preparing a Sterile Field," pp. 279–280.	Initial preparation for procedure.
2. Read contents label on bottle.	Avoids errors in usage.
3. Check expiration date.	Outdated solutions are considered unsafe and unsterile.
4. Inspect intactness of external bottle seal. If unsealed with no opening date noted, discard.	If reclosed properly, sterile solutions for external use are considered sterile for no more than 24 hours after opening.
5. Remove bottle seal by lifting tab, breaking plastic ring, or as directed, and remove cap by unscrewing or lifting off. Listen for sound of vacuum or seal being broken.	Airtight seal holds slight vacuum within unopened bottle.
6. Place bottle cap on table, with top of cap lying on table, open side up. Do not touch bottle rim, edges, or inside of cap.	The bottle rim and inside of cap and bottle are considered sterile, and outsides, clean, but contaminated.
7. Hold bottle firmly with label away from pouring direction and under palm of hand.	Protects label from drips. Stained wet labels are difficult to read clearly and safely.
8. Have sterile receiving container at one side of sterile field. Move container with forceps, sterile gloved hand, or by reaching under and relocating container.	Avoids reaching across sterile field with a nonsterile bottle exterior; avoids dripping on sterile field.
9. Pour solution into receiving container in a slow, steady stream from about 15 cm (10 in) above container (less for smaller bottles). Avoid splashing or touching receiving container rim with bottle neck.	Splashing or dripping causes wet areas in sterile field, with resulting contamination from nonsterile surface underneath sterile area. Bottle neck is considered unsterile and contaminated.
10. Replace cap securely, touching only outsides of cap and bottle.	Preserves sterility of contents.
11. If solution is to be used again, write date, time, and your initials on label.	Provides information for next user regarding sterility of contents. Sterile solutions are considered sterile for 24 hours if cap reseals bottle.

12. Dispose of bottle properly.
   a. If empty, discard in appropriate place.
   b. If for single-client use, place on bedside table or cupboard.
   c. If stock bottle, wipe with disinfectant and return to storage area.
	Assumes responsibility for safe care of supplies.
	
	Decreases changes of cross-contamination.

13. Wash hands.	Prevents cross-contamination.
14. Record procedure and results in client's record.	Provides documentation of care for other professionals and is a legal record of nursing interventions.

RECORDING

When using sterile supplies for a client-care procedure, the nurse is responsible for recording the results of that procedure in the appropriate places in the client's health record. Depending on agency policy, the nurse may need to fill out charge slips for the items used, enter the requisition into the computer, or record the number and kind of items on a unit supply record. This provides a mechanism for charging the client for the supplies used and for resupplying the unit stock of sterile items.

☐ CRITICAL POINTS SUMMARY

1. Sterility is an absolute concept; there is no "almost sterile."
2. Identify actual and potential sources of contamination during use of sterile supplies.
3. Wash hands before and after using sterile supplies.
4. Select the correct package.
5. Identify the nature and purpose of the supplies being used.
6. Inspect the package for identification, dryness, intactness, indicators of sterility, and expiration date.
7. Open the package correctly, following envelope-wrap procedures or manufacturer's directions.
8. Create a sterile field with a package wrapper or sterile drape.
9. Place sterile items more than 1 inch from the edge of a sterile field.
10. Pour solutions without splashing the sterile field or soiling the bottle label.
11. Avoid reaching across a sterile field.
12. Avoid contamination by not touching rims of containers and inner sides of wrappers.
13. Discard single-use items in appropriate trash containers.
14. Return reusable items to central supply without cleaning, using a plastic bag for infectious articles.
15. Remove sterilizing indicator tape before placing reusable wrappers in the laundry.
16. Complete necessary forms or procedures for charging and reordering supplies.
17. Record results of procedure.

☐ LEARNING ACTIVITIES

1. Tour a central service area in a hospital or large clinic setting. Observe the following and discuss your findings with your peers:
   a. Different kinds of sterilizers
   b. Items being sterilized by different methods
   c. Various receiving areas for soiled, clean, and contaminated or infectious items
   d. Clothing and personal hygiene practices of the workers in sterilizing areas
   e. Kinds of packaging materials and package styles available
   f. Storage areas for sterile supplies
2. Examine a sterile supply storage area in a central service or clinical area. Observe the following and compare your findings with your peers:
   a. Types of institutional and commercial packages available
   b. Storage cabinet or shelves (location, dust and vermin protection)
   c. Temperature and humidity of storage area
3. Examine several institutionally and commercially prepared sterile items. Observe the following:
   a. Package label and contents
   b. Sterilizing indicators or sterility labels
   c. Expiration date
4. Observe a surgical procedure in the operating room (through an observation dome or window) and a sterile diagnostic or therapeutic procedure in a clinical area. Discuss with faculty or peers:
   a. Your comparison of the use of sterile technique in these two areas
   b. The ways the integrity of the sterile field is maintained
   c. How contamination was prevented if some items were sterile and others were nonsterile
   d. Your identification of any breaks in sterile technique
   e. A description of concern for and involvement of the client in the procedure
5. Using correct technique, complete these actions:
   a. Open an envelope-wrapped sterile drape
   b. Add an envelope-wrapped sterile basin to the sterile field
   c. Pour sterile normal saline into the sterile basin. Plan to reuse the normal saline in the next activity, and label it accordingly
   d. Drop a sterile 4 × 4 gauze dressing into the basin of sterile normal saline
   e. Add a sterile forceps to the sterile field, placing it in such a way that it can be used with ungloved hands
6. Repeat the activities in 5 above. Have a peer or a faculty member monitor your technique, using the Skill Sequences, pp. 277, 279–281, as guides and the Performance Checklist, p. 284, for evaluation.

☐ REVIEW QUESTIONS

1. Define sterility in your own words.
2. What are the differences between clean, surgically clean, sterile, and contaminated articles?
3. Which method of sterilization and what kinds of wrappers or containers would be most appropriate for:
   a. Fiberoptic bronchoscopes
   b. Petroleum jelly
   c. Stainless steel instruments

d. Cloth or paper items, such as drapes, bandages, or cotton balls
e. Normal saline
4. Which method of sterilization is used most frequently and for what reasons?
5. In addition to the active sterilizing agent, what two other factors play a significant role in achieving sterilization?
6. What four things are to be examined before using any packaged sterile item?
7. What is the best method of detecting breaks in sterile technique?
8. When working with a sterile field, what is the rationale for these practices?
   a. Avoiding reaching across a sterile field.
   b. Regarding sterile field with no waterproof barrier underneath it as being contaminated when it becomes wet.
   c. Placing sterile items within the heat-seal line of a commercially wrapped package and more than 1 inch from the edge of a sterile field.
9. How would you add a basin of sterile saline to an existing sterile field?
10. When carrying out a sterile procedure, what subjective and objective data do you need to gather:
    a. From the client
    b. About the client, the equipment, and the procedure
11. What data might you need to determine whether a procedure would be implemented most safely by using a sterile field for a sterile work area, a sterile supply area, or both?

☐ PERFORMANCE CHECKLIST

OBJECTIVE: To use aseptic technique to open envelope-wrapped and heat-sealed items; prepare a sterile field; add envelope-wrapped and heat-sealed items; and pour sterile solutions.

CHARACTERISTIC	RANGE OF ACCEPTABILITY	SATISFACTORY	UNSATISFACTORY
1. Washes hands.	No deviation		
2. Selects correct sterile package for purpose intended.	No deviation		
3. Explains procedure to client.	No deviation		
4. Inspects package for: • dryness • intactness • indicators of sterility • expiration date	No deviation		
5. Removes all sterilizing indicator tapes.	No deviation		
6. Opens package correctly, without contamination and without reaching across the sterile field.	No deviation		
7. Prepares sterile field without contamination: a. envelope-wrap b. heat-sealed package c. sterile drape	No deviation		
8. Adds sterile items to a sterile field without contaminating the field.	No deviation		
9. Pours sterile liquid into a sterile container without contaminating the field.	No deviation		
10. Writes date, time, and initials on label of reusable bottles of sterile liquids.	No deviation		
11. Uses sterile forceps to transfer a sterile item from one sterile area to another.	Sterile items may be transferred with a sterile gloved hand.		
12. Disposes of used equipment properly: a. Discards single-use items. b. Places reusable items in collecting area. c. Places reusable wrappers in laundry.	No deviation		
13. Washes hands.	No deviation		
14. Records procedure.	No deviation		
15. Reorders or charges for supplies, according to agency policy.	No deviation		

REFERENCES

American Hospital Association: Infection Control in the Hospital, ed 4. Chicago, American Hospital Association, 1979.

Berry EC, Kohn ML: Introduction to Operating Room Technique, ed 4. New York, McGraw-Hill, 1974.

Gruendemann BJ, Meeker MH: Alexander's Care of the Patient in Surgery, ed 7. St Louis, CV Mosby, 1983.

LeMaitre GD, Finnegan JA: The Patient in Surgery, ed 4. Philadelphia, WB Saunders, 1980.

MacClelland DC: Sterilizing by ionizing radiation. AORN Journal 26(4):675-684, 1977.

Mallison GF: Areas of Special Concern: Section F. Central Service. In Bennet JV, Brachman PS (eds): Hospital Infections. Boston, Little, Brown, 1979(a).

Mallison GF: The Inanimate Environment. In Bennett JV, Brachman PS (eds): Hospital Infections. Boston, Little, Brown, 1979(b).

Mallison GF, Standard PG: Safe storage times for sterile packs. Hospitals 48(20):77-78, 80, 1974.

Perkins JJ: Principles and Methods of Sterilization in Health Sciences, ed 2. Springfield, IL, Charles C Thomas, 1969.

Ryan P: Inhospital packaging rationale. AORN Journal 23(6):980-988, 1976.

Sorensen KC, Luckmann J: Basic Nursing: A Psychophysiologic Approach. Philadelphia, WB Saunders, 1979.

Todd DK (ed): The Water Encyclopedia: A Compendium of Useful Information on Water Resources. Port Washington, NY, Water Information Center, 1970.

Wilson ME, Mizer HE, et al.: Microbiology in Patient Care, ed 3. New York, Macmillan, 1979.

Wolff L, Weitzel MH, et al.: Fundamentals of Nursing, ed 6. Philadelphia, JB Lippincott, 1979.

BIBLIOGRAPHY

AORN proposed standards for in hospital sterilization. AORN Journal 29(6):1154-1172, 1979.

Beck WC (guest ed): Abridged sterility: A level of disinfection. AORN Journal 26(2):242, 244, 1977.

Beck WC: Alcohol foam for hand disinfection. AORN Journal 32(6): 1087-1088, 1980.

Brooks SM: Fundamentals of Operating Room Nursing. St Louis, MO, CV Mosby, 1975.

Dixon RE, Brachman PS, Bennett JV (eds): Isolation Techniques for Use in Hospitals, ed 2. US Dept of Health and Human Services publication No. (CDC) 76-8314, Atlanta, Centers for Disease Control, 1975.

DuGas BW: Introduction to Patient Care, ed 3. Philadelphia, WB Saunders, 1977.

Eitzen HE, Ritter MA, et al.: A microbiological in-use comparison of surgical hand-washing agents. Journal of Bone and Joint Surgery 61(A):403-406, 1979.

Ginsberg F: A Manual of Operating Room Technology. Philadelphia, JB Lippincott, 1966.

Gravens DL, Butcher HR, et al.: Septisol antiseptic foam for hands of operating room personnel: An effective antibacterial agent. Surgery 73(3):360-367, 1973.

Gruendemann BJ, Casterton SB, et al.: The Surgical Patient: Behavioral Concepts for the Operating Room Nurse, ed 2. St Louis, CV Mosby, 1977.

Huth ME: Principles of asepsis. AORN Journal 24(2): 790-796, 1976.

Luckmann J, Sorensen KC: Medical-Surgical Nursing: A Psychophysiologic Approach, ed 2. Philadelphia, WB Saunders, 1980.

McLeod DK: Precautions for use of ethylene oxide. AORN Journal 29(2):340-343, 1979.

Miller BF, Keane CB: Encyclopedia and Dictionary of Medicine, Nursing and Allied Health, ed 3. Philadelphia, WB Saunders, 1983.

Ritter MA, French ML, et al.: The antimicrobial effectiveness of operative-site preparative agents: A microbial and clinical study. Journal of Bone and Joint Surgery (AM) 62(5):826-828, 1980.

Rook A: Textbook of Dermatology, ed 3. London, Blackwell Scientific Publications, 1979, vols 1, 2.

Sherman RE: The challenge of barrier testing. AORN Journal 31(2):213-220, 1980.

Standards for inhospital packaging material. AORN Journal 23(6):978-979, 1976.

AUDIOVISUAL RESOURCES

Disinfection: Health Care Principles, Parts I and II
Film. (1973, 15 min. each part)
Available through:
3M Medical Products Division
Dept. ME81, Box 33600
3M Center
St. Paul, MN 55144

Fundamentals of Aseptic Technique
Video. (1976, 22 min., Davis and Geck in cooperation with AAORN)
Available through:
Davis and Geck
American Cyanamid Company
1 Casper Street
Danbury, CT 06810

Infection Control: Disinfection, Sterilization and Asepsis
Filmstrip, slides, cartridge, videotape. (1982, Color, 20 min.)
Available through:
Medcom, Inc.
P.O. Box 116
Garden Grove, CA 92642

SKILL 31 Donning Sterile Gloves

PREREQUISITE SKILLS

Skill 19, "Inspection"
Skill 28, "Handwashing"
Skill 30, "Sterile Supplies"

☐ STUDENT OBJECTIVES

1. Explain the purposes of using sterile gloves.
2. Cite specific situations where sterile gloves are needed.
3. Relate specific principles of aseptic technique to sterile glove use.
4. Don a pair of sterile gloves, using correct aseptic technique.
5. Remove contaminated sterile gloves, avoiding contamination of surroundings.

☐ INTRODUCTION

Sterile gloves are presterilized rubber latex gloves that are worn during sterile procedures to protect the client and sterile equipment from microbial contamination on the nurse's hands.

Sterile gloves are used to handle sterile items when it is not feasible to manipulate them with sterile forceps because of the size or the nature of the equipment or the task. Sterile gloves are worn to avoid introducing microorganisms into the client's body during diagnostic, therapeutic, or surgical procedures, such as urinary catheterization, wound care and dressing applications, and in the operating and delivery room areas. In short, sterile gloves are worn whenever there is a need or desire to decrease the chances of microorganism transfer, bacterial contamination, and possible development of infection.

Donning sterile gloves is perhaps the most common aseptic technique performed by nurses. Correct use of sterile gloves forms the basis for aseptic handling of other sterile items. If the gloves become torn, punctured, or contaminated, everything the nurse handles is automatically regarded as contaminated.

☐ PREPARATION

Since it is impossible to sterilize the skin, sterile gloves serve as a barrier between microorganisms on the worker's hands and the sterile equipment being used. When gloves become punctured or torn, the possibility of contamination from resident and transient hand bacteria always exists. Theoretically, it is estimated that in a 20-minute time period, as many as 40,000 microorganisms can pass through a single glove puncture made by a #18 needle (Perkins, 1969). To decrease this potential for contamination, the hands should always be washed, scrubbed, or massaged with antiseptic foam prior to donning sterile gloves, as this removes transient bacteria and reduces the number of resident bacteria. As soon as sterile gloves are donned, however, the diminished resident bacteria replenish themselves rapidly, since they thrive in the moist, warm environment inside a sterile glove. For this reason, the hands should be washed or scrubbed *after* wearing sterile gloves as well as prior to donning them.

In some sterile procedures, the nurse may use one gloved hand as sterile and the other nonsterile. For example, when doing a urinary catheterization, the hand that is used to separate the labia or position the penis becomes contaminated, and only the other uncontaminated hand may be used to handle the sterile equipment. Some dressing procedures and wound or catheter irrigations require using sterile equipment while handling a nonsterile tube or catch basin for returned irrigating fluid. In these situations, the nurse must plan ahead and think through the procedure to determine how to do the procedure without getting partially finished and finding that a crucial piece of equipment is unopened or not ready for one-handed use. In some instances, the nurse may choose to wear only one sterile glove, as this may make it easier to remember which hand is sterile and which is nonsterile.

As with any sterile procedure, the nurse's keen observation and alertness are the keys to maintaining glove sterility. The only way to ensure sterility and prevent contamination is to pay careful attention to how the gloves are put on and to what is touched with the gloved hand or hands. Whenever sterility is questioned by oneself or others, the gloves must be changed promptly. It is false economy to use a contaminated glove to avoid using additional supplies.

DATA BASE

The choice of when to use sterile gloves generally is left to the nurse's discretion, as it usually is a nursing judgment to determine when and how to implement aseptic technique. To make this judgment, the nurse considers the equipment being used, the procedure itself, the area of the client's body involved, and the client's diagnosis. For example, complex procedures using a number of sterile items are much simpler when using gloves than when using forceps, while a simple wound dressing can be done with forceps. Gloves are needed when applying sterile bandages or dressings on hard-to-dress areas, such as the head and the extremities, or when wound dressings are bulky and need to be held in place with the hand prior to fastening. When a client's resistance is lowered, such as with immunosuppression, aseptic technique may be used for a procedure usually performed with clean technique.

Client History and Recorded Data

The body part involved in a procedure may require the nurse to use sterile gloves, such as with sterile body organs (bladder catheterization) and open wounds. Some clients have a greater need for protection against invading microorganisms. For example, meticulous aseptic technique is crucial for the immunosuppressed client who has the potential for developing an infection from microorganisms that are not pathogenic to the average person.

Physical Appraisal Skills

Inspection. Before using sterile gloves, the nurse *inspects* the glove package for the correct size, intactness, sterility indicators, and expiration date. If the package design is unfamiliar, the opening directions will be helpful.

EQUIPMENT

Sterile gloves are made of thin rubber latex and may be either single-use disposable or reusable. Many institutions have begun to use only prepackaged sterile disposable gloves, but some continue to reprocess reusable gloves.

Sterile gloves are made differently for various purposes. Surgical gloves are sturdy but thin, close-fitting, shaped to fit the right or left hand, sized according to hand sizes, and long enough to extend well up over the wrist. They are packaged singly or in pairs and are used for operative, diagnostic, or therapeutic purposes. Some prepackaged special-use sets, such as dressing trays, urinary catheterization sets, or tracheostomy suction packages, contain one or two sterile gloves. These gloves are shorter, loose-fitting, and fit either hand.

A lubricant is needed to don sterile gloves, especially the fitted surgical gloves. Some gloves have a silicone film that helps eliminate stickiness and increases the ease of donning these gloves. Cream or liquid lubricants are sometimes used; some contain antiseptic or bacteriostatic agents that help reduce bacterial growth on the hands. For many years, powder has been a common glove lubricant. There is some evidence that the use of powder should be discontinued. Perkins (1969) indicates that powder fallout from hands and gloves serves as a vector for microorganism dissemination. The irritant nature of powder can cause postoperative powder granulomata if the powder is not washed off thoroughly before surgery. If powder is used, it should be applied sparingly, preferably before sterilization of the gloves, and residual powder washed off with sterile water prior to using the gloves (Gruendemann and Meeker, 1983).

Presterilized surgical gloves are double-wrapped with an inner paper folder and an outer heat-sealed paper wrapper. In storage areas, sterile glove packages must be protected from excessive natural or artificial light and heat.

When reusable gloves are used, they are washed with cold water before removing them, soaked in cold water (avoiding excess soaking as that causes stickiness), and returned to central supply. Prior to reprocessing, gloves must be machine-washed, tested for leaks, dried, sorted according to size and pairs, powdered, packaged, and finally resterilized.

A major problem with sterilizing reusable gloves is that it is difficult to remove all the air from glove fingers for effective sterilization with steam under pressure, which requires a vacuum. This factor, plus the labor required to prepare them for resterilization, has prompted many institutions to use presterilized single-use sterile gloves.

Hazards. Problems with sterile gloves include accidental contamination during use and excessive reliance on the sterile glove to provide a barrier for bacteria. Health-care workers often ignore the need for handwashing before or after donning sterile gloves, resulting in increased transient and resident bacterial growth on their hands from the warm, moist glove environment. Glove tears or punctures then produce contamination of an aseptic procedure. Long fingernails and rings contribute to the frequency of glove punctures and must be avoided.

☐ EXECUTION

When using sterile gloves to carry out an aseptic procedure, it is important to explain to the client the reason for wearing sterile gloves. Sometimes clients perceive that the use of sterile gloves indicates the nurse's unwillingness to touch them, especially if they have draining wounds, foul-smelling dressings, or disfiguring surgeries. Brief, simple explanations of the need for prevention of infection or protection from bacteria help allay these fears and increase the client's self-care knowledge.

Before opening the correct size sterile glove package, assemble and prepare all other sterile equipment needed for the procedure. Open packages and place them in a clean, appropriate work or client area, as described in Skill 30. Again, plan ahead so that you do not have sterile gloves on, and halfway through the procedure discover a needed item that is unopened. If that does happen, have someone else open the package or break aseptic technique, remove the gloves, open the needed package, and put on fresh sterile gloves.

To open a package of sterile gloves, pull the outer glove wrapper apart by the unsealed flaps and then

288 PROFESSIONAL CLINICAL NURSING SKILLS

discard it or use it as a small sterile field. Find a cleared, clean, flat surface where the inner glove wrapper can be unfolded without being disturbed or contaminating the other sterile items already prepared. The over-bed table, client's bed, or a nearby table or counter may be used for this purpose.

Gloves are packaged in the inner wrapper with the palms upward and thumbs turned laterally. It is easier for the nurse to glove the dominant hand first; that is, a right-handed nurse finds it easiest to put on the right glove first. The gloves and cuffs are adjusted *after* both gloves are donned, being careful not to touch the arms. After the gloves are on the hands, the inner glove wrapper may be left where it is so the nurse can deposit the used gloves on it.

The method of opening inner glove wrappers varies somewhat with the brand of glove. When opening this wrapper, it is crucial to avoid touching the *folded* edge of the turned-back center cuffs. The paper is very stiff and has a strong tendency to return to its original position if not sufficiently back-folded. If you have touched the folded-back edges and one glove remains in the wrapper, contamination will occur if the wrapper springs back to its original position before the next glove is removed. Donning sterile gloves is illustrated in Figure 31–1.

☐ SKILL SEQUENCE

DONNING STERILE GLOVES

Step	Rationale
1. Explain procedure and purpose to client.	Increases client's cooperation and self-care knowledge.
2. Wash hands thoroughly.	Removes transient bacteria and some resident bacteria. Decreases the potential for unknowingly introducing microorganisms into the sterile field if the glove develops a tear or hole.
3. Select glove package of an appropriate size.	Well-fitting gloves are easier to work with.
4. Inspect package for intactness, indicators of sterility, single glove versus a pair of gloves.	Ensures use of correct, safe item.
5. Open outer wrapper according to directions and discard, or use as a small sterile field. (If adding sterile gloves to a sterile field, see Skill 30, Skill Sequence, "Adding Envelope-wrapped Items to a Sterile Field," steps 3 to 4, p. 281).	Continues preparation for procedure.
6. Place inner wrapper on flat, clean surface in convenient location, with labeled cuff edges toward worker.	Provides for convenience and safe donning of gloves.

7. Open inner package completely:
  a. Touching only the outer corners, unfold top cuffed edge of wrapper. Fold slightly backward to unfold the crease.
  b. Unfold lower cuffed edge in the same manner as in previous step.
  c. Grasp <u>single edges</u> of vertical cuffs and completely unfold the remainder of the wrapper. Fold cuffs slightly backward to unfold crease. <u>Do not touch the folded edge of vertical cuffs.</u>
	Avoids reaching across sterile field.
	Folded paper tends to spring back into place.
	
	If folded edge has been touched, and paper wrapper springs back to original position, folded edge contaminates the second glove as it is removed.

8. Touch only the folded-back glove cuff and pick up glove for dominant hand with nondominant hand.	Folded-back cuff will touch hand and is considered nonsterile.
9. Lift glove up and away from wrapper. Stand clear of other objects or people.	Avoids contamination from touching nonsterile items. Avoids working over a sterile field.
10. With glove at or above waist level and own thumb turned toward glove thumb, slide hand downward toward floor and into glove. Pull gently and firmly, inserting thumb and fingers into appropriate openings. If fingers are in wrong openings, do not adjust at this time.	Gravity helps glove fingers open. Anything below the waist is considered nonsterile. Two fingers may enter the same glove finger. This can be adjusted when both gloves are on the hands.
11. Pick up second glove by inserting gloved fingers <u>under</u> turned-back cuff.	Avoids contamination of gloved fingers, since sterile gloved hand is in contact with the part of the glove that is to remain sterile.
12. Hyperextend thumb of gloved hand or fold it tightly across palm.	Protects thumb of gloved hand, which has high potential for contamination from touching ungloved hand or wrist.
13. Insert second hand into glove, as in step 10.	
14. Adjust fingers of both gloves. If necessary, straighten cuffed edges, <u>touching only the outside of glove,</u> and less than 1 inch from top edge.	Correct fit increases working ease. Adjusting cuffs has potential for accidental contamination.
15. Keep gloves in sight and above waist level at all times.	Avoids accidental contamination.
16. Remove gloves when finished with procedure or if accidentally contaminated or torn.	Torn or contaminated gloves allow microorganisms to enter the sterile area.

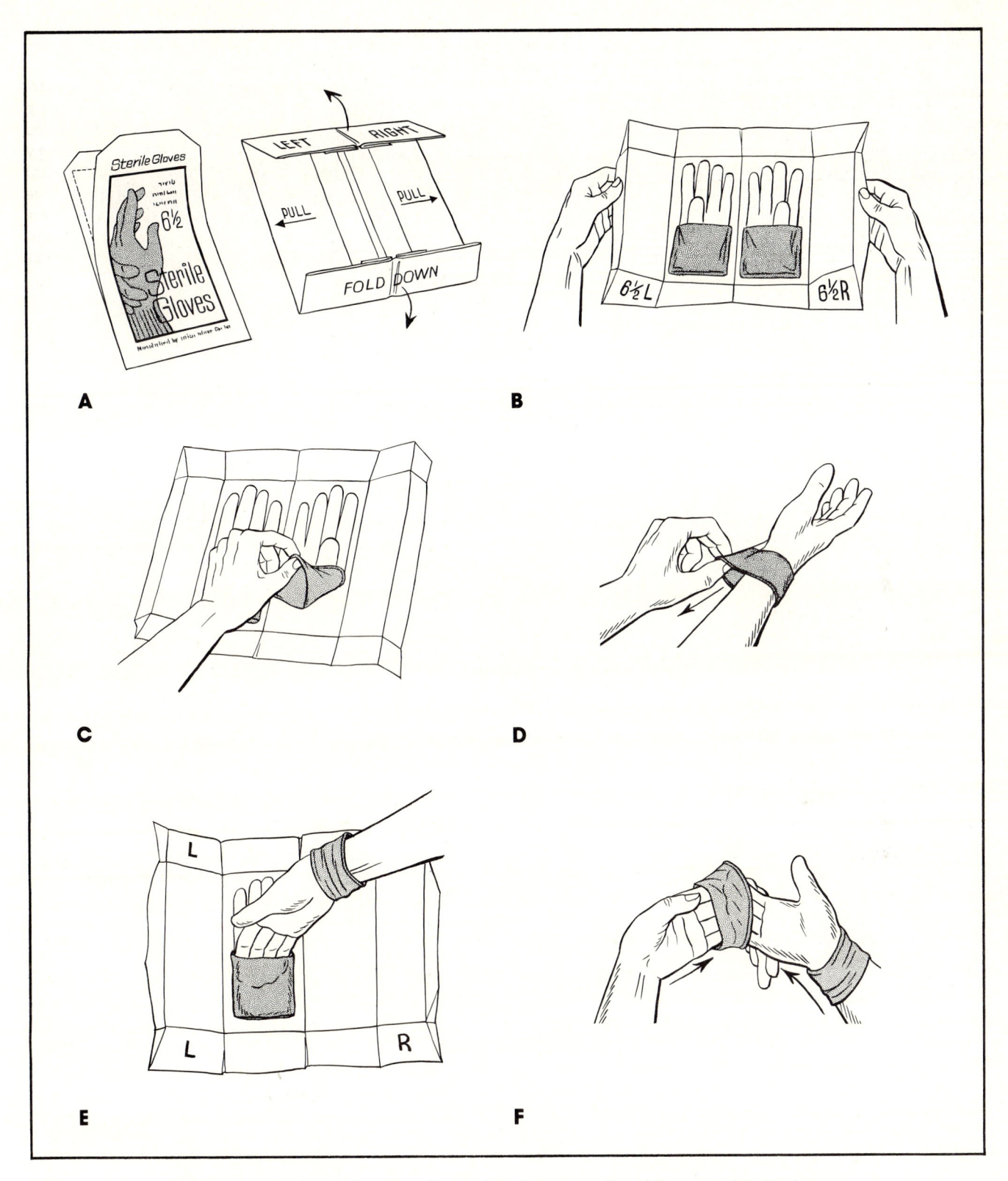

Figure 31-1. Donning sterile gloves. (Drawn from the perspective of the wearer.) **A.** Peel open the heat-sealed wrapper edges and remove the inner glove package. Place inner package on flat, clean surface and unfold first the upper and then the lower folded cuffs. **B.** Unfold wrapper completely, touching only the vertical edges, not the center fold. **C.** Touching only the glove cuff, pick up the glove for the dominant hand. **D.** Holding the glove away from self and the wrapper, direct dominant hand downward into glove, and pull glove onto hand. **E.** Insert gloved fingers under the cuff of the second glove. **F.** Insert nondominant hand into glove. Pull second glove onto hand; keep gloved thumb hyperextended to avoid contamination. Adjust cuffs as needed, avoiding touching arms.

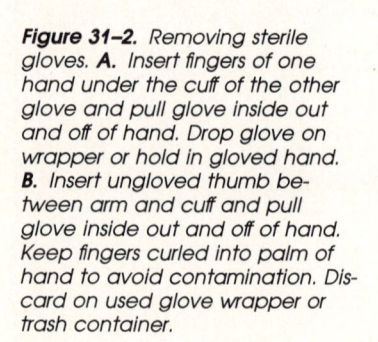

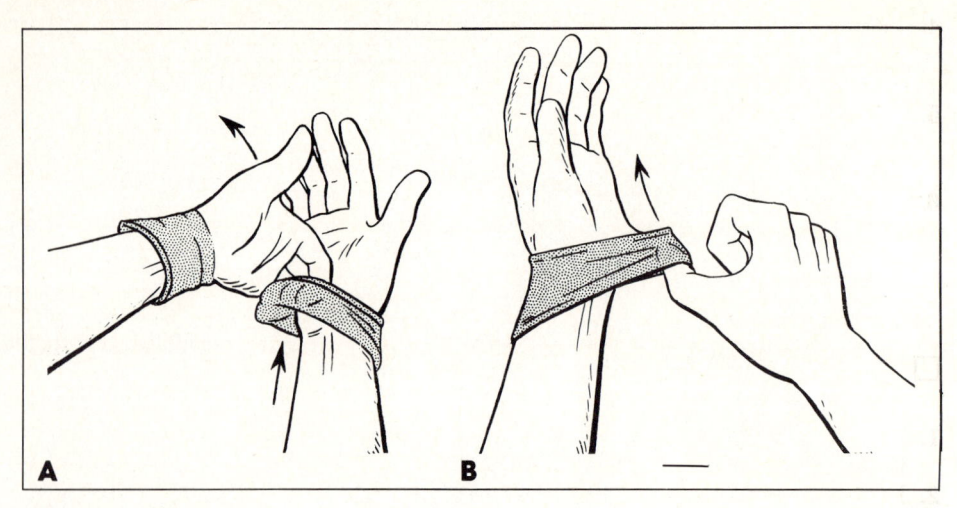

Figure 31–2. Removing sterile gloves. **A.** Insert fingers of one hand under the cuff of the other glove and pull glove inside out and off of hand. Drop glove on wrapper or hold in gloved hand. **B.** Insert ungloved thumb between arm and cuff and pull glove inside out and off of hand. Keep fingers curled into palm of hand to avoid contamination. Discard on used glove wrapper or trash container.

Keep gloved hands at or above waist level and in sight at all times, and carefully monitor what they touch. If there is the slightest question about contamination, reglove with new gloves.

When removing sterile gloves, turn them inside out in order to confine contamination and secretions inside the glove (see Fig. 31–2). Discard the used glove on the inner glove wrapper, used equipment tray, or trash can; or hold the soiled glove in the gloved hand while removing the second glove with the ungloved hand, touching only the inside of the glove and confining the first soiled glove within the inside-out second glove. Because of the presence of transient and resident bacteria and the regrowth of resident bacteria, always wash your hands before *and* after using sterile gloves for any procedure.

☐ SKILL SEQUENCE

REMOVING STERILE GLOVES

Step	Rationale
1. Grasp outside of one glove at least 1 inch from top, or insert fingers under cuff if present. Touch only the outside of glove.	Glove exteriors are contaminated and should not touch the arm.
2. Firmly and steadily, pull glove downward and off the hand, turning glove inside out while removing it.	Confines contamination inside discarded glove.
3. Discard on paper wrapper, in a trash container, or on procedure tray (if the procedure is completed). OR: Hold first glove in gloved hand while removing second glove.	Confines contamination.
4. Place ungloved thumb inside the cuff edge of the gloved hand, next to the wrist.	Glove exterior is contaminated. Glove interior is considered clean.
5. Pull glove off and discard glove(s) as in step 3. (NOTE: If using reusable gloves, wash gloves with cold water prior to removing them and follow agency procedure for the care of used gloves.)	Confines contamination.
6. Wash hands thoroughly.	Resident bacteria thrive and grow in the warm, moist environment of a gloved hand.

☐ CRITICAL POINTS SUMMARY

1. Wash hands before and after using sterile gloves.
2. Avoid touching the folded edges of the inner wrapper.
3. Unfold the inner wrapper completely.
4. Touch only the inside of a sterile glove with your ungloved hand.
5. Touch only the outside of a sterile glove with your gloved hand.
6. Keep gloved hands in sight and at or above the waist level.
7. Constantly mentally and visually monitor where the gloved hands are and what they are touching.
8. Remove gloves by turning them inside out in order to confine the contamination.

☐ LEARNING ACTIVITIES

1. Examine the packaging style of a pair of presterilized surgical gloves. Note indicators of glove placement and how the gloves are arranged in the folder.
2. Try on several pairs of sterile or nonsterile surgical gloves. Determine the best size range for yourself.
3. Practice donning and removing sterile gloves, following the steps in the Skill Sequences, "Donning Sterile Gloves" and "Removing Sterile Gloves."

4. Have a peer monitor you while donning and removing sterile gloves, using the Performance Checklist, to evaluate your technique.
5. Monitor a peer's ability to don and remove sterile gloves, using the Performance Checklist, to monitor the peer's technique.
6. Give specific feedback to each other about observed glove technique.

☐ REVIEW QUESTIONS

1. Which sterile principles from Skill 30 are applicable to donning and removing sterile gloves?
2. Explain the relationship between the principles identified in question 1 and the specific gloving practices.
3. For which of these procedures would the nurse likely need sterile gloves?
   ___ Giving an enema
   ___ Inserting a bladder catheter
   ___ Applying a bandage to a superficial skin abrasion
   ___ Applying a dressing to a draining wound
   ___ Suctioning a tracheostomy tube
   ___ Suctioning an oral cavity
4. What is considered the major problem with reusable gloves?
5. What problems are attributed to the use of glove powder?
6. Why are used sterile gloves turned inside out as they are removed?

☐ PERFORMANCE CHECKLIST

OBJECTIVE: To use appropriate aseptic technique to don sterile gloves and remove them correctly.

CHARACTERISTIC	RANGE OF ACCEPTABILITY	SATISFACTORY	UNSATISFACTORY
1. Explains procedure and purpose to client.	Omit or modify depending on client's condition.		
2. Selects proper glove size.	No deviation		
3. Inspects package for sterility, intactness, and number of gloves.	No deviation		
4. Opens outer wrapper and discards.	May be kept and used as a small sterile field.		
5. Places inner wrapper on flat surface, cuffs toward worker.	No deviation		
6. Completely unfolds inner wrapper without touching folded edges; backfolds folded edges to keep paper wrapper from reclosing.	May reopen wrapper if folded edges were not handled and closed spontaneously.		
7. Puts on dominant glove without touching outside of glove.	Reverse sequence is acceptable.		
8. Puts on nondominant glove without touching inside of glove.	Reverse sequence is acceptable.		
9. Adjusts gloves without contaminating them.	No deviation		
10. Keeps hands at or above waist level and in sight.	No deviation		
11. Removes one glove by turning it inside out, touching only the outside.	No deviation		
12. Removes second glove by turning it inside out, touching only the inside.	No deviation		
13. Discards, singly or together, in appropriate place.	No deviation		
14. Washes hands.	No deviation		

REFERENCES

Gruendemann BJ, Meeker MH: Alexander's Care of the Patient in Surgery, ed 7. St Louis, CV Mosby, 1983.

Perkins JJ: Principles and Methods of Sterilization in Health Sciences, ed 2. Springfield, IL, Charles C Thomas, 1969.

BIBLIOGRAPHY

DuGas BW: Introduction to Patient Care, ed 3. Philadelphia, WB Saunders, 1977.

Kozier B, Erb GL: Fundamentals of Nursing: Concepts and Procedures, ed 2. Reading, MA, Addison-Wesley, 1983.

Sorensen KC, Luckmann J: Basic Nursing: A Psychophysiologic Approach. Philadelphia, WB Saunders, 1979.

Wolff L, Weitzel MH, et al.: Fundamentals of Nursing, ed 7. Philadelphia, JB Lippincott, 1983.

AUDIOVISUAL RESOURCE

Asepsis: Sterile Glove Application
Film loop. (1969, 3 min.)
Available through:
Prentice-Hall Media
150 White Plains Road
Tarrytown, NY 10591

SKILL 32 Dressings and Wound Care

PREREQUISITE SKILLS

Skill 19, "Inspection"
Skill 20, "Palpation"
Skill 28, "Handwashing"
Skill 30, "Sterile Supplies"
Skill 31, "Donning Sterile Gloves"

☐ STUDENT OBJECTIVES

1. Define the terms used to describe various kinds of wounds.
2. Describe the stages and methods of wound healing.
3. Describe assessment data indicative of positive wound-healing status.
4. Compare factors that promote wound healing with those that predispose to delayed wound healing or nonhealing.
5. Compare the signs, symptoms, and treatment of wound dehiscence and evisceration.
6. Explain the functions and uses of various kinds of wound dressings.
7. Describe the purposes and characteristics of various kinds of adhesive tape and other wound closures.
8. Using strict aseptic technique, demonstrate the ability to:
   a. Prepare a sterile field for a dressing change for simple and complex dry sterile dressings.
   b. Tear tape with fingers.
   c. Fasten the dressing with the appropriate adhesive tape or other closure.

☐ INTRODUCTION

A wound is defined as a "bodily injury caused by physical means, with disruption of the normal continuity of structures" (Miller and Keane, 1983, p. 1221).

Wounds may be described as open or closed, depending on whether or not the skin or mucous membranes have been broken. *Closed wounds* include contusions or bruises that result from blunt external force. *Open wounds* involve a disruption of the skin or mucous membranes and varying degrees of underlying tissues. They may result from accidental (traumatic) or intentional (surgical) causes. This skill deals with the care of open rather than closed wounds, primarily those that are caused intentionally through surgical procedures and sutured for primary healing to occur. Many of the principles and practices described here would also be appropriate for the care of accidental wounds.

Wound care refers to all procedures, practices, and observations that support wound healing, for example, wound cleansing and irrigation, suture removal, dressing changes, and assessment of wound status and healing. A dressing is "any of various materials used for covering and protecting a wound" (Miller and Keane, 1983, p. 342). Dressings serve to protect the wound or keep the wound from drying out, depending on the purpose of the dressing, and to absorb drainage. They also have an esthetic value for the client.

A major deterrent to rapid wound healing is a wound infection, which may be caused by either endogenous sources (from the client) or exogenous sources (from the health-care worker or the environment). Scrupulous aseptic technique is needed to decrease the possibility of wound infection from either source. In its 1979 publication *Infection Control in the Hospital,* the American Hospital Association states: "Dressing a wound is a surgical procedure and should be carried out with the precision and care of an operative technique. Thus, each dressing should be applied with sterile precautions as well as with carefully planned methodology" (1979, p. 161).

One of the determinants of the rate and nature of wound healing is the kind of nursing care provided (Cooper and Schumann, 1979). Wound care is a crucial aspect of nursing care, and the nurse needs to know how to provide skilled, safe wound care to clients with diverse kinds of wounds. In addition, the nurse often is asked to give wound-care advice or first aid in a community or social setting and needs to understand basic principles of wound care and the purposes and uses of various dressings and adhesive tapes.

☐ PREPARATION

Wounds are described by the type or extent of disruption to the tissues. For example, an abrasion, floor burn, or subcutaneous tissue cut is described as a *superficial* wound; a gash into a muscle or an abdominal incision is called a *deep* wound. An *incision* is a cut that has sharp, clean, and smooth edges and is made by a sharp instrument, the surgical knife. Incisions may extend only into the skin layers (for example, for grafting or for excision of moles) or through the skin, fascia, muscles, or the peritoneum for more extensive surgery. A *laceration* is an unintentional traumatic cut, and usually has irregular, jagged, and torn edges from the object that caused the cut.

When an incision is made into organs or deep tissue, the wound is described as a *penetrating* wound. If the instrument or object making the incision passes through and exits from the deeper tissues, a body cavity, or an organ, the wound is described as a *perforating* wound. A *puncture* wound is one that is made by a sharp pointed object that pierces deep tissues, leaving behind a very small surface opening. A puncture wound usually bleeds little and seals itself over quickly. This can be a problem, as it provides an excellent environment for anaerobic microorganisms, especially tetanus.

WOUND REPAIR

The process of wound repair involves both regeneration and scar tissue formation. Regeneration (replacement by new cells or tissues that are identical or quite similar to the injured ones) occurs in epithelial, lymphoid, hematopoietic, and parenchymal gland tissues.

Collagenous scar tissue formation (repair by means of fibroblastic activity) may occur in the healing of tendons, fascia, connective tissues, and collagenous structures.

If there are no complications, wound repair occurs in a predictable repair process and time sequence. To facilitate healing, sutures are usually used to draw the wound together, approximating the edges in as normal a fashion as is feasible. The degree to which this is possible depends on the extent of tissue damage or loss at the injury site.

Process of Wound Repair
Initially, the injury to the tissues results in a hemorrhage that becomes a clot and fills the vacancy from the wound. By the end of several hours, a crust begins to form as fibrin and other proteins dry out. This crust helps protect the wound from further fluid loss and bacterial invasion.

Within the first 2 hours, the *local inflammatory response* begins to occur and may last for several days. This is a normal physiologic response to injury and is characterized by reddened swollen wound edges and local warmth and tenderness or pain. The local inflammatory response helps clear debris away from the wound through increased antibodies and defensive white cells and sets the stage for healing through increased presence of fibrinogen. In addition, a *systemic inflammatory response* often occurs, with an elevated body temperature of under 37.7°C (100.0°F) and an increased metabolism which both last for several days and increase the body's repair activity.

Within 24 hours, the epidermis adjacent to the wound begins to thicken and epidermal cells migrate toward the wound. Within 48 hours, this surface layer of epithelial cells is complete, and the wound is sealed from invading bacteria and further fluid loss. This layer of epithelium is fragile and easily broken and provides no strength or support to the wound.

Fibroblastic activity within the dermis begins on the 2nd or 3rd day, followed by collagen formation on about the 4th day as scar formation begins to occur. At this point, the wound has little or no tensile strength and without sutures would separate easily.

About the 4th or 5th day, endothelial cells also begin to multiply, new blood vessels begin to form, and collagen fibers continue to accumulate. This is evidenced by a hard, blunt ridge that begins to develop along the entire length of the incision, known as the healing ridge. This ridge is palpable, but not visible on the skin surface, and results from fascial healing and scar formation. By the 7th day, the healing ridge is quite prominent and easy to palpate. Absence of a healing ridge most likely indicates that healing is delayed for some reason.

By 7 to 10 days, the wound is sufficiently healed so that it is difficult and painful to separate the wound edges. However, the wound continues to be fragile, because most wounds develop less than 15 percent of their ultimate tensile strength by the end of the 3rd week (Auld et al., 1972; LeMaitre and Finnegan, 1980; Madden, 1983).

At the end of 6 weeks, surgical wounds usually have achieved a large percentage of their maximum strength, at which time patients usually are permitted to return to work and their usual activities. However, collagen synthesis and wound healing continue over many months and even years. During this time, the wound continues to increase gradually in strength and the scar usually shrinks in size and becomes pale rather than reddened. During the healing process, absorbable sutures gradually lose their strength and are absorbed by the body. The type of suture selected to close a wound usually corresponds with the anticipated rate of wound healing.

Wound repair is influenced by the type of dressing used. If a nonocclusive dressing (one that allows air to circulate to the wound) is used, or if the wound is exposed to air, the epidermis at the edges and base of the wound becomes dehydrated and incorporated into the crust that covers the wound. This situation is thought by some to be a mechanical barrier to epidermal cell migration, since the cells must cleave between the crust and the underlying dermis. An occlusive dressing (one that keeps air from entering the wound) enhances epithelialization by maintaining hydration on the wound surface. Newer semipermeable and occlusive dressings (discussed later) allow oxygen to penetrate to the tissue and maintain surface moisture, yet also protect the wound from microorganism entry and infection (Schumann, 1982).

Types of Wound Healing

Wound repair may be categorized by the type of healing that occurs, which depends on the nature of the wound, the amount of tissue lost or removed, and the potential for infection. Figure 32-1 depicts the three types of healing. When wounds are made aseptically with a minimal amount of tissue destruction and the edges are approximated carefully, they heal with little tissue reaction or granulation tissue formation and produce minimal scarring. These wounds are said to heal by *first intention* (primary union or closure, Fig. 32-1A).

Wound repair by *second intention,* also known as granulation or indirect union, occurs when the wound edges are not sutured or approximated with tape strips, and granulation tissue (soft, red, sensitive capillary buds) fills in the opening prior to healing (Fig. 32-1B). Healing usually occurs by second intention with decubitus ulcers, abscesses, pilonidal cyst excisions, and gaping, irregular, or torn wounds. Healing by second intention is slower than that by first intention, produces a larger scar, and can result in scar contraction with local deformity or malfunction. It is the method of choice or necessity when tissue is missing or when wound closure would encourage abscess formation.

A third type of repair is that of *third intention* (Fig. 32-1C), which combines the first two types. Wounds that heal by third intention may purposely be left open initially and later approximated, or they may have been sutured initially, followed by a breakdown of the suture line, with later resuturing. Wound edges often are left unapproximated when infection is present or highly probable, such as with abdominal surgery for a ruptured appendix or bowel obstruction. When healthy pink-red granulation tissue begins to grow and no signs of infection or suppuration (pus formation) develop, the wound may then be sutured. Healing by third intention also occurs when a wound infection or an abscess develops in a sutured wound. The wound then separates spontaneously or is opened surgically to allow for drainage and healing. This type of healing is quite lengthy, and produces a large scar with a tendency toward scar contraction.

Delayed Wound Healing

Wound healing may be delayed because of various preexisting increased risk factors: (1) decreased circulation, such as in aged or diabetic persons; (2) lowered nutritional status (especially deficiencies in protein, iron, zinc, vitamin C, and if the injury involves a bone, vitamin D and calcium) as in thin, undernourished persons or those in poor general health; (3) use of certain drugs, such as aspirin and coumadin, that increase bleeding tendencies and steroids that retard the inflammatory process; (4) smoking, which alters respiratory function and causes peripheral vascular constriction and less oxygen supply to the wound; and (5) obesity, since adipose tissue is less vascular than other body tissue and heals more slowly because of reduced oxygen and nutrient supply.

Wound healing may be delayed by specific postoperative events or factors; for example, repeated vigorous vomiting and abdominal distention, which stretch the wound and can delay the formation of the lattice framework within the dermis that supports the fibroblast and endothelial cells. Fluid and electrolyte

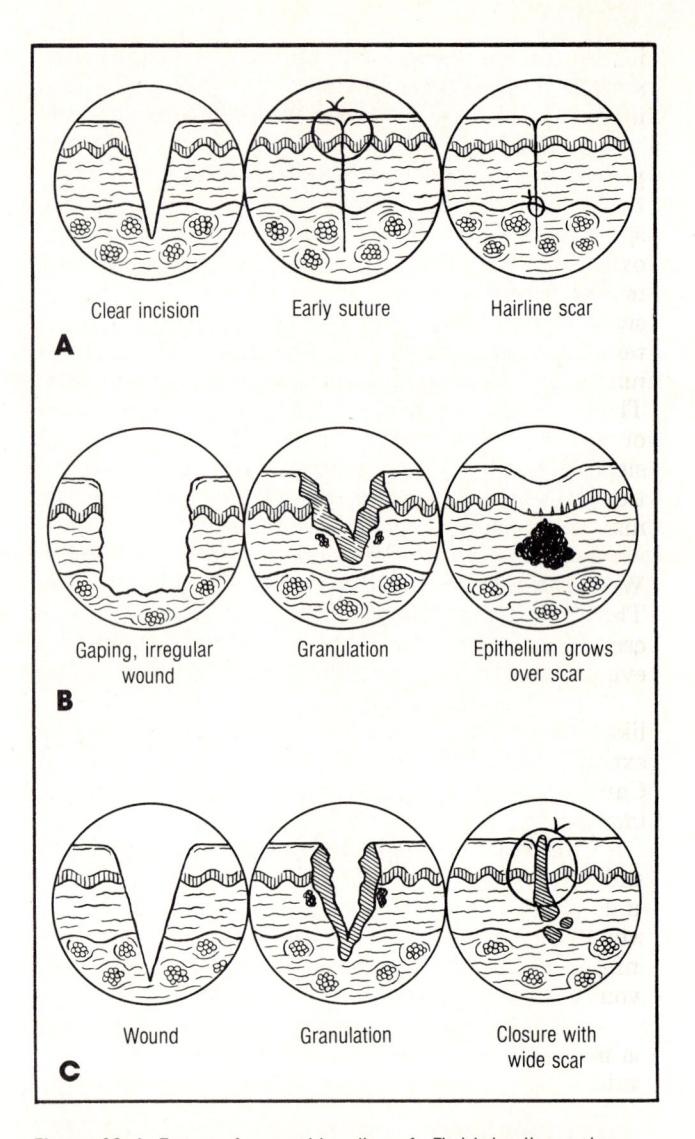

Figure 32–1. Types of wound healing. **A.** First intention, primary union. **B.** Second intention, granulation. **C.** Third intention, secondary suture. (Redrawn from Hardy JD (ed): Rhoads Textbook of Surgery: Principles and Practice, ed 5. NY, JB Lippincott, 1977.)

imbalances can contribute to abdominal distention, and an abnormal pH is known to retard wound healing.

Excessive or unrelieved pain after the immediate postoperative period results in stress, with the production of steroids that decrease the body's natural response to injury. Inadequate systemic and cellular oxygen slows fibroblastic activity. Hematomas or seromas (collections of blood or tissue fluid) at the wound site delay the cellular repair process. Mechanical interference with circulation hinders the transport of nutrients to and waste products from the wound site. This interference may be caused by too tight bandages or poorly fitting casts, improper positioning during sleep, or local edema or hematomas. Bacterial infections delay wound healing by placing additional demands on the body's repair processes.

Wound Complications

The more common wound complications include increased bleeding, infections, and wound dehiscence or evisceration.

Increased bleeding at the wound site is more likely to occur in clients who have blood dyscrasias or extensive malignancies, or in alcoholics with cirrhosis. Careful observation is important for early detection of increased bleeding.

Wound infections cause added pain, disability, and expense for the client; lengthened hospital stays; and increased mortality rates. When to anticipate wound infections and how to assess for the presence of infection are discussed in Skill 34, in conjunction with wound culture specimen collection.

Wound dehiscence and *evisceration* are regarded as medical emergencies and are considered the most serious complications of abdominal wounds. *Dehiscence,* or wound disruption, "generally refers to a separation of an abdominal wound, involving the anterior fascial sheath and deeper layers" (Schwartz et al., 1984, p. 456). In clinical practice, the term dehiscence includes any degree of wound disruption, whether of the skin layers only, or extending through the fascial layers (Fig. 32-2A). Wound disruption generally occurs between 5 and 12 days postoperative, although it may have begun earlier. The primary sign of wound disruption is the presence of a large amount of *serosanguineous* (watery pink-red) drainage on the dressing. If such drainage appears after the first 24 hours postoperative, it is generally considered diagnostic of dehiscence. Madden and Arem (1981, p. 176) indicate that dehiscence is almost always heralded by intraperitoneal fluid leaking through the skin incision.

There is a higher incidence of wound dehiscence in persons over 45 years and clients who are obese, debilitated, poorly nourished, or who have cancer. Postoperative coughing, retching, and hiccups all increase the intraabdominal pressure and strain the incision, making dehiscence more likely. Too tight sutures, local hemorrhage or infection, and vertical incisions (other than midline) are also thought to be contributing factors. Dehiscence sometimes causes the sutures to give way, or it may become evident only when skin sutures are removed. Sometimes when the skin sutures remain intact, the dehiscence manifests itself later as a ventral hernia (Schwartz et al., 1984). According to LeMaitre and Finnegan (1980), wound dehiscence never occurs when a well-defined healing ridge has developed.

Wound dehiscence may or may not be accompanied by *evisceration,* which is the protrusion of abdominal contents through the incision (Figure 32-2B). When evisceration occurs, clients usually experience

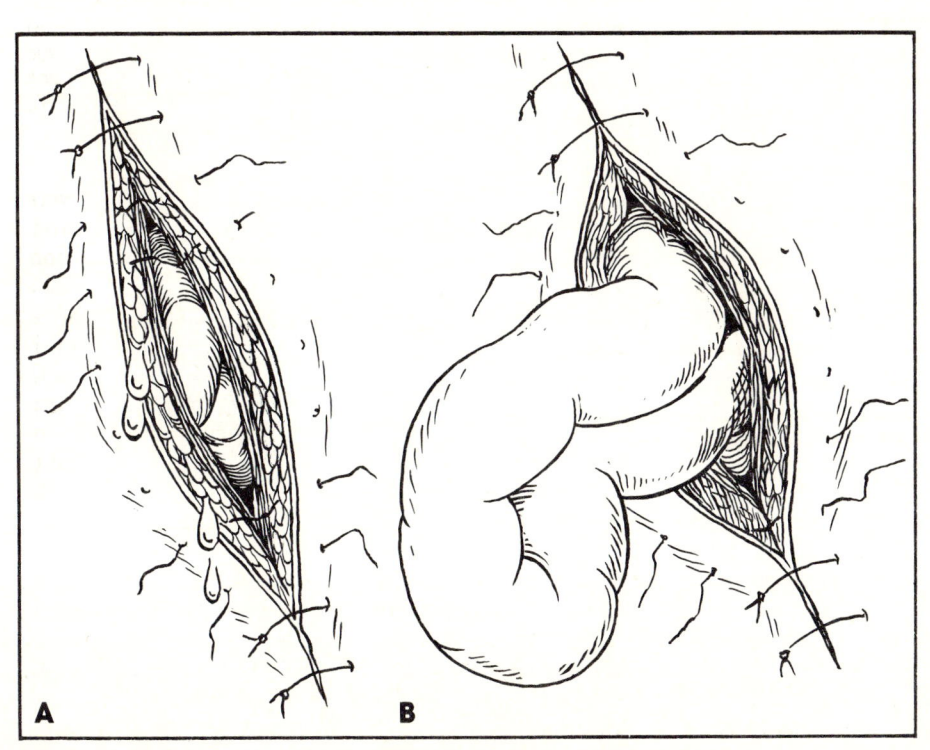

Figure 32-2. Wound disruption: **A.** Dehiscence. **B.** Evisceration.

sudden pain and a sensation of "something giving way," and they may go into shock.

A separated wound should be promptly covered with a dry sterile towel and a binder applied, if this can be done with minimal moving of the client. If abdominal contents are visible, large sterile dressings moistened with sterile normal saline should be applied. The physician must be notified immediately. The client usually is taken to the operating room promptly, so the wound can be reclosed.

Factors That Promote Wound Healing

A general principle in wound healing is that of minimal interference, removing all impediments to normal wound healing and supporting the body's natural healing processes (Madden and Arem, 1981). Wound repair is promoted when the factors that delay wound healing are prevented, counteracted, or minimized. This includes providing pain relief; promoting adequate respiratory exchange; preventing abdominal distention; careful observation to detect incisional infection, hematomas, seromas, and decreased wound approximation; maintaining an adequate fluid and electrolyte balance; and providing increased protein, iron, vitamin C, and for bone injuries, vitamin D and calcium.

Hot and cold packs may be used to promote wound healing. A general rule is to use cold packs early in inflammation and hot packs later. However, careful, frequent observation and assessment of the local circulatory response is necessary, as is knowledge of institutional policy and the physician's preferences. See Skill 46 for a discussion of the use of heat and cold and Skill 36 for a discussion of warm wet dressings.

Gravity can be used to promote wound healing, since elevating an injured body part helps decrease edema formation. Reducing edema often helps relieve pain as well as increase the circulation. Protective dressings, bandages, guards, and slings protect the wound from reinjury.

Because of the prevalence of endogenous sources of wound infection, the nurse must use strict aseptic technique during dressing changes and wound care. Clients and families must also be taught not to touch the surgical wound site.

WOUND CARE

A significant aspect of wound care is the application of a dressing that is acceptable to the client, physician, and nurse, and appropriate to the principles of care for that kind of wound.

Wound dressings serve to: (1) absorb incisional drainage (exudate) and keep the wound dry; (2) protect the wound from further injury by providing support and some immobilization; (3) provide pressure to prevent hematomas; (4) serve as a vehicle for applying medication; (5) help debride (remove devitalized tissue from) infected or open wounds; (6) cover disfiguring injuries or surgeries; and (7) provide psychological rest for people who would rather not see their incision.

The decision whether to use a dressing depends on the nature and location of the wound and the surgeon and client's preferences. After the first 72 hours, the body's natural healing processes have sealed a clean wound from bacterial invasion, making a dressing optional for a nondraining wound with primary closure (Madden, 1983). Some surgeons prefer to leave the wound exposed and undressed immediately after surgery; others dress all wounds. Apparently there is no measurable effect on wound healing from leaving a nondraining, sutured wound exposed to the air. It is considered preferable to leave a wound exposed than to have an inadequate dressing that does not stay in place and cannot maintain a clean wound surface.

Incisions where minimal scarring is desired, such as facial sutures, are often left uncovered so that frequent meticulous suture care can be given and stitch infections avoided.

Unless there is a specific order to the contrary, dressings are changed rather than reinforced when they are saturated. However, many agencies have a policy requiring that a physician do the first postoperative dressing change. A saturated dressing allows bacterial contaminants to enter the wound through capillary attraction from the contaminated outer surface of the dressing and allows wound contaminants to contact the bed linen and clothing. Maintaining a dry wound surface helps decrease the risk of postoperative infection (Alexander, 1983).

Sometimes a drain is placed within a wound to facilitate removal of fluid when accumulation of that fluid would delay healing through hematoma formation and lack of tissue approximation. The role of drains in wound healing and several specific kinds of wound drains are discussed in Skill 35.

Wound drainage is described as sanguineous (bloody), serous (clear and watery, from tissue fluid), serosanguineous (clear fluid mixed with blood), or purulent (thick yellow or white fluid containing pus). It is best to describe the amount of drainage by noting the number and kind of dressings partially or completely saturated, or the specific diameter of the soiled area. Avoid terms such as small, moderate, or large because of their nonspecific nature and subjective interpretation. Increased amounts of drainage are expected when a wound contains a drain that is not connected to suction or gravity drainage. Because of gravity, increased amounts of drainage are found at the dependent edges of the dressing, that is, the lower edges for an ambulatory client or the lateral edges for a bed client who lies primarily on one side.

SELF-CARE OF WOUNDS

Because wound healing is a lengthy process, most clients leave the acute-care setting with wounds that still need some kind of care. To prepare for this, clients should be kept informed about the kind of wound care being provided during their hospitalization. They must understand something about the process of wound healing, factors that promote and hinder wound healing, and the specifics of how to take care of their own particular dressing. For more complex wound dressings, this may include supervised practice sessions in which the nurse assists the client or a family member in developing competence and confidence in home care for the wound. If a dressing is too complex for a client or family member to handle at home, or if they seem unable or unwilling to take proper care of the wound, a referral to a visiting nurse or home-care agency provides needed continuity of care. Clients also need to know what circumstances indicate a need for medical consultation; for example, development of a fever, unusual incisional drainage, increased tenderness or redness around the wound, development of new discomfort with activity, separation of wound edges in a previously closed wound, and a general sense of not feeling well.

DATA BASE

Before providing wound care, it is important to know the purpose for the dressing being used and recall some basic facts about wound healing. For example, most sutured wounds are kept dry to promote healing; thus, a dressing is selected to absorb drainage and allow air to circulate. If the purpose is to prevent fluid loss, such as with a fresh superficial burn or abrasion, a dressing that seals the wound is used, such as a Telfa or Vaseline dressing. The use of an incorrect type of dressing may defeat the purpose of the dressing. For example, sealing a sutured wound tightly with tape or nonporous dressings will cause the wound to remain moist and dark—a perfect culture medium for infection-producing microorganisms rather than allowing air to circulate through a porous dressing. This inappropriate activity sometimes is done for the well-intended purpose of avoiding soiled linens and clothing from wound drainage.

The nurse determines the *time of day* that is most appropriate for wound care and dressing changes, taking into consideration the client's meal and activity schedule. It is not appropriate to plan to change a dressing just prior to mealtime, as that may contribute to anorexia (loss of appetite). Prior to giving wound care or changing a dressing, the nurse determines the client's pain and discomfort level, as well as any need for premedication. Usually, this is not needed except when changing burn or graft dressings, adjusting some drain tubes, or if the client is excessively apprehensive.

The nurse also evaluates the client's physical, mental, and emotional status to help determine if assistance is needed either to hold equipment or to help the client maintain a specific position during the wound care. The health record or kardex indicates whether the client has seen the wound and what response occurred. If the dressing change will give the client a first look at the wound, be prepared to answer questions and offer information about wound healing.

Client History and Recorded Data

Before changing the dressing, the nurse determines the kind of dressing previously used, when it was last changed, and whether there are any drains or tubes in the wound. It also is important to know the location, nature, and extent of the incision, whether the skin edges were approximated or left open, the kind of sutures or skin closure used, and whether any sutures are to be removed. This information is found in the anesthesiologist's report, the surgery report, physician's progress notes, nurses' notes, the kardex, or computer nursing-care plan. To assess the healing process, the nurse considers the number of days postoperative, the current food and fluid intake and output, and whether there are any systemic signs of infection, such as elevated temperature, increased pulse and respiratory rates, or leukocytosis.

Some surgeons have specific requirements about wound cleansing, sometimes including a hands-off policy, allowing nature to take its course. Unless the client's safety is seriously compromised, the nurse respects the surgeon's procedures, even if they differ from the nurse's preferences. In addition to knowing a surgeon's preferences, the nurse needs to know unit and institutional wound-care protocols. The infection control committee in an institution usually develops criteria for wound care.

Physical Appraisal Skills

The decision to apply a specific type of dressing or to change a dressing may arise from an analysis of objective data obtained through inspection and palpation, plus sometimes the sense of smell.

Inspection. *Inspection of the dressing* determines the type of dressing previously applied, whether it was adequate to cover and protect the wound, and the amount and kind of drainage present on the existing dressing. To do this, the nurse must turn back the bed linens or adjust the client's clothing to whatever extent is needed to expose the dressing completely.

Inspection of the wound itself may reveal a healing wound with well-approximated edges; healthy, pink, intact skin adjacent to the wound and at the tape sites; and functioning drain tubes. Inspection may reveal problems with any of these factors.

Palpation. *Palpation of the dressing* reveals a wet or dry outer surface. To assess drainage or frank bleeding, remember to palpate dependent areas of the dressing and to feel underneath the client, as gravity causes fluid to flow toward those areas. Light *palpation of the incision* itself, *while wearing sterile gloves,* reveals the presence or absence of the healing ridge and development of any tender areas. Palpation of the area adjacent to the wound may reveal increased tenderness and warmth, indicating an infection is developing.

Sense of Smell. The sense of *smell* may help determine the suspected presence of some bacteria in the wound drainage, such as foul-smelling staphylococcal infections (see Skill 34).

EQUIPMENT

There are many different kinds of dressings and tape available, with new types constantly being developed for specific purposes or improved function.

Types of Dressings

The dressing placed immediately next to the wound is known as the *primary dressing*. Its purpose is to draw fluid away from the incision, upward toward the *secondary dressing*, which absorbs the fluid. Primary dressings are made of a fine mesh or nonwoven fabric so that granulation tissue cannot penetrate the gauze interstices and begin to bleed when the dressing is removed (Schwartz et al., 1984). They are constructed to function as a wick, drawing the drainage upward and away from the skin surface and allowing it to disperse laterally throughout the dressing. Drainage is then absorbed through direct contact into the secondary dressing, which is thicker, fluffier, and more absorbent.

If wound drainage is slight, primary dressings can be used alone to absorb the drainage. The nurse uses as many primary and secondary dressings as are necessary to absorb the expected drainage, provide protection, and cover the wound and some surrounding skin.

Dressings may be categorized as nonocclusive, occlusive, nonadhering, or medicated. The various categories of dressings have differing properties that promote healing in different ways, depending on the characteristics of the wound. Both primary and secondary wound dressings usually are nonocclusive. Exceptions include burn and graft dressings and moist soaks. In general, unless wound debridement (see Skill 37) is desired, a primary dressing would be nonadherent in nature.

Nonocclusive Dressings. The most common postsurgical dressings are nonocclusive dressings, which allow air to circulate around the wound site. They are also called "hydrophilic" (water-absorbing) contact dressings. Nonocclusive dressings are made of absorbent cotton or synthetic rayon gauze, which serves as a wick to draw the exudate up from the wound surface and into the dressing through capillary attraction. This keeps the wound relatively dry and thus promotes healing. It must be remembered that any nonocclusive dressing can easily be transformed into an occlusive one by adding a plastic, waterproof wrap, or by covering the entire dressing with nonporous tape. This may or may not fulfill the desired purpose for the dressing.

Primary nonocclusive *dressing sponges or flats,* such as the Topper, are made of fine-meshed gauze or nonwoven fabric with an absorbent filler. Flats are available in folded 3 × 3, 4 × 3, or 4 × 4 inch sizes, either two sponges per presterilized heat-sealed package or in bulk nonsterile packages for institutional sterilization. *Unfilled gauze sponges* (without an absorbent filler) are available in similar sizes and packaging. They may be used for wound or skin cleansing or as packing material for an open incision or eroded decubitus ulcer. If a regular dressing sponge was used in these circumstances, the absorbent filler could adhere to the tissues and become a wound irritant.

Secondary nonocclusive dressings, such as Surgipads, ABD's (abdominal pads), or combine dressings, are made of highly absorbent layers of cotton and cellulose. Some are completely absorbent, while others have nonabsorbent outer layers on one surface that delay external saturation of the dressing.

Fluffs are large-meshed gauze sponges that have been opened and fluffed to make them bulkier and more absorbent. They are used for copious wound drainage or in hand dressings for finger support.

Burn dressings are many-layered dressings that have no filler to stick to an open wound. They are used with copious fluid loss or for wet soaks to wounds.

Occlusive Dressings. Occlusive dressings prevent air and moisture from entering the wound and keep tissue fluid from leaving the wound. Occlusive dressings are called "hydrophobic" (water-repelling) contact dressings. Examples of occlusive dressings include medicated dressings such as petroleum (Vaseline) gauze, scarlet-red ointment gauze or furacin gauze, and Telfa dressings; all of which are *nonadherent* in nature. Occlusive dressings are commonly used on graft sites or burns to keep the site from drying out.

Nonadhering Dressings. Nonadhering dressings are primary dressings that do not stick to the wound surface or the surrounding skin. *Nonocclusive nonadherent dressings* may be made from either a petrolatum-coated fabric that allows nonadherence without occlusion (such as Adaptic) or from a flexible microtextured net facing bonded to an absorbent filler (such as Release). As mentioned, Telfa dressings are nonadherent; however, they are occlusive.

Medicated dressings are dressings that have been impregnated with medication or are saturated with a medicated solution or normal saline at the time of use. For example, Furacin gauze dressings contain an antibacterial used for minor burns, and Xeroform gauze dressings deodorize wounds and may promote epithelialization.

Dressing packing strips are made of sterilized nonfraying gauze or fabric, available in 1/4 to 2 inch widths and packaged in jars of 5 to 100 yards. They may be plain, such as those used for packing bleeding nostrils or open or infected wounds, and those used as drainage wicks for abscesses. Or they may be impregnated with medications, such as iodoform or Vaseline. To maintain sterility of the contents and container, the desired length of packing must be removed from the jar with aseptic technique and cut before the dressing change instruments become contaminated with wound drainage.

Sterile, *spray-on dressings*, such as Aeroplast or Resifilm, can be used as a substitute for a dressing on a clean surgical incision. Sprays provide a moisture-proof seal over suture lines and allow complete visualization of the wound. They are quite useful with small wounds or with head lacerations since they permit shampooing. The skin must be completely dry before applying the sealant. Several thin layers usually adhere better than one thick layer. Most sealants last about 5 to 7 days, can be removed by peeling off like tape or by dissolving with acetone or alcohol, and can be reapplied as needed.

A newer development in wound covering is the use of a transparent, semipermeable film, such as Op-Site, Tegaderm, or Ensure. This material is a synthetic, thin, transparent, flexible adhesive membrane that is permeable to air and water vapor but impermeable to water and bacteria. It can therefore protect a wound or injury from outside contaminants but not interfere with the healing process. Described as a "second skin," this membrane "breathes," does not cause skin maceration (wrinkling) or irritation even if left in place up to 14 days, and can be washed with soap and water or worn in the shower without disturbing it. Because they are transparent, these membranes provide ready visualization of a wound. When in place over a wound, no scab forms and epithelialization is said to be more rapid. Some of the many uses for these membranes include: holding intravenous or arterial lines in place; as a graft donor site dressing and a backing for split-thickness grafts; as a postoperative wound dressing; for superficial burns or scalds; as skin protection around a stoma; and to treat or prevent decubitus ulcers (Besst and Wallace, 1979; Chrisp, 1977; Dinner et al., 1979; Remarkable, 1980).

Another new type of wound dressing is Duoderm Hydroactive (Squibb) dressing, which consists of moisture-reactive particles surrounded by an inert, hydrophobic polymer. This dressing is virtually impermeable to atmospheric oxygen, which is thought to stimulate growth of dermal capillaries (Duoderm, 1983; Schumann, 1982). This dressing is placed over the wound and held in place with the hand for a minute or two until warmth from the client's body and the nurse's hand softens the dressing and causes it to adhere to the skin. The Duoderm dressing molds to the skin contours as it warms and remains in place without adhesives. While in place, the hydroactive particles interact with the wound fluid and swell, forming a soft, moist gel-like mass in the wound bed. When the dressing is removed, it does not stick to the wound surface, but the gel remains in the wound. The gel looks very similar to pus, and should be removed by gentle cleansing with saline before evaluating the wound and applying a new dressing. Duoderm dressings are left in place for up to a week as long as they are leak free, and depending on the type of wound, agency policy, or physician preference.

Other new developments in wound coverings include: (1) *silastic foam,* which can be poured into or over open wounds, such as pilonidal sinuses or graft sites, producing a molded form that serves as a close-fitting dressing (Harding and Richardson, 1979); and (2) *human amniotic membrane* combined with nylon silastic and collagen, which keeps wounds, such as burns, from drying out or becoming infected (Encouraging, 1980).

Hazards. A major hazard in the use of dressings is accidental and unnoticed contamination. Improperly applied dressings can defeat the purpose intended. A too-loose dressing may slip and slide, causing contamination from surrounding skin areas. A too-tight dressing decreases circulation and hinders wound healing. When wound dressings are not changed frequently, observations of wound status are decreased, thus decreasing the observation that is a crucial aspect of wound care.

If a nonocclusive dressing is completely covered with tape or plastic, it automatically becomes occlusive and cannot allow air to circulate. When dressings become damp with wound drainage, capillary attraction allows bacterial contaminants from the wound to come in contact with the client's immediate environment and allows environmental contaminants to enter the wound.

Adhesive Tape

Adhesive tape is used in a variety of ways, for example, to hold dressings in place; to provide pressure to prevent fluid loss or hematoma formation; to approximate wound edges; to immobilize body parts, such as fractured ribs; or to stabilize and support a joint, such as prevention or treatment of athletic injuries. Figure 32–3 shows an abdominal dressing held in place with wide adhesive tape.

Adhesive tape consists of a backing material and an adhesive mass. The backing material usually is made of cotton cloth, rayon taffeta, paper, plastic, or

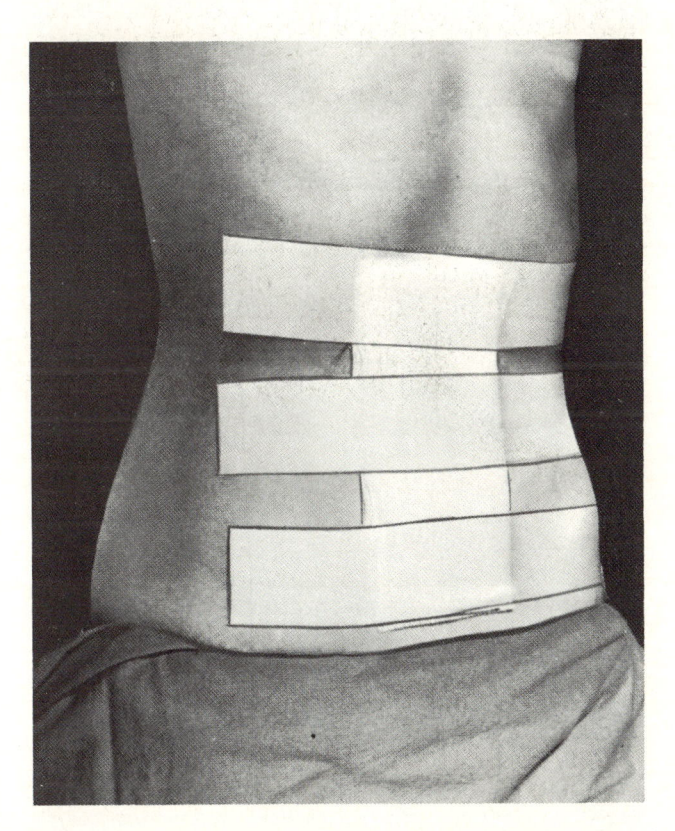

Figure 32–3. Securing an abdominal dressing with wide adhesive tape. (Courtesy of Johnson and Johnson, New Brunswick, NJ.)

foam, and may be porous (nonocclusive) or nonporous (occlusive). Rubber-based adhesives tend to cause irritation and allergic reactions in persons with sensitive skin. Nonallergenic tapes usually have an acrylate-based adhesive and tend to cause less skin irritation. Adhesive tape is available in widths ranging from 1/2 to 3 or 4 inches.

The type of adhesive tape selected depends on the purpose for which it will be used. Heavy *cotton cloth-backed tape* has a rubber base and is strong and economical. Because of the highly adherent quality of this tape, shearing of the skin may occur if the tape is removed too quickly. Since this tape is somewhat occlusive, the underlying skin may become macerated. *Rayon taffeta tape,* such as Dermicel, is a nonallergenic porous cloth-backed tape that works well for holding dressings or for hard-to-tape areas. *Paper tape,* such as Dermalite, is a lightweight nonallergenic porous (nonocclusive) tape that allows the skin to breathe. It is useful for holding dressings in place when strong support and adhesion are not essential. *Plastic tape,* such as Dermiclear, is a strong, transparent, moisture-resistant adhesive tape. This tape adheres well even under moist conditions and can be used to hold intravenous infusions, catheters, and life-support systems in place. Since plastic tape has some elasticity, it can provide some pressure if needed. *Elastic foam tape* has a two-way stretch and can be used to maintain controlled pressure on draining wounds or to prevent hematomas. *Waterproof tape* has a coated backing cloth and can be washed with soap and water. *Strapping tape* is porous and especially designed to immobilize sprains and support body parts while allowing the skin to breathe.

Most kinds of tape can be torn with the fingers when scissors are not available. Hold the tape firmly between the thumbnails and forefingers. Initiate tearing by a quick rotary twisting of the hands in opposite directions (see Fig. 32–4). Paper tape tears easily but not very straight. Plastic tape usually does not tear and needs to be cut.

As much as possible, adhesive tape is applied in such a way that the dressings fit body contours closely but still allow natural body movements to occur. Generally, it is best to apply the center of the tape strip to the dressing first, and then apply the ends laterally and onto the skin. Drawing the tape up too tightly puts undue tension on the skin and contributes to skin irritation. Tape that is too narrow, too long, too short, or improperly spaced does not hold the dressing in a close but flexible position. When cutting or tearing tape and applying it to a dressing, consider movement of body parts and the various positions a client may assume. For example, too-long tape on a chest dressing will loosen with chest expansion, while too-short tape will loosen with a position change. Tape is usually applied near the ends of a dressing and across the center as needed to hold it in place. When taping a dressing to a curved body area such as a shoulder or thigh, the tape should follow body contours. Figure 32–5 shows correct ways to apply adhesive tape.

Liquid or spray skin protectors, such as Skin-Prep or Benzoin, can be applied to the skin before taping a dressing in place. This adherent substance forms a protective coating and is especially helpful when the skin is fragile or thin and when tape must be removed frequently.

To remove tape, loosen and grasp the end of the tape strip. Hold the tape strip upright with one hand and push the skin downward and away from the tape, *removing the skin from the tape.* Do not pull the tape from the skin, as this sometimes strips the skin (removes superficial skin cells or layers) and leaves raw tissue, especially when the skin is fragile, thin, and poorly nourished. Always remove tape *toward* an incision, since tension outward from the wound may disrupt fragile healing structures.

Montgomery straps may be used when repeated dressing changes are necessary. Montgomery straps are cloth adhesive tape strips with reinforced tie-holes in one folded-back nonadherent end. The Montgomery straps are placed on either side of the incision

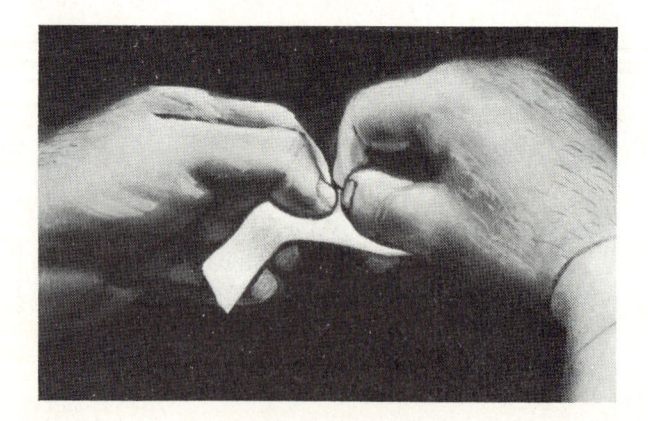

Figure 32–4. Tearing adhesive tape. Hold the tape firmly between the thumbnails and forefingers as shown. Initiate tearing by a quick rotary twisting of the hands in opposite directions. (Courtesy of Johnson and Johnson, New Brunswick, NJ.)

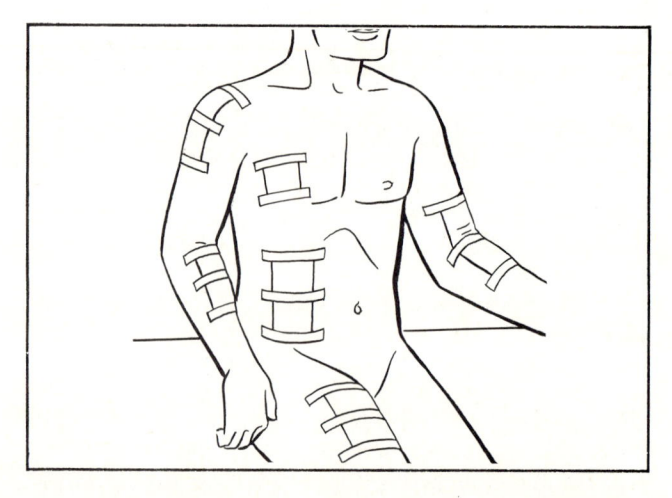

Figure 32–5. Correct length, width, and spacing of adhesive tape.

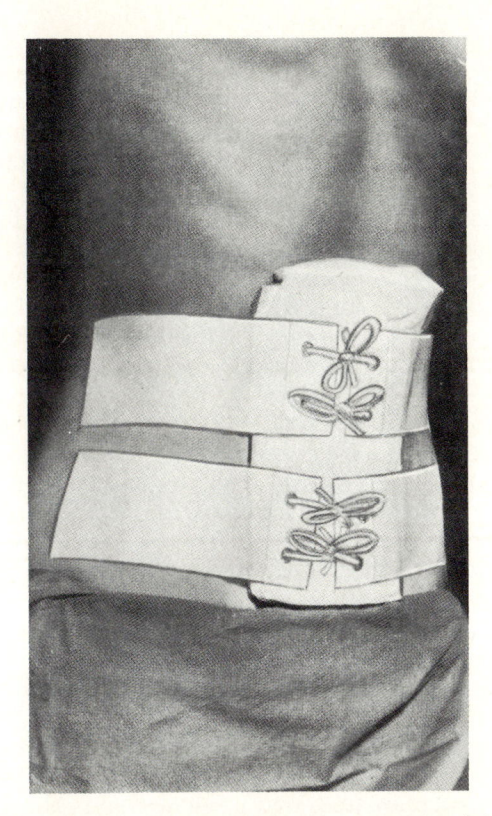

Figure 32–6. Montgomery straps used to secure an abdominal dressing. (Courtesy of Johnson and Johnson, New Brunswick, NJ.)

area, then tapes or gauze strips are attached to the holes and tied over the dressing, keeping them in place (see Fig. 32-6). An alternate method is to place a safety pin in each hole and then connect opposite pins with a strong rubber band. This method has the advantage of flexibility but the disadvantage of needing to be remove the pins before any x-rays are taken because the pins will appear on the x-ray. Unless soiled, Montgomery straps are not changed when the dressing is redone. Using Montgomery straps often increases the client's comfort and decreases the chances for skin damage from repeated tape changes. Montgomery straps are available commercially in large sheets with a number of holes. To use these Montgomery straps, cut the sheets into strips of the width that provides the best contour fit for the body part being bandaged. Montgomery straps also can be made from regular tape of any size by folding back one end of the tape on itself and cutting a tie-hole in the double nonadherent portion.

Hazards. *Allergic reactions* may result from the rubber base on regular adhesive tape; they are indicated by erythema (redness), edema, vesicles (small blisters), and papules (small solid elevated skin lesions). Allergic reactions usually appear within 48 hours. Check with the client or the family about previous tape allergies, or anticipate tape allergies in fair-skinned persons or those with other allergies, and make the tape selection appropriately. Allergies should be noted on the outside of the chart, in the client's record, and on the kardex card.

Chemical reactions occur when components of the backing or adhesive permeate the tissues, or sometimes when occlusive tape is used, causing redness of the skin. *Mechanical reactions* to tape removal include redness from induced vasodilation and skin stripping. The redness from induced vasodilation is temporary, while the redness from skin stripping lasts up to 24 hours.

When taping an extremity or digit, such as an arm or a finger, the tape should not encircle the body part completely, unless it is elastic tape. Constriction and arterial occlusion may occur when nonflexible adhesive tape is used in this way, with damage to body parts. As discussed earlier, if tape is removed incorrectly, suture lines can be weakened and skin layers removed accidentally.

Other Dressing Change Supplies

A *swab* or an *applicator,* which is made of rayon fluff twisted on the end of a stick, may be used to cleanse wounds, apply antibacterial ointment to a wound, or apply protective ointment to a skin surface. *Tongue blades* are thin, flat, lightweight pieces of wood used to apply protective or antibacterial ointment to skin surfaces or large open wound areas.

Several instruments used in changing a dressing are shown in Figure 32-7. A *dressing* or *tissue forceps* is a two-bladed instrument which is compressed at the handle and used to handle surgical dressings or pick

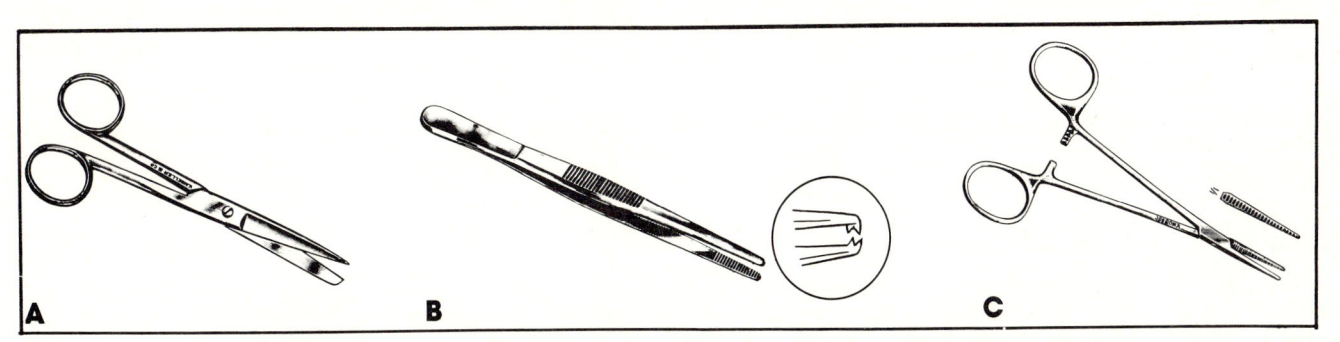

Figure 32–7. Equipment used for changing dressings. **A.** Dressing scissors. **B.** Dressing forceps (insert shows the difference between forceps "with teeth" and "without teeth"). **C.** Small straight hemostat. (Courtesy of American V. Mueller, Chicago, IL, Division of American Hospital Supply Corp.)

up sutures for cutting and removal. Forcep tips are serrated for a more secure grip and may be plain (smooth) or have "teeth." A smooth forceps is usually used for dressing changes, because teeth would catch in the gauze. A *hemostat* is a two-pronged instrument with scissors-style handles. The prongs are usually serrated to provide a more secure grip, and the handles have a ratchet for secure closure and holding. A *dressing scissors* is a straight-bladed scissors with either blunt or straight points. It is used to cut bandages, dressings, or tape.

Impermeable trash bags are made of plastic or waxed paper and are needed for disposal of moist or wet soiled dressings. Plain paper bags are satisfactory for dry soiled dressings.

Single-use *disposable dressing trays* in several sizes for small to large dressings contain all the sterile supplies usually needed for changing a dressing. The outer plastic bag is removed and used for a trash bag.

Institutionally prepared dressing trays often contain a small bowl, sponges used for skin preparation, dressing forceps, hemostat, scissors, and primary (4 × 4) and secondary (ABD or Surgipads) dressings. The wrapper may be used as a sterile field, and sterile gloves and antiseptic solution will need to be added prior to use. Impermeable trash bags and tape are also needed. Additional supplies are needed if sutures are to be removed (Skill 33), cultures taken (Skill 34), wound irrigation performed (Skill 35), or warm wet dressings (Skill 36) or wet-to-dry dressings (Skill 37) applied. If no dressing trays are available, the nurse simply gathers the needed supplies and creates a sterile work area using a sterile towel or barrier drape.

Binders and Bandages

An abdominal binder is sometimes used to hold a dressing in place on the abdomen rather than adhesive tape or Montgomery straps. It also lends support to the incision. Bandages may be used to hold dressings in place on extremities or the head. Binders and bandages are presented in Skill 48.

☐ EXECUTION

Scrupulous aseptic technique is essential when caring for wounds in an institutional setting, because of the significant role exogenous microorganisms play in the development of nosocomial wound infections, and because many clients have lowered resistance to infection. See Skill 34 for a further discussion of wound infections.

DRESSING TECHNIQUE

In the home, clean rather than sterile dressing technique often is acceptable unless the client is at a high risk of infection. The probability of introducing microorganisms foreign to the client is decreased in the client's own home environment. Clean rather than sterile dressings may be used, or sterile dressings may be applied with freshly washed hands. Sterile gloves may be worn if the client is particularly susceptible to infection, or if the care-giver needs protection from the wound drainage.

Careful handwashing always precedes and follows a dressing change so as to decrease the potential for wound contamination or cross-contamination to the nurse or other clients. When changing infected dressings, the risk of cross-contamination can be minimized by using two pairs of gloves: one pair to remove the old dressing and another to apply a new dressing. Clean gloves can be used to remove the infected dressing and sterile gloves to apply the new dressing; or two pairs of sterile gloves may be used. Place all used gloves and dressings in an impermeable trash bag and label as being contaminated. The techniques required for preventing the spread of different kinds of wound infections are discussed in Skill 29.

Dressings are not changed during or immediately after room cleaning. Cleaning sets up air currents that increase circulating particulate matter and bacterial fallout.

When using a dressing cart, remove all needed supplies from the cart before beginning the procedure. If more supplies are found to be needed in the course of the procedure, a second person may obtain them, or you must wash hands and reglove after obtaining the needed supplies. Wound cleansing and application of fresh dressings may be done while wearing one or two sterile gloves. When using one glove, wear the glove on the nondominant hand to handle sterile supplies or hold dressings in place. Use the nonsterile dominant hand to manipulate the handles of the sterile instruments and keep the tips sterile by placing them within the sterile field. The unsterile hand also is available to pour more sterile saline, open a tube of antibiotic ointment, or perform other needed activities. Two sterile gloves may be worn to change a dressing, but if unsterile equipment must be handled during this process, it is preferable to wear only one glove than to try to remember which gloved hand is sterile and which one is unsterile.

Always place a primary dressing (for example, 4 × 4's or Release) directly on the incision to provide a contact dressing that will draw any drainage up and away from the wound, keeping the skin surface fairly clean and dry. The number of primary dressings used will vary depending on the area to be covered and the amount of drainage anticipated. One to three layers of primary dressings often are used. When a stab wound drain is present, place separate primary dressings over the drain and the incision. This draws the drainage upward into the secondary dressings from both separate areas, rather than allowing drainage to flow along the skin which results in cross-contamination between the two areas. Do not place secondary dressings (for example, ABD's or Surgipads) directly on an incision, as they more readily adhere to a wound because of their fluffy filler material. Figure 32–8 diagrams an

EXAMPLE OF A PROPER WOUND DRESSING

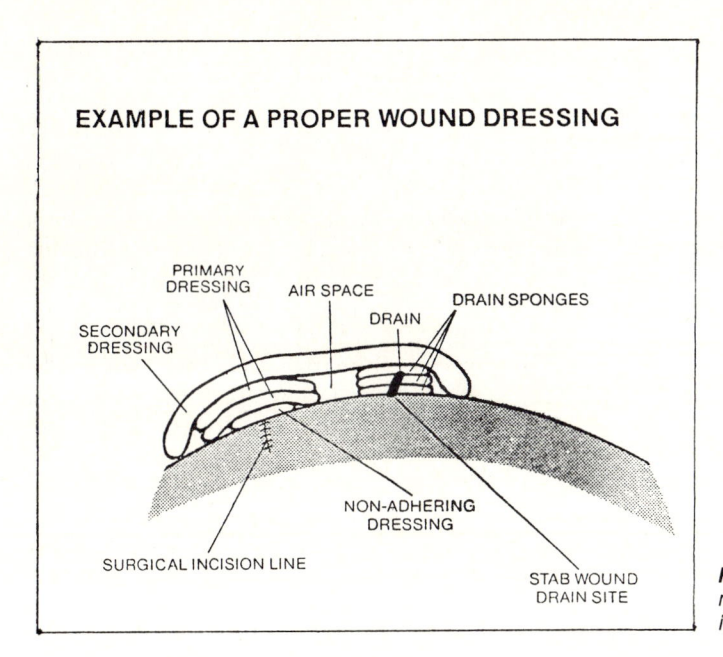

Figure 32–8. Cross section of proper wound dressing. Adapt as needed for different types of wounds. (By Saul Kramer Graphics. Courtesy of Johnson and Johnson, New Brunswick, NJ.)

appropriate way to apply primary and secondary dressings on a wound with a drain. The amount and size of the dressing materials will obviously vary with the specific wound.

WOUND CLEANSING

There are no definitive rules about wound cleansing. Some sources indicate routine cleansing of the incision should be done (Kozier and Erb, 1983; Meshelaney, 1979). Others suggest that removing dried drainage on an adhered dressing may disturb the healing epithelium (Cooper and Schumann, 1979; Noe and Kalisch, 1978).

Many surgeons have specific preferences for cleansing or not cleansing a wound, as well as the type of antiseptic to use. Know and respect the surgeon's preferences for wound care unless client safety is being compromised. In those circumstances, discuss wound care with both the area supervisor and the surgeon.

Wounds may be mechanically cleansed to remove exudate and surface debris by using gauze sponges saturated with an antiseptic, such as povodine-iodine (Betadine) or 70 percent alcohol. Sterile normal saline, water, or half-strength peroxide also may be used. If peroxide is used to oxidize and loosen thickened or crusty exudate, rinse it off with sterile water or saline after the effervescent action is finished.

Always cleanse a wound from an area that is cleaner to an area that is less clean. Because of the high rate of endogenous bacterial infections in which the causative organism comes from the client, the wound is always considered to be cleaner than the surrounding skin, even if there is wound drainage present. Meshelaney (1979) indicates that the bacterial population is lower at the center of the incision and higher at the ends. Because of this, she recommends cleansing the incision from the center outward, and then laterally from the incision (Kozier and Erb, 1983; Sorensen and Luckmann, 1979; Wolff et al., 1983).

To determine the cleansing approach to use for a particular wound, consider where the cleanest part of that wound might be and base the cleansing approach on that assessment. In a vertical incision, the cleanest area probably is at the top, and top to bottom cleansing would be most appropriate. The best way to cleanse a horizontal incision usually is from the center outward. If there is a stitch abscess at one or more sutures, that would be a less clean area than the remainder of the incision. In this situation, cleansing should be done toward the abscess, so that bacteria are not transferred from the abscessed area to the rest of the incision.

A drain site is considered less clean than the incision and is cleansed separately, after the incision. Cleanse a drain or stab wound in a circular spiral pattern, changing swabs after each two rounds. On a vertical or horizontal wound, use a sponge or swab for only one cleansing stroke and then discard it, so as not to transfer bacteria from one area to another. Figure 32–9 shows these wound cleansing methods.

Agency policy may indicate that the suture line itself is cleansed directly only with a specific physician order. In this situation, cleanse the skin area around the wound in the manner described above, omitting the suture line. Cleansing the area around a wound will contribute to a client's psychological well-being and physical comfort.

A common problem for clients with large open draining wounds or wounds with draining fistulae (abnormal tubelike passages between internal organs and the body surface) is the skin irritation and excoriation that comes from constant contact with body tissue

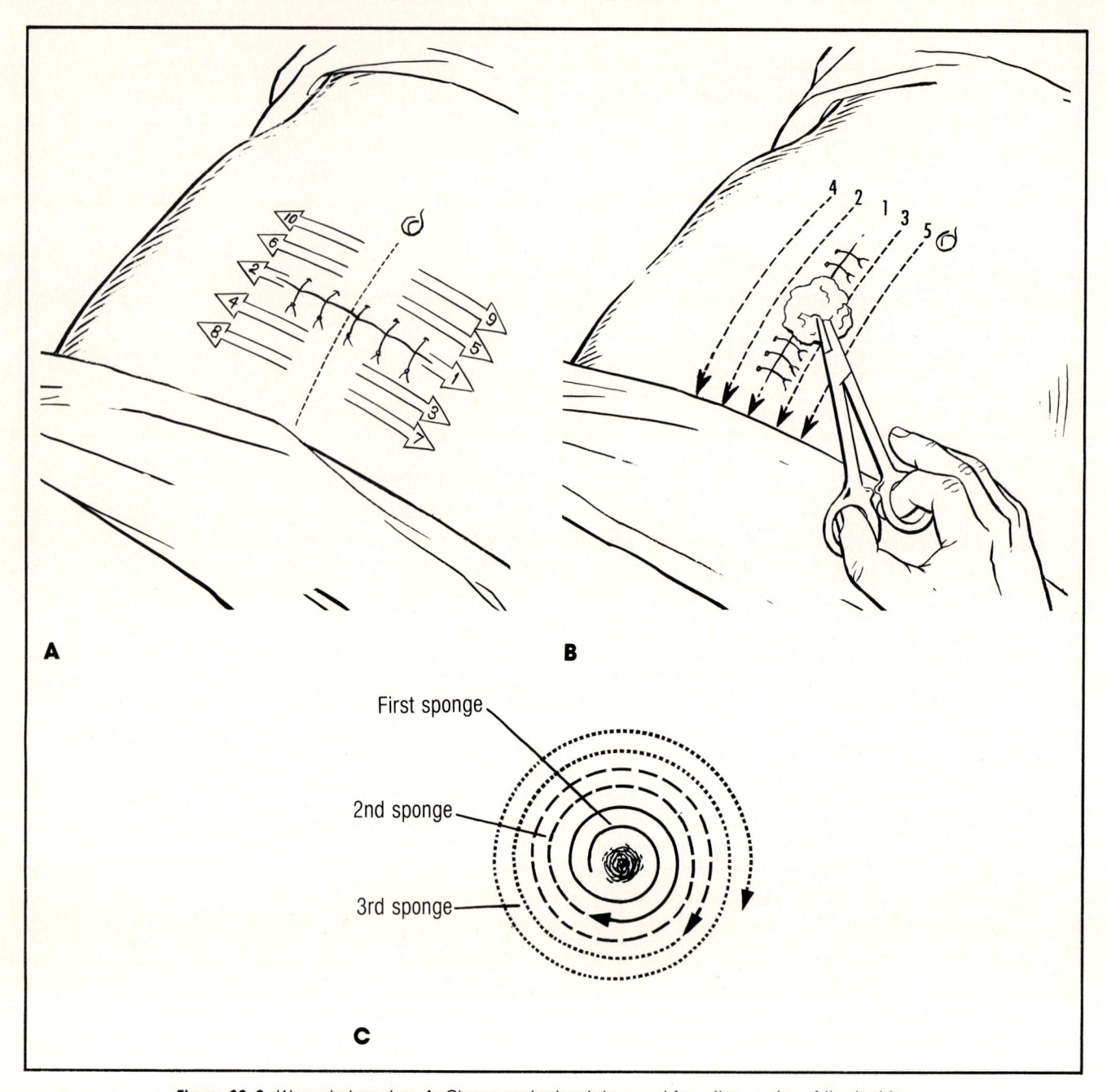

Figure 32–9. Wound cleansing. **A.** Cleanse a horizontal wound from the center of the incision outward and then laterally. Discard swab after each stroke. **B.** Cleanse a vertical wound from top to bottom, and then laterally. Discard swab after each stroke. **C.** Cleanse a drain or stab wound in a circular motion, discarding the sponge after each first or second cycle, depending on the amount of drainage.

fluids, urine, or fecal material. Another common problem is simply containing the drainage and controlling the odor for personal, physical, and psychological comfort and reasons of aesthetics. Many different products have been used to counter these problems. One of these involves the use of Karaya powder, glycerine, and aluminum hydroxide, along with stomal pouches such as ostomy bags (Brubacher, 1982; Manson, 1976). A semipermeable film may be useful for these difficult dressings. Frequent dressing changes, removal of soiled dressings from the room, and air purifiers all help control odor from draining wounds. Buttermilk and normal saline irrigations also have been found to be helpful (Welch, 1982).

☐ SKILL SEQUENCE

DRESSING CHANGE WITH WOUND CARE

Step	Rationale
1. Wash hands thoroughly.	Decreases potential for cross-contamination from transient microorganisms.
2. Select needed equipment: sterile towel or wrapper for sterile field, dressings, tissue forceps, scissors, sterile basin, cleansing solution, swabs, tape, and an impermeable waxed paper or plastic trash bag. Note contents of prepackaged dressing trays.	Planning ahead saves time and extra steps. Soiled and contaminated dressings need to be contained safely.
3. Inspect sterile packages for intactness and sterility.	Ensures use of sterile equipment.
4. Explain procedure to client.	Increases cooperation with procedure; preserves client's right to know; promotes self-care knowledge.
5. Close room door or curtain.	Protects client's privacy and decreases contaminants from air flow.
6. Prepare large, clean, dry area near client to work from, where supplies will be easy to reach without turning the back or reaching across the sterile field.	Keeps the sterile field within sight and avoids accidental contamination.
7. Position client in comfortable manner, exposing entire dressing to worker. Gently adjust clothing and linens for visibility, but avoid unnecessary exposure. Use drapes as needed.	Promotes relaxation and cooperation. Protects personal privacy. Minimizes air currents that disseminate air contaminants. Provides for physical and psychological comfort; protects right to privacy.
8. Open trash bag and place in convenient place near client. Trash bag may be taped to bed rail or bedside table, if removed when dressing completed.	Prevents contamination of work area from soiled items used in wound care.
9. Inspect existing dressing for intactness, drainage, and the amount and kinds of dressings used and the way tape or straps were applied.	Assess if adequate or excessive dressings or tape were used.
10. Tear tape strips of the number and length most likely needed and attach by one end to the overbed table or bed rail. Cut new Montgomery tapes if needed.	Facilitates prompt fastening of dressing when completed.
11. Open prepackaged dressing tray, using aseptic technique (Skill 30, Skill Sequences, "Opening Envelope-Wrapped Sterile Packages," and "Opening Heat-Sealed Sterile Packages," pp. 277–279). OR: Prepare sterile field with double towels or barrier drape (Skill 30, Skill Sequence, "Preparing a Sterile Field," p. 279) and add needed items (Skill 30, Skill Sequences, pp. 281–282).	Maintains sterility of equipment during procedure.
12. Place clean protective pad under client.	Protects bed linen or clothing from accidental soiling.
13. Remove tape or Montgomery straps. To remove tape: a. Hold tape end upward at right angles to the skin and press downward on skin. Pull firmly and gently, removing the skin from the tape. b. Use acetone, alcohol, or oil to remove regular adhesive tape residue or to loosen tape from body hair. c. Wash area with soap and water if acetone is used.	Tape sticks to rubber gloves. Removing tape rapidly, at other than right angles, or pulling tape off skin may tear fragile skin. Removing tape with each dressing change increases comfort and decreases potential for skin breakdown. May cause chemical irritation to skin.
14. Don clean gloves.	Protects self from wound contaminants.
15. Remove old dressings gently, layer by layer, watching for adherence of dressing to the skin, incision, sutures, or drains. Dressing removal: a. Clean dry dressing: May use ungloved hand to grasp outer surface or corners of dressing. b. Soiled, contaminated, or wet dressings: Use clean examining gloves or forceps. c. If dressing adheres to wound, moisten with sterile normal saline, or half-strength hydrogen peroxide (H_2O_2) until dressing removes easily.	Avoids dislodging any drains; gives opportunity to note drainage. Adherent dressings can cause disruption of healing process and fibrin formation. Outside of clean, dry, dressing is considered nonsterile. Avoids transfer of potential pathogens to hands. Avoids unintentional removal of scabs or crusts, which interferes with healing.
16. Note amount and kind of drainage on dressings and any odors present.	Careful observations help document healing process or the development of complications.

(continued)

DRESSING CHANGE WITH WOUND CARE (Cont.)

Step	Rationale
17. Discard dressings in the impermeable trash bag prepared in step 8.	Avoids environmental contamination.
18. Remove clean gloves.	
19. Wash hands or cleanse with antiseptic foam.	Removes contaminants from hands.
20. Inspect wound for incisional exudate, redness, or swelling. Note suture integrity and location and function of drains, if present.	After 2 or 3 days, these signs may be indicative of possible infection.
21. Don one sterile glove on dominant hand.	Used to palpate incision.
22. Gently palpate incision, noting especially tender areas. Note healing ridge development after about the 5th day postoperative. Palpate area adjacent to incision and around drain. <u>Do not return to incision and palpate again.</u>	Unusual tenderness may indicate infection. Indicates adequate healing. Avoids potential for transfer of endogenous bacteria to incision from adjacent skin or drain site.
23. Remove glove and discard.	Glove is contaminated from contact with skin and incision.
24. Culture wound, if indicated. (See Skill 34.)	
25. Don one sterile glove on nondominant hand.	Provides one hand for sterile supplies, with the other available to hold sterile instruments by the handles or to manipulate unsterile equipment.
26. Cleanse wound, using sterile 4 × 4 gauze squares or applicators (not cotton balls or filled sponges).	Cotton ball lint and filler may stick to the sutures.
a. Fold sterile 4 × 4 in quarters with sterile gloved hand and grasp with hemostat held in clean ungloved hand.	Creates a swab to use for cleansing.
b. Dip sterile folded sponge or applicator tips in sterile cleansing solution, squeezing excess against edge of bowl. <u>Hold forceps tips downward at all times.</u>	Moistens sponge without contamination. Avoids contamination. When forceps tips are turned upward, gravity causes the solution to contact the nonsterile handle held by the ungloved hand. When forceps tips are turned downward again, gravity causes the now contaminated solution to run toward the sterile forceps tips and contaminates them and the sponge.
c. Cleanse the incision from the center of the suture line toward the ends, <u>using one stroke per swab.</u> Discard swab after each stroke, as in Figure 32–9A. Alternatives: For a vertical incision, cleanse from top to bottom, as in Figure 32–9B. Cleanse <u>toward</u> any infected or draining part of the incision.	Incision line is considered less contaminated than skin, even if wound is infected. Single use of swabs decreases transfer of organisms from one part of the wound to another. Cleanses from cleaner to less clean area.
d. Using the same method, continue to cleanse laterally from the incision for about 1 to 2 inches, using a fresh swab for each stroke.	Same as above.
e. Cleanse around drains, beginning at the drain and working outward in a circular movement until all surrounding skin area to be covered by dressings is clean. Change swabs after one of circular movements, depending on the amount of drainage (See Fig. 32–9C).	Same as above.
f. Place hemostat on sterile field, keeping tips sterile, handles nonsterile.	Allows hemostat to be used again if needed.
27. To apply antibiotic ointment to an incision:	
a. With ungloved hand, remove cap from tube and place it upright on table.	Avoids contamination of rim of cap.
b. With tube upside-down vertically, discard small amount of ointment into wastebasket, trash bag, or on edge of sterile field.	Removes any contaminants from rim of tube.
c. Squeeze small amount of ointment onto a sterile swab held either in a gloved or ungloved hand.	
d. Apply to incision, from center outward, using a fresh swab and fresh ointment for each stroke.	Avoids transfer of bacteria from one part of the wound to another. Avoids contamination of tube of ointment.
28. Apply tincture of Benzoin or other skin preparation to skin where tape will be applied (optional, depending on skin condition).	Provides protective coating to skin and decreases probability of skin damage with tape removal.
29. Apply protective ointment to skin if ordered or needed, using a sterile gauze pad, tongue blade, or swab.	Helps avoid skin breakdown if urine, feces, or tissue fluid is in prolonged contact with skin.

(continued)

Step	Rationale
30. Using sterile gloved hand and forceps (or donning second sterile glove):	
a. Place a primary dressing of 4 × 4's directly over the incision. Do not shift or slide dressing.	Serves as wicking to draw fluid upward toward outer secondary dressing. Sliding dressings moves contaminants from skin to wound. Protects skin from tissue fluid drainage. Absorbs drain exudate.
b. Place precut dressings around and under Penrose drains (or cut sterile 4 × 4's toward center with sterile scissors). Direct drain away from incision. Add more 4 × 4's on top of the drain.	Wound drainage from the drain could introduce bacteria into the incision.
c. Place secondary combipad over both primary dressing sites. If there is scant drainage, omit secondary dressing.	Provides for increased absorption of wound drainage.
31. Remove glove or gloves and discard in trash. Fasten dressing with prepared tape, Montgomery ties, or binder.	Tape adheres to surgical gloves. Tape or ties prepared in advance facilitates fastening the dressing.
32. Replace client's clothing and bed linens. Reposition for comfort.	
33. Dispose of equipment:	
a. Close soiled dressing bag tightly and place in trash container outside of client's room.	Avoids spread of contaminants, removes them from client's immediate environment, and is more pleasing aesthetically.
b. Discard disposable items.	Appropriate care of equipment.
c. Rinse and return reusable items to central supply for cleaning and resterilization. (EXCEPTION: If patient is on wound precautions, do not rinse before double-bagging and returning to central supply.)	See Skill 29, "Isolation Techniques," pp. 250–253.
34. Wash hands.	Prevents transfer of microorganisms.
35. Document dressing change in health record. Include wound status, amount and character of drainage, and type of dressing applied.	Fulfills nurse accountability and provides ongoing data base.

RECORDING

Record dressing changes and wound care in the nurses' notes, integrated progress notes, or on a flow sheet in the client's health record. Include the amount and kind of drainage; the appearance of the wound; indications of healing or infection; and the client's comments, general reaction, and state of comfort or discomfort. Write any physician and nursing orders about the dressing procedure in the kardex or add them to the computer care plan.

Sample POR Recording

- S—States pain medication lasts 3½–4 hours. Able to turn and cough after pain medication.
- O—Two 4 × 4's and 1 ABD half-saturated with serosanguineous drainage. Wound edges clean and well-approximated.
- A—Wound healing well. Pain relief adequate.
- P—New dressing of two 4 × 4's and 1 ABD applied and clean Montgomery strap ties inserted. Continue dressing change and evaluate volume of drainage q 8 hr.

Sample Narrative Recording

Dressing changed—two 4 × 4's and one ABD half-saturated with serosanguineous drainage. Wound edges clean and well-approximated with no local indications of wound infections. Comfortable with q 3–4 hr pain med. Coughs and turns well after medication.

☐ CRITICAL POINTS SUMMARY

1. Wound healing proceeds in a predictable time sequence of known events.
2. Wound healing occurs by first, second, or third intention.
3. Wound care can promote or hinder wound healing.
4. Use strict aseptic technique for changing wound dressings.
5. Inspect dressing prior to removal.
6. Place soiled dressings in impermeable trash bag.
7. Inspect wound and surrounding area.
8. Cleanse incision from cleaner to less clean areas, then laterally from the wound, ending with any drains.
9. With sterile gloves, palpate the incision for areas of tenderness and for the healing ridge.
10. Apply sterile primary and secondary dressings in amounts and locations appropriate for the wound.
11. Using aseptic technique, cut sterile dressings as needed to fit around any tubes or drains.

308 PROFESSIONAL CLINICAL NURSING SKILLS

12. Fasten dressing securely enough not to slip but not enough to occlude a nonocclusive dressing.
13. Record amount and kind of drainage, appearance of wound, status of sutures and drains.
14. Report signs of healing, infection, wound separation, hematomas, or delayed healing.

☐ LEARNING ACTIVITIES

1. Examine the contents of a dressing cart of a dressing supply area. Indicate the location of these supplies by placing a "C" (dressing *c*art), "S" (*s*torage area), or "NA" (*n*ot *a*vailable) before the item. (NOTE: Availability will vary with the institution.)
   - _____ a. Hypoallergenic paper tape
   - _____ b. Hypoallergenic cloth tape
   - _____ c. Elastic adhesive tape
   - _____ d. Regular adhesive tape
   - _____ e. Butterfly skin closures
   - _____ f. Steri-Strips
   - _____ g. Montgomery straps and ties
   - _____ h. Primary dressings (4 × 4's)
   - _____ i. Nonocclusive abdominal dressings
   - _____ j. Occlusive abdominal dressings
   - _____ k. Nonadhering dressings (specify kind)
   - _____ l. Medicated dressings (specify kind)
   - _____ m. Packing (specify kind)
   - _____ n. Spray-on dressings (specify kind)
   - _____ o. Antiseptic solutions (specify kind)
   - _____ p. Gauze prep sponges (unfilled flats)
   - _____ q. Safety pins
   - _____ r. Rubber bands
   - _____ s. Sterile towels, basins, gloves
   - _____ t. Impermeable trash bags
   - _____ u. List other available dressing supplies

   Indicate where and how these supplies might be available, for example, by special order from central supply.

2. With a marking pen or taped-on line, simulate an abdominal incision and drain location on a peer. With actual equipment (sterile or clean), role-play applying an abdominal dressing, using strict aseptic technique. Have another peer monitor your technique, using the Skill Sequence, "Dressing Change with Wound Care," p. 305, and the Performance Checklist, p. 309, as guides.

3. Apply two pieces of adhesive tape to your own thigh or abdomen. Remove one piece by lifting the end of the tape and pulling the tape off of your skin. Note the directional pull of the skin and tissues. Remove the second piece of tape by lifting the end of the tape and pressing downward on the skin, progressively removing the skin from the tape. Note the directional pull of the skin and tissues. Compare the two methods and determine which would most likely cause less damage to sensitive or fragile skin.

☐ REVIEW QUESTIONS

1. Which of these signs and symptoms of postoperative wound healing would you consider to be expected or unexpected? Place an X in the correct column.

SIGN OR SYMPTOM	EXPECTED	UNEXPECTED
Absence of a healing ridge, day 4	_____	_____
Absence of a healing ridge, day 8	_____	_____
Bright red bleeding, day 1	_____	_____
Bright red bleeding, day 4	_____	_____
Inflamed wound edges, day 3	_____	_____
Inflamed wound edges, day 7	_____	_____
Serosanguineous fluid drainage, day 1	_____	_____
Serosanguineous fluid drainage, day 6	_____	_____

2. How would you describe sanguineous, serous, serosanguineous, and purulent drainage?
3. Why should a wet soiled dressing be changed rather than reinforced?
4. Why is it important to place soiled dressings in a nonpermeable trash bag?
5. What three actions during wound cleansing help decrease the probability of endogenous wound infections?
6. Under what circumstances would occlusive dressings be used?
7. Why is a nonocclusive dressing usually applied to a postoperative wound that is healing by primary intention?
8. How are primary and secondary dressings alike and how do they differ?
9. For what purpose are each of these dressing items usually used?
   - 3 × 3 gauze sponges
   - 4 × 4 gauze toppers (flats)
   - Combine dressings
   - Aeroplast dressings
10. For what reasons might Montgomery straps or a binder be used in a wound dressing?
11. A client's skin reddens when tape is removed. Match the observation in Column 1 with the probable cause in Column 2.

OBSERVATION	PROBABLE CAUSE
_____ Brief, transitory redness	a. Allergic reactions
_____ Redness with vesicles and papules	b. Loss of skin cells
_____ Redness lasting up to 24 hours	c. Loss of skin layers
_____ Weeping, reddened skin	d. Vasodilation

☐ PERFORMANCE CHECKLIST

OBJECTIVE: To use appropriate aseptic technique to change a wound dressing and provide wound care.

CHARACTERISTIC	RANGE OF ACCEPTABILITY	SATISFACTORY	UNSATISFACTORY
1. Washes hands.	No deviation		
2. Collects needed equipment.	No deviation		
3. Inspects for sterility.	No deviation		
4. Prepares clean, dry work area.	No deviation		
5. Positions client for wound visibility and privacy.	No deviation		
6. Inspects existing dressing.	No deviation		
7. Prepares trash bag.	No deviation		
8. Tears tape strips or Montgomery strap ties.	No deviation		
9. Prepares sterile supplies and field without contamination.	No deviation		
10. Removes old tape or ties and dressing, protecting self with gloves as needed.	No deviation		
11. Notes amount and kind of drainage.	No deviation		
12. Inspects wound for signs of healing or infection.	No deviation		
13. Palpates wound, wearing sterile glove.	No deviation		
14. Discards sterile glove and replaces with a new one.	Two sterile gloves may be worn.		
15. Cleanses wound, using correct technique: a. Uses each swab one time. b. Works from center of wound outward. c. Cleanses incision before drains.	No deviation Cleanse vertical wounds from top to bottom. Cleanse toward areas of infection. No deviation		
16. Places primary dressings (4 × 4's) directly on incision site before placing primary dressings around drains; positions drain away from incision.	No deviation		
17. Fastens secondary combipad securely over both primary dressings.	If only scant drainage, a primary dressing is sufficient.		
18. Disposes of equipment: a. Closes dressing bag. b. Disposes in utility room trash. c. Discards disposable items. d. Returns reusable items to central supply.	No deviation		
19. Washes hands.	No deviation		

REFERENCES

Alexander JW: Infection, Host Resistance, and Antimicrobial Agents. In Dudrick SJ, Baue AE, et al: Manual of Preoperative and Postoperative Care, ed 3. Philadelphia, WB Saunders, 1983.

American Hospital Association: Infection Control in the Hospital, ed 4. Chicago, American Hospital Association, 1979.

Auld ME, Craven RF, et al.: Wound healing. Nursing72 2(10):36–40, 1972.

Besst JA, Wallace HL: Wound healing—Intraoperative factors. Nursing Clinics of North America 14(4):701–712, 1979.

Brubacher LL: To heal a draining wound. RN 45(3):30–35, 1982.

Chrisp MA: A new treatment for pressure sores. Nursing Times 73(31):1202–1205, 1977.

Cooper DM, Schumann D: Postsurgical nursing intervention as an adjunct to wound healing. Nursing Clinics of North America 14(4):713–726, 1979.

Dinner MI, Peters CR, et al.: Use of a semipermeable polyurethane membrane as a dressing for split-thin graft donor sites. Plastic and Reconstructive Surgery 64(1):112-114, 1979.

Duoderm® Hydroactive™ Dressings, Technical Booklet. Princeton, NJ, Convatec, E. R. Squibb & Sons, 1983.

Encouraging news on temporary coverings for burn wounds. Journal of the American Medical Association 244(22):2493, 1980.

Harding K, Richardson G: Silastic foam elastomers for treating open granulating wounds. Nursing Times 75(39):1679-1682, 1979.

Kozier B, Erb GL: Fundamentals of Nursing: Concepts and Procedures, ed 2. Reading, MA, Addison-Wesley, 1983.

LeMaitre GD, Finnegan JA: The Patient in Surgery, ed 4. Philadelphia, WB Saunders, 1980.

Madden JW, Arem AJ: Wound healing: Biologic and clinical features. In Sabiston DC (ed): Davis-Christopher Textbook of Surgery, ed 12. Philadelphia, WB Saunders, 1981.

Madden JW: Wound Healing and Wound Care. In Dudrick SJ, Baue AE, et al.: Manual of Preoperative and Postoperative Care, ed. 3. Philadelphia, WB Saunders, 1983.

Manson H: Exorcising excoriation from fistulae and other draining wounds. Nursing76 9(8):57-60, 1976.

Meshelaney CM: Post-op wound dressings: Your guide to impeccable technique. RN 42(5):21-33, 1979.

Miller BF, Keane CB: Encyclopedia and Dictionary of Medicine, Nursing and Allied Health, ed 3. Philadelphia, WB Saunders, 1983.

Noe JM, Kalish S: The problem of adherence in dressed wounds. Surgery, Gynecology, and Obstetrics 148(2):185-188, 1978.

Remarkable advances in wound healing technology. Op-Site Seminar, American Hospital Supply, Indianapolis, IN, June 18, 1980.

Schumann D: The nature of wound healing. AORN Journal 35(6):1068-1077, 1982.

Schwartz SI, Shires GT, et al. (eds): Principles of Surgery, ed 4. New York, McGraw-Hill, 1984.

Sorensen KC, Luckmann J: Basic Nursing: A Psychophysiologic Approach. Philadelphia, WB Saunders, 1979.

Welch LB: Buttermilk and yogurt: Odor control of open lesions. Critical Care Update! 9(11):39-44, 1982.

Wolff L, Weitzel MH, et al.: Fundamentals of Nursing, ed 7. Philadelphia, JB Lippincott, 1983.

BIBLIOGRAPHY

Altemeier WA: Surgical Infections: Incisional Wounds. In Bennett JV, Brachman PS (eds): Hospital Infections. Boston, Little, Brown, 1979.

Altemeier WA, Alexander JW: Surgical Infections and the Choice of Antibiotics. In Sabiston DC (ed): Davis-Christopher Textbook of Surgery, ed 12. Philadelphia, WB Saunders, 1981.

Altemeier WA, Burke JF, et al.: (Editorial Subcommittee of the Committee on Control of Surgical Infections, American College of Surgeons). Manual on Control of Infection in Surgical Patients. Philadelphia, JB Lippincott, 1976.

Bauman B: Update your technique for changing dressings: Dry to dry. Nursing82 (Horsham) 12(1):64-67, 1982.

Brunner LS, Suddarth DS: Textbook of Medical-Surgical Nursing, ed 5. Philadelphia, JB Lippincott, 1984.

Castle M: Wound care: Clear-cut ways to speed healing. Nursing75 5(8):40-44, 1975.

Chang LF: A big payoff for painstaking care. RN 44(8):59-63, 1981.

Cruse PJE, Foord R: A five-year prospective study of 23,649 surgical wounds. Archives of Surgery 107(2):206-210, 1973.

Dudrick SJ, Baue AE, et al.: Manual of Preoperative and Postoperative Care, ed 3. Philadelphia, WB Saunders, 1983.

Groszek DM: Promoting wound healing in the obese patient. AORN Journal 35(6):1132-1135, 1138, 1982.

Hardy JD: Surgical Complications. In Sabiston DC (ed): Davis-Christopher Textbook of Surgery, ed 12. Philadelphia, WB Saunders, 1981.

Humphreys PT, Barthel CS: Power spray cleaning for those hard-to-clean wounds. Nursing83 (Horsham) 13(4):42-43, 1983.

Johnson & Johnson Products Catalog. New Brunswick, NJ, Johnson & Johnson Company, 1979.

Keithley JK: Wound healing in malnourished patients. AAORN Journal 35(6):1094-1099, 1982.

Laughlin VC: Stop the constant drip of draining wounds. Nursing74 4(12):26-27, 1974.

Peacock EE Jr, Van Winkle W Jr: Wound Repair, ed 2. Philadelphia, WB Saunders, 1976.

Rook A: Textbook of Dermatology, ed 3. London, Blackwell Scientific Publications, 1979, vols 1, 2.

Schilling JA: Wound healing. Surgical Clinics of North America 56(4):859-874, 1976.

Westaby S, Everett WG: The wound irrigation device: A new technique for managing troublesome wounds. Nursing Times 75(9):351-353, 1979.

Yordan EL, Bernhard AA: The surgeon's role in wound healing. AORN Journal 35(6):1078-1082, 1982.

SUGGESTED READING

Brubacher LL: To heal a draining wound. RN 45(3):30-35, 1982.

Cuzzell JZ: Wound care forum: Artful solutions to chronic problems. American Journal of Nursing 85(2):163-166, 1985.

Schumann D: The nature of wound healing. AORN Journal 35(6):1068-1077, 1982.

Yordan EL, Bernhard AA: The surgeon's role in wound healing. AORN Journal 35(6):1078-1082, 1982.

AUDIOVISUAL RESOURCES

I Dress the Wound
  Videotape. (1974, Color, 26 min.)
  Available through:
    Johnson and Johnson Products, Inc.
    501 George Street
    New Brunswick, NJ 08903

Draining Wound Management
  Videocassette. (1984, Color, 28 min.)
  Available through:
    American Journal of Nursing Company
    Educational Services Division
    555 West 57th St.
    New York, NY 10019

Wound Care
  Filmstrip. (1978, Color, 6 rolls, 15 min. each.)
  Available through:
    J.B. Lippincott Co.
    10 E. 53rd St.
    New York, NY 10022

Wound Management: The Surgical Dressing
  Filmstrip, slides, cartridge, videotape. (1981, Color, 23 min.)
Principles of Infection Control in Wound Care
  Filmstrip, slides, cartridge, videotape. (1981, Color, 23 min.)
Assessment of Wound Healing
  Filmstrip, slides, cartridge, videotape. (1981, Color, 20 min.)
  Available through:
    Medcom, Inc.
    P.O. Box 116
    Garden Grove, CA 92642

SKILL 33 *Suture Removal*

☐ PREREQUISITE SKILLS

Skill 19, "Inspection"
Skill 20, "Palpation"
Skill 28, "Handwashing"
Skill 30, "Sterile Supplies"
Skill 31, "Donning Sterile Gloves"
Skill 32, "Dressings and Wound Care"

☐ STUDENT OBJECTIVES

1. Explain the role of sutures in wound healing.
2. Compare the composition, durability, and tissue reactivity of absorbable and nonabsorbable sutures.
3. Describe the relationship between sutures and wound infections.
4. Explain the rationale for cutting sutures flush with the skin.
5. Describe the appropriate methods for removing five kinds of skin sutures.

☐ INTRODUCTION

The purpose of sutures is to hold the tissues of a wound together until they heal. Sutures are used inside the body as well as for skin closure.

Suture removal must be appropriately timed within the cycle of wound healing. Sutures that are removed too soon may result in a weakened wound, a wider scar, or even a separation of the wound. Sutures that are left in too long can become a local irritant or cause scars at the stitch sites. They also serve as an entry route for infection-producing microorganisms to enter the wound site.

Agency policy determines who removes sutures. In large teaching institutions, it is often done by medical students, interns, or residents. In smaller acute-care institutions, clinics, or physicians' offices, it may be considered a nursing function.

Suture removal is not a difficult procedure to perform; nor should it be painful for the client. There are some general guidelines and specific actions that will help the nurse accomplish this procedure safely and with minimal trauma to the client.

☐ PREPARATION

Sutures are classified as *absorbable* and *nonabsorbable*. Absorbable sutures are used inside body cavities or tissues and are digested and absorbed during the healing process by the body tissues in which they were placed. Nonabsorbable sutures are not digested by body tissues. They are used on the skin where they can readily be removed or inside the body where more permanent support is desired, such as in blood vessel repair.

The most widely used absorbable suture is a long-used natural substance—*catgut*. Despite its name, catgut is obtained from sheep or cow intestines. Plain catgut remains in the tissues for 3 days to a week before it is absorbed; chromic catgut, which is treated with chromic salts in order to retard its absorbability, does not absorb for 2 to 3 weeks. The absorbability of catgut obviously is an advantage for internal suturing; however, it does induce a marked inflammatory reaction within tissues. In the skin this causes redness and swelling around each suture, which can result in tissue necrosis and excessive scarring. Catgut does not survive well in infected wounds, as infection increases its rate of absorption.

Nonabsorbable sutures are made of *cotton, silk, linen, stainless steel wire,* or *synthetics* such as polyester fiber or polypropylene. Nonabsorbable sutures are either braided or twisted fibers or a single straight strand, known as monofilament sutures. A braided or

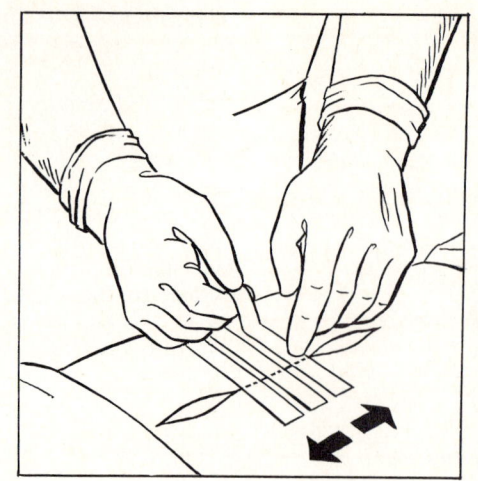

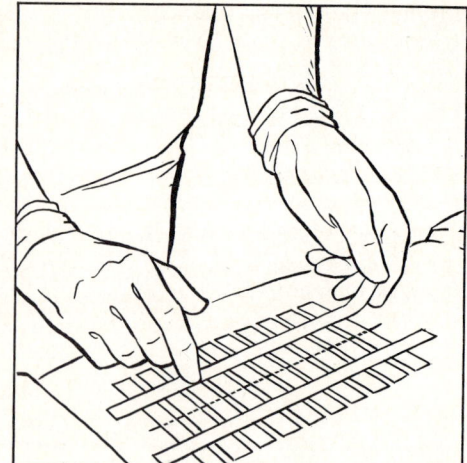

Figure 33–1. Application of Steri-Strips. This microporous sterile surgical tape can be used as a primary wound closure or for added wound stability after suture removal. (Courtesy of 3M Surgical Products Division, St. Paul, MN.)

twisted suture is stronger than a single filament of the same type of suture. If an infection is present, however, only monofilament sutures are used since twists and braids harbor microorganisms and thus may serve as an ongoing source of infection. Sometimes nonabsorbable sutures are extruded (pushed out) spontaneously, even after several years. This "spitting," as it is called, is not serious but can be disturbing to a client.

Sterile skin *staples* or skin *clips* are alternate closures for the skin or for the fascia in a wound that will be left open (Auto Suture, 1981).

Adhesive skin closures such as *Steri-Strips* may be used to maintain wound closure after suture removal or as the primary means of wound closure. Steri-Strips are thin strips of sterile, porous, reinforced, nonwoven fabric tape. They provide a better cosmetic appearance as there are no suture marks, and they are more comfortable for the client. Because they give added wound support, they help avoid widening of the scar, especially where the skin is taut, as on the forehead or a movable joint. Figure 33–1 illustrates the use and application of Steri-Strips. *Butterfly closures* also are used to give support after suture removal or to close small wounds. They have a narrow nonadhering center "bridge" that keeps the closure from sticking to the wound itself (Fig. 33–2).

Retention sutures, which are very heavy nonabsorbable sutures made of nylon, are sometimes used to add extra strength to abdominal incisions. They are stitched in such a way as to encompass all of the layers of the abdominal wall. Protective rubber tubes called bolsters or bumpers are placed around the exposed portions of retention sutures to keep them from cutting into the skin. They are left in place for 2 to 3 weeks, when scar tissue is strong enough to withstand straining and coughing. Retention sutures are nearly always removed by the surgeon, who assumes the responsibility for determining whether adequate healing has occurred.

The length of time for sutures to remain in the wound varies according to the rate of healing of the tissues in which they are placed and the amount of strain the sutures must take. As a general rule, facial sutures can be removed after 3 to 5 days, and other skin sutures after 5 to 7 days. However, in areas of high tension, such as the extensor surfaces of elbows and knees, skin sutures usually are left in place for 10 to 12 days. Sutures usually are left in place for 14 days for slow-healing areas, such as the palms of the hands and the soles of the feet, known as volar surfaces (Luckmann and Sorensen, 1980; Myers, 1971). Rook (1979) indicates that scalp sutures should be left in place for 5 to 8 days, and trunk and limb sutures for 7 to 14 days.

DATA BASE

In most institutions, a surgeon's written order is required when a nurse removes sutures. If the nurse is working in an independent practice or is isolated from medical contacts, the decision to remove sutures becomes a nursing judgment. Before implementing a surgeon's order to remove sutures or before removing them as an independent function, the nurse has the responsibility to assess the state of wound healing that has occurred. Wound healing is discussed in Skill 32.

Client History and Recorded Data

Since wounds heal at different rates in different parts of the body, it is important to determine the wound location and the number of days that have elapsed since surgery or injury. The client's age and diagnosis also affect the rate of healing. Older people heal more slowly than young adults, and patients with cancer or malnutrition often experience delayed healing. In addition to these data, the health record also describes the postoperative recovery period, including any interferences with wound healing.

The client often is able to report symptoms that may indicate an interference with healing (such as localized incisional pain).

SKILL 33: SUTURE REMOVAL

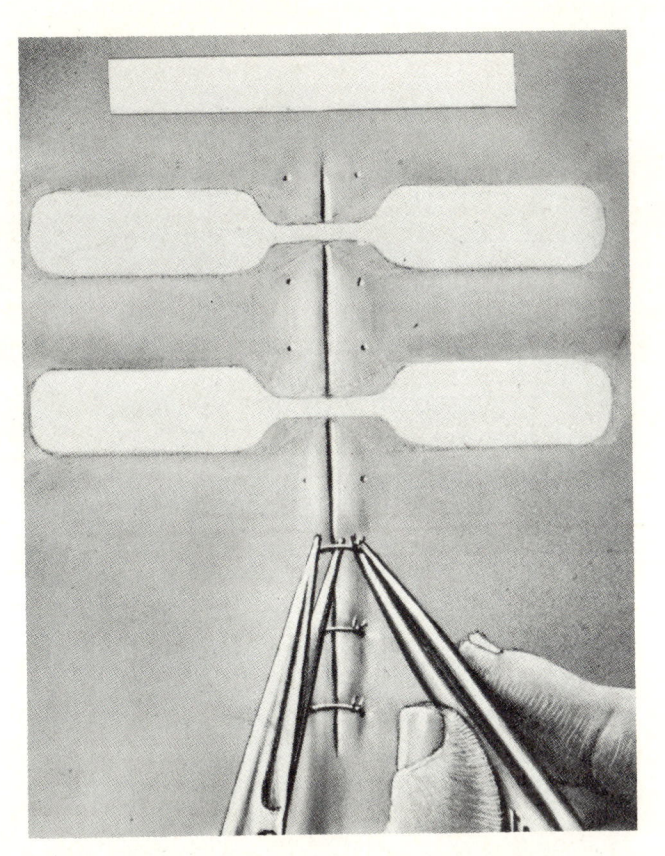

Figure 33–2. Butterfly closures. These sterile waterproof closures can be used to close small wounds or provide support after suture removal. (Courtesy of Johnson and Johnson, New Brunswick, NJ.)

The nurse also assesses the client's understanding of and previous experiences with suture removal. Although it is not usually a painful procedure, many clients fear suture removal, anticipating pain and discomfort or wondering whether adequate healing has occurred.

Physical Appraisal Skills

Inspection. The nurse *inspects* the wound for signs of healing or indications of complications. Presence or absence of a healing ridge, redness, and approximation of wound edges would be evaluated according to known data about wound healing. If signs of infection such as pus are present, if the edges are nonapproximated or weeping, or if the nurse has any questions about the degree of healing that has occurred, the surgeon should be consulted prior to removal of sutures. The nurse also inspects the sutures to determine the correct way to remove them.

Palpation. Palpate the wound to determine any areas of unusual tenderness. Again, the degree of generalized tenderness would be evaluated on the basis of the nurse's knowledge of wound healing.

EQUIPMENT

Suture scissors are small, sharp scissors with curved or pointed tips designed specifically for removing various kinds of sutures or wires. The special tips increase the ease of inserting the scissors under tightly knotted sutures. A *dressing forceps* (also called *thumb forceps*) is used to pick up the individual suture knot for cutting ease. A *small hemostat* sometimes is used to pick up and hold the suture knot while cutting the suture. Forceps and hemostats are illustrated in Figure 32–7, p. 301; a suture scissors is shown in Figure 33–3.

Many agencies have pre-prepared *suture removal sets,* either disposable or reusable. Such kits contain a plastic dressing forceps, plastic suture scissors, and gauze sponges. When opened, the inside of the reusable wrapper or the disposable heat-sealed package can be used as a small sterile field. A *skin staple remover* is a presterilized, single-use tool used to remove skin staples from an incision.

Other equipment needed for suture removal is the same as for a dressing change and cleansing (presented in Skill 32); that is, antiseptic solution, gauze sponges, hemostats, dressings, and tape.

☐ EXECUTION

In areas of tension or slow healing, alternate stitches are removed first. The remaining stitches are then removed one or more days later, depending on the appearance of the approximated edges. To provide addi-

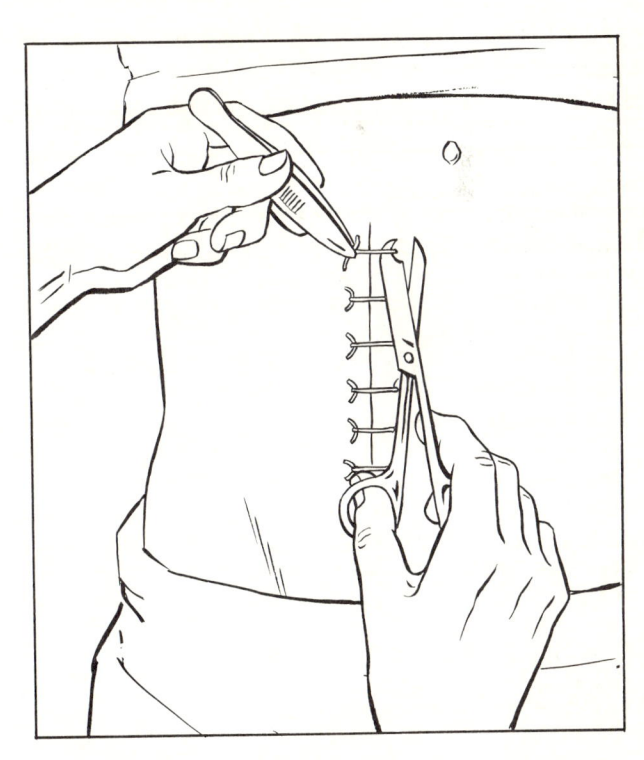

Figure 33–3. Removing plain interrupted sutures, using a curved-tip suture scissors and a fine-pointed tissue forceps.

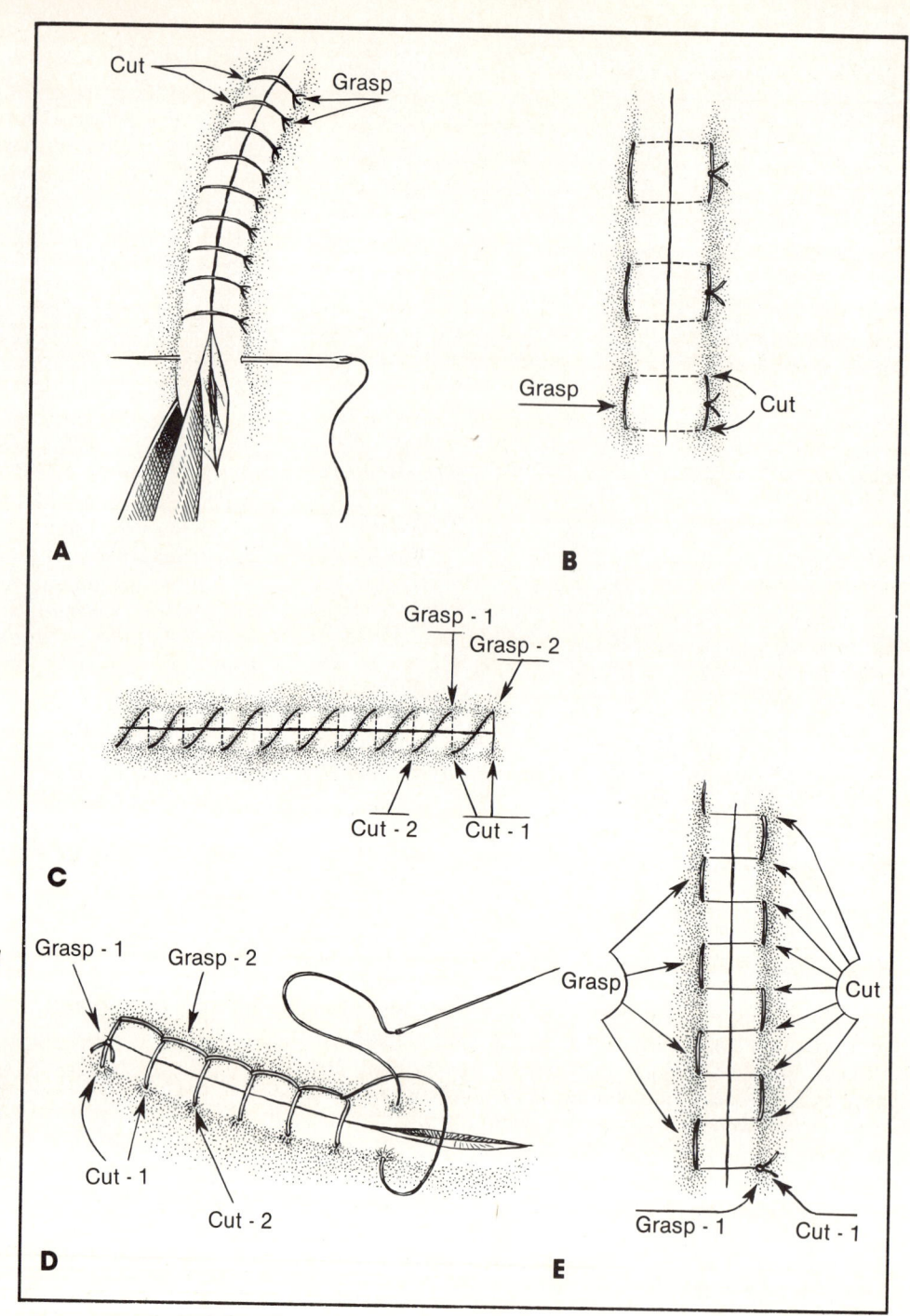

Figure 33-4. Skin suture removal. Appropriate sites for grasping and cutting the suture are indicated. "Grasp 1" indicates the site for grasping the first suture and for pulling to remove that suture. "Cut 1" indicates the site for cutting the first suture. "Grasp 2" and "Cut 2" refer to the second suture and all successive sutures, unless otherwise indicated. **A.** Plain interrupted. **B.** Mattress interrupted. **C.** Plain continuous. **D.** Blanket continuous. **E.** Mattress continuous. (Adapted from Manual of Operative Procedures, ed 10, Ethicon, Somerville, NJ, 1977.)

tional tensile strength and minimize scar widening, Steri-Strips or butterfly closures are frequently used after removal of alternate or all sutures.

Prior to removing sutures, cleanse the incision and stitches with an antiseptic to decrease the resident bacteria and remove dry crusts. Hydrogen peroxide may be used to help remove crusts, followed by a sterile saline rinse and cleansing with an antiseptic. However, even after cleansing, the visible parts of the suture are contaminated with resident skin bacteria and should *not* be pulled through under the skin when removed. The stitch sites may be cleansed again after the sutures are removed if crusts remain.

To remove sutures, grasp the knot with the hemostat or forceps and raise the knot upward from the skin for increased visualization and cutting ease, as shown in Figure 33-3. When lifting sutures for cutting, be sure not to use a directional pull that draws the visible suture down under the skin. Cut the suture flush with the skin to avoid drawing any exposed suture down into and then up out of the skin. Remove sutures from the proximal to the distal end of the incision, which usually is the same sequence in which they were inserted.

The cutting site for safe suture removal varies with the type of suture insertion. The five common skin suture insertion methods are plain interrupted, mattress interrupted, plain continuous, mattress continuous, and blanket continuous (Manual, 1977). Diagrams of these insertion methods are depicted in Figure 33-4, along with the sites for grasping and cutting each type of suture.

Plain interrupted sutures: Raise the knot from the skin, and cut the thread on one side of the incision. Remove sutures.

Mattress interrupted sutures: Grasp the knot with a hemostat to stabilize it. Cut at both sides of the knotted portion of the suture and discard the knotted fragment. Grasp the exposed suture in the opposite side of the incision and pull to remove.

Plain continuous sutures: Cut the suture at two places; opposite the knot and at the thread below on that same side. Remove the first stitch. Grasp and raise the next visible thread, pulling the loose end up and out of the skin. Cut flush with the skin.

Blanket continuous sutures: Grasp the knot and cut the suture opposite the looped side and at the stitch below, also opposite the looped side. Remove the first stitch and discard it. Grasp the next stitch and cut opposite the looped side. Remove the stitch, pulling the suture up and out of the skin.

Mattress continuous sutures: Cut the first suture across from the knot or at one side of the knotted section and remove the first stitch by grasping and pulling the knot. Lift and cut visible sections on one side of the incision. Grasp the suture segment on the opposite side, and pull to remove stitch. If visible sections on one side are very short, cut the longer visible segment at both sides of the segment, grasp the short segment, and remove the remainder of the stitch.

Figure 33-5 illustrates insertion of skin staples and gives directions for removing them.

A small, lightweight dressing may be placed over the wound for a day or so after sutures are removed. The individual usually may shower within a day or two after sutures are removed.

☐ SKILL SEQUENCE

SUTURE REMOVAL

Step	Rationale
1. Confirm the order for suture removal.	Demonstrates accountability.
2. Wash hands.	Avoids transfer of microorganisms from nurse's hands.
3. Select suture removal equipment; check for indicators of sterility.	Ensures use of safe equipment.
4. Explain procedure to client.	Decreases apprehension.
5. Position client for easy exposure of entire wound. Remove clothing or bed linen as needed for complete wound exposure, using additional drapes as needed for privacy.	Involves client in own care. Complete assessment of wound is impossible with only partial visualization.
6. Inspect dressing, remove and dispose of as in Skill 32, Skill Sequence, "Dressing Change with Wound Care," steps 9 to 19, pp. 305–306.	Provides data for evaluating wound healing and for recording in the health record.
7. Inspect and cleanse the wound as in Skill 32, Skill Sequence, "Dressing Change with Wound Care," steps 20 to 26, p. 306, carefully cleansing each stitch site. Use hydrogen peroxide followed by saline to remove crusts as needed.	Provides opportunity to assess wound healing. Decreases potential for introducing endogenous microorganisms into the wound.
8. Grasp the first knot with tissue forceps or hemostat, raise knot from skin and cut suture flush with skin. Pull stitch upward and out of skin. Do not allow the exposed suture to enter the skin tract created by the stitch. Drop stitch on gauze pad.	Increases visualization of the suture and makes it possible to cut suture close to skin surface. Visible sutures are contaminated with resident microorganisms of the skin. Suture may stick to instruments. Sterile gauze square can aid in removal and provides a place to deposit sutures without contaminating the instruments.
9. Remove alternate stitches, unless otherwise indicated. Continuous sutures must be completely removed at one time.	Provides gradual removal of suture support without a sudden increase in tension on wound.
10. Cleanse stitch areas with antiseptic or peroxide to remove remaining crusts.	Promotes comfort and removes sites that may harbor bacteria.
11. Place Steri-Strips or butterfly closures across wound, unless otherwise indicated.	Decreases chances of excessive tension on wound.
12. Apply a small nonocclusive dressing or leave wound exposed, according to client's or physician's preference.	Protects from injury and from catching the remaining sutures on clothing or linen. Air circulation helps keep wound dry and promotes healing.
13. Dispose of equipment correctly.	
14. Reposition client for comfort.	
15. Wash hands.	Avoids cross-contamination.
16. Record procedure in health record.	Provides for accountability and continuity of care.

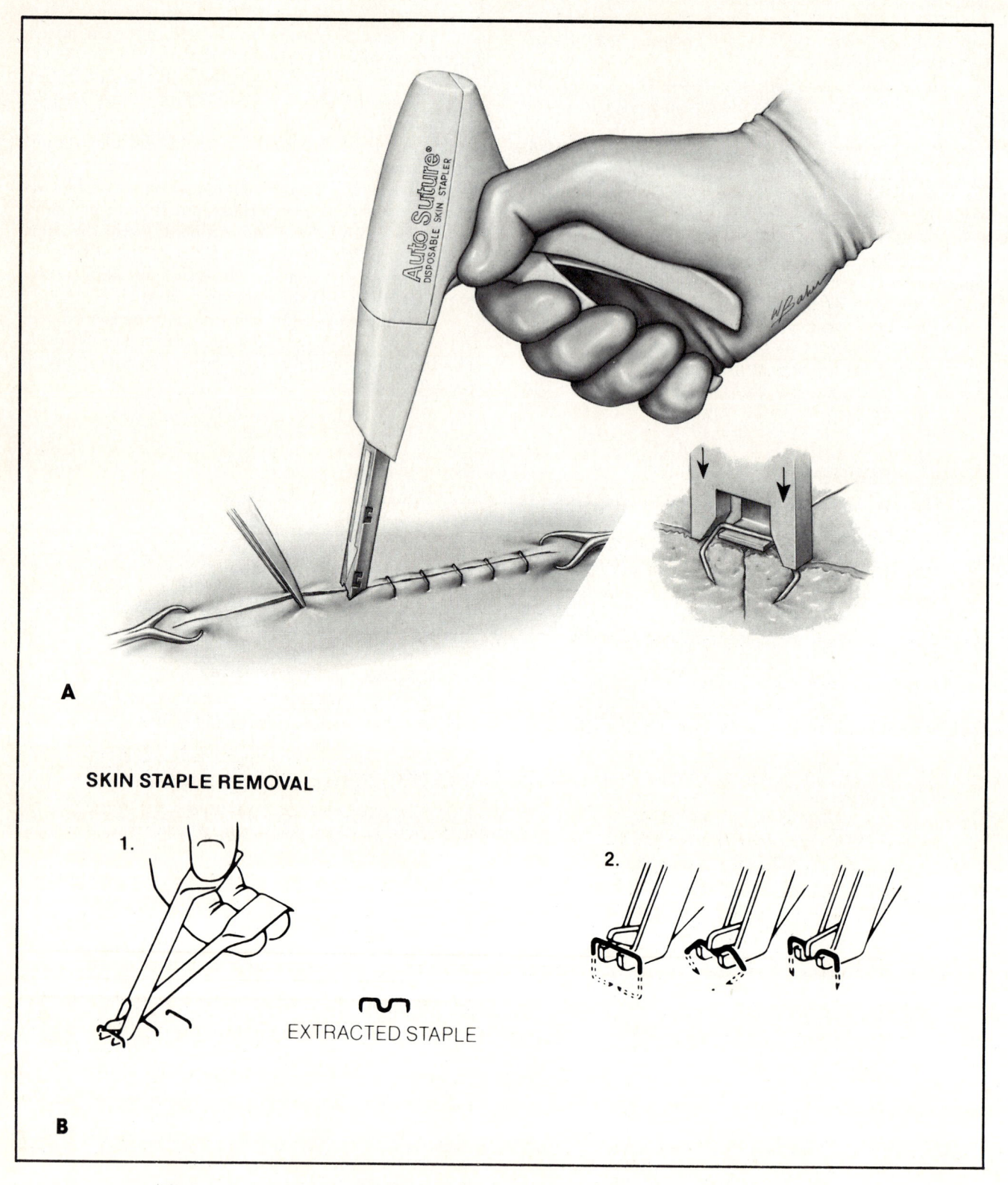

Figure 33-5. **A.** Inserting skin staples for wound closure. Detail insert shows position of staple within tissues. **B.** Removing skin staples with a staple extractor: (1) Place both lower jaws under the staple and close the handles to unbend the staple; (2) Lift the extractor straight up, bringing the staple up and out of the skin. Discard staples on gauze pad or in trash bag, as they are sharp and can cause injury. Discard staple extractor when all staples are removed. (© USSC 1974, 1975, 1980.)

RECORDING

The nurse's anecdotal notes include the appearance of the wound, dressings, and sutures; visible indications of wound healing; number of sutures removed; whether all or alternate sutures were removed; wound reinforcement, such as use of Steri-Strips; dressing application; and the client's response to the procedure.

Sample POR Recording

- S—"I'll be so glad when all those stitches are out!"
- O—Wound edges approximated and clean, except for slight oozing from distal stitch. No redness or tenderness noted.
- A—Wound healing fairly well, but has a potential problem area in distal stitch.
- P—Removed alternate stitches (5) as ordered. Steri-Strips placed on incision where sutures removed. Will observe incision q. shift and remove remaining sutures in 2 days as ordered, unless further drainage occurs.

Sample Narrative Recording

All sutures removed from abdominal wound as ordered. Incision clean and pink; healing ridge present. Steri-Strips applied to incision. Stated "I hope I don't fall apart now!" Wound healing and suture function explained. Seemed relieved and reassured.

☐ CRITICAL POINTS SUMMARY

1. Cleanse incision before and after suture removal, using an antiseptic solution.
2. Assess state of wound healing prior to suture removal.
3. Cut suture flush with skin surface.
4. Do not pull visible exposed portions of suture under and through the skin.
5. Remove alternate sutures or skin staples in areas of tension or slower healing.
6. Reinforce incision with adhesive skin closures or butterfly closures for several days.

☐ LEARNING ACTIVITIES

1. Using the suture insertion diagrams in Figure 33-4 and a needle and thread or yarn, stitch four or five "sutures" of each style on a heavy piece of paper. Remember to work only from the top surface of the paper (which represents the skin surface) and have all knots on that side of the paper. Examine pattern on underside.
2. Using an eyebrow tweezers and manicure scissors (or other small scissors), grasp the knots and cut the sutures at the points indicated in Figure 33-4. Remove each stitch slowly, observing the directional pull. Be sure no surface thread is pulled to the underside of the paper.
3. In a clinical area, locate suture removal equipment. List contents of suture removal sets or the labels of separate instruments needed.

☐ REVIEW QUESTIONS

1. With which type of skin suture would you expect the greatest problem with infection? the least?
2. After how many days postoperative would you expect to have sutures removed from these wounds?
   a. Laceration in the cheek
   b. Excision of mole from the forehead
   c. Abdominal surgery
   d. Knee surgery
   e. Laceration on the palm of the hand
3. What is the rationale for removing alternate sutures, and when is this practice most needed?
4. Why are sutures cut off flush with the skin?
5. Why might pulling exposed sutures downward into the skin predispose toward an endogenous infection?
6. What benefits occur from the use of Steri-Strips or butterfly closures?

☐ PERFORMANCE CHECKLIST

OBJECTIVE: To use aseptic technique to remove skin sutures and clips correctly.			
CHARACTERISTIC	RANGE OF ACCEPTABILITY	SATISFACTORY	UNSATISFACTORY
1. Washes hands.	No deviation		
2. Selects correct equipment.	No deviation		
3. Explains procedure to client.	No deviation		
4. Observes dressing and wound for data about wound healing.	No deviation		
5. Cleanses incision before and after sutures are removed.	Some surgeons may indicate other preferences.		
6. Grasps stitch with tissue forceps or hemostat and raises from skin.	No deviation		

(continued)

OBJECTIVE: To use aseptic technique to remove skin sutures and clips correctly (cont.).

CHARACTERISTIC	RANGE OF ACCEPTABILITY	SATISFACTORY	UNSATISFACTORY
7. Cuts suture flush with skin.	No deviation		
8. Cuts and removes sutures in a way that allows no exposed suture to be drawn downward into the skin.	No deviation		
9. Applies lightweight nonocclusive dressing.	Leave open, if indicated.		
10. Washes hands.	No deviation		
11. Disposes of equipment properly.	No deviation		
12. Records procedure.	No deviation		

REFERENCES

Auto Suture: Information Booklet. Norwalk, CT, Auto Suture Co., 1981.

Luckmann J, Sorensen KC: Medical–Surgical Nursing: A Psychophysiologic Approach, ed 2. Philadelphia, WB Saunders, 1980.

Manual of Operative Procedures, ed 10. Somerville, NJ, Ethicon, 1977.

Myers MB: Sutures and wound healing. American Journal of Nursing 71(9):1725–1727, 1971.

Rook A: Textbook of Dermatology, ed 3. London, Blackwell Scientific Publications, 1979.

BIBLIOGRAPHY

Cooper DM, Schumann D: Postsurgical nursing intervention as an adjunct to wound healing. Nursing Clinics of North America 14(4):713–726, 1979.

Kinney JM, Egdahl RH, et al.: Manual of Preoperative and Postoperative Care, ed 2. Philadelphia, WB Saunders, 1971.

Kozier B, Erb GL: Fundamentals of Nursing: Concepts and Procedures, ed 2. Reading, MA, Addison-Wesley, 1983.

SKILL 34 Wound Culture Specimen Collection

PREREQUISITE SKILLS

Skill 19, "Inspection"
Skill 20, "Palpation"
Skill 22, "Auscultation"
Skill 28, "Handwashing"
Skill 30, "Sterile Supplies"
Skill 31, "Donning Sterile Gloves"
Skill 32, "Dressings and Wound Care"

☐ STUDENT OBJECTIVES

1. Identify the common causes of wound infections.
2. Describe the signs and symptoms of a wound infection.
3. Describe assessment data that indicate a need for culturing a wound.
4. Compare the procedures for obtaining and caring for wound cultures of anaerobic and aerobic microorganisms.

☐ INTRODUCTION

A wound culture specimen is a sample of wound drainage that is collected when a wound infection is suspected or known to exist. The sample is used to inoculate laboratory culture media for the purpose of determining the microorganisms that are present in the specimen.

With the introduction and general use of antibiotic therapy, it was anticipated that postoperative wound infections would virtually be eliminated. Such infections, however, remain a serious problem; the widespread use and misuse of antibiotic therapy has led to a deemphasis of established surgical procedures, relaxation of the "surgical conscience," overdependence on antibiotic use, and development of antibiotic-resistant strains of bacteria that are more difficult to treat. In addition, newer immunosuppressant drug therapy for cancer and an increased incidence of other long-term debilitating illnesses have resulted in larger numbers of persons at increased risk for developing postoperative wound infections.

Regardless of the reason a wound infection develops, a significant aspect of treatment is antibiotic therapy directed specifically at the causative microorganism. Correct methods of collecting the culture specimen are crucial to an accurate laboratory identification of that causative microorganism through a culture and sensitivity or MIC test. Incorrect identification of the causative microorganism can result in incorrect and ineffective therapy.

Because the nurse inspects the wound and the dressing on a regular basis and monitors the client's vital signs, the nurse has the responsibility for noting indications of wound healing and the beginning signs of wound infections. The normal course of wound healing is discussed in Skill 32; This skill explains the process and signs of an infected wound and the methods of obtaining a specimen for culture.

While collection of a wound culture specimen often is specifically ordered by the physician, many agencies have policies that identify this as an independent nursing action when necessary. These policies usually are determined by an infection control committee consisting of nurses or bacteriologists or both.

☐ PREPARATION

The National Nosocomial Infections Study (NNIS), initiated in 1969, estimated the overall postoperative infection rate at 7.4 percent, with a lower rate for clean wounds and a much higher rate for contaminated or dirty wounds (Committee, 1976). The costs of postoperative infections are staggering for both the client and the agency. For the client, such infections mean the direct monetary costs of a lengthened hospital stay, as well as the indirect costs of time lost from productive employment, increased insurance premiums, personal grief and pain, and even loss of life or function. For the agency, they may mean adverse publicity or negative reviews from accrediting agencies.

According to Altemeier (1979), there has been a marked increase in the incidence of gram-negative wound infections since the early 1960s. While the incidence of infections caused by *Staphylococcus aureus* has declined, the NNIS found that the gram-negative *Escherichia coli* was as frequent a postoperative wound pathogen as the well-known *S. aureus,* together comprising 37.3 percent of the 27,000 wound infections in the study. Other common gram-negative pathogens identified in the study included *Pseudomonas aeruginosa* (8.8 percent) and *Proteus mirabilis* (5.6 percent). These bacteria are a common part of the resident and transient microbial flora of the average person.

Recent data from the continuing NNIS indicate that both the median nosocomial infection rate and the rate of surgical wound infections have been declining since 1975. There have been no major shifts noted in the relative frequency of the most common infection sites or the pathogens causing those infections. The reasons for the decline in infection rates are not clear, but it is known that more highly skilled surgeons have lower infection rates and institutions where large numbers of surgical procedures are performed have lower rates than those where few surgeries are performed. Bacteremias (widespread dissemination of pathogenic bacteria by way of the bloodstream) have increased in frequency, as have obstetrical surgical wound infections (Allen et al., 1981).

SOURCES OF WOUND INFECTIONS

Endogenous organisms (those from the client) are known to be a primary source of incisional infections. For example, clients who have nasal colonization of *S. aureus* at the time of surgery have a substantially increased rate of staphylococcal wound infection of the same strain as that found in the nasal area (Altemeier, 1979).

Active infections in other sites of the body increase the chances of wound infections from endogenous sources. Foley catheters, hyperalimentation or intravenous lines, and lower respiratory infections are common foci of infection. Age, obesity, diabetes, general malnutrition, chronic poor health, or debilitation also increase the chances of wound infections.

Clients receiving immunosuppressants, chemotherapy, broad-spectrum antimicrobials, or steroids have an increased risk of wound infections. These clients frequently develop fungal or yeast infections, either alone or concurrent with a bacterial infection. Clients who are hospitalized 3 to 6 days preoperatively are twice as likely to develop an infection in a clean surgical wound than those admitted just prior to surgery. With 14 or more days of presurgery hospital stay, the exposure to hospital flora increases the infection risk four times (Cruse and Foord, 1973; Polk, 1976).

Factors within the wound itself that significantly predispose to infection include the presence of dead, unhealthy, or irritated tissues, or foreign bodies and other irritants.

For purposes of estimating degree of infection risk, surgical wounds are classified as: (1) clean, (2) clean-contaminated, (3) contaminated, and (4) dirty and infected wounds (Altemeier, 1979). Table 34-1 describes and illustrates these categories and their respective infection risk. Categories three and four are combined in this table, since the primary distinction is that category four contains old nonhealing wounds of previously infected body areas, while category three contains fresh wound contamination. It is obvious from this table that location and characteristics of the wound have a direct effect on the probability of infection.

Exogenous (from outside the client) sources of wound infection include intraoperative factors such as airborne bacteria or direct contact spread through breaks in surgical aseptic technique, including glove

TABLE 34-1. Infection Risk According to Wound Category

CATEGORY	DESCRIPTION	EXAMPLES	INFECTION RATE
Clean	Procedures in which the surgeon enters a sterile body cavity and exits through the same cavity, makes no contact with areas having bacterial populations (such as the gastrointestinal and upper respiratory tracts), encounters no inflammation or pus, and experiences no break in sterile techniques.	Open heart surgery, herniorrhaphy, mastectomy.	1-2%
Clean-Contaminated	Surgery, during which no major break in sterile technique occurs, performed on organs or areas with a bacterial population but no inflammation or pus, or on sterile organs or cavities connected with areas containing bacteria. This includes procedures in which the surgeon enters a sterile body cavity and exits through another cavity with a bacterial population.	Appendectomy, gastric and small bowel resections, abdominal hysterectomy, cesarean section (sterile uterus connects to bacterially contaminated vagina), open fractures less than 8 to 10 hours old.	Approximately 5%
Contaminated/Infected	Surgery performed on areas where there is acute inflammation or pus and on wounds containing foreign matter; procedures during which drainage spills from one organ or body cavity to another, or a significant break in sterile technique occurs.	Appendectomy with perforation; colon, rectal, and vaginal surgery; bowel resection with peritonitis or perforation; lacerations or perforation; lacerations and open fractures more than 8 to 10 hours old; oral surgery; incision and drainage of abscesses, boils, and infected pilonidal cysts.	30% or greater

(From Meshelhaney CM: Post-op wound dressings: Your guide to impeccable technique. RN 42(5):21-33, 1979. Used with permission.)

punctures. Inadequate ventilation in clinical areas has also been found to contribute to wound infections (Davidson et al., 1971; Polk, 1976). Preventable sources of exogenous wound infections include inadequate use of aseptic technique during dressing changes and careless handwashing practices, which result in cross-contamination of infectious microorganisms from other clients or staff.

CHARACTERISTICS OF WOUND INFECTIONS

As discussed in Skill 32, the inflammatory response is characteristic of the early phases of wound healing and does not, in itself, necessarily indicate infection. However, when inflammation is prolonged or begins to develop after the 4th or 5th day, the probability of infection needs to be considered. Aerobic wound infections develop about the 5th day postoperative, while anaerobic infections generally develop a little later, between the 6th and 8th day (O'Byrne, 1979). However, a postoperative wound infection may occur even later: 25 percent of all wound infections do not show symptoms until after the patient is discharged (Brachman, 1979).

The body responds to the invasion of pathogens with an inflammatory reaction, which provides an early warning of a developing infection. *Local indications of infection* are heat, redness, swelling, pain, and involuntary limitation of the body part, accompanied by wound drainage. A *generalized body response to infection* also may occur, with fever, increased respiratory and pulse rates, leukocytosis (increased white blood cell count), elevated sedimentation rate, lethargy, general malaise, and anorexia (loss of appetite) or nausea.

Wound infections affect both the degree of temperature elevation and its pattern of elevation. For example, fungal infections tend to manifest low-grade fevers, and aerobic infections produce a pattern of spiking temperatures in the afternoon and evening, dropping to normal by the next morning. A mild temperature elevation for the 1st day or so after surgery is considered a normal physiological reaction. A *persistent* fever or a temperature elevation above 37.7°C (100°F) may indicate a beginning wound infection and needs to be investigated.

When wound drainage is thick and yellow, with large numbers of leukocytes and cellular debris, it is called a *purulent* (*suppurative*) exudate, commonly known as *pus*. When the exudate is thin and contains more plasma than cells, it is called a *serous* exudate. Pus usually is yellowish-white in color, but it may become red-tinged or pink if small vessel bleeding has occurred. *Pseudomonas aeruginosa* produces a green pigment that causes green, yellow-green, or blue-green pus (Fischbach, 1980; Thomas, 1981). The absence of pus in a leukopenic client does not necessarily indicate absence of an infection. Persons with abnormally low white counts may not generate pus when they have an infection, since pus by definition contains numerous white cells.

The *odor* of the drainage from an infected wound gives a clue to the causative organisms. Aerobic organisms such as *Staphylococcus aureus* or *Escherichia coli* have a musty odor, while obligate anaerobic organisms such as the *Bacteroides* or *Peptococcus prevotii* have a highly putrid odor. *Proteus* organisms produce a sulfurlike rotten egg odor and *P. aeruginosa* has a sweet, grapelike odor (Fischbach, 1980).

If a gas gangrene infection develops, crepitation (a dry, crackling sound upon palpation) can be heard when the adjacent tissues are palpated.

A wound infection may develop fairly superficially, where it is more easily visible, or it may be deeper within the wound and less visible. An early sign of a deep wound infection is an area in or near the wound that is especially more tender than the rest of the wound. A wound infection may be generalized throughout the wound, or localized, forming an abscess (localized collection of pus) deeper within the wound. Abscesses often contain anaerobic bacteria, such as *Bacteroides fragilis,* since these organisms thrive in an environment with poor blood and oxygen supply.

TREATMENT OF INFECTED WOUNDS

If a wound is known, suspected, or considered likely to be infected at the time of surgery, it usually is left open and then closed 4 to 6 days later if no infection develops, or whenever the infection clears. This is known as delayed closing, or healing by third intention. If a sutured wound develops an infection, the sutures may be reopened to help drainage. Having an infected wound open rather than closed promotes drainage, which is a key treatment factor. An open wound also facilitates visualization and diagnosis of pathogens, and avoids creating a warm, moist, closed environment conducive to bacterial growth. Nonocclusive dressings usually are used on infected wounds to *allow air to circulate.* Sterile wet dressings may be used to promote drainage or to apply antibacterial solutions.

The infected wound may need debridement, or removal of wound debris through mechanical or chemical methods (see Skill 37). Appropriate antimicrobial treatment of the offending organism should be instituted by the physician as soon as possible after a wound infection develops.

WOUND CULTURE AND SENSITIVITY

The choice of an antibiotic often is determined by a culture and sensitivity test performed on a specimen of wound drainage. In a culture and sensitivity test (commonly referred to as a *C & S*), drainage is collected from the infected wound or abscess and sent to the laboratory for incubation (*culture*) to identify the offending microorganisms. Culture growth then is exposed to antibiotic discs to determine which drug (or drugs) most effectively inhibit growth, that is, to which antibiotics the microorganisms are *sensitive*. Agency culture and sensitivity report forms generally indicate the causative microorganisms and their relative susceptibility to various antibiotics.

Material from infected wounds usually contains both aerobic and anaerobic microorganisms. Most of the microorganisms that cause wound infections in humans are facultative anaerobic microorganisms (exceptions are *P. aeruginosa,* which is a strict or obligate aerobe, and the *Bacteroides,* which are strict or obligate anaerobes). If there is a question of whether to use the aerobic or anaerobic method of collecting a wound culture specimen, the anaerobic method should be used since it is the most likely to result in a viable sample of the largest variety of microorganisms. Another option would be to collect both aerobic and anaerobic specimens, using material from deep inside the wound for anaerobic culture and more superficial material for aerobic culture.

The laboratory usually can give a "looks like" identification of bacteria in 18 to 24 hours and a final identification in about 48 hours. Fungal cultures may take 2 to 8 weeks, however.

Based on past experience and clinical judgment, the physician may choose to institute antibiotic therapy before the laboratory report is completed. And, when the culture and sensitivity report is available, the physician may opt to use an antibiotic that the laboratory report indicates to be marginally effective or noneffective for this particular microorganism, rather than one indicated to be quite effective. There are several reasons for this. Since most laboratory tests are *in vitro* (in a laboratory), the laboratory sensitivity to an antibiotic may or may not always correspond with the effectiveness of that antibiotic in the client (*in vivo,* or in the living body). Laboratory sensitivity results also may not be absolute, and the physician's judgment and experience may determine that an experiential trial use of a given antibiotic is worthwhile. The location of the infection within the body also determines the selection of an antibiotic, because different antibiotics concentrate their effective action in different body tissues.

A newer test, the MIC (Minimal Inhibiting Concentration) test, can predict the client's response to antibiotic therapy more specifically. This test can determine how much antibiotic actually gets to different body areas, as well as the amount needed by the body to inhibit microorganisms to the point where the body's own white cells can deal with them effectively.

DATA BASE

Early diagnosis and treatment of an infection lead to a more rapid resolution of the infection. Nurse observations and assessment are a crucial part of that early diagnosis, since the total clinical picture must be considered, not just the offending microorganisms. To make these judgments, the nurse needs to have a variety of data available.

Client History and Recorded Data

The health record provides data about the kind and location of the wound and the particular client's relative risk for developing an infection. It also indicates the number of days postoperative and the extent and pattern of any temperature elevation, both of which help distinguish between the normal inflammatory response to injury and the development of an infection.

Physical Appraisal Skills

Inspection. Inspection reveals any unusual, prolonged, or localized redness. Inspection also identifies the presence and nature of any wound drainage, including the presence and color of pus.

Palpation. Palpation with a sterile gloved hand is used to determine the presence of unusual, prolonged, or localized wound or drain site tenderness; induration (hardness) around the wound; and the presence or absence of the healing ridge.

Auscultation. Auscultation is used to determine the presence of crepitation (present with gas gangrene), and the sense of smell could assist in identifying the causative microorganism.

EQUIPMENT

Rayon- or polyester-tipped sterile *swabs* are used to collect aerobic culture specimens. Because of the air trapped in these fibers, specially treated swabs must be used for anaerobic culture specimen collection.

Culture tubes are clear sterilized glass or plastic tubes used to provide an appropriate environment for transporting a specimen from a suspected infected area to the laboratory for culturing.

Aerobic culture tubes contain a swab and a transport medium that supports aerobic bacterial life during transport to the laboratory. See Figure 34–1 for directions for one style of aerobic culture equipment.

Gassed-out culture tubes are used to collect anaerobic culture specimens. These glass or plastic tubes are presterilized, filled with carbon dioxide, and have a rubber stopper that is impervious to carbon dioxide. Because carbon dioxide is heavier than air, it keeps the air out when the tube is unstoppered—*if* the tube is kept *upright*. Gassed-out tubes also contain a special transport medium that has its oxygen removed. Together, the carbon dioxide and the transport medium provide a temporary anaerobic habitat during transport to the lab (Marchiondo, 1979). One company provides a single plastic tube system containing two crushable ampules that release a transport medium and hydrogen gas for an anaerobic environment. Some companies provide two gassed-out carbon-dioxide-filled culture tubes for a single specimen collection. One contains the swab; the second has an oxygen-sensitive gel at the bottom. To ensure that the carbon dioxide is not accidentally lost, this second tube is kept stoppered until the specimen is collected on the swab. Then the swab is quickly placed in the second tube, while keeping the tube in an upright position. If carbon dioxide loss does occur, the gel in the culture-tube tip will change color from contact with oxygen. Figure 34–2 shows one style of anaerobic culture equipment.

Sterile syringes can be used to collect wound exudate for either aerobic or anaerobic culture. Sometimes this is the preferable method of collection, because the larger volume of drainage collected provides

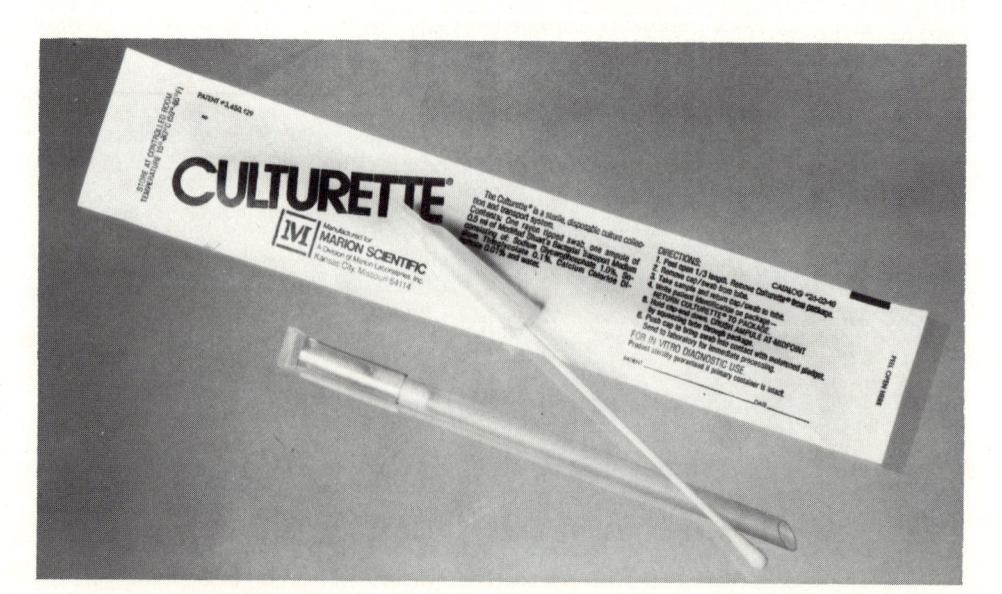

Figure 34–1. Aerobic culture specimen collection equipment. The Culturette's swab/cap assembly eliminates the need for touching the swab, decreasing the potential for contamination. After use, the Culturette is replaced in the paper wrapper, labeled, and sent to the laboratory. (Courtesy of Marion Scientific Corporation, Kansas City, MO.)

SKILL 34: WOUND CULTURE SPECIMEN COLLECTION

☐ EXECUTION

Wound surveillance is a regular part of the care of a postoperative client and includes a careful assessment, with removal of old dressings and an actual inspection, not just a quick look under the old dressing. When clinical symptoms indicate presence of an infection, all existing dressings at *any* site should be removed, the wound inspected for drainage, culture specimens collected as needed, and the wound redressed with a nonocclusive dressing.

Whenever a wound infection is suspected, report observations of wound status to the physician and collect any wound culture specimens ordered by the physician or determined by the nursing staff to be necessary. Agency policy should delineate the specific protocol for nurse-initiated wound cultures.

For a culture and sensitivity test to be worthwhile, the nurse must know how to collect appropriate samples of infected material. The most useful specimens for culture are pus or other wound exudate or excised tissue, although dressings from draining wounds may be cultured. When swabs are used, roll or twist them in the pus to get a thick coating of exudate. A swab with a light smearing of pus dries out quickly, making culture difficult. Insert the swabs into wound crevices, deep into abscess pockets, and under eroded areas such as sometimes occur with large decubitus ulcers. Necrotic wound tissue and debrided material are likely to harbor microorganisms and may be used for culture specimens. If a wound is dry, with no exudate, the swab may be moistened with sterile normal saline and then rolled across the incision.

When a wound has a combination of inflamed, necrotic, and purulent areas, collect a specimen from each of those areas with a separate culture tube, as different microorganisms with varying antibiotic sensitivity may be present. When mixed infections are suspected, both aerobic and anaerobic cultures may be ordered.

The technique for collecting aerobic and anaerobic microorganisms differs. Incorrect collection technique destroys or invalidates culture results, perhaps a reason for limited numbers of documented anaerobic infections and the relatively frequent incidence of "sterile pus" (pus that produces no bacterial growth when cultured because of inadequate collection or culture techniques) (O'Byrne, 1979). When collecting a wound culture specimen, it is important to collect actual wound exudate rather than skin flora. For this reason, cleanse the wound *prior* to obtaining the culture specimen. An iodophor antiseptic or 70 percent alcohol is recommended for cleansing prior to wound cultures (Marchiondo, 1979).

Both aerobic and anaerobic cultures require strict asepsis in the collection process to avoid contamination from extraneous organisms. Exogenous organisms from the nurse's hands, the client's bed clothing, and so on, should not be allowed to contaminate the culture specimen. It also is important not to introduce endogenous organisms from the client into the speci-

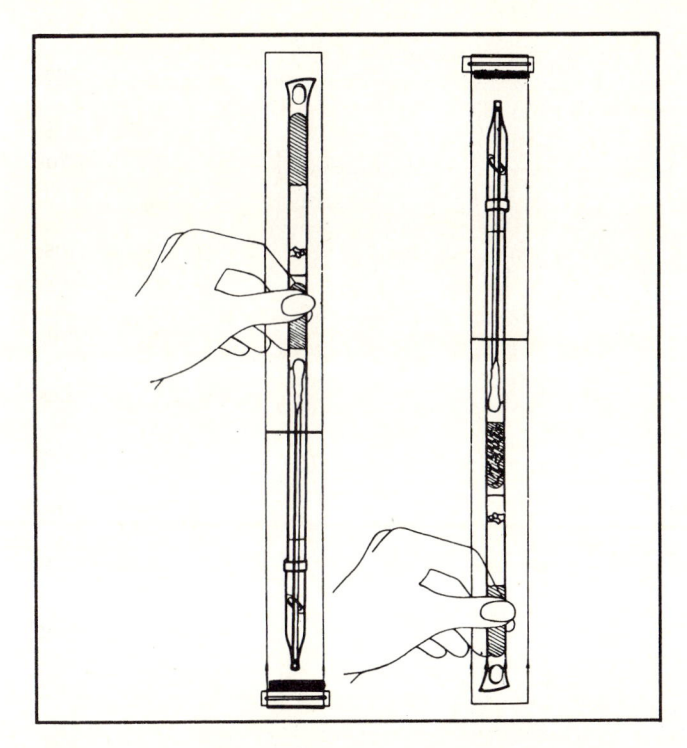

Figure 34–2. Anaerobic culture specimen collection equipment. Anaerobic Culturette. After using according to directions, the inflated Bio-Bag that encases the culture tube indicates presence of an oxygen-free hydrogen gas environment. (Courtesy of Marion Scientific Corporation, Kansas City, MO.)

for better laboratory inoculation. The needle may be removed for aspiration, or a large-bore needle, such as a #18, may be used. After the exudate is aspirated, the air is expelled from the syringe to protect the anaerobic microorganisms. The replaced needle or syringe-tip cap and the syringe plunger serve as effective stoppers and keep air from entering.

Hazards

Contamination of the culture equipment introduces exogenous microorganisms into the specimen. The bed clothes, client's skin, or nurse's hands should not touch the inside of the tube or the swab itself. When returning the swab to the tube, the swab must not touch the outside of the container, as this would cause the swab to become unsterile, and the outside of the tube would be contaminated by specimen material. The cap or stopper must be replaced securely so as not to loosen during transport.

A major problem in culture specimen collection is that of not getting the specimen to the lab in time. Some microorganisms die quickly when removed from the body. Others multiply rapidly at room temperature, and some are killed by refrigeration. Using aerobic containers for anaerobic specimens destroys the specimen and renders the test invalid. The cost to the client in terms of delayed treatment and reculturing can be tremendous.

men, that is, skin flora for an abdominal wound infection or fistula flora when culturing a deep body abscess. The directions accompanying the culture tubes must be followed carefully. If there are no directions with the equipment, call the laboratory for specific instructions, rather than guess, since different brands of equipment are used in different ways.

Culture specimens must be taken to the laboratory promptly so that the specimen can be set up (inoculated and incubated) by the lab within 20 minutes from collection. If the time is delayed, bacterial overgrowth occurs; if refrigeration is used, some bacteria may die. Mishandled or delayed specimens can result in false diagnoses, delays in effective treatment, and repeated specimen collection. When taken promptly to the laboratory, aerobic as well as anaerobic cultures can be inoculated from an anaerobically obtained specimen. Since the majority of wound infection pathogens are facultative, rather than strictly aerobic or anaerobic, those that thrive best in an aerobic environment will survive for a period of time in an anaerobic environment. The reverse is not true, however, because most anaerobic wound pathogens are *not* facultative and do *not* survive in an aerobic atmosphere.

Some anaerobic microorganisms die within a very few minutes after exposure to oxygen. Since the environment is anaerobic, deep wound drainage almost always contains anaerobic microorganisms, which need to be cultured with anaerobic methods.

Correct labeling and accurate completion of the requisition form is another very important aspect of culture specimen collection. Having basic client-identifying data on the label avoids the delay and emotional and physical trauma caused by lost specimens. If the client is receiving antibiotics, include this information on the requisition form or in the computer pathway. Laboratory techniques can be altered to avoid inadequate culture growth from the presence of antibiotics in the specimen. The label also needs to include the specific wound location or site where the specimen was collected. If cultures are taken from more than one area in the same wound or from different areas of the client's body, each specimen tube or syringe must be distinctively labeled for clear identification of its source. The laboratory selects the culture medium according to the body site, and the physician needs to know exactly what site was cultured so as to select the appropriate antibiotic therapy.

☐ SKILL SEQUENCES

AEROBIC WOUND CULTURE SPECIMEN COLLECTION

Step	Rationale
1. Select correct sterile equipment: culture tube with swab or syringe. Inspect for indicators of sterility.	Provides correct care of culture specimen.
2. Wash hands.	Avoids possibility of contamination from the nurse's hands.
3. Explain reason for procedure to client.	Allays apprehension and encourages participation in care.
4. Remove dressing as in Skill 32, Skill Sequence, "Dressing Change with Wound Care," steps 8 to 19, pp. 305–306.	Avoids introducing additional exogenous microorganisms.
5. Inspect, palpate, and cleanse wound and skin around inflamed or infected area. See Skill 32, Skill Sequence, "Dressing Change with Wound Care," steps 20 to 26, p. 306.	Avoids specimen contamination from normal skin flora.
6. With a sterile gloved hand, press gently on wound near infected area if no fresh exudate appears spontaneously. Remove sterile glove.	Fresh exudate produces the most representative microorganism sample.
7. Don fresh clean or sterile gloves.	If hands will be near or touching incision, sterile gloves protect client from transient microorganisms on nurse's hands. Clean gloves protect nurse from microorganisms when sterile gloves are not needed.
8. Remove cap and swab from culture tube without contaminating it.	Avoids introducing exogenous microorganisms into specimen.
9. Carefully, roll swab tip in exudate. Do not allow swab to touch surrounding skin. Insert a separate swab into any boils or abscess pockets.	Ensures actual collection of microorganisms. The best specimens usually are deep within wound or abscess.
10. Return swab or swabs to culture tubes, without touching and contaminating outside of tube with culture material.	Avoids contamination of the environment and those who handle the tube.

11. Alternative syringe method:
   a. Remove needle from a 2–3 ml syringe, or substitute a large-bore needle, such as a #18. Avoid contamination of needle hub or syringe tip.
   b. Place tip of syringe or needle in the exudate and aspirate wound exudate into syringe.
	Larger amount of exudate provides best specimen for culture.
	
	Prevents aspirating air.

(continued)

Step	Rationale
c. With syringe upright, remove the air by pushing plunger into syringe. Avoid expelling exudate. (If only an aerobic culture is desired, some air may be kept in the syringe.)	Aerobic microorganisms can survive temporarily without an air supply. If any question about whether both aerobic and anaerobic cultures are to be done, remove all air.
d. Replace needle cap or syringe-tip cap, tighten, and secure with tape.	Avoids accidental separation during transport, which would result in environmental contamination.
12. Collect additional separate culture specimens from necrotic, inflamed, or infected areas.	Different microorganisms often exist in each of these areas.
13. Remove gloves, turning them inside out as in Skill 31, Skill Sequence, "Removing Sterile Gloves," p. 290.	Specimen collection usually contaminates gloves.
14. Wash hands.	Microorganisms grow on hands inside sterile gloves.
15. Apply new dressing to wound. See Skill 32, Skill Sequence, "Dressing Change with Wound Care," steps 30 to 32, p. 307.	
16. Wash hands.	Decreases potential for cross-contamination from microorganisms within the wound.
17. Label container: client's name, room number, physician's name, date and time collected, specific source of specimen, test ordered.	Avoids lost specimens and provides needed information.
18. Complete lab requisition slip, including all data as in step 17, plus: client's hospital or record number, antibiotics client may be receiving. (NOTE: with computerized systems, enter appropriate data into lab request sequence.)	Aids in correct diagnosis and determination of antibiotic sensitivity.
19. Send to lab within 20 minutes.	Avoids incorrect results from overgrowth or death of representative microorganisms.
20. Record culture specimen or specimens obtained, source, time, appearance of wound and drainage, and client's subjective comments in health record.	Provides written documentation of assessment data and care given.

ANAEROBIC WOUND CULTURE SPECIMEN COLLECTION

Step	Rationale
1. Select correct sterile culture equipment: sterile gassed-out tube or syringe and needle.	CO_2 environment in tube avoids destroying anaerobic microorganisms.
2. Repeat steps 2 to 7, Skill Sequence, "Aerobic Wound Culture Specimen Collection."	
3. Without contaminating swab, remove cap from gassed-out tube, keeping tube upright and near wound site.	Avoids exogenous specimen contamination. Keeps carbon dioxide from leaving tube, since carbon dioxide is heavier than air. As little oxygen as possible should reach specimen.
4. Quickly and carefully, roll swab in exudate or insert into abscess. Replace in tube as rapidly as possible, without contaminating tube or swab. (NOTE: If using dual tube equipment, remove stopper from second tube after specimen is collected. Keep second tube upright and reclose promptly.)	Avoids organism destruction from exposure to oxygen. Avoids loss of correct environment for specimen.
5. Alternative syringe method: a. Remove needle from a sterile 2–3 ml syringe or substitute a large-bore needle, such as a #18. Avoid contamination of needle hub or syringe plunger and tip. b. Place tip of syringe or needle in exudate, aspirate wound exudate into syringe. c. With syringe upright, remove air by pushing plunger into syringe. Avoid expelling exudate. d. Replace needle cap or syringe-tip cap, tighten, and secure with tape.	Same as rationale for steps 3 and 4.
6. Repeat steps 12 to 20, Skill Sequence, "Aerobic Wound Culture Specimen Collection."	

RECORDING

Include in the nurses' notes the data that determined the need for a culture, the specific location or locations cultured, the kind of equipment used, anaerobic or aerobic culture method, and both the time the specimen was collected and the time it was sent to the laboratory. For information purposes, collection of a culture specimen is added to the kardex or computer nursing-care plan.

Sample POR Recording

- S—"I haven't felt well last night and today."
- O—Mucopurulent drainage at 4th and 5th sutures from top of wound. Wound tender to touch just left of those areas. Temp. 99.8°F @ noon.
- A—Wound infection apparently developing.
- P—Notified Dr. Greene. Aspirated 2 ml of drainage c̄ syringe and sent an anaerobic specimen to lab stat. Continue to monitor local and systemic signs of infection q 4°.

Sample Narrative Recording

Incision reddened and inflamed. Mucopurulent drainage at 4th and 5th sutures from the top of the wound. Temp. 99.8°F. Says he doesn't "fell well" today. Aspirated 2 ml of drainage c̄ syringe. Anaerobic specimen sent to the laboratory within 10 minutes for C & S as ordered by Dr. Greene.

☐ CRITICAL POINTS SUMMARY

1. Recognize local and systemic signs of infection.
2. Identify persons or types of wounds with increased potential for wound infection.
3. Have complete visualization when inspecting wounds.
4. Cleanse wound prior to specimen collection so as to collect actual exudate rather than adjacent skin or tissue flora.
5. Examine equipment for indicators of sterility.
6. Aerobic cultures can be grown from anaerobic specimens.
7. Anaerobic cultures *cannot* be grown from aerobic specimens.
8. Keep anaerobic "gassed-out" culture specimen tubes upright when unstoppered.
9. Collect culture specimens from all parts of the wound that have a different appearance, such as inflamed, necrotic, and infected areas.
10. Label culture specimens with name, date, time, source, and tests to be done.
11. Include the name of any antibiotic therapy on the requisition form or in the computer request pathway.
12. Take specimen to the laboratory promptly, within 20 minutes.

☐ LEARNING ACTIVITIES

1. Examine culture tubes for aerobic and anaerobic use. Describe the differences and similarities.
2. Locate laboratory culture and sensitivity reports in a record for a client who is known or suspected to have a wound infection. Indicate the following information:
   a. Type of culture: aerobic or anaerobic
   b. Source of specimen _____
   c. Diagnosis _____
   d. Date and time collected _____
   e. Time received in lab, if indicated _____
   f. Microorganisms isolated _____
   g. Antibiotic sensitivity _____
3. Talk with personnel in a laboratory. Ask them about problems they encounter with specimens and how those problems could be avoided.

☐ REVIEW QUESTIONS

1. Which of these signs and symptoms of postoperative wound healing would you consider to be expected or unexpected signs? Place an *X* in the correct column

SIGN OR SYMPTOM	EXPECTED	UNEXPECTED
Acute local tenderness, day 5	____	____
Generalized wound tenderness, day 3	____	____
Reddened wound edges, day 1	____	____
Reddened wound edges, day 7	____	____
Skin edges unapproximated and wound not sealed, day 3	____	____
Skin edges unapproximated and wound not sealed, day 1	____	____

2. Which of these clients is more likely to develop a wound infection? Place a *+* before those more likely, and a *0* before those less likely to develop an infection. Compare answers with a peer and discuss reasons for differences.
   - ____ 18 year old with a ruptured appendix
   - ____ 48 year old with an uncomplicated appendectomy
   - ____ 50 year old with cancer of the lymphatic system
   - ____ 80 year old with cataract surgery
   - ____ 78 year old with a herniorrhaphy
   - ____ 45 year old with gall bladder surgery and no wound drains
   - ____ 40 year old, admitted one week before surgery

___ 60 year old, admitted one day before surgery
___ 23 year old with tissue lacerations from an automobile accident
___ 72 year old with a repair of a fractured hip
3. What implications does the concept of facultative aerobe have for wound specimen culture collection?
4. Why does an anaerobic culture tube need to be kept upright when opened for use?
5. What is done differently when a syringe is used to collect an anaerobic versus an aerobic wound culture specimen?
6. What kind of problem or problems would you anticipate each of the following labeling situations to cause for the client or staff?
   a. Client's room number is included, but no name.
   b. Physician's name is omitted.
   c. No site specified, simply wound culture.
   d. No collection time indicated.
7. What can cause a wound culture specimen to be nonrepresentative of the actual microorganisms present within the wound?
8. What consequences might occur if a physician receives incorrect information from a wound culture specimen that is collected or labeled incorrectly?

☐ PERFORMANCE CHECKLIST

OBJECTIVE: To use correct aerobic or anaerobic technique and equipment to collect a wound culture specimen.

CHARACTERISTIC	RANGE OF ACCEPTABILITY	SATISFACTORY	UNSATISFACTORY
1. Washes hands.	No deviation		
2. Selects aerobic or anaerobic culture tubes, according to the organism being cultured or test ordered. OR: sterile syringe and needle.	No deviation		
3. Inspects dressing.	No deviation		
4. Removes and disposes of dressing correctly.	No deviation		
5. Cleanses wound.	No deviation		
6. Dons sterile or clean gloves.	No deviation		
7. Collects actual exudate on swab or aspirates into syringe.	No deviation		
8. Keeps gassed-out tubes upright.	No deviation		
9. Returns swab to culture tube without contamination and recloses the tube.	No deviation		
10. Syringe collection: expels all air from anaerobic and aerobic culture specimens.	A purely aerobic culture specimen may have air left in the syringe.		
11. Replaces needle cap or syringe-tip cap tightly and tapes cap, plunger, and syringe together.	No deviation		
12. Applies new dressing.	No deviation		
13. Washes hands.	No deviation		
14. Labels specimen container.	No deviation		
15. Completes requisition form.	No deviation		
16. Takes to laboratory within 20 minutes.	No deviation		
17. Records actions in health record.	No deviation		

REFERENCES

Allen JR, Hightower AW, et al.: Secular trends in nosocomial infections: 1970-1979. American Journal of Medicine 70(2):389-392, 1981.

Altemeier WA: Surgical Infections: Incisional Wounds. In Bennett JV, Brachman PS (eds): Hospital Infections. Boston, Little, Brown, 1979.

Brachman P: Epidemiology of Nosocomial Infections. In Bennett JV, Brachman PS (eds): Hospital Infections. Boston, Little, Brown, 1979.

Committee on Control of Surgical Infections of the Committee on Pre- and Postoperative Care, American College of Surgeons: Manual on Control of Infection in Surgical Patients. Philadelphia, JB Lippincott, 1976.

Cruse PJE, Foord R: A five-year prospective study of 23,649 surgical wounds. Archives of Surgery 107(2):206-210, 1973.

Davidson AIG, Smith G, et al.: A bacteriological study of the immediate environment of a surgical wound. British Journal of Surgery 58(3):326–333, 1971.

Fischbach FT: A Manual of Laboratory Diagnostic Tests. Philadelphia, JB Lippincott, 1980.

Marchiondo K: The very fine art of collecting culture specimens. Nursing79 9(4):34–43, 1979.

Meshelhaney CM: Post-op wound dressings: Your guide to impeccable technique. RN 42(5):21–33, 1979.

O'Byrne C: Clinical detection and management of postoperative wound sepsis. Nursing Clinics of North America 14(4):727–742, 1979.

Polk HC Jr, Fry D, et al.: Dissemination and causes of infection. Surgical Clinics of North America 56(4):817–827, 1976.

Thomas CL (ed): Tabor's Cyclopedic Medical Dictionary, ed 14. Philadelphia, FA Davis, 1981.

BIBLIOGRAPHY

Altemeier WA, Burke JF, et al.: Manual on Control of Infection in Surgical Patients. Philadelphia, JB Lippincott, 1976.

American Hospital Association: Infection Control in the Hospital, ed 4. Chicago, American Hospital Association, 1979.

Bennett JV: Incidence and Nature of Endemic and Epidemic Nosocomial Infections. In Bennett JV, Brachman PS (eds): Hospital Infections. Boston, Little, Brown, 1979.

Castle M: Hospital Infection Control: Principles and Practices. New York, John Wiley & Sons, 1980.

Cooper DM, Schumann D: Postsurgical nursing intervention as an adjunct to wound healing. Nursing Clinics of North America 14(4):713–726, 1979.

Kinney JM, Egdahl RH, et al.: Manual of Preoperative and Postoperative Care, ed 2. Philadelphia, WB Saunders, 1971.

Kozier B, Erb GL: Fundamentals of Nursing: Concepts and Procedures, ed 2. Reading, MA, Addison-Wesley, 1983.

Mallison GF: Areas of Special Concern: Section F. Central Service. In Bennett JV, Brachman PS (eds): Hospital Infections. Boston, Little, Brown, 1979.

Promotional Information. Marion Scientific Corporation, Kansas City, MO.

Schwartz SI, Shires GT, et al. (eds): Principles of Surgery, ed 3. New York, McGraw-Hill, 1979.

Wilson ME, Mizer HE, et al.: Microbiology in Patient Care, ed 3. New York, Macmillan, 1979.

SKILL 35 Wound Drains and Irrigations

PREREQUISITE SKILLS

Skill 19, "Inspection"
Skill 22, "Auscultation"
Skill 28, "Handwashing"
Skill 30, "Sterile Supplies"
Skill 31, "Donning Sterile Gloves"
Skill 32, "Dressings and Wound Care"

☐ STUDENT OBJECTIVES

1. Explain the purpose of using wound drains.
2. Explain the mechanisms by which Penrose, T-tube, and Foley catheter drains and portable wound-suction drainage systems remove exudate from wounds.
3. Describe nursing-care responsibilities associated with the care of clients with drains of various kinds.
4. Identify circumstances under which wound irrigation may be needed.
5. Describe methods used for irrigating open wounds.
6. Explain the use of portable wound suction drainage systems in irrigation of closed wounds.
7. Compare the size, use, and mechanisms for providing negative pressure in different manual suction drainage systems.

☐ INTRODUCTION

Wound drains are tubes and catheters that are placed within a body cavity or surgical wound to encourage the escape of body fluids that can retard healing. (A tube is open at both ends, and a catheter is a tube with a closed tip and one or more perforations at the insertion end.) These body fluids may be blood, lymph, serosanguineous tissue fluid, intestinal juices, or pus. Accumulation of fluid within wound layers delays healing because it puts internal pressure on the suture line and keeps the tissue layers separated, which allows dead space (open space within a wound) to develop, and thus promotes bacterial growth and development of infection. Drains assist in the obliteration of this dead space in an abscess cavity, anatomic space, or wound. This is especially true when a suction apparatus is attached to the drain.

Wound irrigation is the flushing or washing of interior areas of a closed wound or the exposed surfaces of an open wound. Irrigations can be used for mechanical cleansing of excess wound drainage and sloughed tissue or to apply medication locally to the wound.

As the care of wounds generally is the responsibility of the nurse, so is the maintenance of any drains or irrigations associated with that care. There are many different types of wound drainage and irrigation equipment on the market. This skill presents some practices that are basic to open and closed drainage and irrigation systems and describes several examples of these systems. Related skills are presented in Skills 36 and 37.

□ PREPARATION

Wound drains are used postoperatively with radical surgical resections; in axillary, groin, and neck surgery; with amputations; or when leakage is expected postoperatively, such as with gall bladder or pancreatic surgery. Wound drains are frequently inserted into an abscess or fistula (abnormal channel connecting an organ or body area to the body surface) to promote drainage of serosanguineous or purulent exudate. It is important to remember that a drain is a foreign body, and as such it provides an entry for bacteria and can lead to sinus tract formation around the drain or to erosion of tissue adjacent to the drain.

Drains are inserted during surgery. One end is placed within or near the organ or cavity to be drained, and the other end is passed through the body wall adjacent to the incision by means of a stab wound or needle insertion. This avoids a direct route for microorganisms to enter the incision itself. The drain is usually sutured to the skin to prevent accidental removal.

SURGICAL DRAINS

Surgical drains may be used as either an open or a closed drainage system. In an open system, the end of the drain distal to the client is left open and allowed to drain into the dressing through capillary attraction. There is a clear indication that this open end provides an entry route for microorganisms (Alexander, 1983). In a closed system, the distal end of the drain is attached to a drainage tube and a collection container, thus keeping the entire system closed to entry to microorganisms. Drainage is removed from the wound by gravity or suction (negative pressure, that is, pressure less than atmospheric). When a closed system is opened to empty the collection chamber or to reestablish suction, the openings and caps must be handled in an aseptic manner.

Portable Closed Wound Suction Systems

Closed wound drainage and irrigation systems were first used around 1937. In 1960, the first portable closed wound suction drainage system, the Snyder Hemovac, was developed (The Case, 1979). The Hemovac and the newer Surgivac are examples of lightweight portable closed systems that create a vacuum (negative pressure) by means of a manually compressed vacuum chamber. They are lightweight (plastic), quiet (no moving parts), and are pinned to the clothing so the client can move about freely. These systems can be used either for wound suction or irrigation or to alternate between the two. Some portable systems provide suction only, such as the Heyer-Schulte Suction Drain System. Portable manual suction equipment provides negative pressure ranging from 28 to 50 mm Hg, which is not great enough to draw soft tissues into the catheter holes. If a greater negative pressure is desired, an electrical pump (Gomco) or suction from a wall outlet may be attached to these manual systems. Many hospitals have a vacuum system built into the walls, with outlets in the walls where a flow regulator may be plugged in and the suction tubing attached, as described in Skill 56.

A portable wound suction system exerts gentle negative pressure internally in the wound or tissue layers. This suction continuously removes serosanguineous fluid, blood, or lymph, and keeps tissue layers approximated more closely than either gravity drainage or pressure dressings—thus promoting more rapid healing, with fewer problems from accumulated wound debris.

During surgery, several drains may be placed within the same wound to drain different tissue levels. Each wound section being drained must have a separate drainage tube to provide complete evacuation of each area. In the Heyer-Schulte Suction Reservoir System, several "Jackson-Pratt" drains may be connected to a single reservoir. It is not uncommon to have a dozen light-weight Jackson-Pratt drains used with radical neck dissection surgery where large planes of tissue have been separated, dissected, and reclosed. Tissue approximation and removal of serosanguineous fluid is crucial to adequate healing of these wounds.

Gravity Closed Drainage Systems

Closed drainage systems also may drain by gravity through a drainage tube, such as from a T-tube after gall bladder surgery. The drainage tube is attached to a collecting bag of some sort which has a capped or clipped opening for emptying drainage. These openings must be handled with aseptic technique and protected from contamination by hands, clothing, linens, or the floor while they are being emptied.

T-tubes are placed in the common duct after biliary tract surgery to remove bile until postoperative edema has subsided. T-tubes usually drain 300 to 500 ml of bile-colored (yellow-orange) fluid the first 24 hours. This volume decreases to less than 200 ml after 3 to 4 days. A T-tube is left in place for about 10 days and is removed when X-rays indicate there is no obstruction or edema present (Luckmann and Sorensen, 1980).

Penrose Drains

Penrose drains are the oldest type of surgical drain, dating back to 1859 (LeMaitre, 1980). Penrose drains are an open wound drainage system, used to drain abscesses or collections of blood, lymph, or tissue fluid. The fluid is removed from the wound space by capillary attraction along a flat rubber tube. The fluid usually drains directly into the dressing rather than into a collecting bag. However, where there is profuse drainage, an ostomy bag may be placed over the Penrose drain site. Containing profuse drainage helps prevent skin irritation and control odor, and provides for cleanliness (see Skill 61 for application and care of an ostomy bag).

A functioning Penrose drain will cause the dressing to become soiled and wet much more quickly than when no drain is present or when a closed drainage system is used and therefore will need more frequent changing. Dressing replacements should be planned with this in mind, and additional sterile 4 × 4's or absorbable combine pads used in the drain area. Since drainage fluid is irritating to the skin, special protective care must be given to the skin around the wound when the dressing is changed.

If there is profuse drainage, it is important to estimate the amount of Penrose drainage when determining output volume. When recording the dressing change and drainage, include the number and kind of dressings saturated with drainage. Sometimes dressings are weighed before application and after removal. The difference between the weights of the dry and wet dressings is then included in the fluid output figures.

Penrose drains are now used less frequently because of the success of the newer closed wound suction drainage systems. These systems have a much lower rate of infection because they eliminate an open route into the wound and require less nursing care; that is, fewer dressing changes are required and fewer skin problems arise (Cruse and Foord, 1973). The most recent recommendation from the American College of Surgeons is that Penrose drains be used *only* for drainage of pus (Alexander, 1983).

WOUND IRRIGATIONS

Like wound drainage, wound irrigations may be implemented either as an open or closed system. Open irrigations are used with wounds that have been allowed to remain open for delayed closure or healing by secondary intention, and for those wounds that have reopened spontaneously or were reopened due to infection. Fluids used for wound irrigations tend to have an osmotic ionic composition that approximates intracellular fluid.

Closed wound irrigations frequently are used after orthopedic surgery to remove bone fragments and other debris that could cause infections. They also are used preventively when a wound infection is anticipated, or when early signs of wound infection develop.

DATA BASE

When giving care to a client with a drain of any kind, the nurse needs to know the purpose of a specific drain and how to care for it. It also is important to know how much and what kind of wound drainage is expected for a particular client in relation to the diagnosis, the number of days postoperative, any complicating factors, and the client's general condition. Increased amounts of drainage are expected on a dressing when a Penrose drain is present, while very little drainage is expected on the dressing when closed suction drainage systems are used (if the system is functioning correctly). The dependent (lower) areas of a dressing are always checked for drainage, since gravity causes drainage to accumulate there. If fluid is leaking around the stab wound exit of a closed wound drainage tube, the nurse would suspect an obstruction in the tube.

Client History and Recorded Data

Background information from the health record includes the kind of drain present, its location, how it is anchored, and the amount of drainage already evidenced. In the immediate postoperative period, much of this information is available from the anesthesia record or the surgeon's progress report. The operative report usually takes a few days to be processed and typed and generally is not available immediately after surgery. When it becomes available, the nurse enters these data in the kardex or computer nursing-care plan. The record also reflects the pattern of drainage for the past 24- to 48-hour time period. This information helps the nurse determine whether the present amount of drainage is consistent and acceptable, whether irrigation is required, or if the physician must be consulted.

Physical Appraisal Skills

Inspection. Inspection is used to determine the amount, color, and consistency of the exudate on the dressing or within the drainage bag, evacuator, or wall suction container. Body fluids drain at a fairly even rate over a given 8-hour period. Compare the amount of drainage over one 8-hour time period with another. Any substantial decreases may mean drainage tube obstruction. Continued bright red bleeding should be reported to the physician. Inspection reveals whether or not the tube remains fastened securely in the correct place and how well it is functioning. Inspection also reveals whether evacuators in the manually operated portable wound suction drainage system are compressed and are exerting negative pressure (suction) or are decompressed (not exerting suction).

It is important to note whether the drainage tube is kinked. Correct taping at the exit site helps avoid kinking. Continued inspection during wound irrigation provides data about the condition of the wound before and after irrigation, the nature of the debris removed, and the state of wound healing.

Auscultation. When working with manual closed wound drainage systems, *auscultation* indicates whether the unit actually is providing negative pressure or suction. If there is no sound of a vacuum being released when the porthole is opened, no negative pressure was present.

EQUIPMENT

Portable Closed Wound Suction Systems
Portable closed wound suction drainage and irrigation systems consist of presterilized perforated wound tubing, connectors, a connecting tube, and an evacuator. Negative pressure created by manual compression of the evacuator exerts gentle suction within the wound. To function effectively, the systems must be airtight and the evacuator compressed. As the evacuator fills with fluid, it gradually expands and when full, negative pressure is reduced and sometimes absent.

The Snyder Hemovac and Surgivac are examples of portable wound suction drainage systems. They are illustrated later in this skill. These systems have polyvinyl or silicone wound tubings with many perforations ranging in diameter from $3/32$ to $1/4$ inches. Both the Hemovac and the Surgivac are equipped with anti-reflux valves to prevent exudate from returning to the wound. They can be hooked up to wall suction if greater pressure is needed.

The Hemovac evacuator is a circular apparatus with clear side walls that allows clear visibility of the exudate. Steel springs inside the evacuator chamber produce negative pressure when the air inside the evacuator is expressed by manual compression. An attached plug inserted into the pouring spout closes the system and maintains the negative pressure. The Hemovac exerts 50 mm Hg pressure and is available in 200, 400, and 800 ml sizes with graduated markings on the sides for easy measuring. There are some special-purpose 200-ml Hemovac evacuators that produce only 28 mm Hg negative pressure and are designed for use with cranial procedures or hysterectomies, as well as a 100-ml Mini-Snyder Hemovac.

The newer Snyder Surgivac is a translucent, green bellows-type evacuator with a spider-style pump used as an internal vacuum assist. It has a screw-cap opening, with the wound and drainage tubes attached to the cap. The cap rim and tubings rotate to open or close the suction system, and the entire cap is removed to empty the evacuator. The Surgivac is designed to exert a constant, steady 50 mm Hg of negative pressure, even when nearly full.

If wound irrigations are planned when the Surgivac or Hemovac are inserted during surgery, two slender perforated tubes are usually placed parallel to each other within the same tissue plane. This provides an entry for irrigation fluid as well as an exit for returned fluid.

Another brand, the Duval Redi-Vac, creates its negative pressure with an inflatable balloon inside a lightweight translucent container. The balloon is inflated by squeezing a rubber ball on the top of the apparatus and closing a stopcock similar to the Hemovac.

The Heyer-Schulte Suction Drain System is a lighter weight and smaller wound suction drainage system, similar to the Mini-Snyder Hemovac. It consists of either flat or round wound drains attached to a soft, compressible, translucent, calibrated, balloon-shaped reservoir which has a 100 ml capacity. One or more drainage tubes may be attached to one reservoir. Because of their light weight and small size, they are useful when multiple drains are needed (see Fig. 35–1).

T-tubes
T-tube drains are slender red rubber or synthetic T-shaped drains that are used after surgery on the biliary tract. The "T" portion is placed in the common bile duct and the long end is brought out through a stab wound, sutured to the skin, and attached to a gravity drainage system. *Foley catheter* drains are made of soft red rubber or silastic and have an opening in the rounded tip and an inflatable balloon to keep the catheter in place. They are used in the urinary bladder or with surgical wounds such as a gastrostomy or suprapubic prostatectomy. See Figure 35–2 for illustrations of a variety of surgical drains.

Penrose Drains
Penrose drains are soft, flat rubber drain tubes, 25 to 35 cm (10 to 14 in) long, used in abdominal surgery or abscesses. Capillary attraction causes pus and body fluids to flow along the drain's surfaces to the outside where it is absorbed into the dressing or contained in an ostomy bag. A Penrose drain may be sutured to the skin to keep it from spontaneously falling out prematurely, and always has a safety pin or safety clip on the drain to prevent its being drawn completely into the wound. A *cigarette* drain is similar to a Penrose drain, but is narrower and has gauze wicking inside the lumen.

Irrigating Syringes
Glass or plastic *irrigating syringes* may be used to irrigate closed wound drainage systems. These syringes have a plunger and a barrel and may be used with or without the needle, depending on the size of tube being irrigated. The most common size is a 50- or 60-ml (2-oz) syringe.

Bulb or *asepto syringes* are often used for irrigating open wounds. An asepto syringe is a glass or plastic syringe with a red rubber squeeze bulb instead of a plunger. Reusable and resterilizable, they are available in a variety of sizes and styles. The 2- to 4-oz sizes with the catheter tip are commonly used for wound irrigation. Squeezing and releasing the rubber bulb causes water to be drawn into the syringe. Reusable asepto syringes are sterilized unassembled, with the bulb and syringe separated. Dipping the sterile rubber bulb tip into the sterile irrigating solution prior to inserting it into the syringe allows for easier insertion

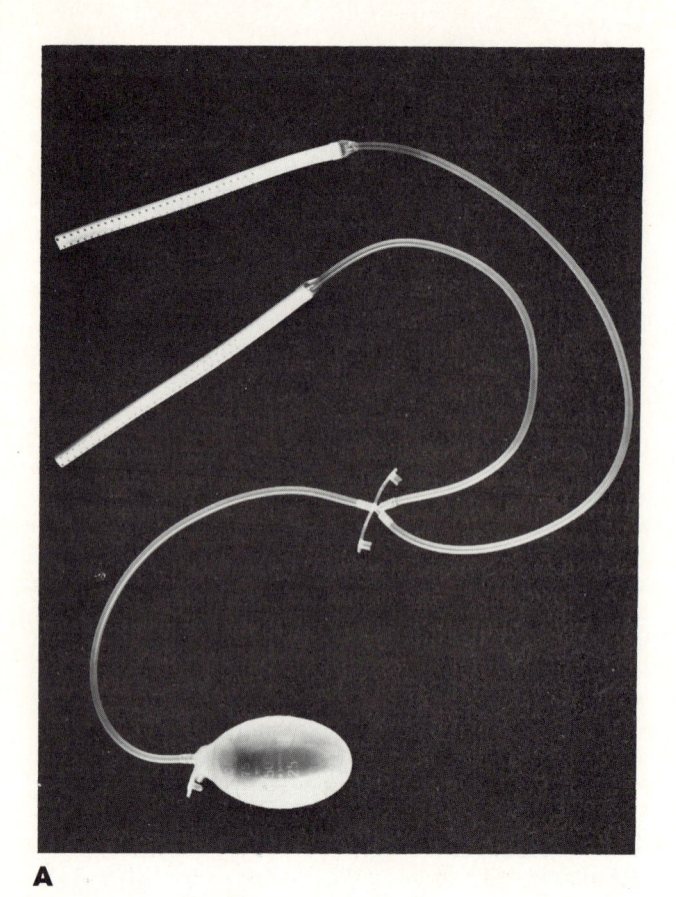

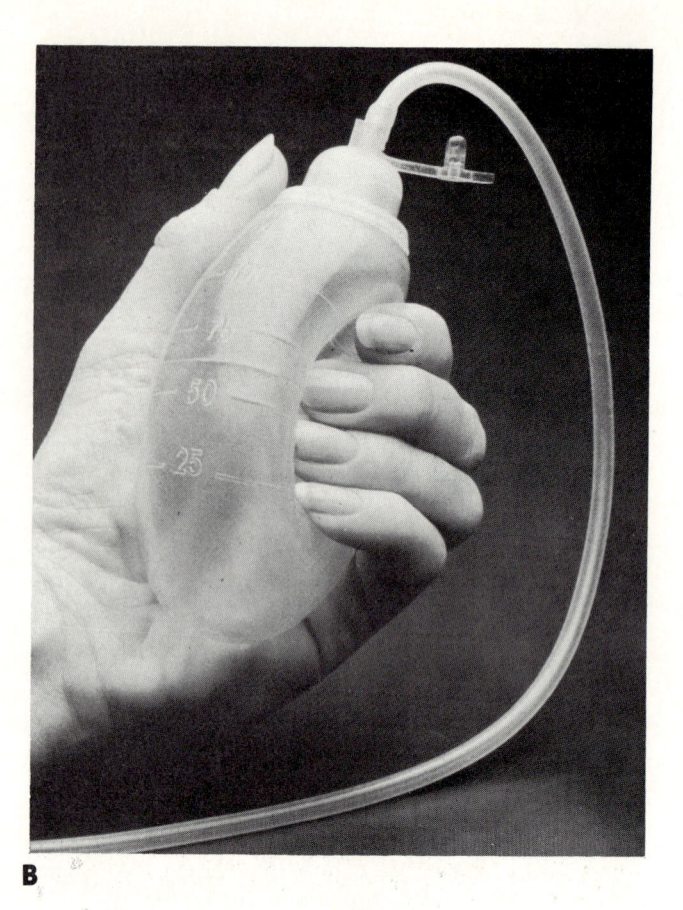

Figure 35–1. Lightweight, small-volume wound suction drainage system. Manual compression creates mild negative pressure. **A.** Heyer-Schulte Suction Drain System; small reservoir with two drains that are inserted into the wound. (Courtesy of American Heyer-Schulte Corporation, Chicago, IL.) **B.** Mini-Snyder Hemovac evacuator. (Courtesy of Zimmer, Inc., Warsaw, IN.)

and a better seal. Figure 35–3 shows syringes used for wound irrigations.

Solutions

Irrigating solutions are used to loosen and remove debris or provide local antibacterial action. Common solutions include sterile normal saline; broad-spectrum, poorly absorbed local antibiotics, such as neomycin; Dakin's solution, an antibacterial, aqueous solution of sodium hypochlorite and sodium bicarbonate; and Alevaire, a wetting agent that thins viscid (glutinous or sticky) secretions and causes bacteria to be more susceptible to antibiotics.

Basins

Two sterile basins are needed for open wound irrigations. A *kidney-shaped* basin is used to catch the returned irrigation solution; its shape allows it to be held closely to the body without leaking. A *round* basin is used within the sterile field to hold the sterile irrigating solution.

Dressings

Dressing supplies, such as a dressing tray, sterile gloves, sterile dressings, and tape are also needed.

When the skin already is irritated or if the solution is irritating to the skin, petroleum jelly (sterile) may be applied around the wound prior to irrigation.

Hazards

While wound drains do provide a necessary exit for excess body fluids and draining pus, thus aiding healing, they also create an additional problem. The tubing itself can serve as an entry for pathogens and a source of infection. Studies have indicated a 34 percent incidence of contamination at the interior ends of Penrose drains, and none at the interior ends of closed wound drainage systems (Cruse and Foord, 1973). The same study noted that Penrose drains require five times as much nursing time for applying dressings than do the closed wound suction drain systems. Since drainage from a Penrose drain usually is absorbed into a dressing rather than collected in a bag, the wet, soiled, contaminated dressings are a potential source of cross-contamination to other clients. Through capillary attraction, they also are a possible avenue for wound infection from environmental contaminants.

Another hazard with drains is the potential for contamination of drain exits, tubing openings, or evac-

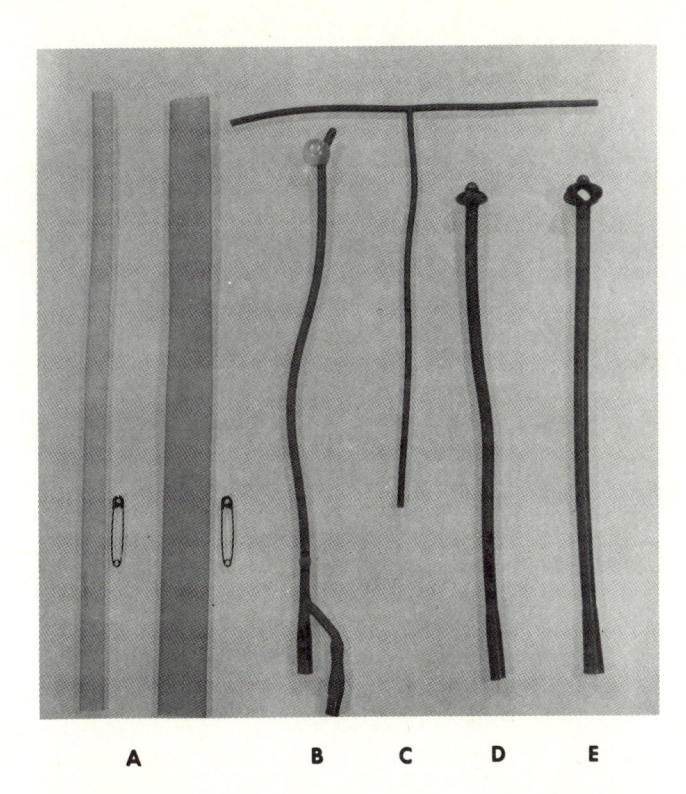

Figure 35–2. Drains commonly used after surgery. **A.** Penrose drains. **B.** Foley catheter. **C.** T-tube. **D.** Mushroom or Pezzer catheter. **E.** Batwing or Malecot catheter. (From Gruendemann B, Meeker MH: *Alexander's Care of the Patient in Surgery*, ed 7. St Louis, CV Mosby, 1983.)

uator portholes, plugs, and caps from direct contact with the worker's hands. These areas are intended to be maintained in an aseptic manner.

☐ EXECUTION

Nursing-care responsibilities when caring for a client with a drain include knowing the presence, location, and purpose of the drain; being able to assess the functioning of the drain; being sure the drain is adequately secured; assessing the nature and volume of the drainage; carrying out specific procedures related to emptying and measuring; and conveying information to other workers.

The nurse may be asked to shorten or remove a Penrose drain, irrigate a Hemovac or Surgivac system,

or irrigate an open wound. It is reassuring to a client when each nurse carries out the procedure as nearly like the previous nurse as possible. Explain changes in the usual wound-care procedure (such as new medical directives), since nonunderstood changes can cause apprehension. Include this new information on the kardex or computer nursing-care plan so it is readily available for the next nurse. When changing a dressing, allow time for questions from the client and provide information as needed.

CARE OF SURGICAL DRAINS

Portable Closed Wound Suction Systems

When emptying a series of evacuators (Hemovac, Surgivac, or Redi-Vac) or reservoirs (Heyer-Schulte) from the same wound or client, separate output figures are tallied. Multiple drains are numbered, with the intake and output record numbered accordingly. This makes it possible to keep a record of drainage from each tube. Usually, drains are left in place until minimal exudate appears in the evacuator or reservoir.

Check portable wound suction evacuators and reservoirs regularly for tubing kinks, degree of compression, and level of exudate. Recompress evacuators whenever they are found expanded, and empty reservoirs before they become completely filled. An evacuator cannot exert negative pressure unless it is compressed, and if not emptied regularly, there is a potential for clogging. A full evacuator also is heavy and clients may find its appearance distressing. When an obstruction in the tubing is suspected, irrigate the system with a firm, but slow, gentle use of sterile normal saline. If standing orders, unit policies, or specific physician directives do not provide for this, contact the physician for an order. If the irrigation does not remove the obstruction and the system continues to malfunction, notify the surgeon at once.

Figure 35–4 depicts the method used to measure, empty, and reestablish suction for the Snyder Surgivac evacuator. Figure 35–5 presents the method used with the Snyder Hemovac.

Gravity Drainage Systems

Drainage or collection bags for gravity systems must always be kept below the level of the wound unless clamped off. Raising the collection bag higher than

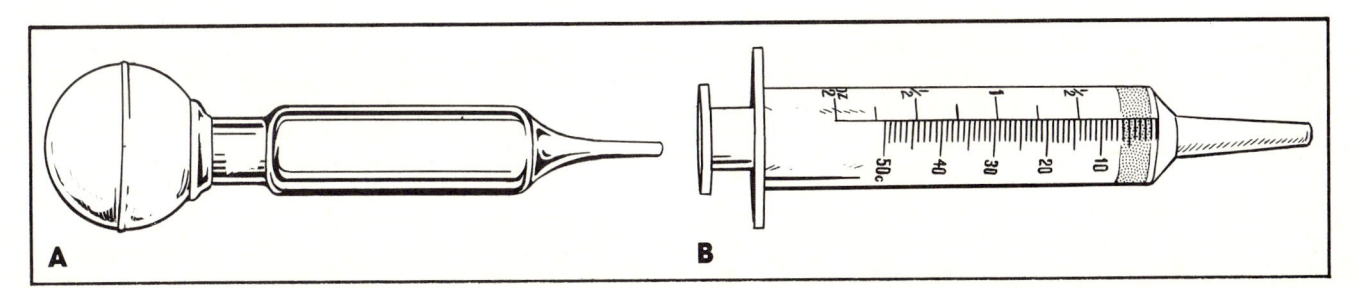

Figure 35–3. Syringe used for wound irrigation. **A.** Asepto syringe. **B.** Plastic plunger syringe with catheter tip.

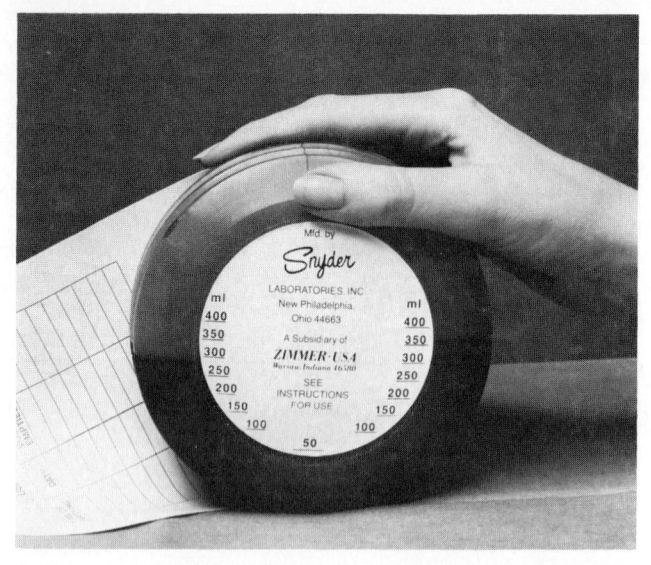

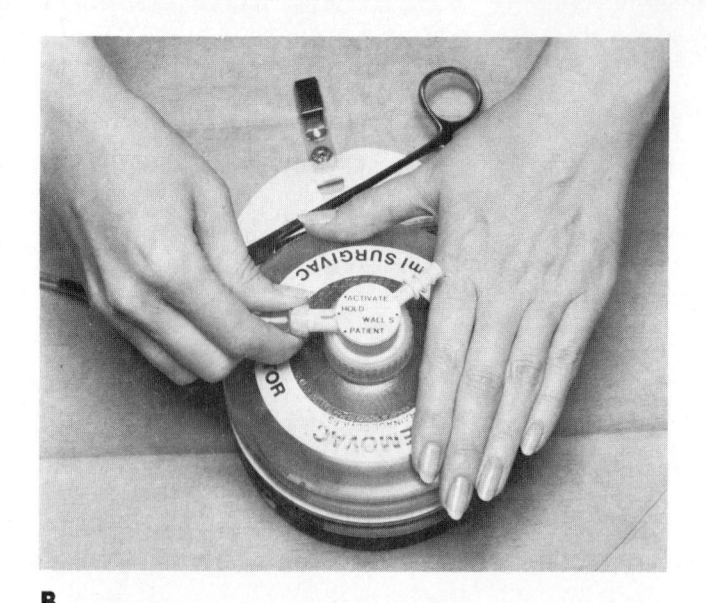

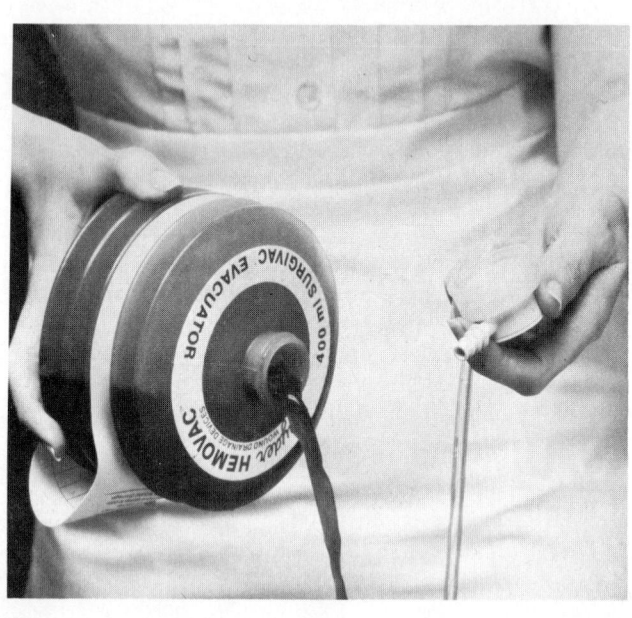

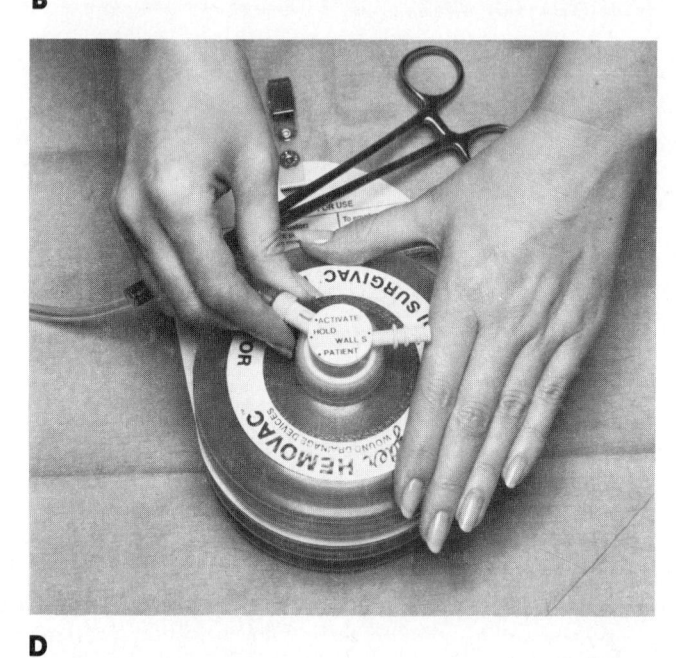

A

B

C

D

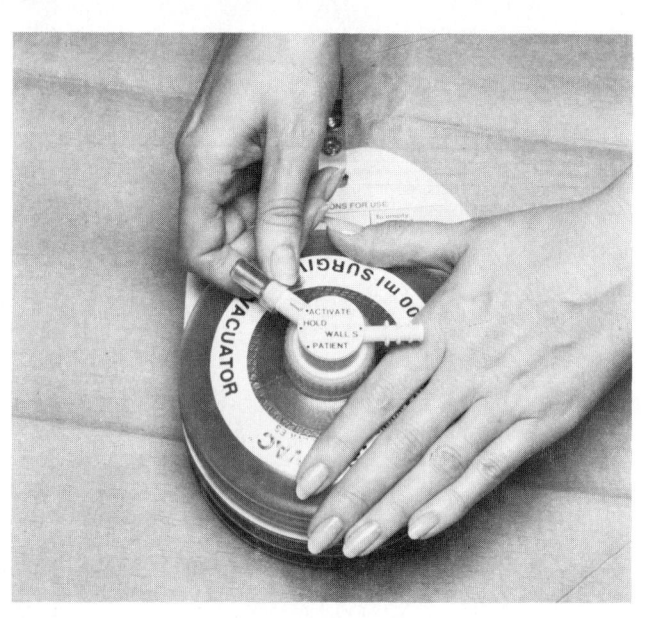

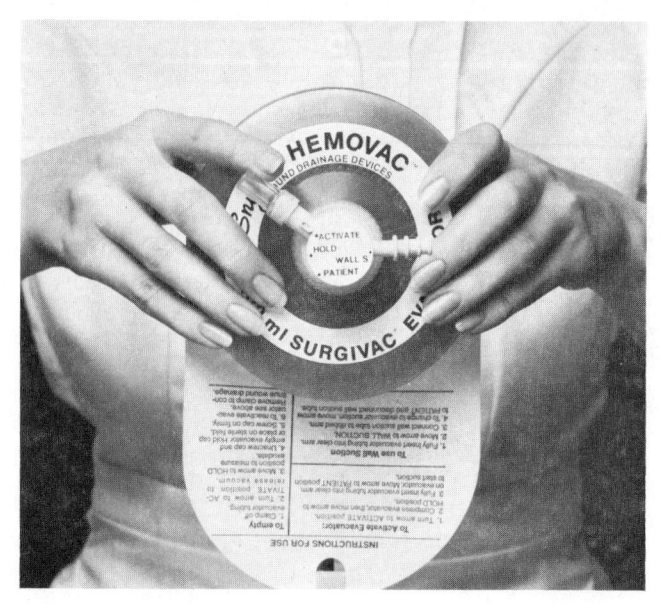

E

F

334

G   H

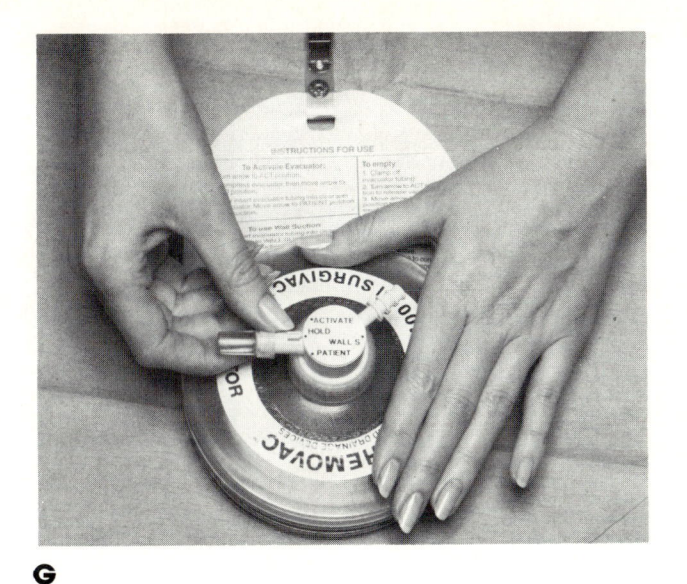

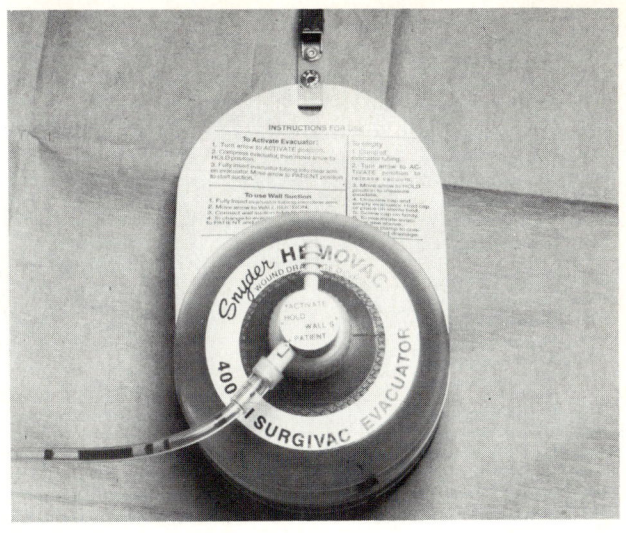

Figure 35-4. Snyder Surgivac Evacuator: Ways to measure and empty exudate and reestablish negative pressure. **A.** Read volume with unit on flat surface. **B.** Set cap to HOLD position before emptying. **C.** Remove cap and empty exudate. **D.** Reset cap to ACTIVATE. **E.** To activate, compress the unit on a tabletop, or **F.** Activate by thumb-to-palm pressure between the hands. **G.** While evacuator is fully compressed, turn sidearm until the arrow points to HOLD. **H.** Set cap to PATIENT. (Courtesy of Zimmer, Inc., Warsaw, IN.)

the wound causes reflux of exudate into the wound. To empty a collection bag from a T-tube or Foley catheter wound drain, open the exit clamp at the lower part of the collection bag and allow the fluid to drain into a measuring container. Collection bags are emptied every shift in the acute- and chronic-care setting, and the amount is recorded on the intake and output record. The color, consistency, and odor are recorded in the nurses' notes or integrated progress notes in the client's health record.

Penrose Drains

Approximately 1 inch of a Penrose drain usually is left extending from the stab wound. A safety pin or special Penrose clamp (such as the Safety Klip) *always* is placed on the Penrose drain next to the skin surface at the point where the drain exits from the skin. The surgeon frequently orders that the drain be advanced (shortened or pulled out) from 2 to 5 cm (1 to 2 in) per day. If the drain has been sutured to the skin, these stitches are removed and the drain advanced, leaving

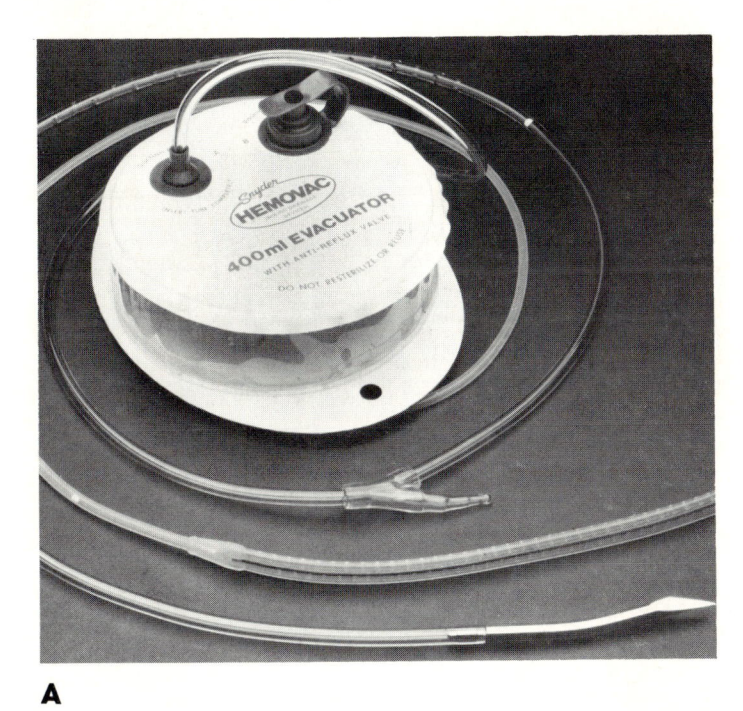

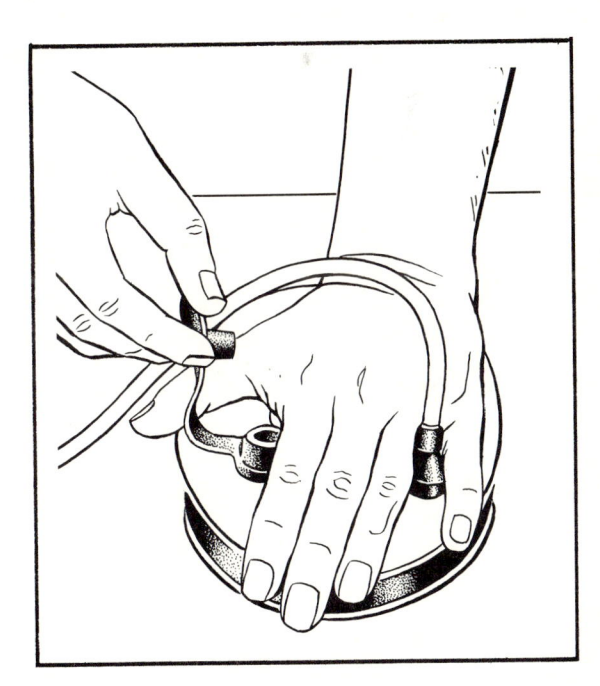

A   B

Figure 35-5. **A.** Snyder Hemovac Evacuator and tubing. **B.** To establish negative pressure, place evacuator on a flat, firm surface (overbed or bedside table), compress evacuator completely with a flat hand, and close pouring spout. (Courtesy of Zimmer, Inc., Warsaw, IN.)

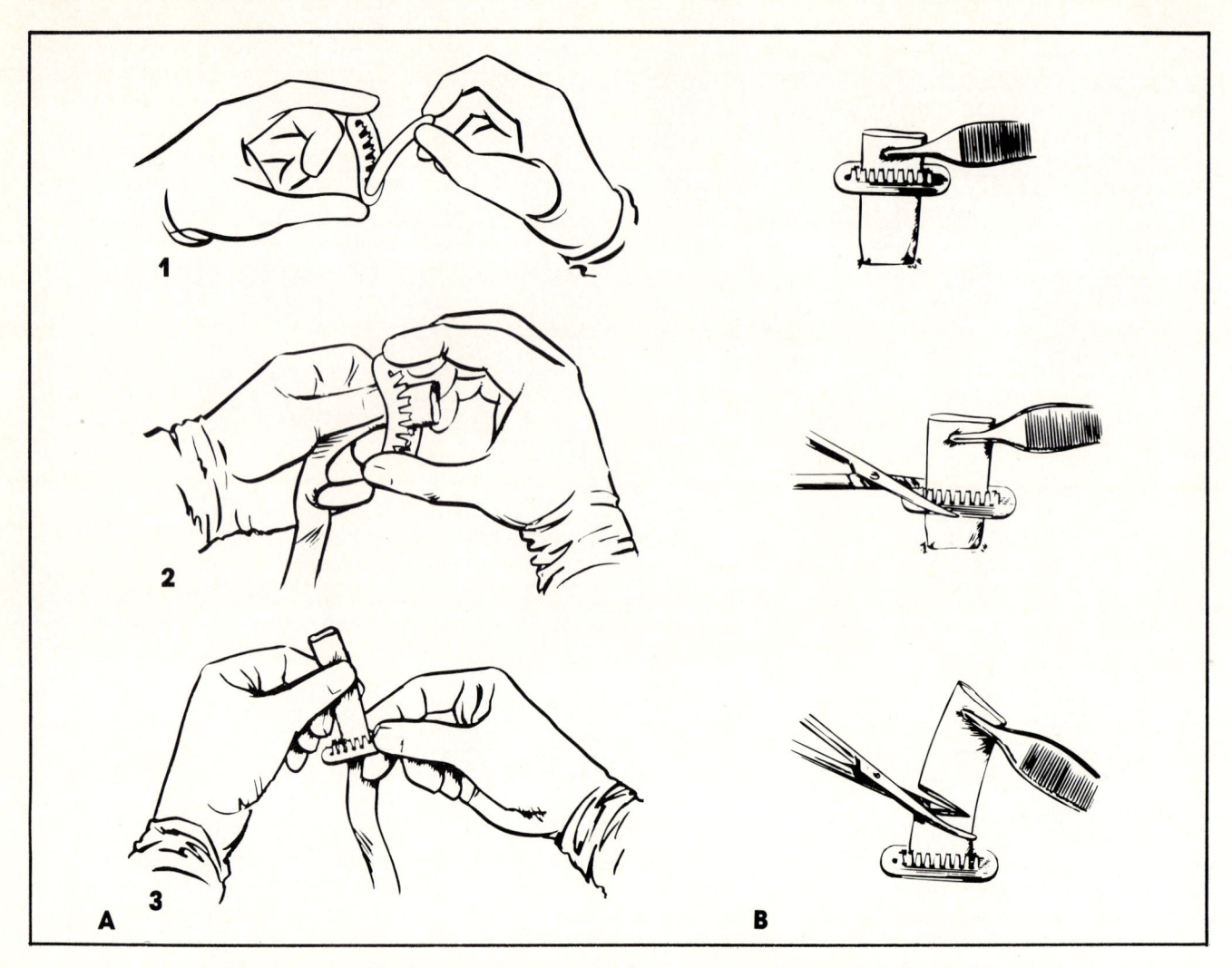

Figure 35–6. Taut Safety "Klip": **A.** Attaching the Klip: (1) Remove plastic tooth protector; (2) Bend Klip—to spread teeth. Push drain through opened teeth; (3) Pull drain through Klip evenly. (Courtesy of Taut, Inc., Geneva, IL.) **B.** Advancing the drain: (1) Advance drain, using tissue forceps or hemostat; (2) Slide down Klip; (3) Cut excess drain. (Courtesy of Taut, Inc., for American Hospital Supply, Geneva, IL.)

the safety pin in place to keep the drain from reentering the wound. Usually, the drain is shortened daily until it is completely removed or falls out spontaneously. This allows the drain tract to heal from the inside out. As with all wound-care procedures, shortening a drain is a sterile procedure. Advancing a Penrose drain using a safety clip is illustrated in Figure 35–6.

☐ SKILL SEQUENCE

ADVANCING A PENROSE DRAIN

Step	Rationale
1. Validate physicians' order for procedure.	Some surgeons prefer to do this themselves; others delegate the task to the nurse.
2. Gather equipment for a dressing change (see Skill 32). Note indicators of sterility. Add sterile scissors, tissue forceps, 2 hemostats, sterile gloves, and a fresh sterile safety pin or Safety Klip.	Provides for aseptic implementation of the procedure.
3. Explain procedure to client.	Allays apprehension; increases client's self-care knowledge.
4. Position client for direct visibility of drain site; drape as needed.	Facilitates manipulation of the drain and protects the client's privacy.

(continued)

Step	Rationale
5. Wash hands.	Avoids introduction of contaminants.
6. Remove dressing; inspect, palpate, and cleanse wound and drain site as in Skill 32, Skill Sequence, "Dressing Change with Wound Care," steps 8 to 26, pp. 305–306.	
7. Grasp drain securely and raise it upright with tissue forceps or sterile gloves and cleanse around drain site, using care not to tug on drain. Use circular strokes from drain outward. Use a fresh swab after each one to two cycles.	Facilitates thorough cleansing around drain before adjusting. Avoids accidental removal of more drain length than desired. Cleanse from area of least contamination (drain site) to area of greater contamination (surrounding skin). (See Fig. 32–9.)
8. Apply protective ointment to skin if wound drainage is irritating, using a sterile tongue blade, gauze pad, or swab.	Urine, feces, and tissue fluid are irritants and can cause skin breakdown.
9. Grasp drain with hemostat; gently and firmly, pull drain out required length, usually 2.5 to 5 cm (1 to 2 in).	Hemostat provides nonslip grip for safe, even pull.
10. Hold drain securely near skin with second hemostat. Using a sterile gloved hand, insert a fresh sterile safety pin through drain, just above the hemostat. Cut off excess drain length, leaving 2.5 cm (1 in) above skin. OR: Remove safety pin and insert drain into a Safety Klip. If Safety Klip already is in place, advance and cut. (See Fig. 35–6.)	Avoids accidentally pulling drain out too far. Holds drain in place and avoids accidental loss within wound. Longer length may get caught and pulled out accidentally.
11. Reapply sterile dressings, dry (Skill 32, Skill Sequence, "Dressing Change with Wound Care," steps 30 and 31, p. 307), or wet (Skill 36, Skill Sequence, "Application of Warm Wet Dressings," p. 347), as ordered. Place precut drain dressings around and under Penrose drain (or cut sterile dressing to midpoint with sterile scissors). Place additional dressings over and under drain. Be sure to point drain away from incision. (See Fig. 32–8.)	Protects the skin from excessive contact with irritating tissue fluid drainage. Increases selective absorbency of dressing at the needed area. Avoids contamination of incision.
12. Remove sterile gloves as in Skill 31, Skill Sequence, "Donning Sterile Gloves," p. 290, and fasten the dressing with adhesive tape, Montgomery straps, or a binder.	Adhesive tape sticks to rubber gloves; binders are applied more easily when gloves are removed.
13. Assist client to a position of comfort.	Conveys caring and promotes rest.
14. Dispose of equipment correctly.	Avoids contamination of environment.
15. Wash hands.	Avoids cross-contamination to other clients.
16. Record procedure in health record, including appearance of wound, drain site, amount of drain removed, method of fastening, and client's reaction.	Provides continuing data base for further nursing action. Demonstrates accountability for care provided.

WOUND IRRIGATIONS

Irrigating Open Wounds

An open wound irrigation is done as part of a dressing change procedure. For comfort reasons, the specified solution (irrigant) is warmed to 34° to 37°C (93° to 98°F) prior to its use. This is the temperature defined as warm by Zislis (1971). To warm the irrigant, place a 250- to 500-ml bottle of irrigating solution in a pan of *hot* tap water and allow it to stand for 10 to 15 minutes. This allows the temperatures of the solution and the water to equalize. Place a thermometer in the *pan* to check the temperature. Loosen the cap of the bottle of solution prior to placing it in the hot water, as this allows for release of pressure as the solution warms. Warm irrigating solution causes local vasodilation with increased blood flow, which aids in healing. A warm solution is also more comfortable for the client than a cool solution.

An average amount of solution used for open wound irrigation is 200 ml, with more or less volume used depending on the size and location of the wound. Use an asepto syringe to direct the solution into all parts of the wound. Position the client so that the fluid can be directed into the wound from the cleanest to the least clean area and so that it will drain into an emesis basin or other receptacle, as shown in Figure 35–7. Continue an open wound irrigation until the wound is relatively free from exudate, sloughed tissue, or other debris. Reapply a fresh sterile dressing after the irrigation is completed.

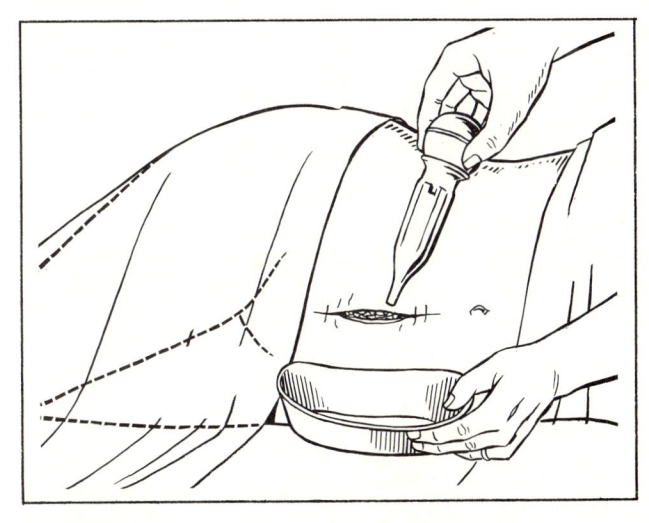

Figure 35–7. Open wound irrigation. Use a syringe to direct the fluid flow from the cleanest to the least clean part of the incision.

Open wound irrigation also can be accomplished by placing a modified stoma bag over the wound (see Skill 61) and attaching it to a drainage collector. Attach intravenous tubing to the container of irrigating solution hung on an IV pole. Insert the end of the tubing or an attached catheter through the entry port in the upper end of the stoma bag and direct it toward the upper aspect of the wound. Allow the fluid to flow by gravity over the wound and out the lower exit port into a drainage collection bag. This allows for a more continuous wound irrigation with less inconvenience to both the nurse and the client.

☐ SKILL SEQUENCE

OPEN WOUND IRRIGATION

Step	Rationale
1. Validate physician's order for procedure.	Provides for correct actions.
2. Gather equipment and note indicators of sterility.	Ensures use of sterile equipment.
3. Explain procedure to client.	Allays apprehension; increases level of self-care knowledge.
4. Wash hands.	Avoids introduction of contaminants from transient bacteria.
5. Label solution bottle with date, time, and initials. Loosen cap.	Reuse for 24 hours is considered acceptable. Loosening cap allows for escape of increased air pressure.
6. Heat solution in pan of hot tap water for 10 to 15 minutes.	Warm solution increases client's comfort and causes some local vasodilation and increased blood flow.
7. Position client so that solution will run downward from wound to catch basin. Expose wound area for maximum visibility by nurse. Drape as needed for privacy. Place waterproof protective pad on bed near wound area.	Facilitates irrigation procedure. Avoids soiling bed linens and clothing.
8. Add sterile gloves, basin, and asepto syringe to dressing tray area.	Sterile gloves are used to palpate and cleanse wound.
9. With label facing the palm, pour normal saline into one round basin and irrigating solution into the other. Recap bottle and place at bedside, not on sterile field.	Avoids soiling the label. Outside of bottle is unsterile. Replacing cap ensures sterility for reuse of solution.
10. Remove dressing, inspect, palpate, and cleanse around wound as in Skill 32, Skill Sequence, "Dressing Change with Wound Care," steps 8 to 26, pp. 305–306. (NOTE: Assemble asepto syringe immediately after donning sterile gloves.) Dip rubber bulb tip in irrigating solution for easy assembly and snug fit. (If no sterile gloves are being worn, be sure to handle only the upper indented flange area of the syringe and the round area of the bulb.)	Have syringe ready for use. Irrigation may be done with or without sterile gloved hands. Avoids contamination of syringe top and bulb tip.
11. Apply protective ointment to skin if solution is irritating, use a sterile tongue blade, gauze pad, or swab.	Protects skin from injury.
12. Using dominant hand, hold tip of syringe in solution; compress and release rubber bulb, drawing solution into syringe. Hold syringe with tip downward.	Avoids contamination by gravity causing solution to flow upward toward ungloved hand and downward to syringe tip as syringe position is changed.
13. Using a firm steady pressure, squeeze asepto bulb, directing solution flow downward from top to bottom of wound. Direct flow into any recesses or pockets within wound.	Avoids having debris flow over freshly washed area. Provides for thorough cleansing.
14. Hold catch basin in place against skin with nondominant hand, so as to contain irrigant return with minimal spillage. Continue irrigating until solution is used up or no more exudate is present.	Avoids contamination of linen or clothing with wound exudate.
15. Dry the skin around wound from incision outward, using sterile gauze.	Minimizes skin maceration.
16. Apply protective ointment if wound drainage is irritating.	Urine, feces, and tissue fluid are irritants and can cause skin breakdown.
17. Reapply sterile dressing, dry (Skill 32, Skill Sequence, "Dressing Change with Wound Care," steps 30 and 31, p. 307) or wet (Skill 36, Skill Sequence, "Application of Warm Wet Dressings," p. 347) as specified. Use sterile gloves, forceps and hemostats as needed.	Protects wound and absorbs drainage.

(continued)

Step	Rationale
18. Remove gloves and fasten dressing with adhesive tape, Montgomery straps, or a binder.	Adhesive tape sticks to rubber gloves; binders are applied more easily when gloves are removed.
19. Assist client to a position of comfort.	Conveys caring and promotes rest.
20. Dispose of equipment correctly.	Avoids contamination of environment.
21. Wash hands.	Avoids cross-contamination to other clients.
22. Record procedure in health record, including kind and amount of solution used, appearance of wound, presence of exudate or sloughed tissues, and client's reaction.	Provides continuing data base for further nursing action. Demonstrates accountability for care provided.

Continuous Irrigation

Figure 35–8 illustrates the use of the Snyder Hemovac or Surgivac system for wound irrigation. Note that the direction of the flow within the wound can be reversed by alternating the clamps. Although manufacturing design minimizes the problem, larger pieces of clots and wound debris may obstruct the tubing system. Reversing the flow at least every 6 hours tends to prevent this problem. It is important not to reverse the flow when visible particulate material is present in the output tubing, as this would cause it to be washed back into the wound. The entire system must be maintained as sterile during use.

RECORDING

After adjusting a tube and irrigating a wound or drain, record the procedure in the nurses' notes. Include date, time, amount, and kind of solution used; the appearance of the wound, drain, or the returned fluid; and the client's reaction to the procedure. Add any modifications and suggestions to the kardex or computer nursing-care plan for future reference.

Sample POR Recordings

- S—States abdomen feels less tender today.
- O—Suture line clean, mildly inflamed. Two 4 × 4's and 1 ABD pad half-saturated with serosanguineous drainage. Penrose drain in place, intact.
- A—Wound healing appropriately.
- P—Penrose drain shortened 2″; new safety pin and dressing applied. Continue observations and shorten more tomorrow as ordered, if drainage decreases.
- S—None
- O—Evacuators found nearly empty. Past 8 hr shift had 200 ml drainage. Slight leakage of serosanguineous fluid around tube exit.
- A—Tube apparently obstructed.
- P—Irrigated drainage tube with 20 ml sterile saline. Several small clots returned. Fluid now flowing into evacuator. Plan to recheck every hour; irrigate p.r.n.

Sample Narrative Recordings

Abdominal wound irrigated with 200 ml Dakin's solution. Returned cloudy fluid with pieces of tissue and mucous shreds. Moist saline dressings applied for wet-to-dry dressings. Says he is more comfortable today.

T-tube clamped for 2 hrs p.c. Reports no abdominal distress or discomfort. Dressing remains dry and intact.

☐ CRITICAL POINTS SUMMARY

1. Surgical wound drains promote wound healing by preventing accumulation of fluid within the wound area.
2. Use aseptic technique to care for wound drains.
3. Cleanse a drain site separately from the incision.
4. Inspect portable closed wound drainage systems for patency, volume of exudate, and degree of compression.
5. Maintain a sustained negative pressure within a portable closed wound drainage system through manual compression of the evacuator.
6. Reverse the flow of continuous closed wound irrigations at least every 6 hours.
7. Penrose drains serve as portals of entry for microorganisms.
8. Open Penrose drains require reinforced dressings to absorb the increased wound drainage.
9. A sterile safety pin or drain clip always is placed on a Penrose drain near the skin surface.
10. Use warm (34° to 37°C; 93° to 98°F) sterile solutions for open wound irrigations.
11. Flush open wounds from cleanest to least clean areas until fluid returns are clear.
12. Apply protective ointment to the skin before or after an open wound irrigation as needed.
13. Record wound drainage volume on the intake and output record.

☐ LEARNING ACTIVITY

In a clinical unit or the central supply of an acute care agency, locate a Snyder Hemovac or Surgivac unit, a Duval Redi-Vac, and a Heyer-Schulte Suction Drain System. Read the directions for use. Locate:

- Evacuator or reservoir
- Exit porthole
- Wound tubing entrance
- Drainage tubing

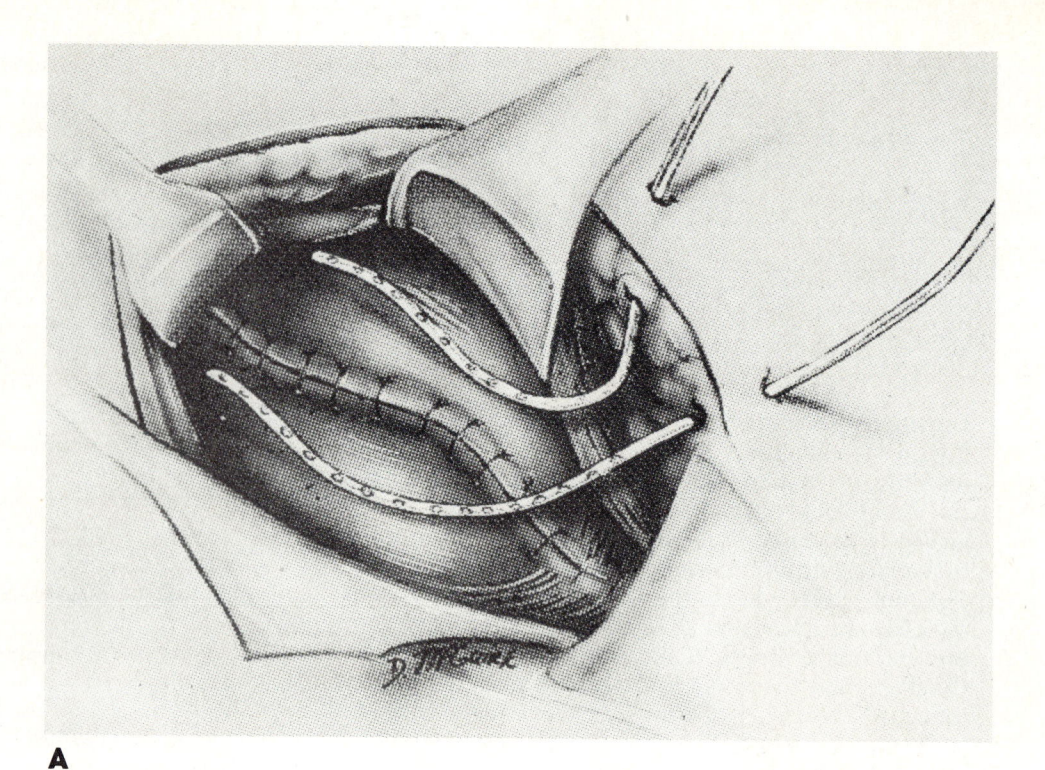

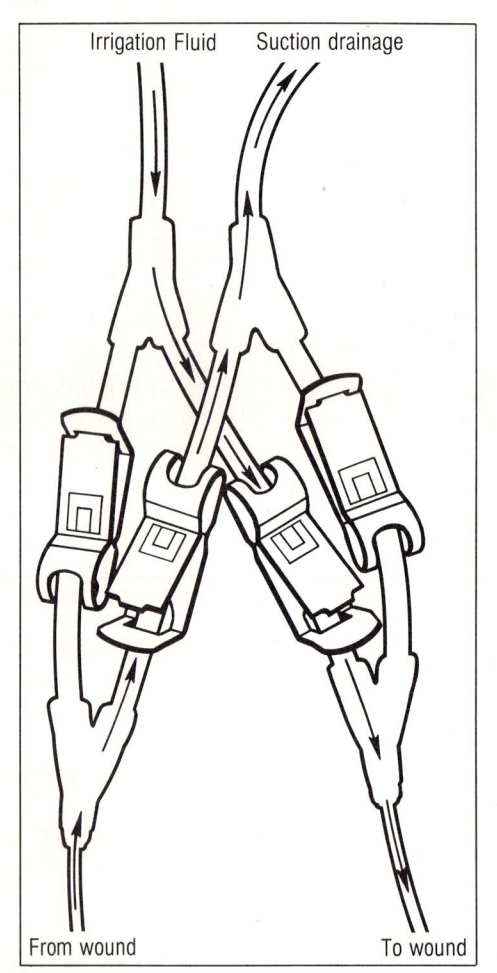

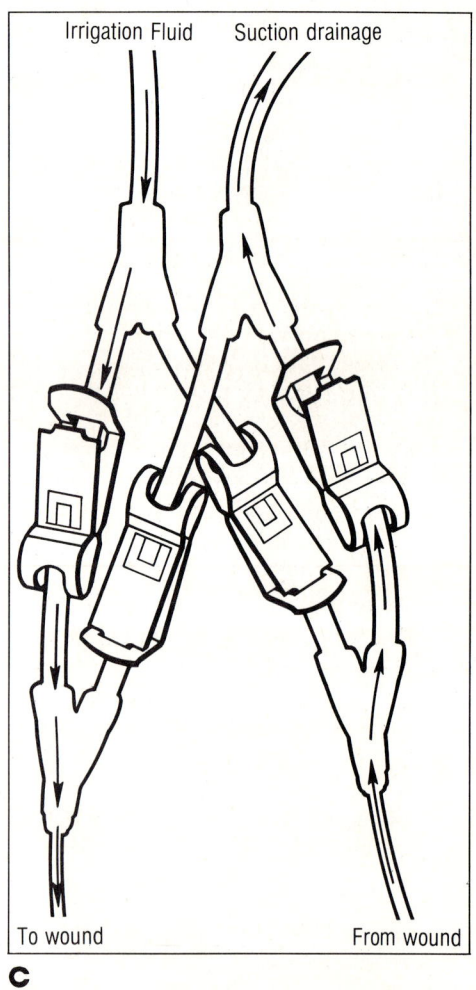

Figure 35–8. Closed wound irrigation with Snyder Hemovac or Surgivac wound drainage system. **A.** Placement of perforated suction drainage tubing within a wound. **B.** Irrigation fluid flows through the wound from right to left through the center unclamped tubes (1). **C.** Closing the center clamps and opening the outside clamps (2) causes the fluid to reverse directions and flow through the wound from left to right. (Courtesy of Zimmer, Inc., Warsaw, IN.)

- Wound tubing
- Volume capacity
- Negative pressure mechanism

☐ REVIEW QUESTIONS

1. What advantages does a closed wound drainage system have over an open drainage system?
2. Which of these drains are considered open? closed?
   _____ Penrose drain
   _____ T-tube with collection bag
   _____ Portable wound suction drain systems
3. Why are additional dressings used over a Penrose drain site?
4. What are the advantages of continuous portable wound suction drainage systems over Penrose drains for the postoperative care of surgical wounds?
5. What actions does a nurse take when finding a noncompressed evacuator?
6. What are two possible reasons for finding no exudate in the evacuator of a Hemovac, Surgivac, Redi-Vac, or the reservoir of a Heyer-Schulte Suction Drain system?
7. What actions might a nurse take if there is no exudate in the evacuator or reservoir of a portable wound suction drainage system?
8. Why is it important not to touch the porthole, plug, or cap with the hands, clothing, or linens when emptying the evacuator or reservoir of a closed wound drainage system?
9. Why are separate output tallies kept for each of the multiple evacuators or reservoirs being used in the same client or wound?
10. Where does the nurse check for dependent wound drainage in the following clients with Penrose drains?
    a. Side-lying client with an abdominal incision
    b. Client with hip surgery who lies on the back
    c. Ambulatory client with an abdominal incision
    d. Client with a perineal abscess who lies on the back
11. For what reason should a gravity flow wound drainage bag be kept below the wound?
12. What precaution would you take prior to carrying out an order to irrigate a portable wound suction drain system being used for continuous wound irrigation?

☐ PERFORMANCE CHECKLISTS

OBJECTIVE: To use aseptic technique to advance a Penrose drain.			
CHARACTERISTIC	**RANGE OF ACCEPTABILITY**	**SATISFACTORY**	**UNSATISFACTORY**
Advancing a Penrose drain: 1. Gathers correct equipment.	No deviation		
2. Explains procedure.	No deviation		
3. Washes hands.	No deviation		
4. Removes dressing and disposes of properly.	No deviation		
5. Uses aseptic technique throughout.	No deviation		
6. Inspects, palpates, and cleanses wound and drain site.	No deviation		
7. Pulls drain outward 2.5 to 5 cm (1 to 2 in) using hemostat.	Degree of advancing drain is variable according to specific order.		
8. Fastens with fresh sterile safety pin or Safety Klip before cutting off excess drain length.	No deviation		
9. Applies new dressing using additional dressings in drain area.	No deviation		
10. Disposes of equipment correctly.	No deviation		
11. Washes hands.	No deviation		
12. Records procedures.	No deviation		

OBJECTIVE: To use aseptic technique to irrigate an open wound.

CHARACTERISTIC	RANGE OF ACCEPTABILITY	SATISFACTORY	UNSATISFACTORY
Open wound irrigation:			
1. Gathers correct equipment.	No deviation		
2. Warms irrigating solution to 34° to 37°C (93° to 98°F).	No deviation		
3. Explains procedure.	No deviation		
4. Positions client.	No deviation		
5. Places protective pad on bed.	No deviation		
6. Washes hands.	No deviation		
7. Removes dressing and disposes of properly.	No deviation		
8. Uses aseptic technique throughout.	No deviation		
9. Dons sterile gloves.	Sterile forceps or hemostats may be used.		
10. Cleanses area around wound.	No deviation		
11. Directs irrigating solution flow downward and into all parts of wound, containing returned fluid in kidney-shaped basin.	No deviation		
12. Applies protective ointment before or after irrigation.	Omit if skin is not likely to become irritated.		
13. Applies new dressing as ordered.	No deviation		
14. Disposes of equipment correctly.	No deviation		
15. Washes hands.	No deviation		
16. Records procedure.	No deviation		

REFERENCES

Alexander, JW: Infection, Host Resistance, and Antimicrobial Agents. In Dudrick SJ, Baue AE, et al.: Manual of Preoperative and Postoperative Care, ed 3. Philadelphia, WB Saunders, 1983.

The Case for Closed Wound Suction. Warsaw, IN, Zimmer, U.S.A., Inc., 1979.

Cruse PJE, Foord R: A five-year prospective study of 23,649 surgical wounds. Archives of Surgery 107(2):206–210, 1973.

Gruendemann BJ, Meeker MH: Alexander's Care of the Patient in Surgery, ed 7. St Louis, CV Mosby, 1983.

LeMaitre GD, Finnegan JA: The Patient in Surgery, ed 4. Philadelphia, WB Saunders, 1980.

Luckmann J, Sorensen KC: Medical–Surgical Nursing: A Psychophysiologic Approach, ed 2. Philadelphia, WB Saunders, 1980.

Taut, Inc.: Advantages of the Taut Safety "Klip®." Geneva, IL, Taut, Medical Division, 1979.

Zislis, JM: Hydrotherapy. In Krusen H (ed): Handbook of Physical Medicine and Rehabilitation, ed 2. Philadelphia, WB Saunders, 1971.

BIBLIOGRAPHY

Christianson F: Closed wound irrigation in orthopedics. ONA Journal 6(9):359–366, 1979.

Heyer-Schulte Brochure. Suction Drain System. Chicago, American Heyer-Schulte Corporation, 1978.

Inservice Guide to Effective Nursing Care: Closed Wound Suction. Warsaw, IN, Zimmer, U.S.A., Inc., 1978.

Kozier B, Erb GL: Fundamentals of Nursing: Concepts and Procedures, ed 2. Reading, MA, Addison-Wesley, 1983.

Sorensen KC, Luckmann J: Basic Nursing: A Psychophysiologic Approach. Philadelphia, WB Saunders, 1979.

Wound suction: Better drainage with fewer problems. Nursing75 5(10):52–55, 1975.

SUGGESTED READING

Neuberger GB, Reckling JB: A new look at wound care. Nursing85 (Horsham) 15(2):34–41, 1985.

AUDIOVISUAL RESOURCES

Wound Irrigation and Specimen Collection
  Filmstrip, slides, cartridge, videotape. (1981, Color, 19 min.)

Closed Suction Wound Drainage
  Filmstrip, slides, cartridge, videotape. (1981, Color, 18 min.)
  Available through:
  Medcom, Inc.
  P.O. Box 116
  Garden Grove, CA 92642

SKILL 36 Wet Sterile Dressings

PREREQUISITE SKILLS

Skill 19, "Inspection"
Skill 20, "Palpation"
Skill 28, "Handwashing"
Skill 30, "Sterile Supplies"
Skill 31, "Donning Sterile Gloves"
Skill 32, "Dressings and Wound Care"
Skill 46, "Thermal Applications"

☐ STUDENT OBJECTIVES

1. Explain the purpose of warm wet dressings.
2. Explain the rationale for alternating warm wet dressings with dry sterile dressings.
3. Describe the cautions needed when applying an external heat source to warm wet dressings.
4. Explain the rationale for the termperatures used for warm wet dressings.
5. Compare the expected and untoward effects of heat.
6. Describe the problems that may result from too-high temperatures or prolonged heat with warm wet dressings.
7. Identify persons who may be at risk from application of heat.
8. Demonstrate the ability to apply sterile warm wet dressings to an open wound correctly.

☐ INTRODUCTION

Wet sterile dressings (also called compresses) are dressings that remain warm and moist during the entire time they are in contact with the wound. They are primarily used to apply local heat to infected wounds and sometimes to increase drainage in wounds that have a highly viscous exudate. Wet sterile dressings are often referred to as "continuous wet dressings"; biologic principles indicate, however, that heat application should be intermittent rather than continuous.

Wet sterile dressings are presented separately from dry dressings or wet-to-dry dressings because the purpose, rationale, and methodology behind their use are quite different. Understanding these differences helps the nurse interpret and implement the physician's order correctly, or if necessary, make the judgment about whether wet or wet-to-dry dressings are required for a particular wound. Because sterile wet dressings are alternated with dry dressings, implementing an order for sterile wet compresses is very time-consuming and requires large amounts of supplies. If the nurse does not understand and value the necessity for strict aseptic technique or the need for alternating wet and dry sterile dressings, shortcuts in time and materials become quite tempting.

Little research has been done on the subject of sterile wet soaks, and the literature is not conclusive in its recommendations for either principles or procedures, nor has much been written about current practices in various agencies. In this skill, and in Skill 37, principles of wound healing, sterility, heat, and physics are used to develop recommendations for these widely used procedures. This skill includes the actions of heat as they affect wounds and wound healing. For a further discussion of the effects of heat, see Skill 46.

☐ PREPARATION

Wound exudate must drain from a wound before healing can occur. When drainage is allowed to accumulate in an open wound, it provides a culture medium for bacteria and delays granulation tissue formation. A wet gauze dressing promotes wound drainage in two ways. Moist gauze enhances capillary attraction through a wicking action. Moisture and warmth cause thin viscous secretions and prevent them from coagulating and drying on the wound surface. Both of these actions encourage drainage to leave the wound. However, if a wound has profuse drainage, a dry dressing generally is a better choice, as it will absorb more drainage (Peacock and VanWinkle, 1976).

Application of heat increases the local inflammatory response to injury by dilating cutaneous arterioles and increasing local circulation to the area. Increased local circulation serves to stimulate new tissue growth, increased suppuration (pus formation), and increased phagocytosis (destruction of bacteria by white blood cells). These actions make application of heat especially beneficial during the early stages of an infection. When an antibacterial solution is used for warm wet dressings, this provides additional local bacteriostatic action.

Warm wet dressings also have a psychologically therapeutic benefit. "There are few wounds, closed or open, which are not made to feel better by the application of moderate wet heat, and thus testimonials are abundant, even though accurately analyzed data are scarce" (Peacock and VanWinkle, 1976, p. 254).

External heat produces its maximal increase in local circulation (from vasodilation) and rise in tissue temperature after approximately 5 to 20 minutes of application, depending on the type of heat used. A rapid rise in tissue temperature is thought to be the most therapeutic. The approximate therapeutic duration of tissue temperature elevation ranges from 5 to 30 minutes. Including the temperature rise time, the usual duration of a heat treatment is from 30 to 45 minutes (Lehman and de Lateur, 1982, pp. 425–426; Stillwell, 1965, p. 236). If local heat applications are continued much longer than this, tissue congestion occurs as a result of the increased vascular permeability associated with vasodilation. Vasoconstriction also occurs after this length of time and, combined with tissue congestion, actually results in a *decreased* blood flow to the area (Gucker, 1965; Jensen, 1976; Sorensen and Luckmann, 1979). The reason for this effect is not clear, although it is known that *temperature changes* stimulate vasodilation or vasoconstriction, but when the new temperature becomes the norm, the vascular size reverts to normal (Fischer and Solomon, 1965). Continuous application of wet dressings can result in skin tissues becoming macerated (wrinkled, waterlogged, and softened from soaking). If the dressing is allowed to become cool, it is quite uncomfortable for the client. For these reasons, warm wet wound dressings should be removed after 45 minutes and a dry sterile dressing applied for at least an hour or until the next ordered time. This allows time for the skin to dry and the tissue temperature to return to normal so vasodilation can again occur with the reapplication of heat.

The temperature recommendations for warm wet dressings vary considerably in the literature. Peacock and VanWinkle (1976) recommend using moderate wet heat on open or closed wounds, which would be between 36.5° and 40.0°C (98° and 104°F) (Zislis, 1971). See Table 46-1 in Skill 46 for classifications of temperatures. According to Waterman et al. (1967), the temperature goal in warm wet dressings is to raise tissue temperatures to around 36° to 38°C (97.0° to 100.5°F), which corresponds to usual body core temperatures. On the other hand, Kottke et al. (1982) and Lehman and de Lateur (1982) indicate that the approximate therapeutic tissue temperature range is from 40.0° to 45.5°C (104.0° to 113.9°F). The effects of heat are discussed more fully in Skill 46.

Preventing loss of heat from warm moist dressings is apparently as successful in maintaining skin and subcutaneous temperatures at therapeutic levels as the application of additional external heat. It is also safer (Fischer and Solomon, 1965; Waterman et al., 1967). Thus, since warm moist dressings are to be removed after 45 minutes, preventing loss of heat seems to be the reasonable approach. Waterman's (1967) studies indicate that placing insulating materials around warm wet dressings is the most successful way to maintain local warmth. He recommends that wool, foam rubber, or a combination foam and polyurethane wrapper be placed over the dressing or around the extremity. Petrello (1973) found that aluminum foil, plastic, and rubber sheeting also serve as effective insulators for warm wet dressings. If these materials are not available, possible substitutes would include several large bath towels covered by a disposable, waterproof, bed-protector pad, or a thermal blanket covered by a spread or towel.

An additional source of external heat is sometimes applied to a warm moist dressing by means of an electric heating pad or hot water bottle (Kozier and Erb, 1983; Petrello, 1973; Sorensen and Luckman, 1979). There are conflicting views about this practice because of the possibility of burns from a hot water bottle that is too hot or a heating pad that is turned too high or malfunctions. When using a heating pad for additional heat, the client or the nurse may be tempted to leave it on continuously or to turn it up too high, with resulting burns and skin damage. In addition, electric heating pads have a potential electric shock hazard if they are not well insulated. The heat receptors within the body readily become adapted to a new temperature, which makes it easy to apply temperatures that cause tissue damage without the person being aware of it. This is especially true for individuals who are at increased risk from application of heat, such as those with decreased cardiovascular status, decreased perception of temperature and pain, altered states of consciousness, and the aged (Jensen, 1976). In addition, some heating pads (especially those designed for home use) do not have adequate thermostatic regulation and generate more heat than is needed. When applying additional external heat sources, the nurse needs to consider both the potential for trauma to the client and the personal and institutional liability and risk of a lawsuit in case of an injury.

HAZARDS OF WET DRESSINGS

Prolonged application of warm wet dressings of any temperature causes skin maceration. In addition, if the dressings are too hot, prolonged erythema (redness), blisters, or discomfort will occur, and tissue damage is possible. The maximum safe skin temperature is considered to be 44°C (111°F) for up to 30 minutes (Millard, 1965: Krusen et al., 1971). There apparently is a close margin of safety between therapeutic tissue temperature levels and temperatures that cause tissue necrosis. If body tissues remain heated at 40°C (105°F) for 4 to 6 hours, tissue necrosis occurs (Stillwell, 1965; Waterman et al., 1967).

While there may be exceptions based on a physician's clinical judgment, in general, heat is not used in these circumstances: (1) with fresh grafts or pedicle skin flaps, because there is insufficient blood flow available and tissue damage will occur; (2) with noninflammatory edema, because heat would simply increase tissue congestion; (3) when the possibility of hemorrhage exists, because vasodilation increases bleeding; (4) with fresh scars, since sensation is diminished; (5) when the vascular supply is inadequate, because the lack of vascular adaptation can cause ischemic necrosis; and (6) over a malignant tumor area, since heat increases the metabolic rate of both normal and abnormal cells (Kottke et al., 1982; Lehman and de Lateur, 1982).

Individuals who need lower dressing temperatures and more frequent observations (including visual inspection) include: (1) elderly persons or those with diabetes, peripheral vascular disease, or neurologic impairment, all of whom have decreased sensitivity to temperature and pain and therefore can be burned without realizing it; (2) the very young, who have unstable temperature-regulating mechanisms and are unable to give accurate feedback about the temperature of the heat being applied; (3) nonresponsive or lethargic clients who are unable to give verbal feedback; (4) clients with paralysis (loss of voluntary movement) or paresthesia (abnormal sensation), who may experience numbness or tingling and are unable to give reliable feedback about the temperature in those areas.

Both physical and psychological responses occur while the warm wet dressings are in place. Expected physical responses include generalized local redness, reflex warming and redness of other parts of the body, that is, consensual vasodilation (Fischer and Solomon, 1965; Lehman and de Lateur, 1982), increased pulse rate without increased blood pressure (Millard, 1965), mild perspiration, and a generalized feeling of warmth and relaxation. Expected psychological responses would include relaxation, relief of discomfort, and reassurance of receiving adequate treatment.

Any indications of discomfort or undesirable reactions during the treatment should be investigated promptly by the nurse. If significant, the treatment should be discontinued and the physician notified. Undesirable local effects of heat applications include blotchy redness of the skin and blisters from too-high temperatures for that particular individual, or local pallor as a result of vasoconstriction. Undesirable systemic effects would include excessive perspiration, increased total body temperature, weakness, and faintness.

DATA BASE

To help evaluate the therapeutic effectiveness of warm wet dressings, the nurse must know the purpose to be achieved by those dressings, the function of the solution being used, and the current status of the wound.

Client History and Recorded Data

The nurse is better able to assess the effectiveness of the warm moist dressings if he or she knows how long the soaks have been used, the number of days postoperative or posttrauma for the client, present and past status of the wound, and the amount and type of wound drainage present. It also is important to consider factors that might increase the individual's risk from heat applications and to consider modifying the temperature or time for the treatment, as well as plan for increased monitoring during application time.

Physical Appraisal Skills

Inspection. When removing the old, dry sterile dressing, the nurse *inspects* the dressing and the wound for the presence, amount, and nature of wound exudate. Inspection also reveals the appearance and color of the exposed subcutaneous tissue, wound edges, and surrounding skin. Inspection determines the presence of any prolonged redness, blotchy redness, blisters, maceration, or other signs of tissue injury or damage.

Palpation. If the skin around the open wound is reddened, palpation is used to assess for specific areas of tenderness or induration (hardness), using a sterile gloved hand.

Sense of Smell. The sense of *smell* can sometimes detect the presence of some kinds of bacteria within the wound (see Skill 34).

EQUIPMENT

Clean examination gloves may be used to remove the soiled dressing, provided the wound is not touched with the unsterile gloves. Wet dressings always are discarded in an *impermeable trash bag* and labeled "Contaminated."

A variety of *solutions* may be used for sterile wet dressings, preferably one that has an ionic and osmotic composition that approximates cellular fluid (Schilling, 1976). *Sterile normal saline* is frequently used, simply as a moistening agent. Weak *acetic acid* provides an acid environment that discourages bacterial growth when urea-splitting organisms are present. *Salicylic acid* and *Dakin's solution* (an antibacterial, aqueous solution of sodium hypochlorite and sodium bicarbonate) are sometimes used to speed up dissolution and separation of necrotic wound debris.

Sterile dressings or *compresses* may consist of *eye pads, 4 × 4's, ABD's* or *Combipads,* depending on the size and location of the wound needing to be soaked. *Sterile barrier drapes* have a moisture-resistant liner or surface and are used for covering the wet dressing. They avoid external contamination of the dressing and help retain heat. *Sterile basins* are used to hold the solutions for moistening the sterile dressings. *Sterile gloves* or sterile *hemostats* are needed to handle and wring out the moist sterile dressings. *Montgomery straps* are the preferred way of keeping wet dressings in place, because they eliminate repeated taping and resultant skin damage. If *adhesive tape* must be used because of size or location of the wound, a piece of tape may be placed on the skin in the appropriate areas and left there. The dressing may then be taped

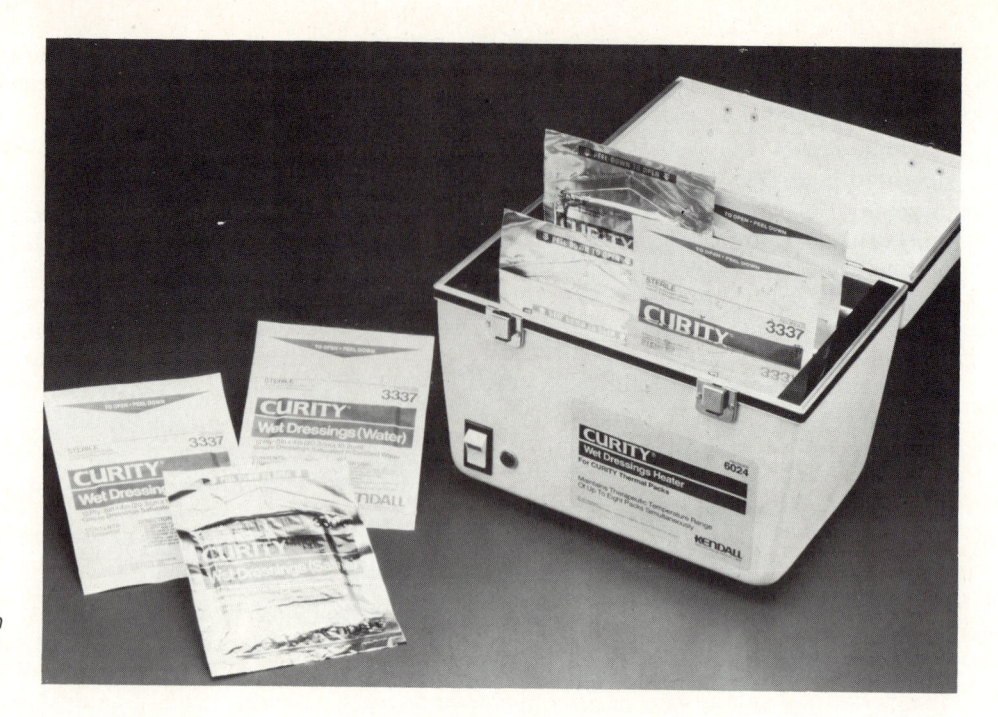

Figure 36-1. Curity Thermal System: A wet dressings heater. (From The Kendall Company, Boston, MA.)

to that adhesive-taped area, thus avoiding frequent removal of tape from the client's skin. See Skill 32 for a further description of these supplies.

A convenient way to prepare sterile hot wet dressings is to use prepackaged sterile wet dressings, such as Curity wet dressings (Kendall). Each peel-open foil package contains a sterile gauze dressing premoistened with either normal saline or distilled water. The unopened packages are placed in a small portable automatic electric heater, as shown in Figure 36-1. The device heats room-temperature packages to 46° to 50°C (115° to 122°F) in approximately 10 minutes and keeps them warm indefinitely, as indicated by the red indicator light. One study (using the older style heater) indicated that these packs sustain heat longer and are less time-consuming and less costly than traditional methods of preparing warm moist dressings (Moore and Winburg, 1975).

Insulating materials include plastic, aluminum foil, heavy bath towels, wool blankets, or thermal blankets with a spread or towel over them. Studies are inconclusive as to which material provides the greatest heat retention with the least heat loss.

Heating pads or *hot water bottles* may sometimes be ordered to accompany warm wet dressings (see Skill 46 for further discussion of these items).

Dry sterile dressings, a *dressing tray*, *sterile gloves* or *hemostats*, and *adhesive tape* are needed to apply the *dry sterile dressing* that alternates with the wet sterile dressing. *Sterile gauze squares*, *sterile hemostats* or *gloves*, and *sterile normal saline* may be needed to cleanse the wound after *removal of the dry dressing*, prior to application of the sterile wet dressings.

☐ EXECUTION

Whether sterile wet dressings are ordered continuously or every 4 hours, they should be removed after 45 minutes and a dry sterile dressing applied. An hour's rest between applications of fresh sterile wet dressings is required when continuous soaks are ordered.

Like all open wound dressings, wet sterile dressings must be applied with aseptic technique, *even if the wound already is infected*. If the wound already is infected, avoid the possibility of adding another, perhaps more serious secondary infection.

Because bacteria travel readily through moist layers and surfaces, a wet dressing provides increased opportunity for environmental contamination to enter the wound and allows wound drainage to reach the surface of the dressing more readily. Therefore, place a sterile barrier drape over the wet dressing before applying the insulating material. If a sterile barrier drape is not available, place a dry sterile dressing over the wet one and add a piece of clean plastic wrap. Although the plastic wrap is not sterile, it is preferable to having the moist dressing in contact with the bed linens and clothing.

Solutions may be heated by placing a bottle of solution (at room temperature) in a pan of water and bringing it to a full boil on a hot plate or stove. Remember to loosen the cap to allow for expansion of air and formation of steam when heated. Remove from heat and allow the temperatures in the pan and the bottle to equalize, as determined by a thermometer placed *in the pan*. If a sterile thermometer is available, this may be used in the bottle. This takes approximately 15 to 20 minutes. The solution temperature should then be approximately 52.5° to 56.0°C (128° to 134°F), which is approximately 16°C (29°F) higher than the desired application temperature of between 36.5° and 40.0°C (98° to 104°F). Approximately 8.0°C (14.5°F) of heat is dissipated to the sterile basin and dressings, with more lost to the atmosphere during the application process.

To help ensure that the temperature will not be too hot, apply the compress so that the lower edge of the first warm dressing initially touches the skin distal to the wound, and ask for the client's perception of the temperature. If necessary, the dressing can be lifted temporarily for cooling and then replaced over the entire wound without contamination (Dison, 1975). Work quickly, because heat is rapidly lost to the surrounding atmosphere.

Because the body's heat receptors adapt to new temperatures readily, the client initially will perceive the dressing as comfortably warm, but fairly soon will perceive it as cooled, even though it is still warm to touch. Clients also sometimes expect a warm wet dressing to feel quite hot initially rather than simply warm. If the nurse explains the temperature rationale and the adaptation process, it helps the client understand why the dressing is not "hot," and why it does not continue to feel as warm as on initial application.

Contour the warm moist dressing to fit closely to the client, and then wrap it completely with insulating material to hold it in close proximity to the body with no air leaks for heat to dissipate. This close wrapping also retains natural body heat, which helps the compresses remain warm.

The process of alternating sterile wet and dry dressings obviously is very time-consuming for the client as well as for the nurse. It also is very confining, especially if the client is ambulatory. As much as possible, schedule the wet dressing applications to avoid meal times, visiting hours, and periods of sleep. It is psychologically reassuring to the client if each nurse implements the moist dressing procedure in a similar manner, and follows the procedural instructions written on the kardex or computer nursing-care plans. Explain the procedure and its purpose to the client and family, as this increases their tolerance and acceptance of the procedure.

When warm wet dressings are removed, they are considered contaminated, because they contain fresh wound exudate of unknown microbial content. Place them in impermeable trash bags, remove them from the client's room, and place them in the designated container for contaminated items.

Remove the alternate dry sterile dressing slowly, as the exudate may have caused the dressing to adhere to the wound. If this has happened, moisten the adherent area with sterile normal saline.

☐ SKILL SEQUENCE

APPLICATION OF WARM WET DRESSINGS

Step	Rationale
1. Validate physician's order for warm wet dressings.	Ensures implementation of correct procedure.
2. Explain procedure to client.	Facilitates cooperation and involves client in self-care.
3. Wash hands.	Avoids cross-contamination.
4. Label solution bottle with date, time, and initials.	Reusing for 24 hours is considered acceptable, if not contaminated.
Loosen cap.	Loosening cap allows for escape of steam and increased pressure and facilitates later one-handed opening.
5. Heat in unsterile pan of water on stove to pan water temperature of 52.5° to 56°C (128° to 134°F). Use towel to transport bottle after it is heated.	Higher temperature than actual application allows for heat loss to equipment and environment. Prevents burning self.
6. Position client for maximum visibility of wound, protecting the client's privacy. Use additional drapes as needed.	Provides for increased work ease and psychological security for the client.
7. Don clean examining gloves.	To protect self when removing dressings.
8. Remove old dry dressing slowly, watching for any adherent areas. Use sterile normal saline to moisten any such areas. Discard dressing in impermeable trash bag.	Avoids disturbing fresh granulation tissue and reduces discomfort to the client.
9. Remove examining gloves and wash hands.	Removes transient microorganisms prior to donning sterile gloves; bacteria multiply inside gloves.
10. Tear tape strips or prepare new Montgomery straps.	Advance preparation for fastening dressing.

11. Prepare sterile field as in Skill 30, Skill Sequence, "Opening Envelope-wrapped Sterile Packages," p. 277.
   a. Add hemostats, gloves, and dressings as needed.
   b. Place gauze dressings in basin.
   c. With label facing palm of hand, pour solution over dressings. Avoid splashing or dripping.
   d. Recap the bottle. Place bottle beside, not on the sterile field.
	Maintains sterility of equipment and solution.
	
	Soiled, wet labels are difficult to read.
	Microorganisms readily pass through wet sterile drapes.
	Outside of bottle is unsterile. Replacing the cap ensures sterility of contents for later use.

(continued)

APPLICATION OF WARM WET DRESSINGS (Cont.)

Step	Rationale
12. Don sterile gloves if desired.	Provides ease in handling dressing.
13. Cleanse wound if loose material or excessive exudate is present in or around wound. Hold folded unfilled gauze pad with gloved hand or hemostat. Use prepared solution to moisten gauze and cleanse wound as in Skill 32, Skill Sequence, "Dressing Change with Wound Care," step 26, p. 306. Avoid contaminating gloves or hemostat. (Allow solution to cool before using for cleansing.)	Allows direct contact of wet dressing to open tissue. Filler material sticks to open tissue. Allows for continued use with dressing. Avoids burning.
14. Check dressing temperature with sterile thermometer, if available.	Ensures correct dressing temperature.
15. Squeeze or wring hot wet dressings with sterile gloved hands or sterile hemostats until not dripping, but still quite wet.	A too wet dressing will leak during application time. A too dry dressing will not provide enough heat or moisture to remain warm.
16. Touch lower edge of hot wet dressing to skin distal to wound and validate temperature with client. Explain that a quite warm, but not burning temperature is desired.	Avoids possibility of accidental burning.
17. Place remainder of dressings gently but firmly over entire wound.	Provides for direct contact of heat and moisture with tissue.
18. Cover with sterile barrier drape.	Prevents contamination of the wet dressings and the environment.
19. Remove sterile gloves.	
20. Secure with Montgomery straps or apply adhesive tape. Apply tape over any previously applied tape that remains in place between dressing changes.	Holds dressing in place without damaging client's skin.
21. Apply thermal blanket, cover with spread or towel, and arrange snugly around the client.	Reduces heat loss and maintains warm temperature.
22. Dispose of equipment properly.	
23. Reposition client for comfort.	
24. Wash hands.	Avoids cross-contamination to other clients.
25. Record procedure in health record. Include type of solution, appearance of wound, and amount and type of drainage. Modify care plan as needed.	Provides for accountability, responsibility, and continuity of care.
26. Plan to remove wet dressings in 45 minutes with clean examining gloves or sterile gloves, and then apply dry sterile dressing.	Avoids vasoconstriction and local tissue congestion.

In the home setting, a warm wet wound dressing can be prepared by placing it in a strainer in a pan of water, along with two hemostats whose handles are kept out of the water. Boil these items for 20 minutes. (For higher altitudes, see Table 30–1 to determine needed time modification.) Lift the strainer out of the water to drain and partially cool the dressing, the time varying with the size of the dressing. Use the hemostats to wring out and apply the dressings to the wound, or use prepackaged sterile gloves. An alternative for the home setting is to heat a prepackaged thermal pack in an oven set at a "warm" temperature for 5 to 10 minutes and then apply it to the wound in an aseptic manner.

RECORDING

Record pertinent data on flow sheets, in the nurses' notes, or in the integrated progress notes. Recorded data include the time and date, the wound and its appearance before and after the soaks, the type of solution used, the length of time the warm wet dressing was left in place, a description of any drainage, the reaction of the client, and the type of dry dressing applied.

Sample POR Recording
- S—Dozed during application of warm wet dressings.
- O—Wound surface clean & pink. Wound edges slightly red and inflamed @ midpoint. Small amt. of purulent drainage @ midpoint.
- A—Infection continues, but improved since yesterday.
- P—Continue warm moist, acetic acid soaks for 45 min. q 4 h. Dry sterile dressing applied between moist soaks, using Montgomery straps.

Sample Narrative Recording
Warm wet acetic acid dressing applied to open abdominal wound for 45 minutes. Wound clean-looking, with healthy pink tissue, except for 3 cm diam. area at midpoint, which has small amt. of mucopurulent drainage. Dry dressing applied c̄ Montgomery straps. Dozed during procedure.

CRITICAL POINTS SUMMARY

1. Use aseptic technique to apply wet dressings, even if wound is infected.
2. Wet dressings are considered contaminated after application to the wound.
3. Moderate heat, 36.5° to 40.0°C (98° to 104°F), is considered appropriate for open wounds.
4. Heat solution to 52.5° to 56.0°C (128° to 134°F) to allow for heat loss during preparation and application.
5. Minimize heat loss through snug application of insulating materials.
6. Use unfilled gauze dressings for direct contact with open tissues.
7. A sterile barrier drape prevents contamination of the dressing and the environment.
8. Application of heat beyond approximately 45 minutes causes tissue congestion and vasoconstriction rather than vasodilation and increased blood flow.
9. Prolonged contact with moisture causes skin maceration, and excessive temperatures cause tissue damage.
10. Persons with impaired cardiovascular or neurologic status, altered states of consciousness, the very young, and the elderly are at a greater than usual risk from application of heat.

LEARNING ACTIVITIES

1. Check the temperature of the hottest water in your home or apartment, using a candy thermometer.
2. Heat a pan of water on the stove, with the candy thermometer in the pan of water. As the temperature rises, use a spoon or baster to apply a small amount of water to the inner aspect of the wrist at each of these temperatures:
   a. 36.5° to 40.0°C (98° to 104°F) (temperature for application of wet dressings)
   b. 52.5° to 56.0°C (128° to 134°F) (temperature for heating the solution)
   Compare the differences in the temperatures. Which one feels warm? Hot? Comfortable? Uncomfortable? Which one caused a withdrawal reaction?
3. Apply three warm wet "dressings" to both forearms and the abdomen of a peer (your "client"), following the directions below.
   The following equipment is needed:
   - Three thick washcloths or 3 hand towels
   - Two bath towels
   - Plastic wrap, aluminum foil, or plastic
   - Thermal or wool blanket
   (NOTE: While there may be no problems, the phenomenon of consensual vasodilation determines this caution: *If you are not feeling well or have abdominal discomfort, or problems with circulatory insufficiency, do not participate in this activity.*)

   a. Saturate one folded washcloth in the hottest tap water your hands can tolerate without discomfort. Squeeze out the washcloth until it is not dripping, but is still quite wet, and apply to your "client's" abdomen, as described in Skill Sequence, "Application of Warm Wet Dressings," p. 347. Validate the perceived temperature with your "client." Immediately, cover the wet cloth with plastic, plastic wrap, or aluminum foil; add a folded bath towel and a thermal blanket, tucking it firmly around the abdomen.
   b. Saturate and squeeze out the second washcloth and place it on your "client's" left forearm. Cover snugly with plastic, aluminum foil, or plastic wrap.
   c. Saturate and squeeze out the third washcloth and place it on your "client's" right forearm. Cover and wrap closely with a dry bath towel.
   d. Ask for feedback from your "client" about initial temperature sensations for each dressing. Ask him or her to rank the temperature on a scale of 1 to 10, with 10 being the highest temperature that was comfortably tolerable, and 1 being cool or room temperature.
   e. During the next 20 minutes, observe your "client" for any systemic reactions to heat, and ask for any subjective symptoms he or she may be experiencing.
   f. After 20 minutes, ask your "client" again to grade the temperature of the dressings. Compare the value with the earlier estimate.

REVIEW QUESTIONS

1. Why are "continuous" warm wet dressings alternated with dry sterile dressings?
2. What helpful local and systemic effects would you expect to occur from application of warm wet dressings to an open wound?
3. What undesirable local and systemic effects may occur from application of local heat?
4. What is the reason for heating the soaking solution for warm wet dressings 16°C (29°F) higher than the desired application temperature?
5. Why is it necessary to use a sterile barrier drape and insulating materials with warm wet dressings?
6. What potential problems can result from excessive or prolonged heat?
7. What precautions would you observe when applying heat to open wounds on these persons?
   a. Three-year-old child
   b. Nonresponsive accident victim
   c. 34-year-old diabetic woman
   d. 74-year-old man with arteriosclerotic peripheral vascular disease
   e. 80-year-old moderately senile woman

☐ PERFORMANCE CHECKLIST

OBJECTIVE: To use aseptic technique to apply warm wet dressings.

CHARACTERISTIC	RANGE OF ACCEPTABILITY	SATISFACTORY	UNSATISFACTORY
1. Assembles equipment.	No deviation		
2. Explains procedure.	No deviation		
3. Washes hands.	No deviation		
4. Heats solution in pan to 52.5° to 56.0°C (128° to 134°F).	No deviation		
5. Slowly removes and discards old dry dressings.	No deviation		
6. Prepares sterile field, adding heated solution in basin, dressings, gloves or hemostats.	Sterile dressing tray may be used.		
7. Uses aseptic technique throughout.	No deviation		
8. Cleanses wound if old exudate present.	No deviation		
9. Squeezes out dressings until not dripping, but still quite moist, using sterile gloves or hemostats.	No deviation		
10. Applies dressings at temperature of 36.5° to 40.0°C (98° to 104°F) to entire wound, exercising initial caution and validating temperature with client.	No deviation		
11. Applies sterile barrier drape.	No deviation		
12. Fastens with Montgomery straps or adhesive tape.	No deviation		
13. Applies insulating material.	No deviation		
14. Disposes of equipment correctly.	No deviation		
15. Washes hands.	No deviation		
16. Records procedure in nurses' notes, indicating any adaptations on nursing-care plan.	No deviation		
17. Observes client for untoward effects of heat.	No deviation		
18. Plans to remove wet dressing in 45 minutes and replaces with dry sterile dressing.	No deviation		

REFERENCES

Dison N: Clinical Nursing Techniques, ed 3. St Louis, CV Mosby, 1975.

Fischer E, Solomon S: Physiological Responses to Heat and Cold. In Licht S (ed): Therapeutic Heat and Cold, ed 2. Baltimore, Waverly Press, 1965.

Gucker T III: The Use of Heat and Cold in Orthopedics. In Licht S (ed): Therapeutic Heat and Cold, ed 2. Baltimore, Waverly Press, 1965.

Jensen JT: Physics for the Health Professions, ed 2. Philadelphia, JB Lippincott, 1976.

Kottke FJ, Stillwell GK, et al.: Krusen's Handbook of Physical Medicine and Rehabilitation, ed 3. Philadelphia, WB Saunders, 1982.

Kozier B, Erb G: Fundamentals of Nursing, ed 2. Menlo Park, CA: Addison-Wesley, 1983.

Krusen FH, Kottke FJ, et al.: Handbook of Physical Medicine and Rehabilitation, ed 2. Philadelphia, WB Saunders, 1971.

Lehman JF, de Lateur BJ: Therapeutic Heat. In Lehman JF (ed): Therapeutic Heat and Cold, ed 3. Baltimore, Williams & Wilkins, 1982.

Millard JB: Conductive Heating. In Licht S (ed): Therapeutic Heat and Cold, ed 2. Baltimore, Waverly Press, 1965.

Moore J, Weinburg M: The case of the warm moist compress. Canadian Nurse 71(3):19–21, 1975.

Peacock EE Jr, Van Winkle W Jr: Wound Repair, ed 2. Philadelphia, WB Saunders, 1976.

Petrello JM: Temperature maintenance of hot moist compresses. American Journal of Nursing 73(6):1050–1051, 1973.

Schilling JA: Wound healing. Surgical Clinics of North America 56(4):859–874, 1976.

SKILL 37: WET-TO-DRY DRESSINGS

C, Luckmann J: Basic Nursing: A Psychophysio-
roach. Philadelphia, WB Saunders, 1979.
General Principles of Thermotherapy. In
Therapeutic Heat and Cold, ed 2. Baltimore,
1965.
toeckinger J, et al.: Effects of various
and subcutaneous temperatures. Ar-
95(3):464–471, 1967.
apy. In Krusen H (ed): Handbook of

Physical Medicine and Rehabilitation, ed 2. Philadelphia, WB Saunders, 1971.

BIBLIOGRAPHY

Dudrick SJ, Baue AE, et al. (eds): Manual of Preoperative and Postoperative Care, ed 3. Philadelphia, WB Saunders, 1983.

Glor BAK, Estes ZE: Moist soaks: A survey of clinical practices. Nursing Research 19(5):463–465, 1970.

Wet-to-Dry Dressings

Gloves"
ound Care"

IVES

f wet-to-dry dressings when

d uses of common solutions
sings.

used by improperly applied

ion wound healing to the
gs.

lement in secondary inten-

tic technique when caring

that help determine the
ent.

We   ings that are saturated
with   a medicated solution,
plac   wed to dry. Their function   ue (remove) necrotic tissue from an
open wound. They also serve to inhibit the growth of
bacteria. They are used for open surgical, traumatic,
or chronic wounds (such as decubitus ulcers) that need
to heal by second intention with granulation tissue
(Chang, 1979).

The nurse must know how to apply wet-to-dry
sterile dressings in such a way that they will achieve

debridement when removed and will promote rather
than hinder the healing process. The nurse must also
be able to recognize when a wound could benefit from
debridement and when granulation tissue and epithelialization occurs. These observations are recorded and
reported for physician evaluation.

☐ PREPARATION

During the process of wound healing by second intention, granulation tissue forms within the wound. Epithelial cells within the epidermis migrate from the
wound edges over the granulation tissue until the
wound is completely closed.

Granulation tissue is soft, red, sensitive tissue
that bleeds easily. It fills the space created by the
wound, produces a barrier to bacteria, and serves as a
bed for advancing epithelial cells. It is composed of
minute thin-walled capillaries that grow off the parent
blood vessels. These capillary buds enlarge and become surrounded and supported by connective tissue
cells and are gradually transformed into connective
tissues that close and fill the wound. By this time,
surface epithelialization is complete, and a scar has
begun to form. Anything that interferes with granulation tissue formation or epithelial cell migration interferes with wound healing. In open wounds, this interference is most likely to be an infection (Madden and
Arem, 1981).

For granulation tissue to develop, a wound must
be clean and free from infection-prone necrotic tissue
or other debris. Debridement is the process by which
this necrotic debris or infected material is removed
from an open wound. While debridement of large
amounts of dead tissue needs to be done surgically in
the operating room, superficial debridement can be accomplished through the use of wet-to-dry dressings.
Debridement also may be achieved through the use of
enzymes such as Elase or Travase.

When a layer of moistened gauze is placed on the
wound surface, it traps necrotic material in its meshes
as it dries. The necrotic debris is then removed along

with the gauze unless the gauze layers are too thick or were too wet or not wet enough when applied. If the gauze layers are too thick or were too wet, they do not dry out enough to trap the debris, and may cause tissue maceration and breakdown, which produces an ideal culture media for bacterial growth. If the gauze layers were not moist enough, they will dry before wound debris can be trapped.

Generally, a wet-to-dry dressing should be moist enough to dry thoroughly in 4 to 6 hours, or by the time it is due to be changed. When removing the previous dressing, the nurse can determine whether the right amount of moisture was used. If the dressing is completely dry and has little or no enmeshed debris, it was probably too dry when applied. If the dressing is still damp, the gauze layers were too thick or too wet, or both (Chang, 1979).

Medicated solutions are sometimes used in wet-to-dry dressings for debridement purposes or to inhibit the growth of bacteria. Hydrogen peroxide mechanically debrides through its effervescent action. Acetic acid and povidone-iodine (Betadine, BPS, Final Step, Isodine) are antibacterial solutions that reduce bacterial growth and also produce mechanical debridement when the dried gauze is removed. However, some surgeons believe antibacterial solutions are too irritating for open wounds and use only normal saline or peroxide.

Any open wound will have some drainage, whether it be serous tissue fluid, tissue fluid with some bleeding (serosanguineous), or the mucopurulent exudate associated with an infection. Even though an open wound contains necrotic tissue that needs debridement, it also will have some drainage. However, large amounts of drainage and purulent exudate usually are not associated with wounds that are healing well.

All wet-to-dry dressings on open wounds must be done with strict aseptic technique. Because the wound is most likely already contaminated or infected, introducing additional contaminants can produce a second, more serious infection.

DATA BASE

Before applying wet-to-dry dressings, the nurse will want to know the expected action of the ordered solution and the wound characteristics for which debridement is appropriate. This information helps evaluate the therapeutic effectiveness of the wet-to-dry dressings.

Client History and Recorded Data
Baseline data for evaluating the status of the wound and the effectiveness of wet-to-dry dressing therapy would include the date of surgery or trauma, past treatment of the wound, whether infection is present and when it developed, and whether the wound is healing or regressing. The nurses' notes or progress notes in the health record usually contain this information.

Physical Appraisal Skills

Inspection and Palpation. Before removing the old dressing, the nurse *inspects* and *palpates* it for dryness. If the gauze was too damp when applied, it will not have dried. The nurse also notes the color of the dried drainage on the dressing so it can be recorded and, if unusual, reported to the physician. As the dried gauze is pulled off, the nurse *inspects* the exposed wound surfaces for the presence of necrotic material still needing debridement and looks for evidence of granulation tissue formation or wound epithelialization, which would mean those areas require no further debridement. The nurse also notes the amount of necrotic tissue trapped in the dried gauze dressing.

EQUIPMENT

Unfilled gauze squares or pads of a medium mesh are used for wet-to-dry dressings. A too-fine mesh does not permit necrotic tissue to become trapped, and a too-coarse mesh does not hold the wound debris. Filled gauze pads (with an inner absorbent filler layer) are never used for this purpose. If only filled gauze pads are available, they can be unfolded and the filler removed, using aseptic technique. *Tape,* preferably silk (which usually is less irritating to the skin), is needed to hold the outer edges of the gauze in place. Tape must not cover the entire dressing, so that drying can occur.

Sterile normal saline is the most common solution for wet-to-dry dressings. Opened bottles should be marked with the date, time, and initials of the nurse. An opened bottle of sterile saline may be reused for 24 hours and is considered sterile if the cap and rim have not been contaminated. *Hydrogen peroxide* (H_2O_2), usually in a 3 percent solution, is used on grossly contaminated wounds. Its effervescence speeds the separation of necrotic material from wound surfaces and crevices. It is *not* used on wound surfaces with fresh epithelial tissue.

There is some controversy about the use of antibacterial solutions in open wounds, because of their irritant nature. *Acetic acid,* usually in a 0.25 percent solution, sometimes is used with infected wounds. It is effective against a variety of pathogenic microorganisms, including *Pseudomonas aeruginosa,* but may not be effective with *Staphylococcus aureus* or anaerobic bacteria. *Povidone-iodine,* usually in a 10 percent solution (9 percent povidone and 1 percent iodine), sometimes is used on purulent draining wounds. It is considered particularly effective against *Staphylococcus* and anaerobic bacteria.

A *sterile basin, sterile gloves, sterile field,* and sometimes a *sterile hemostat* or *tissue forceps* are needed. The equipment needed varies with the size, nature, and location of the wound.

Hazards
Filled gauze pads are not used because the filler material sticks to open wound surfaces and becomes a

breeding ground for bacteria. The filler deters the trapping of necrotic debris, and filled sponges dry slowly, defeating the purpose of wet-to-dry dressings. Completely covering a dressing with tape results in a nonocclusive dressing becoming occlusive and nondrying.

Acetic acid solution tends to excoriate the skin around the wound edges. The effervescent action of hydrogen peroxide removes newly epithelialized tissue as well as necrotic tissue.

☐ EXECUTION

The solution used for wet-to-dry dressings should be at room temperature or warmed slightly for the client's comfort. This can be done by placing the bottle of solution in a pan of hot tap water for 10 to 15 minutes. Temperatures comparable to those used for wound irrigation would be appropriate, that is, 34° to 37°C (93° to 98°F). See Skill 35.

Using sterile gloves or hemostats, carefully insert a saturated and wet but not dripping single layer of unfilled gauze into all parts of the wound. A hemostat may be needed to tuck the gauze into wound crevices or eroded areas, such as exist with some massive decubitae. Debridement occurs only if there is direct contact between the gauze and the wound surface. Add enough slightly moistened fluffed dressings to fill the wound space. If the moistened gauze does not completely fill the wound, the unfilled empty or dead spaces will not have contact with the antibacterial-soaked gauze and will not be debrided. These dead spaces then become breeding grounds for infection to develop. If the gauze is packed in too tightly, it will not dry readily. Excessive pressure on the open wound also decreases local circulation.

When removing the dried gauze dressing, pull it firmly and slowly toward the center of the wound. Wound debris will be removed with the dressing. Observe carefully for new granulation tissue, and avoid disturbing these fresh pink-red areas (Madden and Arem, 1981). If the dressing has adhered to granulation tissue, moisten that area with a small amount of sterile normal saline so it can be removed with minimal bleeding. When most of the wound surface has become free of necrotic debris, debridement with wet-to-dry dressings should be discontinued.

☐ SKILL SEQUENCE

APPLICATION OF WET-TO-DRY DRESSINGS

Step	Rationale
1. Wash hands.	Avoids cross-contamination from transient microorganisms.
2. Select needed sterile equipment; inspect for intactness and sterility.	Avoids introducing exogenous microorganisms.
3. Write date, time, and initials on bottle label. Loosen cap.	Reusing sterile solutions for 24 hours is considered acceptable. Loosening cap allows for escape of increased pressure and facilitates later one-handed opening.
4. Place bottle of solution in a pan of hot tap water for 10 to 15 minutes.	Warmed solution provides increased comfort for client.
5. Explain procedure to client.	Facilitates cooperation and involves client in self-care.
6. Prepare room, client, sterile area, and sterile supplies as in Skill 30, Skill Sequences "Preparing a Sterile Field", pp. 279–280. "Adding Heat-sealed Items to a Sterile Field", p. 281; and "Adding Envelope-Wrapped Items to a Sterile Field," steps 5 to 12, pp. 281. Place gauze pads and basin on the sterile field.	Maintains sterility of equipment during procedure.
7. Remove tape or untie Montgomery straps; remove old dressings with clean gloves and discard in impermeable trash bag; inspect wound. See Skill 32, Skill Sequence, "Dressing Change with Wound Care," steps 19 to 23, p. 306.	Protects self from wound contaminants.
8. Pour solution into basin with label facing palm as in Skill 30, Skill Sequence, "Pouring Sterile Solutions," p. 282.	Avoids soiling the label. Avoids contaminating the sterile field.
9. Don sterile gloves.	Avoids introducing exogenous microorganisms.
10. Remove cotton filler from gauze pad if not using unfilled gauze pads.	Avoids introducing exogenous microorganisms.
11. Place gauze pad in solution and squeeze out excess; have pad neither dripping wet nor damp dry.	
12. Pack single layer of medium-mesh wet gauze into or over entire wound surface, pressing gauze into any depressions. Avoid touching surrounding skin. Add dampened fluffed gauze to fill wound space loosely and keep gauze in contact with surface.	Effective debridement depends on direct contact with wound surfaces. Dead air space contributes to bacterial growth.
13. Unfold a dry sterile unfilled gauze pad and arrange it loosely over wet wound packing. Do not use ABD's or Combipads.	Absorbs any excess drainage and holds wet dressing in place. Heavy dressings do not allow wet dressings to dry readily.

(continued)

APPLICATION OF WET-TO-DRY DRESSINGS (Cont.)

Step	Rationale
14. Tape edges of gauze pad in place, but do not cover the entire dressing with tape.	Complete taping would result in an occlusive dressing that cannot dry.
15. Write date, time, and initials on tape.	Provides ready data for spacing dressing changes. Indicates accountability for actions.
16. Dispose of equipment correctly.	
17. Wash hands.	
18. Record procedure in health record, including type of solution, appearance of wound, and any drainage. Use flow sheets as available. Update care plan as needed.	Provides ongoing data base for continuity of care; fulfills nurse accountability and responsibility.

RECORDING

After the procedure is finished, record pertinent data in the health record. Depending on the record system, this might be on a flow sheet, in the nurses' notes, or in the integrated progress notes. Recorded data include time and date, solution used, number of dressings used, approximate size of wound, appearance of wound, effectiveness of debriding action, and any client reactions or comments.

Sample POR Recording
- S—"How does it look today?" "It doesn't hurt anymore!"
- O—Grey-white material encrusted in old dry dressing. One area of fresh pink tissue (2-cm diam.) present in upper third of wound. Remainder of wound surface partially covered with white cheesy debris and some healthy pink tissue visible.
- A—Wet-to-dry dressings accomplishing some wound debridement.
- P—Continue wet-to-dry soaks q 4° for several days and reevaluate.

Sample Narrative Recording
Dry dressing removed—encrusted with dried gray-white material. Minimal amount of bleeding from upper edge of wound where fresh pink tissue (2-cm diam.) is present. Remainder of wound is partially covered with cheesy white debris, with some healthy tissue visible. No pain with procedure.

☐ CRITICAL POINTS SUMMARY

1. Wet-to-dry dressings are used to debride necrotic tissue from wounds that are healing by second intention.
2. Use aseptic technique with wet-to-dry dressings on any open wound.
3. Place a single layer of unfilled gauze in close contact with all surfaces and aspects of the wound, including erosions and crevices.
4. Use a lightweight, nonocclusive dressing that allows the gauze to dry.
5. A wet-to-dry dressing that is applied properly will be dry within 4 to 6 hours.
6. Remove dried dressing by pulling toward the center of the wound.
7. Necrotic tissue trapped in the single gauze layer is removed along with the dried dressing.

☐ LEARNING ACTIVITIES

1. Moisten three unfilled gauze squares. Squeeze one square until quite dry, leave one square dripping wet, and partially wring out the third one. Spread on a flat, moisture-proof surface. Observe and note the variable length of drying time.
2. Moisten one unfilled and one filled gauze square to the same degree of wetness. Spread out as in activity 1 and compare the drying times.
3. What conclusions can you draw about degree of moisture and filled versus unfilled gauze for wet-to-dry dressings?

☐ REVIEW QUESTIONS

1. In what ways are the purposes and techniques of warm wet dressings similar to those of wet-to-dry dressings? How do they differ?
2. If a wound already is infected, why is it necessary to use aseptic technique for wet-to-dry dressings?
3. What function does debridement play in secondary intention wound healing?
4. How does a wet-to-dry dressing achieve debridement?
5. Describe problems that occur if wet-to-dry dressings: (a) dry too quickly; (b) are too wet; (c) are too thick; (d) are applied too tightly.
6. What solution would you choose for a noninfected decubitus ulcer with loosened pieces of necrotic tissue?
7. Why would you choose the solution in question 6 in preference to one of the other four common solutions?
8. Explain the reasons for taping only the edges of a wet-to-dry dressing.
9. Why are filled gauze sponges never used for wet-to-dry dressings on an open wound?

☐ PERFORMANCE CHECKLIST

OBJECTIVE: To use appropriate aseptic technique to apply sterile wet-to-dry dressings.

CHARACTERISTIC	RANGE OF ACCEPTABILITY	SATISFACTORY	UNSATISFACTORY
1. Washes hands.	No deviation		
2. Collects needed sterile equipment and checks for sterility and intactness.	Prepared dressing tray may be used.		
3. Labels solution bottle with date, time, and initials.	No deviation		
4. Loosens cap and warms bottle in pan of hot tap water for 10 to 15 minutes.	No deviation		
5. Explains procedure to client.	No deviation		
6. Positions and drapes client for visibility of wound and privacy.	No deviation		
7. Prepares sterile work area.	No deviation		
8. Removes old dressing with clean gloves.	No deviation		
9. Inspects wound and old dressing.	No deviation		
10. Packs wet (not dripping) gauze into all aspects of the wound, using sterile gloves or equipment.	No deviation		
11. Adds damp fluffed gauze and flat dry gauze pad.	Fluffed gauze may be omitted if little drainage is present and if wound space is small.		
12. Tapes at edges only.	No deviation		
13. Writes date, time, and initials on tape.	No deviation		
14. Disposes of equipment correctly.	No deviation		
15. Washes hands.	No deviation		
16. Records procedure.	No deviation		

REFERENCES

Chang LF: How to succeed with wet-to-dry dressings. RN 42(1):63–66, 1979.

Madden JW, Arem AJ: Wound healing: Biologic and clinical features. In Sabiston DC (ed): Davis-Christopher Textbook of Surgery, ed 12. Philadelphia, WB Saunders, 1981.

BIBLIOGRAPHY

Brunner LS, Suddarth DS: Textbook of Medical–Surgical Nursing, ed 5. Philadelphia, JB Lippincott, 1984.

Kottke FJ, Stillwell GK, et al.: Krusen's Handbook of Physical Medicine and Rehabilitation, ed 3. Philadelphia, WB Saunders, 1982.

Krusen FH, Kottke FJ, et al.: Handbook of Physical Medicine and Rehabilitation, ed 2. Philadelphia, WB Saunders, 1971.

Luckmann J, Sorensen KC: Medical-Surgical Nursing: A Psychophysiologic Approach. Philadelphia, WB Saunders, 1980.

Waterman NC, Stoeckinger J, et al.: Effects of various dressings on skin and subcutaneous temperatures: A comparison. Archives of Surgery 95(3):464–471, 1967.

SUGGESTED READING

Cuzzell JZ: Wound care forum: Artful solutions to chronic problems. American Journal of Nursing 85(2):163–166, 1985.

AUDIOVISUAL RESOURCE

Wound Management: The Surgical Dressing
Filmstrip, slides, cartridge, videotape. (1981, Color, 23 min.)
Available through:
Medcom, Inc.
P.O. Box 116
Garden Grove, CA 92642

10 Personal Hygiene

☐ INTRODUCTION

Personal hygiene practices serve to maintain health and prevent disease of the skin and its accessory organs. They are an important part of most people's daily routine because they provide a sense of physical and psychological well-being. The ways in which each individual attends to his or her own hygiene needs is a matter of personal preference, social and cultural values, and financial status. Personal hygiene habits are instilled in each of us during early childhood from our family's beliefs and practices. These habits may be changed later in life to accord with different beliefs, new information, or changes in financial status.

Personal hygiene practices have a significant effect on the extent to which disease is prevented and health is maintained. For example, bathing too often can cause drying of the skin and result in breaks in its integrity, and the use of inappropriate soaps and lotions can irritate the skin.

Personal hygiene practices generally involve bathing, toothbrushing, shampooing, hair grooming, and shaving. For some, manicures, pedicures, and the use of vaginal douches, lotions, and cosmetics may also be routines that contribute significantly to self-concept.

When we are unable to perform all or part of our routine practices because of illness, we become dependent on others to assist us. The nurse assumes the responsibility for the cleanliness and comfort of clients confined to a hospital or receiving nursing care at home. The extent to which the nurse performs personal hygiene care for a client depends on the degree of illness and incapacity as well as the attitude and preference of the client. Because the skin and its appendages provide the first line of defense for disease prevention, the nurse's activities are designed to maintain the skin in a healthy condition or to restore it to as near normal as possible. The decisions the nurse makes about the frequency of care and the agents used are made on the basis of an analysis of the data collected from the client history and by physical appraisal.

Teaching clients about good hygiene practices is also an integral part of providing care. Nurses are frequently sought out as consultants about personal hygiene practices and the merits of various hygiene products. To respond effectively, the nurse needs to have a basic understanding of the main components of these products.

The skills in this chapter include those required to maintain the integrity of the skin and its appendages: "Skin Care" (Skill 38), "Perineal Care" (Skill 39), "Oral Care" (Skill 40), "Hair Care" (Skill 41), "Nail Care" (Skill 42), "Vaginal Irrigation" (Skill 43), "Breast Examination" (Skill 44), and "Care of the Corpse" (Skill 45).

To understand the normal variations of the skin and its appendages and the factors and agents that enhance or impede its health, the nurse uses basic knowledge of the anatomy and physiology of the integumentary system. Answering the entry test questions will facilitate this.

☐ ENTRY TEST

1. What are the functions of the skin?
2. What are the functions of each of the three layers of the skin?
3. What are the locations and functions of the sebaceous, apocrine, and eccrine glands?
4. What are melanocytes?
5. What are the external structures of the female genitalia?
6. What glands lubricate the female genital area and where are they located?
7. Where are the urethral and vaginal orifices located?
8. What is the anatomic location of the vagina?
9. What are the structural characteristics of the vagina?
10. What causes the development of the female breasts?
11. What type of tissue is in the female breast?
12. Where is the largest amount of breast tissue located?
13. How is the female breast tissue supported?

14. What type of tissue composes the areola and nipple?
15. What is the physiologic function of the female breasts?
16. What is the function of the lymph nodes?
17. Where are the lymph nodes located?
18. What are the external structures of the male genitalia?
19. How many teeth are in the child and adult mouth?
20. What are the names and location of the salivary glands?

SKILL 38 Skin Care

PREREQUISITE SKILLS

Skill 19, "Inspection"
Skill 20, "Palpation"
Skill 28, "Handwashing"
Skill 51, "Monitoring Fluid Balance"

☐ STUDENT OBJECTIVES

1. Describe the purpose and effects of bathing.
2. Explain the role of the stratum corneum in maintaining skin health.
3. Associate the types of skin changes with the appropriate method of appraisal.
4. Differentiate between the factors that affect the barrier integrity of the skin.
5. Describe the skin changes associated with aging.
6. Explain the rationale for each item of equipment used for bathing.
7. Differentiate between the types of hygiene care provided for bed clients.
8. Use the appropriate physical appraisal techniques to appraise the skin.
9. Summarize the factors that promote good skin health.
10. Select the appropriate method to bathe a client safely.

☐ INTRODUCTION

Bathing clients is a basic nursing responsibility. Although the primary purpose of bathing is to remove soil, body odor, and dead epithelial cells from the skin surface, routine bathing has other beneficial effects for clients. Physiologically, the movements and friction in the washing and drying processes act to exercise muscles and joints and stimulate circulation. Transient bacteria are also removed from the skin, so that the potential for infection is reduced. Psychologically, bathing serves to refresh and relax clients.

Baths may also be given for specific therapeutic purposes. Baths of varying temperatures are used to calm excited clients, reduce body temperature, and promote wound healing. Medicated baths may be used to treat skin conditions.

The nurse can use bathing time to converse and develop a rapport with clients. Bathing time also provides an opportunity to collect data from clients and counsel and teach them, as well as to appraise the condition of the skin. The nurse gives or assists a client with a partial or complete bath in bed, at a sink, from a small basin, or in a shower or bathtub.

Too frequent bathing for any purpose has some negative effects. Dry skin can become more dry and cause itching that can result in breaks in the skin from scratching.

All people do not necessarily value cleanliness highly, and it is important for nurses to be sensitive to clients who may feel this way. More frequent bathing while in the hospital must be tactfully explained, in a manner that conveys respect for the client's feelings.

☐ PREPARATION

Maintaining the integrity of the skin is a basic responsibility of the nurse, particularly when the client is confined to an institution for care. In order to judge the condition of the skin and provide appropriate care, the nurse needs an understanding of some aspects of its structure and function.

THE STRUCTURE AND FUNCTION OF THE SKIN

Genetic makeup is a major factor in determining skin color, texture, and thickness. It also significantly influences how the skin responds to physical and chemical trauma and bacteria (Rook et al., 1979).

The Epidermis
The epidermis, the visible layer of skin, is about as thick as a page in this book. It transmits light and is transparent. The outermost layer of the epidermis, the stratum corneum (known also as the horny layer), consists of dead tissue which serves as the principal barrier for the skin. The epidermis contains 20 layers

or more of tightly packed cells and has a lipid surface from sebum excreted by the sebaceous glands. The outer layer of dead cells is constantly scaling and sloughing off and being replaced by new cells. The balance of cell loss and replacement is important. If the loss occurs faster than the cells can be replaced, then the skin becomes thin, eroded, and wasted. If cells are formed faster than the dead cells are sloughed off, then scales or thickened skin results. The stratum is normally thicker on the palms and soles and on any other site that is subjected to repeated friction or pressure. Callus formation is an example of the skin's response to friction and pressure.

The Dermis
The dermis is a thick layer of tissue under the epidermis that contains blood, lymph vessels, and nerves. There are three types of fibers included in the dermis: collagen, reticulum, and elastin. Collagen, a major protein of connective tissue, allows stretching and contraction and is a major source of skin strength. Reticulum fibers help to link the collagen fibers together, and elastin is believed to play a role in the elastic quality of the dermis. Much of the substance and feel of the skin comes from the dermis. A significant amount of the body's water is stored in the dermis. The turgor, or fullness, of this tissue reflects the body's fluid balance. Turgor is discussed in Skill 51.

Skin Color
Skin color is largely dependent on the amount of melanin produced by the melanocytes. It is normal to have some variation in the pigmentation of the skin. An excessive amount of melanin is called *hyperpigmentation*. A freckle is a tiny area of hyperpigmentation. Certain physiological disorders of the adrenal or pituitary gland can cause melanocyte stimulation that produces a generalized darkening of all skin and mucous membranes.

Hypopigmentation is a decrease in the amount of pigment normally present. It makes the skin lighter than the person's normal skin color. Hypopigmentation may be caused by genetic, endocrine, or nutritional abnormalities or by trauma, infection, or inflammation that damages the melanocytes (Parrish, 1975). The size of the hypopigmented area depends on the cause. For example, a light skin area caused by a burn or inflammation would be apt to be small, while a genetic abnormality could cause the entire skin surface to be light.

In persons of dark complexion, the pigmentation of dead epidermal cells becomes quite apparent when a light-colored washcloth is used for bathing. Because the dark-colored sloughed skin cells are dark on the washcloth and may be mistaken for dirt, the uninformed nurse may question the cleanliness of the client or the thoroughness of the previous bath (Block and Hunter, 1981).

In addition to normal skin color due to pigmentation of the epidermis, the skin has a reddish hue that comes in part from the underlying blood vessels in the dermis. The volume of blood flow and the oxygen and carbon dioxide content of the blood contribute to the skin color and provide an important index of tissue perfusion.

Pallor (paleness) of the skin occurs when vessels are constricted and fail to deliver sufficient oxygenated blood to a specific or generalized area. Pallor is most easily detected in body areas where the capillary beds are superficial and the normal pigmentation is decreased, such as the earlobes. Decreased pigmentation in the epidermis permits better visualization of the capillary beds. *Erythema*, a red skin color, is caused by dilation of the blood vessels, which brings more blood to the skin surface. *Cyanosis* refers to a skin color that is dusky blue-gray. It occurs when the tissues are perfused with deoxygenated hemoglobin. When blood vessels are broken and blood seeps into the subcutaneous tissues, the skin becomes purplish; this is called *ecchymosis*. *Jaundice* is a change in skin color that results from excess accumulation of bile pigments in the blood plasma and body tissues, causing the skin to become yellow. The techniques used to detect changes in the color of the skin are described later in this skill; techniques used to detect changes in the fullness of the skin are described in Skill 51.

Barrier Property of the Skin
The barrier property of the skin comes from the stratum's resistance to diffusion. Seventy percent of the epidermis is water, and without the stratum present to hold in the water, the outward diffusion of water increases by about 30 times. If the complete layer of the stratum is removed, as might occur by abrasion or stripping off by adhesive tape, the barrier function is significantly reduced and damage or disease may occur in the living epidermis. An increased inward penetration of a variety of molecules also occurs, thus providing an opportunity for harmful substances to permeate the protective barrier (Baker, 1979).

The water content in the stratum itself is between 10 and 20 percent, and the barrier integrity of the stratum depends on maintaining this percentage. When hydration falls below 10 percent, the stratum becomes brittle and cracks easily, allowing an increased amount of irritants to penetrate it. This causes inflammation, which results in chapping. Water is the only known softener of the stratum corneum, and different parts of the body are permeable to water in varying degrees. Excessive hydration softens the stratum and reduces its effectiveness as a barrier. Areas with thicker stratum such as the palms and soles appear wrinkled after prolonged immersion in water because the stratum has absorbed a great deal of water.

The ambient (room) humidity is considered to be the single most important factor affecting the hydration of the stratum corneum. *Lowered humidity* causes water to evaporate from the skin until a balance is reached between the external environment and the skin. Lowered ambient temperature also decreases the amount of water in the stratum, regardless of humidity changes, because the blood vessels become constricted and normal physiological processes are depressed. Even in an environment with a favorable humidity and temperature, water loss and trauma occur to the skin from *friction, rubbing, scrubbing,* and *scratching,* as well as from excessive exposure to fat solvents, soaps, and detergents. When the lipid surface of the stratum corneum is removed by a solvent, water can dissolve substances in the stratum that hold water in and keep it pliable (Baker, 1979).

In the daily course of an individual's personal and occupational life, the skin comes in contact with many substances that act as *irritants*. Skin and equipment cleansers used in the home and workplace have organic solvents that change the pH and dissolve fat from the skin. Minerals, such as iron in hard water, and chemicals, such as chlorine in swimming pools, act as mechanical irritants when they become deposited in skin fissures. Alkalies, acids, oxidizing agents, plant and animal products, metal dust and particles, textile particles, and cement and wood dust are examples of some of the irritants in our environment (Fregert and Hjorth, 1979).

Exposure to *cold, heat, steam, sunlight,* and *ultraviolet rays* also damages the skin. The ultraviolet rays that cause sunburn and tanning can, over a period of years, cause premature aging of the skin. Degenerative changes in the connective tissue in the dermis and changes in the epidermis result in a loss of tone, with the skin appearing wrinkled and leather-like. Melanin absorbs ultraviolet rays and reduces the amount that penetrates the lower epidermis and dermis. The more melanocytes an individual has, the more the skin is protected from burning and premature aging. However, even blacks, who have the most protection due to large amounts of melanin, can become sunburned. Skin cancer is related to sun exposure and is rare in blacks because of the protection they receive from the melanin in their skin (Parrish, 1975).

Pressure Sores

A common skin problem in people who do not change their body position to relieve pressure is the pressure sore, or decubitus ulcer. A pressure sore is an area of erythema that progresses to tissue necrosis (death) and a skin ulcer. This problem may occur in a person of any age, either ambulatory or bedridden, whose sensory responses to discomfort or pain are absent or dulled, or a person who is unable to change position voluntarily. Some of the factors that increase the potential for skin breakdown and the development of pressure sores include poor nutrition, anemia, loss of body fat and atrophied muscles, incontinence, and moist skin. Sustained external pressure against the skin and subcutaneous tissue over bony prominences in any body area causes ischemia and anoxia, particularly over bony prominences such as the heel, sacrum, and shoulder blade. This results in mechanical obstruction of the blood supply to the tissues with deprivation of oxygen. While the pressure is present, the overlying skin area appears pallid in color. Figure 38–1 depicts the usual pressure point areas.

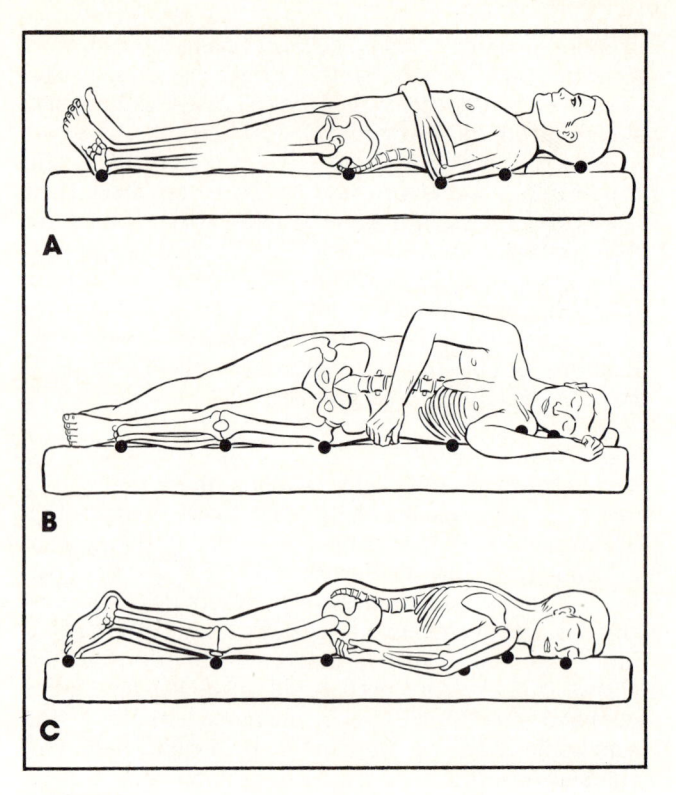

Figure 38–1. Pressure point areas to be appraised by inspection and palpation: **A.** Supine position areas, **B.** Lateral position areas, and **C.** Prone position areas.

The three skin lesions that may occur during the development of a pressure sore are vesicle, crust, and ulcer. A *vesicle* (blister) is an elevated bubble that contains clear fluid. *Crust* consists of dried exudative material such as serum, pus, and blood. It may be thick or thin. An *ulcer* is a lesion that extends through the epidermis to the dermis. Ulcers are caused by the destruction of tissue. Figure 38–2 depicts these skin lesions.

The processes that take place in the skin during the progression from the intact state to the ulcer state are described in five stages by Tepperman et al. (1977). Each of these stages may not always be discerned and observed by the nurse, but it is important that they be recognized whenever possible so that appropriate interventions can be implemented to prevent the subsequent stage from developing, thus avoiding the ultimate formation of an ulcer.

Stage I, *blanching hyperemia,* occurs when the external pressure is removed from the skin. The pressure area becomes erythematous (reddened) because there is an increased blood flow (hyperemia) in compensation for the lack of circulation while the pressure was present. This erythema will blanch when light finger pressure is applied to the skin.

Stage II, *nonblanching hyperemia,* occurs if the tissue ischemia and anoxia persist. The capillaries become unstable and tissue damage begins. The skin does not blanch with finger pressure but remains erythematous.

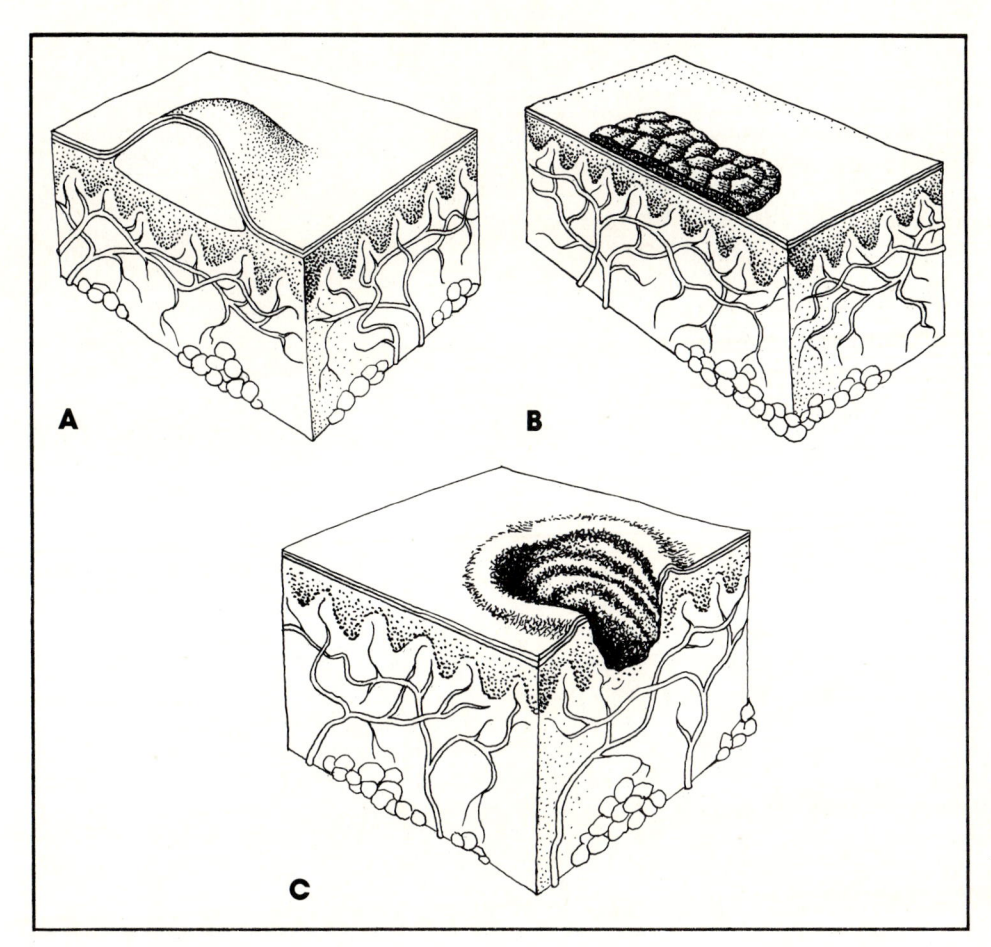

*Figure 38–2. **A.** A vesicle is a small elevated bubble that contains clear fluid. It is less than 1 cm in size. **B.** Crust consists of dried exudate such as serum, blood, or pus on the skin. **C.** An ulcer is a lesion that extends through the epidermis to the dermis.*

Stage III, *vesicle and eschar formation,* follows as a result of the passage of fluid from the damaged capillaries into the tissues. At the same time, the tissue cells die since the capillary damage deprives them of oxygen. The necrotic (dead) tissue separates from the healthy tissue and a well-defined margin develops around the pressure area. The necrotic tissue becomes dehydrated, and a thick black crust known as eschar is formed.

Stage IV, a *clean ulcer,* results when the eschar separates from the underlying tissues because of the action of tissue enzymes. Various agents used to treat decubitus ulcers may also promote the eschar separation.

Stage V, an *infected ulcer,* is relatively common because of the opportunity for pathogenic bacteria to invade the broken skin. With an infection, the border and tissues around the ulcer are erythematous, swollen, and warm, and purulent discharge drains from the ulcer.

THE EARS, MUCOUS MEMBRANES, AND NOSE

The Ears

Skin also lines the external acoustic meatus of the ear. Cerumen is earwax and is produced in the outer third of the auditory canal by modified apocrine glands called cerumen glands. The ducts of these glands open either directly onto the skin surface, or into the hair follicles along with the sebaceous glands.

The cerumen that collects in the canal normally flows out toward the external ear where it can easily be removed with the corner of a damp washcloth placed over the finger. It is not a safe practice to clean the canal with cotton-tipped applicators, hairpins, or any object that fits into the canal. The canal may be injured and there is real potential for puncturing the tympanic membrane. Persons who produce a large amount of earwax may have problems with the impacted earwax. This impaction is seldom removed by the nurse because of the danger of puncturing the tympanic membrane, traumatizing the canal, and causing an infection. The client is therefore referred to a physician to have the impacted cerumen removed.

The Mucous Membranes

Mucous membranes line all of the body's tubular and hollow organs. They are continuous with the skin in areas such as the nose, mouth, and vagina. Like the skin, they also serve as a barrier, preventing loss of body fluids and invasion by pathogenic microorganisms that could cause an infection. This tissue has a surface layer of nonkeratinized epithelium that is supported by loosely woven connective tissue. The surface of the membranes is kept moist and lubricated by mucus-secreting glands.

The Nose

The nose has an extremely vascular mucous membrane lining. Mucus and cilia trap and remove dust and other fine particles from inspired air. Extremely dry air may be humidified by the mucus during inhalation. Mucous membranes may also become dry in environments with low humidity, and thus become less effective in humidifying the inspired air. Environmental dryness may also cause some discomfort and even lead to breaks in the tissue that may result in crust formation. Mucus secretions that are normally removed by blowing the nose can accumulate when a person is physically unable to blow his or her nose. Because these secretions may block the airflow on both inspiration and expiration, it is important that they be removed.

AGING SKIN

The skin changes as an individual ages. The changes modify the pattern and incidence of skin reactions to endogenous (internal) and exogenous (external) influences.

Over time, the skin contains less water and collagen loses its flexibility. Skin aging actually begins gradually at birth. These gradual changes become more marked as the levels of sex hormones begin to subside in middle age. The cumulative effects of years of sun exposure begin to be apparent. Aging skin gradually becomes dry, wrinkled, yellow, and blemished. It may also become more transparent with thinning of the epidermis. Bruises from minor injury readily occur because of easily broken capillaries. The aging skin is more easily dehydrated, and its effectiveness as a barrier is reduced because of the thinner stratum corneum. The number of active eccrine glands is decreased; and as a result of the reduced hormonal output, the apocrine sweat glands and sebaceous glands become less active. The collagen in the dermis becomes stiffer and may also become thinner. This change in the collagen, along with a decrease in the amount of subcutaneous tissue, causes the sagging appearance of aging skin. The skin stretches easily because of decreased elasticity. Sun-exposed areas have increased dermal changes due to long-term damage.

The dry skin of the elderly frequently causes *pruritis* (itching), which is aggravated by the low ambient humidity often present in the air of centrally heated homes and dry climates. Cold or warm wind causes evaporation of moisture from the skin. The use of humidifiers with central heating helps to reduce the dry ambient air. Chronic diseases such as diabetes and liver disease or blood dyscrasias can also add to the dryness problem. Bathing with detergent soaps, taking bubble baths, or using hot water also increase skin dryness. Although bathing helps to hydrate the stratum corneum, the skin actually becomes more dry because of evaporation. Soap, which has a drying effect, must be thoroughly rinsed off the skin. The water holding capacity of the skin can be improved by using skin lubricants after bathing that help to trap the moisture. Mineral oils such as Alpha Keri bath oil can be added to the bathwater to reduce the drying effect. Natural fiber undergarments such as cotton help to reduce skin irritation that may be caused by synthetic fabrics.

BATHING

There are several factors the nurse considers before bathing a client: purpose (cleansing or therapeutic), location (shower, bathtub, sink, or bed), amount of body to be bathed (part or all), and extent to which the client requires assistance in actual bathing. These factors are interrelated. For example, a client who is able to shower may require some help with part of the bathing process. Another client may be fully capable of bathing all of his or her body in bed except for the back. A client requiring a warm bath may require help in getting in and out of the bathtub.

General Principles for Bathing

Three basic principles apply to any type of bathing: asepsis, safety, and body mechanics.

In accord with the fundamentals of medical asepsis, washing always proceeds from the most clean body area to the least clean. This means that the face is bathed before the trunk, the trunk before the feet, and the perineal area last. Even if it is not feasible to progress systematically from the most clean area to the least clean, the linen, bathwater, and basin used to bathe the least clean areas should not be used to bathe the cleaner body areas. Washing clean areas with equipment used on less clean areas transfers potentially pathogenic microorganisms.

Ensuring the safety of the client is a primary responsibility of the nurse. When the nurse prepares the client for a bath, all supplies and equipment are arranged so that the client can reach them easily without risk of falling or unnecessary exertion. If the client is able to be out of bed, the height of the bed is positioned at its lowest level so that the client can get in and out without risk of falling. The path to the bathroom is clear of hazards that could cause the client to slip or fall. Bathtubs and showers need to have safety nonslip surfaces and handrails. The nurse adjusts the water temperature so that it neither burns nor chills the client.

Therapeutic Baths

Therapeutic baths are used to produce specific physical responses. They may consist of water alone or have some medication added to the water.

When water alone is used, the *temperature* is therapeutic. (An in-depth discussion of the therapeutic effects of heat and cold is presented in Chapter 11.) A client with an elevated body temperature may be bathed with cool water either in a bathtub or by a sponge bath to lower the temperature. Cool water on the skin promotes heat loss from the body through evaporation of the moisture and through direct conduction, thereby reducing the body temperature.

Cool-water baths begin with the water temperature at 22°C (71.6°F). The temperature is gradually decreased as the client is able to tolerate a lower temperature without chilling. Immersion of the entire body in a bathtub of neutral-temperature water at 33.5° to 35.5°C (92° to 96°F) in a quiet environment produces sedation, muscle relaxation, and general vasodilatation. This type of bath is used to calm excited clients. Hot baths of 36.5° to 40°C (98° to 104°F) promote wound healing by relieving vascular congestion and reducing inflammation, and also relieve muscle spasms and pain. Hot baths may be given to the entire body or to a specific body part.

Medicated baths are most commonly used in the home, but there are instances when they are ordered in the hospital by the physician. The most frequent purpose of medicated baths is to relieve discomfort from skin disorders. The value of these baths lies in the residue of the medication left on the skin, and also in the relaxing and sedative effects the water may have on the client. The skin is patted dry after the bath to preserve the film of medication left on the skin and to prevent irritation from rubbing the skin dry. A medicated bath may be given either in the bathtub or by sponge. The ability of the client to bathe himself or herself and the amount of skin to be treated usually determine which method is selected.

The agent used in a medicated bath may be either a common household product such as oatmeal, cornstarch, or baking soda (sodium bicarbonate), or a pharmaceutical preparation. Rambo and Wood (1982) describe the types of medicated baths used to reduce pruritis (itching) and inflammation. An *oatmeal bath* can be prepared by adding instant oatmeal directly to hot water (36.5° to 40°C [98° to 104°F]). The amount used depends on the desired consistency. When old-fashioned oatmeal is used, 3 cups of oatmeal is cooked in 2 quarts of water until it turns into a paste. The cooked oatmeal is placed in a cheesecloth bag, tied securely, and swished around in a bathtub half full of water until the desired consistency is obtained. The desired consistency is usually a thin gelatinous liquid that feels silky to the touch. A *cornstarch bath* is prepared by dissolving 1 pound of cornstarch in cold water and then adding boiling water to dilute the mixture to a thin solution. The solution is then boiled again for a few minutes to reheat it before adding it to a half-filled bathtub. A *sodium bicarbonate bath* is prepared by dissolving the sodium bicarbonate in water in a 1-to-500 ratio. One teaspoon of sodium bicarbonate mixed in 500 milliliters of water provides the correct concentration, but since a half-filled bathtub holds about 15 gallons of water, 2 cups of sodium bicarbonate are needed to make a 1:500 solution.

DATA BASE

Prior to bathing a client, the nurse identifies the level of self-care possible or permissible. The client's preferences are considered as well. The method selected for bathing a specific client depends on a combination of factors, including the client's medical diagnosis, physical and mental capabilities; the physician's order; the available physical facilities; and the available nursing personnel.

In addition to cleansing, therapeutic, and communication purposes, bathing provides an excellent opportunity for the nurse to gather data by appraising the condition of the skin. This is especially true when the client requires partial or total assistance with bathing.

Client History and Recorded Data

Information obtained by the nurse and medical staff from the skin appraisals is made available on the client's health record. Data that affect the frequency and method of bathing are also included on the kardex. For example, if a client has a rash in an intertriginous area and an absorbent powder is used to reduce the effects of moisture, this information should be recorded so that the condition can be frequently monitored and the intervention evaluated.

A nursing history or assessment interview can be used to gather data related to bathing. The interview relates specifically to the client's age, life style, and medical diagnosis and includes questions about allergies and problems with changes in skin pigmentation, texture, rashes, and pruritis (itching). The length of time the problem has existed and the effects of any treatment used are determined. The relationships of the problem with seasonal, environmental, and occupational irritants are established. The nurse also finds out if the skin problem has any effect on the client's self-concept and socialization behavior.

Since bathing practices contribute to the health of the skin, the nurse also interviews clients about their bathing routine, including usual frequency, time of day, and method of bathing. This information may provide opportunities for the nurse to engage in some health teaching about skin care. It also provides a means for reducing some of the stress of institutionalization as the nurse plans with the client how aspects of this routine can be incorporated into the plan of care. Unfortunately, much care is provided at the convenience of the staff and serves to depersonalize the client. When it is possible to include at least some of the client's normal routine in the care plan, the client is more apt to feel cared for as an individual.

Physical Appraisal Skills

A client's skin is appraised at the time of admission to the institution or program of care. After the initial appraisal, the frequency of subsequent appraisals depends on the client's health status and any concerns that may arise about the way in which the skin is responding to internal and external forces. It is usually most convenient to appraise the entire skin during the bath.

Inspection. An adequate inspection of the skin requires a good light source, particularly for dark-skinned persons. Daylight is the best light, but when it is not available, Roach (1977) suggests that a 60-

watt lamp be used since ceiling and over-bed lights are usually inadequate. The inspection begins with a general survey of the skin for pigmentation color, cleanliness, and the presence of any obvious lesions. As with any appraisal, it is best to develop a systematic approach to look for lesions, evidence of rubbing or scratching, or other breaks in the skin. The location and characteristics of any lesion or wound must be fully described. It is particularly important for the student to validate what is seen with other more experienced staff.

The smooth skin areas of the back, chest, abdomen, and extremities are inspected before proceeding on to the deep fold areas where the skin is in opposition to itself. Creases and folds are smoothed out for full and careful scrutiny. One side of the body is compared with its counterpart.

The normal skin pigmentation is noted as well as any areas that are hyperpigmented or hypopigmented. It is important to become familiar with an individual's normal skin color to establish a baseline reference for any future color changes.

Pallor and cyanosis are best detected in areas that have the least amount of pigmentation, such as the lips, tongue, earlobes, palms, soles, and nail beds. Pallor may appear as yellowish-brown in brown-skinned persons and as ashen gray in black-skinned persons. There are occasions when the nurse is not familiar enough with the normal skin color of a client to detect accurately the presence of cyanosis. Roach (1974) recommends a technique of applying light pressure to the skin to create a pallor and then observing the color return. Cyanosis is present when color returns from the periphery to the center. In the absence of cyanosis, the normal color returns in less than 1 second and appears from below the epidermis as well as from the periphery.

Jaundice is best seen in the sclera of the eye in both light- and dark-skinned people. However, in dark-skinned people, carotene in the fatty deposits located under the conjunctiva can mimic jaundice. Roberts (1975) suggests that the sclera located at the junction of the lids be inspected for the most accurate color.

Erythema is usually apparent in light skin, but not in dark skin. When erythema is caused by an inflammation, the skin will have increased warmth and possibly some swelling. When there is a question of whether erythema or a rash is present in dark skin, Roach (1977) recommends that the skin be stretched with the thumb and forefinger to cause the skin to blanch. The resulting decrease in red tone emphasizes the presence of a rash. Ecchymosis may also be detected in the same manner.

Edema may be apparent on inspection because the skin is tight, smooth, and shiny due to the accumulation of fluid in the subcutaneous tissues.

Inspection of the Ear and Nose. The skin on the pinna and in the external ear canal is inspected before bathing. The external ear canal must be straightened to permit inspection. This is done on adults by pulling the ear lobe up and back and on children by pulling the ear lobe down and back. The techniques are somewhat different because the canal is shaped differently. The ear canal, particularly in children or confused adults, may have foreign bodies that need to be removed. If this is not done the foreign bodies may be inadvertently pushed farther into the canal or may become wet from bathing. Vegetative matter like peas or beans swell when wet and can occlude the canal, causing hearing loss. They are also a potential source of infection. When foreign bodies are not easily accessible for removal by the nurse, the client must be referred to a physician.

The mucous membranes of the nose are also inspected on clients who are unable to remove or expel accumulated secretions by themselves. The daily bath provides an appropriate time for this inspection, although clients who have large accumulations may require more frequent appraisals. To inspect the nasal mucous membranes, direct the beam of a flashlight into each nasal passage while gently elevating the tip of the nose with a finger to expose the interior membranes. The healthy membrane is smooth, pink, and glistening with a mucous film over the tissues. As with the ear canal, the nose is a place where children and confused adults may place foreign bodies. Foreign bodies have the potential for blocking the nasal airway or for being inhaled into the trachea or bronchi, thus causing more acute respiratory embarrassment and presenting a significant problem for removal. Attempts at removing them involve a risk of pushing the foreign body farther into the nasal cavity. Therefore, the nurse refers the client to a physician as soon as possible, so that the object can be safely removed.

Palpation. Light stroking palpation with the dorsum of the hand is used to determine skin texture. The texture may be smooth, rough, dry, or moist.

Skin temperature is also checked with the dorsum of the hand. Increased warmth occurs on areas of inflammation. Decreased temperatures are usually caused by circulatory disorders in the hands, lower legs, and feet. The extremities are checked for temperature simultaneously, so that one side may be compared with the other. To do this, it is best to start palpating with the dorsum of both hands at the distal (fingers and toes) aspect of the extremities and slowly progress upward. Light palpation will detect warmth and tightness of the skin as well as any hardening of the deep tissues that may occur with inflammation.

Inspection and Palpation of Pressure Points. Pressure points must also be appraised in any client who has the potential for developing pressure sores. Persons at highest risk include those with neurologic disorders such as spinal cord injuries, cerebral vascular injuries, and multiple sclerosis; persons with rheumatoid arthritis; persons with chronic substance abuse of alcohol and drugs; and persons with fever or bladder or bowel incontinence ("Four Proven Steps," 1977). The areas of the body at particular risk for development of pressure sores are dependent on the client's body position. The danger points include: the occiput, the rim of the ear, the side of the head, the shoulder, the shoulder blade, the dorsal thoracic area, the elbow, the hip, the ischium, the sacrum, the ischial tuberosity, the trochanter, the perineum, the posterior and anterior knee, the inner and outer ankle, and the heel ("Four Proven Steps," 1977). These points are shown in Figure 38-1. Each area should be carefully scrutinized using both inspection and palpation to detect the presence of any stage of tissue change as described previously: blanching hyperemia, nonblanching hyperemia, vesicle and eschar formation, clean ulcer, or infected ulcer.

Smell. The sense of smell is useful in detecting body odor from poor hygiene or draining lesions or wounds, and these data can direct the nurse to investigate the cause.

EQUIPMENT

Bathing may be done in a shower or bathtub, at a bathroom sink, or with a basin at the bedside or in bed. Bathtubs and showers must have *nonslip strips* on the floor and *safety bars* located in places that are within the client's grasp. A safety rail may be mounted on the side of the bathtub and on the wall behind the bathtub. Chairs and seats are available for placement in the shower and bathtub for persons unable to use the facility safely without modification. A nurse call signal must be available for the client to use in case assistance is needed. Showers eliminate the problems of infection spreading between clients using a common bathtub. Ayliffe et al. (1975) recommend the addition of an antiseptic solution to the bathtub water to protect clients with uninfected wounds and to prevent the spread of infection from clients with infected wounds. Since the scum left in the bathtub may have microorganisms that survive even with the use of a disinfectant, the bathtub surface is cleaned with an abrasive preparation after each use. For the same reasons, the bathroom sink is also scrubbed and disinfected after each use for a client bath. Bath basins are often disposable and a part of the supply kit issued to each client upon admission. Since this basin is used for only one client, there is no danger of contamination from other clients. Even so, the basin still needs to be scrubbed with a disinfectant after each use, because resident microorganisms from different parts of the body and pathogenic microorganisms from wounds will survive in the sink after the water is emptied and present a potential for infection or reinfection.

Washcloths, towels, and *bath blankets* of cotton are the most absorbent. A thin, lightweight bath blanket is used to cover a client during a bed bath and may also be used for sink baths. The bath blanket prevents unnecessary exposure during the bath, avoids chilling, and may also be used to partially dry the client upon exit from a bathtub or shower. In the bed bath it replaces the top sheet and bedspread, thereby preventing the bed linen from becoming damp.

Sponges or commercially made *bath mitts* may be used as washcloths and are particularly helpful for use with clients who can bathe themselves but have limited use of one hand. A washcloth may be folded around the hand for form a mit. This technique is illustrated in Figure 38-3.

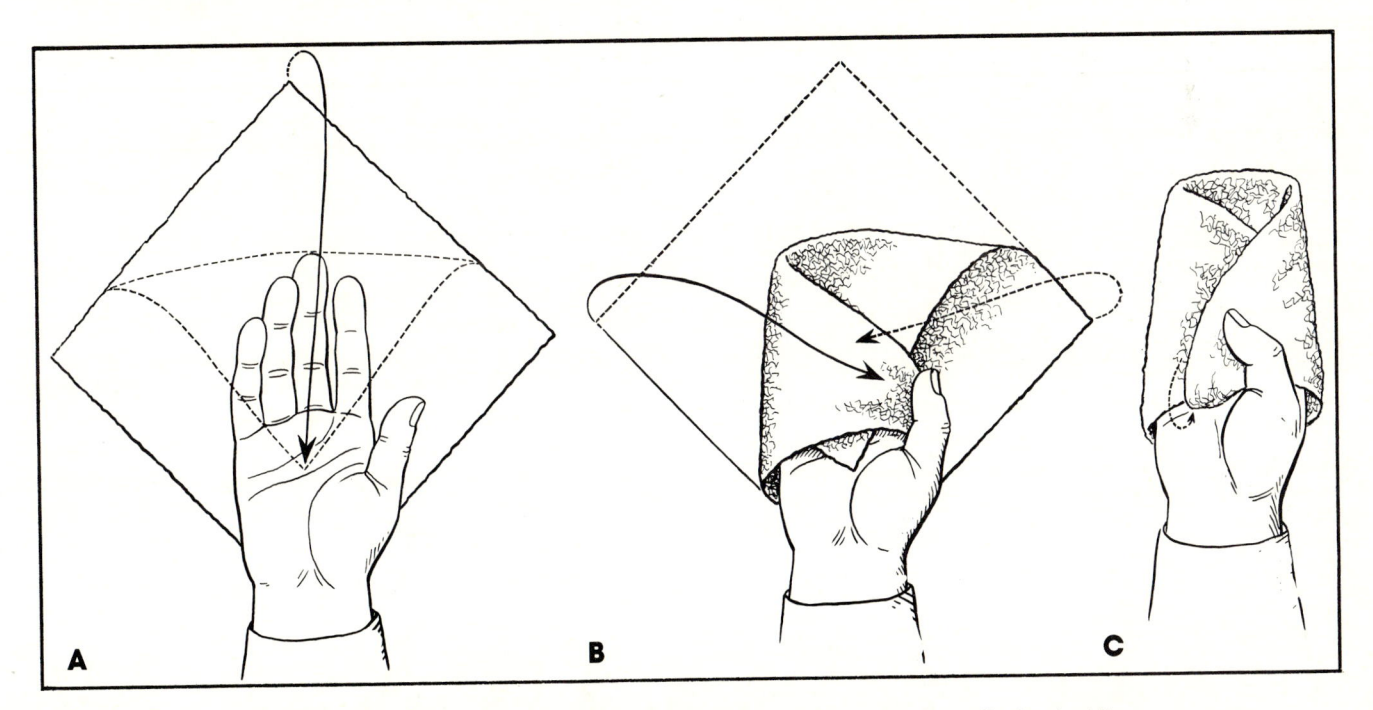

Figure 38-3. The washcloth mitt is made by the triangular method. **A.** Place the back of the dominant hand on the cloth having one corner aimed at the wrist, then bring the opposite corner over the palm. **B.** Fold both of the other corners across the palm. **C.** Tuck under the top corner to fasten and hold mitt in place with the thumb.

The *water temperature* for a cleansing bath is adjusted according to the medical condition and skin texture of the client. Warm water, 35.5° to 36.5°C (96° to 98°F), is used for dry skin to prevent further loss of skin moisture. Hot water, 36.5° to 40°C (98° to 104°F), is used with caution, according to the client's tolerance and preference. In the shower or bathtub hot water can cause vasodilatation of vessels in the skin surface, thereby diverting blood away from the brain and other vital organs. This provides an extremely unsafe situation because the client can become weak, faint, and fall.

Soaps used for bathing in hospitals and other inpatient settings are frequently antibacterial. These provide some protection against gram-positive bacteria if they are used over a period of several days (MacKenzie, 1970). Soap dries the skin because it disrupts the surface tension and removes the protective layer of sebum. When dry skin is a problem for a client (as with the elderly), superfatted soaps such as Dove, Tone, or Basis help to reduce the dryness because they do not remove as much lipid from the stratum corneum. All soap should be used sparingly and should be rinsed off. A soap dish that drains the soap should be provided for each client. Leaving the soap in the bathwater during the bath makes the water too soapy and prevents adequate rinsing.

Moisturizing preparations that dissolve in water and adhere to the skin (such as Alpha Keri) may be placed directly in the bathwater. Other preparations, such as Lubriderm applied to the skin after bathing while the skin is still moist increase the water-holding capacity of the stratum corneum by leaving a film that retards evaporation of the skin water. Baby lotion that is smooth and nongreasy may be used in place of soap and water to bathe dry skin of the elderly person, since the lotion leaves the skin soft. Highly perfumed preparations such as bath salts and bubble baths are drying to the skin because of their high alcohol content and should not be used in bathing dry skin.

Creams are emulsions of oil and water. They are more effective than lotions because they contain more oil per volume than do lotions. Creams vanish into the skin because the water evaporates and the oil does not leave an unpleasant, greasy film. *Ointments* have less water than creams. They also lubricate the skin, but some have so much oil that they leave an uncomfortable, greasy film. Hydrogenated vegetable shortenings such as Crisco or Spry are inexpensive and nonscented products that are good skin moisturizers.

Powders are minute, insoluble particles of dry substances such as calcium carbonate, zinc stearate, talc, and starch. One preparation may include one or more types of substances. Powders can be used to reduce friction, soothe, and absorb moisture from the skin. There are basically two types of powders: adsorbable and nonadsorbable. Adsorbable powders act by adsorbing (attracting and holding) secretions through a capillary attraction. Cornstarch is an example of an adsorbable powder, and in pure form it should be used sparingly because it can become pasty when it adsorbs fluid. Nonadsorbable powders (also called absorbent), such as talc, are useful for protecting irritated skin surfaces because they do not cake on moist skin and they reduce friction. However, they should not be applied to denuded or oozing skin surfaces because they cake and form a crust that can encourage bacterial growth.

☐ EXECUTION

The information available on the kardex about the bathing plan should be validated with the charge nurse and the client before beginning the bath. The frequency and type of bathing varies with the individual. To determine whether a client should be bathed and if the bath should be complete or partial, with water, lotion, or a combination of both, the nurse needs to consider the client's physical comfort, energy level, skin condition, and the amount of soil and perspiration present on the skin. It is not uncommon for people to overestimate their ability to bathe themselves independently. Therefore, it is necessary for the nurse to assess the client's stamina before allowing him or her to bathe without assistance. There is often no need for the traditional complete bath that seems to be given routinely in many hospitals.

It is essential that privacy be ensured for bathing by closing the room door, cubicle curtains, or both. Room doors should not be locked; rather, a "Do not enter" or "In use" sign may be hung on the door.

The nurse is responsible for the client's safety at bath time. This includes providing protection from injury and drafts, exercising good judgment in determining the method used, and adequately instructing the client on how to use whatever devices are deemed necessary, such as a shower chair and safety rails. To prevent accidental burns or chilling, the nurse adjusts the water temperature in the shower before the client enters it, or half fills the bathtub before the client enters the bathtub and then adds water to the appropriate level. Be careful to avoid hot spots while adding water to the bathtub by agitating the water and cautioning the client about adding water himself or herself. The nurse stays close at hand while the client is bathing to check on his or her progress and status. The call signal must be readily available in case the client needs assistance. Set a limit of 15 to 20 minutes for a tub bath and less for a shower, to prevent weakness and fatigue that is caused by vasodilatation from heat and steam as well as from the physical exertion of bathing. Use moisturizing preparations with caution in the shower or bathtub, because they make the surfaces slippery and can cause the client to fall. When assisting the client to bathe in the shower or bathtub it may be necessary to wear a protective apron to prevent your uniform from getting wet.

When bathing a client, nursing personnel can use

a washcloth more effectively and efficiently by folding it into a mitt that covers the hand. This not only prevents it from flapping and dripping over the client, but also prevents the client from getting scratched or poked by the care-giver's fingers and nails. There are two ways to make a mitt: triangular and rectangular. The method selected depends on the size of the washcloth and personal preference. Figure 38-3 depicts the triangular method, which is usually more suitable for a small washcloth.

THE BED BATH

Bathing in bed is reserved for clients who are unable to be up because of illness or disability. Clients with cardiovascular or respiratory conditions which require conservation of energy, clients with restricted mobility due to disease or injury, clients with neurologic and orthopedic conditions, and clients who have just had surgery must all bathe in bed. Clients usually dislike bathing in bed because it reinforces their limitations and dependence on others and it is difficult to bathe thoroughly. Even with closed doors or cubicle curtains, privacy is a problem and a client is vulnerable to disruptions from personnel who simply walk in without knocking or seeking permission.

The types of bathing in bed that the nurse must assist with include early morning care, evening care, and the bed bath. Early morning care is provided before breakfast and consists of providing a basin with water, washcloth, towel, and soap so that the client can wash the face and hands before the meal is served. Some clients may need the bedpan or urinal before washing and others may want equipment for mouth care. Evening care refreshes and relaxes clients before they retire for the night. It includes washing the face and hands and a back massage. The linen is also straightened so that the bed is more comfortable for sleep.

Clients who are confined to bed also need to have handwashing equipment provided to them after each time they use the bedpan or urinal and before each meal is served. Nursing personnel frequently forget these basic hygiene measures, and clients are reluctant to ask when they perceive the staff as being busy.

Collect all of the necessary supplies before beginning a bed bath. Place personal items such as soap, powders, lotions, and deodorant within easy reach on the bedside table. In addition to the bath equipment, have fresh linen available and ready for the linen change that normally follows the bath. When clients bathe themselves, advise them to call for a change of bathwater when the water becomes soapy or soiled and when they are ready to have their lower legs, genital area, and back washed if they are unable to do this for themselves. Clients may also need to be told not to leave the soap in the bathwater but to use the soap dish to prevent the water from becoming too soapy, making it difficult to rinse adequately after bathing.

The sequence for washing the body during the bed bath is the same as that used for any other type of bath. It progresses from the cleanest body area to the least clean. If the lower extremities are to be washed after the perineal area, disinfect the basin and use fresh water and a clean washcloth, to prevent the transfer of potentially pathogenic microorganisms from the genital area to the skin on the lower extremities. In the event that the client is incontinent of urine or feces, use tissues to wipe the perineal area before bathing. A grossly soiled perineal area may have to be washed with two sets of equipment to remove completely all of the secretions and excretions. The method for cleansing the perineal area is presented in Skill 39.

Although rubbing the skin with the washcloth and towel stimulates the circulation, washing and drying should be done gently. Because the skin can be damaged by vigorous drying, it is advisable to pat it dry with an absorbent towel. This is particularly important for the elderly and others who have fragile skin. When clients dry themselves they may need to have these points mentioned to them.

Remove the top linen carefully with a minimum of shaking and movement to prevent the dispersion of microorganisms into the room. Bedmaking is presented in Skill 66. Some institutions change all of the bed linen every day, while others use the unsoiled top sheet as a bottom sheet to conserve on linen. When the linen is to be reused, fold it and place it on a clean chair or other surface to prevent it from becoming contaminated. Place soiled linen in a linen bag or hamper.

The Skill Sequence, p. 368, describes one of several ways to bathe a client in bed. While bathing a client be aware of the principles of medical asepsis and use them in the bathing sequence. Observing these principles means it is acceptable to wash the face before the arms, the arms before the body, and the axillae as part of the arms or as part of the chest. The groin may be washed as part of the legs or the abdomen; however, the legs and perineal area are left until last because they are considered to be the least clean. Since the perineal area is the most contaminated area of the entire body it should be bathed last; otherwise the care-giver must acquire all clean equipment before proceeding with the bath.

It is also important to observe the principles of good body mechanics so as to prevent injury to self and to the client during the bath. Raising the level of the bed reduces the strain on the nurse's back by eliminating the bending over that would otherwise be necessary to reach the client. Shifting the client to the side of the bed nearest the care-giver makes it easier to reach the opposite side of the body without excessive stretching and reaching. Standing erect with the knees bent slightly and facing the client without having to twist the body are aspects of good body mechanics that reduce unnecessary fatigue and prevent injury.

☐ SKILL SEQUENCE

BED BATH

Step	Rationale
1. Check kardex for bath plan.	Provides directions for special care needs.
2. Explain procedure to client.	Allays anxiety; enlists cooperation.
3. Wash hands.	Prevents cross-contamination from microorganisms on hands.
4. Prepare equipment and supplies and place on bedside stand and over-bed table.	Prevents delays and interruptions during care.
5. Elevate bed level and lower side rail on side nearest care-giver.	Prevents back strain for care-giver and protects client from falling out of bed.
6. Close door and cubicle curtains.	Ensures privacy.
7. Place bath blanket over top of bed linen. Hold blanket in place while pulling down linen to foot of bed.	Preserves client's modesty and prevents chilling.
8. Remove and fold linen with a minimum of movement. Place it on a clean surface if it is to be reused. (Discard it in a linen bag if it is not reusable.)	Controls the dispersion of microorganisms into the air. Prevents additional contamination of linen.
9. Remove client's gown or pajamas.	Permits inspection of skin.
10. Position client at side of bed nearest to care-giver.	Eliminates need to stretch to reach client.
11. Position over-bed table at side of bed.	Places supplies in an accessible location.
12. Raise side rail and half fill basin with warm water.	Protects client from falling while care-giver is away from bedside. Prevents spilling and splashing water.
13. Wash client's face and ears:	
a. Place towel under client's head.	Prevents pillow from getting wet while face is being washed.
b. Moisten washcloth and clean eyes with washcloth over finger. Movement should be from the inner canthus to the outer canthus. Use a different section of the washcloth to bathe each eye. Do not use soap near eyes.	Prevents moving secretions and debris toward tear duct. Avoids transferring microorganisms from one eye to the other. Avoids burning sensation from soap in eyes.
c. Form a mitt with washcloth and wash face with or without soap, according to client's preference. Rinse all soap off. Pat skin dry.	Controls washcloth from flapping over client.
d. Using caution, clean inside of nose with a moistened cotton-tipped applicator if inspection indicates this is needed.	Clients who are unable to blow out nasal discharges must have them removed or nasal passage may become occluded, reducing air exchange. Inserting applicator too far can damage mucosa.
e. Use a damp washcloth around a finger to cleanse front and back of outer ear. Gently cleanse outer aspect of ear canal. Dry in the same manner.	Removes cerumen. Small objects such as cotton-tipped applicators should not be placed in ear canal because of danger of trauma to canal or tympanic membrane.
14. Wash client's arms:	
a. Relocate towel lengthwise under client's arm farthest from care-giver. Extend it from axilla to wrist. Raise arm by holding at the elbow. Wash and rinse arm using long strokes toward the axilla. Pat dry.	Facilitates return of venous circulation from periphery. Client may be unable to hold arm up without help.
b. Place towel under the hand. Place basin of water on bed on towel. Immerse hand in water and wash all surfaces, moving fingers at all joints.	Cleanses hands more thoroughly and refreshes client. Joint movement maintains full range of motion to keep fingers from becoming stiff.
c. Repeat step 14 for opposite arm and hand.	
15. Wash client's chest: Place towel on chest and then pull down bath blanket. Raise part of towel to wash and rinse sections of chest. Use one hand to hold towel up and wash with the other. Lift breasts, if necessary, to wash under them. Pat skin dry. Leave towel over chest.	Protects modesty by preventing exposure. Pendulous breasts create intertriginous areas. Moisture accumulates and tissue damage can occur.
16. Wash client's abdomen: Place second towel across abdomen. Pull bath blanket down to client's pubic area. Wash, rinse, and dry abdomen. Use corner of washcloth or a cotton-tipped applicator to cleanse umbilicus. Draw up bath blanket to cover and then remove towels.	Prevents unnecessary exposure and avoids chilling.
17. Wash client's legs and groin:	
a. Remove blanket from one leg, taking care to keep perineal area covered. Place towel lengthwise under leg.	Protects modesty.
b. Wash, rinse, and dry front and back of leg.	
c. Pull towel down under foot.	
d. Wash, rinse, and dry all surfaces of foot and toes. If client can bend the knee, place basin on towel and immerse foot in basin and wash. Support leg with one arm as shown in Figure 38–4. Remove foot from basin; move basin to over-bed table and dry foot.	Cleanses feet more thoroughly, refreshes client. Client may be unable to hold leg in place without help.
e. Wash opposite leg in same manner. Change water as necessary when it becomes soiled or soapy.	Both sides of the body may be bathed sequentially.

(continued)

SKILL 38: SKIN CARE

Step	Rationale
18. Wash client's back: a. Position client on the side facing away from care-giver. b. Drape blanket so it exposes the back but covers the rest of the body. Place towel lengthwise on bed parallel to the back. Tuck towel edge under the back. c. Wash, rinse, and dry back with long, gentle strokes. Buttocks are bathed as part of the back. A back massage (Skill 47) may follow this step. NOTE: If lotion is used to bathe dry skin areas, the bath is done in the same manner. Perineal area may be washed after the back to eliminate need to disinfect bath basin before bathing the back. Perineal care is presented in Skill 39.	Long strokes follow contour of muscles and are relaxing. Bathing perineal area before the back eliminates turning client onto his or her side more than once. The nurse must consider client's tolerance for activity when deciding when to wash perineal area during the bath, keeping aseptic principles in mind.
19. Replace bath supplies and equipment. Disinfect bath basin by washing it with a disinfectant. Discard used linen in the laundry bag. Make bed with clean linen (Skill 66). Tidy bedside tables.	

RECORDING

To maintain an accurate and up-to-date data base, record any changes in the skin color and condition at the time the changes are observed, whether daily or more often. Record specific and complete data so that subsequent changes can be easily detected.

The type of bath and the client's physical and pyschological responses to it, either positive or negative, are included in the bathing plan and any subsequent changes in it on the kardex to alert nursing personnel to the type of care each client requires. Examples of the type of entry on the kardex regarding bathing are: self-care shower; self-care at the sink—needs assistance with back and legs; bed bath—needs full care; and bed bath—needs assistance with back and legs.

Sample POR Recording
- S—"I'd rather give myself a bath—I'll feel like a helpless baby if you do it."
- O—Tired quickly; unable to wash own face.
- A—Needs assistance with bath although prefers not to.
- P—Partial bath given to conserve energy.

- S—NA
- O—Skin intact; generalized pallor present; blanching hyperemia present over sacrum.
- A—Decreased peripheral circulation present.
- P—Reposition q hour to avoid excessive pressure; keep skin clean and dry.

Sample Narrative Recording
Reluctant to have nurse give bath: "I feel like a helpless baby." Partial bath given. Very weak, unable to wash own face. Generalized pallor present; skin intact; blanching hyperemia present over sacrum. Repositioned to relieve pressure on sacrum.

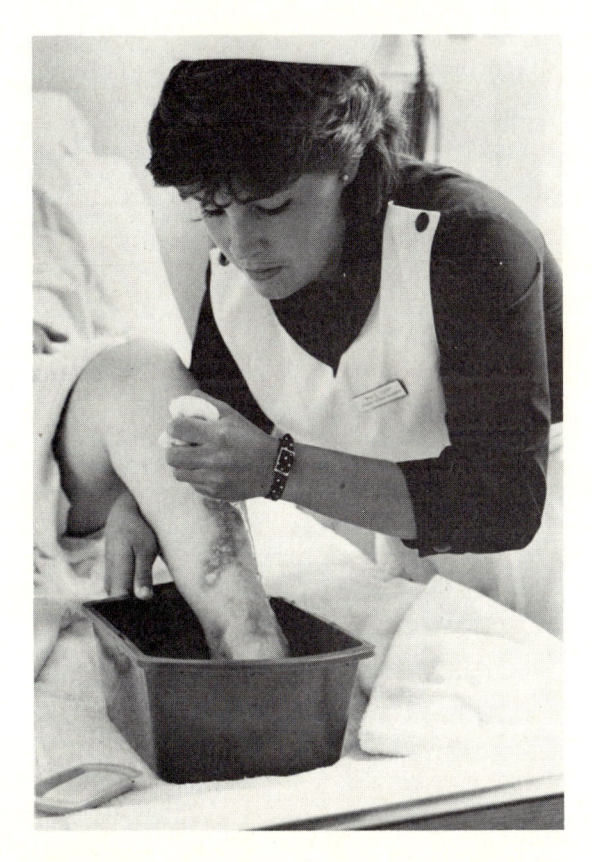

Figure 38–4. The nurse supports the leg while the foot is immersed in the bath basin.

☐ CRITICAL POINTS SUMMARY

1. Environmental temperature and humidity can alter the integrity of the skin.
2. Special techniques are necessary to appraise accurately the skin color and tissue changes in blacks.

3. Appraisal of the skin includes color, integrity, and the presence of lesions.
4. Safety precautions required for safe bathing include: warm water temperature, safety rails, non-slip surfaces, available call signal, and frequent checking on the progress and condition of the client.
5. Rinse all soap off thoroughly to prevent drying the skin.
6. Not every client needs a complete soap and water bath every day.
7. The bathing sequence progresses from the most clean to the least clean body area to prevent transfer of potentially infectious organisms.
8. Change bath water when it becomes soiled or soapy.
9. Protect the client's privacy during bathing.
10. Bathing is individualized according to the client's needs.

☐ LEARNING ACTIVITIES

1. Apply alcohol, powder, lotion, and soap to different areas of your own skin and leave it on for a few hours. Periodically note the sensation and effect each has on the skin.
2. List the changes you observe in your skin in winter and summer and from exposure to wind and sun.
3. Talk with several people about the concerns they have about their skin, and how the appearance of their skin affects their self-concept. Try to find out what those persons with skin problems believe are the causes and what they are doing to resolve the problems.
4. Practice inspecting and palpating the skin of persons of different races and ages to identify color and tissue differences.
5. Practice giving a complete bed bath to a peer. Role play being both the nurse and the client. Discuss your sense of physical and psychological comfort during the bath and how it feels to have someone else bathe you.

☐ REVIEW QUESTIONS

1. What are the positive and negative effects of bathing?
2. Why is it important to keep the stratum corneum intact?
3. How do environmental factors affect the barrier integrity of the skin?
4. What are the skin color and tissue changes that the nurse should be alert for?
5. How can color changes be detected in dark-skinned persons?
6. What are the tissue characteristics you would expect to find in a person with normal, decreased, and increased fluids? How would you detect them?
7. What specific abnormal conditions would you expect to find on the skin of an aged person? What would you do or recommend for these conditions?
8. What types of clients are vulnerable to pressure sores? What conditions promote the development of pressure sores?
9. How would you differentiate between each stage of pressure-sore development?
10. What information should be recorded about a client's personal hygiene habits and skin condition? How should the data be used in the nursing-care plan?
11. What precautions would you use to prevent a client from injury while bathing in a shower, bathtub, or bed?
12. In what way would you alter your bathing-care plan for a client with mildly dry skin and for one with extremely dry skin?
13. What specific principles in regard to bathing should be observed by the nurse, client, or both?

☐ PERFORMANCE CHECKLIST

OBJECTIVE: To use the correct method to give a bed bath safely.

CHARACTERISTIC	RANGE OF ACCEPTABILITY	SATISFACTORY	UNSATISFACTORY
1. Checks kardex for bath plan.	No deviation		
2. Explains procedure to client.	No deviation		
3. Washes hands.	No deviation		
4. Prepares equipment and supplies and places on bedside stand and over-bed table.	No deviation		
5. Closes door and cubicle curtains.	No deviation		
6. Elevates bed level; keeps opposite side rail up.	No deviation		
7. Places bath blanket over linen.	No deviation		

(continued)

CHARACTERISTIC	RANGE OF ACCEPTABILITY	SATISFACTORY	UNSATISFACTORY
8. Removes linen, folds it, and places it on clean surface or discards it in linen bag; removes client's gown.	No deviation		
9. Positions client near care-giver; positions over-bed table at side of bed.	No deviation		
10. Raises side rail; obtains warm bathwater.	No deviation		
11. Washes face and ears: a. Places towel under head. b. Cleanses eyes without soap. c. Makes mitt to wash and rinse face. Pats dry. d. Uses moistened cotton-tipped applicator to cleanse nose. e. Cleanses front and back of outer ear. Uses damp cloth around finger to clean outer aspect of external ear canal. Dries in same manner.	Client may prefer to wash own face and ears. Not necessary for all clients. No deviation		
12. Washes arm: a. Places towel lengthwise under arm. Raises arm by holding at wrist. Washes, rinses and dries arm. b. Places towel and basin under hand. Immerses hand, cleanses all surfaces of hand. Removes basin and dries hand. c. Repeats step 12 a and b for opposite arm and hand.	No deviation Hand may be washed with washcloth.		
13. Washes chest: a. Places towel on chest then pulls down bath blanket. b. Washes and rinses chest in sections; lifts breasts if necessary; pats dry; leaves towel over chest.	No deviation No deviation		
14. Washes abdomen: a. Places second towel over abdomen and pulls down bath blanket. b. Washes, rinses, and dries abdomen and cleans umbilicus. c. Pulls up blanket and removes towels from chest and abdomen.	No deviation No deviation No deviation		
15. Washes legs and groin: a. Removes blanket from one leg; places towel lengthwise under leg. b. Washes, rinses, and dries front and back of leg. c. Pulls towel down under foot. Washes, rinses, and dries all surfaces of foot and toes. d. Washes opposite side in same manner.	Groin may be washed with abdomen. No deviation No deviation May immerse foot if client can bend the knees. Both sides may be washed sequentially.		
16. Changes bathwater as often as necessary.	No deviation		
17. Washes back: a. Positions client on side facing away from care-giver and drapes blanket to expose back only. b. Places towel lengthwise on bed parallel to back; using long strokes, washes, rinses, and dries back and buttocks.	No deviation No deviation		
18. Completes bath with perineal care and back rub.	Perineal care may be given before washing the back.		
19. Replaces all supplies and equipment; disinfects bath basin.	No deviation		
20. Discards used linen in laundry bag.	No deviation		
21. Makes bed (Skill 66).	No deviation		
22. Tidies bedside stand.	No deviation		

REFERENCES

Ayliffe GA, Babb JR, et al: Disinfection of baths and bathwater. Nursing Times 71(36, suppl):22–23, 1975.

Baker H: The skin as barrier, Chap 11, pp 249–255. In Rook A, Wilkinson DS, Ebling FJG (eds): Textbook of Dermatology, vol 1, ed 3. London, Blackwell Scientific Publications, 1979.

Block B, Hunter ML: Teaching physiological assessment of black persons. Nurse Educator 6(1):24–27, 1981.

Four proven steps for preventing decubitus ulcers. Nursing77 7(9):58–61, 1977.

Fregert S, Hjorth N: The principal irritants and sensitizers, Chap 15, pp 443–484. In Rook A, Wilkinson DS, Ebling FJG (eds): Textbook of Dermatology, vol 1, ed 3. London, Blackwell Scientific Publications, 1979.

MacKenzie A: Effectiveness of antibacterial soaps in a healthy population. Journal of the American Medical Association 211(6):973–976, 1970.

Mitchell P, Loustau A: Concepts Basic to Nursing, ed 3. New York, McGraw-Hill, 1981.

Parrish JA: Dermatology and Skin Care. New York, McGraw-Hill, 1975.

Rambo B, Wood L: Nursing Skills for Clinical Practice, vol 1. Philadelphia, WB Saunders, 1982.

Roach LB: Assessing skin changes: The subtle and the obvious. Nursing74 3(3):64–67, 1974.

Roach LB: Color changes in dark skin. Nursing77 7(1):48–51, 1977.

Roberts SL: Skin assessment for color and temperature. American Journal of Nursing 75(4):610–613, 1975.

Rook A, Wilkinson DS, Ebling FJG: Textbook of Dermatology, vol 1, ed 3. London, Blackwell Scientific Publications, 1979.

Tepperman PS, DeZwirek CS, et al: Pressure sores: Prevention and step-up management. Postgraduate Medicine 62(3):83–89, 1977.

BIBLIOGRAPHY

Cahn MM: The skin from infancy to old age. American Journal of Nursing 60(7):993–996, 1960.

Carney RG: The aging skin. American Journal of Nursing 63(6):110–112, 1963.

Cripps DJ: Skin care and problems in the aged. Hospital Practice 12(4):119–127, 1977.

Davis ED: Give a bath? American Journal of Nursing 70(11):2366–2367, 1970.

Friberg H: Holding moisture stores in the skin. Patient Care 11(17):153–161, 1977.

Hardy J: Bathing patients without soap and water. Nursing Care 7(2):25–27, 1974.

Kenney JA: Treatment of skin diseases of the adolescent. Journal of School Health 40(1):7–10, 1970.

Lenininger M: Transcultural Nursing: Concepts, Theories, and Practices. New York, John Wiley & Sons, 1978.

Mitchell P, Loustau A: Concepts Basic to Nursing, ed 3. New York, McGraw-Hill, 1981.

Sana JM, Judge RD: Physical Appraisal Methods in Nursing Practice. Boston, Little, Brown, 1975.

Uttley M: Sweat glands and perspiration. Nursing Mirror 133(22):35–38, 1971.

Wells TJ: In geriatrics patients: That 'minor' skin problem could be trouble. RN 41(7):41–46, 1978.

Williams-LeMaile RL: The clinical and psychological assessment of black patients. In Luckroft D (ed): Black Awareness: Implications for Black Patient Care. New York, American Journal of Nursing, 1974.

Zeller WW: Adolescent attitudes and cutaneous health. Journal of School Health 40(3):115–120, 1970.

AUDIOVISUAL RESOURCES

Basic Nursing Care, Bed Bath
Filmstrip and cassette. (1982, Color, 20 min.)
Available through:
Medicom, Inc.
P.O. Box 116
Garden Grove, CA 92642

Fundamental Skills/Bed Bath
Videotape (½, ¾ in). (1978, Color, 17 min.)
Available through:
Indiana University School of Nursing
NICER Department
1100 West Michigan Street
Indianapolis, IN 46223

How to Give Your Patient a Bed Bath
Filmstrip and cassette. (1975, Color, 32 min.)
Available through:
Techniques Learning Council
921 Green Street
Pasadena, CA 91106

How to Give a Partial Bed Bath
Videorecording (¾ in). (1974, Color, 5 min.)
Available through:
Professional Research, Inc.
930 Pitner Ave.
Evanston, IL 60202

The Bed Cath Procedures.
Videorecording (¾ in). (1976, Color, 19 min.)
Available through:
Comprenetics, Inc.
5805 Uplander Way
Culver City, CA 90230

SKILL 39 Perineal Care

PREREQUISITE SKILLS

Skill 19, "Inspection"
Skill 28, "Handwashing"
Skill 38, "Skin Care"

☐ STUDENT OBJECTIVES

1. Describe the purposes of perineal care.
2. Describe the types of stimuli that induce penile erection.

3. Identify ways the nurse can reduce embarrassment and the potential for penile erection while giving perineal care to a male.
4. Describe the characteristics of the skin that are appraised at the time perineal care is given.
5. Differentiate the methods used to care for the perineum.
6. Describe the aseptic principles used in cleansing the perineum.
7. Cleanse the perineal area using appropriate aseptic technique.

☐ INTRODUCTION

Anatomically, the perineum extends from the symphysis pubis to the tip of the coccyx and includes the urinary and genital orifices and the anus. The care given to the perineal area may be referred to as genital care or perineal care. There are different hygienic and therapeutic purposes for giving care to the different parts of the perineum.

Daily cleansing of the perineal area is an integral part of bathing and is necessary to prevent odor, infection, and physical discomfort. Although a client may not require a complete bath daily, the perineal area should be cleansed with soap and water at least once daily. More frequent cleansing may be required for clients who are incontinent of urine or feces or who have concentrated urine or excessive secretions from the vagina or penis.

Special cleansing of the perineum after obstetric delivery or surgical procedures involving the area may require the use of medical or surgical aseptic procedures. Irrigations may be used to rinse off secretions or excretions. A special therapeutic bath referred to as a sitz bath may be used to cleanse and provide moist heat to the perineum. Sitz baths relieve irritation and promote tissue healing.

☐ PREPARATION

The area included in perineal care has a high potential for bacterial growth and unpleasant odor in both males and females. The dark, warm, moist environment in the perineal zone provides an environment conducive to bacterial growth. Normal secretions from the Bartholin's glands and the glands around the cervix, as well as from the sebaceous and apocrine glands on the labia majora, discharge onto the external tissues. Smegma, a product of apocrine-gland secretion combined with dead epithelial cells, is a thick, white cheesy substance that collects between the folds of the labia and clitoris and under the prepuce of the penis.

Most clients prefer to cleanse their genital areas themselves, but when they are acutely ill, easily tired, unconscious, or physically unable to do so, the provision of perineal care becomes the responsibility of the nurse. Providing perineal care can be a source of embarrassment or anxiety to the nurse and the client. This discomfort may arise from the sexual overtones associated with touching the genital area and may be increased when the nurse is caring for someone of the opposite sex or of the same age. It is important, therefore, that the nurse adopt a matter-of-fact attitude and contain his or her negative feelings lest they be communicated to the client. Understanding some aspects of normal sexual response may help the nurse to cope better with this aspect of perineal care.

SEXUAL RESPONSE

A penile erection is a rapid process that can occur within 5 to 10 seconds. It is caused by an engorgement of blood in spongy tissue that results in the erectile tissue in the organ becoming hard and erect. Penile erection may be induced by reflexive action or by psychic stimuli. Reflexive erections may occur soon after birth and are not dependent on higher centers of the brain or emotions. It is believed that they are mediated through the lumbosacral spinal cord. They occur when highly sensitive erectile tissue in the glans penis, scrotum, or rectum is stimulated. Reflexive erections are involuntary and may be induced by touching the glans penis, scrotum, or rectum, by a full urinary bladder, or by contact with cool bath water. Psychic erections are initiated through the brain by thinking, feeling, or seeing something that arouses the sexual response. A psychically induced erection, sometimes referred to as a voluntary erection, is less likely to occur if the nurse adopts a matter-of-fact attitude. In actual practice, the incidence of penile erections during bathing is rare because the clients are so ill (Hogan, 1980).

In the female, the clitoris is homologus to the penis. The erectile tissue is well supplied with sensory nerve endings that respond to physical manipulation, but the observable reaction is more subtle than that of the male. Thus, it may go unnoticed by the nurse and, therefore, not induce anxiety (Hogan, 1980).

DATA BASE

Client History and Recorded Data
The data obtained during the admission appraisal and interview concerning the skin should include information about the perineal area. All relevant information is incorporated into the nursing-care plan and appropriately entered in the kardex. An accurate and complete data base enables the nurse to evaluate changes in the skin and appropriately adjust the nursing interventions to promote healthy tissue and prevent deterioration of the skin. A teaching plan for self-care can easily be developed from the data base. This is particularly important for clients who have poor hygiene habits, who are obese and have deep skin folds that provide conditions for intertriginous (areas of opposing skin) problems, or who are incontinent or immobilized.

Clients who have had surgery in the perineal area are subject to normal postoperative edema of those tissues. Information about the nature and extent of the surgery is available on the surgery report in the health record and should be reviewed before care is given.

Physical Appraisal Skills

Inspection. The condition of the perineal area may be inspected before or during washing or treatment. Even if the client is capable of self-care, the nurse inspects the skin between the thighs and labia, and between the labia and all other areas of the perineum if the client is incontinent; has concentrated urine, urinary catheters, or unusual or large amounts of discharge or itching; or has had surgery in the perineal area. It is important to look for breaks in the skin, lesions, and chapping, and to note skin color. The character of any secretions or discharges needs to be noted, as well as any odors present.

EQUIPMENT

Routine washing of the perineal area is done with the same equipment used for the bath (Skill 38). The washcloth and towel may be used for the perineum if it is not soiled. After cleansing the perineum, the washcloth and towel are discarded in the laundry. The bath blanket is arranged to prevent unnecessary exposure and chilling during the procedure. Disposable gloves are worn by the care-giver when there are breaks in the skin on the hands or when there is known contaminated matter on the client's skin.

Various methods are used to give special care to the perineum. The method used will vary with the institution, even for the same perineal conditions.

Premoistened pads such as Tucks are frequently used either by the nurse or by the client for routine cleansing after obstetrical delivery. They may also be used to cleanse the perineum after each voiding or defecation for clients who have had surgical procedures such as hemorrhoidectomy. These pads are saturated with a solution of 50 percent witch hazel and 10 percent glycerin. Witch hazel is an astringent that serves to dry up secretions on the skin because it shrinks the tissue. It also has a cooling effect because it evaporates readily. The glycerin leaves a soothing film on the skin.

A clean or sterile *irrigation* may also be used for cleansing. For a perineal irrigation, tap water or an antiseptic solution may be poured from a pitcher or dispensed by an irrigating bag with an attached tubing and perforated nozzle. When the perineum is irrigated, the client is placed on either the toilet or a bedpan to collect the solution. Clean or sterile gloves are worn when the perineum is wiped or patted dry. The cotton balls or gauze squares used to dry the skin are disposed of in an impervious bag and placed in the trash. A *sitz bath* may be taken in a regular bathtub

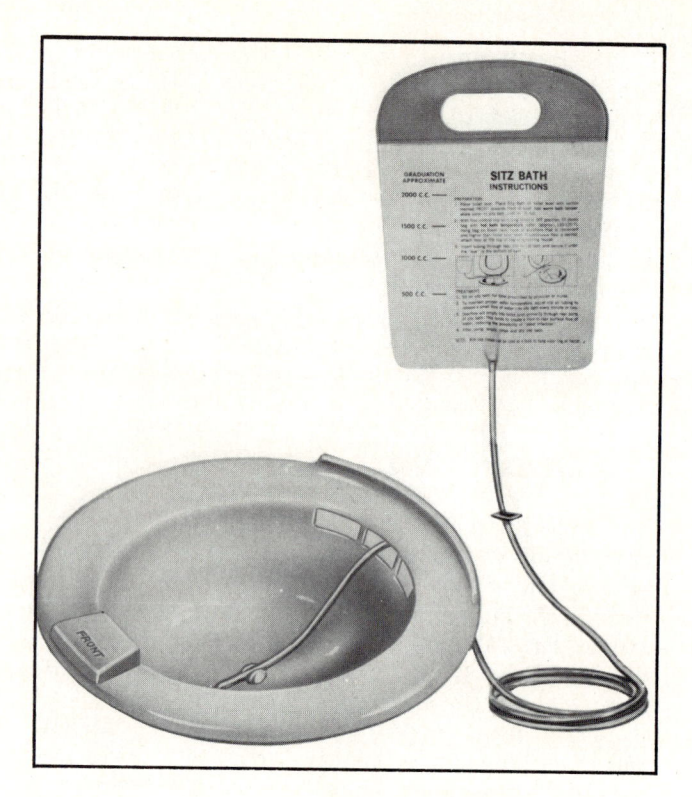

Figure 39–1. Disposable sitz bath with irrigating bag. (Courtesy of the Vollrath Company, Sheboygan, WI 53081.)

or a specially designed permanent or disposable tub or basin. A disposable sitz bath is shown in Figure 39–1. The warm solution is placed in the plastic container, which is hung from a hook or an intravenous pole. The pan rests on the toilet seat, thus allowing the fluid to drain into the toilet. A permanent sitz bath tub accommodates the hip and perineal areas. The legs, torso, and arms are not submerged. Both permanent and disposable sitz baths provide for a continuous inflow and outflow of warm water, thus ensuring that the correct temperature is maintained for the required time.

☐ EXECUTION

Daily washing of the perineum is usually done as the last part of the bath because the perineum is the most contaminated area of the body. This eliminates the need to disinfect the bath basin during the bath. If clients are capable of self-care, the nurse initiates perineal care by providing the supplies and telling them that he or she will leave while they finish their baths. For clients who need more specific direction, the nurse chooses any common term used to identify the perineal area, such as private parts or crotch. When the client is unable to wash the area, use tact and a matter-of-fact attitude in preparing the client to accept the care. Help to preserve privacy and reduce the client's anxiety by closing the cubicle curtains and the room door, and adequately covering the client's perineal area with the bath blanket and towels. Nurses unable to conceal their own embarrassment from clients should probably enlist the assistance of others to give the care. This is also appropriate if a client objects to a particular nurse giving the care. Sometimes a nurse of the same sex as the client is more acceptable to the client. However, some male clients may become anxious if the care-giver is male.

When clients are capable of giving self-care, it is the nurse's responsibility to instruct them in the procedure. Clients also need to learn how to use special equipment and sterile technique when it is required following some surgical procedures.

WASHING THE PERINEAL AREA

It is vital to observe the principles of asepsis in caring for the perineal area. The sequence of bathing is always from the most clean area to least clean; the mons pubis is considered the most clean area, and the anus is considered the least clean. The washcloth is folded into thirds so that a clean side is used only once, with a single stroke. This reduces the potential for transferring microorganisms from the lower perineum to the cleaner parts of the genital area. Thus, washing proceeds from the anterior perineum toward the posterior perineum. Use a clean part of the washcloth for each section of the genitalia. The same sequence is applicable for cleansing the perineum after voiding or defecation.

Prior to washing the perineal area provide the client with an opportunity to use the bedpan or urinal. During washing, remove the top linens and place a bath blanket diagonally to cover the upper body and drape the perineal area and legs. For maximum exposure, position the client in the dorsal recumbent position: on the back, with the legs spread apart and the knees flexed. Place a towel under the buttocks to prevent getting the bed wet. Facing away from the client and avoiding eye contact helps to reduce embarrassment during the cleansing. The condition of the skin can be appraised before and during washing.

Female Care

If the client is female, wash the mons pubis first. Then separate the labia with the finger and thumb of one hand and use the other hand to wash down over the urethral and vaginal orifices. Each fold between the labia majora and minora is washed separately, with a clean area of the washcloth for each section as shown in Figure 39-2. When using cotton balls, use a fresh one for each wipe and then discard it. Use a minimum amount of soap and rinse and dry after the entire area has been washed. Cleansing does not extend below the posterior aspect of the labia. For better exposure and access, cleanse the area between the posterior labia and anus while the client is turned on the side, facing away from the nurse. It is easier for the client to maintain this position if the upper knee is flexed and extended somewhat over the lower leg. Wash, rinse, and

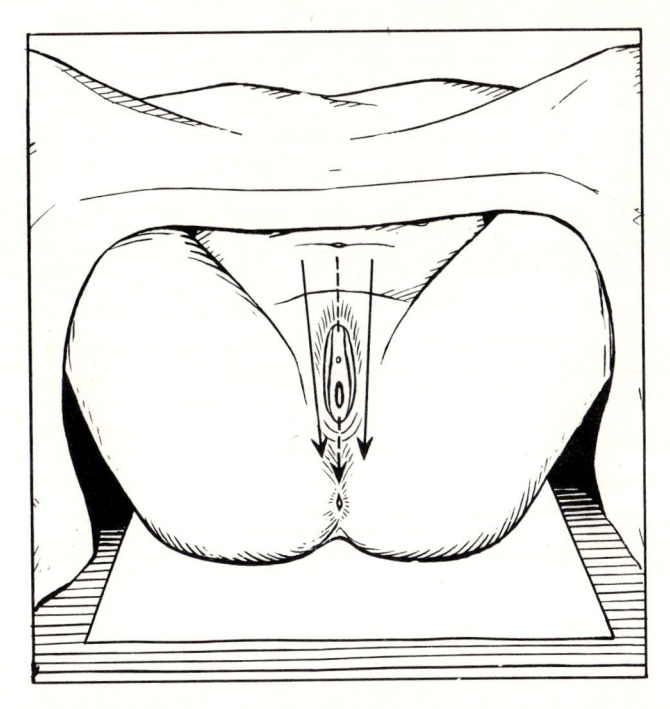

Figure 39-2. The client is placed in the dorsal recumbent position with a bath blanket draped over the legs to prevent unnecessary exposure. After separating the labia, each fold between the labia is washed separately with a single stroke, moving from top to bottom.

dry the posterior perineum with strokes that move from anterior to posterior. Cornstarch or talcum powder may be sprinkled on a gauze square and applied lightly to the skin folds on the inner aspect of the thighs and between the buttocks to reduce friction and absorb moisture.

Male Care

Preparation for cleansing the male perineal area is similar to preparation for cleansing the female, but a second towel is placed over the lower abdomen so that the genital area will be covered when the bath blanket is pulled down to the thighs for bathing. Wash the mons pubis first, since it is the cleanest area. To wash the penis, use one hand to raise the penis up and away from the scrotum, and use the middle finger and thumb of the opposite hand to retract the foreskin on uncircumcised males so that the smegma collected under it can be removed. Take care not to over-retract the foreskin, as this can be painful. Use a clean section of the washcloth to cleanse each section of the penis. Wash the tip of the penis around the urethra in a circular direction beginning with the center and moving toward the edge to remove the smegma. After rinsing and drying the tip return the foreskin to cover the tip of the penis. If the foreskin is left retracted, it can interrupt circulation and cause edema. Wash, rinse and dry the shaft of the penis with single wipes down toward the scrotum and then cleanse the anterior of the scrotum in the same manner. The posterior of the scrotum and the remaining perineum can be washed by raising the scrotum in the cupped palm of the hand. The anal and gluteal fold areas are cleansed in the same manner as on the female. If an erection occurs while cleansing the genital area, the nurse may elect to ignore it, to acknowledge it and complete the care, or to indicate to the client that he or she is leaving for a few moments and will return. Hogan (1980) cautions that leaving abruptly may cause the client who has had an involuntary erection to feel ashamed. The Skill Sequence, "Washing the Perineal Area," specifies the procedures for female and male care.

☐ SKILL SEQUENCE

WASHING THE PERINEAL AREA

Step	Rationale
1. Check kardex for nursing and medical orders.	Provides directions for special care needs.
2. Wash hands.	Prevents cross-contamination from microorganisms on hands.
3. Prepare equipment and supplies.	Prevents delays and interruptions during care.
4. Explain procedure to client.	Allays anxiety; provides opportunity for discussion.
5. Close door and cubicle curtains.	Prevents drafts and chills, and provides privacy.
6. Position client on his or her back.	Permits exposure of area.
7. Female care:	
a. Arrange bath blanket diagonally with one corner at the chin to cover body and legs.	Provides privacy and prevents chilling.
b. Raise client's buttocks and place a towel lengthwise over bed, under client's buttocks.	Prevents getting bed wet.
c. Have client spread legs apart and flex knees.	Provides maximal exposure of perineal area.
d. Wrap side corners of bath blanket around client's legs and anchor under feet.	Prevents drape from slipping out of place.
e. Raise center corner of blanket up to mons pubis.	Exposes perineal area.
f. Wash, rinse, and dry mons pubis.	Cleanest section is washed first to prevent transferring microorganisms.
g. Fold washcloth into thirds.	Provides three clean surfaces, one for each area to be washed.
h. Moisten washcloth with warm water and a scant amount of soap.	Soap can be difficult to rinse thoroughly and causes dryness and irritation.
i. Separate both the majora and minora labia with forefinger and thumb of your nondominant hand.	Exposes tissues between labia.
j. Take one stroke down the center over the clitoris and the urethral and vaginal orifices.	Prevents transferring microorganisms from less clean area.
k. Turn washcloth to clean side and moisten with warm water and scant amount of soap.	Avoids transferring microorganisms on washcloth to skin.
l. Separate labia majora and minora on one side.	Exposes tissue in fold.
m. Wash once down the fold between labia on same side.	Prevents transferring microorganisms from less clean area.
n. Follow steps 7l through m for opposite side. Rinse and pat the area dry, being certain to separate labia minora.	Prevents tissue damage.
o. Turn client on her side facing away from care-giver.	Provides care-giver exposure to perineum.
8. Bend client's upper knee and extend it in front of her lower leg.	Helps client to maintain position.
9. Raise client's upper buttocks with one hand.	
10. Wash, rinse, and dry area between gluteal folds.	
11. Wash perineum, including anus, from front to back with single stroke. Rinse and pat dry.	Prevents transferring microorganisms to least clean area.
12. Apply powder to a gauze square and pat it onto intertriginous areas.	Reduces friction and absorbs moisture.
13. Return client to her back, replace bed linen, and remove bath blanket. (Change bed linen if necessary.)	
14. Male care:	
a. Follow steps 1 to 6.	
b. Place a second lengthwise towel over chest and genital area under bath blanket. Pull down bath blanket to thighs, holding towel in place.	Prevents unnecessary exposure.

(continued)

Step	Rationale
c. Fold washcloth into thirds.	Provides three clean surfaces, one for each area to be washed.
d. Remove towel and use nondominant hand to raise towel, then lift penis up away from scrotum.	Exposes all surfaces of penis.
e. Moisten washcloth with warm water and scant amount of soap.	Soap is drying to skin.
f. Retract foreskin on uncircumcised male, using forefinger and thumb of dominant hand. Hold in retracted position with nondominant hand.	Permits removal of smegma.
g. Start at center of tip of penis and wipe in circular direction around end of penis.	Cleanest area of penis is washed first to prevent spread of microorganisms.
h. Rinse and pat dry.	
i. Replace retracted foreskin.	Retracted foreskin can act as a tourniquet on shaft of penis and cause edema.
j. Turn washcloth to clean side, moisten, and apply soap.	Prevents transferring microorganisms.
k. Wash down shaft of penis using single strokes.	Prevents tissue damage.
l. Rinse and pat dry.	Avoids transferring microorganisms on washcloth to skin.
m. Turn washcloth to clean side, moisten, and apply soap.	
n. Wash, rinse, and dry anterior scrotum.	
o. Cup nondominant hand and gently raise scrotum.	Rapid and vigorous movement may stimulate an erection.
p. Wash, rinse, and dry scrotum and perineum.	
q. Turn client onto his side and complete care as in steps 8 to 13. (NOTE: When client has fecal excreta on the perineum, use tissues to remove excreta before providing perineal care. If the tissue fails to remove all of excreta, use warm, soapy water. Disinfect the basin, obtain a clean washcloth and water, and begin perineal care. Some institutions have disposable washcloths and disposable gloves that may be used to remove fecal excreta.)	

PERINEAL IRRIGATIONS AND SITZ BATHS

Perineal irrigation for a bedridden client is done with the client on a bedpan. If possible, the client is sitting, to prevent the solution from running up the thighs and groin area. Clients who can be out of bed may sit on a bedside commode or the toilet. Have the client void (empty the bladder) before the irrigation. Pour a warm solution of 35.5° to 36.5°C (96° to 98°F) over the client's anterior perineal area from a height of about 6 inches or less, to direct the flow properly and to prevent discomfort or trauma from excessive water pressure. Use cotton balls or gauze squares to remove accumulated secretions and dry the skin. Use each cotton ball for only one wipe and then discard it. The cotton ball may be held in the hand or with a forceps. Some situations (such as perineal surgery) require that sterile technique and equipment be used to prevent the transfer of microorganisms to the perineum.

☐ SKILL SEQUENCE

PERINEAL IRRIGATION

Step	Rationale
1. Check kardex for nursing and medical orders.	Provides directions for special care needs.
2. Wash hands.	Prevents cross-contamination from microorganisms on hands.
3. Prepare equipment and supplies.	Prevents delays and interruptions during care.
4. Explain procedure to client.	Allays anxiety; provides opportunity for discussion.
5. Close door and cubicle curtains.	Prevents drafts and chills, and provides privacy.
6. Prepare 500 milliliters (or amount indicated) of prescribed solution at warm temperature 35.5° to 36.5°C (96° to 98°F).	
7. Test solution temperature on client's inner thigh prior to pouring solution over perineum.	

(continued)

PERINEAL IRRIGATION (Cont.)

Step	Rationale

8. a. Using an irrigating bag:
   (1) Clamp tubing prior to filling bag.
   (2) Attach perforated nozzle to tubing.
   (3) Hold nozzle over sink or bedpan.
   (4) Release clamp on tubing to permit solution to fill tubing. Reclamp tubing.
  b. Using a pitcher: Fill pitcher with solution.
	Prevents solution from leaking from tubing.
	
	Prevents wetting the bed or floor.
	Removes air from tubing.

9. Position client on his or her back, cover with bath blanket, and fold linen down to foot of bed. (Cover client as described in Skill Sequence, "Washing the Perineal Area," step 7a.)	
10. Position client on bedpan. Elevate head of bed so that client is sitting. Raise center of blanket up to pubic area. Spread client's legs apart and flex knees. (NOTE: If client is seated on toilet, spread legs apart in a way that allows adequate space for solution to flow over client's genital area and into toilet bowl.)	Prevents solution from running up thighs. Exposes genital area.

11. Using an irrigating bag:
  a. Hold irrigating bag with one hand.
  b. Raise nozzle above bag level and place it in the same hand holding bag.
  c. With free hand, release clamp on tubing; kink tubing with free thumb and forefinger.
  d. Keep tubing pinched and use remaining fingers of free hand to grasp nozzle from other hand.
  e. Hold nozzle about 1 to 2 inches above mons pubis, keeping tubing pinched.
  f. Raise bag 6 inches above genital area.
  g. Release kinked tubing and direct nozzle so that solution flows down over center and sides of perineal area.
(NOTE: If client is male, place penis on mons pubis so that solution will flow over scrotum and perineum.)
	Prevents solution from flowing out before nozzle is in position.
	
	Prevents direct contact with skin, which would contaminate nozzle.

12. Using a pitcher: Hold pitcher 6 inches above mons pubis area and slowly pour solution over perineal area, directing flow down the center and sides.	Pitcher will become contaminated if it contacts skin. If pitcher is held higher, water pressure is greater than necessary and is difficult to direct. It also splashes and is uncomfortable.
13. Dry the skin from anterior to posterior using one cotton ball or gauze square for each stroke.	Prevents transferring microorganisms.
14. Discard cotton balls or gauze squares in an impervious bag and place in the trash. Or use a clean towel to dry area as described in Skill Sequence, "Washing the Perineal Area," steps 7 and 14.	Disposal in the toilet may stop up plumbing.
15. Remove bedpan.	
16. Dry buttocks area with a towel.	Solution drains to buttocks area.
17. Replace bed linen and remove bath blanket.	
18. Empty bedpan and rinse irrigation bag or pitcher. Discard bag.	
19. Record skin condition, any discharge, and results of irrigation in client's health record.	

A sitz bath is taken in a clean regular or sitz bathtub or a disposable sitz bath pan. The required water temperature may be hot, 36.5° to 40°C (98° to 104°F), or warm, 35.5° to 36.5°C (96° to 98°F), according to the purpose of the bath and the client's tolerance to the temperature. Position the client comfortably, without pressure on the posterior perineum, legs, or back. An inflated rubber ring may be used for the client to sit on in a regular bathtub to prevent pressure on the perineum. When using a permanent sitz bathtub, folded towels may be used to pad the lower back and under the knees to make the client comfortable. Bath blankets are used to cover the client's upper and lower body while the client is sitting in the bath. Maintain the water at a fairly constant temperature for 20 minutes. After that time, the beneficial effects of moist heat are lost, as discussed in Skill 46. Monitor the client's response during the bath, so that early signs of weakness or fainting from vasodilation are detected.

☐ SKILL SEQUENCE

SITZ BATH

Step	Rationale
1. Check kardex for nursing and medical orders.	Provides directions for special care needs.
2. Wash hands.	Prevents cross-contamination from microorganisms on hands.
3. Prepare equipment.	Prevents delays and interruptions during care.
4. Explain procedure to client.	
5. Close door and cubicle curtains.	Prevents drafts and chills, and provides privacy.
6. Fill bathtub about one-sixth full, or sitz tub about one-quarter full, with correct temperature of water. Regulate water inflow on sitz tub.	Avoids overflow when client sits in basin. Water level should not be above iliac crest.
7. Have client remove underwear or pajama pants. Remove any dressings and binders.	
8. Seat client in water, checking water temperature on client's skin before full immersion. (NOTE: When using bathtub, assist client into bathtub, using safety rails.)	Prevents burning client. Prevents client from falling.
9. Place folded towels in lumbar sacral area and under knees if necessary.	Avoids pressure and discomfort when using permanent sitz bathtub.
10. Cover client's upper and lower body with a blanket.	Avoids chilling and protects modesty.
11. Check client's pulse rate and observe for signs of weakness about every 5 minutes. Leave call signal with client. Stay with client if necessary to ensure safety.	Movement of blood to pelvic area may cause weakness or fainting.
12. Assist client out of bath after 15 to 20 minutes. Assess his or her response; check pulse.	Maximum effect of heat is attained within 20 minutes.
13. Pat skin dry. Inspect tissue area.	
14. Replace surgical dressing if necessary.	
15. Assist client in dressing and return to bed for rest.	Provides time for blood circulation to return to normal. Avoids chilling after bath.
16. Disinfect bathtub or sitz tub. Place used linen in laundry bag.	Prevents transfer of organisms.
17. Record client's reaction to bath, skin condition, and amount and characteristics of discharge.	Documents client's status.

Hazards

It is important to check the temperature of the water used for perineal irrigation and sitz bath with a thermometer to be sure that it is not too hot. What may seem to be a satisfactory temperature to the nurse may be too hot for the client, especially if the skin is tender from swelling or trauma. Even after checking the water with a thermometer, it is wise to test the client's reaction to the solution temperature by putting some of the solution on the inner aspect of the thigh or buttocks before using it on the perineum. When adding hot solution to maintain the proper temperature, agitate the water or add the solution slowly to prevent hot areas from occurring and burning the client.

Cleaning the Sitz Bath

The supplies used to disinfect the bathtub, sitz tub, basin, or bedpan after each use should be those recommended by the infection-control practitioner or committee.

RECORDING

Entries for routine perineal care are not usually made on the client health record. However, changes in the skin condition and the presence of any discharge, as well as any change in the type of care needed, are documented on the health record. New interventions are noted on the kardex so that subsequent care-givers will know the current interventions and be able to evaluate them.

Sample POR Recording

- S—"My crotch is sore and feels swollen. It feels better after the irrigation."
- O—Slight edema and mild erythema present in the posterior third of the perineum.
- A—Perineal inflammation present; discomfort partially relieved by irrigation.
- P—Continue perineal irrigations with 500 ml warm H_2O PRN as ordered.

Sample Narrative Recording

States "crotch is sore and swollen." Warm perineal irrigation with 500 ml of tap water given. Slight edema and mild erythema present in the posterior third of the perineal area. Some relief of discomfort after the irrigation.

☐ CRITICAL POINTS SUMMARY

1. The perineal area extends from the mons pubis to the area between the gluteal folds.
2. Cleanse the perineal area at least once a day, and more often if the client's condition requires it.
3. Washing, premoistened pads, irrigations, and sitz baths are alternative means for cleansing the perineum.
4. Ensure the client's privacy during perineal care.
5. Reduce or avoid embarrassment while giving care by adopting a matter-of-fact attitude and by facing away and avoiding eye contact with the client.
6. Principles of aseptic technique require that only one stroke be taken at a time, working from the most clean area to the least clean.
7. Appraise the condition of the skin for integrity and the presence of odorous secretions.
8. Penile erection is less apt to occur if the urinary bladder is empty and warm water is used for bathing.
9. Return a retracted foreskin over the glans after cleansing.
10. Protect the client from burns from hot water.

☐ LEARNING ACTIVITIES

1. List the terms used by your family and friends to describe the perineal area. Compare your list with the list of a peer.
2. Select a peer to role play how you would approach clients of the same sex and of the opposite sex who need to have you give them perineal care. Discuss your level of comfort with this responsibility.
3. Reflect on your own attitude regarding sexuality and intimacy.
4. Discuss with a peer how you would respond to a client who had a penile erection while you were giving care.
5. Practice giving perineal care to a model in the classroom laboratory before cleansing a client.

☐ REVIEW QUESTIONS

1. Why is perineal care necessary?
2. What types of stimuli induce a penile erection?
3. How can a nurse reduce embarrassment and the potential for a penile erection?
4. What changes in the skin should a nurse look for when giving perineal care?
5. What are the different ways perineal care can be given? How would you explain each of the ways to a client?
6. What specific actions are used to incorporate aseptic technique in cleansing the perineal area?

☐ PERFORMANCE CHECKLISTS

OBJECTIVE: To use the correct procedure to cleanse the perineal area.

CHARACTERISTIC	RANGE OF ACCEPTABILITY	SATISFACTORY	UNSATISFACTORY
1. Checks kardex for nursing and medical orders.	No deviation		
2. Washes hands.	No deviation		
3. Prepares necessary equipment and supplies.	No deviation		
4. Explains procedure to client.	No deviation		
5. Closes door and cubicle curtains.	No deviation		
6. Positions client on his or her back.	No deviation		
7. Female care: a. Covers client with bath blanket.	No deviation		
b. Positions legs and secures blanket.	No deviation		
c. Raises center of blanket to expose area.	No deviation		
d. Washes, rinses, and dries mons pubis.	No deviation		

(continued)

CHARACTERISTIC	RANGE OF ACCEPTABILITY	SATISFACTORY	UNSATISFACTORY
e. Folds washcloth into thirds and moistens; applies small amount of soap to washcloth.	No deviation Soap may be omitted if skin is dry or itchy.		
f. Separates both labia with thumb and forefinger of nondominant hand.	No deviation		
g. Uses a different cloth surface for every stroke from anterior to posterior: one each for center and each side of labia. Rinses and dries afterward.	No deviation		
h. Turns client on side facing away from care-giver, flexing upper leg to help client hold client's position.	No deviation		
8. Cleanses and dries area between gluteal folds.	No deviation		
9. Raises upper buttock with one hand; wipes perineum from front to back with single strokes; rinses and dries.	No deviation		
10. Applies powder to intertriginous areas.	No deviation		
11. Replaces top linen; removes blanket or changes bed linen.	No deviation		
12. Cleanses and replaces equipment.	No deviation		
13. Male care: a. Follows steps 1 to 6; places towel lengthwise over chest and genital area; pulls down bath blanket to thighs.	No deviation		
b. Folds washcloth into thirds.	No deviation		
c. Raises towel and lifts penis away from scrotum.	No deviation		
d. Moistens washcloth with warm water; applies soap.	No deviation		
e. Retracts foreskin with forefinger and thumb; cleanses with circular stroke, starting at center; rinses and dries.	Omit if client is circumcised.		
f. Replaces retracted foreskin.	No deviation		
g. Changes to clean area of washcloth; moistens and applies soap.	No deviation		
h. Washes, rinses, and dries anterior scrotum.	No deviation		
i. Raises scrotum with cupped hand; washes, rinses, and dries posterior scrotum and perineum.	No deviation		
14. Turns client on side away from care-giver, flexing client's leg to maintain position.	No deviation		
15. Cleanses and dries area between gluteal folds.	No deviation		
16. Raises upper buttock with one hand and washes perineum from front to back with single strokes; rinses and dries.	No deviation		
17. Applies powder to intertriginous areas.	No deviation		
18. Replaces bed linen; removes blanket or changes bed linen.	No deviation		
19. Cleanses and replaces equipment.	No deviation		

OBJECTIVE: To use the correct method to give a perineal irrigation safely.

CHARACTERISTIC	RANGE OF ACCEPTABILITY	SATISFACTORY	UNSATISFACTORY
1. Checks kardex for nursing and medical orders.	No deviation		
2. Washes hands.	No deviation		
3. Prepares equipment and supplies.	No deviation		
4. Explains procedure to client.	No deviation		
5. Closes door and cubicle curtains.	No deviation		
6. Prepares and checks temperature of solution. Tests solution temperature on client's inner thigh prior to pouring.	No deviation		
7. Attaches nozzle, fills bag and tubing with solution, and clamps tubing; or fills pitcher. Positions client on back and covers with blanket.	No deviation		
8. Positions client on bedpan; elevates client to sitting position.	Not necessary if client on toilet.		
9. Raises center of blanket to pubic area.	No deviation		
10. a. Holds bag 6 inches above mons pubis; with tubing pinched, holds nozzle 1 inch above mons pubis; releases tubing and directs flow over center and sides of perineal area. OR:			
b. Holds pitcher 6 inches above mons pubis and slowly pours solution over center and sides of perineal area.	No deviation		
11. Dries the skin from anterior to posterior with one stroke; uses a clean cotton ball for each stroke; discards cotton balls in impervious bag and disposes in trash.	No deviation		
12. Removes bedpan and dries buttock area with a towel.	No deviation		
13. Replaces bed linen and removes blanket.	No deviation		
14. Empties bedpan.	Not necessary if client on toilet.		
15. Records skin condition, any discharge, and results of irrigation in client's health record.	No deviation		

OBJECTIVE: To use the correct method to give a sitz bath safely.

CHARACTERISTIC	RANGE OF ACCEPTABILITY	SATISFACTORY	UNSATISFACTORY
1. Checks kardex for nursing and medical orders.	No deviation		
2. Washes hands.	No deviation		
3. Prepares equipment and supplies.	No deviation		
4. Explains procedure to client.	No deviation		
5. Closes door and cubicle curtains.	No deviation		
6. Fills bathtub or sitz tub with correct temperature water; adjusts water temperature controls.	No deviation		
7. Has client remove clothes. Removes surgical dressings.	No deviation		
8. Assists client to sit in bath, using safety precautions; pads pressure areas.	No deviation		

(continued)

CHARACTERISTIC	RANGE OF ACCEPTABILITY	SATISFACTORY	UNSATISFACTORY
9. Covers client with blanket.	No deviation		
10. Checks client often for signs of weakness or fainting.	No deviation		
11. Assists client out of bath after 15 to 20 minutes.	No deviation		
12. Pats skin dry; inspects tissue area; replaces dressings and clothes.	No deviation		
13. Assists client back to bed.	No deviation		
14. Disinfects bathtub or sitz tub.	No deviation		
15. Records reaction to bath, skin condition, amount and characteristics of discharge.	No deviation		

REFERENCE

Hogan R: Human Sexuality: A Nursing Perspective. New York, Appleton-Century-Crofts, 1980.

BIBLIOGRAPHY

Gibbs GE: Perineal care for the incapacitated patient. American Journal of Nursing 69(1):124–125, 1969.

Rambo BJ, Wood LA: Nursing Skills in Clinical Practice, vol 2. Philadelphia, WB Saunders, 1982.

AUDIOVISUAL RESOURCES

Vaginal Douche and Perineal Care
 Filmstrip. (1970, Color, 25 min.)
 Available through:
  Robert J. Brady Company
  Route 197
  Bowie, MD 20715

Peri Care
 Filmstrip. (1974, Color, 22 min.)
 Available through:
  Medcom, Inc.
  P.O. Box 116
  Garden Grove, CA 92642

SKILL 40 Oral Care

PREREQUISITE SKILLS

Skill 19, "Inspection"
Skill 20, "Palpation"
Skill 28, "Handwashing"

STUDENT OBJECTIVES

1. Describe the purpose and effects of oral care.
2. Explain the role of saliva in promoting oral health.
3. Explain the factors that affect oral health.
4. Describe changes in the oral cavity associated with illness, medical therapies, and medications.
5. Describe the normal characteristics of each of the structures in the oral cavity.
6. Describe the characteristics of the oral structures included in an oral appraisal.
7. Identify factors that determine the degree of needed assistance with oral care.
8. Identify the precautions to be observed while giving oral care to clients unable to swallow adequately.
9. Administer safe oral care to clients.

INTRODUCTION

Oral-care practices are an essential component of daily personal care in both health and illness. Maurer (1977) refers to the oral cavity as one of the most significant areas of the body because of its function in relation to nutrition, speech, and emotional expression. The quality of an individual's oral health depends on nutrition, the use of preventive oral-care practices, the presence or absence of oral infections or systemic disease, and the presence or absence of trauma to the teeth and soft tissues of the mouth. Oral care helps to prevent dental caries, stimulate the gingiva, keep the oral mucosa soft and moist, prevent halitosis, and provide physical and psychological comfort.

An evaluation of the oral health of clients admitted to one hospital over a period of 8 months revealed that 89 percent had some form of oral disease that required treatment. It was found that most of these patients were not aware of the problems they had and did not have a family dentist (Block, 1976). Because additional oral problems can be generated by illness, and because we tend to discontinue our usual oral-care practices while we are ill, the role of the nurse in providing oral care is crucial. Nurses are in a unique position to affect the quality of oral health because they are the decision makers for the type of personal care an institutionalized client receives. Nurses either give direct care themselves or supervise the care given by others. Regardless of the setting in which nurses work, a major focus of nursing practice is teaching preventive health-care practices and helping people to become more responsible for their own health. Nurses working in community settings such as clinics, schools, and homes with the well and the ill have numerous opportunities to teach good oral-care practices that prevent oral disease. Klocke and Sudduth's (1969) study demonstrates that nurses can help clients improve their oral health and reduce plaque formation with a one-time instruction in a standardized method of toothbrushing. The components of an adequate oral-care program include the following (Block, 1977):

1. Detecting obvious oral disease
2. Educating clients about their oral problems
3. Referring to a dentist for treatment
4. Teaching effective oral care
5. Performing oral care for clients unable to care for themselves
6. Helping to reduce the adverse effects of disease and medications on the oral structures

□ PREPARATION

Before undertaking any aspect of an oral-care program the nurse needs a basic understanding of the structures and function of the contents of the oral cavity. Saliva, the soft oral tissues, tongue, palate, and tonsils, and the teeth affect and are affected by nutrition, disease, treatment, and care practices.

THE ORAL CAVITY

Saliva
Saliva consists of two types of secretions: a serous secretion containing the enzyme ptyalin, which digests starches, and a mucous secretion, which lubricates the oral structures (Guyton, 1981). Speaking, eating, and swallowing are facilitated by the presence of saliva. In combination with jaw movements, saliva also cleans the teeth by removing food particles. The normal saliva pH of between 6 and 7 helps to decrease the acidity of the mouth, and interferes with the processes involved in dental decay. Saliva may be watery, ropy, or mucoid. Factors that reduce the amount and quality of saliva and influence its consistency include the following:

1. Organic and functional disturbances such as aging
2. Inability or refusal to eat
3. Reduced fluid intake
4. Dental prostheses
5. Drugs such as atropine, reserpine, chlorpromazine, and antihistamines
6. Mouth breathing
7. Obstructed salivary gland ducts
8. Radiation therapy to the head or neck

The reduction or absence of saliva from these disturbances of the salivary glands is known as xerostomia. When saliva is reduced in amount, it becomes thickened and sticky, with a lowered pH, making it more acid. Increased acidity of the saliva is a factor in dental decay. Dry mucous membranes cause discomfort in the soft tissues of the mouth, which makes wearing dentures difficult. Swallowing becomes difficult and modifications in the diet may be necessary to ensure adequate nutrition.

An artificial saliva substitute developed by the Veterans Administration Oral Disease Research Laboratory is used to treat persons who have xerostomia (Smith, 1983). This preparation is available at local pharmacies and does not require a prescription. It consists of several minerals combined with sorbitol, methycellulose, water, and flavoring. The person applies a few drops of the solution to the tongue or between the lip and the teeth, then distributes it around the mouth with the tongue. It may be used as often as necessary to relieve oral dryness.

Excessive amounts of saliva may result from an overproduction of saliva due to stimulation of the nerve impulses in the brain or reflexes in the upper gastrointestinal tract. A client with a normal volume of saliva may retain excessive amounts in the mouth because of difficulty in swallowing (DeGowin and DeGowin, 1981). Excess saliva has some positive effects on the teeth because it bathes the teeth surfaces and acts to clear carbohydrates from the oral cavity (Menaker, 1980). When the increased amount of saliva interferes with speech, nutrition, and general personal comfort, it may be controlled by anticholinergic drugs or tranquilizers that reduce the salivary flow. Suctioning provides another alternative; it can be done intermittently, or, depending on the severity and duration of the condition, a small mushroom catheter can be implanted in the floor of the mouth, exited through an incision under the jaw, and connected to a suction machine.

Soft Oral Tissues
Periodontal tissue includes the gingiva, which in health is firmly attached to the neck of the tooth; the gingival papilla, which is the projection that fills the space between the teeth; and the periodontal ligament, which attaches the tooth to the gingivae and bone. Periodontal tissue is vulnerable to several types of disease.

Healthy *gingiva* (gum tissue) is coral pink in whites but may be much darker in blacks. It is moist and may have a stippled appearance like that of an orange peel. The gingiva frequently recedes with aging, but the process may be hastened by poor brushing habits or disease. When the gingiva recedes, the rough, lusterless border of the root near the enamel is exposed, which can cause a hypersensitive reaction to hot or cold substances in the mouth.

An ascorbic acid (vitamin C) deficiency may cause the gingivae to become swollen, tender, and spongy; turn deep red or purple; and bleed easily. *Hyperplasia* of the gingival tissue is an increase in the amount of tissue. The condition progresses over time and may result in the teeth being covered with gingival tissue. Hyperplasia is sometimes related to phenytoin sodium (Dilantin) therapy for seizures and to leukemia, which causes an infiltration of leukocytes into the tissue. Anticoagulant therapy may cause the gingivae to bleed easily from very slight irritation, such as brushing.

Periodontal disease is caused mainly by the presence of irritating agents in the crevice between the gingiva and the crown of the tooth. Clients with an increased vulnerability for periodontal disease include those with diabetes, thyroid imbalance, malnutrition, alcoholism, hormonal imbalance, and blood dyscrasia, and those who are being treated with chemotherapy (Levine and Grayson, 1973). *Gingivitis* is a mild, superficial inflammation of the tissue that can be identified by blood on the toothbrush or bleeding gums. When gingivitis extends to all of the adjoining mucosa or includes the pharyngeal structures, it is known as stomatitis. *Periodontitis* is present when the teeth are mobile, the tissue is severely receded from the tooth, and purulent exudate is present at the gingival margin. Gingivitis and periodontitis are often asymptomatic and may go unnoticed by the client. The following are signs of periodontal disease (Perlitsh, 1974):

1. Bleeding gums
2. Bad breath
3. Soft, swollen, or tender gums
4. Pus from the gum line when pressure is applied
5. Loose teeth
6. Gums shrinking away from the teeth

More teeth are lost after age 40 because of periodontal disease than because of dental decay, so the nurse should be alert to the clinical signs of disease in the client's mouth (Levine and Grayson, 1973).

The Tongue
The tongue is a moist, flexible organ, which is pink in whites and bluish in blacks. In addition to serving as an accessory organ of the digestive tract and producing articulation of speech, the tongue provides some cleansing of the teeth by its movement within the mouth. With aging, the tongue may become flabby and lose some of its strength and mobility, thus reducing its cleansing effectiveness. The papillae on the dorsum of the tongue collect cells that are shed from the oral tissues, bacteria, and food particles. These all form a normal coating on the tongue. A hairy tongue, sometimes referred to as a furry or black tongue, is sometimes due to an overgrowth of organisms within the papillae. This may be caused by treatment with antibiotics that inhibit the growth of normal bacteria and allow the overgrowth of fungi. It may also be found in debilitated clients.

The tongue is subjected to trauma from hot or cold substances, irritation from smoking, inflammation, ulcers, and infections. Some vitamin deficiencies can cause changes in the size and texture of the tongue. For example, vitamin B_{12} deficiency can cause a decrease in tongue size, thinning of the mucosa, and a slick and smooth surface. With pellagra, a niacin deficiency, the tongue first becomes reddened at the tip and borders. The redness eventually spreads and the tongue swells. A riboflavin deficiency can cause burning of the tongue. Edema of the papillae and the bases of the papillae creates dark red elevations that give the name of cobblestone tongue (DeGowin and DeGowin, 1981).

The Palate
The palate forms the roof of the mouth and separates the oral cavity from the nasal cavity and the pharynx. Mucous glands in the palate help to keep it moist. The anterior palate is pink and hard and has ridges. It is subject to burns and abrasions from food. The posterior palate is soft with a darker pink mucosa. The palate is important in speech formation. Pressure of the tongue against the soft palate helps to force the food bolus into the pharynx.

The Tonsils
Tonsils are almond-shaped masses of lymph tissue that can be seen on either side of the back of the mouth at the junction of the oropharynx. They are a frequent site of infection in children. When infected, tonsils are easily seen. Although tonsils are not considered part of the oral cavity, infected tonsils contribute to unpleasant mouth odor, cause oral discomfort, and interfere with good oral health. When working with a child, the nurse needs to inspect the condition of the tonsils and consider their influence on the child's oral health.

The Teeth
A tooth consists of a hard outer shell of enamel covering the crown and the dentin. Dentin provides the bulk of the tooth and its roots, and is similar to bone. Pulp, which is in the center of the tooth, contains blood and lymphatic vessels and nerves that enter the tooth through openings in the root tips. The dentin of the root is covered with a thin layer of cementum.

The first set of teeth, known as deciduous teeth, is equally divided between the upper and lower jaws. They begin erupting at about age 6 months, and all 20 of them are usually in place between the 20th and 30th months. The deciduous teeth are shed between ages 7 and 13. The 32 permanent teeth are usually in place by age 21. Oral care should begin as soon as the teeth begin to erupt. Dental caries in a child under age 3 are usually due to milk or juice held in the child's mouth for prolonged periods of time. This commonly results from the habit of taking a bottle to bed and drinking from it while sleepy. Tooth decay at such an early age can have long-term effects. It can predispose the child to other oral infections, affect the spacing of the permanent teeth if it causes loss of deciduous teeth, and interfere with good nutrition if the child is unable to chew solid food. Speech development may also be impeded if teeth are missing while the child is learning to form words.

Tooth decay is a decalcification of the mineral components and dissolution of the organic matrix of the tooth. Tooth decay involves softening of the hard tooth tissue and results in cavity formation (dental caries). For dental decay to occur, microorganisms, carbohydrates (primarily sucrose), and a susceptible tooth surface must be present. An individual's susceptibility to tooth decay depends on several indigenous factors: saliva composition and flow rate, tooth form and alignment, the physicochemical nature of the tooth surface, and the composition of bacterial plaque. There is also a weak familial pattern to dental decay; the genetic factor that determines tooth form may produce teeth that have pits and fissures, which are susceptible to decay because they provide areas for entrapped food debris and a protected environment for bacterial growth (Menaker, 1980). However, a family pattern of dental decay is related more to the family's dietary habits, routine dental care, and emphasis on oral care than it is to a genetic factor (Menaker, 1980). In addition, the physicochemical nature of the tooth surface can be influenced by the ingestion of various trace elements in the diet or through the topical effect of substances such as fluoride.

Dental plaque is a soft mass of bacterial colonies that adhere to the natural teeth as well as to removable or fixed restorations. The microorganisms in dental plaque set up a chain reaction that is responsible for initiating dental caries, promoting inflammatory responses by the periodontal tissue, and forming calculus on the teeth. Dental plaque contains many microorganisms capable of producing acids when they are combined with sucrose. These acids act on and dissolve the tooth surface (Menaker, 1980). Plaque forms on tooth surfaces even in the absence of any oral nutrition.

Calculus is calcified dental plaque. It is a hard material that forms on natural and artificial teeth and oral appliances. Calculus plays an important role in the progress of periodontal disease.

☐ NUTRITION

Good teeth begin with a balanced diet that includes food from the milk, meat, vegetable and fruit, and grain groups. The substance considered most responsible for dental decay is sucrose. However, its role in causing dental caries is significantly reduced when it is consumed as part of the meal and then cleared from the mouth by other foods. When taken as a snack, sucrose remains in the mouth for a longer period of time. Uncooked crisp, juicy fruits and vegetables are considered to be ideal snacks and desserts because of their detergent (cleansing) action. These foods help stimulate the gingivae, and are quickly cleared from the mouth. Soft foods tend to adhere to the teeth and leave considerable debris around the teeth.

Fluoride is an essential micronutrient and is found in most soils, natural water supplies, and foods. It is normally present in the body in high concentrations in the skeleton and teeth and in low amounts in the blood stream. Fluoride inhibits the development of dental caries by: (a) protecting against demineralization of the teeth and enhancing the rate of remineralization, (b) remineralizing dental lesions with a deposit of fluoride salts, and (c) influencing the ecology of dental plaque through its antimicrobial activity (Menaker, 1980).

About one-half of the United States population now benefits from fluoride that has been added to the water supply in a concentration of 1 part per million (ppm). This concentration has a systemic effect on unerupted and erupted teeth and is valuable for preventing dental caries in children up to age 13, until all of the permanent teeth are erupted except the third molars. Continuous use of fluoridated water from birth results in a 60 to 70 percent decrease in caries (Wilkins, 1983).

DATA BASE

Client History and Recorded Data

In order to provide appropriate oral care, the nurse finds out

1. If the client has dentures
2. If there is any alteration of the taste sensations
3. If there is any soreness of the tongue or mouth
4. If there is any bleeding or receding of the gingival tissue
5. If any lesions are present in the oral cavity

The nurse also finds out what the client's normal oral-care routine is, and how often and what type of dental services the client uses. This information helps the nurse to identify what kind of teaching may need to be done, if any, and to integrate the client's regular oral-care practices into a plan of care while hospitalized. The plan of care must also take into account the client's level of consciousness, state of mental alertness, and ability to cooperate during oral care.

Information on the client's health record can alert the nurse to potential oral problems. Certain diseases, conditions, and treatments are often accompanied by specific oral problems. For example, uremia or chemotherapy may cause stomatitis. Clients with fever, dehydration, and respiratory illnesses often have dry mucous membranes. Radiation therapy reduces the activity of the salivary glands; the resulting decreased flow of saliva causes the normal pH of the mouth to become lower and thus more acidic, and the scanty amount of saliva present is thick and ineffective in cleansing the tooth surfaces and lubricating food for easier swallowing. Tranquilizers and anticholinergic drugs ordered for specific illnesses can also reduce the flow of saliva, and antibiotics administered to fight infections can change the normal flora of the mouth and thus result in fungal or yeast superinfections. Thick antacid preparations taken for gastric disturbances may leave a cumulative residue in the mouths of clients who have dry mucous membranes.

Physical Appraisal Skills

A daily appraisal of the oral cavity is needed for clients who are having actual or potential oral-health problems as just described. Any hospitalized person who has an altered fluid or food intake is a potential candidate for oral health problems to some degree. A daily appraisal enables the nurse to detect any changes that will require revisions in the plan for oral care.

Inspection. A light source and tongue depressor are essential for adequate inspection of the oral cavity. The presence and consistency of the saliva are determined by inserting the tongue depressor into the mouth and touching the palates and floor of the mouth, then slowly withdrawing the depressor to look at the amount and consistency of the saliva. Care needs to be taken not to press on the distal aspect of the tongue; this can evoke the gag reflex and is very unpleasant for the client. The nurse also looks at the amount of moisture present in all areas of the mouth. Then the color and texture of the gingival tissue and the mucous membranes covering the palates and tonsillar pillars are determined. The teeth are inspected for soft debris. If the client's condition permits, this can be done after he or she has used a disclosing solution that stains the dental plaque. The lips are inspected for texture and moisture.

Palpation. The tongue and lips are palpated to determine texture and moistness. The nurse wears clean disposable gloves while doing this to avoid direct contact with the microorganisms in the mouth and to prevent transferring microorganisms into the mouth. The client should be made aware of what is going to be done so that he or she will not unintentionally bite down on the nurse's hands.

Guide for Oral Appraisal. An objective appraisal of the oral cavity is possible by use of a guide and rating scale devised by DeWalt (1975) for appraising nine different aspects of the oral cavity. By scoring each of the nine variables that affect oral health, the nurse develops a data base from which to detect changes in the oral cavity. When this tool was used in a study designed to determine the effect of oral-care measures, DeWalt (1975) was able to substantiate positive and significant changes in the oral tissues of patients who received oral care designed to meet their individual needs. DeWalt's (1975) guide for oral appraisal is presented in Table 40-1.

EQUIPMENT

Oral-Care Devices

Toothbrushes are available in electric and manual models. Electric toothbrushes consist of a handle and a detachable brush. They may have low and high speeds that control the number of strokes per minute. The brush tends to be smaller than the manual toothbrush, which may serve as an advantage for persons who require a smaller brush to reach all of the tooth surfaces. Electric toothbrushes do not require the user to apply pressure, which is an advantage to the handicapped user and to the care-giver. The electric toothbrush has been shown effective in removing dental plaque and reducing the incidence of gingivitis (Wilkins, 1983).

Manual toothbrushes are available in a wide variety of sizes and designs. The American Dental Association (1979) recommends that a toothbrush should be easily and efficiently manipulated, lightweight, easily cleaned and treated, durable, and inexpensive. Manual toothbrushes can be adapted for handicapped persons by increasing the size of the handle or by attaching the brush handle to a device that they are able to hold (Maurer, 1977).

The toothbrush bristles should be straight and of equal length to permit access to all areas. Bristles of uneven lengths are less efficient and may cause injury to the gingiva when hard pressure is applied on the brush in an effort to use all of the shorter bristles (Wilkins, 1983).

Hard and medium bristles are currently contraindicated because of the potential damage to the gingival tissue. If they are used, care must be exercised to prevent tissue damage. Soft-bristle toothbrushes have the advantage of producing more effective cleaning because they can be directed into the grooves of the teeth and the interproximal areas, and are less traumatic to the gingival tissue. The condition of the bristles affects the efficiency and effectiveness of brushing. A toothbrush should be replaced when the bristles lose their alignment and rigidity. It is recommended that a person own two toothbrushes for alternate use, permitting one to dry out while the other is in use.

Denture brushes should not have hard bristles because of the damage they can cause to the dentures. Some denture brushes have two types of bristle arrangements: one set of bristles is arranged in a round group of tufts for access to the inner, curved surface, and another set of bristles is arranged in a rectangle for use on the biting surfaces.

The *toothette* is a disposable device used as a toothbrush. It consists of a soft, round sponge attached to a stick, similar to a lollipop in appearance. The toothette does not enter into the space between the teeth or slide under the gingival borders as do the bristles of a brush. DeWalt (1975) found that the toothette was less abrasive to the oral tissues of the elderly, and that a significant improvement in the tongue color and condition of the mucous membranes and lip texture occurred when the toothette was used

TABLE 40-1. Guide for Oral Appraisal

VARIABLE	TOOLS FOR DATA COLLECTION	METHOD OF MEASUREMENT	NUMERICAL AND DESCRIPTIVE RATINGS[a] 1	2	3
Salivation	Tongue blade	Insert blade into mouth, touching gums, palates, and floor of mouth. Slowly remove and observe.	Ropy or viscid	Dry or scanty	Moist
Tongue moisture	Visual and palpatory assessment	Feel and observe appearance of tissue	Coated	Dry	Moist
Tongue coloring	Visual assessment	Observe appearance of tissue	Red and blistered	Red	Pink
Palates	Visual assessment	Observe appearance of tissue	Dry and coated with debris	Dry	Moist
Gingival tissue	Tongue blade and visual assessment	Gently press tissue with tip of blade	Red, shiny, edematous, bleeding	Red, shiny, edematous	Pink and resilient
Membranes (palates, uvula, and tonsillar fossa)	Visual assessment	Observe appearance of tissue	Red with general inflammation (includes two of the membranes)	Red with local inflammation (includes one of the membranes)	Pink
Lip texture	Visual and palpatory assessment	Observe and feel tissue	Rough, large amount of debris	Rough, small amount of debris	Smooth and soft
Lip moisture	Visual and palpatory assessment	Observe and feel tissue	Cracked or bleeding	Dry	Moist
Soft tooth debris	Disclosing solution	Apply solution to all tooth surfaces as directed on package	Soft debris covers more than two-thirds total teeth surface	Soft debris covers one-third, but less than two-thirds total teeth surface	Soft debris covers less than one-third, or edentulous

[a] Scoring the findings for each of the 9 variables is done on the following 3-point scale: 1 = poor condition; 2 = fair condition; and 3 = good condition. After collecting the data for a variable, assign the number that corresponds most closely with the data. When the appraisal is completed, add up the 9 scores. You will have a final score between 9 and 27 that enables you to determine the client's oral health status at the end of each appraisal.

Developed by Evelyn M. DeWalt R.N., M.S., Associate Professor, University of Arizona College of Nursing, Tucson. Published in: Effect of time hygienic measures on oral mucosa in a group of elderly subjects. Nursing Research 24(2):104–108, 1975. Reproduced with permission from Nursing Research.

to cleanse and massage the oral tissues. However, the toothette was not as effective as a toothbrush in removing dental plaque.

A mechanical *water irrigation device* consists of a motor-driven pump irrigator that generates an intermittent stream of water, with the water pressure adjusted by a control dial. The unit includes a reservoir to hold the water and a hand-held interchangeable tip that can be rotated 360 degrees for use at different angles. Irrigation devices have been shown to be valuable aids in maintaining the health and cleanliness of the oral cavity. They remove loose debris from the teeth and interdental areas but do not remove attached deposits of plaque. Other benefits of the irrigator include reduced numbers of organisms in the mouth, decreased incidence of gingivitis, and promotion of tissue healing. Because infections could be induced by forcing debris under the gingiva, a power-driven water irrigator should not be used on a person who has untreated gingivitis or periodontitis, deep periodontal pockets, or tissue flaps covering unerupted or partially erupted third molars. Use of an irrigation device is not considered to be a substitute for toothbrushing (Wilkins, 1983). Oral irrigation may also be performed with a bulb syringe that has an attached rubber tip.

Dental floss is available in two varieties: waxed and unwaxed. Waxed floss slides between the teeth more easily and is less apt to snag on rough tooth edges. Unwaxed floss is thinner than waxed floss and is easier to place between teeth that are close together. It is more absorbent than waxed floss and thus holds the plaque as it is removed.

Denture cups are small containers with a lid that fits securely. They are made of plastic or coated cardboard that will hold water without leaking. Dentures should be stored in these cups when they are not in use. The denture cups used in health-care facilities have a place either on the lid or side of the container in which to write the client's name and room number. Denture cups protect the client's dentures from loss and damage.

Oral-Care Agents

Dentifrices are substances used with a toothbrush to remove dental plaque debris from the oral tissues and teeth. They may also serve as vehicles for applying special therapeutic agents such as fluoride to the teeth. A dentifrice is not required for plaque removal, since brushing with only water is effective. The most inexpensive dentifrice available is a combination of sodium bicarbonate (baking soda) and salt. Sodium bicarbonate has a slight abrasive action that helps to remove stains from the teeth as well as plaque and debris. Sodium bicarbonate also helps lossen oral debris and removes thick mucus by thinning it. Since it does not foam, it is easier to remove from the mouth than a commercial dentifrice. Salt is very abrasive to the tooth enamel and should be used only in combination with sodium bicarbonate in a mixture of one-third salt and two-thirds sodium bicarbonate.

Commercial dentifrices are available in pastes and powders, and are used to polish the teeth and leave a pleasant taste in the mouth. Commercial dentifrices that are promoted on the basis of their ability to whiten teeth have an abrasive agent that may be excessively harsh for routine use by the general public (American Dental Association, 1979).

Oxygenating agents are chemical agents capable of releasing molecules of oxygen when in contact with tissue enzymes. They are useful in oral care, because the liberated oxygen exerts a mechanical cleansing action and loosens and cleans adherent debris (American Dental Association, 1979). Hydrogen peroxide has limited germicidal power because it readily decomposes when it comes in contact with organic matter. It must be kept in a cool, dark place and tightly stoppered to prevent deterioration. Its chief value is as a cleansing agent for purulent wounds and inflamed mucous membranes. Hydrogen peroxide should not be used on fresh granulation tissue because it breaks down the fresh granulation growth. When used as a mouthwash, hydrogen peroxide is diluted to half strength with an equal part of water. It is effective in removing thick, sticky mucus from the mouth and the coatings on the tongue caused by dryness. To be effective, a fresh solution must be mixed immediately before use, and the solution must be kept in contact with the tissues for a minimum of 1½ minutes. Hydrogen peroxide is a 3 percent solution with a pH of 4. Even at half strength it remains an acid, and there is some concern about the decalcifying effect this acid has on tooth enamel with frequent and long-term use. Extensive use can also result in a hairy tongue, because the normal flora of the mouth are destroyed by its germicidal effect.

Carbamide Peroxide 10 percent *(Gly-oxide),* another nonirritating bactericidal oxygenating agent, consists of 10 percent carbamide peroxide in anhydrous glycerol. Tassman et al. (1963) found Gly-oxide to be an effective oral-care aid for use by disabled clients who are unable to provide their own oral care. The client can rub Gly-oxide saturated gauze on the tooth and soft-tissue surfaces once a day and then use Gly-oxide as a mouth rinse after each meal and at bedtime. In the study by Tassman et al. (1963) this plan of care removed soft plaque, helped to flush food deposits from the teeth, and improved the tone and firmness of the soft tissues.

Glycerin is a sweet, oily fluid used as an ingredient in numerous products such as skin lotions and medications, as a sweetening agent, and on oral mucous membranes to reduce surface tension. It soothes and relieves irritation, especially on the mucous membranes, because it coats the surface and protects irritated tissue from further irritation. Glycerin is water soluble and has a neutral pH. In 1969 Wiley noted that a solution of glycerin and lemon juice has been cited in nursing texts as an oral-care agent for cleansing and relieving dryness for at least 35 years. However, in her study, preparations of glycerin and lemon juice did not meet the criteria she established for a safe and effective agent, because the pH of a variety of combinations of lemon and glycerin ranged from 2.6 to 3.9, which is well below the normal 6.2 to 7.6 pH of the oral cavity. Since acids chemically demineralize the tooth surface and since demineralization is part of the dental-caries process, Wiley concludes that lemon and glycerin solutions are unsafe and questions the value in using it. Drimmelen and Rollins (1969) found that a 1:1 solution of lemon and glycerin had a drying effect on the oral tissues of elderly clients included in their study.

Mouthwashes are not considered to contribute substantially to oral health. When using a mouthwash, the label should be checked to determine if the mouthwash should be used full or half strength. Several commercial mouthwashes have a high percentage of alcohol and can be drying to the soft oral tissues. The label of ingredients should be read before use, because if the client already has dry mucous membranes such as occurs with radiation therapy, then mouthwashes with a high percentage of alcohol will further dry and irritate the tissues. Some commercial mouthwashes are promoted on the basis of a germicidal effect, but there is no adequate evidence that the oral cavity benefits from killing the normal flora with antiseptic solutions. The efficiency of any mouthwash depends on the amount of time it is held in the mouth (American Dental Association, 1979). Alkaline aromatic mouthwash has a 5 percent alcohol content and a pH of 6.7, which is close to the normal pH of the oral cavity and therefore does not contribute to creating an acid climate in the mouth (Passos and Brand, 1966). Sodium bicarbonate may be used as a mouthwash in a solution of 1 teaspoon to 8 ounces of water. It is effective in thinning thick mucus and has a deodorant effect. Flavored mouthwashes may help temporarily relieve unpleasant taste sensations or mouth odors. After surgery during which mucolytic agents are used, mouthwashes relieve dryness and refresh the mouth, especially when the client is unable to drink or eat.

Fluoride supplements are available in pills, chewable tablets, drops, and mouthwash preparations. When the water supply is not fluoridated, children should receive a dietary fluoride supplement. Adults also benefit from fluoride. The use of a fluoridated dentifrice is not considered an adequate substitute for a topical application. Fluoride mouthwash with a .05 percent sodium fluoride solution can be used as a topical application for adults. Ten milliliters of the solution is swished about the mouth for 30 seconds and then expectorated. Food and drink should not be ingested for 30 minutes after the rinse (Block, 1976).

Fluoride preparations should be kept in a child-proof container to prevent accidental ingestion and overdose. The symptoms of an acute overdose include vomiting, nausea, and retching. Chronic fluoride overdoses result in enamel fluorosis, which varies in severity. Mild fluorosis causes the enamel to develop small, opaque white areas, while severe fluorosis causes the entire enamel to develop brown stains and become pitted.

Assistive Agents and Devices

Disclosing preparations are dyes in liquid or tablet form that color plaque deposits. The stained plaque can be removed only by effective brushing and flossing. A disclosing solution may be used before and after toothbrushing and is helpful in identifying areas that require special attention.

A *bulb (asepto) syringe* can be used to flush out the oral cavity with water or mouthwash when a client is unable to rinse with a glass. A suction machine should be kept readily available to remove the fluid in the event that the fluid cannot be safely drained from the mouth.

A *tongue depressor* is needed to appraise the oral cavity. When one end of a depressor is wrapped and padded with gauze squares and secured with adhesive tape, it can be used to wipe and remove debris from the mouth. When a mouth prop is not available, the padded depressor can also be used to prop open the mouth while care is being given.

A *mouth prop* or *bite block* is a firm plastic or rubber block-like wedge that is placed between the upper and lower teeth to keep the mouth open during oral care. It is a valuable device for use with clients who are unable to keep their mouths open without assistance for the time required for oral care. A string should be attached to the block so the block can be easily retrieved from the mouth.

Petroleum jelly is an emolient that can be used to keep the lips from drying and cracking. A thin film prevents evaporation of water from the skin.

An *emesis basin* is a small, curved receptacle that fits comfortably under the lips and is used to catch material and fluid expectorated or drained from the mouth.

☐ EXECUTION

The nurse may need to assist clients who are unable to perform part of their own care or administer complete care to clients who are unable to do so. The degree of knowledge about oral care and attitudes toward it vary among clients, and the nurse must adopt an individualized approach for each client. The frequency of care, the type of oral agent, the technique used, and the duration of a specific oral-care plan must all be individualized. The basic principle of oral care is to provide oral care as often as the client's condition requires it, on the basis of an appraisal of the oral tissues. This care includes: (a) keeping the mucous membranes clean and moist at all times, and (b) cleaning the tooth surfaces.

All clients should have their teeth and mouth cleaned at least twice a day, in the morning and before retiring. The supplies needed routinely for oral care can be set up on a tray and kept at the bedside. Basic supplies generally needed for most clients include a toothbrush, dental floss, a disclosing preparation, tongue depressors, gauze squares, and petroleum jelly. Additional items depend on the specific requirements of the client.

Whenever possible it is best to have clients participate in oral care. The emphasis and value the nurse places on oral care can influence clients positively to improve their self-care practices. Clients capable of giving their own care can be observed to determine their toothbrushing technique, so that instruction can be given if needed for complete removal of dental plaque.

If the client is able to sit up, elevate the head of the bed to the highest position of comfort. If the client must lie flat, turn him or her on the side facing the care-giver. Place a towel and an emesis basin under the chin. First, use the disclosing preparation according to the specific directions, so that the areas of dental plaque will be revealed. After rinsing out the excess disclosing solution, floss the teeth. Flossing is done before brushing so that the proximal tooth areas will be clean for the application of fluoride in the dentifrice or mouthwash.

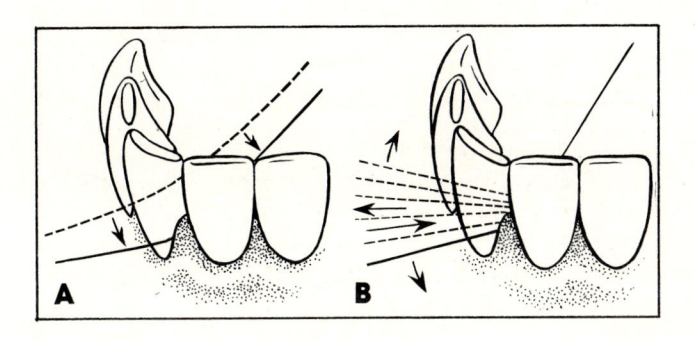

Figure 40-1. Flossing the teeth. **A.** Slowly direct the floss between the teeth and hold it in place firmly in a C shape. Then move it beneath the gingiva until resistance is felt. **B.** Slide the floss horizontally and vertically with pressure against the tooth to remove plaque.

FLOSSING THE TEETH

To floss the teeth, break off a 12- to 15-inch strand of floss, which is ample for flossing all of the teeth. Wrap the floss around the third finger of each hand and hold it firmly between the thumb and index finger of each hand, allowing 1 to 1½ inches between the fingers. Begin at the back of the teeth and slowly direct the floss between the teeth with a sawing motion. Avoid snapping the floss through the contact area between the teeth to help prevent injury to the gingiva. Curve the floss around the tooth in a C shape, holding it against the side of the tooth firmly before moving it gently beneath the gingiva until tissue resistance is felt. Slide the floss horizontally and vertically, using pressure against the tooth to remove plaque. Work systematically around all of the teeth in the upper and lower arch, using a clean section of floss for each tooth. Have the client rinse out his or her mouth after the flossing is completed. The technique for teeth flossing is shown in Figure 40-1.

TOOTHBRUSHING

There have been several toothbrushing techniques devised over the years, but the Bass or *sulcular method* is currently recommended as least traumatic to the tissues while still being effective in removing plaque near and under the gingival margin and in massaging the gingivae (Smith, 1983). With this method the bristle tips are directed toward the gum line at a 45-degree angle, which permits the tips of the bristles to enter under the gingival margin. Slight pressure and short strokes are used to vibrate the toothbrush horizontally over two to three teeth at a time for a count of ten. The toothbrush is then moved to the next set of two to three teeth, allowing some overlap with the previous teeth. This is continued until all of the teeth are brushed on both the lingual (tongue) and buccal (cheek) sides, except the lingual side of the front teeth. These surfaces are brushed by holding the toothbrush the long, narrow way and using short strokes with the toe of the toothbrush. The biting surfaces of the teeth are cleaned by using slight pressure and short strokes to vibrate the bristle tips across and into the pits and fissures of the tooth surface. Long scrubbing strokes permit the bristles to contact only the highest points of the tooth surface. Figure 40-2 depicts the position of the toothbrush for the sulcular brushing method.

There are certain oral conditions for which toothbrushing is contraindicated, such as acute inflammatory or traumatic lesions of the oral mucosa, recent periodontal surgery, and when jaws are wired after injury or surgery. For clients with these conditions, warm normal saline rinses are effective in removing debris from the mouth and help to promote healing.

BRUSHING THE TONGUE

The papillae on the tongue create areas that hold debris and microorganisms. Brushing the tongue reduces oral debris, retards plaque formation and accumulation, reduces the number of microorganisms, and improves the overall cleanliness of the mouth (Wilkins, 1983). To brush the tongue, have the client open the mouth wide and protrude the tongue. Hold the toothbrush at a right angle to the tongue with the bristle tips directed toward the throat. Use light pressure to

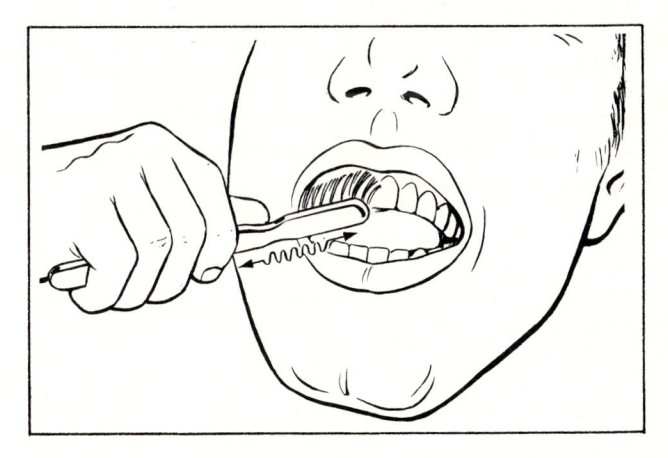

Figure 40-2. Toothbrushing with the sulcular method. Direct the bristle tips toward the gum line at a 45-degree angle to permit the bristles to enter under the gingival margin. Using slight pressure and a vibratory motion over two to three teeth at a time for a count of ten to remove the plaque. Move the toothbrush to the next set of two to three teeth, allowing for some overlap.

draw the side of the bristles forward and over the tip of the tongue; repeat this three to four times and then rinse the mouth. The tongue should not be scrubbed with the tips of the bristles, for this will irritate the papillae and be uncomfortable for the client. Applying too much pressure on the posterior aspect of the tongue can stimulate the client's gag reflex.

DENTURE CARE

Dentures are artificial substitutes for teeth. They may be complete, partial and removable, or partial and fixed to the natural teeth. Unconscious clients should not wear their removable dentures because of the potential for the dentures to fall out of place and obstruct the airway.

Complete and partial dentures must be removed for cleaning. A paper tissue and a denture cup are needed when removing dentures. When they are able, most clients prefer to remove and clean their own dentures. The maxillary (upper) denture may be held in place by a vacuum; if so, then this seal must be broken before the denture can be removed. Having the client blow into his or her own mouth with the lips closed tightly sometimes breaks the seal, and the denture can then be lifted out. If the client is unable to do this, or if this method is ineffective, the nurse can remove the denture. Don a pair of disposable gloves and grasp the facial (front) surface of the maxillary denture with the thumb and forefinger, using the opposite hand to retract the lip away from the denture. Move the denture up and down slightly to break the seal, and then slide it out of the mouth and place it in the denture cup. Because the mandibular (lower) denture is not held in place by a vacuum, it can be lifted out by grasping it in the same manner as the maxillary denture. Use the opposite hand to retract the lip away from the denture before removal. Use the paper tissue to wipe away the saliva drawn from the client's mouth with the dentures. Figure 40–3 shows how dentures are removed. To remove a partial denture, don a pair of gloves and grasp both sides of the denture at the point at which it is clasped to the natural teeth, exert even pressure simultaneously, lift the denture vertically, remove it from the mouth, and place it in a denture cup.

After the dentures are removed, rinse the mouth thoroughly with warm water. Cleanse the gingiva and mucosa with a soft toothbrush or toothette, using long, straight strokes from front to back.

To clean the dentures, hold them low over a basin of water or a towel so they will not break if dropped. Hold them securely in the palm of one hand without squeezing them. Use warm water and a nonabrasive dentifrice to brush all areas, giving special attention to the surface area that contacts the oral tissue. Rinse the dentures thoroughly before returning them to the client. Wet the dentures for easy insertion. The denture cup should be labeled as such and have the client's name on it. When not in the mouth, store the dentures in water of room temperature. Hot water warps the dentures. Commercial cleanser and soaking agents may be added according to the directions on the package. Paste cleansers are not recommended for denture care because they are too hard to rinse off and can be abrasive to the dentures. Scratches on the dentures can be irritating to the tissues, can affect the way they fit, and can provide areas for debris to accumulate.

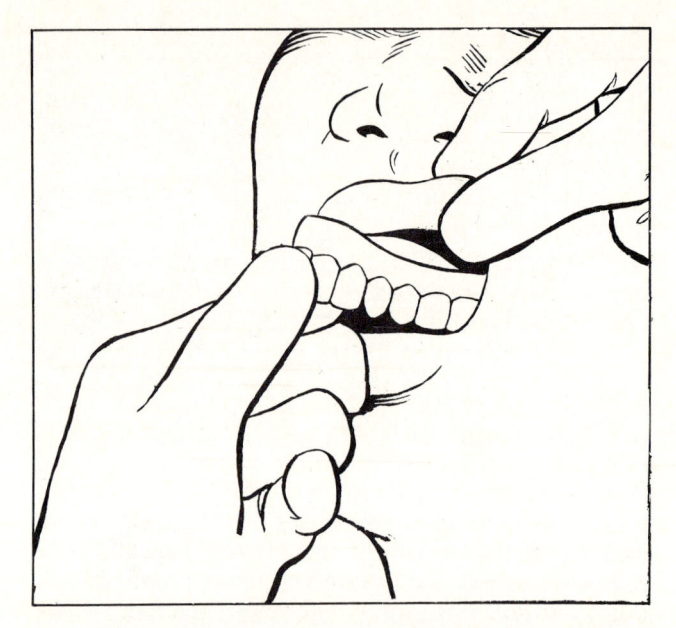

Figure 40–3. Denture removal. To remove the maxillary denture, grasp the facial surface of the denture with the thumb and forefinger of one hand; use the opposite hand to retract the lip away from the denture. Move the denture up and down slightly to break the seal, and then slide it out of the mouth and place it in a denture cup.

Fixed dentures are brushed along with the natural teeth. It is helpful to precede brushing with an oral irrigation or a vigorous mouth rinse to remove loose debris from the mouth. Abrasive dentifrices should not be used on fixed dentures because of the potential for scratching the denture surfaces. The area where the denture attaches to the natural teeth requires special brushing and flossing attention so that plaque does not accumulate.

THE UNCONSCIOUS CLIENT

Clients who are not fully conscious or able to swallow adequately are at risk for aspirating fluids into the lungs. To prevent this, exercise special precautions while giving oral care. Place the client on his or her side so that fluid in the mouth will drain out into an emesis basin. Have a soft rubber catheter and suction machine available at the bedside, so that fluids can be removed from the mouth. Before beginning the oral appraisal, don a pair of disposable gloves and coat the lips with petroleum jelly if they are dry to prevent the lips from cracking. Insert a gauze-padded tongue depressor into the mouth and wedge it between the upper and lower teeth on one side of the mouth to keep the mouth open if the client is unable to open it. If it is available, insert a bite block between the teeth on the opposite side of the mouth and then remove the padded tongue depressor. Use a tongue depressor and light to conduct the oral appraisal. Irrigate the mouth with small amounts of warm water or normal saline and an asepto syringe to flush out the loose debris, and then suction out the fluid. Use a gauze-covered tongue depressor or a folded gauze square held by a surgical clamp and gently wipe the mucous membrane surfaces free of mucus. Sordes, an accumulation of brown crustlike material on the mucous membranes, teeth, gums, and tongue, can be loosened with half-strength hydrogen peroxide or other oxygenating agent applied with cotton-tipped applicators. Remove the debris with a gauze-covered tongue depressor and suction, and then flush the mouth again. Floss the teeth and rinse the mouth before brushing the teeth. After toothbrushing and thoroughly rinsing the mouth, suction out the fluid. Shift the bite block or tongue depressor to the other side of the jaws and clean the other side of the mouth in the same manner. Brush the tongue and remove the bite block or padded tongue depressor. Dry the lips and apply another thin coat of petroleum jelly. Figure 40–4 shows the positioning for giving oral care when the client cannot sit up or is unable to manage his or her own secretions. It also shows how a bite block is placed between the jaws to keep the mouth open.

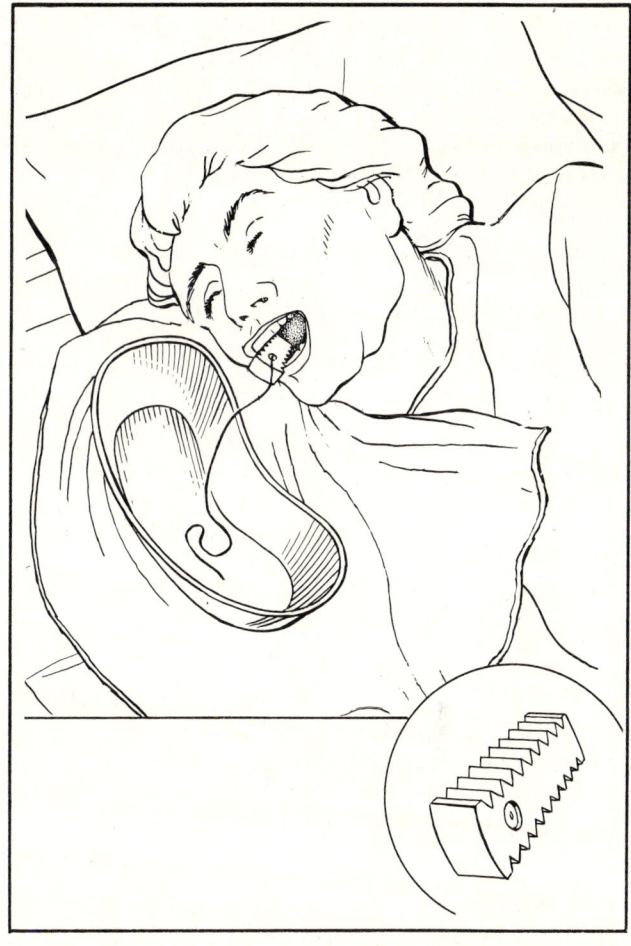

Figure 40–4. When complete oral care must be provided position the unconscious client on the side, lying flat, with a bite block placed between the jaws to keep the mouth open.

☐ SKILL SEQUENCE

PROVIDING ORAL CARE FOR THE CLIENT WHO NEEDS COMPLETE ASSISTANCE

Step	Rationale
1. Check kardex for nursing and medical orders.	Provides direction for special care needs.
2. Wash hands.	Prevents cross-contamination from microorganisms on hands.
3. Prepare equipment and supplies at bedside.	Prevents delays and interruptions during care.
4. Explain procedure to client.	Allays anxiety; enlists cooperation. A comatose client may be able to hear.
5. Close door and cubicle curtains.	Prevents drafts and chills, and provides privacy.
6. Position client on his or her side, facing care-giver with head turned to side. May sit client up if he or she is able to swallow.	Prevents aspiration of fluid into lungs.
7. Place a towel and emesis basin under chin.	Collects debris and fluid from mouth.
8. Don disposable gloves.	Prevents cross-contamination from microorganisms on hands.
9. Coat client's lips with thin layer of petroleum jelly.	Prevents lips from cracking during care.
10. Separate lips and teeth and insert padded tongue depressor between upper and lower teeth on one side of mouth. Place a bite block on opposite side (if available) and remove padded depressor.	Bite block stays more securely in place than tongue depressor.

(continued)

PROVIDING ORAL CARE FOR THE CLIENT WHO NEEDS COMPLETE ASSISTANCE (Cont.)

Step	Rationale
11. Use "Guide for Oral Appraisal" (Table 40-1) to inspect and palpate oral structures.	Provides data for determining agents and techniques to be used.
12. Obtain additional equipment and supplies if necessary. Remove bite block or padded tongue depressor if oral care will not be given promptly.	Appraisal data may indicate a need for additional items.
13. Cleanse oral cavity:	
a. Flush loose debris with small amounts of warm solution, using an asepto syringe or mechanical irrigator.	Removes loose debris to prevent aspiration. Enables nurse to see oral structures.
b. Insert catheter to suction out fluid if necessary.	Prevents aspiration of fluids.
c. Remove mucus and debris with moist, gauze-covered tongue depressor or covered forceps.	Gauze traps debris better than cotton-tipped applicators.
d. Wipe all surfaces with a clean, moist applicator, or gauze-covered tongue depressor, or a gauze square held by a surgical clamp.	Provides additional cleansing, massage, and lubrication to tissues.
e. Repeat steps 13a to d as needed to remove all debris.	
14. Apply disclosing preparation to teeth according to directions, if available. Flush oral cavity with warm solution and remove by suctioning.	Reveals dental plaque. Removes excess disclosing solution.
15. Floss all upper and lower teeth beginning at back of mouth. Flush and suction mouth or have client expectorate fluid.	Cleans plaque from proximal tooth areas to permit flouride contact.
16. Brush all upper and lower teeth, using sulcular method; rinse mouth; suction or have client expectorate.	Removes plaque.
17. Insert a second padded tongue depressor between front upper and lower teeth, then switch the padded tongue depressor or bite block to the cleansed side. Remove tongue depressor from between front teeth.	Keeps the mouth open while changing the tongue depressor or bite block to cleansed side. Exposes noncleansed side for cleansing.
18. Clean the second side of the mouth and teeth as in steps 13 to 16.	
19. Brush tongue; rinse and suction mouth; have client expectorate if able.	Removes debris.
20. Remove padded tongue depressor or bite block; wipe lips.	
21. Coat lips with thin layer of petroleum jelly.	Keeps lips smooth.
22. Clean and replace supplies and equipment.	Ensures readiness for subsequent oral care.
23. Record appraisal findings, agents, and techniques used.	Promotes accountability; provides ongoing data base.

RECORDING

The data obtained from the oral appraisal performed before giving care, as well as the specific agents and techniques used to cleanse the oral cavity, are entered on the health record.

Sample POR Recording
- S—NA
- O—All mucous membrane surfaces dry; saliva thick and tenacious. Numerous sordes present on buccal and palate surfaces; tongue coated with white material; lips dry; soft debris on a few teeth.
- A—Needs continuing assistance with oral care.
- P—Half-strength H_2O_2 to remove sordes; rinsed with disclosing solution before teeth flossed and brushed, tongue brushed, and oral cavity rinsed. Lips coated with petroleum jelly. Continue oral care q 2 hrs.

Sample Narrative Recording
All mucous-membrane surfaces dry; saliva thick and tenacious. Sordes present on buccal and palate surfaces. Soft debris on a few teeth. H_2O_2 used to remove them. Teeth flossed and brushed after rinse with disclosing solution. Tongue brushed. Lips coated with petroleum jelly. Oral care to be repeated in 2 hrs.

☐ CRITICAL POINTS SUMMARY

1. Oral care prevents periodontal disease, infection, and halitosis, and also keeps the mucosa soft and moist.
2. Oral-care practices, nutrition, specific illnesses, and specific treatments affect the quantity and quality of saliva and the texture and moistness of the soft tissues.
3. The type of saliva, dietary intake, and mechanical cleansing are factors in dental decay.
4. More teeth are lost in adults because of periodontal disease than because of dental decay.
5. The type of oral care, the agents used, and the frequency with which care is given are determined by the client's illness, medication and treatment regime, and level of self-care.

6. Inspection and palpation of the oral cavity provide data for selecting the equipment and agents used in oral care and for determining the frequency of oral care.
7. Encourage clients to participate in their own care to whatever extent they are capable.
8. When dentures are worn, the gingivae and soft tissues need to be cleaned to remove plaque.
9. Unconscious clients and clients unable to swallow adequately must be positioned on the side to prevent fluid aspiration into the lungs while receiving oral care.
10. When giving complete oral care, use a bite block or padded tongue depressor to separate the jaws.
11. Regular use of petroleum jelly prevents cracked lips.
12. Complete oral care includes using disclosing solution, flossing, and brushing the teeth and tongue.

☐ LEARNING ACTIVITIES

1. Examine your own oral-care practices and dietary habits, and identify those that enhance good oral health and those that impede it.
2. Interview persons of various ages to determine their practices, knowledge, and attitudes about oral care, and the frequency with which they use preventive dental services.
3. Compare the differences in the appearance of your own teeth after eating a chocolate snack versus a fresh fruit snack.
4. Investigate the variety of oral-care equipment and agents in your local drugstore.

☐ REVIEW QUESTIONS

1. What are the purpose and effects of daily oral care?
2. How does saliva promote oral health?
3. What are the factors that affect oral health?
4. How does fluoride inhibit development of dental caries?
5. What changes might you expect to find in the oral cavity of clients who:
   a. Have a reduced salivary flow?
   b. Have vitamin C, B_{12}, niacin, and riboflavin deficiencies?
   c. Have periodontal disease?
   d. Are taking antibiotics?
6. How would you describe the normal appearance of the oral cavity?
7. What would you inspect and palpate during an appraisal of the oral cavity?
8. What information would you need to determine the degree of assistance a client might require with oral care?
9. What precautions would you take while giving oral care to clients who are unable to swallow adequately?
10. What is the sequence of activities you would use in giving complete oral care?

☐ PERFORMANCE CHECKLIST

OBJECTIVE: To use the appropriate method to give oral care safely to a client needing complete assistance.			
CHARACTERISTIC	RANGE OF ACCEPTABILITY	SATISFACTORY	UNSATISFACTORY
1. Checks kardex for nursing and medical order.	No deviation		
2. Washes hands.	No deviation		
3. Prepares equipment and supplies at bedside.	No deviation		
4. Explains procedure to client.	No deviation		
5. Closes door and cubicle curtains.	No deviation		
6. Positions client on his or her side with head turned toward side facing caregiver. Places towel and emesis basin under chin.	May sit client up if client is able to swallow.		
7. Dons disposable gloves.	No deviation		
8. Coats lips with layer of petroleum jelly.	No deviation		
9. Separates lips and inserts padded tongue depressor between upper and lower teeth on one side of mouth.	Omit if client is able to open own mouth.		
10. Places bite block on opposite side and removes padded tongue depressor.	Omit if bite block is not available.		

(continued)

OBJECTIVE: To use the appropriate method to give oral care safely to a client needing complete assistance (cont.).

CHARACTERISTIC	RANGE OF ACCEPTABILITY	SATISFACTORY	UNSATISFACTORY
11. Uses "Guide for Oral Appraisal" (Table 40-1) to appraise mouth systematically.	No deviation		
12. Obtains additional equipment and supplies after removing bite block or padded tongue depressor from mouth.	Omit if all needed items are available at bedside.		
13. Cleanses oral cavity: a. Flushes loose debris with small amounts of solution, using asepto syringe or mechanical irrigator. b. Inserts catheter into mouth and suctions out fluid. c. Removes mucus and debris with moist gauze-covered tongue depressor or forceps. d. Wipes all surfaces with clean, moist applicators, gauze-covered tongue depressor, or gauze square held with a surgical clamp. e. Repeats steps 13a to d as needed to remove all debris.	No deviation Omit if client is able to expectorate. Omit if all debris is removed by irrigation. Omit if mucosa is clean. No deviation		
14. Applies disclosing preparation to teeth according to directions; flushes oral cavity with warm solution; removes with suction.	Omit if disclosing preparation is not available.		
15. Flosses all upper and lower teeth beginning at back of mouth; flushes and suctions mouth or has client expectorate.	No deviation		
16. Brushes upper and lower teeth using sulcular method; rinses mouth; suctions or has client expectorate.	No deviation		
17. Inserts second padded tongue depressor between front teeth and then moves bite block or padded tongue depressor to cleansed side; removes tongue depressor from between front teeth.	Omit tongue depressor if client is able to open mouth.		
18. Cleans second side of the mouth and teeth as in steps 13 to 16.	No deviation		
19. Brushes tongue; rinses and suctions mouth or has client expectorate.	No deviation		
20. Removes padded tongue depressor or bite block; wipes lips.	No deviation		
21. Coats lips with thin layer of petroleum jelly.	No deviation		
22. Cleans and replaces supplies and equipment.	No deviation		
23. Records appraisal findings, agents, and technique used.	No deviation		

REFERENCES

American Dental Association: Accepted Dental Therapeutics, ed 38. Chicago, American Dental Association, 1979.

Block PL: Dental health in hospitalized patients. American Journal of Nursing 76(7):1162–1164, 1976.

DeGowin EL, DeGowin RL: Bedside Diagnostic Examination, ed 4. New York, Macmillan, 1981.

DeWalt E: Effect of timed hygienic measures on oral mucosa in a group of elderly subjects. Nursing Research 24(2):104–108, 1975.

Drimmelen J, Rollins HF: Evaluation of a commonly used oral hygiene agent. Nursing Research 18(4):327–332, 1969.

Guyton A: Textbook of Medical Physiology, ed 6. Philadelphia, WB Saunders, 1981.

Klocke JM, Sudduth AG: Oral hygiene instruction and plaque formation during hospitalization. Nursing Research 18(2):124–130, 1969.

Levine P, Grayson BH: Safeguarding your patients against periodontal disease. RN 36(7):38–41, 1973.

Maurer J: Providing optimum oral health. Nursing Clinics of North America 12(4):671–685, 1977.

Menaker L: The Biologic Basis of Dental Caries. Hagerstown, MD: Harper & Row, 1980.

Passos JY, Brand LM: Effects of agents used for oral hygiene. Nursing Research 15(3):196–202, 1966.

Perlitsh MJ: Seven warning signs of gum disease. Journal of Periodontology 45(8):542–546, 1974.

Smith J: Salivary gland reaction in the dying patient. In Kutscher AH, Goldberg IK (eds): Oral Care of the Aged and Dying Patient. Springfield, IL, Charles C Thomas, 1973.

Smith R: Personal communication. Chief of Dental Services, Richard L. Roudebush, Veterans Administration Medical Center, Indianapolis, 1983.

Tassman G, Zayon GM, Zafran JN: When patients cannot brush their teeth. American Journal of Nursing 63(2):76, 1963.

Wiley SB: Why glycerol and lemon juice? American Journal of Nursing 69(2):342–344, 1969.

Wilkins EM: Clinical Practice of the Dental Hygienist, ed 5. Philadelphia, Lea & Febiger, 1983.

Meissner JE: A simple guide for assessing oral health. Nursing80 10(4):84–85, 1980.

Reitz M, Pope W: Mouthcare. American Journal of Nursing 73(10):1728–1730, 1973.

Slattery J: Dental health in children. American Journal of Nursing 76(7):1159–1161, 1976.

Weisz AS: The use of a saliva substitute as treatment for xerostomia in Sjögren's syndrome—A case report. Oral Surgery 52(4):384–386, 1981.

SUGGESTED READING

Gannon EP, Kadezabek E: Giving your patients meticulous mouth care. Nursing80 10(3):70–75, 1980.

BIBLIOGRAPHY

Battles CE: Nursing management of the radiation therapy client. In Marino LB (ed): Cancer Nursing. St Louis, MO, CV Mosby, 1981.

Buckingham RW: Dental care policies for treating the terminal cancer patient. Dental Hygiene 55(4):23–26, 1981.

Dyer ED, Monson MA, Cope MJ: Dental health in adults. American Journal of Nursing 76(7):1156–1158, 1976.

Gannon EP, Kadezabek E: Giving your patients meticulous mouth care. Nursing80 10(3):70–75, 1980.

Ginsberg MK: A study of oral hygiene nursing care. American Journal of Nursing 61(10):67–69, 1961.

AUDIOVISUAL RESOURCES

Oral Hygiene
Videorecording (¾ in). (1974, Color, 15 min.)
Available through:
Professional Research, Inc.
930 Pitner Ave.
Evanston, IL 60202

Oral Hygiene
Filmstrip and cassette. (1972, Color, 25 min.)
Available through:
Medcom, Inc.
P.O. Box 116
Garden Grove, CA 92642

Oral Hygiene for the Total Care Patient
16 mm film. (1970, Color, 16 min.)
Available through:
National Audiovisual Center
Order Section EQ
Washington, DC 20409

SKILL 41 Hair Care

PREREQUISITE SKILLS

Skill 19, "Inspection"
Skill 20, "Palpation"
Skill 28, "Handwashing"

☐ STUDENT OBJECTIVES

1. Describe the purposes of hair care.
2. Explain why head hair grows longer than body hair.
3. Identify the reasons for alopecia.
4. Differentiate between head lice and crab lice.
5. Describe the complete treatment necessary to control head lice and crab lice.
6. Describe the characteristics of the hair that are included in an appraisal.
7. Explain the procedure for combing the hair.
8. Explain the various methods used to shampoo hair safely.
9. Describe how to give care to a beard.
10. Differentiate the methods used to shave a male client.
11. Groom and shampoo the scalp and facial hair safely and completely.

INTRODUCTION

Hair, like the skin, requires daily care. Cleansing and grooming of the hair serve to:

1. Prevent the accumulation of organisms that can cause infection.
2. Maintain the scalp in a healthy condition.
3. Stimulate circulation to the hair follicles.
4. Loosen and remove dead cells from the skin.
5. Distribute sebum from the scalp to the hair shaft.
6. Remove soil.

Daily hair care also has psychological benefits for the client. Clean, well-groomed hair can enhance an individual's appearance and contribute to his or her general sense of comfort and well-being.

PREPARATION

THE STRUCTURE AND CHARACTERISTICS OF THE HAIR

Hair is a protein product of specialized epithelial cells. Hair follicles, which are tubes that extend into the dermis, develop during the 3rd month of fetal life. Hair is formed on the face and scalp as early as the 4th fetal month. New hair follicles do not develop after birth. If hair follicles are destroyed, no new hairs can be formed to replace those that are lost. Sebum, a fatty secretion of the sebaceous glands of the skin, lubricates the hair, preventing it from drying and becoming brittle. It also limits the amount of absorption and evaporation of water from the hair and scalp.

Humans have two types of hair: terminal and vellus. Terminal hair is usually coarse, long, and thick, but these characteristics vary according to the body area. For example, terminal hair is found on the scalp, pubic area, arms, legs, chest, abdomen, and face, but the length of these hairs varies considerably. Vellus hair is shorter, finer, and a lighter color than terminal hair. Vellus hair is the fuzz that covers all of the other body areas, and it is frequently almost invisible.

At birth, all body hair is growing; but in the first few weeks of life, all hair follicles go into a telogen, or resting phase. Thus, a life cycle of growth and nongrowth phases for each hair follicle begins. The duration of the anagen, or growth phase, depends on where on the body the hair is located and determines the length of each hair. Short hair on the limbs and pubic area has an anagen phase that lasts only a few months before the telogen phase begins. Long hair on the scalp is the result of an anagen phase that lasts for years. The telogen phase begins when the hair stops growing and terminates when a hair is pushed out by a new hair that begins to grow in the same hair follicle.

Hair growth is cyclical, but not all of the hair follicles are in the same phase at the same time. The normal adult has about 85 to 90 percent of scalp hair in an anagen phase and 10 to 15 percent in the telogen phase at any one time. Telogen hairs may rest for months before they are pushed out by a new anagen hair. About 75 to 100 hairs are lost daily through normal hair shedding (Parrish, 1975). The rate of hair growth is influenced by extremes of environmental temperatures; warm weather stimulates growth and cold weather retards it.

Before puberty, scalp hair grows more rapidly in boys than in girls; after puberty, the reverse is true. In both sexes, the rate of growth peaks between the ages of 50 and 69 years. The large terminal hairs seen on the male face, chest, and body are the result of androgens. Pubic hair begins to grow as a result of androgen stimulation during puberty, followed about 2 years later by facial hair.

The form of hair varies widely between races, and there is considerable variation within races. There are four gross forms of hair: straight, wavy, helical (having coils of constant diameter), and spiral (having coils that diminish in diameter outward). The shape of the follicle affects the form of the hair; for example, spiral hair grows from curved follicles. The number and distribution of hair follicles is essentially the same in all races, but the genetic factors determine variations in hair pattern and the rate of growth. For example, whites have earlier and greater beard and axillary hair development than do the Japanese. The hair of whites has a wide variation in form; it may be straight, wavy, or helical. The hair of blacks is usually helical or spiral (Rook and Wilkinson, 1979).

Hair color is inherited independently from form. Graying of hair follows a genetic pattern in terms of age and location on the head. It usually appears after age 40 and occurs earlier in whites than in blacks.

DISORDERS OF HAIR GROWTH

A *premature halt in hair growth* and a conversion to the telogen (resting) phase can occur after pregnancy, severe illness, high fever, or heparin therapy. As new hair replaces the old hair, thinning may occur before the new hair becomes visible. Decreased hair growth or hair loss may be caused by either *infection* or *inadequate pituitary gland function* (hypopituitarism). Decreased hair luster and growth occur with the *protein deprivation* of starvation. The hair of a person who receives *chemotherapeutic drugs* for cancer may appear to become thinner, because of a decrease in the caliber of the hair shaft. The caliber of the hair shaft increases with phenytoin sodium therapy (for seizure disorders), making the hair seem thicker (Ebling and Rook, 1979).

Sometimes a male pattern of hair distribution known as *hirsutism* occurs on females and children. Mild or moderate hirsutism may be a familial trait, while marked hirsutism is due to abnormalities of the adrenal glands. Elderly women typically have hair growth on the upper lip and chin. This may be due to decreased levels of estrogen or a cumulative effect of androgens. Corticosteroid therapy also can cause a secondary hirsutism.

Alopecia, or baldness, is present when there is a sufficient loss of hairs to be noticeable. This is a hereditary characteristic commonly seen in males. The front hair recedes first, and then the hair is lost from the top of the head, with additional thinning at the temples. This type of baldness may also occur in females as part of the normal aging process. Alopecia may also occur in patches on any body part. In young people, alopecia is associated with severe emotional stress; the hair regrows unless the loss is extensive and prolonged. Baldness may also occur as a result of rubbing or traction on the hair, such as the use of tight curlers and hair styles such as the pony tail. Disturbed persons may inflict baldness on themselves by pulling their hair out (Parrish, 1975).

Hair texture may become altered for a variety of reasons. Dry, brittle hair can result from excessive washing, as well as from the use of chemicals such as dyes or detergents. An increased silkiness and fineness of the hair may be caused by too much thyroid hormone, while too little thyroid hormone can produce dry and coarse-textured hair.

Ingrown hairs are a common problem with male facial hair. They may also occur on the back of the neck. Ingrown hairs can result from shaving too closely, which causes the angular ends of the hair to be trapped under the stratum corneum. This results in the formation of a pili incarnati, a pustule, within a follicle that has a buried hair. Black males are affected by ingrown hairs more often than nonblacks because of the curliness of their hair. Shaving with the grain and avoiding stretching the skin too tightly before stroking with the razor or using an electric razor may help to reduce the problem. Depilatories designed for use on facial hair may provide an alternative to shaving (LeMaile-Williams, 1974). When the problem is extensive or becomes chronic, growing a beard may be an alternate solution.

PEDICULOSIS

Body infestation of lice is known as pediculosis. Body hair provides a harbor for two types of lice: head lice *(Pediculus humanus capitis)* and pubic or crab lice *(Phthirus pubis).*

Head lice are blood-sucking insects that are usually confined to the scalp. The severe itching they cause provokes intense scratching, which can result in breaks in the skin that become infected. As few as ten lice may be present on the hair at any one time, thus making it difficult to determine if pediculosis is present. The diagnosis is usually made by finding nits, or eggs, on the hair shaft very close to the scalp. Nits are most commonly found at the nape of the neck or behind the ears. Head lice are transmitted either by close contact with an infested person or from fomites recently used by an infected person. Fomites include items such as combs, brushes, garments, and bedding that serve as vehicles for transferring lice. Blacks are rarely infested with head lice, but all other persons are equally susceptible (Juranek, 1976). Head lice can become an acute problem in elementary schools, and this sometimes results in temporary school closings.

Head lice are controlled by early treatment of infested persons. Infested hair is shampooed with over-the-counter preparations such as A-200 Pyrinate, or a prescription shampoo, Kwell. Fomites must also be treated. Hot water of 60°C (140°F) is used to wash personal items; combs are soaked in a 2 percent Lysol solution (also at 60°C) for 5 to 10 minutes. Nonwashable items can be sealed in an impermeable plastic bag for 10 days to destroy both lice and eggs. Lice die within 48 hours without a blood meal and the eggs will not hatch after 10 days at room temperature. It is necessary to vacuum thoroughly the home and rooms used by the infested person (Juranek, 1976). It is necessary to examine all family members and close contacts for lice and nits so that they can be treated and not infect each other.

Crab lice mainly infect the pubic hair but may also be found in the axillae, eyelashes, eyebrows, mustache, and beard. They also cause severe itching. Crab lice are transmitted by close contact such as during sexual intercourse. They may also be transmitted by wearing infested underwear or using infested bedding. Crab lice die within 24 hours of being separated from the host. Kwell is the most effective treatment for crab lice. The fomites are disinfected in the same manner as for head lice (Juranek, 1976).

DATA BASE

Client History and Recorded Data

Client concerns about changes in their hair, scalp, or beard can be elicited as part of the admission interview or before assisting with personal hygiene.

Changes in hair color, luster, quantity, texture, or strength may be due to any of the systemic illnesses, treatments, or conditions just mentioned. The nurse may be able to explain to the client what the changes are related to, so that the client is able to understand the relationship between the condition and the cause. These changes also are important data that need to be communicated to the physician, because they may indicate a need for reevaluation of the treatment plan.

The client's hygiene and grooming habits should be incorporated into the plan of care. Although most clients prefer to care for their own hair, restrictions on activity may prevent them from doing so. When the hair requires a shampoo or any special care, any plan to provide such care must be developed in accord with the medical regime and the institution's policies and must be entered on the kardex. Many institutions require a physician's order to shampoo clients' hair or to allow clients to use a beauty salon service.

Physical Appraisal Skills

Inspection. Scalp and facial hair is inspected for cleanliness, color, luster, amount, texture, distribution, and the presence or absence of waves and curls. The skin on the scalp (and face, when a beard is present) is appraised for the presence of lesions and bald spots. When there is evidence from history or observation of itching or scratching, the nurse needs to consider the possibility of lice infestation. Prior to examining for lice, the nurse explains to the client why the procedure is necessary.

Palpation. The texture of the hair is determined by rubbing a few strands between the finger and thumb.

EQUIPMENT

Equipment used to groom the hair must be selected with care. Sharp edges on combs or brushes can damage the hair and scalp. Combs should have wide teeth with dull edges, and brushes should have nonmetal, firm bristles. Very curly hair may require the use of a pick comb, which has very widely spaced low teeth that can easily draw through tangled curly hair. Lotions or jellies applied to dry scalps and hair facilitate grooming and relieve dryness. Hair-care tools should be cleaned before a shampoo, and any other time it seems necessary, with detergent and water.

Electrical Appliances

Safety regulations in institutions usually require that electrical appliances such as hair dryers and curlers be checked by the maintenance department for electrical safety before they can be used by a client on the clinical unit. It is the nurse's responsibility to inform the client of this and to contact the maintenance department. Loose connections and ungrounded appliances pose electrical hazards and may cause the client to receive an electric shock. Care should also be taken not to use electrical appliances where they may fall into water, such as at a basin, sink, or tub.

The Shampoo

When it is not possible to shampoo a client's hair at a basin, sink, or shower, dry or wet no-rinse shampoos may be used to remove the excess soil and oil. The type of equipment needed for a wet shampoo varies with where the shampoo is given. When the shampoo is done in the shower, a chair, towels, bath blanket, and shampoo are sufficient. A shampoo at the sink requires a shampoo spray (a length of tubing that connects to the faucet and has a spray nozzle attached); pitchers, large cups, or an irrigating bag (for pouring water over the hair); a chair with a seat high enough for the client's head to reach the sink edge; and several towels.

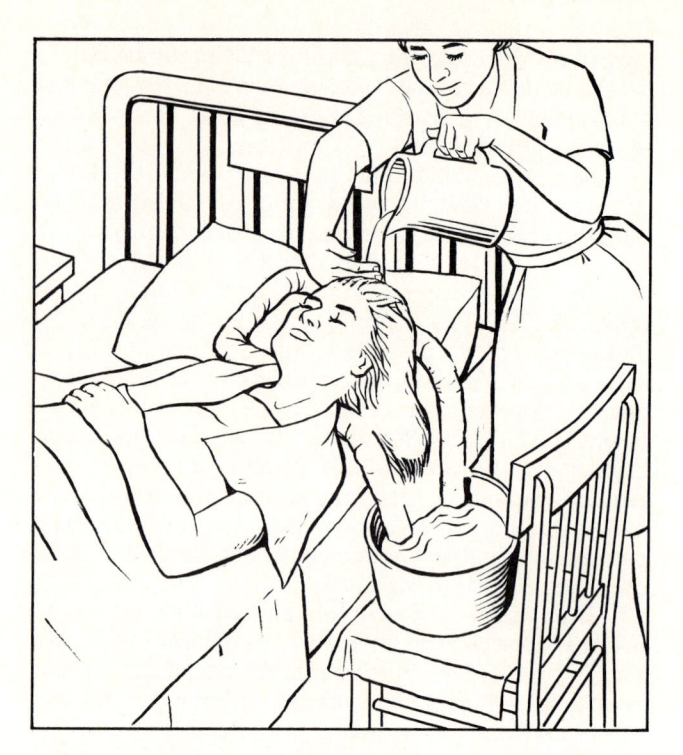

Figure 41-1. For a bed shampoo, position the client on the bed diagonally, with the head near the edge. The shampoo tray and trough collect and drain the water into a pail at the bedside.

To shampoo hair in bed, it is necessary to protect the bed from getting wet. A waterproof tray and trough are placed under the client's head, so that the water is collected and drained into a receptacle at the bedside. Commercially made *shampoo trays* to collect water are available but they may also be improvised as follows: Fold a bath blanket into quarters, place it on a flat surface, and roll three sides to form a rim. Anchor the rim in place with pins. Place a sheet of plastic larger than the tray over the surface to create a large, shallow basin. Part of the plastic hangs down the unrolled side of the blanket to form a trough. The basin and trough will collect water used in the shampoo and drain it into a pail or large basin placed on a chair at the bedside as shown in Figure 41-1.

At least two pitchers are needed to hold water for the shampoo: one with warm water and another with hot water that is used to add to and maintain the proper warm temperature. Water temperature used for a shampoo is warm to hot (35.5° to 40°C [96° to 104°F]), depending on the client's tolerance to heat and his or her skin condition. At least two towels are required; one is place around the client's shoulders, and the other is used to blot dry the wet hair. Paper towels may also be used effectively to blot the wet hair. As in the bed bath, the client is covered with a bath blanket and the top of the linen is removed.

Shaving Equipment

Shaving a male client may be done with either an electric shaver or a safety razor. A preshave lotion prepares the face and beard for an electric shave. For a safety-razor shave, a basin of hot water, shaving soap, a washcloth, and a towel are needed.

☐ EXECUTION

GROOMING THE HAIR

It is the nurse's responsibility to ensure that the hair and beard are groomed at least once a day to prevent tangles and snarls and to enhance the client's sense of comfort and well-being. Grooming is usually done after the bath is completed. If the client is confined to bed, it is best to groom the hair before the linen is changed. If the client is fatigued after the bath, it may be necessary to allow a short rest before proceeding with hair care. Grooming the hair is easier for both client and nurse when the client is able to sit up on the side of the bed or in a chair, but this is not always possible.

Before grooming the hair, spread a towel across the shoulders to collect the loose hair and any scale fallout from the scalp. Consult the client about the way the hair is to be styled for appearance and comfort. A client with long hair may be more comfortable with the hair arranged off the neck and shoulders. When combing long hair, parting the hair down the center from front to back, and then again into smaller sections on each side, makes it easier to deal with tangles or snarls because it enables the combing of hair in small sections. Hold each section firmly by the fingers and thumb of one hand near the scalp to prevent pulling on the hair and hurting the client. Begin combing and brushing at the ends of the hair with gentle strokes and gradually progress up to the scalp, until all of the snarls are removed and all of the hair is groomed. Black clients with dry, very curly hair need to have mineral oil or olive oil applied to their hair to prevent dryness, which results in split ends and hair breaking off at the follicle (Grier, 1976). Very curly hair may be tamed and controlled by using a slightly damp comb.

Snarls and *matted* areas are never cut from the hair. Apply small amounts of water, vinegar, or alcohol to the hair to help loosen the tangles. When the hair is in a complete mass of snarls, it may be necessary to work with it periodically for a few days to remove all of them. Many clients are not able to tolerate in one session the amount of care needed to remove all snarls. In fact, an overzealous attack on badly snarled hair can be so uncomfortable for a client that he or she refuses to allow any further attempts at grooming, thus compounding the problem. Although it is best not to let the hair get into such a state, clients are sometimes admitted to a clinical unit with their hair in an unkempt condition.

Braiding is a way to keep long hair in a comfortable style for someone confined to bed. Braids should be woven loosely so that they do not pull on the scalp, and should be formed so that they do not create a bulky mass at the nape of the neck or the sides of the head. Loose pony tails placed on each side of the head are an alternative to braids. Ribbons or covered elastic bands are preferred fasteners for the hair ends, since hairpins and barrettes can press on and damage the scalp and can be uncomfortable.

SHAMPOOING THE HAIR

A shampoo should be planned for a time when the client is rested and is not scheduled for other treatments or expecting visitors. Clients able to bathe themselves may require some assistance with shampooing. Care must be taken to protect the client from exposure to drafts and chilling during the shampoo and while the hair is being dried.

The Shower Shampoo
The easiest method for a shampoo is in the shower. If the client is unable to stand long enough for a shower, a shower chair can be used. While the hair is being shampooed, position the shower chair so that the client is facing away from the water flow, and the client's head is tilted back to keep soap out of the eyes.

The Sink Shampoo
When hair is washed at a sink, the client is seated with the back to the sink and the neck extended and resting on the edge of the sink. Elevate the seat pillows if necessary to permit a comfortable position for the client. Place a folded towel between the neck and the sink edge to cushion the neck. Use a bath blanket to prevent chilling, and drape a towel around the shoulders to help keep the client dry. Clients who may be out of bed but who are unable to sit or stand may lie on a stretcher for a shampoo at the sink. The safety precautions for a stretcher shampoo include strapping the client to the stretcher, covering him or her with a bath blanket, and locking the wheels on the stretcher during the transfer and the shampoo (transfer of a client from the bed to a stretcher is described in Skill 65).

Pitchers, a shampoo spray, or an irrigating bag are used to pour water over the head if the flow from the tap is not adequate to reach the scalp and hair. Pour water over the front hairline and sides toward the back. After the hair is thoroughly wet, massage shampoo gently into the hair and scalp with the fingertips to create a lather, proceeding from the front to the back and sides. Add water as needed to maintain an adequate lather until all of the hair and scalp is washed. Excessive lather can be removed from the hair by smoothing the flat of the hands over the scalp and hair, and gently scraping the lather into the sink before starting to rinse the hair. Do not massage the hair and scalp vigorously if the client has a sensitive scalp. Rinse hair thoroughly to remove all of the soap. This may require more than two pitchers of water. A second shampoo may be necessary to get the scalp and hair thoroughly clean. A conditioner or rinse may help to remove some of the tangles. Lemon and vinegar rinses are helpful in removing shampoo.

Prior to shampooing a black client's hair, the nurse determines if the hair has been temporarily or permanently straightened. This is important because temporarily straightened hair returns to its natural curly state when water is applied. If the patient is confused or unconscious and is unable to tell the nurse about his or her hair, a few strands obtained from the combing can be placed in a cup of water to find out if they curl. Use a dry shampoo if the hair is temporarily straightened.

Natural or permanently straightened hair is washed in the manner described above. It is preferable to use an alkaline or protein shampoo, because an alkaline shampoo does not undo the effect of permanent straightening and a protein shampoo helps to reinforce and smooth the hair surface. Grier (1976) suggests shampooing very curly dry hair with a warm mixture of alcohol and mineral oil. The alcohol helps to remove the old oil and the mineral oil cleanses and acts as an emollient. This mixture must be shaken vigorously to create an emulsion before it is poured on the hair and massaged into the scalp and the full length of the hair. Use a pick or wide-toothed comb to comb the saturated hair gently. When all of the tangles are removed, towel dry the hair. If the hair texture is dry after the shampoo, apply additional oil and remove the excess with a clean towel. Arrange the hair according to the client's preference or braid it.

The Bed Shampoo

If the client is unable to get out of bed, a shampoo can be given in bed with additional equipment as shown in Figure 41-1 and as just described. Protect the linen and bed from getting wet by using a waterproof tray and trough. Prepare the client as for a bed bath (Skill 38), and remove the pillow. Then, position the client diagonally across the bed with the head near the edge. Place the shampoo tray under the head, with the trough running from the tray and draped over the edge of the bed. Place the end of the trough in a pail or basin large enough to hold the water that will drain off the head. Next, place the pail on a chair so that the water will not spill on the floor, and cover the chair seat with a piece of plastic so it does not get wet.

Before beginning the shampoo, prepare several pitchers of water, some at the correct temperature and some slightly hotter, so they can be used to reheat the water being used on the client as it cools. Place the pitchers on the over-bed table, together with the shampoo and other needed items. During the shampoo, turn the client's head to both sides so that the entire scalp and all of the hair is washed and rinsed. Be careful not to get water and shampoo in the client's eyes; a small towel or washcloth over the eyes can prevent this. When the shampoo is completed, blot the hair dry with a towel. Some clients will not tolerate vigorous rubbing of the hair and scalp, and coarse, heavy hair or curly hair can become very tangled from towel drying. Instead, section the hair and comb out the tangles; then proceed with gentle rubbing of sections of the hair between the folds of the towel. This is more time-consuming but produces a better result than trying to dry all of the hair at one time. A hair dryer can be used to finish the drying. Then, comb the hair, as described above, using clean utensils.

GROOMING THE BEARD

The beard needs to be combed daily and washed as often as necessary. Washing may be needed more or less often than a head shampoo, depending on the amount of oil, perspiration, and debris in the beard. Covering the beard with a napkin or towel during meals may help to keep food from falling into it, which is a particular problem for clients who are fed by someone else or who have difficulty managing eating utensils. The beard may be washed with the face, using soap and then rinsing and towel drying. If the beard is long enough, it can be washed by enclosing it in a folded soapy washcloth or towel and massaging it, then rinsing it in the same manner. All of the soap should be rinsed off before the beard is dried.

SHAVING

Male clients require shaving while in the hospital. It is usually done after the bath, but it may be deferred if the client is fatigued. The client who is unable to shave himself may prefer to use a barber service if it is available. Relatives and friends are also sometimes enlisted for this task. However, sometimes the nurse must do the shaving, either with an electric shaver or a safety razor.

Before using the electric shaver, check the cord to be sure it is not frayed. Open the razor head and remove the accumulated hair. Position the client comfortably, in an erect position if possible, with the head well-supported by pillows. Drape a towel across the chest and around the neck to collect the hair. The skin and beard should be completely dry. An electric preshave lotion is often used, since it has an astringent ingredient that removes oil from the skin and hair, dries perspiration, closes the pores, and causes the hair to stand more erect. When using a shaver with rotary blades, one hand moves the electric shaver in a circular direction over the skin with gentle pressure, while the fingers and thumb of the opposite hand hold the skin taut. The circular movement directs the shaver with and against the grain of the hair and thus provides a close shave. A shaver with straight blades is used in a back and forth direction. Some clients have hair growth extending down the neck and under the chin. If these areas are more sensitive than the face, it may be necessary to use strokes that move in the direction of the hair growth to prevent irritation of the skin. During the shave, the nurse inspects the hair carefully to determine its direction of growth. An electric shaver is safer than a safety razor because it eliminates the potential for cutting the skin. However, abrasions can occur on sensitive skin from a dull electric shaver and the application of too much pressure on the shaver head.

Prior to shaving with a safety razor, it is necessary to soften the skin and beard. Place a washcloth or towel in a bath basin half full of hot water at 36.5° to 40°C (98° to 104°F). Wring out the washcloth and steam the face and neck, being careful not to burn the skin. Leave the washcloth in place for several minutes until the face and beard are soft. Apply a small amount of shaving cream to the face and massage it in to create a lather, which reduces the surface tension and enables the razor to glide over the skin and hair without pulling. Even though shaving against the hair growth results in a closer shave, when shaving someone else it is safer to shave in the direction of the hair growth. Since the facial hair has no set pattern of growth over the face and neck, the nurse needs to scrutinize the hair to determine the direction of growth before starting to shave. Hold the razor at about a 10 degree angle to the skin and move it with short, gentle strokes while holding the skin taut. Rinse the razor in the basin of water as the lather accumulates on it. When the shaving is complete, rinse the face thoroughly with clean fresh water and then pat dry with a towel. Apply after-shave lotion if the client wishes.

Clients who have problems with blood clotting due to disease or anticoagulant drugs are at risk for hemorrhaging from minor cuts. Shaving with a razor blade may be prohibited for such clients, and it may be necessary for the nurse to explain this to them.

☐ SKILL SEQUENCE

BED SHAMPOO

Step	Rationale
1. Check health record and kardex for nursing and medical orders.	Provides directions for special care needs.
2. Explain procedure to client.	Allays anxiety; enlists cooperation.
3. Wash hands.	Prevents cross-contamination from microorganisms on hands.
4. Prepare equipment at bedside.	Prevents delays and interruptions during care.
5. Close door and cubicle curtains.	Prevents drafts and chills, and provides privacy.
6. Prepare client: a. Cover client with a bath blanket. b. Fold top linen at foot of bed.	Keeps client warm and prevents linen from getting wet.
7. Position client diagonally across the bed with head at edge of bed.	Provides better access to head without stretching.
8. Remove pillow from under client's head.	Enables placement of shampoo tray on a flat surface.
9. Place shampoo tray under head.	Prevents bed from getting wet.
10. Drape plastic trough down side of bed and into pail.	Drains water into receptacle.
11. Provide client with small towel to wipe face, or keep nearby for care-giver's use.	Water or soap may splash onto client's face.
12. Check water temperature and add hot water if necessary.	Precaution against chilling or burning client's scalp.
13. Begin at hairline and slowly pour water over hair, saturating all of hair.	Prevents splashing and wetting client's face and bed.
14. Apply shampoo; spread over hair.	Facilitates distribution of shampoo for thorough washing.
15. Massage scalp with pads of fingers and rub hair to create a lather.	Long nails cause discomfort and may injure scalp. Massage stimulates and cleanses scalp.
16. Turn client's head to each side to reach all of scalp and hair areas, adding water as needed to maintain lather.	Provides access to all areas.
17. Stroke hair with hands to remove excess lather; deposit lather in trough or pail.	Facilitates rinsing hair.
18. Pour enough warm water over hair to rinse thoroughly all scalp and hair.	Shampoo must be thoroughly removed from hair.
19. Rub strands of hair between fingers to determine if adequately rinsed and clean.	Hair squeaks when thoroughly rinsed.
20. Check client's fatigue level.	Shampooing can be very tiring even though client is passive during procedure.
21. Repeat shampoo if necessary and if client is able to tolerate.	Soil and oil may not be completely removed with one lather.
22. Apply conditioner or other rinse to hair.	Helps remove soap and tangles.
23. Squeeze out excess water from hair.	Prevents water from dripping on client.
24. Dry client's ears, neck, and face.	
25. Wrap a towel around head and blot wet hair.	Excess water is quickly absorbed by the towel without causing unnecessary snarls by rubbing.

(continued)

BED SHAMPOO (Cont.)

Step	Rationale
26. Remove towel from shoulders if damp and replace with a dry towel.	Prevents discomfort and chills.
27. Remove shampoo tray and trough from bed.	Prepares head of bed for upright position.
28. Raise client to a sitting position if feasible.	Hair is easier to dry and groom with client in sitting position.
29. Section hair and comb thoroughly before drying.	Avoids tangling hair.
30. Section hair again and gently rub each section in a folded towel.	Facilitates drying and prevents retangling hair.
31. Blow dry hair with electric dryer if available.	
32. Comb hair by sections as before.	Makes it easier to untangle hair, is more comfortable for client.
33. Style or set hair according to client's preference.	
34. Remove all shampoo equipment and dispose of wet linen in laundry bag.	
35. Replace top bed linen and assist client into a comfortable position to rest.	Client may be fatigued from procedure.
36. Record shampoo, scalp and hair condition, and client's response.	Close inspection of scalp and hair may reveal reportable conditions. Documents action on health record.

RECORDING

Routine grooming of the hair is not usually recorded unless there are abnormal conditions of the hair and scalp that should be described. Scalp lesions, abnormalities of the hair, and badly snarled or matted hair are noted. The interventions used and the client's response are entered on the record, and the subsequent plan of action is also noted on the kardex. Shampoos are always recorded.

Sample POR Recording
- S—"I don't like people fussing with my hair! It makes my head hurt."
- O—Hair severely matted and tangled, especially at back of head.
- A—Reluctant to have hair-care given.
- P—Comb out tangles for brief intervals 2 to 3 times per day until they are all removed.

Sample Narrative Recording
Hair severely matted, particularly at the back of the head. Able to tolerate combing only for short periods. Will comb out snarls 2 to 3 times per day until hair is in satisfactory condition.

☐ CRITICAL POINTS SUMMARY

1. The amount and quality of hair is affected by pregnancy, high fever, severe illness, protein deficiency, heparin therapy, and chemotherapy.
2. Females with marked male-like hair distribution may have gonadal or adrenal abnormalities or may be receiving corticosteroid therapy.
3. Alopecia may be hereditary, self-inflicted, or result from emotional stress or traction on the hair.
4. Detergents and dyes can cause dry, brittle hair.
5. The nurse must be alert for signs of head lice or crab lice or nits.
6. Persons infested with head and crab lice must be treated early to prevent the spread of the lice. The fomites of infected persons must also be disinfected.
7. Black males are more prone to chronic ingrown hairs from shaving than are whites.
8. An appraisal of the hair is as important as an appraisal of the skin.
9. Preventing hair from snarling and matting is part of the nurse's responsibility.
10. A physician's order is usually required to shampoo a client's hair.
11. The client must be protected from drafts, chills, and burns during a shampoo.
12. Clients with bleeding problems may be prohibited from shaving with a razor blade.
13. Beards, as well as scalp hair, require combing and washing.
14. Skin and beard must be softened prior to shaving with a razor blade.

☐ LEARNING ACTIVITIES

1. Inspect and palpate the scalp and hair of persons of different ages. Note the similarities and differences.
2. Consider how your own self-concept is related to the appearance of your hair.
3. Select a peer with whom to practice giving and receiving a shampoo. Discuss your reactions to the shampoo.
4. Ask a male relative or friend to let you shave him. If he is afraid to have you use a safety razor rather than an electric shaver, what could you say to instill him with confidence in your ability to shave him safely?
5. Talk with a public health nurse or elementary schoolteacher about the incidence of head lice he or she encounters and what treatment is used.

REVIEW QUESTIONS

1. Why is hair grooming important?
2. Why is scalp hair longer than body hair?
3. What are some of the causes of alopecia?
4. How would you explain the difference between head lice and crab lice?
5. What steps make up the complete treatment to control head lice and body lice?
6. What characteristics are included in an appraisal of the hair?
7. How would you comb badly snarled hair?
8. What precautions must be taken to shampoo a client's hair safely?
9. How would you shampoo the hair of a client who cannot be out of bed?
10. How is shaving a client with an electric shaver different from shaving him with a safety razor?
11. How would you groom and wash a beard?

PERFORMANCE CHECKLIST

OBJECTIVE: To use the correct method to shampoo a client's hair safely in bed.

CHARACTERISTIC	RANGE OF ACCEPTABILITY	SATISFACTORY	UNSATISFACTORY
1. Checks health record and kardex for nursing and medical orders.	No deviation		
2. Explains procedure to client.	No deviation		
3. Washes hands.	No deviation		
4. Prepares equipment at bedside.	No deviation		
5. Closes door and cubicle curtains.	No deviation		
6. Covers client with blanket and folds down top linen.	No deviation		
7. Positions client diagonally across bed with head at edge of bed.	No deviation		
8. Removes pillow from under head and replaces with shampoo tray.	No deviation		
9. Drapes plastic trough into pail.	No deviation		
10. Has small towel nearby to wipe client's face.	No deviation		
11. Mixes water to correct temperature.	No deviation		
12. Slowly wets hair and applies shampoo.	No deviation		
13. Spreads shampoo over hair and massages all of scalp and hair.	No deviation		
14. Removes excess lather before thoroughly rinsing hair.	No deviation		
15. Checks hair for adequate rinsing.	No deviation		
16. Repeats shampoo.	Omit if client is fatigued or if hair is clean.		
17. Applies rinse or conditioner and squeezes out excess water from hair.	Use if available.		
18. Dries client's face and neck, wraps head with towel, and blots hair.	No deviation		
19. Removes shampoo tray and trough; replaces damp towel on shoulders.	No deviation		
20. Repositions client if feasible; sections, combs, and gently dries each section of hair; blows dry if possible.	No deviation		
21. Combs hair in sections to remove snarls and styles or sets hair.	No deviation		
22. Positions client comfortably for rest.	No deviation		
23. Removes all shampoo equipment and disposes of wet linen in linen bag.	No deviation		
24. Records shampoo, scalp and hair condition, and client's response.	No deviation		

REFERENCES

Ebling FJG, Rook A: Hair. In Rook A, Wilkinson DS, Ebling FJG (eds): Textbook of Dermatology, ed 3, vol 2. Oxford, England, Blackwell Scientific Publications, 1979.

Grier ME: Hair care for the black patient. American Journal of Nursing 76(11):1781, 1976.

Juranek DD: The nuisance diseases: Pediculosis and scabies. APIC Newsletter 4(1):1–5, 1976.

LeMaile-Williams RL: The clinical and psychological assessment of black patients. In Luckraft D (ed): Black Awareness: Implications for Black Patient Care. New York, American Journal of Nursing, 1974.

Parrish JA: Dermatology and Skin Care. New York, McGraw-Hill, 1975.

Rook A, Wilkinson DS: The prevalence, incidence and ecology of diseases of the skin. In Rook A, Wilkinson DS, Ebling FJG (eds): Textbook of Dermatology, ed 3, vol 1. Oxford, England, Blackwell Scientific Publications, 1979.

BIBLIOGRAPHY

Rambo BJ, Wood LA: Nursing Skills in Clinical Practice, vol 2. Philadelphia, WB Saunders, 1982.

Rook A: The ages of man and their dermatoses. In Rook A, Wilkinson DS, Ebling FJG (eds): Textbook of Dermatology, ed 3, vol 1. Oxford, England, Blackwell Scientific Publications, 1979.

SUGGESTED READING

Grier ME: Hair care for the black patient. American Journal of Nursing 76(11):1781, 1976.

AUDIOVISUAL RESOURCE

Patient Grooming: How to Shave a Male Patient
Videorecording (3/4 in). (1974, Color, 5 min.)
Available through:
   Comm Sales/Minnesota Association of Health Care Facilities
   Professional Research Inc.
   930 Pitner Ave.
   Evanston, IL 60202

SKILL 42 Nail Care

PREREQUISITE SKILLS

Skill 19, "Inspection"
Skill 20, "Palpation"
Skill 28, "Handwashing"

☐ STUDENT OBJECTIVES

1. Explain the purpose of nail care.
2. Indicate the components of nail care.
3. Describe the appearance of normal nails.
4. Describe the common abnormalities of nails.
5. Describe the characteristics of nails that are included in an appraisal.
6. Indicate the precautions observed in cutting nails.
7. Provide safe nail care to clients.

☐ INTRODUCTION

Like hair, nails are an appendage of the skin and require regular care. Nails are subject to neglect and abuse from inadequate cleansing, exposure to excessive moisture, harsh chemicals, and trauma. Nail care is usually provided as part of the bath and includes cleansing, trimming the nail length, and attention to the soft tissues surrounding the nail. Cleansing removes organisms harbored under and around the nails, thereby eliminating potential sources of inflammation and infection for the surrounding tissues. Cleansing also prevents the transfer of microorganisms to other parts of the body. Trimming the length of the fingernails prevents injury from scratching. Long toenails receive pressure from the end of the shoe and can cause trauma to the nail bed.

The quality, color, and shape of the nails provide important information about the individual's health status. DeGowin and DeGowin (1981) refer to the fingernails as windows through which signs of physical disease may be seen. The alert nurse is in a position to identify many of these changes and to assist the client in understanding them. The nurse can also teach the client appropriate nail care to improve the quality of the nails.

☐ PREPARATION

THE STRUCTURE AND FUNCTION OF THE NAILS

Nails correspond to the claws of lower animals. The flattened plate-like structure of the nail consists of an exposed body of dead cells and a root that is embedded in the skin. The free end of the nail extends be-

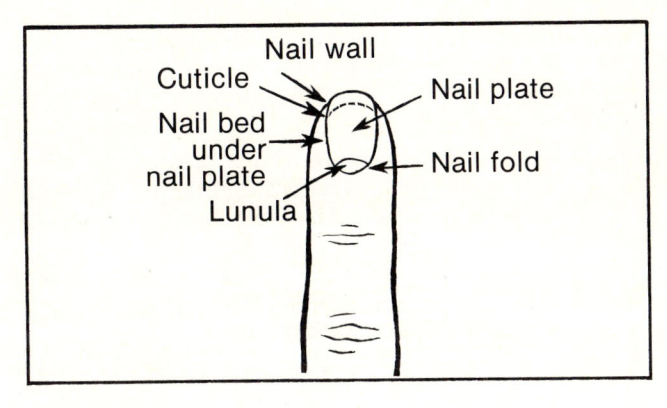

Figure 42-1. The fingernail and its related structures.

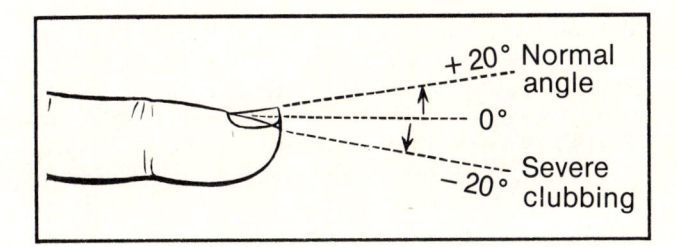

Figure 42-2. Changes in the angle of the fingernail with clubbing.

yond the tip of the digits. This protects the digits and also serves as a tool for defense and for picking up objects. Anatomically, the nail includes the nail walls, which are the folds of skin along the lateral edges of the nail; the nail plate, which is the nail; the nail fold, which is the fold of skin over the root of the nail; the nail bed, which is the epithelial layer of tissue under the nail plate; and the nail root, which is the site of nail growth that lies under the lunula. The cuticle is the hardened rim of skin that accumulates at the periphery of the nail walls and nail fold. Figure 42-1 shows a fingernail and its related structures.

Nails are the product of specialized epidermal tissue that begins to form during the 3rd fetal month. By the 9th fetal month they extend to the end of the digit. Nail growth is continuous but slow, and if a nail is lost it will be replaced. Nail growth occurs through the addition of cells to those already at the nail root. This growth pushes the nail plate distally over the nail bed without losing the attachment of the nail plate to the nail bed. Nail growth originates 3 to 5 mm below the edge of the cuticle. Fingernails grow about 1 mm per week, and it takes about 3 to 5 weeks before new growth is visible. Toenails grow at a rate that is one-third to one-half slower than the growth rate of fingernails. The rate of nail growth is greatest during childhood and decreases slowly with aging; the decrease in the growth rate may be accompanied by an increase in the thickness of the nail.

NORMAL APPEARANCE OF THE NAILS

The normal nail plate is usually transparent and smooth with a convex shape. The color of the nail beds reflects vasomotor function and the quality of peripheral circulation. When these are normal, the nail bed has an excellent blood supply, which provides a pink color to the nail in light-skinned persons, and a dusky pink color in dark-skinned persons. The free end of the nail is white at the point of separation from the nail bed. The white moon (lunula) seen at the base of the nail is the distal part of the matrix containing the nail cells. The moon is not always visible on all fingers but is usually seen on the thumb (Parrish, 1975).

DISORDERS OF THE NAILS

Nails may become brittle, thin, and flattened from impaired circulation. Decreased peripheral circulation such as occurs in the elderly may cause the nails to become thickened. Clubbing of the nails occurs when there is long-term impairment of the circulation, such as occurs with chronic obstructive lung disease or chronic cardiac insufficiency. With clubbing, the normally obtuse angle between the nail plate and the posterior nail fold decreases over time until the angle is lost and the nail is on the same plane with the digit. Figure 42-2 shows changes in the angle of the fingernail with clubbing. Slowed nail growth, exaggerated nail curve, and a pale yellow or yellow-green color occurs with obstructed lymphatic circulation. Color changes may also occur as a result of certain drugs such as antimetabolites, cholesterol-lowering drugs, or high doses of vitamin A. Nails become brittle and concave with a ridged nail plate as a result of malnutrition, iron deficiency, calcium deficit, excess thyroid hormone, or constant immersion of the hands in water (DeGowin and DeGowin, 1981).

Hemorrhages under the nail plate and detachment or loss of the nail may result from a contact dermatitis. Exposure to household or industrial chemicals and the excessive use of nail hardeners are common causes of contact dermatitis. The nail bed may also become irritated from the use of artificial nails. When artificial nails are removed, small pieces of the nail plate surface may be pulled off, disrupting the nails' integrity.

Most of these disorders may be seen in both toenails and fingernails, although most of the signs are less pronounced in toenails. However, the pain resulting from some of these disorders may be greater in the toenails because of the weight borne by the feet (Saman, 1979).

TRAUMA TO THE NAILS

Trauma to the nails may be self-induced or accidental. *Fingernail biting* is a common habit and tends to occur among several members of one family. It is thought to be related to restlessness and insecurity. With fingernail biting, the free edge of the nail is absent and the cuticles may also be so bitten that they become irregular and broken. *Hangnails* are frequently due to biting but may also be caused by minor injuries to the fingernail or toenail. With a hangnail, hard pieces of the epidermis in the lateral fold of the nail break away. This can be very painful, particularly when the split extends into the underlying tissues. Infections can occur at these sites.

Toenails are subject to various traumas. Pressure on the toes from footwear that is too tight affects the way the nails grow. *Ingrown nails,* which result from compression of the side of the toe, usually occur on the great toe. The lateral nail fold is penetrated by a portion of the edge of the nail plate that may have become separated from the main part of the nail. The soft tissues of the nail fold become painful and red, and then swollen and infected. Cutting the nail in a half-circle manner instead of straight across is considered to be a main contributory cause of ingrown toenails. Overcurvature of the nails may be the result of tight-fitting shoes, psoriasis, or congenital anomalies. The great toe is most commonly affected, but other nails may also be affected. With an overcurved nail, the long axis of the nail curves so that the edges of the nail press into the lateral nail folds. When the nail penetrates the epidermis, it looks like an ingrown nail (Saman, 1979).

DATA BASE

Client History and Recorded Data

The nurse needs to be knowledgeable about the client's medical diagnosis before providing nail care, since the diagnosis may call for special nail care. Special care is often required when cutting the nails of persons with impaired peripheral circulation, such as elderly and diabetic clients, because impaired circulation may affect their ability to perceive pain that would alert them to the presence of infection. Wound healing is also impeded by impaired circulation. An example of other persons with an increased risk for infection are those receiving antimetabolite therapy. Many institutions prohibit nurses from cutting a diabetic client's toenails unless they have had special training by a physician or a podiatrist. With the current trend toward self-care, many diabetic persons are taught how to cut their own nails correctly. Cutting ingrown, thick, or infected nails is not considered to be a nursing responsibility.

Physical Appraisal Skills

Inspection. The nails are inspected for cleanliness, grooming, integrity, swelling, and presence of any infection. The nail beds also provide a readily accessible area to detect the presence of pallor and cyanosis. The color, shape, quality, and thickness of the nail plate are inspected. Because the presence of colored nail polish prevents an accurate inspection of the nail, it must be removed. The color of the nail beds is compared with that of the nurse. (This assumes that the nurse has a normal color and has no problems with adequate perfusion of oxygenated blood in the fingers.) To determine if the nail is *thin* or *thick,* the free edge of the nail is inspected.

Inspection and Palpation. *Pallor* and *cyanosis* are detected best by performing the capillary filling test. The results of this test are also compared with the nurse's own nail color. To determine if pallor is present, the free edge of the second or third finger nailplate is pressed to induce blanching. After the pressure is released slowly, the rate of color return should be the same as that of the nurse; a slower return indicates reduced vasomotor function. In cyanosis the nail beds appear a dusky-blue prior to palpation, and after the nail plate is pressed the color returns slowly by spreading from the periphery to the center. In the absence of cyanosis, normal color returns in less than 1 second and appears to return from under the pale area as well as from the periphery (Roach, 1974).

Pressing the free edge of the nail plate also reveals whether the nail is pliable or brittle.

EQUIPMENT

Prior to giving nail care the nurse identifies the type of equipment required. Many clients do not usually bring nail-care equipment with them to the hospital. The nurse may request the family to bring the items from home or obtain them from the hospital gift shop. Nail clippers are usually available from the central supply department. Borrowing items from other clients is not a safe practice, because potentially infective organisms can be transferred from one client to another.

Orange sticks are used to clean under the nails. They are safer than a nail file because they are softer and less apt to damage the nail bed. *Nail clippers* trim nails more evenly than scissors. *Emery boards* are used to shape and smooth the edge of the nails and do not leave burrs that will snag on clothing or scratch the skin. *Nail brushes* may be necessary if the client has excess and embedded soil under and around the nails. Dry, hard cuticles can be softened by applying and massaging a *lubricating lotion* into the tissues.

☐ EXECUTION

Nail care is usually given as part of the bath, but it is appropriate to give it at another time. It is easier to clean the nails during the bath, because immersing them in soap and water helps to soften the soil and make it easier to remove. Brittle and tough nails are also easier to cut after they have been softened. When a nail brush is used to remove excess soil that is embedded under and around the nail, the brush bristles should be softened in hot, soapy water to prevent injury to the tissues. While cutting the nails it is impor-

SKILL SEQUENCE

NAIL CARE

Step	Rationale
1. Wash hands.	Prevents cross-contamination from microorganisms on hands.
2. Obtain permission from client; explain procedure.	Nails are cut only with client's permission; allays anxiety.
3. Prepare equipment and supplies.	Prevents delays and interruptions during care.
4. Cleanse nails:	
a. Immerse hand or foot in warm, soapy water.	Softens soil for easier removal and nails for easier trimming.
b. Use an orange stick to remove soil from under nails or brush gently with a nail brush.	Less damaging to tissues than a nail file.
c. Remove hand or foot from water.	
d. Use a towel to gently retract cuticles and to dry all skin surfaces.	Cuticles should not be trimmed.
e. Place a towel under hand or foot.	Collects nail trimmings.
f. Massage lotion into cuticles.	Softens tissues.
5. Clip nails with a nail clipper, keeping the length of nails beyond the distal aspect of the lateral nail fold. Clip toenails straight across. Smooth and round free end of fingernails with an emery board according to client's preference.	Prevents splitting nails as would scissors. Prevents hangnail and ingrown nail. Eliminates rough edges of cut nails. Client may prefer straight nails.
6. Collect towel with clippings and dispose of the clippings in wastebasket.	Keeps clippings away from client, where they may irritate skin.
7. Empty bath basin and replace equipment.	
8. Record procedure on health record.	Documents action on health record.

tant that the sides of the nail be left long enough to extend beyond the lateral fold; otherwise, hangnails and ingrown nails can develop. Fingernails can be rounded or left straight, depending on the client's preference. Toenails are not trimmed with curves into the lateral folds or shaped to be rounded because of the problem of ingrown nails. Cuticles should not be cut. Gently pushing them back with the washcloth while they are soft, plus using a lubricating lotion, helps to keep them from tearing and splitting.

RECORDING

Recorded information includes the color of the nail plates and nail beds. When nail plates and nail beds are abnormal, information is also included on the integrity of the nails and cuticles, and any abnormal characteristics of the nail. When the nails are trimmed by the nurse, or require trimming that the nurse is unable to perform, that information is also recorded.

Sample POR Recording
- S—"I usually have a podiatrist trim my toenails. Could I have one see me here?"
- —Fingernails thin, brittle, and ragged. Cuticles dry but intact. Toenails long and very thick.
- A—Needs assistance with toenail care.
- P—Discuss podiatrist referral with Dr. Jones. Fingernails trimmed and cuticles lubricated with petroleum jelly.

Sample Narrative Recording
Fingernails thin, brittle, and ragged. Cuticles dry but intact. Nails trimmed at patient's request, cuticles lubricated with petroleum jelly. Toenails long and very thick. Normally has a podiatrist care for feet and would like to have one visit her now. Will discuss with Dr. Jones.

CRITICAL POINTS SUMMARY

1. Nail care helps protect the client from injury and infection.
2. Normal nails are transparent, pink, convex, and smooth.
3. The color of the nail beds indicates the quality of the client's vasomotor function and peripheral circulation.
4. Alterations in the color, quantity, and quality of the nails are related to systemic illness or environmental factors.
5. Improperly fitting shoes and incorrect cutting of the toenails traumatize the toes and predispose the person to infection.
6. Cleaning and proper trimming of the nails are the responsibility of the nurse. However, the nurse does not routinely cut the toenails of clients who have diabetes or impaired peripheral circulation.
7. Teaching proper self-care of nails is an important aspect of client care.

LEARNING ACTIVITIES

1. Compare the hands and nails of persons of different ages and races. Note the characteristics that are normal and abnormal.
2. Note the similarities and differences between the fingernails and toenails of hospitalized clients.
3. Interview persons with impaired peripheral circulation and diabetes to determine how much they know about caring for their own toenails.

REVIEW QUESTIONS

1. Why is nail care given as part of personal hygiene?
2. What is included in nail care?
3. How would you describe the appearance of a normal nail?
4. What are some of the common disorders of the nails caused by systemic disease and environmental factors?
5. What are the common injuries of fingernails and toenails?
6. What characteristics of the nails are examined in an appraisal?
7. What precautions must be observed while cutting the nails?
8. How would you deal with diabetic persons who need to have their toenails cut?
9. What equipment would you use to give a client complete nail care?

PERFORMANCE CHECKLIST

OBJECTIVE: To use the correct method to cleanse and trim nails safely.

CHARACTERISTIC	RANGE OF ACCEPTABILITY	SATISFACTORY	UNSATISFACTORY
1. Washes hands.	No deviation		
2. Obtains permission and explains procedure.	No deviation		
3. Prepares equipment and supplies.	No deviation		
4. Cleanses nails: a. Immerses in warm, soapy water. b. Cleanses under nails with orange stick or nail brush. c. Uses towel to retract cuticles and to dry hands. d. Messages lotion into cuticles.	 No deviation No deviation No deviation Omit if cuticles not dry.		
5. Clips nails without cutting into nail fold; keeps nail length beyond distal part of nail fold; trims toenail straight across; smooths and rounds edge of fingernail.	Omit according to client perference.		
6. Replaces equipment.	No deviation		
7. Records procedure on health record.	No deviation		

REFERENCES

DeGowin EL, DeGowin RL: Bedside Diagnostic Examination, ed 4. New York, Macmillan, 1981.
Parrish JA: Dermatology and Skin Care. New York, McGraw-Hill, 1975.
Roach LB: Assessing skin changes: The subtle and the obvious. Nursing74 3(3):64–67, 1974.
Saman PO: The nails. In Rook A, Wilkinson DS, Ebling FTG (eds): Textbook of Dermatology, ed 3, vol 2. Oxford, England, Blackwell Scientific Publications, 1979.

BIBLIOGRAPHY

Simko MV: Foot welfare. American Journal of Nursing 67(9):1895–1897, 1967.
Ventura E: Foot care for diabetics. American Journal of Nursing 78(5):886–888, 1978.
When nails are ingrown, injured or infected. Patient Care 8(18):168–196, 1974.

SKILL 43 Vaginal Irrigation

PREREQUISITE SKILLS

Skill 19, "Inspection"
Skill 28, "Handwashing"

☐ STUDENT OBJECTIVES

1. Describe the purposes of a vaginal irrigation.
2. Identify the controversial issues associated with douches.
3. Explain the factors affecting the health of the vagina.
4. Identify some conditions for which a douche may be indicated.
5. Describe the characteristics of a safe douche solution.
6. Describe the precautions that must be observed for a douche to be safe.
7. Administer a safe vaginal irrigation.

☐ INTRODUCTION

A vaginal irrigation, commonly referred to as a douche, is a flushing of the vagina with a solution. Douches are used clinically to cleanse the vagina prior to surgery, to treat certain vaginal infections, or to flush out excessive discharge that is present with such disease conditions as cancer of the cervix.

Many women douche for hygienic purposes, especially after menses and intercourse. However, the value of doing so has been widely disputed; in fact, it has been found to be harmful. Many women also use douching as a means of contraception. However, the failure rate of douching as a contraceptive is high. Studies have found sperm in the fallopian tubes as early as 5 minutes after exposure to cervical mucus (Hogan, 1985). The practicality of a woman douching within 5 minutes of the time sperm is deposited in the vagina is poor; it would require that the douche equipment be ready and that the woman move to the bathroom immediately after the man has ejaculated.

☐ PREPARATION

The media have barraged women with the idea that they should douche to feel clean and smell good. However, there has been controversy among medical professionals as to the merits of douching when it is used regularly for cleansing purposes, as many women are in the habit of doing. Currently there seems to be consensus that regular douching is unnecessary. Kaminetzky (1965) believes that the normal cleansing action in the vagina eliminates the need for women to douche for hygiene purposes. Green (1977) supports this belief and adds that even when the most physiological solutions are used, douching may in some instance be harmful because the normal protective mucus and bacterial flora of the vagina are washed away. Additional arguments against regular douching include possible trauma to the vaginal wall if unnecessary force is used to insert the douche nozzle, irritation to the vaginal tissues from concentrated chemicals, burns from excessively hot solutions, and the risk of embolism produced by the fluid or air forced into the uterus (Kilroy, 1977).

FACTORS AFFECTING THE HEALTH OF THE VAGINA

The Vaginal Environment

The vagina is affected by normal physiological processes that occur as a result of hormonal changes. The normal adult vagina has an acid pH ranging between 3.5 and 4.2, largely because of high levels of estrogen and the presence of Döderlein's bacilli, which, along with anaerobic streptococci and diphtheroids, is a normal flora found in the vagina. The amount and variety of organisms in the vagina is controlled by the lysozyme ingredient in cervical secretions and the acidity of the normal adult vagina. At the time of menses, and after menopause, estrogen levels are lower, and the pH becomes more alkaline, at 5.7. When this occurs the thin tissue surfaces of the vulva (external genitalia) and the vagina are more susceptible to bacterial invasion.

With aging, the alkaline pH is combined with the normal atrophy of the genital tract and a decrease in the production of mucus. Döderlein's bacilli are replaced with a mixed flora or one in which cocci dominate, thus encouraging local infection of the vagina (Karnaky, 1961).

The major source of normal moisture in the vagina is mucus secreted by the cervix, which mixes with bacteria and the cells shed from the tissues. The discharge is normally thin or mucoid in texture, and clear or cloudy in color. It may contain some whitish creamy material. Normal vaginal discharge is odorless and nonirritating to the skin and usually does not cause itching or burning. As the secretions flow out toward the introitus (vaginal entrance) by gravity, they constantly cleanse the vagina by a normal physiological cleansing process. This discharge is normally present in small amounts on the vulva. Large amounts of cervical mucus are produced when there are high levels of estrogen, for example, during pregnancy. Sexual or other emotional stimulation also increases the amount of cervical mucus. Under the influence of maternal estrogen, the newborn female infant has a normal vaginal discharge until the hormones are cleared from the system (Benson, 1971).

The term *leukorrhea* means a white or yellowish vaginal discharge containing mucus and pus cells, and is frequently used to refer to normal physiological vaginal discharge as just described as well as to abnormal discharge. The increased estrogen level that occurs during cyclic ovarian activity can cause leukorrhea. Leukorrhea may occur at any age and affects most women at some time during their life. It can also be a symptom of a local or systemic disorder, although it is not a disease itself. Leukorrhea can be caused by douching (especially if irritating substances are used), high levels of estrogen or estrogen depletion, vaginal or cervical infection, or cervical cancer. Excessive vaginal discharge should be investigated by a physician when it occurs at noncyclical times. The client may believe that all vaginal discharges are normal. However, when the amount of discharge is sufficient to soil the underwear, the discharge may be abnormal and should be treated. A specimen of the vaginal discharge obtained during a pelvic examination is sent to the laboratory for smear or culture and sensitivity. The nurse can check the record for the result.

VAGINAL INFECTIONS

Vaginal infections may occur at any age when the pH of the vagina becomes more alkaline. Bacterial growths are most abundant at a pH of 7.6 to 8.0, and decrease as the pH becomes more acidic (Karnaky, 1961). When douches are used to treat vaginal infections, the solution should be buffered so that it will be acid within the vagina.

Vaginal discharge caused by an infection may be called leukorrhea, but the character and odor of the discharge is different from that caused by normal physiological processes. *Monilial infections* (candidiasis) produce a thick, white curdy discharge; *trichomonal infections* produce a watery, gray or green, frothy, odorous profuse discharge, and *bacterial infections* are characterized by gray discharge of moderate amounts (Malasanos et al., 1981). The most common sites of origin of vaginal discharge are the cervix, vagina, vulva, and upper genital tract.

DATA BASE

Client History and Recorded Data
Information about vaginal discharge and discomfort may be obtained during the admission interview and recorded on the health record. Often, however, there is little or no information on the record because of the reluctance of women to discuss vaginal problems unless a significant problem exists or the care-giver raises the subject. Unfortunately, many nurses are reluctant to initiate a discussion about vaginal discharges or concerns unless the client is admitted with a pelvic disorder.

The nurse can elicit basic information about the health status of the vagina by asking the client if she has a discharge and finding out about the nature, amount, and consistency of it and if she has burning, itching, or discomfort of the perineal area with intercourse. The client's self-care practices such as douching, the use of vaginal deodorants, and the use of vaginal inserts such as tampons, diaphragms, and spermicidal preparations should be investigated also because they may cause irritation of the vaginal tissues. It is important for the nurse to find out if and how the client has been treating the vaginal discharge, so that appropriate teaching may be implemented.

Vaginal irrigations given in the hospital are ordered by a physician.

Physical Appraisal Skills

Inspection. Prior to performing a vaginal irrigation, the vulvar tissue and the remaining perineum are inspected for redness, inflammation, and the presence of discharge. When a discharge is present, the amount, consistency, and color are noted and recorded.

Smell. The odor of the discharge and of any clothing soiled with discharge is noted and recorded.

EQUIPMENT

Disposable or reusable equipment is available for vaginal irrigation. A douche kit or tray usually includes the items shown in Figure 43–1: an irrigating bag or can with a connecting tubing, a long, slightly curved perforated douche nozzle made of glass or plastic, disposable gloves, an antibacterial solution, cotton balls, and drapes. A water-soluble lubricating jelly is also needed, although it is not included in most douche kits or trays. Sterile equipment and aseptic technique are used if there are any open wounds or lesions present in or around the vagina, to prevent the introduction of microorganisms that could cause an infection. If there are no wounds or lesions, clean technique may be used.

The irrigating bag or can should hold at least 1000 ml of fluid. Gloves are worn to protect the client from microorganisms that may be on the nurse's hands as well as to protect the nurse. The cotton balls are saturated with the antibacterial solution and used to cleanse the outer vulva, to prevent the introduction of organisms into the vagina when the douche nozzle is inserted. One of the drapes is used to cover the perineal area and to provide a clean or sterile area around the vagina during the douche. The other drape is used as a clean or sterile field on which to place the equipment. The water-soluble jelly is used as a lubricant on the douche nozzle to facilitate the insertion. A mobile or bed intravenous pole is used to hang the bag or can from during the irrigation, so that the nurse's hands are free to do the irrigation.

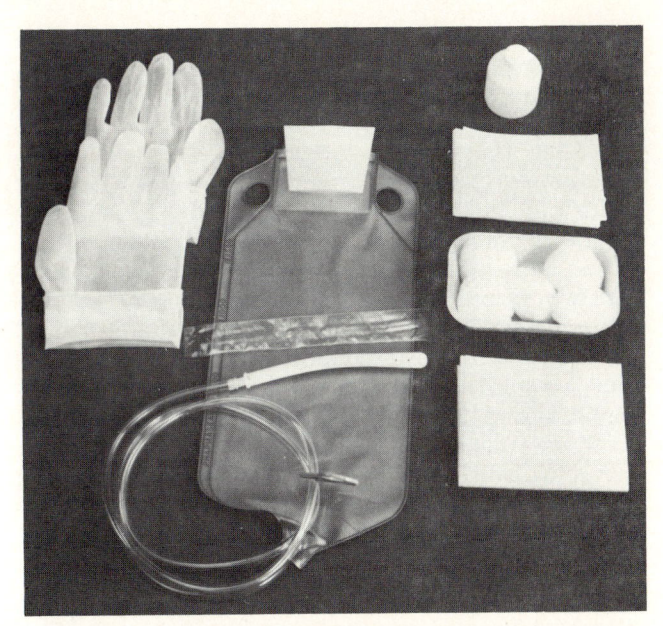

Figure 43-1. A disposable vaginal douche kit contains disposable gloves, irrigating bag with tubing and douche nozzle, a small tray, cotton balls, paper drapes, and an antibacterial solution. (Courtesy of American Pharmaseal Laboratories, Glendale, CA 91209.)

Irrigating Solutions

The pH of any vaginal irrigating solution needs to be properly buffered to keep it within a narrow acid range and to have it conform to the properties of the normal vaginal secretions. The pH of a solution will change when it is introduced into an infected vagina. A solution that is too acidic can cause irritation and burning of the vaginal and perineal tissues (Karnaky, 1961). In a hospital setting, the physician prescribes the irrigating solution used for the douche. Povidone-iodine douche is a commonly used antiseptic solution, because it has a low surface tension that assists in the penetration of the solution into the vaginal folds and crevices. A ½-ounce packet of povidine-iodine douche is mixed with 1 quart of warm water.

Beyers (1974) states that many of the ingredients found in the douche preparations that women purchase have no beneficial effects and that some are harmful to the tissues. A buffered acidified physiological solution is recommended by Beyers (1974) and Karnaky (1961).

Neither water nor a weak vinegar solution is considered to be an effective cleansing agent, although these are used commonly by many women. The benefits may be more in terms of psychological comfort than actual cleansing.

The Food and Drug Administration has taken measures to attempt to remove many commercial douche preparations from the market because of their association with the incidence of vaginitis. Preparations that include perfumes have been found to be irritating to vaginal tissue.

☐ EXECUTION

Prior to administering a douche, have the client empty her bladder to prevent abdominal discomfort during the procedure. For the irrigating solution to flush the vagina properly, the client must lie on her back (in the dorsal recumbent position). The douche may be administered with the client in bed sitting on the bedpan, or lying in a bathtub without water. In hospitals, a douche is usually given in bed. Remove the bed linen or pull it down to the foot of the bed, and use a bath blanket to drape the client. If the client has never had a douche before, explain the procedure to her. If the client wishes to and is capable of doing so, she may insert the nozzle herself after first washing her hands. If the procedure is to be done using aseptic technique, follow the procedures described in Skills 30 and 31.

About 1000 ml of solution is generally required to flush the vagina adequately. A warm temperature of 35.5° to 36.5°C (96°F to 98°F) is usually appropriate for most irrigations. If the purpose is to provide heat to the pelvic tissues, then solution at a hot temperature of 36.5° to 40°C (98° to 104°F) is used.

After washing the hands, don disposable gloves and cover the perineal area with drapes. Soak the cotton balls with the antibacterial solution, and cleanse the vulva to remove any organisms that could be transferred into the vagina when the douche nozzle is inserted. Inspect the nozzle for cracks, chips, or burrs, since defects in the nozzle can injure the tissues. The can or bag holding the irrigant should be elevated 30 to 60 cm (12 to 24 in) above the hips. If it is held higher, the greater pressure exerted could force infected debris into the uterus, cause trauma to the tissues, or initiate a fluid or air embolism into the peritoneal cavity by way of the fallopian tubes.

Allow a small amount of the solution to flow over the external genitalia to determine the client's tolerance for the temperature. Insert the nozzle slowly, with the solution flowing, inward and downward toward the coccyx, since this is the direction of the vagina. Figure 43-2 depicts how the nozzle is inserted into the vagina. During the irrigation, rotate the nozzle 180 degrees to facilitate the flow and to ensure that the entire vagina is flushed.

When all of the solution has been used, withdraw the nozzle. Elevate the client to a sitting position to help expel the irrigant before removing the bedpan. If it is not possible for the client to sit up, have her strain as if she were having a bowel movement, as this helps to expel more of the fluid. (However, this action is contraindicated for clients with myocardial infarctions or any other condition in which the Valsalva maneuver would be dangerous.) Observe the color of the expelled fluid and the characteristics of any debris flushed from the vagina. After drying the external genitalia, remove the bedpan, replace the bed linen, and remove the bath blanket. Place all of the disposable equipment in an impervious bag and put it in a

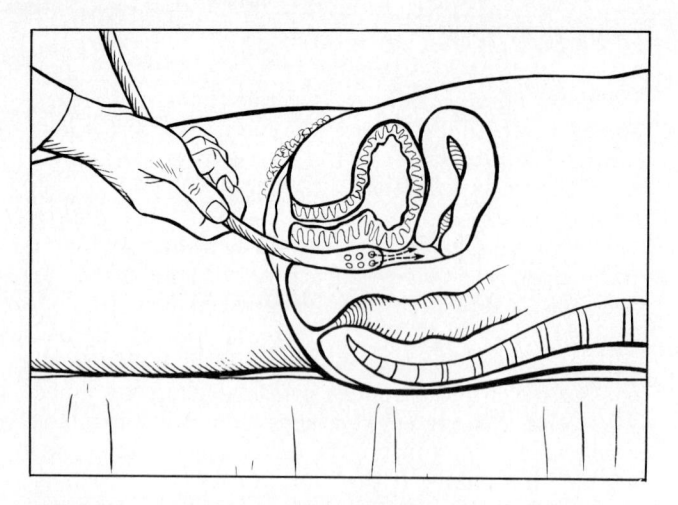

Figure 43–2. The douche nozzle is inserted gently into the vagina backward and downward toward the coccyx, while the client is in the dorsal recumbent position.

trash receptacle. Rinse all reusable equipment and return it to central suppy.

HAZARDS

Injury to the vaginal tissues can occur if the douche nozzle is damaged or inserted with too much force. Excessively hot solutions can burn the tissue. Incorrectly prepared douches with a high chemical concentration can cause irritation and ulceration of vaginal tissue, resulting in discomfort and leukorrhea. Solutions that are not compatible with the normal physiology of the vagina can irritate the tissues or adversely alter the vaginal environment, thus resulting in infections. Irrigant flowing under too much pressure can force infected material into the uterus, and also has the potential for creating air or fluid emboli in the peritoneal cavity.

☐ SKILL SEQUENCE

VAGINAL IRRIGATION

Step	Rationale
1. Check health record or kardex for nursing and medical orders.	Provides directions for special care needs.
2. Wash hands.	Prevents cross-contamination from microorganisms.
3. Prepare equipment and supplies.	Prevents delays and interruptions during care.
4. Close door and cubicle curtains.	Prevents drafts and chills, and provides privacy.
5. Explain procedure to client.	Allays anxiety; enlists cooperation.
6. Place client in the dorsal recumbent position.	Facilitates flow of irrigant to all parts of vagina.
7. Open irrigating kit or tray, using clean or sterile technique as appropriate.	Items can become contaminated with incorrect technique.
8. Fill irrigating bag or can with proper solution at correct temperature, keeping tubing clamped.	Prevents irrigant from leaking.
9. Hang irrigating bag on an intravenous or bed pole so bag is not more than 60 cm (24 in) above hips.	Avoids excessive force of fluid into vagina.
10. Cover client with bath blanket arranged diagonally, and then pull down top bed linen to foot of bed.	Prevents linen from getting wet.
11. Place bedpan under buttocks.	Catches irrigant.
12. Bend client's knees, spread her legs apart, and raise corner of blanket to pubis.	Exposes perineal area.
13. Don gloves.	Prevents transfer of microorganisms.
14. Place one drape from kit over perineal area and the other on the bed near client's feet.	Provides clean/sterile field around perineal area.
15. Place douche tray or kit on drape.	Makes supplies easily accessible.
16. Open antibacterial solution and pour over cotton balls.	
17. Cleanse center and each side of vulva using one stroke from top to bottom. Discard cotton balls on corner of tray.	Avoids introducing bacteria from vulva into vagina.
18. Grasp nozzle and inspect for defects. Lubricate nozzle with a water-soluble jelly.	Cracks or chips in nozzle can cause injury to the tissues. Water-soluble lubricant facilitates insertion into vagina.
19. Open clamp on tubing and allow a small amount of solution to flow over the vulva.	Determine client's tolerance to temperature to avoid burns.

(continued)

Step	Rationale
20. Insert the nozzle gently into the vagina, backward toward the coccyx.	Follows anatomic direction of the vagina.
21. Slowly rotate nozzle 180 degrees, moving it in and out while the solution is flowing.	Helps to flush all areas of vagina.
22. Withdraw nozzle when all solution is used and place it on the tray. Remove tray from bed.	
23. Elevate client to sitting position.	Helps to expel remaining solution.
24. Return client to flat position and dry external genitalia with tissues. Discard tissues in bedpan.	Prevents chafing of skin.
25. Remove bedpan; dry buttocks area if necessary.	Buttocks may become wet from solution in bedpan.
26. Replace top bed linen, remove blanket, position for comfort.	
27. Discard disposable equipment in an impervious bag. Rinse reusable equipment and return it to central supply department.	
28. Record client's reaction and results of procedure on health record.	Nurse is accountable for recording actions and adding to data base.

RECORDING

The amount and type of irrigant used, the client's tolerance of the procedure, the color of the returned fluid, and the nature of the expelled debris are recorded in the health record.

Sample POR Recording
Unless the client had problems unrelated to the irrigation at the time of the procedure, and there were additional data, a SOAP note would not be done on this procedure. Instead, the procedure would be recorded on a flow sheet, along with the characteristics of the returned fluid and debris.

Sample Narrative Recording
1000 ml warm Povidone-iodine douche given with the client lying in bed. Solution returned clear with a few mucous shreds.

☐ CRITICAL POINTS SUMMARY

1. Normal physiological processes alter the vaginal environment, changing the pH throughout the life cycle.
2. An acid vaginal pH and high estrogen levels help to control the growth of potentially harmful microorganisms.
3. The healthy adult vagina is self-cleansing.
4. The consistency, color, amount, and odor of vaginal discharge vary with the cause.
5. The douche must be given in the dorsal recumbent position to be effective in cleansing the vagina.

☐ LEARNING ACTIVITIES

1. Examine the ingredients in various douche preparations available in your local pharmacy. Identify the ones you believe conform to the normal physiology of the vagina.
2. Examine the various types of irrigation equipment available in local pharmacies and discount stores. Identify the advantages and disadvantages of the various types.
3. Select women from the ages of 20 to 60 to interview about their knowledge of and experiences with douches. Compare their varying levels of knowledge about douches, and their misconceptions and lack of factual information, if any. Consider what you would include in a teaching plan for them.

☐ REVIEW QUESTIONS

1. Why are vaginal irrigations used?
2. What are some of the controversial issues associated with douching?
3. What changes in the vaginal pH would you expect during menses and after menopause?
4. What factors contribute to the development of a vaginal infection?
5. What are the characteristics of a safe douche solution?
6. What precautions must be observed in giving a vaginal irrigation?
7. What equipment is needed to give a vaginal irrigation?

PROFESSIONAL CLINICAL NURSING SKILLS

☐ PERFORMANCE CHECKLIST

OBJECTIVE: To administer a vaginal irrigation safely.

CHARACTERISTIC	RANGE OF ACCEPTABILITY	SATISFACTORY	UNSATISFACTORY
1. Checks health record or kardex for nursing and medical orders.	No deviation		
2. Washes hands.	No deviation		
3. Collects equipment and supplies.	No deviation		
4. Closes door and cubicle curtains.	No deviation		
5. Explains procedure to client and places her in dorsal recumbent position.	Omit if client is familiar with procedure.		
6. Opens irrigating kit or tray using appropriate technique.	No deviation		
7. Fills irrigating bag or can with proper solution at correct temperature.	No deviation		
8. Hangs bag or can not more than 60 cm (24 in) above hips.	No deviation		
9. Drapes client with bath blanket arranged diagonally; pulls top linen down to foot of bed.	No deviation		
10. Places bedpan under buttocks.	No deviation		
11. Bends client's knees, spreads client's legs, and raises blanket to pubis.	No deviation		
12. Dons gloves and places one drape over perineal area and other on bed near client's feet.	No deviation		
13. Places douche kit or tray on drape.	No deviation		
14. Opens antibacterial solution and pours over cotton balls.	No deviation		
15. Cleanses center and each side of vulva, using one stroke from top to bottom.	No deviation		
16. Grasps nozzle and inspects for defects; lubricates with water-soluble jelly.	No deviation		
17. Opens clamp on tubing and allows a small amount of solution to flow over vulva.	No deviation		
18. Inserts nozzle gently into vagina backward and upward toward coccyx.	No deviation		
19. Slowly rotates nozzle 180 degrees moving it in and out while solution is flowing.	No deviation		
20. Withdraws nozzle when all solution is used and places it on tray; removes tray from bed.	No deviation		
21. Elevates client to sitting position.	Omit if client is unable to sit up. (Have her expel fluid by straining unless contraindicated by medical diagnosis.)		
22. Returns to flat position; dries external genitalia with tissues; discards tissues in bedpan.	No deviation		
23. Removes bedpan, dries buttocks, replaces top linen, and removes blanket; positions client for comfort.	No deviation		
24. Discards disposable equipment in impervious bag; rinses reusable equipment and returns it to central supply department.	No deviation		
25. Records client's reaction and results of procedure on health record.	No deviation		

REFERENCES

Benson RC: Handbook of Obstetrics and Gynecology, ed 4. Los Altos, CA, Lange Medical Publications, 1971.

Beyers JF: To douche or not to douche. American Family Physician 10(3):135–139, 1974.

Green TH: Gynecology: Essentials of Clinical Practice, ed 3. Boston, Little, Brown, 1977.

Hogan RM: Human Sexuality, ed 2. Norwalk, CT, Appleton-Century-Crofts, 1985.

Kaminetzky HA: Vaginal biology and the douche. Journal of the American Medical Association 191(11):154–155, 1965.

Karnaky KJ: Normal physiologic vaginal douches. American Journal of Surgery 101(4):456–462, 1961.

Kilroy PA: Feminine hygiene products—Issues and answers. Journal of Obstetrics, Gynecologic and Neonatal Nursing 6(1):37–41, 1977.

Malasanos L, Barkauskas V, et al: Health Assessment, ed 2. St Louis, MO, CV Mosby, 1981.

BIBLIOGRAPHY

Benson RC (ed): Current Obstetric and Gynecologic Diagnosis and Treatment, ed 4. Los Altos, CA, Lange Medical Publications, 1982.

Stock RJ, Stock ME, Hult JM: Vaginal douching: Current concepts and practices. Obstetrics and Gynecology 42(1):141–145, 1973.

AUDIOVISUAL RESOURCE

Vaginal Douche and Perineal Care
Filmstrip and cassette. (1970, Color, 25 min.)
Available through:
Robert J. Brady Company
Route 197
Bowie, MD 20715

SKILL 44 Breast Examination

PREREQUISITE SKILLS

Skill 19, "Inspection"
Skill 20, "Palpation"
Skill 28, "Handwashing"

☐ STUDENT OBJECTIVES

1. Explain the reasons why a breast examination should be performed.
2. Identify women who are at greater risk for developing breast cancer.
3. Differentiate the factors that influence the size and consistency of breast tissue.
4. Identify specific nonmalignant disorders of the breast.
5. Describe the characteristics of the breast that are appraised by inspection and palpation.
6. Define the terms used to describe breast masses.
7. Use the correct techniques to appraise male and female breasts.

☐ INTRODUCTION

Breast examinations are performed to detect signs and symptoms of cancer at an early stage, so that early treatment can be effective in extending life expectancy. When breast cancer is detected at an early stage, current treatment results in about an 87 percent rate of 5-year survival. But once cancer has spread to the axillary nodes, the 5-year survival rate may be reduced to 47 percent (American Cancer Society, 1984a). Breast cancer remains the leading cause of death for women. One out of every 11 women will have breast cancer during her lifetime (American Cancer Society, 1984a). Less than 1 percent of all breast cancers occur in males (Case, 1984).

Bullough (1980) reports data obtained from a 1973 Gallup survey that reveal that only 50 percent of the women in the sample had a breast examination within the previous year, and 24 percent had no breast examination by a physician for 5 years. When the respondents had visited a physician for some reason other than a breast problem, a breast examination was seldom performed. Some of the reasons why women do not practice breast self-examination include (a) lack of knowledge about the practice, (b) lack of understanding on how to perform the examination, (c) inability to remember how the breast feels from one examination to another, and (d) lack of knowledge about what abnormal tissue feels like.

The frequent contact nurses have with clients puts them in a position to have a significant impact on the early detection of breast cancer. They can do this by examining their own breasts and those of their clients and by teaching clients how to perform the examination themselves. Breast examination should be an integral part of every woman's routine health-care practices because information from the American Cancer Society (1984b) reveals that about 90 percent of breast cancers are first detected by the client. Regular breast examinations should begin in the teen years. The American Cancer Society (1984b) recommends that breast examinations be done monthly about 7 to 10 days after the beginning of the menstrual period starting at age 20. Women between the ages of 20 to 40 without symptoms of breast disease should have an examination by a physician every 3 years. In addition, women between the ages of 35 to 40 should have a baseline mammogram (breast X-ray) performed. Because of the increased risk for breast cancer associated with advancing age, after age 40 breast examinations by a physician and mammography should occur every 1 to 2 years.

Currently, there is no known method for preventing breast cancer. All women must be considered at appreciable risk for breast cancer (Seidman et al., 1983).

☐ PREPARATION

CHARACTERISTICS OF NORMAL BREASTS

The Female Breast
Heredity, nutrition, and individual sensitivity to hormones influence breast size. In the female, it is normal for the left breast to be slightly larger than the right. The largest amount of breast tissue occurs in the upper outer quadrant of the breast, and some of this tissue extends into the axilla. The portion of glandular breast tissue located in the axillary area is referred to as the axillary tail of Spence. About half of all breast cancers develop in the upper outer and axillary tail tissue (Case, 1984). Breasts vary in size, shape, and consistency during the menstrual cycle, pregnancy, and lactation. They are normally smallest during the 4th to 7th days of the menstrual cycle. In many women they are largest during the 3rd to 5th days before the onset of menses, and it is during this time that the breasts become full, tense, and tender. In pregnancy and lactation, the breasts may become two to three times their normal size.

In young women the breasts tend to be firm, somewhat elastic, and cone shaped with the border clearly delineated. In pregnancy they are firmer and larger, and the lobules become more distinct, making it confusing to differentiate them from masses. In older women after menopause, the breasts develop an irregular consistency, the sharp borders disappear, and large breasts may become pendulous. The breast form becomes flattened and flabby, because the glandular tissue atrophies and the proportion of fatty tissue increases. Breasts sag and become pendulous because of the loss of elasticity in *Cooper's ligaments* (Martin, 1978).

In young females the normal color of the areola is pink, but after the 2nd month of the first pregnancy the color changes permanently to brown. One or both nipples may become inverted in puberty. When inversion occurs later in life, it is due to retraction of the tissue; this is abnormal and should be investigated.

The Male Breast
The normal male breast consists of scattered ducts with strands of collagenous tissue for support.

CHARACTERISTICS OF BREAST MASSES

Breast masses are described according to the location, size, and other characteristics of the lesion, the presence of tenderness, and the retraction of tissue over the mass.

The *location* of a lesion is described by identifying the quadrant in which it is found, that is, upper outer, lower outer, upper inner, and lower inner. The findings can be communicated more precisely when the narrative description of a lesion includes a circular diagram of the breast divided into quadrants (with the areola and nipple in the centers) as in Figure 44-1. The *size* of the lesion is approximated in all of its dimensions in centimeters. The lesions may be multiple or single. Multiple lesions may be separate or matted together.

The *shape* of a lesion may be round, oval, or irregular. The *consistency* may be hard and solid, or soft. The lesion borders are described in terms of *discreteness;* that is, the borders may be sharply defined or may be encapsulated with discrete borders or indiscrete and nonencapsulated with borders. The lesion may be fixed or may have some degree of movement with palpation. This is referred to as *mobility*. *Erythema* may be present in the skin over the lesion; *tenderness* may be elicited during palpation. When retraction is present, breast tissue is dimpled or has a depression because Cooper's ligament is shortened.

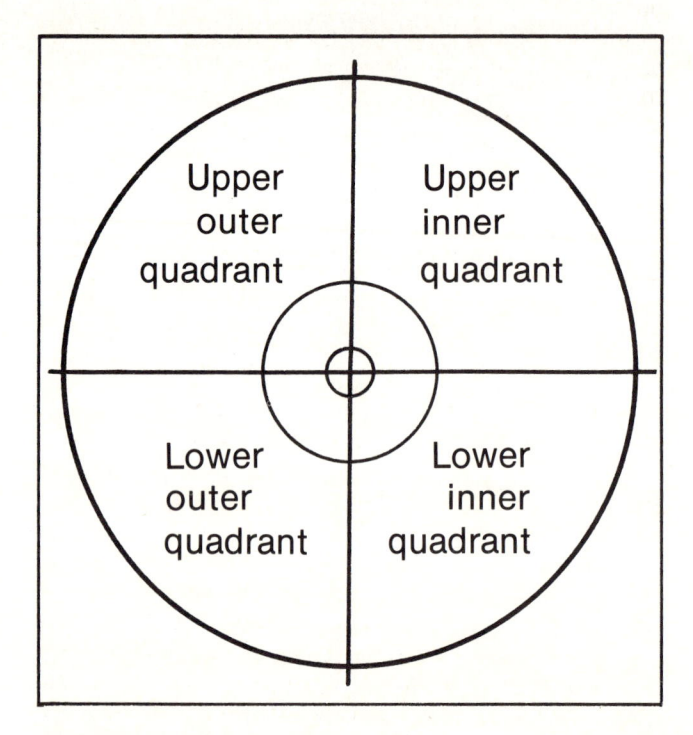

Figure 44-1. Diagram of the four quadrants of the right breast.

Retraction of tissue over the mass may be elicited when the skin over the lesion is squeezed together.

BENIGN CONDITIONS OF THE BREASTS

It is important for the nurse and the client to know that there are several benign (noncancerous) conditions of the female breast that need to be differentiated from malignant disease (cancer). These conditions may cause tenderness, lumps, or discharge. Some of these conditions are fibrocystic disease, fibroadenoma, breast abscess, fat necrosis, warty growths in a duct, mastitis, and chronic mastitis.

Certain medications such as estrogens, some antihypertensive drugs, and some tranquilizers can cause breast pain, tenderness, irregular swelling, and secretions from the nipples (Green, 1977). Therefore questions about the type of medications that are being taken should be asked when interviewing the client. When the breasts secrete fluid other than during pregnancy or lactation, it may be caused by mechanical stimulation, drugs, disorders of the hypothalamus or pituitary glands, or benign or malignant tumors.

In males, breast tissue may be increased enough to look like female breasts. This is known as *gynecomastia* and may be present in one or both breasts. The breast tissue is smooth, firm, and mobile, and is located under the areola. Gynecomastia can be caused by a large amount of fatty tissue in the breasts or by systemic disease that alters the level of estrogens and promotes the development of breast tissue. Other causes of gynecomastia include familial trait, drugs such as digitalis, or gonadal disorders. Temporary gynecomastia is normal in about 50 percent of males at puberty.

When the nurse detects a lump in a client's breast, or discovers a nipple discharge that is not due to pregnancy or lactation and that was previously unknown to the client or the physician, it is important that the client be examined promptly by a physician, so that the cause of the abnormality can be diagnosed.

DATA BASE

Client History and Recorded Data

When a nurse is caring for a client who has been admitted for reasons other than a breast problem, information about the breasts is obtained during the admission interview or while discussing routine hygiene practices. If a breast examination was included with the client's physical examination, the results of the examination are available on the health record.

In seeking information about the breasts, the nurse finds out if the client has had a breast examination by a professional, how often, and whether the client knows how to examine her own breasts and how frequently she does this. These are points that the nurse should include during the interview, so that an appropriate teaching plan can be developed. It is also important to question the client about the presence of any discharge from the nipples, masses in the breasts, and any tenderness, pain, or discomfort.

Physical Appraisal Skills

During the appraisal, the nurse must keep in mind the client's age, weight, and stage of menstrual cycle or pregnancy, because these factors significantly influence both the size and consistency of the breasts.

Inspection. The client must be uncovered to the waist to permit complete inspection. A good light source is essential so that shadows will not distort the appearance of the breasts. This aspect of the examination is best performed with the client sitting on the side of the bed or examining table. Observations include the symmetry of the shape and size of the breasts, and the color of the skin. Note any area of local erythema, hyperpigmentation, moles, or nevi. If edema is present, the pores of the skin will be more pronounced and the skin will look like the texture of an orange peel. Inspect the areolar size, shape, symmetry, and color; the nipple size, shape, and color; and the presence of any discharge or lesions. Discharges from the breast may be milky, watery, purulent, serous, or bloody. If the breasts are symmetrical, the nipples should point in the same direction. Asymmetry in the size and position of the breasts may be due to developmental differences or may indicate an abnormality such as a mass or inflammation.

Palpation. All of the tissue palpation in a breast examination is done with the palmar surfaces of the index and middle fingers held together, moving gently in a smooth back-and-forth direction or a circular direction.

First to be palpated are the accessible lymph nodes that lie within the axillary area. These lymph nodes are a major component of the lymph drainage system of the breasts and therefore are of clinical significance, because cancer development and the spread of cancer disease cells occurs along the lymph vessels to the lymph nodes. The areolar areas of the breasts are palpated next to detect the presence of any underlying mass, and the nipples are gently squeezed to detect the presence of any masses or discharge. After palpating the areolar area, procede to finish palpating all of the remaining breast tissue.

When a client reports having a breast mass, the nurse appraises the opposite breast first, so that a baseline is established before the abnormal breast is palpated.

EQUIPMENT

The only equipment required for a breast examination is a good light source, a bed or examining table, and a bath blanket or sheet. If the client has large breasts, a small pillow, folded sheet, or blanket is placed under the shoulder during palpation.

☐ EXECUTION

Breast examination is performed with the client's chest bare; therefore, it is essential that privacy be ensured during the appraisal. The nurse must keep in mind that clients have widely varying degrees of comfort about their bodies, and that some may view breast examination as an invasion into a very private and intimate body area. Assessing the client's attitude prior to initiating the appraisal helps the nurse to select an acceptable approach. Explaining the purpose of each maneuver during the appraisal not only helps to put the client at ease, but also helps the client understand the rationale for each aspect of the examination. This explanation can also serve as the basis for teaching self breast examination.

During the inspection phase of the appraisal, have the client sit on the side of the bed or examining table. A complete visual appraisal requires that the client assume four different positions. Three of these positions involve maneuvers with the arms that create a tension on Cooper's ligaments which permit early detection of retraction of breast tissue. Stand in front of the client as she sits with her arms resting at the sides. First conduct a general inspection for symmetry of the size and shape of the breasts, the color of the skin, and the presence or absence of changes previously described. Then have her abduct her arms over the top of the head as shown in Figure 44-2. This position permits observation of upward movement of the breasts which can be restricted due to loss of function of the suspensory ligaments. Next have the client push with both hands against the hips to elicit contraction of the pectoral muscles. This maneuver permits detection of any dimpling in the breast that may result from either an infiltrated mass or shortened suspensory ligaments. Finally, have her lean forward to permit the breasts to move outward away from the body. Leaning forward provides an additional opportunity to note changes that might be created by restriction of the suspensory ligaments. Support her in this position if necessary to prevent her from falling forward.

Palpate the axilla first to detect the presence of any enlarged lymph nodes. This is done best with the client seated as for inspection. When palpating the lymph nodes in the axillae, Malasanos et al. (1981, p. 283) suggest that the nurse consider each axilla as a four-sided pyramid, so that each lymph node area will be thoroughly palpated. Figure 44-3 shows the area encompassed in the axillary pyramid. Beginning at 12 o'clock and moving in a clockwise direction, the sides of the pyramid to be systematically palpated are: the upper part of the humerus for the brachial axillary nodes; the edge of the pectoralis major muscle for the mammary nodes; the thoracic wall for the intermediate nodes; and the anterior edge of the latissimus dorsi muscle for the subscapular nodes. Sana and Judge (1975) recommend that each group of lymph nodes also be palpated with the arm placed in all positions that encompass complete range of motion, so the nodes that might be hidden by muscle or fat can be detected. To keep the client relaxed for maximum evaluation of the tissues on the four sides of the pyramid, support the arm on the side being palpated. This is done by holding the arm away from the chest wall with one hand while the other hand is palpating the lymph nodes. Use the palmar surface of the fingers with a gentle but firm massaging motion, moving the hand across the skin to cover the skin in each separate area. To appraise the lymph nodes that might be hidden by muscle or fat, use one hand to support the arm and move it toward the head, then down and across the chest, and then back toward the scapula. At the

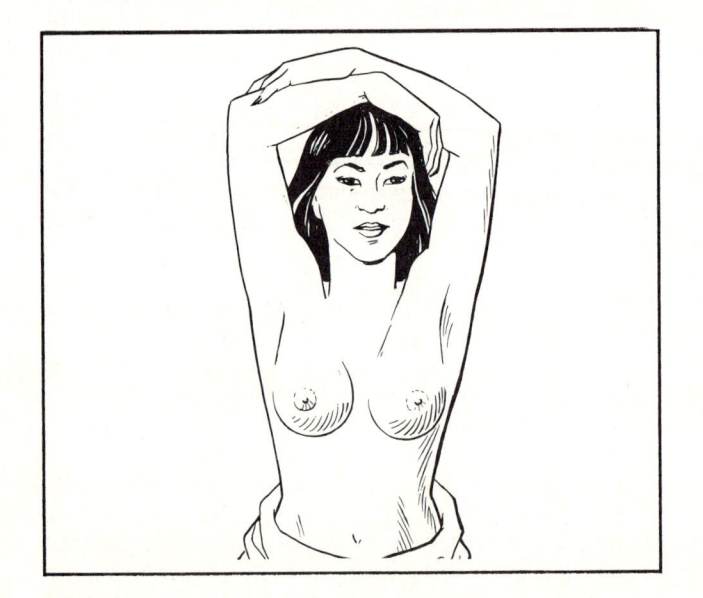

Figure 44-2. Inspection of the breasts with the arms raised over the head. This position places tension on the suspensory ligaments and permits early detection of tissue retraction.

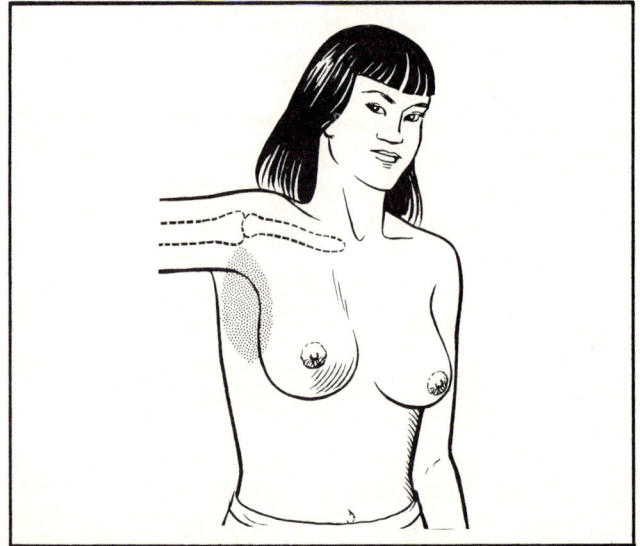

Figure 44-3. Area within the axillary pyramid that is palpated for enlarged lymph nodes.

same time, use the other hand to palpate the lymph nodes on each side of the axilla.

Although breast tissue is normally palpated in the supine (lying) position, there are special circumstances that call for palpation to be done while the client is sitting and then again while supine. These include the examination of women who have complaints of masses and women with pendulous breasts. To palpate breasts in the sitting position use a bimanual technique: place one hand under the breast to support the tissue, and the other hand on top to palpate the tissue against the underlying hand. When a client has pendulous breasts this method ensures that all of the breast tissue is adequately appraised. Figure 44-4 depicts bimanual palpation.

To palpate the breasts with the client in the supine position, raise the arm on the side to be appraised and place the client's hand at the back of her neck. This flattens and spreads the breast tissue over the rib cage. When the client has large breasts, place a small pillow under the shoulder of the side being examined. This helps to distribute the tissue toward the center of the chest wall. Slightly abduct the upper arm to permit palpation of the axillary area of the breast. Begin by palpating the areolar area of the breast to detect the presence of any underlying mass, and gently squeeze the nipples to detect the presence of any masses or discharge. When a discharge is expressed from the nipple, each lobe of the breast must be milked along its radii to determine the lobe producing the discharge. When the appropriate lobe is milked, the discharge will drain from the nipple. Figure 44-5 depicts the palpation technique with the client in the supine position.

There is no specific starting point for palpating the remaining breast tissue, but it is best for each nurse to develop a systematic method that will be

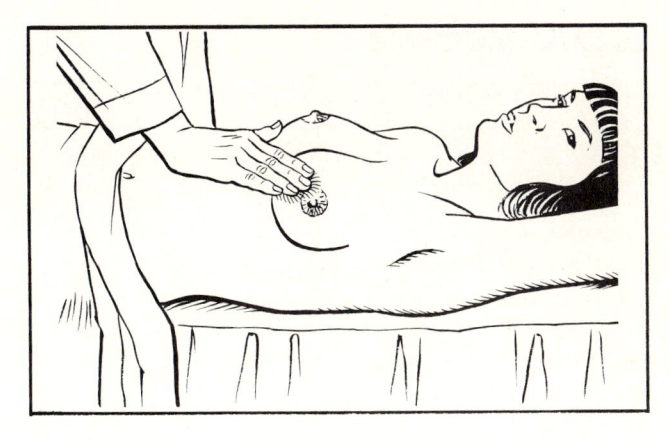

Figure 44-5. Palpation of the breast with the client in the supine position.

used for each appraisal. Malasanos et al. (1981) suggest that the breast be viewed either as having a series of concentric circles or as a bicycle wheel with six to eight spokes that divide it into areas for appraisal. Whichever approach is used, palpate each imaginary line to ensure covering the entire breast. It is important that the upper outer quadrant and the axillary area be given particular attention. If a mass is detected during palpation, pinch the tissue over the mass to determine if retraction is present.

MALE BREAST EXAMINATION

The same technique used to examine the female breast is used also for the male breast, with some minor adaptations appropriate for the amount of breast tissue present. The majority of male breast cancers occur in the areolar area, so special attention should be taken with this area.

TEACHING BREAST SELF-EXAMINATION

Prior to teaching a client breast self-examination (BSE), the nurse needs to know if and how often the client examines her own breasts and what types of questions or concerns she might have about the procedure. This information should be incorporated into the teaching plan. A breast simulation model can be used to supplement BSE instruction.

The procedure for breast self-examination recommended by the American Cancer Society (1975) is slightly modified from that used by the professional and is divided into three stages: one inspection stage and two palpation stages. Inspection is performed in front of a mirror and in good light. Palpation of the axillae and breasts is done in the shower or bathtub while the body is wet, and then again while supine on a bed. In the shower or bathtub, one arm is elevated and the hand held behind the head, while the opposite hand palpates all areas of the first axilla and then the

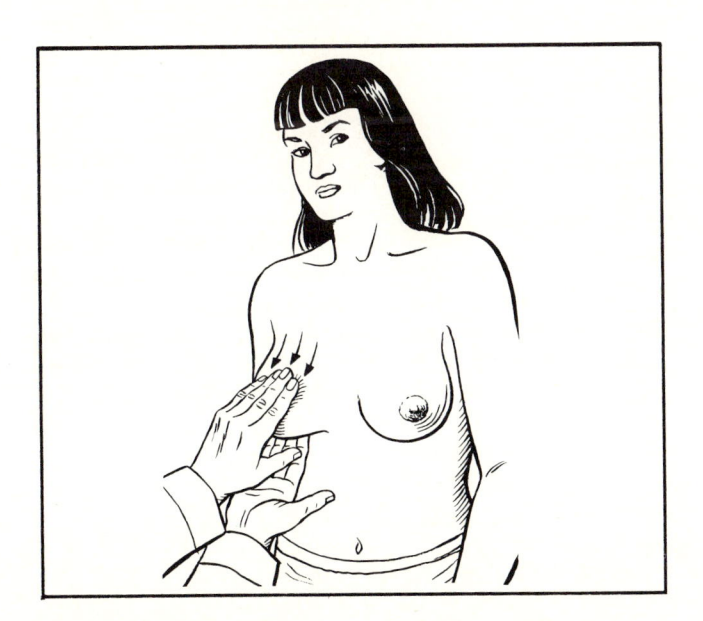

Figure 44-4. Palpating the breast in a sitting position, using the bimanual technique.

SKILL SEQUENCE

BREAST EXAMINATIONS

Step	Rationale
1. Wash hands.	Prevents cross-contamination from microorganisms on hands.
2. Explain procedure to client.	Allays anxiety; provides opportunity for discussion.
3. Close door and cubicle curtains.	Prevents drafts and chills, and provides privacy.
4. Remove clothing from client's upper body.	Chest must be fully exposed for appraisal.
5. Have client sit on edge of bed or examining table.	
6. With client's arms resting at sides, inspect breasts for symmetry, size, and shape. Note color and presence of erythema, lesions, and edema. Note characteristics of areolae and nipples.	May reveal differences in breasts; may alert nurse to specific areas needing special attention.
7. Have client raise arms straight up above head. Note any areas of retraction.	Retraction is revealed with pull exerted on Cooper's ligaments.
8. Have client push hands forcibly against sides of hips, or put hands together and push against them.	Retraction is revealed with pull exerted on Cooper's ligaments.
9. Abduct arm away from body and palpate each side of axillary pyramid, while holding arm with one hand.	Facilitates palpating axillary lymph nodes.
10. Shift client's arm position to above head, across chest, and back toward scapula, and examine axillary pyramid in each position.	Permits access to deep lymph nodes.
11. Have client assume supine position on bed or examining table. Place a small pillow under shoulder on side to be palpated, if breasts are large. Raise client's arm and place hand at back of neck on side to be examined.	Shifts breast tissue toward center of chest and flattens it against chest wall.
12. Establish image in your mind of breast as concentric circles or a bicycle wheel with six to eight spokes.	Establishes landmarks for systematic palpation of breasts.
13. Place the fingers of palpating hand together and use palmar surface to palpate all areas of breast tissue. Include axillary tail in upper outer quadrant.	
14. Palpate areola and compress nipple. (NOTE: If discharge is expressed from nipple, milk each lobe along its radii until discharge source is identified.)	Common area of cancer in males.
15. Palpate opposite breast in same manner.	
16. Record findings on the health record.	Nurse is accountable for reporting actions and findings.

breast. While lying down, a small pillow is placed under the shoulder on the side being examined; both the axillae and breasts are again palpated.

Although the American Cancer Society recommends that breast self-examination be performed once a month during the week following the menstrual period, many women may remember to adopt the practice if it is done more often. Associating the examination with a weekly practice such as shampoo or manicure helps the client become more familiar with the normal changes that occur in the breasts throughout the month, and also helps the client remember what each breast feels like when it is normally its smallest and its largest, and makes the examination part of a client's hygienic routine (Howe, 1981).

If a client finds a lump or dimple or has a discharge, it is important that the client know that a physician should be promptly contacted, so that a more complete investigation can be conducted. Not all lumps or discharges are a sign of cancer, and a physician will be able to make the differentiation.

RECORDING

The normal and abnormal findings of a breast examination are entered on the health record, as well as the amount of teaching that has been completed and that which remains to be done.

When a mass has been identified, include a drawing showing each quadrant of the breast (or breasts), as shown in Figure 44-1. Indicate the location of the mass on the drawing, and label the breasts in the drawing as right and left. Also include a narrative description of the characteristics of the lesion itself.

Sample POR Recordings
- S—"I want to learn how to examine my own breasts."
- O—Attentive and asked questions while nurse performed exam.
- A—Interested in learning SBE.
- P—Help to do own exam tomorrow and repeat until she is comfortable.

- S—NA
- O—Breasts pendulous; no tissue retraction; axillary nodes not palpable. Breasts firm, nontender; no masses felt; no discharge from nipples.
- A—Normal breasts.
- P—No interventions needed.

Sample Narrative Recording

Breast exam included as part of bath. Breasts pendulous; no tissue retraction; axillary nodes nonpalpable. Breasts firm, nontender; no masses felt; no discharge from nipples. Wants to learn BSE. Method reviewed today; will begin BSE tomorrow and repeat until she is comfortable with technique.

CRITICAL POINTS SUMMARY

1. One in every eleven women will have breast cancer during her lifetime.
2. Ninety percent of all women with breast cancer detect the lesion themselves.
3. Less than 1 percent of all breast cancers occur in men.
4. A breast examination should be performed at least once a year by a professional and monthly by each woman, beginning in the teen years.
5. Inspection can reveal changes in the symmetry, size, and color of the breasts.
6. Palpation of the axillary nodes helps detect lymph-node involvement and is an essential part of a complete breast examination.
7. Palpation of breast tissue is done in a systematic manner that includes the axillary tail of Spence.
8. Teaching a client breast self-examination should be an integral part of every professional breast examination.
9. Not all lumps, dimples, and discharges are caused by cancer.
10. To be complete, a recording of abnormal findings in breast tissue should include a diagram that shows the location of the mass.

LEARNING ACTIVITIES

1. Examine your own breasts at different times during the month to determine normal changes.
2. Use a Betsy Breast simulation model to practice palpating the breasts and to become familiar with different types of lesions.
3. Interview hospitalized women and men who have had benign and malignant breast disorders to determine how the disorders were identified.

REVIEW QUESTIONS

1. Why should the breasts be examined?
2. Which women are at greatest risk to develop breast cancer?
3. What are the factors that influence the size and consistency of the breasts?
4. What are some of the benign conditions found in the breasts?
5. What characteristics of the breasts are noted by inspection? by palpation?
6. How would you describe a breast mass in a health record?
7. What would you include in a teaching plan for breast self-examination?

PERFORMANCE CHECKLIST

OBJECTIVE: To appraise the breasts accurately and completely.

CHARACTERISTIC	RANGE OF ACCEPTABILITY	SATISFACTORY	UNSATISFACTORY
1. Washes hands.	No deviation		
2. Explains procedure to client.	No deviation		
3. Closes door and cubicle curtains.	No deviation		
4. Removes clothing from upper body.	No deviation		
5. Has client sit on edge of bed or examining table.	No deviation		
6. Inspects breasts for symmetry, size, shape, skin color, and presence of erythema, lesions, and edema; notes characteristics of areolae and nipples.	No deviation		
7. Has client raise arms above head and notes areas of retraction.	No deviation		
8. Has client push hands forcibly against side of hips or put hands together and push against them.	No deviation		

(continued)

OBJECTIVE: To appraise the breasts accurately and completely (cont.).			
CHARACTERISTIC	RANGE OF ACCEPTABILITY	SATISFACTORY	UNSATISFACTORY
9. Palpates each side of axillary pyramid while holding client's abducted arm.	No deviation		
10. Moves arm into range of motion positions for additional palpation of axillary pyramid.	No deviation		
11. Has client assume supine position; places small pillow under shoulder if breasts are large.	No deviation Omit if breasts are small.		
12. Raises client's arm and places hand at back of neck.	No deviation		
13. Palpates all areas of breast tissue systematically.	No deviation		
14. Palpates areola and squeezes nipple.	No deviation		
15. Palpates opposite breast in same manner.	No deviation		
16. Records findings on health record.	No deviation		

REFERENCES

American Cancer Society: How to Examine Your Breasts. American Cancer Society, 777 Third Ave, New York, NY 10017, 1975.

American Cancer Society: Cancer 1984 Facts and Figures. American Cancer Society, 777 Third Ave, New York, NY 10017, 1984a.

American Cancer Society: Facts on Breast Cancer. American Cancer Society, 777 Third Ave, New York, NY 10017, 1984b.

Bullough B: Discovery of the first signs and symptoms of breast cancer. Nurse Practitioner 5(6):31–47, 1980.

Case C (ed): The Breast Cancer Digest, ed 2. (NIH Publication No. 84-1691). National Cancer Institute, U.S. Department of Health and Human Services, Public Health Service, National Institutes of Health, Bethesda, MD, 1984.

Green TH: Gynecology: Essentials of Clinical Practice, ed 3. Boston, Little, Brown, 1977.

Howe HL: Enhancing the effectiveness of media messages promoting regular breast self-examination. Public Health Reports 96(2):134–142, 1981.

Malasanos L, Barkaukas V, et al: Health Assessment, ed 2. St. Louis, MO, CV Mosby, 1981.

Martin LL: Health Care of Women. Philadelphia, JB Lippincott, 1978.

Sana J, Judge R: Physical Appraisal Methods in Nursing Practice. Boston, Little, Brown, 1975.

Seidman H, Stellman SD, Mushinski MH: A different perspective on breast cancer risk factors: Some implications of the nonattributable risk. Reprinted from A Cancer Journal for Clinicians 32(5), 1982. In Professional Education Publications, American Cancer Society, 777 Third Ave, New York, NY 10017, 1983.

BIBLIOGRAPHY

King RC: Detailed guidelines for a thorough examination of the breast. RN 45(7):57–63, 1982.

Turnbull E: Prevention: Breast examination practices. American Journal of Nursing 77(9):1450–1451, 1977.

AUDIOVISUAL RESOURCES

How to Examine Your Breasts
Film (16mm). (1975, Color, 7 min.)
Available through:
American Cancer Society
777 Third Avenue
New York, NY 10017

Examination of the Breasts and Axillae
Videorecording (3/4 in.) (1974, Color, 6 min.)
Available through:
JB Lippincott Company
227 South 6th Street
Philadelphia, PA 19148

Male Breasts: Examination Techniques & Procedures
Videorecording (3/4 in.) (1978, Color, 4 min.)
Available through:
Medical Electronic Educational Services
954 West Grant
Tucson, AZ 85705

Teaching Self-Examination of the Breasts
Slides with cassette. (1975, Color, 20 min.)
Available through:
University of Michigan
School of Nursing
Ann Arbor, MI 48109

SKILL 45 Care of the Corpse

PREREQUISITE SKILL

Skill 65, "Transfer Activities"

☐ STUDENT OBJECTIVES

1. Describe the purpose of care of the corpse.
2. Identify the activities associated with care of the corpse.
3. Explain the physiological changes that occur in the body after death.
4. Describe the ways in which the nurse can comfort the survivors of the deceased.
5. Identify the health record forms that must be completed upon the death of a client.
6. Specify the information the nurse needs to obtain upon the death of a client.
7. Describe the steps involved in providing care to the corpse.
8. Provide care to the corpse in a dignified manner.

☐ INTRODUCTION

Care of the corpse (postmortem care) is given after the client has been pronounced dead by a physician. The purpose of giving care to the deceased client is to help preserve the appearance of the corpse by keeping the tissues in the best possible condition. There are several important activities that the nurse must perform in connection with the death of a client that are considered part of this skill, although they are not directly related to the care of the corpse. These include preparing the deceased for viewing by the survivors, comforting the survivors, collecting and protecting all of the deceased's personal possessions, and assembling the health record forms required at death.

☐ PREPARATION

It is generally the nurse's responsibility to notify the physician of the death of a client, so that an examination can be done to confirm the death. Death occurs when all bodily tissues cease to function. Under normal circumstances, the complete absence of cardiac and respiratory activity indicates that death has occurred. However, there are some circumstances in which the usual indicators of death are inadequate. These include situations in which the client had been maintained on life-support systems such as mechanical ventilators or cardiac pacemakers, or in which the client is a victim of near drowning. For example, for a client who has been sustained on a mechanical ventilator, the absence of respiratory activity could not be used as a criterion for death because the ventilator is breathing for the client. Similarly, the cardiac pacemaker causes the heart to beat. Persons who are victims of near drowning may have both respiratory and cardiac functions so depressed that they are not apparent. To determine death for persons in these situations, the physician must use different criteria and conduct supplementary examinations. These examinations may include serial tests to detect the presence of sensory and motor responses to stimuli, observations to detect spontaneous respiratory activity and reflex activity, and electroencephalograms to determine the presence of brain life (DeGowin and DeGowin, 1981). Nurses must be aware of the policies for such situations that are in use by the institution where they practice nursing.

THE PHYSIOLOGICAL CHANGES IN DEATH

Pennington (1978) describes how the physiological changes that occur in death provide the rationale for the actions included in care of the corpse.

Algor Mortis

The first change that occurs after death, *algor mortis*, is the loss of heat from the corpse as it gradually cools to the environmental temperature. This cooling begins after circulation stops and the center for temperature control in the hypothalamus no longer functions. Cooling progresses at an approximate rate of 1°C (1.8°F) per hour depending on the amount of insulation provided by adipose tissue, the amount and type of clothing worn, and whether the corpse has been immersed in water or exposed to a warm or cool environment. As the corpse temperature approaches that of the environment, it feels cool to the touch. Because this may be stressful for the survivors, the nurse should prepare them for the change. The skin of the deceased loses its elasticity when the corpse is cool and may be easily torn or damaged by slight trauma induced by such activities as removing adhesive tape.

Livor Mortis

The second change, *livor mortis*, begins within about 2 to 3 hours after death. Red blood cells break down and hemoglobin is released into the surrounding tissues. This causes the skin on the gravity-dependent areas of the body to become mottled or bruised, and the body may have the appearance of having been beaten. Recognition of this condition as a normal change is important so that it is not misinterpreted. Where the cause of death is unknown or where foul play is suspected, the changes associated with livor mortis need to be differentiated from abuse. Cases of Sudden Infant Death Syndrome (SIDS) can sometimes be interpreted by health or legal workers as abuse, causing unnecessary additional problems for the grieving family.

Rigor Mortis
The third change, *rigor mortis,* begins 2 to 4 hours after death. The absence of the enzyme adenosine triphosphate (ATP), which is responsible for relaxation of the muscle fibers, results in muscle contraction, causing immobilization of the body joints. The process of muscle contraction begins first in the involuntary muscles of the heart, arteries, gastrointestinal tract, and bladder, and then progresses in sequence to the voluntary muscles of the head, neck, trunk, and lower extremities. The maximum rigidity of the muscles is achieved in 48 hours, when usually the corpse is with the mortician. When all of the chemical activity in the muscles is exhausted, the stiffness begins to recede.

COMFORTING THE SURVIVORS

The nurse's actions can influence the way in which the survivors will cope with loss, and can help make that loss more bearable. Rinear (1975) suggests that the nurse listen to the survivors carefully, in order to understand and attempt to meet their needs. Small acts of kindness, such as providing the survivors with privacy, helping them to make phone calls, and permitting them to spend time with the deceased while the corpse is still warm, whenever possible, can be valuable. The survivors may want to have a report of the deceased's last moments and hear of any last words spoken. However, it is inappropriate for the nurse to tell the survivors about any pain and discomfort experienced by the deceased before death. Survivors obtain a great deal of comfort when the nurse acknowledges the help and support the survivors gave to the deceased prior to death. When the nurse also experiences a sense of personal loss, sharing this with the survivors can help to affirm the dignity and worth of the deceased.

DEATH PAPERS

There are several forms that need to be completed when a client dies. Those that must be completed by the physician include the death certificate, request for postmortem examination, and gift of the corpse to a state anatomic board if applicable; however, the nurse may be expected to have these forms available and to enter the client's name and other identifying information on them. The nurse is usually responsible for ensuring that the form for the release of the corpse to the mortuary is completed and signed by the mortician when the corpse is taken from the room.

DATA BASE

Client History and Recorded Data
When the client is pronounced dead by the physician, the nurse needs to find out if there are any specific wishes of the deceased or the survivors that must be attended to promptly. Information concerning the nature of these wishes may be written on the health record or the kardex, or the nurse may have to ask the survivors if they are present. These directives include contacting survivors or persons of religious or cultural significance, or making plans for organ donations. Persons of religious or cultural significance to the deceased and the survivors can provide a great deal of support and comfort, so it is important that the nurse not overlook this means of helping the survivors. In the event that the deceased has donated specific body organs to an organ bank, that agency must be contacted so that the appropriate procedures may be implemented to preserve the viability of the organs. Information regarding organ donation is frequently not available on the health record or the kardex. The nurse may need to ask the survivors, search the deceased's wallet for a donor card, or check the deceased's driver's license to find this information.

EQUIPMENT

Shroud packs usually include the following:

1. A plastic, waterproof shroud sheet that is used to wrap the corpse.
2. Ties to secure the extremities and the shroud.
3. A chin strap, which is a piece of fabric with two pairs of strings attached, used to keep the mouth closed.
4. Two large pads that are used to wrap the ankles and wrists to keep the ties from cutting or damaging the skin.

Shroud packs are available in child, adult, and extra large sizes.

If the corpse is to be cleansed for viewing by the family or transferred to the mortician or morgue, the nurse also needs to collect equipment for bathing and give a partial bath prior to opening the shroud pack.

☐ EXECUTION

Before beginning care of the corpse, the nurse closes the cubicle curtains or the room door to provide privacy for others in the area. The nurse needs to find out if the deceased's survivors are present or will be arriving within a short time, in order to plan the work of preparing the corpse for viewing by the family and subsequent transfer to the morgue or mortician. Whenever possible, it is best to do these activities while the corpse is in the stage of algor mortis, so that the tissues receive minimal damage. The corpse is placed in the cool environment of the morgue refrigerator as soon as possible, to maintain the tissues in the best possible condition. Cooling retards the progress of the physiological changes of death.

To prepare for viewing by the family, the nurse partially bathes the corpse, closes the eyes and mouth, grooms the hair, places a pillow under the head and arranges the corpse in the bed as if asleep, and provides clean top linen. When time permits, remove any equipment used to provide care before death such as intravenous solutions, pacemakers, or oxygen therapy. If this is not possible, move them away from the deceased to permit the survivors access to the deceased. Catheters and tubes inserted into external orifices and tracheostomy tubes can be removed. Prosthetic devices such as dentures are usually removed, placed in a container, and labeled with the deceased's full name and identification number. Institutional policy may direct that they be enclosed with the shroud or given to the mortician. Drains and catheters inserted into surgical incisions are usually left in place. They will be removed either by the pathologist during a postmortem examination or by the mortician. Cover open wounds with dry dressings. Remove all nonessential dressings and adhesive tape. The hospital identification bracelet is left on the corpse.

COLLECTING THE VALUABLES

It is imperative that all of the deceased's personal possessions be handled with care to prevent loss or damage. Collect all of the items and label them with an identification tag that includes the deceased's full name, identification number, age, and the date. If a survivor assembles the personal possessions, the nurse inventories all of the items collected before they are removed. Valuables are not to be left unattended in the room; they are either kept in the nurses' office or sent to the institution's registrar office. All possessions are listed on the health record in an inventory manner. The deceased's personal possessions include all jewelry, prostheses, eyeglasses, cards, letters, religious articles, clothing, plants, and food. Rambo and Wood (1982) suggest that rings that cannot be removed because they are too tight be padded with cotton if they have stones and then taped in place on the finger. A description of the ring and the action taken with it is then entered on the health record. If the survivors take the deceased's possessions from the nurse, their names are noted on the health record.

SHROUDING AND TRANSFERRING THE CORPSE

Since legal and mortuary procedures vary from area to area, the specific procedures need to be determined. The following procedure is generally acceptable for care after death; it is done after the survivors have viewed the deceased. First, place sterile pads over the eyes and secure them in place with a bandage to preserve the tissue in the event that they will be used for

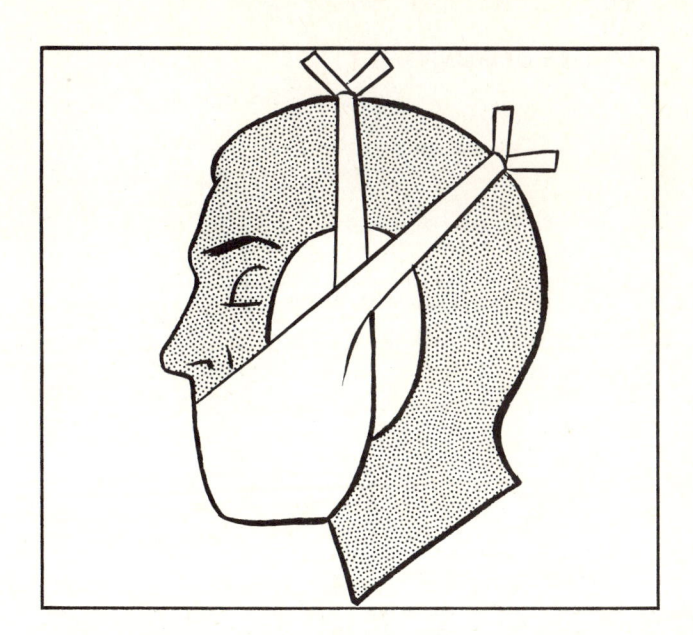

Figure 45–1. The chin strap is placed under the jaw and the ties are crossed over the top of the head and secured.

an organ transplant. When it is known that the eyes have been donated to an eye bank, the information is recorded on the release to the mortuary form. To prevent the extremities from falling away from the body during transfer to the stretcher, pad the wrists and ankles with large cotton pads and tie together. If the jaw will not stay closed, place the chin strap under the jaw and cross the ties over the top of the head and secure them as shown in Figure 45–1. Attach an identification tag to the wrists or ankles. Wrap the corpse completely in the shroud, and tie the shroud in place. Attach another identification tag to the outside of the shroud as shown in Figure 45–2.

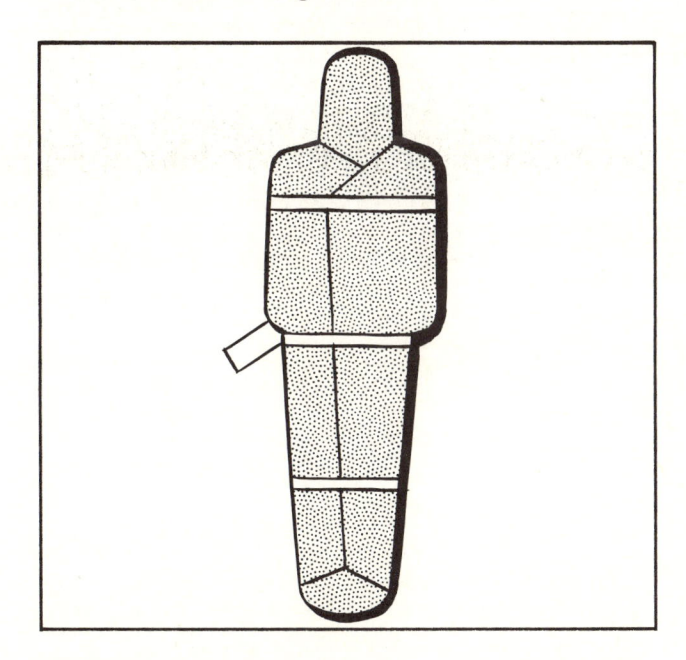

Figure 45–2. The shroud is tied in place, and an identification tag is attached to the outside.

SKILL SEQUENCE

CARE OF THE CORPSE

Step	Rationale
1. Verify that client has been pronounced dead by a physician.	Avoids premature preparation of the corpse.
2. Collect equipment and supplies. Write all required information on three identification tags.	Prevents delays in procedure.
3. Close door and cubicle curtains.	Provides privacy for others in same room or general vicinity.
4. Elevate bed to high position and place it in flat position.	Facilitates good body mechanics for care-giver.
5. Position corpse in supine position. Close eyes. Replace dentures if required by agency policy. Close mouth.	Corpse is placed in good alignment before rigor mortis occurs.
6. Prepare deceased for viewing:	
a. Remove tubes and catheters from external orifices. Leave all surgical drains and tubes in place.	Makes deceased more presentable. Important for postmortem examination.
b. Remove all jewelry and prosthetic devices. Wrap and tape rings that cannot be removed.	Protects valuables from loss or damage.
c. Bathe corpse with clear water; pat skin dry. Groom hair.	Makes deceased more presentable.
d. Place a clean gown on corpse.	Makes deceased more presentable.
e. Place one pillow under head; use clean linen on top of bed if necessary.	Makes deceased more presentable.
f. Remove equipment from room.	Provides room for survivors.
7. Assemble and inventory all personal possessions and list them on health record. Attach a completed identification tag. Indicate to whom the personal possessions are given.	Prevents liability for lost valuables. Possessions may be taken by survivors, kept in nursing office, or taken to registrar's office.
8. Prepare corpse for shrouding:	
a. Place a chin strap under jaw, cross ties over top of head, and tie securely.	Keeps mouth closed.
b. Cover eyes with sterile pads and secure in place with bandages according to agency policy.	Preserves eyes for future use.
c. Remove all casts, nonessential dressings, and adhesive tape.	May be done when corpse is prepared for viewing if time permits.
d. Cover open or draining wounds with dry dressings. Place gauze or abdominal pads over vagina, urethra, and rectum if leakage of secretions occurs.	Prevents soilage of corpse. Relaxation of muscle sphincters permits leakage.
e. Wrap pads around wrists, place arms over abdomen, and tie them together.	Prevents tissue damage from ties. Holds arms close to body, preventing them from falling during transfer.
f. Wrap pads around ankles then tie them together.	Keeps legs from separating during transfer.
g. Attach one identification tag to wrists or ankles according to agency policy.	Prevents mistaken identity of corpse.
9. Shroud corpse:	
a. Turn corpse on the side away from care-giver.	Good body mechanics help prevent injury to care-giver.
b. Place opened shroud flat on bed, parallel to corpse.	
c. Roll corpse back onto shroud.	
d. Turn corpse toward care-giver and pull shroud across bed to opposite side of corpse.	
e. Wrap shroud around head and body, secure with ties, tape, or pins.	Keeps shroud in place.
10. Attach a completed identification tag to outside of shroud.	Prevents need to open shroud to identify corpse.
11. Transfer corpse to morgue:	
a. Secure adequate help to transfer corpse to stretcher. Secure with straps and cover with a sheet.	
b. Transport corpse to morgue in an inconspicuous manner. (NOTE: Agency policy may require that the corpse be left in the room for removal by a mortician or coroner.)	
12. Return stretcher to unit and dispose of soiled linen. Place clean linen on stretcher.	Prepares stretcher for future use.
13. Remove all remaining supplies and equipment from room. Dispose of items appropriately.	Prepares room for terminal cleaning by housekeeping staff.
14. Record date and time of all relevant activities.	Documents action on health record.
15. Assemble and complete all health record forms.	

The corpse is then transferred to a stretcher, secured with straps, and, if the mortician is not expected to remove it from the unit, covered with a clean sheet for transport to the morgue. Frequently a staff member closes all of the room doors that are on the route between the deceased's room and the elevator, to provide privacy and avoid distress for other clients and visitors in the area. Clients and visitors in the halls are asked to clear the area. To expedite the transfer, another staff person obtains the elevator and if necessary asks visitors and clients to vacate the elevator, so that the corpse can be transported without onlookers whenever possible. Some agencies use a specially designed stretcher that has a frame rather than a solid top. Suspended from the frame is a long shelf on which the corpse is placed. A clean sheet is then placed over the top of the stretcher, resulting in the appearance of a conventional empty stretcher as it is being wheeled to the elevator and morgue. This eliminates the need to close doors and vacate the halls and elevator.

The service elevator is used whenever it is available. The stretcher is returned to the unit and the linen from it placed in a linen bag and replaced with clean linen. All remaining items in the deceased's room are removed and either discarded or sent to the appropriate department for cleaning. Housekeeping is notified that the room is ready for terminal cleaning.

RECORDING

All of the events that occur from the time the client died to the completion of transfer to the mortician or morgue are entered in the health record. These include: the date and time the client died; the name of the physician and the time he or she was contacted about the death (if not present to pronounce the client dead at the time the death occurred); and the survivors present or who was notified of the death. Information about organ transplant and the inventory and disposition of all of the deceased's possessions are also placed in the record, as well as the date and time of the transfer of the corpse to the mortician or morgue.

Sample POR Recording
- S—NA
- O—No respirations or pulse perceptible. Pronounced dead by Dr. Green at 10:00 A.M.
- A—Expired at 10:00 A.M.
- P—Wife notified by physician of the death. Corpse prepared for mortician. Ring with red stone on 3rd finger L hand padded and taped in place. Inventory of personal possessions included in health record. Wife to collect them from the registrar's office. Corpse removed by Gurney's Funeral Home at 11:00 A.M.

Sample Narrative Recording
10:00 A.M.   Respirations and pulse not perceptible. Pronounced dead by Dr. Green. Physician notified wife of death. Ring with red stone on 3rd finger L hand padded and taped in place. Inventory of personal possessions attached to health record. Wife to collect them from registrar's office. Corpse prepared for mortician.

11:00 A.M.   Corpse removed by Gurney's Funeral Home.

☐ CRITICAL POINTS SUMMARY

1. Care of the corpse is best given while the corpse is in the algor mortis stage.
2. The nurse can significantly affect how the survivors deal with loss.
3. Catheters and tubes in surgical wounds are not removed by the nurse after death.
4. The corpse is transferred from the unit in a discreet manner.
5. The deceased's corpse and personal possessions must be accurately inventoried and identified.
6. The nurse may need to search for information that identifies the deceased as an organ donor.

☐ LEARNING ACTIVITIES

1. Interview nurses employed at different health-care facilities to find out the various ways in which care of the corpse is implemented.
2. Talk with family members who have experienced a death to determine what type of support nurses provided them at the time of death.
3. Examine the forms available in a hospital that are completed upon the death of a client.
4. Interview nurses and physicians in a hospital unit to find out about the procedures used for different types of organ donations and transplants.

☐ REVIEW QUESTIONS

1. Why is care given to a corpse?
2. Match the name of the physiological change in Column B with the sign (or signs) associated with that change listed in Column A.

   COLUMN A
   ___ Skin cool to touch
   ___ Bruises on gravity-dependent body areas
   ___ Joint stiffness
   ___ Tears on previously intact skin

   COLUMN B
   1. Rigor mortis
   2. Livor mortis
   3. Algor mortis

3. How can the nurse help to make the loss more bearable for the deceased's survivors?

4. What are the forms that must be completed by the physician upon the death of a client?
5. Which form is the nurse responsible for completing?
6. What persons and agencies have to be contacted upon the death of a client?
7. Where would the nurse find information about organ donation?
8. What responsibilities does the nurse have for the deceased's personal possessions?
9. List in sequence the steps taken to provide care to the corpse.

☐ PERFORMANCE CHECKLIST

OBJECTIVE: To provide care to the corpse in a dignified manner.

CHARACTERISTIC	RANGE OF ACCEPTABILITY	SATISFACTORY	UNSATISFACTORY
1. Verifies that client has been pronounced dead by a physician.	No deviation		
2. Collects equipment and supplies; completes identification tags.	No deviation		
3. Closes door and cubicle curtains.	No deviation		
4. Elevates bed to high position; places it flat.	No deviation		
5. Positions corpse supine, closes eyes, replaces dentures, and closes mouth.	Omit dentures according to agency policy.		

6. Prepares deceased for viewing:
  a. Removes all appropriate tubes and catheters.
  b. Removes all jewelry and prosthetic devices.
  c. Bathes corpse and grooms hair.
  d. Places clean gown on corpse, puts a pillow under head, and covers corpse with clean linen.
  e. Removes equipment from room.
	Follow agency policy.
	
	No deviation
	
	No deviation
	No deviation
	
	No deviation		

7. Inventories and lists all personal possessions; assembles and attaches an identification tag; adds inventory and disposition on health record.	No deviation		

8. Prepares corpse for shrouding:
  a. Attaches chin strap.
  b. Covers eyes with sterile pads.
  c. Removes nonessential casts, dressings, and tape from corpse.
  d. Covers open wounds and external body orifices.
  e. Pads and ties wrists and ankles.
  f. Attaches identification tag to wrists or ankles.
	Omit if mouth stays closed.
	Follow agency policy.
	Follow agency policy.
	
	No deviation
	
	No deviation
	No deviation		

9. Shrouds corpse:
  a. Turns corpse to side away from care giver and places open shroud parallel to corpse; turns corpse back onto shroud; turns corpse toward care giver and pulls shroud across bed to opposite side of corpse.
  b. Wraps shroud around head and corpse; secures in place.
	No deviation
	
	No deviation		

10. Attaches identification tag to shroud.	No deviation		

11. Transfer body to morgue:
  a. Uses adequate help to transfer corpse to stretcher; secures corpse with straps and covers with clean sheet.
  b. Transfers corpse to morgue in inconspicuous manner.
	Omit according to agency policy.		

(continued)

CHARACTERISTIC	RANGE OF ACCEPTABILITY	SATISFACTORY	UNSATISFACTORY
12. Returns stretcher to unit and prepares it for future use.	No deviation		
13. Disposes of all remaining items in room appropriately; notifies housekeeping.	No deviation		
14. Records date and time of all relevant activities.	No deviation		
15. Assembles and completes all health record forms.	No deviation		

REFERENCES

DeGowin EL, DeGowin RL: Bedside Diagnostic Examination, ed 4. New York, Macmillan, 1981.

Pennington EA: Postmortem care: More than a ritual. American Journal of Nursing 78(5):846–847, 1978.

Rambo BJ, Wood LA: Nursing Skills in Clinical Practice, vol 2. Philadelphia, WB Saunders, 1982.

Rinear E: Helping the Survivors of Expected Death. Nursing75 5(3):60–65, 1975.

11 Supportive and Protective Treatments

☐ INTRODUCTION

Since the general goal of nursing is to help the client return to a maximum level of wellness, all direct client-care activities that are part of nursing practice can be considered to be either *supportive* or *protective* for the client. There are nursing interventions that have a primary focus, however, of either supporting normal physiological and psychological processes or protecting the client from the negative effects of those normal physiological and psychological processes. *Supportive interventions* stimulate and enhance normal processes, such as the use of heat applications to promote the normal inflammatory response, massage to stimulate circulation to the skin and muscles, and bandages to support body tissues during the healing process. *Protective interventions* shield the client from injury, danger, or some loss of normal function. Interventions in this category include those that help to impede normal physiological processes, such as the use of cold applications to reduce the normal inflammatory response, and those that protect the client from altered psychological processes, such as the use of restraining devices to protect the client or others from injury.

It is the nurse's responsibility to anticipate a client's need for supportive or protective interventions. The nurse is the person who has the most frequent contact with the client and is in the best position to detect changes in the client's physical and psychological condition. Some interventions used to support or protect the client may be initiated by the nurse, and others may require a physician's order. However, a physician is often dependent on the nurse's evaluation of the client's status as well as on the nurse's judgment regarding the need for a particular type of intervention.

Skills presented in this chapter have both supportive and protective aspects. These skills include "Thermal Applications" (Skill 46), "Massage" (Skill 47), "Applying Bandages and Binders" (Skill 48), "Mechanical Restraints" (Skill 49), and "Cast Care" (Skill 50).

☐ ENTRY TEST

1. Which layers of the skin have blood vessels?
2. What type of blood vessels are located in each skin layer?
3. What are the names, sites of origin, directions of fibers, and insertions of the major superficial muscles of the back of the neck, shoulders, back, and buttocks?

SKILL 46 Thermal Applications

PREREQUISITE SKILLS

Skill 19, "Inspection"
Skill 20, "Palpation"
Skill 28, "Handwashing"
Skill 51, "Monitoring Fluid Balance"

☐ STUDENT OBJECTIVES

1. Describe the normal physiological responses to heat and cold.
2. Identify the therapeutic purposes of heat and cold.

3. Explain why the adaptive mechanisms of the thermal receptors can work to the disadvantage of the client.
4. Explain the relationship between the rebound phenomenon and the therapeutic effect of thermal applications.
5. Describe the adverse systemic effects of heat and cold.
6. Identify the types of conditions and diseases for which heat and cold are contraindicated.
7. Explain each of the mechanisms by which heat is exchanged.
8. Identify the data that are collected by inspection and palpation.
9. Identify the precautions required for safe use of various types of thermal devices.
10. Specify the appropriate temperature range and the duration of thermal applications with different devices.
11. Administer thermal applications safely.

□ INTRODUCTION

Heat applied to the body for therapeutic purposes is known as *thermotherapy*. Heat may be applied to a small body area such as a wound, to a larger body part such as an extremity, or to the entire body. Application of heat to a specific body area is commonly used to promote soft tissue healing, to increase the suppurative process (pus formation), to decrease pain, and to decrease muscle tone. Heat applied to the entire body, as with a bath, is used to promote relaxation and sedation.

Cold applied to the body for therapeutic purposes is known as *cryotherapy* and, like heat, may be applied to part or all of the body. Application of cold to a specific body area is used most commonly to relieve pain, to reduce extravasation of blood and fluids into tissues after trauma, and to preserve the viability of tissue when blood circulation is inadequate or interrupted for a short period of time. Tepid water, classified within the cold category, is used to sponge-bathe clients with an elevated body temperature. Hypothermia, a body temperature below 37°C (98.6°F), may be intentionally induced. This extracorporeal cooling of the bloodstream is used primarily for clients who are undergoing surgery and will not be presented in this skill.

Applications of heat and cold may be either moist or dry, and the temperatures used vary, depending on the desired therapeutic purpose.

MECHANISMS OF HEAT TRANSFER

There are four mechanisms by which heat is transferred from one source to another: convection, conduction, conversion (also known as radiation), and evaporation. None of these mechanisms is mutually exclusive. Internal body heat is transferred by convection and conduction. External body heat is transferred from the body by convection, conduction, conversion, and evaporation. Heat is also transferred to the external body surface by convection, conduction, and radiation. These mechanisms must be understood before the nurse applies either heat or cold.

Convection

When the body surface is warmer than ambient air, heat flows from the body surface to the air. The amount of heat lost depends on the temperature difference between the body and the air. If they are both equal no heat is exchanged. The body gains heat when it is cooler than the air and loses it when it is warmer than the air. The rate of heat transfer from the body depends on the amount of body surface exposed and the speed of the air movement. Natural convection refers to the natural environment; forced convection occurs when the wind or a fan contributes to air movement.

Heat transfer within the body occurs primarily by forced convection of the circulatory system. The rate of blood circulation affects the internal distribution of body heat. This is the process by which the temperature from an external application is disseminated to other body areas.

Conduction

When there is contact between two objects, heat flows directly (is conducted) from one object to the other. Conduction occurs in gases, liquids, and solids by a diffusion of heat from the surface of the greater temperature to that of a lesser temperature. In the body, heat is transferred from the internal tissues by conduction outward to the skin and from the skin to any cooler object with which it comes in contact. When a temperature is applied locally, it is transferred by conduction directly to the skin and the underlying tissues. A disadvantage of using conduction for a thermal application is that the skin cannot be observed without removing the application. Fat and muscle are poor conductors and therefore provide good insulation for other body tissues.

Conversion

Heat transfer by conversion (radiation) occurs through the transmission of radiant energy that is absorbed and converted to heat without physical contact. People gain or lose heat from and to objects and the air in the environment by conversion. A heat lamp is an example of a therapeutic source of radiant energy.

Evaporation

Evaporation is a process by which a liquid is changed into a vapor (gas). This process occurs when heat is absorbed into a liquid's molecules. When a gram of water evaporates from the skin surface, 0.58 kilocalories of body heat are lost (Guyton, 1981). Evaporation of perspiration is the chief mechanism the body has for cooling itself, because evaporation of moisture on the skin draws heat from the body and disperses it into the air in the form of a vapor. The process of evaporation is used therapeutically when sponge baths are given with water or alcohol to reduce an elevated body temperature. Alcohol has a lower surface tension than water and therefore vaporizes more rapidly, thus increasing the rate of heat loss.

☐ PREPARATION

PHYSIOLOGICAL EFFECTS OF HEAT AND COLD

The rationale for the therapeutic effects of heat and cold is based on the physiological responses body tissues have to different temperatures.

The primary effect of heat applied to the skin is to raise the temperature of the underlying tissues, which initiates a series of physiological responses from the cutaneous circulation. Heat inhibits the normal vasoconstrictor impulses from the sympathetic nervous system, thus permitting the subcutaneous blood vessels to dilate. Heat also increases tissue metabolism, thereby increasing the oxygen requirement. An increased blood flow through the dilated vessels brings more oxygen, nutrients, antibodies, and leukocytes to the tissues and increases the removal of metabolic wastes. These physiological changes promote soft tissue healing and increase the suppurative process. An adverse effect of the blood-flow rate increase occurs from the rise in the capillary hydrostatic pressure, which causes an increased permeability of the blood vessel walls. This permits extracellular fluid to flow into the tissues, causing either edema formation or an increase in preexisting edema (Fischer and Soloman, 1965; Millard, 1965; Lehmann and De Lateur, 1982).

The primary effect of cold applied to the skin is to lower the temperature, which causes vasoconstriction of the cutaneous blood vessels. The series of physiological responses that evolve from vasoconstriction are the opposite of those that occur from vasodilatation. Metabolism, blood flow, supply of oxygen, nutrients, antibodies, and leukocytes are reduced, as is the removal of waste products. These responses prevent or reduce edema formation and the extravasation of blood or fluid into the tissues after trauma. They also help to preserve the viability of a portion of the body that is gangrenous or has a septic wound because the septic process is retarded. An adverse effect of cold occurs when surface body tissue that is exposed to extremely low temperatures becomes frozen. Prolonged freezing causes permanent damage to the tissues and the circulation (Fischer and Soloman, 1965).

Both heat and cold relax skeletal muscle tone by their effect on nerve conduction. Heat stimulates the cutaneous thermal receptors and increases the speed with which the sensory nerve impulses are conducted and the speed of cutaneous circulation. Cold decreases the speed with which the sensory nerve impulses are conducted and the speed of cutaneous circulation. Muscle relaxation results from an increase and decrease in sensory nerve conduction and vasodilatation and vasoconstriction (Griffin and Karselis, 1978; Lehmann and De Lateur, 1982). When the pain of muscle spasm is caused by ischemia (occluded blood vessels preventing adequate blood flow), vasodilatation induced by heat provides pain relief.

Application of cold enhances control of muscle activity and decreases nervous system irritability that produces painful muscle spasms (Lehmann and De Lateur, 1982). An adverse effect of cold may occur with the reduction in the efficiency of muscle function when it is applied to persons who already have moderate muscle weakness (Stillwell, 1971).

Consensual Response
When heat or cold is applied to a specific body area, changes in the rate of blood flow also occur in other body areas, but to a lesser degree. For example, a consensual response to a thermal application placed on one arm can occur in the opposite arm or in the lower extremities. The speed with which the response occurs indicates that it is due to a reflex phenomenon and not a change in the core temperature of the body. The occurrence of a consensual response depends on the intensity of the temperature of the thermal application and the area of skin (Fischer and Soloman, 1965; Lehmann and De Lateur, 1982).

Rebound Phenomenon
There is a point at which the maximum degree of therapeutic effect is attained from the applied temperature and then the opposite effect begins. This is known as the rebound phenomenon. When heat is applied, the maximum increase in cutaneous circulation from vasodilatation is reached after 20 to 30 minutes. Continuation of the heat application beyond 30 to 45 minutes results in tissue congestion (Lehmann, 1965, p. 359; Stillwell, 1965, p. 236). The blood vessels then begin to constrict for some unknown reason. When vasoconstriction is present during continued heat application, the therapeutic effects are absent and the client is at risk for being burned because the constricted vessels are not able to dissipate heat adequately by their normal convective process (Schliephake, 1965).

With cold applications, the maximum degree of vasoconstriction is achieved when the cutaneous blood vessels reach about 15°C (59°F). With a temperature less than 15°C, vasodilatation begins because of the direct effect of cold on the vessels. The belief is that this is either because the mechanism that contracts the vessel wall becomes paralyzed or because the nerve impulses to the vessels are blocked. This protective mechanism helps to prevent freezing tissue of body parts normally exposed to cold such as the ears and nose (Guyton, 1981, p. 354). Thermal applications must be removed before the rebound phenomenon occurs.

Systemic Effects of Heat and Cold

The application of heat to a localized body area may result in a generalized effect that significantly increases cardiac output and pulmonary ventilation. The greater the size of the body area treated, the more potential there is for the effect to occur. Generalized vasodilatation may divert a large enough supply of blood to the cutaneous circulation from the internal organs to produce a drop in blood pressure. This effect may be more pronounced in persons who have coronary or pulmonary disease and those with circulatory disturbances, such as arteriosclerosis, than in persons who are healthy. Even healthy but very young or elderly persons may not be able to tolerate heat because of poor regulatory temperature mechanisms.

There are normal protective physiological responses to prolonged cold that may occur or become more pronounced if a cold application is prolonged. These include shivering and shunting of blood. Shivering is a normal attempt of the body to produce heat to warm itself. Shunting of blood from the peripheral to internal blood vessels occurs in an attempt to maintain the core body temperature. The vasoconstriction induced by cold increases blood pressure.

Influence of Temperature on the Physiological Response

The extent of an individual's physiological response to a thermal application and the degree to which the application is therapeutic depend on the environmental temperature and humidity and the client's skin temperature prior to the application. The effect of a heat application is enhanced in a warm and humid environment, because the body is unable to dissipate heat by its normal evaporative mechanism and because the conductive heat loss from the application is reduced when the environmental temperature is equal to or greater than the application. The amount of time required to raise the tissue temperature to a therapeutic level is thus reduced and the application duration is less. To prevent the client from having a systemic effect or incurring tissue damage, the nurse observes the client closely for any adverse reaction.

The effect of a cold application is also enhanced when it is administered in a cold, dry environment because the body is losing heat to the environment. In the event that a cold application must be administered, the nurse keeps the client warm with blankets to prevent shivering and an increase in blood pressure.

PERCEPTION OF THERMAL SENSATION

An individual perceives different thermal sensations according to the degree of stimulation acting on different types of thermal receptors. When extreme degrees of heat or cold stimulate the nerve endings, a burning type of pain is perceived because thermal pain receptors are responding to the stimuli. Persons who have sensory nerve deficits may not be able to feel the pain of an application that is hot or cold enough to cause skin damage.

There is also an adaptative mechanism in the thermal receptors that accounts for the short duration of the initial response to sudden changes in temperature. Warm and cold thermal receptors are strongly stimulated by a temperature that is extremely different from the body surface. This strong stimulation fades rapidly at first, then more slowly as the receptor adapts to the new temperature (Guyton, 1981). This adaptive mechanism explains why we initially feel very warm when entering a room after being outside in a cold environment but then soon feel comfortable. Nurses and clients may be tempted to change the temperature of a thermal application to hotter or colder because of the difference in thermal sensation after adaptation occurs.

CONTRAINDICATIONS IN THE USE OF HEAT AND COLD

Since heat increases cellular metabolism, it is not used with clients who have a malignant disease because it has the potential for spreading the disease. Clients who have disorders or disease of the cardiovascular, respiratory, and renal systems may have the function of these systems seriously compromised when heat is applied to a large body area. Heat is not applied to clients with disorders affecting either the venous or lymphatic circulation, because these clients already have limited excretion of metabolic waste and a tendency for edema formation. Nor is heat applied to an area where diffusion of fluid is restricted, as occurs with clients who have poor circulation. Any client who has limited or absent sensory perception may not be aware of the applied heat and therefore is at risk for being burned. The sedative effect of heat can also be hazardous if the client is unable to respond appropriately. Acutely inflamed areas on any client have an increased danger of edema formation, and heat should not be applied. For example, an inflamed appendix could rupture if heat was applied.

Cold is contraindicated for clients who have impaired circulation because they already have reduced tissue nourishment. Cold also increases arterial spasm in clients who have Raynaud's disease. Some persons have an allergy to cold, in which an inflammatory response consisting of erythema, swelling, joint pain, and occasional muscle spasm occur (Lehmann et al., 1974). When cold is applied to an athletic injury, pain is masked and continuation of intense physical activity can predispose the person to additional injury. Some persons react excessively to cold with a sudden increase in blood pressure. This could be hazardous for those with hypertension.

CLINICAL USES OF HEAT AND COLD

The media most commonly used by nurses to administer superficial thermal applications are water and the radiant energy from heat lamps. *Water,* an excellent thermal conductor, is used in the form of packs, compresses, soaks, and baths to transfer dry or wet heat or cold. It is important to keep in mind that heat and cold are relative and that there are gradients of temperature between heat and cold. The temperature ranges involved in classifying water are shown in Table 46-1. *Radiant energy* is used as a dry heat source. The energy emitted from a heat lamp is converted into heat in the superficial skin layers. The amount of heat output of a lamp depends on the type of heating element of the lamp and its radiating area. The lamp used most often by nurses is a common 40-watt electric light bulb.

Dry versus Wet Thermal Applications

Although moist dressings serve a specific purpose when used for open wounds as presented in Skills 36 and 37, there appears to be no scientific basis for the common belief that wet heat is more effective in achieving therapeutic results than dry heat (Stillwell, 1971). Dry heat is usually tolerated at a higher temperature than moist heat, but the amount of heat transferred to the skin depends on which thermal transfer mode is used (conduction, convection, or conversion) and the method of application.

There are advantages and disadvantages associated with both dry and moist applications. For many persons moist heat is more comfortable than dry heat; it is not as drying to the skin and causes less sweating and therefore less loss of body fluids. On the other hand, prolonged application of moist heat causes skin maceration, and evaporation of the moisture results in more rapid cooling of the application than with dry heat. There is also a greater potential for burning tissues with moist heat because the water serves as an excellent thermal conductor.

TABLE 46-1. Classification of Temperature Ranges of Water

	FAHRENHEIT	CENTIGRADE
	Degrees	Degrees
Very cold	34–55	1.0–13.0
Cold	55–65	13.0–18.0
Cool	65–80	18.0–27.0
Tepid	80–92	27.0–33.5
Neutral	92–96	33.5–35.5
Warm	96–98	35.5–36.5
Hot	98–104	36.5–40.0
Very hot	104–115	40.0–46.0

From Zislis JM: Hydrotherapy. In Krusen FH (ed): Handbook of Physical Medicine and Rehabilitation, ed 2. Philadelphia, WB Saunders, 1971. Used with permission.

Body heat is transferred from the tissues to both dry and moist cold applications. Moist cold conducts a more intense temperature because of the thermal conductivity of water, thus posing a greater risk of burning the tissue or freezing the tissues. When extreme wet cold applications are placed over a large body area there is the additional risk of significantly lowering body temperature.

Heat versus Cold Applications

There are some diseases and conditions for which either heat or cold are used. The decision to use one or the other depends on whether the disease or condition is in the acute or chronic stage, or on the client's response to a particular temperature. For example, during the acute stage of rheumatoid arthritis and gout, heat may aggravate swollen tissues and pain. It is recommended that heat be applied *only after* the swelling and tenderness begin to subside (Schleiphake, 1958). Some groups of clients with the same disease process may have a beneficial response to heat, while others may not. Kangilaski (1981) found that individuals who had synovitis in their knees with rheumatoid arthritis obtained no pain relief from heat but did from cold. The effective treatment consisted of ice cubes in a plastic bag placed above and below the knee three times a day for 20 minutes. The outside of the bag was 6.7°C (44°F). Although only one knee was treated, both knees obtained pain relief from the therapy and improved range of motion, presumably from the consensual effect.

The choice of heat or cold to reduce edema must be made with consideration for the underlying cause. Edema caused by traumatic tissue injury is treated with cold immediately following the injury for about 48 hours until the edema is no longer forming. Heat applied after this period increases capillary permeability and helps the reabsorption of the extravasated fluid (Griffin, 1978).

DATA BASE

Client History and Recorded Data

Before initiating any type of thermal application, the nurse finds out the purpose of the application and its desired effect. That information and the client's age, general health status, and specific disease are obtained from the health record, so that any need for caution or any contraindications can be identified. The client is asked about his or her response to previous thermal applications and the existence of an allergic reaction to cold if that is the temperature prescribed. The nurse also determines if the client has any deficit in perception of thermal sensations due to fatigue, level of consciousness, or neurologic impairment that would prevent adequate reaction to applications that are too hot or too cold. The medical diagnosis provides clues about the potential for such problems. In hospitals the physician orders thermal applications; a complete order includes the type of application and the duration and frequency of the application.

Physical Appraisal Skills

Inspection. Skin on the body area where the application is to be placed is first inspected to determine the color, presence of edema, skin irritation, open lesions, scars, or stoma that would influence using a thermal application. The tissue reaction to the thermal application is evaluated both during and after the application. A normal response to the rapid flow of arterial blood into the tissues causes the skin to have an evenly distributed pink or red color. Persistent mottling of the skin is an indication that the tissues are too hot. Cold tissues normally slow blood flow, and the absence of nutrients and oxygen gives the skin an evenly distributed bluish hue, which is followed by a pink blush. This occurs because with severe vasoconstriction of the cutaneous blood vessels, the skin assumes the color of connective tissue in the subcutaneous layer, which is either a whitish hue or a white ashen pallor. Inspection would also reveal skin maceration (waterlogged, having a wrinkled appearance) from moist or wet heat applications left on for a prolonged period of time and erythema, blisters, or skin damage from applications that are too hot or too cold.

Palpation. The presence of edema before and after the application of heat or cold is determined by palpation as described in Skill 51. When edema is present before the application, it is also important to evaluate the amount of change after the application is removed.

EQUIPMENT

Many of the devices available for superficial thermal applications may be used for either hot or cold applications.

Thermal Transfer Devices: Conduction

Leakproof rubber bags with secure stoppers may be filled with either hot water or ice. They are available in various sizes and shapes. A rubber bag is always checked for leaks prior to use. This is done by filling the bag, securing the stopper, drying the outside, and then inverting the bag to see if the water leaks out from the cap or from punctures in the bag itself. When using a bag for a heat application, the bag is preheated with hot water. This prevents loss of heat from the water that will be used for the application to warm the bag. Water of the correct temperature is placed in a pitcher and the temperature is measured with a utility thermometer. A temperature of between 40.5° and 43.3°C (105° to 110°F) is considered safe for infants and for children under 2 years, the elderly, the diabetic, and the unconscious client. A range of 46.1° to 51.6°C (115° to 125°F) is used for older children and adults (Dodd, 1979).

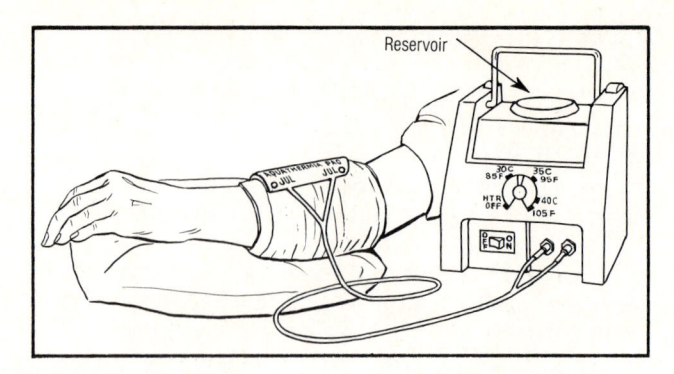

Figure 46–1. Aquathermia pad and water reservoir.

A rubber or vinyl surgical glove is sometimes used as a substitute for a bag, particularly when the area to be treated by cold is small or has contours that will be difficult to cover. After filling the glove, a knot is tied in the wrist portion to prevent leakage.

An *aquathermia pad* consists of a control unit that houses a motor, a heating element, a reservoir to hold distilled water, a temperature gauge, a thermostatic control, and two lengths of rubber tubing that are connected to a vinyl pad, as shown in Figure 46–1. The pads are available in various sizes and may be used for dry or moist applications. The pad has channels through which water circulates, providing a constant temperature. When using an aquathermia pad, the water compartment (reservoir) is filled two-thirds full of distilled water, and the control unit is placed on a stable surface at the bedside that is slightly higher than the level of the body area where the pad will be applied. The force of gravity facilitates the water flow through the pad.

The air bubbles in the tubing in the pad are eliminated by tilting the control unit from side to side while the pad is filling. Failure to remove the air before beginning the treatment can result in air locks in the tubing that can impede the water circulation and cause stress on the motor. If the water is to be heated, the thermostat is set at 40.5°C (105°F) for a few minutes before the pad is to be applied to the client. A thermometer gauge in the water compartment indicates when the correct temperature is reached. If it is to be cold, the compartment is filled with water of the correct temperature, 15°C (59°F). Since this is an electrical unit, safety precautions required for all electrical equipment are observed. The cord is checked for fraying, the unit is placed so that the cord is not in the path of traffic, and the cord is plugged into a grounded outlet with dry hands. Pins or adhesive tape are never used to hold the pad in position on the client, because they damage the vinyl pad. A gauze bandage can be tied loosely around the pad to keep it in position.

An *electric heating pad* consists of a waterproof pad with an electric coil inside and a heat control switch on the cord. The heat control has high, medium, and low settings. The high control may be removed by the institution to prevent use of the pad on the high setting. The medium setting provides a temperature in the range of 46° to 52°C (115° to 126°F). Since the temperatures considered safe for a heating pad are the same as for a hot water bag, the medium setting is hotter than is considered safe for persons other than older children and some adults. Although the pad is of waterproof material, it is not wise to use the pad over a moist dressing or compress as discussed in Skill 36.

Disposable chemical packs consisting of a prefilled plastic pack or bottle are available in two types, one for heat and another for cold. The device has two compartments of chemical compounds that are mixed immediately before using by squeezing, striking, or kneading the pack. The hot pack is designed to maintain a constant temperature between 40.5° and 46°C (105° to 115°F) for 20 to 30 minutes. The cold pack provides a constant temperature between 10° and 26.1°C (50° to 80°F) (Dodd, 1979, p. 1158). Reusable ice packs filled with a semiliquid gel are also available. These packs may be kept in a freezer and refrozen when they thaw.

Moist compresses may be devised by using a washcloth, a towel, or gauze dressings saturated with tap water, normal saline, or medicated solution ordered by a physician. They may be hot or cold. When the compress is to be kept hot, an insulating material such as plastic, aluminum foil, or a heavy towel or thermal blanket is placed over the compress. An external source of heat (either a hot water bag or an aquathermia pad) is sometimes used to maintain the desired temperature. Cold compresses are prepared using ice to chill the solution. Ice chips or cubes may be placed in the water or in a basin to chill a bottle of prescribed solution. An ice bag may be placed over a cold compress to keep it cold.

Hydrocollator packs also provide a source of moist heat. They are made of fabric filled with a dried silica gel which absorbs a great deal of water. These packs are immersed in distilled water heated in a thermostatically controlled container that can be raised up to a maximum temperature of 79.4°C (175°F) (Lehmann and De Lateur, 1982). Tongs or insulated rubber gloves are used to remove the hot packs from the hydrocollator. The heated packs are wrapped in several layers of turkish towel covers or bath towels to reduce the heat intensity before they are applied. The number of layers of terry cloth determines the amount of heat conducted to the skin. Some institutions require that the pack be covered with 8 to 10 layers of toweling. Hydrocollator packs have the advantage of slowly releasing heat (Lehmann et al., 1974, p. 227). They are used most often by physical therapy departments to relieve pain and promote muscle relaxation before exercise therapy. Figure 46-2 shows a hydrocollator and pack.

Thermal Transfer Devices: Conversion

A *heat cradle* is a frame consisting of several metal bands that are shaped and soldered like a half moon, as shown in Figure 46-3. The heat source is one or more 25-watt electric light bulbs that are inserted into sockets built into the frame at its highest points. A thermostat is often fixed to the frame. A heat cradle is used when a large body area must be warmed. Bed linen is placed over the cradle to retain the heat inside, but it must be placed so that it does not contact the light bulbs. The heat is reduced by loosening some of the light bulbs and increased by adding blankets. The cradle must be allowed to warm up before use.

A *heat lamp* is probably the most common source of dry heat used by nurses on clinical units. A heat lamp consists of a regular light bulb in a gooseneck lamp without a reflector. (Infrared and ultraviolet lamps are most often used by physical therapy departments.) A reflector on the lamp increases the amount of heat output; therefore, it is safer to use the lamp

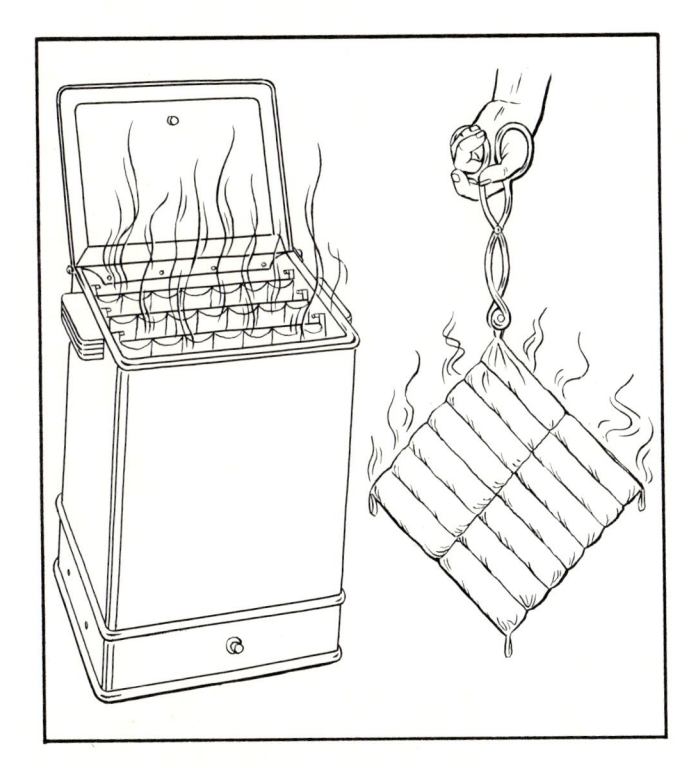

Figure 46-2. Hydrocollator and pack.

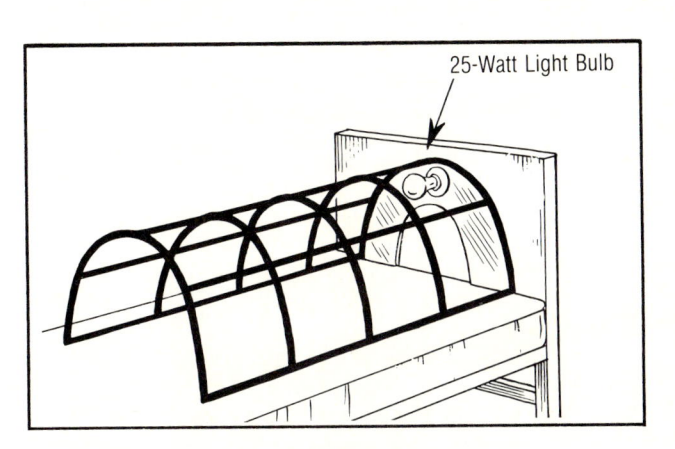

Figure 46-3. Heat cradle.

without the reflector. The strength of the bulb and the distance of the bulb from the client determine to some extent the amount of radiant heat transferred. It is important to be aware that a lamp's heat output increases until it is tripled at the end of 1 hour (Lehmann et al., 1974, p. 229). Bower and Bevis (1979) recommend that a bulb stronger than 40 watts not be used and that it be placed at least 35 cm (18 in) away from the area to be treated.

Thermal Transfer Devices: Convection
A *hubbard tank, whirlpool bath,* and *hot tub* permit immersion of the entire body or a part into a bath of agitated water. The water temperature usually ranges between 32° and 38°C (90° and 100°F), with the temperature set according to the purpose of the treatment. These baths are most often used by physical therapy departments for relaxation, physical exercise, and pain relief. Clients who have burns over a large area may be immersed for debridement of burn tissue (Dodd, 1979; Lehmann and De Lateur, 1982).

Thermal Transfer Devices: Evaporation
Tepid water or a combination of *water with 70 percent isopropyl alcohol* diluted to half strength is used to bathe clients with a prolonged elevated body temperature. In addition to the alcohol solution, a bath thermometer, six washcloths, two bath blankets, a towel, and a bath basin are needed. A rectal thermometer for determining the client's body temperature before and after the sponge bath is also necessary. A fan may be used in conjunction with the sponge bath to increase the rate of evaporation.

☐ EXECUTION

Before applying any type of thermal application, the nurse gives the client a clear explanation of the purpose of the treatment, how the application is to be made, the temperature that will be used, how the application should feel, and its duration and frequency. This explanation is important because most people are not aware of the normal physiological response of tissue to heat or cold. They tend to believe that a strong intensity of temperature and prolonged application are necessary to achieve a beneficial effect. Without an explanation, the client may be tempted to modify the temperature, duration, or frequency of the application and thus risk tissue damage.

In addition to the precautions required with the devices mentioned above and the contraindications previously described, there are some key points that the nurse must know and observe to prevent discomfort or injury to the client and the risk of legal liability.

1. Thermal packs and pads are always covered with an insulation material, preferably flannel, or if it is not available, a towel or pillowcase. This reduces the intensity of the temperature and prevents the accumulation of moisture on the skin.

2. Moisture on the skin serves as an additional conductor and increases the intensity of the thermal application to the client.
3. Local thermal applications are always placed on top of the body area to be treated. If the client lies on the application, the amount of skin contact is increased, intensifying the temperature of the local tissue. Placement of the application on the top of the body area provides the opportunity for the temperature of the application to dissipate to the environment and permits the body area to disperse some of the applied temperature. (These temperature transfers occur by a combination of conduction and conversion.)
4. Thermal applications are removed promptly whenever the nurse observes adverse tissue reactions or the client complains of burning or painful sensations.
5. The temperature of a solution used is measured with a utility thermometer whenever possible. In the absence of a thermometer, the nurse checks the solution temperature by placing some on the inner aspect of the nurse's forearm before using it on the client.
6. The client's skin is always dried when the application is removed.
7. Thermal applications are prepared and applied using medical or surgical aseptic technique.

APPLYING THERMAL DEVICES

Hot Water and Ice Bags
Fill a hot water bag one-third to one-half full and an ice bag two-thirds to three-fourths full to reduce the weight of the bag on the client. Express all of the air from the bag by folding it upon itself or squeezing it before securing the cap. This reduces the volume of the bag; removes air, which is a poor conductor of temperature; and increases the bag's flexibility so that it better fits the body contours. When the treatment is finished, empty and drain the bag, dry the outside, and separate the sides of the bag to permit it to fill with air before securing the cap. This keeps the bag slightly inflated and prevents the rubber from sticking to itself.

Moist Compresses
Nonsterile moist compresses are prepared with a material suitable for the size and location of the site. For example, to prepare a moist compress to the eye, either a gauze dressing or a washcloth may be used, but for an arm or leg a towel is more suitable.

When hot water is used, partially fill a basin from the faucet and measure the temperature to ensure that it is between 38° and 43°C (100.4° and 109.4°F). When saline or a medicated solution is used, heat the bottle containing the solution by placing it in a pan of water and heating it on a stove. Heating a bottle of solution takes about 15 to 20 minutes. Heat the solution to about 52.5° to 56°C (128° to 134°F), which is higher than the desired temperature. Approximately

8°C (14.5°F) of the heat is dissipated to the basin and the compress, and more is lost to the environment during the application. For cold compresses, add ice chips or cubes to the water, and place other solutions in the refrigerator or in a basin with ice chips.

To keep the bed linen from getting wet, place a piece of plastic under the area to be treated. Saturate the compress with the solution in the basin and wring out the excess moisture before placing it on the client. Use an insulating material over a hot or warm compress to keep the heat loss at a minimum. Without an insulating cover, a heated compress must be changed every 5 to 15 minutes to maintain the temperature. A hot or cold pack or an aquathermia pad may be used to maintain the moist compress temperature. Inspect the skin for color and tissue changes about every 15 minutes during the treatment.

See Skill 36 for further information on moist sterile compresses. Cold moist sterile compresses are prepared in the same manner as warm moist sterile compresses, but with a chilled solution.

Heat Lamp

Before using a heat lamp, check the bulb to be sure that it is not stronger than 40 watts. Position the client so there is no danger of the client accidentally moving too close to the bulb. In lieu of actually measuring the distance between the bulb and the body area to be treated, measure the length of your own arm to find out where 35 cm (18 in) is up from the fingertips. Use this as a convenient means of judging the distance to place the lamp. Fully expose the body area to be treated but preserve the privacy of the client; for example, place a "Do Not Disturb" sign on the room door or close the cubicle curtains. Heat lamps are often used to dry moist incisions and wounds in body areas that are considered private, such as an episiotomy (which is performed during obstetrical delivery) or a decubitus ulcer. Resist the temptation to create a tent over the lamp and client, because this prevents dispersion of heat and provides a potential for burning the client. Inspect the skin every 5 minutes during the duration of the treatment to detect signs of overheating of the tissues and to prevent burning. The usual duration of a heat lamp treatment is 20 to 30 minutes (Dison, 1975). However, it is wise to limit the first treatment to half of this time so the client's response to the heat can be evaluated. When the treatment is finished, turn off the bulb, disconnect the lamp, and return it to the proper storage area.

The Sponge Bath

Sponge baths given with tepid water (27° to 33.5°C) or a half-strength solution of tepid water and 70 percent isopropyl alcohol help to dissipate body heat by stimulating the cutaneous circulation and promoting evaporation. There is general agreement that water in the tepid range should be used for sponge baths (Dodd, 1979; King et al., 1981; Lewis, 1980). This temperature facilitates vasodilatation and reduces the potential for shivering, which only increases body temperature. Cold water is not used because it produces vasoconstriction and decreases peripheral circulation, which decreases the body's ability to transfer heat to the environment.

Before beginning the bath, explain to the client its purpose and acknowledge that the client will probably feel somewhat uncomfortable during the bath. When alcohol is used, the client may find the fumes unpleasant. Some children become nauseated and vomit from the odor of the alcohol. Prepare the client for a bed bath as described in Skill 38. Have additional blankets available in the event that the client begins to chill and requires warming. Since alcohol makes the skin feel cooler, the client may be more apt to chill during an alcohol bath. Plastic sheeting or bed protectors may be placed under the client to keep the bed from getting wet during the bath. The bed is apt to get wet because the skin is not dried during the course of the bath, since this would reduce the evaporating effect. Obtain the client's vital signs before beginning the bath, so that a baseline of data is available for comparison.

Bathe the client's face with clear water and then place a cool moist sponge or washcloth over the forehead and in both axillae and groins to increase the heat loss from the large superficial arteries. Place a warm water bottle at the client's feet to reduce the generalized sensation of coolness. Expose each body area as it is bathed, then cover it lightly with a part of the blanket used over the rest of the body. Bathe each extremity for 5 minutes and the chest, abdomen, back, and buttocks for about 10 minutes. Use firm strokes to help stimulate the cutaneous circulation, thus bringing more blood to the skin to enhance heat loss. Do not dry the skin, but let the moisture evaporate. A complete sponge bath takes about 30 minutes. Change the water and compresses on the head, axilla, and groin when it is no longer tepid. If alcohol is used for the bath, the solution may have to be changed more often because it warms up more quickly due to evaporation. When using alcohol, avoid bathing the client too close to the perineal area because alcohol causes burning when in contact with the mucous membranes.

Monitor the client's tolerance of the procedure during the bath and periodically check the pulse to determine if the rate is decreasing, which is an indication of a reduction in temperature. At the completion of the bath, cover the client lightly with a dry blanket. Measure the vital signs 15 and 45 minutes after the first bath is completed and before beginning another. This interval is important because continuous sponging without permitting time for the thermostatic center in the hypothalamus to become reset at a lower temperature can result in too great a drop in body temperature.

Hydrocollator Packs

New hydrocollator packs must be immersed in distilled water for at least 1 hour to permit complete saturation and even distribution of the silicone gel. Once the packs have been wet, they are not permitted to dry out because their effectiveness will be diminished. They can be kept moist by placing them in a plastic bag or returning them to the hydrocollator machine. The water in the machine is maintained at an adequate level to cover the packs completely at all times.

When initiating a treatment, allow about 20 minutes for the water to heat to a temperature of 60°C (140°F) and 5 minutes for a cooled pack to reheat. When the pack is heated, use tongs or insulated rubber gloves to handle its corners, and let the pack drain over the water compartment of the machine. Wringing out the pack can break the stitching and release the silicone gel.

Before applying packs, wrap them in an insulation material so the client is not burned. The institution may have a policy that specifies the minimum number of layers that must be used. Prepare a sufficient number of towels for use before removing the pack from the machine. To cover one pack with nine layers of cloth requires three towels. Prior to beginning a series of treatments, make sure that an ample supply of dry towels is available for all of the packs, because wet towels are not reused. When using towels, place them open on a flat surface in layers so that they are easily available. Wrap packs quickly after removal from the machine to keep heat loss at a minimum. To wrap a pack, place it in the center of the towel and fold each of the four sides of the towel over the pack so that the pack is completely covered, as shown in Figure 46–4. Then turn the pack over, place it on a second towel, and wrap it in the same way; turn the pack over and place it on the third towel and wrap it as before. This equalizes the number of layers of toweling on each side of the hot pack and holds the towel wrap securely in place.

Place the client in a comfortable position so that the pack can be placed on top of the body area to be treated. The client must remain stationary during the duration of the treatment to prevent moving the pack. Expose the area to be treated and remove any jewelry present, because metal heated by the pack could burn the client. If the pack is to be applied to a joint such as a wrist, elbow, or shoulder, it may be necessary to place a rolled towel under the joint to provide it with support during the treatment. Rolled towels are placed on each side of a narrow body area to help

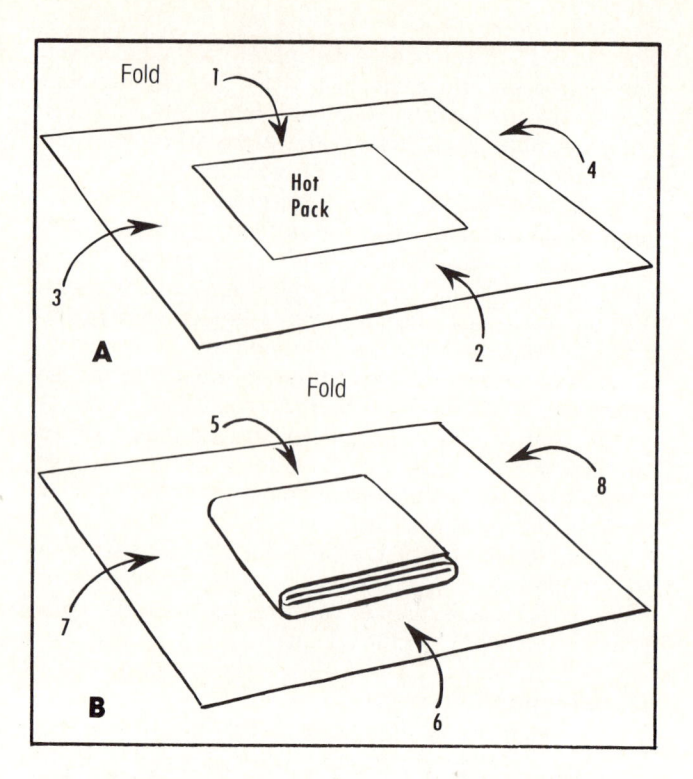

Figure 46–4. Wrapping hydrocollator packs. **A.** Wrap the pack in a single layer of toweling, and **B.** add successive layers, one at a time.

support the weight of the pack. Hydrocollator packs are hottest during the first 10 minutes. Inspect the client's skin for redness every 5 minutes for the first 10 minutes of the treatment. Remove the pack if the skin is red during this interval because this indicates low tolerance of the hot pack. Check clients who have sensitive skin more frequently than every 5 minutes. Stay with the client for the full duration of the first treatment, so that early signs of adverse reactions can be detected. For subsequent treatments on clients who are alert and cooperative, it is permissible to leave the client with the signal light and instructions to call the nurse promptly if any sign of overheating occurs or the pack gets displaced (Indiana University Hospitals, 1980).

□ SKILL SEQUENCE

APPLYING HYDROCOLLATOR PACKS

Step	Rationale
1. Check kardex for nursing order and medical orders.	Ensures appropriate intervention.
2. Prepare necessary equipment and supplies.	Avoids delays and interruptions during treatment.
3. Wash hands.	Prevents transferring microorganisms.
4. Explain procedure to client.	Allays anxiety and indicates how client can cooperate with treatment.
5. Fill hydrocollator with distilled water. Set thermostat control at 60°C (140°F) and place packs in machine.	Allows time to prepare client while packs are heating.
6. Assist client into comfortable position, expose body area to be treated, and remove any jewelry present.	Client needs to be comfortable to maintain position for duration of treatment. Metal conducts heat and may burn client.

(continued)

Step	Rationale
7. Place rolled towels on side (sides) of joint and under joint.	Reduces full weight of pack on joint.
8. Prepare covers or towels for hot packs.	Makes covers readily available.
9. Remove pack from hydrocollator machine by holding tab corners with tongs or insulated rubber gloves. Hold pack over water compartment to drain.	Prevents direct contact with hot packs and burning hands. Wringing wet pack may break stitched seams on pack and release silicone gel.
10. Place pack in center of towel and sequentially fold each side of towel over pack.	All areas of pack must be covered to prevent burning nurse and client.
11. Invert pack and place on second towel and wrap as in step 10. Continue to invert and wrap pack until required number of layers are added.	Equalizes number of towel layers on each surface of pack.
12. Place wrapped pack on body area. Remind client not to move while pack is in place.	Movement can shift pack from designated area and loosen wrap on pack.
13. Cover client with bed linen. Place call signal within reach of client.	Helps to retain heat. Enables client to notify nurse of adverse reactions.
14. Remove pack and check skin reaction every 5 minutes for first 10 minutes. (NOTE: Remain with client for duration of first treatment.)	Prevents burning client. Reassures client and enables nurse to take prompt action if adverse reactions occur.
15. Remove pack after 20 minutes and replace with fresh wrapped pack if prescribed by physician.	Heat loss after 20 minutes makes pack no longer effective. If prescribed duration of treatment is longer than 20 minutes, apply a fresh hot pack.
16. Remove wet towels and place pack in machine or securely closed plastic bag.	Keeps packs moist.
17. Place wet towels in laundry.	Dry towels must be used for each hot pack treatment.
18. Appraise skin condition, evaluate therapeutic effect, and record results on client health record. (NOTE: Report adverse reactions promptly to the physician.)	Provides ongoing data base for continuity of care.

RECORDING

After removal of a thermal application, note the client's local skin and systemic reactions and the effectiveness of the treatment in relation to the purpose on the client's health record. A specific, detailed account of any adverse reaction or complication is also recorded, as well as reported to the physician promptly.

Sample POR Recording

- S—"My ankle feels better after that ice bag! It was throbbing like a toothache!"
- O—L. ankle 1+ edema reduced to trace edema after application of ice for 20 min.
- A—Subjective and objective relief obtained from ice bag.
- P—Continue observation and repeat ice bag application in 1 hr.

Sample Narrative Recording

Ice bag applied for 20 min to l. ankle.
Edema reduced from 1+ to trace.
States ankle less painful after treatment.

☐ CRITICAL POINTS SUMMARY

1. The effect of a local application of heat or cold extends to other body areas by consensual and systemic action.
2. The maximum effect from applying heat or cold is reached in 20 to 30 minutes.
3. The risk of burning a client increases when vasoconstriction occurs.
4. Knowledge of existing disease processes is important to prevent adverse physiological reactions to heat or cold.
5. Convection, conduction, conversion, and evaporation help to regulate body temperature and affect the therapeutic actions of thermal applications.
6. Inspect the treated body area for color and integrity before, during, and after the thermal application.
7. Use a cover over the application to protect the skin from direct contact with the heat or cold.
8. To avoid burning a client, measure the temperature of the application before using it.
9. Interrupt a tepid or alcohol bath when the client complains of being cold, before shivering begins.
10. Use electrical equipment safely.

☐ LEARNING ACTIVITIES

1. Obtain separate samples of tap water that feel very hot, hot, warm, cool, cold, and very cold to your hand. Measure the temperature of each sample and compare the measurements and the thermal sensation you felt with the classification of water temperature ranges presented in Table 46–1.
2. Step into a hot or cold shower or bathtub and note the amount of time it takes you to adapt to the temperature.

3. Fill a hot water bag three-fourths full of hot water; do not expel the air before securing the cap. Place the uncovered bag on your forearm. Note how hot the bag feels and how comfortable the weight of the bag is on your arm. When you remove the bag, note how much perspiration collects on the skin. Reduce the water in the bag to half, expel the air, cover the bag, and replace the bag on your forearm. Compare the difference in fit, weight, and comfort.
4. Put several ice cubes in a plastic bag and close it securely. Place it on the back of your hand and note how long you can tolerate the cold before it becomes very uncomfortable.
5. Blow across the back of your wrist. Moisten the back of your wrist with water and blow again. Use alcohol to moisten your wrist and blow again. Compare the subjective perception of coolness (degree of heat loss) with dry skin, water, and alcohol.

☐ REVIEW QUESTIONS

1. Match the physiological responses listed below with the corresponding temperature application:

PHYSIOLOGICAL RESPONSE	TEMPERATURE APPLICATION
___ Vasodilation	A. Heat
___ Vasoconstriction	B. Cold
___ Increased capillary hydrostatic pressure	C. Heat and cold
___ Decreased edema formation	
___ Decreased cutaneous circulation	
___ Increased removal of metabolic wastes	
___ Skeletal muscle relaxation	
___ Increased voluntary control of muscle activity	
___ Reduced efficiency of muscle function	

2. Select the temperature (temperatures) that would provide therapeutic effects for the following conditions:

	HEAT	COLD
Initial stage of traumatic edema	___	___
Muscle spasms due to nerve irritability	___	___
Muscle spasms due to ischemia	___	___
Cutaneous wound healing	___	___

3. Why does the perception of a temperature change soon after the initial contact?
4. Why is there a limited time period within which a therapeutic response to heat or cold occurs?
5. Give examples of the systemic adverse effects that can result from heat or cold.
6. What are some types of conditions or diseases for which heat and cold are contraindicated?
7. How do convection, conduction, conversion, and evaporation affect body temperature and thermal applications?
8. What information does the nurse collect by inspection and palpation before, during, and after a thermal application?
9. Describe the precautions required for the safe use of each of the following devices:
   a. Hot water bag
   b. Aquathermia pad
   c. Electric heating pad
   d. Hydrocollator pack
   e. Heat lamps
10. Indicate the correct temperature and duration of treatment for each of the following thermal devices:

DEVICE	TEMPERATURE	DURATION
Hot water bag (adults)		
Aquathermia pad		
Moist compresses		
Ice bag		
Tepid water bath		

☐ PERFORMANCE CHECKLIST

OBJECTIVE: To apply moist heat by hydrocollator pads safely.

CHARACTERISTIC	RANGE OF ACCEPTABILITY	SATISFACTORY	UNSATISFACTORY
1. Checks kardex for nursing-care and medical orders.	No deviation		
2. Prepares equipment and supplies.	No deviation		
3. Washes hands.	No deviation		
4. Explains procedure to client.	No deviation		

(continued)

CHARACTERISTIC	RANGE OF ACCEPTABILITY	SATISFACTORY	UNSATISFACTORY
5. Fills hydrocollator with distilled water; sets thermostat control on 60°C (140°F); and places packs in machine.	No deviation		
6. Positions client; exposes designated body area; removes jewelry present.	No deviation		
7. Places rolled towels on sides and under joint.	Not necessary for large body areas.		
8. Prepares covers for packs.	No deviation		
9. Removes and drains packs using tongs or insulated rubber gloves.	No deviation		
10. Centers packs on dry towel and sequentially folds each side of towel over pack.	No deviation		
11. Inverts pack and centers it on second towel; wraps as above and repeats in same way for third wrapping.	No deviation		
12. Positions pack on designated area, covers client with bed linen and places call light within client's reach.	No deviation		
13. Removes pack and checks skin reaction every 5 minutes for first 10 minutes.	No deviation		
14. Removes pack after 20 minutes and replaces with fresh pack if necessary.	No deviation		
15. Removes wet towels; places pack in securely closed plastic bag or hydrocollator machine.	No deviation		
16. Places wet towels in laundry.	No deviation		
17. Records skin condition, therapeutic results on health record. Reports adverse reactions promptly.	No deviation		

REFERENCES

Bower FL, Bevis EO: Fundamentals of Nursing Practice: Concepts, Roles and Functions. St Louis, CV Mosby, 1979.

Dison N: Clinical Nursing Techniques, ed 3. St Louis, CV Mosby, 1975.

Dodd MJ: Caring for a Person Requiring Applications of Heat and Cold. In Sorensen KC, Luckman J (eds): Basic Nursing: A Psychophysiologic Approach. Philadelphia, WB Saunders, 1979.

Fisher E, Solomon S: Physiological Responses to Heat and Cold. In Licht S (ed): Therapeutic Heat and Cold, ed 2. Baltimore, Waverly Press, 1965.

Griffin JE, Karselis TC: Physical Agents for Physical Therapists. Springfield, IL, Charles C Thomas, 1978.

Guyton AC: Textbook of Medical Physiology, ed 6. Philadelphia, WB Saunders, 1981.

Indiana University Hospitals. Nursing Services. Application of moist heat via hydrocollator steam packs. Unpublished. Indianapolis, IN, 1980.

Kangilaski J: "Baggietherapy": Simple pain relief for arthritic knees. Journal of the American Medical Association 246(4):317–318, 1981.

King EM, Wieck L, et al.: Illustrated Manual of Nursing Techniques, ed 2. Philadelphia, JB Lippincott, 1981.

Lehmann JF, DeLateur BJ: Diathermy and Superficial Heat and Cold Therapy. In Kottke FJ, Stillwell GK, et al. (eds): Krusen's Handbook of Physical Medicine and Rehabilitation, ed 3. Philadelphia, WB Saunders, 1982.

Lehmann JF, Warren CG, et al.: Therapeutic Heat and Cold. In Urist MR (ed): Clinical Orthopedics and Related Research 99 (Mar–Apr): 207–245, 1974.

Lewis LW: Fundamental Skills in Patient Care, ed 2. Philadelphia, JB Lippincott, 1980.

Millard JB: Conductive Heating. In Licht S (ed): Therapeutic Heat and Cold, ed 2. Baltimore, Waverly Press, 1965.

Schliephake E: General Principles of Thermotherapy. In Licht S (ed): Therapeutic Heat and Cold, ed 1. Baltimore, Waverly Press, 1958.

Stillwell GK: Therapeutic Heat and Cold. In Krusen FH, Kottke FJ, et al. (eds): Handbook of Physical Medicine and Rehabilitation, ed 2. Philadelphia, WB Saunders, 1971.

Zislis JM: Hydrotherapy. In Krusen FH, Kottke FJ, et al. (eds): Handbook of Physical Medicine and Rehabilitation, ed 2. Philadelphia, WB Saunders, 1971.

BIBLIOGRAPHY

McMaster WC: A literary review on ice therapy in injuries. American Journal of Sports Medicine 5(3):124–126, 1977.

Rambo BJ, Wood LA: Nursing Skills in Clinical Practice. Philadelphia, WB Saunders, 1982, vol 2.

Rocks JA: Intrinsic shoulder pain syndrome: Rationale for heating and cooling in treatment. Physical Therapy 59 (2):153–159, 1979.

Ruck TC, Patton HD (eds): Physiology and Biophysics, ed 20. Philadelphia, WB Saunders, 1973.

446 PROFESSIONAL CLINICAL NURSING SKILLS

AUDIOVISUAL RESOURCES

Local Applications of Heat and Cold
 Filmstrip and cassette. (1984, Color, 17 min.)
 Available through:
  Medcom, Inc.
  P. O. Box 116
  Garden Grove, CA 92642

Hot and Cold Applications
 Film (16mm). (1972, Color, 12 min.)
 Available through:
  National Audiovisual Center
  Order Section E Q
  Washington, DC 20409

SKILL 47 Massage

PREREQUISITE SKILLS

Skill 19, "Inspection"
Skill 20, "Palpation"
Skill 28, "Handwashing"
Skill 38, "Skin Care"
Chapter 14, "Introduction"

☐ STUDENT OBJECTIVES

1. Describe the purposes of massage.
2. Indicate the effects of massage on the skin, skeletal muscles, and circulation.
3. Compare the manner in which each type of massage movement is performed.
4. Indicate the rhythm and rate used for massage movements.
5. Describe the effects of each type of massage movement.
6. Specify the information the nurse collects before giving a massage to a client.
7. Describe the data collected by inspection and palpation.
8. Give a back massage using a combination of massage movements.

☐ INTRODUCTION

The word *massage* refers to various manipulations of the soft tissues of the body with the hands for the purpose of some therapeutic effect (Wood and Becker, 1981, p. 3). Massage may be both stimulating and relaxing and may be viewed as a passive form of exercise because of its effect on body tissues. Massage can improve the circulation and movement of nutritive elements, increase the elimination of waste products from the tissues, and soothe the central nervous system and peripheral nerves (Wakim, 1980). Massage also communicates caring through the emotional effect of touching. The body area most often massaged is the back, although other body areas that are subject to pressure-sore formation are also frequently massaged to stimulate cutaneous circulation.

The use of massage as a form of therapy dates back for centuries and has been included within the scope of nursing practice for many years.

☐ PREPARATION

PHYSIOLOGICAL EFFECTS OF MASSAGE

The desired physiological effects of massage on the skin, skeletal muscles, and circulation are achieved only if the massager has a good working knowledge of the body, its parts, and its movements. It is important that the location of muscles and muscle fibers, tendons, blood vessels, and direction of blood flow be recognized (Wakim, 1980).

The Skin
Massage has a soothing effect on the skin and makes it softer and more supple. Once the skin adapts to the prolonged use of massage, it becomes more flexible, more elastic, and tougher.

Skeletal Muscle
Although massage does not increase the strength or size of skeletal muscle, when given intermittently it does help to prevent atrophy of inactive muscle. Rhythmic activation of muscle stimulates the propulsion of venous blood and lymph through the mechanical force of the muscle action that is artificially induced by massage. This helps relieve muscles that are fatigued from either overexertion or prolonged inactivity. Massage promotes elimination of metabolic wastes and an increase in the nutritive elements distributed by an increase in blood flow.

Circulation
Massage facilitates the mechanical flow of blood and lymph and stimulates the circulation in the veins as

well as in the arteries and arterioles. A gentle stroking massage toward the center of the body stimulates the vasomotor nerves that supply the cutaneous blood vessels. Prolonged massage causes a hyperemic reaction in the skin and muscle being massaged. This occurs because of an increase in arterial circulation resulting from an increased blood flow in the veins. It has been shown that the numbers of erythrocytes in the superficial blood vessels increase by 40 to 50 percent during active hyperemia (Wakim, 1980). One study showed that after a 20-minute back massage, systolic and diastolic blood pressure tended to decrease; but there was a delayed effect of a slight increase in systolic pressure and an additional decrease in diastolic pressure. Subjects in the study also had an increase in heart rate (Wood and Becker, 1981, p. 26).

MASSAGE MOVEMENTS

The three basic massage movements are stroking, compression, and tapotement. The movements used for stroking and compression are of the same rhythm and rate; a rate of 15 movements per minute is recommended by Wood and Becker (1981). It is important that the same rhythm and rate be used when changing from stroking to compression, so that the desired physiological effects can be achieved. The rate at which the massage movements are performed affects the amount of massage a client receives. Tapotement is performed more rapidly than stroking and compression.

Stroking is a slow, rhythmic movement in which the hands apply a fairly consistent amount of pressure over a body area. The entire palmar surfaces of the hands and fingers are used. The fingers are held together, and the thumb may be placed in either an abducted position or an adducted position, according to the amount of hand surface required to cover the body area. One or two hands may be used. The hands are warm, relaxed, and flexible so that they conform to the body contour and can apply an equal amount of pressure. The strokes are made in long sweeps, and the time between the beginning and end of each stroke is equal. The amount of pressure used during stroking depends on the purpose of the massage and the condition of the underlying tissues. There are two kinds of stroking: effleurage and deep stroking.

Effleurage, derived from the French word *effleurer* ("to touch lightly"), is a stroke that is barely perceptible to the client. It soothes and lessens muscle tension, so it is used at the beginning and end of a massage. The stroke may be done in any direction because it affects only neurologic reflexes and not circulation. However, on body areas covered with visible hair, the stroke follows the growth pattern because stroking against the hair growth produces unpleasant sensations (Wood and Becker, 1981). The very light touch of effleurage permits the massager to obtain information about the state of relaxation and contour of the muscles.

Deep stroking, as compared with effleurage, is any stroke that is given with enough pressure to affect the neurologic reflexes and the venous and lymphatic circulation. The amount of pressure used to affect the circulation need not be heavy or forceful. When muscle relaxation has been achieved by using effleurage first, the subsequent strokes given with slightly more pressure are transmitted directly to the blood and lymph vessels. The direction of movement of deep strokes is centripetal (toward the center of the body and following venous blood flow). At the completion of a deep stroke movement, the hands are returned to the distal area, using effleurage to prevent interference with the effect of deep stroking on the circulation. Wood and Becker (1981) suggest that there be no interruption in the contact of the hands with the skin, because the nerve endings respond to the reflex stimulus when contact is disrupted. At least one hand remains in contact with the skin during the course of the massage.

Compression movements are used to stimulate circulation. There are two types: kneading and friction. They differ from stroking in that the movements are performed intermittently instead of continuously.

Kneading or petrissage is more forceful than stroking. It must be performed on a relaxed muscle for its circulatory effects to be achieved. Kneading consists of alternately grasping or compressing muscle tissue. It is performed by using the thumb and other fingers to grasp and raise a rather large fold of skin, subcutaneous, and muscle tissues, then rolling the fold in a circular motion. Pressure on the skin fold is tightened, loosened, and released before advancing to an adjacent area to repeat the kneading. The palm, palmar surfaces of the fingers, the thumb, or the thumb and fingers of one or both hands may be used for kneading. Care is taken not to pinch the skin and subcutaneous tissues and to reduce the amount of applied pressure as the bulk of the tissues diminishes. Kneading is done with the same rhythm and rate used for stroking.

Friction provides deep static pressure to the underlying tissues. It is started with light pressure and gradually progresses to a firmer pressure. The pressure used will depend on the state and condition of the underlying tissues. With friction movements, the superficial tissues are moved over the underlying tissues. Friction is performed by using the thumb, fingers, or palm of one or both hands, moving them in a slow circular direction, with little movement, over a small area of skin while keeping contact with the skin. The pressure is firm but not heavy enough to cause discomfort (Wood and Becker, 1981). The pressure is released after several circles have been completed and the hand is moved on the skin to the next area. The same rhythm and rate of movement is used for friction as for the other massage techniques.

Tapotement is a percussive movement in which brief, brisk, gentle blows are applied to the body area, alternately with each hand. In healthy persons, tapotement may be used to stimulate muscle contraction by reflex action and to increase the capillary circulation. However, Wood and Becker (1981) suggest stroking and compression are more appropriate for this purpose. Tapotement is not used on clients who are emaciated and have little subcutaneous or muscle tissue because it will be uncomfortable. Tapotement is performed by using either the ulnar border of each hand in a hacking movement, or by a gentle tapping with the tips of the fingers against the body area while the wrist is flexed, or by clapping the body area with the fingers, while the palm of the hand is held in the form of a concave cup. When performed on the chest wall, the alternating rapid blows generate vibrations in the lung that loosen mucus plugs in the bronchial tree. Physical therapists most often use tapotement on clients who have respiratory disease.

DATA BASE

Client History and Recorded Data

Before massaging a client, the nurse reviews the health record to determine if there are contraindications for a massage. Clients who are on bed rest, who have reduced physical activity, or who have impaired circulation are more vulnerable to thrombus formation in the veins of the extremities, particularly the legs. Massage could dislodge a thrombus and permit it to travel to another area in the circulatory system, thus blocking a major vessel and causing a serious obstruction of blood flow or death. As a general rule, it is not wise to massage the extremities of any client. Clients who have either superficial or deep tissue trauma could have increased tissue damage or hemorrhage as a result of massage. Children with Wilms tumor or malignant abdominal masses are not massaged because of the potential for dispersing the tumor cells through the lymph system. There is no basis for contraindications for massaging other clients who have malignant disease. There is a common misconception that clients who have either a suspected or confirmed myocardial infarction should not have a back massage. There is not convincing evidence currently available to support the assertion that any deleterious effects could occur from the moderate stimulation of a back massage (Fisch, 1983).

Massage is seldom ordered by a physician as part of the treatment regime of a nurse. A physician may, however, write a specific order prohibiting massage. It is the nurse's responsibility to include massage within the context of nursing orders for a client. It is not routine practice to see massage entered in a plan of care or on a kardex because there is a general assumption that if a client requires a massage, it will be given. This approach leaves too much to chance and deprives clients of benefits they could obtain from regularly scheduled massages. In establishing priorities for the care of clients, the nurse determines carefully which clients have a particular need of regular massage for relaxation and stimulation of circulation. Such clients include those who are on continuous bed rest, those who are obese, and those who are emaciated and may develop pressure sores. These clients may have decreased circulation to the muscles, increased skin irritation, and general fatigue from muscle disuse. The frequency of a massage is determined by talking with the client to find out general feelings of comfort and muscular fatigue as well as by observing cues that indicate restlessness, discomfort, and fatigue. It is important to keep in mind that being confined to a bed can be very tiring, although clients are apt to feel that they have no reason for fatigue since they have not been physically active.

Physical Appraisal Skills

Inspection. The skin over bony protuberances requires inspection for integrity and color to determine the need for regular massage and stimulation of circulation to pressure areas. The general condition of the skin on other body areas, the amount of subcutaneous tissue, and the muscle mass are also evaluated by inspection before, during, and after a massage. Skin appraisal and information about pressure-sore development are presented in Skill 38.

Palpation. Stroking and compression may be viewed as forms of palpation that enable the nurse to collect data about the texture of the skin and the condition of the underlying subcutaneous and muscle tissues. The state of relaxation or tension present in muscle tissue is determined before, during, and after the massage.

EQUIPMENT

The medium used for a massage depends somewhat on personal preference, the purpose of the massage, and the condition of the skin and underlying tissues. Oil lubricants make the skin soft, smooth, and slippery and also prevent pain that results from pulling on body hair. The oil lubricants most commonly used include olive oil, mild glycerin, mineral oil, or coconut oil. Most institutions provide clients with a body lotion as part of the admission kit, and this is often used as a massage lubricant. A fine talcum powder also can be used to reduce the friction on the skin unless contraindicated because of dry skin, as may occur with the elderly.

In addition to lubricant, a bath blanket or bed linen is used to cover the client during the massage. A towel may be needed to dry any lotion remaining on the client's skin when the massage is finished.

☐ EXECUTION

Most clients welcome massage, particularly a back massage, but have come to believe that it is a luxury because of the busy pace at which they perceive their nurses working. Unfortunately, nurses also frequently view a massage as luxury when in fact it is an integral part of nursing care. The most opportune time for the nurse to schedule a massage is during or after a bath and before the client is prepared for sleep. However, clients who require frequent turning for relief of pressure over bony protuberances should at least have the pressure areas massaged with each position change. The nurse is mindful that a client may refuse a massage because of a "busy nurse" perception. The nurse who believes that a massage is an integral part of nursing care will tell the client, "It's time for your massage now" or, "I'd like to massage your back (neck, feet, etc.) now," rather than "Would you like your back massaged now?"

BASIC PRINCIPLES OF MASSAGE

There are some basic principles that are to be observed when performing massage:

1. Observe medical aseptic technique through handwashing before and after the massage and by reserving a bottle of lotion for each client.
2. Place the client in a relaxed position with the arms at the sides when prone and in good body alignment, whenever possible.
3. Observe good body mechanics while giving the massage to prevent muscle strain and injury and excess fatigue.
4. Keep the environment quiet and free from distractions that interfere with relaxation.
5. Do not massage painful areas.
6. Massage should not be painful.
7. Observe the client's response to each type of massage movement and change it if the client finds it unpleasant or uncomfortable.

In preparation for a massage, elevate the bed to a height that facilitates massaging the client without undue stretching. If the oil or lotion is to be prewarmed, place it in a basin of water to raise it to a neutral temperature between 33.5° and 35.5°C (92° to 96°F). A neutral temperature promotes relaxation while cold causes vasoconstriction and increases muscle tension. Place the client in a comfortable position in good body alignment and fully expose the area to be massaged. If necessary, use a bath blanket or the bed linen to cover the rest of the client, providing privacy and preventing the client from chilling. Assume a position facing the area to be massaged. Stand at the bedside with the back straight and the feet about 30 cm (12 in) apart to establish a solid base of support and maintain balance. Advance the foot closest to the bed and place the other foot slightly behind the first. Keep both knees and ankles flexed so that the body can sway forward and backward, shifting the weight from one foot to the other with each massage movement. This permits free movement of the hands and arms and requires very little movement of the hips or spine, thus reducing fatigue. Swaying with each movement helps to establish a rhythm and also helps to control the rate with which the movements are given.

Pouring the lubricating lotion directly on the client usually startles the client. Instead, pour it into your hand and rub both hands together to distribute the lotion before beginning a massage. Inform the client of what you are doing or are about to do so that the client can anticipate what is going to happen. This is particularly important when the client is unable to see what is going on.

When *massaging pressure areas,* begin with effleurage strokes to relax the tissues before applying firmer pressure. Friction can be used over small areas but follow it with stroking or kneading to stimulate the circulation and to relieve any discomfort the client may feel from the pressure or heat generated by the friction.

For a *back massage,* place the client close to the edge of the bed nearest you. If possible, have the client prone with the bed flat. Help the client to assume a passive attitude to facilitate relaxation, and try to minimize the number of times the client must change positions during the massage. When a client is unable to lie prone, place him or her on the side facing away from you, so that part of the back, shoulders, and buttocks can be exposed and massaged. Then reposition the client on the opposite side of the body and complete the massage from the other side of the bed. Clients who cannot assume either the prone or side position can still have their backs massaged, but the massage may not be as complete and may require the assistance of a second person. The second person can assist by pushing down on the mattress to allow space for the nurse massaging the client to reach between the mattress and the client's back.

As with other areas, begin a back massage with effleurage and use this movement to apply a light film of lotion evenly over the shoulders, the entire back, and the buttocks. Placing the hands on the shoulders to begin the back massage is less invasive of the client's intimate space than beginning the massage at the buttock area. It also facilitates relaxation. These light strokes also provide data about the condition of the skin and the state of the muscles. These data help to determine the amount of pressure to use for subsequent movements. Use long, gliding strokes that follow the contour of the muscles of the back, the shoulders, and the buttocks. Once the client is relaxed, combine the deeper stroking, kneading, and friction movements, keeping in mind the purpose of the massage and the effects of each type of movement. Be sensitive to the client's response to each type of movement and the massage of different areas. At the completion of each movement, remember to keep at least one hand in contact with the skin and make changes from one type of movement to another smoothly. Avoid applying pressure on the spine and other bony areas lacking muscle tissue, because this is uncomfortable for the client. If additional lotion is required for lubrication, pour it into the hand that remains in contact with the skin.

450 PROFESSIONAL CLINICAL NURSING SKILLS

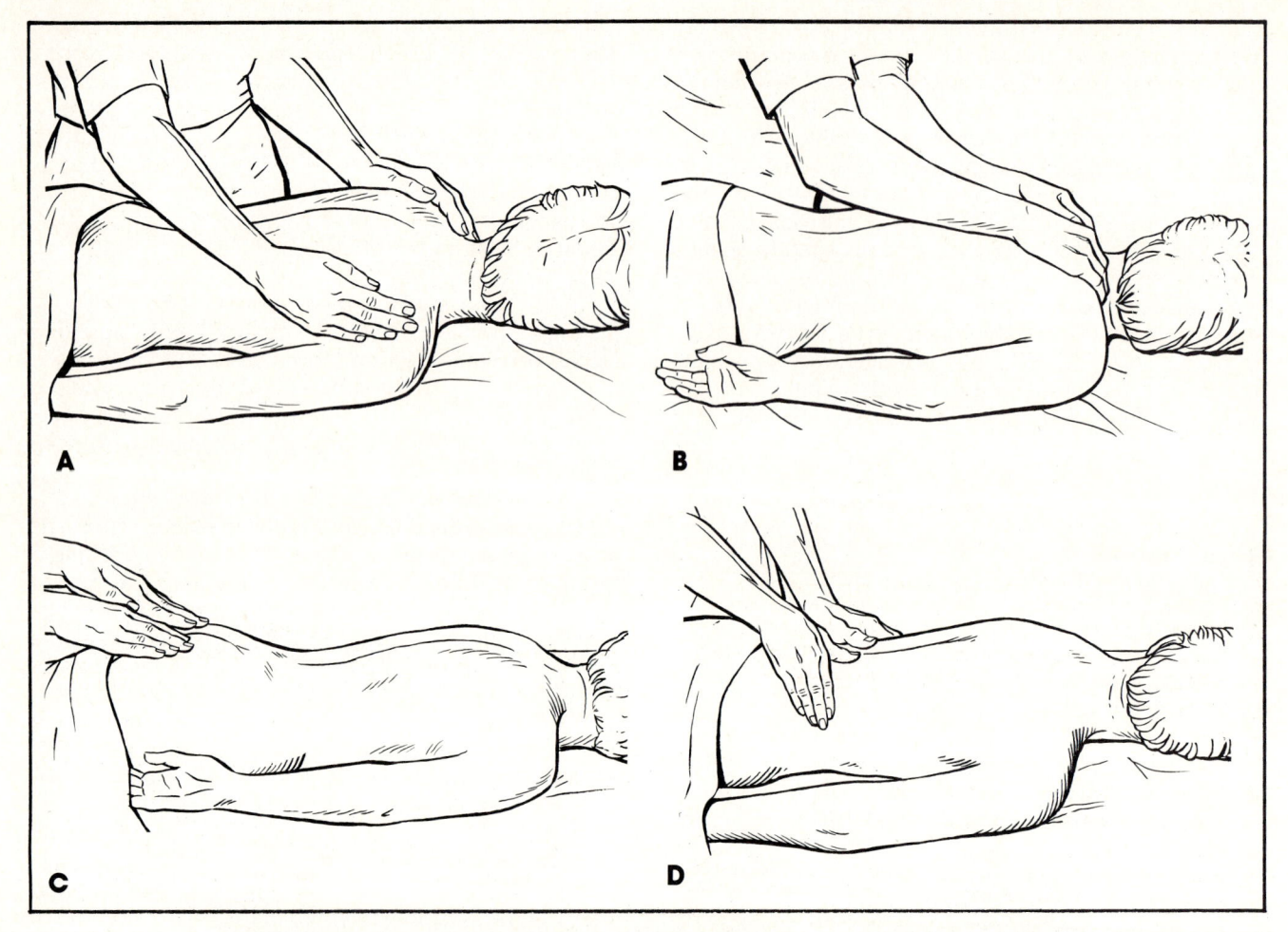

Figure 47-1. Hand positions and sequence of back massage movements. **A.** The fingers are held together and the thumb is either adducted or abducted according to the contour of the body area being massaged. **B.** The hands are placed on the shoulders with the thumbs lateral to the spinous processes of the cervical vertebrae. **C.** The deep stroke is started at the lower border of the sacrum using the fingers of both hands. **D.** The hands with the thumbs adducted at waist level stroke the midline of the lower back.

A massage for therapeutic effects of relaxation and stimulation of circulation lasts between 10 and 20 minutes. Use effleurage for the final massage movements, so that the client feels relaxed after the stimulating effects of deeper stroking or kneading and friction. If any lotion remains on the skin, pat the skin dry with a towel to prevent the client from feeling wet or sticky.

There are several ways in which a massage may be given. Figure 47-1 shows the hand positions and sequence of strokes that may be used for a back massage.

☐ SKILL SEQUENCE

BACK MASSAGE

Step	Rationale
1. Check kardex for nursing and medical orders.	Specifies medical prohibition for massage.
2. Explain procedure to client.	Enables client to anticipate what is to happen.
3. Collect necessary equipment.	Prevents interruptions during procedure.
4. Wash hands with warm water.	Prevents cross-contamination. Cold hands stimulate vasoconstriction and muscle tension.
5. Place liquid lubricant in basin of warm water.	Cold lubricant stimulates vasoconstriction and muscle tension.
6. Adjust bed to height appropriate for massage and lower side rail on side nearest care-giver.	Prevents strain and unnecessary fatigue.

(continued)

Step	Rationale
7. Place client in prone or side-lying position close to edge of bed nearest care-giver and expose back, shoulders, and buttocks.	Makes client more accessible. Exposes area to be massaged.
8. Cover client with bed linen or bath blanket.	Protects privacy and prevents chilling.
9. Pour lubricant on one hand and rub hands together to distribute it evenly.	Warms lubricant and makes hands glide easily over skin.
10. Place palmar surface of each hand on outer aspect of both shoulders and use long effleurage strokes down lateral aspect of back to buttocks. Glide hands toward center of back on each side of spine and return to base of neck and repeat several times. (NOTE: Keep hands parallel to spine with fingers pointed toward head. As muscles relax, increase amount of pressure slightly.)	Placing hands on shoulders less invasive of client's intimate space than beginning massage at lumbosacral or buttocks. Initial movements are used to distribute lotion, relax tissues, and collect data. Conforms to direction of major muscles. Slight pressure is easily transmitted through relaxed muscles and stimulates circulation.
11. Gently knead each area on top of shoulders and near base of neck several times.	These are body areas where muscle tension is often concentrated.
12. Glide hands down back to buttocks and use palmar surface of hands and fingers to apply friction movement to buttocks, moving in circles until all of buttocks area is massaged; then use petrissage or stroking movements over same area.	Keeps hands in contact with skin while transferring to another area. Buttock area is subject to fairly constant pressure while lying in bed.
13. Return hands to shoulders and gently knead shoulders and upper arms.	
14. Glide hands down to waistline and massage each side of lumbosacral area using firm strokes.	This area usually has weak muscles that become easily fatigued and is also where high muscle tension often occurs.
15. Repeat massage over areas of client's preference, using strokes that are most effective.	Client often has specific areas that need additional massage.
16. Complete massage by using effleurage over entire back, shoulders, and buttocks.	Enhances relaxation effect.
17. Use towel to pat skin dry if necessary.	Provides for comfort.
18. Reposition client if necessary for comfort and replace bed linen.	Client may be relaxed and comfortable and wish to remain in same position assumed for massage.
19. Return lotion to client's bedside stand and wash hands.	Keeps lotion available for next massage. Prevents transfer of organisms to next client.
20. Record client's response and condition of skin and muscles on health record.	

RECORDING

The client's response to the massage and the condition of the skin before and after the massage are entered on the health record. The type and frequency of the massage is also included in the plan of care noted on the kardex, so that a consistent plan is executed by all nursing staff personnel.

Sample POR Recording

- S—"I can't imagine why I feel so tired just lying in bed all day. My back is really stiff and I just can't relax."
- O—Moving restlessly in bed; unable to find a comfortable position.
- A—Generalized tension and fatigue due to anxiety and inactivity.
- P—Give back massage now and include with A.M. and P.M. care.

Sample Narrative Recording

Restless and unable to find a comfortable position. States back feeling stiff and unable to relax. Back massage given, more relaxed and less stiff. Plan to give back massages with A.M. and P.M. care.

☐ CRITICAL POINTS SUMMARY

1. Circulatory stimulation from massage occurs without heavy or forceful pressure.
2. The rhythm and rate of massage movements are slow and consistent.
3. Clients with myocardial infarction or circulatory impairments in the extremities should not have massage.
4. A client's extremities are not massaged without a specific medical order.
5. Massage is an important nursing intervention that is included as a component of client care.
6. The condition of the skin and muscles is appraised before, during, and after massage.
7. Hands and lubricating lotions are warmed before contact with the client.

8. Effleurage is used for the initial and final massage movements.
9. Friction is always followed by kneading or stroking.

☐ LEARNING ACTIVITIES

1. Role play the following exercises with a peer, taking turns at being the nurse and the client:
   a. Chill your hands and apply a cool lubricating lotion to the client's skin with two or three effleurage strokes. Assess the response of the client to the cool temperature. Then, warm your hands and the lotion and repeat the strokes and compare the client's response to each temperature.
   b. Use effleurage over the entire back, shoulders, and buttocks to appraise the condition of your client's skin and muscles. Note the differences you perceive in the state of relaxation and tension in various muscle groups.
   c. Use very firm strokes over the spine and note the client's response.
2. Give a complete back massage to a peer, practicing each type of massage movement several times and alternating the sequence of the movements.

☐ REVIEW QUESTIONS

1. What are some reasons why massage is used?
2. What are the effects of massage on the skin, skeletal muscles, and circulation?
3. Explain how you would perform stroking, kneading, and friction.
4. How rapidly are stroking, kneading, and friction movements done?
5. What are the different effects produced by effleurage, deep stroking, kneading, and friction?
6. What information would you obtain before massaging a client?
7. What data are collected by inspection and palpation before, during, and after a massage?
8. Describe how you would give a client a back massage.

☐ PERFORMANCE CHECKLIST

OBJECTIVE: To give a relaxing and stimulating back massage using a combination of massage movements.

CHARACTERISTIC	RANGE OF ACCEPTABILITY	SATISFACTORY	UNSATISFACTORY
1. Checks kardex for nursing and medical orders.	No deviation		
2. Explains procedure to client.	No deviation		
3. Collects equipment.	No deviation		
4. Washes hands with warm water; warms lubricating lotion.	No deviation		
5. Adjusts level of bed to appropriate height; lowers side rail nearest care-giver.	No deviation		
6. Positions client for massage close to edge of bed nearest care-giver; exposes client's back, shoulders, and buttocks.	No deviation		
7. Covers client with bath blanket or bed linen.	No deviation		
8. Pours lubricant on hand and rubs hands together.	No deviation		
9. Places palmar aspect of each hand on outer aspect of each shoulder and uses effleurage down lateral aspect of back and buttocks. Glides hands toward center of back on each side of spine and returns to base of neck. Repeats several times.	No deviation		
10. Gently kneads each area on top of shoulders and near base of neck several times.	No deviation		

(continued)

CHARACTERISTIC	RANGE OF ACCEPTABILITY	SATISFACTORY	UNSATISFACTORY
11. Glides hands down back to buttocks and uses palmar surface of hands and fingers to apply friction to small areas of buttocks, eventually covering entire buttocks. Uses petrissage or stroking over same area.	Adjust amount of hand surface to conform to size of buttocks.		
12. Returns hands to shoulder area; kneads shoulders and upper arms.	No deviation		
13. Glides hands to waistline; massages each side of lumbosacral area using strokes.	No deviation		
14. Repeats massage movements that are most effective over areas of client's preference.	No deviation		
15. Completes massage using effleurage over entire back, shoulders, and buttocks.	No deviation		
16. Pats skin dry.	Omit if skin is dry.		
17. Positions client for comfort.	No deviation		
18. Returns lotion to bedside stand and washes hands.	No deviation		
19. Records client's response and condition of skin and muscles on health record.	No deviation		

REFERENCES

Fisch C: Personal communication. Director, Krannert Institute of Cardiology, Indianapolis, April 1983.

Wakim KG: Physiologic Effects of Massage. In Rogoff JB (ed): Manipulation, Traction and Massage, ed 2. Baltimore, Williams & Wilkins, 1980.

Wood EC, Becker PD: Beard's Massage, ed 3. Philadelphia, WB Saunders, 1981.

Michaelsen D: Giving a great back rub. American Journal of Nursing 78(7):1197–1199, 1978.

Niland M: Providing Basic Patient Hygiene. In Sorensen KC, Luckmann J (eds): Basic Nursing: A Psychophysiological Approach. Philadelphia, WB Saunders, 1979.

Temple KD: The back massage. American Journal of Nursing 67(10):2102–2103, 1967.

BIBLIOGRAPHY

Beakey BM: An overlooked therapy you can use ad lib. RN 45(7):50–54, 1982.

SKILL 48 Applying Bandages and Binders

PREREQUISITE SKILLS

Skill 19, "Inspection"
Skill 20, "Palpation"
Skill 28, "Handwashing"
Skill 38, "Skin Care"
Skill 51, "Monitoring Fluid Balance"

☐ **STUDENT OBJECTIVES**

1. Identify the purposes for which bandages and binders are used.
2. Explain why porousness, flexibility, and extensibility are important properties of materials used to make bandages and binders.
3. Describe the relationship between body alignment and effectiveness of a bandage or binder.
4. Indicate the measures used to protect the skin from the effects of bandages and binders.
5. Indicate the data that are collected by inspection and palpation when using binders or bandages.
6. Describe the different types of bandages and binders.
7. Execute each type of bandage application technique.
8. Apply bandages and binders safely.

INTRODUCTION

Bandages are strips of material in various lengths and widths, available in rolled form for convenient application. They are used to cover or bind a body area or part. Binders are a type of bandage used to cover or bind a larger body area than would be feasibly accomplished with a bandage. Bandages and binders are used for similar purposes: (a) to hold a dressing in place, (b) to provide support to the tissues, (c) to provide pressure to an area, (d) to limit the range of motion of a part, and (e) to protect an injured part or to aid in the return of venous circulation from the extremities to the heart. The choice of using either a bandage or a binder depends on the purpose and the particular area to be treated. Bandages and binders can be applied directly to the skin or over a dressing; again the choice of using either depends on the purpose and the area to be treated.

PREPARATION

FACTORS AFFECTING THE USE OF BANDAGES AND BINDERS

Porousness, Flexibility, and Extensibility

The gauze, muslin, cotton flannel, and elastic material from which bandages and binders are made vary in the degree of porousness and extensibility, and these properties are important when selecting the appropriate type of bandage or binder. *Porousness* is determined by the type of fibers and looseness of weave used to make the material. A loosely woven material permits more air to circulate to the skin and thus decreases the warmth and moisture on the skin. Applying more layers of bandage than are needed serves to increase the warmth and moisture on the skin. Loosely woven materials are also more absorbent. Gauze, an example of an absorbent material, is appropriate for use when a wound has a large amount of drainage or when a bandage needs to be kept moist or wet.

Flexibility is affected by the density of the fabric weave. The more flexible a material is, the more it can be molded to fit the contour of the body area or part. Loosely woven flexible materials do not provide much support to the tissues. Muslin or cotton flannel are less flexible and absorbent and therefore more appropriate for providing support.

Extensibility of a bandage or binder depends on the elastic properties of the material. Stretch can be the result of the type of elastic fibers used or the type of weave used to make the material. It is important to know that there are variable amounts of stretch in different types of bandages and binders, because stretch helps to determine the tension a bandage or binder possesses and therefore affects the amount of pressure it will apply to the covered tissues. The more tension and stretch a material has, the more potential it has for compressing the tissues. A body part requiring a low amount of pressure would need a bandage or binder capable of providing low compression, whereas a body part requiring high compression would need a bandage or binder capable of providing high compression. It is important that the compression used on the tissues be less than the hydrostatic vascular pressure, because a compression greater than that would impede blood flow and could result in edema formation. The actual amount of compression applied to the tissues depends on both the extent to which the material is stretched when it is applied and the diameter of the body part. Although the stretch may remain constant, the pressure on the tissues increases as the diameter of the part decreases (Thomas et al., 1980). For example, more pressure is applied to a narrow area such as a wrist than would result from an equally stretched bandage applied to the forearm.

Body Alignment

Bandages and binders are applied snugly so that they stay in place but do not interfere with desired normal function and alignment of the body area, part, and joints. The proper position of the part is determined individually for each client, because the normal degree of movement and function and the potential for the loss of function varies with each client. For example, a bandage required to hold a dressing in place on an elbow could be applied with the elbow flexed and the arm in an aligned position of rest or with the elbow straight and the arm fully extended. If this same client has normal function of the elbow and no existing disease or condition that requires the elbow to be straightened then the flexed position is most appropriate. However, if the client has a neurologic disease or arthritic condition where a flexed elbow would promote contracture of the tendons and ligaments at the joint, it would be better to bandage the elbow in a straight position with the arm extended to prevent loss of function due to the development of contractures. Joints are not bandaged in a hyperextended position because this places stress on the joint, ligaments, and tendons.

Body alignment is also important when using binders. Chest and abdominal binders cannot be applied properly and without wrinkles if the client is not positioned in straight alignment. Binders can interfere with respiratory function if they are not secured in place or if they are applied too tightly. Proper positioning of the client before applying the binder enables the nurse to see where the binder needs to be placed and allows the nurse to check the placement once it is secured.

Skin Protection

Skin that is covered by a bandage or binder needs to be protected from the effects of warmth, moisture, and pressure. Warmth and moisture can be kept at a minimum by the choice of bandage material. The potential for the growth of infection-producing microorganisms can be reduced by providing skin care and by using medical aseptic technique to handle all clean bandages and binders. Whenever possible, the skin is bathed and dried before it is covered with a bandage or binder. Adjacent skin areas that contact each other are separated by absorbent gauze that will help to promote air circulation and absorb the perspiration. In some instances it is appropriate to use a light dusting of an absorbent talcum powder to help to keep the skin dry and to reduce the friction of the opposing areas of skin. Because it is an irritant to nonintact skin, powder is not used on open skin areas or near wounds. It is important to keep in mind that bandages and binders themselves can be a source of skin irritation and discomfort for the client if the nurse does not provide basic hygienic skin care when using bandages and binders.

To help protect the skin from the effects of prolonged pressure, padding must be placed over bony protuberances that are subject to pressure, such as the ankle, heel, or scapula. This is particularly important when the client's movement is restricted, because it is not possible to note changes in the skin's condition when it is covered with a bandage or binder. Pins and metal fasteners used to secure the bandage or binder in place are located in a position that will not apply pressure to the underlying tissues. They are not put over bony protuberances or wounds.

Wrinkles in the bandage or binder can also cause pressure on the underlying tissues. This occurs when the bandage or binder is too snug or becomes dislodged from the intended position. Bandages and binders are applied with an even amount of tension over the entire area to be covered so as to minimize the potential for an increased amount of pressure over any one area or part.

Soiled and damp bandages and binders are another source of skin irritation. Soiled and damp bandages and binders are changed at least once a day to protect the skin.

DATA BASE

Client History and Recorded Data
Before applying a bandage or binder, the nurse needs to understand its purpose and desired effects. This information is usually available on the client's health record, but the nurse may need to draw on his or her own knowledge of the specific condition or disease to be able to relate the effect of the bandage or binder to the therapeutic need of the particular client. When the bandage or binder is to be applied to an extremity, the nurse determines if the client has any deficits in neurovascular status, to avoid further impairment of these systems. It is also important to know if the client has a decreased level of consciousness or neurologic impairment that might prevent him or her from reporting symptoms such as tingling, numbness, or discomfort caused by the bandage or binder.

There are many types of bandages and binders that the nurse can apply on the basis of his or her own nursing judgment. Many institutions, however, require a physician's order for the application of chest and abdominal binders, elastic bandages, or elastic hose. The nurse stays abreast of the clinical unit's practices regulating the application of these bandages and binders. Sometimes there are policies that specifically prescribe or prohibit the use of a particular type of binder or bandage for specific types of clients.

Physical Appraisal Skills

Inspection. The condition of the skin is inspected for color, presence of lesions, and edema before the application of the bandage or binder and upon its removal. If the bandage or binder has been used over a dressing, the amount, color, and consistency of the wound drainage present on the dressing is noted. Inspection is also used to apply the bandage or binder in the correct manner and to check on its security and safety once it is in place.

Palpation. The temperature of the skin and the quality of those pulses that are covered are palpated periodically. These data provide a baseline from which to determine subsequent changes before applying the bandage or binder. The same data are obtained when the bandage or binder is removed.

EQUIPMENT

Types of Bandages
Bandages range in width from 1 to 6 inches. *Cotton gauze* bandages are often referred to as roller bandages to differentiate them from the gauze squares that are used for dressings. Gauze bandages are most commonly used to hold dressings in place. There are many types of gauze bandages that vary considerably in porousness and extensibility. The oldest and least expensive type is plain, single-layer gauze. It has a very limited absorbency and extensibility and the edges fray easily. Other types of gauze such as Kling, Kerlix, and Sol-band are more absorbent, flexible, and somewhat extensible. They are woven so that the layers cling to each other and therefore are much easier to apply securely without using special wrapping techniques. These bandages can be used to apply firm pressure to a body part. Gauze bandages are not washable, so their reuse depends on their cleanliness in relation to the purpose for which they are used. For example, an intact, clean gauze bandage may be reused when it is not necessary that the bandage be sterile, as may occur when the bandage is used to provide support or pressure to a body part.

Muslin and *cotton flannel* bandages are firm, fairly inflexible, durable, and washable, but much less porous than gauze. They are used for support and to provide warmth to the tissues.

Stockinet is a tubular knit material that is somewhat flexible and is used to encase a body part or hold a dressing in place. It is washable and durable. *Tubegauze* is a loosely woven, fine tubular gauze that can be shaped to fit any body part and is often used to hold dressings in place. *Elastic bandages,* often referred to as ace bandages, are firm, somewhat flexible, and also durable and washable. They are used to support injured parts, to immobilize joints, and to increase venous return to the heart from the extremities.

Types of Binders

Abdominal binders are made in two basic styles and types of fabric. Rectangular abdominal binders may be made of elasticized fabric or several thicknesses of sturdy nonstretch cotton or muslin. Elasticized binders may have stays placed at intervals to prevent wrinkling or curling of the borders. Rectangular cotton binders are fastened in place with pins or tape, while elasticized binders have self-adherent or hook-and-eye closures. The second style of abdominal binder is a scultetus binder, which consists of a rectangular piece of sturdy cotton or muslin that has many tails attached to two opposite sides. Both styles of binders are commercially available in several sizes. Abdominal binders may be used to hold dressings in place instead of adhesive tape or Montgomery straps. They are also used to provide support after surgery.

Breast binders may be either flat, straight, and rectangular-shaped or designed in the form of a sleeveless jacket or vest. They are made of muslin or cotton flannel. Breast binders are used either to hold dressings in place or to apply pressure to the breasts after childbirth to help decrease production of milk by the mammary glands.

T-binders are belts that have one or two lengths of fabric attached to the center. They are made of muslin or cotton flannel and are used to hold rectal or perineal dressings in place. The single T-binder is used for females and the double for males.

Slings are another form of binder. They are usually a triangular piece of muslin or cotton flannel material and are used to help support the weight of a paralyzed or weak arm as well as a cast or to limit the movement of a shoulder or arm.

Elastic stockings, also commonly referred to as antiembolism stockings or TED hose (a brand name), are often used in lieu of elastic bandages to promote the return of venous blood to the heart by supporting the veins in the legs. They are used with clients who have reduced muscle activity as occurs during bed rest or restricted ambulation, and also persons who have impaired circulation. Elastic stockings are often applied preoperatively to prevent pooling of blood in the legs during and following surgery. Elastic stockings are available in a variety of sizes and lengths: below the knee, midthigh, or full length. Most full-length stockings have a variable stretch, with the tightest stretch below the knee and less stretch above the knee. Some brands have a circular opening in the foot near the toes that provides access to the toes for appraisals of the circulatory status.

☐ EXECUTION

APPLYING BANDAGES

Select the type and width of bandage that is most appropriate for the part to be bandaged and the purpose to be achieved. For example, plain gauze is adequate to hold a dressing in place when compression is not desired, but if compression is needed, one of the nonreusable extensible bandages is used. Always handle a clean bandage with freshly washed hands.

The easiest way to control a roll of bandage during application is to hold it in the dominant hand with the free end of the fabric coming off of the roll clockwise. This keeps the nondominant hand free to position and hold the bandage in place on the client. Before applying a bandage, unroll a short length and stretch it between both hands to determine the amount of extensibility in the fabric. This will help to judge the amount of stretch to exert on the bandage during application. Bandages that have a large degree of extensibility can be stretched too much during application and thereby exert too much compression on the tissues, resulting in interference with neurovascular function.

To apply a bandage, assume a position in relation to the body area to be bandaged that permits access and good visibility. Position the body area or part in good alignment before beginning the application and check with the client while applying the bandage to make sure it is comfortable and evenly snug but not tight.

When applying a bandage to an extremity, begin at the distal portion and wrap toward the proximal to avoid interference with circulation. Leave a small part of the distal aspect of the extremity exposed, so that periodic appraisal of the neurovascular status can be made. Leaving large portions of the distal end of an extremity uncovered permits edema formation, thus increasing the compression of the underlying tissues and neurovascular systems. Applying a bandage too tightly also compresses these tissues. When using elastic bandages to enhance venous return from the legs, cover the heel with the bandage. When placing a bandage over a wet dressing or applying a dressing that is apt to become wet from a draining wound, apply it more loosely so that it will not constrict the tissues when the material shrinks as it dries.

Remove bandages at the first signs of neurovascular impairment and appraise the skin and neurovascular status before reapplying the bandage or binder more appropriately.

Bandaging Techniques

The techniques used to apply bandages are referred to as turns. Selection of the type of turn to use depends upon the type of bandage material and the body part to be bandaged. One or more types of turns may be necessary to apply a bandage securely.

The *circular turn* is the most basic technique and is used to anchor the initial end of the bandage around

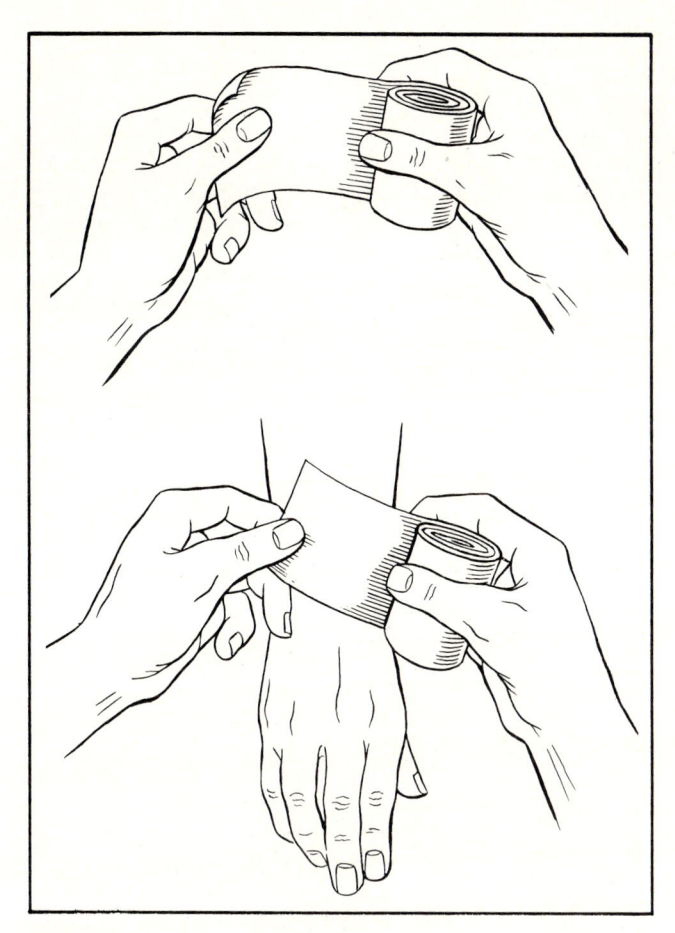

Figure 48-1. To apply a roller bandage, hold the bandage in the dominant hand and place the loose end at an oblique angle to serve as an anchor for the first turn.

a part as well as to complete the application. To execute the circular turn, place the initial end of the bandage on the part at a slight angle, hold it in place with the thumb, and circle the part with the roll held in the opposite hand, gradually unrolling the bandage as needed from the roll until one complete layer of bandage is in place, as shown in Figure 48-1. Repeat the complete circle as often as necessary, overlapping each layer evenly until the number of layers is adequate for the desired purpose. Cut the bandage at the desired length and secure the terminal end with adhesive tape or a safety pin. When the circular turn is used as the initial anchoring for a more extensive bandage, two circles are usually adequate to hold the initial end in place.

The *spiral turn* is a variation of the circular turn and is used to shape the bandage to a cylindrical part such as an arm or leg. Anchor the bandage at the initial point with two circular turns and then begin to overlap each turn over the previous layer about one-half to three-fourths the width of the bandage, depending on the thickness desired. Place each layer of bandage at about a 30-degree angle to take up the slack on the lower border of the bandage. Figure 48-2A shows the spiral turn.

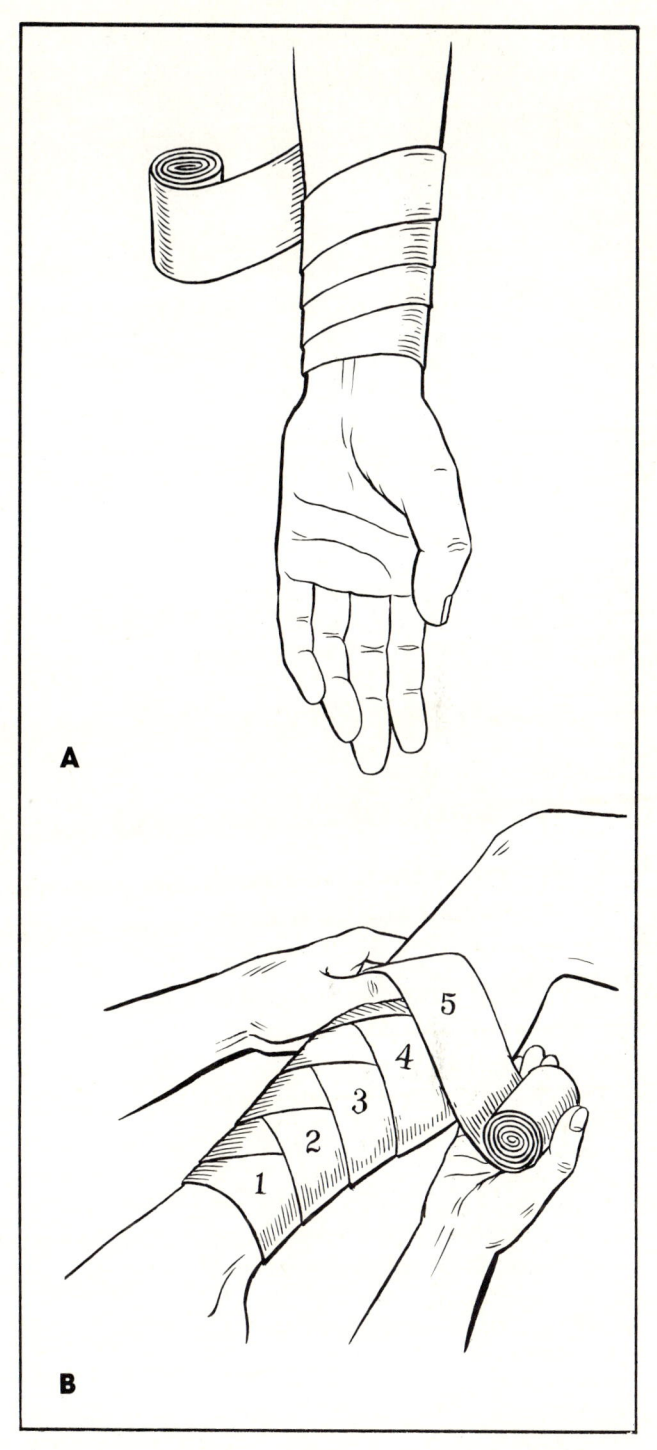

Figure 48-2. Wrapping an extremity. **A.** The spiral turn is used on areas with slight variance in circumference. **B.** The spiral reverse turn is used on areas with a more pronounced variance in circumference.

The *spiral reverse turn* is used to apply inflexible gauze to circumferential areas that change in diameter, such as an entire arm or leg. This turn takes up more slack on the lower border of the bandage than the plain spiral turn does. To execute this technique, anchor the initial end of the bandage with two circle turns and then begin a spiral turn, but stop at the center of the turn and place the free thumb at that

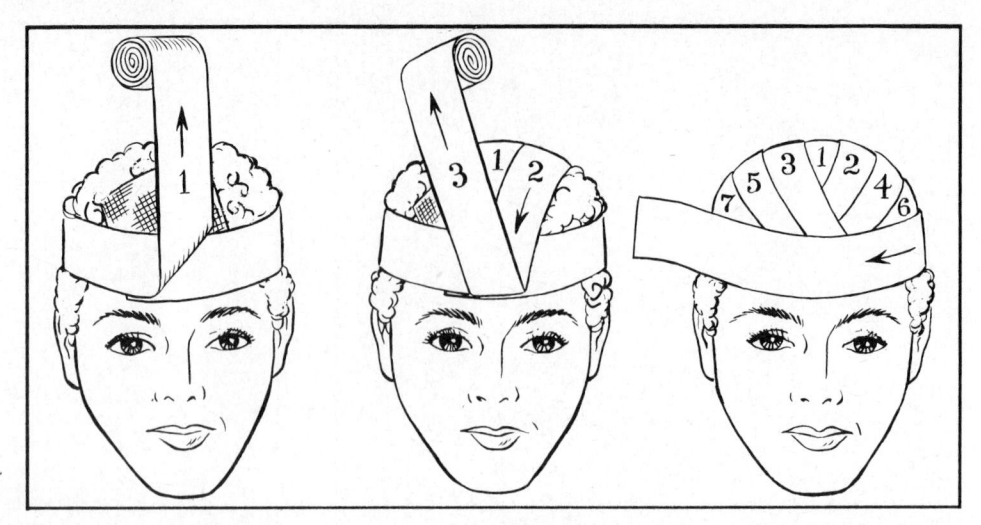

Figure 48-3. Recurrent turns are used to shape the bandage to a rounded part.

point on the upper border of the bandage. Reverse the bandage upon itself over the thumb while continuing around the extremity in the same direction, bringing the bandage around to the same center point as before. Use the same angle and amount of overlap as with the spiral turn. Remove the thumb and relocate it to the new layer for the next reverse turn. Continue until the part is completely bandaged, and finish by using one or two circular turns at the end of the part. Figure 48-2B shows how to execute the spiral reverse turn.

Recurrent turns are used to bandage a rounded part such as the head, a finger or thumb, or the stump of an amputation. Although the circular turn is used to anchor the beginning and end of the bandage, it is not always appropriate on a part such as a finger or an amputated stump because it may interfere with blood flow from the proximal to the distal part. To make a recurrent turn dressing on a head, begin with one or two circular turns around the circumference of the head, then stop at the center of the area to be bandaged and bring the bandage up at a 90-degree angle and hold the turn in place. Pass the bandage back and forth over the head, alternating placement of the bandage from side to side, creating a fold at each point where the bandage meets and overlaps the circular turn. Use the thumb to hold each fold in place. Continue until all of the head is covered. Finish the bandage by making circular turns around the head to anchor the recurrent turns, as shown in Figure 48-3.

The *figure-of-eight turn* is used to immobilize joints such as the elbow, knee, and ankle either partially or completely. To make a figure-of-eight turn, begin with one or two circular turns at a point below the joint and continue with the spiral turns up to the joint. Then bring the bandage above the joint and make one or two more circular turns; continue alternating the bandage wrap above and below the joint until the joint area is adequately covered. Terminate the bandage above the joint with a circular turn. The amount of skin area below and above the joint covered by the bandage depends on the purpose and the amount of support required. Figure 48-4 shows the figure-of-eight turn.

The *spica turn,* a variation of the figure-of-eight turn, is used to bandage a thumb, shoulder, groin, or breast. It is also used in combination with recurrent and spiral turns to apply elastic bandages to a residual stump of an amputated limb. Because of the difficulty in keeping bandages snugly in place on these sites, the bandage is wrapped around an additional adjoining part. To make a spica turn, place the bandage on the diagonal and make spiral turns over both body parts, overlapping each ascending and descending layer. Make circular turns on the diagonal, as shown in Figure 48-5, to prevent constricting the circulation.

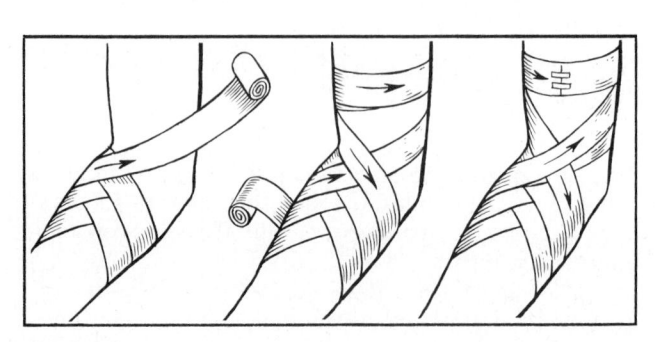

Figure 48-4. The figure-of-eight turn is used when bandaging across a joint.

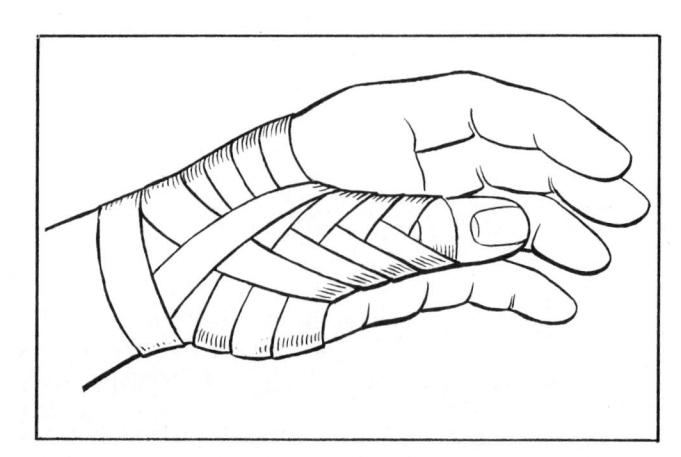

Figure 48-5. The spica turn is used to anchor a bandage to another body part.

APPLYING BINDERS

Prior to applying a binder, assess the type and size needed to ensure that the purpose will be achieved and that the client will not have normal physiological functions impeded.

Abdominal Binders

To apply an abdominal binder, place the client in a flat, supine position and in straight body alignment. Center the binder under the client's lower back with the edge of the binder at the level of the pubis symphysis. A binder that is placed too low can interfere with elimination and ambulation, and a binder that is placed too high can interfere with respiration. Pull on each side of the binder to straighten it and remove all wrinkles. When applying an *elasticized binder*, securely hold one side in place over the abdomen and pull the opposite side across it and fasten it in one location. Proceed to approximate the remaining edges and secure them.

Begin securing the binder at a point that is not directly over a wound and then work above and below the wound to avoid applying too much pressure over the wound, adjusting the overlap to fit the body contour. It is often easier to apply this type of binder more evenly and with less discomfort to the client when two persons work together. One person holds one side of the binder while the other person pulls and positions the opposite side over the abdomen and secures it in place.

To apply a *scultetus binder,* begin at the lower border of the binder and pull one tail snugly across the midline of the abdomen at a slight upward angle. Hold the first tail in place with one hand while bringing the opposite tail over it, then hold that tail in place or secure it with a safety pin. Continue to alternate wrapping each pair of tails over the abdomen until the binder is in place. Check with the client to determine if the binder feels comfortable and if the pressure is evenly distributed. Secure the last tail with a safety pin. If the tails of the binder are too long for the width of the abdomen, fold the tail back upon itself or obtain a smaller size. A completed wrapped scultetus binder is smooth and has an even pattern of overlapped ties, as shown in Figure 48–6.

Breast Binders

To apply a flat breast binder, place the client in a flat, supine position, center the binder under the back of the client's chest, and straighten out the sides to remove all wrinkles. If the client has pendulous breasts, place an absorbent gauze square between the breast and chest wall to absorb perspiration. This helps to prevent skin irritation from the increased moisture and warmth that result from the presence of the binder. Pull each side of the binder over the midline of the chest and secure in place with safety pins. If the client has large pendulous breasts, enlist the help of the client or a second person to hold the breasts in place over the front of the chest wall. With pins, make darts in the front and sides of the binder to ensure a comfortable and effective fit. After the binder is in place, observe the client's respiratory function to detect any interference.

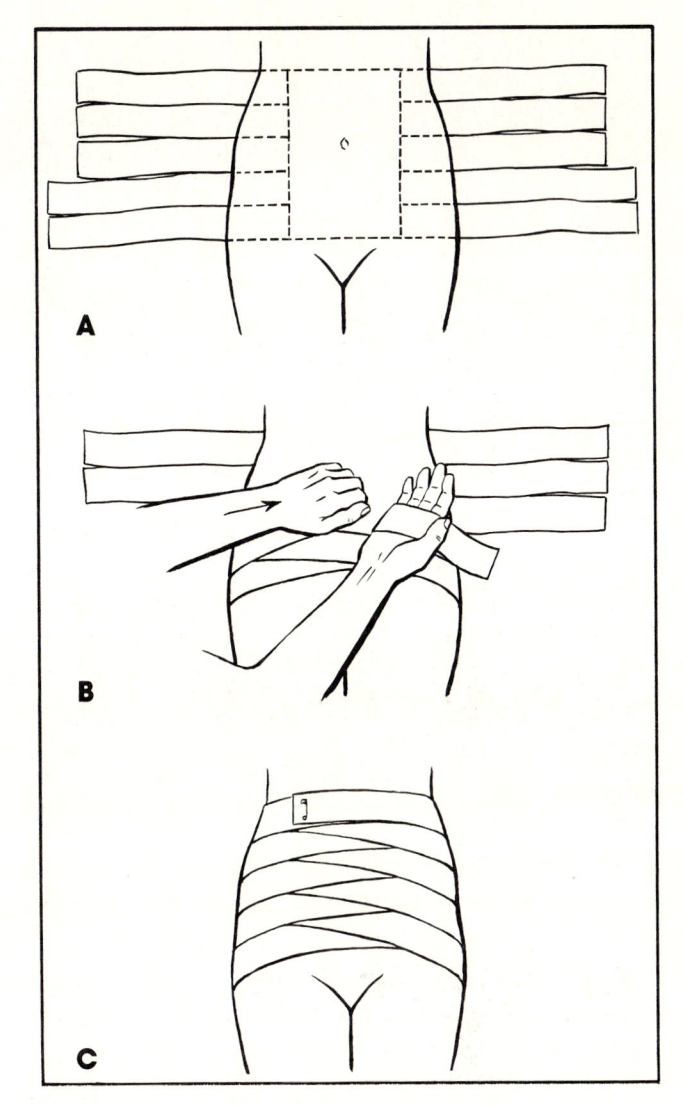

Figure 48–6. Applying a scultetus binder. **A.** Place the client in the center of the binder. **B.** Wrap the alternating tails around the abdomen. **C.** Anchor the tails with a safety pin.

T-Binders

To apply a T-binder, place the belt around the waist with the T-tail in alignment with the client's gluteal fold. Bring the T-tail between the legs over the dressing and secure it with safety pins. When using the double T-binder on male clients, be sure to position one T-tail on each side of the scrotum to prevent pressure on the scrotum and discomfort to the client.

Slings

To apply a triangular sling for support of an arm or shoulder, place one of the nondiagonal borders of the fabric flat across the front of the chest with the corners extending out to the side of and under the arm. Place the arm that needs to be supported in a 90-

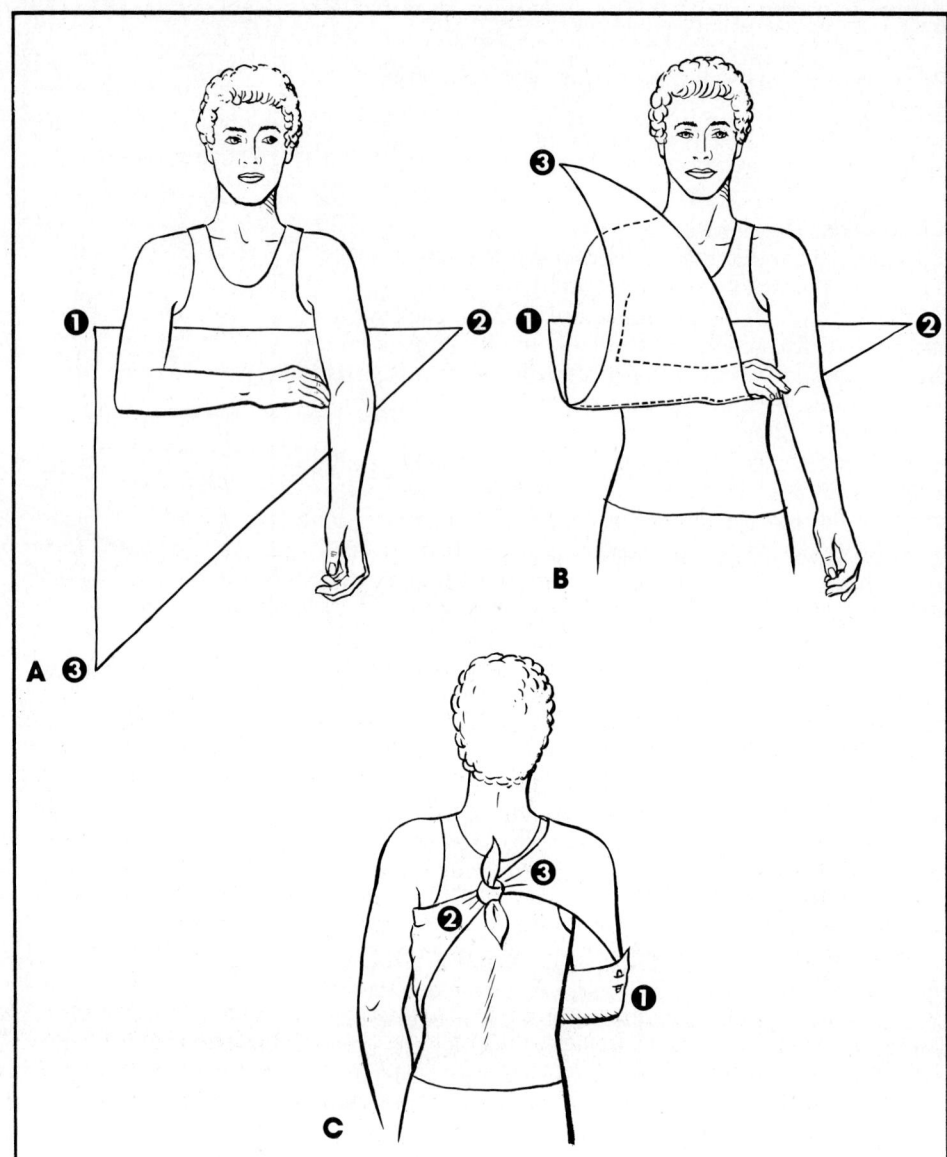

Figure 48–7. Applying a sling. **A.** Place the sling under the arm needing support. **B.** Bring the lower front corner of the sling up over the shoulder. **C.** Use a square knot to tie a knot at the back to one side of the spinal column.

degree flexed position. To distribute the weight of the arm across the shoulders and back evenly, bring the lower front corner of the sling up over the shoulder on the affected side and pull the other corner of the straight edge diagonally across the back. Use a square knot to tie these corners together securely. Position the knot to one side of the spinal column to avoid pressure over the bones. Avoid tying the sling at the base of the neck, because this places too much pressure on the back of the neck and can be uncomfortable as well as detrimental to a client with arthritis or neck injuries. It can also result in poor posture and cause the person to alter a normal gait. Once the sling is tied at the back, fold the free borders of the sling at the side of the arm and secure them in place at and above the elbow with safety pins. Figure 48–7 shows how to apply a sling.

Elastic Stockings

Elastic stockings are applied before the client gets out of bed for the day, because there is the least amount of blood in the leg veins at this time. Elastic stockings must be properly fitted to the client so that they will produce an even compression on the legs and avoid excessive pressure that can result from stockings that are too tight, too long, or too short. For proper fit, expose the client's legs and measure them with a measuring tape. For below-the-knee stockings, measure the largest diameter of the calf and the length from the sole of the heel to the top of the calf. The stocking should not extend up into the popliteal space because of the potential for increasing pressure over the veins. For midthigh or full-length stockings, measure the diameter of the midthigh and the length from the sole of the heel to the midthigh or the gluteal fold. Use these

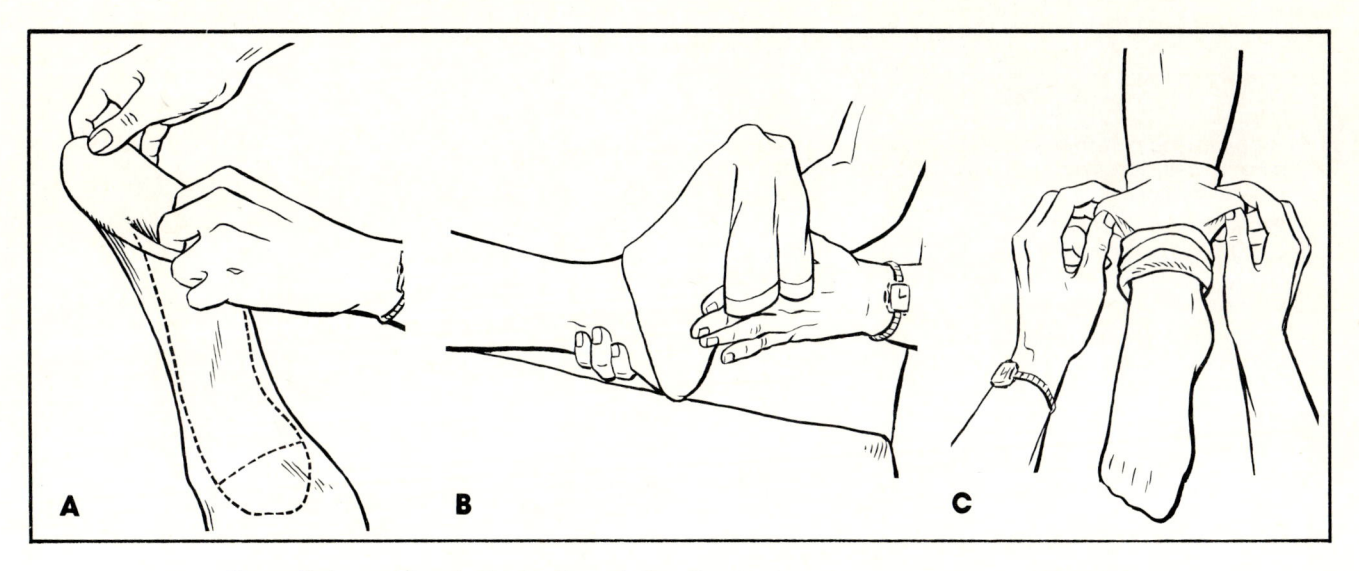

Figure 48–8. Applying elastic stockings. **A.** Turn the stocking inside out with the heel properly folded. **B.** Insert the foot into the folded-down stocking. **C.** Use both hands on opposite sides of the leg to pull the stocking up at about mid-calf.

measurements to determine the correct size of stockings according to the guide on the manufacturer's package.

To be effective, elastic stockings are put on smoothly and straight so that they conform to the natural contours of the leg. They cannot be pulled on like regular hosiery. Wrinkles in the stockings act as tourniquets and impede blood flow as well as being uncomfortable for the client. The stocking heel pocket must be centered over the client's heel and the full area of the calf properly aligned. Figure 48–8 shows how the stocking is applied. Full-length stockings have a gusset located at the top of the inner thigh that has more stretch. This is placed over the femoral area, so that there is no pressure on the artery and vein that would impede blood flow.

Before applying the stockings, wash and dry the legs, then apply a light dusting of talcum powder over the entire surface of the leg, using light, gentle strokes. This helps the stockings to glide over the skin more easily. If the client has dry skin, omit the powder because it makes the skin drier. Do not massage the legs, because there is a potential for dislodging a thrombus (blood clot) from the leg veins into the systemic circulation. Pull back the opening near the toes every 2 to 4 hours to check the neurovascular status of the toes. Signs of impaired neurovascular status include: (a) pale skin color, (b) skin cool to the touch, (c) inability to feel or flex the toes on request, (d) inability to perceive pressure, and (e) presence of numbness or tingling. Remove the stockings once every 12 hours to appraise the circulatory status and skin color and texture. Clients who do not understand the purpose of wearing elastic stockings or bandages have the misconception that they need to be worn only while ambulating. Since the purpose is to facilitate venous return, it is important that stockings or bandages be worn when the client is inactive or on bed rest. It is sometimes appropriate that they be removed when the client is ambulating.

☐ SKILL SEQUENCE

APPLYING ELASTIC STOCKINGS

Step	Rationale
1. Check physician's order on nursing kardex.	Ensures appropriate intervention.
2. Wash hands.	Prevents transferring microorganisms.
3. Expose one leg at a time and wash, dry, and powder legs.	Removes dead skin cells and facilitates putting on stockings.
4. With one hand, hold stocking by top cuff and use dominant hand to reach inside and grasp center of heel pocket. Pull heel pocket up through stocking to top cuff. Fold heel pocket across center. Leave stocking foot inside stocking. (NOTE: Stocking is now inside out with foot portion left inside stocking.)	Pulls stocking inside out in preparation for application.
5. Insert client's foot into stocking foot, centering and aligning heel.	

(continued)

APPLYING ELASTIC STOCKINGS (Cont.)

Step	Rationale
6. Pull remaining portion of stocking up over foot and ankle, clearing heel. Stocking is now right side out, gathered around the ankle.	Prepares remaining portion for application.
7. Recheck position of heel.	Ensures proper alignment.
8. Pull all of stocking down around ankle so that it is inside out, with a folded-over edge at ankle. Smooth out all wrinkles.	Prepares remaining portion for application.
9. Use fingers and thumbs of each hand to grasp both sides of inverted stocking about 2 inches below top border of folded-over edge and pull it up leg a few inches.	Facilitates application and permits removal of wrinkles.
10. Pull stocking back down about 1 inch to smooth out wrinkles.	Permits removal of wrinkles; helps to keep stocking in proper alignment for fitting to leg contours. Distributes stretch of stocking more evenly over entire leg than when pulled on in one motion. Stimulates venous return.
11. Continue alternating steps 9 and 10 until stocking is gradually and fully pulled in place. (NOTE: When applying full-length stockings, check location of gusset for proper alignment over femoral area when stocking has been pulled up to midthigh. Check location of knee area of stocking for proper placement at client's knee.)	Important that gusset be centered over femoral artery to prevent compression of artery. Tighter stretch from lower leg portion of stocking should not extend over popliteal area because this would cause excessive pressure in that area.
12. Remove stockings: Grasp top band of stocking with hands on each side of leg and gently pull stocking off inside out.	
13. Stockings should be washed or aired. Apply a second pair of elastic stockings.	Hygienic measures; tends to prolong stretch of stockings.
14. Record findings from skin and neurovascular appraisal and the type of elastic stockings applied.	Documents client's status and nursing actions.

ANCHORING BANDAGES AND BINDERS

It is possible for the client to be pricked or stabbed by the safety pins or metal clips that are often used to hold bandages and binders in place. This may occur either when they are inserted or if they become displaced. To insert a safety pin without pricking the client, place a finger between the client's skin and the bandage or binder at the point of insertion, and use the finger to guide the pin back out to the surface of the fabric. Apply metal clips over at least two layers of bandage, so that the clip points are grasping the bandage material and not the client's skin.

Adhesive tape is commonly used to secure the terminal end of a gauze bandage. However, it is not used on reusable bandage or binder materials such as muslin, cotton flannel, or elastic bandages, because it leaves a gummy residue on the fabric that cannot be removed by washing.

CARE OF BANDAGES AND BINDERS

Bandages and binders made of durable fabrics such as muslin or cotton flannel can be washed in the laundry or by hand. Elasticized materials are washed by hand in mild soap, rinsed thoroughly, and air dried flat to prevent them from stretching. After they are thoroughly dry, elastic bandages are rolled evenly without wrinkles so they are ready for reuse.

CLIENT TEACHING

When a client must continue to use a bandage or binder after discharge, it is the nurse's responsibility to ensure that the client or a family member knows how to observe and care for the skin and apply, remove, and care for the item. The client is given an adequate supply of bandages or is informed where they might be obtained.

RECORDING

The type of bandage or binder and the location are noted on the client health record. The results of neurovascular and skin appraisals and any signs of compromised neurovascular function are carefully described.

Sample POR Recording

- S—"My legs don't swell up so much since I've been wearing these stockings."
- O—Toes pink, no edema in the feet or ankles.
- A—Venous congenstion in legs decreased.
- P—Continue to apply full-length elastic stockings.

Sample Narrative Recording

States that her legs are not swelling up as much since she has been wearing the full-length elastic stockings. Toes pink and no edema present in the feet or ankles. Will continue to apply stockings.

CRITICAL POINTS SUMMARY

1. The porousness of a bandage affects the amount of air circulation to the skin.
2. Flexible materials mold to fit the body contours.
3. The degree of extensibility of a bandage affects the amount of pressure exerted on the tissues.
4. The amount of pressure exerted on the tissues must not exceed the hydrostatic vascular pressure.
5. The body area or part to which a bandage or binder is applied is placed in good body alignment to prevent interference with normal function.
6. Skin areas covered by bandages and binders are protected from the effects of heat, moisture, and pressure.
7. The body area is inspected for color, presence of lesions, and edema before the bandage or binder is applied and after it is removed.
8. Palpation is used to detect skin temperature and pulse quality.
9. The nurse checks with the client while applying a bandage or binder to ensure that it is not tight.
10. A bandage on an extremity is wrapped beginning at the distal aspect.
11. Safety pins and metal clips are inserted so that they do not prick the client; they are placed in a location that will not cause pressure against the tissues.
12. Medical aseptic technique is used to handle and apply bandages and binders.

LEARNING ACTIVITIES

1. Visit the central supply department and ask to see the types and sizes of bandages and binders available. Find out which ones are ordered most frequently. Compare the degree of porousness, flexibility, and extensibility of several types of bandages.
2. Observe the techniques used by nurses and physicians to apply bandages and binders, noting the appropriateness and correctness of each application.
3. Interview the nurse in charge of a general surgical unit to find out the policies governing the use of abdominal binders.
4. With a peer, practice making each type of bandage turn with plain gauze.
5. Have a peer apply elastic bandages to both of your legs below the knees. Wear the bandages for at least 30 minutes while remaining inactive in bed or sitting in a chair. Note how comfortable they are and if you feel any constriction in your legs. Have the peer palpate the quality of your dorsalis pedis pulses.
6. Practice measuring a peer's leg for below-the-knee, midthigh, and full-length elastic stockings. If stockings are available, apply the stockings.

REVIEW QUESTIONS

1. What are some of the purposes for using bandages and binders?
2. Match the properties of bandage and binder materials listed below with the corresponding effects. Each property may be used more than once.

PROPERTIES	EFFECTS
a. Porousness	____ Tissue compression
b. Flexibility	____ Absorbency
c. Extensibility	____ Molds to body contours
	____ Air circulation
	____ Tissue temperature

3. What is the effect on the tissues when the compression from a bandage exceeds the hydrostatic vascular pressure?
4. Why is it important to position the body area, parts, and joints in good alignment before applying a bandage or binder?
5. List the specific measures the nurse uses to protect the skin under a bandage or binder from the effects of warmth, moisture, and pressure.
6. What data does the nurse collect before and after applying a bandage or binder?
7. Why does wrapping a bandage begin at the distal aspect of an extremity?
8. Why is it important to leave a small part of the distal aspect of a bandaged extremity exposed?
9. How can the nurse prevent a client from being pricked by a safety pin or metal clip?

PERFORMANCE CHECKLIST

OBJECTIVE: To apply elastic stockings safely.			
CHARACTERISTIC	RANGE OF ACCEPTABILITY	SATISFACTORY	UNSATISFACTORY
1. Checks physician's order.	No deviation		
2. Washes hands.	No deviation		
3. Exposes, washes, dries, and powders both legs.	No deviation		

(continued)

OBJECTIVE: To apply elastic stockings safely (cont.).			
CHARACTERISTIC	RANGE OF ACCEPTABILITY	SATISFACTORY	UNSATISFACTORY
4. Turns stocking inside out, leaving stocking foot inside stocking with heel pocket folded across center.	No deviation		
5. Inserts client's foot into stocking foot, centering and aligning heel.	No deviation		
6. Pulls remaining portion of stocking right side out up over foot and ankle; then rechecks position of heel.	No deviation		
7. Pulls all of stocking down around ankle inside out, with a folded-over cuff at ankle. Smooths out all wrinkles.	No deviation		
8. Grasps both sides of inverted stocking below folded cuff and pulls it up leg a few inches.	No deviation		
9. Pulls stocking back down about 1 inch and smooths out wrinkles; alternates pulling stocking up then down until stocking is gradually pulled fully into place.	No deviation		
10. Checks stocking for proper placement of knee area and gusset over femoral area for midthigh and full-length stockings.	No deviation		
11. Removes stocking inside out by pulling down on both sides of top band.	No deviation		
12. Records skin condition and results of neurovascular appraisal, and type of elastic stockings applied.			

REFERENCE

Thomas S, Dawes C, Hay P: A critical evaluation of some extensible bandages in current use. Nursing Times 76(26): 1123–1132, 1980.

BIBLIOGRAPHY

Lewis LW: Fundamental Skills in Patient Care. Philadelphia, JB Lippincott, 1980.

McMahon MM: Providing Physical Protection and Bodily Support. In Sorensen KC, Luckman J (eds): Basic Nursing: A Psychophysiologic Approach. Philadelphia, WB Saunders, 1979.

AUDIOVISUAL RESOURCES

Application of Bandages and Binders
  Filmstrip and cassette. (1976, Color, 20 min.)
  Available through:
    Medcom, Inc.
    PO Box 116
    Garden Grove, CA 92642

Applying Anti-Embolism Stockings/Ace Bandages; Application of Applying Binders. Videorecording (3/4 in). (1981, Color, 19 min.)
  Available through:
    Robert J. Brady Company
    Route 197
    Bowie, MD 20715

Care and Wrapping of a Below-the-Knee Stump
  Videorecording (3/4 in). (1979, Color, 7 min.)
  Available through:
    Health Sciences Consortium
    200 Eastowne Drive, Suite 213
    Chapel Hill, NC 27514

SKILL 49 Mechanical Restraints

PREREQUISITE SKILLS

Skill 19, "Inspection"
Skill 20, "Palpation"
Skill 28, "Handwashing"
Skill 38, "Skin Care"
Skill 51, "Monitoring Fluid Balance"

☐ STUDENT OBJECTIVES

1. Explain the purpose in using restraints.
2. Describe the adverse psychological and physiological effects of mechanical restraints.
3. Explain how acts of negligence can result from the use of restraints.

4. Indicate the type of information about the use of restraints that is specified by state laws and institutional policies.
5. Specify the type of data about a client that would help a nurse anticipate a need to restrain the client.
6. Describe the type of data the nurse collects before, during, and after using restraints.
7. Specify the nursing actions that are used to protect a client from injury while restrained.
8. Indicate the types of knots that are most appropriate to secure restraints.
9. Demonstrate the procedure used to restrain a client safely.

☐ INTRODUCTION

Physical restraints are mechanical devices that are used to ensure the safety of a client by restricting and controlling freedom of movement. They are used therapeutically when it is absolutely necessary to prevent a client from harming himself or herself or, in the case of mentally ill clients, from harming others. Restraints should not create problems for the client by interfering with the plan of treatment or health status. Clients who require restraint are mentally confused, have an altered level of consciousness, or for some reason are unable to cooperate with the plan of treatment, as is often the case with infants and children.

Mechanical restraints are categorized as *soft* or *hard*. Soft restraints are made of fabric and are designed to be tied or buckled in place. Hard restraints are made of leather or firm plastic and are designed to be locked in place. Mechanical restraints are applied either to a body part such as a wrist, ankle, or chest or to the entire body. For example, a wrist restraint may be used to restrict the movement of an arm when a client has an intravenous infusion, and a chest restraint may be used to prevent a client from getting out of bed and falling.

Restraints that are not applied to the body are referred to as environmental restraints because they contain a client within a confined area. Environmental restraints include side rails, canopies that enclose the client in the bed, or a private room that may be or may not be locked. On psychiatric units a locked private room is called a seclusion room.

When considering the use of restraints, the nurse keeps in mind that the purpose of any type of restraint is to protect the client from harm and to facilitate the client's recovery. Restraints are never to be used as a form of punishment.

☐ PREPARATION

Even though mechanical restraints are used to protect the client and facilitate recovery, they also are often responsible for creating some adverse psychological and physiological effects.

PSYCHOLOGICAL EFFECTS

A client who is physically restrained may become restless, anxious, fearful, suspicious, or angry and lose trust in the care-giver. Even when only one arm and leg are restrained, clients may perceive themselves as helpless and childlike, since they often need assistance to meet some very basic needs such as taking a drink of water or changing body position. Clients may feel dehumanized and try to escape the restraints by untying or manipulating them to gain freedom. Clients may also plead with family members, visitors, or passersby to release them.

Seeing a loved one restrained often has a negative effect on the family and visitors. Restraints convey the message that the client is not capable of self-control or of cooperating with the plan of care and, therefore, the behavior must be controlled by some external means. Family members may also feel embarrassed about the behavior of their relative, and visitors may feel pity for the client and anger at the staff for what may be perceived as unkind treatment. If family members do not understand the reason for restraints or the precautions that nurses use to ensure the client's safety while in restraints, they too may become angry.

PHYSIOLOGICAL EFFECTS

Because mechanical restraints restrict movement, they can cause minor or severe damage under and near the restraint. The skin may become irritated, and temporary or permanent damage to the circulation or nerve supply may occur from the pressure of the restraint on the tissues. Restriction of body movement can cause loss of motion or dislocation of joints and can hamper normal physiological function. For example, when an arm is restrained for an extended period of time for the purpose of avoiding dislocation of an intravenous needle or catheter, a client may lose some range of motion in the shoulder, elbow, and wrist joints; or if a client struggles against the restraint, the client could dislocate a joint. Chest or body restraints that are applied too tightly may contribute to pulmonary infection such as pneumonia, because the restraints can interfere with normal respiratory function by restricting the depth of inspiration and expiration. Clients who are unable to swallow properly can aspirate mucus, fluids, or food into the lungs and thus are vulnerable to pneumonia.

LEGAL ASPECTS OF RESTRAINTS

Since the use of restraints is fairly common in nursing and medical practice, it is important for the nurse to be aware of the legal aspects that are involved with both the inappropriate use of restraints and the failure to use restraints appropriately when needed. During all client-care activities, a nurse is expected to make necessary observations and take appropriate action to protect the client from harm. A nurse is also expected to exercise reasonable judgment in providing care. To avoid negligence, the nurse always applies both of these principles when considering and using restraints. Situations in which the client is at risk of physical harm include those in which the nurse fails to use restraints when they are needed, applies the restraints in such a way that the client suffers damaging physical effects, and fails to observe the client for adverse effects of the restraints. Creighton (1981), Murchison and Nichols (1970), and "Restraining" (1974) describe cases in which clients were awarded large sums of money in damage suits against hospitals for injuries that resulted from either the inappropriate use of restraints or the failure to use restraints appropriately.

State laws address the use of both mechanical and environmental restraints, particularly for the mentally ill. Some laws indicate that, except in the case of emergency, restraints of any form cannot be used unless the need for them is determined by a physician. The law may also state that in an emergency, restraints may be used for a maximum of 12 hours without the determination of a physician. The law may also specify that a restrained client must be observed frequently and that the time and condition of the client must be periodically recorded on the client's health record. State law may require that each separate use of restraints and the reason for using them must also be entered on the health record. Even with the absence of state law requirements, professional standards of care require frequent observations and documentation on the health record.

Hospital policies that address the use of restraints usually follow closely the points included in the laws of that state. However, they may be much more specific. The nurse needs to know the law pertaining to restraints in the state in which the nurse is practicing nursing and also the specific policies of the institution in which he or she is working. Some institutions require a written order by a physician before any type of restraint may be used; others permit the nurse in charge to exercise his or her clinical judgment and use soft restraints for a specified period of time pending a written order. Most institutions specifically prohibit the use of hard, locked restraints without a written order by the physician. Institutional policy may also require that the renewal order for restraints be written every 24 hours.

DATA BASE

Client History and Recorded Data

In anticipation of the potential need to restrain clients, a nurse is always alert for conditions and events that can precipitate the need to use restraints. Clients' ability to cooperate with the treatment plan or control themselves can be affected by physiological factors such as age (the very old or very young), electrolyte imbalances, drugs that alter the level of consciousness, and diseases that affect the neurologic system. Psychological factors that affect self-control and cooperation include psychiatric conditions, the ability to understand and accept treatment, and anxiety or fear. The medical diagnosis and the treatment plan may also provide indicators of a need for restraints. The nurse keeps informed about the client's current level of consciousness and ability to cooperate.

Information about these factors is normally available on the client health record or the nursing kardex, or it can be obtained by speaking to and observing the client's behavior. In addition to gathering data from these sources, the nurse keeps abreast of changes in a client's status that could require the use of restraints, such as changes in either the client's level of consciousness, contact with reality, or behavior. The nurse recognizes that a client may verbally indicate a sincere desire to cooperate but may be unable actually to do so for either physiological or psychological reasons. For example, mentally alert clients with a neurologic disease may be unable to control involuntary movements and clients who are having misperceptions of reality such as occur with hallucinations or psychosis misinterpret what they hear and see and may need some form of external control.

Physical Appraisal Skills

Inspection. An initial inspection provides a baseline of data that can be used to evaluate any changes noted in subsequent inspections. Additional inspections are made during and after the application of mechanical restraints. The skin and tissues to which the restraint is to be applied are always carefully inspected for color, the presence or absence of lesions, and edema. The range of motion of joints above and below the restraint are appraised before, during, and after the use of restraints. Respiratory rate and depth is evaluated before and during the use of chest restraints.

Palpation. Palpation is also used before, during, and after use of restraints to determine the presence of edema, numbness, discomfort, or pain in the body area under and near the restraint.

EQUIPMENT

Mechanical restraints may be either improvised or commercially manufactured. Improvised restraints include folded bed linen, bathrobe belts, stockinet, woven strips of fabric or webbing, or gauze bandages. Commercial restraints are made of tightly woven twill fabric, leather, or firm plastic. A restraint must be strong enough to restrain the body part and large enough to prevent constriction of the tissues.

TYPES OF RESTRAINTS

Safety belts made of webbing, twill, or leather with a buckle on one end are available in various lengths for

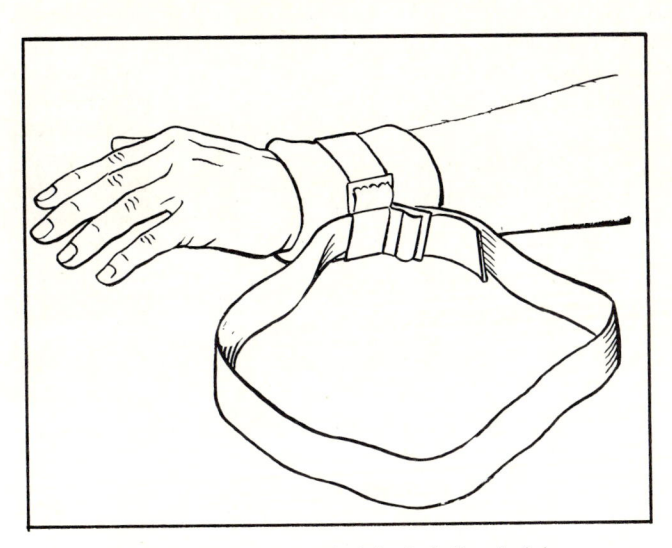

Figure 49-1. Limb restraints. **A.** *Soft restraint.*

use on different body areas. They are used to secure a client to a stretcher, chair, or bed. Safety belts are also used when turning clients who are on a Stryker frame or Circo-electric bed.

Limb restraints consist of cuffs that are applied to the wrists or ankles and straps that are used to secure the extremity to the bed or chair frame. Commercially available limb restraints may be soft or hard, as shown in Figure 49-1. The cuff of a soft restraint consists of a rectangular soft-padded fabric that is applied directly to the skin and has long straps attached. The cuff on a leather or plastic limb restraint often is not sufficiently padded to protect the skin from abrasion, so a soft pad of flannel, toweling, or an abdominal dressing must be wrapped around the skin before the cuff is applied. Long straps are provided for securing the extremity. Improvised cuff restraints can be created by wrapping and securing an abdominal dressing or washcloth around the wrist or ankle with adhesive tape and using a long strip of gauze bandage to secure the extremity to the bed or chair frame. Limb restraints are used when it is necessary to restrict the movement of an extremity to prevent a client from pulling on intravenous infusions, tubes, or dressings, or to control a client's movement while a procedure is performed.

Chest restraints are made of either a tightly woven fabric in the form of an open jacket that wraps across the back or front of the chest and covers the major portion of the chest, or straps designed in the form of a halter that fits around the chest, as shown in Figure 49-2. Straps attached to the sides of the chest restraint may or may not have buckles to secure the client in the bed or chair. An improvised chest restraint can be fashioned from a tightly rolled or folded bed sheet that can be applied as a halter. Chest restraints are used to prevent a client from getting out of the bed or chair when this activity would likely result in a fall.

Elbow restraints are made of thick cotton or flannel fabric. They are about 12 inches long and have 6 to 8 pockets into which tongue blades or plastic slats can be inserted to make the restraint rigid, as shown in Figure 49-3. Several ties attached to one edge of the restraint are used to tie the restraint around the elbow. Sometimes there are additional double ties at the top of the restraint that can be used to secure the restraint to the client to reduce the mobility of the arm. Elbow restraints are used most often on children to prevent them from pulling on tubes and dressings or picking at skin lesions.

Commercial *mitt restraints* are made from a tightly woven fabric with attached straps that secure the mitt to the wrist, as shown in Figure 49-4. Improvised mitts can be made from tubular stockinet but these must be taped in place at the wrist. Mitts are used to prevent a client from using the hands to pull on or pick at tubes, dressings, or skin lesions. Wrist restraints may also be used in conjunction with the mitts to control arm movement if necessary.

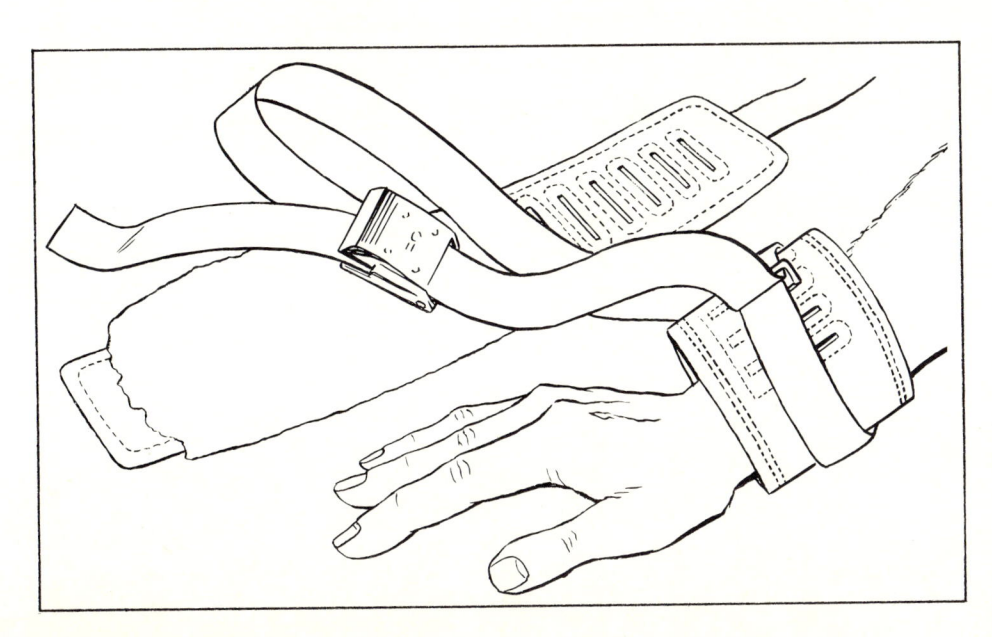

Figure 49-1. **B.** *Hard restraint.*

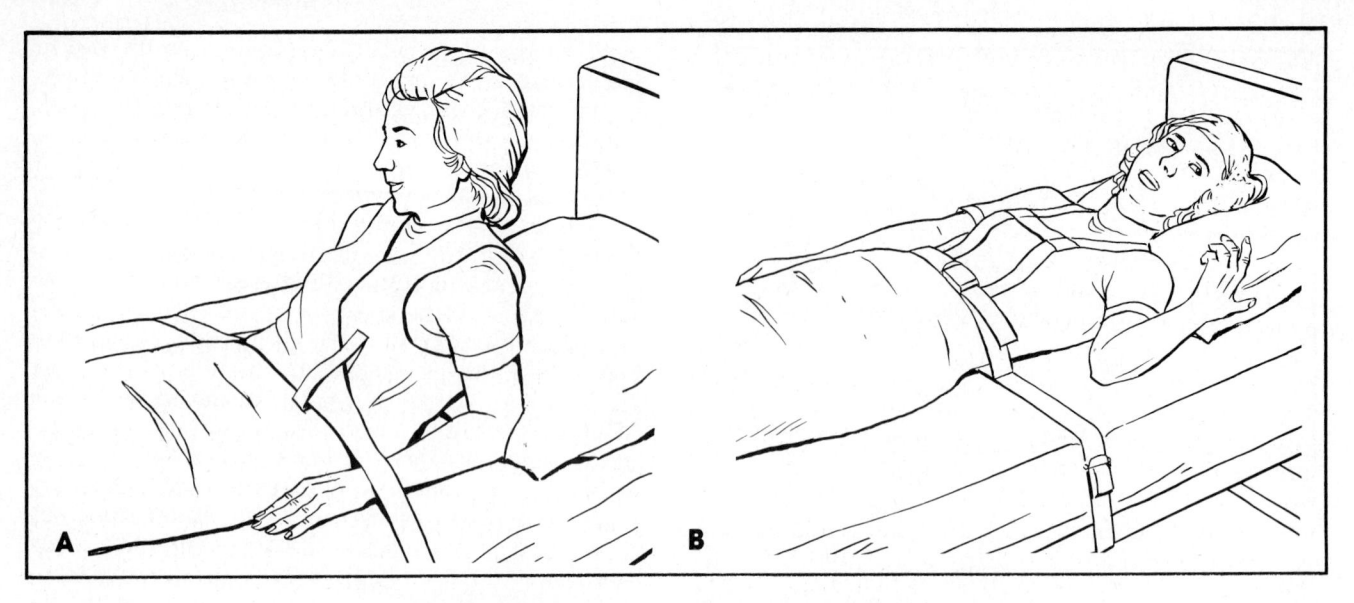

Figure 49-2. Chest restraints. **A.** Jacket restraint. **B.** Halter restraint.

☐ EXECUTION

When it is necessary to restrain a client, consider carefully the degree of restraint required and select the most appropriate type of restraint to achieve the desired purpose. The degree of restraint required varies with the desired purpose. Permit a client as much freedom of movement as possible. For example, an alert and cooperative client who is unable to keep an arm correctly positioned while receiving an intravenous infusion may need to have that arm loosely restrained only as a reminder to prevent dislodging the infusion. On the other hand, a client who pulls out or attempts to pull out an intravenous infusion may need to have both arms restrained. If this same client also attempts to get out of bed against medical orders, the client may need to be contained in bed with a chest restraint and an additional restraint on the opposite ankle.

The size and the strength of the restraint must be adequate for the size and physical strength of the client. Restraints that are too large do not provide the necessary restriction of movement; restraints that are too small constrict the tissues and cause damage. The physical power of the client who struggles against a soft improvised restraint may be sufficient to break it.

Explain the reason for the restraint and the extent to which the client is to be restrained carefully to both the client and the family. Reassure the client and family that frequent observations will be made while the restraints are in place, that the restraints will be periodically released, and that whatever assistance the client requires to meet basic needs such as eating, drinking, using the bedpan, and changing position will be provided by the nursing staff. Also let them know that the restraints will be used only as long as is abso-

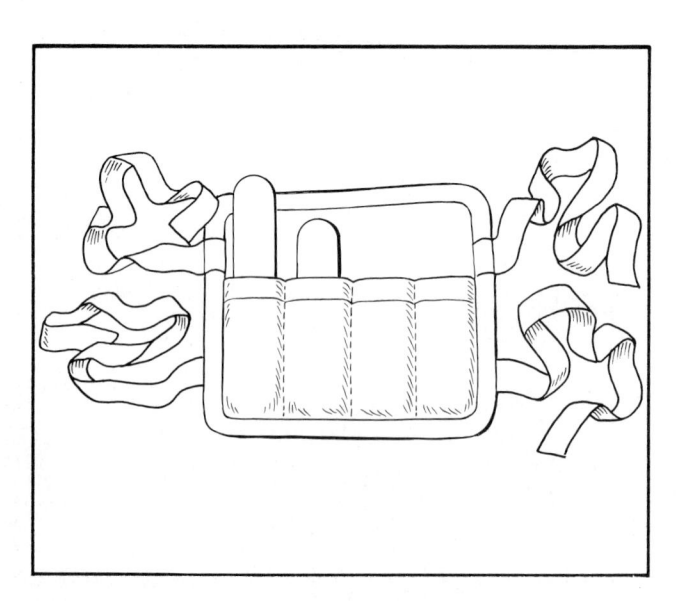

Figure 49-3. Elbow restraint.

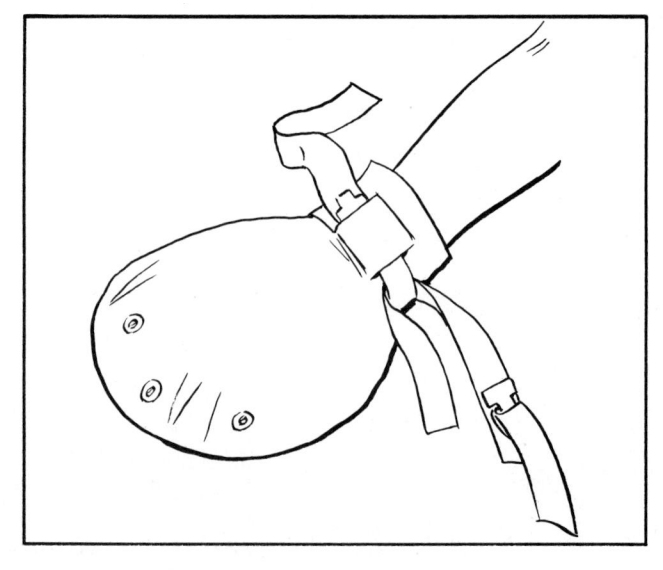

Figure 49-4. Mitt restraint.

lutely necessary. Be prepared to provide frequent reinforcement of this information and reassurance to the client and the family.

APPLYING THE RESTRAINTS

Before applying the restraint, bathe, dry, and powder the skin that is to be covered by the restraint and appraise the condition of the tissues. Do not apply the restraint directly on the client's bare skin, since friction of the restraint against the skin can cause abrasions and lacerations. Place a soft padding of flannel, toweling, or an abdominal dressing under the cuff of unpadded limb restraints, and a hospital gown or shirt without buttons under a chest restraint. Eliminate all wrinkles in the clothing worn under the chest restraint to prevent pressure against the skin. Before securing the restraint on the client, place the client in a position with good body alignment and comfort. If a client needs to have mitts applied to prevent him or her from using the fingers or hands, place hand rolls in the palms so that the fingers can grasp the roll in a position of function. This helps to prevent loss of mobility while the mitt is in place.

Never apply limb restraints to only one side of the body, because this allows a client to use the free side to escape from the restraints or to get partially out of the bed or chair, thus providing the opportunity for injury. Depending on the client's condition, apply limb restraints in the following patterns:

1. One wrist and the opposite ankle
2. Both wrists and one ankle
3. Both ankles and one wrist
4. Both wrists and both ankles

Do not apply a limb restraint to an extremity that has an arteriovenous shunt or an arterial or venous line in place. Use an intravenous board to splint the extremity and then attach the restraint to the board.

There are two types of knots that are considered most appropriate for securing a limb restraint cuff in place on a client: the clove-hitch knot and the square knot. Both of these knots provide some degree of safety in that they stay in place and will not tighten and constrict the circulation. It is also difficult for a client to release them accidentally or intentionally. The half-bow knot is recommended to secure the free end of the restraint to the bed or chair frame, because it is easily untied by merely pulling on the loose end and it will not slip when tension is applied to the secured part of the tie. Figure 49–5 shows how these knots are made. Wetting the knot makes it difficult for a client to untie.

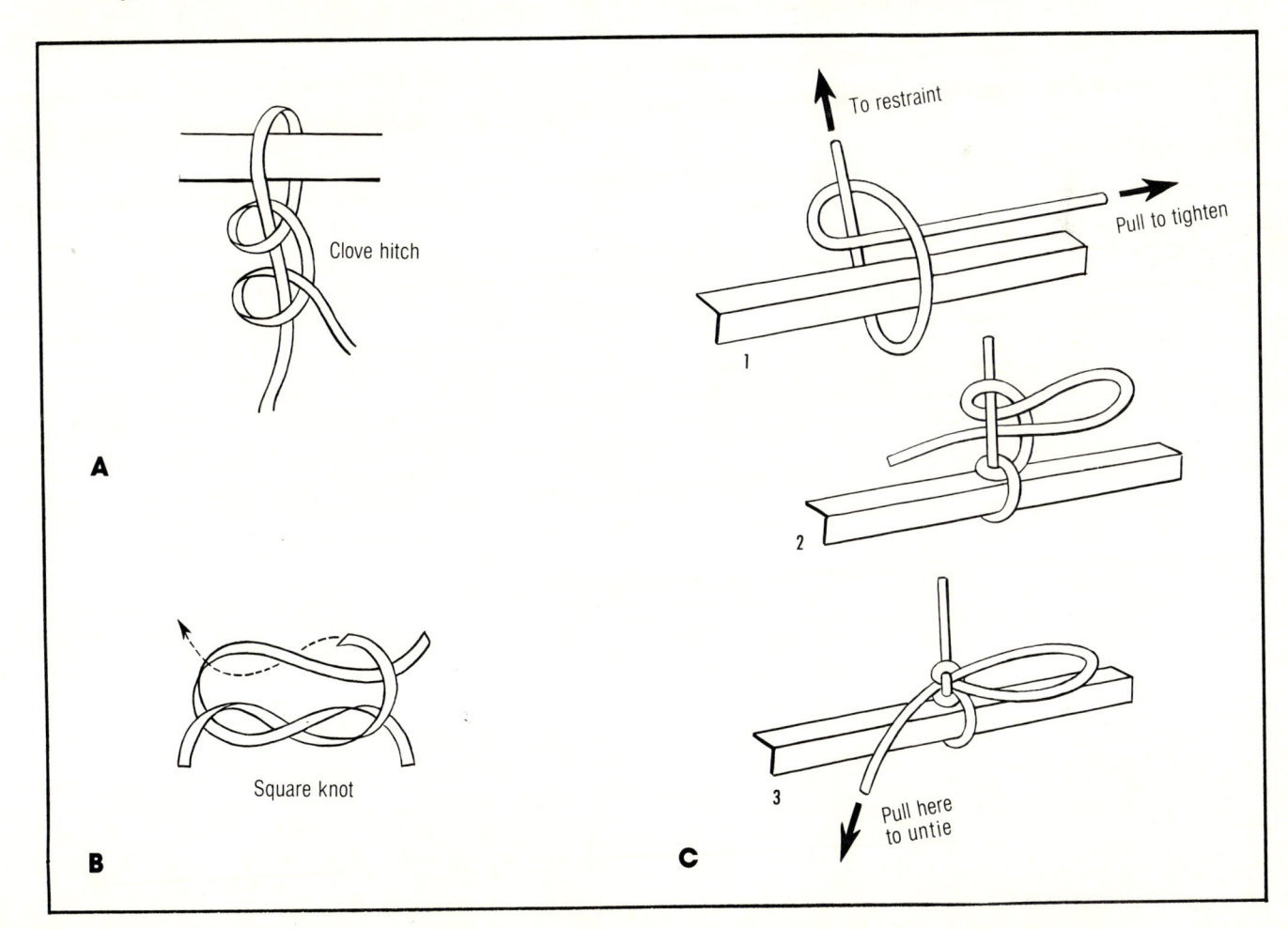

Figure 49–5. Making knots. **A.** The clove-hitch knot. **B.** The square knot. **C.** The half-bow knot.

Place the knots and buckles that secure the restraint on the client in locations that prevent the client from lying on them, to avoid having continuous pressure applied against the skin. They need to be inaccessible to the client to prevent escape. When dealing with a client who proves to be an escape artist, resist the temptation to tape the restraint closures. This makes it difficult to release the client promptly in the event of an emergency and leaves a gummy residue on the restraint.

Once the restraint is in place on the client, determine the best location to secure the free end. Keep in mind the maximum degree of freedom the client can be allowed and still have the purpose of restraint achieved. For example, if the goal is to prevent the client from pulling off a dressing on the upper part of the body, it would be best to anchor the restraint at or below the client's waist level. Attach the free end to a part of the bed or chair that is permanently fixed. A restraint that is secured to a bed side rail can become too tight or too loose when the side rail is raised or lowered. The most secure place to anchor the restraint for a client confined to bed is the bedsprings under the mattress. Use of this area prevents the client from reaching and releasing the knot or buckle.

Care of the Restrained Client

When the client is restrained, make sure that the call light is within grasp. This provides reassurance that someone can be reached and makes the client feel more at ease. Observe the client *at least* every 2 hours and (a) attend to his or her personal needs such as nutrition and elimination, (b) check on the restraints to make sure that they are not too tight or too loose, (c) appraise the skin condition under and distal to the restraint, and (d) reposition the client if the client is unable to do so himself or herself. Remove the restraints every 2 hours and give skin care to the areas under and around the restraints as well as to any pressure points on other parts of the body. If possible, rotate the restraints frequently, using alternate body parts. While the client is restrained, frequently reevaluate the client's willingness and ability to cooperate with the medical and nursing-care plan, so that the duration of the restraints is not unnecessarily prolonged.

COMBATIVE AND PSYCHIATRIC CLIENTS

Restraining a combative or suicidal client requires a different approach than that for other clients. Recognize and accept the possibility that a combative client may cause physical harm to the staff during the application of restraints. When a decision has been made to restrain a combative client, plan in advance and have an adequate number of staff available. Have the staff approach the client simultaneously with the needed restraints in hand, so that the restraints are applied quickly and with minimal struggle.

When a client is known or suspected to be suicidal, be aware that restraints can be used as a weapon by which a client can commit suicide. Secure the restraints so that there is no possibility of the client releasing them or repositioning them so that they can be used for strangulation. When it is necessary to restrain a psychotic client mechanically, leather or plastic locked restraints are most often used to decrease the possibility of the restraints coming loose or released. Keys for locked restraints are kept either taped to the client's bed or carried by all personnel on the unit. The key must be readily available so that a client can be promptly released, if necessary, for emergency medical care (such as cardiopulmonary resuscitation) or evacuation from the unit because of a disaster such as a fire. Have adequate personnel available when it is time to release the restraints to provide care and perform appraisals. Whenever possible, release only one extremity or body area at a time to enable the staff to control the client's movements. When psychiatric clients' restraints are not in use, remove them from the room so that they cannot be used for purposes that are destructive to the client or others.

☐ SKILL SEQUENCE

APPLYING A LIMB RESTRAINT

Step	Rationale
1. Check physician's order on health record or kardex.	A legal requirement to protect client (except in emergency).
2. Wash hands.	Prevents cross-contamination from microorganisms on hands.
3. Obtain restraints.	Avoids delay in executing procedure.
4. Explain procedure and reason to client and provide reassurance.	Allays anxiety.
5. Bathe, dry, and powder skin area to be restrained.	Protects skin by reducing friction created by movement of restraint over skin.
6. Place client in position of comfort with good body alignment.	Minimizes discomfort and potential for injury while restrained.

(continued)

SKILL 49: MECHANICAL RESTRAINTS

Step	Rationale

7. To apply a commercial restraint:
   a. Wrap padded side of cuff snugly around wrist or ankle.
   b. Secure cuff in place either by pulling tie end through slit on cuff, by fastening Velcro straps, or by tying a clove-hitch or square knot.
   (NOTE: Place knot on top part of extremity.)
To apply an improvised restraint:
   a. Wrap an abdominal dressing or folded washcloth snugly around wrist or ankle.
   b. Secure cuff pad in place with adhesive tape.
   c. Wrap a 3- to 4-foot long gauze bandage around cuff and tie in place using a clove-hitch or square knot to hold tie snugly.
	Padded cuff provides additional protection for skin. Method of fastening cuff varies with product design.
	
	Prevents pressure against tissues.
	
	Padding protects skin from friction of safety strap.
	
	Gauze bandage serves as safety tie to secure extremity to stationary object. These knots will not tighten to cause constriction or loosen to allow escape.

8. Slip a finger under secured cuff to check for appropriate amount of ease.	Ensures proper fit to avoid constriction or escape.
9. Place extremity in position of alignment and comfort.	Prevents physical distortion and discomfort.
10. Wrap each end of safety tie around immovable part of bed or chair at a location that permits maximum safe movement for client while achieving purpose of restraint.	Securing tie to a movable part poses potential for tightening or loosening tension on extremity.
11. Move extremity within maximum range of freedom permitted before securing tie with a half-bow knot.	Establishes maximum, safe range before securing tie. Allows for prompt release if necessary.
12. Apply restraints to other limb or limbs following steps 1 to 11.	
13. Place call light within client's reach.	Enables client to call nurse when necessary.
14. Record relevant data on health record.	Nurse is accountable for documenting use of restraints.

RECORDING

The potential for injury and legal liability associated with the use of any type of restraint requires that the use of restraints be completely documented on the client health record. Each separate use of the restraints must be clearly recorded as well as the reasons for their use. This documentation includes: the client behavior that precipitated the need for restraint, the type of restraint used, the time it was applied, the client's reaction to the restraint, and the time it was removed. A description of the client's physical condition is essential, including the presence or absence of edema or lesions on the skin. In the event of an emergency when restraints must be used without a physician's order, the recording includes notification of the physician about the use of restraints.

Restraints on psychiatric and nonpsychiatric clients may be recorded in different ways. Psychiatric units may use a flow sheet because observations may be required every 15 to 30 minutes. Flow sheet data usually include: information about the location, security, and rotation of the restraints, and the client's status. Data relevant to the client include: nutrition, elimination, hygienic needs, emotional needs, circulation, skin condition, signs of mental and physical exhaustion, and the need for additional medication. This information is also relevant for the restrained nonpsychiatric client and is included in the recording whenever the client's condition and length of time in restraints provide data pertinent to these areas.

Sample POR Recording

- S—"Mary, you need to collect all of the dirty clothes. I'm going to get up and start the laundry."
- O—Pulling at the IV tubing; trying to get out of bed over the side rails. Did not recognize the nurse.
- A—Mentally confused and disoriented.
- P—Two soft wrist restraints and a jacket restraint applied. Dr. Gene notified by telephone about the change in mental status and restraint application. Observe closely for continued confusion, disorientation, and physical responses.

Sample Narrative Recording

Found pulling at IV tubing, talking to persons not present, and expressing a need to get up and start doing the laundry. Trying to get out of bed over the side rails. Does not understand that she is in the hospital. Soft restraints applied to both wrists and jacket restraint at 7:30 P.M. Quiet and resting after restraints applied. Dr. Gene notified by telephone.

☐ CRITICAL POINTS SUMMARY

1. Restraints are used only to ensure the safety of a client.
2. Mechanical restraints may cause a client to become restless, fearful, and angry.
3. Mechanical restraints can cause skin abrasions, temporary or permanent damage to the circula-

tory or nervous system, loss of motion, or joint dislocation.
4. The potential for acts of negligence with the use of mechanical restraints requires that a nurse make frequent observations, take appropriate action, use reasonable judgment, and record each observation and action.
5. The nurse must be knowledgeable about state laws and institutional policies regarding the use of restraints.
6. To anticipate the need for restraints, the nurse continuously evaluates a client's physiological and psychological status.
7. Restraints can be used for destructive purposes by mentally ill clients.
8. The key for locked restraints must be readily available to all personnel on the unit.
9. Use a restraint adequate in size and strength to prevent injury to the client.
10. Protect the client's skin from friction caused by the restraint.
11. Use knots to secure the restraint to a client which do not constrict the tissues.
12. Never secure a restraint to a movable part of the bed or chair.
13. Release restraints periodically to permit skin care, mobility, and position change.

☐ LEARNING ACTIVITIES

1. Visit the central supply department of a hospital to compare the different types of soft and hard restraints available. Ask one of the employees how often each type is requisitioned for use on the clinical units.
2. Read all of the restraint policies used in the institution in which you are working. Note the differences you find between policies that address the use of restraints for psychiatric and nonpsychiatric clients.
3. Enlist the help of a peer to restrain you in bed with full limb restraints for 2 hours. Make a mental note of how many different activities you are unable to perform while restrained.
4. Obtain a length of cord or rope about ½ inch in diameter and about 3 feet long and practice tying the clove-hitch, square, and half-bow knots.
5. Apply a wrist restraint to a peer, using a clove-hitch knot to secure the restraint at the wrist. Secure the free end of the straps to a stationary object with a half-bow knot. Have the peer struggle against the restraint and observe whether the restraint tightens on the wrist. Remove the restraint and repeat the exercise using a square knot at the wrist.

☐ REVIEW QUESTIONS

1. List the reasons why clients may need to be restrained.
2. What are some of the psychological and physiological effects mechanical restraints can have on a client?
3. What actions would minimize the adverse effects of restraints on the client and family?
4. How can a nurse avoid acts of negligence when caring for the client who is mechanically restrained?
5. Where can a nurse learn the specific policies that must be followed when restraints are used?
6. What types of data about a client would permit the nurse to anticipate the need for restraints?
7. What types of data does a nurse collect by inspection and palpation before, during, and after the use of restraints?
8. When using restraints, what are the nursing actions for:
   a. Skin care?
   b. Securing knots and buckles?
   c. Applying limb restraints?
   d. Rotating restraints?
   e. Observing the physical and emotional aspects of the client?

☐ PERFORMANCE CHECKLIST

OBJECTIVE: To use the correct procedure to restrain a client safely.			
CHARACTERISTIC	RANGE OF ACCEPTABILITY	SATISFACTORY	UNSATISFACTORY
1. Checks physician's order.	No deviation		
2. Washes hands.	No deviation		
3. Obtains restraints.	No deviation		
4. Explains procedure and reason to client; gives reassurance.	No deviation		
5. Bathes, dries, and powders skin area to be restrained.	Omit during emergency situation.		
6. Positions client comfortably with good body alignment.	No deviation		

(continued)

CHARACTERISTIC	RANGE OF ACCEPTABILITY	SATISFACTORY	UNSATISFACTORY

7. To apply a commercial limb restraint:
   a. Wraps padded cuff snugly around wrist or ankle and secures in place.
   b. Places knot on top part of extremity.
To apply an improvised limb restraint:
   a. Wraps an abdominal dressing or folded facecloth snugly around wrist or ankle and secures in place with adhesive tape.
   b. Wraps a 3- to 4-foot length of gauze bandage around cuff: ties in place with a clove-hitch or square knot.
	No deviation
	
	No deviation
	
	No deviation
	
	No deviation		

8. Slips a finger under secured cuff to check for fit.	No deviation		
9. Places extremity in position of alignment and comfort.	No deviation		
10. Wraps each end of safety tie around immovable part of bed or chair at a point that provides maximum safe movement of extremity.	No deviation		
11. Moves extremity within maximum range of freedom; secures tie with half-bow knot.	No deviation		
12. Places call light within client's reach.	No deviation		
13. Records relevant data on health record.	No deviation		

REFERENCES

Creighton H: Law Every Nurse Should Know, ed 4. Philadelphia, WB Saunders, 1981.

Murchison I, Nichols TS: Legal Foundations of Nursing Practice. New York, Macmillan, 1970.

Restraining patients: Duty to observe results. Nursing Digest 2(2):95–96, 1974.

BIBLIOGRAPHY

McMahon MM: Providing Physical Protection and Bodily Support. In Sorensen KC, Luckman J (eds): Basic Nursing: A Psychophysiologic Approach. Philadelphia, WB Saunders, 1979.

Rambo BJ, Wood LA: Nursing Skills for Clinical Practice. Philadelphia, WB Saunders, 1982, vol 2.

SUGGESTED READING

Yarmesch M, Sheafor M: The Decision to Restrain. Geriatric Nursing 5(6):242–244, 1984.

AUDIOVISUAL RESOURCES

Applying Restraints
　Videorecording (¾ in). (1981, Color, 12 min.)
　Available through:
　　Robert J. Brady Company
　　Route 197
　　Bowie, MD 20715
Use of Restraints
　Filmstrip and cassette. (1979, Color, 14 min.)
Long-Term Care Restraints
　Filmstrip and cassette. (1982, Color, 14 min.)
　Available through:
　　Medcom, Inc.
　　P.O. Box 116
　　Garden Grove, CA 92642

SKILL 50 Cast Care

PREREQUISITE SKILLS

Skill 19, "Inspection"
Skill 20, "Palpation"
Skill 21, "Percussion"
Skill 28, "Handwashing"
Skill 38, "Skin Care"
Skill 46, "Thermal Applications"
Skill 51, "Monitoring Fluid Balance"

☐ STUDENT OBJECTIVES

1. Identify reasons why casts are applied.
2. Describe the purposes of cast care.

3. Describe the actions a nurse uses to facilitate drying the cast.
4. Describe the signs and symptoms characteristic of problems with a cast.
5. Describe the actions necessary to prevent complications from occurring to a client with a cast.
6. Describe the elements of data the nurse collects while providing care to a client with a cast.
7. Provide safe care to a fresh cast.
8. Bind the edges of a cast correctly.

☐ INTRODUCTION

A cast is a rigid mold that encases an extremity or body area. It is formed by applying and shaping several layers of bandage made of a plaster of paris, fiberglass, or plastic to the contour of the body area. Some of the reasons why casts are applied include keeping bone fractures aligned; immobilizing a body part, such as a knee, after surgical reconstruction; maintaining a corrected deformity; and permitting an injured or weakened body structure to rest and be supported during the healing process. Casts may be applied over either intact skin or a surgical incision (Farrell, 1978a).

There are three general groups of casts: cylindrical casts, used for limbs; spica casts, used to immobilize an appendage to the main body part or extremity, such as a hip or shoulder; and a body cast, used to immobilize the spine. Figure 50–1 shows examples of these types of casts.

The basic purposes of cast care are to preserve the integrity of the cast and to prevent the occurrence of physiological complications. Although this type of care is often referred to as cast care, it is important to realize that the care always includes care of the client as well as the cast. One cast procedure that the nurse has responsibility for is binding the cast edges with adhesive tape. This prevents skin irritation from the rough cast edges and avoids crumbling of the cast.

☐ PREPARATION

To understand the aspects of care required for a client and the cast, the nurse reviews basic knowledge of the materials and the general procedure used to apply a cast.

PROPERTIES OF CASTS

The most commonly used casting material is plaster of paris. It consists of anhydrous calcium sulfate, a white chalky powder that is made by dehydrating gypsum with intense heat. Open-weave bandages impregnated with the powder are saturated with water immediately prior to a cast application. The bandages are then wrapped and molded around the body part.

Heat generated by a chemical reaction that occurs as the wet plaster begins to dry can be felt by the client. The amount of heat generated depends on the size and thickness of the cast and the temperature of the water used to wet the bandages. A fresh plaster cast is always left exposed so that the heat can dissipate; otherwise, the client could be burned or become overheated (Roaf and Hodkinson, 1980). Plaster of paris casts are hot, take several hours to dry, and are heavy.

Lightweight alternatives to plaster of paris are fiberglass and plastic. These materials are considerably more expensive than plaster, and so they are used primarily for casts that do not require frequent changing. Compared with plaster of paris, these casts are cooler, less apt to cause skin problems, easier to keep clean, and do not deteriorate when they become wet. They also dry within a few hours (Meredith, 1979).

APPLYING THE CAST

Before the cast is applied, stockinet, sheet wadding, or both are placed directly over the skin. Stockinet is a tubular cotton knit material that conforms to the

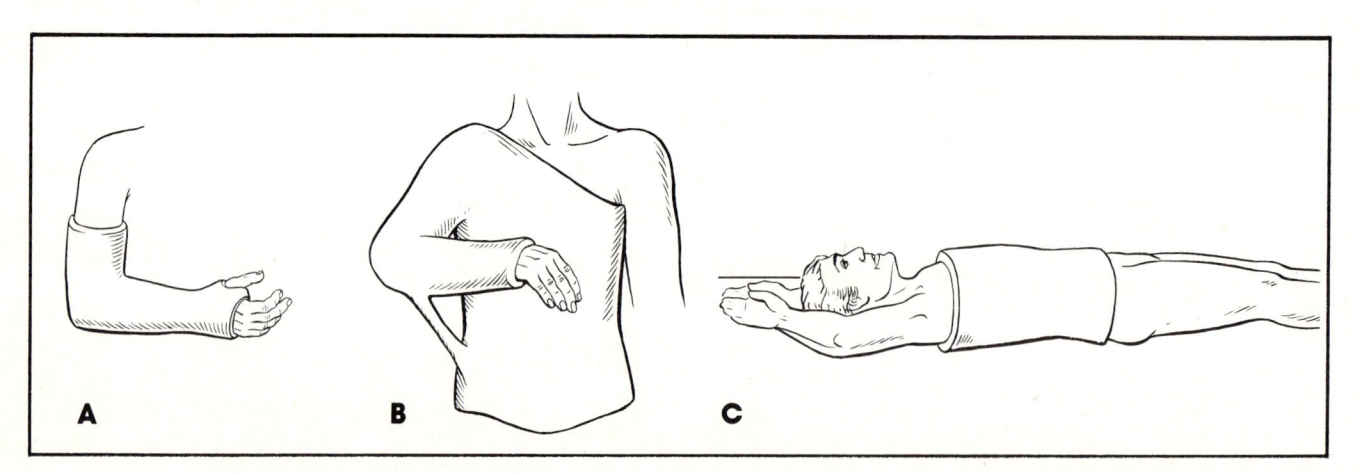

Figure 50–1. Types of casts: **A.** Cylindrical cast. **B.** Spica cast. The client's body is used to stabilize and maintain the cast position. **C.** Body cast.

shape of the body area. Sheet wadding is a soft, thin fluffy strip of material that is wrapped around the body area and applied so that it is wrinkle-free. These materials prevent the cast material from coming in direct contact with the skin and provide some padding over the bony protuberances, thus providing protection from pressure from the cast. The cast is applied snugly; however, there is usually space enough to insert one or two fingers between the cast and the skin (Farrell, 1982). When a plaster cast begins to set, the physician uses a knife to trim the rough edges of the cast. The underlying sheet wadding or stockinet is left intact to provide a protective band between the cast edge and the client's skin.

DRYING THE PLASTER CAST

Until it dries, a fresh plaster of paris cast is called a green cast. It gets this name because the damp cast is a gray-green color. It also has a dull sheen and a musty smell. A cast dries by evaporation of water; a fresh cast may take anywhere from 12 to 48 hours to dry, depending on the thickness and size. The nurse is responsible for ensuring that the cast dries thoroughly as it was originally molded. A wet or damp cast is handled with the open palms of the hands to prevent finger indentations, which would create pressure points on the underlying skin or bony protuberances. The cast should dry from the inside out. If the client is to be discharged soon after the cast is applied, a fan may be used to facilitate drying. The use of hair dryers and heat lamps is discouraged because they add to the existing heat emanating from the cast and pose a risk for burning the client or causing overheating. If the cast dries too quickly it can crack.

While the cast is drying, the pillows or bed area under the cast are covered with absorbent material. Plastic or rubber coverings retain heat and reduce evaporation from the cast, thus impeding the drying process. Repositioning the client and the casted body area every 3 hours helps to prevent flat areas and indentations and also exposes other sides of the cast to the air. Moving a client in a large cast requires careful handling to prevent breaking the cast. While it is drying, portions of a cast that extend away from the body, as shown in Figure 50–1B, must be supported. It may require three persons to move a client in a large cast safely.

A dry cast is white, has a sheen, feels like the room temperature, and has a resonant sound when percussed. When the cast is dry, the rough edges of it are bound with tape to prevent skin irritation, fraying, and accumulation of debris under the cast (Luckmann and Sorensen, 1980).

THE CLIENT AND THE CAST

Teaching the client how to maintain the cast and live with it is an important role of the nurse. Clients generally consider casts a nuisance. Casts are heavy and somewhat uncomfortable, limit mobility, restrict independence, and require modification of a person's routine activities. When a cast is first applied, the client may be in pain and may be apprehensive about his or her well-being. The nurse is sensitive to these feelings and responds appropriately. Explanations as to why the cast is necessary, why it looks as it does, and how the client's basic needs will be met are carefully given. The nurse assesses the client's readiness and ability to listen. Lengthy explanations are not given while the client is in pain or semiconscious as the result of anesthesia. Brief, clear explanations are usually most appropriate immediately after the cast has been applied.

PHYSICAL PROBLEMS RESULTING FROM CASTS

The nurse needs to be alert for signs of neurovascular damage and drainage through the cast when caring for a client in a cast (Farrell, 1982).

Traumatized tissue normally responds with edema formation. When edema forms under the cast it can make the cast too tight, thus causing pressure on blood vessels and nerves. A cast may also become too tight as a result of shrinkage as it dries. The impaired circulation from increased pressure results in the sequential development of increased edema, skin pallor or cyanosis, pain, and numbness. Pressure on nerves can cause temporary or permanent loss of sensation and function.

It is the nurse's responsibility to appraise the *neurovascular status* of the body area distal to the cast every 30 minutes for several hours after the cast is applied and to report promptly signs of persistent edema and pressure to the physician. This appraisal includes skin color, temperature, mobility, and sensation. Data from an appraisal that indicate normal functioning include pink skin (or brown or black depending on the normal skin color), skin that is warm to the touch, and the ability to move the fingers or toes and to identify pressure points and pinpricks on the skin. Abnormal findings include pale or colorless skin (gray for dark-skinned persons), fingers or toes cold to the touch, an inability to flex or extend the fingers or toes on request, and numbness or tingling. When there is a great deal of edema, the frequent appraisals are done for a longer period of time. Once the cast is dry and the potential for immediate complications from the cast is no longer of concern, the nurse continues monitoring the status of the client and the cast at least once every 8 hours. As long as the cast is in place, there is the risk that physical activity and body position can cause pressure areas under the cast and edema formation.

Positioning the casted extremity to promote gravity drainage of lymphatic fluid and venous return helps to reduce the potential for pressure areas and edema formation. When the client cannot move the muscles under the cast, the normal muscle action that facilitates the return of venous blood from the periphery is lost or significantly decreased. A client who is ambulatory and has the extremity in a dependent position needs to elevate the extremity periodically to prevent edema formation and unnecessary pressure on the tissues.

Stains on the cast indicative of tissue drainage may be due to the normal oozing of blood and serum from a surgical incision, an infection of a wound, or necrotic tissue. Seepage from a surgical wound is normal, but the nurse must carefully note the color and the amount. Bright red drainage from an incision may increase for 28 to 48 hours after surgery. As the amount decreases, the color changes to brown. The color and amount of drainage are recorded every 3 hours and brought to the attention of the physician. Drawing a light circle around the stain, marking the time and date, helps to measure the change in the volume of drainage.

The first signs of a wound infection or presence of necrotic tissue caused by pressure from the cast may be in the form of complaints from the client of pain or pressure and a warm area on the outside of the cast. A musty offensive odor may precede the appearance of drainage.

The client needs to be informed about the purpose and the importance of each aspect of these appraisals, so that the client is able to report promptly sensations of pain, of pressure, and of changes in the size of stains on the cast from drainage. This is particularly important when the client is discharged soon after the cast is applied.

SKIN CARE

To prevent irritation, the skin near and under the edge of the cast requires careful attention. Immediately after the cast is applied, plaster on the skin is removed with a damp washcloth. All loose bits of plaster and debris around the edge and under the cast are removed. Also, the bed linen is straightened frequently to prevent wrinkles and remove crumbs and other debris. It is important to keep the client comfortable in bed. During a bath, the skin adjacent to the cast may be cleansed with a moist washcloth. Plaster is very porous and will absorb fluid easily. When the cast is wet, it becomes soft. To protect the cast from getting wet during a bath or while using the bedpan, plastic may be tucked under the cast edge and over the outside. A client with a leg or arm cast may shower or take a tub bath with the cast enclosed in a large plastic trash bag tied securely above the cast. Alcohol is often used to cleanse the skin around and under the edge of the cast, because it removes oil and perspiration and evaporates so quickly it does not cause the cast to become wet. Skin lotions are not used under the cast because they tend to build up and become sticky.

Casts are warm and prevent the skin from ventilating. Dry skin under the cast often causes the client to feel itchy. Some physicians insert a long gauze strip under the cast to be used as a scratcher. It is pulled back and forth to gently massage the skin. Other devices are never to be poked under the cast because of the risk of creating skin irritation and open lesions. Skin irritation under the cast may be caused by wrinkles in the sheet wadding or stockinet. Gently pulling on the edge of the sheet wadding or stockinet may remove the wrinkles and source of irritation. Frequent position changes help to relieve constant pressure over one area. The skin around bony protuberances near the cast also requires special attention to prevent pressure sores and discomfort (Farrell, 1982).

MOBILITY

Unless contraindicated, the client who is in a cast begins exercising all of the joints and muscles as soon as possible. This prevents loss of strength and joint stiffness. Moving the joints above and below the cast while the cast is still damp reduces stiffness and helps to improve circulation and reduce edema formation.

Maintaining and increasing strength and mobility helps clients to become more independent and prepares them to turn in bed, transfer to a wheelchair, and use crutches. It is also important that the client be kept in good body alignment to prevent strain on muscles, tendons, and ligaments. The body part that is in a cast must also be positioned in proper alignment to prevent unnecessary pressure areas on the tissue under the cast. When the client is moved in bed, the cast is securely supported with pillows. Clients who are able to get out of bed also need to have the cast properly supported (Luckmann and Sorensen, 1980). The client is told that swelling may occur with increased activity and that this can cause pain. To reduce the swelling, the casted extremity is elevated above heart level.

CAST REMOVAL

Clients need to be prepared for removal of the cast and the appearance of the skin and muscles. A cast is removed with a vibrating saw that may be attached to a vacuum cleaner type of hose and bag. Since a client may be fearful of being cut, he or she needs to be reassured that the blade does not cut the skin, only the cast. The blade is removed as soon as it cuts through the plaster and the underlying padding. At the most it may scratch the skin. The skin under the cast is scaly and yellow, and the muscles are weak and flabby from disuse. When the cast is removed, warm water or oil is used to cleanse the skin gently so as to prevent abrasion of viable tissue. A limb that has been casted is moved with care because the bone is brittle. It is supported with pillows in a similar position to the one in which it was cast until the client has had an opportunity to become accustomed to the change in body balance and loss of muscle strength. Joints are exercised without force within the limits of stiffness and pain. The physician may request a physical therapist to initiate an exercise program. The client needs to be aware that it takes time after the cast is removed for the body part to return to full function. An extremity may continue to swell when it is in a dependent position. Frequent elevation helps to reduce the edema. Healed fractures need to be protected from stress, so the client needs to know to what extent activity must be restrained. Normally the physician explains what the client can and cannot do.

DATA BASE

Client History and Recorded Data

The nurse reviews information in the health record about the type of injury or surgery and the type, size, and location of cast applied is reviewed before planning care for the client. The nurse also needs to know if the cast is still wet, if the client is experiencing pain or has areas of pressure, and if edema is present. The recorded pattern of temperature, pulse, respiration, and blood pressure measurements provide data relevant to the client's physiological and psychological status before and after the cast application. It is important to continue to monitor these vital signs for early indications of infection and stress. Specific medical and nursing orders for appraisals and interventions are recorded on the nursing kardex. These orders include the time intervals for appraisals, for turning the client and the cast, for changing the position of the cast, and for the amount of activity permitted.

The nurse becomes familiar with basic information about the client, such as age, sex, role in family, and life style, so that the teaching plan can include information relevant to the individual.

Physical Appraisal Skills

Inspection. The integrity of the cast is determined by inspection. This is an important component of cast care that is done immediately after the cast is applied and then frequently thereafter until the cast is removed. The body of the cast is inspected for cracks and softening and the cast edges for crumbling. The skin around and under the cast edges is inspected for irritation and the presence of crumbs and foreign bodies. Skin color and the presence of edema are carefully scrutinized. Edema that is not relieved by elevation of the body part is reported to the physician. The mobility of joints above and below the cast is also noted while the client moves each joint.

Palpation. Skin temperature and the adequacy of capillary filling in the nail beds in areas distal to the cast are detected by palpation. The techniques used for these appraisals are described in Skill 38. The amount of edema present in an area distal to the cast also is determined by palpation. The technique for this is presented in Skill 52.

Sensory and motor nerve function in areas distal to the cast is detected by pinching or lightly pricking the skin with a pin and having the client move each of the parts. These appraisals are particularly important with clients who have arm or leg casts, because the superficial branches of the radial, median, and ulnar nerves in the arm and the peroneal and tibial nerves in the leg may be compressed by the cast. To determine sensory function of nerves in the arm, the dorsal side of the web space between the thumb and index finger, the volar (palm) side of the index finger, and the volar side of the little finger are tested. Motor function is determined by having the client hyperextend the thumb or wrist, place the thumb and little finger in opposition, and flex the wrist and abduct all of the fingers. Sensory function of the nerves in the leg is tested by pricking the dorsal side of the web space between the great and second toe and the volar (sole) surface of the foot. Motor function is determined by having the client dorsiflex (turn upward) the foot and extend the toes and plantarflex (turn downward) the foot and flex the toes.

Percussion. Direct percussion of the cast yields a resonant sound when the cast is dry and a dull sound when it is still damp.

EQUIPMENT

Additional pillows are needed to support the client in a cast in good body alignment and to elevate a casted extremity to prevent or reduce edema formation. *Adhesive tape* 2½ cm (1 in) wide is used to bind the raw edges of the cast, and *scissors* are needed to cut the tape.

☐ EXECUTION

The first steps in caring for a client in a cast involve facilitating drying and preventing edema formation. Keep the cast fully exposed to the air and use linen to cover the uncasted parts of the client. Maintain the client in a position that permits the cast on an extremity to be elevated higher than heart level. Support body casts with pillows placed under the body and cast to maintain the client in proper body alignment and protect the cast from indentations. Reposition the client and the cast every 2 to 3 hours to permit exposure of all of the cast surfaces to the air. Advance planning is needed before moving a client in a large body cast. At least three persons are needed so that the cast and the client are adequately supported to prevent undue stress on the cast and to keep the client in good body alignment.

During the first 24 to 48 hours, ice bags may be applied to the cast area near the location of the injury to reduce edema formation. Fill the ice bags as described in Skill 46. To prevent indentations in the cast from the weight of the ice bags, place the ice bags so that they lean against the cast rather than lay on top of it. Check the condition of the cast frequently for indentations from the ice bags.

FINISHING THE EDGE OF THE CAST

When the cast is dry, the rough edges of the cast are bound with strips of adhesive tape. Binding the edges of the cast serves several purposes: It helps to prevent skin irritation from the cast edges; it helps to reduce wrinkles in the sheet wadding or stockinet by holding it in place; and it prevents the cast edges from crumbling. The limited amount of space between the edge of the cast and the skin around arms, fingers, and toes makes it difficult to place the tape binding properly. The edge of the cast may be bound with either long pieces of adhesive tape 2½ to 5 cm (1 to 2 in) wide or with shorter 5 to 7½ cm (2 to 3 in) strips that have the corners on one end rounded as in a flower petal. The petaled edge helps to place the tape and prevent the tape edges from curling up. The width of the petals depends on the amount and contour of the cast edge to be covered. In some areas, wide strips are difficult to place properly without wrinkles, and wrinkles in the tape provide a source of skin irritation. To expe-

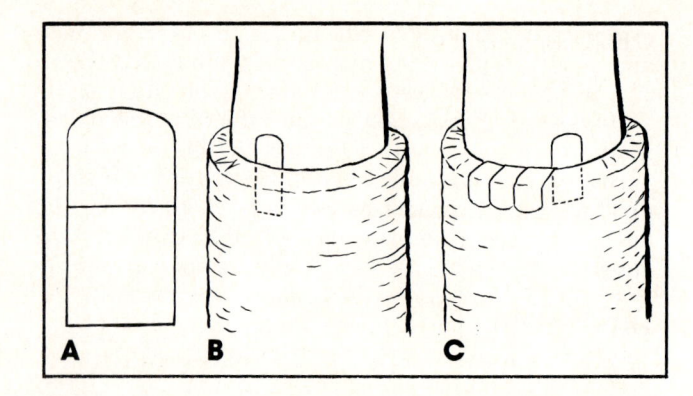

Figure 50–2. Preparing adhesive tape petals. **A.** The corners of one end of the tape are rounded. **B.** The squared end of the petal is inserted inside the cast edge. **C.** Each petal is slightly overlapped to prevent gaps.

dite the procedure, use the greatest width of tape that can be contoured to the cast edge without wrinkles. Figure 50–2 shows how to cut and apply the tape petals. The steps for binding a cast edge with adhesive tape are presented in the following Skill Sequence. (If the client is discharged while the cast is still damp, the nurse tells the client how to bind the cast edge with tape.)

☐ SKILL SEQUENCE

BINDING THE CAST EDGES

Step	Rationale
1. Percuss cast to ensure that it is dry.	Tape will not securely adhere to a damp cast and will prevent cast from drying.
2. Explain procedure to client.	Allays client's anxiety.
3. Wash hands.	Prevents transferring organisms.
4. Collect appropriate width (widths) of adhesive tape and bandage scissors.	Two and one-half cm (1 in) tape is usually used for small areas and 5 cm (2 in) for large areas.
5. Place client in a position of comfort so that cast edges are accessible.	Facilitates completion of task.
6. Cut several lengths of adhesive tape 2 to 3 inches long (tape petals). Round corners of one end of strip of tape. Tape petals may be placed on a sheet of wax paper or hung on edge of over-bed table.	Tape length must be adequate to extend from inside cast, over edge, and to outside. Rounded corners help prevent corners from curling. Keeps tape available for use.
7. Press tape end with square corners firmly to inside of cast; pull tape taut and press it to outside surface. (NOTE: Excess sheet wadding or stockinet under cast edge may be trimmed or lapped over outside edge of cast.)	Fixes tape securely to cast.
8. Slightly overlap successive tape petals and change position of client and cast as necessary to permit access to all cast edges.	Reduces potential for edges curling and avoids gaps.
9. When all cast edges are bound, properly align client in a comfortable position.	Position required for binding cast may not be good body alignment or comfortable.
10. Return supplies to appropriate storage area.	Makes supplies available for next user.
11. Record procedure on health record.	Nurse is accountable for recording actions.

RECORDING

Notations on the client health record regarding the status of the cast and the client include: any complaints the client has of pain or pressure, or both; the position of the casted part and the results of neurovascular and skin appraisals; and the time when the cast was bound. Evidence of stains and changes in the size and color of stains are also recorded. It is important that the nurse specifically note the time and the content of verbal reports to the physician. The nurse also records the client's acceptance of immobility, cooperation with the plan of care, and response to teaching. The plan of care documented on the kardex includes the schedule for neurovascular checks, for repositioning the client and cast, and for special skin-care needs, as well as the amount of and type of mobility prescribed. Notes indicating any special care or positioning preferred by the orthopedic specialist are entered on the kardex so that they can be incorporated into the care plan.

Sample POR Recording

- S—"My little toe is tingling and feels like something is pressing on the side of my foot."
- O—Toes and nail beds pink. Able to feel pinprick on all surfaces of toes and move toes in full range. Cast still damp, elevated on two pillows.
- A—Pressure from cast causing tingling.
- P—Notify Dr. James immediately of tingling in little toe unrelieved by position change. Continue frequent appraisals.

Sample Narrative Recording

L. leg cast elevated on two pillows. States presence of pressure on lateral side of foot and slight tingling in little toe. Able to feel pinprick on all toe surfaces; can move toes in full range; skin and nails pink. Pressure and tingling not relieved by position change. Cast still damp. Dr. James called. Will continue hourly NV checks.

☐ CRITICAL POINTS SUMMARY

1. Keep the cast exposed to the air and well supported until it is dry.
2. Reposition the cast and body or body part every 3 hours.
3. Keep the client in good body alignment.
4. Conduct appraisals on the neurovascular status of the body area distal to the cast every 30 minutes until the cast is dry and then at least every 8 hours.
5. Be alert for the presence of unexpected stains on the cast.
6. If cast becomes stained, carefully inspect the color and amount of stain, circle its boundaries, and record the date and time.
7. Find out if the client has pain or sensations of pressure from the cast.
8. Bind the cast edges with tape when the cast is dry.
9. Protect the cast from getting wet during bathing or elimination.
10. Instruct the client and the family about how to care for the cast and the signs and symptoms that need to be reported immediately.

☐ LEARNING ACTIVITIES

1. Visit a cast room to observe how a cast is applied.
2. Interview persons who have had a cast. Find out what kind of instruction they received from the physician and nurse about care of the cast and the symptoms that should be reported.
3. Find out what type of modifications each person had to make in his or her daily life while the cast was on.
4. Weigh a discarded cast and consider how you would cope with wearing it.

☐ REVIEW QUESTIONS

1. What are some reasons why a cast is applied?
2. Why is cast care necessary?
3. What does the nurse do to facilitate drying the cast?
4. Why could a client be burned or become overheated from a wet or damp cast?
5. What are the signs and symptoms indicative of pressure on superficial nerves? on blood vessels?
6. How does a nurse use inspection, palpation, and percussion to appraise the cast and the related body areas?
7. How would you explain the reason for each aspect of cast appraisal to a client?
8. What general principles are observed while handling a cast and positioning the client?
9. Why are the edges of a cast bound with adhesive tape?

☐ PERFORMANCE CHECKLIST

OBJECTIVE: To bind the edges of a cast correctly.			
CHARACTERISTIC	RANGE OF ACCEPTABILITY	SATISFACTORY	UNSATISFACTORY
1. Percusses cast to ensure it is dry.	No deviation		
2. Explains procedure to client.	No deviation		
3. Washes hands.	No deviation		
4. Collects supplies.	No deviation		
5. Positions client comfortably, making cast edges accessible.	No deviation		
6. Prepares tape in appropriate lengths and petal edges.	No deviation		
7. Presses petaled tape edge under cast, pulls taut, and presses to outside edge. Overlaps successive petals. Repositions client as necessary.	No deviation		
8. Leaves client properly aligned and comfortable.	No deviation		
9. Returns supplies to storage area.	No deviation		
10. Records procedure.	No deviation		

REFERENCES

Farrell J: Illustrated Guide to Orthopedic Nursing, ed 2. Philadelphia, JB Lippincott, 1982.

Farrell J: Casts, your patients, and you. Part I: A review of basic procedures. Nursing78 8(10):65–69, 1978(a).

Luckmann J, Sorensen KC: Medical–Surgical Nursing: A Psychological Approach, ed 2. Philadelphia, WB Saunders, 1980.

Meredith S: Preparing your patient to live with his cast. RN 42(7):37–43, 1979.

Roaf R, Hodkinson LJ: Textbook of Orthopaedic Nursing, ed 3. Oxford, England, Blackwell Scientific Publications, 1980.

BIBLIOGRAPHY

Farrell J: Casts, your patients, and you. Part II: A review of arm and leg cast procedures. Nursing78 8(11):57–61, 1978(b).

Lane PL, Lee MM: Special care for special casts. Nursing83 (Horsham) 13(7): 50–51, 1983.

12 Nutritional Care

☐ INTRODUCTION

Ingestion of food and fluids (nutrients) is essential to life. Ingestion of adequate amounts and appropriate kinds of nutrients is necessary for maintenance of health, recovery from illness, and restoration to health.

Nutritional status refers to a person's current state of health and reflects the adequacy or inadequacy of that person's diet in supplying nutrients essential for life. *Nutritional assessment* involves a systematic gathering of subjective and objective data about a person's nutritional status, perceptions about food and eating, and understanding of current illness-related aspects of food and eating. Inseparable from nutritional assessment, *fluid balance assessment* involves a systematic gathering of subjective and objective data about fluid gains and losses in health and illness, including the measurement of weight and intake–output. *Nutritional support* involves use of one or more alternate methods of feeding for clients who will not, cannot, or do not take adequate nourishment through usual eating patterns. This support may be *supplemental* (additional) to the client's usual diet, or it may comprise the client's total nutritional needs. This support may be provided *orally, enterally* (directly into the stomach or small intestines), or *parenterally* (directly into the venous circulation). *Self-care* refers to the ability to eat independently. Assistance in eating is provided in a way that promotes and uses maximum self-care capabilities.

In any work setting, nurses are closely involved in helping clients meet their basic need for food and fluids, usually working in cooperation with the dietitian and physician. In acute- and chronic-care agencies, this assistance often means direct hands-on care, that is, serving food, helping clients with eating, giving tube feedings, and administering total parenteral nutrition (TPN) fluids intravenously. In home and community settings, this may mean teaching and assisting family members to provide nutritional support for the client. Nurses in these settings, as well as those who work in clinics and physicians' offices, need both to assess nutritional and fluid balance status and to teach clients and family members how to meet their particular nutritional needs.

In recent years there has been increasing attention paid to nutritional aspects of client care. Several studies have described the wide extent of malnutrition among hospitalized clients, as identified in Skill 52. Medical and nursing literature contain more frequent references to nutritional support and the problem of hospital malnutrition. Much of this interest has coincided with the trial-and-error development of TPN in the early 1970s. Many hospitals now have a TPN department or interdisciplinary team, and supplemental or total nutritional support is instituted much more readily than in years past. It is possible that some of the added attention to nutritional needs of clients reflects an increasing interest in healthful eating habits and fitness in the general population.

There is a good deal of symbolism associated with food and eating. Eating is a social event shared with family and friends, as well as a means to express religious and cultural traditions. Food choices reflect a person's socioeconomic status and personal decision making. Eating is the earliest independent self-care activity mastered by most people. Difficulty with eating (such as the inability to eat or to feed oneself) generally has a profound, usually negative, psychological and emotional impact. Attending to nutritional needs has a positive effect on clients' physical and psychological well-being.

This chapter presents "Monitoring Fluid Balance" (Skill 51), "Nutritional Assessment and the Serving of Food" (Skill 52), "Assistance with Eating" (Skill 53), "Enteral Nutritional Support" (Skill 54), and "Total Parenteral Nutrition" (Skill 55). The focus of these skills is on the consumption of nutrients (including fluids) through a variety of approaches. Elimination of fluids is considered only from the perspective of fluid balance assessment; assisting with intestinal and urinary elimination is presented in Chapters 13 and 15.

ENTRY TEST

1. Name the two body fluid compartments, the percent of total body water in each, and the major electrolyte components of each.
2. Explain the relationship of sodium and water to fluid balance.
3. What is a kilocalorie (kcal)?
4. How many kcal are produced when 1 g of carbohydrate is metabolized? One g of protein? One g of fat?
5. What foods are included in each of the Basic Four food groups, and how many servings of each are required to meet the basic adult nutrient requirements?
6. What is meant by RDA (Recommended Dietary Allowance) and U.S. RDA (U.S. Recommended Daily Allowance)?
7. Compare anabolism and catabolism.
8. What structures are needed for normal swallowing?
9. What digestive functions occur when food is chewed?
10. What is the function of the tongue in the process of swallowing?
11. Identify the anatomic location of the pharynx, esophagus, larynx, and trachea.
12. What is the role of the stomach in digestion?
13. What is the role of the small intestine in digestion and absorption?
14. In what form are proteins, fats, and carbohydrates absorbed into the bloodstream?
15. Describe the appearance and composition of gastric fluid.
16. Trace the flow of blood from the brachial, cephalic, internal and external jugular, subclavian, and femoral veins to the pulmonary circulation.
17. Identify the intrathoracic pressure changes occurring during inspiration and expiration.

SKILL 51 Monitoring Fluid Balance

PREREQUISITE SKILLS

Skill 19, "Inspection"
Skill 20, "Palpation"
Skill 22, "Auscultation"
Skill 24, "Pulse Appraisal"
Skill 26, "Blood Pressure Appraisal"
Skill 27, "Height and Weight Appraisal"
Skill 28, "Handwashing"

STUDENT OBJECTIVES

1. Describe subjective and objective assessment data indicative of fluid balance, excess, and deficit.
2. Describe changes that occur in fluid requirements during illness.
3. Identify situations and data that indicate a need for monitoring fluid balance.
4. Contrast nursing responsibilities in fluid restriction and forcing fluids.
5. Discuss the reliability and significance of fluid intake and output measurement and daily weight as indicators of fluid balance.
6. Discuss common sources of error in recording intake and output.
7. Correctly monitor and record a client's fluid intake and output.

INTRODUCTION

Fluid balance refers to the relationship between the amount of fluid and electrolytes taken into the body (intake) and the amount of fluid and electrolytes that leave the body (output). Fluids may be ingested orally, inserted via nasogastric or gastrostomy tubes, infused parenterally into a central or peripheral artery or vein, or administered subcutaneously by hypodermoclysis. In health, fluid intake and output are approximately equal, while an imbalance usually accompanies or indicates illness. Illness almost always increases the body's need for fluids and causes a decrease or loss of the body's ability to ingest or tolerate fluid through the usual oral route. Illness also may interfere with the body's ability to eliminate fluid or it may cause the body to excrete excessive amounts of fluids. Therefore, signs and symptoms of fluid imbalance may either serve as diagnostic clues for illness or occur as a result of the drugs and therapies used to treat illness.

Monitoring fluid balance is an important nursing activity because of the significant role fluid balance plays in health and illness and because direct client observations are the most reliable and accurate way to do this monitoring. The changes representing fluid imbalance are sometimes extremely subtle; the observations of the nurse are thus valuable, because the nurse spends more time observing the client than does the physician.

The primary technical skills used to monitor fluid balance are intake–output measurement (often called I&O) and daily weight; according to Pflaum (1979) and Metheny and Snively (1983), both are necessary for adequate fluid balance monitoring. The process of obtaining accurate weights is presented in Skill 27, and this skill focuses on obtaining accurate intake–output measurement. However, there are other aspects of fluid balance monitoring that must be considered in conjunction with those measurements, such as vital signs, turgor, and skin appraisal for edema. Therefore, the nurse must understand and be alert for clinical signs and symptoms of fluid imbalance as well as be able to measure intake–output and weight accurately.

Measuring intake and output is an important yet relatively simple procedure that sometimes becomes so commonplace it loses its significance. Unfortunately, accurate accounts of intake and output are often difficult to obtain in the average hospital. There are multiple possibilities for error in both the measuring and recording of fluid gains and losses, and persistent and consistent efforts are needed to ensure that errors and omissions are minimized.

Although a physician may request that fluid intake and output be monitored for specific clients, it is generally considered a nursing responsibility to determine when clients need to have fluid balance monitored and to implement that monitoring as a nursing order, without a specific physician directive. The nurse may be responsible for direct implementation of intake–output measurement or for delegating, supervising, or teaching that activity.

This skill focuses on monitoring fluid balance through assessment of clinical signs and symptoms of imbalance in conjunction with the technical skill of measuring fluid intake and output. Fluid balance is considered only from the perspective of the role of water in the plasma and interstitial components of the extracellular fluid compartment (ECF). Although not discussed in this skill, it is well known that electrolytes are an integral part of maintaining fluid volume and balance. It is assumed that the student has acquired a basic understanding of the physiology of fluid and electrolyte balance, and the student is referred to basic medical–surgical or fluid–electrolyte textbooks for review and further study as needed.

□ PREPARATION

Water is a universal component of all living matter, both plant and animal. Because of its nearly universal solvent characteristics, Metheny and Snively (1983, p. 4) write, "Since the adult body is from 60–70% water, each one of us is, in a real sense, a bag of more or less solid materials dissolved in water." Within the body, water serves as an aqueous environment for cell metabolism, a transport vehicle to and from cells, a regulator of body temperature, a solvent, a medium for excretion of wastes, and an aid to digestion through hydrolysis of foodstuffs (breakdown of molecules through addition of water). Water also maintains plasma volume and the concentration of intracellular and extracellular fluid.

Survival is impossible without water. Adults can live for several months without food, but for only 10 days without water, providing the weather conditions are moderate. Children can survive about half that long, depending on their age.

BODY FLUID BALANCE

The percentage of water in the human body varies with age, sex, and body fat content. Infants have a higher proportion of body water (77 percent) and the elderly have a lower proportion (47 percent). After approximately the age of 16, males begin to acquire a greater proportion of body water, until they have about 17 percent more than females. The average adult woman is about 50 to 54 percent water, by weight, while the average adult male is about 60 to 70 percent water. As we age, our total body water percentage decreases, but some sex difference remains and the elderly man has about 5 percent more body water than the elderly woman (Luckman and Sorensen, 1980, p. 175; Metheny and Snively, 1983, p. 21).

Women have a lower proportion of body water because they have proportionately more body fat than men, and adipose tissue has very little water content. In obese adults the percentage of body water, by weight, may be as low as 45 to 50 percent (Guyton, 1981, p. 392; Metheny and Snively, 1983, p. 21).

Water and electrolytes combined are taken into the body through food and most liquids, including drinking water. Softened, well, mineral, and city water all contain electrolytes; only distilled water provides pure water. All foods contain water and electrolytes; water also is produced during the oxidation of foods within the body. Together, the water in food and the water produced by the oxidation of food account for about half of the adult fluid intake.

To meet body requirements, the average healthy adult needs an intake of approximately 2600 ml of fluid per day, with a range of 2000 to 3000 ml per day considered normal. This amount includes the ingestion of liquids (1300 ml) and food (1000 ml), and oxidation (300 ml) (Metheny and Snively, 1983, p. 105).

In a healthy person, water is lost through the kidneys as urine, through the intestines in the feces, through the lungs as breath, and through the skin as perspiration. Water loss from the skin is of two types: sensible and insensible. *Sensible* water loss refers to visible water loss (sweat) that contains sodium, potassium, chlorides, and magnesium. *Insensible* water loss includes both evaporation of water vapor from the body that does not appear as visible moisture on the

TABLE 51-1. 24-Hour Average Intake and Output of Water in a Healthy Adult

INTAKE (milliliters)		OUTPUT (milliliters)	
Oral Liquids	1300	Urine	1500
Water in foods	1000	Stool	200
Water of oxidation	300	Insensible:	
		Lungs	300
		Skin	600
Total	2600		2600

From Metheny NM, Snively WD: Nurses' Handbook of Fluid Balance, ed 4. Philadelphia, JB Lippincott, 1983, p 105.

skin, and water loss from the lungs. Only water is lost during insensible water loss; electrolytes are not lost. Together with the water in feces, these insensible losses through evaporation from the skin and in expired air are known as *obligatory* fluid loss; that is, these losses occur regardless of fluid intake. The amount of water lost as urine, on the other hand, is variable, depending on the intake of fluids.

Urine volume ranges from 1000 to 2000 ml per 24 hours (40 to 80 ml per hour) in adults in a basal state. A minimum urine output of 500 ml per 24 hours is needed to excrete daily metabolic wastes; less than this amount is considered oliguria (Condon and Nyhus, 1985, p. 209; Metheny and Snively, 1983, p. 104).

For an average healthy adult whose daily fluid intake is 2600 ml, fluid losses would be approximately as follows: urine (1500 ml), insensible perspiration (600 ml), breath (300 ml), and feces (200 ml) (Metheny and Snively, 1983, p. 105). Average adult fluid intake and output are summarized in Table 51-1.

FLUID IMBALANCES

A fluid imbalance exists when there is either an excess or deficit of fluid volume, first in the extracellular compartment and then in the intracellular compartment. Fluid imbalances vary widely in severity. If the imbalance—whether an excess or deficit of fluid—is severe enough, it can be fatal.

Clinical fluid balance problems are a mix of water and solute (primarily sodium) imbalances. However, in the clinical setting, it is far easier to determine if a client has a normal, excessive, or deficient total body water volume than it is to determine if the sodium and potassium levels are normal, excessive, or deficient (Condon and Nyhus, 1985). Therefore, fluid loss and gain sometimes is described in terms of only water loss and gain. However, when fluid loss occurs, the type of fluid used to replace a particular fluid deficit would be determined by an estimate (or laboratory evaluation) of the solutes (primarily sodium) lost along with the water. A distinction between water excess and deficit and sodium excess and deficit is beyond the scope of this text.

Fluid Deficit

A fluid deficit occurs when body fluids become depleted through excessive losses or decreased intake of fluids. If uncorrected, dehydration develops, with clinical signs and symptoms reflecting the severity of the fluid deficit. Fluid losses commonly occur as a result of fever, vomiting, diarrhea, nasogastric suctioning, increased perspiration, burns, and osmotic diuresis. Water or fluid depletion also can result from decreased intake, such as occurs with nausea, inability to swallow, or being on nothing-by-mouth (NPO) status.

The amount of fluid lost in illness varies with the type and severity of the factor causing the loss. To avoid dehydration and fluid deficit, fluid replacement must equal fluid losses, both in volume and composition. The following examples illustrate these concepts.

Temperature elevation increases insensible water losses through accelerated metabolic activity, increased respiratory rate, and the added water needed for temperature regulation and evaporation. Metabolic activity increases by 13 percent for each degree Celsius (7 percent for each degree Fahrenheit) above the normal level (Bennett and Petersdorf, 1974). For a temperature of 38.4° to 39.4°C (101° to 103°F), the 24-hour fluid intake should be increased by at least 500 ml above the usual 2000 to 3000 ml; and for a temperature of above 39.5°C (103°F), an additional 1000 ml of fluid are needed every 24 hours above the usual amount (Condon and Nyhus, 1985, p. 214).

Fluid loss through perspiration varies with the degree of sweating. Moderate, intermittent sweating requires that fluid intake be increased by 500 ml; moderate, continuous sweating requires that fluid intake be increased by 1000 ml; and profuse, continuous sweating requires intake of 2000 ml or more additional fluid. These replacement fluids may contain sodium. Postoperative nasogastric suctioning results in variable volumes of lost secretions that must be measured and replaced with a water and electrolyte solution (Condon and Nyhus, 1985).

If fluid replacements cannot be tolerated by the oral route, they may be given intravenously. Because nasogastric suctioning is intended to keep the stomach empty, those replacements are always given intravenously.

When daily total fluid losses consistently exceed total fluid gains even by as little as 500 ml per 24 hours, serious deficits can occur over time in a cumulative manner. When losses are excessive and rapid, a person can become seriously ill from a fluid volume deficit within a few hours.

Although it involves only the extracellular compartments initially, a water deficit eventually results in decreased fluid volume in all body fluid compartments; the primary symptoms and signs are thirst, oliguria, and hypernatremia. To some extent, the degree of water deficit can be estimated by the clinical signs and symptoms present. Table 51-2 presents a summary of these clinical indicators of water depletion.

TABLE 51-2. Clinical Signs of Water Depletion in Adults

MAGNITUDE OF DEFICIT (liters)	CLINICAL FEATURES
1.5 or less	Thirst
1.5 to 4.0	Marked thirst
	Dry mouth, groin, axillae
	Serum sodium increased
	Urine specific gravity increased
	Hematocrit, skin turgor, and blood pressure normal
4.0 or more	Intolerable thirst
	Marked hypernatremia
	Oliguria
	Decreased body weight
	Slightly increased hematocrit
	Apathy, stupor
	If not corrected, hyperosmolar coma, death

From Condon RE, Nyhus LM: Manual of Surgical Therapeutics. Boston, Little, Brown, 1985, p 197. Reproduced with permission.

Fluid Excess

An excess of body water often is iatrogenic (resulting from medical treatment), as occurs with administration of electrolyte-free fluids or from excessive parenteral fluid administration. An excess of body water leads to an increase in the volume of all fluid compartments with a state of hypoosmolarity. Signs and symptoms depend on the degree of overload and the rate at which it develops. Moderate degrees of water excess often are asymptomatic clinically except for increased urine volume, increased body weight, and decreased serum sodium concentration. Water intoxication can occur if overload is quite marked and renal excretion or ADH function is impaired.

An excess of body water and sodium is associated with increased interstitial fluid volume and edema formation. Edema is discussed below.

ASSESSMENT OF FLUID BALANCE

To assess fluid balance, the nurse considers specific measurements of fluid intake and output, weight, and vital signs, and appraises pulses, vein filling, edema, turgor, skin and mucous membrane dryness, thirst, face and eyes, urine and stool, speech, and level of consciousness. Laboratory data provide additional objective data for fluid balance assessment. A summary of the clinical signs of fluid excess (hypervolemia) and fluid deficit (hypovolemia) in the plasma component of the ECF is presented in Table 51-3.

Fluid Intake and Output Measurement

"Most discrepancies between gains and losses of body fluids can be detected when an accurate record is kept of the total fluid intake–output" (Metheny and Snively, 1983, p. 106). However, both the literature and common experience acknowledge that intake and output records are notoriously inaccurate (Grant and Kubo, 1975; Metheny and Snively, 1983; Nursing78 Books, 1978). In a study of routine intake and output measurements in a general hospital, Pflaum (1979) found a mean daily error of 800 ml per day when compared with daily weight calculations of fluid loss. She recommends that body weight calculations and intake–output measurements be compared and the causes of any variance greater than plus or minus 250 ml be investigated. Pflaum indicates that intake should be monitored when there is a need to assure

TABLE 51-3. Clinical Signs of Hypervolemia and Hypovolemia

	HYPERVOLEMIA	HYPOVOLEMIA
Cardiovascular system		
Blood pressure	Increased	Decreased
Pulse	Increased	Increased
Postural changes	No	Yes
Neck veins	Distended	Flat
Peripheral pulses	Bounding	Weak; thready
Venous filling	Fast	Slow
Urine output		Low
Specific gravity	Less than 1.010	More than 1.030
Body weight	Increased	Decreased
Intake and output	Intake is greater than output	Output is greater than input
Respiratory system		
Respiratory rate	Often increased or variable	Increased
Rales	Yes	Rarely
Secretions	Moist	Dry; thick
Integumentary system		
Skin turgor	Good	Poor
Edema	Yes	Infrequently
Mucous membranes	Moist	Dry
Thirst	No	Yes
Speech	Normal	Thick; slurred

From Menzel LK: Clinical problems of fluid balance. Nursing Clinics of North America 15(3):557, 1980. Reproduced with permission.

adequate hydration or limit fluids, and that output should be monitored when there is altered urine formation, gastrointestinal losses, or acute bleeding.

A fluid intake value that is greater than the output value usually reflects excess fluid retention, although it may also be compensatory following temporary fluid restriction or dehydration. A fluid intake value that is less than the output value can alert the nurse to a hypovolemic or dehydrated state.

Intake Measurement. All fluids taken into the body by all possible routes are included when fluid intake is measured. In addition to eating and drinking, this includes enteral fluids given through nasoenteric and gastrostomy tubes directly into the stomach or small intestine, total parenteral nutrition formulas given intraarterially, fluids and electrolytes given intravenously or subcutaneously, and any irrigants or instillations that are not withdrawn from the body. Liquids used to administer medications also are included in intake values. One study found that fluid intake with medications ranged from 240 to 472 ml for some clients, and that the water intake with medications actually exceeded by 30 percent the total daily fluid intake for a client (Holmes, 1965).

Output Measurement. All possible routes by which fluids leave the body are included in the measurement of fluid output, such as vomitus, nasogastric suction, illeostomy or colostomy drainage, liquid feces, and draining wounds that are attached to suction or collection bags. Some fluid losses are often estimated, such as incontinent urine and liquid feces, uncaught vomitus, burn fluid loss, wound drainage in dressings, and perspiration. The necessity for estimating these fluid losses is demonstrated by Metheny and Snively's (1983, p. 109) estimate that one necessary bed linen change from excessive perspiration represents at least 1 liter of lost fluid.

The frequency with which output is measured depends on the severity of the client's fluid balance problem. A 4- to 8-hour summary may be adequate for some clients; others may require an hourly accounting of gains and losses so that the treatment plan can be tailored to their immediate needs for medications or fluid intake. When hourly monitoring of an adult's urine output is being done, urinary output of less than 30 ml per hour must be reported immediately to the physician.

Weight
Daily weighing is one of the most effective methods of monitoring fluid balance, since rapid body weight variations closely reflect fluid volume changes (Luckmann and Sorensen, 1980). When caloric intake remains relatively stable, a gain or loss of 1 kg (2.2 lb) of body weight represents a gain or loss of 1 liter of fluid (or 1 lb represents approximately 1 pt of fluid). Even under starvation conditions, a person loses only 0.7 to 1 kg (⅓ to ½ lb) per day (Metheny and Snively, 1983, p. 111). A rapid weight loss or gain of 2 percent is indicative of a mild fluid volume deficit or excess; a 5 percent weight loss or gain indicates a moderate volume deficit or excess; and a weight loss or gain of 8 percent or more indicates a severe volume deficit or excess (Metheny and Snively, 1983, p. 111). Condon and Nyhus (1985) indicate that barely perceptible pitting edema indicates an increase of at least 2.7 liters of water and sodium.

The client's weight prior to the onset of illness is identified by consulting the health record, the client, or his or her family. If this is not possible, the nurse usually can determine the client's admitting weight, last date weighed, and the pattern of weight lost or gained. All clients are to be weighed at regular intervals and the weight recorded on a flow sheet or graphic record, so that patterns of weight gain or loss may be visualized readily. Isolated or occasional weights do not provide a pattern or trend and are relatively meaningless for evaluating fluid loss or gain. For accuracy, daily measurements of body weight are obtained at the same time of the day using the same balance-beam scales and with the client wearing the same clothes and having an empty bladder, as discussed in Skill 27. Daily measurement of weight often is used to assess the effectiveness of diuretic therapy in clients with congestive heart failure. It is not unusual for an edematous client to lose 2.5 kg (5 lb) or 2.5 liters (2.5 qt) of fluid in response to high potency diuretics such as furosemide (Lasix).

Vital Signs
Vital signs reflect fluid balance status. A *temperature* elevation can reflect a fluid deficit and indicate dehydration, or, as discussed earlier, it can produce a deficit. A bounding *pulse rate* may reflect a fluid volume excess; an increased rate combined with easy obliteration indicates a fluid volume deficit. *Respirations* affect fluid status, and an increased respiratory rate causes increased loss of fluid through the lungs, with a potential for imbalance. Water loss through expired air is increased when clients on mechanical ventilators do not receive adequate humdification. Fluid volume excess can produce shortness of breath and moist rales (associated with pulmonary edema) in clients who have no cardiopulmonary disease. In the absence of pulmonary disease, moist rales represent at least a 1500 ml accumulation of excess body fluids (Condon and Nyhus, 1985, p. 206). *Blood pressure* also may reflect fluid volume changes; for example, postural hypotension may occur as a result of fluid deficit. When the standing systolic blood pressure is 10 mm Hg less than the supine blood pressure, a fluid volume deficit usually exists (Metheny and Snively, 1983, p. 94).

Peripheral Pulses. With fluid volume deficit, peripheral pulses become weak, thready, and easily obliterated when the client is in an upright position, since the force of gravity tends to keep the existing volume in more dependent locations, such as the legs. With fluid volume excess, the pulse is full and bounding, not easily obliterated, and there are no positional changes.

Vein Filling

Peripheral Vein Filling. The rate of *peripheral vein filling* reflects the plasma fluid volume status. In a normally hydrated person, peripheral veins usually will empty in 3 to 5 seconds when the extremity is elevated above heart level, and refill in the same amount of time after being placed in a dependent position; that is, below heart level. With fluid excess, the veins will take longer than 3 to 5 seconds to empty. When a fluid deficit exists, the veins refill slowly and may not become readily evident, even in the dependent position. Figure 51-1 shows the vein filling and emptying associated with positional changes. Another way to appraise vein filling is to occlude and release a small vessel on the hand or foot while it is positioned on the same level as the heart. With normal fluid volume, the vein refills immediately, but refilling is delayed in the presence of a volume deficit.

Jugular Vein Filling. Jugular vein filling is considered to be a reliable indicator of central venous pressure, which is determined in part by the plasma volume. In the supine position, the external jugular veins usually fill to the anterior border of the sternocleidomastoid muscle. Flat neck veins in a supine position may indicate a plasma volume deficit. When a healthy person is in a semirecumbent position at a 30- to 45-degree angle, external venous distention extends no higher than 2 cm above the sternal angle and disappears in an upright position. If the client does not have congestive heart failure, changes in neck vein filling reflect plasma volume changes. For example, blood volume depletion is suspected if the neck veins remain flat even when the client is horizontal, and volume excess may be suspected when the veins are distended with the client in a slightly elevated position (Metheny and Snively, 1983, p. 94).

Edema

An abnormal retention of fluid (both water and sodium) within the body is called edema. It commonly develops in the interstitial spaces (*interstitial edema*), in the lung tissue (*pulmonary edema*), or within the peritoneal cavity (*ascites*). It may also develop in the pleural space or the pericardial cavity. When fluid accumulates in the interstitial spaces, the overlying skin becomes smooth, shiny, taut, and cool to touch. In dark-skinned people, edematous areas have a lighter color than other areas because of the stretched skin (Mitchell and Loustau, 1981). Edema may result in visible or measurable increase in the size of a body part.

Subjectively, clients with edema may report tightness of shoes, rings, and belts, especially near the end of a day. They may also report weight gain and dyspnea.

Edema is not usually evident clinically until 2.5 to 5 kg (5 to 10 lb) of excess fluid have accumulated and the interstitial fluid volume is about 30 percent above normal. The degree of edema is often estimated on a scale of one plus (1+) to four plus (4+), with 1+ indicating barely perceptible edema and 4+ indicating severe edema in which the limbs are swollen to a diameter of 1¼ to 2 times normal. In seriously edematous tissues, the interstitial fluid volume increases to several hundred percent above normal (Guyton, 1981, p. 376; Metheny and Snively, 1983, p. 97).

Edema may be *pitting* or *nonpitting*. It is known as *pitting edema* when a depression remains after two fingers or the ball of the thumb are pressed into an edematous area overlying a bony prominence as shown in Figure 51-2. The bone keeps the thumb or fingers from sinking into the soft underlying tissues. This pressure causes the fluid to move to another area, leaving an indentation in the skin that will persist until the interstitial space gradually refills with fluid.

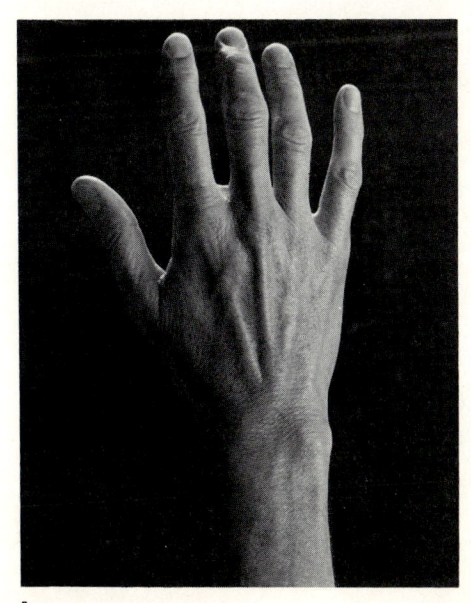

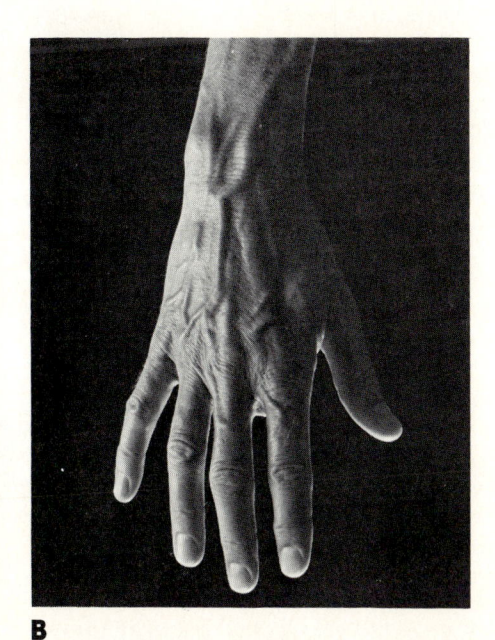

A **B**

Figure 51–1. Vein filling. **A.** With normal plasma volume, elevation of the hand causes the hand veins to empty in 3 to 5 seconds. **B.** Placing the hands in a dependent position causes the veins to fill in 3 to 5 seconds. (Photo by James Haines.)

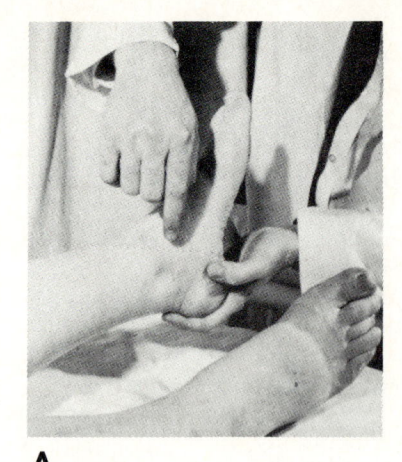

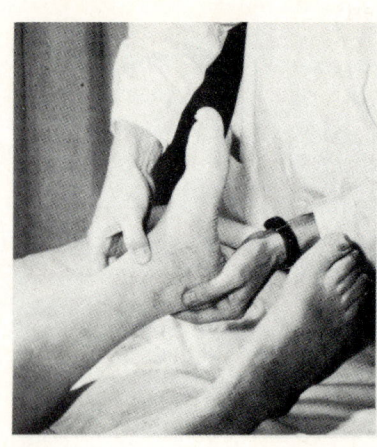

Figure 51–2. A. Pitting edema of the feet and lower legs. **B.** The same client after edema has been relieved by treatment. (Courtesy of CIBA-Geigy Pharmaceutical Co., Summit, NY.)

The depth of indentation indicates the severity of the edema, with 1+ pitting edema being a slight depression that disappears quickly, and 4+ a depression that disappears very slowly. Pitting edema usually is not evident until at least a 10 percent increase in body weight has occurred (Metheny and Snively, 1983, p. 97). This would be 6 kg (13 lb) for a 59-kg (130-lb) person. Edema may occur in areas where soft tissues rather than bone underlies the skin. Since there is nothing firm to press against, this edema is more difficult to evaluate.

As the name implies, *nonpitting edema* leaves no indentation when the tissues are pressed. The presence or absence of pitting does not necessarily reflect the severity of the edema. Sometimes seriously edematous tissues do not pit, such as in infected or traumatized areas (Guyton, 1981, p. 376).

Edema is known as *dependent edema* when it shifts its location with changes in body position, the fluid collecting by gravity in dependent (lower) areas. In ambulatory clients, the feet, ankles, and lower legs are in a dependent position. In bedridden clients, the pretibial and sacral areas are dependent, or if the client is turned on the side, the lower side of the body becomes dependent.

When excess body fluid is retained in the peritoneal cavity, it is known as ascites. To aid in the evaluation of ascites, abdominal girth is often measured on a regular (perhaps even daily) basis, using a nonstretchable measuring tape made of paper or metal, rather than cloth.

Turgor

Turgor reflects fluid volume in both the subcutaneous tissues and the dermis, since a significant amount of body water is stored in the dermis, giving the skin a feeling of fullness and elasticity. Turgor often is described as good, fair, or poor and is evaluated by pinching and releasing a fold of skin. Normal turgid skin returns to its normal shape almost immediately after being released. With a fluid deficit, the skin remains slightly pinched and wrinkled for a variable length of time, depending on the degree of fluid deficit. With decreased turgor, the skin also has a sticky, doughy feeling. In Figure 51–3 the skin has not returned to its normal position 30 seconds after pinching, indicating a moderately severe extracellular fluid volume deficit (Moyer, 1952). In the elderly, loss of subcutaneous tissue and skin elasticity decreases skin turgor; evaluation of tongue turgor is therefore considered to be a better indicator of fluid balance in el-

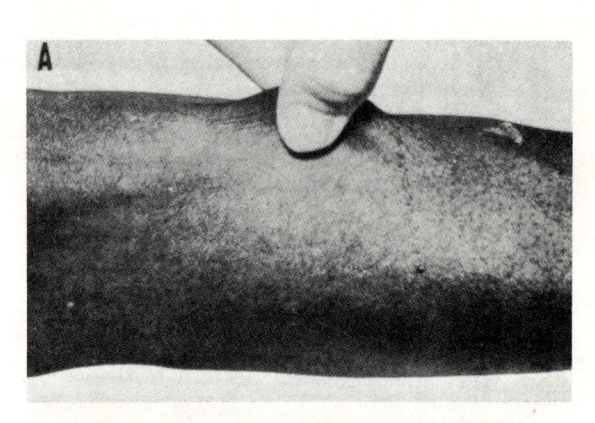

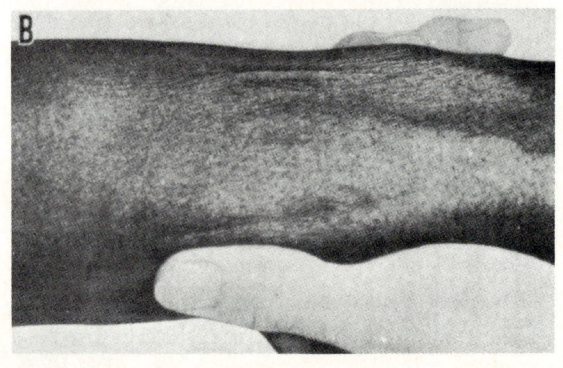

Figure 51–3. Poor skin turgor. **A.** Skin of forearm is picked up. **B.** It does not return to its normal position 30 seconds later. (From Moyer CA: Fluid Balance: A Clinical Manual. Chicago, Year Book Medical Publishers, Inc., 1952, with permission.)

derly clients than is skin turgor. The normal tongue is firm and full, but with fluid deficit, longitudinal fissures develop.

Skin and Mucous Membrane Dryness

Normal mucous membranes appear moist and glistening with thin secretions. Dry mucous membranes may reflect a fluid volume deficit but also may be the result of mouth breathing. To distinguish between the two, Metheny and Snively (1983, p. 96) recommend that the nurse run a clean ungloved finger inside the oral cavity where the gums and cheek meet and feel those mucous membranes. Dryness in this area indicates a volume deficit rather than dryness from mouth breathing. Another way to distinguish the dryness of fluid deficit from that associated with mouth breathing is for the client to rinse his or her mouth or hold water in the mouth and spit it out without swallowing (sham drinking). Both of these measures will temporarily relieve thirst deriving from mouth dryness but not the thirst deriving from fluid deficit.

The amount and character of saliva may reflect fluid volume. When oral fluid intake is decreased the amount of saliva is reduced and it becomes thickened and sticky. However, if total fluid intake through all routes (oral, parenteral, and enteral) is adequate, this finding could indicate a fluid volume deficit.

Complete lack of perspiration on the skin in the axillary and groin areas may also indicate a major fluid volume deficit, unless there is a malfunction of the sweat glands. In the normal individual, apocrine sweat glands provide constant moisture in these areas.

Thirst

Thirst is sometimes an indicator of volume deficit. In the healthy individual, the subjective symptom of thirst (awareness of the need to drink) serves as a stimulus for maintaining normal fluid balance. In illness and aging, thirst is not a reliable indicator of fluid needs. Drugs, altered states of consciousness, cardiovascular disease, renal damage, and severe burns also alter the reliability of thirst as an indicator of fluid volume status.

Face and Eyes

When fluid imbalance occurs, facial appearance sometimes changes. With extreme extracellular fluid deficit, a person may have a drawn facial expression with sunken eyes. The eyeballs may feel soft when gentle pressure is applied to the upper eyeball area, because of loss of fluid from the vitreous humor within the posterior portion of the eye. The firm lens in the anterior portion of the eye does not reflect fluid volume changes. With excess extracellular fluid, a person may have puffy eyelids, swollen circumorbital areas, or cheeks that are fuller than usual, and may complain of his or her face feeling puffy.

Urine and Stool

When the number of stools increases and the consistency becomes soft or liquid, there is a corresponding increased loss of body fluid. This may occur in clients who have diarrhea or those with right (ascending) colostomies (located proximal to the absorption of water from the stool). Tube-fed clients are also known to have soft or liquid stools (Walike et al., 1975). Clients with fluid volume deficit frequently have constipation, with small, hard, dry stools.

Urine becomes darker and more concentrated when fluid volume deficit occurs, since the kidneys conserve fluid in an attempt to maintain normal fluid balance.

Speech

Dry mucous membranes and lips can cause a person to have difficulty forming words, and the tongue may seem to stick to the mouth.

Level of Consciousness

Both fluid excesses and deficits can alter a client's level of consciousness. Inadequate water intake is known to contribute to mental confusion; excessive body fluids may cause confusion as well as lethargy, seizures, and coma, leading to death (Grant and Kubo, 1975). However, the correlation between fluid imbalance and cerebral symptoms is imprecise and must be evaluated in light of the other data.

Laboratory Data

In a healthy person, common urine specific gravity varies between 1.015 and 1.025, although it may range from 1.003 to 1.030 depending on the diet (Corbett, 1982). When oliguria (decreased urine output) from water deficit occurs, the urine is concentrated and has a high specific gravity. A dilute urine with a low specific gravity implies adequate hydration or even overhydration. Low specific gravity also accompanies acute renal failure (Metheny and Snively, 1983, p. 101). A specific gravity of 1.025 to 1.030 represents concentrated urine; 1.001 to 1.010 represents dilute urine (Fischbach, 1980, p. 788).

Urine osmolality varies between 400 and 1500 mOsm/L in a healthy person. In oliguria due to total body water deficit, the urine has a high osmolality, usually above 1200 mOsm/L because of maximal tubular resorption of water. However, the *serum osmolality* usually remains unaffected, and simultaneous measurement of serum and urine osmolality provides the most useful information about renal function (Condon and Nyhus, 1985).

The *blood urea nitrogen* (BUN) may rise with dehydration. If the elevation is due to dehydration, increased fluid intake will lower the BUN without any additional treatment. The normal range of BUN is 10 to 15 ml per 100 ml (Fischbach, 1980, p. 758).

INCREASING AND DECREASING FLUID INTAKE

In illness states, fluid intake often is limited or increased to help maintain fluid balance. Fluid orders are often written as "Limit fluids to _____ ml per day" or "Force fluids to _____ ml per day." When fluids are to be increased and encouraged, a water pitcher is placed in an obvious and convenient location for easy client access, and is kept refilled with cold water. Serving additional juices or other beverages of the client's preference between meals helps increase the total fluid intake.

When fluids are to be restricted, water pitchers are either located inconspicuously or removed from the room. Decreased allotments of oral fluid can be made more acceptable to the client by providing small drinking containers, serving beverages hot or cold rather than at room temperature or lukewarm, substituting ice chips for water, and serving fluids at pre-established times. Sham drinking, frequent rinsing of the mouth, oral care, and lubrication of dry lips also help the client tolerate decreased fluid intake. Decreased fluid allotments are to be divided among all three shifts and must include fluids taken with meals and medications. The day and evening shift allocations usually are equal, with the night shift receiving less. An allocation of 1600 ml per 24 hours might be as follows: 600 ml for meals, 200 ml with medications, 300 ml for the day shift, 300 ml for the evening shift, and 200 ml for the night shift. This division of fluids is planned with the client, considering his or her preferences.

SELF-CARE AND INTAKE–OUTPUT MEASUREMENT

Clients and their families are encouraged to help maintain intake–output records whenever possible. When they are involved in their own care and understand the reasons for keeping track of intake and output, most clients and families do a good job, since they have a vested interest in the accuracy of the results.

When clients are expected to record their own intake and output, the nurse assesses their ability to do so and provides sufficient instruction so they are able to perform the task accurately. To measure their own fluid balance, clients must have adequate eyesight to see the container calibrations and read the intake and output forms. They also need to have sufficient strength and coordination to handle the output measuring containers, the mental ability to understand and carry out the task, and the interest and willingness to participate in their own care. If there is some question about the accuracy of client-kept intake–output records, the nurse will need to determine if the problem is related to physical or mental difficulties or is a psychological issue related to nonacceptance of illness.

DATA BASE

To make a decision about the methods used to monitor a client's fluid volume status, the nurse uses information about the conditions that contribute to fluid imbalance and about clients who are at increased risk of developing fluid imbalance. Illness conditions that contribute to fluid imbalance include vomiting, diarrhea, renal disease, burns, congestive heart failure, ulcerative colitis, cirrhosis of the liver, severe diabetes, hormonal disturbances, and pulmonary disease. Fluid imbalance may also be caused by surgery, diuretic therapy, low-sodium diets, hormone therapy, and intravenous therapy. Some clients need their fluid balance monitored because they are not able to meet their own fluid needs unassisted. These clients include confused, nonresponsive, weak, or neurologically impaired persons, and the elderly and the very young.

Client History and Recorded Data

Knowing the client's diagnosis and past history helps the nurse to evaluate the significance of any variations in clinical signs and symptoms. Significance of signs and symptoms depends on the magnitude of the imbalance, the rapidity of its onset, the length of time it has been present, and the efficiency of the client's compensatory homeostatic mechanisms. Knowing the diagnosis and the reason for monitoring fluid balance also helps the nurse answer questions and explain about intake–output measurement to the client and his or her family, or teach the client how to carry out this task for himself or herself. The diagnosis itself may be a sufficient indicator for the nurse to institute intake–output measurement as a nursing action; for example, clients with a diagnosis of congestive heart failure invariably have their fluid balance measured because of the actual or potential fluid imbalance associated with that diagnosis.

The nurse may elicit subjective data about symptoms of fluid imbalance during an assessment interview or while giving direct care. When total body fluid increases, a person may notice that rings, shoes, and clothing become too tight. With fluid deficit, a person may report weight loss, thinner facial appearance, loose clothing, decreased perspiration, dry mouth, difficulty forming words, and comments of concern from family or friends.

Actual *intake and output data* and *serial weights* are obtained from flow sheets or the nurses' notes in the health record. Although these values are important, they are not evaluated in isolation but are considered as one part of the clinical picture. Whenever a client's intake and output are being measured, the nurse is alert for other indicators of fluid imbalance and conducts a partial or complete fluid balance assessment as the client's condition indicates. A guide for assessing fluid balance, presented in Table 51-4, can be used for this purpose.

Metheny and Snively (1983, p. 87) suggest that the nurse ask a series of questions to help create a nursing diagnosis associated with fluid balance:

- Is there a disease state present that can disrupt fluid balance, and what kind of imbalance is anticipated? (For example, a fever would cause a fluid deficit.)
- Is the client receiving medications or therapies that disrupt fluid balance, and in what way is the bal-

TABLE 51-4. Guide for Assessment of Fluid Balance

A. General observations
  1. Visible signs of fluid deficit or fluid overload in face, eyes, hands, feet, and respiratory effort (shortness of breath)
  2. Subjective comments of tight shoes, rings, and clothing; dyspnea; weight loss; and thirst (include response to rinsing mouth and sham drinking)
  3. Speech—ease with which words are formed
  4. Color of skin
  5. Level of consciousness—confusion, lethargy, seizures
B. Normal patterns of fluid intake and output in 24 hours
  1. Usual amount, type, and frequency of fluids ingested
  2. Usual urine output, including amount, frequency, and color
  3. Usual number and character of stools
  4. Usual amount of perspiration
C. Current fluid intake and output measurements for 24 hours
  1. Fluid intake—type and amounts
    a. Oral
    b. Enteral
    c. Parenteral
  2. Fluid output
    a. Urine—amount and appearance
    b. Liquid stools—frequency, amount, and appearance
    c. Excessive perspiration—amount and duration
    d. Wound drainage—source, amount (or estimate), and appearance
D. Fluid intake and output changes due to illness
  1. Medical diagnosis
  2. Nursing diagnosis
  3. Fluid prescription
  4. Drugs affecting fluid balance
E. Weight
  1. Admission, pre-illness, and serial weights
  2. Gains or losses in a specific time frame
F. Vital signs
  1. Temperature—elevation and duration of elevation
  2. Pulse—rate and quality
  3. Respirations—rate, depth, presence of rales
  4. Blood pressure—supine and upright
G. Vascular observations
  1. Peripheral pulses—sites, volume, and ease of obliteration
  2. Jugular vein filling—appearance when flat, elevation, and level of vein filling
  3. Peripheral vein filling—site, position, and rate of filling
H. Skin and mucous membranes
  1. Turgor
    a. Age, sex of client
    b. Site checked
    c. Length of time to return to normal
  2. Moisture
    a. Dryness/moistness at junction of gums and cheeks
    b. Dryness/moistness in the groin and axillae
    c. Amount and character of saliva
I. Edema
  1. Location, severity, and degree of pitting
  2. Color and temperature of skin in edematous areas
  3. Serial measurements of limb or abdominal circumference
J. Laboratory data (Fischbach, 1980)

	Normal Values	Client's Values
1. Urine specific gravity	Normal Range: 1.003–1.040 Common Values: 1.010–1.025 Concentrated urine: >1.025 Dilute urine: 1.001–1.010	
2. Urine osmolality	400–1500 mOsm/L	
3. Blood urea nitrogen (BUN)	10–15 mg/100 ml	

ance likely to be upset? (For example, thiazide diuretics cause sodium and fluid loss, whereas steroid therapy results in retention of sodium and water.)
- Is this loss normal or abnormal? What is its source, and what imbalance is usual from this source? (For example, increased perspiration and nasogastric suction both cause abnormal extracellular fluid and electrolyte loss.)
- Are there any dietary restrictions, and how do they affect fluid balance? (For example, low-sodium diets usually help decrease excessive retention of fluids.)
- Has the client been taking adequate amounts of nutrients and fluid orally or by alternate routes? If not, how long has intake been inadequate? (For example, nausea and anorexia associated with influenza result in decreased oral intake. If not replaced, these losses can become quite serious over a period of several days or less, depending on the person's age and general health. If increased fluid loss from vomiting and diarrhea accompanies the decreased intake, the deficit rapidly becomes more dangerous, even fatal.)
- How does the total fluid intake compare with the total fluid output? Since intake and output should be approximately equal, differences in these values require careful assessment to determine whether the differences represent measurement error or actual imbalance.

Physical Appraisal Skills

Inspection. Inspection of the skin for fluid volume changes requires a good light source, such as daylight or a 60-watt light, since ceiling and overbed lights usually are inadequate. Inspection begins with a general survey of the client's overall appearance for signs of fluid overload or fluid deficit, such as facial expression, appearance of the eyes and cheeks, tight rings, visibly swollen ankles, or shortness of breath.

Vein Filling. There are two ways to inspect and appraise the rate and volume of *peripheral vein filling:* (1) Instruct or assist the client to raise the hands above the heart level for 3 to 5 seconds and then place the hands in a dependent position. Bedfast clients should lower their hands below the level of the bed to create adequate positional change. Observe the rate at which the veins empty and refill, and the fullness of the venous return. (2) Occlude a superficial vein with one finger and empty the vein distally from the pressure point with a second finger. Use a firm, smooth stroke for a distance of 2 to 3 inches. With the first finger remaining in place, lift the second finger quickly, allowing the blood to return into the emptied vein. Observe the rate and degree of refilling.

To inspect for *jugular vein filling,* position the client in a semi-Fowler's position (30- to 45-degree angle), with the head slightly elevated on a pillow. Remove any clothing that might constrict the neck or upper chest, and direct a light source in an oblique direction toward the neck, first on one side and then the other. Keep the neck straight and the head turned slightly away from the side being inspected, as shown

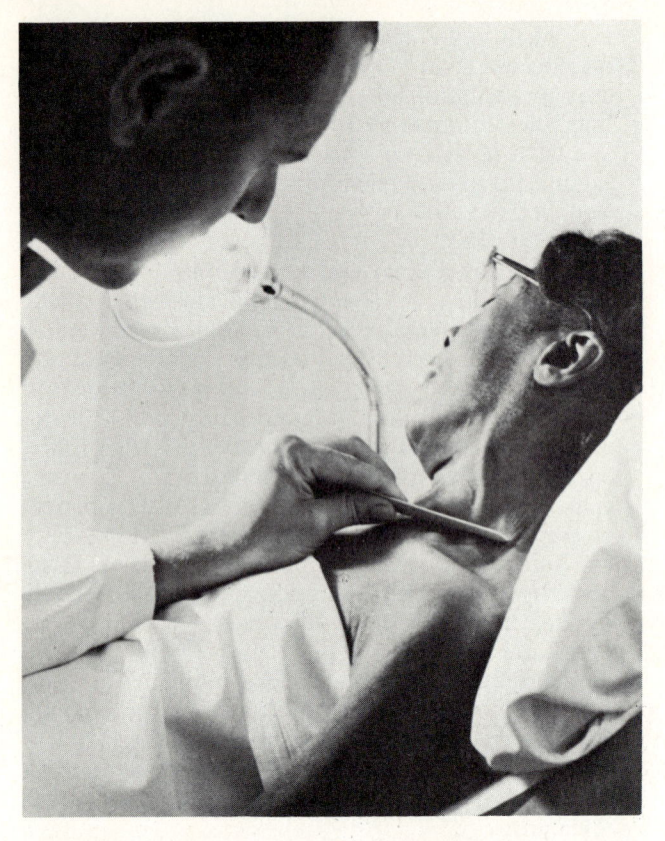

Figure 51-4. When lying in a partly-reclined position, this client has distended neck veins. Note the position of the head and the placement of the lamp for increased visualization. (©Reproduced with permission of the American Heart Association.)

in Figure 51-4 (Bates, 1983; Metheny and Snively, 1983). Look for the highest point at which the jugular vein pulsations are evident, or the point above which the jugular vein appears collapsed or flattened. It may be necessary to adjust the client's position in order to see jugular vein distention; in some instances, the bed may have to be elevated as much as 90 degrees before the venous distention becomes visible (Bates, 1983, p. 187).

Other Uses for Inspection. Inspection is also used to identify the skin characteristics associated with edema, to examine the facial appearance, the urine color, the rate of skin return when testing for turgor, and to gather data about abdominal girth and weight.

Palpation

Peripheral Pulses. Palpation is used to appraise the volume of the *peripheral pulses,* preferably while the client is in an erect position.

Edema. The presence, type, and degree of edema is determined with varied degrees of palpation. Use light to moderate palpation with the flat fingertips to determine the presence of edema. To detect the skin surface changes associated with edema, use light palpation with the dorsum of the hand. To examine the arms and legs for edema, palpate the two extremities simultaneously, beginning with the dorsal aspects of the hands and feet. This technique makes comparisons possible. It is especially important to palpate for edema in dependent body areas, that is, feet, ankles, and lower legs for ambulatory clients and the pretibial (over the tibia) and presacral (over the sacrum) areas for bedfast clients.

To palpate for pitting edema, press the ball of the thumb (or the palmar surfaces of the distal phalanges of the first two fingers) slowly and firmly into the skin for 5 to 15 seconds. This may be painful for the client, so it is best to explain in advance what is going to be done. Since estimation of pitting edema is a subjective measurement, it is wise to validate the findings with more experienced staff until confidence in one's own judgment develops. The amount and location of the edema is recorded on the client health record.

Turgor. To appraise skin turgor, pinch the skin over the sternum, forehead, or inner aspect of the forearm. Note the quality of the skin tissues, release the skin, and observe the rate of return to normal, as was shown in Figure 51-3. Use a flashlight to inspect the tongue for excessive longitudinal furrows associated with decreased tongue turgor.

Skin and Mucous Membranes. After palpating to appraise oral dryness, wash your hands thoroughly for self-protection and prevention of cross-contamination of microorganisms. If you have any breaks in the skin of the hands, someone else should be asked to do this palpation.

Use the flat fingertips to palpate for dryness in the groin and axillae. Handwashing before and after this palpation provides for cleanliness.

Eyeballs. To appraise the firmness or softness of the eyeballs, have the client look down and then palpate with the flat fingertips. Apply gentle pressure to the upper eyeball in the vitreous humor area, avoiding pressure over the sensitive and easily injured corneal area.

Auscultation. Auscultation is used to detect *moist rales* that occur with fluid volume excess when the excess fluid begins to accumulate in the lungs. As the fluid accumulation increases, pulmonary edema may develop.

Sense of Smell. The sense of smell helps identify the concentrated strong-smelling *urine* that often accompanies fluid deficit and dehydration.

EQUIPMENT

To measure intake and output when monitoring fluid balance, the nurse uses a system of record keeping, knows the capacity of various food and beverage containers, and has appropriate calibrated containers available for measuring output.

SKILL 51: MONITORING FLUID BALANCE

Intake–output records are dated and timed listings of the kinds and amounts of all fluids taken into the body by all routes, plus the kinds and amounts of fluids lost from the body by all routes. It may be necessary to calculate hourly totals for acutely ill clients with a severe fluid imbalance. For less acutely ill clients, 4- or 8-hour summaries are adequate. Twenty-four hour totals are always calculated so that patterns of losses and gains can be noted. Intake–output record forms vary from agency to agency, and sometimes within the agency itself. For example, critical-care areas require more detailed intake–output flow sheets than general-care areas; urologic units would need precise ways to record continuous bladder irrigations; and burn units would need to evaluate fluid losses in dressings. Intake–output record forms have separate columns for various categories of fluid intake and output. Intake columns usually are on the left side of the page and output columns on the right. Space is provided for the date, time, amount of fluid, and 8- and 24-hour totals. Intravenous fluid records often are kept on separate record forms at the bedside and then combined with other intake routes in the 8- and 24-hour totals.

Some agencies use separate intake–output flow sheets or small cards at the bedside and record only the 8-hour totals on a flow sheet, such as is shown in Figure 51–5. At the agency represented in Figure 51–5, the parenteral fluids are recorded on a separate flow sheet. The bedside intake card is colored and includes the capacities of the various beverage containers, whereas the output card is white, in order to avoid confusion with the intake card (Figure 51–6.) The figures are tallied at the end of each 8- and 24-hour period, and the totals are placed on the flow sheet in the permanent record. The cards are kept for several days as a reference and then destroyed.

A *pen or pencil* is always kept at the bedside when bedside intake–output records are being used. A clipboard with an attached pen helps avoid lost pens.

"Measure Intake and Output" signs are placed on the client's bed and in the bathroom to serve as reminders for the staff, client, or family to measure and record all intake and output.

Calibrated drinking glasses are helpful in measuring amounts of liquids consumed. This is especially true for between-meal drinking, since clients frequently drink only small amounts of water at a time. If noncalibrated cups are used, staff tend to estimate amounts. Estimates of intake increase the margin of error and are to be avoided unless it is not possible to measure the volume directly, such as with a spilled urinal or uncaught vomitus. If commercially calibrated glasses are not available, for example, in the home, various fluid levels in the glass may be identified by using a measuring cup and then marked with tape, colored nail polish, or a felt-tip marking pen.

Calibrated containers or pitchers made of plastic, metal, or cardboard are available for measuring output. These containers are rinsed with cold water after each use and usually are stored in the client's bathroom or bedside table. If not well rinsed, containers used to measure urine, gastric secretions, and vomitus soon become unsightly and develop unpleasant odors. Many drainage collection bags, such as Foley catheter drainage bags, are calibrated for ease in measuring. If this is the case, the output pitcher may simply be used to drain the collection bag. Small amounts of fluid are always poured into a calibrated container for measurement, as the calibrations on most collection bags are imprecise. However, some urine drainage collection sets are calibrated for small amounts, such as are shown in Skill 60.

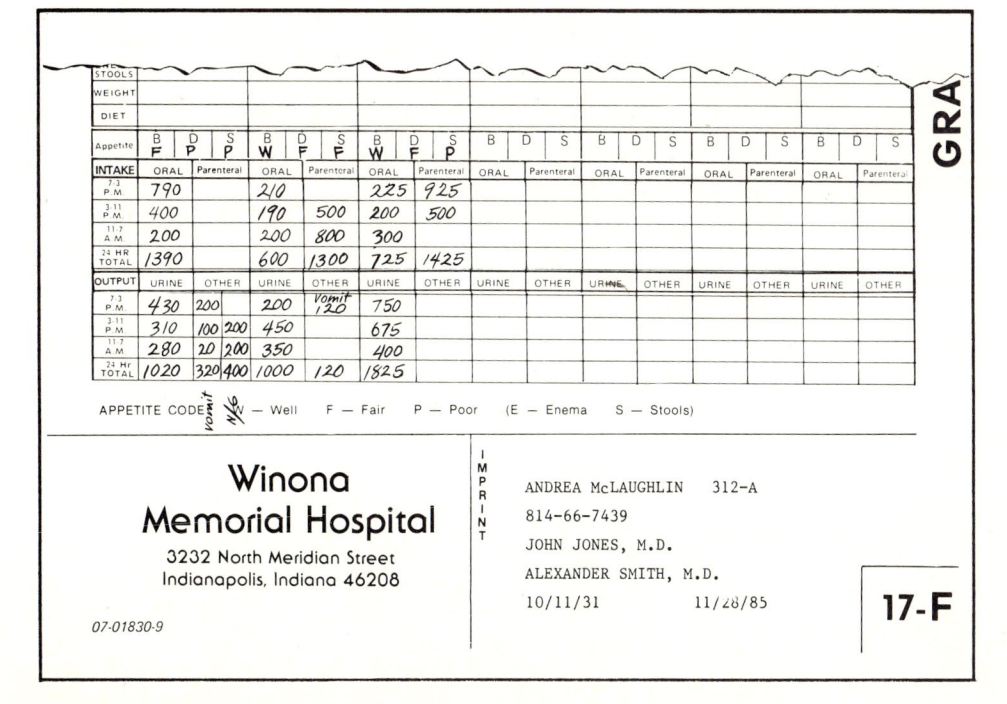

Figure 51–5. Flow sheet in health record. Note the 8- and 24-hour totals for oral and parenteral intake and urine, vomitus, and suction output. A more detailed flow sheet might be needed in an intensive-care setting. (Courtesy of Winona Memorial Hospital, Indianapolis, IN.)

WINONA MEMORIAL HOSPITAL
INDIANAPOLIS, INDIANA 46208

DAILY FLUID OUTPUT RECORD

HOUR	TYPE OF FLUID	AMOUNT IN C C
7 A.M.	Lt. yellow urine	120
8 A.M.	yell-gr vomitus	150
9 A.M.		
10 A.M.		
11 A.M.		
12 N.	Amber urine	180
1 P.M.		
2 P.M.	Amber urine	200
3 P.M.	green N/G suction	250
	TOTAL TO 3 P.M.	(900)
4 P.M.		
5 P.M.		
6 P.M.	lt. yellow urine	250
7 P.M.		
8 P.M.	"	220
9 P.M.		
10 P.M.	"	100
11 P.M.	green N/G suction	200
	TOTAL TO 11 P.M.	(770)
12 M.		
1 A.M.	Amber urine	200
2 A.M.		
3 A.M.		
4 A.M.	lt. yellow urine	150
5 A.M.	"	100
6 A.M.	green N/G suction	100
	TOTAL TO 7 A.M.	(550)

Patient's Name Julie Miller

Room No. 652 Bed 2 Date Day 1 Post op

07-03920-6

WINONA MEMORIAL HOSPITAL
INDIANAPOLIS, INDIANA 46208

DAILY FLUID INTAKE RECORD

Ice Tea Glass	360c.c.	Ice Cream	120c.c.
Conex Plastic Glass	210c.c.	Coffee Cup	130c.c.
Juice Glass	120c.c.	Bouillon Cup	160c.c.
Water Glass	210c.c.	Jello	90c.c.
Milk Carton	240c.c.	Styrofoam Cup	150c.c.

HOUR	TYPE OF FLUID	AMOUNT IN C C
7 A.M.		
8 A.M.	Tea	60
9 A.M.		
10 A.M.	Water	30
11 A.M.		
12 N.		
1 P.M.	Water	45
2 P.M.		
3 P.M.	bouillon	60
	TOTAL TO 3 P.M.	(195)
4 P.M.	Water	30
5 P.M.	bouillon	60
6 P.M.	Milk	120
7 P.M.	Jello	100
8 P.M.		
9 P.M.	ice cream	120
10 P.M.		
11 P.M.	Water	45
	TOTAL TO 11 P.M.	275
12 M.		
1 A.M.	7-up	100
2 A.M.		
3 A.M.		
4 A.M.	Water	60
5 A.M.		
6 A.M.	Tea	100
	TOTAL TO 7 A.M.	(260)

Patient's Name Julie Miller

Room No. 652 Bed 2 Date Day 2 Post op

07-03910-8

Figure 51–6. *Bedside record cards for recording intake and output. Note the capacities of eating utensils on the intake card and the spaces for 8- and 24-hour totals. This agency uses a separate form for recording intravenous infusions. (Courtesy of Winona Memorial Hospital, Indianapolis, IN.)*

Specially designed *toilet adapter pans* are also available for clients who are ambulatory and able to use the bathroom. The single-use plastic containers fit over the toilet rim under the seat and enable female clients to void more normally. Many are calibrated for ease in measurement.

☐ *EXECUTION*

ASSESSMENT OF FLUID BALANCE

Responsible, professional monitoring of fluid balance includes an assessment of a wide variety of clinical signs and symptoms. To become familiar with the scope of data that can be gathered about fluid balance status you will find it helpful to collect complete information about fluid balance from several clients. Once you have become competent in gathering these data, you will be more readily aware of clinical signs and symptoms of fluid imbalance. Because of the subtle and complex nature of many of the clinical indicators of fluid imbalance, continued practice in these assessments is needed.

INTAKE MEASUREMENT

Record both the kind and the amount of oral, enteral, and parenteral fluids in the client health record. These data make it possible to examine electrolyte and kilocalorie consumption as well as fluid intake.

Measurement of oral intake includes all fluids and foods that are liquid at room temperature, such as gelatin dessert, ice cream, ice, soup, and soft puddings. Except for ice, the volume of these solid foods does not change significantly between the solid and liquid state. Ice melts to one-half its original volume. Recording of intake is inaccurate if this melting factor is not considered or if unmelted ice in iced beverages is considered part of the amount consumed. Sometimes clients share their food trays with their family or friends. When collecting a tray after mealtime, validate that the client actually consumed the contents of the empty containers.

Intravenous fluids and irrigation solutions pose special problems for accurate intake measurement. Intravenous fluid bottles or bags often contain more than the designated amounts. For example, a 1000-ml bottle may actually contain 1100 ml, and a 500-ml bottle often contains 600 ml (Luckmann and Sorensen, 1980). This overfill problem can be avoided by carefully monitoring fluid levels and changing the container when the fluid level reaches the zero mark rather than waiting until it is completely empty.

When tubes or drains are irrigated, if the amount inserted is greater than the amount withdrawn, the difference is intake. If the amount withdrawn is greater than the amount inserted, the difference is regarded as output. Intake from irrigations may be recorded by adding the total amount of irrigant inserted to the intake column of the input–output record and the total amount withdrawn to the output column. Alternatively, the difference in the two amounts may be compared and the difference added to the intake or output column, as appropriate.

OUTPUT MEASUREMENT

Measure output from all routes as accurately as possible and record it in separate categories. Separate totals of fluid loss make it possible to estimate or calculate electrolyte and kilocalorie losses and plan replacements accordingly. For example, equal volumes of urine and nasogastric suction fluid have vastly different electrolyte compositions. When estimates of losses are necessary, their accuracy is increased by giving specific descriptions of the amount of linen, clothing, or dressings saturated with blood, urine, vomitus, or perspiration. Perspiration can be estimated on a scale of one plus (1+) to four plus (4+), with 1+ representing barely visible sweating and 4+ representing profuse sweating.

When output is being measured, instruct clients to use a bedpan, urinal, or toilet collection device. Toilet tissue preferably is placed directly in the toilet or in the wastebasket. Otherwise, it is left in the urine, as a greater measurement variance occurs when it is removed than when it is left in.

Collection containers for suction apparatus and urinary catheters often are calibrated for ease of measurement. However, when small amounts of fluid are being measured, more accurate measurements are obtained if they are poured into a small calibrated container, unless the specially designed small urine collection chambers are used.

PROMOTING ACCURATE INTAKE–OUTPUT MEASUREMENT

Each person involved in the care of a client on intake and output measurement assumes responsibility for recording all intake and output promptly and accurately. Use calibrated containers or containers of known volume. Hold calibrated containers at eye level, reading the volume level at the center, rather than at the edge, of the meniscus.

Use the volumes listed on the bedside record form for intake measurement, since these vary with the institution. Although clients and their families may have been taught to monitor fluid intake and output, it is the nurse's responsibility to evaluate the kind and amount of fluid intake and output, to make some determination of how well the client or family is performing the task, and to take time to answer questions or provide additional information as needed.

Being aware of potential problem areas in measuring both intake and output can help the nurse institute measures to avoid or minimize these errors. The following is a listing of common sources of staff error in recording fluid balance, adapted from Metheny and Snively (1982, pp. 108–109):

1. Inadequate explanations to clients and their families about the importance of measuring intake and output, and the method of doing so.
2. Well-meant, forgotten intentions to record a drink or voiding at a more convenient time.
3. Assumptions that clients have consumed the contents of empty containers on a food tray, without verification from them or their families.
4. Failure to consider volume displacement of ice in iced drinks or the melted volume of ice chips.
5. Estimation of measurements that should be directly measured, because it takes less time.
6. Failure to record the amount of unreturned fluids used for irrigations.
7. Failure to estimate losses through perspiration, wound exudate, incontinent urine and liquid stool, and uncaught vomitus.
8. Failure to record accurately the amount of parenteral fluids received on each shift.
9. Failure to include water taken with medication administration.
10. Failure to include intravenous bottle overfill.

Inaccurate intake–output records appear to be related to a combination of institutional, unit, and staff policies, practices, and circumstances. For example, an institution may not provide adequate in-service educational programs for all levels of personnel, and the system of record keeping for intake and output measurement may be cumbersome or unworkable. A nursing-care unit may be understaffed, so that the personnel directly responsible for the care of seriously ill clients are not well qualified, supervision may be lax, the staff may be poorly motivated to provide quality care, or the method of communicating to the

496 PROFESSIONAL CLINICAL NURSING SKILLS

staff which clients need to have intake and output measured may not be adequate. The staff may not always comprehend the value in measuring intake and output, recognize the need for accurate records, or implement the procedure correctly.

There are several organizational practices on a clinical unit that can promote more accurate intake-output measurement. These practices include:

1. Current listings of clients on intake and output (I & O) posted on the nursing unit or placed in the kardex
2. Consistent use of intake-output signs on clients' doors, beds, or in the bathroom
3. Adequate and easily located bedside records with attached pencil
4. Frequent updating of kardex orders
5. Regular reevaluation of clients' need for intake-output measurements, so that staff do not regard intake-output measurements as busy work.

☐ SKILL SEQUENCE

MEASUREMENT OF FLUID BALANCE

Step	Rationale
1. Validate nurse or physician order for intake-output measurement.	Ensures necessity of monitoring fluid balance.
2. Explain reason for intake-output measurement to client and family.	Promotes increased accuracy of intake-output records by involving client in his or her own care.
3. Wash hands.	Avoids cross-contamination.
4. Place bedside intake-output record and a pen or pencil in a convenient, clean, and dry place.	Ready availability of recording forms and pen increases use and accuracy.
5. Provide calibrated drinking glass and urine measuring container (pitcher or toilet seat adapter).	Readily available measurement containers increases probability of staff recording intake and output values. Calibrated containers increase speed and ease of measuring.
6. Instruct client and family about measuring intake and output: a. Reading and using metric measures b. Written notations of sizes of beverage containers and calibration of drinking glasses c. Location, use, and calibration of output containers d. Intake includes all ice and liquids, as well as foods that are liquid at room temperature e. Seperate recording of various routes for output loss f. Need for accuracy of measurement g. Importance of immediate recording of all intake and output h. Goal for intake—increase, limit, or primarily monitoring	Clear understanding of why and how to measure intake and output increases ability to complete task accurately.
7. If fluids are to be increased, place water pitcher in readily available location and provide additional beverages selected by client and consistent with dietary prescription.	Increased availability of preferred beverages increases likelihood of reaching desired fluid intake goals.
8. If fluids are to be restricted, remove water pitcher. Plan fluid allocation with client, dietitian, and medical nurse.	Adherence to fluid limitations is facilitated by self-care involvement and reminders.
9. Promptly enter all intake and output values on bedside record form, using metric measurements; indicate kind of beverages consumed; describe appearance of urine, vomitus, drainage, or other body fluids.	Ensures that need to record is not forgotten later. Containers are usually calibrated in metric measures. Helps determine electrolyte gains and losses and, therefore, need for specific types of fluid replacement.
10. Calculate separate totals for each route of intake and output at end of an 8-hour shift—or more often if client is critically ill—and record in client health record.	Provides current, ongoing data about fluid balance.
11. Calculate total 24-hour intake and output and place in client health record. Totals to include: a. Each intake and output route b. All combined routes of intake c. All combined routes of output	Provides data for evaluating gains and losses and need for fluid replacement, additional therapies, or alteration of fluid prescription.
12. Evaluate balance/imbalance in intake and output, assess other quantitative and qualitative measurements of fluid balance status, and report to physician as needed.	Fulfills accountability and responsibility and provides ongoing data base.

RECORDING

Record all fluids on the bedside record form promptly, regardless of the route by which they enter the body. Include the kind of fluids consumed or infused to help monitor electrolyte intake, and indicate the route by which they were given. Record all forms of output promptly, including a description of the fluid loss. Calculate both intake and output totals at least every 8 and 24 hours. Urine output may need to be monitored on an hourly basis for acutely ill persons.

Narrative or POR recordings would include other clinical indicators of fluid balance or imbalance as appropriate for the client's circumstances. Sample recordings are shown in Figures 51-5 and 51-6.

□ CRITICAL POINTS SUMMARY

1. For adequate fluid balance in health, ingested fluids approximately equal excreted urine.
2. Illness increases the body's need for fluid, increases fluid losses, and often decreases oral fluid intake.
3. Fluid balance assessment includes appraisal of intake-output, weight, vital signs, pulses, vein filling, edema, turgor, skin and mucous membrane dryness, thirst, face and eyes, urine and stool, speech, level of consciousness, and selected laboratory data.
4. Fluid gains and losses are directly reflected in intake and output values and body weight.
5. Accurate intake-output records depend on:
   a. Accurate understanding of the reasons for fluid balance measurement by staff, client, and family
   b. The value placed on intake-output measurement by nursing staff
   c. Clinical unit policies that support consistent measuring of fluid balance for appropriate clients
   d. Availability of complete recording equipment
   e. Consistent, prompt recording of all intake and output
   f. The use of calibrated containers for fluid intake and output measurement
   g. Actual measurement of intake and output
   h. Careful estimation of all losses that cannot be measured directly
   i. Inclusion of liquids given with medications, volume change when ice melts, and consideration of intravenous fluid container overfill

□ LEARNING ACTIVITIES

1. Examine fluid intake-output records in a client health record in an acute-care or long-term agency. Look for:
   a. Length of time intake and output has been measured
   b. Completeness of entries
   c. Eight- and 24-hour intake and output totals
   d. Routes indicated for fluid intake and type of fluid
   e. Routes indicated for fluid loss and nature of losses

   From the total health record, determine the reason for having intake and output measured.
2. Ask a staff nurse, team leader, or unit manager about the most common reasons for inaccurate and incomplete intake-output records, and the degree of difficulty that unit experiences in obtaining complete and accurate intake-output records.
3. Fill a glass measuring cup or drinking glass with crushed or chipped ice. Note level or volume of ice. Allow to melt. Note level or volume and compare the two values.
4. Prepare two iced beverages, one with a large amount of ice, the other with a small amount of ice. Pour the liquid from each one and measure the volume. Note the different liquid volumes from the two beverages. Allow the ice to melt, measure, and compare.
5. How do the activities in 2 and 3 relate to accurate fluid balance measurement?
6. Weigh yourself on the morning after a meal with a high salt intake, such as pizza, popcorn, or the like. During the day, observe your thirst level, fluid intake, increased or decreased urinary output, tightness of rings, and so on. What indications of fluid retention (excess) did you notice? When? Discuss your observations with your peers. How do these observations relate to fluid balance measurement for clients?

□ REVIEW QUESTIONS

1. Why is intake and output measurement a reliable indicator of fluid balance?
2. What is the relationship between fluid gains and losses and weight gain and loss?
3. What kinds of clients are at increased risk for developing fluid imbalance?
4. What factors does the nurse consider when determining which clients need intake and output measured?
5. What signs, symptoms, or changes in each of the following would indicate fluid volume excess or deficit?

	FLUID EXCESS	FLUID DEFICIT
Weight		
Temperature		

(cont.)

	FLUID EXCESS	FLUID DEFICIT
Pulse		
Respirations		
Blood pressure		
Stools		
Skin turgor		
Mucous membranes		
Peripheral vein filling		
Jugular vein filling		
Peripheral pulses		
Thirst		
Urine		
Facial expression		
Speech		
Level of consciousness		
Eyeballs		

6. What changes would be expected in the following laboratory values with fluid excess or deficit?

	FLUID EXCESS	FLUID DEFICIT
Serum osmolality		
BUN		
Urine osmolality		

7. What categories of foods are included with liquids as intake, and why?
8. Why are totals recorded separately for each output route?
9. Why are the kind of fluids consumed included in the intake record?
10. How can fluid restrictions be made more acceptable to clients?
11. What nursing actions would help a client increase his or her fluid intake?
12. What nursing actions increase the likelihood of accurate client-kept intake–output records?

☐ PERFORMANCE CHECKLIST

OBJECTIVE: To measure, record, and tally fluid intake and output values correctly.

CHARACTERISTIC	RANGE OF ACCEPTABILITY	SATISFACTORY	UNSATISFACTORY
1. Validates medical or nursing order.	No deviation		
2. Explains rationale to client and family.	No deviation		
3. Washes hands.	No deviation		
4. Places bedside intake–output records and a pen in a convenient place.	No deviation		
5. Provides required equipment.	No deviation		
6. Explains methods of measuring intake and output.	No deviation		
7. Plans for fluid increases or restrictions.	No deviation		
8. Instructs patient and family.	Omit if unable to assist.		
9. Promptly enters all intake and output on bedside record.	No deviation		
10. Uses metric measures throughout.	No deviation		
11. Records types of intake fluids and nature of output losses.	No deviation		
12. Calculates totals for each intake and output route: a every 8 hours b every 24 hours	May be more often for critically ill clients. No deviation		
13. Records intake and output totals in client health record.	No deviation		
14. Evaluates fluid balance/imbalance; reports to physician as needed.	No deviation		

REFERENCES

Bates B: A Guide to Physical Examination, ed 3. Philadelphia, JB Lippincott, 1983.

Bennett J, Petersdorf R: Alterations in body temperature. In Wintrobe M, et al. (eds): Harrison's Principles of Internal Medicine, ed 7. New York, McGraw-Hill, 1974.

Condon RE, Nyhus LM: Manual of Surgical Therapeutics, ed 6. Boston, Little, Brown, 1985.

Corbett JV: Laboratory Tests in Nursing Practice. Norwalk, CT, Appleton-Century-Crofts, 1982.

Fischbach F: A Manual of Laboratory Diagnostic Tests. Philadelphia, JB Lippincott, 1980.

Grant MM, Kubo WM: Assessing a patient's hydration status. American Journal of Nursing 75:1306–1313, 1975.

Guyton AC: Textbook of Medical Physiology, ed 6. Philadelphia, WB Saunders, 1981.

Holmes JH: Fluid intake with medication. Archives of Internal Medicine 116:(6)813, 1965.

Luckmann J, Sorensen KC: Medical-Surgical Nursing: A Psychophysiologic Approach, ed 2. Philadelphia, WB Saunders, 1980.

Menzel LK: Clinical problems of fluid balance. Nursing Clinics of North America 15(3):549–576, 1980.

Metheny NM, Snively WD: Nurses' Handbook of Fluid Balance, ed 4. Philadelphia, JB Lippincott, 1983.

Mitchell PH, Loustau A: Concepts Basic to Nursing, ed 3. New York, McGraw-Hill, 1981.

Moyer CA: Fluid Balance. A Clinical Manual. Chicago, Year Book, 1952.

Nursing78 Books: Monitoring Fluid and Electrolytes Precisely. Nursing78 Skillbook Series. Horsham, PA, Intermed Communications, 1978.

Pflaum SS: Investigation of intake–output as a means of assessing body fluid balance. Heart and Lung 8(3):495–498, 1979.

Walike BC, Padilla G, et al: Patient problems related to tube feeding. In Batey MV (ed): Communicating Nursing Research. Boulder, CO, Western Interstate Commission for Higher Education, 1975, vol 7.

BIBLIOGRAPHY

Beland IL, Passos JY: Clinical Nursing: Pathophysiological and Psychosocial Approaches, ed 4. New York, Macmillan, 1981.

Krause MV, Mahan LK: Food, Nutrition and Diet Therapy, ed 7. Philadelphia, WB Saunders, 1984.

Maxwell MH, Kleeman C: Clinical Disorders of Fluid and Electrolyte Metabolism. New York, McGraw-Hill, 1980.

Roberts A: Body water and its control. Nursing Times 74(47):69–72, November 23, 1978.

Sorensen KC, Luckmann J: Basic Nursing: A Psychophysiologic Approach. Philadelphia, WB Saunders, 1979.

Suitor CW, Crowley MF: Nutrition: Principles and Application in Health Promotion, ed 2. Philadelphia, JB Lippincott, 1984.

Thomas CL: Tabor's Cyclopedic Medical Dictionary, ed 14. Philadelphia, FA Davis, 1981.

Urrows ST: Physiology of body fluids. Nursing Clinics of North America 15(3):537–547, 1980.

SUGGESTED READING

Metheny LK, Snively WD: Nurses' Handbook of Fluid Balance, ed 4. Philadelphia, JB Lippincott, 1983.

Nursing78 Books: Monitoring Fluid and Electrolytes Precisely. Nursing78 Skillbook Series. Horsham, PA, Intermed Communications, 1978.

AUDIOVISUAL RESOURCES

Fluids and Electrolytes: Fluid Balance
  Slides, filmstrip, videotape, film. (1984, Color, 24 min.)
Fluids and Electrolytes: Isotonic Volume Changes
  Slides, filmstrip, videotape, film. (1984, Color, 25 min.)
Fluid Balance: Assessment, Maintenance, Intervention
  Slides, filmstrip, videotape, film. (1981, Color, 21 min.)
  Available through:
  Medcom, Inc.
  P.O. Box 116
  Garden Grove, CA 92642

SKILL 52 Nutritional Assessment and the Serving of Food

PREREQUISITE SKILLS

Skill 19, "Inspection"
Skill 20, "Palpation"
Skill 22, "Auscultation"
Skill 28, "Handwashing"

☐ STUDENT OBJECTIVES

1. Summarize physiological and psychological factors that regulate food intake.
2. Distinguish between hunger and appetite; satiety and anorexia.
3. Identify physical findings that indicate nutritional balance and imbalance.
4. Distinguish among malnutrition, undernutrition, and overnutrition.
5. Explain various factors that affect the consumption of food.
6. Identify illness-related factors that alter a person's usual consumption of food.
7. Describe factors that help determine the type of diet a client receives.

8. Identify foods included on and excluded from clear and full liquid and mechanical soft diets.
9. Discuss the role of the dietitian in meal preparation and serving.
10. Describe ways the nurse and the dietitian work together in promoting adequate nutrition for clients.
11. Describe various ways food is kept at proper temperatures during delivery to clinical areas.
12. Describe preparation of clients for mealtimes.
13. Correctly assess and record a client's nutritional intake.

☐ INTRODUCTION

This skill has two basic components; the process of serving meals to clients and the assessment of their nutritional status. *Serving meals* includes the distribution of meal trays, the provision of assistance with eating as needed, and the evaluation and recording of food consumption. Although the nurse may be involved in serving meals, in more and more agencies this function is being assumed by the dietary department. Nurses, rather than dietary staff, however, are responsible for monitoring clients' food consumption. *Nutritional status* refers to an individual's health condition as influenced by the utilization of nutrients. Nutritional status is assessed through a correlation of information from medical, nursing, and diet histories, physical examination, and laboratory findings (Robinson and Lawler, 1982; Whitney and Cataldo, 1983). Information about clients' food intake patterns, food tolerance, and nutritional status is a vital part of client health status appraisal.

Adequate nutrition is an integral part of both the maintenance of good health in a well person and the care of an ill person. When food consumption is inadequate, health status decreases, resistance to disease is lowered, illness recovery time is lengthened, recovery from surgery is delayed, postoperative infections and delayed wound healing are more common, and energy levels drop.

Although illness usually increases a client's nutritional needs, it decreases his or her ability to meet those needs. Nutritional needs increase during illness because catabolic processes are accelerated over anabolic processes. Recovery from surgery, infection, or illness requires that the rate of anabolism exceed the rate of catabolism. Although an adequate intake of nutrients is crucial for a return to a balanced metabolic state, the increased losses and decreased intake of nutrients that accompany illness make this difficult to achieve. For example, nutrient losses may occur through diarrhea or vomiting, and decreased intake of nutrients may occur from anorexia, inability to ingest or digest food, or enforced deprivation of food for diagnostic or therapeutic purposes.

Food intake often is modified for therapeutic purposes, such as a low-sodium diet for a hypertensive person or a clear liquid diet the day after surgery. A client may be completely deprived of food for a period of time before and after surgery or for some diagnostic procedures. For a variety of reasons, clients sometimes refuse to eat or eat very little food. For example, food consumption decreases when a person is nauseated, angry, tired, confused, or is too poor to purchase adequate food; or a person may dislike the food or find it unacceptable for religious or ethnic reasons.

Because nutritional intake and status are closely allied with health and illness, nurses must be able to (a) assess the client's nutritional status and ability to ingest and digest food, (b) identify areas of nutritional deficits or excesses, (c) recognize nutritional problems that may be related to illness, diagnostic tests, or therapeutic measures, (d) evaluate the success of therapeutic regimes, (e) and initiate actions to modify food intake. In a hospital, the nurse performs some of these actions, for example, evaluating the ability to ingest and digest food. Other actions are carried out collaboratively with the physician or dietitian, for example, modifying a diet order or evaluating nutritional status.

The nurse who works in a clinic or public health agency may have a nutritionist available for consultation or direct client work, but the nurse also is expected to make nutritional evaluations and provide nutrition teaching. The public health nurse frequently is asked about infant formulas, food preparation for an ill person or for a person with poor appetite, food budgeting, and how to adapt a prescribed diet to the individual client or family's religious and ethnic preferences and economic necessities.

Primary prevention of illness includes promotion of wellness and good health, and nutrition is a major component of that wellness promotion. With the general public developing an increasing interest in wellness, nutrition, and self-care, nurses are being asked to provide nutritional evaluation, consultation, and teaching.

☐ PREPARATION

REGULATION OF FOOD INTAKE

Food intake is regulated by a combination of physiological and psychological cues. The physiological sensation of *hunger* causes physical discomfort that motivates a person to obtain and eat food, even if it does not taste good. Physiological cues for eating include uncomfortable stomach contractions and a shaky, anxious, weak feeling associated with a lowered blood sugar.

Appetite is a more pleasurable sensation that involves a desire for food and drink motivated by the person's perception of the palatability of the food. Appetite often is related to psychogenic factors and may or may not be related to hunger. The internal environment of the body plays a role in food regulation. When the body needs food, the lateral nucleus of the hypothalamus (the feeding center) sends out signals that stimulate the person to seek food. When the person has consumed enough food, the ventromedial hypothalamus (the satiety center) sends out signals that inhibit the lateral hypothalamus and cause the person to stop eating. The absence of a normal desire for food is known as *anorexia*. Anorexia is often associated with fever, illness, drug ingestion, certain psychological states, and even some vitamin deficiencies.

Satiety represents a state of satisfaction or a lack of desire for further food following its ingestion, commonly known as "being full." When a person responds only to internal cues for eating, food intake and weight are kept in balance with minimal or no effort. However, external cues for eating often exert more influence on eating behaviors than do internal cues. For example, food habits, the taste of food, emotions, and social pressure influence us to eat even when we actually are not hungry. The body tends to self-correct in that weight lost in illness is usually regained to the point of normal weight.

Exercise is known to help curb the appetite, in spite of popular beliefs to the contrary. Exercise increases energy expenditures, results in a feeling of well-being, and releases tension. We usually avoid food before moderately vigorous exercise, and our appetite tends to be curbed following exercise because of a temporary decrease in blood supply to the gastrointestinal tract (Suitor and Crowley, 1984).

MALNUTRITION

Malnutrition is a general term that indicates an excess, deficit, or imbalance of one or more of the essential nutrients (Mitchell & Loustau, 1981; Suitor and Crowley, 1984). *Primary malnutrition* occurs when a person habitually eats in a way that does not meet his or her nutritional requirements. *Secondary malnutrition* results from faulty body function, such as malabsorption syndrome or the lack of intrinsic factor in gastric juice, which is needed for vitamin B_{12} absorption. *Undernutrition* occurs when a person does not consume an adequate amount of nutrients. *Overnutrition* occurs when a person consumes more food than needed, often of inappropriate kinds. *Protein–calorie malnutrition* (PCM) is a marked deficiency in both calories and proteins, which results in symptoms ranging from marasmus (wasting of subcutaneous fat and muscle tissue) to the severe kwashiorkor syndrome of edema, apathy, skin and hair changes, and metabolic alterations.

Early (subclinical) undernutrition generally has few clinical signs and symptoms, and it is quite possible to be undernourished without being aware of it. As deprivation persists, however, body reserves are depleted and overt signs and symptoms develop. In the United States, teenage girls are highly vulnerable to being undernourished as a result of eating habits and dieting to achieve or maintain thinness. In addition, the high rate of teenage pregnancies contributes to this rate of undernutrition among adolescent girls because of the added nutritional demands of pregnancy.

Overnutrition is a common problem among adults in the United States, indicated in part by the prevalence of illnesses associated with being overweight, such as hypertension, heart disease, and diabetes. Overnutrition occurs as a result of an intake of kilocalories that exceeds the amount expended for meeting energy needs. Over a period of days or weeks, an intake of 3500 kcal beyond that needed for energy expenditures results in a weight gain of 0.45 kg (1 lb). Conversely, an intake of 3500 kcal less than what is needed for energy expenditures results in a weight loss of 0.45 kg (1 lb).

On a worldwide basis, PCM is a serious nutritional problem, especially for infants and children in developing countries. Although not as common in children in North America, repeated studies indicate malnutrition is a significant problem among hospitalized clients in acute-care settings. Using the indices of weight/height, triceps skinfold, arm muscle circumferences, serum albumin, and hematocrit, several studies found a 50 and 60 percent incidence of PCM among medical and surgical patients (Bistrian et al., 1974, 1976). They found that a combined calorie and protein deficiency was significantly more common in medical patients than in surgical patients, whereas surgical patients experienced more severe protein deficiency, reflecting the more catabolic nature of surgical diseases. They also found that PCM was widely distributed among broad disease categories and believe that nutritional support of hospital patients has been quite lacking.

Institutional factors contributing to these deficiencies include inadequate nutritional preparation for surgery, prolonged use of glucose and saline intravenous feedings, frequent venipunctures, failure to observe food intake, withholding of meals because of diagnostic tests, inadequate amounts or lack of appropriate nutrients in the composition of tube feedings, and diffusion among many care-givers of the responsibility for client care (Bistrian et al., 1974; Butterworth and Blackburn, 1975). When individual factors causing decreased food consumption also are considered, some degree of the magnitude of the problem of hospital undernutrition can be appreciated.

FACTORS AFFECTING FOOD CONSUMPTION

Physical Strength and Functional Abilities

A person's ability to shop for, prepare, and consume food is affected by physical strength and functional abilities. An elderly woman living alone in a second-floor walk-up apartment may be able to prepare and consume food, but not have enough strength to shop. Friends, family, or a homemaker service may be able to provide the latter service, enabling her to be relatively self-sufficient. A healthy person confined to bed with a broken leg would be able to consume food but not shop for or prepare it. A person who has had a stroke with resulting paralysis would need help with all three of these aspects of food consumption.

The ability to chew food may be affected by the number of healthy teeth present, or the presence and fit of dentures. The ability to swallow may be altered because of neurologic impairment, such as occurs after a stroke. Individuals with cardiac and respiratory problems often need to eat more slowly, resting periodically. If made to feel rushed or pushed to hurry, these individuals will usually simply stop eating and say they are full or finished. Individuals with arthritic conditions or limited vision may have trouble opening milk cartons and salt and pepper packages, pouring beverages, or removing protective covers from food dishes.

Mental and Emotional Status
Retarded and mentally ill persons generally are able to consume food independently, but may not be able to manage shopping for and preparation of food. Persons hospitalized for severe depression or anorexia nervosa might not be able or willing to feed themselves. Emotions may cause people to overeat or to lose their interest in food, especially in times of high stress.

The fear, worry, insecurity, and frustrations that accompany being ill often are expressed through food and eating behaviors such as anorexia, fussiness, and demands for extra attention. Babcock (1952, p. 222) says that "it is easier to show discouragement through anorexia than it is to explain that one is feeling inadequate and depressed in the presence of a frightening disease or disheartening experience." Rather than being due to uncooperativeness, refusal to eat certain foods may be caused by unpleasant associations with food. For example, some adults associate milk, custards, cooked cereals, and strained foods with childhood and either the dependency or security of that period of time. This may cause them either to refuse those foods (even when needed therapeutically) or to cling to them beyond the time they are needed. For some clients, having food withheld or having restrictive diets offered may be associated with childhood reward–punishment food experiences, causing them to regard the nurse as being punitive.

Appetite and Hunger
In illness, appetite and hunger do not regulate food intake as reliably as they usually do in health. Anorexia in a hospitalized person often is due to the combined effects of illness, the stress of being hospitalized, and fears about diagnosis or prognosis. Some of the factors contributing to anorexia include altered taste sensations (such as from some drugs), decreased ability to digest food (with symptoms of nausea, vomiting, flatulence, and bloating), a bad taste in the mouth (such as from fever, decreased oral intake, poor oral care, or some drugs), and having abstained from food for several days. When a person is ill, it is not uncommon for the sight and smell of food to trigger nausea and vomiting. In addition, unfamiliar or unpalatable food, overly large servings, fatigue, or disagreeable odors can cause a decreased appetite. Clients often are unaccustomed to hospital food, and there are many unusual and unpleasant odors in a hospital, such as those from dressings, drainage tubes, or human waste.

Economic Factors
A special diet may cause a problem in a family's food budget. Specialty foods such as low-sodium dietetic foods or increased amounts of protein, fruits, and vegetables are more costly than many families' usual fare. Undernutrition is more common among lower-income people, partly because of the higher cost of well-balanced meals. Education also has a strong relationship to nutritional status and levels of health, since education is positively correlated with affluence and negatively correlated with low incomes (Blum, 1974). The less well educated people are, the less they are likely to know about nutrition and balanced diets.

Especially when teaching clients about therapeutic diets, it is important for the nurse to consider whether their economic resources are sufficient for basic food purchases plus any special foods needed, and what kinds of storage and cooking facilities are available in the home. Nurses come from predominantly middle-class backgrounds and they often are unaware of or forget that some low-income families (both urban and rural) do not have refrigerators, freezers, ovens, or a car for easy access to grocery stores, or that they may live in an apartment without cooking facilities.

Cultural Factors
Racial or ethnic heritage, family background, religious practices, and social status help determine the kinds of foods a person is accustomed to eating, and how those foods are prepared. These factors also influence a person's willingness to eat hospital food or to follow a therapeutic diet. For example, a Seventh Day Adventist probably would not be willing to eat a high-protein diet that included meat, since many persons of this religious group are vegetarians. Orthodox Jews will not eat pork or shellfish, although Reformed or Conservative Jews may do so.

In general, a person will be much more likely to follow a therapeutic diet if it incorporates usual and familiar foods. This may mean planning a diabetic exchange or low-sodium diet that includes chicken, fish, rice, and vegetables for persons with Vietnamese or Chinese food preferences, rice and beans for a Puerto Rican, beans and tortillas for a Mexican–American, or meat and potatoes for a midwestern American farmer (Whitney and Cataldo, 1983).

The Food Itself
The appearance, odor, taste, texture, temperature, preparation, and type of food all influence a person's perception of the acceptability of that food, particularly when ill or hospitalized. We often reject without

tasting food that looks unattractive or has a strange or unusual smell, and also tend to eat less food when the taste or texture is unfamiliar. In addition, if hot foods are not served hot and cold foods cold, they are regarded as unpalatable and unappetizing. Moreover, institutional preparation of food is different from home preparation, so even familiar foods may become unfamiliar to a hospitalized person.

The appearance of the food tray itself may influence the person's consumption of food. Spilled beverages and poorly organized, cluttered trays have a negative effect on the appetite.

Illness Conditions
Food is prohibited before and after surgery; individuals are placed on NPO status (nil per os, or nothing per mouth) for 6 to 10 hours before surgery because of the danger of vomiting and aspiration during anesthesia. After surgery, fluids are not given until the effects of anesthesia have passed and may be delayed even longer if there is nausea or vomiting. The physician's order may be written as, "Sips of water as tolerated." Foods other than clear liquids are not given until bowel sounds are heard, indicating that gastrointestinal motility has returned after being suspended by anesthesia.

An acutely ill person has less desire for food (anorexia), less energy for eating, and a decreased ability to digest food. Illness and decreased oral intake often result in an altered sense of taste and smell, both of which affect the desire for food.

Modification of the diet may be necessary to provide additional amounts of nutrients that are lacking. For example, a person with simple iron-deficiency anemia needs increased amounts of iron-rich foods, such as liver, egg yolks, and whole grains; a person who is deficient in vitamin C needs additional amounts of foods rich in vitamin C, such as citrus fruits, strawberries, tomatoes, dark green leafy vegetables, and so on. It is beyond the scope of this text to discuss deficiency states, and the student is referred to nutrition textbooks for this information.

Surgery, trauma, or severe burns increase the body's need for kilocalories (energy), proteins, vitamin C, and a variety of minerals because the body is in a negative nitrogen balance. This negative nitrogen balance results from an increased tissue protein breakdown, a decreased synthesis of protein, or both. As much as 30 g nitrogen (equivalent to 2 lb of muscle tissue) can be lost in 1 day when severe trauma is present (Dudrick and Rhoads, 1981). Immobility also causes a negative balance, resulting from atrophy of bone and muscle.

Some medical diagnoses require therapeutic diets as part of the treatment regime. Examples of this include hypertension (low-sodium diets), coronary artery disease (low-cholesterol diets), diabetes (diabetic exchange or weighed diets), or gallbladder disease before surgery (low-fat diets). These dietary modifications usually are prescribed specifically by a physician.

Some medications require dietary modifications. Monoamine oxidase (MAO) inhibitors (such as Marplan, Nardil, and Parnate) used to treat severe depression require a tyramine-free diet. Tyramines occur naturally in aged cheeses, liver, dried fish, and in fermented alcoholic beverages. Ingestion of tyramine-containing foods by persons taking MAO inhibitor drugs results in severe, sometimes fatal, hypertension with intracranial hemorrhages.

Other medications or treatments may cause nutritional problems. For example, cancer chemotherapeutic agents frequently cause nausea, vomiting, gastritis, stomatitis, malabsorption of nutrients, and a decreased ability to utilize proteins, vitamins, and minerals. Salicylates and antibiotics may cause nausea, vomiting, and gastritis with hemorrhage; anticonvulsants often cause gum hyperplasia; and some antacids interfere with absorption of nutrients.

NUTRITIONAL SERVICES IN HEALTH-CARE AGENCIES

Nutritional services within a health-care agency include both food services and dietary services, which usually are the responsibility of a registered dietitian who is accountable to the agency administration. An agency may have complete dietary and food services, or it may contract with outside companies or persons for some or all of these services. For example, the agency may prepare all its own food, purchase some convenience prepackaged foods, or contract with a catering service for all food.

Food Service
Food service includes preparation and service of food for clients, employees, and sometimes family members. Food service systems for clients may be centralized or decentralized. In a centralized system, the individual food trays are assembled in the central kitchen area and either placed in a food service cart for transportation by staff to nursing units or transported via a conveyor system or dumbwaiter.

In a decentralized system, food is prepared in a central location and then transported in bulk to smaller service kitchens near the nursing unit. The individual trays are assembled there by either dietary or nursing personnel. Some decentralized systems involve actual preparation of the food in the nursing units, although this duplication of equipment and personnel tends to be expensive. In some agencies, food is served to clients in a dining room, either cafeteria style or with prepared plates of food or trays for those on therapeutic diets. Agencies with centralized kitchens usually have small kitchen areas on a nursing unit where beverages and light food are kept for between-meal feedings (often called nourishments) or snacks.

In acute-care agencies, meals are often served three times per day, with bedtime or between-meal snacks available on request, at the physician's order, or at the nurse's discretion. Some agencies have adopted a four-to-five meal per day schedule, with a light early breakfast and later evening meal, plus a larger brunch and late afternoon dinner. This practice of spreading food intake more widely over a 24-hour period accommodates early morning diagnostic tests without the client having to miss or delay a meal. Because smaller, more frequent meals are often better tolerated by ill or aged persons, this schedule frequently is used in nursing homes.

The actual serving of trays to clients and the collection of used trays may be done by the nursing staff or the dietary department, and either staff may be responsible for recording the kind and amount of food actually consumed by the client. Flow sheets in the client's health record usually contain space for these data, and most dietary department meal lists include space for food consumption and appetite.

Dietary Services
Dietary services may include the planning of regular and modified diets, the assessment of nutritional needs of clients, and the provision of individualized and group nutritional teaching and planning. In agencies certified to receive Medicare or Medicaid payments, a qualified dietitian must be involved in planning and implementing client food services.

In smaller agencies, only part-time dietitian services may be available, and the nurse learns how best to utilize the dietitian's knowledge and services, what kind of problems to refer to the dietitian, and how to provide adequate nutritional care when the dietitian is not present. In larger health-care agencies, nurses, dietitians, and physicians work together as an interdisciplinary team to provide comprehensive nutritional and dietary services. A registered dietitian (R.D.) has college or graduate preparation in dietetics, nutrition, or food services, and has passed a national examination. A dietitian may specialize as a clinical, administrative, consultant, community, research, or teaching dietitian. A cooperative, reciprocal relationship between the nurse and the dietitian is essential for clients' nutritional needs to be met adequately.

Agency routines generally provide channels for new diet orders, delayed trays, omitted meals, food allergies, and discharge diet orders to be communicated from the medical and nursing staff to the dietary department. Agency policies provide for such things as meal schedules or the method of ordering late trays. To provide adequately for clients' nutritional intake, the nurse becomes familiar with the food service policies and dietary services in the particular agency.

Most agencies, especially acute-care agencies, offer a daily menu from which clients may select foods for each meal. These menus include only the foods available for that person's dietary prescription. This practice allows for consideration of individual likes, dislikes, and appetite variations. The nurse, dietitian, dietetic technician, or dietetic assistant is responsible for monitoring clients' dietary selections and offering assistance as needed to ensure adequate variety and amounts of food selection.

A NORMAL DIET

A normal diet is "one whose aim is to maintain a healthy person in a state of nutritive sufficiency, providing amounts of energy, protein, vitamins, minerals, and other nutrients sufficient to meet the needs of the individual in his particular stage of the life cycle" (American Dietetic Association, 1981, p. A3). A healthy diet also avoids excesses of any nutrients that increase the risk of diet-related disease, such as excessive kilocalories with resultant obesity and possible hypertension, diabetes, and heart disease.

Diagnostic and Therapeutic Modifications
Dietary intake frequently needs to be modified for diagnostic or therapeutic purposes. This modification may be for a specific medical condition or health problem, such as a diabetic diet for a person with diabetes, a low-calorie diet for an overweight person, or a controlled potassium, sodium, and protein diet for a person with renal failure. The student is referred to medical–surgical and nutrition textbooks for discussions of those types of dietary modifications. The nurse needs sufficient knowledge about what foods are included in various diets to be able to scan a tray being served and judge the appropriateness of its contents for the specified diet label.

Consistency and Texture Modifications
Other dietary modifications relate specifically to consistency and texture. They are used when the client has difficulty ingesting or digesting a standard or regular diet or as a transition from NPO status following surgery to a resumption of a regular diet. Every health-care agency has its own set of standard or house diets that determines the consistency and texture modifications for that agency. The nurse becomes familiar with the standard diets at whatever agency he or she is practicing nursing. A brief description of standard hospital diets is included here, but the student is referred to a nutrition textbook written for nurses for complete information about both standard and therapeutic diets.

Standard Hospital Diets
The basic standard hospital diets include clear liquid, full liquid, mechanical soft, and regular (or selective).

A *clear liquid* diet includes only those fat-free foods that are liquid or will liquefy at room temperature. Highly restrictive and inadequate in kilocalories and most nutrients, its primary function is to provide a source of oral fluids. A clear liquid diet includes fluids such as broth, bouillon, gelatin dessert, and tea.

A *full liquid* diet consists of any food that is liquid or will liquefy at room temperature. If well-planned and balanced, it can provide adequate nutrition for a fairly substantial length of time. A full liquid diet includes any foods on a clear liquid diet, plus foods such as plain ice cream, sherbet, pudding, custard, or yogurt; milk, milkshakes, and eggnogs; and refined cooked cereals.

A *mechanical soft* diet is often used as a transition between a full liquid and a regular diet. It is highly individualized according to the client's ability to chew, swallow, and digest food. This diet contains soft, easy-to-chew, and nonirritating foods, which are chopped, ground, or pureed as needed. A mechanical soft diet sometimes is referred to as "diet as tolerated" or "regular diet as tolerated."

A *regular* or *selective* diet is a usual diet, with no restrictions other than the client's own preferences.

NUTRITIONAL ASSESSMENT

Assessment of nutritional status is accomplished in a variety of ways and often in collaboration with a dietitian or physician. Table 52-1 presents a nutrition evaluation guide that can be used as a framework for gathering data about dietary adequacy and practices, illness status, ability to ingest and digest food, and laboratory values that reflect general nutritional status. The guide requires the use of an assessment interview (Skill 15), the physical appraisal skills of inspection (Skill 19) and auscultation (Skill 22). Although it is not feasible to do such a thorough assessment of all clients, practice in using this guide gives the nurse some familiarity with the purpose and scope of a complete nutritional assessment and helps the nurse identify other clients that need either a complete or a partial nutritional assessment. Some parts of the guide are more relevant to an acutely ill person, such as identifying sources of protein and fluid loss, level of consciousness, or the ability to swallow. Other areas are especially relevant when teaching about a new diet or planning home care, such as identifying the client's activity level, food preferences, and restrictions, evaluating the client's understanding of the therapeutic diet, and determining who shops for and prepares food at home. Most of the content areas covered by Table 52-1 have already been discussed in this or other skills. Two aspects of this guide are discussed in more detail here: a food history and the use of laboratory data.

Food History
In larger agencies, a food history is taken by the dietitian, but in smaller agencies or in the home setting, the nurse often needs to do this. A food history may involve asking the person to recall what he or she has eaten during the past 24 hours or report what would normally be consumed during a 24-hour period. Alternatively, the person may be asked to keep a food diary for several days to a week, accurately recording all food and fluids consumed.

A third method, the activity-associated food history, often helps individuals more accurately identify all the foods they eat during the day (Williams, 1981). For most of us, eating is associated with activity or work throughout the day. During this type of interview, a general pattern of a day's activity and food intake is obtained. Specific meals are not usually mentioned by the interviewer, since some people may eat at other than formal meals. A basic assumption of this food history approach is that we *do* eat at varying times throughout the day, and the interviewer simply inquires about *what is eaten* rather than *whether* the person eats a specific meal. This approach is especially useful for people who snack between meals, who do not eat regular meals, or who are obese, since these people tend to underreport what they eat.

In an activity-associated food history, the interviewer would ask questions such as the following:

- "About what time do you usually get up in the morning? After you get up, do you usually have something to eat? What kinds of food might you have at this time?"
- "In the middle of the morning do you usually take a break? What kind of food do you have with your morning coffee or coke break?"
- "In the middle of the day, do you usually have something to eat? Can you give me some examples?"
- "What about in the middle of the afternoon?"

The questions continue in this manner through the entire day until bedtime.

The interviewer also inquires about serving sizes; where the noon meal is eaten (for example, cafeteria, restaurant, vending machines, or brown bag lunches); and specific activities that often involve foods, such as television-watching, reading, ballgames, movies, and coffee breaks. A question such as "When you watch television or read, what kind of snack foods do you usually eat?" is more likely to elicit accurate information than, "Do you eat any snack food when watching television or reading?" People who snack between meals are more likely to respond truthfully to the less judgmental tone of the former; those who do not snack between meals will say so.

Laboratory Data
Elevated or depressed levels of certain body substances may indicate actual or potential nutritional problems, particularly if serial measurements are taken. Some cautions are needed in interpreting laboratory data for nutritional evaluation purposes. Normal laboratory values are based primarily on healthy white adults and may not represent all ethnic or racial groups, and the ranges of normal vary from laboratory to laboratory and with the method of analysis used. Pathology may alter a laboratory test result; for example, blood loss that causes hypovolemia can result in decreased red blood cell counts.

Some acute-care institutions have the capacity for doing complex laboratory studies that are helpful in identifying specific nutritional alterations. These tests generally are not available in smaller institutions or in community or home-care settings. The laboratory tests discussed here as part of nutritional assessment are common ones; the nurse is accustomed to looking at the results of these tests when evaluating the overall status of the client. It is important that the nurse also think of these tests as potential indicators of nutritional problems and a need for more com-

TABLE 52-1. Nutrition Evaluation Guide[a]

A. Dietary adequacy
  1. Overt general appearance (thin, obese, normal); appearance of hair, skin, eyes, and nails.
  2. Individual's perception and evaluation of own state of health and dietary adequacy, including energy levels for usual daily activities, considering age.
  3. Weight in relationship to height, age, sex, body build, and ideal weight (overweight: > 10% over ideal weight; underweight: < 20% under ideal weight).
  4. Weight gain-loss patterns, including past or present use of weight-loss or fad diets.
B. Dietary practices
  1. Person who is responsible for shopping for and preparing food in home setting.
  2. Number and timing (spacing) of meals.
  3. Frequency of meals eaten away from home.
  4. Favorite or preferred foods; excessive ingestion of any foods.
  5. Extent of inclusion of Basic Four food groups in diet.
  6. Special diet, prescribed by physician, self, or other.
  7. Food history: activity-associated food history; 24-hour self-recall; food diary.
  8. Dietary preferences or restrictions: religious dietary practices; ethnic and cultural preferences; use of health or organic foods; use of vegetarian diet; allergies.
C. Perceptions and attitudes about food and eating
  1. Judgment about importance of food: How important are regular meals, hot food, and correct preparation of food? Does the individual "eat to live" or "live to eat?" Does the individual like to eat most all kinds of foods?
  2. Judgment about significance of food: What foods are eaten when lonely, sad, depressed? What foods are eaten as a celebration? What celebrations or holidays center around food and eating? How are birthdays, anniversaries, etc., celebrated?
D. Current dietary status
  1. Diet order or prescription: purpose of special diet; foods limited or prohibited.
  2. Projected duration of dietary modifications.
  3. Individual's perception and understanding of diet modifications.
E. Current illness status
  1. Medical and nursing diagnoses.
  2. Sources of protein loss (blood loss through menses, wounds, or injuries, occult or frank blood in stool, blood in vomitus, and other protein losses through burns or wound drainage).
  3. Sources of fluid loss (vomiting, diarrhea, nasogastric suctioning, burns, wound drainage).
  4. Present activity level and self-care ability.
F. Ingestion of food
  1. State of teeth and gums: dentulous (having teeth); partially or completely edentulous (absence of teeth); fitted with dentures; presence of gum or tooth disease.
  2. State of mouth: appearance and condition of mucous membranes; degree of salivation; presence of mouth odors or debris.
  3. Ability to chew and swallow (observed or self-reported).
  4. Level of consciousness.
  5. Medications or illness states that affect ingestion of food.
G. Digestion of food
  1. Problems with digestion: nausea, vomiting, eructation (belching), diarrhea.
  2. Bowel sounds.
  3. Degree of gastrointestinal motility.
  4. Medications or illness states that affect digestion of food.
H. Common laboratory data[b]

		Normal Level	**Client Level**
1.	Red blood count	Women: 3.6–5.0 million/cu mm	
		Men: 4.2–5.4 million/cu mm	
2.	Hematocrit	Women: 37–47/100 ml	
		Men: 40–54/100 ml	
3.	Hemoglobin	Women: 12–15 g/100 ml	
		Men: 14–16 g/100 ml	
		Newborns: 14–20 g/100 ml	
4.	Serum albumin level	4–4.5 g%	

Questions for analysis of nutritional data:

1. How does this individual's nutritional status affect or reflect his or her health/illness status?
2. What are this individual's primary nutritional needs?
3. What interventions would help meet this individual's nutritional needs (and be compatible with his or her diagnosis, plan of care, functional capabilities, and psychosocial orientation)?
4. Which nutritional needs require resolution through collaboration with the dietitian or physician? Why?
5. What nutritional teaching needs does this individual have?

[a] This guide would require modification when used with a small child, infant, or anyone else where the primary respondent would be other than the specified client.
[b] Normal values from Fischbach FT: A Manual of Laboratory Diagnostic Tests. Philadelphia, JB Lippincott, 1980.

plete nutritional assessment or referral to the physician.

Common laboratory tests with nutritional significance are measures of *hematologic status, protein levels,* and *blood lost* through the gastrointestinal tract. *Red blood cell count, hemoglobin,* and *hematocrit* provide hematologic data. When these values are reduced, the body's ability to carry nutrients and oxygen to the cells and waste products from the cells is decreased. It is important to keep in mind that dehydration will increase these values and may mask significant problems. Many factors, such as blood loss, iron deficiency, or blood dyscrasias, may cause reduced hematologic values. In the absence of disease, reduced *serum albumin* levels represent a serious protein deficiency or a loss of blood proteins. Protein is an essential component of all body tissues and is needed for growth, repair, and health maintenance. A decreased serum albumin level is one indicator of PCM and considered more reliable than total serum protein levels. Blood lost through the gastrointestinal tract may be visible (frank or gross) or hidden (occult). Occult blood can be detected through laboratory tests or by using a screening test such as *Hematest* or *Occultest.* Loss of blood through the stool or vomitus represents loss of blood proteins and other nutrients.

Anthropometric Measures

Anthropometric measures are not included in Table 52-1, although they may also be used to assess nutritional status. *Arm muscle circumference* is considered a good indication of lean body mass and thus of skeletal protein reserves, which is important in evaluating PCM (Bistrian et al., 1974, 1976; Krause, 1984). Arm muscle circumference is calculated from the *triceps skinfold* and *arm circumference* measurements. The method is described in several current nutrition textbooks (Suitor & Crowley, 1984; Whitney & Cataldo, 1983). Skinfold measurements also are discussed in Skill 27.

In addition to appraising a client's current nutritional status, the nurse monitors changes in that status on a daily and weekly basis. This is done primarily through (a) observing and recording food and fluid intake and fluid and nutrient losses and (b) regular weighing of clients. In addition to a record of height, these two basic factors are considered the most crucial aspects of combating hospital malnutrition (Butterworth and Blackburn, 1975).

DATA BASE

To assist a client with a food tray and to evaluate nutritional status, the nurse needs data about the client's diagnosis, diet prescription, ability to feed himself or herself, and any problems associated with eating. These data can be obtained from the health record, through a medical, nursing, or dietary history, through laboratory data, and through direct observations.

Client History and Recorded Data

The medical diagnosis and history provides information about any medical or surgical problems that might alter nutritional status or the ability to ingest or digest food. For example, a person receiving cancer chemotherapy has some degree of malnutrition associated with a decreased intake due to anorexia, nausea, vomiting, and stomatitis (inflammation of the mouth). Knowing the client's diagnosis and diet prescription helps the nurse evaluate the appropriateness of the contents of the food tray as it is served. Knowing the client's activity status (physician's orders for ambulation and activity) and positional restrictions helps the nurse and client decide whether a meal will be eaten while sitting in bed, in the chair, in the dining room, or lying flat in bed.

The client's health record includes the client's weight, height, and food consumption. It also contains information on the client's self-care ability (the degree of independence in performing activities of daily living) and the amount of assistance needed at mealtime. Some factors that affect self-care ability are readily evident, such as dressings or casts on the hands or arms, weakness, recent blindness, or deformed hands from arthritis.

A nursing or dietary history elicits information about past and present eating habits, food consumption, problems with ingestion and digestion, food allergies, religious, ethnic, or cultural preferences or requirements, and some sense of the role food plays in the person's life.

Laboratory data found in the health record can be used to confirm nutritional problems or identify areas needing further exploration.

Physical Appraisal Skills

Signs and symptoms of malnutrition often are nonspecific in that they usually are the result of combined or even multiple deficiencies and necessitate multiple nutritional treatment. For example, even in as specific a deficiency as iron-deficiency anemia, where the primary symptom is fatigue, increased amounts of vitamin C as well as iron are needed to increase the body's available iron and replace iron stores. The nurse needs to be alert to signs and symptoms that may represent nutritional deficiencies, to initiate further investigation with a dietary history, and to make a referral to a physician or a nutrition counselor.

The skills of *inspection, palpation,* and *auscultation* are used to identify indicators of general nutritional status. Table 52-2 presents methods used to appraise various body areas, the physical signs that indicate normal appearance and function (that is, adequate nutritional status), and the physical signs that are associated with malnutrition.

EQUIPMENT

The equipment used for providing food service to clients includes menus for food selection, trays of covered foods, temperature-control mechanisms, and transportation devices.

TABLE 52-2. Physical Signs Indicative or Suggestive of Malnutrition

BODY AREA	NORMAL APPEARANCE	APPRAISAL TECHNIQUE	SIGNS ASSOCIATED WITH MALNUTRITION
Hair	Shiny; firm; not easily plucked	Inspection	Lack of natural shine; hair dull and dry, thin and sparse; hair fine, silky, and straight; color changes (flag sign); can be easily plucked
Face	Skin color uniform; smooth, pink, healthy appearance; not swollen	Inspection	Skin color loss (depigmentation); skin dark over cheeks and under eyes (malar and supraorbital pigmentation); lumpiness or flakiness of skin of nose and mouth; swollen face, enlarged parotid glands; scaling of skin around nostrils (nasolabial seborrhea)
Eyes	Bright, clear, shiny; no sores at corners of eyelids; membranes a healthy pink and are moist. No prominent blood vessels or mound of tissue or sclera	Inspection	Eye membranes are pale (pale conjunctivae); redness of membranes (conjunctival injection); Bitot's spots; redness and fissuring of eyelid corners (angular palpebritis); dryness of eye membranes (conjunctival xerosis); cornea has dull appearance (corneal xerosis); cornea is soft (keratomalacia); scar on cornea; ring of fine blood vessels around cornea (circumcorneal injection)
Lips	Smooth, not chapped or swollen	Inspection	Redness and swelling of mouth or lips (cheilosis); especially at corners of mouth (angular fissures and scars)
Tongue	Deep red in appearance; not swollen or smooth	Inspection	Swelling; scarlet and raw tongue; magenta (purplish color) of tongue; smooth tongue; swollen sores; hyperemic and hypertrophic papillae; atrophic papillae
Teeth	No cavities; no pain; bright	Inspection	May be missing or erupting abnormally; gray or black spots (fluorosis); cavities (caries)
Gums	Healthy; red; do not bleed; not swollen	Inspection	"Spongy" and bleed easily; recession of gums
Glands	Face not swollen	Inspection Palpation	Thyroid enlargement (front of neck); parotid enlargement (cheeks become swollen)
Skin	No signs of rashes, swellings, dark or light spots	Inspection	Dryness of skin (xerosis); sandpaper feel of skin (follicular hyperkeratosis); flakiness of skin; skin swollen and dark; red swollen pigmentation of exposed areas (pellagrous dermatosis); excessive lightness or darkness of skin (dyspigmentation); black and blue marks due to skin bleeding (petechiae); lack of fat under skin
Nails	Firm, pink	Inspection	Nails are spoon-shaped (koilonychia); brittle, ridged nails
Muscular and skeletal systems	Good muscle tone; some fat under skin; can walk or run without pain	Palpation	Muscles have "wasted" appearance; baby's skull bones are thin and soft (craniotabes); round swelling of front and side of head (frontal and parietal bossing); swelling of ends of bones (epiphyseal enlargement); small bumps on both sides of chest wall (on ribs)—beading of ribs; baby's soft spot on head does not harden at proper time (persistently open anterior fontanelle); knock-knees or bowlegs; bleeding into muscle (musculo-skeletal hemorrhages); person cannot get up to walk properly
Internal systems Cardiovascular	Normal heart rate and rhythm; no murmurs or abnormal rhythms; normal blood pressure for age	Auscultation Palpation	Rapid heart rate (above 100 bpm—tachycardia); enlarged heart; abnormal rhythm; elevated blood pressure
Gastrointestinal	No palpable organs or masses (in children, however, liver edge may be palpable)		Liver enlargement; enlargement of spleen (usually indicates other associated diseases)
Nervous	Psychological stability; normal reflexes		Mental irritability and confusion; burning and tingling of hands and feet (paresthesia); loss of position and vibratory sense; weakness and tenderness of muscles (may result in inability to walk); diminishment and loss of ankle and knee reflexes

Adapted with permission from: Christakis G (ed): Nutritional assessment in health programs: Clinical assessment of nutritional status. American Journal of Public Health 63 (Suppl.):18–26, 1973.

Menus

Many agencies provide menus from which clients select their desired beverages, main course, salad, and dessert from the choices available within their prescribed dietary limitations.

Food Trays

To avoid airborne contaminants and for aesthetic reasons, all food items are covered during transportation from the food preparation area to the client's bedside. Some food is available in prepackaged containers.

Bowls, cups, or glasses are covered with lids or plastic wrap. Ventilated plastic or metal covers are placed over plates of food. Eating utensils may be wrapped in a napkin or enclosed in a waxed bag. Food service dishes may consist of disposable paper or plastic, pottery, or even fine china and crystal in some settings. All items are placed on a tray and transported to the bedside.

Temperature-Control Mechanisms

During transit, food may be kept at the proper temperature in several ways. Heated and refrigerated food service carts are designed to keep foods at optimum temperatures. The refrigerated side is maintained at 7°C (45°F), and the heated side is kept at 71° to 77°C (160° to 170°F). In some carts, all hot foods are placed in the heated side, and all cold foods in the refrigerated side, with the final assembly of the tray done in the clinical area. Some carts accommodate divided trays, with the side containing hot foods kept hot and the side containing cold foods kept refrigerated, as in Figure 52-1. With these carts, all trays are assembled in the central food preparation area and arrive at their destination already completely assembled.

Insulated containers of several varieties are in use in some health-care agencies. In the Cambro Caddy System, trays are assembled on a conveyor belt, using insulated containers for hot and cold foods and beverages. Trays are then placed in unheated and unrefrigerated enclosed carts for transport to client-care areas. In the Aladdin Temp Rite System, hot and cold foods are placed in disposable dishes in an insulated compartmented tray. The trays are then stacked so that hot and cold thermal columns are created, with hot foods remaining hot and cold foods remaining cold without external heating or cooling. The trays are delivered to clinical areas on open carts, as in Figure 52-2.

Pellets are doughnut-shaped pieces of metal that are heated to 204°C (400°F) and placed in a metal container. The covered hot food plate is positioned over this metal container, placed on the individual tray with other items, and delivered to clinical areas by unheated and unrefrigerated enclosed carts.

Transportation Devices

Depending on the method of temperature control, either enclosed or open carts are used to transport food trays to clinical areas. Enclosed, unheated, and unrefrigerated carts are used to transport food trays containing insulated containers or heated pellets. Enclosed temperature-controlled carts are used when individual food containers are not insulated or heated. Open carts are used to transport insulated tray systems such as the Aladdin Temp Rite System.

Dumbwaiters and vertical conveyors may be used instead of carts for transportation of food trays from the central food preparation area to clinical areas.

☐ EXECUTION

IMPLEMENTING THE DIET ORDER

The type of diet received by a client in a health-care agency is determined by the physician, nurse, or dietitian, with the physician having the ultimate responsibility. The physician may write an order for a specific diet, such as "regular diet," "2-g sodium diet"; or the order may be nonspecific, such as "diet as tolerated" or "usual diet." The latter type of diet order allows the nurse or the dietitian to select the kind of diet appropriate for the client's functional abilities and preferences. For example, when an elderly client with

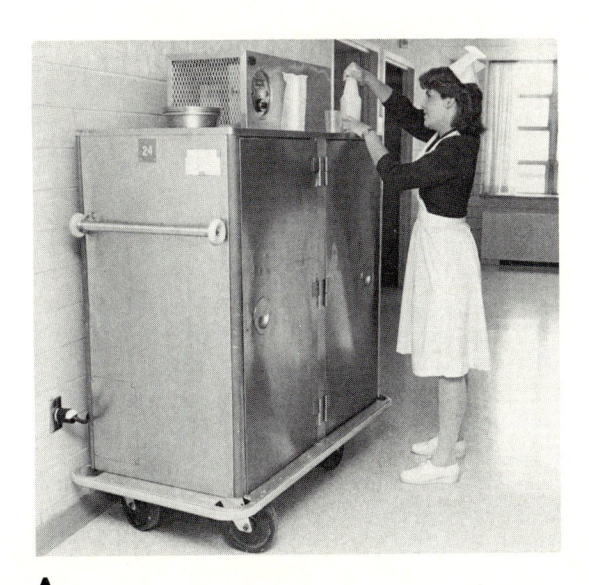

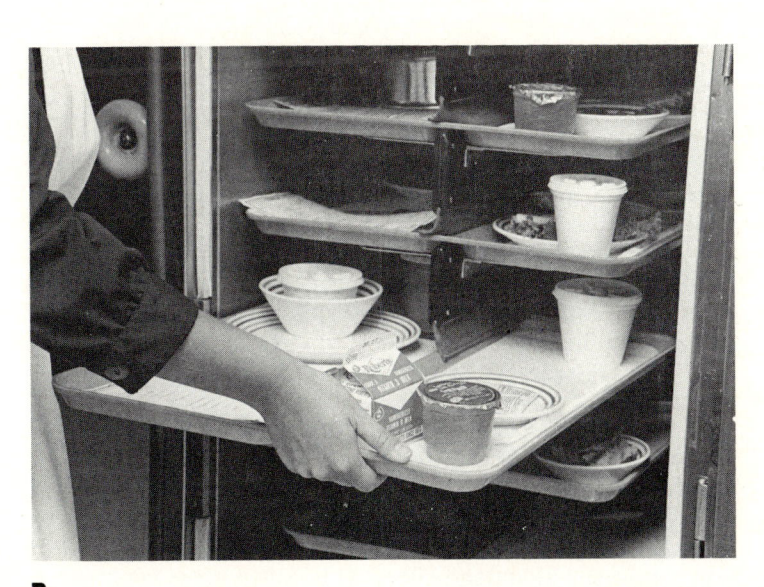

A

B

Figure 52-1. **A.** *Insulated meal cart.* **B.** *Divided compartments keep hot foods hot and cold foods cold. (Photo by James Haines.)*

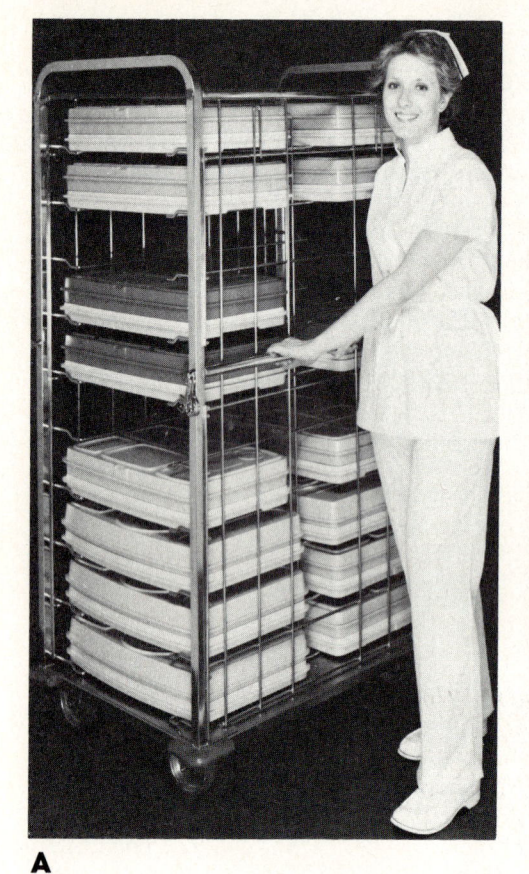

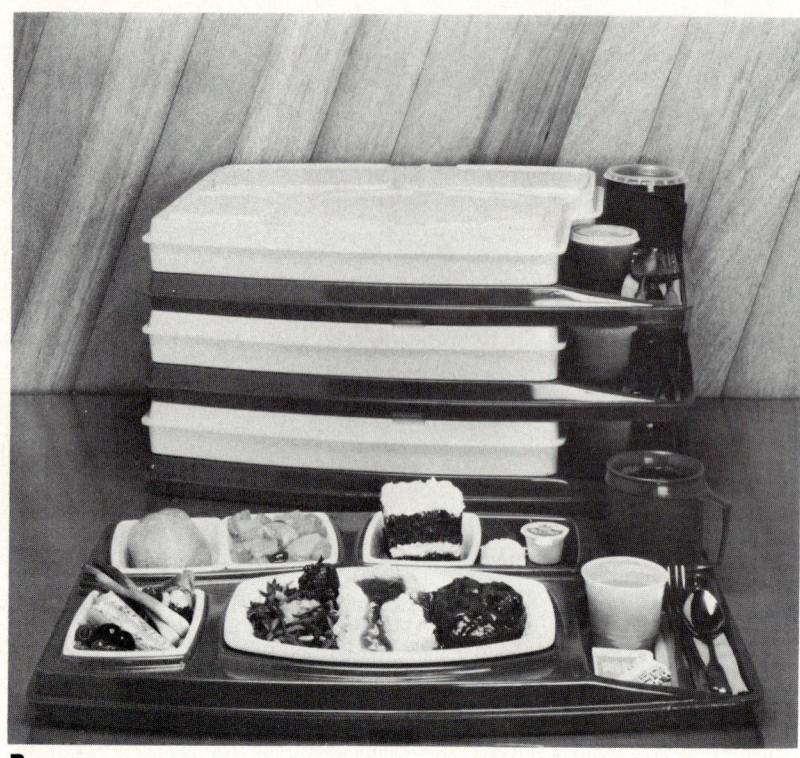

Figure 52-2. Insulated food servers. **A.** Transported on open carts. **B.** Provide hot and cold areas for individual foods. (From Aladdin Synergetics, Inc., Nashville, TN, with permission.)

poorly fitting dentures is admitted to an agency, the nurse may determine that this client needs easy-to-chew foods and will order a mechanical soft diet, select easily chewed foods from the menu, or request special foods according to client or family requests. Alternatively, as a result of an interview with a client who has decreased tolerance for milk products, the dietitian may choose to try a lactose-free diet.

All agencies have routine policies for transmission of diet orders to the dietary department, which the nurse needs to know. The nurse is responsible for updating kardexes and care plans so that they contain current dietary information, including the amount of assistance needed with eating, food allergies, or special requests. Some agencies also have dietary kardexes for use by the dietary department.

Menu Selection
Clients may need help selecting their food from the menu selector. Some may be unable to mark their own menus because they are too ill or tired, have difficulty seeing, or need to lie in a position that makes writing difficult. In these cases, it is helpful for the nurse to read the menu aloud and allow the client to make verbal choices. Before the menu selectors are sent to the dietary department, it is often advisable for nursing or dietary personnel to check the menu selectors for completeness or duplication, since sometimes clients do not understand the selection process and mark all items on the menu.

MEALTIME CARE

Environment and Personal Hygiene
Every effort is made to remove unneeded, unsightly equipment, used linens, and soiled dressings from the client's immediate area prior to serving a food tray. Minimizing or eliminating unpleasant odors at mealtime can increase appetite and food consumption. This may require that a client be removed from his or her room, if possible; or an air purifier might be obtained. Before mealtime, offer the client an opportunity for handwashing or at least to wipe his or her hands with a damp washcloth. If the client has a bad taste, or has sordes, providing oral care before meals will usually increase the palatability of the food and, therefore, generally increase food consumption. It often is helpful to acknowledge verbally the presence of altered taste sensations, associate them with the client's illness state, and encourage the client to try to eat to assist in his or her own recovery.

Positioning the Client

For mealtime, assist the client to assume as nearly a normal sitting position as is medically and functionally feasible, since this contributes toward easier chewing and swallowing and more closely approximates the usual eating posture. As much as possible, encourage the client to be out of bed for meals, since this more nearly approximates usual eating habits and helps counteract the dependency and helplessness some people associate with eating in bed. When the client is eating in a chair, place the meal tray on the over-bed table, which can be adjusted to the proper height. If a dining room is available for clients, encourage ambulatory clients to eat there, since socialization is an important part of eating and tends to increase the appetite. Assisting clients who are able to walk or ride in a wheelchair to the dining room can provide needed exercise. Together with the client, judge whether the client's fatigue level from this exercise will stimulate the appetite or make the client too tired to eat. Judgment about the degree of assistance clients need is discussed further in Skill 53.

Fatigue levels may dictate that the client remain in bed, either sitting on the edge of the bed or lying in bed with the head of the bed elevated. A few minutes spent repositioning the client in bed before elevating the head of the bed is time well spent in terms of increased comfort, ability to chew and swallow, expanded respiratory capacity, and decreased fatigue. Figure 52-3 illustrates the difference made when an individual is moved higher in bed before the head of the bed is elevated.

Identifying the Tray

Before food trays are removed from the food cart and distributed to clients, a member of either the dietary or nursing staff checks each tray against a master list to make certain that all diet changes have been implemented, that the correct trays have been prepared, and that all delayed or withheld trays are so identified. Each tray is checked to be sure that everything necessary is present. The person serving the tray identifies the recipient to ensure that each person receives his or her proper tray. This is done by checking the room number, bed label, and arm identification band, and by calling the client by name.

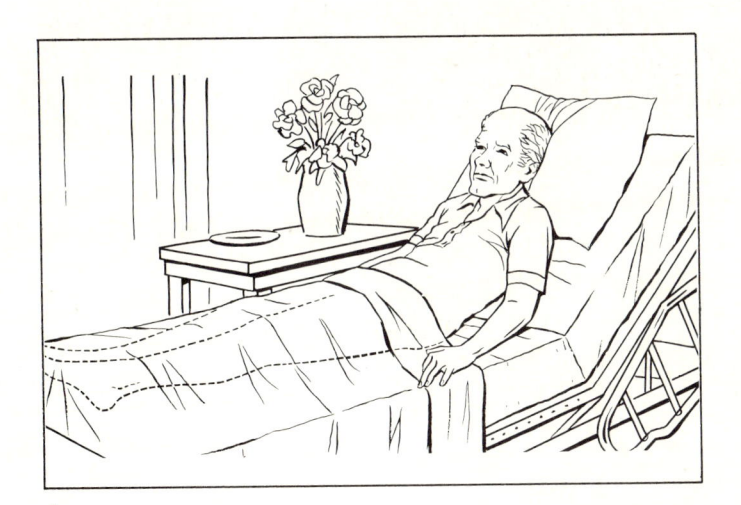

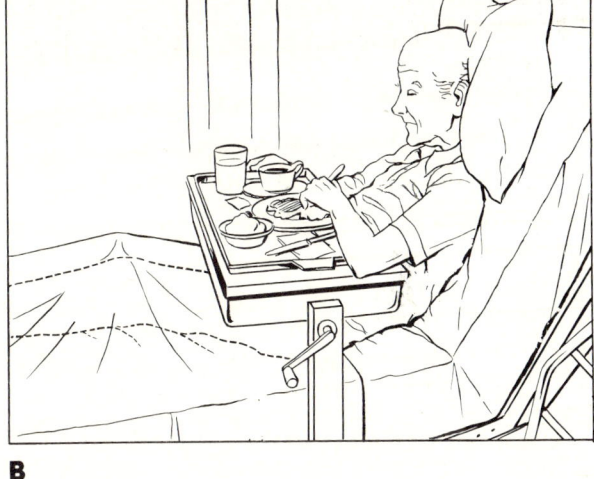

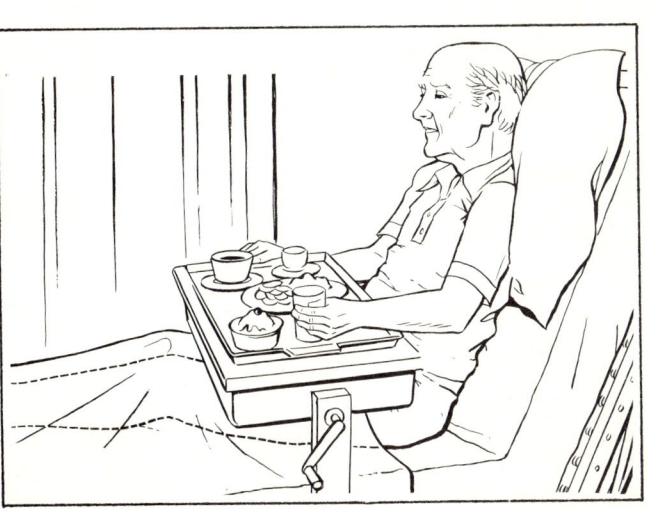

Figure 52-3. Positioning for eating in bed. **A.** A client in a Fowler's position often slides down in bed. **B.** Elevating the head of the bed without repositioning the client places the client in an awkward, hunched position. **C.** Assisting the client to reposition before elevating the head of the bed allows for increased comfort, ease in eating, and increased lung and stomach capacity.

Serving the Tray

When serving a food tray, be sure that it is delivered on time, that it is arranged conveniently and attractively, with no spilled foods or messy dishes, and that it contains the foods selected by the client. Serve hot foods hot and cold foods cold. Offer to open cartons and containers, cut meat, pour beverages, or butter bread. If the client needs more assistance than you can provide at that point, return the tray to the food cart or unit kitchen until adequate assistance can be obtained. Never leave a noninsulated food tray to cool at the bedside of a client who is waiting for assistance with eating.

Mealtime Observations

Whether or not the nurse actually feeds a client, mealtime provides an excellent opportunity to make observations about the client's color and general appearance, attitude toward consumption of food, and general nutritional status. Mealtime also is a good time to evaluate clients' understanding of the role of diet in their illness, recovery, and promotion of health, as well as to answer questions about diet and food. These observations may prompt the nurse to undertake a more complete dietary appraisal at a later time.

AFTER-MEALTIME CARE

Once the client has finished eating, offer or provide oral care and handwashing and return the client to a comfortable position. Many ill people benefit from a period of rest after meals, allowing digestion to proceed undisturbed.

☐ SKILL SEQUENCE

MEALTIME CARE OF CLIENTS

Step	Rationale
1. Inform client that meal is ready to be served.	Prepares client for mealtime.
2. Provide opportunity for client handwashing. a. Suggest handwashing in the bathroom. b. Provide pan of water and towel. c. Offer wet facecloth. d. Provide foam handwashing agent. e. Offer disposable wet wipes.	Promotes aesthetics and personal cleanliness.
3. Provide oral care for clients with unpleasant mouth taste, odor, or sordes.	Increases appetite and intake of food.
4. From kardex or personal assessment, determine level of self-care and ability to feed self.	Enhances self-concept; provides for assistance as needed.
5. Wash own hands.	Avoids transfer of transient microorganisms.
6. Check all food trays with master list of ordered diets.	Ensures that specified diets have been prepared.
7. Remove food tray from food cart. Check for completeness; add missing items.	
8. Serve trays first to clients who need only minimal assistance or none at all.	A more efficient use of time, with least delay for most people.
9. Identify individual client by checking room number, bed label, and arm band, and call client by name.	Ensures that each person receives intended tray.
10. Assist client to as near a sitting position as possible, in bed, on side of bed, in chair, or in a dining room. Position on side if client cannot have head elevated.	Approximates physiological position for chewing and swallowing; "normal" position is psychologically beneficial. Swallowing is easier on side than when supine.
11. Place tray in front of client, with utensils and food plate facing him or her. Adjust position of tray for ease in eating.	Facilitates manipulation of utensils.
12. Remove covers of hot food or insulated tray cover. Observe client's reaction to food.	Provides data for assessment of appetite and interest in food.
13. Offer assistance in rearranging items and utensils, opening cartons and containers, cutting meat, buttering bread, etc.; assist as needed. (NOTE: Do NOT leave an uninsulated food tray on bedside table if a nursing-care procedure is being carried out, or if client needs more help than can be given at that time.)	Ensures that client is able to feed self or that adequate assistance is obtained. Food will not remain at proper temperatures if it is held outside insulated food cart.
14. Evaluate nutritional status as necessary.	
15. Remove tray when client is finished eating; note amount and type of food consumed. Inquire about reasons for uneaten food, degree of satiety, and satisfaction with food service and type and amount of food.	Provides data for kardex or nursing-care plans and for dietary modifications.
16. Offer or provide oral care.	Removes food particles from mouth and teeth; helps prevent caries and periodontal disease.
17. Position client for comfort and allow to rest.	Enhances digestion.
18. Record appetite on dietary master record and in client health record.	Fulfills nurse's accountability and responsibility; contributes to ongoing data base.

RECORDING

Record dietary intake on the master dietary record for the dietary department and in the client health record for the nursing staff. Most health records have flow sheets for appetite to be recorded as G (good), W (well), F (fair), or P (poor). (See Figure 51-5.) Because these terms reflect a subjective judgment and their use varies from nurse to nurse, include a more detailed record of appetite and food intake in the nurses' notes or progress notes, particularly when problems with eating exist or are anticipated. It is possible for a client to have a quite inadequate intake of balanced nutrients and be listed as eating well. For example, it is possible for a client to eat half of the food served and be listed as eating well, when he or she has eaten only starches and no proteins or fruits. When this continues over time, clients can become undernourished. It is also important to determine what the *client* actually ate, since family members sometimes will consume uneaten food rather than have it wasted. When you are uncertain if the client actually consumed the food, it is appropriate to explain to the family the need to know the foods the client actually ate, thus providing an accurate record of intake.

When clients are on intake–output measurement, always include liquids from the food tray on those records.

Sample POR Recording

- S—"I'm not hungry today, just thirsty." "No, I don't feel sick to my stomach and haven't vomited."
- O—Drank only milk (240 ml), tea (130 ml), and broth (160 ml) from soft diet tray.
- A—Anorexia, accompanied by thirst, from unknown cause.
- P—Monitor food and fluid intake carefully for next few meals and observe for additional problems.

Sample Narrative Recording

Drank only liquids (milk, tea, and broth) from soft diet tray. States she is "not hungry today, just thirsty." Denies nausea or vomiting.

□ CRITICAL POINTS SUMMARY

1. In health, hunger and appetite are generally adequate regulators of food intake.
2. Food consumption usually is decreased during illness because of altered appetite, hunger, taste, sense of smell, and ability to ingest and digest food.
3. A normal diet (which includes the Basic Four food groups) requires modification during illness for medical reasons or to provide needed alterations in consistency and texture.
4. A clear liquid diet contains fat-free foods that are clear and liquid (or liquefy) at room temperature.
5. A full liquid diet contains clear liquids plus other foods that are liquid (or liquefy) at room temperature.
6. A mechanical soft diet is individually modified to meet ingestion and digestion needs.
7. Nursing and dietary personnel collaborate to provide adequate food and dietary services.
8. Hot food is kept hot and cold food is kept cold during transport to clinical areas and until actually served.
9. Handwashing and oral care before and after meals provide for personal hygiene, comfort, and increased appetite.
10. Assisting clients in assuming as near an upright seated position as is possible facilitates chewing and swallowing and focuses on wellness.
11. The person who serves a food tray is responsible for offering and providing basic assistance with food tray items.
12. Mealtime is an appropriate time for assessing appetite, nutritional status, teaching needs, perception of dietary modifications, and attitudes toward food.
13. Assessment of nutritional status includes dietary adequacy and practices, diet prescription, ability to ingest and digest food, current illness state, perceptions of food and eating, and selectively used laboratory data.
14. Food intake and appetite are recorded on both dietary and nursing record forms.

□ *LEARNING ACTIVITIES*

1. Keep a personal food diary for 1 week, and analyze it for the inclusion of the Basic Four food groups.
2. Conduct an activity-associated diet history with one individual and a 24-hour food recall with another individual. Recognizing individual differences, compare the two diet histories in terms of relative completeness, accuracy of reporting, and usefulness for identifying a need for nutrition education.
3. Interview several hospitalized clients to determine their perception of the food served:
    a. What is their perception of food temperatures, taste, variety, visual appeal, and method of serving?
    b. Do they look forward to mealtime? Why or why not?
    c. How has illness or hospitalization modified their interest in food?
    d. How has illness or hospitalization modified their ability to ingest or digest food?
    e. Was assistance with the food tray offered and given willingly?
    f. Do they know what type of diet they are receiving?
    g. What is their understanding of the reason (or reasons) for the types of diets they are receiving?

4. Look through a nursing kardex or care plan. Identify the number of clients who have been:
   a. On NPO status for at least one meal in the past 2 days.
   b. Receiving only intravenous fluids (with perhaps water by mouth) for 2 days or more.
   c. Receiving only clear liquids for 2 days or more. As a staff or charge nurse on a unit such as this, are there any interventions you might want to make that would improve the nutritional status of the clients? If so, what would they be?

☐ REVIEW QUESTIONS

1. What physiological and psychological functions are served by food and eating?
2. How does physiological regulation of food intake differ from psychological regulation?
3. Under what circumstances would you expect to find undernutrition, overnutrition, and PCM?
4. What personal and institutional factors contribute to malnutrition of hospitalized clients?
5. Indicate which of the following foods would be appropriate for a clear liquid or a full liquid diet by placing a C or F before the item. If appropriate for both, place a B; if not included in either a clear or full liquid diet, place an N for neither.

   _____ Apple juice
   _____ Bouillon
   _____ Butter pecan ice cream
   _____ Coffee with cream and sugar
   _____ Cream of potato soup
   _____ Cream of wheat
   _____ Eggnog
   _____ Instant Breakfast in milk
   _____ Lemon gelatin
   _____ Vanilla pudding
   _____ Vegetable beef soup
   _____ Seven-Up

6. For what purposes are clear liquid, full liquid, and mechanical soft diets used?
7. Under what circumstances should handwashing and oral care be provided for clients prior to mealtime?
8. What benefits occur from approximating an upright seated position during mealtime?
9. What are several ways food can be maintained at proper temperatures during transportation and serving?
10. What two nursing actions ensure that a client receives the correct food tray?
11. What kind of assistance is offered to the client when a food tray is served?
12. How do the functions of the nurse and the dietitian complement each other in providing food and nutritional services to clients?
13. What factors are to be included in a complete nutritional assessment?
14. What is the role of laboratory test data in a nutritional assessment?

☐ PERFORMANCE CHECKLIST

OBJECTIVE: To demonstrate the ability to serve trays to clients correctly, including evaluation of nutritional status and intake.

CHARACTERISTIC	RANGE OF ACCEPTABILITY	SATISFACTORY	UNSATISFACTORY
1. Tells client meal is about to be served.			
2. Provides for client handwashing or cleansing.	No deviation		
3. Offers or provides oral care as needed.	No deviation		
4. Determines self-care ability.	No deviation		
5. Washes own hands.	No deviation		
6. Checks food trays with master list.	No deviation		
7. Checks food tray for completeness and adds needed items.	No deviation		
8. Identifies client.	No deviation		
9. Assists client to as near sitting position as possible.	Side-lying position is appropriate if head cannot be elevated.		
10. Places tray in convenient position.	No deviation		
11. Assists client as needed.	No deviation		
12. Assesses nutritional status.	May be done at times other than meals.		
13. Removes tray.	No deviation		
14. Offers or provides oral care.	No deviation		
15. Positions client for comfort and rest.	No deviation		
16. Records appetite and intake in dietary master record and in health record.	No deviation		

REFERENCES

American Dietetic Association: Handbook of Clinical Dietetics. New Haven, Yale University Press, 1981.

Babcock CJ: Problems in sustaining the nutritional care of patients. Journal of the American Dietetic Association 28:222–227, 1952.

Bistrian BR, Blackburn GL, et al: Protein status of general surgical patients. Journal of the American Medical Association 230(6):858–860, 1974.

Bistrian BR, Blackburn, GL, et al: Prevalence of malnutrition in general medical patients. Journal of the American Medical Association 235(15):1567–1570, 1976.

Blum HL: Planning for Health, Development and Application of Social Change Theory. New York, Human Science Press, 1974.

Butterworth CE, Blackburn GL: Hospital malnutrition and how to assess the nutritional status of a patient. Nutrition Today 10:8–18, 1975.

Christakis G (ed): Nutritional assessment in health programs: Clinical assessment of nutritional status. American Journal of Public Health Supplement 63(Suppl.): 18–27, 1973.

Dudrick SJ, Rhoads JE: Metabolism in surgical patients: Protein, carbohydrate, and fat utilization by oral and parenteral routes. In Sabiston DC Jr (ed): Davis–Christopher Textbook of Surgery, ed 12. Philadelphia, WB Saunders, 1981.

Fischbach FT: A Manual of Laboratory Diagnostic Tests. Philadelphia, JB Lippincott, 1980.

Krause MV, Mahan LK: Food, Nutrition and Diet Therapy, ed 7. Philadelphia, WB Saunders, 1984.

Mitchell PR, Loustau A: Concepts Basic to Nursing, ed 3. New York, McGraw-Hill, 1981.

Robinson CH, Lawler MR: Normal and Therapeutic Nutrition, ed 16. New York, Macmillan, 1982.

Suitor CW, Crowley MF: Nutrition: Principles and Applications in Health Promotion, ed 2. Philadelphia, JB Lippincott, 1984.

Whitney EN, Cataldo CB: Understanding Normal and Clinical Nutrition. St Paul, MN, West Publishing, 1983.

Williams SR: Nutrition and Diet Therapy, ed 4. St Louis, CV Mosby, 1981.

BIBLIOGRAPHY

Beyers M, Dudas S: The Clinical Practice of Medical–Surgical Nursing, ed 2. Boston, Little, Brown, 1984.

Blackburn GL, Bistrian BR, et al: Nutritional and metabolic assessment of the hospitalized patient. Journal of Parenteral and Enteral Nutrition 1(1):11–22, 1977.

Brunner LS, Suddarth DS: Textbook of Medical-Surgical Nursing, ed 5. Philadelphia, JB Lippincott, 1984.

Chapell ML: The language of food. American Journal of Nursing 72(7):1294–1295, 1972.

Green ML, Harry J: Nutrition in Contemporary Nursing Practice. New York, John Wiley & Sons, 1982.

Luckmann J, Sorensen KC: Medical-Surgical Nursing: A Psychophysiological Approach, ed 2. Philadelphia, WB Saunders, 1980.

Newton ME, Folta J: Hospital food can help or hinder care. American Journal of Nursing 67(1):112–113, 1967.

SUGGESTED READING

Christakis G (ed): Nutritional assessment in health programs: Clinical assessment of nutritional status. American Journal of Public Health Supplement 63(Suppl.):18–27, 1973.

Newton ME, Folta J: Hospital food can help or hinder care. American Journal of Nursing 67(1):112–113.

AUDIOVISUAL RESOURCES

A Nursing Role in Nutritional Assessment
Slide/cassette. (1978)
Available through:
Ross Laboratories
Educational Services Department
625 Cleveland Avenue
Columbus, OH 43216

Basic Nursing Care: Feeding the Patient
Slides, filmstrip, videotape, film. (1982, Color, 17 min.)

Concepts in Nutrition: Cultural Foundations of Diet
Slides, filmstrip, videotape, film. (1979, Color, 15 min.)
Available through:
Medcom, Inc.
P.O. Box 116
Garden Grove, CA 92642

SKILL 53 Assistance with Eating

PREREQUISITE SKILLS

Skill 19, "Inspection"
Skill 20, "Palpation"
Skill 22, "Auscultation"
Skill 28, "Handwashing"
Skill 52, "Nutritional Assessment and the Serving of Food"
Skill 67, "Chest Therapy Exercises"

☐ STUDENT OBJECTIVES

1. Describe ways to promote a normal mealtime atmosphere when a client must be fed.
2. Explain the nurse's role in facilitating clients' acceptance of needing to be fed.
3. Identify clients who are likely to need to be fed.
4. Discuss assessment data that help determine the degree of feeding assistance needed.

5. Describe techniques that facilitate chewing and swallowing in a dysphagic client.
6. Describe assistive devices the nurse or client may use at mealtime.
7. Safely feed clients requiring varying degrees of assistance.

INTRODUCTION

Assisting someone with eating includes a wide range of activities. It may include pouring beverages, cutting meat, and buttering bread so a client can feed himself or herself more readily, or actually placing the food in the client's mouth and facilitating swallowing. Assisting a client with food and fluid intake is a very common nursing activity in both acute-care and long-term settings. In the community setting, the nurse may need to teach family members how to cope with a client's anorexia and demonstrate special feeding techniques.

In general, clients who need assistance with eating include those who avoid eating and those who are unable to feed themselves adequately. A person may avoid eating for either physical or psychological reasons. When a person repeatedly experiences pain, choking, or other disturbing symptoms while eating, he or she eventually begins to avoid food even if the brain and stomach send hunger signals. This aversion to eating usually persists long after the physical problem is resolved. Persons with psychological aversions to food include adolescent girls with anorexia nervosa who refuse to eat because they perceive themselves as too heavy, seriously depressed clients who do not have enough energy to eat, and clients with poor self-images who do not feel worthy of eating.

There are many reasons why some persons are unable to feed themselves adequately or at all. Persons with severe neurological disorders or quadriplegia (paralysis of all four extremities) do not have the neuromuscular control needed for the activities of self-feeding. Some neuromuscular conditions interfere with the ability to chew, suck, or swallow, such as after a cerebrovascular accident or with advanced multiple sclerosis, Parkinsonism, and some brain tumors. Persons with severe mental retardation or senile dementia often lack the mental ability to implement self-feeding activities. The very young may not yet have developed self-feeding ability and the very old may have partially lost that ability. Physical illness combined with a weakened, debilitated condition often leaves insufficient energy for self-feeding.

The inability to feed oneself may be temporary, such as when both arms are in casts or traction, or when the hands are injured or bandaged. However, the ability to feed oneself also may never have been developed (such as with a severely retarded person) or may have been permanently lost (such as with advanced neurologic disorders or complete quadriplegia). The ability to feed oneself is one of the primary aspects of self-care. When a person cannot do this for himself or herself, someone else must assume that function or implement alternate ways of providing nutrients, such as enteral or parenteral feedings (discussed in Skills 54 and 55).

PREPARATION

Feeding someone is one of the most basic of all caring activities and may be a symbol of parental care and nurturing. From the perspective of the person being fed, however, this care also may be a symbol of dependence and helplessness. Developmentally, feeding oneself is the earliest independent activity a person achieves. Once this task is mastered, most people resent being fed unless they are too ill or tired to care. When people have difficulty feeding themselves, they may be too frustrated, angry, or embarrassed to ask for or accept help willingly, and instead may refuse help by saying that they are not hungry or they may even resist being fed. Some sense of independence and control over basic life functions can be promoted if clients can help feed themselves, even in small ways, as is discussed later in this skill.

SELF-WORTH AND BEING FED

Self-worth is promoted through self-care and through the nurse's approach to the feeding process. The most helpful approach to feeding someone is to use a matter-of-fact yet caring manner and negotiate with the client the degree and kind of help provided. If a client is too ill to care, a simple statement of intent is helpful, such as, "I'm going to help you eat your lunch today." In most instances it is more helpful to acknowledge the client's distress about being fed ("It's hard to have to be fed" or, "Being fed often makes a person feel quite helpless") than to discount his or her concerns through comments like, "It's okay, it's part of my job" or, "Don't worry about it—I don't mind." Following the client's usual feeding patterns also helps decrease the distress associated with being fed. For example, some people eat salad first and others eat it just before dessert; some people eat all of one food item before beginning the next one on their plate, whereas others eat a little from each item; and some people drink a beverage only after the meal is completed, while others alternate solid and liquid food.

DETERMINATION OF NEED FOR ASSISTANCE IN EATING

The physician may decide that a client needs to be fed because of his or her medical condition, such as when a person with a cerebral aneurysm is placed on aneurysm precautions. In many instances, however, the nurse makes the decision about how much and what kind of eating assistance is given. For example, the nurse may decide to feed a client so as to conserve his or her energy for other activities such as sitting in a chair or ambulating. Clients who need help with bathing and intimate personal care may or may not have the strength to feed themselves. Clients with some neuromuscular disorders may lack adequate coordination and therefore need to be fed, as will clients with both arms in traction.

Clients are often able to feed themselves if the food is cut, if the dishes are arranged and spread out to avoid spilling, and if enough time is given. It is generally an inappropriate nursing decision to feed someone rather than allowing self-feeding simply in the interests of time and tidiness. If the person is a messy eater, the nurse provides privacy and clothing protection and cleans up afterward.

Clients with neurologic impairment (such as follows a stroke) or with degenerative diseases (such as arthritis, Parkinsonism, and multiple sclerosis) often need assistance with the acts of grasping utensils and placing food in their mouths or with the processes of chewing, sucking, and swallowing. These clients need the specialized services of a physiatrist, a rehabilitation specialist, or an occupational, speech, or physical therapist. These members of the health-care team often work together to evaluate a person's abilities, and plan and implement an assistance program for a specific person. They may work directly with the client as well as leave instructions for the nurse to implement on the nursing unit. It is the nurse's responsibility to know what that assistance program is, to execute it consistently, and to evaluate its effectiveness. It is helpful if the same nurse provides this care on a regular basis, and if the family also is involved, especially if the client will need continued assistance at home.

ASSISTANCE WITH EATING

Clients who are fed orally need to be able to chew and swallow without aspirating food or fluids. A major nursing responsibility associated with feeding clients is to assess their ability to chew and swallow and be alert for potential problems. Swallowing and chewing problems usually do not occur in isolation from each other, and often involve problems with tongue control and sucking as well. Chewing involves the grinding surfaces of the teeth and the masseter and buccinator muscles; sucking uses those muscles as well as the orbicularis oris. The term *swallowing dysfunction,* rather than the term *dysphagia,* is used to describe problems with these interrelated functions (Zimmerman and Oder, 1981). Dysphagia refers to the "sensation of food being hindered in its normal passage from mouth to stomach," which primarily involves the esophagus (Castell, 1979).

Physiology of Swallowing
The act of swallowing (deglutition) requires the functioning of the medulla oblongata, 5 cranial nerves, and 25 different skeletal muscles. Swallowing occurs in three stages: the voluntary oral or buccal–pharyngeal stage, and the involuntary pharyngeal and esophageal stages. When swallowing is initiated as a voluntary action, it becomes a reflex action as the food reaches the pharyngeal area and continues into the esophagus. Swallowing also can be initiated as a reflex action when food is placed in the pharynx. A normal swallow takes 5 to 10 seconds, with less than 1 second each required for the oral and pharyngeal stages and 3 to 7 seconds for the esophageal stage. Sensory input is a necessary triggering mechanism for stimulating swallowing. Sensory input comes from salivation and the presence of food or fluids within the mouth. Salivation is stimulated by the taste, temperature, texture, and olfactory perception of food.

During the predeglutition phase, the food is chewed, condensed, and mixed with saliva to form a bolus. During the oral stage, the tongue moves backward, carrying the bolus toward the pharynx, as the soft palate elevates. In the pharyngeal stage, the tongue propels the bolus downward through the oropharynx, as the larynx elevates and moves forward, the hyoid bone elevates and moves posteriorly, and the vocal cords close. These actions close off the trachea and protect the airway from the entrance of food or fluid, which is known as aspiration. Contrary to common belief, the epiglottis is relatively unimportant in airway protection during swallowing (Dobie, 1978). Pharyngeal constrictor muscles cause the hypopharynx to contract, the pharyngoesophageal sphincter relaxes, and the bolus enters the final esophageal stage. Problems with swallowing can occur at any of the three stages, but nursing interventions are directed primarily toward the first two, which involve the acts of sucking and chewing as well as the actual swallowing of the food.

Swallowing Dysfunction
Transient swallowing dysfunction, such as choking or aspiration, occurs with surprising frequency in awake, normal individuals, but rarely causes difficulty because of prompt reflex correction. During deep sleep, about 45% of healthy persons aspirate pharyngeal secretions. The bacterial content of these secretions causes no apparent harm because of rapid removal by normal pulmonary clearance mechanisms.

—Zimmerman and Oder, 1981, p. 1756

Sudden, severe choking is life-threatening and may respond dramatically to obstructed airway techniques as presented in Skill 76.

Although less dramatic, the inability to eat and to protect the airway from aspiration is equally life-threatening. Swallowing dysfunction may occur as a result of decreased muscle strength or from a loss of sensation that interferes with the initiation and coordination of the reflex motor activities involved in swallowing. It results in (a) a decreased oral intake and (b) an increased likelihood of aspiration due to inadequate separation of the airway from the digestive tract. When the swallowing reflex is diminished, aspiration of food, fluids, saliva, pharyngeal secretions, and other foreign substances is increased, which increases the potential for bacteria to enter the lungs. The decreased intake results in weakness, which further decreases the ability to swallow, and in malnutrition, which decreases the client's immunity to foreign substances. Thus, a negative, cyclical process occurs. Zimmerman and Oder (1981) believe that swallowing dysfunction is often overlooked and is an unsuspected source of bronchitis, bacterial pneumonia, or chemical pneumonitis.

Swallowing dysfunction may occur in clients who have decreased levels of consciousness or are unconscious, such as with drug overdose or seizure disorders; from iatrogenic causes, such as with nasogastric tubes or from sedatives; as a result of neuromuscular conditions, such as head injury, cerebrovascular accidents, or multiple sclerosis; and from anatomic reasons, such as after facial injury or radical neck resection. It also may occur in elderly and debilitated persons with no specific illness, or in persons recovering from an illness that decreased their level of consciousness. Nasogastric tubes reduce pharyngeal sensory input and contribute to or aggravate existing swallowing dysfunction, and aspiration can occur from the gastric reflux that often occurs with enteral feedings through a nasogastric tube. Swallowing dysfunction also occurs in clients with fluctuating levels of consciousness, since they may have adequate swallowing and airway protective reflexes when alert but aspirate their own secretions when less responsive.

Recognizing Swallowing Dysfunction. For the general hospital unit, Zimmerman and Oder (1981) recommend identifying clients who may have swallowing dysfunction by looking for the following clinical features: fluctuating level of consciousness; periodic difficulty following simple commands; constantly open mouth; gurgling oral secretions; nasogastric tube in place, especially larger ones; drooling or using large amounts of tissues; and the need for very frequent nasotracheal suctioning.

Other identifying clinical features are associated with common neurologic disorders such as those associated with a cerebrovascular accident (stroke), for example, paralysis of the extremities of one side, tongue deviation to the nonparalyzed side, facial drooping, drooping of the corner of the mouth, drooling, inability to smile, and difficulty forming words.

Evaluating Swallowing. Swallowing and chewing functions need to be evaluated before feeding is begun. Before beginning this evaluation, an initial auscultation of the lungs is done as a baseline for later evaluation in case of aspiration. Feeding must not be initiated if there is no cough or gag reflex present. These reflexes can be elicited by inserting a suction catheter into the pharynx or pressing a tongue depressor lightly on the posterior portion of the tongue for 3 to 7 seconds. To test for swallowing, a small amount (10 ml) of water is placed into the client's mouth, using either a syringe or a straw with a clean finger over the tip. The client is asked to hold the water in the mouth and then swallow. If a swallowing dysfunction is present and aspiration occurs, the client will cough, choke, and perhaps have altered breath sounds. However, aspiration of such a small amount of water is considered harmless in comparison to an unrecognized swallowing dysfunction and aspiration of food and fluids (Zimmerman and Oder, 1981). If there is no difficulty swallowing, the client is given more water with the syringe or straw and asked to drink water from a cup or through a straw. Clients who can drink water easily will rarely have a significant swallowing problem with food. The ability to drink water is evaluated with the client in a nearly upright position, which is described below. While giving water, the nurse observes for both volitional and spontaneous swallowing and for the elevation and forward movement of the larynx.

If the client is able to swallow water, a small amount of soft-textured food such as applesauce is placed in the client's mouth and the strength of the chewing action and tongue control is observed. Sometimes clients are able to swallow but have weak chewing musculature or poor tongue control.

Sucking ability can be evaluated by asking the client to drink liquids through a straw. Closure of lips around the straw and the height the liquid rises in the straw are observed. If the lips do not close well, the nurse manually assists closure and observes any difference in the level of fluid drawn into the straw.

A physical or occupational therapist or rehabilitation specialist can do a more complete evaluation of the ability to chew and swallow; can evaluate motor control of the head, mandible, lips, soft palate, and tongue; and can plan a treatment or exercise program that will involve the client, family, nurse, and therapist. It is important to include the medical diagnosis on the referral to the therapist, as that aids in planning the treatment.

Facilitating Eating
The following general nursing interventions are appropriate for the nurse to use in facilitating eating and swallowing with clients in a general hospital setting (Buckley et al., 1976; Gaffney and Campbell, 1974; Griffen, 1974; Hargrove, 1980):

1. Place the client in a nearly upright seated position (80- to 90-degree elevation) in bed or in a chair. Flex the neck forward about 25 degrees. Avoid placing a firm pillow at the base of the neck, since this may stimulate a tonic neck reflex. Allow the client to remain in this position or partially elevated for about 15 to 30 minutes after being fed, unless contraindicated. Pillows or rolled towels may be placed beside the head for stabilization if needed. Avoid hyperextension of the neck, since swallowing is more difficult in that position and the likelihood of aspiration is increased.
2. Inspect the mouth before feeding; remove debris

and give oral care as needed. A toothbrush or a washcloth over a gloved finger may be used to loosen thick tongue debris. If the client wears dentures, put them in place and check their fit.
3. Use graduated feedings, beginning with pureed or minced foods such as applesauce, tapioca, or pudding, since these foods provide the most sensory stimuli and are easy to swallow. As swallowing improves, advance the diet to thick or jellied liquids, chowders, cooked cereals, or pureed vegetables. The next stage is offering soft solids such as canned fruit, and, finally, regular solid food may be given. Although the usual hospital dietary progression is from clear liquids to solids, do not offer clear liquids to clients with swallowing dysfunction until after they can manage soft solid foods, since liquids do not offer adequate sensory stimulation and these clients generally have difficulty controlling liquids within the mouth.
4. Give small portions of food and pause after each swallow before giving the next bite. Sometimes a gentle cough or clearing of the throat after a swallow will facilitate swallowing.
5. Serve appetizing, attractive foods and let the person see and smell them to stimulate salivation.
6. Offer foods at somewhat warmer or cooler than room temperatures, but not very hot or cold, as that tends to have an anesthetic effect on the mouth structures and decreases both sensory input and taste sensation and salivation.
7. When feeding someone, bring the utensil to the mouth from below the chin level rather than at eye level to encourage neck flexion.
8. While the client is eating, remind him or her to think about the food being eaten and verbally direct him or her to chew and swallow, since this brings the process under volitional control.
9. If the client has difficulty swallowing, it sometimes helps to place the forefinger above the lips and the thumb below, causing the lips to purse outward.
10. When sucking is weak, manually close and hold the lips around the straw or enlarge the diameter of the straw by placing a disc around it, or use a shortened straw to decrease sucking effort.
11. Create a quiet and relaxed atmosphere whenever possible, as this makes it easier for the client to concentrate on chewing and swallowing, and relaxation increases swallowing ease.
12. Avoid allowing the client to become overly fatigued, as fatigue makes chewing and swallowing more difficult and increases the likelihood of aspiration.
13. If the client can swallow liquids but has decreased salivation and inadequate oral lubrication, give occasional sips of liquids during the feeding. Avoid having the client make rapid and successive, unsuccessful swallowing attempts without adequate lubrication, since this tends to inhibit the swallowing reflex.
14. Use a fresh lemon, ice, flavored popsicles, or sweet liquids to stimulate increased saliva production. Oily liquids such as beef broth also help thin oil secretions, while milk and milk products thicken them.
15. To offer liquids with a cup, place the cup ring on the client's lower lip so that it touches both corners of the lips and, holding the client's head steady in a slightly forward tilted position, slowly tilt the cup toward the client, allowing a small amount of liquid to flow into his or her mouth. Pause and instruct him or her to swallow after each mouthful. A transparent cup makes it easier to see the liquid and adjust the rate at which it is given.
16. For clients who have the pharyngeal reflex stage of swallowing intact but not the oral stage (as occurs after radical neck or mouth surgery), use a large syringe with a short rubber tubing to place liquids directly into the pharynx. Special pusher spoons are available that can place semisolid food directly into the pharynx.

Neurosensory Facilitation Techniques for Eating

Much work currently is under way on facilitation techniques for various kinds of neurologically impaired persons. Some techniques may facilitate eating in clients with neurologic conditions such as a cerebrovascular accident (CVA), Parkinson's disease, myasthenia gravis, or amyotropic lateral sclerosis. These techniques are based on the physiological effects of quick-stretch, vibration, tapping, and stretch pressure on muscles (Farber, 1982, pp. 148–152).

When a firm, very quick stretch (elongation) is given to a muscle, the sensory receptors in the muscle spindle send excitatory messages to the stretched muscle and inhibitory messages to the antagonist muscle, resulting in contraction of the stretched muscle. *Quick-stretch* is done in the direction of the muscle fibers. *Vibrating* a muscle or tendon stimulates the muscle spindles to contract; *tapping* the belly of a muscle facilitates its contraction; and *stretch pressure* combines pressure into a muscle belly with a stretching motion. A mechanical vibrator is sometimes used to stimulate muscles, but its use is not recommended for the face because of the potential for overstimulation.

To vibrate muscles manually, place three fingertips adjacent to each other on a muscle belly; hold the fingers, wrist, and forearm rigid and move the fingers back and forth rapidly without shifting the finger placement on the skin. To quick-stretch a muscle, place the index and middle fingers (slightly separated) over the muscle belly, press firmly, separate the fingers quickly and firmly without shifting the finger placement on the skin, and release quickly. This combination of actions stretches and releases both the muscle and the overlying skin. To exert a more sustained stretch pressure on a muscle, place two or three

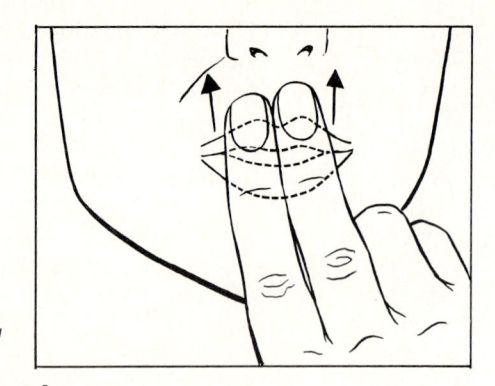

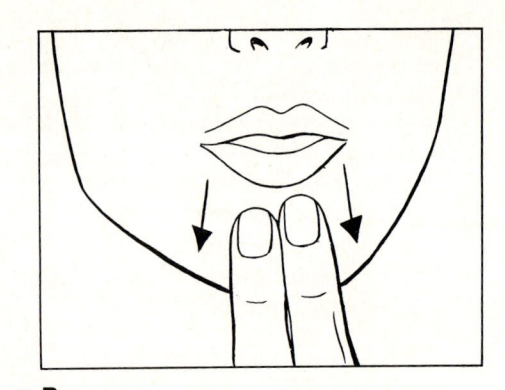

*Figure 53–1. Use quick-stretch pressure to facilitate mouth closure. **A**. Use upward pressure above the lips. **B**. Use downward pressure below the lips.*

fingers on the muscle and stroke firmly and gently from its origin to its insertion.

The following facilitation techniques provide neurosensory stimulation for eating, chewing, sucking, and swallowing:

1. To facilitate opening the mouth: Touch the lips lightly with a spoon or apply intermittent, caudally directed pressure on the upper lip.
2. To facilitate closing the mouth: Use the index and middle fingers to produce an upward-directed quick-stretch pressure above the lips and downward directed quick-stretch pressure below the lips, as shown in Figure 53–1.
3. To facilitate chewing action:
   a. Vibrate or tap the masseter muscle for about 15 to 20 seconds, as shown in Figure 53–2A.
   b. Give a quick-stretch to the masseters by placing the index and middle fingertips on the cheek and quick-stretch toward the zygomatic bone and mandible, following the direction of the muscle fibers, as shown in Figure 53–2B.
   c. Apply firm, caudally directed pressure on the masseter muscle, as shown in Figure 53–3A.
4. To facilitate eating with lateral tongue displacement and weak facial muscles: Place the food slightly posterior and laterally on the tongue on the same side as the displacement or weak facial musculature, since the tongue is pulled to that side by the unaffected tongue muscles. If food is placed on the side opposite to the displacement, food accumulates there ("squirreling"), because the weakened musculature cannot move the food out of the cheek. Slight downward pressure on the tongue with the spoon helps elevate the tongue and initiate swallowing.
5. To facilitate a functional tongue position: For a protruding tongue, facilitate tongue retraction by exerting gentle but firm outward and downward traction on the tongue. Place a gauze square or facecloth around the tongue for a firm grasp. For a tongue that is withdrawn into the mouth, facilitate tongue protraction (outward protrusion) by placing a spoon or tongue blade on the distal portion of the tongue and give a firm, quick inward and downward stretch motion. (See Figure 53–4.)
6. To enhance the gag reflex and thus promote swallowing ease:
   a. Have the client open the mouth and extend the tongue slightly; assist as necessary.
   b. Place a spoon or tongue blade on the posterior portion of the tongue and maintain moderate downward pressure for 5 to 7 seconds, as shown in Figure 53–5.
7. To facilitate swallowing: With the fingertips, stroke lightly but firmly down each side of the larynx, being careful to avoid bilateral pressure on the carotid arteries, which can cause a decrease in the heart rate. (See Figure 53–3B.)

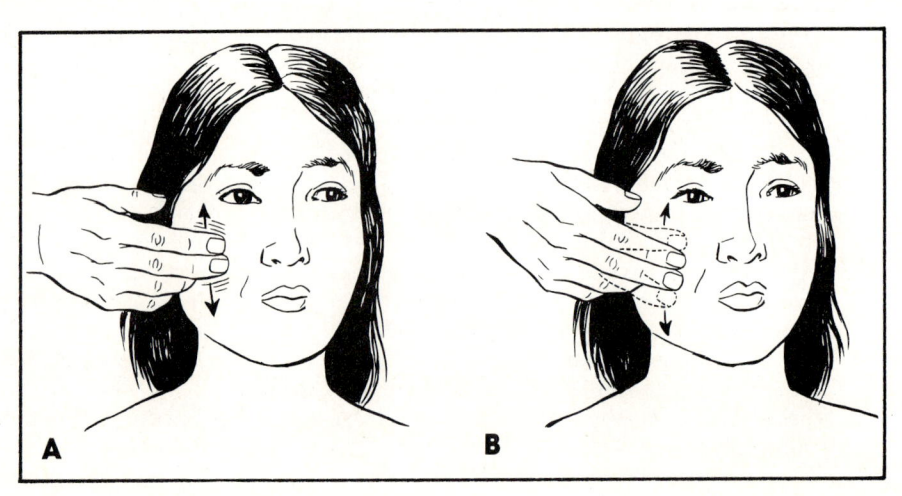

*Figure 53–2. Facilitate chewing action by **A**. vibration, and **B**. quick-stretching the masseter muscle.*

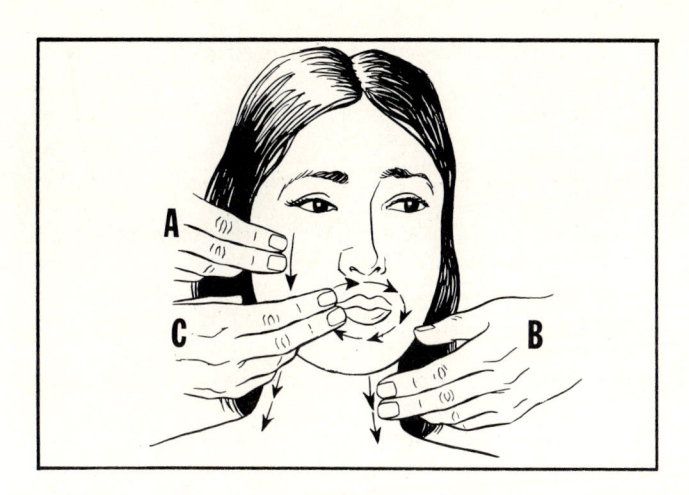

Figure 53–3. *Use firm, gentle pressure from muscle origin to insertion to facilitate* **A.** *chewing, and* **B.** *swallowing. Use circumoral pressure to facilitate* **C.** *sucking.*

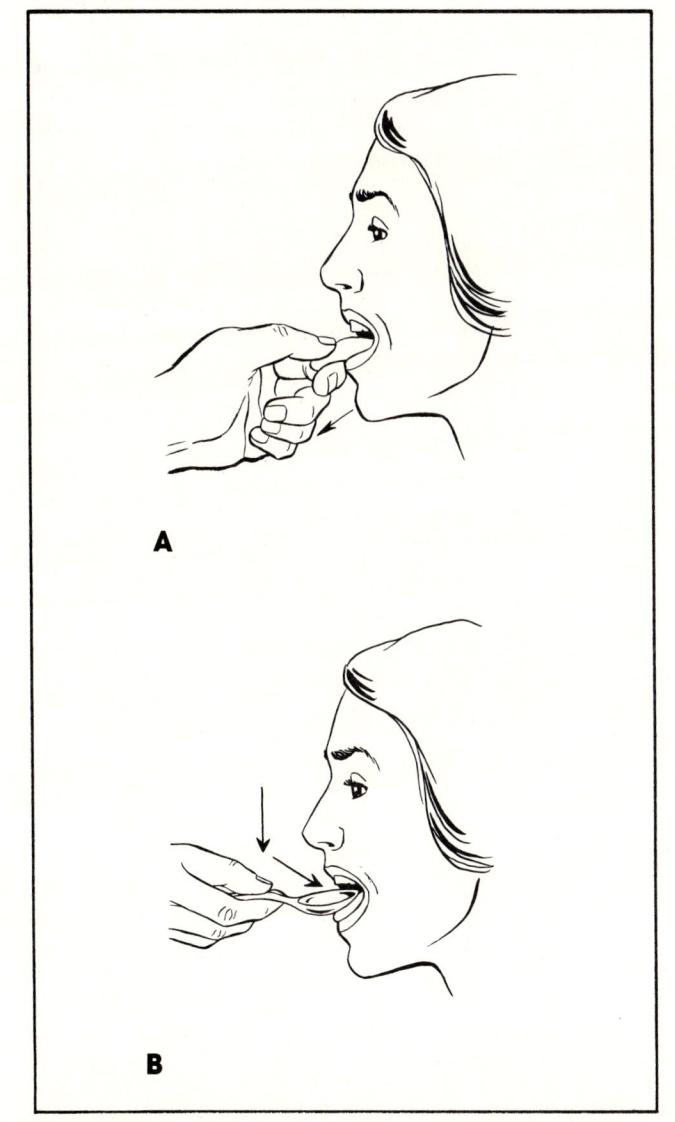

Figure 53–4. *Facilitate functional tongue position by* **A.** *using outward and downward quick-stretch pressure for a protruding tongue, and* **B.** *using inward and downward quick-stretch pressure for a retracted tongue.*

8. To facilitate sucking action:
   a. Vibrate or use a rapid gentle tapping action on the orbicularis oris (muscles around the mouth).
   b. Quick-stretch the orbicularis oris by first placing the index and middle fingers beneath the nostrils and quick-stretch upward and laterally; second, quick-stretch the lower lip with a downward and lateral movement, as shown in Figure 53–6.
   c. Use a firm, steady pressure in a circular motion around the mouth, as shown in Figure 53–3C.
   d. Provide intermittent quick-stretch action at intervals while the client is sucking through the straw.

The techniques just described are most helpful if the nurse takes time to first vibrate and then quick-stretch the masseters and orbicularis oris and vibrate and stroke the neck before beginning to feed the client. Since the effects are short-term, they will need to be repeated intermittently throughout the meal. Because these techniques are fairly specialized, it is helpful to have a more experienced person, such as a physical therapist, demonstrate their use and provide supervised practice.

For more information about additional feeding and facilitation techniques and sensory-motor stimulation used for rehabilitation, the student is referred to Farber (1982), Silverman and Elfant (1979), and Gallender (1979).

DATA BASE

Client History and Recorded Data

Prior to feeding a client, the nurse reviews basic information about the client's diagnosis, diet prescription, and self-care ability, as discussed in the Data Base section of Skill 52. In addition, the nursing kardex or health record includes the use of assistive devices for feeding, swallowing facilitation techniques that are successful for this client, any previous problems with feeding, chewing or swallowing difficulties, refusal to be fed, past level of food consumption, appetite, or excessive fatigue. If a rehabilitation specialist, physical therapist, or occupational therapist has evaluated or is seeing the client regularly, the health record will contain a report or progress notes about what the client should be expected to do, assistive devices used, and suggested facilitative techniques for eating and swallowing. The nurse also uses data from the health record, personal observation, and subjective comments from the client to assess level of comfort and need for relief from pain or nausea. Admitting data (occupation, family position, residence) and the nursing history (recreational and avocational interests) can give the nurse ideas for conversation during mealtime.

Physical Appraisal Skills

Inspection. Inspection is used to observe for chewing capability and for the presence of both voluntary and spontaneous swallowing. When feeding a client, in-

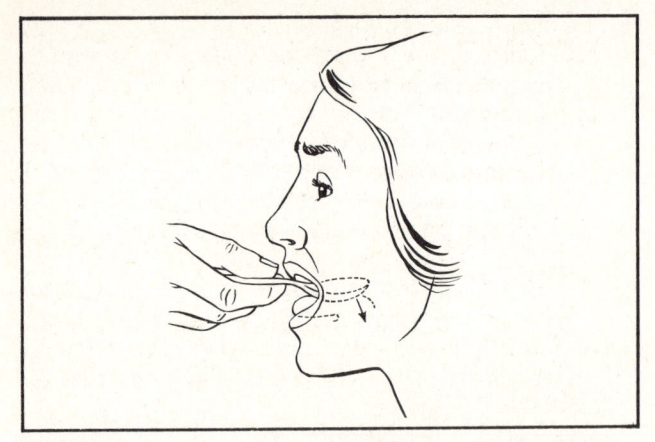

Figure 53–5. To enhance the gag reflex, maintain downward posterior tongue pressure for 5 to 7 seconds.

spection reveals clinical indicators of potential swallowing dysfunction such as drooling, open mouth, and gurgling oral secretions. It also is used to appraise the condition of the mouth and to identify objective signs of fatigue, such as pallor and shortness of breath.

Palpation. Palpation is used to identify elevation and displacement of the larynx during swallowing. This is done by placing the flat fingertips on the larynx and asking the client to swallow. Note the extent of elevation and forward displacement. Place the thumb and index finger on the lateral aspects of the hyoid bone just below the angle of the jaw and ask the client to swallow. Note the elevation and posterior displacement.

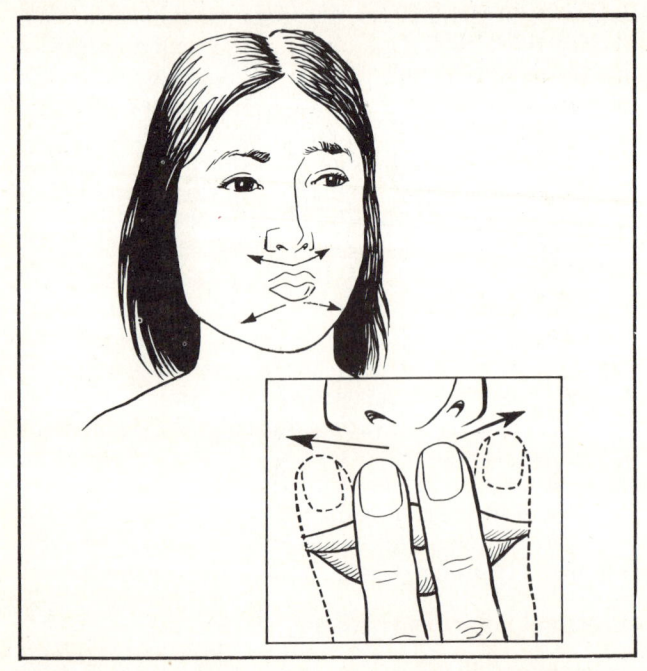

Figure 53–6. Facilitate sucking action by a quick-stretch pressure above and below the lips. Note movement of fingers shown in insert.

Auscultation. Auscultation is used to gather baseline data about pulmonary status prior to determining swallowing capability.

EQUIPMENT

A wide variety of *assistive feeding devices* can be purchased or improvised. These devices may be as simple as bending a spoon to make a curved handle or as complex as a powered hand splint that aids in grasping a fork. Physical or occupational therapy and rehabilitation departments frequently design assistive devices to meet a particular client's specific need. Sometimes simply placing foam or a knitted coaster on a slippery glass prevents the glass from slipping out of the hands. A spoon or fork handle can be enlarged with a soft hair curler for easier gripping or a universal cuff can be added to the handle. A long handle can be attached to a utensil for clients who have difficulty reaching their mouths. Suction cup bases keep plates and cups from sliding. Plastic mugs with T-shaped handles are easy for clients with arthritis to use. A plate guard provides a vertical edge to push food against and more readily load a spoon or fork. A piece of bread or toast also serves as a pusher to help load a utensil. Figure 53–7 shows some common assistive eating devices.

Most acute- and chronic-care agencies will have feeding equipment such as plastic cups, transparent straws of varying diameters and lengths, and rubber tubing to attach to large asepto or plunger syringes.

☐ EXECUTION

Before beginning to feed a person, it is important to alleviate problems that could decrease the appetite. This might involve removing unpleasant sights and smells, changing the ventilation, changing soiled dressings or linen, or providing oral care for a client

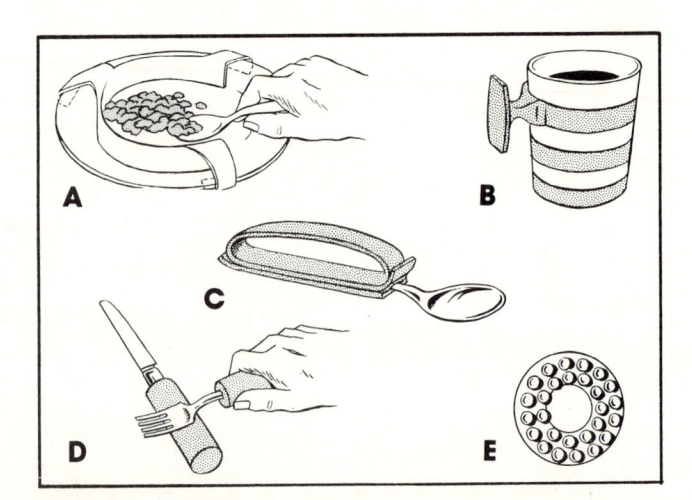

Figure 53–7. Common assistive devices for eating. **A.** Plate guard. **B.** T-handle mug. **C.** Universal cuff attached to a utensil. **D.** Padded utensil handle. **E.** Nonslip pad used to stabilize a plate.

with poor oral hygiene or a bad taste in his or her mouth. It also involves relief of pain and nausea through use of prescribed medication, position change, or relaxation.

When feeding clients, follow their usual eating patterns as much as possible. This includes handwashing, oral care, grace before meals, sequence of eating, and socialization. Avoid hurrying clients or urging them to eat quickly. These actions tend to cause clients to feel rushed, to tire too quickly, and possibly to stop eating before they have had as much food as they would like. Therefore, try to avoid frequent glances at the clock or having another bite of food poised and ready before the client has even begun to swallow the previous bite. Careful planning of staff work load can help provide adequate time for feeding without undue interruptions. Patience, understanding, and conversation (even if it is only the nurse talking!) help the mealtime pass more quickly and pleasantly, and generally help increase food consumption and digestion.

Whether you provide minimal or complete help with eating, there are many ways the client can assist in feeding himself or herself. The following suggestions range from situations where the nurse provides minimal assistance to those where nearly complete assistance is required.

1. Place the tray at a convenient height and location, cut the food into bite-size portions, open containers, arrange all items for easy reach, and return regularly to see if additional help is needed.
2. Have the client feed himself or herself for the first part of the meal; then assist the client before the point of fatigue is reached.
3. Alternate with the client in feeding bites of food, using separate utensils.
4. Place a bite of food on the utensil and ask the client to place it in his or her mouth.
5. Encourage the client to manage finger foods such as bread, toast, or crackers, feeding him or her those items requiring a utensil.
6. Hold the beverage container and encourage the client to hold the straw.
7. Encourage the client to assist in holding the beverage container or guiding the eating utensil.

While feeding a client, observe the ability to chew and swallow, the amount of self-feeding he or she is capable of doing, and the degree of fatigue experienced. Periodically check inside the client's mouth to see if food has actually been swallowed. If the client fatigues quickly, increase the amount of help given, or allow him or her to rest before finishing the meal.

To evaluate fatigue, look for an increase in pulse and respiration, shortness of breath, flushed face from overexertion, or pallor from weakness. It may be helpful to ask the dietitian to plan more frequent and smaller meals, which would tend to decrease client fatigue, require shorter blocks of nurse time, and possibly increase total food consumption.

When a therapist has developed planned feeding techniques for a given client, it is important to follow that plan with each meal, since consistency increases successful implementation. The therapist may feed the client at one meal, but nursing staff will need to feed the client at the other meals. Describe the feeding plan clearly in the kardex or nursing-care plan and post it at the bedside. When a nursing assistant does the feeding, the role of the professional nurse is to provide adequate instruction and supervision so that the plan is correctly implemented.

☐ SKILL SEQUENCE

FEEDING PATIENTS

Step	Rationale
1. Consult kardex or nursing-care plan for feeding assistance plans and amount of assistance needed. If no information is available, assess client's abilities prior to and during feeding.	Implements therapeutic plan; provides continuity of care. Provides for appropriate assistance given.
2. Arrange own work load to remain with client during entire mealtime.	Supportive of client; reassuring to client.
3. Remove unpleasant sights and odors from room.	Helps decrease nausea and anorexia and increase appetite.
4. Provide for relief of pain and nausea if possible.	Helps decrease nausea and anorexia and increase appetite.
5. Gather equipment for oral care, handwashing, and any assistive devices used by client. Obtain extra towels, wet washcloth, or wet wipes.	Increases time-efficiency. Additional linen is used for clothing protection and clean-up of drooling or spills.
6. Explain own role in assisting with feeding.	Increases cooperation; decreases client's concern over enforced dependence.
7. Provide opportunity for client to empty bladder and to cleanse hands.	Increases comfort and promotes personal hygiene and cleanliness.
8. Provide oral care; check fit of dentures.	Promotes salivation and increases appetite; identifies potential chewing problems.
9. Assist client to a secure position of comfort, approximating a sitting position, in a semirecumbent position, or on side. Avoid hyperextension of neck.	Increases ability to swallow; decreases probability of choking and aspiration.

(continued)

FEEDING PATIENTS (Cont.)

Step	Rationale
10. Wash hands.	Avoids cross-contamination.
11. Check name of client and type of diet with master dietary list; scan tray for appropriateness of contents.	Ensures correct diet has been ordered.
12. Check contents of tray for completeness; obtain any needed items.	Increases time-efficiency.
13. Compare name on tray with room number, bed label, and arm identification band; call client by name.	Ensures that client receives correct tray.
14. Place napkin or towel across chest or bed as needed. Place tray on over-bed table in front of or beside client.	Avoids soiling clothing and linens. Facilitates nurse feeding and client assisting.
15. Position self in comfortable position, preferably seated and facing client and within his or her visual field.	Decreases nurse fatigue; gives nonverbal message of relaxation and lack of time pressure; implies a more equal status.
16. Allow time for saying grace if client desires.	Provides for continuation of usual religious practices.
17. Prepare food or adjust containers on basis of degree of assistance needed and client's ability to chew.	Increases sense of independence and self-worth.
18. Offer sip of water and observe for swallowing or choking.	Helps identify swallowing dysfunction.
19. Offer bite-size portions of food; observe for chewing and swallowing. Offer food in order of client preference. Describe food if client cannot see.	Decreases potential for choking. Familiar routine increases food consumption; enables nonsighted client to anticipate what is being fed.
20. Allow sufficient time for chewing and swallowing. <u>Do not hurry client.</u>	Feelings of being hurried discourage client from eating as much as he or she otherwise might. Tension decreases digestion.
21. Use facilitative swallowing techniques as needed or as prescribed by therapist.	Assists client with eating; provides consistency for therapeutic plan.
22. Initiate pleasant conversation.	Increases digestion; enhances self-worth.
23. Provide for hand and face cleansing and oral care.	Removes food particles that could be aspirated; keeps oral cavity clean and hydrated.
24. Return used tray to meal cart or tray rack, according to agency policy.	Provides appropriate care of equipment.
25. Record amount of fluids consumed on bedside record or health record. Record client's appetite, food consumption, degree of self-care, and reaction to being fed.	Provides ongoing data for nutritional status assessment. Assumes professional responsibility.

RECORDING

After feeding a client, note and record the amount of food eaten, the length of time required, the degree of assistance provided, the client's interest in food and reaction to being fed, and any problems with manipulation of utensils, chewing, swallowing, or sucking.

Sample POR Recording

- S—"If I weren't so tired, I wouldn't let you do this for me." "I'm really not very hungry today."
- O—Fed self several bites of food and then allowed nurse to feed about half of contents of lunch tray. Chews slowly, with no swallowing problems. Pale, looked tired; had pulse of 102 after self-feeding.
- A—Unable to feed self completely because of fatigue; has decreased appetite.
- P—Plan to continue to assist with meals. Explore what foods might be appealing.

Sample Narrative Recording

Slowly fed self several bites and allowed nurse to feed about half of lunch. Says he's not very hungry and is "so tired." Pale, looked tired, and had pulse of 102 after feeding self.

☐ CRITICAL POINTS SUMMARY

1. Evaluate the nature and degree of feeding assistance needed by each client.
2. Provide for relief of pain and nausea before feeding.
3. Enhance appetite and digestion through environmental management and provide a relaxed, pleasant, unhurried mealtime.
4. Determine client's ability to swallow before feeding.
5. When feeding a client:
   a. Plan to remain with the client throughout the feeding.
   b. Follow the client's usual eating routines.
   c. Avoid hurrying the client.
6. When assisting a client to eat:
   a. Follow the planned feeding assistance program consistently.
   b. Use assistive devices to facilitate as much self-feeding as possible.
7. Provide for oral care before and after feeding.
8. Use appropriate facilitative measures to promote sucking, chewing, and swallowing.
9. Report and record intake, appetite, and any problems with eating.

LEARNING ACTIVITIES

1. Feed another person and be fed.
   a. Equipment needed for each person: Small bowl of cereal with milk, cup of hot tea or coffee, glass of cold juice, spoon, straw, and a towel or napkin.
   b. Procedure
      (NOTE:—the "client" should not assist in any way with the following activities):
      (1) Position your "client" in bed or in a chair.
      (2) Protect clothing with napkin or towel.
      (3) Use the spoon to feed the entire bowl of cereal.
      (4) Assist the "client" to drink the juice through the straw.
      (5) Assist the "client" to drink the hot liquid directly from the cup.
      (6) Exchange places with your partner and repeat the procedure.
   c. Evaluation:
      (1) Identify your feelings and reactions to being fed. (You might have felt uncomfortable, embarrassed, eager to be finished, hurried, out-of-control, or relaxed and comfortable.)
      (2) Identify your feelings and reactions to feeding someone else. (You might have felt awkward, uncertain, hesitant, or confident and comfortable.)
      (3) Compare your reactions with those of your partner.
      (4) What does this activity say to you about the experience of feeding a client?
2. Visit an occupational therapy or rehabilitation department and observe assistive devices for persons with permanent or temporary difficulty eating or observe facilitation techniques used for dysphagic individuals.

REVIEW QUESTIONS

1. How would you enhance the self-worth of a client who needs to be fed?
2. What factors determine whether or not a client needs to be fed?
3. How would you determine the appropriate amount of self-feeding for a client?
4. What functions does oral care serve, both before and after feeding?
5. List ways to enhance appetite and decrease nausea and anorexia.
6. How would you determine whether or not a client is able to swallow?
7. Why should food and fluid not be given to a client with an absent or diminished swallowing reflex?
8. In what ways can mealtime be made a pleasant time for a client being fed?
9. What assistive devices might be used to help a client hold a spoon or fork? Hold a glass? Place food on a spoon? Suck through a straw?
10. Match each facilitation technique listed below with the appropriate eating action or actions:

FACILITATION TECHNIQUE	EATING ACTION
Downward pressure on the tongue with a spoon	____ Chewing
Forward and downward quick-stretch on the neck	____ Head positioning
Intermittent downward pressure on the upper lip	____ Mouth opening
Lateral upward and downward quick-stretch to the orbicularis oris	____ Sucking
Light bilateral stroking on the larynx	____ Swallowing
Light touching of the lips with a spoon	____ Lateral tongue displacement
Placing firm pressure on base of the neck	____ Not applicable
Placing food on the opposite side from tongue displacement	
Placing food on the side of tongue displacement	
Quick-stretch to the facial muscles	
Vibrating or tapping the facial muscles	

PERFORMANCE CHECKLIST

OBJECTIVE: To use appropriate feeding methods, swallowing facilitation measures, and assistive devices to feed a client safely, either partially or completely.

CHARACTERISTIC	RANGE OF ACCEPTABILITY	SATISFACTORY	UNSATISFACTORY
1. Consults kardex or care plan for feeding assistance plans and amount of help needed.	No deviation		
2. Arranges workload to allow adequate time.	No deviation		
3. Prepares environment.	No deviation		
4. Provides relief for pain and nausea.	No deviation		

(continued)

OBJECTIVE: To use appropriate feeding methods, swallowing facilitation measures, and assistive devices to feed a client safely, either partially or completely (cont.).

CHARACTERISTIC	RANGE OF ACCEPTABILITY	SATISFACTORY	UNSATISFACTORY
5. Gathers needed equipment including assistive devices and protective linen.	No deviation		
6. Explains own role in feeding.	No deviation		
7. Provides for emptying the bladder, handwashing, oral care; checks fit of dentures.	No deviation		
8. Places client in upright or semireclining position of comfort and stability, with neck slightly flexed.	If not feasible, position client comfortably and securely on side.		
9. Checks tray for completeness and correct diet for particular client.	No deviation		
10. Compares tray name with client's room number, identification band, and bed label; calls client by name.	No deviation		
11. Protects clothing and linen from accidental food spills.	No deviation		
12. Positions tray in front of client and self in client's visual field.	No deviation		
13. Observes ability to swallow and chew.	No deviation		
14. Follows client's mealtime rituals and preferences.	No deviation		
15. Remains with client during entire mealtime.	Plan in advance for relief, if needed.		
16. Allows sufficient time for chewing and swallowing; DOES NOT HURRY.	No deviation		
17. Uses assistive devices as needed.	No deviation		
18. Uses facilitative chewing, sucking, and swallowing techniques as needed.	No deviation		
19. Cleanses face and hands and provides oral care.	No deviation		
20. Returns tray to appropriate place.	No deviation		
21. Records intake, appetite reaction, and any problems.	No deviation		

REFERENCES

Buckley JE, Addicks CL, Maniglia J: Feeding patients with dysphagia. Nursing Forum XV(1):69–85, 1976.

Castell DO: Clinical conference on dysphagia. Gastroenterology 76(5, Part 1):1015–1024, 1979.

Dobie RA: Rehabilitation of swallowing disorders. American Family Physician/GP 17(5):84–95, 1978.

Farber SD: Neurorehabilitation: A Multisensory Approach. Philadelphia, WB Saunders, 1982.

Gaffney TW, Campbell RP: Feeding techniques for dysphagic patients. American Journal of Nursing 74(12):2194–2195, 1974.

Gallender D: Eating Handicaps: Illustrated Techniques for Feeding Disorders. Springfield, IL, Charles C Thomas, 1979.

Griffin KM: Swallowing training for dysphagic patients. Archives of Physical Medicine and Rehabilitation 55(10):467–470, 1974.

Hargrove R: Feeding the severely dysphagic patient. Journal of Neurosurgical Nursing 12(2):102–107, 1980.

Silverman EH, Elfant IL: Dysphagia: An evaluation and treatment program for the adult. American Journal of Occupational Therapy 33(6):382–392, 1979.

Zimmerman JE, Oder LA: Swallowing dysfunction in acutely ill patients. Physical Therapy 61(12):1755–1763, 1981.

BIBLIOGRAPHY

Brill EL, Kilts DF: Foundations for Nursing. New York, Appleton-Century-Crofts, 1980.

Kottke FJ (ed): Krusen's Handbook of Physical Medicine and Rehabilitation. Philadelphia, WB Saunders, 1982.

Lewis LuVW: Fundamental Skills in Patient Care, ed 2. Philadelphia, JB Lippincott, 1980.

Luckmann J, Sorensen KC: Medical–Surgical Nursing: A Psychophysiological Approach, ed 2. Philadelphia, WB Saunders, 1980.

Mitchell PH, Loustau A: Concepts Basic to Nursing, ed 3. New York, McGraw-Hill, 1981.

Suitor CW, Crowley MF: Nutrition: Principles and Applications in Health Promotion, ed 2. Philadelphia, JB Lippincott, 1984.

SUGGESTED READING

Silverman EH, Elfant IL: Dysphagia: An evaluation and treatment program for the adult. American Journal of Occupational Therapy 33(6):382–392, 1979.

Zimmerman JE, Oder LA: Swallowing dysfunction in acutely ill patients. Physical Therapy 61(12):1755–1763, 1981.

SKILL 54 Enteral Nutritional Support

□ PREREQUISITE SKILLS

Skill 19, "Inspection"
Skill 20, "Palpation"
Skill 22, "Auscultation"
Skill 28, "Handwashing"
Skill 40, "Oral Care"
Skill 52, "Nutritional Assessment and the Serving of Food"
Skill 53, "Assistance with Eating"

□ STUDENT OBJECTIVES

1. Identify the advantages of nutritional support by the enteral route as compared with the parenteral route.
2. Define gastrostomy, esophagostomy, and jejunostomy.
3. Differentiate among the nasogastric, orogastric, and nasojejunal routes for enteral feedings in terms of anatomic location, rationale for use, and types of tubing and formulas used.
4. Compare the composition, purposes, benefits, and disadvantages of commercial and blenderized feedings.
5. Describe care and precautions with enteral feeding formulas administered by both continuous and intermittent methods.
6. Explain the time framework and rationale for aspirating and measuring gastric contents with both continuous and intermittent feedings.
7. Describe the process of physiological and psychosocial adaptation to enteral feedings.
8. Safely administer an enteral feeding through a feeding tube.

□ INTRODUCTION

Enteral formulas are specially prepared liquid nutrients that can be administered directly into the gastrointestinal tract through a tube or ingested orally. They may be used for total nutritional support or as an adjunct to conventional oral diets, parenteral feedings, or both. A variety of commercially prepared formulas currently are used as enteral feedings, and occasionally blenderized foods may be used. Nasogastric tube feedings were first used in the early 1880s. During the first half of the 20th century, milk product formulas were used for tube feedings, and in the 1950s, Barron developed blenderized diets and a pump to ensure accurate flow rates for those viscous formulas (Cataldo and Smith, 1980).

Nurses are responsible for administering enteral feedings in acute, chronic, and home settings. As part of discharge planning or in the home environment, nurses may also need to teach clients and families about preparation or administration of a formula. The nurse who understands the types and purposes of various formulas, the problems and concerns likely to be encountered by clients, and the manner of successfully administering these formulas will be better able to provide direct care and teaching for clients and families.

Enteral feedings, sometimes called gavage feedings or tube feedings, are used when the client is unable to ingest, digest, or absorb conventional food through the oral route. This may be because of an inability to swallow, as occurs with clients who are comatose or neurologically impaired or have an obstruction of the upper alimentary canal, such as a tumor, lesion, or stricture; or those persons who have a decreased ability to absorb nutrients, such as after radiation therapy or with inflammatory bowel disease. Enteral feedings also are used when normal ingestion of food is not possible, as may occur after radical neck dissection and throat or oral surgeries; when the caloric demands of illness are greater than the client can consume in the usual manner, such as after severe burns or during an overwhelming infection or debilitating illness; or when appetite and food consumption are less than needed for maintenance of health or recovery from illness, such as in elderly or immobilized persons and cancer patients. Studies indicate that the majority of tube-fed clients have either head and neck surgery or neurologic deficits, that more males than females receive tube feedings, and that most are over

45 years of age (Heitkemper et al., 1978; Walike et al., 1975). Feedings often are ordered as a palliative treatment for clients with terminal cancer. This brings the additional dimension of coping with a terminal illness and grieving for both the client and the family.

Decreased food intake contributes to anorexia, which contributes to further decreases in food intake, with malnutrition an inevitable result. An unintentional weight loss of 10 percent places a person at risk for malnutrition and secondary illnesses. If a person has lost more than 20 to 30 percent of his or her desired weight, it is very difficult to recover that weight with ordinary meals, and enteral or parenteral feedings are likely to be required (Buergel, 1979). Preferably, this level of inadequate nutritional status can be avoided by careful assessment and early initiation of nutritional support. Assessment of nutritional status is discussed in Skill 52.

Unless there are major contraindications, nutritional support via the enteral route is preferred over the parenteral route for the following reasons. The presence of nutrients within the intestinal tract has an "intraluminal effect" that helps maintain the integrity of the bowel mucosa (Driscoll and Rosenberg, 1978). The enteral route is safer than total parenteral nutrition (hyperalimentation), which is discussed in Skill 55, since the risk of infection and fluid–electrolyte imbalance is less when the gastrointestinal tract is used. The cost of enteral feeding is substantially lower than the cost of parenteral feeding, in terms of the feeding itself, the equipment, and the staff time for administering and monitoring. Enteral feeding may also be more pleasant for the client, especially if conventional foods can be blenderized and used.

☐ PREPARATION

ENTERAL FEEDING ROUTES

Enteral feedings can be infused into the stomach, distal duodenum, or the proximal jejunum. The feeding tube may be inserted through the nose (nasogastric, nasoduodenal, or nasojejunal routes) or mouth (orogastric route), or through a surgically created stoma (opening or ostomy) directly into the esophagus (esophagostomy), stomach (gastrostomy), or jejunum (jejunostomy).

Figure 54-1 illustrates the various routes by which tube feedings may be administered. Insertion and care of these tubes is discussed in Skill 56. The *nasogastric, orogastric,* and *nasojejunal* routes are usually used for short-term tube feedings because they do not necessitate a surgical incision. A nasogastric tube is not usually used for long-term feeding because of nasal irritation, interference with swallowing secretions, and other potential complications. Also, visible nasal feeding tubes are not usually considered socially and psychologically acceptable for home use.

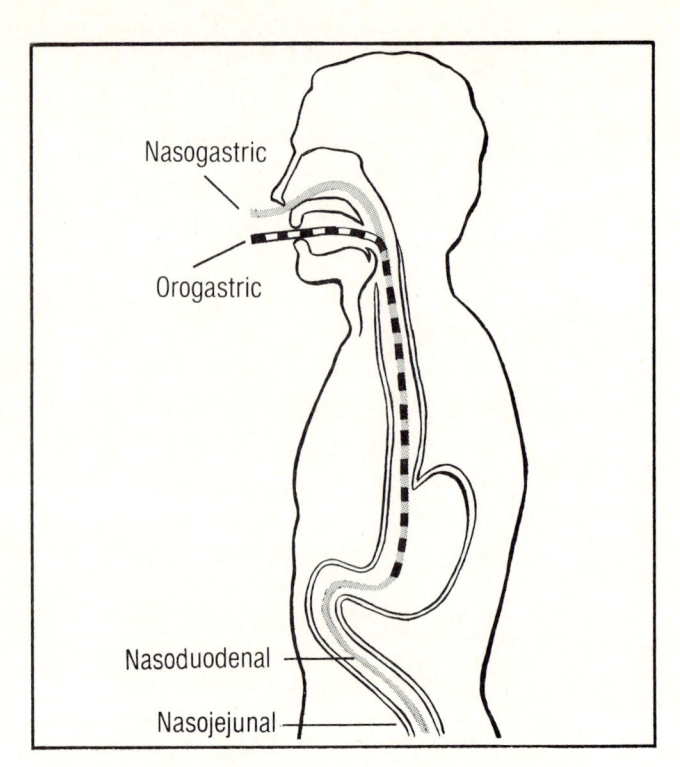

Figure 54–1. Administration routes for enteral feedings. **A.** Nonsurgically created routes. Nasogastric route: *The tube is inserted through the nose and into the stomach and then secured in place.* Orogastric route: *The tube is inserted through the mouth and into the stomach at mealtime and removed after the meal.* Nasoduodenal and nasojejunal routes: *The tube is inserted through the nose and beyond the stomach into the duodenum or jejunum and secured in place.*

Because of the problems associated with long-term use of nasogastric tubes, gastric feedings are usually given through a gastrostomy, esophagostomy, or by means of an orogastric tube inserted for each meal.

An *esophagostomy* is a surgically created skin-lined canal leading from the surface of the lower neck or chest directly into the esophagus. A fairly large-diameter feeding tube is passed through the stoma into the stomach for each feeding and then removed. With this route, there is less risk of developing an infection or skin excoriation than with a gastrostomy, and the client does not have to undress or loosen clothing for the feeding as with a gastrostomy.

A *gastrostomy* is a surgically created temporary or permanent opening (stoma) into the stomach, connecting the stomach with the abdominal wall. A gastrostomy tube may be sutured or taped in place for short-term use. After the stoma has healed, the tube may be inserted by the nurse or client for each feeding and then removed.

A *jejunostomy* is a surgically created opening providing direct access to the jejunum. This may be done by inserting a small-lumen needle catheter for short-term use. For longer-term use, a larger catheter or tube may be sutured in place or a stoma similar to a colostomy or ileostomy may be created. The stoma is particularly useful for confused and uncooperative

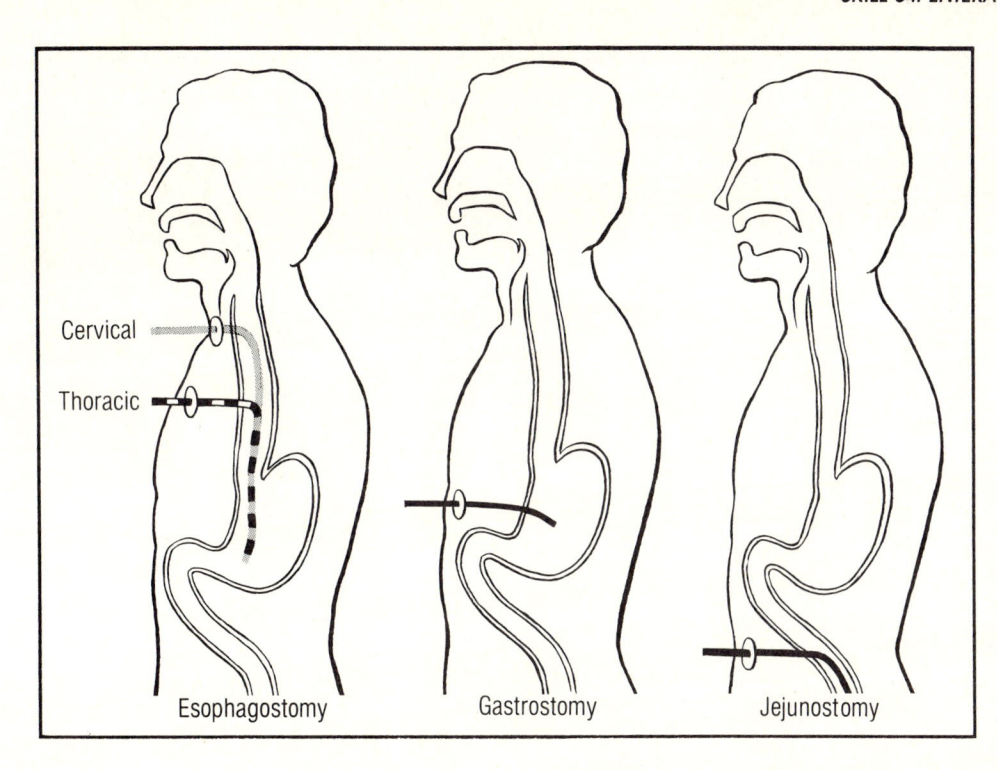

Figure 54-1. B. *Surgically created routes.* Esophagostomy: *a stoma through the neck or thorax, allowing a tube to be passed into the stomach at mealtimes and removed after the feeding.* Gastrostomy: *A stoma that allows a tube to be inserted directly into the stomach and sutured or taped in place.* Jejunostomy: *A stoma that allows a tube to be inserted directly into the jejunum and sutured in place.*

persons who might remove a tube left in place. The jejunal route is used when the stomach must be bypassed or has been removed.

Both a gastrostomy and a jejunostomy require special skin care to prevent excoriation from seepage of gastric or jejunal fluids onto the skin. The skin around the abdominal opening requires washing with a gentle soap and thorough drying twice a day, or whenever secretions leak. Zinc oxide or petroleum jelly can be applied to the skin for protection against maceration and irritation. Formula is not usually infused through the gastrostomy or jejunostomy tube until 3 days after initial insertion, which allows time for the stomach or intestine to seal around the tube.

For a hospitalized client, the gastrostomy or jejunostomy tubing is secured to the abdomen with tape, sutured in place, or both. Methods for securing larger-lumen gastrostomy tubes and small-lumen jejunostomy tubes are shown in Figure 54-2. Secure taping avoids accidental tugging on the tubing, with potential dislodging and discomfort for the client. If necessary or desired, a dressing may be placed over the gastrostomy or jejunostomy insertion site or the abdominal incision after the tube has been taped in place. The end of a jejunostomy tube is kept readily accessible for attaching a continuous tube feeding set. The end of a gastrostomy tube is kept covered with a small dressing that is secured with a rubber band, in case of leakage, as shown in Figure 54-2. The ends of gastrostomy and jejunostomy tubes are kept clean, not sterile, since they open into the stomach and intestines, which are not sterile.

The dumping syndrome occurs when food and fluid from the stomach empty rapidly into the small intestine and cause distention within 5 to 30 minutes after a meal. It can occur when highly concentrated formulas are administered directly into the jejunum too rapidly. The dumping syndrome often is described as a feeling of fullness and nausea and frequently is accompanied by sweating, pallor, headaches, vertigo, and feelings of warmth. A sharp increase in blood glucose levels accompanies the rapid gastric emptying, with a compensatory oversecretion of insulin. This results in hypoglycemia 2 to 3 hours after the meal, manifested by weakness, sweating, anxiety, and tremors (Jones et al., 1978).

ENTERAL FEEDING METHODS

Enteral feedings may be given as intermittent bolus (batch) feedings or as a continuous drip feeding. Because it has fewer side effects, continuous enteral feeding is considered preferable to intermittent feeding (American Dietetic Association, 1981; Dobie and Butterick, 1977; Griggs and Hoppe, 1979; Krause and Mahan, 1979). Continuous feedings are given through the nasogastric, nasoduodenal, jejunostomy, and gastrostomy routes. Intermittent feedings are given through nasogastric, orogastric, esophageal-gastric, gastrostomy routes, and sometimes through a jejunostomy, if the client can tolerate it. Continuous feedings are administered by a gravity flow or with an infusion pump that delivers a more constant rate of flow, both measured in milliliters per hour. Intermittent feedings involve giving a larger volume of formula (200 to 350 ml) in a relatively short period of time (5 to 15 minutes) and at 2- to 4-hour intervals.

Figure 54–2. A. To secure a gastrostomy tube: (1) Place one end of the tape on the abdomen, encircle the tube with the tape strip so that it meets beneath the tube, and place the other end of the tape on the abdomen. Repeat, overlapping the tape strips until the tube is secure. (2) Split one-half of an 8-inch strip of tape lengthwise. Place the nonsplit end of the tape on the abdomen with the split opening adjacent to the tube. Wrap the split ends around the tube in opposite directions. (3) When not in use, cover the end of the gastrostomy with a small, clean dressing and secure with a rubber band. When an abdominal dressing is used, tape the tubing to the dressing as well as to the skin. **B.** To secure a small-lumen catheter inserted in the jejunum: (1) Loop the tubing near the insertion site and apply overlapping tape strips, beginning at the insertion site and leaving the catheter hub exposed. (2) Place a second tape strip lengthwise from the insertion point down to and securely around the hub. (NOTE: The knots at the bases of the tubes in **A.** and **B.** represent sutures holding the tubes in place.)

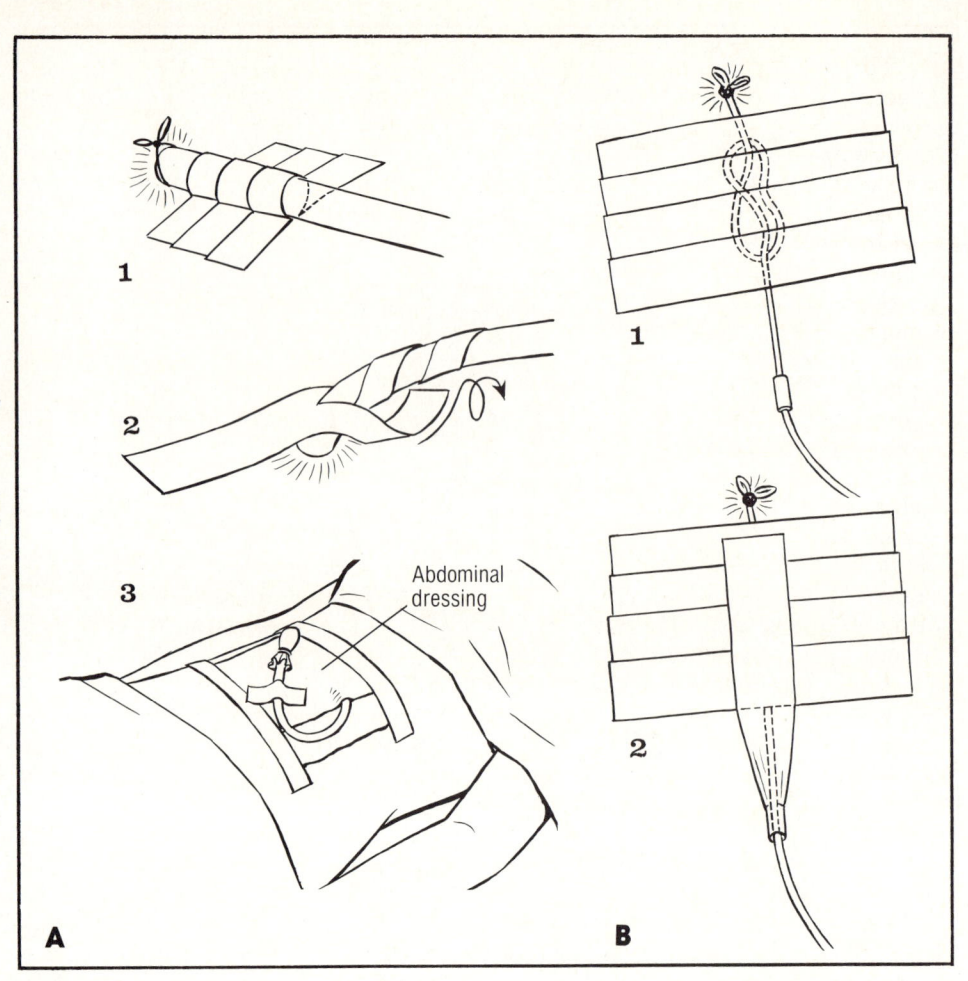

ENTERAL FEEDING FORMULAS

Numerous liquid nutritional products are available commercially, with new products being marketed at a rapid rate. Nutrition texts, journal articles, and manufacturer's written materials provide information about the characteristics of specific formulas. Although it is not possible to learn detailed information about specific formulas, the nurse can understand clients' fluid needs and can recognize potential sources of adverse reactions when he or she understands basic characteristics of enteral formulas. These characteristics include concentration; lactose, protein, and fat content; residue; and viscosity. In addition to commercially prepared products, enteral formulas may be made by blenderizing conventional foods, as sometimes is done in the home setting. A light green food dye is often added to enteral formulas to distinguish them from other gastric contents if vomiting occurs, or when aspirating for residual, as described later.

Commercial Formulas

Commercial formulas are available in ready-to-use liquid form or in powder that is reconstituted just before use. These products have the advantages of having a consistent nutrient content, sterility before containers are opened, ease of preparation, and low risk in terms of mixing error. They are nonperishable at room temperature if unopened but must be refrigerated after opening. Commercial formula products are of four types: intact formulas, hydrolyzed formulas, supplemental formulas, and specialty formulas.

Intact Formulas. These formulas are sometimes called balanced complete formulas with intact protein or meal replacement formulas. They generally contain about 15 percent protein, 35 percent fat, 50 percent carbohydrates, and if given in calorically adequate amounts, contain enough vitamins and minerals to meet daily needs. Examples of meal replacement formulas include Isocal and Sustacal (Mead Johnson), Ensure, Ensure Plus, Osmolite (Ross), and Travasol (Travenol). They work well for clients who are able to digest and absorb nutrients fairly well. Some formulas contain blenderized conventional foods and therefore have more fiber, such as Vitaneed (Organon) and Compleat-B and Compleat-Modified (Doyle) (which contains no lactose). Meal replacement formulas are preferred when digestion and absorption are intact. They are the least expensive type of feeding and are often less costly than blenderizing conventional foods at home or in an institution (Comparison, 1981).

The *concentration* of these enteral formulas ranges from 1 to 2 kcal per ml and from near-physiological osmolality, which is approximately 300 mOsm per kg water (Whitney and Cataldo, 1983, p. 754), to more than twice that. A higher kilocalorie composition sometimes mean a higher osmolality, so careful label reading is necessary. For example, Sustacal contains 1 kcal per ml and has an osmolality of 625 mOsm per kg water; Isocal contains 1 kcal per ml and has an osmolality of 300 mOsm per kg water; Ensure contains 1 kcal per ml and has an osmolality of 450 mOsm per kg; and Ensure Plus contains 1.5 kcal per ml and has an osmolality of 600 mOsm per kg water. The greater kilocalorie composition allows for greater caloric needs to be met without using large volumes of formula, such as is necessary to meet the high caloric and protein needs of persons who have been burned or to fit the fluid restrictions of persons with cardiac or renal disease. It is especially important to dilute formulas with a higher osmolality during the initial adaptation period, as discussed later.

Lactose content may be a cause of the common side effect, diarrhea. If lactose intolerance is known or suspected, a lactose-free formula such as Ensure, Isocal, Prosobee (Mead Johnson), or Compleat-Modified can be used. High *protein* levels increase the formula osmolality and can contribute to or cause dehydration unless adequate additional fluids are given.

Except for the blenderized types of formulas, most of these formulas leave little *residue* (material left in the colon following digestion). Low residue contributes to development of constipation. Some formulas have a high *viscosity,* such as the blenderized formulas, which are very thick, while others are less thick. An infusion pump is needed when thicker formulas are administered through small-lumen feeding tubes.

Hydrolyzed Formulas. These formulas are chemically defined complete formulas and can provide total nutritional support. They contain hydrolyzed (partially digested) proteins or free amino acids, few fats, high concentrations of carbohydrates, and vitamins and minerals to meet nutritional needs. They are used for persons who have limited digestive and absorptive capabilities (such as with enzyme deficiencies or a surgically shortened intestinal tract) or those who require minimal colonic residue (such as in colitis). Examples are Critcare HN (Mead Johnson), Vital (Ross), Vivonex (Norwich-Eaton), and Travasorb High Nitrogen (Travenol).

Chemically defined formulas are expensive, have a high osmolality (460 to 850 mOsm per kg), are very thin, and leave very little colonic residue.

Supplemental Formulas. Supplemental formulas or nutrient modules can be used as adjuncts to a regular diet or they may be added to a prepared formula to alter its composition for special nutritional needs. Examples of these modular supplements include Polycose (Ross) (carbohydrates), Casec (proteins), and MCT Oil (fats) (Mead-Johnson).

Specialty Formulas. Some formulas are created for specific illness conditions, such as liver or renal failure. Examples include Hepatic-Aid and Travasorb Renal (Travenol). They are expensive, with a high osmolality.

Noncommercial Blenderized Formulas

Noncommercial blenderized formula feedings are made from regular foods liquefied in a blender and then strained and refrigerated prior to use. They are most often used at home. The advantages of these feedings are that they simulate a normal diet, contain the trace minerals and vitamins found in regular foods, and can be planned to fit the individual's specific nutritional needs. Some persons on long-term enteral feedings prefer to have the regular family diet blenderized and even served in courses (Boucher, 1977; Rains, 1981). For long-term home use, blenderized feedings may be somewhat less expensive, may allow the person to participate more completely in mealtime, may provide more bulk for normal bowel function, and may be more palatable.

There are some disadvantages of noncommercial blenderized formulas. They tend to separate and need frequent agitation during administration. If the particles are not sufficiently small in size, they may clog a feeding tube. Using strained baby food eliminates this problem but adds to the cost of feedings. Because of the perishable ingredients used and the potential for bacterial overgrowth from accidental introduction of contaminants during preparation, the refrigerated shelf-life of blenderized formula is only 24 hours. After that time has transpired, these formulas must be discarded.

CALORIC AND FLUID NEEDS WITH ENTERAL FEEDINGS

Enteral formulas must be provided in sufficient volume and concentration to meet the body's usual needs and the increased demands of illness. This can mean caloric requirements of between 1800 to 2200 kcal, or as high as 5000 kcal per day with major trauma or burns (Krause and Mahan, 1984, p. 711). This would mean that a minimum of 1800 to 2000 ml of formula with a concentration of 1 kcal per ml must be administered every 24 hours. Unfortunately, this does not always happen. For example, one study reported that the average daily intake of 121 tube-fed persons was approximately 1300 ml per day (Walike et al., 1975).

If as many as 2500 to 3000 ml of formula are administered daily, the average adult's fluid requirements are met. When a client receives less than 2500 ml of formula per day or has fluid losses in excess of the usual (see Skill 51), additional water should be given through the feeding tube or an intravenous infusion (Kubo et al., 1976). Tube-fed clients need more water when they complain of thirst (either with or without mouth dryness), or when their protein intake is greater than 1 g per kg of body weight. Elderly persons need increased water intake since their kidneys are less able to concentrate urine.

Condon and Nyhus (1985) recommend that for every 1 ml of tube feeding, at least an additional 0.5 ml of water be given, and Krause and Mahan (1984) recommend adding water (one half the formula volume) to bolus feedings. These general rules require modification when fluid intake is restricted for therapeutic reasons, such as occurs with persons who have renal disease or heart failure.

ADMINISTRATION OF ENTERAL FEEDINGS

Rate and Volume of Administration

Continuous enteral feedings are given at a rate of 80 to 150 ml per hour, either by gravity or through a pump. The lower the osmolality, the more rapidly the formula may be infused. However, jejunal feedings always are given slowly to avoid the dumping syndrome and diarrhea.

Intermittent enteral feeding volume ranges from 200 to 300 ml of formula given over a 10-minute period at 2-, 3-, or 4-hour intervals. Some agency policies may require a longer infusion time of 20 to 30 minutes. There are conflicting research data about the effect of *rate of administration* on client tolerance. Hanson (1974) found that rapid feeding (syringe-fed in less than 10 minutes) was associated with increased incidence of accelerated heart rate, nausea, gagging, and regurgitation. However, Heitkemper et al. (1978) found that 250 ml of formula given in 5 minutes produced minimal adverse responses. In a study by Walike et al. (1975) of 121 clients for 1730 study days, tube feedings were administered in less than 5 minutes in 61 percent of the 778 study days for which data concerning duration were available, in 5 to 15 minutes in 30 percent of the study days, and more than 15 minutes for the remaining 9 percent. Although they did find the rate of administration of feedings was positively associated with the number of stools per day, the study provided no clear indications of the effect of rate of administration on client symptoms in general.

In a 1981 study, 14 volunteers were given bolus feedings of 250 to 750 ml at rates of 30 to 85 ml per minute. The findings indicated that *rate* rather than volume influences symptomatic tolerance of enteral feedings. Volumes of up to 750 ml were well tolerated when the rate of administration was maintained at 30 ml per minute, although smaller volumes were tolerated without subjective distress at more rapid rates (after the first feeding experience). There was no significant interaction effect of rate and volume on the time required for gastric motility to return after feedings. The researchers indicated that their findings suggest that symptoms decrease and tolerance improves with repeated feedings, and that the first feeding is best given slowly and in small volumes (Heitkemper et al., 1981). Other authors associate increased rate of feeding with nausea and recommend decreasing the rate if nausea occurs (Metheny and Snively, 1983).

A recommended approach is to begin by allowing the feeding to flow in by gravity over a 10 minute period of time. If a particular client experiences distress in this time period, the administration time should be gradually increased.

Temperature of Enteral Feedings

There is disagreement about the effect of *formula temperature* on tolerance to tube feedings. Williams and Walike (1975) found that administering cold intermittent enteral formulas (5° to 7°C [41° to 45°F]) delayed gastric motility but did not significantly affect gastrointestinal tract transit time when compared with warm (36° to 38°C [97° to 100°F]) or room-temperature (24°C [75°F]) formulas. As a result of his clinical study, Hanson (1974) concluded that warming formula was an unnecessary step. Kagawa-Busby et al. (1980) found that adverse symptoms of cramping pain and diarrhea occurred primarily after cold, as opposed to warm or room-temperature, feedings. They recommend continuing the practice of warming intermittent feedings to room temperature prior to administration.

With continuous feedings, the formula container is often cooled with ice, but the formula itself warms to room temperature as it passes slowly through the administration tubing to the stomach. It is considered safe to hang an unrefrigerated 8-hour supply if (a) single-use containers are attached directly to the administration set or (b) the reusable formula container is *empty* before additional formula is added. If some formula that has been at room temperature for 8 hours is left in the container, it becomes mixed with new formula and can be a source of bacterial overgrowth and souring. If the room temperature is quite warm, such as during the summer in rooms without air conditioning, 8 hours probably is too long for formula to hang unrefrigerated.

Generally recommended practices for continuous feeding include (a) keeping the formula cool during administration by using equipment with an ice container or (b) hanging only a 4- to 8-hour supply if no cooling equipment is available, being careful not to mix old and new formula.

Generally recommended practices for intermittent feedings include (a) warming refrigerated formulas prior to administration and (b) optional warming of room-temperature single-use containers of formula.

ADAPTATION TO ENTERAL FORMULA FEEDINGS

When enteral formulas are initiated, a process of physiological adaptation must occur. This may take 3 to 5 days. Attempting to hurry the adaptation process to increase the nutritional intake is likely to result in formula intolerance.

Intolerance to the formula feedings is demonstrated primarily by such adverse reactions as nausea and vomiting, diarrhea, and abdominal cramping. When diarrhea occurs, the adaptive process must be restarted. Possible causes for the adverse reactions include the administration rate, the formula temperature (both of which are discussed in the preceding section), and the lactose content of the formula. *Lactose intolerance* is an inability to digest milk sugar and is characterized by abdominal cramps, flatus (gas), abdominal distention, and diarrhea. These symptoms develop within ½ to 4 hours after milk ingestion. Lactose intolerance occurs in a large percent of the nonwhite adult population in the United States. Persons with this intolerance require a lactose-free formula, as indicated earlier.

Physiological adaptation is achieved by diluting the formula initially, introducing small amounts, and increasing the rate of administration gradually. After the desired rate of infusion or the volume of formula has been achieved with client tolerance, the formula concentration is increased. The volume and the concentration are never increased at the same time. Highly osmolar formulas are diluted initially to one-quarter strength, whereas formulas with a more physiological osmolality are diluted to one-half strength. If no diarrhea or other signs of intolerance occur in 24 hours, the concentration is increased by 25 percent until full strength is reached, with 24 hours allowed for the client to adjust to each increase.

Continuous enteral feedings administered either by gravity flow or infusion pump are initiated with a flow rate of 40 to 60 ml per hour (Griggs and Hoppe, 1979; Krause and Mahan, 1984). If no diarrhea or other signs of intolerance develop within 12 to 24 hours, the rate may be increased by 25 ml per hour each day until the desired rate is attained.

Intermittent enteral feedings are initiated with a volume of 50 to 100 ml per feeding, with the bottom of the range used if the client has experienced difficulty retaining or digesting food prior to the introduction of the formula. This volume is increased by approximately 50 ml per day until the desired volume is reached.

Psychosocial adaptation to tube feedings is also necessary, since the inability to eat in a normal way drastically influences a person's life style and self-concept. Research indicates that common and distressing experiences of hospitalized tube-fed clients include being deprived of tasting food, chewing, and drinking liquids; being thirsty; and having an unsatisfied appetite for specific foods. Hospitalized clients considered these problems more significant than deprivation of socialization when eating (Padilla et al., 1979; Rains, 1981). Rains (1981) found that social isolation and withdrawal was a greater problem for long-term, tube-fed clients living at home. These clients may also feel tied down to the equipment and self-conscious about having a tube in the nose or having to remove clothing for gastrostomy feedings, especially after they leave the sheltered hospital environment.

GENERAL PHYSIOLOGICAL PROBLEMS WITH ENTERAL FEEDINGS

A number of physiological problems associated with enteral feedings may occur even when formula tolerance has developed.

Glucosuria often occurs because of the concentrated carbohydrates in enteral formulas, and both diabetic and nondiabetic clients often need to be given insulin. Diabetic clients are monitored for urine glucose and acetone throughout the duration of tube feeding therapy, preferably with a double-voided specimen. Nondiabetic clients have their urine monitored during adaptation to formula and for 48 hours after the required concentration and rate are achieved. If glucose and acetone are consistently negative, urine checks may be discontinued.

Aspiration pneumonia often develops after regurgitation of formula (gastric reflux). It is much more likely to occur in persons who are comatose, in debilitated persons whose cough reflex is depressed, and in the elderly, especially if the head of the bed is not elevated during and after formula administration. In a prospective study of 30 tube-fed clients with artificial airways, correct feeding techniques resulted in no formula aspiration (Clinical, 1985). The use of jejunal feedings also helps prevent regurgitation.

Constipation may develop after the client has become stabilized on the enteral feeding because of the low-fiber and high-milk content of many formulas. Additional fluids help, but stool softeners and cathartics may be needed.

Heartburn may accompany an intermittent feeding and is thought to be due to irritation of the esophageal mucosa from gastric regurgitation into the esophagus. Elevating the head of the bed for several hours after a feeding, seeing that the client avoids a slumped position, and promoting relaxation often help reduce this discomfort.

Nausea may develop if too large a total volume per feeding is given, if feedings are initiated sooner than 30 minutes after insertion of a nasogastric tube, if the tube tip is improperly located, or if lactose intolerance exists.

Fluid and electrolyte imbalance may occur with prolonged use of enteral feedings and can become severe enough to cause impaired consciousness or even death. This imbalance is more likely to occur with persons who cannot perceive or communicate thirst, such as confused or unconscious clients; with persons whose fluid and electrolyte regulating mechanisms are impaired or damaged, for example, clients with cerebrovascular accidents, cardiac or renal disease, and the elderly; and with persons whose total fluid intake is restricted or who receive concentrated formulas in a volume of less than 2500 ml per day (Hoppe, 1980).

Hyperosmolar dehydration can result from excessive diarrhea or from fluid compartment shifts caused by osmotic diuresis, glucosuria, excessive protein intake, or hyperosmolar formulas.

SELF-CARE WITH ENTERAL FEEDINGS

Clients receiving long-term enteral feedings are usually taught to administer their own feedings, care for a stoma or gastrostomy, and insert their own oral gastric or esophagostomy tubes. Additionally, at least one responsible family member is taught how to provide the needed care, so that illness or fatigue will not interrupt the feeding pattern.

Clients who are to receive enteral feedings after discharge are referred to the local visiting nurses service, public health department, or home-care agency for continued nursing supervision, evaluation, and teaching. This is especially important immediately after discharge. It is not uncommon for both clients and families to be able to manage the needed care adequately in the hospital, where supplies and assistance are readily available, but to have many questions and uncertainties once they are solely responsible.

The hospital discharge planning services should be involved in home-care planning as soon as it is known that the client will be sent home requiring enteral feedings, because time is needed to arrange for equipment and supplies, and to help prepare the client and family for what will be required in caring for the client. In many cities, there are home-care agencies which provide a package service that includes delivery of an enteral pump, equipment, and formula for a given fee. These companies often are able to bill the client's insurance company, Medicare, or Medicaid for reimbursement, which provides substantial economic relief for families.

Families who consider homemade blenderized formulas should be encouraged to compare those costs with the cost of case prices of commercial formulas or costs through a home-care agency where insurance reimbursement is available. An intake of 1500 kcal each day would require six 8-oz cans or one and one-half cans of the larger 32-oz size. Costs of equipment are the same for both kinds of formulas. Time factors and individual preferences are often the deciding factors for a family.

DATA BASE

Client History and Recorded Data

When the prescribed formula contains lactose, the nurse determines if the client has a lactose intolerance before administering it. The formula prescription should include the type and amount of the feedings, the frequency and rate of feeding, and the amount of water to be included. If the prescription does not include the amount of water, the nurse consults the physician to obtain guidelines for the total fluid intake. The nurse may also need to consult the dietitian to plan the frequency, amounts, and flow rate for the feedings if they are not included in the physician's order. All of this information is entered on the client's health record, the nursing-care kardex or nursing-care plan, and the diet therapy record if one is used.

To monitor a client's nutritional status adequately, the nurse finds out the purpose for which the formula is given, that is, whether supplementing or replacing the traditional diet. Age, sex, weight, diagnosis, vital signs, and laboratory hematology and protein values provide data about the client's nutritional status and needs. Temperature and pulse are of significance because they reflect the metabolic rate. Flow sheets in the health record or at the bedside contain daily weight values and results of urine tests for glucose and acetone. These data help to evaluate the adequacy of the formula, the body's utilization of the formula, any potential need for insulin, and any fluid balance problems.

The client's physiological and psychological adaptation to the tube feedings are determined by detecting symptoms of formula intolerance or other problems and eliciting feelings of satisfaction, satiety, general degree of comfort, and acceptance of the presence of the tube and the need for the feedings. Knowledge of the length of time the client has been receiving the tube feeding and whether there have been any problems will help the nurse evaluate these reactions.

Physical Appraisal Skills

Inspection. The nurse uses inspection to determine whether or not the tape and tape-string anchoring of the feeding tube remain intact. Inspection also reveals the cleanliness of the tube itself, the condition of the nares (presence of crusts, redness, irritation), the status of oral hygiene, and any dryness of the lips. When aspirating to determine placement of the tube in the stomach or to measure residual gastric contents, the nurse uses inspection to distinguish between retained feedings (which would resemble curdled formula and may be colored light green) and normal gastric secretions (which are clear with brown flecks). Abdominal distention can be observed by inspecting the abdomen from above and from the side of the client.

Palpation. The nurse uses palpation to detect abdominal distention, which may or may not be accompanied by abdominal cramping.

Auscultation. The nurse uses a stethoscope to auscultate for air inserted into the stomach as a gastric tube placement check.

EQUIPMENT

The equipment used for tube feeding administration is presterilized but used in a medically aseptic manner, since the stomach is not a sterile body cavity.

Formula Containers

Commercial formulas are available in liquid or powder form. Formula is packaged in 240- to 250-ml (8-oz) containers for single-use feedings, or in 1000-ml (1-qt) sizes that may be used for several feedings. Glass or plastic bottles have a screw-top cap that can be removed and attached directly to a feeding set. They also have a metal or plastic hanger attached to the bottom so they can be inverted and hung from an intravenous pole. Aluminum cans open with a pull tab and must be poured into a reusable container attached to a feeding set. Institutionally prepared formula containers usually are large glass bottles with screw-top caps. It is important to clean the top of a can with soap and water or an alcohol wipe, since the formula comes into contact with the can top as it is poured.

Administration and Feeding Sets
An administration set includes a *container* and a *feeding set*. The feeding set consists of a drip chamber, tubing, flow regulator, and connector. It may be preattached to a container (usually a plastic feeding bag) or have an adaptor or screw cap for use with single-use formula containers. Figure 54–3 shows a feeding set with a preattached feeding bag. The transparent or translucent drip chamber provides visualization of flow rate from the container through the tubing. The tubing itself is about 125 cm (50 in) long to allow the client freedom of movement. The tapered connector at the proximal end of the tubing fits into the feeding tube opening. When a feeding pump is not used, the flow rate is regulated by roller or screw clamps through which the tubing passes and a time tape applied to the container (see below). Roller clamps provide more accurate regulation and are easier to operate with one hand. Some administration sets designed specifically for use with a feeding pump do not have a drip chamber, since drip rate monitoring is not necessary for adequate pump functioning.

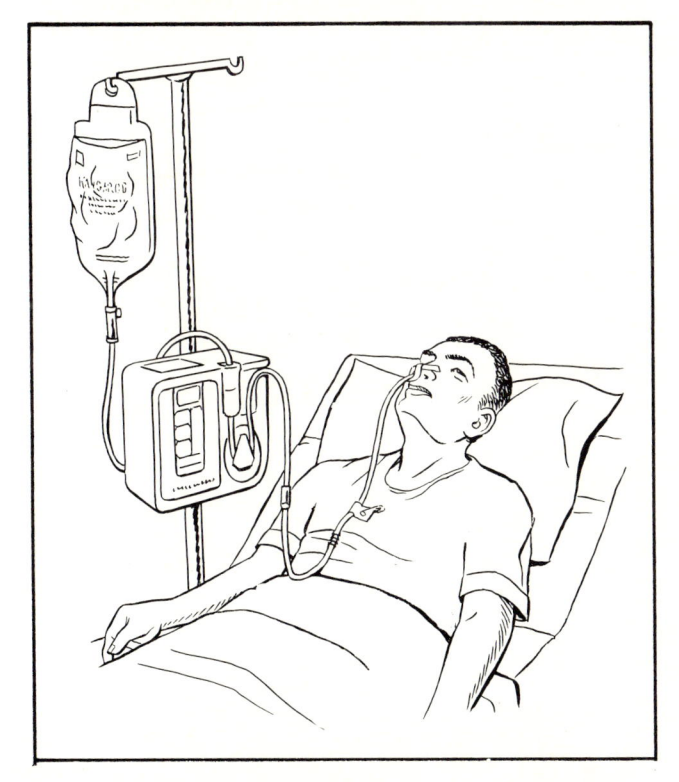

Figure 54–3. Continuous tube feeding using an enteral pump and plastic bag formula container with a side pouch that holds ice for cooling the formula.

Single-use containers can be inverted and removed from the feeding set so that water may be added to flush the tubing or increase the fluid intake. When a single-use container is empty, the tubing is clamped until the next scheduled feeding, and then a new formula container is attached.

Reusable administration containers are usually heavy plastic bags with an attached feeding set. They have a snap-cap or foldover opening at the top of the container, which makes it easy to add more formula and yet keep room contaminants out of the formula. Some containers, such as the Kangaroo Tube Feeding Set (Chesebrough-Pond's, Inc.) have a side pouch for adding ice to keep the formula cold when continuous feedings are given, thus minimizing the potential for bacterial overgrowth. A drain plug at the bottom provides easy draining of melted ice. Some pumps, such as the Barron pumps, are equipped with their own reusable containers for formula and ice.

Sometimes improvised containers and tubing are used. The tubing of a clean and unused enema bag may be cut off a few inches below the bag and an intravenous tubing adaptor inserted and taped in place. Some institutions use empty resterilized glass intravenous fluid bottles or plastic irrigation bags to contain the formula, and use intravenous tubing as the feeding set. Since tube feeding is not a sterile procedure, as long as medically aseptic techniques are carefully followed these containers are considered safe.

All equipment used for intermittent feedings is thoroughly rinsed with cold water after each use and positioned in such a way that it can dry (such as hanging a feeding bag upside down to drain or separating the parts of a syringe). The equipment is then covered with a clean towel or wrapper rather than placed in a plastic bag. These practices discourage microorganism growth in any residual formula left in the equipment. Tube feeding equipment used for either continuous or intermittent feedings is changed every 24 hours for cleanliness and aesthetic purposes.

A large bulb syringe or a catheter *syringe* is used to aspirate gastric contents for checking tube placement and residual gastric volume. This same syringe may be used to administer an intermittent tube feeding by removing the plunger or rubber ball and reattaching the syringe to the feeding tube. A *funnel* may also be used for this purpose. The warmed formula is poured into the syringe or funnel from the single-use container, or from a *graduated measuring pitcher* if blenderized formula or large-sized commercial containers are used. The amount of formula must be measured. Use of this equipment for intermittent enteral feeding is illustrated in Figure 54–4.

Feeding Tubes
Feeding tubes usually are single-lumen tubes available in varying diameters and lengths. They may have open or closed tips, and usually are perforated with four or more openings at the distal end. Tube diameters are designated in French (F) sizes, as illustrated in Figure 54–5. The French size represents the diameter of the tube lumen, with one unit on the French

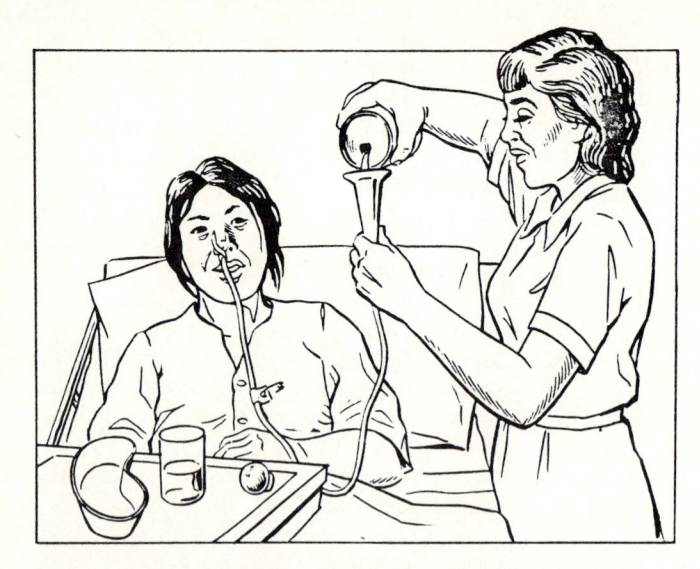

Figure 54–4. Administering an intermittent tube feeding with a syringe and container of warmed formula. The flow rate is regulated by the height at which the syringe is held.

scale roughly equivalent to 0.33 mm (Miller and Keane, 1983). Feeding tubes usually are fitted with a cap, plug, or clamp to close the open end between feedings or when the feeding is being temporarily suspended, as may be necessary during transport of the client within the hospital.

Older, Larger Tubes. Until recent years, the most commonly used feeding tubes were firm plastic (polyvinyl chloride) or red rubber Levin tubes of French sizes 12 to 18 F. Although there are numerous problems associated with the use of these large-diameter tubes for enteral feedings, unfortunately they still are frequently used. These problems include discomfort from the large diameter; irritation, ulceration, and necrosis of the nares; esophageal reflux, irritation, and stricture; and oral complications stemming from mouth breathing and dry mouth. With continued use, the tubes tend to harden, thus increasing nasal irritation. It is also often difficult for clients to swallow food and fluids around the tube on a supplemental basis, or even to swallow their own secretions. These problems are particularly common with red rubber tubes, which should never be used for other than very short-time purposes.

Small-Lumen Feeding Tubes. Recently, *small-lumen feeding tubes* have been developed; these are more pliable and soft and are made of silicone rubber, such as the Keofeed (IVAC) tube, or polyurethane such as the Dobhoff (Biosurg) tube. These tubes do not harden readily, thus minimizing the problems associated with the more rigid tubes. Secretions can readily be swallowed and clients can even eat and drink with this type of tube in place. However, they are more readily dislodged with vomiting than are larger tubes, and aspiration for gastric residual is more difficult. These tubes are available in two lengths, 90 cm (36 in) for nasogastric feedings and 125 cm (42 in) for nasoenteric feedings, and French sizes ranging from 5 to 12 F.

Small feeding tubes often have a mercury-weighted tip or a tungsten tip to aid in insertion and help maintain placement. An example is the 42-inch Keofeed tube. Longer feeding tubes have a larger mercury bolus at the tip that allows the tubing to pass from the stomach to the small intestine, if duodenal or jejunal rather than gastric feedings are required. These longer tubes are radiopaque so that correct placement can be determined by x-ray.

When removing mercury-weighted feeding tubes, the nurse follows special precautions for disposal of the mercury. The mercury tip is clipped off, placed in a container with a lid, and returned to central supply. Mercury is never placed in a trash can; it must be destroyed in a special incinerator that prevents emission of noxious gases (Cataldo and Smith, 1980).

Feeding tubes have indelible markings printed at evenly spaced intervals distal from the insertion tip. These markings provide points of reference for insertion and for visual inspection of tube placement. When a feeding tube is left in place, it is always carefully anchored in place. Tube markings and anchoring are discussed in Skill 56.

When selecting a feeding tube for a gravity-flow tube feeding, the diameter selected is the smallest one through which the feeding will flow. Generally, more viscous formulas require a size 10 F tube, while thinner formulas will readily flow through a 5 or 6 F tube. If a smaller tubing is desired for a viscous formula, a pump may be used to facilitate the flow.

There are a few disadvantages to these newer, smaller-lumen feeding tubes. The smaller tube lumen makes aspiration of gastric contents more difficult, thus requiring more time and patience when checking tube position or residual prior to feeding. They also are more likely to be coughed, sneezed, or vomited up out of the mouth or into the back of the throat. Tube

French size (F)	Inside diameter (inches)	Cross section (to scale)
Tube no. 8	1/16	◎
Tube no. 12	7/64	◎
Tube no. 14	1/8	◎
Tube no. 16	9/64	◎

Figure 54–5. French sizes and inside diameters of commonly used nasogastric tubes. The most comfortable French size for the adult client is 8 F. (From Gormican A: Tube feeding: A few common oversights. Dietetic Currents 2(2):1–6, 1975, with permission.)

position always is checked prior to the next feeding if the client has vomited or experienced severe coughing.

Feeding Pumps
Mechanical pumps deliver a constant flow rate of formula regardless of the client's position. Most pumps operate by a peristaltic pumping action. A portion of the tube leading from the food source usually is made of flexible latex or silicone. This flexible tubing is stretched over a rotor assembly, and as the rotor turns the tubing is stretched and alternately occluded and released. This action moves the formula in small, intermittent amounts into the stomach or jejunum. Some pumps are volumetric and can be set to deliver a steady flow of fluid over a given period of time, similar to an intravenous infusion pump.

Pumps designed specifically for enteral use are considerably less expensive than the more sophisticated intravenous infusion pumps, because the monitoring needed for enteral feedings is much less precise than for intravenous infusions. Intravenous infusion pumps are discussed in Skill 74. Although intravenous infusion pump rates usually can be adjusted in 1-ml increments, enteral pumps have larger increments or a series of rates from which to select. Enteral pumps have a flow rate accuracy of about plus or minus 10 percent, while intravenous infusion pumps are generally accurate within about plus or minus 2 percent. Enteral pumps have no air bubble detection, may or may not have a built-in battery, and usually have no volume administered readout—all of which are crucial for pump monitoring of intravenous fluids. Enteral pumps also are easier to operate and have fewer alarms—usually only occlusion, empty bag, and rate change alarms. The Kangaroo 330 Feeding Pump (Ross Laboratories) shown in Figure 54–6 is an example of an easy-to-operate enteral pump. It operates on either alternating current or built-in batteries, thus allowing for client ambulation. A built-in alarm system provides audiovisual signals (flashing lights and beeping) when the feeding container is empty or the tubing occluded, if the flow rate changes from its setting, or if the battery charge becomes low.

The Barron pumps are peristaltic volumetric pumps used to deliver either intermittent or continuous feedings. In the original model that was first developed in 1949, the flow rate is controlled by a series of pulleys and a belt that is shifted between pulleys to adjust the flow rate in milliliters per hour. For example, using a small groove on the motor side and a larger groove on the roller side will give a slow delivery rate, while a larger groove on the motor side combined with a smaller groove on the roller side will give a rapid delivery rate (Friedrich, 1962). Many of these original pumps are still in use and functioning well. The newer model, the Ethox/Barron Enteral Feeding Pump, has a dial selector for six different flow rates, indicated in both milliliters per 24 hours and milliliters per hour. The Barron pumps are illustrated in Figure 54–7. The formula bottle or feeding bag is placed on ice inside an insulated container and connected to the pump with a flexible tubing. The pump is then attached to the feeding tube. If the pump needs to be disconnected for more than a few minutes, the end of the tube coming from the pump to the client can be placed in the formula container and the motor left running. This keeps the formula circulating and prevents the formula in the tube from either spoiling or clogging the tubing.

Feeding pumps need to be wiped off with a damp cloth whenever formula is spilled on them. If this is not done, formula can sometimes leak into the pump mechanism and cause damage, and the pumps become sour-smelling and unpleasant to clients, families, and staff.

☐ EXECUTION

MONITORING TUBE PLACEMENT

Tube placement must be checked in several ways before giving each intermittent gastric feeding and every 4 hours for clients with continuous tube feedings. First, check the placement and taping of the tube visually, looking for intactness and location of markings. Second, insert 10 to 15 ml of air into the tube while listening to the epigastric area with a stethoscope. Third, aspirate the gastric contents with a bulb syringe or a large catheter syringe. The sound of air entering the stomach is clearly audible as a bubbling or gurgling sound. All three placement checks must be used, since only one check may give misleading information.

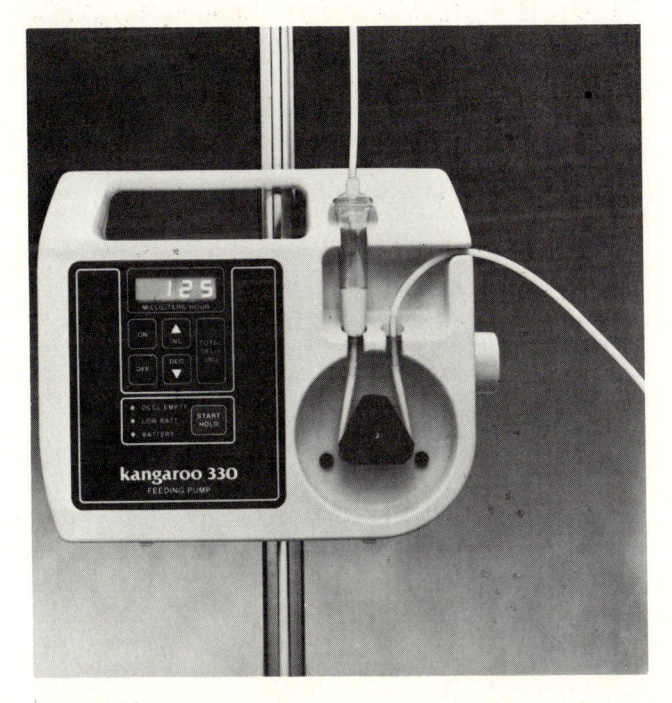

Figure 54–6. Kangaroo 330 Feeding Pump for enteral feedings. Note feeding set drip chamber, tubing in place around the rotor mechanism, flow rate indicators (ml per hour), operating buttons, and alarms. (Reproduced courtesy of Chesebrough-Pond's, Inc., owner of registered trademark "KANGAROO.")

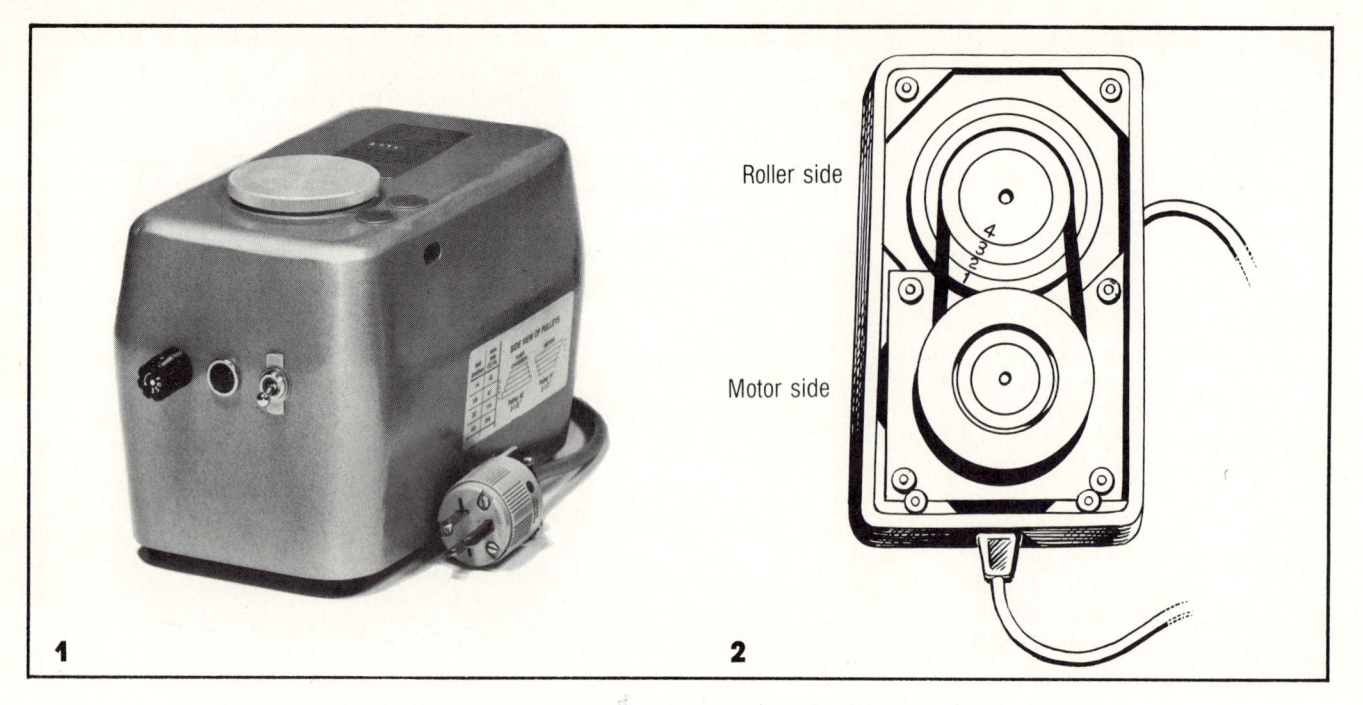

Figure 54-7. A. (1) The original Barron Food Pump for enteral feedings. (2) This pump uses a belt-drive mechanism to make four flow-rate adjustments: First speed (very slow), 43 ml per hour; second speed (slow), 65 ml per hour; third speed (moderate), 113 ml per hour; fourth speed (fast), 200 ml per hour. Using a small groove on the motor side combined with a larger groove on the roller side gives a slow delivery rate and vice versa. Formula container is placed in ice bucket near pump. (Courtesy of Ethox Corporation, Buffalo, NY.)

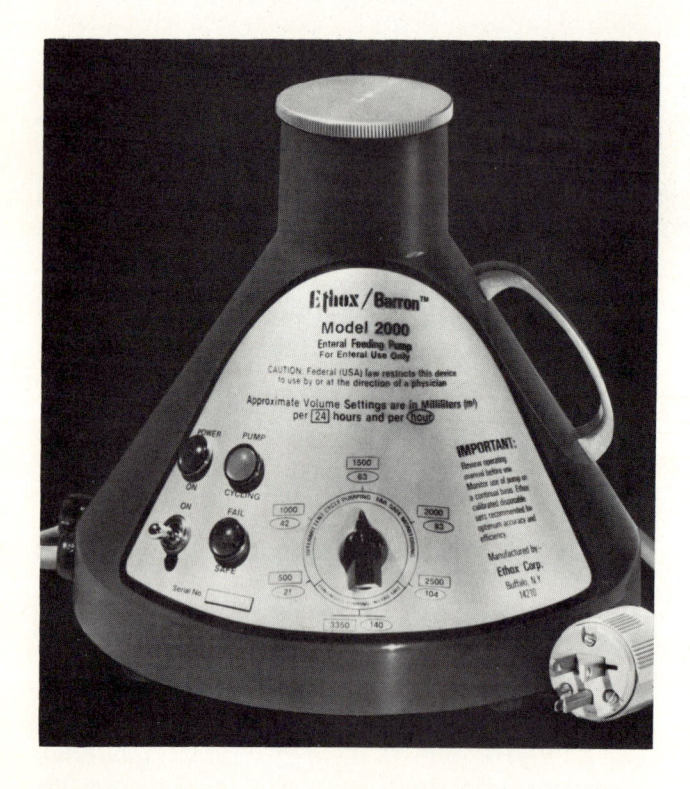

Figure 54-7. B. The Ethox/Barron Enteral Feeding Pump (Model 2000) has six dial-selected rates, ranging from 500 ml per 24 hours (21 ml per hour) to 3350 ml per 24 hours (140 ml per hour). Specially designed formula bags can be placed upright in ice bucket during use. (Courtesy of Ethox Corporation, Buffalo, NY.)

At the same time tube placement is checked, aspirate the *entire gastric contents,* measure them, and then return them to the stomach to prevent loss of vital electrolytes. If the aspirated volume exceeds 150 to 200 ml, the current feeding usually is not given as scheduled. Agency policy would determine whether the feeding is decreased by the residual over 150 to 200 ml, postponed for reassessment in 1 hour, completely omitted, or if the physician is to be consulted. If the client is alert, avoid emphasizing the presence of excessive amounts of residual, as it may cause concern to the client.

If a gravity-flow continuous or intermittent feeding does not flow properly, insert water through the tube, or move the tube in or out 1 inch or so, recheck for correct gastric placement, and reanchor.

SKIN CARE

Clients with nasogastric tubes require frequent and careful *oral and nasal care* because of the irritation of the tube in the external nares and the lack of normal oral stimulation from food and fluids. Remove and replace a feeding tube with a clean tube as needed for comfort and hygienic purposes. Wash the skin with a mild soap, rinse, and dry it. If there is drainage around the tube, zinc oxide or a vitamin A and D ointment may be applied to prevent or clear up skin irritation.

Precautions for giving medications through a feeding tube are discussed in Skill 71.

GIVING CONTINUOUS ENTERAL FEEDINGS

Clients receiving continuous enteral feedings need to have the head of the bed elevated to about 30 degrees at all times to prevent gastric reflux and aspiration of any regurgitated formula. Flush the tube with tap water every 4 hours and whenever the feeding is disconnected for more than a few minutes to mechanically cleanse the lumen of residual formula. This action avoids clogging and ensures tube patency.

Monitor continuous feedings by direct observation of the drip or pump rate and with a time tape. A *time tape* reflects the time span over which a given amount of formula is to be infused, and the amount of formula already infused. To prepare a time tape, determine the number of milliliters per hour, write the beginning time parallel to the inverted fluid level, the ending time at the near empty point, and the hourly markings at the appropriate milliliter level, as illustrated in Figure 54-8. A time tape is needed because a gravity flow drip rate varies as the feeding tube moves during activity and position change, and these flow rate variations can easily result in too much or too little formula being administered. Although a pump more reliably controls the amount of formula being infused, pumps do malfunction. Having the amount and elapsed time readily visible helps the nurse monitor the actual flow rate and plan when more formula needs to be added.

If a continuous enteral feeding falls behind its scheduled timetable, do not attempt to catch up. Either readjust the flow to the appropriate rate or reset the pump and make a new time tape, since too rapid an infusion rate may cause symptoms of intolerance or contribute to hyperosmolar dehydration.

Label a reusable formula administration container with the type of formula being administered, so that staff and physicians have that information readily available.

Agency policy usually indicates whether a 4- or 8-hour supply of formula is hung at one time and whether ice is used. If iced containers are used, check the supply at least every 8 hours, depending on the room temperature. Drain water and replace with new ice as needed. Remember to allow a reusable container to empty completely before adding more formula; otherwise the old formula can cause bacterial overgrowth. Obtain new enteral feeding equipment daily or at least 3 to 4 times a week to avoid residual formula contributing to microorganism overgrowth. Both gravity and pump alarms will allow only partial emptying of the tube after the container is empty. This small amount of air is not likely to cause gastric distress, since it is no greater than that used for tube placement checks.

GIVING INTERMITTENT ENTERAL FEEDINGS

Warm the formula to room temperature by placing the single-use container or measured amount in a pan

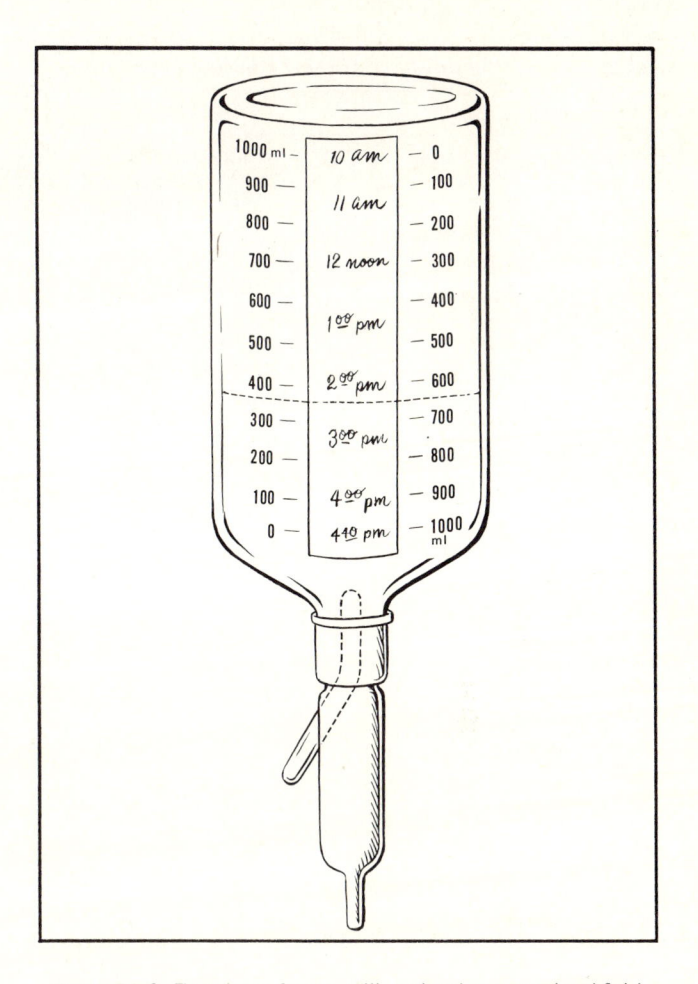

Figure 54-8. Time tape for use with enteral or parenteral fluid administration. This time tape was prepared for infusing 1000 ml of fluid at a rate of 150 ml per hour. It was hung at 10:00 A.M. and will end at approximately 4:40 P.M. The milliliter markings on the right side of the container represent volume levels of fluid used with the bottle inverted for administration; the markings on the left represent volume levels when the container is in an upright position. In this bottle, 650 ml have been infused, 350 remain, and the time should be about 2:20 P.M.

of hot tap water for approximately 15 minutes. Do *not* heat formula on a stove, because the higher, direct heat can cause protein coagulation and a clogged tubing, as well as destroy vitamins. Do not warm opened commercial or blenderized formulas by allowing them to stand at room temperature, since the length of time needed for warming would allow microorganisms to grow. Milk products are excellent culture media.

Position the client in at least a 45° elevation before beginning the feeding. If possible, increase this elevation to nearly upright for 30 minutes to 1 hour after the feeding, as this facilitates gastric emptying and decreases the potential for gastric reflux and heartburn.

After checking tube placement, hold or hang the formula container 12 to 18 inches above the stomach, and then raise or lower it as needed to cause the feeding to infuse within a 10-minute period. As would be expected, raising the container increases the flow rate, whereas lowering it decreases the flow rate.

TABLE 54-1. Summary of Enteral Feeding Monitoring

CHARACTERISTIC	FREQUENCY
Inspect nasogastric tube taping and check placement and residual	When initiating a new or intermittent feeding; q 4 hr with continous feeding
Check gravity drip rates	q 30 min-1 hr
Check pump drip rates	q 1-2 hr
Check glucose and acetone	q 4-6 hr for diabetic clients and all clients with glucosuria
Refill ice container, if used	q 4-6 hr (depending on room temperature)
Refill feeding container	q 4-8 hr
Provide oral care	q 4-8 hr and PRN
Measure intake and output	q 8 hr
Weigh client	q day
Rinse and dry feeding equipment	After each use for intermittent feedings
Change feeding container and tubing	q day
Check vital signs	According to agency routine
Change nasogastric feeding tube	As needed or ordered
Observe for untoward responses	PRN

Remain with the client during an intermittent feeding. If the client is alert and interested in helping, he or she may hold the syringe or pour the formula. This shared experience provides socialization and allows time to observe the client's reaction to the feeding. Conversation and a pleasant atmosphere increase the flow of digestive juices, resulting in increased tolerance of the formula. Flush a feeding tube with 30 to 90 ml of water after an intermittent feeding to prevent the formula from clogging in the tube. If the formula flow is sluggish, the tube may be flushed before administering the feeding to help start the flow of liquid. Some agency policies may require initial flushing to determine patency of the tube. The additional fluid also helps maintain an adequate fluid intake and increases the client's tolerance of more concentrated formulas.

After a feeding, rinse the equipment, allow it to air-dry, cover with a towel, and then reuse it for the next feeding. Obtain fresh equipment daily.

MONITORING ENTERAL FORMULA ADMINISTRATION

Table 54-1 presents a summary of the factors that need monitoring during administration of both continuous and intermittent tube feedings. Clients receiving continuous feedings are monitored regularly, day and night. Using a feeding pump decreases some of the need for frequent formula monitoring, but the *client* still needs to be monitored regularly.

☐ SKILL SEQUENCES

GIVING CONTINUOUS ENTERAL FEEDINGS

Step	Rationale
1. Validate physician's order for tube feeding and fluids, including type, amount, strength, and frequency.	Ensures that correct person receives correct feeding.
2. Wash hands thoroughly.	Avoids transfer of microorganisms.
3. Inspect cleanliness and anchoring of feeding tube. Change tubing if needed.	Soiled feeding tubes have an unpleasant appearance and odor, and can be sources of microoganism growth. Perspiration may loosen tape, allowing tube to slip.
4. Check equipment at bedside for completeness and cleanliness. Obtain new equipment as needed.	Conserves energy and time. Equipment does not need to be sterile since nose, throat, and stomach are not sterile body cavities.
5. Select correct formula: a. Note date and time on opened or blenderized formulas. Discard after 24 hours. b. If not using entire contents, label newly opened can with date and time opened and store in refrigerator. c. Note consistency of formula. Shake or mix exactly according to directions. d. Clean top of can before opening.	Potential for microorganism growth after opened more than 24 hours or is unrefrigerated. Provides data for next nurse. Ensures safety of remaining formula. Presence of lumps or curdling may interfere with flow through tubing. Correct mixing provides proper calories and fluids. Prevents contamination of contents.
6. Prepare new feeding set: a. Pour 4- to 8-hour supply of unwarmed formula into administration container and hang it from an IV pole. b. Squeeze drip chamber, filling it halfway. Allow tubing to fill with formula and close clamp. c. Attach administration set tubing to feeding tube and open clamp. d. Add ice to side pouch or ice container.	Avoids excessive warming of formula and growth of microorganisms. It is not possible to count drip rate if chamber is completely full. Keeps formula cool and prevents growth of microorganisms.
7. Prepare a time tape and apply to formula container.	Aids in monitoring flow rate.
8. Identify client by room and bed number, name, and identification band.	Ensures correct person receives ordered feeding.

(continued)

Step	Rationale
9. Attach new administration set tubing to feeding tube, or pour additional formula into existing container.	Maintains continuous formula flow.
10. Adjust flow rate manually with roller clamp or set pump to deliver desired rate.	Ensures giving correct amount of formula.
11. Keep head of bed elevated 30 degrees at all times.	Minimizes potential for gastric reflux.
12. Every 4 hours, clamp off tubing or shut off pump, disconnect feeding tube, and check tube placement: a. Inspect tape holding tube in place. b. Use asepto or large catheter syringe to aspirate gastric contents. c. Measure and return gastric contents to stomach. Do not give feeding if more than 150 to 200 ml gastric residual. Contact physician for further orders or consult agency policy, or both.	Loose tape may indicate incorrect tube placement. Presence of light-green gastric fluid helps identify delayed gastric emptying. Helps prevent electrolyte imbalance from lost gastric contents. Greater than 150 to 200 ml residual is considered delayed gastric emptying.
13. Add formula when container is empty.	Avoids clogged tubing from formula stasis. If container not allowed to empty completely, residual formula becomes culture medium for microorganism growth.
14. Remove water from side pouch or ice container and add more ice as needed.	Keeps formula cool and avoids growth of microorganisms.
15. Provide nasal or oral care as needed.	Increases client's comfort and sense of well-being.
16. Record placement checks and amount of residual; record type and volume of formula, rate of flow, and tolerance of feedings on flow sheets or in nurses' notes or progress notes.	Provides ongoing data base; indicates accountability for actions.

GIVING INTERMITTENT ENTERAL FEEDINGS

Step	Rationale
1. Follow steps 1 to 6 and 8, "Giving Continuous Enteral Feedings."	Same as in steps 1 to 6 and 8, "Giving Continuous Enteral Feedings."
2. Warm required amount of formula to no more than 36° to 38°C (97° to 100°F) by placing it in a pan of hot water for about 15 minutes. Do not heat on stove.	Warmed formula seems to cause less gastrointestinal distress. The body normally warms foods before they reach the stomach.
3. Close doors or draw curtains around bed unless client prefers otherwise.	Provides privacy.
4. Elevate head of bed to high Fowler's position, or at least 30 degrees. If not feasible, turn client on right side and elevate head of bed as tolerated.	Upright or right-side position helps fluid reach lower part of stomach, reducing potential for overfill and reflux.
5. Provide nasal or oral care as needed.	Increases client's comfort and sense of well-being.
6. Place a towel over the client's chest and bed linens nearest nurse. (NOTE: For gastrostomy feedings, fold linens below ostomy site and place towel over upper part of body.)	Prevents soiling and need to change linens or clothing. Provides ready access to tubing and privacy for client.
7. Remove clamp, cap, or plug from feeding tube.	
8. Check position of nasogastric or orogastric tube as in step 12, "Giving Continuous Enteral Feedings." (NOTE: For gastrostomy feeding, remove dressing, check anchor sutures and tube placement.)	Ensures correct tube placement.
9. Flush tubing with 30 to 60 ml of room-temperature tap water if flow is sluggish.	Clears tubing of any residual formula present and aids formula flow.
10. To administer formula using a syringe: a. Remove rubber bulb from asepto syringe or plunger from catheter syringe and attach to feeding tube. b. Gradually pour warmed formula into syringe (or funnel). Hold syringe at 45 degree angle when initially beginning to pour formula. c. Hold syringe 30 to 45 cm (12 to 18 in) above the stomach, adjusting height so as to administer formula in 10 to 15 minutes. (NOTE: Some clients are able to hold the syringe and participate in the feeding.) d. Pinch tubing over end of syringe to interrupt formula flow when adding more formula, or pour slowly and continuously. e. Avoid allowing syringe to empty completely. Do not force feeding with rubber squeeze bulb or syringe plunger.	Decreases amount of air that enters tubing. Allows fluid to enter stomach by gravity. Raising syringe increases force of gravity and lowering syringe reduces it. Prevents air from entering stomach. Allows unnecessary air to enter stomach. Forcing feeding may overdistend or rupture stomach.

(continued)

GIVING INTERMITTENT ENTERAL FEEDINGS (Cont.)	
Step	Rationale
11. To administer formula with a feeding set, pour warmed formula into administration container or attach feeding set to warmed single-use container. Follow steps 6, 9, and 10, "Giving Continuous Enteral Feedings." (NOTE: If administration set has a container that closes tightly, formula may be warmed after being poured into that container.)	Warmed formula seems to cause less gastrointestinal distress.
12. Remain with client; have an unhurried approach and engage in pleasant conversation.	More nearly simulates socialization of mealtime and enhances digestion.
13. Flush tubing with 30 to 90 ml water (more if ordered) at room temperature. Be sure to add water when formula level reaches bottom of syringe or container, <u>before</u> level drops into tubing. If necessary, fold and pinch feeding tube or close clamp on administration tubing while adding water.	Rinses tubing, prevents clogged tubing, and provides needed fluid volume. Prevents introducing air into the stomach.
14. Close or replace clamp on feeding tube. Repin to client's clothing.	Prevents leakage between feedings. Helps prevent inadvertent removal and increases client's comfort level.
15. Allow or encourage client to remain elevated for 30 minutes to 1 hour.	Facilitates gastric emptying.
16. Rinse and clean reusable equipment. Cover and leave in convenient location at bedside. Discard or return to central supply every 24 hours.	Prevents microorganism growth; clean equipment is aesthetically pleasing.
17. Record placement checks and amount of residual; record type and volume administered, time spent administering formula, and client's tolerance of feeding in health record.	Provides ongoing data base; indicates accountability for actions.

RECORDING

Record the kind and amount of tube feeding and additional water *actually* administered. Most agencies use either a specific flow sheet or an intake–output record for this purpose. Include at least a daily entry in the nurses' notes about the client's tolerance of the feeding and any problems that exist. Record tube position checks and the amount of residual obtained. If the feeding is held or delayed, record the amount of time and the reason. Tabulate fluid balance every shift and also every 24 hours for clients receiving tube feedings (see Skill 51).

Sample POR Recording

- S—Reported slight nausea and temporary heartburn after previous intermittent tube feeding. States "I feel full after the tube feeding."
- O—Tube taping intact; 25 ml residual obtained prior to feeding. No vomiting or abdominal distention noted after feeding.
- A—Adapting satisfactorily to tube feeding per nasogastric tube.
- P—Continue to increase the 100 ml feeding of Ensure by 75 ml per day rather than by 150 ml; increase administration time from 10 to 15 minutes; increase elevation of head of bed.

Sample Narrative Recording

Ensure, 100 ml given per N/G tube, c̄ only slight nausea and some heartburn. N/G tube remains in place; 25 ml residual prior to feeding. No abdominal distention or vomiting after feeding. Says, "I feel full after the tube feeding," and reported slight nausea and temporary heartburn after previous feeding.

☐ CRITICAL POINTS SUMMARY

1. When enteral feedings are initiated, increase the rate and concentration gradually and separately over 3 to 5 days.
2. Monitor fluid balance for all clients receiving enteral formulas.
3. Write the date and time on the label when formula is opened.
4. Store opened and unused formula in the refrigerator no longer than 24 hours.

CONTINUOUS ENTERAL FEEDINGS

5. Pour enough unwarmed formula into the administration container to last for 4 to 8 hours.
6. Allow the administration container to empty completely before adding more formula.
7. Drain water and replenish ice as needed, if iced containers are used.
8. Check the tube placement and gastric residual and flush the tubing every 4 hours.
9. Keep the head of the bed continuously elevated to a 30 degree angle.

INTERMITTENT ENTERAL FEEDINGS

10. Elevate the head of the bed to a 45 degree angle or higher.

11. Check the position of the nasogastric feeding tube prior to feeding.
12. Check for gastric residual and return all contents to the stomach unless greater than 150 to 200 ml.
13. Warm feeding prior to administration.
14. After feeding, flush the tubing with room temperature tap water.
15. Administer formula over a 10- to 15-minute time span.
16. Provide a pleasant mealtime environment.
17. Rinse the equipment thoroughly, cover with a towel, and leave at bedside.

LEARNING ACTIVITIES

1. Examine several varieties of enteral formulas in the utility room or supply area of a clinical unit that uses enteral feedings, or in the central supply area. Compare the sizes, ingredients, flavors, and container styles. Identify whether each container is for single-use or is refillable, and the type of feeding set that would be needed for administration. Read the labels to identify the kcal per ml and osmolality of each one.
2. Obtain an enteral pump and the administration equipment commonly used in your clinical facility. Assemble the equipment and fill the feeding container with colored water. Attach the tubing to the pump according to the directions and practice operating the pump. Allow the fluid to flow into a sink or pan. Observe the peristaltic mechanism (if visible), trigger the occlusion alarms by pinching the tubing, and reset the pump. Adjust the flow rate to various speeds.
3. In a clinical setting, observe enteral pumps being used to administer enteral feeding formulas. Note whether the container is reusable or single-use, if ice is being used, the type of formula, the amount infused over the last several hours, and the individual's position. Also note the size of the feeding tube and the security with which it is anchored. If the person is alert and willing, ask about the comfort level of the tube and feeding.
4. Interview several staff nurses for their perceptions of the advantages and disadvantages of continuous feedings given with and without pump monitoring and of continuous versus intermittent feedings.

REVIEW QUESTIONS

1. List three advantages of enteral nutritional support over parenteral nutritional support.
2. What are the advantages and disadvantages of commercial formulas as compared with noncommercial blenderized formulas?
3. For what reason (or reasons) are formulas warmed for intermittent bolus feedings and kept cool for continuous flow feedings?
4. Why are gastric contents aspirated and measured before an intermittent feeding? During continuous feedings?
5. How frequently is feeding tube placement checked with intermittent and continuous feedings? Why?
6. During the process of adaptation to formula feedings, why is the rate of feeding not increased simultaneously with the concentration of the formula?
7. What factors are evaluated to determine the amount of water given in addition to formula?
8. When administering enteral feedings, how can the following symptoms and problems be minimized or avoided?

   Nausea and vomiting Aspiration pneumonia
   Diarrhea   Fluid–electrolyte imbalance
   Heartburn   Hyperosmolar dehydration
   Glycosuria   Constipation

9. Why is the urine of both diabetic and nondiabetic tube-fed persons checked for glucose and acetone? How long does this monitoring continue for both kinds of clients?
10. How does the formula composition and rate of administration differ when jejunal feedings are given instead of gastric feedings?

PERFORMANCE CHECKLISTS

OBJECTIVE: To use correct medical aseptic technique to administer a continuous enteral feeding.			
CHARACTERISTIC	RANGE OF ACCEPTABILITY	SATISFACTORY	UNSATISFACTORY
1. Validates physician's order for formula and fluids.	No deviation		
2. Washes hands thoroughly.	No deviation		
3. Inspects anchoring and cleanliness of feeding tube.	No deviation		
4. Inserts new tube if needed.	No deviation		

(continued)

OBJECTIVE: To use correct medical aseptic technique to administer a continuous enteral feeding (cont.).			
CHARACTERISTIC	**RANGE OF ACCEPTABILITY**	**SATISFACTORY**	**UNSATISFACTORY**
5. Inspects tube feeding equipment for adequacy and cleanliness.	No deviation		
6. Obtains new equipment if needed.	No deviation		
7. Notes the date and time on opened or blenderized formula; discards outdated formula.	No deviation		
8. Follows directions for mixing or shaking formula.	No deviation		
9. Labels container.	No deviation		
10. Prepares time tape and applies to container.	No deviation		
11. Attaches new administration set with formula.	Pours additional formula into existing administration set.		
12. Identifies client by room and bed number, name, and identification band.	No deviation		
13. Adjusts flow rate manually or sets pump to correct rate.	No deviation		
14. Keeps head of bed elevated to 30 degrees at all times.	No deviation		
15. Every 4 hours, checks tubing placement. (Clamps tubing or turns off pump.) a. Inspects tape. b. Aspirates gastric contents. c. Measures and returns contents to stomach.	No deviation No deviation No deviation If gastric residual is more than 150 to 200 ml, hold feeding and consult with physician, agency policy, or both.		
16. Adds formula when container is empty.	No deviation		
17. Empties water and replenishes ice as needed.	No deviation		
18. Provides nasal or oral care as needed.	No deviation		
19. Records placement checks, amount of residual, type, volume, and flow rate of formula, and tolerance of feeding.	No deviation		

OBJECTIVE: To use correct medically aseptic technique to administer an intermittent enteral feeding.			
CHARACTERISTIC	**RANGE OF ACCEPTABILITY**	**SATISFACTORY**	**UNSATISFACTORY**
1. Validates physician's order for formula and fluids.	No deviation		
2. Washes hands thoroughly.	No deviation		
3. Inspects anchoring and cleanliness of feeding tube.	No deviation		
4. Inserts new tube if needed.	No deviation		
5. Inspects tube feeding equipment for adequacy and cleanliness.	No deviation		
6. Obtains new equipment if needed.	No deviation		
7. Notes date on formula container; discards if outdated.	No deviation		
8. Follows directions for mixing or shaking formula.	No deviation		
9. Warms formula to correct temperature.	No deviation		
10. Identifies client and provides privacy.	No deviation		

(continued)

CHARACTERISTIC	RANGE OF ACCEPTABILITY	SATISFACTORY	UNSATISFACTORY
11. Elevates head of bed to high Fowler's position.	Use at least 30 degree elevation. Follow medical restrictions on position.		
12. Provides nasal or oral care as needed.	No deviation		
13. Protects client's clothing and linens with towel.	For gastrostomy, cover upper body and expose gastrostomy site.		
14. Removes clamp, cap, or plug from feeding tube.	For gastrostomy, remove dressing, check sutures and tube placement.		
15. Checks tube placement: a. Inspects tape. b. Aspirates gastric contents. c. Measures and returns contents to stomach.	No deviation No deviation If gastric residual is more than 150 to 250 ml, hold feeding and consult with physician, agency policy, or both.		
16. Flushes tubing with 30 to 60 ml room-temperature tap water.	No deviation		
17. Administers formula with syringe: a. Holds syringe at correct angle to pour formula. b. Holds syringe at correct height. c. Maintains continuous flow of formula. d. Allows formula to flow in by gravity, allowing minimal air to enter stomach. e. Adjusts flow rate by raising and lowering container.	Client may hold syringe. No deviation No deviation No deviation No deviation No deviation		
18. Administers formula with feeding set: a. Fills container and tubing correctly. b. Adjusts gravity flow rate correctly.	No deviation Set pump correctly.		
19. Remains with client for observation and socialization.	Judgment may be exercised.		
20. Flushes tubing with 30 to 60 ml room-temperature tap water.	No deviation		
21. Records placement checks and amount of residual, type and volume of formula, length of administration time, and client's tolerance of feedings.	No deviation		

REFERENCES

American Dietetic Association: Handbook of Clinical Dietetics. New Haven, CT, Yale University Press, 1981.

Boucher M: Broken jaw cookbook. American Journal of Nursing 77(5):831–833, 1977.

Buergel N: Monitoring nutrition status in the clinical setting. Nursing Clinics of North America 14(2):215–227, 1979.

Cataldo CB, Smith L: Tube Feedings: Clinical Applications. Columbus, OH, Ross Laboratories, 1980.

Clinical News: Are tube feedings safe for patients with artificial airways? American Journal of Nursing 85(2):128, 1985.

Comparison shopping: Common commercial formulas. RN 44(11):36–38, 1981

Condon RE, Nyhus LM (eds): Manual of Surgical Therapeutics, ed 6. Boston, Little, Brown, 1985.

Dobie RP, Butterick OD: Continuous pump/tube enteric hyperalimentation—Use in esophageal disease. Journal of Parenteral and Enteral Nutrition 1(2):100–104, 1977.

Driscoll RH, Rosenberg IH: Total parenteral nutrition in inflammatory bowel disease. Medical Clinics of North America 62(1):185–201, 1978.

Friedrich HN: Oral feeding by food pump. American Journal of Nursing 62(2):62–64, 1962.

Griggs BA, Hoppe MC: Nasogastric tube feedings. American Journal of Nursing 79(3):481–485, 1979.

Hanson RL: Effects of administering cold and warmed tube feedings. Communicating Nursing Research 6:136–140, 1974.

Heitkemper ME, Hanson R, Hansen BW: Effects of rate and volume of tube feeding in normal subjects. In Batey MV (ed): Communicating Nursing Research. Boulder, CO, Western Interstate Commission for Higher Education, 1978, vol 10.

Heitkemper ME, Martin DL, et al: Rate and volume of intermittent enteral feeding. Journal of Parenteral and Enteral Nutrition 5(1):125–129, 1981.

Hoppe M: The new tube feeding sets: A Nursing80 product survey. Nursing80 10(3):79–85, 1980.

Jones DA, Dunbar CF, Jirovec MM: Medical-Surgical Nursing: A Conceptual Approach, ed 2. New York, McGraw-Hill, 1982.

Kagawa-Busby KS, Heitkemper MM, et al: Effects of diet temperature on tolerance of enteral feedings. Nursing Research 29(5):276–280, 1980.

Krause MV, Mahan LK: Food, Nutrition, and Diet Therapy, ed 7. Philadelphia, WB Saunders, 1984.

Kubo W, Grant M, et al: Fluid and electrolyte problems of tube-fed patients. American Journal of Nursing 76(6):912–916, 1976.

Metheny NM, Snively WD: Nurses' Handbook of Fluid Balance, ed 4. Philadelphia, JB Lippincott, 1983.

Miller BF, Keane CB: Encyclopedia and Dictionary of Medicine, Nursing and Allied Health, ed 3. Philadelphia, WB Saunders, 1983.

Padilla GV, Grant M, et al: Subjective distresses of nasogastric tube feeding. Journal of Parenteral and Enteral Nutrition 3(2): 53–57, 1979.

Rains BL: The non-hospitalized tube-fed patient. Oncological Nursing Forum 8(2):8–13, 1981.

Walike BC, Padilla GV, et al: Patient problems related to tube feeding. In Batey MV (ed): Communicating Nursing Research. Boulder, CO, Western Interstate Commission for Higher Education, 1975, vol 7.

Whitney EN, Cataldo CB: Understanding Normal and Clinical Nutrition. St Paul, MN, West Publishing, 1983.

Williams KR, Walike BC: Effect of the temperature of tube feedings on gastric mobility in monkeys. Nursing Research 24(1):4–9, 1975.

Williams SR: Nutrition and Diet Therapy, ed 4. St Louis, CV Mosby, 1981.

Luckmann J, Sorensen KC: Medical-Surgical Nursing: A Psychophysiologic Approach, ed 2. Philadelphia, WB Saunders, 1980.

Sorensen KC, Luckmann J: Basic Nursing: A Psychophysiologic Approach. Philadelphia, WB Saunders, 1979.

Suitor CW, Crowley MF: Nutrition Principles and Application in Health Promotion, ed 2. Philadelphia, JB Lippincott, 1984.

SUGGESTED READING

Cataldo CB, Smith L: Tube Feedings: Clinical Applications. Columbus, OH, Ross Laboratories, 1980.

Griggs BA, Hoppe MC: Nasogastric tube feedings. American Journal of Nursing 79(3):481–484, 1979.

Heitkemper ME, Martin DL, et al: Rate and volume of intermittent enteral feeding. Journal of Parenteral and Enteral Nutrition 5(1):125–129, 1981.

Metheny NM: 20 ways to prevent tube-feeding complications. Nursing85 (Horsham) 15(1):47–50, 1985.

Rains BL: The non-hospitalized tube-fed patient. Oncological Nursing Forum 8(2):8–13, 1981.

AUDIOVISUAL RESOURCES

Nasal Intubation for Enteral Feedings
  Film (1981, 20 min.)
Principles of Enteral Tube Feedings
  Part 1: Nutrient Needs and Formula Selection
  Part 2: Administration and Monitoring
  Part 3: Metabolic Monitoring
  Slide/cassette. (1982)
  Available through:
    Ross Laboratories
    Education Services Department
    625 Cleveland Avenue
    Columbus, OH 43216
Gavage
  Slides, filmstrip, videocassette, film. (1977, Color, 12 min.)
    Available through:
    Medcom, Inc.
    P.O. Box 116
    Garden Grove, CA 92642

BIBLIOGRAPHY

Adams MM, Wirching RG: Guidelines for planning home enteral feedings. Journal of the American Dietetic Association 84(1):68–71, 1984.

Arnold C: Why that liquid formula diet may not work (and what to do about it). RN 44(11):34–39, 1981.

Bayless TM, Rothheld B, et al: Lactose and milk intolerance: Clinical implications. New England Journal of Medicine 292(22):1156–1159, 1975.

Billings D McG, Stokes LG: Medical-Surgical Nursing. St Louis, MO, CV Mosby, 1982.

Brunner LS, Suddarth DS: The Lippincott Manual of Nursing Practice, ed 3. Philadelphia, JB Lippincott, 1982.

Gormican A: Tube feeding: A few common oversights. Dietetic Currents 2(2):1–6, 1975.

SKILL 55 Total Parenteral Nutrition

PREREQUISITE SKILLS

Skill 19, "Inspection"
Skill 28, "Handwashing"
Skill 30, "Sterile Supplies"
Skill 31, "Donning Sterile Gloves"

Skill 32, "Dressings and Wound Care"
Skill 51, "Monitoring Fluid Balance"
Skill 54, "Enteral Nutritional Support"
Skill 74, "Intravenous Fluid and Medication Administration"

STUDENT OBJECTIVES

1. Explain the purposes for which total parenteral nutrition (TPN) is used.
2. Identify situations where TPN is a useful therapy.
3. Describe the general composition of TPN solutions.
4. Describe potential complications from administration of TPN solutions.
5. Explain the relationship of complications associated with TPN administration to the composition of TPN solutions.
6. Explain nursing measures used to prevent complications and promote client safety during administration of TPN solutions.
7. Describe indications for using intravenous fat emulsions.
8. Explain precautions associated with administration of intravenous fat emulsions.
9. In the clinical setting, (a) add TPN solution to an existing central venous line, change the intravenous tubing and the subclavian dressing in a safe manner, (b) add fat emulsions to an existing peripheral venous line in a safe manner, and (c) monitor the infusion of TPN solutions and fat emulsions correctly.

INTRODUCTION

Parenteral nutritional feedings refer to nutrients provided by a route other than the gastrointestinal tract (enteral route). Although some nutrients can be given subcutaneously (such as fluids and glucose) or intramuscularly (such as vitamins), the primary parenteral route used for nutritional purposes is intravenous, normally via central veins.

Parenteral nutrition may be given as a supplement and provide only part of a client's nutritional needs, such as when clients who are dehydrated or unable to drink for a brief period of time are given glucose and electrolyte solutions. Alternatively, it may be used as the exclusive source of nutrients when other feeding routes are unavailable or are not feasible, that is, it is used to provide total parenteral nutrition.

Total parenteral nutrition (TPN) is the intravenous infusion of amino acids (nitrogen), hypertonic glucose, and other essential nutrients (vitamins, electrolytes, fats, minerals, and trace elements) in amounts great enough to meet the body's total nutritional needs for maintenance or to meet the additional demands of illness or debilitation. Insulin may be added to aid in glucose metabolism. Total parenteral nutrition is commonly called *hyperalimentation,* although this is technically incorrect. The latter term indicates nutritional support given in amounts that are in excess of usual requirements; however, this may or may not be true for TPN, depending on the specific client's requirements.

Total parenteral nutrition may be used in a variety of situations, such as with clients who have severe burns and a negative nitrogen balance; chronically malnourished clients being prepared for surgery; clients who will not be able to eat for 7 days or more postoperatively; clients with gastrointestinal disorders such as fistulas, enteritis, pancreatitis, or short bowel syndrome requiring that the gastrointestinal system be at rest; clients who are preparing for gastrointestinal surgery; clients with anorexia nervosa; clients suffering acute flare-ups of Crohn's disease; and some clients with cancer (Colley and Wilson, 1979a; Dietel et al., 1978; Ivey, 1979; Ladefoged, 1981; Mitchell and Scott, 1982). Almost any kind of undernourished, debilitated, or cachectic (malnourished with wasting) client can benefit from TPN, although the enteral route is preferred if it is possible to use. The enteral route is cheaper, safer, and has a more physiological utilization of nutrients. Some authors are beginning to question whether TPN sometimes is used as a life-support and life-prolonging measure rather than as a therapy directed toward recovery. They propose that clients who are to receive TPN ought to have a reasonable possibility for recovery or, as in the case of cancer clients, would receive significant palliation from radiotherapy or chemotherapy (Dietel et al., 1978; Hüshen, 1982; Steiger and Fazio, 1976).

Successful administration of TPN requires the joint efforts of an interdisciplinary team that includes the physician, pharmacist, nurse, dietitian, epidemiologist, social worker, discharge planning nurse, client, and family. In most agencies where TPN is administered regularly, interdisciplinary teams have established specific policies and procedures to ensure that catheter care and TPN administration are implemented precisely and consistently.

First developed in the late 1960s by Dr. Stanley J. Dudrick, TPN has become an increasingly common therapy and no longer is confined to intensive-care settings; clients are often sent home for long-term maintenance on TPN (Hales, 1979). Although the equipment and procedures are basically similar to those used in any intravenous infusion, the nature of the formula being infused and the insertion site mandate additional knowledge and skill for the nurse who is caring for a client with TPN in any setting. This skill focuses both on the administration of TPN formulas and the nursing care specific for clients receiving TPN.

PREPARATION

TPN CATHETER SITES

Total parenteral nutrition is administered through a polyvinyl or silastic catheter inserted into the subclavian vein and threaded into the vena cava with the tip near or in the right atrium, as shown in Figure 55–1. The rapid blood flow in a central vein readily dilutes the hypertonic TPN solution, minimizing the phlebi-

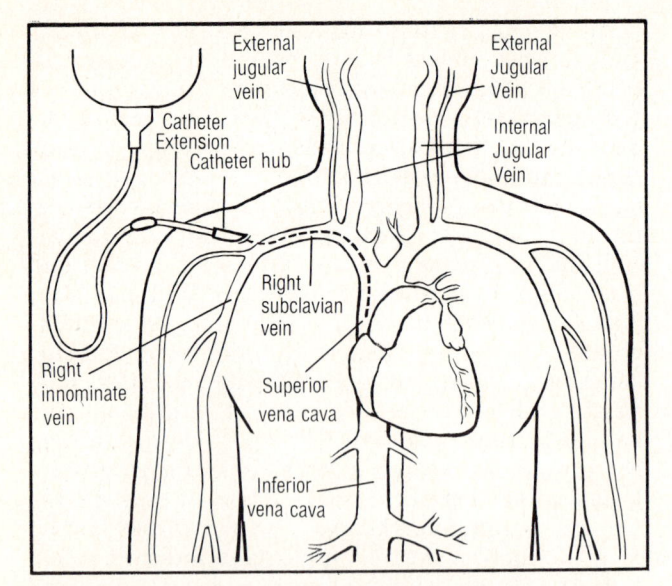

Figure 55–1. *The TPN catheter is usually inserted in the right subclavian vein and threaded into the superior vena cava, just outside the right atrium, or into the atrium itself.*

tis and thrombosis that would develop in 4 to 8 hours if the solution were administered in a peripheral vein. Although the catheter usually is inserted in the neck area through the subclavian or jugular vein, longer catheters sometimes are inserted peripherally, threaded through the vein, and the tip positioned similarly. The solution thus is delivered into a central location. For example, a right atrial Swan–Ganz catheter may be inserted in the brachial or cephalic (occasionally the femoral) vein, or an atrial catheter may be inserted through a subcutaneous tunnel on the chest or abdomen and into the external jugular vein. With a double-lumen right atrial catheter such as the Broviac–Hickman catheter, the small-lumen catheter (Broviac) is used for the TPN solution and the larger-lumen catheter (Hickman) is used for blood samples, monitoring pressure, or provision of other fluids and medications (Anderson et al., 1982). Insertion sites in the arm and femoral sites tend to have problems with phlebitis and more infusion problems because of increased fluid flow resistance in the longer tube.

The TPN catheter is inserted by the physician, using strict surgically aseptic technique and sutured in place at the insertion site to avoid accidental dislodging. A single-lumen TPN catheter is not used for any other purpose, such as blood sample withdrawal, central venous pressure (CVP) monitoring, or administration of drugs. This central line also is not irrigated, except by specific physician order, since that could cause contamination or dislodge any clots that may have formed.

During subclavian or jugular catheter insertion, the client is placed in the Trendelenburg position, which facilitates visualization of the area and helps prevent air emboli. A sheet rolled into a 3-inch cylinder and placed between the shoulder blades and down to the waist provides hyperextension of the shoulders and increased visualization. Additionally, the client is asked to perform Valsalva's manuever (breathing in and holding the breath while bearing down). Together with the positioning, this action helps keep air from rushing into the vena cava through the catheter (Colley and Wilson, 1979a). After the catheter is inserted, a chest X-ray is routinely taken to check the placement of the catheter tip. Administration of TPN is begun only after this position is confirmed by X-ray. Monitoring of vital signs is a crucial nursing responsibility during and immediately after catheter insertion.

TPN SOLUTIONS

The basic purpose of TPN is to achieve a positive rather than negative nitrogen balance, thus providing for anabolic rather than catabolic metabolism. A negative nitrogen balance and catabolism are characteristic of protein–calorie malnutrition, as discussed in Skill 52. A positive nitrogen balance is anabolic and promotes tissue repair, normal wound healing, and weight gain (Kaminski et al., 1977). Therefore, the TPN solution must provide for basic nutritional maintenance, restore previous losses in debilitated persons, and compensate for ongoing nutrient losses. A normal TPN solution contains approximately 1 kcal per ml, which is comparable to the usual enteral feeding formula. After initial adaptation, the usual volume administered is 3 liters, or 3000 kcal per 24 hours. To meet the caloric needs of some clients receiving TPN, more concentrated solutions may be used. For example, clients who have been burned may require up to 5000 to 7000 kcal per day. Intralipids (fats) may be given through a peripheral vein in addition to the TPN formula. When additional calories are needed, fats rather than glucose are preferred since there is less likelihood of the client developing hyperglycemia with glucosuria and osmotic diuresis, or of developing respiratory distress since the respiratory quotient (the ratio of the volume of expired carbon dioxide to oxygen) is lowered. Sufficient calories are given for the client to gain 0.1 to 0.2 kg per day (0.25 to 0.5 lb per day). If able, the client may take oral food in addition to receiving TPN.

Total parenteral nutrition solutions contain a balance of protein (amino acids) and hypertonic glucose (20 to 50 percent dextrose) that provides for optimal protein synthesis and anabolism within the body. Because of their high osmolarity, TPN solutions are always given through a central vein or a shunt. The maximum glucose concentration that is tolerated peripherally is 10 percent for adults (Mitchell and Scott, 1982). Solutions are prepared daily using strict aseptic technique, preferably in the pharmacy under a laminar-flow hood to prevent airborne contamination. It is preferable to add all needed electrolytes, vitamins, and the like at the time of preparation, but it is sometimes necessary to add more ingredients or insulin on the nursing unit. If this is done, the nurse must work in a clean, nonturbulent area, be extremely careful about dosages, and use strict aseptic technique. Because of their highly perishable nature, TPN solutions must be refrigerated until they are used.

RATE AND METHOD OF ADMINISTRATION

Similar to enteral feedings, the rate of TPN formulas needs to be initiated gradually so the body can adapt to the high concentration of dextrose. In adults, the flow rate is begun at 50 to 60 ml per hour and remains constant for nearly the first 24 hours (approximately 1 L per 24 hours). If the client does not develop glucosuria greater than 1 g per 100 ml, the rate is increased to 80 ml per hour for the second 24-hour period (2 L per second 24 hours), and then to 125 ml per hour for the third 24-hour period (3 L per third 24 hours). Sometimes the amount is increased to 4 L per 24 hours (166 ml per hour), but this is considered the maximum most clients can tolerate (Ivey, 1979; Krause and Mahan, 1984). Gradual initiation and careful monitoring of the client's responses are especially important when he or she has severe malnutrition or is severely stressed. Several deaths have been attributed to too much glucose given too rapidly and without proper monitoring to semistarved clients. It is recommended these persons be allowed more time (5 to 7 days) to adapt to TPN and that 20 to 30 percent of the kilocalories be supplied as fats (Aggressive TPN, 1981, pp. 97–98).

Glucosuria is generally transient and occurs only for the first 2 to 3 days, or when the dosage is increased. If glucosuria develops, the rate may be decreased or exogenous insulin administered to both diabetic and nondiabetic clients. Insulin must be given to correct the glucosuria and thus avoid osmotic diuresis, which results in fluid loss, weight loss, and electrolyte imbalance. The required amount of insulin may be added to the formula or given subcutaneously at intervals, on the basis of urine glucose tests. Adding the insulin to the TPN formula is thought to provide more even and adequate glucose metabolism and more stable blood glucose levels.

When TPN formulas are discontinued, the rate must again be lowered to 50 ml per hour for several hours to 1 day so that the body can readapt to the lower glucose levels (Blackburn, 1979; Hodges, 1979; Ivey, 1979; Kaminski et al., 1977). However, if the client's blood sugar levels are higher than 200 mg%, the physician will probably order a fairly rapid decrease in TPN flow rate to avoid excessive glucosuria and osmotic diuresis. Sometimes a 10 percent dextrose solution is used to help a client adapt to or become weaned away from TPN, since a 10 percent dextrose solution at 125 ml per hour is the dextrose equivalent of a TPN solution with 25 percent dextrose at a rate of 50 ml per hour. If for some reason the next bottle of TPN solution is not ready when needed, 10 percent dextrose in water ($D_{10}W$) can be safely used as a temporary emergency substitute to avoid having the line clot or the client develop hypoglycemia (Suitor and Crowley, 1984).

It is extremely important that a constant flow rate is maintained, because the client can develop hypoglycemia when the rate drops. An infusion pump or controller, rather than gravity flow, is always used for administering TPN. (See Skill 74 for a description of these devices.) Common mechanical causes for decreased flow rates include clogged filters, kinked tubing, or a malfunctioning catheter. If the flow rate of a TPN solution has been slowed inadvertently, no attempt should be made to catch-up. Rather the problem causing the slower rate is corrected and the pump reset at the prescribed rate. Ivey (1979) indicates that the flow rate should never be increased by more than 50 percent, even if the rate has dropped considerably below the prescribed rate, because most clients are unable to tolerate such a rapid increase in dextrose and respond by developing glucosuria. They may also become dehydrated from osmotic diuresis and may experience a sense of ill-being or impending doom.

TPN solutions may be administered in a continuous or cyclic manner, with glucose omitted for several hours while the protein solution continues to infuse. This is thought to promote utilization of fat and glycogen that are stored during glucose infusion, thus decreasing the likelihood of the client developing a fatty liver (Krause and Mahan, 1984; Suitor and Crowley, 1984). Another form of cyclic TPN involves infusing the TPN only at night while the client is asleep. The catheter is clamped, separated, and capped, and heparin is injected to avoid clogging of the tube. This method is often used for clients who are receiving TPN at home.

ADVERSE REACTIONS

Infections
The major complication associated with TPN administration is infection resulting from bacteria such as *Staphylococcus aureus, S. epidermis,* and *Klebsiella,* and from fungi such as *Candida albicans* (Giordano et al., 1981). The catheter provides an entry for pathogens; the concentrated glucose solution provides an excellent medium for bacterial growth; the occlusive dressing provides a warm, dark environment; and the client is usually already debilitated. Infections may develop from contamination of the catheter, insertion site, tubing, filters, or solution. Bacteria from anywhere on the body can attach to the catheter tip where they become a point of origin (nidus) for continued infection. Total body infection (septicemia) may also occur. Unexplained, persistent fever should be suspected as indicating a TPN-associated infection. If a sudden dramatic temperature spike occurs, it probably means that the solution has been contaminated. A temperature of 38.5°C (101°F) or a 1°C (2°F) increase in temperature elevation must be reported to the physician promptly. The development of glucos-

uria in clients who have been stable is usually followed by an infection within 18 to 24 hours. If infection is suspected, the entire intravenous equipment system must be changed, including the catheter hub. If an unexplained fever continues, the physician will probably remove the catheter and reinsert a new one. Potentially infected catheter tips are always cultured. To do this, the last few inches of the catheter are snipped off with a sterile scissors, placed in a sterile glass tube, and taken immediately to the laboratory.

Venous Complications

Thrombosis or thrombophlebitis may occur, partially due to irritation of the vein from traumatic insertion of the more stiff polyvinyl tubing and from hypertonic solutions. Signs and symptoms such as pain and swelling at the arm and neck or at the insertion site must be reported promptly.

Metabolic Complications

Hyperglycemia may occur from too rapid an infusion of a highly concentrated TPN formula, resulting in glucosuria and osmotic diuresis. If not corrected, serious dehydration and eventual loss of consciousness may occur. *Hypoglycemia* may result if the TPN formula is stopped abruptly or the rate is slowed drastically. Hypoglycemia results from the endogenous insulin that is secreted in response to the concentrated glucose solution. *Fluid and electrolyte imbalances* may occur, especially when TPN is first begun. Initially, low potassium and phosphorus levels are common because these minerals move back into the cells as anabolic metabolism replaces catabolic metabolism. Although these imbalances rarely last longer than 1 week and stabilization usually occurs, phosphorus, potassium, and other electrolytes such as calcium, magnesium, sodium, and chlorides are usually monitored on a twice-weekly basis. A *fatty acid deficiency* may occur after 2 or 3 months of TPN therapy if no fats are given concurrently.

Air Embolism

If the infusion system separates accidently, such as during client activity or position change, an air embolism may occur because of the open tubing and the lower pressure in the central venous system. The symptoms of this air embolism include coughing, shortness of breath, and chest pain. If separation and embolism occur, the infusion system must be reconnected immediately (or clamped with a padded hemostat if this is not possible), the client must be positioned on his or her left side, and the physician must be notified. If detected promptly, the symptoms will usually subside in 10 to 20 minutes (Sattler et al., 1978).

Because of the potential for air embolism with accidental separation, all tubing connections require careful taping. Locking connectors such as Luer-Lok may also be used.

FAT EMULSIONS

Fat emulsions are often given concurrently with TPN solutions, both to prevent fatty acid deficiency and to increase the client's total calorie intake beyond what is possible with TPN solutions. One bottle of fats per week will generally prevent this deficiency from occurring in clients who are receiving nothing by mouth. The benefits from giving fats rather than increasing glucose intake have already been discussed. There are two commercial brands of fat emulsions available: Intralipid 10 percent and 20 percent (derived from soybean oil) and Liposyn 10 percent and 20 percent (derived from sunflower oil). Both solutions are isotonic; the 10 percent solution provides 1.1 kcal per ml and 0.1 g of fat per ml and the 20 percent solution provides twice those amounts. Lipids do not need to be refrigerated. Some types of intralipids can be mixed with TPN solutions. Hospital policy will indicate when this is possible.

An emulsion is a mixture of two liquids that are not mutually soluble, with one dispersed throughout the other in small droplets or globules. If a fat emulsion separates or becomes frothy, it is not safe for intravenous administration and must be discarded. An emulsion must be totally homogenized. Fat emulsion separation is visible as oiling out (separation into layers) or creaming (separation into fat globules).

As with TPN solutions, the first time a fat emulsion is administered, it is given slowly so that any allergic reactions may be noted. These reactions are similar to blood transfusion reactions, with symptoms of dyspnea, cyanosis, nausea and vomiting, flushing, perspiration, elevated temperature, and headache. An initial rate of 1 ml per minute in 15 to 30 minutes for 10 percent lipids or 0.5 ml per minute in 30 minutes for 20 percent lipids is recommended. The maximum rate for 10 percent lipids is considered to be 500 ml over a 4-hour period, whereas the maximum rate for 20 percent lipids is considered to be 500 ml in 8 hours (Hutchison, 1982).

Additives are *never* put into a fat emulsion, since they may be incompatible and cause the emulsion to separate. Povidone iodine or alcohol is used to cleanse the bottle stopper before inserting the adaptor spike straight into the stopper. The adaptor spike may be twisted to seal it *after* it is inserted, but a twisting motion during insertion may dislodge minute particles from the stopper. Tubing is primed very slowly to avoid introducing air bubbles, and a filter is *never* used because it could also break down the emulsion. Fat emulsions are intended to be single-dose solutions; unused portions of a container must be discarded rather than saved for a later dose.

Some clients may experience an unpleasant taste sensation during the infusion of lipids. This taste can be diminished by slowing the infusion rate, giving the lipids during sleep, or by changing from a soybean to a sunflower product (Hutchison, 1982).

DATA BASE

Client History and Recorded Data

The health record contains information about the client's diagnosis, the reason the TPN solutions are being given, the type of solution and flow rate ordered, and progress notes about the client's response to TPN therapy. The nurse would want to know the results of urine testing for glucose, the temperature pattern, the intake and output values, and the laboratory results for blood glucose and phosphorus. Phosphorus is monitored because hypophosphatemia can occur when large amounts of glucose are metabolized (Hodges, 1979).

The nurse observes the client's color, skin condition, appearance, and orientation, since changes may indicate development of hyperglycemia or hypoglycemia, electrolyte or mineral imbalance, or various deficiencies. Any subjective complaints about discomfort or feeling ill must also be thoroughly investigated.

Since TPN formulas are administered to correct or avoid nutritional problems, the nurse assesses the client's nutritional status, both initially and at least on a weekly basis during therapy. Assessment of nutritional status is discussed in Skill 52.

Physical Appraisal Skills

Inspection. Inspection is used to determine intactness of the arterial catheter dressing, the security of the tape on the tubing and catheter junctions, and of the tape that holds the filter in place. Inspection also reveals any local signs of infection that may be evident when the dressing is changed. Inspection will reveal any cloudiness, precipitates, or particulate matter evident in TPN solutions, any separation and frothing in fat emulsions, and any glass cracks in the bottles. The nurse also inspects the flow rate of the TPN solution or fat emulsion and visually compares the actual rate of delivery with the time tape. Inspection is also used for order verification. This can be done by comparing the label on the prepared solution with the physician's order as it appears in the computer system, nursing-care kardex or care plan, or on the order sheet in the client health record. This comparison is always done carefully because of the variety of similar abbreviations used in labeling, such as mmol (millimoles), min (minutes), ml (milliliters), mg (milligrams), and mcg (micrograms).

SELF-CARE

When the subclavian site is used, clients and family members often find the insertion of a large needle into a vein near the neck more frightening than a peripheral intravenous infusion with a smaller needle. Other frightening aspects of TPN therapy include the mask that is worn for dressing changes, the extra care and monitoring the infusion setup receives, and the special instructions (Valsalva's maneuver and position) for tubing changes with the subclavian site. Clear yet simple explanations and instructions can help alleviate this distress and increase the client's level of understanding and cooperation. Some institutions have developed client information sheets that briefly explain what TPN is, where and why it is given, and what kind of food value they are receiving. One information sheet explains that a standard bottle of TPN contains a little over 1/2 lb of sugar and the protein equivalent of seven slices of beef liver (Connor and DiTrapano, 1981).

Clients are sometimes sent home while still requiring TPN solutions and have been able to return to productive work, infusing their solutions at night during sleep (Ivey, 1979; Sattler et al., 1978; Suitor and Crowley, 1984; Whitney and Cataldo, 1983). When clients are sent home with a TPN catheter in place, the family must be instructed about all aspects of TPN administration and given ample time to practice under nurse supervision (Schneider and Mirtallo, 1981).

EQUIPMENT

Standard *intravenous infusion equipment* is used to administer TPN solutions. This equipment is described in Skill 74. Scrupulous technique is needed when changing bottles or bags of solution, because systemic infection can easily result from poor technique. Some agencies require that a bacterial filter and a 0.22-micron air filter be added to the intravenous tubing; others require the less expensive 5-micron air filter (Colley and Wilson, 1979a; Ivey, 1979). A filter is not used with fat emulsions, except when administered in combination with a TPN solution. In that event, at least a 1.2-micron filter must be used to avoid breaking the fat molecules.

Although no adverse reactions have been reported with conventional tubing, some sources recommend that a tubing with a lower phthalate concentration be used to administer lipids because of the possibility of phthalate extraction into the emulsion (Hutchison, 1982). Such tubings may come with the lipid solution or are available from pump manufacturers.

A short extension tubing may be inserted between the catheter hub and the filter. This makes it possible to change the filter and tubing without disturbing the dressing.

As indicated earlier, an *infusion pump* or *control device* is used to administer TPN solutions. Fat emulsions may be delivered with pump devices through a *gravity-flow infusion*. If gravity flow is used, a monitoring device is needed to monitor the flow rate accurately. These devices, described in Skill 74, are useful because the built-in audible or visual alarm systems promptly alert the nurse to either decreased or increased flow rates. Thus, it is possible to detect and remedy problems readily, and to avoid the hypoglycemia and hyperglycemia often associated with variable infusion rates of TPN.

Commercially prepared sterile disposable *subclavian dressing kits* are available for changing the dressing on the catheter insertion site. A typical sterile kit would include the following:

- Presaturated acetone, alcohol (or an acetone–alcohol combination), and povidone–iodine swabs for skin cleansing
- Sterile gauze sponge and povidone–iodine ointment for application at the catheter insertion site
- Sterile gauze and occlusive tape for the final dressing
- Face masks for the nurse and the client
- Disposable sterile gloves
- Scissors and forceps for manipulating the dressing (optional)

Some institutions prepare their own subclavian dressing trays to fit their specific protocols. Instead of presaturated swabs, the tray may contain many gauze squares, several forceps, and small cups. Acetone, alcohol, and povidone–iodine are poured from larger stock bottles into the cups, and the gauze squares are held with forceps and used as sponges for cleansing the skin. If no trash bag is included in the kit, the outer plastic bag container or a wastebasket may be used to discard the soiled dressing and used wet swabs.

A gauze dressing is used over the insertion site, and then a piece of adhesive-backed elasticized bandage, surgical foam, or 2-inch silk tape is used to cover both that dressing and an additional 1-inch skin area on all sides. This procedure creates a well-sealed occlusive dressing, as shown in Figure 55–2.

Another option for a subclavian dressing is to use a transparent semipermeable dressing such as Op-Site, Tegaderm, or Ensure instead of gauze. Because the incision site is visible and can be monitored, this dressing can be changed less often, such as on a weekly basis. However, one study of 261 persons receiving TPN found a consistent but not statistically significant increase in catheter-related sepsis with this type of dressing (Powell et al., 1982).

Adhesive tape is used to seal all tubing and catheter junctions to avoid accidental separation. Some institutions use special tubing tags to record the date,

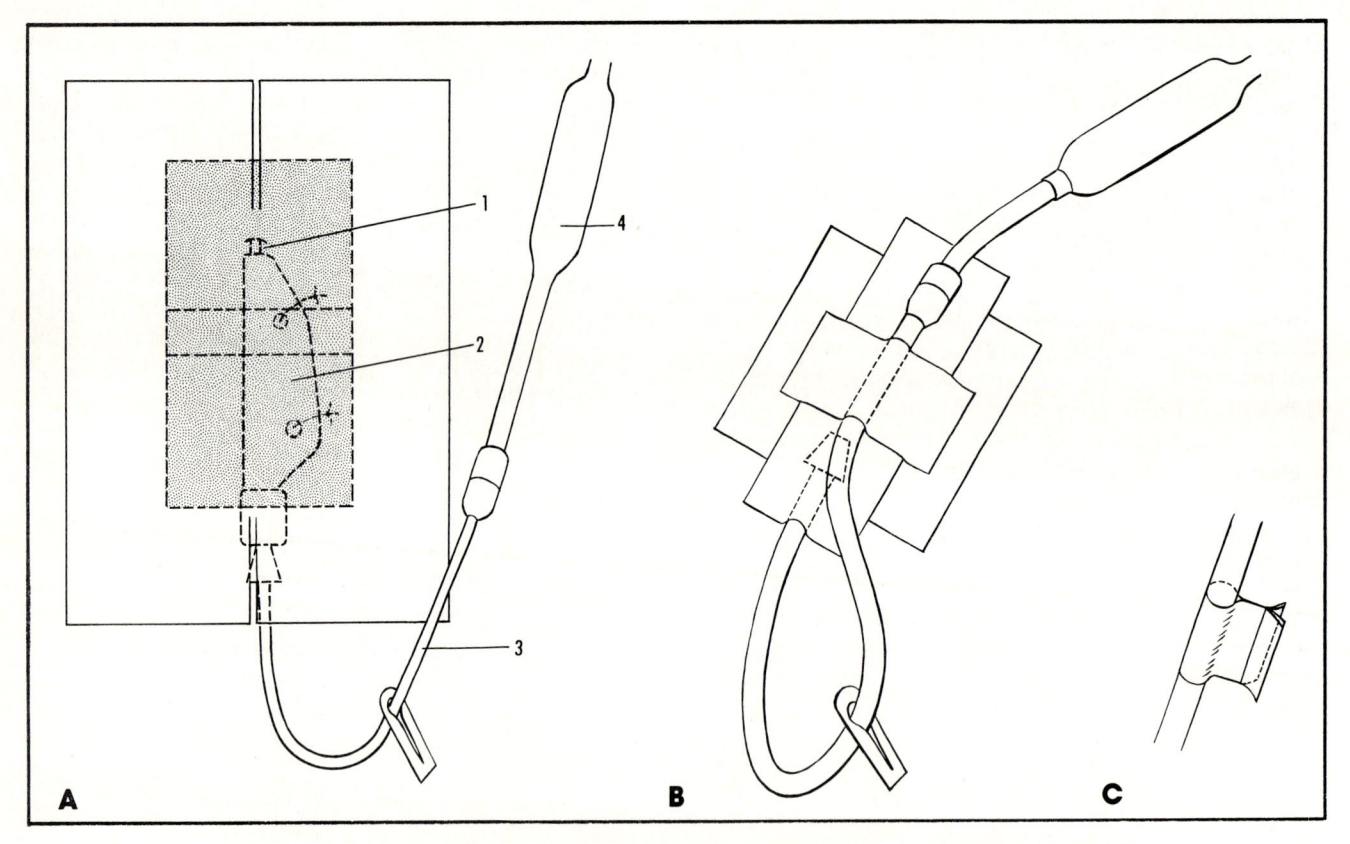

Figure 55–2. Occlusive dressing for subclavian insertion site. **A.** Partially completed dressing shows (1) catheter insertion site, (2) plastic catheter guard sutured in place to avoid accidental dislodging, (3) extension tubing with slide clamp, used to facilitate tubing change without disturbing dressing, and (4) filter set. The shaded areas represent 2 × 2 inch gauze sponges placed beside and over the insertion site and the solid lines represent two strips of 2-inch silk tape placed over the gauze squares. **B.** Completed dressing showing third strip of 2-inch tape placed over the center of the dressing and securing the junction between the catheter and the extension tubing, with the extension tubing looped back over the dressing and taped in place. The filter set–extension tubing junction has not yet been taped. **C.** Method for taping tubing connections securely: A 4-inch strip of 2-inch tape with turned-back ends is placed securely around connections. The turned-back tabs face each other and are ready for removal.

time, and the nurse's initials when tubing is changed. In other institutions this information is written on adhesive tape and attached to the tubing. Adhesive tape is also used to anchor the filter to the dressing for security purposes. *Time tapes* may also be used to help monitor the flow rate for both TPN solutions and fat emulsions, since they provide an overall time perspective. These tapes are described in Skills 54 and 74.

☐ EXECUTION

GOALS OF CARE

Major nursing goals in the care of a client receiving TPN solutions are to (a) prevent infection, (b) maintain a constant flow rate, and (c) detect glucosuria and electrolyte imbalance.

Prevention of Infection
Prevention of infection is best achieved by paying strict attention to every detail involved in changing the tubing, bottles, and dressing. No shortcuts are permissible, and even the slightest break in aseptic technique may be the cause of a local infection or a septicemia. Monitor the client at least every 8 hours for systemic signs of infection, such as elevated temperature and pulse rate. Inspect the insertion site for signs of local infection whenever the dressing is changed.

Maintenance of Constant Flow Rate
To maintain a constant flow rate, use an infusion-control device or a pump and a time tape, and personally check the flow rate frequently.

Detection of Glucosuria and Electrolyte Imbalances
To detect *glucosuria*, monitor urine glucose every 6 hours throughout the course of TPN therapy, using Tes-Tape paper or Clinitest tablets for this purpose. A 2 percent glucose is reported to the physician as soon as possible, so that temporary insulin adjustments may be made. Smaller amounts of glucosuria may be reported during regular physician visits.

Urine glucose is reported in percentage, not with a 1+ to 4+ scale because of the discrepancy in the value of those units in the two commonly used glucose tests—Tes-Tape and Clinitest tablets. A 2 percent glucose is measured as a 4+ when using either method, but a 1+, 2+, or 3+ with Tes-Tape is less than or equivalent to a 1+ with Clinitest tablets. It is also to be remembered that some drugs, such as aspirin and the cephalosporins (Keflin, Ceclor), can cause false-positive Clinitest results.

It is not generally considered necessary to monitor urine acetone levels because ketonuria does not occur unless the client is diabetic and receiving insufficient insulin (Kaminski et al., 1977). Electrolyte imbalances can be detected early by regular monitoring of laboratory analyses of electrolytes, which is usually done three times per week.

TUBING AND DRESSING CHANGES

The Centers for Disease Control (CDC) suggest that tubing be routinely changed every 24 to 48 hours (Simmons et al., 1981, p. 5).

During tubing change for a subclavian site, the client must be placed in a flat or slight Trendelenburg position (unless contraindicated). Before disconnecting the old tubing, ask the client to perform Valsalva's maneuver (hold breath and bear down) while the tubing is being changed. The flat or Trendelenburg position (rather than a semireclining position) increases the venous pressure at the insertion site, and Valsalva's maneuver provides a positive intrathoracic pressure (a negative pressure occurs on expiration). The combination of these two factors prevents air from rushing into the central venous line when it is opened, which would result in an air embolism. Air embolism is a rare but often lethal complication (Coppa et al., 1981). If the client has an endotracheal or tracheal tube and is unable to perform Valsalva's maneuver, a second nurse is needed to ventilate the client with a

TABLE 55-1. Monitoring Patients with TPN Solutions

CHARACTERISTIC	FREQUENCY
Monitor flow rate	q 30 min–1 hr
Examine the dressing and tubing connections	q 2–4 hr
Take temperature, pulse, and respirations	q 4–8 hr or as ordered
Measure urine glucose	q 6 hr or as ordered
Measure intake and output	q shift and q 24 hr
Read formula label	When delivered to unit or when adding to the infusion set up
Weigh client	Daily
Take calorie count (by dietitian)	Daily
Observe color, appearance, and orientation	Daily or when changes occur
Change intravenous tubing	q 48 hr or as ordered
Change subclavian dressing	Three times per week or as ordered
Record findings	As needed

mechanical breathing bag. The tubing is changed while the inspiratory phase is held, and before it is released (Colley and Wilson, 1979b). To help prevent an air embolism, the procedure is done quickly, but not so quickly as to cause contamination of the catheter and equipment. Because of the meticulous attention to detail that is required, it generally takes an experienced nurse about 15 minutes to change a subclavian dressing.

The dressing at the insertion site is changed two or three times per week, depending on institutional policy. The Centers for Disease Control recommend inspecting and redressing the insertion site every 48 to 72 hours (Simmons et al., 1981, p. 5). Either alcohol, acetone, or a combination of the two, is used to cleanse the skin of debris and surface fats, followed by a gentle povidone–iodine (Betadine, Isodine, PVP-1) scrub. If the person is sensitive to iodine, another antibacterial agent might be used, but iodine is preferred because of its antifungal action against the most common source of infection—*Candida albicans*. If a tincture of iodine is used, it must be removed with alcohol because of its irritant action on the skin. Povodine–iodine is an iodophor, which is less irritating to the skin and should be allowed to dry on the skin.

Labeling the tubing and dressing with the date, time, and nurse's initials helps avoid additional expense, energy, and increased potential for infections from unnecessary changes. All tubing connections must be taped securely to avoid accidental separation during activity or nursing care, as shown in Figure 55–2.

MONITORING TPN THERAPY

Clients receiving TPN therapy are weighed daily, using the same scales at the same time of the day and with the client wearing the same clothing. A weight gain that is greater than ½ lb per day may be due to fluid retention. Intake and output are always monitored when clients receive TPN. The many factors that require regular monitoring when clients are receiving TPN solutions are summarized in Table 55–1.

☐ SKILL SEQUENCES

TUBING AND SOLUTION CHANGE

Step	Rationale
1. Validate physician's order for solution, including type, amount, strength, and flow rate.	Ensures correct person receives correct feeding.
2. Gather needed equipment.	Increases time-efficiency.
3. Raise bed to a convenient working height; clear over-bed table.	Facilitates use of good body mechanics; provides adequate work space.
4. Inspect solution for precipitate; compare ingredients on label with health record and IV record.	Indicates unacceptable solution, as precipitates would clog filter. Ensures use of correct solution.
5. Identify client by checking room and bed numbers, identification band, and call by name.	Ensures solution is given to correct patient.
6. Explain procedure to client.	Decreases client's apprehension; increases client's self-care knowledge.
7. Place client in a flat or slight Trendelenburg position, depending on agency or physician policy.	Helps avoid air embolism when changing tubing.
8. Wash hands.	Prevents transfer of microorganisms.
9. Use flawless aseptic technique to attach new tubing to new bottle of TPN solution, prime (fill) tubing and filter and replace tubing cap as in Skill 74, Skill Sequence, "Preparing an Intravenous Infusion," steps 11 to 15, p. 947. (NOTE: New bottles of TPN solution are added to the existing tubing, except at the q 48 hour tubing change.)	Aseptic technique avoids contamination and infection. Advance preparation facilitates rapid tubing change. More frequent tubing change does not significantly decrease infection rates.
10. Remove old tubing from pump or rate controller, decreasing rate to "keep open." Place new tubing in pump.	Prepares for rapid changeover to new tubing.
11. Remove any tape or dressing covering catheter hub or extension set and tubing junction site. Swab junction of catheter hub and tubing with povodine–iodine or alcohol.	Provides access to junction site. Decreases potential for bacterial contamination.
12. Place sterile gauze square beneath junction.	Provides small sterile field.
13. Hold new tubing between first and second fingers with cap slightly loosened.	Readies new tubing for quick changeover.
14. Ask client to perform Valsalva maneuver (bear down and hold breath); clamp off old tubing; quickly remove it and insert new tubing. Use hemostat if connection is snug (or have a second nurse insert the new tubing).	Holding breath and bearing down increases intrathoracic pressure, preventing air from rushing into opened catheter. Having catheter open for a minimal time decreases potential for air embolism.
15. Open tubing, turn on pump, set at desired rate.	Reinstates flow promptly to prevent clogging the catheter.

(continued)

Step	Rationale
16. Secure all connections with adhesive tape; tape filter to dressing.	Prevents accidental separation of tubing with air embolism. Prevents tugging on catheter from filter being caught on clothing or linen with possible dislodging of catheter.
17. Check entire setup to be sure all clamps are open, pump or flow rate is set correctly, all junctions are taped, and no leaks are present.	Final check avoids serious problems (decreases flow or openings into system) going undetected.
18. Tag tubing with date, time, and own initials.	Indicates accountability. Provides data for ongoing nursing care.
19. Return client to a position of comfort.	Promotes rest.
20. Dispose of used equipment in appropriate manner.	Demonstrates responsibility for own clean-up.
21. Wash hands.	Avoids cross-contamination.
22. Record tubing change on kardex, in nurses' notes, or in progress notes in health record, or on appropriate flow sheet indicating date, time, and any problems.	Indicates accountability; provides data for ongoing care.

DRESSING CHANGE

Step	Rationale
1. Gather needed equipment.	Increases time-efficiency.
2. Raise bed to a convenient working height; clear over-bed table.	Facilitates use of good body mechanics; provides adequate work space.
3. Explain procedure to client.	Decreases client's apprehension, increases client's self-care knowledge.
4. Position client flat on back; expose client's shoulder area.	Provides adequate visualization; helps avoid air embolism if tubing is also changed.
5. Wash hands.	Prevents cross-contamination.
6. Inspect dressing for drainage and intactness. Remove old tape that holds filter and extension tubing onto dressing. Loosen taped edges of old dressing.	Prevents tugging on catheter, with accidental dislodging.
7. Change tubing and extension set as on pp. 955–956.	Increases time-efficiency and avoids later additional interference in system.
8. Open prepackaged kit or assemble needed items on sterile field.	Provides sterile equipment and work area.
9. Don face mask and give face mask to client to wear.	Decreases chances of contamination from respiratory secretions.
10. Remove and discard old dressing; use a clean, ungloved hand or wear a disposable clean glove. Inspect insertion site for indications of infection; inspect anchoring of catheter.	Infection is most frequent complication with TPN administration. Inspecting catheter anchoring is a caution against accidental removal of tubing.
11. Don sterile gloves.	Maintains sterility of equipment.
12. Cleanse skin around catheter with three successive acetone-soaked or acetone alcohol sterile gauze sponges or swabs. Use gentle scrubbing action with circular movements from insertion site outward, as in Skill 32, Skill Sequence, "Dressing Change with Wound Care," step 26e, p. 312, and Figure 32–9. Area should be clean and free of debris. Avoid direct contact with catheter.	Acetone is a defatting agent that removes debris, bacteria, and old tape residue from skin. Cleansing is always from most clean to least clean part, without retracing movements and contamination. Acetone has corrosive action on newer silastic catheters.
13. Cleanse catheter with one povidone–iodine-soaked sterile gauze sponge or presaturated swab, as in step 12. Cleanse skin area with remaining two swabs. Allow to dry or remove with alcohol according to agency policy.	Use of antibacterial and antifungal agent minimizes possibility of infections, especially Candida albicans infections.
14. Apply povidone–iodine ointment to a 2-inch square gauze sponge and transfer to insertion site. Fit two 2-inch square gauze sponges beside catheter; place one over insertion site.	Use of antibacterial and antifungal agent minimizes possibility of infections, especially Candida albicans infections. Larger dressings can allow an unsutured catheter to work itself out.
15. Apply a 4 × 6 inch piece of elasticized adhesive to form an occlusive dressing covering gauze square but leaving part of catheter hub exposed. To do this, begin at midpoint of catheter hub and apply dressing with a smooth, continuous movement as the backing is being removed. Do not touch back side of elastic or stretch dressing excessively. (ALTERNATE: If 2-inch silk tape is used, apply several overlapping 6-inch strips in a similar location.) (NOTE: A liquid or spray skin protector such as Skin Prep or Benzoin may be used before applying tape.)	Occlusive dressing excludes moisture and bacterial contaminants. Secures catheter hub but leaves it accessible for tubing changes. Motion promotes smooth application. Underside of elastic adhesive must remain sterile. Excessive stretching decreases occlusive characteristics and may cause catheter to kink. Decreases potential for skin stripping; increases adhesiveness of tape.

(continued)

DRESSING CHANGE (Cont.)

Step	Rationale
16. Seal all edges of taped dressing with 1-inch nonporous adhesive tape. Cut a ½-inch slit into side of one tape strip to accommodate catheter hub. Cut tape strips as they are applied.	Secures dressing and provides occlusive seal. Anchors catheter hub and maintains occlusive seal when tubing is changed and hub manipulated. Keeps tape strips clean.
17. Remove gloves and masks.	No longer needed; tape is easier to handle with ungloved hands.
18. Secure the junction between the catheter hub and tubing with adhesive tape. Tape extension tube and filter to dressing. Check all other junctions for secure taping if tubing is not being changed at this time.	Prevents accidental separation of tubing with air embolism. Prevents tugging on catheter if filter gets caught on clothing or linens.
19. Label dressing with date, time, and own initials.	Indicates accountability. Avoids unnecessary dressing changes. Provides data for ongoing nursing care.
20. Return client to a position of comfort.	Promotes rest.
21. Dispose of used equipment in appropriate manner.	Demonstrates responsibility for own clean-up.
22. Wash hands.	Avoids cross-contamination.
23. Record on kardex, in nurses' notes or progress notes in health record: time and date of dressing change, skin condition, catheter anchoring, and any problems.	Indicates accountability for ongoing care.

RECORDING

Record solution, tubing, and dressing changes in the client's health record on flow sheets, in the nurses' notes, or in the progress notes. A written narrative or SOAP (POR) recording would include the date, the time, the activity performed (bottle, tubing, or dressing change), the appearance of the catheter insertion site if the dressing was changed, the kind of solution added, any infusion problems, and the client's general status.

Sample POR Recording

- S—NA
- O—Subclavian dressing intact, clean, and dry prior to removal for dressing change. No redness or pus evident at insertion site. Able to do Valsalva's maneuver with tubing change.
- A—Nonproblematic TPN infusion.
- P—Dressing and tubing changes. 1000 ml TPN solution with 100 mg ascorbic acic added to subclavian line. Plan to continue present protocol and orders for TPN care.

Sample Narrative Recording

TPN tubing and dressing changed. 1000 ml of TPN solution with 100 mg Vit. C added to TPN infusion. Old dressing intact, clean and dry. Insertion site clean, no signs of infection. Offers no complaints of discomfort re subclavian site.

☐ CRITICAL POINTS SUMMARY

1. Prevent infection by using strict aseptic technique during all tubing and dressing changes and during addition of new bottles or bags of solution.
2. Maintain constant flow rate to avoid hyperglycemia or hypoglycemia.
3. Monitor urine glucose every 6 hours and electrolyte levels several times per week.
4. Avoid air embolism during tubing change of a subclavian line by:
    a. Placing the client in a flat or slight Trendelenburg position.
    b. Having the client perform Valsalva's maneuver when the tubing is disconnected.
    c. Working quickly.
5. Tape all tubing junctions to avoid accidental separation.
6. Use occlusive dressings over the catheter insertion site to help avoid contamination and infection.
7. Use acetone to remove skin debris and bacteria, and povidone–iodine to provide antibacterial and antifungal actions.
8. Label tubings and dressings with the date, time, and own initials each time they are changed.

☐ LEARNING ACTIVITIES

1. Choose any hospital and locate the policies and procedures for TPN tubing and dressing changes. Where are they posted or found? Who helped write them? How are they reviewed or revised?
2. Contact the infection control department in any hospital and inquire about the epidemiologic monitoring done with TPN therapy.
3. On a nursing unit where clients receive TPN:
    a. Locate TPN formula bottles to be administered that day. Where did you find them? Read the label of ingredients, noting the protein and glucose sources and the additives contained in the solution.

b. Look at the nursing kardex and note the diagnoses of clients receiving TPN. Can the diagnoses be categorized in any manner?
c. Locate a TPN or subclavian dressing change kit and examine the contents listed on the label. Identify the purpose for which each is used.

REVIEW QUESTIONS

1. What purposes do the two major components of TPN solutions serve?
2. Why is infection the most common complication of TPN?
3. What nursing actions help reduce the potential for an infection developing in a client receiving TPN?
4. What is the relationship between the composition of the TPN solution, the rate of flow, and the development of hyperglycemia or hypoglycemia?
5. How does the nurse prevent an air embolism from occurring?
6. Why are acetone and povidone–iodine used for skin cleansing with a dressing change for TPN catheter sites?
7. What purpose does an occlusive dressing serve for a TPN catheter site?
8. Why is secure taping of all junctions and the filter absolutely crucial with TPN administration equipment?
9. Why is meticulous aseptic technique imperative for tubing and dressing changes?
10. Why is it crucial for the client to perform Valsalva's maneuver when TPN tubing is changed?

PERFORMANCE CHECKLISTS

OBJECTIVE: To use strict aseptic technique and correct procedure to change the IV tubing and TPN solution container.

CHARACTERISTIC	RANGE OF ACCEPTABILITY	SATISFACTORY	UNSATISFACTORY
1. Validates physician's order.	No deviation		
2. Gathers all needed equipment.	No deviation		
3. Identifies and inspects solution.	No deviation		
4. Identifies correct client.	No deviation		
5. Explains procedure.	No deviation		
6. Positions client properly.	No deviation		
7. Washes hands.	No deviation		
8. Uses flawless aseptic technique to attach and prime new tubing.	No deviation		
9. Swabs catheter hub-tubing junction with povidone–iodine or alcohol.	Agency policy may require different antibacterial agent.		
10. Decreases flow rate to a keep-open rate.	Tubing may be completely clamped and closed.		
11. Instructs client to do Valsalva's maneuver when tubing is changed.	No deviation		
12. Uses flawless aseptic technique and small sterile field to remove old tubing and insert new tubing.	No deviation		
13. Reestablishes flow to desired rate.	No deviation		
14. Secures all catheter and tubing junctions with tape.	No deviation		
15. Tapes extension set and filter to dressing.	No deviation		
16. Rechecks all connections and functions.	No deviation		
17. Indicates time, date, and initials on tape tag.	No deviation		
18. Returns client to position of comfort.	No deviation		
19. Disposes of equipment correctly.	No deviation		
20. Washes hands.	No deviation		
21. Records pertinent data.	No deviation		

OBJECTIVE: To use strict aseptic technique and correct procedure to change a dressing on a TPN catheter insertion site.			
CHARACTERISTIC	RANGE OF ACCEPTABILITY	SATISFACTORY	UNSATISFACTORY
1. Gathers all needed equipment.	No deviation		
2. Identifies client and explains procedure.	No deviation		
3. Positions client properly.	No deviation		
4. Washes hands.	No deviation		
5. Inspects and loosens old dressing.	No deviation		
6. Opens sterile supplies.	No deviation		
7. Nurse and client don masks.	No deviation		
8. Removes old dressing in appropriate manner.	No deviation		
9. Inspects skin and catheter insertion site for infection.	No deviation		
10. Dons sterile gloves.	No deviation		
11. Uses strict aseptic technique throughout.	No deviation		
12. Cleanses site: a. Uses 3 acetone-soaked swabs on skin around catheter. b. Uses 1 povidone-iodine swab on catheter insertion site and 2 swabs on skin around catheter.	May use acetone-alcohol swabs. No deviation		
13. Prepares skin by applying skin sealant.	Agency policy may omit.		
14. Applies sterile dressing: a. Places povidone-iodine ointment on insertion site. b. Covers insertion site with gauze squares. c. Applies elasticized adhesive dressing. d. Seals edges of taped dressing.	No deviation No deviation No deviation May use silk tape strips. No deviation		
15. Removes own gloves; removes own and client's masks.	No deviation		
16. Secures catheter-tubing junction with tape.	No deviation		
17. Labels dressing with date, time, and own initials.	No deviation		
18. Returns client to position of comfort.	No deviation		
19. Disposes of equipment properly.	No deviation		
20. Records time and date of dressing change and any untoward reactions on kardex, in nurses' notes, or progress notes in the health record.	No deviation		

REFERENCES

Aggressive total parenteral nutrition can be lethal. Nurses Drug Alert V(13):97-98, 1981.

Anderson MA, Aker SN, Hickman RO: The double-lumen Hickman catheter. American Journal of Nursing 82(2):272-273, 1982.

Blackburn GL: Hyperalimentation in the critically ill patient. Heart and Lung 8(1):67-70, 1979.

Colley R, Wilson J: Meeting patients' nutritional needs with hyperalimentation: How to begin hyperalimentation therapy. Nursing79 9(5):76-83, 1979a.

Colley R, Wilson J: Meeting patients' nutritional needs with hyperalimentation: Managing the patient on hyperalimentation. Nursing79 9(6):57-61, 1979b.

Connor KM, DiTrapano VC: Demystifying TPN. RN 44(8):30, 1981.

Coppa GF, Gouge TH, Hofstetter SR: Air embolism: A lethal but preventable complication of subclavian vein catheterization. Journal of Parenteral and Enteral Nutrition 5(2):166-168, 1981.

Dietel M, Vasic V, Alexander MA: Specialized nutritional support in the cancer patient: Is it worthwhile? Cancer 41(6):2359-2363, 1978.

Giordano C, Conly D, Masoorli S (consultant): Toward impeccable IV technique: Taking the worry out of hyperal. Part 2. RN 44(7):50-55, 1981.

Hales DR: Parenteral nutrition: First decade, trends. Hospitals 53(23):100-102, 1979.

Hodges RE: Total parenteral nutrition: An important therapeutic advance. Postgraduate Medicine 65(3):171-180, 1979.

Hüshen SC: Questioning TPN as the answer. American Journal of Nursing 82(5):852-854, 1982.

Hutchison M McG: Administrations of fat emulsions. American Journal of Nursing 82(2):275-277, 1982.

Ivey MF: The status of parenteral nutrition. Nursing Clinics of North America 14(2):285-304, 1979.

Kaminski MV, Burke WA, Blackburn GL: Intravenous Hyperalimentation in Modern Hospital Practice (Forward by JM Ling). Tuckahoe, NY, USV Laboratories, Division USV Pharmaceutical Corp, 1977.

Krause MV, Mahan LK: Food, Nutrition, and Diet Therapy, ed 7. Philadelphia, WB Saunders, 1984.

Ladefoged K: Quality of life in patients on permanent home parenteral nutrition. Journal of Parenteral and Enteral Nutrition 5(2):132-137, 1981.

Mitchell C, Scott S: Total parenteral nutrition: A nursing perspective. Heart and Lung 11(5):426-429, 1982.

Powell C, Regan C, Fabri PJ, Ruberg RL: Evaluation of Opsite catheter dressings for parenteral nutrition: A prospective, randomized study. Journal of Parenteral and Enteral Nutrition 6(1):43-46, 1982.

Sattler L, Wateska LP, et al: Cleveland Clinic Foundation Home TPN Manual. Irvine, CA, McGaw Laboratories, 1978.

Schneider PJ, Mirtallo JM: Home parenteral nutrition programs. Journal of Parenteral and Enteral Nutrition 5(2):157-160, 1981.

Simmons BP, Hooton TM, et al: Guideline for prevention of intravascular infections. In Guidelines for the Prevention and Control of Nosocomial Infections. Atlanta, Centers for Disease Control, 1981.

Steiger E, Fazio VW: Total Parenteral Nutrition: A Clinical Manual of Principles and Techniques. Irvine, CA, McGaw Laboratories, 1976.

Suitor CB, Crowley MF: Nutrition Principles and Application in Health Promotion, ed 2. Philadelphia, JB Lippincott, 1984.

Whitney EN, Cataldo CB: Understanding Normal and Clinical Nutrition. St Paul, MN, West Publishing, 1983.

BIBLIOGRAPHY

American Dietetic Association: Handbook of Clinical Dietetics. New Haven, CT, Yale University Press, 1981.

Borgen L: Total parenteral nutrition in adults. American Journal of Nursing 78(2):224-228, 1978.

Feldtman RW, Andressy RJ: Meeting exceptional nutritional needs: 1. Total parenteral nutrition. Postgraduate Medicine 64(2):64-77, 1978.

Jacobson NT: How to administer those tricky lipid emulsions. RN 42(6):63-64, 1979.

Juliani LM: Trouble-free administration of hetastarch and TPN. RN 44(8):64-65, 1981.

Luckmann J, Sorensen KC: Medical-Surgical Nursing: A Psychophysiologic Approach, ed 2. Philadelphia, WB Saunders, 1980.

Munro-Black J: The ABC's of total parenteral nutrition. Nursing84 (Horsham) 14(2):50-56, 1984.

Nursing Photobook: Managing IV Therapy. Nursing80 Photobook. Horsham, PA, Intermed Communications, 1980.

Williams SR: Nutrition and Diet Therapy, ed 4. St Louis, CV Mosby, 1981.

Wilson J, Colley R: Meeting patients' nutritional needs with hyperalimentation: Administering peripheral and enteral feedings. Nursing79 9(5):62-69, 1979.

SUGGESTED READING

Colley R, Wilson J: Meeting patients' nutritional needs with hyperalimentation: How to begin hyperalimentation therapy. Nursing79 9(5):76-83, 1979.

Colley R, Wilson J: Meeting patients' nutritional needs with hyperalimentation: Managing the patient on hyperalimentation. Nursing79 9(6):57-61, 1979.

Wilhem L: Helping your patient "settle in" with TPN. Nursing85 (Horsham) 15(4):60-64, 1985.

Wilson J, Colley R: Meeting patients' nutritional needs with hyperalimentation: Administering peripheral and enteral feedings. Nursing79 9(5):62-69, 1979.

AUDIOVISUAL RESOURCES

Total Parenteral Nutrition
  Videocassette. (1980)
  Available through:
    Biomedical Media Production Unit
    University of Michigan Medical Center
    Ann Arbor, MI 48109

TPN: The Dual-Energy System
  Slides and audiocassette. (1980)
  Available through:
    Cutter Biological
    Division of Cutter Laboratories, Inc.
    2200 Powell Street
    Emeryville, CA 94608

Total Parenteral Nutrition: An Overview
  Filmstrip, slides, videocassette, film. (1980, Color, 13 min.)

Total Parenteral Nutrition: Preparing the Patient
  Filmstrip, slides, videocassette, film. (1980, Color, 11 min.)

Total Parenteral Nutrition: Nursing Care—The Administration Set
  Filmstrip, slides, videocassette, film. (1980, Color, 12 min.)

Total Parenteral Nutrition: Nursing Care—The Protocol
  Filmstrip, slides, videocassette, film. (1980, Color, 10 min.)
  Available through:
    Medcom, Inc.
    P.O. Box 116
    Garden Grove, CA 92642

13 *Elimination Assistance*

Elimination of waste products through the urinary and gastrointestinal systems is necessary to prevent accumulation of toxic substances and damage to the body organs. When clients receive appropriate assistance with elimination processes and adequate management of elimination problems, their physical and psychological comfort is increased and their recovery from illness is facilitated.

One way the nurse facilitates clients' elimination processes is by helping them increase their capabilities for *self-care* in ways that are acceptable to each individual, while at the same time helping promote independence. When doing an *abdominal appraisal,* a nurse uses the skills of inspection, auscultation, percussion, and palpation to collect data about the functional status of the abdominal organs. For example, nasogastric and intestinal tubes are inserted for the purpose of relieving or preventing abdominal distention. Abdominal appraisal provides data to evaluate both the need for gastrointestinal tubes and their effectiveness as a therapeutic measure. Abdominal appraisal also provides data about common problems associated with elimination, such as bladder distention, retention with overflow, diarrhea, constipation, or fecal impactions.

When assisting clients with bowel and bladder elimination, the nurse implements a variety of nursing measures, such as offering bedpans and urinals, inserting a urinary catheter, giving an enema, or developing innovative and appropriate ways to manage urinary and fecal incontinence. In addition to assisting with urinary and gastrointestinal system function, these same procedures are often used to administer medications or to prepare clients for diagnostic or surgical procedures. Functional problems of the urinary or intestinal system require either temporary or permanent diversions that provide for elimination through routes other than the normal routes, such as a colostomy or ileostomy. In addition to providing care for these clients, the nurse teaches them to manage those alternate elimination routes.

Nurses also work with clients who require gastrointestinal tubes for diagnostic purposes or to prevent and relieve complications due to dysfunction of the gastrointestinal system. Insertion, care, and maintenance of these tubes are included in this chapter because of their role in maintaining adequate gastrointestinal system functioning.

As with other aspects of client care, the nurse works in cooperation with the physician and other health-care team members to provide assistance with urinary and gastrointestinal procedures in acute-, chronic-, and home-care settings. This care may include direct hands-on care, appraisal of the abdomen, or teaching clients and their families how to provide care, make relevant observations, and prevent elimination problems.

□ PRINCIPLES OF PRESSURE AND FLUID MOVEMENT

Many of the therapies and procedures associated with the gastrointestinal tract involve gravity or suction drainage of body organs or the use of fluids for irrigating those organs. There are basic principles of pressure and fluid movement that help the nurse both understand the way those therapies operate and how to implement them correctly so as to use pressure and fluid movement principles to the best advantage. For these reasons, this introduction includes basic principles of fluid movement and some pressure dynamics involved in suction and drainage.

Common uses of positive and negative pressures in the clinical setting include the measurement of blood pressure and the use of suction and drainage. Pressure is measured in millimeters of mercury (mm Hg) or centimeters of water (cm H_2O), that is, the amount of pressure needed to support a column of mercury or water to a certain height. Positive or negative pressure refers to any pressure greater or less than atmospheric pressure (760 mm Hg or 14.7 psi at sea level). For example, a blood pressure of 140 mm Hg is 140 mm Hg of pressure above atmospheric pressure and a suction setting of 90 mm Hg is 90 mm Hg of pressure less than atmospheric pressure. Negative pressure is created by partially removing air from a space, creating a partial vacuum. Because the pressure of the atmosphere outside the space is greater than the pressure within the space, air or liquid moves into the partial vacuum until the pressure is equal to that of the atmosphere.

A variety of technical procedures involve fluid movement into and out of body cavities or orifices. Some of the principles that govern fluid movement are given here, along with some examples of their clinical application.

1. The pressure exerted by a liquid depends in part on the depth of that liquid, that is, on the height of the column of that liquid, regardless of the shape of the liquid column. Pressure gradient is directly related to the difference between two pressures. Fluids flow from an area of greater pressure to one of lesser pressure. Increasing the pressure gradient increases the rate of fluid flow.

   Clinical Application: The column of liquid in an enema or enteral feeding setup extends from the surface level of the fluid in the container to the level at which the distal end of the attached tubing is placed. Raising or lowering the height of the enema or tube feeding container without changing the level of the tubing outlet increases or decreases the total height of the column and the pressure gradient. Therefore, raising the container increases the pressure and rate of flow at the tubing outlet and lowering the container produces the opposite result.

2. Fluid movement is affected by the viscosity of the liquid, that is, by its tendency to resist flow, or its relative thickness. A highly viscous solution flows more slowly than a less viscous one.

   Clinical Application: Thick milk-based enteral feeding formulas flow more slowly than thinner formulas or water.

3. Fluid movement varies inversely with the length of the tubing through which it flows, that is, doubling the length will halve the flow rate and tripling the length will decrease the flow rate to one third of its original rate.

   Clinical Application: Long gastrointestinal suction drainage tubing decreases the amount of pressure actually exerted by a given vacuum setting as compared with shorter drainage tubing.

4. Fluid movement in a tubing increases to the fourth power as the tubing diameter increases. That is, a 2-cm-diameter tube has flow rate 16 times as rapid as a 1-cm-diameter tube.

   Clinical Application: Large-diameter gastrointestinal suction drainage tubing or urinary catheter drainage collection tubing will remove gastric contents or drain urine more efficiently than a narrow-diameter tubing.

The skills in this chapter include "Insertion and Care of Gastrointestinal Tubes" (Skill 56), "Bedpans and Urinals" (Skill 57), "Bowel Elimination Procedures" (Skill 58), "Urinary Incontinence Care" (Skill 59), "Urinary Catheterization" (Skill 60), and "Ostomy Care" (Skill 61).

☐ ENTRY TEST

1. What are the body organs and structures through which food passes from the point of ingestion to the point of elimination?
2. Where are the internal and external sphincters of the colon located?
3. What are the mechanisms that move food through the gastrointestinal tract?
4. What are the functions of the stomach and the large and small intestines?
5. Explain the process of normal defecation.
6. Describe the characteristics and locations of the urinary sphincters.
7. Explain the process of normal micturition.
8. What is the length, configuration, and location of the urethra in the female and the male?
9. What are the characteristics of the various sections of the male urethra?
10. Where and how do the ureters and the urethra enter the bladder?

SKILL 56 *Insertion and Care of Gastrointestinal Tubes*

PREREQUISITE SKILLS

Skill 19, "Inspection"
Skill 20, "Palpation"
Skill 21, "Percussion"
Skill 22, "Auscultation"
Skill 28, "Handwashing"
Skill 40, "Oral Care"
Skill 51, "Monitoring Fluid Balance"

☐ STUDENT OBJECTIVES

1. Identify reasons for using gastrointestinal drainage and suction.
2. Differentiate among the various tubes used for both gastric and intestinal suction and drainage.
3. Describe two common sources of suction used for gastrointestinal purposes.
4. Distinguish between continuous and intermittent suction in terms of actual and potential problems.

5. Describe how to insert, irrigate, and remove a nasogastric tube.
6. Describe four methods used to check for correct placement of a nasogastric tube.
7. Describe the purposes and procedure for a gastric lavage.
8. Specify nursing care required by clients with nasogastric and gastrointestinal tubes.
9. Identify the quadrants, areas, and landmarks used in physical appraisal of the abdomen.
10. Identify the abdominal organs located in each quadrant or area.
11. Specify data collected through a physical appraisal of the abdomen.
12. Indicate the signs and symptoms of abdominal distention.
13. Insert, irrigate, and remove nasogastric tubes in a correct and safe manner.

☐ INTRODUCTION

Gastrointestinal tubes are long hollow tubes with perforations at the end and are designed for insertion into the gastrointestinal tract. They are available in different lengths that permit entry into the stomach or the small and large bowel. These tubes may be inserted for a variety of purposes and may or may not be attached to suction to provide for drainage. For example, a nasogastric tube often is inserted into the stomach to obtain a gastric fluid specimen for laboratory analysis or to monitor the acidity level of clients who have extensive burns or trauma because of the possibility of their developing stress ulcers. It may also be used to administer oral medications (Skill 71) or enteral feedings (Skill 54). A nasogastric tube is used for a lavage (washing out) of the stomach after ingestion of poisons or an overdose of medications. When gastric bleeding occurs, an iced lavage sometimes is used to control the bleeding. Nasogastric tubes often are inserted before surgery and attached to suction during and after surgery to keep the stomach empty until peristalsis is reestablished and the stomach can empty normally. They also are used with suction when there is delayed gastric emptying and gastric distention occurs. Clients with gastric distention are at risk for vomiting and aspiration of foreign material, as well as being quite uncomfortable.

Longer tubes are inserted into the small or large bowel for decompression (removal of pressure, such as from intestinal gases), either with or without suction. These tubes may be used before and after surgery or to relieve the distention, edema, and inflammation that occurs in the bowel proximal to an intestinal obstruction.

Nasogastric tubes are inserted and removed by either a physician or a nurse, while longer intestinal tubes usually are inserted and removed only by a physician. Some agencies may have selective restrictions on nurse insertion of nasogastric tubes, such as situations in which clients are unconscious, delirious, hemorrhaging, or have had recent oral, esophageal, or gastric surgery.

When used with suction for drainage purposes, gastrointestinal tubes require frequent monitoring and irrigation. This is necessary because the mucous secretions, blood, or debris that are often contained in gastrointestinal drainage tend to clog the tube and interfere with suction and drainage. The nurse is held accountable for making pertinent observations of the client's status, monitoring the suction tube function, irrigating the tube to maintain patency and adequate suction, and observing and recording the amount and character of the drainage. In some agencies, irrigation is initiated as a nursing order, whereas in other agencies a physician's order is required. It is important to become familiar with agency policy regarding these activities.

The length of time a gastrointestinal tube is left in place depends on the purpose for which the tube is being used. For example, when a nasogastric tube is used to prevent postoperative distention, it may be removed within 2 or 3 days. If the return of peristalsis is delayed, the tube will be left in place longer. An intestinal tube used to relieve a bowel obstruction may be in place for a number of days, and feeding tubes are sometimes left in place for months at a time.

This skill presents the techniques of inserting, irrigating, and removing nasogastric tubes as well as the monitoring and special care required when clients have drainage tubes connected to suction. Physical appraisal of the abdomen is also included because abdominal distention often accompanies the conditions for which intubation is used and may reflect problems with the suction system.

☐ PREPARATION

Gastrointestinal contents are removed from the stomach and intestines through the use of mechanical suction or a siphon action.

Suction is the use of negative pressure to move liquids, air, or solids from one place to another. Suction functions according to the basic principles that govern fluid movement (both gas and liquids) as discussed in the introduction to this chapter. Negative pressure is created by partially removing air from a space, resulting in a partial vacuum. Because the pressure of the atmosphere outside the space is greater than the pressure within the space, air or liquid moves into the partial vacuum until the pressure inside is equal to that of the atmosphere. To produce gastrointestinal suction with drainage, a pumping mechanism creates a partial vacuum in a drainage collection container that is attached to the gastrointestinal tube. This causes the fluid to be pushed up from the stomach or intestines through the gastrointestinal tube and into the collection bottle.

Negative pressure used for gastrointestinal suction is provided either by a centrally created vacuum that is piped throughout the agency and accessible through wall outlets near the bedside or by portable thermotic pumps that allow for greater freedom of movement for the client. Short-term negative pressure can also be created with a handheld asepto or catheter syringe. Pipeline suction provides either continuous or intermittent suction, depending on the type of pressure regulator being used. Thermotic pumps provide intermittent suction. Intermittent suction is the use of brief alternating periods of negative pressure and release, whereas continuous suction is a constant negative pressure. Intermittent suction is generally preferred for gastrointestinal suction since the on–off cycle releases the suction on any gastrointestinal mucosa that may have been drawn into the inlet ports of the tube tip. Additionally, the fluid in the tube tends to drop backward into the stomach with gravity during the off cycle, which helps clear the inlet ports.

A *siphon action* is used when a gastric lavage is done. A siphon is used to move liquid from a higher to a lower level through a tube without an external suction source. For a siphon to function, the tube connecting the two containers must be completely filled with fluid and the end of the tubing leading from the upper container (called the short tube) must remain beneath the level of fluid. As the liquid falls through the longer tube leading to the lower container, a partial vacuum is created, and air pressure on the surface of the upper fluid forces fluid into the upper short tube to fill the vacuum. The fluid will continue to move up the short arm and down into the lower container until the upper container is empty, unless more fluid is added or the direction of the flow is reversed. A siphon action is used to evacuate or lavage the stomach, such as after drug overdosage.

PROBLEMS ASSOCIATED WITH THE USE OF GASTROINTESTINAL TUBES

Whether the nurse inserts a nasogastric tube or assists the physician in inserting an intestinal tube, he or she is alert to the problems associated with insertion of tubes. Once the tube is in place, similar care and maintenance is needed, regardless of whether the distal end of the tube is in the stomach or the intestines. An exception is that a nasogastric tube is stabilized at the nose whereas an intestinal tube is allowed to advance through the intestines.

The insertion of a gastrointestinal tube is an uncomfortable experience for most people. Once the tube is in place, the discomfort diminishes, but, to some extent, it continues for the duration the tube is in place. The presence of a tube in the nose, throat, esophagus, and stomach is a potential source of a number of problems, many of which can be minimized or prevented by careful, thorough nursing care and observations. Fortunately, minimal problems are associated with long-term use of the small-lumen feeding tubes that are in common use.

Problems Associated with Insertion

Nasal turbinate injury with bleeding may occur during the insertion of any gastrointestinal tube if the client has a deviated septum, obstructed nares, or if the tube is inserted upward rather than downward toward the ear. A more serious insertion problem, however, is inadvertent tracheal entry with the tube. Tracheal entry causes additional discomfort to the client because of the respiratory distress and the fact that the insertion procedure must at least partially be repeated. If tracheal entry is not identified before enteral feedings or tube irrigations are done, the client will develop respiratory complications.

A nasogastric tube must be inserted into the stomach to a depth that clears the esophageal sphincter and reaches into the fundus of the stomach. Incorrect placement contributes to inadequate drainage of stomach contents and problems with enteral feedings, such as decreased tolerance and esophageal reflux, as discussed in Skill 54.

Problems after Insertion

The problems that occur after the tube is inserted range from minor concerns such as sore throat and dry mouth to life-threatening problems such as esophageal erosion.

Sore throat and dry mouth can be eased by gargling with warm saline tap water or topical anesthetic solutions, or using a topical anesthetic spray. Occasionally, clients are allowed to chew gum or use hard candy or anesthetic throat lozenges (as directed) to relieve mouth dryness and sore throat. Sometimes a sore throat can be eased by retaping the tube, thus changing the position of the tube in the throat and increasing comfort.

Frequent oral care is essential, and sometimes must be done every hour. A sore nose can be avoided by carefully cleansing the nares around the tube to remove secretions and crusts. A cotton-tipped applicator moistened with water or half-strength hydrogen peroxide can be used for this purpose, followed by application of a water-soluble lubricant. Dry lips can be relieved with a lip pomade or cream.

Hoarseness and earache may occur because of tube placement in the pharynx and larynx. Careful oral care helps decrease these problems, and explanations of why they occur will help clients tolerate these discomforts.

Erosion of the nares can occur if the tube is taped in such a way that pressure is applied to the external naris. It can also occur if nasal secretions are allowed to accumulate and form a crust around the tube for an indefinite length of time.

Parotitis, an acute staphylococcal infection of the parotid gland, may occur and the eustachian tubes can become blocked by the tube position. Nasal breathing is difficult with a tube in a nostril, and the resulting mouth breathing plus inadequate oral care contributes to parotitis and other oral infections, especially in debilitated or immunosuppressed clients. In addition, the tube serves as a wick for bacteria to travel upward from the stomach or the intestines to the oral cavity. This is a particular problem when an intestinal tube has entered the colon, since colon bacteria can then migrate to the oral cavity. An antibiotic mouthwash or gargle sometimes is prescribed for these clients.

Fluid–electrolyte imbalances may occur, since nasogastric and intestinal suction can remove substantial amounts of electrolyte-rich fluids. The bowel secretes 7 to 8 liters of fluid each day, most of which is normally reabsorbed (Luckmann and Sorensen, 1980, p. 1451) and about 2000 to 3000 ml of gastric secretions are normally secreted each day, but this is decreased when gastric suction is in place (Luckmann and Sorensen, 1980, p. 1392; Metheny and Snively, 1983, p. 218). Nasogastric suction may result in chloride, potassium, and hydrogen depletion, and intestinal suction may produce sodium depletion. Gastric losses are compounded when the client is allowed to have more than small amounts of water or ice chips. Both melted ice and water essentially serve as a gastric lavage when suction is operating, and because they are hypotonic, they contribute to fluid and electrolyte losses. Metheny and Snively (1983) recommend that clients with nasogastric tubes receive nothing by mouth since gastric secretions are greatly reduced when the stomach is at rest. In many agencies, both gastric and intestinal losses are calculated and replaced by intravenous administration of an electrolyte-rich solution, such as lactated Ringer's solution. The nurse can minimize the potential for an electrolyte imbalance to occur by a judicious use of oral fluids, ice chips, and irrigations and by a regular assessment of fluid balance, including careful monitoring of intake and output.

Esophageal problems may occur because the tube is inserted through the gastroesophageal junction. These problems include esophageal reflux, esophagitis, and esophageal erosion and stricture.

Gastric distention may occur if peristalsis is not present or if the nasogastric tube becomes obstructed with gastric mucosa, mucus plugs, or debris and causes gastric contents to be retained in the stomach. Clinical indicators of gastric retention and delayed emptying include gastric distention, decreased suction drainage output, nausea, and vomiting around the suction tube. Gastric distention can be detected through regular appraisal of the abdomen and careful output monitoring.

Respiratory problems may occur. It is difficult for a client to cough and breathe deeply with a tube passed into a nostril and through the pharynx. The resulting compromised ventilation is especially important for the pre- and postoperative client. Aspiration pneumonia is a potential problem, especially if tube placement is incorrect and if clients are less than fully alert or have difficulty swallowing their own oral secretions.

Injury to the gastric mucosa may occur when the mucosa is drawn into the sucking ports or inlets of a nasogastric tube, sometimes resulting in ulcers and perforation. Excessive negative pressure will contribute to this problem, especially with continuous unvented suction or if the tube tip is lodged against the gastric wall. Gastric injury can be minimized by checking the function of the suction and irrigating the tube with normal saline, air, or both at frequent intervals, as described later.

PHYSICAL APPRAISAL OF THE ABDOMEN

Whenever possible, the nurse appraises the abdomen before a gastrointestinal tube is inserted for suction and drainage. This information provides a data base for later comparison of the effectiveness of the therapy. Appraising the abdomen during the time the tube is in place helps the nurse assess its effectiveness. Appraisal before and after removing a tube helps determine the client's ability to function adequately without the tube.

To describe appraisal findings in a way that others will understand, two different systems are used to divide the abdomen into sections visually. One system uses four areas, referred to as follows: left upper quadrant (LUQ), right upper quadrant (RUQ), right lower quadrant (RLQ), and left lower quadrant (LLQ). The vertical axis for determining the quadrants is a line extending from the xiphoid process down the midline to the symphysis pubis; the horizontal axis crosses directly through the umbilicus. To understand and interpret appraisal findings, the nurse must be able to have a mental picture of the location of the abdominal organs within each of the four quadrants, as shown in Figure 56–1.

The second system uses nine regions. The three most commonly used regions are the epigastric, umbilical, and suprapubic (hypogastric) regions. A variety of anatomic landmarks are used to locate and describe appraisal findings. Identifying landmarks and three abdominal regions are shown in Figure 56–2.

Before beginning a physical appraisal of the abdomen, ask the client to void so that a distended bladder will not interfere with the examination. Explaining what will be done during the appraisal will help the client to relax and make the examination easier. Position the client in a supine position with a pillow under the head, the arms at the sides over the chest, and the knees slightly flexed, with a pillow under the knees. These actions promote relaxation of the abdominal musculature and facilitate more accurate appraisal. Clients often want to put their arms above their heads, but this position tends to increase muscle tension in the abdomen. Note the client's facial expression and general comfort level in the examining position. Restlessness and discomfort can alert the nurse to problem areas. Continue to monitor facial expression at intervals throughout the examination.

Appraisal of the abdomen begins with inspection, followed by auscultation. Percussion and palpation always follow auscultation because these activities increase or decrease peristalsis and alter auscultatory findings. The abdomen is appraised in a systematic

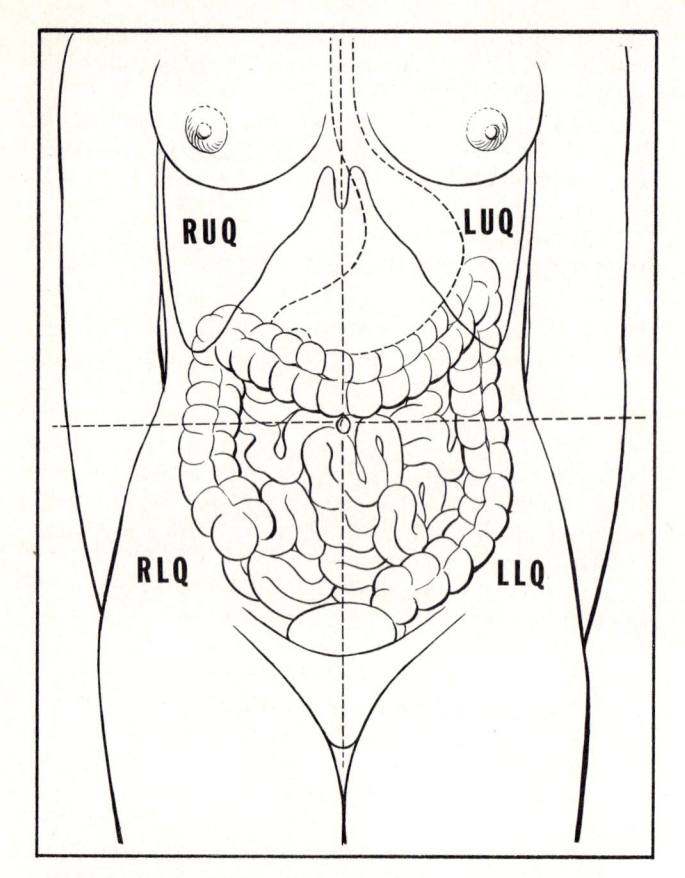

Figure 56-1. Four quadrants used to describe physical appraisal findings, and the gastrointestinal organs located in each. **RUQ** (right upper quadrant): contains the pyloric portion of the stomach, the duodenum, the hepatic flexure of colon, and parts of the ascending and transverse colon. **LUQ** (left upper quadrant): contains the body and esophageal portion of the stomach, the splenic flexure of the colon, and parts of the transverse and descending colon. **RLQ** (right lower quadrant): contains the cecum and portions of the small intestines. **LLQ** (left lower quadrant): contains part of the descending colon, the sigmoid colon, and parts of the small intestines. (NOTE: The bladder lies in the midline, behind the symphysis pubis when empty and above if full.)

way, beginning in one quadrant and progressing to the others, using the same sequence with each appraisal technique.

Inspection

Inspection is an important part of an abdominal appraisal; unfortunately, it is often either hurried or omitted. Inspection includes appraisal of the appearance of the skin, contour and symmetry, distention, the position of the umbilicus, abdominal elevation during respiration, and the presence of peristaltic movements.

Since the skin over the abdomen is generally covered and protected, it usually has a lighter color and smoother texture than skin on other areas. The skin over the abdomen becomes thin and glistening when it is stretched from gross abdominal distention.

Abdominal contour is described as flat, scaphoid (concave), rounded, or protuberant. The abdomen usually is symmetric, that is, the shape and size of both sides are similar. Abdominal distention alters the contour of the abdomen and may alter its symmetry. Generalized abdominal distention is usually symmetric and often results from gas in the intestines, free fluid in the abdominal cavity, or pregnancy. The abdomen becomes assymmetric with localized distention from tumors, enlarged organs, or distended loops of bowel. Abdominal distention is discussed later in more detail. Normally, the umbilicus is inverted. It becomes deeply sunken in the obese abdomen, flattened or slightly everted with abdominal distention, and develops a pronounced eversion with an umbilical hernia.

Abdominal elevation often occurs with inspiration. In general, males tend to breathe with the abdomen when at rest, and females tend to breathe with only costal movements. Inspiratory elevation of the abdomen is decreased when abdominal distention is present.

In very lean individuals, peristaltic activity can sometimes be seen as waves or ripples on the abdominal wall. When strong peristaltic contractions are visible in an average individual, the possibility of bowel obstruction should be considered. Peristaltic waves of the stomach and small intestine can sometimes be seen as elevated oblique bands that move downward from the upper left quadrant toward the right.

To inspect the abdomen, use a portable free-standing lamp with a directional shade for a light source. Place the light so that it will shine across the abdomen toward the nurse or lengthwise over the client, since this provides the best visualization of contour. Position yourself on the client's right side and first inspect the abdomen from above while standing and then sit down to inspect across the surface of the abdomen. From these positions, even small irregularities in contour will create shadows and any protuberances will be visible.

Auscultation

Auscultation is used to detect the presence and nature of bowel sounds. Bowel sounds are produced as the gas and fluid in the intestines intermingle and are moved throughout the gastrointestinal tract by peristaltic waves.

Normal bowel sounds in the small intestine are heard as medium-pitched, gurgling or clicking sounds. In the large intestine, they are lower pitched and more rumbling in character. The duration of a single bowel sound may range from less than 1 second to several seconds at a rate of approximately 5 to 34 times per minute.

Bowel sounds can be heard at any location in the abdomen because sounds are transmitted throughout the abdomen. However, bowel sounds in the small intestine are usually more active and prominent in the auscultation center, which is 1 to 2 cm below and to the right of the umbilicus. Bowel sounds are louder and more frequent after a meal. The best time to hear bowel sounds in the small intestine is about 1 to 2 hours after a meal. Bowel sounds can usually be heard

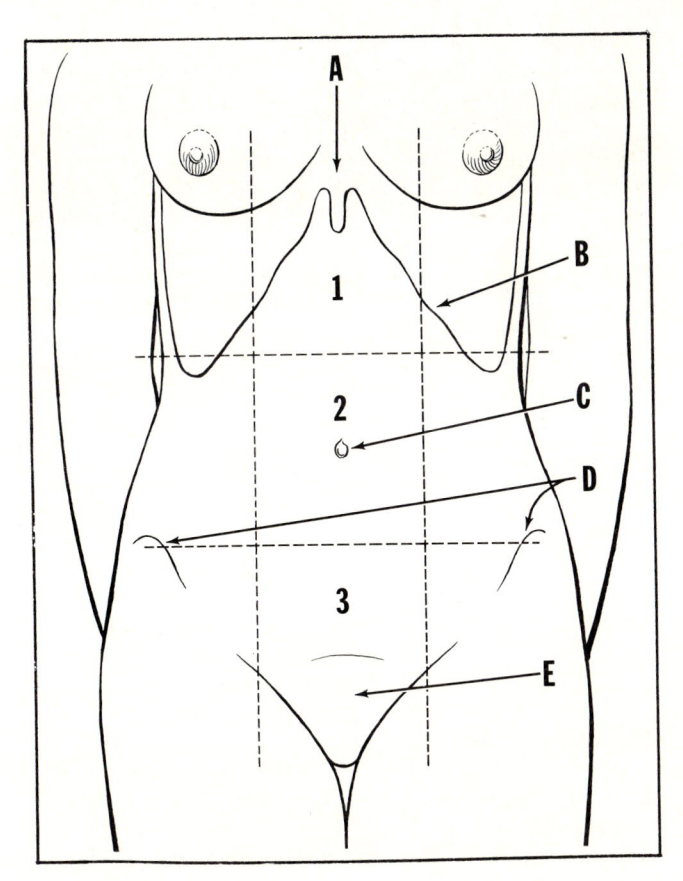

Figure 56–2. Three abdominal regions used to describe physical appraisal findings: (1) epigastric, (2) umbilical, and (3) suprapubic (hypogastric). Identifying landmarks used to describe physical appraisal findings: A. xiphoid process, B. costal margin, C. umbilicus, D. anterosuperior iliac spines, and E. symphysis pubis.

in the ileocecal valve area (RLQ) about 4 to 7 hours after a meal as the intestinal contents pass through that valve.

Hypoactive or diminished bowel sounds indicate inhibited motility, such as occurs with inflammation, paralytic ileus, late bowel obstruction, and following abdominal surgery. Following abdominal surgery, bowel sounds normally reestablish themselves within 1 to 3 days, while longer than 3 or 4 days may be indicative of complications (Sana and Judge, 1982, p. 297). Because of the variable rate at which bowel sounds occur, it is important to listen for bowel sounds for 5 minutes by the clock before deciding that no bowel sounds exist.

Hyperactive bowel sounds are associated with hypermotility of the bowel, such as occurs with irritable colon, acute gastroenteritis, diarrhea, and early mechanical bowel obstruction. Hyperactive bowel sounds are usually more high pitched, loud, rushing, and tinkling. Occasionally loud prolonged gurgles of hyperactivity are heard, called borborygmi, or the familiar "stomach growling." High-pitched tinkling sounds may accompany early bowel obstruction and are reported to the physician.

Auscultation of bowel sounds is done with the diaphragm of the stethoscope because it can detect faint sounds and accentuate higher-pitched sounds. Before beginning, warm the diaphragm by rubbing it between the hands and place it gently on the client's abdomen in the auscultation center. Allow it to rest in position without touching it, since additional pressure can stimulate increased bowel sounds. Leave the stethoscope in place for several minutes before lifting it and moving it to the adjacent quadrant. Listen in each quadrant, and spend a total of 3 to 5 minutes listening.

Percussion

When in a supine position, the air in the stomach and intestines rises above the liquid contents and can be percussed. The normal percussive sound in the abdomen is tympany. The tympanic note of the stomach is relatively low pitched and varies with the gastric contents. A variable-sized gastric air bubble can be percussed in the area of the left lower anterior rib cage. The percussive note is loudest over this air bubble, and more faint over the area containing gastric contents. A highly tympanic stomach suggests gastric dilatation and may represent a pyloric obstruction.

The note of tympany is high pitched over the small intestines and of an intermediate pitch over the colon (Robins, 1974, p. 49). High-pitched tympany over the upper abdomen may reflect small bowel obstruction, and increased tympany over the lower abdomen may represent large bowel obstruction. When greater resonance is heard with abdominal percussion, it usually represents gaseous distention. Dullness with percussion may represent the presence of fluid or a tumor.

Palpation

Palpation is the last part of an abdominal appraisal because the pressure stimulates involuntary muscle contractions and makes further examination difficult. A normal abdomen feels soft, supple, and flexible to light palpation. In lean muscular individuals, however, the abdominal surface will feel quite hard, even when fully relaxed. The normal stomach cannot be palpated, even after a meal. However, it is possible to palpate the upper abdominal and epigastric distention that may occur with delayed gastric emptying or pyloric valve obstruction.

When the abdomen is palpated, tensing of the muscles often occurs from fear or ticklishness. This voluntary guarding usually relaxes somewhat with expiration. Involuntary guarding occurs when a painful area is palpated. Rigidity is an extreme form of guarding that may be seen in conjunction with absent bowel sounds and may be associated with bowel obstruction, peritonitis, or intraabdominal bleeding.

Before beginning to palpate the abdomen, ask the client to identify any sore or tender areas in the abdomen and plan to examine them last. Since cold hands cause abdominal tensing and withdrawal from the examiner's hands, warm your hands before beginning to palpate by rubbing them together or by washing them in warm water.

Palpate the abdomen in a systematic manner, with a light to moderate pressure and a gentle touch. Note any localized areas of tenderness, rigidity, or protuberances, and be alert for indications of distention. Deep palpation generally is needed for appraising gastrointestinal function.

Abdominal Distention

When the abdomen is distended from gas or fluid, it feels firm and full to light palpation. Since a grossly distended abdomen can be quite painful and sensitive to touch, light palpation is used to examine a distended abdomen.

Generalized abdominal distention results from either free fluid in the peritoneal cavity (ascites) or from intestinal gases. Upper abdominal and epigastric distention may occur with delayed gastric emptying or pyloric valve obstruction. If the distention is due to ascites, the abdomen will appear symmetrically rounded and distended, with the distention extending laterally to the flanks, causing them to bulge. With distention from intestinal gases, the abdominal walls slope upward toward the midline rather than being rounded, and the flanks do not bulge. When distention is pronounced, the skin becomes tight and glistening, the umbilicus may become everted, and abdominal elevation with respirations decreases.

Bowel sounds may be intensified with moderate ascites since the gases in the intestines cause them to float. With severe ascites, however, bowel sounds are decreased or subdued.

When the abdomen is percussed with the client in a supine position, ascites will produce tympany in the center of the abdomen around the umbilicus and dullness laterally and in the flanks. This happens because ascitic fluid seeks the lowest point in the abdomen and the bowels tend to float on top of the fluid. When the client is turned on the side, the fluid settles with gravity and the area of tympanic dullness shifts toward the dependent side, while the superior portion of the abdomen becomes tympanic. Visually, the point of greatest protuberance also shifts with gravity toward the dependent side of the abdomen. This positional change in abdominal dullness is known as the test for shifting dullness.

DATA BASE

Knowledge of the medical and nursing diagnoses and usual therapeutic plans helps the nurse explain the purpose and care of a gastrointestinal tube to the client and family. This knowledge also forms a basis for making nursing judgments about whether the amount and character of drainage is expected or unexpected. Prior to irrigating or inserting a nasogastric tube, it is helpful to read the nursing history or interview the client to determine his or her past experiences with these procedures. This information allows the nurse to incorporate the client's life experiences into explanations and reassurances offered.

Client History and Recorded Data

The health record provides the specific information about the client's past history, diagnostic findings, therapeutic plan, and prognosis. It also provides data about current and past problems with any existing gastrointestinal tubes, such as problems with tube clogging, crusting of nares, or abdominal distention. The record also indicates when a nasogastric tube was changed most recently and the rate of progress of a long intestinal tube through the intestines.

The record contains the physician's orders for inserting or removing a nasogastric tube, any restrictions on irrigating either gastric or intestinal tubes, and sometimes the type and frequency of irrigation. An irrigation order is often written "Irrigate N/G tube p.r.n. to maintain patency," leaving the decision about type of solution and frequency of irrigation to nursing judgment. Nursing orders on the kardex or in the nursing-care plan must reflect nursing observation of the status of both the client and the suction device and indicate the frequency of irrigation, the type and frequency of oral and nasal care, and any other particular care an individual client requires. Nurses' notes also describe the client's status prior to insertion of a gastrointestinal tube, such as the presence of nausea, vomiting, abdominal distention, gastric bleeding, or anticipated surgery to provide a baseline for evaluating later data. Postinsertion data will then reflect any changes in the client's status after intubation and drainage have been initiated.

Inspection. Inspection is used to determine the correct insertion length for a nasogastric tube. It also reveals the patency of the nostrils prior to insertion of a tube, the presence of the tube in the throat, the client's reaction during insertion, and the amount and characteristics of the gastric drainage returned after the tube has been inserted. During regular care of the client with a gastrointestinal tube, the nurse uses inspection to appraise the mouth, lips, and nares for crusts, sordes, and dry mucous membranes. Inspection is used to evaluate the functioning of the suction apparatus by noting the amount of fluid in the collection bottle, the movement of fluid in the suction tubing, and the presence of vomiting or abdominal distention. It also reveals the characteristic light–green color and mucoid appearance of gastric contents. The appearance of intestinal contents will vary with the location of the distal tip of the tube and the client's problem; that is, it may contain bile or fecal material. Fresh or old blood may also be noted.

When appraising the abdomen, inspection identifies the appearance of the skin, the contour and symmetry of the abdomen, and the position of the umbilicus. It is also used to detect the degree of distention present, the abdominal elevation with respirations, and the presence of any peristaltic movements. Other findings, such as striae or scars, may be significant for a particular client.

Auscultation. Auscultation is used to determine the presence or absence, frequency, and pitch of bowel sounds. Auscultation for bowel sounds is done before the gastrointestinal tube is inserted in order to provide a baseline for later comparison, and prior to removal of the tube to identify if peristalsis is reestablished. Auscultation is also used to detect the air as it enters the stomach during tube placement checks, and the sense of hearing identifies the hissing sound of a patent vented sump tube.

Percussion. Percussion is used to identify the presence of free fluid within the abdominal cavity and gas within the intestines. When doing the fluid-shift test for ascites, percussion differentiates areas of dullness and tympany. Percussion is also used to detect the size of the gastric air bubble and the presence of gastric dilatation.

Palpation. Light palpation is used to appraise the abdomen for distention prior to insertion of gastrointestinal tubes to provide a data base for later comparison. The abdomen is also appraised during the time the tube is in place to help evaluate the success of the therapy, and after it is removed to evaluate intestinal functioning.

Sense of Smell. The characteristic odor of gastric or intestinal secretions is identified through the the sense of smell.

EQUIPMENT

Gastrointestinal Tubes

Tubes used for gastrointestinal drainage are either short or long, depending on whether they are placed in the stomach or allowed to move on into the intestines. Some are single-lumen tubes, while others have two or three lumens. The additional lumens are used as air vents or for inflating a stabilizing balloon.

Short Tubes. Examples of different types of short nasogastric tubes are shown in Figure 56–3.

Levin tubes (Fig. 56–3A) are used for nasogastric suction or gastric analysis. They are single-lumen

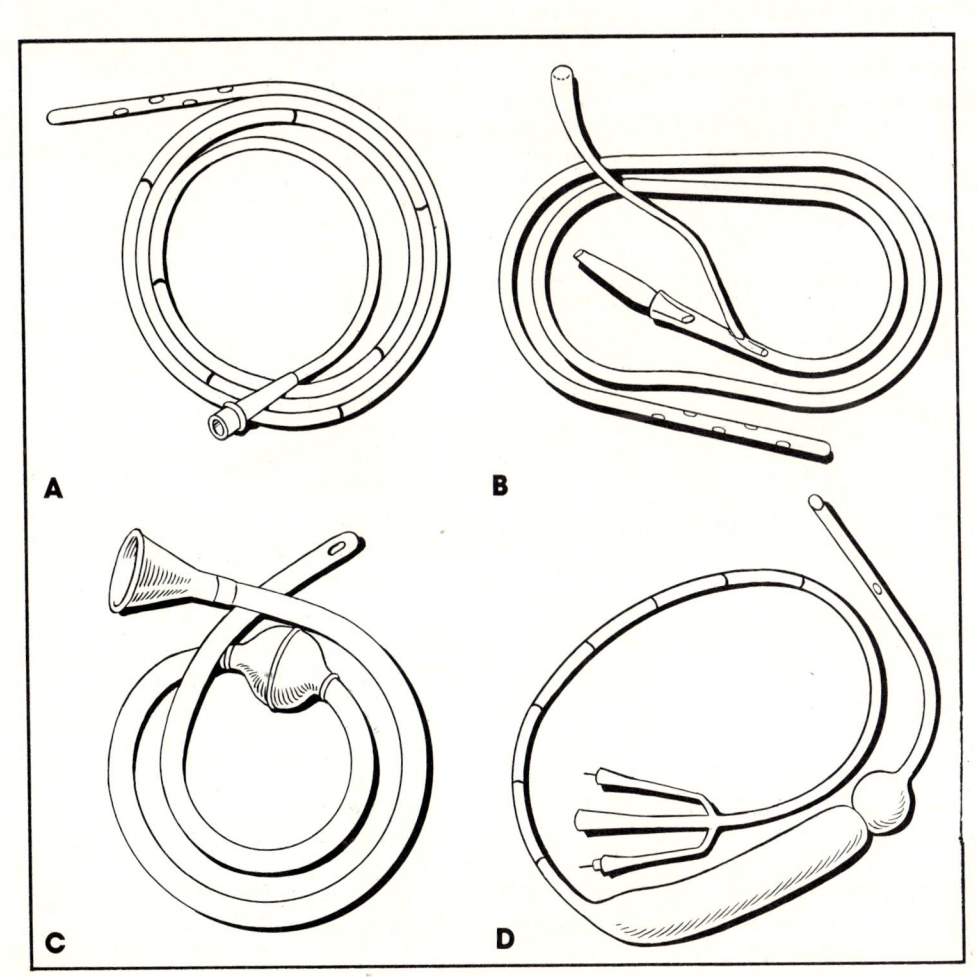

Figure 56–3. Short nasogastric tubes. **A.** Levin tube. **B.** Salem Sump tube with vent tube lumen pigtail. Both Levin tube and Salem Sump are used for gastric drainage. **C.** Ewald large-diameter tube with squeeze bulb, used for gastric lavage. **D.** Sengstaken–Blakemore tube, used for esophageal and gastric bleeding.

tubes made of clear plastic (polyvinyl chloride) or opaque red rubber, and are commonly available in French sizes 14 to 18 and 91 cm (36 in) and 122 cm (48 in) lengths. Tubes made of plastic are far less irritating to the nasal passages and esophagus than are those made of red rubber. In fact, Condon and Nyhus (1985, p. 173) clearly state, "A red rubber nasogastric tube should *not* be used." Some plastic tubes are thermosensitive, meaning that they are firm when inserted and soften at body temperature, thus decreasing irritation and discomfort after the tube is in place. Levin tubes usually have an open tip with four to six perforations (inlet ports or eyes) in the distal 15 cm (6 in) of the tube. They often have distance markings for ease in insertion. For example, the Argyle Stomach tube has markings at 46 cm (18 in), 56 cm (22 in), 66 cm (26 in), and 76 cm (30 in) from the distal end.

Sump tubes (Fig. 56–3B) are used for nasogastric suction. They are plastic double-lumen tubes, generally available in French sizes 10 to 18, and in the same lengths as Levin tubes. A commonly used sump tube, the Salem Sump tube (Argyle), is made of thermosensitive material and has distance markings similar to the Argyle Stomach tube. Sump tubes usually have a closed tip and more perforated inlet ports than do Levin tubes; some have radiopaque lines for x-ray identification of tube placement. The larger of the two lumens serves as the suction lumen and the smaller tube as an air vent. The smaller tube usually ends in a 6- to 8-inch colored extension tubing, commonly called a pigtail. In addition to its venting function, the small-lumen pigtail may be used for water and air irrigation, but it is *never* clamped or occluded in any way. The Anderson tube is similar in length, size, and function to the Salem Sump tube, but it is actually two tubes riding beside each other. The larger-lumen clear plastic tube is for suction, and the smaller opaque white tube serves as the air vent tube.

Ewald tubes (Fig. 56–3C) are large single-lumen plastic or red rubber tubes used for gastric lavage, generally available in French sizes 16 to 40. Some, such as the Edlich Gastric Lavage tube (Argyle), are made of thermosensitive plastic and have depth markings for insertion ease like those of nasogastric tubes. Because of their large diameter, these tubes often are inserted into the stomach through the mouth. Some orogastric tubes have a funnel tip for pouring lavage fluid and a built-in squeeze bulb that is used to initiate a siphon action.

The *Sengstaken–Blakemore tube* (Fig. 56–3D) is a triple-lumen, double-balloon-tipped tube that is used almost exclusively for esophageal or upper gastric bleeding. It usually is 91 cm (36 in) long, size 20F, and made of red latex rubber. After insertion, the physician inflates the distal gastric balloon with 150 to 400 ml of air, and the proximal elliptical esophageal balloon to a pressure of 20 to 25 mm Hg. Before insertion, both balloons are tested by inflating them under water and watching for escaping air bubbles. The use of this tube is well described by McConnell (1975). Short tubes used for feeding were discussed in Skill 54.

Long Tubes. Examples of several types of long intestinal tubes are shown in Figure 56–4.

Miller–Abbott tubes (Fig. 56–4A) are used for intestinal decompression. A Miller–Abbott tube is a long double-lumen rubber tube with one lumen leading to a thin latex rubber balloon that is attached just proximal to the metal tip and again 4.5 cm higher on the tube. The metal tip has numerous perforations; there

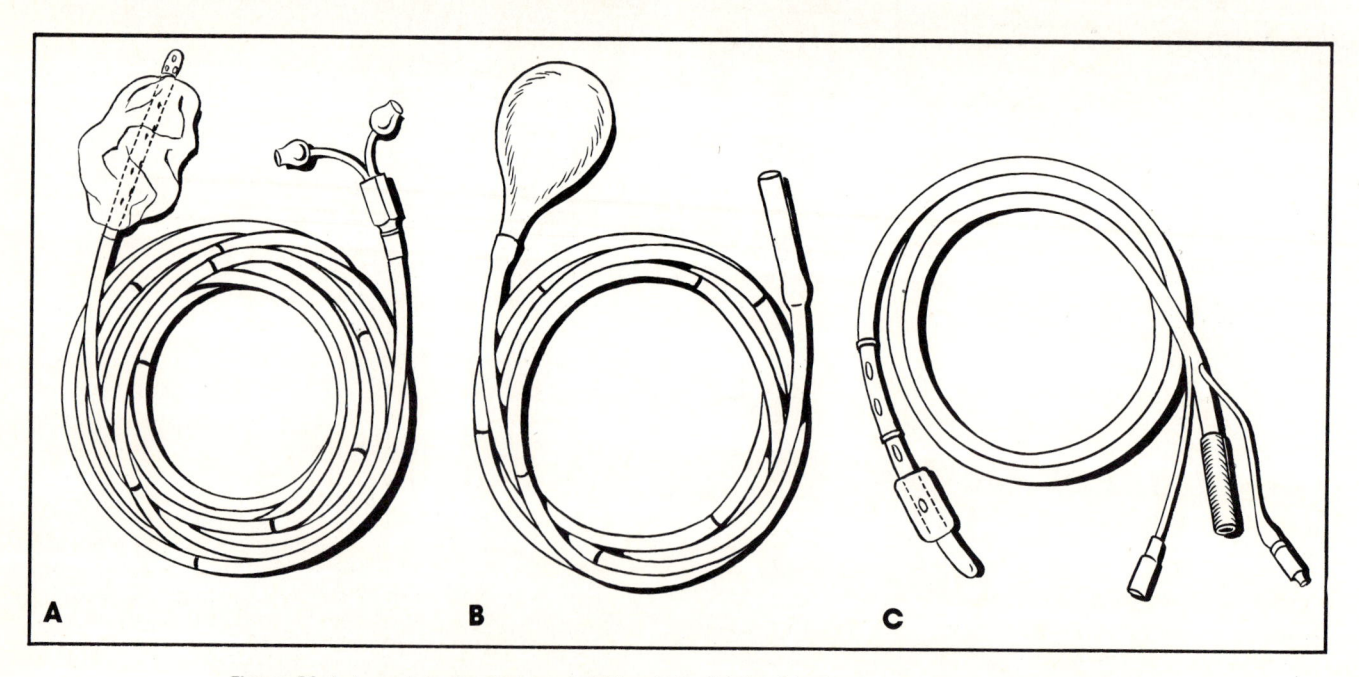

Figure 56–4. Long intestinal tubes. **A.** Miller–Abbott tube (double lumen). **B.** Cantor tube (single lumen). **C.** Dennis tube (triple lumen).

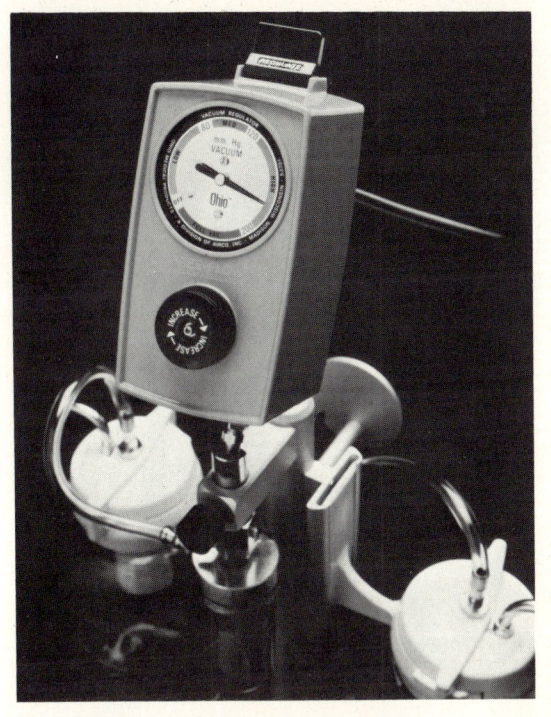

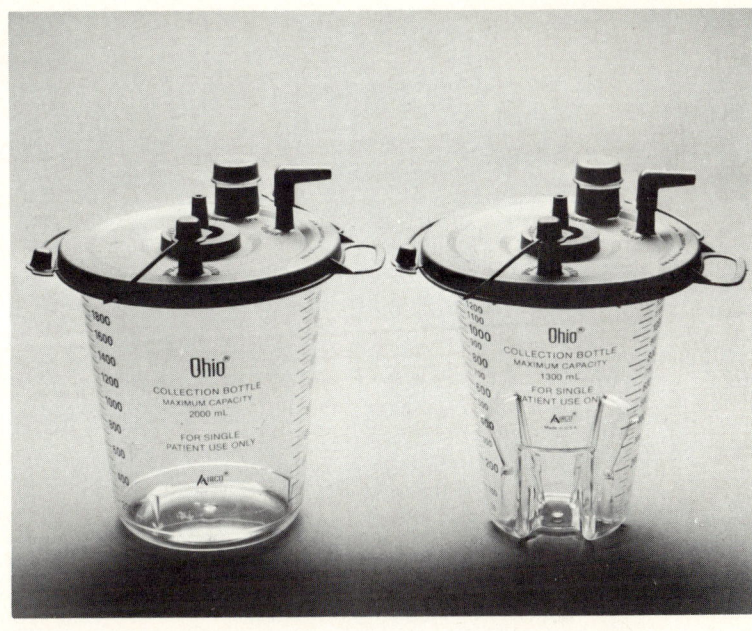

Figure 56–5. Wall suction equipment. **A.** Vacuum regulator, pressure gauge, and safety overflow trap bottle. **B.** Collection bottle. (With permission from Intertech/Ohio, a division of Intertech Resources Inc.)

are several perforations within the balloon, and additional perforations proximal to the balloon. The proximal end of the tube has a Y-shaped metal tip; the longer one is for suction and drainage and the shorter one for insertion of mercury. To avoid confusion, these tips are usually labeled. Miller–Abbott tubes are generally available in several French sizes and in 180 cm (6 ft), 244 cm (8 ft), and 360 cm (12 ft) lengths. Marked intervals on the tube help keep track of its progress through the intestines. Beginning at 45 cm (18 in) from the distal tip, markings are located every 15 cm (6 in) to the 150 cm (5 ft) point and every 30 cm (12 in) from that point to the 330 cm (11 ft) point. Because they are difficult to clean and sterilize, Miller–Abbott tubes are discarded once they have been used.

Cantor tubes (Fig. 56-4B) are also used for intestinal decompression. A Cantor tube is a single-lumen plastic or rubber tube with a latex balloon attached at the distal tip. Cantor tubes are generally available in similar sizes and lengths as Miller–Abbott tubes. The balloon is filled with 4 to 8 ml of mercury prior to insertion into the stomach, using a small-gauge needle and syringe. Occasionally, additional holes are made in the balloon to avoid distention from intestinal gases that may diffuse into the balloon; the mercury does not escape through these tiny holes. Because of the size of the mercury bag at the tip of a Cantor tube, this tube is inserted into the nose and pharynx and brought out through the mouth with a hemostat. The mercury is then placed in the bag, reinserted into the mouth and swallowed by the client.

Some newer intestinal tubes have three lumens, such as the *Dennis tube* (Argyle). The third lumen is used for irrigation or venting. The Dennis tube (Fig. 56-4C) is made of thermosensitive polyvinyl and has x-ray opaque and distance markings.

Suction Equipment
Equipment used for gastrointestinal suction is used and maintained in a clean, medical aseptic manner.

Pipeline Suction. Pipeline suction is created by centrally located rotary pumping mechanisms with piped connections to reservoirs of negative pressure located near the individual wall outlets in client rooms, providing a continuous and ready supply of suction. A pipeline vacuum system generally produces negative pressure within a range of 380 to 500 mm Hg negative pressure, which is too great for most clinical purposes.

Regulators are attached to the pipeline vacuum to modify the vacuum and control the amount of negative pressure actually used for gastrointestinal suction. A regulator may provide continuous or intermittent pressure and usually has a full vacuum setting that will bypass the regulator mechanism and provide full pipeline suction for emergency use, such as is needed in severe hemorrhage. A regulator usually is

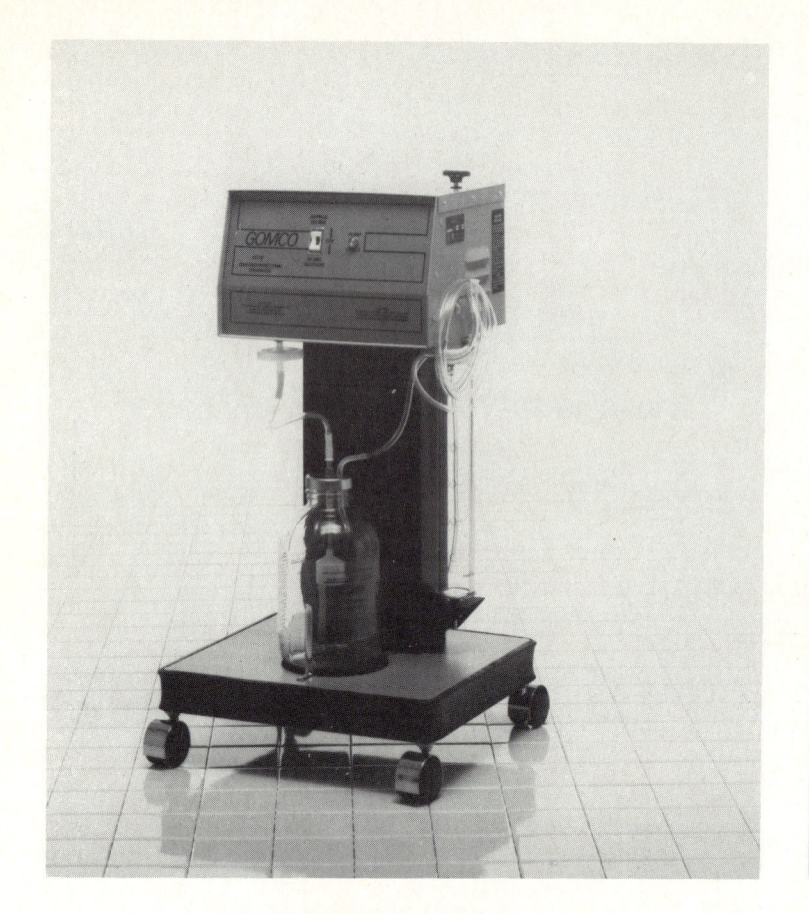

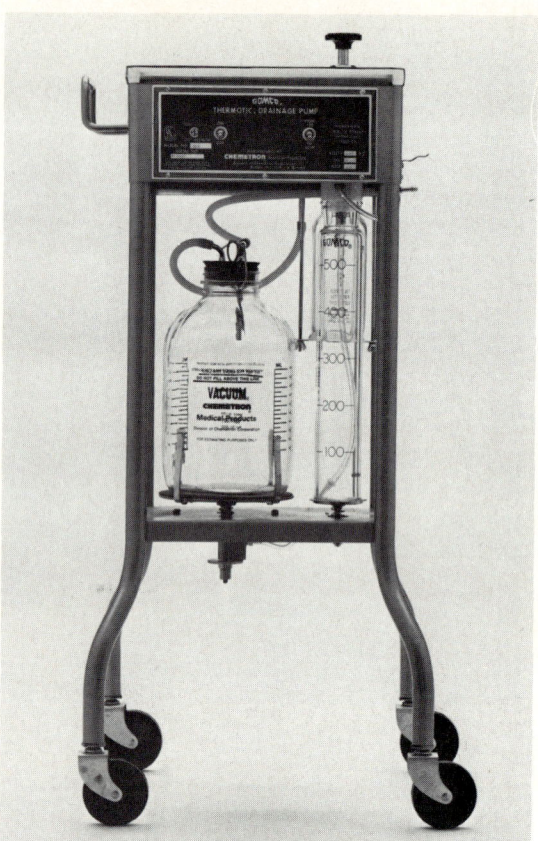

Figure 56–6. Gomco Thermotic pumps for gastrointestinal drainage. Newer style pump (left). Older style pump (right). Note collection bottle, overflow trap bottle, and weight-sensitive platforms. (Courtesy Gomco Division, Allied Healthcare Products, Inc., Buffalo, NY.)

inserted into the pipeline system and serviced by agency maintenance personnel or the central service department. To adjust a regulator to the desired level of negative pressure, occlude the suction tubing or place a finger over the collection bottle orifice where the tube is to be attached and turn the suction on to the desired level. Because the system then is closed to the atmosphere, the gauge will indicate the maximum pressure available at that setting. Regulators usually have a round dial calibrated from 0 to 200 mm Hg, with a setting for full vacuum.

Collection chambers may be made of disposable plastic or reusable glass. They have a variable capacity of 500 to 2000 ml, are calibrated for measurement ease, and have a float shutoff that closes off the vacuum supply when the fluid level rises to a given point. When emptying the collection chamber, turn off the suction or clamp the tubing between the vacuum outlet and the collection chamber, thus releasing the vacuum in the chamber. If drainage has gotten into the float mechanism, rinse thoroughly with hot water, as dried secretions will interfere with the float's function.

The collection chamber for pipeline suction is placed level with or somewhat above the client. As with positive pressure, the amount of negative pressure required to raise a column of liquid varies with its height. In gastrointestinal suction, this means that the higher the collection bottle is placed above the client, the greater the amount of negative pressure needed to raise drainage from the gastrointestinal tract to the collection bottle. If the collection chamber is located below the client, intermittent suction to some degree becomes continuous because the siphon effect begins to function during the off cycle.

An *overflow safety device* is always located between the drainage collection chamber and the regulator in the event that the float shutoff valve in the collection bottle fails to function properly, allowing drainage fluid to pass out of the collection chamber toward the regulator. A filter in this safety device traps lint and dust. If drainage fluids, lint, and dust enter the regulator, the regulator may malfunction and pathogens may enter the suction system. As an added precaution, pipeline suction systems have a safety tank to trap any debris that might enter the system accidentally. The safety device is not meant to be an additional collection chamber. If drainage appears in the collection chamber, replace it with a new one. Figure 56-5 shows a wall regulator with a collection chamber and safety device.

Thermotic Pumps. Gastrointestinal suction is most often achieved with a portable thermotic pump. The *Gomco Thermotic pumps* shown in Figure 56-6 are the most commonly used thermotic pump. They are quiet, efficient, and can easily be moved around the room when the client sits in a chair or goes to the bathroom. In addition, if the agency has pipeline suction only in intensive- or critical-care areas, a thermotic pump may be the only available suction source.

The Gomco Thermotic pump is nonmechanical and electric powered; like all electrical equipment, it must be connected to a grounded electrical source. It provides intermittent suction by alternately expanding and contracting air within a cylinder at regular intervals. Within the closed pump cylinder, a given volume of air is heated. As it expands, some of it is forced through the outlet valve. This outlet valve closes, the heat stops, the air cools, and a negative pressure is created. Gomco Thermotic pumps have only two suction settings: low (90 mm Hg) and high (120 mm Hg). A green light appears when the pump is turned on, and an amber light blinks intermittently to indicate the pump cycle. Four to five minutes are required to exhaust the air from the drainage collection receptacle before adequate negative pressure is created and drainage begins (Operating, 1969).

The *collection chamber* in a Gomco Thermotic pump is a large 2600 ml glass bottle, capped with a plug that is sealed in place with a metal loop spring. The plug contains two bent metal tubes; the suction tubing leading to the client is attached to the metal tube that extends the farthest into the bottle, while the tubing leading to the safety trap bottle and the suction source is attached to the shorter metal tube. The collection chamber rests on a bottle plate that serves as a weight-operated safety device. When the combined weight of the bottle and its contents reaches a given point, the system vents to the atmosphere, shuts off the suction but not the pump, and thus avoids drawing fluid up into the pumping mechanism. Some models have a safety trap bottle suspended from the pump and located above and lateral to the collection chamber. It serves to protect the pump in case the weight-operated shutoff malfunctions. If fluid appears in the safety trap, a new pump must be obtained.

Some Gomco Thermotic pump models have an automatic flushing device that enables the nurse to irrigate the nasogastric tube with 35 to 50 ml of irrigant without opening the system. These models have an additional glass bottle, a 500-ml flushing solution reservoir.

A thermotic pump's suction is tested by placing the end of the suction tubing in a glass of water and observing for suction. If a thermotic pump is creating no suction, the following factors should be checked: (1) the machine, to see if it is plugged in and the lights are operating, (2) tubing attachments to pump and bottles, (3) the closure of the bottle cap, and (4) the suction tubing for obstruction. If all of these are functioning adequately and there is still no suction, a new pump must be obtained.

To remove the glass collection bottle for emptying, the nurse unhooks the coil spring from one side of the bottle neck, removes the cap, and then removes the bottle. If any fluids are spilled onto the bottle plate, it is important to clean them off promptly since foreign material interferes with the automatic shutoff safety feature.

Suction Tubing. Tubing used with suction apparatus is sturdy and thick-walled and usually made of clear plastic for easy visualization of material being suctioned. Suction tubing should have at least a 7-mm (5/16-in) inner diameter, since a smaller lumen decreases the amount of suction delivered and clogs more readily. Since tubing size influences the rate at which drainage will flow, the length of the suction tubing from the client to the collection bottle should be short as is feasible and still allow for adequate patient movement. A longer tubing decreases the efficiency of the negative pressure.

Insertion Equipment

Commercially prepared nasogastric insertion kits are available, or the nurse may need to gather the separate items. The following equipment is always needed to insert a nasogastric tube. The type of tube will be determined by the physician.

Water-soluble lubricant is used to lubricate the distal portion of the tube for easier insertion. A *large syringe,* either bulb (asepto) or plunger style with a capacity of 20, 30, or 50 ml is needed to insert air into the stomach and to aspirate gastric contents as tube placement checks. A *stethoscope* is used to auscultate for the sound of air entering the stomach during tube placement check. A *bath towel* or *moisture-resistant drape* is placed across the client's chest to protect clothing and linen from gastric contents or vomiting. A *flashlight* is used to inspect the patency of the nares and, along with a *tongue blade,* is used to check for gag reflex prior to insertion of the tube. An *emesis basin* is kept near at hand in case the client vomits during tube insertion. *Tissues* are needed because tearing generally occurs. *Two glasses of water* and a *drinking straw* are used to help the client swallow the tube. *Adhesive tape strips,* 1/2 inch wide and 2 or 4 inches long, are used to fasten the tube to the nose, upper lip, or cheek after it is inserted. To avoid uncomfortable tugging and accidental dislodging, a *rubber band* is looped around the tube and fastened to the client's clothing with a *safety pin*. Alternatively, a piece of adhesive tape is placed around the tube and pinned to the clothing.

Irrigation Equipment

A *graduated container* of approximately 500 ml capacity is used to contain the irrigant. An *emesis basin* or other pan is used to contain the aspirated fluid. A *large syringe* of the type described earlier is used to insert the irrigant. A *towel* or *protective drape* is used to protect the bed linen at the connection to the suction tubing. Commercially prepared kits may contain all of the above items, with the carton serving as a receptacle for aspirated solution, or the kit may consist simply of a graduated container and a large bulb syringe.

A *tube clamp hemostat* may be used to clamp off the suction tubing before disconnecting a single-lumen suction tube for irrigation, or when a "T" connector is used between the nasogastric tube and the suction tubing. A second clamp or catheter cap is used to close the end of the nasogastric tube when it is disconnected temporarily.

Normal saline is the usual solution used for irrigating gastrointestinal tubes, although an electrolyte solution may be used. An isotonic solution helps avoid the additional fluid and electrolyte loss that may occur if hypotonic water is inserted into the stomach or intestines on a frequent basis.

Removal Equipment

A *towel* or moisture-resistant drape is used to protect the clothing and bed linens. A *hemostat* or *tube clamp* is used to clamp the tube and avoid leakage during removal. The client will need *tissues* to wipe and blow his or her nose after the tube has been removed.

☐ EXECUTION

Insertion of a nasogastric or nasointestinal tube is an uncomfortable procedure; irrigation is usually done when clients are quite ill, and removal of the tube usually indicates they are recovering. The way the nurse carries out these procedures can be reassuring or frightening for the client, depending on the nurse's technical skill and ability to explain the procedures in ways that each individual can understand.

All of these procedures are done using medical aseptic technique, since the stomach and intestines are nonsterile body cavities. Agencies often have specific policies that designate who may carry out these procedures and indicate the type and frequency of irrigations.

INSERTING A NASOGASTRIC TUBE

Before beginning to insert a nasogastric tube that is to be attached to suction, check the suction operation by turning the suction on and placing the tubing in a glass of water. This amount is subtracted from the output record tally.

Although nasogastric tubes often have distance markings for insertion guides, be sure to measure the

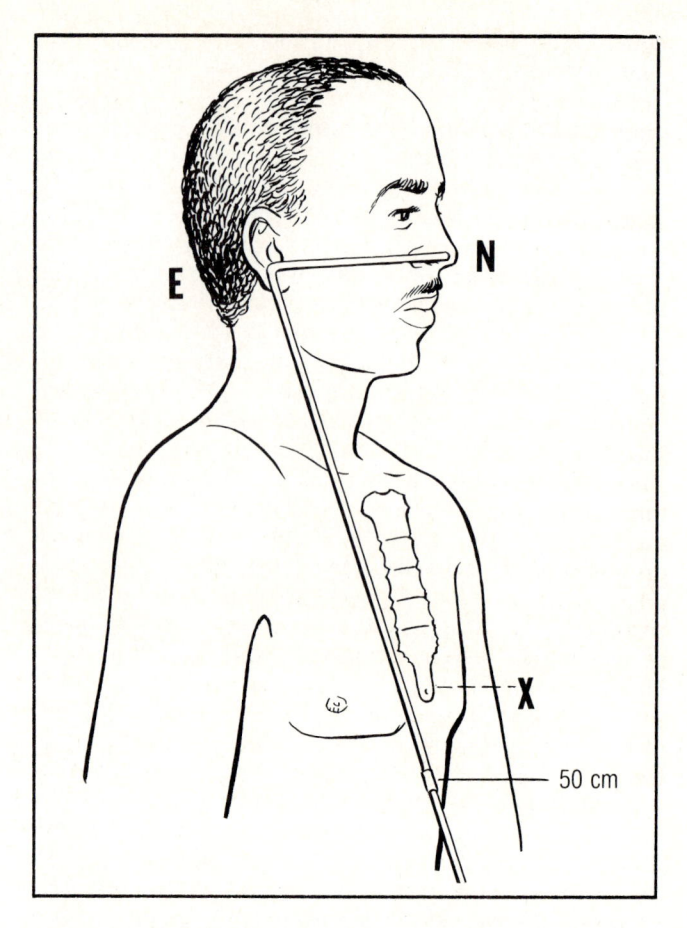

Figure 56–7. Mark the nasogastric tube with ink or a piece of tape 50 cm from the distal tip. With the client's head in a neutral position, place the tip of the tube at the tip of the nose (**N**), extend the tube to the tip of the ear (**E**) and then to the tip of the xiphoid (**X**). Mark the distance halfway between that point and the 50-cm mark, and insert to that depth. This point varies with the individual.

needed length for each person, since body length and build make a standard insertion distance inaccurate and inappropriate. Place a piece of tape or an ink mark at this point, which is usually somewhere between the second and third markings on a Levin or Salem Sump tube.

The traditional way to measure length for nasogastric tube insertion is to place the distal tip of the tube at the tip of the nose and measure to the earlobe and to the tip of the xiphoid process (NEX). However, this method was found to be inaccurate in nearly 28 percent of the subjects in Hanson's 1979 study of tube placement in 104 subjects (99 cadavers and 5 laboratory subjects), using 1 to 10 cm insertion distance within the stomach as an acceptable range. On the basis of his study, Hanson recommends marking a nasogastric tube at a point 50 cm from the distal tip and measuring the NEX with the face forward and the neck in a neutral position. The insertion point is halfway between the 50 cm point and the NEX distance, as shown in Figure 56–7. He describes a specially designed tape measure based on these calculations that may be used for this calculation. One margin has centimeter markings and the other margin has angled shadow markings that reflect the insertion distances (Hanson, 1979).

To prepare a firm plastic nasogastric tube for insertion, place it in a pan of warm tap water to soften it for easier insertion. Place limp red rubber tubes in ice water or a bowl of ice to make them firm enough for easy insertion.

Small-lumen feeding tubes create some special insertion problems. Some tubes are made sufficiently rigid for insertion by a metal stylet inside the lumen and others are encased in a firm plastic shield. The stylet or shield is removed after the tube is in place. Another method is to place both the tip of a small-lumen tube and a larger nasogastric tube into half of an empty gelatin capsule and insert as if they were one tube. Check placement through the larger tube and anchor the feeding tube in place. Leave both tubes in place for a half hour to dissolve the gelatin, after which the larger one is removed (Griggs and Hoppe, 1979). Unfortunately, the gelatin capsule sometimes swells before it reaches the stomach and at other times it does not always dissolve and is withdrawn with the larger tube (Robinson and Cox, 1979).

Since single-use nasogastric tubes are packaged in a coiled position, there may be a natural curve to the distal portion of the tube. If not, a temporary curve can be created by wrapping the distal 15 to 20 cm (6 to 8 in) of the tube around a finger tightly and then releasing it. Lubricate the distal 7.5 to 10 cm (3 to 4 in) of the tube with water-soluble lubricant. Avoid filling the inlet ports with lubricant, as it can drip out and into the larynx during insertion. An oil-based lubricant is *never* used. If the tube enters the trachea accidentally, a pneumonia is much more likely to occur from an oil-based than a water-soluble lubricant.

Before inserting a nasogastric tube, instruct the client about his or her role in helping with the insertion; that is, to swallow water through a drinking straw once the tube is in the oropharynx. Inform the client about tearing during insertion of the tube and provide tissues for that purpose.

Position the client in a high Fowler's position (Fig. 56–8), since that makes insertion easier. Place a pillow behind the shoulders so that the head can lean backward easily, hyperextending the neck. Work from the right side of the bed if you are right-handed, and from the left if left-handed. Agree on a signal the client can use to ask you to pause during the procedure for a brief rest, such as raising a hand.

Inspect the nares for patency and indications of a deviated septum. Light upward pressure on the tip of the nose often straightens the septum and increases visibility. Use a flashlight or adjust the over–bed light for an adequate light source. Ask the patient if he or she has a deviated septum, blocked sinuses, or a preference for having the tube in one side of the nose. To determine which naris has the most free flow of air,

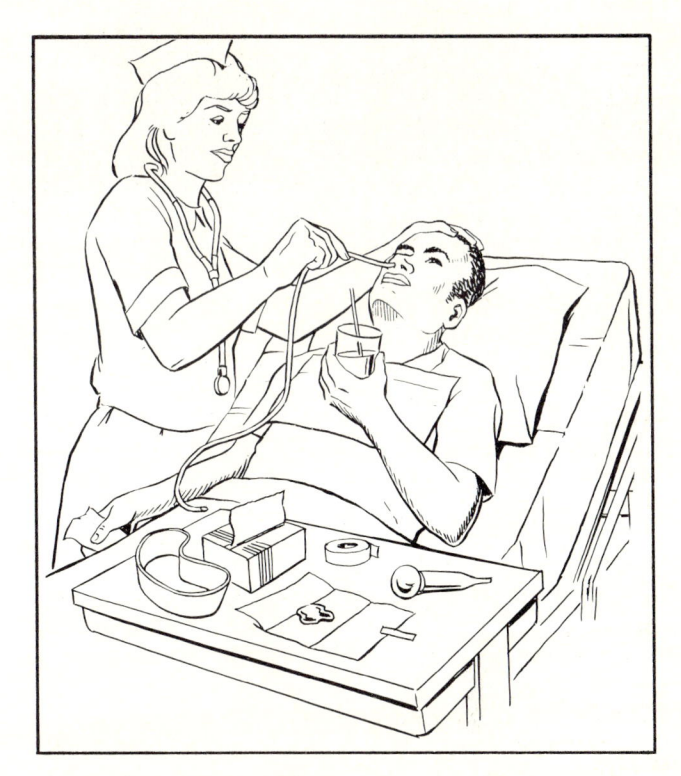

Figure 56–8. Inserting a nasogastric tube. Note client's and nurse's positions and equipment ready for use.

gently and alternately occlude each naris with one finger and feel the flow of air on another finger. Select the nostril with the greatest airflow.

With the client's neck hyperextended slightly, insert the tube in a downward direction toward the ear, not up toward the top of the nose, so as to avoid injuring the tender nasal turbinates. An alternate position is with the lower jaw thrust forward in a "sniffing" position. Both positions are shown in Figure 56–9A. Use a gentle, rotating motion until the tube reaches the oropharynx. Gagging and coughing are very common at this point. To decrease these problems, ask the client to take short panting breaths and allow him or her to rest briefly. Before advancing the tube farther ask the client to flex the neck, dropping the head forward, since this helps close the trachea and open the esophagus (Fig. 56–9B). Rotate the tube 180 degrees, which redirects the curve toward the esophagus. Begin to advance the tube while the client drinks water or dry-swallows air through a drinking straw (Fig. 56–9C). Swallowing helps the tube move into and through the esophagus and sipping water helps decrease gagging and choking. Advance the tube from the oropharynx between respirations, since it is less likely to enter the trachea at that time. Do not try to force the entire tube down quickly, since this is quite uncomfortable. Clients may be able to insert the tube after it reaches the oropharynx, since they can better coordinate their swallowing with the tube advancement. If this is done, coach continuously, such as by

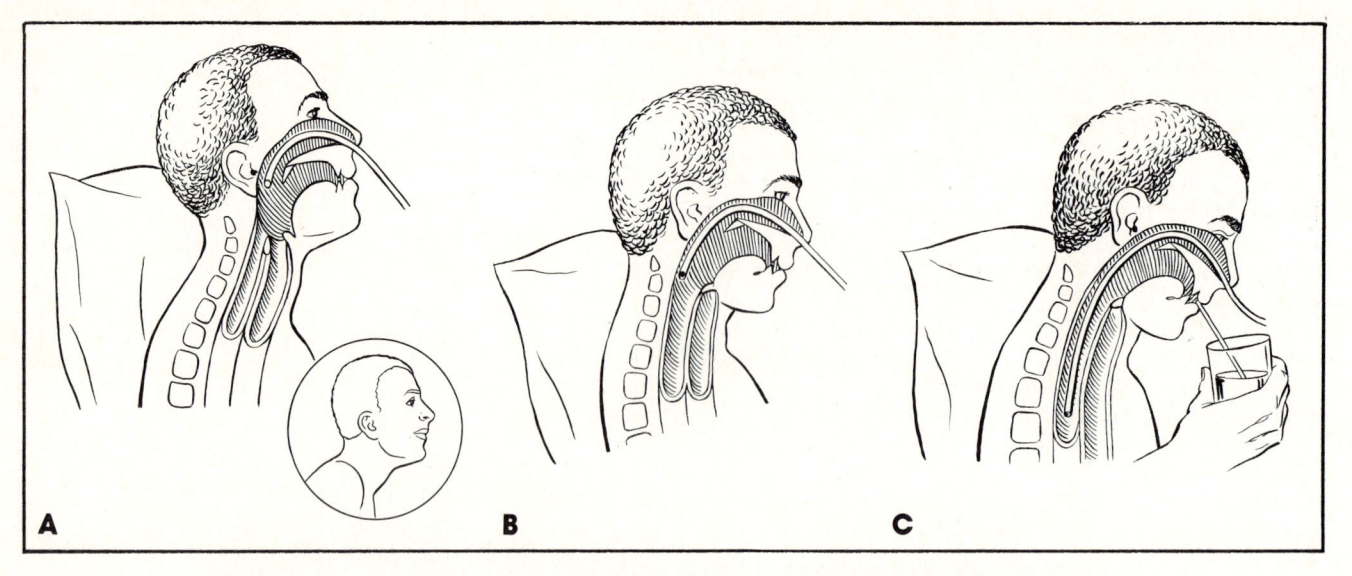

Figure 56–9. **A.** Hyperextend the neck slightly and insert the nasogastric tube downward toward the ear. (Alternate "sniffing" position shown in insert.) **B.** When the tube reaches the oropharynx, flex the neck to help direct the tube toward the esophagus. **C.** Advance the tube as the client swallows, since swallowing closes the glottis over the trachea.

saying: "Swallow now and push the tube in some more . . . and now some more . . . you're doing great! . . . swallow again." After the tube is inserted, much of the swallowed air will be released and water can be removed with a syringe or suction. If the client is unconscious or too lethargic to swallow, stroke the neck downward on either side of the larynx, during insertion, as this will help advance the tube.

If an alert client begins to cough and choke, or a less than alert client becomes dusky and cyanotic during insertion, withdraw the tube to the pharynx, evaluate the technique used, enlist the client's cooperation, rotate the tube, and try inserting it again. Alternatively, it may be necessary to remove the tube completely and allow the client to rest while preparing the tube for reinsertion.

After the tube is inserted, the client or an assistant may hold the tube in place without movement while the nurse checks for correct placement. Keep the distal end of the tube higher than the level of the abdomen to avoid fluid backflow and leaking.

Placement of a nasogastric tube is checked in several ways. For the first check, attach a bulb (asepto) or catheter syringe to the nasogastric tube. Place the diaphragm of the stethoscope over the epigastric area and insert 10 to 15 ml of air into the tube while listening for the "whoosh" of air entering the stomach (Fig. 56–10). If the tube is in the esophagus, the client may belch fairly promptly and no sound will be heard over the epigastric area. If the tube is in the trachea, the client will not be able to speak or hum. For the second placement check, use the attached syringe to aspirate gastric contents. If no gastric contents can be aspirated, advance the tube slightly or reposition the client on the left side and aspirate again. If neither of these checks indicates correct placement, use a flashlight and tongue blade to look in the back of the mouth to see if the tube is visible leading to the esophagus or if it is curled up in the throat, as this is not unusual when inserting small-lumen feeding tubes. Alternatively, if the client is unconscious, the tube may not have entered the esophagus. Another reliable way to confirm tube placement is using x-rays, although this is not necessary routinely and is quite costly. However, it is an appropriate nursing decision

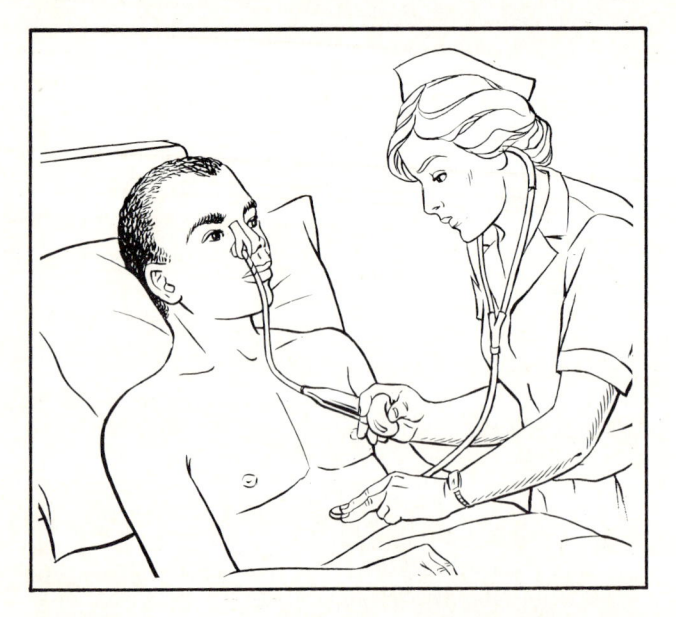

Figure 56–10. Check nasogastric tube placement with an asepto or catheter syringe. Insert 15 to 20 ml of air and listen with a stethoscope in the epigastric area for the "whoosh" of air entering the stomach.

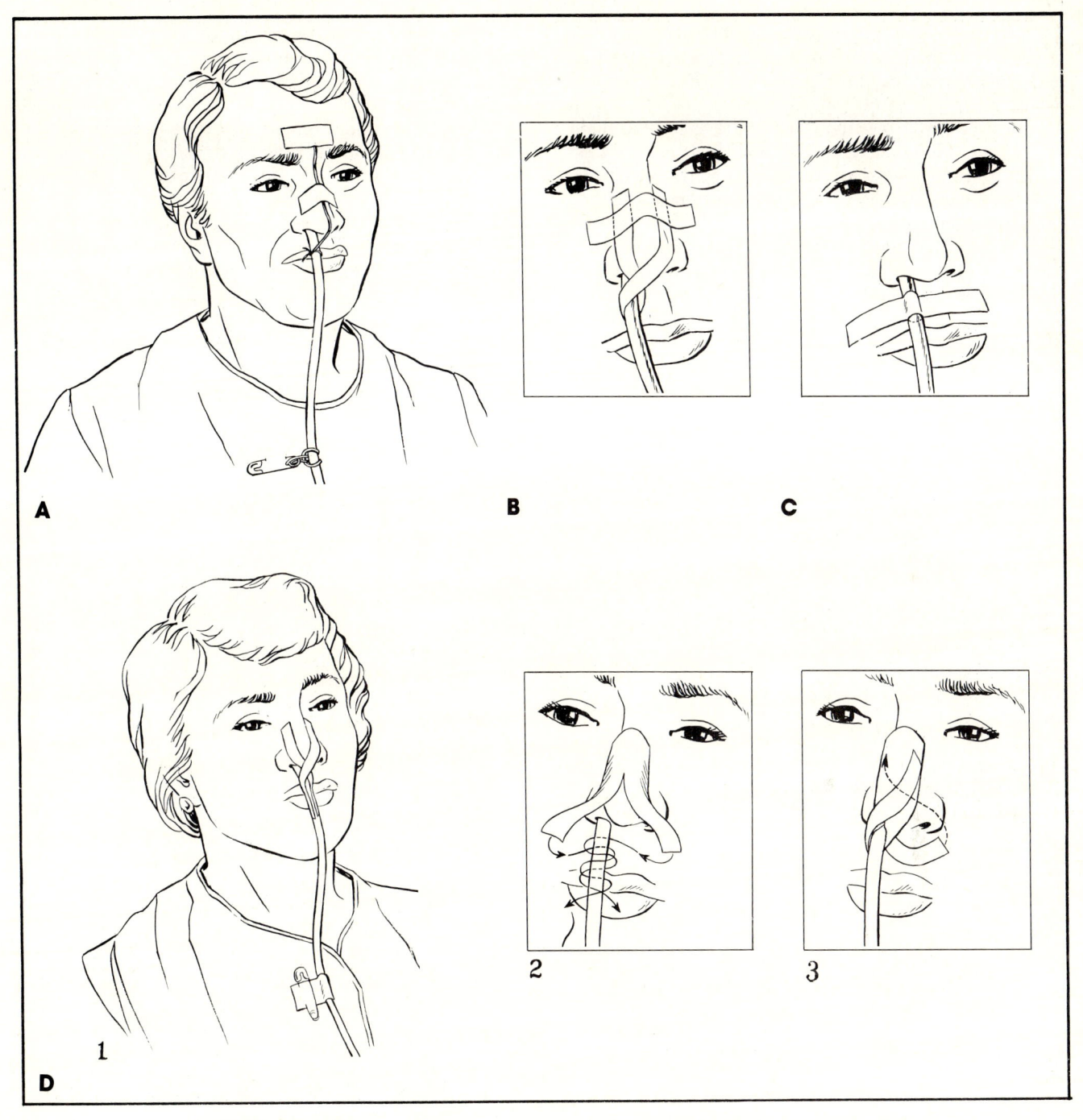

Figure 56–11. Securing a nasogastric tube. **A.** Tie a heavy thread around the tube and fasten it to the nose and forehead with adhesive tape strips. Allow enough thread length between the tube and the tape to allow for inward and outward movement of the tube with swallowing. **B.** Place the center of a 15 to 20 cm (6 to 8 in) long strip of ½-inch adhesive tape under the tube about 2 cm (¾ in) from the nares. Wrap tape ends around the tube in opposite directions and secure to the bridge of the nose. **C.** Place the center of a 10 to 12 cm (4 to 5 in) strip of ½-inch adhesive tape under the center of the tube about 2 cm (¾ in) from the nares. Crimp the tape together beneath the tube and anchor the tape to the upper lip. **D.** Use a single 12.5 to 13 cm (5 to 6 in) strip of adhesive tape (½ or ¾ in) to anchor the tube in one of three ways. For each, cut a lengthwise split in the tape to within 5 cm (2 in) of the end. **1.** Place the uncut end on the back of the tube; cross the ends over each other on the front of the tube and anchor them to the nose. Add a lateral adhesive strip across the nose as needed for additional security. **2.** Place the uncut end on the nose and wrap the split ends in opposite directions around and over the tube, back onto the nose. **3.** Place the uncut end on the nose and wrap the split ends in opposite directions, spirally down the tube. Secure the tube to the client's gown with a rubber band and pin as in **A** or a tape tab and pin as in **D1**.

to ask the physician for x-ray confirmation of tube placement if nursing judgment indicates an uncertain placement after performing all the other placement checks.

An outdated method of checking tube placement is to place the proximal open end of the tube in a glass of water and observe for air bubbles with exhalation. Lack of air bubbles does not necessarily mean the tube is in the stomach; it could be curled in the trachea. The potential danger in this procedure is that if the tube is in the respiratory tract, it can function as a straw if the person inhales while the proximal end is in the water (McConnell, 1979; Hirsch and Hannock, 1981). Unfortunately, some nurses continue to use this method.

After the tube is determined to be in correct position, anchor it over the bridge of the nose in such a way that no pressure is put on the external naris and so it can move in and out slightly when the client swallows. Figure 56–11 shows several safe ways to tape a nasogastric tube. Connect the tube to suction if ordered. If no suction is being used, clamp the tube with a metal tubing clamp or insert a tubing plug to prevent backflow and leakage.

Inserting a nasogastric tube is most easily done with an assistant. The assistant can stabilize the client's head if necessary, hold the glass of water and straw, offer the tissues or wipe the tearing, hold the emesis basin if the client vomits, or provide reassurance by holding the client's hand, patting the shoulder, and giving verbal encouragement.

☐ SKILL SEQUENCE

INSERTING A NASOGASTRIC TUBE

Step	Rationale
1. Confirm physician's order for insertion of tube.	Ensures correct implementation of physician's instructions.
2. Identify client and explain procedure.	Involves client in own care; increases cooperation; allays apprehension. Avoids error.
3. Prepare equipment.	Time-efficient nursing action.
4. Wash hands.	Avoids cross-contamination.
5. Pull curtain around bed or close door.	Provides privacy.
6. Check suction pump operation using a glass of water; include on intake–output record. Obtain new pump if needed.	Identifies nonfunctioning equipment before starting procedure.
7. Elevate bed to comfortable work height and prepare equipment in convenient location. Work on right side of bed if right-handed, and vice versa.	Conserves nurse energy; time-efficient activity. Facilitates manipulation of tube.
8. Examine tubing for rough or sharp edges.	Can cause irritation or injury.
9. Chill red rubber tubing in a pan of ice water; warm plastic tubing in a pan of warm water.	Chilling firms the rubber tubing, making it easier to insert. Warming softens the plastic tubing, making it more flexible and easier to insert.
10. Elevate head of bed to highest position; place pillow behind shoulders.	Aids insertion of tube; allows for hyperextension of neck.
11. Measure tubing and mark with tape or ink, as described in text. Identify tubing's natural curve or create a curve.	Determines correct length for individual client. Provides identifying landmark for insertion; a curved tube follows the curve of the pharynx more readily, making insertion easier.
12. Remove client's eyeglasses and dentures.	Tearing is common during insertion; dentures may become loosened and interfere with insertion.
13. Place a towel over chest, provide client with tissues, have emesis basin available.	Protects clothing and bed linen from water spillage or emesis.
14. Check patency of nostrils with flashlight; check for comparative breathing ease in each nostril. Select most patent nostril. (NOTE: If replacing existing tube, clean old tape from nose and face with small amounts of tape remover.)	If replacing an existing tube, choose the opposite nostril. Promotes comfort and aesthetics.
15. Use a tongue blade to check for gag reflex; if none present, contact physician.	If gag reflex is diminished, client will have difficulty swallowing tube; if absent, danger of incorrect placement is increased.
16. Lubricate the distal 10 to 15 cm (4 to 6 in) of the tube with water-soluble lubricant; avoid filling the holes with lubricant.	Facilitates insertion and minimizes trauma to nasal passages. Water-soluble lubricant less likely to cause aspiration pneumonia if tube enters the trachea. Lubricant in holes of tube may drop into the larynx during passage of tube through pharynx.
17. Arrange with client for a signal to indicate a need for a rest during procedure. Give client tissues and glass of water with straw.	Gives client some sense of security and control. Prepares client for procedure.

(continued)

Step	Rationale
18. Have client hyperextend neck slightly. With curved end pointing downward, slowly and gently insert tube into nostril, directing it downward and toward ear, not up nose. Do not force; try other nostril if firm resistance. Rotate tube 180 degrees while advancing it to the pharynx.	Opens and straightens nasopharynx. Avoids the discomfort of contacting nasal turbinates. Slight resistance when tube reaches nasopharynx is usual, but severe resistance is not expected. Rotation sometimes helps direct tube posteriorly toward esophagus.
19. Allow client to rest briefly after tube reaches oropharynx.	Tearing and discomfort is usual at this point as a result of pressure in nasopharynx.
20. Have client flex neck and take big swallows of water or suck on an empty straw, advancing tube with each swallow until previously marked point is reached. (NOTE: If client alert and cooperative, have him or her advance own tube, with nurse holding water and giving verbal instructions to swallow.)	Position helps trachea close and esophagus open. Swallowing aids in passage of tube as it causes trachea to close and directs tube into esophagus. Water helps avoid gagging and choking. Inserting own tube is more comfortable, as client can coordinate advances with swallowing more readily.
21. Check tube placement (assistant or client holds tube in place temporarily). a. Observe for cyanosis, choking, coughing. b. Place diaphragm of a stethoscope over epigastric area. Insert 10 to 15 ml of air with syringe and listen for sound of air entering stomach. c. Aspirate stomach contents, using gentle suction with catheter. NOTE: If no gastric contents return: (1) Advance tube 2.5 to 5 cm (1 to 2 in) and aspirate again. (2) If still no gastric contents return, turn client on left side and aspirate again. d. If in doubt about placement, ask client to talk or hum; look in back of mouth and throat with a flashlight to see if tubing is curled up there; or request to confirm placement with x-ray.	Determines whether tube is in lungs or stomach. If tube is in lungs, a conscious client will cough or choke; an unconscious or lethargic client will become cyanotic. If tube is in trachea, nothing will be heard; if tube is in esophagus, air will not be heard and client will most likely belch promptly. Presence of gastric fluid is most certain placement check. Tube may be above level of gastric fluid in stomach. Brings stomach contents into greater curvature of stomach, making it easier to aspirate fluid. If tube has passed through vocal cords, client will be unable to speak or hum. In unconscious clients, tube may not have entered esophagus. Tube position readily visible on x-ray.
22. Connect tubing to suction if ordered, or clamp or plug tube.	Initiates ordered treatment; avoids leakage during taping of tube.
23. Anchor tubing in place, avoiding pressure on external naris. Attach to clothing with rubber band or tape and safety pin, leaving enough slack to avoid pulling on the tube.	Pressure on naris can cause irritation and necrosis. Helps prevent discomfort from tube tugging on nose with movement.
24. Return client to position of comfort.	Provides for rest.
25. Explain expected sensations in throat, fluid restrictions, and use of ice or other palliative measures.	Increases cooperation with treatment regime.
26. Dispose of single-use items and return reusable items to central service according to agency policy.	Assume responsibility for care of equipment and client's environment.
27. Wash hands.	Avoids cross-contaminaton.
28. Record procedure in health record, noting time, placement checks used, size and type of tube used, method of anchoring tube, client's response and ability to cooperate, amount and characteristics of gastric fluid, any problems encountered, and amount and kind of suction attached.	Provides a base line for further evaluation; fulfills nurse accountability.
29. Initiate intake–output procedures.	Fluid balance monitoring is mandatory with gastrointestinal suction.

IRRIGATING NASOGASTRIC TUBES

Nasogastric tubes are irrigated to check for patency, to flush for cleanliness, and to dislodge material that may be drawn into the inlet ports. If the tube is clogged and needs to be irrigated, the following will be noted: a decrease in the amount of drainage fluid over what has been occurring or is expected, lack of movement of contents in the suction tube, abdominal distention, nausea and vomiting around the tube, absence of a hissing sound from the vent tube, and drainage from the vent tube.

Nasogastric tubes usually need irrigating every hour or two and sometimes more often (Condon and Nyhus, 1985; Metheny and Snively, 1983). Preventing clogging with regular irrigation is usually more effective than unclogging a clogged tube. The frequency of irrigation and the type and amount of solution to be used may be specified by the physician, determined by agency policy, or based on nursing judgment. It is generally expected that the nurse will irrigate a nasogastric tube sufficiently often that it does not become clogged and lose its effectiveness. However, when the client has had gastric or esophageal surgery, irrigation is done *only* with a specific order from the physician.

Although, in theory, vented nasogastric tubes clog less readily and need less irrigation than single-lumen Levin tubes, the actual need for irrigation is quite variable and depends on the nature of the secretions being removed, the placement of the tube tip, and the type of tube used.

Either normal saline or air may be used to irrigate a nasogastric tube. Irrigating with air avoids loss of electrolytes and inaccurate intake-output records, although it may cause abdominal distention and bloating. Normal saline is more effective than air in maintaining tube patency when thick secretions or blood is in the tubing.

Before beginning an irrigation, place the client at a 30 to 45 degree elevation since this helps avoid gastric reflux of irrigant. Explain the process and purpose of the irrigation. Clamp the suction tubing on a Gomco Thermotic drainage pump before separating the connection tubing, since this pump takes some time to reestablish its suction after the system is disrupted. Place the end of the suction tubing in a safe place, such as over the handles or in the clip of a portable pump, or under the pillow, so that it does not fall on the floor.

Irrigate the suction lumen by inserting 30 to 50 ml of water or air slowly and gently into the tube with a large syringe. (Some agency policies specify that the irrigant flow in by gravity.) If possible, aspirate the irrigant with the syringe. If all the irrigant does not return, add the retained amount to the intake-output record as additional intake. If no irrigant can be aspirated, reposition the client or adjust the tube position in and out slightly and aspirate again. A word of caution: if the client had the nasogastric tube inserted during gastric or esophageal surgery, do *not* reposition the tube without specific physician direction.

When irrigating a vented tube, keep the open end of the vent tube above the client's midline to help keep gastric fluid from escaping from the vent. When gastric drainage is found leaking from a vent tube or the vent is not hissing, the suction lumen probably is clogged. When this happens, irrigate the suction lumen. If gastric leakage continues or no hissing sound is heard, irrigate the vent tube with 10 ml of normal saline followed by 10 to 20 ml of air. The saline flushes the vent tube and the air clears it of fluid so that it can again function as an air vent. Sometimes leakage can be prevented by inserting 10 to 20 ml of air into the vent tube every 8 hours (Hirsch and Hannock, 1981). The vent tube on a Salem Sump tube is *never* clamped, as is sometimes done when leakage occurs, since this converts the suction to a single-lumen system. Leakage will not usually occur if the suction lumen is kept patent and if air is inserted into the vent tube regularly. Leakage occurs when the vent tube begins to function as a siphon instead of an air vent. The on-off action of intermittent suction at times may contribute to leakage of a vented tube, and in some agencies policy may indicate that continuous suction is always used with sump tubes (McConnell, 1975).

After the irrigation is completed, rinse the equipment in hot water unless frank blood is present. Hot water removes gastric secretions more readily than cold water but will coagulate blood proteins. Cover the equipment with a towel and keep it at the bedside close to the suction source. Replace the equipment every 24 to 48 hours, depending on agency policy, or any time it cannot be rinsed clean.

☐ SKILL SEQUENCE

IRRIGATING A GASTROINTESTINAL TUBE

Step	Rationale
1. Confirm medical or nursing order for type and amount of fluid and frequency of irrigation.	Ensures correct implementation of therapeutic plan.
2. Prepare equipment or inspect existing equipment for cleanliness. Replace equipment every 24 to 48 hours or as needed.	Time-efficient nursing activity; stomach is a nonsterile body cavity.
3. Explain procedure to client.	Enlists client cooperation; allays apprehension; involves client in own care.
4. Wash hands.	Avoids cross-contamination.
5. Pour irrigant solution into graduated container provided in the irrigation set and draw up 30 to 50 ml in large syringe.	Baseline data for accurate intake-output records.
6. Disconnect suction tubing from nasogastric tube. (NOTE: If using a thermotic pump, clamp suction tubing first. If using a T-connector, shift the clamp to the suction tubing. Place tubing in a secure place.)	Thermotic pumps require 4 to 5 minutes to reestablish suction. Avoids directing irrigant toward the suction source. Provides for cleanliness of tubing.
7. Position client at a 30 to 45 degree elevation, unless contraindicated or not tolerated.	Helps avoid gastric reflux from irrigation.

(continued)

Step	Rationale
8. Insert solution slowly and steadily into nasogastric tube (or allow to flow in by gravity, based on agency policy or physician directive).	Avoids causing discomfort.
9. Aspirate fluid (unless contraindicated by agency policy or physician order) and discard in emesis basin or second graduated container. Do not use excessive force. If no fluid can be aspirated:	Force may draw gastric mucosa into sucking ports of tube.
a. Reposition client and aspirate again.	Tip of tube may be above fluid level in stomach.
b. Reposition tube, moving it in or out 1 to 2 inches and aspirate again. (NOTE: Do NOT reposition tubing if it was placed there during gastric or esophageal surgery.)	May cause damage to gastric suture lines.
If irrigating a Salem Sump tube:	
c. Keep air vent pigtail above client's midline during irrigation.	Minimizes likelihood of gastric fluid escaping through air vent.
d. Insert 10 to 20 ml saline into air vent, followed by 10 ml of air.	Achieves purpose of irrigation.
Repeat insertion and aspiration until desired amount of fluid is used or tube patency is assured.	
10. Reestablish suction and fasten tubing to clothing as needed.	Continues therapeutic plan.
11. Rinse equipment in hot water (use cold water if drainage contains frank blood) and cover with towel.	Promotes cleanliness and esthetics and inhibits overgrowth of microorganisms; hot water removes gastric secretions, but coagulates blood.
12. Record procedure in client's health record; include time, type and amount of irrigant, amount and character of return, problems encountered, and client's response. Add amount of retained fluid to intake-output record.	Provides data base for comparison with other irrigations; fulfills nurse accountability. Promotes correct intake-output measurement.

CARE OF THE CLIENT WITH GASTROINTESTINAL SUCTION AND DRAINAGE

When a gastrointestinal tube is in place, a client's comfort and tolerance for the tube can be increased by meticulous nursing care. Give oral and nasal care frequently, sometimes every 2 hours, depending on the oral status and level of discomfort. Remove the tape, cleanse the nose, and reapply fresh tape every few days or when it becomes soiled or loosened. Check the suction operation and tube patency frequently, sometimes as often as every half hour, depending on the thickness of the drainage and the size of the particles it contains. If suction is not maintained adequately, gastric retention, discomfort, distention, and even vomiting may occur. Encourage coughing and deep breathing at regular intervals, as this will help avoid a decreased respiratory exchange. Because highly acidic gastric contents are corrosive to the mucosa, Hirsch and Hannock (1981) recommend testing gastric secretions for pH several times a day. If the pH is less than 3.5, they suggest that the physician be asked for an antacid order.

Since suction is less effective when collection bottles become fairly full, empty the collection bottles at least every 8 to 10 hours, and more often as needed. Do not allow the collection bottles to overfill and trigger the cutoff valve or automatic air vent, because all suction is lost. If any drainage fluid appears in the overflow safety bottle with either pipeline or thermotic suction, arrange for immediate replacement of the pipeline collection chamber or the thermotic pump, since overflow indicates malfunction of the safety devices. Large amounts of drainage can be measured with the calibrations on the collection bottles; smaller amounts are measured with a graduated measuring container. Note and record the amount, color, consistency, and odor of the drainage. Flush the drainage down the toilet, rinse the collection bottle and graduate with hot water, return to the suction apparatus, and reestablish suction.

When emptying the collection bottle on a Gomco Thermotic pump, remember to remove the plug before removing the bottle from its base. This prevents drainage from accidentally being drawn into the suction tube in the plug as the bottle is tilted. Suction will be reestablished within 4 to 5 minutes after the system is reconnected.

Accurate intake-output records are a very important part of nursing care when clients have gastrointestinal tubes, both to monitor fluid-electrolyte balance and to provide data for planning replacement intravenous fluids. A summary of nursing care for these clients is presented in Table 56-1.

Sometimes suction has to be interrupted temporarily, such as for ambulation, diagnostic tests, or when determining whether the client can tolerate being without the tube. If it is to be a short interruption, clamp the suction tubing on a portable thermotic pump because of the time needed to reestablish suction. For longer periods of time, or with pipeline suction, turn off the suction source. Clamp the nasogastric tube with a tubing clamp or hemostat to prevent

TABLE 56-1. Nursing Care for Clients with Nasointestinal Tubes

NURSING ACTIVITY	FREQUENCY
Inspect nares for discharge and irritation.	q 4–8 hr and p.r.n.
Cleanse nostrils; apply water-soluble lubricant.	q 4–8 hr and p.r.n.
Inspect taping and check tube placement.	q 4–8 hr and p.r.n.
Replace tape p.r.n. for cleanliness and comfort.	Every 2–3 days or p.r.n.
Inspect mouth for dryness, sordes, and thick secretions.	q 4–8 hr and p.r.n.
Give thorough oral care.	Several times per day and p.r.n.
Check tube patency.	Hourly and p.r.n.
Irrigate tube.	Hourly and p.r.n.
Empty collection bottle.	q 8–10 hr
Monitor suction apparatus function.	q 8–10 hr and p.r.n.
Fasten tubing to clothing or bed.	At all times
Record intake and output.	q 8–10 hr or p.r.n.
Replace drainage volume with intravenous fluids.	As ordered by physician
Appraise abdomen for distention.	Daily or p.r.n.
Auscultate and record bowel sounds.	Daily or p.r.n.
Answer family and client questions and explain activities.	p.r.n.

leaking. If no clamp is available, pinch the tube on itself and insert the pinched portion into the distal end of the tube. Do *not* use a sump vent tube as a cap for the suction lumen, since fluid backflow can enter the air vent and impair the venting function.

ASSISTING WITH INSERTION OF INTESTINAL TUBES

Although the physician inserts intestinal tubes, the nurse is often asked to assist with the procedure by preparing the equipment, positioning the client, and providing explanations. The insertion procedure is similar to that for nasogastric tubes. However, after an intestinal tube has been inserted into the stomach, do not fasten it firmly to the nose since it is expected to progress into the intestinal tract. Instead, tape the tube to the forehead or cheek, allowing a fair amount of slack between the tape and the client's nose. As the tube advances and the slack is taken up, retape the tube. Coil the excess tubing and pin it to the client's clothing.

After the client has been intubated with an intestinal tube, the head of the bed is usually kept elevated at 30 degrees and the client is turned onto the right side or to a prone position, since this helps the tube advance into the intestines (Condon and Nyhus, 1978; McConnell, 1975). Once the tube has passed through the pyloric sphincter (usually confirmed by x-ray), the client may be encouraged to ambulate to speed the tube's progress through the intestines. Intestinal tubes can be used for decompression only if the client has active peristalsis, since that is how they move through the intestinal tract to the point of obstruction.

Long intestinal tubes can be irrigated like nasogastric tubes, although it takes longer to insert the fluid and it can be difficult to aspirate the fluid because of the length of the tube. When the tip of an intestinal tube has traveled far down into the intestines, a clear liquid diet may be allowed if there is no nausea or vomiting. These liquids will be absorbed by the upper small intestine.

REMOVING GASTROINTESTINAL TUBES

Before removing a gastrointestinal tube, position the client at a 30 or 45 degree elevation, since that will help avoid gastric reflux. Explain the procedure, provide tissues, remove the tape holding the tube in place, and then remove the tube as described below. For the first 24 to 48 hours after the tube is removed, monitor the client for signs and symptoms of abdominal distention and discomfort, nausea and vomiting, bowel sounds, and passage of flatus. If problems develop, contact the physician about reinserting the tube.

Nasogastric Tubes

Nasogastric tubes are removed either for the purpose of reinserting a fresh tube in the opposite naris or because there is no longer a need for the tube. Before removing a nasogastric tube for reasons other than changing tubes, clamp the tube to determine whether the stomach is emptying normally. The physician may order that the tube be clamped for several 30-minute to 1-hour time periods every 3 to 4 hours, or for a continuous time period of 6 to 24 hours. If bowel sounds are actively present, the physician may decide to remove the tube without a waiting period. Monitor the client carefully during these time intervals. If acute discomfort or vomiting occurs, reestablish suction and notify the physician.

Pull a nasogastric tube out steadily and slowly so as not to cause discomfort and irritation. Provide the client with tissues, since tearing usually occurs. To avoid having fluid leak from the proximal end of the tube as it is being removed from the nose, clamp the tube or leave it attached to the suction tubing until it is completely removed. Since mucus and debris cling to a nasogastric tube as it is removed, wrap the tube in a towel as you remove it. Keep it out of the client's sight as much as possible.

Intestinal Tubes

Intestinal tubes are not usually removed until after peristalsis has been reestablished throughout the bowel, as indicated by a bowel movement or passing flatus. The physician usually removes an intestinal tube or leaves specific instructions for its removal. An intestinal tube is removed slowly, since it must be pulled against peristaltic action. The client will feel the resistance and may become nauseated. When the distal end of the tube reaches the pharynx, it is often brought out through the mouth with a forceps, the balloon removed, and then withdrawn the rest of the way through the nose. The tube may have a distinct fecal odor as it is removed. The client's distress can be decreased by explaining the odor, removing the tube from view promptly, and giving oral care as soon as possible. If the tube has passed the ileocecal valve, it will not be withdrawn through the mouth or nose because of fecal contamination. Instead, the tube is cut off at the nares after the distal tip has appeared rectally and the tube is allowed to pass through the entire gastrointestinal tract. When this occurs, the tubing is coiled and anchored to the skin as it extrudes from the rectum, or sections may be cut off and kept to later determine that all the tube has been eliminated.

☐ SKILL SEQUENCE

REMOVING A NASOGASTRIC TUBE

Step	Rationale
1. Confirm physician's order for removal of nasogastric trube.	Ensures correct implementation of physician's instructions.
2. Evaluate client status.	Fulfills nurse accountability for own actions.
3. Explain procedure to client.	Enlists cooperation; allays apprehension.
4. Prepare equipment.	Time-efficient nursing activity.
5. Wash hands.	Avoids cross-contamination.
6. Turn off suction machine or wall suction regulator. Disconnect tube from suction equipment.	Suction during removal could injure esophageal lining.
7. Elevate head of bed to approximately 45 degrees or turn client on right side.	Helps avoid gastric reflux.
8. Remove tape securing tube from nose and remove pin holding tube to clothing.	Frees tube for removal.
9. Don nonsterile gloves.	Nasopharyngeal secretions have a high bacteria content, and mucus and small amounts of gastric contents usually exit with tube.
10. Have client breathe in and hold breath.	Prevents aspiration of drainage from tube.
11. Remove tube quickly and steadily, but not forcibly; curl tube in hand or enclose it in a towel as it is removed.	Avoids damage to tissues; tube is often unsightly when removed.
12. Offer tissues and have client blow nose. Offer mouthwash or provide oral care.	Removes accumulated secretions. Provides for comfort and esthetics; provides needed care for oral tissues.
13. Remove suction equipment; discard single-use suction apparatus and tubings; return reusable equipment to central service according to agency policy.	Assumes responsibility for care of equipment and client's environment.
14. Wash hands.	Prevents cross-contamination.
15. Record procedure in health record, noting time, amount of drainage in collection bottle, client's reaction, and any problems encountered.	

GASTRIC LAVAGE

Gastric lavage is most often done in an emergency-room setting. Either the physician or the nurse may pass the large-diameter orogastric tube.

Use a funnel to pour irrigating fluid into the stomach. After the stomach is filled with fluid, turn the end of the tube downward below the stomach, forming the long arm of a siphon. If no fluid returns, remove the air with the built-in squeeze bulb or a large syringe. Allow the gastric contents to drain and repeat the procedure until the poison or medication is removed. If the tube is kept full of fluid during the alternating filling and emptying, the siphon will continue to function (Flitter, 1976; Jensen, 1976).

RECORDING

If not already in the nurses' notes, record pertinent data about the need for the nasogastric or intestinal tube; for example, continued nausea and vomiting, abdominal or gastric distention, or as preparation for surgery or diagnostic tests.

After inserting a nasogastric tube, record the time, the type and size of tube inserted, the placement checks used, the amount and kind of drainage returned, how and where the tube is taped, the client's ability to participate in and tolerate the procedure, and the kind and amount of suction used (if applicable). Record the same kind of data in the nurses' notes after assisting a physician with insertion of an intestinal tube.

When irrigating a nasogastric tube, record the amount and kind or irrigant used, the amount and character of fluid returned, and add the amount of retained fluid to the intake-output record. Include the frequency with which the tube needs to be irrigated in order to maintain its patency, and whether air was inserted into a vent tube. Much of this information can be included on flow sheets in the health record.

After removing a nasogastric tube, record the time, length of time the tube was clamped before removal, and the presence or absence of abdominal distention, nausea, vomiting, and any indication of discomfort.

Sample POR Recording

- S—"No, I'm not nauseated and my stomach feels OK. Yes, I've passed some gas."
- O—Abdomen soft; N/G tube has been clamped for 12 hr; bowel sounds present in the RLQ & LLQ; no vomiting.
- A—Peristalsis reestablished; no apparent problems while N/G tube clamped.
- P—N/G tube removed per order of Dr. Smith @ 8:30 P.M. Monitor for abdominal distention and nausea and vomiting for next 24 hr.

Sample Narrative Recording

N/G tube clamped since 8:30 A.M. States he is not nauseated, has not vomited, and has been passing gas. Abdomen soft; bowel sounds heard in RLQ & LLQ. No apparent problems while N/G tube clamped. Tube removed @ 8:30 P.M. per order of Dr. Smith.

□ CRITICAL POINTS SUMMARY

1. A nasogastric tube must be placed correctly to avoid respiratory complications.
2. Nursing-care measures will minimize the problems associated with having a nasogastrointestinal tube in place.
3. Intermittent gastrointestinal suction may be provided by a portable thermotic pump or with a wall regulator and pipeline vacuum.
4. Physical appraisal of the abdomen provides data for evaluating abdominal distention.
5. Physical appraisal of the abdomen is done in the following sequence—inspection, auscultation, percussion, and palpation.
6. Insert a nasogastric tube with the client in a high Fowler's position.
7. Insert a nasogastric tube to a depth of halfway between 50 cm from the distal tip and the NEX length (nose–ear–xiphoid).
8. Check nasogastric tubing placement by:
   a. Observing for cyanosis or respiratory difficulty
   b. Inserting air into the stomach and listening for its sound, and
   c. Aspirating gastric contents.
9. Secure a nasogastric tube without causing pressure on the external nares.
10. Allow an intestinal tube to advance through the intestines.
11. Irrigate nasogastric tubes frequently to maintain patency, unless contraindicated.
12. Instill air in the vent of a sump tube at regular intervals to help maintain its patency and function.
13. Measure and record the amount and characteristics of all gastrointestinal drainage.
14. Maintain accurate intake and output records for all clients with gastrointestinal tubes.

□ LEARNING ACTIVITIES

1. Work with a partner and examine each other's abdomen, using the skills of inspection, auscultation, percussion, and light palpation. Repeat with another partner and compare findings.
2. Examine various kinds of tubes used for gastrointestinal intubation. Note the different sizes, lengths, perforations, number of lumens, and composition. Relate those characteristics to the clinical use of each tube.
3. Obtain a Gomco Thermotic pump from central service.
   a. Practice removing the rubber stopper and taking the collection bottle out of its holder.
   b. Place the end of the suction tubing in a large bottle or pail of water (water source) that is placed below the level of the collection bottle.

Turn on the suction machine and note the length of time before water enters the collection bottle. Note which glass tube in the collection bottle stopper is for suction and which is for drainage. Observe the intermittent flashing light and listen to the sound of the suction, noting the relationship to the water being drawn into the collection bottle.

c. When some of the water has been drawn into the collection bottle and the suction tubing is full of water, raise the water source above the level of the glass tube from which drainage exits. Then raise the center of the drainage tubing above the level of the water source while keeping the end of the tubing submerged under water. Turn off the suction and observe the siphon action that causes the water source to continue to empty into the collection bottle. Explain this action. Lower the water source below the level of the glass tube and note the water flow. Turn on the suction and note the water flow.

d. Observe the rate of flow into the collection bottle as it becomes full and compare it with the initial flow rate. Gently press down on the collection bottle to trigger the weight-controlled shutoff mechanism.

4. Observe both a Gomco Thermotic pump and a wall suction regulator in use in a clinical area.
5. Talk with several staff nurses who care for clients with nasogastric tubes on a regular basis. Inquire about the most common problems they have encountered inserting or maintaining nasogastric tubes and how they have managed those problems.
6. Talk with clients who have had nasogastric tubes. Inquire about their perceptions of the insertion procedure and the experience of having a tube in the nose. What discomforts and problems did they encounter?
7. In a clinical or simulated setting, observe insertion and removal of a nasogastric tube.
8. Under supervision of an experienced person, insert a nasogastric tube in a peer. Remove the tube. Reverse roles, using a clean tube. Compare your experiences.

☐ REVIEW QUESTIONS

1. Explain the sequence in which physical appraisal skills are used when appraising the abdomen.
2. Match the organs in Column II with the quadrant or region of the abdomen in which they are located in Column I. The organs in Column II may be used more than one time.

COLUMN I	COLUMN II
_____ LUQ	A. Ascending colon
_____ LLQ	B. Bladder
_____ RUQ	C. Cecum
_____ RLQ	D. Descending colon
_____ Epigastric	E. Duodenum
_____ Suprapubic	F. Pyloric valve
_____ Umbilical	G. Sigmoid colon
	H. Stomach
	I. Transverse colon

3. What physical appraisal data would you expect to find when the abdomen is distended from free fluid in the peritoneal cavity?
4. What data would accompany distention with intestinal gases?
5. What is the most accurate way to measure insertion distance for nasogastric tubes?
6. Why is a client placed in a 30 to 45 degree elevation prior to irrigating or removing a nasogastric tube?
7. Circle the correct option in the following statements about *inserting* a nasogastric tube:
   a. Place the client in a (semi-Fowler's position/nearly upright position/on the right side).
   b. Initially, the client's neck should be (flexed/hyperextended).
   c. Direct the insertion force (downward toward the ear/up into the nose).
   d. As the tube moves down toward the pharynx, (hold tube steady without rotation/rotate tube 180 degrees).
   e. Before advancing the tube into the esophagus, have the client (flex/hyperextend) the neck.
   f. While advancing the tube, have the client (deep breathe/pant/swallow water).

   Explain each of your choices.

8. What are two reasons a nasogastric tube is advanced into the esophagus between the client's respirations and while the client is swallowing?
9. Describe the most accurate way to check placement of a nasogastric tube after insertion or prior to irrigation.
10. What principle is involved in taping a nasogastric or intestinal tube in place?
11. How do continuous and intermittent suction differ?
12. What nursing actions should be taken if drainage appears in the overflow trap bottles of either wall suction systems or a Gomco Thermotic pump?
13. What potential danger exists when clients with nasogastric tubes consume large amounts of ice chips and tap water or when tap water irrigations are used?
14. Why is normal saline or an electrolyte solution used to irrigate a nasogastric tube?
15. What function is served by the vent tube in a sump-style tube?
16. What are the most common reasons for air vent leakage in a sump-style tube?
17. For what reasons are intake and output monitored when gastrointestinal suction is used?

PERFORMANCE CHECKLISTS

OBJECTIVE: To use the correct measuring, insertion, and placement check techniques to insert a nasogastric tube.

CHARACTERISTIC	RANGE OF ACCEPTABILITY	SATISFACTORY	UNSATISFACTORY
1. Prepares equipment.	No deviation		
2. Identifies client and explains procedure.	No deviation		
3. Checks pump function.	Applicable only if suction to be used.		
4. Washes hands.	No deviation		
5. Warms plastic tubing in warm water. OR: chills soft rubber tubing.	No deviation		
6. Places client in near-upright position.	Modify if contraindicated by physician.		
7. Selects nostril with greatest patency.	Use opposite nostril to replace existing tube.		
8. Checks gag reflex.	No deviation		
9. Lubricates distal tip of tube.	No deviation		
10. Provides client with straw and glass of water and tissues.	Use empty straw if water contraindicated.		
11. Has client hyperextend neck.	No deviation		
12. Inserts tube with curved tip down, directs force toward ear and rotates tube inward 180 degrees.	Rotation may not be helpful.		
13. Allows client to rest before inserting tube into esophagus.	No deviation		
14. Has client flex neck.	No deviation		
15. Inserts with swallows and between respirations.	No deviation		
16. Checks tube placement: a. Inserts air into stomach b. Aspirates gastric contents c. Asks client to talk or hum	No deviation		
17. Anchors tube to client's nose with no pressure to external naris.	No deviation		
18. Fastens tube to clothing.	No deviation		
19. Returns client to position of comfort.	No deviation		
20. Disposes of equipment correctly.	No deviation		
21. Washes hands.	No deviation		
22. Records pertinent data.	No deviation		

OBJECTIVE: To use the correct technique to irrigate a nasogastric or intestinal tube.

CHARACTERISTIC	RANGE OF ACCEPTABILITY	SATISFACTORY	UNSATISFACTORY
1. Prepares equipment.	If equipment is in room, check for cleanliness; change every 24 to 48 hr.		
2. Explains procedure.	No deviation		
3. Washes hands.	No deviation		
4. Draws solution into syringe.	No deviation		
5. Positions client in 30 to 45 degree elevation.	Modify if contraindicated by physician.		
6. Disconnects suction (if thermotic pump, clamps suction tubing).	With T-connector, clamp suction tubing leading to pump.		
7. Inserts fluid slowly into suction lumen.	No deviation		

(continued)

CHARACTERISTIC	RANGE OF ACCEPTABILITY	SATISFACTORY	UNSATISFACTORY
8. Alternately inserts and aspirates fluid until tube is patent.	Fluid may return through suction tubing.		
9. Repositions tube and client as needed.	Avoid respositioning tube if inserted during gastric or esophageal surgery.		
10. Inserts air into vent lumen of a vented sump tube.	No deviation		
11. Reestablishes suction.	No deviation		
12. Rinses equipment with hot water, stores for reuse.	Use cold water if frank blood present.		
13. Repositions client for comfort.	No deviation		
14. Records pertinent data.	No deviation		

OBJECTIVE: To use the correct technique to remove a nasogastric tube.

CHARACTERISTIC	RANGE OF ACCEPTABILITY	SATISFACTORY	UNSATISFACTORY
1. Evaluates client status.	No deviation		
2. Explains procedure.	No deviation		
3. Prepares equipment.	No deviation		
4. Washes hands.	No deviation		
5. Shuts off suction.	No deviation		
6. Positions client to 45 degree elevation.	Turn on right side if unable to elevate.		
7. Removes anchoring tape and pin.	No deviation		
8. Dons nonsterile gloves.	Use a towel to handle tube.		
9. Has client breathe in and hold.	No deviation		
10. Removes tube steadily.	No deviation		
11. Offers tissues and mouth care.	No deviation		
12. Removes equipment; discards or returns to central service.	No deviation		
13. Washes hands.	No deviation		
14. Records pertinent data.	No deviation		

REFERENCES

Condon RE, Nyhus LM (eds): Manual of Surgical Therapeutics, ed 6. Boston, Little, Brown, 1985.

Flitter HH: An Introduction to Physics in Nursing, ed 7. St Louis, CV Mosby, 1976.

Griggs BA, Hoppe MC: Update: Nasogastric tube feeding. American Journal of Nursing 79(3):483–485, 1979.

Hanson RL: Predictive criteria for length of nasogastric tube insertion for tube feeding. JPEN 3(3):160–163, 1979.

Hirsch J, Hannock L (eds): Mosby's Manual of Clinical Nursing Procedures. St Louis, CV Mosby, 1981.

Jensen JT: Physics for the Health Professions, ed 2. Philadelphia, JB Lippincott, 1976.

Luckmann J, Sorenson KC: Medical-Surgical Nursing: A Psychophysiologic Approach, ed 2. Philadelphia, WB Saunders, 1980.

McConnell E: All about gastrointestinal intubation. Nursing75 5(9):30–37, 1975.

McConnell E: Ten problems with nasogastric tubes . . . and how to solve them. Nursing79 9(4):78–81, 1979.

Metheny NM, Snively WD: Nurses' Handbook of Fluid Balance, ed 4. Philadelphia, JB Lippincott, 1983.

Operating Instructions and Spare Parts Manual, Gomco Thermotic Drainage Pumps, Models 764 and 765-A. Buffalo, NY, Gomco Surgical Manufacturing, 1969.

Robins AH: G.I. Series: Physical Examination of the Abdomen. Richmond, VA, AH Robins, 1974.

Robinson EP Jr, Cox PN: Feeding tube introduction—An easier way. Critical Care Medicine 7(8):349–350, 1979.

Sana JM, Judge RD: Physical Assessment Skills for Nursing Practice, ed 2. Boston, Little, Brown, 1982.

BIBLIOGRAPHY

Bates B: A Guide to Physical Examination, ed 3. Philadelphia, JB Lippincott, 1983.

Beyers M, Dudas S: The Clinical Practice of Medical-Surgical Nursing, ed 2. Boston, Little, Brown, 1984.

Brunner LS, Suddarth DS: The Lippincott Manual of Nursing Practice, ed 3. Philadelphia, JB Lippincott, 1982.

Beyers M, Dudas S: The Clinical Practice of Medical-Surgical Nursing, ed 2. Boston, Little, Brown, 1984.

Erickson R: Tube talk: Principles of fluid flow in tubes. Nursing82 (Horsham) 12(7):54–62, 1982.

Guyton AC: Human Physiology and Mechanisms of Disease, ed 3. Philadelphia, WB Saunders, 1982.

Kozier B, Erb G: Techniques in Clinical Nursing. A Comprehensive Approach. Menlo Park, CA, Addison-Wesley, 1982.

Lindberg JB, Hunter ML, Knuszeuski AZ: Skills Manual for Introduction to Person-Centered Nursing. Philadelphia, JB Lippincott, 1983.

Malasanos L, Barkauskas V, et al: Health Assessment, ed 2. St Louis, CV Mosby, 1981.

Miller BF, Keane CB: Encyclopedia and Dictionary of Medicine, Nursing, and Allied Health, ed 3. Philadelphia, WB Saunders, 1983.

Sader AA: New way to stabilize nasogastric tubes. The American Journal of Surgery 130(1):102, 1975.

Smith CE: Abdominal assessment—A blending of science and art. Nursing81 (Horsham) 11(2):42–49, 1981.

VanWay CW III, Buerke C: Gastrointestinal intubation. In Bucci SL (ed): The Principles of Vacuum and Its Use in the Hospital Environment. Madison, WI, Ohio Medical Products, 1978.

Volden C, Grinde J, Carl D: Taking the trauma out of nasogastric intubation. Nursing80 10(9):64–67, 1980.

SUGGESTED READING

Griggs BA, Hoppe MC: Update: Nasogastric tube feeding. American Journal of Nursing79(3):483–485, 1979.

McConnell E: All about gastrointestinal intubation. Nursing75 5(9):30–37, 1975.

McConnell E: Ten problems with nasogastric tubes and how to solve them. Nursing79(4):78–81, 1979.

Smith CE: Abdominal assessment—A blending of science and art. Nursing81 (Horsham) 11(2):42–49, 1981.

Volden C, Grinde J, Carl D: Taking the trauma out of nasogastric intubation. Nursing80 10(9):64–67, 1980.

AUDIOVISUAL RESOURCES

Nasal Intubation for Enteral Feedings
Film. (1981, Color, 20 min.)
Available through:
Ross Laboratories
Educational Services Department
625 Cleveland Avenue
Columbus, OH 43216

Nasogastric Intubation
Videocassette. (1976, 7 min.)
Available through:
Health Sciences Learning Resources Center
University of Washington
Seattle, WA 98195

Nasogastric Intubation
Videocassette. (1973, 30 min.)
Available through:
Institute for Continuing Physician Education
4530 W. 77th St.
Edina, MN

Gastric and Gastrointestinal Decompression
Filmstrip. (1977, Color, 20 min.)

Nasogastric Intubation
Filmstrip. (1977, Color, 15 min.)
Available through:
Medcom, Inc.
P.O. Box 116
Garden Grove, CA 92642

Nasogastric Intubation
Film. (1973, 8 min.)
Available through:
National Medical Audiovisual Center
Order Section E-Q
Washington, DC 20409

SKILL 57 Bedpans and Urinals

PREREQUISITE SKILLS

Skill 19, "Inspection"
Skill 20, "Palpation"
Skill 21, "Percussion"
Skill 22, "Auscultation"
Skill 28, "Handwashing"
Skill 34, "Wound Culture Specimen Collection"
Skill 39, "Perineal Care"
Skill 56, "Insertion and Care of Gastrointestinal Tubes"

☐ STUDENT OBJECTIVES

1. Identify normal and abnormal characteristics of urine and stool.
2. Describe physiological positions for voiding and defecating.
3. Describe common elimination problems that result from physiological and psychosocial factors.
4. Describe nursing measures that enhance the ability to respond to voiding and defecation reflexes.

5. Describe data indicative of urinary retention with bladder distention.
6. Differentiate techniques used in offering bedpans and urinals to alert clients, to clients needing assistance, and to helpless clients.
7. Explain ways to promote client comfort, safety, and privacy and avoid embarrassment when offering and removing bedpans and urinals.
8. Offer and remove a bedpan and urinal in a safe manner, using appropriate medically aseptic techniques.
9. Identify the nurse's responsibility in collecting and testing urine and stool specimens.

□ INTRODUCTION

Bedpans and urinals are used as alternative receptacles for urine and feces when either the client is not able to use a toilet or when urine and stool specimens need to be collected. Examples of reasons a person may be unable to go to the bathroom include immobility, such as with body casts, traction, or recent spinal fusion; medical restrictions on the amount of activity permitted, such as after a heart attack, threatened abortion, or with aneurysm precautions; or physical weakness, such as in terminal illness or immediately after surgery.

The degree of assistance required in using bedpans and urinals varies. Some clients are able to use bedpans or urinals independently and only need to have them available for use and then have someone empty and return the utensil. Some clients, such as those recovering from recent surgery or those who are weak, tired, or lack neuromuscular coordination, need assistance in using a bedpan or urinal but are able to identify their need to eliminate and ask the nurse for assistance. Others may know when they need to void (urinate) or defecate but have difficulty communicating that need to the nurse—for example, persons with tracheostomies, oral surgery, and some neuromuscular conditions have difficulty verbalizing their needs. Language differences can create similar problems. Lastly, there are clients who need assistance but are unable to identify when they need to void or defecate and therefore cannot ask the nurse for the bedpan and urinal—for example, persons who are mentally or emotionally impaired or confused or those who have lost neuromuscular control over their elimination processes.

Offering bedpans or urinals is a very common yet essential nursing procedure. Assisting clients with bowel and bladder elimination helps them meet a basic human need, and observations of urine and stool provide valuable information about their health status. Urine and stool are collected in bedpans and urinals for the purpose of measuring output volumes and obtaining specimens for testing. Urine and stool specimens are tested by the nurse or the client or are sent to the laboratory for analysis. These specimens are used for diagnostic purposes, to monitor health status, and to evaluate the effect of some therapies. The accuracy of the test results often is dependent on whether the nurse has followed correct collecting and testing procedures.

In addition to being sources of information, feces and urine can also be the cause of problems such as wound and bladder infections. Microorganisms that are normal for the colon become pathogens when introduced into wounds and the bladder. Although normal urine is sterile, it usually contains perineal microorganisms. Both urine and stool can carry pathogenic microorganisms, and handling urine and stool is considered a contaminated activity (see Skill 28). Therefore, the nurse is careful to handle bedpans and urinals in a medically aseptic manner, and wash hands carefully afterwards. Ordinary sewer systems provide adequate disposal of urine and stool, even when they contain pathogens.

□ PREPARATION

The frequency, timing, and actual capability of voiding or defecating are quite variable with different persons and depend on a number of physiological and psychosocial factors.

PHYSIOLOGICAL FACTORS AFFECTING ELIMINATION

Most people experience an urge to void when the bladder contains about 150 ml of urine and have marked sensations of bladder fullness at about 400 ml (Luckmann and Sorensen, 1980). However, the timing of bladder emptying varies with the person's tolerance for stretch sensations within the bladder, as well as with both physiological and psychosocial factors. Voiding may occur every 2 hours or as infrequently as two or three times per day. If urination occurs more often than every 1.5 hours or less than once in every 12 hours, it probably should be investigated (Sorensen and Luckmann, 1979).

Normal physiological voiding for females occurs in the seated or squatting position; for males, it occurs in the standing position. In these positions, gravity and increased intraabdominal pressure from abdominal muscle contractions aid voiding. Leaning forward, flexing the knees, or pressing on the abdomen also is sometimes helpful. Relaxation of the perineal muscles is essential for voiding to occur, and general muscular tension interferes with this relaxation. However, an overly relaxed or weak perineal musculature makes it difficult to inhibit the micturition reflex voluntarily and therefore contributes to sensations of frequency and urgency as well as dribbling of urine.

Voiding frequency is increased by drugs such as diuretics, by increased fluid intake, especially of caffeine-containing liquids like coffee or tea, by irritation from urinary tract infection, in advanced pregnancy when the fetus exerts pressure on the bladder, and when decreased sphincter control exists, as with a neurogenic bladder.

Voiding frequency is decreased when fluid intake is decreased and when people have developed an increased tolerance for bladder stretch pressure.

Bowel Elimination

The normal frequency of defecation varies from one to three bowel movements per day to one bowel movement one to three times a week, without the individual experiencing either diarrhea or constipation. In both males and females, the normal physiological position for defecation is the squatting position, where gravity and increased intraabdominal pressure from muscle contraction and leaning forward aid in expelling the feces.

Consistent *habit patterns* of defecation contribute greatly toward normal bowel elimination. Mass peristaltic movements, rather than the peristaltic waves of the small intestine, move the fecal contents through the large intestine. These movements usually occur only a few times each day and are most common for about 15 minutes during the first hour or so after breakfast. They are stimulated in part by the gastrocolic and duodenocolic reflexes that result from distention of the stomach and duodenum with food, particularly after an overnight fast. A rhythmic pattern of elimination can be established if the person responds consistently to the defecation reflex that occurs when the feces are forced downward into the rectum by these movements. If the reflex is ignored when it occurs, it will cease after a few minutes and return again when more stool enters the rectum, perhaps several hours later. It is sometimes possible to initiate the defecation reflex at a convenient time by taking a deep breath and performing Valsalva's maneuver (forcible exhalation against a closed glottis), thus forcing fecal contents into the rectum and eliciting a new reflex. However, Guyton (1982, p. 497) indicates that "unfortunately, reflexes initiated in this way are never as effective as those that arise naturally, for which reason people who inhibit their natural reflexes too often are likely to become severely constipated."

A high-fiber *diet* increases fecal bulk and gas-forming foods distend the intestinal wall, thus providing increased stimulation for the defecation reflex. A low-fiber, high-carbohydrate diet produces less fecal bulk and diminishes the defecation reflex. Increased *fluid intake* increases the bulk and softness of the stool, while an overall decreased intake of either food or fluid decreases fecal bulk. General *exercise* increases body muscle tone, and specific abdominal and perineal muscle exercises will strengthen the muscles used in defecation. Some *medications,* such as narcotics, cause constipation; others, such as antibiotics that destroy normal bacterial flora in the intestines, cause diarrhea. *Irritants* such as spicy foods, poisons, or bacterial toxins increase intestinal motility, decrease transit time in the large bowel, and usually result in an increased frequency of softer or liquid stools since there is less time for reabsorption of water. *Surgical procedures* affect bowel motility; for example, handling of the bowel during surgery stops peristalsis for up to several days. Surgery in the perineal area produces edema and may cause pain with defecation, which often causes the client to avoid defecation. Some *diagnostic tests* interfere with bowel function; for example, when a barium enema is administered, the colon is cleared with laxatives and enemas, an x-ray-opaque dye is inserted, and then more laxatives must be taken to clear the barium from the colon. *Increasing age* often causes decreased ability to maintain normal bowel elimination, *psychosomatic or functional stress-related factors* affect bowel elimination, and motor and sensory control for elimination may be disturbed by *neuromuscular conditions* such as spinal cord injury or stroke.

PSYCHOSOCIAL FACTORS AFFECTING ELIMINATION

For most people, urinating and defecating are very private processes. In the American culture, bathrooms have doors and locks. Public restrooms are separate for men and women and always have at least some cubicles with doors or curtains, especially in women's restrooms. Elimination is seldom discussed other than in slang terms or vulgarities. Children often do not learn the correct terminology for elimination or for the body organs and orifices associated with elimination functions. Many people never look at their own urine and stool, and often regard it with disgust. On the other hand, some people are quite open and comfortable in discussing elimination, and still others are overly preoccupied with bowel function, a concern promoted by American advertising.

The process of micturition is quite responsive to the power of suggestion through audio, visual, and mental channels. For example, thinking and talking about urination and knowing someone else is going to the bathroom are capable of initiating the micturition reflex. Conscious thought and a decision to urinate also can initiate micturition. Even though the urge to urinate becomes quite strong, the person who has been successfully toilet-trained and has no neurologic impairment usually can inhibit the micturition reflex for quite some time until a socially acceptable time and place are found.

Many people develop habit patterns surrounding defecation, such as drinking hot and cold liquids upon arising, and reading or drinking coffee in the bathroom. In addition to the psychological benefits of these practices, spending a relaxed and quiet time in the bathroom facilitates responding to the defecation impulse. Habit patterns associated with defecation are often interrupted by travel and inflexible or stressful work settings, and some people are unable to use any other than their own familiar bathroom for defecation.

In the hospital setting, lack of accustomed privacy often inhibits the ability to respond to voiding and defecation reflexes. The bathroom is shared with a stranger; the nurse may be of the opposite sex and may remain in the bathroom to help or wait just outside the door; and the person may need to use a commode, bedpan, or urinal while a roommate, nurse, or physician is on the other side of a curtain.

When people are acutely ill, they may welcome the assistance of a nurse with elimination, or at least accept it as necessary, although still preferring to do it independently. At other times, clients are quite uncomfortable with nurse assistance. Many nursing activities associated with elimination run counter to the mores instilled during the toilet-training period and early childhood. When giving bedpans and urinals, nurses often touch people in private body areas and perform functions considered personal; they ask questions about voiding and defecating and what urine and stool look like, sometimes within the hearing of other clients, relatives, or personnel; and they may ask clients to save and handle their own urine and stool for purposes of specimen collection.

For similiar reasons, nurses often are uncomfortable initially about discussing elimination, helping people with bedpans and urinals, and handling urine and stool for cleansing and testing purposes. A matter-of-fact, direct attitude, coupled with explanations of what has to be done, usually is helpful to both the nurse and the client. Out of necessity, nurses generally overcome this initial discomfort quite readily. Unfortunately, they sometimes forget that what has become commonplace to them still is uncommon for most clients.

APPRAISAL OF URINE AND FECES

Appraisal of urine and feces includes gross appraisal of the appearance and character of these substances, testing done by the nurse, and reports of laboratory analysis of specimens.

Appraisal of Urine

Color. Normal urine is sterile and light yellow to dark amber in color. Urine becomes concentrated and dark when urine output is decreased as a result of decreased fluid intake or dehydration. Medications may alter the color of urine. For example, the urinary antiseptic phenazopyridine (Pyridium) produces orange-colored urine, the anticonvulsant phenytoin (Dilantin) produces a urine that is pink, red, or red-brown in color, and iron preparations cause urine to become dark brown or black on standing (Slawson, 1980).

Foods such as blackberries, beets, and rhubarb can cause red urine, and large amounts of carotene produce bright yellow urine. When there is *bleeding* in the upper urinary tract, the urine becomes dark red or smoky-grey; bleeding in the lower tract produces red urine. Changes in urine color are discussed in greater detail in various laboratory reference manuals and medical-surgical textbooks.

Opacity. Normal freshly voided urine is transparent and becomes cloudy when standing. If freshly voided urine is cloudy, a urinary tract infection or inflammation may be suspected. A small amount of blood in the urine may also turn the urine cloudy or smoky.

Odor. Freshly voided urine has a characteristic aromatic odor. The ammonia odor of old urine results from bacterial splitting of urea molecules. A foul odor in freshly voided urine may be caused by a urinary tract infection, some drugs, or dietary intake of foods such as asparagus.

Specific Gravity. Normal urine specific gravity ranges from 1.003 to 1.030 (Metheny and Snively, 1983). A higher specific gravity often reflects dehydration, increased glucose concentration, or presence of a dye after x-ray. A dilute urine (1.001 to 1.010) may reflect overhydration, diuretic therapy, water intoxication, or diabetes insipidis (Fischbach, 1980).

pH. Normally, urine is slightly acidic, with a pH ranging from 4.3 to 8.0, depending on diet and acid-base balance. A higher pH represents a more alkaline urine and a lower pH, a more acidic urine. Maintaining urine pH is an important aspect of therapy for clients with urinary tract infections in which urine may be acidified with an acid-ash diet or large doses of vitamin C; and in the prevention of renal calculi when urine pH is made either more acidic with an acid-ash diet or more alkaline with an alkaline-ash diet, depending on the type of renal calculi.

Sediment. Urine sediment normally contains a few epithelial cells, a few white blood cells (<5 per high-power field (hpf)), occasional red blood cells (2 to 3 per hpf), a few hyaline or granular casts, and sometimes a few bacteria or yeast from perineal contamination (Condon and Nyhus, 1985, p. 163; Corbett, 1982, p. 71).

Abnormal Components. Normal urine contains no protein, glucose, or ketones. Urine is frequently tested for these substances since their presence or absence is used to detect or monitor illness conditions. For example, protein may be present in acute stress or renal disease, glucose in diabetes mellitus, and ketones in diabetic ketoacidosis.

Appraisal of Feces

Normal Components. Approximately 150 g of feces is produced each day. The feces are composed of about 25 percent solid material and 75 percent water. The solid material consists of about 30 percent dead bacteria, 10 to 20 percent fat, 10 to 20 percent inorganic material, 2 to 3 percent protein, and 30 percent undigested roughage of food and dried constituents of digestive juices, such as bile pigments and sloughed epithelial cells (Guyton, 1982, p. 517). Since food residues comprise only a part of the fecal contents, even clients who receive no oral intake will continue to have bowel movements.

Color. Normal feces are brown in color, due to the presence of bile pigments. White or clay-colored stools, known as *acholic stools,* indicate lack of bile pigments or a biliary obstruction. Pale stools with visible fat and mucus are called *steatorrhea* and are associated with malabsorption of fats. *Black stools* occur with supplemental iron, increased dietary intake of foods high in iron such as spinach, or upper gastrointestinal bleeding. *Melena* refers to black stools with a tar-like consistency that occur because of digested blood in the stool. Black stools and melena are not the same as the normal dark green mucilagenous first stools of full-term newborn infants. *Red stools* can be caused by lower gastrointestinal bleeding and undigested blood, or from excessive ingestion of beets. Red blood smeared on the outside of the feces is usually a sign of hemorrhoidal bleeding and red blood mixed in with the feces represents bleeding from the colon.

Consistency. Feces are normally soft formed from the shape of the rectum. Depending on the amount of water in the feces, they may also be soft and unformed liquid or hard. Very hard stools are sometimes described as marbles, pellets, or rock-like. Liquid stools are referred to as diarrhea.

Odor. The characteristic odor of feces comes from the action of intestinal bacteria on the fecal contents. The odor varies with the individual's own colonic bacterial flora and with the food eaten. The presence of bleeding or gastrointestinal infections produces more foul odors than usual. The odor of stool also changes with the pH, which is dependent on bacterial fermentation and putrefaction within the bowel (Fischbach, 1980).

Abnormal Components. Sometimes the feces contain substances that normally are absorbed in digestion, such as the fecal fat that occurs in the stools of people who have malabsorption problems. Other abnormal components of feces may aid in diagnosis of illness, for example, bacteria, parasites, pus, blood, and unusually large amounts of colonic mucus.

COMMON PROBLEMS THAT INTERFERE WITH VOIDING AND DEFECATION MECHANISMS

A variety of urinary and bowel problems and symptoms may reflect specific illness conditions or a more general lack of good health. Common urinary problems and symptoms include

- dysuria (painful or difficult urination)
- difficulty voiding
- frequency (urination at short intervals without an increase in total daily urine output)
- urgency (a sudden, compelling desire to void)
- nocturia (excessive urination at night)
- dribbling (leading urine between voidings)
- retention (inability to urinate)
- hematuria (blood in the urine)
- hesitancy (difficulty starting the urine stream)
- decrease in size and force of the urinary stream

Common bowel problems and symptoms include

- constipation (hard stools that are difficult to pass)
- diarrhea (liquid stools)
- flatulence (excessive intestinal gas)
- fecal impaction (inability to defecate, accompanied by seepage of liquid stool)

Difficulty Voiding

Clients may experience difficulty voiding because of physiological reasons such as the aftereffects of anesthesia or from the general muscle tension associated with pain. Clients are generally able to void 8 to 16 hours after surgery. However, after perineal or gynecologic surgery, postoperative edema and anticipated fear of pain often cause difficulty voiding for a longer period of time. Unfamiliar surroundings and any strong emotions such as fear, excitement, or embarrassment can also interfere with the ability to respond to the micturition reflex. Generally these problems with voiding are temporary and will respond to nursing measures to induce voiding.

Voiding Inducement Measures. If the client is in pain, medication to relieve pain may induce voiding. If permitted, increased fluid intake often aids in voiding. Although it is sometimes difficult, providing maximum privacy in the bathroom or at the bedside may help. Clients who are sensitive about the sounds of elimination in a shared room may be helped by turning on the television, radio, or water faucet to mask these noises. Placing the hands in warm water or listening to the sound of running water will sometimes induce voiding. Male patients generally can void if assisted to a standing position, and females will find it easier to void in a near-squatting position, which can usually at least be partially achieved in bed when using a bedpan. Moist heat applied to the female perineum, such as with a warm wet washcloth, can sometimes induce voiding; or warm water may be poured over the perineum while the client sits on the toilet or bedpan. A warm tub bath, Sitz bath, or shower may decrease general muscle tension and relax the perineal muscles sufficiently enough to induce micturition. Sometimes drugs such as neostigmine (Prostigmin) or bethanecol (Urecholine) are ordered by the physician to induce voiding.

The common problems of difficulty voiding, urinary retention, and diarrhea are discussed here. Constipation, flatulence, and fecal impaction are discussed in Skill 58. Information about these and other problems can be found in medical–surgical and fundamentals textbooks and other sources.

Urinary Retention
Urinary retention exists when urine is being produced and the bladder fills with urine, but the person is unable to void. It is not to be confused with anuria (lack of urine) and oliguria (decreased amounts of urine). One of the most common causes of urinary retention in males is prostatic hypertrophy, since 30 to 50 percent of all males over 50 years have some degree of prostatic hypertrophy with varying degrees of urethral constriction (Luckmann and Sorensen, 1980). Other causes of retention for both sexes include anesthesia; medications such as opiates, sedatives, antihistamines, and antipsychotics; injury to the sensory or motor nerves involved with micturition, such as with spinal cord injury; urethral stricture; bladder calculi; or fecal impaction. Poor fluid intake also contributes to retention because the detrusor stretch receptors are not activated when the bladder fills at a slow rate. On the other hand, when the detrusors are stretched beyond a certain point, they become incapable of contracting and micturition does not occur; thus, urinary catheterization becomes necessary.

As the bladder continues to fill, it rises above the symphysis pubis. A full, distended bladder often is visible, palpable, and can be percussed. Subjectively, the client experiences discomfort and fullness and an almost continuous desire to void without being able to do so. The discomfort increases as the bladder distends and may become quite acute and associated with diaphoresis and restlessness. In some conditions, the bladder may distend to accommodate 3000 to 4000 ml of urine (Elhart et al., 1978, p. 572).

When the bladder reaches a certain degree of fullness, the pressure forces some of the urine out through the urethra, resulting in what is called *retention with overflow*. The person continues to experience the need to urinate, and as the bladder continues to fill, it again overflows. When small amounts of urine (30 to 60 ml) are voided at frequent intervals (15 or 20 minutes to 1 hour), the nurse suspects retention with overflow and appraises the abdomen for bladder distention.

Urinary retention with excessive bladder distention is a potentially serious problem. The overstretched bladder wall is susceptible to ischemia and breaks in the mucosa, both of which predispose to bladder infections. Also, the distention straightens the protective oblique entry of the ureters into the bladder and predisposes to urine reflux into the ureters and possibly even a kidney infection (Beland and Passos, 1981; Sorensen and Luckmann, 1979).

Deep bimanual palpation is used for detecting a distended bladder. Place the palmar surfaces of the fingers between 2.5 to 5 cm (1 to 2 in) above the pubic bone, and gently but firmly press downward, curving the fingers back toward the hands (Burns and Johnson, 1980, p. 211). If the bladder is not palpable at that point but other signs and symptoms indicate a possible distention, relocate the hands higher on the abdomen and palpate again. The bladder sometimes distends as high as the umbilicus. A distended bladder feels round, smooth, and like a tense mass (Malasanos et al., 1981, p. 372). In thin or relaxed persons, palpation of the abdomen may identify the presence of stool in the sigmoid colon or cecum, as described in Skill 58. Obesity obscures the findings obtained through palpation of both bladder and bowel. To percuss the borders of the bladder, begin just above the symphysis pubis and percuss caudally and laterally, noting where the sounds change to the normal tympany of the abdomen. As with palpation, percussion is difficult on obese persons.

Diarrhea
Diarrhea, or liquid stools, can be caused by many factors. Emotions such as anxiety are common causes of diarrhea, and for some people, it can result from spicy and greasy foods or water that contains microorganisms to which they have not developed immunity. Other causes include infectious organisms such as staphylococci, streptococci, or salmonella, medications such as laxatives, thyroid preparations, or some antibiotics, and hyperosmolar tube feedings when the adaptation process is hurried.

Consistency rather than frequency of stools is usually used to define diarrhea. Diarrhea occurs when intestinal motility is greatly increased, intestinal transit time is reduced substantially, and less water is absorbed from the feces. Combined with secretions from intestinal irritation, the result is feces that are still liquid when they reach the rectum.

Along with liquid stools, people often experience abdominal cramps, distention, flatus, urgency of defecation, or symptoms of malaise, anorexia, vomiting, and temperature elevation. If diarrhea continues, fluid and electrolyte depletion can occur. Diarrhea stools are acidic in nature and contain intestinal enzymes that readily cause irritation and excoriation if they remain in contact with the skin. When someone has diarrhea, it often is helpful to apply a protective ointment around the anus, such as zinc oxide or, if irritation has already developed, a vitamin A and D ointment.

SPECIMEN TESTING AND COLLECTION

Urine and stool specimens are frequently collected for diagnosis, monitoring of health and illness status, and evaluation of the effectiveness of therapy. Specimens may be tested by the nurse or client in the home, clinic, or hospital setting to determine the presence or absence of substances such as glucose, acetone, protein, and blood. These tests use enzyme reagent strips (often called dipsticks) or reagent tablets and provide an almost immediate estimate of the amount of the substance present in the urine or stool specimen.

It is important to follow instructions precisely when using reagent tables and dipsticks. Beaumont

(1975) estimated that approximately 10 percent of all test readings using diagnostic test kits are incorrect due to human error in testing. Williams's 1971 study of 122 nursing personnel revealed that significant errors in urine testing for glucose and acetone were made by staff persons of all educational levels. Errors were more likely to occur when staff members performed those kinds of tests frequently and when they knew the results of the client's previous tests. Apparently, familiarity with the procedure decreased the care and precision used, and nurses tended to obtain the results they were anticipating. Specific directions for using testing materials are included on product containers and in test kits and package inserts, and laboratory manuals give detailed descriptions of testing procedures, precautions and safeguards regarding product use, and interpretation of the results.

If more complex and precise evaluations of urine and stool are required, specimens are sent to a laboratory. The method used to collect a specimen may vary with the type of test to be performed. For example, when a urine culture is ordered, a sterile urine specimen must be collected to isolate the offending organism. The nurse's role in collecting a variety of urine and stool specimens is described in laboratory manuals, hospital procedure books, and medical–surgical nursing textbooks. It is important to identify the proper procedure for collection, storage, and transportation to the laboratory before collecting the specimen because the accuracy of test results often depends on the accuracy of the collection procedure. For example, a major problem in diagnosing urinary tract infections is the number of false positives due to improper collection techniques (Sorensen and Luckmann, 1979, p. 731). If there is any uncertainty about specimen collection procedure, consult the laboratory that will be doing the analysis.

A method known as a clean-catch midstream technique is used to collect a sterile urine specimen. A urinary catheter is inserted only if the client is unable to assist with the technique. The nurse's role in collecting a clean-catch specimen is to teach the person how to collect the specimen correctly. It is important for the client to understand that accurate culture results depend on following the technique exactly as directed so that unwanted microorganisms are not introduced into the specimen. Instruct the client to carry out the following steps:

1. Open the sterile urine container and place it near the toilet.
2. *Females:* Remove all clothing from the waist down, sit on the toilet with the legs spread apart widely, separate the labia with the fingers and keep them separated.
   Males: Stand in front of the toilet; retract the foreskin, if needed, to expose urethral meatus.
3. Cleanse meatus with antiseptic wipes. Females are to cleanse front to back with 3 tissues as for urinary catheterization (Skill 60).
4. Start the urine stream into the toilet.
5. Hold specimen cup a few inches from the meatus and catch enough urine to fill the container about two-thirds full.
6. Finish voiding in the toilet.
7. Place lid on the specimen container.

DATA BASE

When offering a bedpan or urinal or when collecting urine and stool specimens, it is helpful to inquire about previous experiences with these activities. The nurse is then able to take this information into consideration when explaining the process to the client. It is important to know the institution's policies for cleaning and storing bedpans and urinals if each client is not provided with a personal one. Before giving a bedpan or urinal to a client, the nurse identifies whether or not a specimen is to be collected, the purpose for collecting the specimen, and how to conduct the test or collect the specimen and transport it to the laboratory. If the nurse is performing the test, the directions for that specific test and any needed color charts should be available before the specimen is collected.

Client History and Recorded Data

The health record provides background information to help the nurse judge whether the appearance, consistency, and amount of urine and stool are within normal limits for this person. This judgment is based on the medical diagnosis, diagnostic tests, therapeutic plans, general health status, and conditions that are being monitored, such as diabetes mellitus or gastrointestinal bleeding.

The health record may include activity restrictions that affect bathroom use, such as "up ad lib," "bathroom privileges," "stand to void," or "BR for BM only." However, the nurse is often responsible for determining whether the client uses the bathroom, a commode, a bedpan, or a urinal. To make this decision, in addition to the medical diagnosis, age, and activity restrictions, the nurse uses information from the nursing history, kardex, or nurses' notes about the client's general health status and functional abilities. That is, the nurse would consider the client's strength, coordination, mental status, physical limitations, aids needed for elimination, and problems such as nocturia, urgency, or difficulty starting the urine stream.

In addition to written information, it is important also to appraise directly the client's physical ability to go to the bathroom or to lift himself or herself onto the bedpan, and determine the most beneficial and feasible position for elimination. Although this kind of information may be recorded appropriately, client status and abilities often change rapidly and require current appraisal.

Physical Appraisal Skills

Inspection. The nurse uses inspection to determine the amount, color, appearance, and opacity of urine and the amount, color, and consistency of stool. Inspection is used to determine the correct position of a client on the bedpan and to compare the results of specimen testing with color charts. Sometimes inspection will reveal the presence of a distended bladder in the suprapubic area.

Palpation. Palpation is used to identify the presence of a distended bladder and the presence of feces in the sigmoid colon.

Percussion. The outline of a distended bladder may be defined by percussion. A full bladder has a dull or kettle-drum sound.

Auscultation. The presence or absence of bowel sounds is determined by auscultation.

Sense of Smell. The characteristic aromatic odor of urine and the pungent odor of stool are evident through the sense of smell. Abnormal or unusual odors may be noted, as identified earlier.

EQUIPMENT

Bedpans

Bedpans are used for defecation by both men and women. Women also use a bedpan for voiding, whereas men usually prefer to use a urinal. Bedpans are used in bed, on a chair, or may be placed in a commode beside the bed for clients who have difficulty using them in bed and cannot go to the bathroom.

Bedpans are made of plastic or metal and are available in two styles, as shown in Figure 57-1. The standard, high-backed bedpan has one open end and a three-sided flat rim that is placed under the client's buttocks (Fig. 57-1A). Standard bedpans are available in adult and pediatric sizes. Small, thin, or emaciated clients often find the pediatric bedpan more comfortable. The fracture or slipper bedpan has one low flattened end that is placed under the buttocks and a handle on the higher end that is used to help place and remove the pan (Fig. 57-1B). This pan is used for clients who cannot be turned safely, such as those who have spinal injuries, or those who are difficult to lift or turn onto a standard bedpan, such as clients who have body casts or who are immobilized with some types of traction.

Plastic bedpans may be included as part of the admission equipment kit given to a client or obtained later if needed. They are cleaned between use and either sent home with the client upon discharge or discarded. Metal bedpans may be kept in the bedside stand as part of the standard equipment. After the client is discharged, they are cleaned and sterilized by the central supply department. In some health-care facilities, individual bedpans are not provided; instead, metal bedpans are kept in a centrally located soiled utility room. With this system, after the bedpan has been emptied, cleaned and resterilized, it is returned to the common supply. An institution may use this method on units where bedpans are seldom needed, such as on primarily ambulatory, self-care, or psychiatric units.

Bedpan Covers. Bedpan covers are pieces of sturdy cloth or flexible paper that are used to cover the bedpan or urinal while it is being carried to the bathroom or utility room. In addition to an aesthetic function, these covers diminish objectionable odors and decrease client embarrassment.

Cleaning Bedpans. Bedpans are rinsed after each use, either in the client's bathroom or in the soiled utility room. Many institutional bathrooms have a flexible hose or hinged arm attached to the toilet plumbing that is used to rinse the bedpan after it has been emptied into the toilet. A sink that is used for handwashing is never used for this purpose. A disinfectant solution and brush may be kept in the bathroom for cleaning fecal material from the bedpan. The bedpan is stored in the bedside unit out of sight. If a client is experiencing urgency or diarrhea and wishes to have the bedpan more readily accessible, it is covered and placed on a chair or at the foot of the bed. When bedpans are used for a long period of time or frequently become heavily soiled, metal ones are replaced occasionally with a newly sterilized one, and plastic ones are disinfected or discarded. When cleaning a bedpan, rinse and brush up under the rim where liquid feces can sometimes accumulate.

Bedpan Flushers. When bedpans are used for more than one client, the utility room contains a large square open hopper or a bedpan flusher. The large open hopper flushes like a toilet and usually has an attached spray nozzle on the end of a hose for rinsing the bedpan. A brush and disinfectant solution also may be available. A bedpan flusher is a device that automatically empties the bedpan and scrubs it with a cold water scrub cycle, followed by a steam heat cycle. The flusher is opened with a foot pedal that spreads the locking clamps that hold the bedpan or urinal in place during the cleaning cycle, as shown in **Figure**

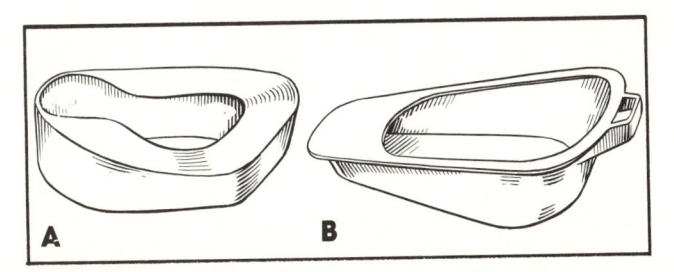

Figure 57-1. A. Regular style bedpan. Available in adult and pediatric sizes. The rounded flat rim is placed under the buttocks. B. Fracture or slipper pan. The flattened end is placed under the buttocks and the handle used to assist placement and removal.

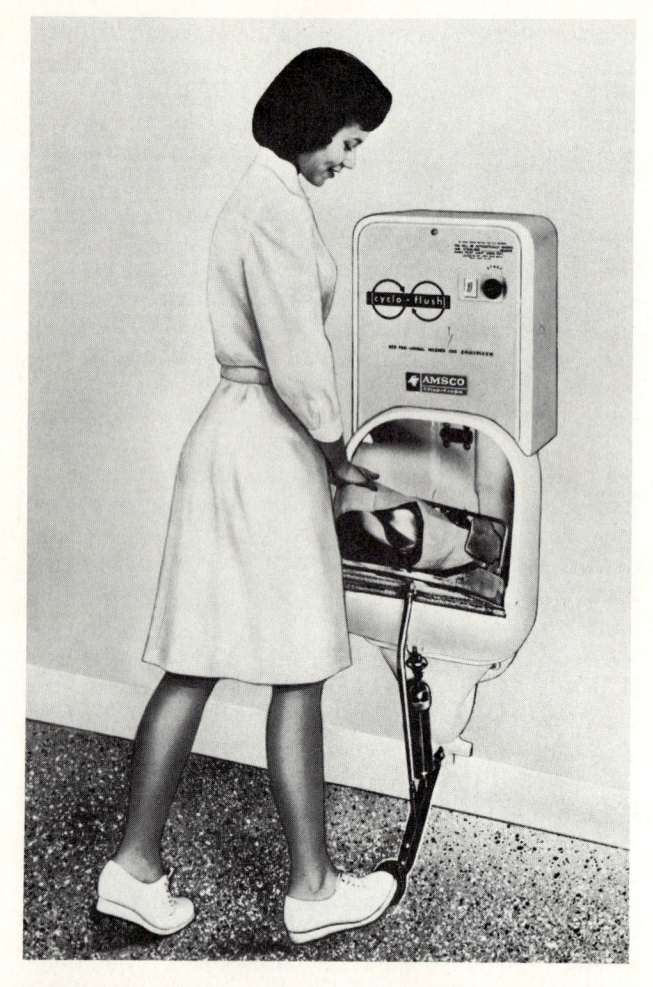

Figure 57–2. Cycloflush bedpan flusher/sanitizer. (Courtesy of American Sterilizer Company, Erie, PA.)

57–2. The start button should be pushed with the arm rather than with hands that are contaminated from handling the bedpan (AMSCO, 1981).

Urinals

A urinal is a plastic or metal container with an open top, a handle, a flat bottom, usually one flattened side, and sometimes a hinged cap. Urinals designed for women have a more oval opening and a larger flattened side area than those designed for men, as shown in Figure 57–3. Most male clients will use a urinal for urination if they are confined to a bed or are limited to standing at the bedside. Urinals are useful for women when using a bedpan is very difficult, such as with gross obesity or pain with moving; when lifting onto a bedpan is prohibited, as may occur with some injuries or surgeries; or when the sacral area is open and pressure would be harmful, such as with sacral decubitae.

Like bedpans, urinals are emptied in the bathroom, rinsed, and returned to the bedside stand. Some urinals have an open-ended handle that serves as a hook to attach it to the bed or a specially designed bar on the lower edge of the overbed table.

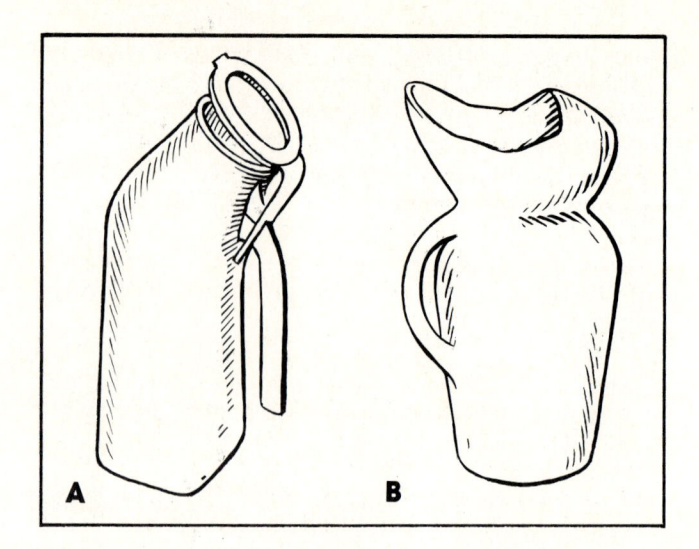

Figure 57–3. A. Male urinal with attached cap. B. Female urinal.

☐ EXECUTION

Bedpans and urinals are usually offered to clients in the morning upon arising, before morning care or bathing, before and after meals, and again at bedtime. If a bladder training program is being implemented, bedpans are offered every 2 or 3 hours around the clock. Offering a bedpan or urinal before providing other hygienic care increases the client's comfort and avoids interrupting the care for elimination needs. As much as possible, assist the client to carry out the usual routines associated with defecation and voiding.

When emptying bedpans or urinals, always inspect the urine for abnormalities, even if none are suspected. Report and record unusual characteristics of urine and stool. If those characteristics cannot be accounted for by drugs, diet, or other readily identifiable factors, save the urine or stool for the physician to inspect.

Preferably, store a bedpan or urinal in the bedside unit when it is not in use. However, male clients frequently prefer to have the urinal more accessible, and clients who have diarrhea or female clients with urinary frequency or urgency often want the bedpan to be more accessible. If so, choose a safe, convenient location, such as the foot of the bed or a chair at the bedside. For aesthetic reasons, cover bedpans and urinals when not in use, and instruct clients to call the nurse to empty them after each use. When bedpans or urinals are used for successive voidings without emptying, spills are more likely, odors increase, and bacteria have a chance to grow. *Never* place bedpans and urinals on the overbed table since that is used for the meal tray, personal hygiene activities, and for equipment used in both surgical and medical aseptic procedures.

Provide handwashing equipment after using the bedpan for bowel elimination, and preferably after urination as well. Some diseases are spread through the fecal-oral transmission route, and handwashing after defecation is the most effective way to interrupt this cycle. As discussed elsewhere, a nurse's own careful handwashing is a crucial aspect of preventing disease transmission among clients or to himself or herself.

ASSISTING WITH BEDPANS

When using bedpans in bed, clients are often anxious about having an accident and are afraid of soiling the bed linen. This is less likely to happen if the bedpan is the right size and shape for the client and if it is placed correctly. When accidental spills do occur, a matter-of-fact attitude and a prompt linen change will help minimize embarrassment. Sometimes accidents are almost unavoidable, such as when clients have diarrhea, have had an enema, or are difficult to position on the bedpan. In these circumstances, avoid unnecessary and tiring linen changes by placing a waterproof pad under the client's hips before giving the bedpan.

The discomfort and embarrassment of using a bedpan in bed can be minimized by increasing the client's privacy, comfort, and safety.

To provide for *privacy,* close the door or draw the curtains, use background music or noise as needed, and avoid unnecessarily exposing the genital area. Minimize genital exposure by turning the top bed linen back at a diagonal across the abdomen and thighs, since this exposes only the side and not the pubic area.

To provide for *comfort,* warm metal bedpans, pad the back edge of the bedpan with washcloths or surgical dressings when the client is thin, support the lower back with folded towels as needed, and use robes and blankets for warmth. To enhance psychological comfort, have toilet paper available, place the call signal within reach, provide handwashing equipment, and use a room deodorizer or air freshener after the client has a bowel movement.

To provide for *safety,* raise the siderails and place the bed in a low position after the client is on the bedpan if you will be leaving the room. Clients who do not ordinarily need side rails find them helpful to hold onto while sitting on or turning on and off of the bedpan.

To help prevent ducubitus formation for susceptible clients, pad the bedpan and position the client correctly on the bedpan to avoid the shearing force that occurs when clients slide in a downward and forward direction (Sorensen and Luckmann, 1979, p. 791).

Sometimes clients who have diarrhea or urinary frequency will want to remain on the bedpan for long periods of time rather than call the nurse frequently. This practice should be discouraged because pressure from the hard bedpan interferes with circulation in the sacral area and legs and can contribute to decubi-

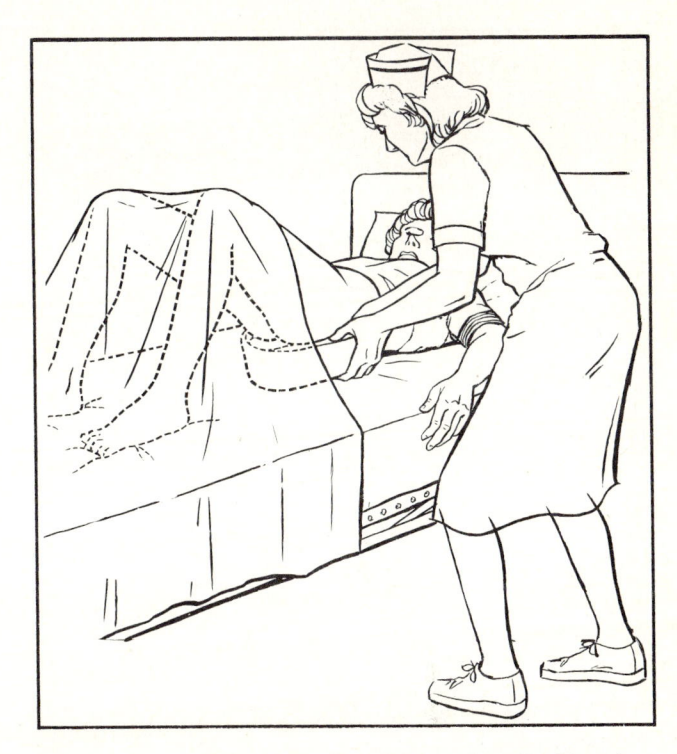

Figure 57-4. Lifting a client onto a bedpan. The client bends the knees and lifts the buttocks while the nurse places the bedpan.

tus formation in clients with poor nutrition and compromised circulation.

For your own safety, place the bed in a high position to give and remove a bedpan since it is impossible to use correct body mechanics with the bed in the low position. To place bedpans under patients who can lift themselves, ask them to bend their knees and lift their buttocks off the bed, and place the bedpan in a correct position under the buttocks. If the client needs help, place your hand under the small of the back, help lift the buttocks, and place the bedpan under the buttocks, as shown in Figure 57-4. It may be helpful to rest your elbow on the bed and use it for additional leverage. If the client is helpless or heavy, ask someone to help you place the bedpan. If the bed has an overbed frame with a trapeze bar, the client can use this to help raise the buttocks.

An alternative method for placing a bedpan is to have the client turn on and off the bedpan. To do this, first turn the client on the side facing away from yourself, making certain that the siderail on that side is raised and secure. Place the bedpan against the client's buttocks in a correctly aligned position (Fig. 57-5A). As the client turns back onto the bedpan, press downward on the upper side of the bedpan and hold it against the buttocks firmly, as shown in Figure 57-5B. This method is particularly useful for clients who are helpless, heavy, have difficulty lifting themselves, or need to avoid Valsalva's maneuver, which is involved in raising the buttocks.

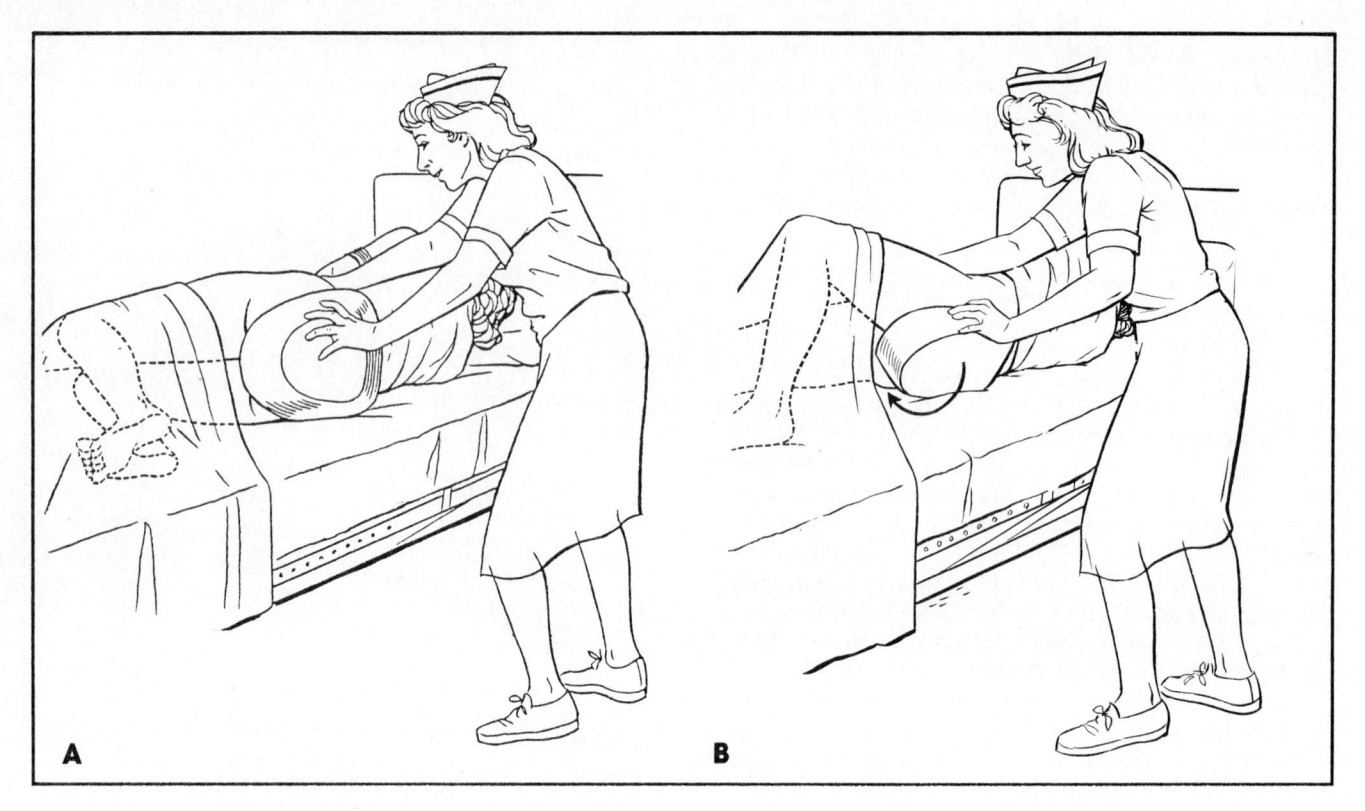

Figure 57–5. Turning a client onto a bedpan. **A.** The client turns away from the nurse. The nurse places the bedpan in the correct position. **B.** The nurse holds the bedpan firmly in place while the client turns back into it.

Before placing the client on the bedpan, take a few minutes to reposition him or her so that the hip joints are at the breaking point in the bed. This will avoid having the bedpan at a tilt under the client after the head of the bed is elevated. To avoid strain or injury, use correct body mechanics when repositioning clients or placing them on bedpans.

After placing the client on the bedpan, elevate the head of the bed as nearly upright as possible to take advantage of gravity and to approximate the normal physiological position for voiding and defecating. Lowthian (1975) points out that it is quite difficult for a woman to void into a bedpan or female urinal when lying in a supine position, as this position causes the urethra to direct urine upwards. He suggests that if necessary, the urine stream can be diverted downward by closing the labia majora anteriorly. Since this wets the entire vulva and perineum with urine, wiping with toilet tissue is especially necessary.

A female client who is alert usually prefers to wipe or cleanse her own vulvar area. If she needs help, wipe between the labia from front to back, using fresh toilet tissue for each stroke. The area around the anus also becomes wet when a woman urinates into a bedpan and must also be wiped. The anal area needs to be wiped or cleansed whenever a client has a bowel movement and it is very difficult for a client to do this while in bed. To wipe and cleanse the anal area, first turn him or her on the side away from yourself. Lift the upper buttock to visualize the area. Use toilet tissue and wipe from front to back. Work gently and carefully, particularly when external hemorrhoids are present. If the area is heavily soiled with feces, use gloves to protect yourself from direct fecal contact. If a urine specimen is needed or intake and output needs to be measured, place the toilet tissue in a moisture-resistant bag rather than in the badpan. Remove residual fecal deposits by washing the perianal area with soap and water and rinsing well. When the client has diarrhea, wash the anal area after each liquid stool to decrease the amount of time the acidic feces and digestive enzymes are in contact with the skin.

For several reasons, toilet paper is not placed in the bedpan when a urine or stool specimen is being collected. When wet toilet paper remains in the bedpan after emptying, the volume of urine is decreased and for some 24-hour urine tests the total volume is an important part of the laboratory analysis. Perfumed or colored toilet paper can alter some chemical analyses of urine, and the particulate shreds from toilet paper can influence microscopic examination. Toilet paper that is mixed in with a stool specimen can interfere with the mechanical emulsification of the feces prior to examination.

☐ SKILL SEQUENCE

ASSISTING WITH A BEDPAN

Step	Rationale

A. Placing a Bedpan

1. Wash hands.
2. Obtain appropriate style and size bedpan.
3. Close door or draw curtains.
4. Warm metal bedpan.
5. Raise bed to comfortable working position and lower head of bed to an almost flat position when possible.
6. Place bedpan on foot of bed or on adjacent chair in convenient location.
7. Fold top bed linen back diagonally over client.
8. Ask the client to bend knees and raise buttocks. If needed, assist by placing the hand nearest client's head under small of back and lift. Use your elbow against bed as a lever if needed. Use your other hand to place bedpan under client. Check and adjust bedpan's position. Pad bedpan as needed.
9. For a helpless or heavy client:
   a. Turn client on side, facing away from nurse.
   b. Place protective pad under hips.
   c. Place bedpan against buttocks in appropriate alignment. Press upper edge of bedpan downward toward bed and turn client onto his or her back. Keep bedpan pressed firmly in place while turning. Check and adjust bedpan position as needed. Use correct body mechanics. (NOTE: Work with another person to turn heavy or helpless clients.)
10. Replace top bed linen.
11. Raise head of bed as high as is permitted or is comfortable. Support back and sides with pillows as needed.
12. Raise side rails as needed and return bed to low position. Provide client with call signal and toilet tissue. (NOTE: If client is on intake–output measurement or a urine or stool specimen is needed, instruct him or her to place toilet tissue in a moisture-resistant bag.)
13. Wash hands.

Rationale:
- Avoids transfer of microorganisms.
- Increases client comfort.
- Provides privacy.
- Reflex reaction to cold bedpan inhibits micturition reflex.
- Promotes safe body mechanics for nurse; distributes client's weight more evenly and facilitates lifting onto bedpan.
- Bedpan is within nurse's reach.
- Minimizes client exposure.
- Distributes work effort more evenly.
- Correct placement helps avoid accidental spilling.

- Preparatory for bedpan placement.
- Prevents soiling bed linen.
- Places bedpan in correct position for use without spilling.

- Correct body mechanics provide for nurse safety.
- Decreases client energy expenditure and nurse effort.

- Minimizes client exposure.
- Provides nearly physiological position for voiding or defecating.

- Provides for client safety.
- Alerts nurse when client is finished; promotes self-care.
- Tissue in urine makes measurement more difficult and alters some test results.
- Prevents cross-contamination.
- Avoids transfer of microorganisms.

B. Removing a Bedpan

1. Wash hands.
2. Determine need for assistance in wiping vulvar area.
3. Raise bed to comfortable working position. Lower head of bed to almost flat position.
4. Fold to bed linen back diagonally across client.
5. Assist client to lift himself or herself as in step A(8). Stabilize front of bedpan while lifting. Alternate method: Place firm downward pressure on near edge of bedpan and turn client away from nurse, off bedpan.
6. Remove bedpan, cover it, and place it on a chair or at foot of bed.
7. Assist in cleansing female vulvar area as needed. Use several thicknesses of toilet tissue and wipe between labia from urethra toward anus. Use fresh tissues for each stroke. Place soiled tissues in bedpan. (See exceptions in step A(12).)
8. Cleanse anal area. Spread buttocks and wipe from front to back as for perineal cleansing. Wash perianal area with soap and water as needed and dry area thoroughly. Apply protective ointment if there is potential for excoriation.

Rationale:
- Avoids transfer of microorganisms.

- Promotes safe body mechanics for nurse; distributes client's weight more evenly and facilitates lifting onto bedpan.
- Minimizes client exposure.
- Promotes safe body mechanics. Avoids spilling contents.

- Minimizes odor and decreases patient embarrassment.

- Vulvar wiping is difficult to do when client is in bed.
- Avoids urethral contamination with fecal matter.
- Provides for client safety.

- Avoids urethral contamination with fecal matter in female. Prevents accumulation of microorganisms and helps prevent skin irritation. Protects skin from irritants.

(continued)

ASSISTING WITH A BEDPAN (Cont.)

Step	Rationale
9. Change linens as needed; return client to position of comfort and safety. (NOTE: Bed must always be in low position when nurse is out of room.)	Provides for comfort and safety.
10. Observe contents of bedpan; measure if client is on intake-output; remove specimen if needed.	Gathers needed data; implements diagnostic or therapeutic plan.
11. Empty bedpan in appropriate place, rinse, scrub as needed according to agency policy, and return to correct storage place.	Provides medically aseptic care for equipment.
12. Provide for client handwashing; use aerosol deodorant spray as needed for odor control.	Hygienic measure; avoids potential self-contamination; decreases embarrassing odors.
13. Wash own hands.	Avoids transfer of microorganisms.
14. Record amount and characteristics of urine and stool in health record and on flow sheets according to agency policy. Report unusual findings. Label any specimens correctly and send to laboratory.	Provides ongoing data base; fulfills nurse accountability.

ASSISTING WITH A URINAL

For voiding, male clients who are alert require only that a urinal be left in a convenient place or handed to them with instructions to call the nurse when finished, so that the urinal may be emptied. Many male clients have difficulty voiding in a lying down position, and it is not uncommon to assist an otherwise bedfast male client to his feet simply so that he can use a urinal. To do this, one nurse stands on either side of the client for support. Either the client or one of the nurses holds the urinal in place, with the client's gown usually providing adequate privacy. If this physiological position does not result in urination, voiding inducement measures are often helpful.

Sometimes a bedfast male client is unable to place the urinal for himself because of fatigue, traction, casts, immobility, or inability to use one or both hands. In those circumstances, lift the penis and place it completely in the urinal, positioning the bottom of the urinal lower than the opening. Avoid scooping the penis into the urinal instead of lifting and placing it, since that may cause discomfort or actual injury to the penis.

Since there is no toilet paper provided at male urinals in public restrooms, many males shake the penis to remove the urine drops that remain on its tip after voiding. However, since some men may prefer to wipe the penis tip after voiding, it is a courtesy to have facial or toilet tissues available when a male client uses the urinal in bed or at the bedside. If the client is helpless and you are placing and removing the urinal for him, dry the tip of the penis with tissues, since this will decrease odors and avoid dampness in the genital area and potential skin problems.

A male client is generally able to use a urinal when lying on the back, in a lateral recumbent position, or when turned on the abdomen on a CircOlectric bed. However, most female urinals are useful only when the woman is in a supine or semirecumbent position. Lowthian (1975) discusses problems involved in devising an adequate female urinal and describes some of the devices in use in the United Kingdom.

To place a female urinal, ask the client to spread her legs apart, place the oval opening over the entire vulva, and hold the urinal in place firmly. Since most females are unacquainted with urinals, explain that the oval opening is designed to fit the female perineal anatomy and will contain the urine. As is the case when a bedpan is used, the entire vulvar area will probably need to be wiped with toilet tissue after female clients void into a urinal.

☐ SKILL SEQUENCE

OFFERING A URINAL

Step	Rationale
1. Wash hands.	Avoids transfer of microorganisms.
2. Obtain appropriate type of urinal.	Preparatory step.
3. Close door or draw curtains.	Provides privacy.
4. Warm metal urinal.	Cold metal inhibits micturition reflex.

(continued)

Step	Rationale
5. Provide toilet or facial tissue as needed.	Female clients will need to be wiped. Some male clients prefer to dry penis after voiding.
6. Male urinal: Hand urinal to clients who are alert. If client is unable to void, assist to standing position unless contraindicated. Hold urinal in place as needed. (NOTE: For nonalert client: with one hand, place penis inside urinal. Use other hand to position urinal between legs, placing bottom of urinal lower than top.)	Most males are able to use urinal independently. Standing is physiological for male voiding. Ensures correct placement and avoids trauma to penis. Avoids accidental overflow and spilling.
7. Female urinal: Spread client's legs and place urinal over vulva; hold in place firmly during voiding.	Correct placement avoids spilling.
8. Provide nurse call signal and instruct client to call when finished with urinal.	Prompt emptying decreases potential for accidental spills.
9. Remove urinal when client is finished voiding. For female clients: Assist with vulvar wiping as in Skill Sequence, "Assisting with a Bedpan," step B(7). Wipe anal area if needed. For male clients who need assistance: wipe tip of penis with toilet tissue.	Same as 8. Same as Skill Sequence, "Assisting with a Bedpan," step B(7). Avoids damp linen and perineal area. Same as Skill Sequence, "Assisting with a Bedpan," step B(8). Promotes comfort; avoids damp perineal area.
10. Cover urinal to carry it to bathroom or utility room.	Minimizes odor and decreases embarrassment.
11. Observe contents of urinal; measure contents if client is on intake-output; remove specimen if needed.	Gathers data; implements plan of care.
12. Empty urinal, rinse with cold water, and return to appropriate storage place.	Rinsing after each use decreases odors and bacterial growth.
13. Provide for client handwashing.	Basic hygiene measure.
14. Wash own hands.	Same as step 1.
15. Record amount and characteristics of urine as in Skill Sequence, "Assisting with a Bedpan," step B(14).	Same as Skill Sequence, "Assisting with a Bedpan," step B(14).

RECORDING

Measure and record the volume of urine and liquid stools when clients are on intake-output measurement, and include a description of urine and stool characteristics and any problems associated with elimination. Flow sheets are often used for this purpose. Although not all clients who use bedpans and urinals need to have their output measured, include basic information about urine and stool, such as "used bedpan to void clear yellow urine X 3" or "to BR for BM; reports usual movement." Include the degree of assistance required when using the bedpan or urinal and whether a male client was helped to stand by the bedside. Include collection of specimens for laboratory analysis or nurse testing, although flow sheets are often used for this purpose as well. Suggestions for increasing the ease, safety, or comfort of giving the bedpan are recorded in the health record or the nursing care plan, kardex, or computer.

Sample POR Recording

- S—"I can't go in bed! I really need to pass my water! Please help me get up!"
- O—Has not voided for 10 hours. Bladder palpable 5 cm above symphysis pubis. Voided 400 ml clear yellow urine after being helped to stand at bedside.
- A—Positional inability to void.
- P—Assist client to stand and void every 4 to 6 hrs.

Sample Narrative Recording

Unable to void while lying in bed. Has not voided for 10 hr. Bladder palpable 5 cm above symphysis pubis. Voided 400 ml clear yellow urine while standing at bedside with help.

☐ CRITICAL POINTS SUMMARY

1. The ability to void and defecate is influenced by physiological and psychosocial factors.
2. Ensure privacy, safety, and comfort for the client using a bedpan or urinal.
3. Place a bedpan in correct alignment and position the client in a nearly physiological position.
4. Wipe the female vulvar area from front to back after urinating.
5. To remove irritant fecal matter from the skin, wipe the anal area from front to back after defecating.
6. Appraise the amount and characteristics of urine and stool when emptying bedpans and urinals.
7. Do not place bedpans and urinals on overbed tables.
8. Identify urinary retention through appraisal for bladder distention.
9. Use voiding inducement measures when clients have difficulty urinating.

10. Standing often helps a male client urinate.
11. Accurate urine and stool test results depend on correct methods of specimen collection.

☐ LEARNING ACTIVITIES

1. Work with a peer and role play placing and removing both a regular and fracture bedpan.
   a. Have the peer himself or herself lift onto the bedpan without any help.
   b. Assist with lifting, using your hand under the small of the back.
   c. Turn the peer on and off of the bedpan, both with and without the help of a second person.
   d. If using a hospital-style bed, elevate the head of the bed to a nearly upright position.
   e. Reverse roles and compare experiences and perceptions.
2. Examine male and female urinals. Note the difference in the shape and size of the opening and consider how the styles relate to male and female anatomy.
3. Visit a clinical unit; determine whether bedpans are kept in the bedside unit or in a central soiled utility area. Ask several staff members about the policies for cleaning bedpans and urinals after individual use and between use by different clients.
4. Locate an open hopper and a bedpan flusher/sanitizer in a clinical area. Read the directions on the flusher, insert a bedpan, and activate the flusher. Note any signs indicating precautions for using the flusher.

☐ REVIEW QUESTIONS

1. Identify the following characteristics of urine and feces as normal (N) or abnormal (A).

   URINE
   ____ Bright yellow color
   ____ Dark amber color
   ____ Foul odor when fresh
   ____ Foul odor on standing
   ____ Light straw color
   ____ pH of 5.6
   ____ Pink or red–brown color
   ____ Specific gravity of 1.019

   FECES
   ____ Bright red color
   ____ Clay-colored, or acholic, stools
   ____ Large amounts of mucus
   ____ Melena
   ____ Occult blood mixed in the feces
   ____ Red blood on the surface of the feces
   ____ Soft formed and shapeless
   ____ Steatorrhea

2. How does the physiological position for voiding differ between males and females?
3. In what ways do physiological positions facilitate voiding and defecation?
4. What factors contribute to difficult voiding and defecation?
5. Identify five voiding inducement measures and the basis for their effectiveness.
6. What subjective symptoms would be reported by a client with a distended bladder?
7. What objective data about bladder distention would the nurse obtain through physical appraisal skills?
8. What data about bladder distention would be obtained through the nursing or medical history and direct observation and interview?
9. In what circumstances is it more advisable to turn, rather than lift, a client on and off a bedpan?
10. In what ways can the nurse decrease the likelihood of having accidental urine spills when bedpans and urinals are used in bed?
11. What problems are associated with the use of female urinals?
12. What factors does a nurse consider when deciding how much assistance a client needs in using a bedpan or urinal?
13. When giving a bedpan, what nursing interventions will help (a) protect the client's privacy, (b) provide comfort, and (c) ensure safety?
14. When clients do not have their own personal bedpan or urinal, what cleaning methods are considered appropriate?
15. For what reasons is it important to follow correct urine and stool specimen collection and testing procedures?

☐ PERFORMANCE CHECKLISTS

OBJECTIVE: To use appropriate technique to give and remove a bedpan safely.			
CHARACTERISTIC	RANGE OF ACCEPTABILITY	SATISFACTORY	UNSATISFACTORY
A. Placing a Bedpan			
1. Washes hands.	No deviation		
2. Obtains appropriate bedpan.	No deviation		

(continued)

CHARACTERISTIC	RANGE OF ACCEPTABILITY	SATISFACTORY	UNSATISFACTORY
3. Provides privacy.	No deviation		
4. Warms metal bedpan.	No deviation		
5. Raises bed to working height.	No deviation		
6. Lowers head of bed to nearly flat position.	Modify position based on medical restrictions or patient comfort.		
7. Folds top linen back diagonally.	No deviation		
8. While placing bedpan, asks client to bend knees and lift buttocks.	Assist in lifting as needed.		
Or:			
9. Asks client to turn on side, places and holds bedpan, and has client turn back onto bedpan.	Assist or turn as needed; use assistant as needed.		
10. Uses correct body mechanics.	No deviation		
11. Replaces top linen.	No deviation		
12. Elevates head of bed to nearly upright position.	Modify position based on medical restrictions or client comfort.		
13. Checks and adjusts bedpan position.	No deviation		
14. Raises siderails.	No deviation		
15. Places bed in low position.	Omit if nurse remains with client.		
16. Provides call signal.	Remain with client if needed.		
17. Provides toilet tissue for alert, able clients.	No deviation		
B. Removing a Bedpan			
1. Washes hands.	No deviation		
2. Raises bed to working height.	No deviation		
3. Lowers bed to nearly-flat position.	Modify position based on medical restrictions or client comfort.		
4. Asks client to lift buttocks.	Assist as needed.		
Or:			
5. Asks client to turn away from nurse and off bedpan.	Assist or turn as needed; use assistant as needed.		
6. Stabilizes bedpan when lifting or turning.	No deviation		
7. Uses correct body mechanics.	No deviation		
8. Wipes and cleanses vulvar and anal areas.	Client may be able to do this.		
9. Changes linens if damp or soiled.	No deviation		
10. Returns client to position of comfort and safety.	No deviation		
11. Places bed in low position.	No deviation		
12. As ordered: a. Measures urine. b. Removes urine or stool specimen. c. Conducts appropriate test.	No deviation		
13. Empties and cleans bedpan; returns to appropriate storage area.	No deviation		
14. Provides for client handwashing.	No deviation		
15. Washes own hands.	No deviation		
16. Records and reports relevant data.	No deviation		

OBJECTIVE: To use appropriate technique to give a urinal to males and females.

CHARACTERISTIC	RANGE OF ACCEPTABILITY	SATISFACTORY	UNSATISFACTORY
1. Washes hands.	No deviation		
2. Obtains appropriate urinal.	No deviation		
3. Warms metal urinal.	No deviation		
4. Provides privacy.	No deviation		
5. Assists male client to a standing position.	Use assistant as needed, omit if contraindicated.		
6. Hands urinal to male client.	Place penis in urinal and hold urinal in place if necessary.		
7. Provides call signal.	Remain with client if needed.		
8. Places female client in semirecumbent position.	Omit if contraindicated.		
9. Spreads female client's legs and holds urinal firmly over vulvar area.	If no assistance needed, provide call signal.		
10. Wipes female perineal area.	Client may be able to do this.		
11. Returns client to position of comfort and safety.	No deviation		
12. As ordered: a. Measures urine. b. Removes urine specimen. c. Conducts appropriate test.	No deviation		
13. Empties, rinses, and returns urinal to appropriate storage area.	No deviation		
14. Provides for client handwashing.	No deviation		
15. Washes own hands.	No deviation		
16. Records and reports pertinent data.	No deviation		

REFERENCES

AMSCO Operating Manual, Bedpan Washer-Sanitizer and Bedpan Washer: Cycloflush and Aeroflush: Equipment Instructions, Erie, PA, American Sterilizer, 1981.

Beaumont E: Diagnostic kits. Nursing75 5(4):28–33, 1975.

Beland IL, Passos JY: Clinical Nursing: Pathophysiological and Psychosocial Approaches, ed 4. New York, Macmillan, 1981.

Burns KR, Johnson PJ: Health Assessment in Clinical Practice. Englewood Cliffs, NJ, Prentice-Hall, 1980.

Condon RE, Nyhus LM: Manual of Surgical Therapeutics, ed 6. Boston, Little, Brown, 1985.

Corbett JV: Laboratory Tests in Nursing Practice. Norwalk, CT, Appleton-Century-Crofts, 1982.

Elhart D, Firsich SC, et al: Scientific Principles in Nursing, ed 8. St Louis, CV Mosby, 1978.

Fischbach FT: A Manual of Laboratory Diagnostic Tests. Philadelphia, JB Lippincott, 1980.

Guyton AC: Human Physiology and Mechanisms of Disease, ed 3. Philadelphia, WB Saunders, 1982.

Lowthian PT: Portable urinals for women. Nursing Times 71(44):1739–1741, 1975.

Luckmann J, Sorensen KC: Medical–Surgical Nursing: A Psychophysiologic Approach, ed 2. Philadelphia, WB Saunders, 1980.

Malasanos L, Barkauskas V, et al: Health Assessment, ed 2. St Louis, CV Mosby, 1981.

Metheny NM, Snively WD: Nurse's Handbook of Fluid Balance, ed 4. Philadelphia, JB Lippincott, 1983.

Slawson M: Thirty-three drugs that discolor urine and/or stools. RN 43(1):40–41, 1980.

Sorensen KC, Luckmann J: Basic Nursing: A Psychophysiologic Approach. Philadelphia, WB Saunders, 1979.

Williams SM: Diabetic urine testing by hospital personnel. Nursing Research 20(5):444–447, 1971.

BIBLIOGRAPHY

Beyers M, Dudas S: The Clinical Practice of Medical–Surgical Nursing, ed 2. Boston, Little, Brown, 1984.

Brunner LS, Suddarth DS: Textbook of Medical–Surgical Nursing, ed 5. Philadelphia, JB Lippincott, 1984.

Chavigny K, Nunnally D: A comparison of methods for collecting clean-catch urine specimens in a clinic population of obstetric patients. American Journal of Obstetrics and Gynecology 122(1):34–41, 1975.

Kozier B, Erb G: Techniques in Clinical Nursing. Menlo Park, CA, Addison-Wesley, 1982.

Lindberg JB, Hunter ML, Krusewski AZ: Introduction to Person-Centered Nursing. Philadelphia, JB Lippincott, 1983.

McGuckin MB: Getting better urine specimens with the clean-catch midstream technique. Nursing81 (Horsham) 11(1):72–73, 1981.

Nordmark MT, Rohweder AW: Scientific Foundations of Nursing, ed 3. Philadelphia, JB Lippincott, 1975.

Pinel C: Disorders of micturition in the elderly. Nursing Times 71(51):2019–2021, 1975.

Potter PA, Perry AG: Fundamentals of Nursing: Concepts, Process, and Practice. St Louis, CV Mosby, 1985.

Sorensen KC, Luckmann J: Basic Nursing: A Psychophysiological Approach. Philadelphia, WB Saunders, 1979.

AUDIOVISUAL RESOURCE

Basic Nursing Care: Urinary Care
Filmstrip, slides, videocassette, film. (1982, Color, 20 min.)
Available through:
Medcom, Inc.
P.O. Box 116
Garden Grove, CA 92642

SKILL 58 Bowel Elimination Procedures

PREREQUISITE SKILLS

Skill 19, "Inspection"
Skill 20, "Palpation"
Skill 28, "Handwashing"
Skill 56, "Insertion and Care of Gastrointestinal Tubes"
Skill 57, "Bedpans and Urinals"

STUDENT OBJECTIVES

1. Differentiate among large- and small-volume cleansing enemas, oil-retention enemas, carminative enemas, and colonic irrigations in terms of mode of action, intended effect, and method of administration.
2. Identify the hazards associated with different types of enemas and enema solutions.
3. Describe assessment data indicative of the need for a cleansing enema.
4. Explain physiological and pyschological factors that contribute to development of constipation.
5. Describe nursing interventions that promote bowel regularity and relieve constipation.
6. Describe causative factors in the development of normal and excessive amounts of flatus.
7. Identify nursing actions that can relieve and prevent the negative effects of flatus.
8. Describe factors that promote the development of fecal impactions.
9. Identify nursing measures to relieve existing impactions and prevent recurrences.
10. Describe nursing interventions that promote safety and comfort during an enema.
11. Administer cleansing and retention enemas, using appropriate medical aspetic technique.

INTRODUCTION

An enema is the introduction of a fluid into the rectum and colon through a tube inserted in the anus. Enemas are given to stimulate peristalsis and the defecation reflex, thus artificially inducing defecation. They are given for the purpose of cleansing the lower bowel before surgery, childbirth, or diagnostic procedures; to remove barium after x-ray procedures; to relieve constipation; to soften hard feces; to relieve gas pains; and sometimes to establish regular patterns of bowel elimination during bowel training.

Enemas have been given since ancient times and are often considered a very commonplace procedure. Many people use them at home on a regular basis to promote "regularity" or relieve temporary constipation. When admitted to a health-care setting, they usually want this practice continued, either by the nursing staff or by themselves.

Miller (1975) describes an enema as the most unglamorous, misunderstood, and improperly performed procedure in clinical medical practice. He points out that giving an enema is often delegated to the newest and most uninformed member on the nursing team, who may or may not be properly trained in the procedure. A study of 50 clients in Great Britain confirmed that nurses with more experience in giving enemas gave more successful enemas (Duffin et al., 1981). It is especially important that a cleansing enema given prior to diagnostic studies of the colon or abdomen actually achieve cleansing of the bowel. Miller (1975), a radiologist, considers a clean colon the most important factor in diagnosing cancer of the colon and other abdominal structures because fecal matter mimics colonic lesions and can also mimic or hide renal stones and bone metastasis. He reports that nearly one in five cancers of the colon are missed on the initial barium enema because they are mistaken for fecal matter. Giving cleansing enemas preoperatively for general surgery seems to be practiced primarily in the United States. Except as preparation for large-bowel surgery, Burkitt (1982) indicates that enemas are not used as routine preoperative preparation in most other Western countries.

Enemas are administered by the professional nurse or by ancillary personnel for whom the nurse is responsible. Enemas are often used in home-care or long-term care settings, where clients are often relatively inactive or immobile. In these settings, physicians' orders for enemas generally are on a p.r.n. basis, allowing the nurse the opportunity of using professional judgment about the client's current elimination needs.

Although enemas are quite beneficial and useful, they can easily be overused and misused, and, in some circumstances, can actually be quite damaging. Because they are considered a simple procedure, some basic principles of administration are often ignored. Major nursing responsibilities associated with the use of enemas are teaching clients and their families safe techniques for administering enemas, discussing the problems associated with enemas as long-term management of constipation, and offering alternative ways of promoting normal elimination.

☐ **PREPARATION**

COMMON BOWEL PROBLEMS

Enemas are used to relieve common problems associated with elimination, such as constipation, fecal impaction, and flatus, or sometimes to provide bowel training for clients with fecal incontinence.

Constipation
Constipation is the passage of dry, hardened stools, accompanied by considerable voluntary muscle effort. Consistency of stool, rather than frequency of elimination, determines whether constipation exists, although frequency is often decreased. Associated symptoms that result from the continued presence of constipated stool and prolonged rectal stimulation include headache, bloated feelings, lethargy, and anorexia. Straining to pass a constipated stool usually involves using Valsalva's maneuver. This action can cause untoward reactions such as bradycardia, angina, or cardiac arrest in cardiac patients, can increase intracranial pressure in clients with head injury, and can disrupt recent bowel or perineal sutures.

A variety of physiological and psychological factors are implicated in constipation. For example, constipation is likely to occur when no regular defecation habits have been established and the defecation reflex is repeatedly ignored. It also results from inadequate dietary bulk and fluid, insufficient exercise, emotional disturbances, medications such as codeine or some antacids, and overuse of laxatives, suppositories, and enemas. Problems such as intestinal adhesions, cancer, hemorrhoids, and anal lesions contribute to or exacerbate existing constipation. Constipation is a particular problem for immobile or elderly persons, especially the institutionalized elderly. This is so because they have decreased activity levels and muscle strength, inadequate dietary habits, many medical problems, and, often, long-established habits of using laxatives or enemas. Institutional practices regarding diet and activity may contribute to constipation. On one geriatric unit, the gradual addition of fiber to 17 clients' diets resulted in a 27 percent decrease in the number of laxatives given. Those who were on regular diets had a 46 percent decrease in laxative use, those on soft diets had a 24 percent decrease, and those on pureed diets, a 7 percent decrease. On this unit, laxative use was used to determine enema frequency because laxative administration always preceded administration of an enema and was easier to monitor (Bass, 1977).

Fecal Impaction
A fecal impaction is a collection of putty-like or hardened feces in the rectum that prevents normal defecation. Impaction is caused by retention of feces in the rectum, such as occurs with prolonged constipation, from barium used for diagnostic x-rays, or whenever the defecation reflex has not resulted in expulsion of feces over a period of time.

Small amounts of liquid incontinent feces usually seep around the impacted fecal mass and are sometimes mistaken for diarrhea. When accompanied by a history of no bowel movements for more than 3 or 4 days, this seepage is considered to be a quite definitive symptom of impaction. A digital examination confirms the presence of hardened stool. Additional symptoms include an unsuccessful desire to defecate, rectal pain, anorexia, and abdominal fullness. The abdomen may become visibly distended, and hard stool is sometimes palpable in the lower left quadrant of the abdomen.

Impactions can sometimes be removed by using oil-retention enemas to soften the stool, followed by a cleansing enema to stimulate defecation. If the impaction is very large, or does not respond to enemas, it will need to be broken up digitally and removed manually, as described later. Laxatives will also help lubricate and moisten the hardened stool but usually act too slowly to relieve immediate distress.

Flatulence
Flatulence refers to the presence of excessive amounts of intestinal gas that may be expelled as flatus. If the gases are not expelled, abdominal distention occurs, accompanied by abdominal discomfort and cramping pain, and sometimes respiratory distress and referred shoulder pain from pressure on the diaphragm. On appraisal, the abdomen is usually visibly distended and is tympanic with percussion.

Intestinal gas comes from three sources: swallowed air (nitrogen and oxygen), gases produced by bacterial action in the colon (carbon dioxide, methane, and hydrogen), and the diffusion of gases from the bloodstream into the colon. The large intestine forms 7 to 10 liters of gases per day, but usually all except 0.6 liters is reabsorbed through the intestinal mucosa. When people pass large amounts of flatus rectally, it is often because of excessive motility of the large intestine from irritation, causing the gases to move through more rapidly than they can be absorbed (Guyton, 1982, p. 520).

A variety of factors contribute to flatulence. Anxiety and tension are common causes. Constipation allows the gases to accumulate, since they are not expelled regularly. Although most swallowed air is expelled by belching, excessive amounts contribute to intestinal flatulence. An increase in swallowed air results from rapid eating and drinking; chewing gum; drinking through a straw; postnasal drip and increased swallowing; chlorinated beverages, beer, champagne, and foods containing excessive ingestion of large amounts of air such as milk shakes and sponge cakes; or deliberate swallowing of air so as to promote belching and relieve gastric fullness. Specific foods are gas forming on an individual basis, for example, cabbage, beans, cauliflower, and spicy dishes. Flatulence and distention also occur when gastrointestinal motility is decreased, such as after surgery, with lower bowel obstruction, inactivity, immobility, and some medications.

Relief from the discomfort of flatulence comes as gas is reabsorbed or expelled. Activity and exercise are considered the best and most natural way to relieve flatus. Rectal tubes, carminative enemas, return-flow enemas, or medications containing simethicone are also helpful.

Fecal Incontinence

Fecal incontinence refers to a lack of voluntary control of the rectal sphincters, resulting in spontaneous defecation whenever the defecation reflex occurs. Physiological reasons for incontinence include anything that interferes with anal sphincter function, such as lacerations, fistulas, or sensory loss. Diarrheal stools can sometimes be so explosive and voluminous that the sphincter cannot contain them. Sometimes clients are incontinent because their call signal is not answered soon enough. Mental and emotional problems may cause incontinence, and it is not uncommon that institutionalized elderly people simply give up and stop trying to be continent.

Since feces are irritating to the skin, faithful and careful washing with soap and water after each defecation will help prevent skin breakdown. Bowel training programs are often successful in reestablishing continence and are discussed in various medical–surgical texts. In some agencies, enemas are a part of this training to help establish regular defecation times. When alleviation of diarrhea or incontinent stools is not possible, such as in some terminal illnesses, a fecal incontinence collector may be useful, as described later.

TYPES OF ENEMAS

Enemas are generally of four types—cleansing, retention, carminative, or irrigations of the colon.

Cleansing Enemas

Large-Volume Enemas. *Tap water* and *normal saline* are considered relatively safe solutions for cleansing enemas. These enemas stimulate peristalsis and the defecation reflex by producing rectal distention with 500 to 1000 ml of fluid. For a saline enema, 8 ml (2 tsp) table salt is added to 1 L (qt) of plain tap water, or commercially prepared normal saline can be used.

Soap-solution enemas stimulate defecation both by distention of the colon and by chemical irritation of the mucosa from the soap. A soap solution for enema purposes consists of 5 ml of liquid castile soap in 1000 ml of water.

Although there is considerable negative evidence regarding their use, soap-solution enemas continue to be used rather widely. They have been criticized since the early 1900s because of their negative effects (No Soap, 1971). Irritation of the colon persists for 3 weeks after a soap-solution enema, and there are numerous reports of proctatitis and rectal mucosa damage, as well as some nearly fatal complications (No Soap, 1971; Pike et al., 1971; Sorensen and Luckmann, 1979).

If a soap solution is used, the above concentration (1 part soap to 200 parts water) should not be exceeded and only liquid castile soap is used. Green soap and dish detergent are too harsh, bar soap harbors microorganisms, and soft soap prepared from unused soap scraps has an unknown concentration (Hogstel, 1977).

Small-Volume Enemas. Small-volume *phosphate enemas,* such as Fleet Brand Enema, are commercially prepared hypertonic solutions of sodium biphosphate and sodium phosphate. They stimulate peristalsis and defecation by a mild chemical irritation and by producing bulk and colonic distention as the small amount of hypertonic solution (135 ml) draws water into the colon. Another small-volume cleansing enema, Fleet Bisacodyl Enema, contains 10 mg of bisacodyl rather than phosphates. Bisacodyl is a contact laxative that increases the fluid content of the colon.

Advantages of small-volume enemas include the convenience and ease of administration, the fact that the solution need not be warmed, the safety of having a premeasured volume of a known concentration, client comfort associated with a small volume, and their almost universal effectiveness with relatively few complications.

Hazards with Cleansing Enemas. Although often a safe procedure, various hazards may occur with cleansing-enema administration in addition to the problems with soap solutions mentioned above.

Physiological and pyschological *dependence* can occur, similar to that which occurs with overuse of laxatives and suppositories. After an enema is given and the colon is cleared of stool, 2 to 3 days are required for the bowel to fill with enough stool to stimulate the defecation reflex again. By this time, the individual is concerned about not having had a bowel movement and has taken another enema, laxative, or suppository—and so the cyclic process continues. The use of laxatives and suppositories is discussed in various medical–surgical, pharmacology, and nutrition textbooks.

Vagus nerve stimulation occurs when the anal sphincters are stretched and the bowel is distended with fluid. Persons with cardiac problems may develop cardiac arrhythmias, and myocardial infarctions (heart attacks) have been known to occur as a direct result of an enema. *Local tissue trauma* can occur when a hard enema tube tip is rough or chipped, such as the tip on a small-volume enema, or from a solution that is too hot or is given under too great a pressure.

Fluid and electrolyte imbalances may develop from the enema solution. Water from hypotonic tap water is absorbed by the body. In healthy persons, this causes few problems; however, water excess can occur in infants or persons with inadequate cardiac or renal function. Because of the potential for this problem to occur, the number of consecutive tap water enemas is usually limited to three when enemas are ordered "till clear." Even the relatively safe normal saline solution can cause fluid imbalance by increasing sodium retention in people with congestive heart failure or cirrhosis of the liver. Hypertonic solutions draw water from interstitial spaces and contribute to fluid depletion and dehydration, especially in children and other susceptible persons. Moreover, electrolyte imbalances have occasionally been known to occur after small-volume phosphate enemas (Davis et al., 1977).

Contraindications for Cleansing Enemas. In some circumstances, enemas are contraindicated or given only with a specific physician's order. For example, Valsalva's maneuver (used to expel the enema solution) is contraindicated in clients with increased intracranial pressure or a recent myocardial infarction; enemas given during pregnancy may stimulate premature labor; and increased local pressure from the enema can cause damage to perineal, rectal, or vaginal sutures. Enemas are not generally given when abdominal pain, nausea, and vomiting are present; when bowel sounds are absent, such as occurs during the first few days following an operation; or when abdominal distention associated with bowel obstruction or paralytic ileus is present.

Retention Enemas

A retention enema is one in which a small amount of solution is instilled into the rectum and allowed to remain there for varying lengths of time. To avoid stimulating the defecation reflex, the solution is administered slowly, under low pressure, and using a smaller diameter rectal tube or tip (sizes 14F to 20F for adults).

Oil-Retention. *Oil–retention enemas* usually consist of 100 to 200 ml (4 to 8 oz) of mineral, cottonseed, or olive oil or a commercially prepared oil solution. The oil is warmed to body temperature before administration, as solutions that are either warmer or cooler than body temperature stimulate peristalsis and the defecation reflex. The oil is retained in the rectum for 30 to 60 minutes or overnight so that it can soften the feces. Although softening does occur and the oil acts as a lubricant, it is usually necessary to follow an oil-retention enema with a cleansing enema. A fecal softening agent and surfactant such as diocytl sulfosuccinate may be added to the oil-retention enema or given by itself as a retention enema to soften the feces.

Other, less common types of retention enemas include *medicated enemas,* such as rectal neomycin, which may be used prior to bowel surgery to destroy colonic bacteria; *nutritive enemas,* such as dextrose and water given in serious volume depletion and shock; *anthelmintic enemas* used to destroy intestinal parasites; *emollient enemas,* such as starch to soothe irritated rectal mucosa; and some *carminative enemas* for relief of flatulence.

Carminative Enemas

Carminative enemas are given to relieve intestinal distention and flatulence. A variety of solutions may be used to release the intestinal gases and stimulate their expulsion. The *Mayo enema* consists of 240 ml warm water, 60 ml white sugar, and 30 ml sodium bicarbonate. A *milk and molasses enema* consists of equal amounts of milk and molasses, using from 90 to 120 ml of each. The milk is warmed to 43.3°C (110°F) and the molasses is then added. A *glycerin and water enema* (sometimes called a G and W enema) consists of 30 to 90 ml (1 to 3 oz) of glycerin in 500 ml of warm water. A *1-2-3 enema* contains 30 ml (1 oz) of a 50 percent solution of magnesium sulfate, 60 ml (2 oz) of glycerin, and 90 ml (3 oz) of water. If magnesium sulfate crystals are used, they are dissolved in boiling water, the glycerin is added, and the solution is cooled to 40.6°C (105°F). Because of the availability of drugs that stimulate peristalsis, these enemas are used infrequently.

Irrigations of the Colon

A *return-flow enema,* or Harris flush, is sometimes used to relieve intestinal distention and flatulence. With this procedure, 250 to 300 ml of normal saline or tap water is instilled into the rectum and colon while the enema container is held at the usual 45 cm (18 in) above the anus. When the solution has entered the rectum and colon, the can is lowered below the rectal level, allowing the fluid to drain out of the rectum and back into the container, using a siphon action. As the fluid returns, gas bubbles up into the container. When the return flow ceases, the container is again raised and then again lowered after another 250 to 300 ml is instilled. The alternate raising and lowering is continued five or six times or until minimal gas is returned. The alternating inflow and outflow of solution stimulates peristalsis and brings the gas further down in the intestinal tract so it can be expelled. As the enema solution becomes thick with feces, it may be replaced, using a total of approximately 1000 ml of solution.

Colonic irrigations are sometimes used to flush out the large intestine. Two rectal tubes are used to insert and drain fluid from the colon simultaneously, using a total of about 3000 to 4000 ml of solution.

DATA BASE

Before giving an enema, the nurse knows the action and purposes of various types of enemas, how to prepare them, and the different administration procedure required for each. The nurse also becomes familiar with agency protocols that include enemas as part of routine preparation for diagnostic tests or surgical procedures. In addition, the nurse identifies the reason (or reasons) a client is being given a particular kind of enema.

Client History and Recorded Data

The physician's order includes the type of enema, the amount of solution, and the time or frequency with which it is to be given. The medical diagnosis, history, or diagnostic plans may provide information about the reason for the enema, for example, a cleansing enema prior to a barium enema to detect cancer of the colon or a postoperative enema to aid in relief of flatulence. If recent rectal surgery has been done or if rectal pathology is present, the physician may indicate the size rectal tube to be used.

To determine whether the client can expel the enema in the bathroom or will need a commode or bedpan, the nurse considers the physician's activity orders as well as the client's limitations on movement, his or her strength, coordination, mental alertness, and ability to cooperate. Although the client's capabilities may be reported in the health record and kardex, it is important to make direct observations because client status can change quickly.

When the enema order is listed as a p.r.n. order, the nurse gathers data about the time, amount, and character of the person's last bowel movement. Before giving a p.r.n. enema, the client is reevaluated to determine if any change in status would cause the enema to be contraindicated. When the enema is being given to reduce flatulence, data about abdominal distention and discomfort are needed before the enema is given so that the results can be evaluated. Knowing the client's previous experience with enemas makes it easier for the nurse to explain the procedure in an understandable manner. Knowing the client's past ability to retain an enema solution helps the nurse and client plan where the enema will be expelled and whether it will need to be given while the client is on the bedpan.

Health records indicate the type of diet, fluid prescription, the client's actual food and fluid consumption, and medications affecting the intestinal tract. This information will help the nurse evaluate the results from the enema and plan further interventions, including teaching. Vital signs provide base-line data to evaluate any changes that may occur during administration of the enema.

Physical Appraisal Skills

Inspection. Abdominal distention from flatulence or large amounts of stool may be visible on inspection, either by viewing the abdomen from the side or from above. Peristaltic waves are sometimes visible when large amounts of intestinal gas are present. Strong contractions that are visible through an abdominal wall of average thickness may represent a bowel obstruction.

Inspection reveals the seepage associated with fecal impaction, the presence of incontinence, and the status of the perianal area. Inspection of this area may identify hemorrhoids, cracks, or fissures and determine the degree of healing after surgery or a need for cleansing. Inspection of the enema administration tip may reveal a cracked or chipped nozzle. The nurse inspects the results of the enema so that he or she can report and record descriptions of those results.

Auscultation. Auscultation will indicate whether bowel motility is present.

Percussion. Flatulence with abdominal distention produces more pronounced tympany over the anterior surface of the abdomen (Robins, 1974).

Palpation. When a person is thin and relaxed, hard stool can sometimes be palpated in the lower left quadrant of the abdomen. The feces-filled cecum and ascending colon are palpated as a soft, boggy, rounded mass. The presence of a fecal impaction is determined by digital palpation within the rectum.

Sense of Smell. Along with inspection, the sense of smell is used to identify the presence of fecal incontinence or seepage with impaction. It also identifies passage of flatus.

EQUIPMENT

Enema equipment is used in a medically aseptic manner. The equipment is washed and rinsed thoroughly before being used again for the same person. Reusable equipment is sterilized between use by different persons and disposable equipment is either discarded or sent home at discharge time.

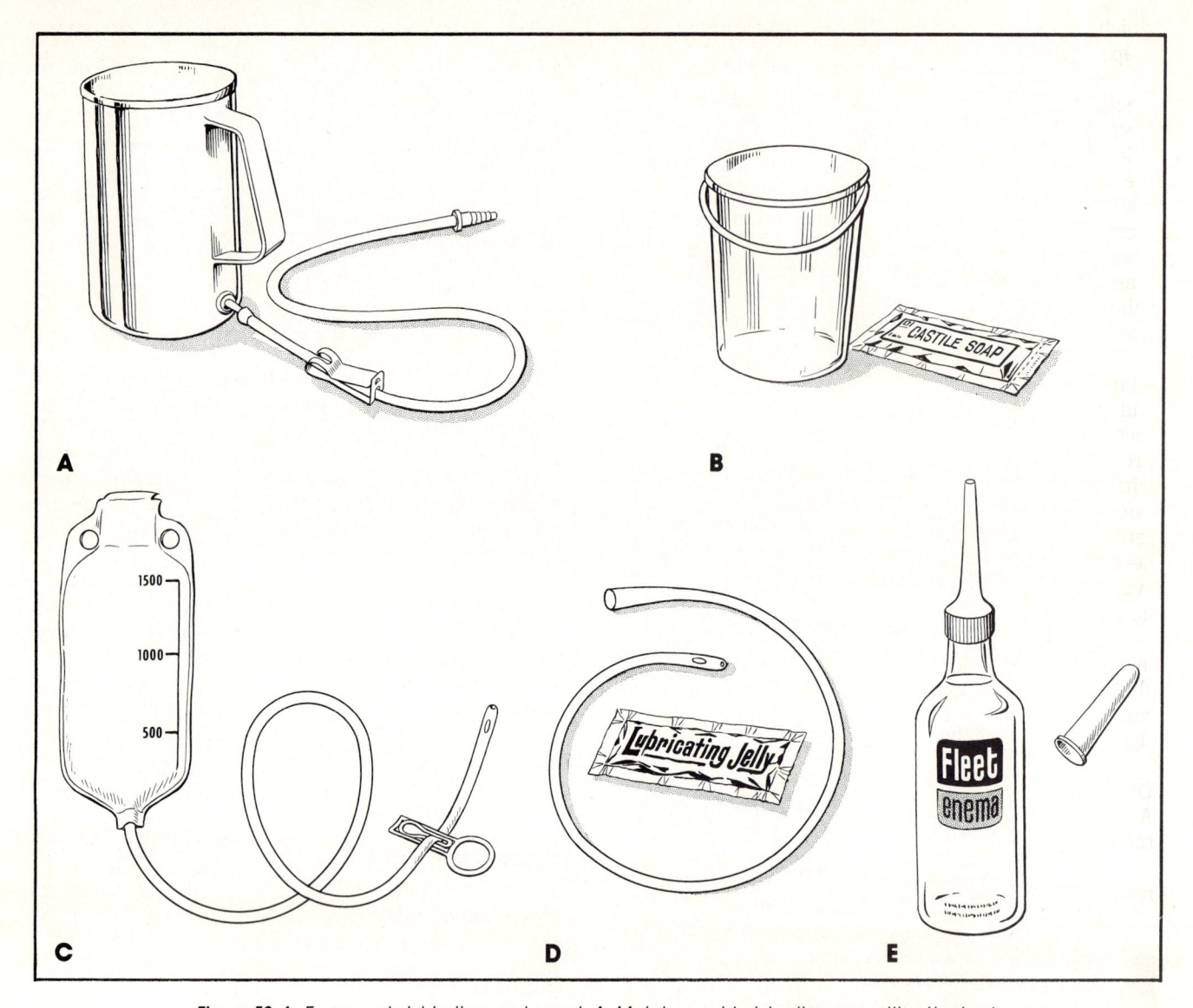

Figure 58–1. Enema administration equipment. **A.** Metal, reusable irrigation can with attached tubing, connector, and snap clamp. **B.** Plastic, disposable enema bucket and packet of castile soap. **C.** Plastic, disposable flip-top enema bag with attached catheter-tipped tubing and sliding clamp. **D.** Red rubber rectal tube and packet of water-soluble lubricant. **E.** Small-volume enema.

In addition to one of the solutions described earlier, the following equipment is needed to administer an enema—a solution container, connecting tube, rectal tube, tubing clamp or hemostat, and lubricant. Other equipment that may be needed includes disposable gloves, a bedpan, a protective pad, toilet tissue, a bath blanket, and possibly a robe and slippers and stool specimen container.

Commercially prepared enema kits include a solution container, connecting tubing with an administration tip, lubricant, protective drape, clamp, and perhaps even the solution. Small-volume, ready-to-use enemas are self-contained and need no additional equipment. Common types of enema equipment are shown in Figure 58–1.

Enema Solution Containers

Most cleansing-enema containers have a 1500 to 2000 ml capacity. Reusable *metal cans* have a handle and a bottom opening for attaching the connecting tubing and rectal tube. *Enema bags* are made of polyvinyl chloride. They have an attached connecting tubing with administration tip and built-in handles so that they can be hung from an intravenous infusion pole or hook. Some have filling ports with a snap-cap closure and others have a fold-over top closure to prevent spilling. *Plastic buckets* with attached handles are freestanding for easier filling. They have an opening at the bottom and may or may not have an attached plastic connecting tubing and administration tip. Some buckets have a retaining notch on one edge in which to insert the rectal tube for stabilization while preparing the client.

Rectal Tubes and Tubing
Rectal tubes are made of disposable clear polyvinyl chloride or red opaque vinyl. Some clear plastic tubes are thermosensitive and become soft and pliable at body temperature. Approximately 51 cm (20 in) long, rectal tubes are available in sizes 18F to 32F, with sizes 18F to 20F being the most commonly used. Some plastic rectal tubes are marked at 13 cm (5 in). Rectal tubes usually have an opening on the distal tip plus one large opening just proximal to the tip.

Clear polyvinyl chloride *connecting tubing* has an adaptor on one end to attach a rectal tube, or it may end in a rectal administration tip that is similar to a rectal tube tip. The tip may be prelubricated with a protective sheath. Some enema kits have a tubing with an administration tip already attached to a container, so that there is no need to assemble the enema setup. Some administration tips on the end of connecting tubing are quite blunt and can be painful and even cause tissue trauma, particularly for clients with hemorrhoids.

Tubing clamps are either flat sliding clamps or metal snap-open clamps that latch securely in the closed position. If no clamps are available, a *hemostat* can be used. Clamps are used to keep the solution in the container until the rectal tube is inserted.

Other Needed Items
A *water-soluble lubricant* is used to lubricate the rectal tube prior to insertion.

Disposable plastic gloves are used to protect the nurse's hands from direct contact with fecal material. They are especially important when clients cannot retain the solution and it must be administered while the client is on the bedpan. A *bedpan* is used to contain the overflow fluid when the tubing is filled prior to insertion, as a receptacle for soiled toilet tissue, and for expelling the enema solution.

A *protective or waterproof pad* is always used unless a linen change is planned immediately after the enema. *Toilet tissue* is used to compress the anus if the solution leaks out of the anus, to wipe the rectal tube as it is withdrawn, and to dry the anus.

A *bath blanket* is used to provide warmth and prevent soiling of the top bed covers; a *robe and slippers* are needed for the client's safety, warmth, and privacy when walking to the bathroom. If a stool specimen is to be collected after the enema, the appropriate *specimen container* is needed.

Ready-to-Use Enemas
Ready-to-use small-volume enemas, such as Fleet Brand Enema, are supplied in a disposable plastic squeeze bottle with a prelubricated tip. Some enemas are available in small plastic bags with an attached tubing and prelubricated tip.

Incontinence Protection
The Hollister TM Male–Female Fecal Incontinence Collector, shown in Figure 58–2A, is a device similar to an ostomy pouch. It is designed to contain liquid feces and minimize contact of liquid feces with the skin. This device is made of an odor barrier film; it is held in place with an adhesive foam ring designed to fit either the male or female perianal area (Fig. 58–2B) and it contains a gas vent and port for taking rectal temperatures (Fig. 58–2C).

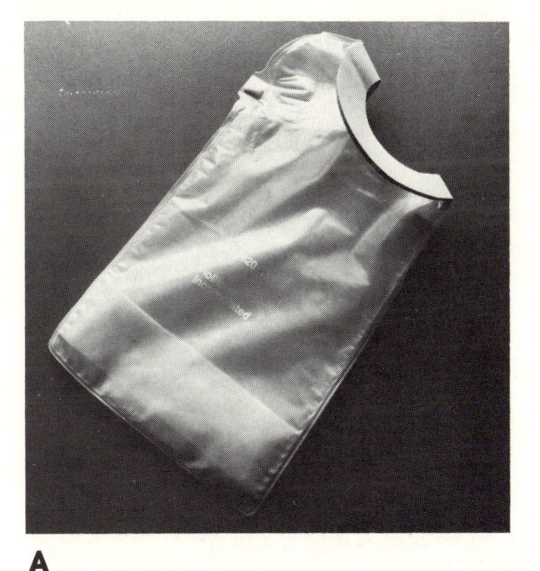

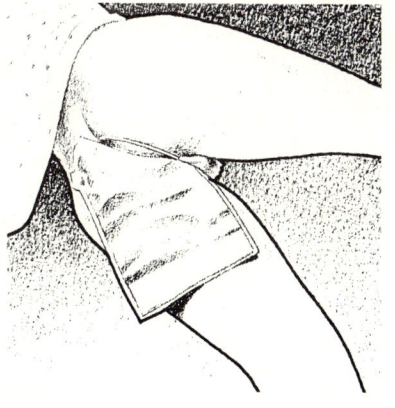

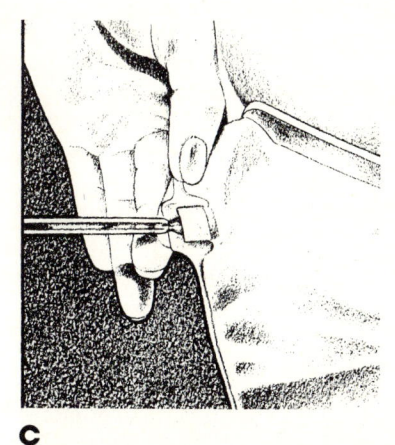

Figure 58–2. **A.** Male–Female Fecal Incontinence Collector. **B.** Place the client on the side, apply the adhesive-backed ring around the anal area. **C.** Rectal temperature may be taken through the port without removing the collector. (Reprinted with permission of copyright owner, Hollister, Inc., Libertyville, IL.)

☐ EXECUTION

Administering enemas, inserting rectal tubes, and removing impactions are some of the least desirable tasks nurses do for clients. Although they provide substantial relief for clients suffering from constipation, flatulence, and impaction, these procedures may also be a source of considerable embarrassment, discomfort, and anxiety. It is embarrassing to need help with such a basic personal function as having a bowel movement. The procedures are uncomfortable, sometimes even painful, and involve exposure of private body areas. Many clients worry about being able to "hold the enema" and are fearful of soiling the bed or having accidents, since they have been taught from early childhood that these actions are socially unacceptable.

There are other sources of anxiety and worry associated with bowel elimination procedures; for example, cleansing enemas often precede diagnostic tests or surgical procedures that may have uncertain outcomes, and intestinal gas and impaction may mean a less than optimal recovery from illness. The individual's anxiety can be reduced considerably when the nurse is skillful and comfortable in administering bowel elimination procedures and adopts a matter-of-fact approach. Explain the purpose of the procedure and how the client can be of help while it is being performed. As much as possible, plan these procedures before daily care is given and before bed linen is changed. If this is not possible, protect the bed thoroughly, and if accidental soiling occurs, change the linen promptly.

A successful cleansing enema involves inserting an adequate amount of solution far enough into the colon to stimulate peristalsis and produce evacuation of stool along with expulsion of fluid. To a great extent, the success depends both on the techniques used by the nurse and the degree of relaxation the client can achieve during the procedure—and relaxation is influenced by the nurse's approach, skill, and manner.

ADMINISTERING LARGE-VOLUME CLEANSING ENEMAS

Preparing the Solution

Prepare the designated solution in the soiled utility room or client's bathroom, out of the client's view, since the preparation is often anxiety producing. Enema containers, tubing, and connectors assemble more easily and tightly if the connections are wet. Close the clamp in the connecting tubing or place a hemostat about 30 cm (12 in) above the rectal tube. Since cold metal absorbs heat, warm metal enema cans with hot water before adding the solution.

Adjust the water temperature at the faucet to 40.5° to 43°C (105° to 110°F) and fill the container to the 1000-ml mark. Temperatures greater than 43°C (110°F) can injure the rectal mucosa and temperatures below 21°C (70°F) cause abdominal cramping (Sorensen and Luckmann, 1979; Tillery and Bates, 1966). The usual amount given is 500 to 1000 ml, with 1000 ml generally considered the maximum, although the adult colon can hold up to 2000 ml (Miller, 1975). For a normal saline enema, add 8 ml (2 tsp) of table salt to 1000 ml of water; for a soap-solution enema, add one 5-ml package of liquid castile soap to 1000 ml of water. Greater concentrations can have a harmful effect. Bottled normal saline may be used for an enema, but it is more expensive and more difficult to use because it must be warmed to the correct temperature whereas the temperature of tap water can be adjusted as needed. Before going to the bedside, close the caps or ports of plastic bags securely to avoid spilling.

Preparing the Client

Explain the type and purpose of the enema, including whether it is to be expelled or retained. Explain ways the client can facilitate insertion of the rectal tube and what can be done about cramping, and instruct him or her to take deep, regular, and slow breaths during the procedure. Discuss with the client where the enema is to be expelled. If the bathroom is to be used, be sure it will be available and have a robe and slippers ready.

Position the client in a comfortable and convenient position in the right or left lateral Sims position or on the back. The traditional position has been the left lateral, but fluid flow and the success of an enema apparently are not directly related to position, as long as the person is lying down (Dison, 1979; Lewis, 1984; Sorensen and Luckmann, 1979; Tillery and Bates, 1966). Enemas are not given with the client sitting on the toilet; in this position, gravity causes the solution to distend the rectum rather than flowing up into the colon and therefore stimulates premature defecation.

Cover the client with a bath blanket in such a way that the buttocks and anus remain exposed. Protect the bed with a waterproof pad and place the bedpan on the bed near the buttocks. Figure 58–3 shows a client in a left lateral Sims position, with the nurse preparing to insert the rectal tube.

Giving the Enema

The enema container may be placed on the overbed table, hung from an intravenous pole, or held in the nurse's hand. Most inexperienced nurses find it is easiest to have both hands free. Adjust the table or pole so that the fluid level is 45 cm (18 in) above the anus. This height will provide an adequate amount of pressure for the solution to reach the cecum in 2 to 5 minutes (Sorensen and Luckmann, 1979; Tillery and Bates, 1966). Place the rectal tube in a secure place so that it does not fall to the floor.

It is usually a good idea to wear disposable gloves when giving an enema. The tube needs to be held in place the entire time that the enema is being given. It is not always possible to predict which individuals will be able to retain the solution and which will not.

Before inserting the rectal tube, lubricate the distal 5 to 7.5 cm (2 to 3 in) of the tube. Open the clamp and allow solution to flow into the bedpan to remove

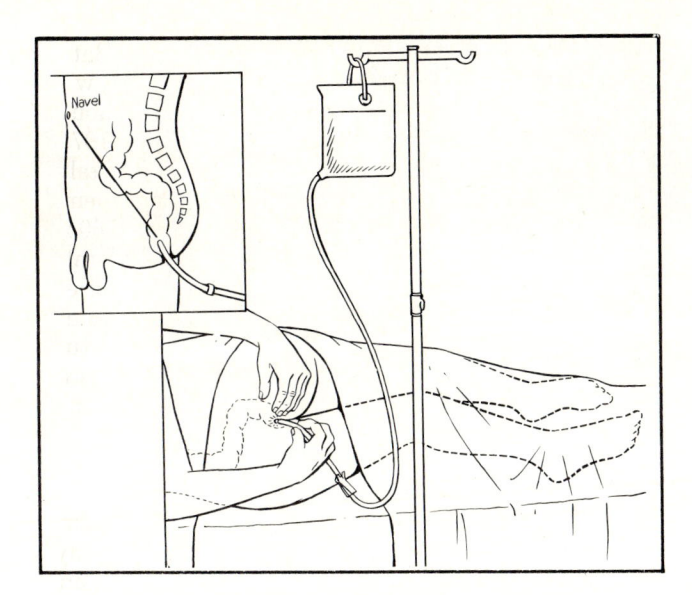

Figure 58-3. Administering a large-volume enema. Note client's and nurse's position and equipment being used. Enema container is placed 45 cm (18 in) above the client's rectum. Direct rectal tube 5 cm (2 in) toward the umbilicus as shown in the insert. Note the direction of the anal canal as compared to the rectum.

air from the tubing. Although it is not harmful for air to enter the colon, it prevents the fluid from flowing in as readily, especially if there is much flatus or constipated stool present; moreover, air seems to stimulate the defecation reflex more quickly. Allowing the enema fluid to flow into the bedpan also warms the rectal tube.

The rectal tube is inserted into the anus in the direction of the umbilicus. The preferred insertion depth is 5 cm (2 in), which is just past the internal sphincter. The anal canal itself is only 2.5 to 5 cm (1 to 2 in) long, and a deeper insertion can cause injury to the anterior rectal wall or may simply coil the tube within the rectum. Tillery and Bates (1966, p. 535) point out that "in order to avoid the possibility of perforation, the person who gives the enema needs to appreciate the angle between the direction of the anal canal, pointing from the anus forward to the umbilicus, and the rectum which points upward and back." This relationship is shown in Figure 58-3.

Before attempting to insert the tube, separate the buttocks so that you can see the anus. If large external hemorrhoids obscure the anus, be especially generous with lubrication and gentle with insertion. In this circumstance, a lubricated gloved index finger can sometimes locate the anus more easily than the rectal tube tip.

There are several ways to relax the anal sphincter and decrease the client's discomfort as the rectal tube is being inserted. Touching the rectal tube tip to the anal sphincter causes an initial reflex contraction, which is followed by relaxation of the sphincter. The sphincter will also relax when the client bears down as if to move the bowels or exhales after taking a deep breath. Rotate the tube as you gently and slowly insert it, as this may produce relaxation by avoiding involuntary sphincter contractions.

After the tube is inserted, open the clamp or hemostat and allow the fluid to flow in slowly. Raise or lower the container to adjust the pressure and rate of delivery so that it takes 10 minutes to give 1000 ml. This allows the fluid enough time to flow up into the colon and stimulate peristalsis. If the fluid is given more rapidly, the rectum distends with fluid and causes pain and an immediate urge to defecate.

If the fluid does not flow in readily, temporarily raise the container to 50 to 60 cm (20 to 24 in). The increased pressure may open a tip that is clogged with stool, but a sustained greater elevation and pressure rarely clears the tube and causes a dangerously increased pressure if it does clear suddenly (Tillery and Bates, 1966). If the solution does not flow, remove the rectal tube, clear the openings manually with toilet paper, reinsert the tube, and allow the fluid to flow in slowly as soon as the tip passes the external sphincter (Hogstel, 1977).

It is important to help the client relax while the fluid is flowing into the colon, because relaxation decreases the pressure within the colon and increases the amount of solution that the client can retain. Relaxation is promoted by a comfortable position, warmth, privacy, and by having the client breathe in and out through the mouth. Having the bedpan or robe and slippers near at hand is reassuring and therefore also relaxing.

Since the goal for a cleansing enema is to introduce fluid fairly far into the colon and thereby stimulate peristalsis, it is important to avoid the premature stimulation of the defecation reflex from distention of only the rectum. This can be done by having the client in a lying-down position, instilling the fluid over approximately a 10-minute time period, and having him or her remain lying down for 5 to 10 minutes after the enema fluid has been inserted. An upright position and rapid introduction of the fluid simply distends the rectum and does not stimulate peristalsis sufficiently enough to produce thorough evacuation.

Two common problems in giving enemas are *cramping* and *leaking*. When cramping occurs, lower the container below the level of the colon to allow some fluid to flow back into the container, thus decreasing the pressure and the pain. When the cramp passes, raise the container and continue the enema. Clamping the tube does not reduce the pressure in the colon (Hogstel, 1977; Miller, 1975).

To counteract leaking around the tube, (1) decrease the rate of flow, (2) apply firm pressure with a pad of eight to ten layers of toilet tissue held against the anus and around the tube, and (3) compress the buttocks together over the tube. Chisholm (1974) suggests cutting the tip off a baby bottle nipple and inserting the enema tube through the nipple as shown in Figure 58-4. When inserted into the anus, the nipple rim acts as an anal sphincter. Another way to control leakage is to use a large-diameter Foley catheter with a 30-ml inflatable bag instead of a rectal tube. After

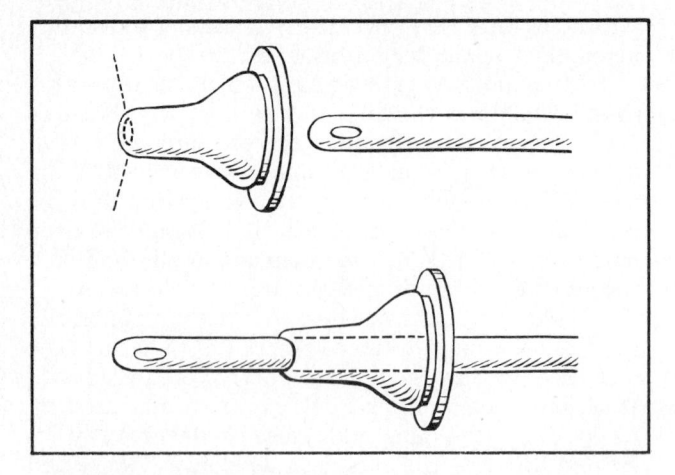

Figure 58–4. Nipple guard for rectal tube to minimize leakage during enema. Cut off tip of nipple and insert rectal tube; nipple forms a supplemental sphincter when tube is inserted into the rectum.

insertion, the balloon is inflated. Gentle tension on the catheter presses the balloon against the inside of the anus.

Observe the client's level of discomfort during the procedure and decrease the rate of flow as needed. Observe color and general condition, being alert for any pallor, diaphoresis, or respiratory distress. If necessary, caution the client to avoid hyperventilating when mouth-breathing.

When the client's tolerance for solution has been reached, or 1000 ml has been given, clamp the tube so that it does not leak as it is withdrawn. Place a pad of toilet tissue around the tube next to the anus and pull the tube out through the tissue while pressing against the anus. This cleanses the tube and helps avoid leaking. Ask the client to remain lying down for 10 minutes so that the solution can spread through the colon. If the client turns on the right side after the enema is given, it may help the solution flow into the transverse and ascending colons and give more thorough cleansing (Hogstel, 1977).

If the client is left alone after the solution is administered, place the call signal within easy reach and be sure to answer it promptly. Assist the client to a physiological position in the bathroom or on the commode or bedpan and provide toilet paper, privacy, and a call signal. Instruct the client to expel the enema solution in the same way as having a bowel movement, to report passage of flatus, and not to flush the toilet until you have inspected the results.

Assist with cleansing and washing the anal area and buttocks as needed and provide for client handwashing. Explain that during the next hour or so the client will most likely feel the need to have several more bowel movements. Discard disposable equipment or rinse and store it appropriately for a later reuse for the same client. Return reusable materials to central supply according to agency policy.

ADMINISTERING SMALL-VOLUME CLEANSING ENEMAS

Prepare the client and the bed as described above. Small-volume enemas are not warmed, but are given at room temperature to avoid cramping from cold solution. Small-volume enemas may be given with the client in any position other than seated. Sometimes the knee–chest position is recommended. For this position, the client kneels and then lowers the chest and head forward until the side of the face rests on the bed, using the arms for support. Sometimes the enema is given in the bathroom, with the patient in the knee–chest position on a pad on the floor. Regardless, absolute privacy is essential when using this position because of its embarrassing nature. Generally, it is not safe to use this method with elderly or weak persons.

Insert the prelubricated tip of the small-volume enema container into the anus and instill the solution by rolling the container tightly on itself. This keeps the fluid from being drawn back into the container when compression is released. Use 1 to 2 minutes to insert the fluid. Ask the client to retain the fluid without changing position for 2 to 5 minutes, after which time the urge to defecate is usually quite strong. Assist the client to the bathroom, bedpan, or commode to expel the solution as described earlier. Discard the container.

GIVING A RETENTION ENEMA

Prepare the equipment in the same manner as for a cleansing enema. Explain the purpose of the enema and the need to retain rather than expel the enema. There are several ways to diminish stimulation of the defecation reflex and increase retention time. A body-temperature solution (37°C or 98.6°F) is less likely to stimulate peristalsis, using a small-size rectal tube reduces sphincter stimulation, and elevating the container only slightly above the anus avoids rectal distention and a desire to defecate.

Oil-retention enemas are retained 30 to 60 minutes to overnight. Nutritive enemas are not expelled, and carminative enemas may or may not be expelled.

INSERTING A RECTAL TUBE

A rectal tube is used to stimulate peristalsis and move the flatus down so that it can be expelled. To insert a rectal tube, use a commercially prepared flatus bag (Fig. 58–5A) or gather the following equipment: rectal tube, container or pad to cover the end of the tube, water-soluble lubricant, and adhesive tape (Fig. 58–5B).

Use a rectal tube the same size as would be used to give an enema to that particular person. Since fluid as well as gas often escapes from the colon, place the end of the tube in a container, such as through the cap of a stool- or urine-specimen container. Add a vent for

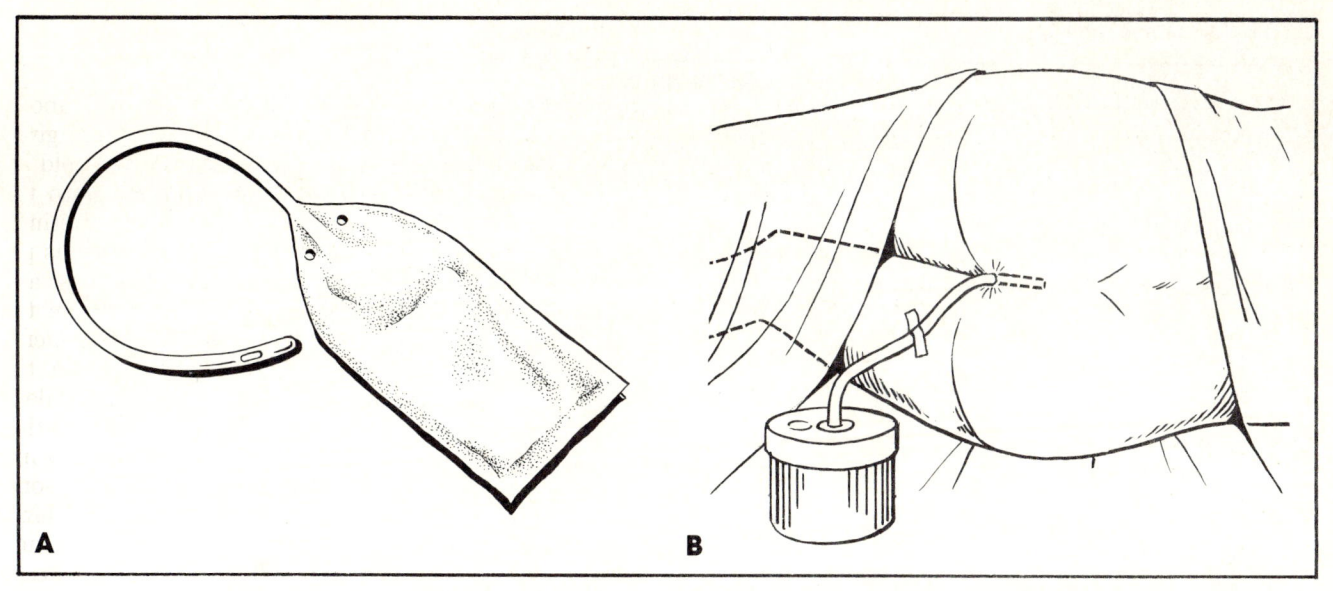

Figure 58–5. A. Vented flatus bag, with prelubricated tip. **B.** Improvised flatus bag using a rectal tube, waxed cardboard stool specimen container, and water-soluble lubricant. Note vent hole in container cap.

gas to escape. Alternatively, wrap a surgical dressing such as an ABD pad around the tube and anchor it with rubber bands. Insert the tube in the same manner as for an enema. Use generous lubrication. After insertion, anchor the tube to the buttocks with nonirritating tape and place the flatus container on the bed near the client. Sometimes one end of a connecting tube is attached to the rectal tube and the other end is placed in a flatus bottle that contains a measured amount of water. The bottle is suspended from the bed frame with the end of the tube under the water level. Bubbling indicates that flatus is being expelled. When using other equipment, expulsion of flatus is determined by client self-reports of passing flatus and of increased comfort, as well as the presence of the characteristic odor of flatus.

Leave the rectal tube in place for 20 to 30 minutes and reinsert it every 2 or 3 hours as needed. Insertion of the tube stimulates peristalsis and if left in place for longer times, stimulation no longer occurs. In addition, the anal sphincter becomes less responsive to stimulation and can become permanently damaged (Dison, 1979; Lewis, 1980; Sorensen and Luckmann, 1979).

FECAL DISIMPACTION

To remove a fecal impaction (disimpaction), gather the following equipment: disposable glove, water-soluble lubricant, bedpan, toilet tissue, and cleansing materials.

Before a fecal impaction can be removed manually, the large, hard fecal mass must be broken into smaller pieces. To do this, insert a heavily lubricated gloved index finger into the rectum in the direction of the umbilicus. Massage around the fecal mass and work the finger into it. Break the mass into small pieces and then bring them down toward the anus; remove the pieces one at a time, and place them in the bedpan. After the feces are removed, cleanse the perianal area as needed and assist the client to a comfortable and safe position.

This procedure must be performed very gently because it can easily cause anal and rectal injury. It is also very fatiguing and embarrassing for the client. Stop the procedure if the client becomes too fatigued and continue after he or she has rested. To decrease embarrassment, provide adequate explanation, absolute privacy, and approach the task in a matter-of-fact manner. Removing an impaction is sometimes easier and more successful if an oil-retention enema is first given to soften the stool.

In addition to knowing agency policy about disimpaction, validate the findings of an impaction and the decision to remove it with the nurse in charge. A specific physician's order is needed before an impaction is removed from clients with several kinds of illness conditions. For example, cardiac patients, such as those with myocardial infarctions, heart block, or congestive heart failure, may develop serious arrhythmias from vagal stimulation resulting from anal stretching and rectal distention and stimulation. Injury and additional bleeding can occur when the client has local bleeding tendencies, such as rectal polyps or lower intestinal and vaginal bleeding. Disimpaction also has the potential for loosening or tearing suture lines in clients who have had recent rectal, gynecologic, or genitourinary surgery. A physician's order is also recommended in pregnant clients and in clients undergoing pelvic irradiation.

☐ SKILL SEQUENCE

GIVING AN ENEMA

Step	Rationale
1. Document physician's order.	Implements therapeutic and diagnostic plans.
2. Explain purpose and procedure of the enema. Instruct as to how client can assist with procedure.	Enlists client cooperation; increases comfort and ease of enema administration.
3. Wash hands.	Prevents transfer of microorganisms.
4. Prepare equipment and ordered solution away from client's view. Select rectal tube size appropriate for the type of enema being given. Have solution at 40.5° to 43° (105° to 110°F).	Avoids causing anxiety. Small-diameter rectal tube prevents anal sphincter stimulation. Too cool temperature causes cramping; too warm, injury.
5. Provide privacy.	Decreases embarrassment, encourages relaxation, and increases success of enema.
6. Raise bed to comfortable working height.	Allows for correct body mechanics and promotes nurse safety.
7. Hang enema bag on IV pole; place can or bucket on overbed table; stabilize tubing.	Equipment is ready for use; allows both hands free for working. Avoids having rectal tube fall to floor.
8. Adjust height of pole or table so fluid level in container is 45 cm (18 in) above anus.	Provides optimal pressure gradient.
9. Replace top linen with bath blanket. Assist client to a lying-down position of comfort and preference.	Provides warmth and protection. Position does not affect administration significantly.
10. Drape with bath blanket, exposing anal area.	Avoids exposure and embarrassment.
11. Place waterproof pad under client.	Protects bed linen from moisture and soiling.
12. Don clean gloves.	Protects hands from fecal contamination.
13. Lubricate rectal tube from tip to 5 cm (2 in) proximal to tip.	Provides for ease in insertion and avoids sphincter trauma.
14. Place bedpan on bed near buttocks. Open clamp slightly, allow fluid to flow into bedpan, and reclose clamp.	Removes air from tubing and fills tubing with warm water.
15. Separate buttocks to visualize anus.	Blind entry can traumatize tissues, causing pain and injury.
16. Touch rectal tube tip to anus and briefly wait for sphincter to relax.	Stimulates normal rectal closure reflex, which is followed by relaxation of anal sphincter. Avoids injury and discomfort.
17. Use a rotating motion and insert rectal tube gently and smoothly in the direction of umbilicus to a distance of 5 to 7 cm (2 to 3 in).	Rotation relaxes sphincter. Anal canal is directed anteriorly and is 2.5 to 5 cm (1 to 2 in) long.
18. Open tubing clamp and allow fluid to flow in slowly; adjust container height so that fluid flows in over a 10-minute period. Remind client to breathe deeply. Caution against hyperventilating as needed. (NOTE: For retention enema: Hold fluid container slightly above anus; allow fluid to flow in slowly, over 2 to 3 minutes.)	Rapid administration causes rectal distention and premature desire to defecate. Time is needed to allow fluid to reach upper colon. Hyperventilation can cause faintness. Lower pressure gradient decreases rectal distention and stimulation of defecation reflex.
19. If cramping occurs during enema: a. Ask client to breathe deeply through the mouth or pant. b. Lower enema can below rectum until cramp eases, but do not stop fluid flow.	Promotes relaxation and increases capacity to hold fluid. Decreases pressure within colon.
20. If fluid leaks from anus during enema: a. Leave rectal tube in place. b. Lower container slightly. c. Compress buttocks around anus. d. Apply pressure around anus with a pad of toilet tissue. (NOTE: If leakage is anticipated or occurs immediately after fluid begins to flow, use a baby bottle nipple over rectal tube, or use a Foley catheter with a 30-ml balloon instead of a rectal tube.)	Removing tube can stimulate defecation reflex. Decreases pressure in colon; helps retain fluid. Acts as a secondary anal sphincter.
21. When solution is instilled or client has reached tolerance point: a. Clamp tubing b. Place pad of 5 to 10 layers of toilet tissue around rectal tube and apply firm pressure around tube and against anus while withdrawing tube. c. Withdraw tube gently, with tube continuing to point toward umbilicus.	Avoids leaking from tube when it is withdrawn. Helps client maintain control of sphincter and cleanses rectal tube. Changing direction stimulates defecation reflex.
22. Discard toilet tissue in bedpan, place tube and tubing in can or bucket, and wrap tube in paper towels if using enema bag. Discard disposable single-use small-volume enema container.	Avoids contamination of environment. Interior of enema can is already contaminated from backflow.

(continued)

SKILL 58: BOWEL ELIMINATION PROCEDURES 617

Step	Rationale
23. Remove and discard gloves.	Avoids contamination of environment.
24. Ask client to retain enema for 10 to 15 minutes while lying quietly in bed. Place bed in low position. (NOTE: For retention enema: Remind client not to attempt to expel solution.)	Increases effectiveness of enema. An upright position increases gravity pressure in colon and causes premature desire to defecate. Solution is intended to be absorbed or have a local action.
25. Provide nurse-call signal and instruct to call for help to go to bathroom.	Provides for client safety.
26. Rinse equipment if it is to be used again by same client. Store in bedside stand in bedpan storage area or in bathroom, not with personal care items.	May be safely reused for same client. Equipment is considered contaminated from contact with fecal material.
27. Assist client to bathroom, commode, or onto bedpan. Elevate head of bed to nearly upright position. Provide privacy and instruct not to flush toilet and to report passage of flatus.	Nurse needs to observe results of enema.
28. Observe results and remove specimen if needed.	Provides data; implements plan of care.
29. Discard contents of bedpan or flush toilet. Cleanse bedpan according to agency policy.	Provides appropriate disposal of feces.
30. Assist with perianal cleansing as needed. Provide handwashing equipment for client.	Promotes client comfort, provides for personal hygiene needs, and prevents skin irritation.
31. Remove bath blanket and replace top linen; change linen as needed. Return client to position of comfort and safety.	Provides for client comfort and safety.
32. Wash own hands.	Prevents transfer of microorganisms.
33. Report and record amount and type of solution administered, length of time fluid was retained, where fluid was expelled, approximate amount of solution returned, amount and character of stool returned, client's reports or nurse observations of passage of flatus, any untoward reactions, and any specimens sent to the laboratory.	Provides ongoing data base. Provides for nurse accountability.

RECORDING

Record the data that indicated an enema was needed, the type and amount of solution used, and the results obtained. Describe the color, consistency, and amount of stool, color and amount of solution, and the client self-reports or your observations about flatus expelled. Include any problems that occurred during administration, such as leakage, inability to retain an adequate amount of fluid, and cramping that did not respond to usual nursing measures. Record any pallor, diaphoresis, respiratory distress, or other untoward reaction that may have occurred, what was done about it, and the client's current status. If a stool specimen was obtained, record the time it was sent to the laboratory.

Sample POR Recording

- S—"I feel so much better since that enema! I passed a lot of gas too!"
- O—Approx. 800 ml tap water given as enema; expelled in BR. Returned dark brown fluid, large amounts of dark brown, hard-formed stool and audible flatus. To BR X 2 since enema; expelled more formed stool and solution.
- A—Adequate results from cleansing enema given to relieve constipation.
- P—Discuss c̄ client, physician, & dietitian ways to avoid recurrent constipation.

Sample Narrative Recording

Approx. 800 ml TWE given. Expelled dark brown solution c̄ large amount dark brown hard formed stool & large amounts of flatus in BR. Stated, "I feel so much better!" To BR x 2 since enema; expelled mod. amount formed stool & small amt. of solution each time. Plan consult c̄ physician & dietitian about how to help client avoid recurrent constipation.

☐ CRITICAL POINTS SUMMARY

1. Large-volume cleansing enemas stimulate peristalsis and the defecation reflex by creating bulk within the colon.
2. Small-volume hypertonic cleansing enemas produce bulk and cause irritation.
3. Tap water and normal saline are the preferred solutions for large-volume enemas.
4. An oil-retention enema is usually followed later by a cleansing enema.
5. Colonic irrigations use an alternating in-and-out flow of solution to cleanse the bowel or relieve flatus.

6. Fecal impactions are broken up digitally and removed manually.
7. Rectal tubes used for relief of excessive flatulence are left in place for no more than 20 to 30 minutes at a time.
8. Anal and rectal stimulation during an enema can precipitate serious cardiac arrhythmias.
9. Enema solutions are more easily instilled when the client and the anal sphincter are relaxed.
10. An enema can be given successfully with the client in any lying-down position.
11. Nursing interventions can counteract the problems of leaking and cramping.
12. Avoid premature stimulation of the defecation reflex when giving cleansing enemas.
13. Minimize stimulation of the defecation reflex when giving retention enemas.
14. Provide for privacy, comfort, and safety during an enema.

☐ LEARNING ACTIVITIES

1. Interview a person who needed an enema during a hospital stay. Ask him or her to describe the experience of receiving an enema; identify whether it was a large-volume or small-volume enema (if possible); describe the actions the nurse took that helped him or her to feel relaxed, comfortable, and safe; and inquire about negative experiences with the enema. Ask the person how he or she felt after the enema was finished and what suggestions he or she would make to nurses about giving enemas.
2. Interview several nurses who give enemas regularly. Inquire about their preferences for giving large- as opposed to small-volume enemas and their reasons for those preferences. Ask about methods they have found helpful in coping with leaking and cramping and how they help clients accept the desired amount of solution. Also inquire about their experiences with and suggestions for relieving flatus and removing fecal impactions. How would you describe these nurses' feelings about giving enemas?
3. In the central supply department or clinical unit, examine several types of disposable and reusable enema equipment. Identify advantages and disadvantages of each.

☐ REVIEW QUESTIONS

1. List four purposes for which enemas are most commonly given.
2. Compare the mechanism that stimulates peristalsis in large- and small-volume enemas.
3. How do colonic irrigations differ from large-volume cleansing enemas?
4. How can you avoid the following hazards when giving an enema?
   a. Local tissue trauma and colon irritation
   b. Intestinal perforation
   c. Fluid–electrolyte imbalance
   d. Cardiac arrhythmias
   e. Dependence
5. What factors contribute to the development of constipation, excessive flatulence, and fecal impaction?
6. Describe subjective and objective data that would indicate that a client has
   a. Constipation
   b. Fecal impaction
   c. Flatulence
7. Identify data gathered by inspection and palpation prior to:
   a. Giving a cleansing enema
   b. Inserting a rectal tube for flatulence
   c. Removing a fecal impaction
8. What data would indicate whether a client could retain enema fluid or be able to go to the bathroom to expel the fluid?
9. What effect does the client's position during and after an enema have on the successful outcome of both cleansing and retention enemas?
10. Why is a temperature of 40.5°C (105°F) used for a cleansing enema and a temperature of 37°C (98.6°F) used for a retention enema?
11. What nursing interventions help promote client relaxation during an enema?
12. List four ways to stimulate anal sphincter relaxation when inserting the rectal tube tip.
13. What can the nurse do to prevent premature stimulation of the defecation reflex while giving a cleansing enema?
14. In what ways do rectal tubes, flatus bags, and carminative enemas relieve flatulence?
15. What effect does an oil-retention enema have on fecal impaction?

☐ PERFORMANCE CHECKLIST

OBJECTIVE: To use medical aseptic technique to administer an enema safely and comfortably.			
CHARACTERISTIC	RANGE OF ACCEPTABILITY	SATISFACTORY	UNSATISFACTORY
1. Explains procedure, type, and purpose of enema.	No deviation		
2. Washes hands.	No deviation		

(continued)

CHARACTERISTIC	RANGE OF ACCEPTABILITY	SATISFACTORY	UNSATISFACTORY
3. Prepares equipment and solution, and selects appropriate sized tube.	Physician may determine size.		
4. Provides privacy.	No deviation		
5. Positions bed at appropriate height.	No deviation		
6. Hangs or places solution at 45 cm (18 in) above anus.	No deviation		
7. Protects bed linens with pad, positions client, and covers with bath blanket.	No deviation		
8. Dons clean gloves.	No deviation		
9. Lubricates distal 5 cm (2 in) of rectal tube.	No deviation		
10. Removes air from tubing.	No deviation		
11. Visualizes anus to insert tubing; touches tube tip against anus.	Instruct client to bear down or take a deep breath and exhale.		
12. Promotes relaxation of client.	No deviation		
13. Adjusts container to appropriate height and administers solution for desired time interval.	No deviation		
14. Indicates verbally how to manage cramping and leakage.	No deviation		
15. Wipes tube and compresses anus while removing tube.	No deviation		
16. Discards tissue in bedpan.	No deviation		
17. Instructs client to retain enema for desired time interval.	No deviation		
18. Provides call signal.	No deviation		
19. Removes and discards gloves.	No deviation		
20. Cleans or disposes of equipment.	No deviation		
21. Assists client to bathroom and instructs not to flush toilet.	May need to use bedpan or commode.		
22. Observes results.	No deviation		
23. Discards bedpan contents or flushes toilet.	No deviation		
24. Assists with perianal and hand cleansing; returns client to position of comfort and safety.	No deviation		
25. Washes own hands.	No deviation		
26. Reports and records enema and results.	No deviation		

REFERENCES

Bass L: More fiber—less constipation. American Journal of Nursing 77(2):254–255, 1977.

Burkitt DP: Procedures of unproved value. Journal of the American Medical Association 247(9):1278–1279, 1982.

Chisholm R: From the mouths of babes. Nursing74 4(1):68, 1974.

Davis R, Eichner JM, et al: Hypocalcemia, hyperphosphatemia, and dehydration following a single hypertonic phosphate enema. Journal of Pediatrics 90(3):484–485, 1977.

Dison N: Clinical Nursing Techniques, ed 4. St Louis, CV Mosby, 1979.

Duffin HM, Castleden CM, Chaudhry AY: Are enemas necessary? Nursing Times77(45):1940–1941, 1981.

Guyton AC: Human Physiology and Mechanisms of Disease, ed 3. Philadelphia, WB Saunders, 1982.

Hogstel M: How to give a safe and successful cleansing enema. American Journal of Nursing 77(5):816–817, 1977.

Lewis LW: Fundamental Skills in Patient Care, ed 3. Philadelphia, JB Lippincott, 1984.

Miller RE: Opinion: The cleansing enema. Radiology 117(2):483–485, 1975.

No soap. Emergency Medicine 3(11):151–154, 1971.

Pike BF, Phillippi PJ, Lawson EH: Soap colitis. New England Journal of Medicine 285(4):217–218, 1971.

Robins AH: G.I. Series: Physical Examination of the Abdomen. Richmond, VA, AH Robins, 1974.

Sorensen KC, Luckmann J: Basic Nursing: A Psychophysiologic Approach. Philadelphia, WB Saunders, 1979.

Tillery B, Bates B: Enemas. American Journal of Nursing 66(3):534–537, 1966.

BIBLIOGRAPHY

Blackwell AK, Blackwell W: Relieving gas pains. American Journal of Nursing 75(1):66–67, 1975.

Condon RE, Nyhus LM (eds): Manual of Surgical Therapeutics, ed 6. Boston, Little, Brown, 1985.

Corbett JV: Laboratory Tests in Nursing Practice. Norwalk, CT, Appleton-Century-Crofts, 1982.

Fischbach FT: A Manual of Laboratory Diagnostic Tests. Philadelphia, JB Lippincott, 1980.

Kozier B, Erb G: Techniques in Clinical Nursing: A Comprehensive Approach. Menlo Park, CA: Addison-Wesley, 1982.

Malasanos L, Barkauskas V, et al: Health Assessment, ed 2. St Louis, CV Mosby, 1981.

Potter PA, Perry AG: Fundamentals of Nursing: Concepts, Process, and Practice. St Louis, CV Mosby, 1985.

Sana JM, Judge RD: Physical Assessment Skills for Nursing Practice, ed 2. Boston, Little, Brown, 1982.

When the problem is intestinal gas. Patient Care 7(6):81–92, 1973.

SUGGESTED READING

Hogstel M: How to give a safe and successful cleansing enema. American Journal of Nursing 77(5):816–817, 1977.

Tillery B, Bates B: Enemas. American Journal of Nursing 66(3):534–537, 1966.

AUDIOVISUAL RESOURCES

Administering a Cleansing Enema
  Videorecording. (1981, Color, 10 min.)
  Available through:
    Robert J. Brady Company
    Route 197
    Bowie, MD 20715

Bowel Elimination
  Filmstrip and cassette. (1978, Color, series of 10 cassettes, 15 min. each.)
  Available through:
    J. B. Lippincott Company
    227 South 6th Street
    Philadelphia, PA 19148

Administration of Enemas
  Filmstrip and cassette. (1970, Color, 25 min.)
  Available through:
    Career Aids
    8950 Lurline Avenue
    Chatsworth, CA 91311

Basic Nursing Care, Cleansing Enema
  Filmstrip and cassette. (1982, 22 min.)
  Available through:
    Medcom, Inc.
    P.O. Box 116
    Garden Grove, CA 92642

SKILL 59 Urinary Incontinence Care

PREREQUISITE SKILLS

Skill 19, "Inspection"
Skill 28, "Handwashing"
Skill 58, "Bowel Elimination Procedures"

☐ STUDENT OBJECTIVES

1. Explain common causes of urinary incontinence.
2. Identify problems resulting from incontinence.
3. Identify nursing measures used to counteract the negative effects of incontinence.
4. Differentiate between incontinence problems for men and women.
5. Explain the principles of correct application of a male external urinary drainage system.
6. Identify various ways to protect the skin when a person is incontinent of urine.
7. Describe hazards associated with incorrect application of a male external urinary drainage system.
8. Apply a male external urinary drainage system safely and correctly.

☐ INTRODUCTION

Incontinence is the inability of the urinary or anal sphincters to control the passage of urine or feces. Fecal incontinence is discussed in Skill 58. Urinary incontinence may be complete, with total involuntary emptying of the bladder, or partial, with dribbling of urine. Urinary incontinence may be permanent, as with spinal cord injury and some neuromuscular conditions. It may also be temporary or intermittent, such as the stress incontinence that occurs with pregnancy or coughing.

Anything that interferes with sphincter control can cause incontinence. For example, spinal cord injury interferes with bladder innervation; drugs such as narcotics, sedatives, and alcohol decrease a person's awareness of the need to void; and weak perineal muscles decrease the efficiency of the external sphincter. Incontinence can also occur with urinary tract infections, tumors, urethral strictures, fecal impaction, loss of consciousness, and regression. In the elderly, incontinence may be associated with "giving up" and fulfilling expectations of being incontinent. Incontinence can also occur when the client needs to urinate and the call signal is not answered quickly enough.

Depending on the reason for incontinence, continence can sometimes be regained through bladder retraining or surgery. When this is not feasible, incontinence in males can be managed quite successfully by using external drainage devices. Unfortunately, no comparable device is available for females, and absorbent pants or pads are the best option. Because of the high rate of urinary tract infections associated with indwelling catheters, they are not generally used for incontinence in the acute-care setting. Sometimes urinary diversion with a permanent ostomy is used to achieve control of urinary elimination (see Skill 61).

When caring for clients who are incontinent, the nurse often applies and monitors external drainage devices, provides protection and absorbency when external drainage is not feasible, and implements skin-care practices that are designed to minimize the problems associated with urinary incontinence. Although procedures for care of incontinence may be ordered by the physician, decisions about the kind of care needed are more often determined by the professional nurse and based on careful assessment of the client's needs and capabilities.

☐ PREPARATION

TYPES OF INCONTINENCE

Incontinence can be categorized as stress, urge, neurogenic, psychogenic, and iatrogenic incontinence.

Stress incontinence is the most common type of urinary incontinence. It usually occurs in women, although it may also occur in men with prostatic hypertrophy. In stress incontinence, urine dribbling occurs in response to a physical stressor, such as laughing, coughing, or sneezing. It may also occur when a client strains with a bowel movement, stoops to pick up something from the floor, or rises from a seated position or sits down from a standing position. Stress incontinence is often the result of childbirth trauma, loss of tissue tone, and aging. These factors weaken the pelvic muscles that support the bladder and straighten the urethrovesicular angle, thus decreasing the normal mechanisms for maintaining urine within the bladder. Stress incontinence is also more likely to occur in women whose urethras are shorter than the average.

Urge incontinence refers to the inability to hold back the urine flow after experiencing a sudden urge to urinate. A person with urge incontinence lacks voluntary control over the voiding reflex and often does not get to the bathroom in time to avoid an accident. Urge incontinence is usually caused by an infection or an inflammatory condition and is often accompanied by frequency, burning, or pain with urination, and fever. It may also occur premenstrually or with some drugs, such as antihistamines and epinephrine.

Neurogenic incontinence, or neurogenic bladder dysfunction, results from an interference with the innervation of the bladder. It is usually caused by a neurologic disease such as multiple sclerosis or trauma such as a spinal cord injury. Depending on the type of dysfunction, there may be uncontrolled voiding on the first urge to urinate, reflex incomplete voiding without sensations of bladder fullness, or an inability to perceive sensations of bladder fullness, resulting in chronic retention with overflow.

Psychogenic incontinence may be associated with depressive illness, agitated hypomanic states, regression, sensory deprivation, or severe retardation. It may also represent dependence, insecurity, manipulative attention-getting, or rebellion.

Iatrogenic incontinence refers to incontinence that occurs as a result of treatment of illness conditions, such as the side effects of drugs. For example, some diuretics such as furosemide (Lasix) have such a rapid action that incontinence occurs because of inability to get to the bathroom or bedpan in time. Hypnotics such as the barbiturates and psychotropic drugs such as diazepam (Valium) or promazine hydrochloride (Sparine) can produce such a deep sleep that the usual micturition reflex stimuli do not waken the person. Tricyclic antidepressants such as imipramine hydrochloride (Tofranil) may also cause incontinence.

The unfamiliar environment of a hospital may cause incontinence, especially for elderly or confused clients. Sometimes incontinence is simply the result of impaired manual dexterity, an overly long distance to the bathroom, or failure of the nursing staff to answer a call signal promptly.

PROBLEMS ASSOCIATED WITH INCONTINENCE

Incontinence produces sociopsychological, skin, odor, and laundry problems for clients in both the hospital and home settings.

Sociopsychological Problems
Being incontinent can be a distressing experience. Not only is it uncomfortable to be wet with urine, but it usually produces shame and embarrassment. Urinary control is learned in early childhood as a child gains independence and self-control. For most people, loss of urinary control signifies helplessness and childishness.

In our society, the odor of urine on clothing is socially unacceptable, and many persons with incontinence are sensitive and fearful about this. They tend to withdraw from social contacts and often refuse to leave their homes.

Skin Problems
The continued or frequent presence of urine causes the perineal area to be damp much of the time, causing maceration and increasing the likelihood of skin breakdown. In addition, the ammonia produced from urine breakdown is an irritant and often causes a dermatitis similar to diaper rash in infants. It is important to remember that clients who are incontinent are often quite ill or have some impairment of circulation or innervation, which predisposes them to tissue breakdown. When these persons are not kept dry or turned frequently, pressure sores (decubitus ulcers) are likely to occur.

Laundry and Odor Problems
At home, clients improvise many ways to keep their clothing dry. They may use sanitary napkins to absorb smaller amounts of incontinent urine, or towels and old rags for greater absorbency. If not changed often enough, clothing still becomes wet and odors develop, especially if the skin is not cleansed thoroughly each time. Bedfast, incontinent clients need special bed protection and frequent linen changes. Both at home and in an institution, incontinent clients can generate very large amounts of laundry. The odor from the soiled laundry becomes a problem unless urine-soaked clothing and linen are promptly removed from the environment. Continuing odors of ammonia in clinical areas usually indicate that urine-soaked linen and clothing are not changed promptly and cared for appropriately.

MANAGEMENT OF INCONTINENCE

Nursing management of clients who are incontinent is directed toward protecting the skin, clothing, and bed linen, decreasing odors, and keeping the skin as clean and dry as possible. The most successful way to achieve these goals is to help clients become continent or to prevent the urine from contacting their skin, by using specially designed absorbent pants or pads or external urinary drainage devices.

A complete diagnostic evaluation may reveal causes of incontinence that can be corrected. Drug therapy can be modified or instituted, surgery may correct an anatomic problem that causes stress incontinence, urinary tract infections and chronic coughs can be treated, and, sometimes, electrical stimulation is used to inhibit the micturition reflex. When incontinence does not respond to treatment, it can be managed in a variety of ways, such as pelvic exercises, bladder training, external catheters, and protecting bed linen and clothing. In obese clients, weight reduction will often decrease or eliminate stress incontinence.

Pelvic Exercises
Pelvic exercises (Kegel exercises) will help reduce or prevent female stress incontinence. Kegel exercises are particularly beneficial in younger women who have good muscle tone and have had only one or two children. To do these exercises, have the client sit in a chair with her knees spread and feet planted on the floor. Instruct her to squeeze or contract her perineal muscles as if she were suddenly attempting to stop urinating. The body position ensures that the client will contract the perineal rather than the gluteal muscles. The exercise should be repeated ten times in succession and at least four times daily. In addition, instruct the client to try to stop and start the urine stream several times whenever she voids. It is particularly important to teach these exercises to younger mothers and pregnant women as a long-term preventive measure.

Bladder Training
Bladder training helps some clients achieve continence, depending on the cause of the problem. The physician will usually indicate when bladder training is to be initiated for neurologically impaired persons. Nurses often initiate bladder training for elderly, confused, or retarded clients. Bladder training consists of providing the opportunity to void at regular intervals that are shorter than the interval between incontinent voidings. The intervals are determined by careful observation of the client's pattern of incontinence. Initially this interval may be as often as every 30 minutes to 1 hour and then gradually lengthened. Fluid intake is encouraged, not restricted, and offered on a regular basis. Diapers are avoided since they tend to give permission to be incontinent and are demoralizing to an adult. Further discussions of bladder training may be found in various medical–surgical textbooks.

External Catheters
Incontinence in males can often be easily managed by attaching an external collection device to the penis. These devices consist of a collector and a drainage system and are known as external, condom, Texas, or X-dwelling catheters. The collector is held in place on the penis with flexible adhesive strips or tape and the lower end is attached to a bedside drainage system like that used with indwelling catheters (see Skill 60) or attached to a leg bag for greater mobility.

Although often quite successful, there are problems associated with the use of external catheters. If the external catheter is positioned so that the tip of the penis is too close to the distal inner end of the collector, friction can occur, with irritation and trauma to the penis. When the lower end of the collector twists around itself, urine outflow is obstructed and urine backup can cause the collector to loosen, leak, and come off. In addition, this improper positioning and twisting cause the urinary meatus and penis to be continually wet with urine. Tissue maceration and breakdown can occur if the penis is always damp inside the collector (Steinhardt and McRoberts, 1980).

A pool of urine in constant contact with the meatus is also a source of bladder infection. A British study indicated that urine cultures from condom catheters showed bacterial counts in a range of 10^5 to 10^6 organisms per milliliter while urethral samples showed counts of less than 10^4 per milliliter (Lawson and Cook, 1977).

When the penis is too short for an external catheter to be applied, incontinence pants may be worn, or a two-piece wafer-style ostomy appliance may be used. In order for the ostomy appliance to be used, it is necessary to shave the pubic hair around the penis. Occasionally a device known as a pubic pressure urinal is used. It holds the penis securely in place within a condom but can cause pressure problems because of its snug fit around the abdomen and pubic area (Baum, 1978).

Protection of Clothing and Linen
Clothing may be protected with specially designed disposable or reusable incontinence pants. A Florida study of 276 "persistently incontinent" clients in seven nursing homes found that the use of a fitted disposable brief was judged to improve the quality of life in 75 percent of those individuals who were sufficiently alert for their responses to be interpreted. The briefs ranked consistently higher than other methods of incontinence care in factors such as bedding and clothing protection, skin dryness, client comfort, convenience, ease of application, ease of removal, and odor containment (Beber, 1980).

Bed linen and mattresses can be protected by placing a rubber or plastic draw sheet under a regular draw sheet or by using a lightweight plastic-backed protective pad such as the commonly used blue Chux incontinence pads. Although these thin pads do protect the linen, their absorbency is limited. When used immediately next to the skin, the skin remains damp with urine after an incontinent voiding, and if not changed fairly promptly, the pads sometimes stick to the skin. Some of these problems can be avoided by placing the incontinence pad inside a pillowcase.

DATA BASE

The health record documents the history of incontinence, including onset and duration of the problem, the frequency of incontinent voiding, and whether the client is incontinent only at night or around the clock. The health record or nursing-care plan includes actions already undertaken to manage the incontinence problem, including ways to protect the bed and clothing. If an external catheter is not feasible because the penis is too small, that information is noted. Because the data in the record may be incomplete and a client's health status may change frequently, information about incontinence is obtained or validated directly through interviews with the client or family.

The diagnosis, age, and general state of health can alert the nurse to the possibility that a given client may be incontinent. For example, an elderly woman who is newly hospitalized for cataract surgery has an increased probability of being incontinent because of age, the unfamiliarity of her surroundings, and decreased mobility after surgery. Information about usual voiding frequency can be used to determine how often to offer a bedpan or take the client to the bathroom, thus avoiding incontinence. Additional data about the problem of incontinence come from an assessment of fluid intake, mental status, manual dexterity, and the ability to use the bedpan, urinal, or bathroom.

Physical Appraisal Skills

Inspection. Whenever an incontinent client's linen or clothing are changed, the perineal area and surrounding skin are inspected for breaks, erythema, maceration, or rashes. Before applying an external catheter, the nurse inspects the penis size to determine the type and size of collector that would provide the best fit. The condition of the skin on the penis is inspected whenever the catheter is changed, or at least once in every 24 hours. Inspection will also reveal whether the external collector is securely attached, loosened, leaking, or twisted. When this inspection is done every 2 or 3 hours, wet clothing and linen can often be avoided.

Sense of Smell. The odor of urine breakdown may alert the nurse to a wet bed or clothing that need changing.

EQUIPMENT

External Urinary Catheters
External catheters have either a condom or a sheathlike collector. Thin, flexible latex condom-style collectors allow for spontaneous erections without impeding the circulation in the penis. However, the distal end can easily become twisted when the client moves. Sheath-style catheters are made from heavier, less flexible latex. They seldom become twisted, but can cause discomfort, skin irritation, and impaired circulation when spontaneous erections occur. External collectors are available in several sizes to provide adequate fit without leakage or constriction.

There are a wide variety of commercially manufactured disposable external catheters on the market, two of which are shown in Figure 59–1. A number of the newer designs combine a thin stretchable condom with a specially designed tip that prevents twisting and kinking. For example, some have a stiff rubber connector tip that does not readily twist or kink, and others are designed with convoluted ridges or a bubble design at the distal end of the collector.

If a commercial catheter is not available, an external catheter can be improvised from an ordinary condom, a piece of ⅜-inch rubber tubing, and a small rubber band or a short piece (½ inch) of ⁹⁄₃₂-inch plastic tubing (Whyte and Thistle, 1976). Figure 59–2 provides a description of this procedure.

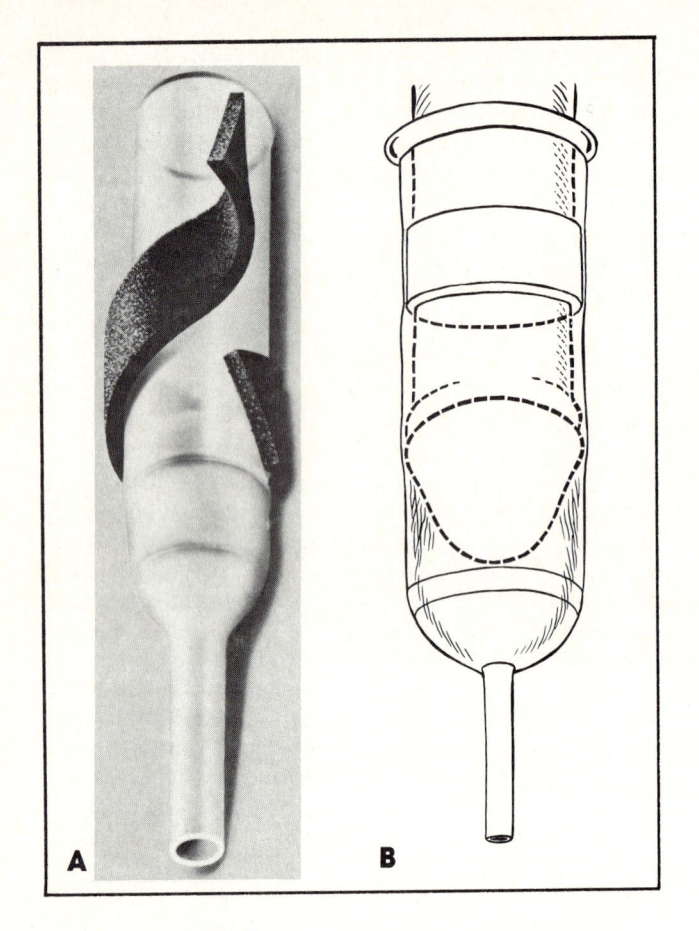

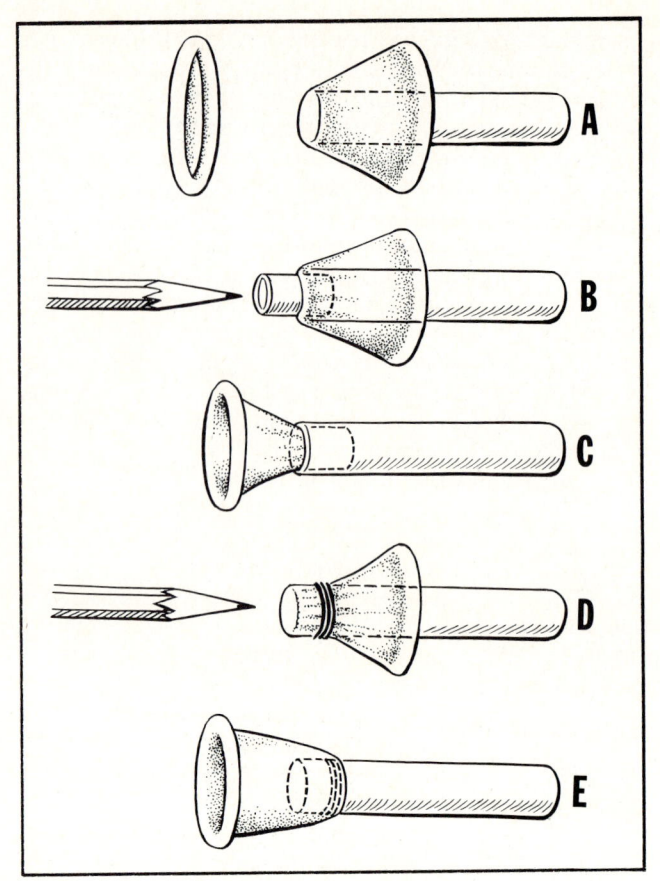

Figure 59–1. External urinary catheters. **A.** Uri-Drain is anchored outside the collector with a flexible foam strip. (From Chesebrough-Ponds, Inc., Greenwich, CT, with permission.) **B.** External catheter anchored with flexible strip inside the collector.

Figure 59–2. Improvised external condom catheter. **A.** Place a partially unrolled condom over a piece of ³/₈-inch rubber tubing. **B.** Press a short (¹/₂-in) piece of ⁹/₃₂-inch tubing inside the ³/₈-inch tubing, forcing the condom inside. Make a hole in the condom with a pencil or other sharp object. **C.** Partially unrolled condom catheter ready for application. **D.** Condom may also be secured with a small rubber band. **E.** Condom catheter ready for application.

External catheters are held in place with various types of flexible adherent strips, either inside or outside the collector. Those strips or patches that are placed on the inside of the collector are often made of a self-adherent substance similar to ostomy skin barriers (described in Skill 61) or of stretchable self-adhesive foam. One external catheter has an adhesive-lined collector that needs no additional adhesive strips; it works fairly well on clients who do not have sensitive skin. A note of caution: If the skin on the penis is irritated, the only kind of adhesives or self-adherent strips or patches that can be used inside a collector are those made of a skin-barrier substance. Some collectors are held in place with flexible adhesive strips placed around the outside of the collector. Nonflexible tape is *never* used to hold an external catheter in place because of the possibility of impeding circulation if a spontaneous erection occurs.

Incontinence Pants and Pads

A variety of reusable and disposable pants and pads is available commercially. They are designed to absorb and draw urine away from the skin, with the layer adjacent to the skin remaining fairly dry while the external waterproof layer protects the linen and clothing. Some incontinence pants are pull-on lined briefs with an elasticized waist and legs; some designs are similar to an elasticized leg style disposable infant diaper and can be adjusted to fit most body sizes and shapes by using adhesive-strap or gripper-snap waist closures; other styles have an absorbent disposable pad, similar to a sanitary napkin, inside a reusable moisture-resistant brief.

Another method of incontinence protection involves using a reusable pad that is folded and pinned or taped in place on the client, similar to a cloth diaper. In addition, a variety of reusable and disposable pads is available for bed and chair protection. The selection of a specific type of incontinence protection will vary with the degree of incontinence, size and physical condition, and the convenience and economy needed.

☐ EXECUTION

One of the most significant aspects of working to resolve an incontinence problem is communicating hope to the client and family. Incontinence is very demoralizing and it is not uncommon for people to give up hope of ever being dry again. It is important to have a positive attitude, assume continence is possible, give positive feedback for successes, and be matter-of-fact about lapses and accidents.

Before initiating any activities designed to keep the incontinent client dry, explain the procedures that will be used and what they are to accomplish. Doing this in a matter-of-fact, direct way helps the client accept the interventions with minimal distress and embarrassment. Clients and their families often do not know about some of the newer products, devices, and approaches that make management of incontinence easier and they will welcome this information. The newer incontinence pants are virtually leakproof and often make it possible for clients to resume social activities. Families need to know that incontinence pants, bladder training, or a well-fitted external urine collection device will decrease the amount of work involved in home care of an incontinent client. These measures will also decrease skin problems associated with prolonged contact with urine and improve self-image. If the client will need incontinence pants, encourage the family to compare the cost, comfort, and work involved in both disposable and reusable styles.

When caring for someone who is incontinent, remember to wash and dry the skin after each voiding, so that ammonia from urine breakdown does not remain in contact with the skin for a prolonged period of time. Always provide privacy when changing linens and clothing and avoid unnecessary exposure, such as completely stripping and uncovering the client. Send urine-damp linens to the laundry immediately after removing them. In the home, the family can use a vinegar solution or products designed for infant diaper care to soak reusable pads and pants liners prior to washing them. This practice decreases odors and stains.

EXTERNAL CATHETERS

Successful use of an external catheter involves careful preparation of the penis, correct application, and daily hygienic care and inspection. Before applying an external catheter, assess the size and shape of the penis and select a size and style of catheter that will fit and remain in place.

Preparation of the Penis
Wash the penis and surrounding area with soap and water, rinse, and dry thoroughly. This will remove urine, perspiration, secretions, and transient bacteria from the penis. An external catheter fits closely around the penis, forming a warm environment that is conducive to microorganism growth. In addition, dampness contributes to skin maceration and breakdown, and the collector will stay in place longer if the penis is clean and dry when it is applied. If there is excessive hair at the base of the penis, shave a small area so that it does not interfere with secure anchoring of the collector. Use scissors to clip the hair for clients who would be especially prone to skin breakdown from razor nicks, such as paralyzed clients. If the collector has been applied carefully but still does not remain in place, a skin adhesive (such as is used for ostomy care) can be applied to the penis. If adhesives are used, be sure they are removed before applying a new collector. To do this, use an adhesive remover of the same brand as the adhesive and wash the penis afterward with soap and water to avoid skin irritation (see Skill 61). Before using a spray skin adhesive, protect the pubic hair from the adhesive by cutting a hole in the center of a paper napkin or paper towel and slipping the penis through the hole.

Applying the Catheter
When applying a catheter collector with a flexible self-adherent strip, remove the protective paper from one side of the strip and apply it circumferentially or spirally around the penis approximately 4 to 5 cm (1½ to 2 in) proximal to the glans. Hold it in place for about 1 minute, so that body and hand warmth will cause the self-adherent strip to adhere to the skin. The ends of the strip meet but do not overlap. To apply a cloverleaf adhesive skin protector, remove the backing, stretch the opening, slip it over the penis, and press it into place at a similar point on the penis. Figure 59–1 shows two ways to secure an external catheter.

Roll a sheath or condom-style collector outward on itself, if it is not already pre-rolled. Roll the collector onto the penis, leaving a 1- to 2-cm (½- to ¾-in) space between the tip of the penis and the internal end of the collector. This space prevents irritation of

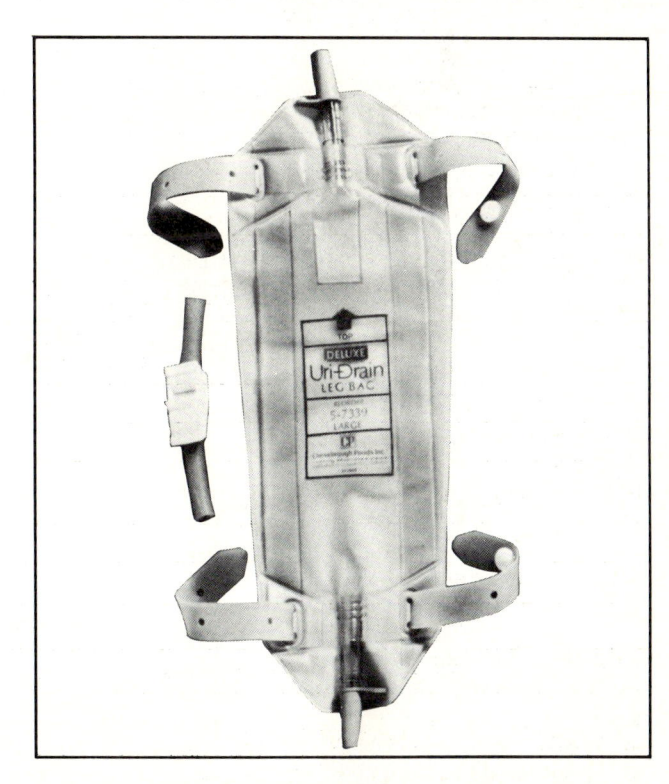

Figure 59–3. Reusable leg bag for urinary drainage with external or indwelling catheters. (From Chesebrough-Ponds, Inc., Greenwich, CT, with permission.)

the glans and keeps the tip of the penis from being bathed in urine. If a self-adherent strip or patch is used, press the collector onto the self-adherent strip in a smooth, even manner to avoid leakage in the event of inadvertent backflow of urine. When self-adherent strips or patches are not used inside the collector, apply elastic adhesive tape to the outside in a nonconstrictive manner. One way to do this is to wrap the tape in a spiral fashion around approximately three quarters of the length of the penis. Another way is to encircle the penis with the elastic tape and have the ends either abut or approximate each other. This allows the tape to separate upon pressure from a spontaneous erection. Do not overlap the tape strips, since the overlap will not separate readily and allow for increased penis size in the event of an erection. Never use nonstretchable tape to anchor an external catheter. Since it is not possible to predict accurately which clients will have spontaneous erections, always plan for that possibility when selecting and applying an external catheter. Depending on the relative lengths of the penis and collector, a roll of rubber may be left near the base of the penis. If so, Whyte and Thistle (1976) recommend cutting this excess off carefully to avoid possible constriction of the penis. After the collector is in place, connect the distal end of the external catheter to a closed drainage system (see Skill 60) or leg bag as shown in Figure 59–3.

Maintenance Care with an External Catheter

After attaching the drainage tubing, position it in such a way as to avoid having it twist around itself and cut off the outflow of urine. Check the tubing position whenever changing the client's position. Remove the external catheter daily and wash, rinse, and dry the penis and surrounding area. Inspect the penis carefully to detect any irritated areas or problems with circulation. Keep the drainage bag below the level of the bladder at all times to prevent reflux of urine into the collector and around the penis.

☐ SKILL SEQUENCE

APPLICATION OF EXTERNAL CATHETER

Step	Rationale
1. Determine need for an external catheter or verify physician's order.	Ensures implementation of appropriate treatment plan.
2. Explain procedure to client and family.	Enlists cooperation; improves client's self-image.
3. Wash hands.	Avoids transfer of microorganisms.
4. Gather appropriate style and size of external catheter.	Time-saving nursing activity.
5. Draw curtains or close room door.	Provides privacy.
6. Place bed at a correct working height, using siderails as needed.	Essential for correct body mechanics and client safety.
7. Position client on his back in a flat or semi-Fowler's position. Fold linen back to expose genital area. Cover upper part of body with blanket.	Facilitates application of collector. Avoids chilling.
8. Wash penis with soap and water, rinse and dry. (NOTE: If there is an excessive amount of pubic hair at base of penis, cut hair with scissors or shave area before washing.)	Prepares penis for application of collector; removes perspiration, secretions, and microorganisms. Hair interferes with adherence of collector.
9. Apply flexible, self-adherent strip or cloverleaf around penis in a circumferential or spiral manner. Avoid overlapping ends of strip.	Holds collector in place from inside; avoids constriction of penis and impaired circulation.
10. Roll collector outward on itself.	Prepares collector for application.
11. Roll collector onto penis, leaving 1 to 2 cm (1/2 to 3/4 in) between tip of penis and distal inner end of collector.	Avoids irritation and trauma to tip of penis; avoids having meatus continuously bathed with urine.
12. Attach collector onto penis: a. Press collector firmly against self-adherent strip or patch and hold in place for 1 minute. OR: b. After applying collector, place elastic adhesive tape around penis and collector in a spiral fashion or with ends approximated or abutted, rather than overlapped.	Provides leakproof seal between adhesive and collector. Body warmth causes collector to adhere to strip. Holds collector in place without constricting penis and impeding circulation in event of a spontaneous erection.
13. Connect collector to bedside drainage or leg bag. Instruct client to avoid kinking or twisting collector tip.	Provides for collection of urine; avoids urine backflow into collector.
14. Return client to a position of comfort and safety, with bed in low position.	Fulfills responsibility for safe care.
15. Wash own hands.	Avoids transfer of microorganisms.
16. Record condition of penis, type of collector and skin preparation used, any problems encountered during application, and client's reaction to procedure.	Fulfills nurse accountability and provides ongoing data base.

RECORDING

Record observations about the condition of the penis and the type of skin preparation used before applying the external catheter. Record the kind of catheter applied, whether it was anchored on the inside or outside of the collector, and the kind of adherent strips, patches, or adhesive tape used and the manner in which they were placed around the penis. Also record the client's reaction to the procedure, as well as his or her mental status and ability to assist with maintaining correct positioning of the catheter.

Sample POR Recording

- S—"That's a little tender there!" "I'll be glad to not be wet anymore!"
- O—Reddened area 0.5 cm in diameter distal to glans on lower aspect of penis. Has been incontinent of urine q 1–3 hrs. at unpredictable intervals.
- A—Continues to be incontinent, with potential for skin breakdown on penis.
- P—1. Urihesive System X-catheter applied and connected to bedside drainage. Applied skin protector and used flexible self-adherent strip inside collector.
  2. Plan to remove catheter and inspect skin condition q 24 hrs.
  3. Observe for kinks and twists in collector each time position is changed, or at least q 2 hrs.

Sample Narrative Recording

Urihesive System X-catheter applied and attached to bedside drainage. Noted reddened area 0.5 cm in diameter just distal to glans on lower aspect of penis. Perineal area washed and dried; skin protector applied. States he will be glad to not be wet anymore and that the area is slightly tender. Catheter anchored with flexible self-adherent strip inside collector and positioned to avoid twisting or kinking of collector.

☐ CRITICAL POINTS SUMMARY

1. Incontinence causes problems of skin irritation and breakdown, odor, increased laundry, reduced self-image, embarrassment, and social withdrawal.
2. Incontinence may have treatable causes.
3. A positive expectation that incontinence problems can be managed gives a client and family the hope of being dry again.
4. Incontinence may improve with bladder training or pelvic exercises.
5. If incontinence cannot be improved, incontinence pants are used for female clients and external catheters are used for male clients.
6. Wash and dry the perineal area of an incontinent client after each incontinent voiding to remove irritant urine products.
7. Apply an external catheter to a clean, dry penis.
8. Leave a 1- to 2-cm (1/2- to 3/4-in) space between the tip of the penis and the internal end of the collector.
9. Always use flexible tape to anchor an external catheter.
10. Apply flexible elastic tape outside the collector in a nonconstrictive manner.
11. Apply flexible self-adherent strips inside the collector in a spiral or circumferential manner.
12. Adhesive strips used on irritated skin must be made of a skin-barrier material.
13. Remove the catheter; wash, dry, and inspect the penis; apply a clean catheter daily.

☐ LEARNING ACTIVITIES

1. Examine several different types of external catheters. Identify features that diminish or contribute to twisting and kinking. Compare different ways of anchoring the catheters, and identify advantages of each.
2. Interview several staff nurses who frequently care for clients who have external catheters. Inquire about their experiences with different types of catheters, problems with maintenance, and methods of coping with those problems.
3. Examine disposable and reusable incontinence pants. Compare the size, shape, and method of fastening. Consider which might be more comfortable to wear, easiest for the nurse to put on a bed client, and least visible under regular clothing. If possible, pour 200 ml of water onto each type of pants. Compare the absorbency in terms of the wetness of the pants and liners on the inside surface and the dryness on the outside.
4. Interview several nurses who work regularly with clients who wear incontinence pants. Inquire about their preferences for different types and styles of incontinence pants.

☐ REVIEW QUESTIONS

1. What nursing measures can be used for each of the following problems associated with urinary incontinence?
   a. Skin irritation and breakdown
   b. Tissue maceration
   c. Odors
   d. Embarrassment
   e. Social withdrawal
   f. Excessive amounts of laundry
2. How would you instruct a client to perform Kegel exercises?
3. How is management of incontinence different for males and females?
4. Why is nonflexible tape never used to hold an external catheter in place?
5. What are safe ways to apply flexible self-adherent anchoring strips inside a collector? Explain.

6. What are safe ways to apply elastic tape on the outside of the collector? Explain.
7. Identify five components of daily care when an external catheter is in place.
8. When an external catheter is in place, what problems would be most likely to occur in each of the following situations?

a. An overly tight collector
b. Kinks or twists in the lower end of the collector
c. Collector placed so that the distal inner end is less than 1 to 2 cm (½ to ¾ in) from the tip of the penis
d. Nonflexible tape used to anchor the collector

☐ PERFORMANCE CHECKLIST

OBJECTIVE: To apply an external catheter safely.			
CHARACTERISTIC	**RANGE OF ACCEPTABILITY**	**SATISFACTORY**	**UNSATISFACTORY**
1. Explains procedure.	No deviation		
2. Washes hands.	No deviation		
3. Obtains appropriate size and style of catheter.	No deviation		
4. Raises bed to working height.	No deviation		
5. Positions client on back.	No deviation		
6. Washes, rinses, and dries penis.	If excessive pubic hair, shaves area at base of penis before washing.		
7. Applies flexible, self-adherent strip or cloverleaf patch in circumferential manner, without overlapping ends.	Omit if catheter is to be anchored on outside of collector.		
8. Rolls collector outward on itself.	No deviation		
9. Rolls collector onto penis, leaving 1 to 2 cm (½ to ¾ in) space at penis tip.	No deviation		
10. Attaches collector onto penis: a. Presses collector against adhesive strip. OR: b. Places elastic adhesive around penis in a nonconstrictive manner.	Omit if using outside anchor strips. Omit if using inside anchor strips.		
11. Connects collector to bedside drainage.	Leg bag may be substituted.		
12. Returns client to position of comfort and safety.	No deviation		
13. Washes own hands.	No deviation		
14. Records and reports relevant data.	No deviation		

REFERENCES

Baum ME: "I want to be dry!" Nursing78 78(2):75–78, 1978.
Beber CR: Freedom for the incontinent. American Journal of Nursing 80(3):842–844, 1980.
Lawson SD, Cook JB: Condom urinals. Nursing Mirror 145(22):19–21, 1977.
Steinhardt G, McRoberts JW: Total distal penile necrosis caused by condom catheter. JAMA 244(11):1238, 1980.
Whyte JF, Thistle NA: Male incontinence: The inside story on external collection. Nursing76 76(9):66–67, 1976.

BIBLIOGRAPHY

Beland IL, Passos JY: Clinical Nursing: Pathophysiological and Psychosocial Approaches, ed 4. New York: Macmillan, 1981.
Beyers M, Dudas S: The Clinical Practice of Medical–Surgical Nursing, ed 2. Boston, Little, Brown, 1984.
Brunner LS, Suddarth DS: Textbook of Medical–Surgical Nursing, ed 5. Philadelphia, JB Lippincott, 1984.
Butts PA: Assessing urinary incontinence in women. Nursing79 79(3):72–74, 1979.
Luckmann J, Sorensen KC: Medical–Surgical Nursing: A Psychophysiologic Approach, ed 2. Philadelphia, WB Saunders, 1980.
Product Information. Princeton, NJ, ER Squibb & Sons, 1982.
Product Data Sheet: Incontinence. Libertyville, IL, Hollister Incorporated, 1982.
Sorensen KC, Luckmann J: Basic Nursing: A Psychophysiologic Approach. Philadelphia, WB Saunders, 1979.
Willington FL: Incontinence: The prevention of soiling. Nursing Times 71(14):545–548; 1975.

SKILL 60 Urinary Catheterization

PREREQUISITE SKILLS

Skill 19, "Inspection"
Skill 20, "Palpation"
Skill 21, "Percussion"
Skill 28, "Handwashing"
Skill 30, "Sterile Supplies"
Skill 31, "Donning Sterile Gloves"
Skill 32, "Dressings and Wound Care"
Skill 39, "Perineal Care"
Skill 57, "Bedpans and Urinals"
Skill 59, "Urinary Incontinence Care"

☐ STUDENT OBJECTIVES

1. Identify the purposes for which urinary catheterization is used.
2. Describe nursing interventions that promote psychological comfort and safety during catheterization and while clients have indwelling catheters in place.
3. Differentiate the characteristics and purposes of different types of urinary catheters.
4. Describe the problems associated with the use of urinary catheters.
5. Explain the need for using surgical asepsis when inserting urinary catheters and medical asepsis when caring for them.
6. Describe the three routes by which microorganisms can enter the bladder when an indwelling catheter is in place.
7. Explain the rationale for various measures used to decrease the incidence of catheter-associated urinary tract infections.
8. Describe the principles underlying the use of a closed, preconnected urinary catheter drainage system.
9. Explain the correct ways to secure a catheter to a leg or abdomen.
10. Describe ways to avoid urine reflux into the bladder while an indwelling catheter is in place.
11. Identify the advantages and disadvantages of the dorsal recumbent and lateral positions for female catheterization.
12. Explain the rationale of and the procedure for clean intermittent self-catheterization.
13. Use surgical aseptic technique to insert an in-and-out and an indwelling urinary catheter.
14. Remove an indwelling catheter in a safe manner.
15. Describe two techniques for irrigating the bladder or for instilling medications into the bladder.

☐ INTRODUCTION

Urinary catheterization is the insertion of a catheter through the urethra into the urinary bladder for the purpose of removing urine. This procedure has been known since the earliest recorded history. The Egyptians used bronze or tin tubes; flexible catheters were developed in the eighteenth century, and rubber catheters have been used since the early nineteenth century after B. F. Goodrich developed the vulcanizing process (Morel, 1972). Glass catheters were also in common use for many years.

Catheterization may be accomplished using a plain catheter that is inserted and removed after the urine is drained from the bladder. It may also be done using an indwelling catheter that is inserted into the bladder and left in place either to keep the bladder empty or to monitor urinary output continuously. The specific purposes for which catheterization is performed are (1) to relieve urinary tract obstruction such as occurs with benign prostatic hypertrophy, (2) to provide urinary drainage for clients with neurogenic bladder dysfunction and urinary retention such as paraplegic or quadriplegic persons, (3) during surgery on the bladder or structures adjacent to the bladder such as the rectum, uterus, and vagina so as to avoid inadvertent injury to the bladder as well as after those surgeries to avoid increased pressure on sutures, and (4) to obtain accurate measurement of urinary output with critically ill patients. At times it is also used to determine the amount of urine left in the bladder after voiding, that is, the residual urine.

Although urinary catheterization is a useful procedure, and is sometimes essential, it carries with it the risk of urinary tract infection and possible injury to the mucous membranes. The urinary tract is the most common site of nosocomial infections, accounting for more than 40 percent of those reported by acute-care hospitals and affecting an estimated 600,000 patients per year. Between 66 and 88 percent of these infections follow some instrumentation applied to the urinary tract, primarily the use of an indwelling urinary catheter (Wong, 1981). In one study, catheter-associated urinary tract infections were found to add an average of 4 days to a hospitalization (Haley et al., 1981). Increased costs for nosocomial urinary tract infections are not as great as those associated with wound infections or bacteremia (Sheckler, 1980). Nevertheless, the increased number of days required for hospitalization due to catheter-associated infections contributes to increased costs because of fixed levels of reimbursement for specific diagnostic groups.

Because of the high incidence of urinary tract infections associated with urinary catheterization, this procedure is reserved for specific purposes, rather than used routinely for obtaining a sterile urine specimen for culture, emptying the bladder, or keeping incontinent persons dry.

Prevention of nosocomial catheter-associated infections is directly related to the kind of nursing care clients receive and is based on the known routes by which microorganisms enter the bladder—with the catheter at the time of insertion and around or through the catheter after insertion. Therefore, it is crucial that the nurse follow surgical aseptic technique when inserting a urinary catheter and know how to care for an indwelling catheter and its drainage system in such a way that the potential for infection around and through the catheter is minimized. The nurse also is responsible for teaching clients and their families how to care for the catheters, both in the hospital and in the home, as well as for teaching and supervising ancillary agency personnel who work with clients who have indwelling catheters, such as transportation personnel, technicians, or nursing assistants. In addition, the nurse often needs to exercise professional judgment about the use of indwelling catheters as a therapeutic measure. For example, a common postoperative order is "Catheterize p.r.n. if unable to void" or "Insert Foley catheter if incontinence continues." Before implementing these orders, it is the nurse's responsibility to do a careful assessment of the client's fluid intake and voiding patterns and then implement voiding inducement measures, bladder training procedures, or try alternative methods of keeping an incontinent person dry. An indwelling catheter is not used primarily for the convenience of the nursing staff or as a substitute for adequate nursing care.

This skill discusses the insertion and removal of plain and indwelling catheters in both males and females, the collection of urine specimens from a catheter, the process of self-catheterization, and the irrigation of a catheter.

☐ PREPARATION

The process of inserting a plain catheter into the bladder and removing it as soon as the urine is drained is known as an in-and-out straight catheterization. It is used for a temporary condition that interferes with micturition, such as recent surgery or childbirth, or when checking for residual urine after voiding. Residual urine results when a person is able to urinate but unable to empty the bladder completely. The residual urine that remains within the bladder can cause bladder infection and calculi. Residual urine is often associated with partial bladder obstruction, such as from an enlarged prostate gland.

On rare occasions, a one-time catheterization is ordered to obtain a urine specimen for laboratory analysis. Most of the time, however, a clean-catch technique will produce an adequate specimen for culture purposes. In-and-out catheterization may also be done on a regular basis three or four times a day as the only method of emptying the bladder. This method is known as intermittent catheterization, and may be used with clients who have neurogenic bladders after cerebrovascular accidents, spinal cord injuries, or dysfunctional bladders from any cause. When properly performed, the rate of infection with this technique is lower than it is with indwelling catheters, as discussed later.

When a catheter is left in the bladder to provide continuous drainage of urine, an indwelling catheter is used. This type of catheter has an inflatable balloon proximal to the catheter tip; the inflated balloon holds the catheter securely in the bladder. The catheter is aseptically connected to drainage tubing and a collection bag that can be opened at the bottom to drain the urine. These catheters are quite useful for short periods of time, such as during and after surgery, to monitor renal function during shock or acute illness, whenever there is bleeding within the bladder or urethra, or when the urethra is obstructed. Indwelling catheters may be used on a long-term basis for those clients with neurogenic bladders who are unable to achieve bladder control. As an alternative, a male can be fitted with an external catheter or taught self-catheterization. Sometimes a urinary diversion is performed, or a catheter may be inserted directly into the bladder just above the symphysis pubis (suprapubic catheter). Infection rates for these other routes are generally lower than they are with an indwelling catheter. For long-term care of a bedfast client in the home, an indwelling catheter is often used when intermittent catheterization is not feasible and other methods of incontinence care are unsuccessful.

There is some controversy as to whether an indwelling catheter should drain continuously or intermittently. With intermittent drainage the catheter is alternately clamped and released; this is thought to mimic the normal filling and emptying of the bladder and flush the catheter as it drains (Blannin, 1982; Williamson, 1982). Other sources, however, indicate that this procedure is useless, a waste of time, and possibly harmful as it can contribute to bladder overdistention and infection if it is not adequately monitored (Bates, 1981; Kinney et al., 1980). In general, the practice is not currently regarded as appropriate by urologists (Steele, 1983).

CATHETER-ASSOCIATED URINARY TRACT INFECTIONS

The primary problem associated with urinary catheterization is infection. The infection rate is quite low (1 to 2 percent) when a catheterization is done as a single in-and-out procedure using strict aseptic technique. When indwelling catheters are used, the infection rate is between 20 and 25 percent for catheters in place more than 3 or 4 days. Although this is a substantial decrease from the 98 to 100 percent infection rate that preceded the initiation of a closed drainage system in the 1960s, it is still unacceptably high. A closed drainage system is one in which the catheter remains connected to the drainage tubing at all times (Kunin, 1979; Wong, 1981). Unfortunately, the closed system is often opened for a variety of reasons, with a corresponding increase in infection. For example, in several studies, placing a special plastic wrap seal around the catheter tubing junction decreased the infection rate by about two thirds (Andriole, 1975; Parrott et al., 1982).

Urinary tract infections associated with indwelling catheters have been found to occur significantly more often in women than in men, particularly in women over 50 years old. Other groups of clients who are at increased risk for developing catheter-associated urinary tract infections are postpartum women, elderly, debilitated, or critically ill clients, and those with urinary retention due to structural or neurologic abnormalities (Cunha, 1982; Garibaldi et al., 1974, 1980; Wong, 1981).

In healthy clients, a catheter-related infection usually clears spontaneously once the catheter is removed. This is not necessarily true for clients who are at increased risk for infection. For example, urinary tract infections were thought to have played a role in the renal failure that was found to be the cause of death in 73 percent of 117 paraplegic clients (Warren et al., 1981). Other studies indicate a strong association between increased mortality and the occurrence of a nosocomial catheter-associated urinary infection (Parrott et al., 1982; Platt et al., 1982).

Urinary tract infections are caused by either endogenous contamination from the perineal area or exogenous microorganisms transferred from other clients on the hands of personnel or through contaminated equipment. Microorganisms enter the urinary tract of a client with a catheter through any one or a combination of the following routes: (1) they may be introduced with the catheter at the time of insertion; (2) they may ascend around the exterior of an indwelling catheter (*extraluminal route*); or (3) they may ascend through the lumen of an indwelling catheter (*intraluminal route*).

If microorganisms are accidentally introduced during an in-and-out single catheterization, apparently the body's natural defenses and regular voiding remove the offending organisms promptly. When a catheter remains in place, however, it serves as a foreign body, stimulating the mucous membranes to produce additional secretions. These secretions provide a mechanism for microorganisms to ascend to the bladder from the perineal area by way of the outside of the catheter. This is particularly a problem for women because of a short urethra and the proximity of the anus to the urethral meatus. Intraluminal contamination of the catheter system occurs when the catheter–drainage tubing junction is separated or when the collection bag becomes contaminated. Common reasons given for opening the catheter–drainage tubing junction include obtaining a urine specimen, irrigating the catheter, or convenience in turning, positioning, and transferring. Catheter drainage bags may become contaminated if the drainage port is contaminated when the bag is emptied. If the bag is not completely emptied each time, any microorganisms that may be present in the urine will multiply and increase the risk of an ascending intraluminal contamination.

Prevention of Urinary Tract Infections

Catheter-associated urinary tract infections can be minimized by taking care to avoid contamination when inserting the catheter and taking steps to decrease the potential for contamination through the extraluminal and intraluminal routes. Figure 60–1 shows the common sites for microorganisms to enter the catheter system.

Insertion of Catheters. When inserting the catheter, strict aseptic technique is used to prevent microorganisms from being introduced with the catheter. This is particularly important when inserting an in-

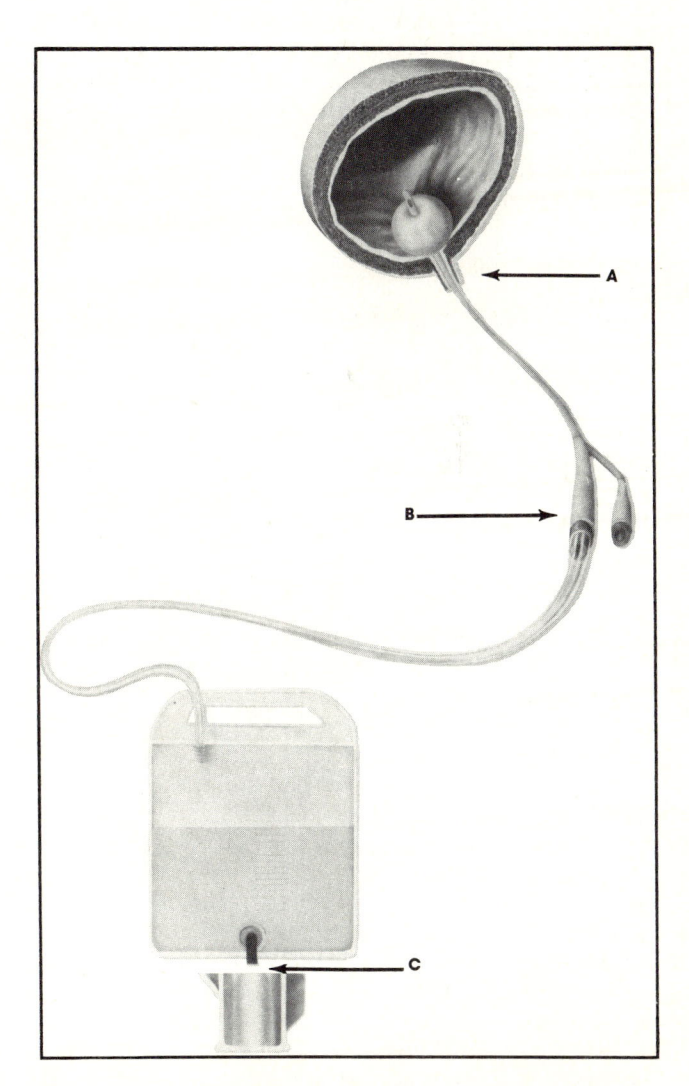

Figure 60–1. Microorganisms can enter the catheter system: **A.** Around the catheter. **B.** At the catheter–tubing junction if separated and contaminated. **C.** Through the drainage port, if contaminated. (Courtesy of Bard Urological Division, C. R. Bard, Inc., Murray Hill, NJ.)

dwelling catheter, since that client will not be flushing the urethra by voiding when the catheter is in place.

Intraluminal Contamination. *The primary way to reduce the incidence of catheter-associated infections is to maintain a sterile, closed drainage system* to prevent intraluminal contamination (Kunin, 1979). For example, the drainage system should not be separated to obtain a urine specimen and if a catheter irrigation is necessary, it must be done with strict aseptic technique. To remind the staff to avoid disconnecting the catheter simply for convenience, the junction can be taped or a preconnected catheter system with a "tamper-evident" seal can be used. This seal cannot be replaced once it has been removed, thus clearly indicating that the system has been opened. One study indicated that sealed catheter–tubing junctions resulted in significantly fewer catheter disconnections by hospital staff and a significantly lower rate of urinary tract infections (Platt et al., 1982).

It is important to remember that the *drainage collection bag* represents a reservoir of infection-producing organisms; about 20 percent of catheter-associated infections have been found to result from bag contamination (Parrott et al., 1982). The drainage port itself is a potential source of intraluminal infection. Contamination may occur when personnel empty the collection bag with unwashed hands and contaminate the drainage port. Cross-contamination may occur between clients who share a room if personnel do not wash their hands before handling each catheter system or if they use the same emptying container for several clients (Maki et al., 1972; Wong, 1981). It is therefore essential that the nurse wash his or her hands before handling a catheter or the drainage system, use medical aseptic technique when emptying the collection bag so as to avoid contaminating the drainage port, and use a separate emptying container for each client. Do not allow the collection bag to rest on the floor, as the drainage port may become contaminated. It has been demonstrated that urine in the collection bag becomes contaminated 1 to 6 days before the bladder does and that the cultured organisms are the same in both the bag and the bladder (Andriole, 1975). Therefore, do not turn the bag upside down and always keep it lower than the bladder level to avoid reflux of urine from the collection bag into the tubing. Microorganisms may travel from the drainage bag to the catheter and bladder by reflux or by capillary attraction. In addition to these precautions with the collection bag, position the drainage tubing to promote straight drainage to the bag and avoid dependent loops of tubing where urine can collect, become stagnant, and foster growth of microorganisms.

Extraluminal Contamination. Extraluminal contamination is generally associated with endogenous microorganisms from the perineal area. The most common offending microorganisms are intestinal in origin, such as *Escherichia coli, Enterobacter, Klebsiella, Proteus,* and *Enterococcus.* To lessen the probability of endogenous microorganisms from the perineal area ascending into the bladder along the catheter, cleanse the entire perineal area with soap and water on a daily basis. This procedure includes cleansing of the catheter from the meatus downward with soap and water or povidone–iodine (Betadine). For female clients, the preferable way to provide adequate perineal and catheter care is to place the client on the bedpan and alternately soap and rinse the perineal area and catheter. This method produces less manipulation of the catheter within the meatus and urethra, decreasing the potential for injury; it also flushes debris away from the meatus. If the catheter becomes heavily soiled with vaginal or fecal drainage and cannot be cleaned thoroughly, it is best to remove the catheter and reinsert a new one. Avoid using powder in the perineal area when an indwelling catheter is in place, as it tends to cake and form additional debris.

Routine urinary meatal care is not included in the latest recommendations from the Centers for Disease Control (Wong, 1981). In recent prospective, controlled studies, special cleansing of the urinary meatus with povidone–iodine solution followed by povidone–iodine ointment or daily meatal cleansing with green soap and water were demonstrated to be ineffective in decreasing the frequency of catheter-associated urinary tract infections in clients with closed indwelling catheter systems. There is some thought that the manipulation of the catheter during meatal care can injure the mucous membrane or force microorganisms into the urethral orifice (Cunha, 1982).

An indwelling catheter is anchored securely to the leg or abdomen as described later in this skill. In-and-out movement of the catheter apparently increases the potential for microorganisms to ascend the exterior of the catheter. It also creates traction on the urethra, which can cause irritation and trauma to the mucous membranes, and sometimes causes actual necrosis of the internal sphincter.

Other Preventive Factors
In addition to careful maintenance of the catheter system itself, there are other aspects of care that relate to the use of catheterization as a therapeutic measure. For example, when indwelling catheters are used in the postoperative or postpartal period, the nurse monitors not only the client's progress, but the length of time the catheter is left in place. The maximum limit for adults is thought to be 48 to 72 hours unless a longer period is required in order to avoid undue pressure after perineal or pelvic surgery. The time limit for infants and children varies considerably with age, size, physical status, and illness condition. It is also important that the client maintain a fluid intake of 2000 to 2500 ml per day unless contraindicated for other reasons, have adequate nutrition and exercise, and avoid constipation since this can contribute to poor catheter drainage. Sometimes the urine is acidified with drugs or very large doses of vitamin C, since an infection is less likely to occur in an acid urine (Blannin 1982: Kinney et al., 1980).

Another measure that may help decrease the incidence of infection associated with indwelling catheters relates to the room placement of clients. Nursing personnel apparently are more likely to wash their hands when moving between rooms than when moving between clients within the same room (Maki et al., 1972). Therefore, clients with indwelling catheters who are at particular risk of infection (such as immunosuppressed or debilitated clients) are not placed in the same room with clients who have an infection of any kind.

Manufacturers have introduced many modifications in indwelling catheter equipment to alleviate some of the above-mentioned problems, such as designing contamination-free drainage ports or developing ways of inserting a disinfectant into the drainage bag. Unfortunately, carefully controlled studies have not been done to determine the efficacy of most of these modifications, other than the preconnected tamperproof catheter–drainage tube junction.

Based on clinical experience, the relatively new Foley catheter with Tamper-Evident Seal has some promise of decreasing urinary tract infections. The hydrophilic BN-74 catheter coating apparently causes less irritation within the urethra and also absorbs the povidone–iodine used for daily cleansing of the external portion of the catheter. The collection bag drainage port is also hydrophilic and absorbs the Lugol's iodine that is inserted into the port each day by means of a crushable ampule. It is believed that the povidone–iodine and Lugol's solution provide an antimicrobial barrier at the catheter site and the collection bag drainage port (Product, 1982). In addition, the catheter–tubing junction is protected with a bright red seal that cannot be replaced once it has been removed to separate the junction. This makes any separation and infection potential readily identifiable.

Catheter Size. Sometimes the physician will designate the size of the catheter to be used and at other times the nurse will need to make that judgment. The usual size for adult females is 14F or 16F; for adult males it is 16F or 18F. Catheter size is determined by the size of the urinary meatus, since the meatus is the smallest part of the urethra. Thus, a catheter that enters the meatus easily will readily traverse the entire urethra, unless some kind of obstruction exists, such as a tumor or as occurs with benign prostatic hypertrophy in males.

A catheter that is too large causes undue pressure on the meatus, with the potential for tissue erosion to occur. In addition, a catheter that is too large can cause pressure in the male urethra where the catheter bends over the penosacral junction, sometimes causing an abscess, sloughing, and strictures. On the other hand, a catheter that is too small is more likely to become obstructed from mucus, blood, or other debris.

The preferred balloon size for an indwelling catheter is 5 to 10 ml. It is not an acceptable practice to overinflate the balloon, since that may cause it to rupture. The resulting balloon fragments can become the nuclei for bladder calculi (Kinney et al., 1980). The larger (30-ml) balloons are often used in the immediate postoperative period after a transurethral resection of the prostate. Sometimes personnel will choose to insert a catheter with a 30-ml balloon in the belief that it will deter a confused person from pulling out the catheter. Although a 5-ml balloon *is* fairly easily pulled out, as Blannin (1982, p. 438) points out, "the determined patient will pull the catheter out even with a 30 [-ml] balloon so the smaller the balloon the better as there will be less trauma to the urethra."

Using a larger catheter or a larger balloon does not prevent urine leakage (bypassing) around the catheter, since that is due primarily to catheter obstruction or to urine collecting under a too-large balloon. Large, 30-ml balloons often cause the bladder to become irritable. This irritability causes the bladder to contract, forcing the small amount of urine that lies beneath the balloon to exit from the bladder around the catheter (Blannin, 1982; Ferrie et al., 1979; McGill, 1982).

CATHETER AND BLADDER IRRIGATION AND INSTILLATION

An irrigation is a mechanical flushing with a liquid. Catheters and bladders are irrigated to remove mucus shreds, blood clots, or other debris for the purpose of keeping the catheter from becoming obstructed. Irrigation may be needed when a catheter is kept in place for prolonged periods of time or after surgery for a transurethral resection of the prostate gland. Although not recommended for general use, occasionally an antibiotic irrigation or instillation may be ordered for a bladder infection. The instillation is performed for the purpose of applying a local medication to the bladder mucosa. It is done in the same way as an irrigation except that instead of permitting the fluid to drain out immediately, the catheter is clamped so that the medication will remain in contact with the bladder mucosa for the specified length of time. The bladder must be empty when the medication is instilled, so that the medication can be in contact with the mucosa.

PSYCHOLOGICAL ASPECTS OF CATHETERIZATION

The psychological aspects of needing help with urination were discussed in Skill 57. Privacy, control, and self-esteem also are important for the client who is being catheterized. For example, when an indwelling catheter is in place, the drainage collection apparatus is usually clearly visible to everyone in the environment. Hospital personnel become quite accustomed to seeing this equipment, but many clients find it quite distressing and embarrassing to have their bladder status advertised in this way.

Catheter insertion generally causes distress for both men and women because a private area of the body is exposed. This distress may be increased when more than one person is present, or the nurse is not of the same sex as the client. A female in the dorsal recumbent position often feels particularly exposed and vulnerable. In addition, since the procedure may take 5 to 10 minutes or more even for an experienced person, the client may become fatigued, have difficulty lying still, and experience leg cramps.

A situation that generally arouses much anxiety in both the nurse and the client is a young female nurse catheterizing a male client who is her own or her father's age. Occasionally a male client will have an erection while the penis is being cleansed prior to the insertion of the catheter, which can cause embarrassment for both the client and the nurse. This is less likely to occur if a firm rather than a light touch is used to hold and cleanse the penis. If an erection does occur, it is helpful to acknowledge what has happened in a matter-of-fact way and indicate that you will wait a few minutes for it to subside. Talking about something else, even the weather, is usually distracting for both the nurse and the client, and the erection soon subsides. Do not try to insert the catheter while the penis is erect. It is more difficult to insert a catheter when the penis is erect and there is increased potential for the catheter to be forced outside the urethra into a blind passage.

LONG-TERM USE OF INDWELLING CATHETERS

In the home and long-term care settings, clients often need to have indwelling catheters for long periods of time, even for years, because of such conditions as neurogenic bladder or incontinence that are not manageable in other ways. The incidence of catheter-associated urinary tract infections is considerably lower in the home than the institutional setting, because clients generally are tolerant of microorganisms in their own environment. Clients and their families are taught how to provide perineal care, empty the drainage system, irrigate the catheter, and know the signs and symptoms of catheter obstruction and urinary tract infection. The catheter may be connected to a leg bag (portable drainage bag attached to the leg) or to a conventional drainage collection system. A visiting or home-care nurse changes the catheter as needed, using surgical aseptic technique.

It is generally recommended that a catheter be changed as needed, rather than on a scheduled routine. When clients have an indwelling catheter in place for months or years, sediment often develops within the bladder, collects within the lumen of the catheter, and eventually obstructs the catheter. A catheter is to be changed when concretions (granular materials) are felt when the catheter is rubbed between the thumb and fingers. If the tip of the catheter has crustations and a partially clogged eye when it is removed, plan to change the catheter several days earlier the next time to minimize the chance of obstruction. Latex catheters will generally remain patent about 2 weeks, while silastic catheters may remain patent 4 to 6 weeks or even up to 6 months. When sediment is present, irrigation is not recommended because that would simply wash the sediment back into the bladder. If the catheter tends to become obstructed from mucus plugs, it may be aseptically irrigated on a regular basis, either by a nurse or by a family member who has been taught the procedure. Boiled water, sterile saline, or 0.25 percent acetic acid solution may be used for irrigation. The drainage collection system is changed whenever the catheter is changed, and more often if it begins to leak, develops a foul odor, or if contamination is suspected.

More clinical studies need to be done on the frequency of catheter changes, since there is some indication that regularly scheduled catheter changes may be beneficial for some persons. A recent 6-month prospective study of a small (17) group of clients in a Veterans Hospital indicated that regular monthly catheter changes resulted in fewer symptomatic urinary tract infections (Priefer et al., 1982).

In addition to the problem of obstruction when long-term indwelling catheters are used, urine may bypass the catheter and leak around the exterior of the catheter. Bypassing is more likely to occur if fluid intake is inadequate and the urine becomes concentrated, if the catheter becomes clogged, or if a large-size balloon such as a 30-ml balloon is used, as discussed earlier.

INTERMITTENT SELF-CATHETERIZATION

Intermittent self-catheterization refers to the regular emptying of the bladder with a plain catheter and an in-and-out clean technique. It is performed by the client and is increasingly used for both adults and children who are temporarily or permanently unable to empty the bladder. Although this procedure has been used extensively in other countries since World War II, it began to be used in the United States only in the late 1960s. Long-term follow-up of persons using clean intermittent self-catheterization indicates improved urinary continence, decreased incidence of infection, increased bladder function, and improved mental and emotional status (Lapides et al., 1976). Since intermittent self-catheterization allows clients to control their own voiding, they generally experience an increased sense of independence, self-worth, and well-being. When used as an alternative to an indwelling catheter, many clients feel more socially acceptable because they no longer need external drainage equipment. They also find personal hygiene is simpler and there is no interference with sexual relations.

Clean technique has been found to be quite adequate for use outside the hospital because people tend to be tolerant of microorganisms in their own environment. In addition, the simplicity of the clean technique encourages clients to adhere to their scheduled emptying times. Regular emptying of the bladder is apparently the most important factor in preventing urinary tract infections, and clients are advised to catheterize on schedule even if handwashing facilities are not available. Commercial wet wipes are considered an acceptable substitute for handwashing, and clients are advised to carry extra catheters in case they are unable to wash the catheter after use.

While in the hospital, the client is taught how to catheterize himself or herself and demonstrates the ability to do this correctly, as described in the execution section of this skill. At least one family member is also taught the procedure in case the client is unable to do so. In the hospital, sterile equipment and aseptic technique are used because microorganisms in hospital settings are more resistant to antibiotic therapy and more likely to cause infections. A "no-touch" technique is often used for cathertization. This procedure involves using a red rubber catheter encased in a plastic bag with a specially designed opening that allows the catheter to be inserted aseptically directly from the bag, which also serves as the collection chamber for the urine. As of yet, there are no cost comparisons of intermittent catheterization and indwelling catheters in the hospital setting (Champion, 1976; Kinney et al., 1980; Lapides et al., 1976; Wong, 1981).

DATA BASE

Before inserting a catheter, the nurse gathers information about the client's ability to assume the needed position for the catheterization, willingness to cooperate and comply with requests, and ability to lie quietly during the procedure. This information helps determine the amount of help needed during the procedure. In addition, the nurse determines if supplementary light is required for good visualization during the procedure.

To determine whether to implement a p.r.n. order for a catheter irrigation, the nurse identifies existing problems with the catheter, such as bypassing or blockage. Before changing an indwelling catheter, document the need for change by identifying the presence of granular material in the catheter, the frequency with which obstruction occurs, and the physician's orders.

Before inserting a catheter to relieve urinary retention, evaluate voiding frequency, overflow voiding, and signs and symptoms of bladder distention. It also is important to know agency policy regarding the amount of urine to be withdrawn at any one time, as discussed in the execution section of this skill.

Client History and Recorded Data

The kardex, computer care plan, or health record includes the physician's orders for insertion of an indwelling catheter, a plain catheter for residual urine, the amount of residual urine considered acceptable, the frequency of intermittent catheterization, any irrigations ordered, and possibly the size of the catheter to be used. The health record also indicates the reason a catheterization or irrigation is being performed, whether any perineal or pelvic surgery has been done recently, if a female client has recently given birth, or if a male client has a history of urinary obstruction, such as from benign prostatic hypertrophy. The nursing history, nurses' notes, or an interview with the client or his or her family reveals previous experiences with catheterization and usual voiding patterns, including frequency and amount of urine. This information can be used as a basis for explanations offered to the client and family.

Physical Appraisal Skills

Inspection. Inspection is used to determine the state of perineal cleanliness before the catheter is inserted and during the time the indwelling catheter is in place. It is also used to detect any kinks or dependent loops in the position of the drainage tubing, to check that the catheter has been secured correctly and firmly, to examine the condition of the skin at the taping or catheter strap site, and to determine whether a tamper-evident catheter–tubing junction seal has been broken, which would indicate that the system has been opened. The nurse also inspects the drainage collection bag or urine meter to identify the character and amount of urine produced in a given amount of time. Inspection also reveals whether the collection bag is appropriately fastened to the bed or chair, and not touching the floor.

Palpation and Percussion. Palpation and percussion are used to distinguish bladder distention from retention before a catheter is inserted.

Sense of Smell. The sense of smell may detect a leakage of urine around the catheter or a soiled drainage collection system that needs to be discarded and replaced.

EQUIPMENT

Catheters

Urinary catheters are firm yet flexible tubes made of latex, red vinyl, or clear plastic. They have a smooth round closed tip with two drainage eyes on either side of the catheter just distal to the tip. Some latex catheters are coated with Teflon or silicone to make them less irritating to the body. Catheters may be made of silicone, which is an inert substance that apparently decreases the body's reaction to having a catheter in place and reduces the amount of granular encrusting that is common with long-term use of indwelling catheters. Plastic catheters are usually used for a one-time catheterization; latex catheters can remain in place up to 2 weeks, and a silicone (silastic) catheter may remain in place up to 6 months without problems. Since silicone catheters are more expensive than latex ones,

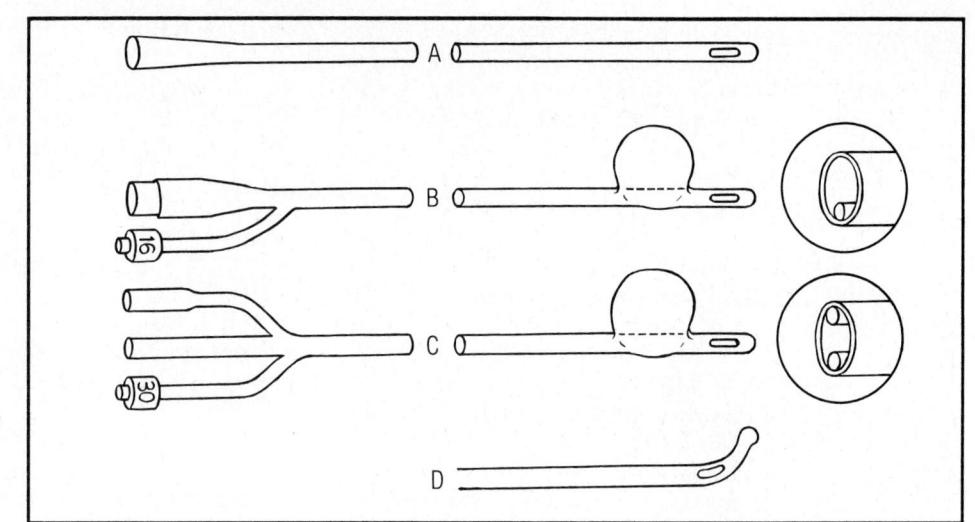

Figure 60-2. Urinary catheters (Note cross-section of lumens). **A.** Plain, single-lumen catheter for in-and-out use. **B.** Indwelling, double-lumen catheter for continuous bladder drainage. **C.** Indwelling, three-way triple-lumen catheter for continuous bladder irrigation. **D.** Coudé tip.

they are best reserved for this longer-time use and for clients who have problems with latex catheters. Another type of catheter is made of silicone and coated with a hydrophilic substance (such as the BN-74, from Bard) that absorbs body fluid and is compatible with body tissue in a way similar to a soft contact lens.

Urinary catheters are available in different styles and sizes, several of which are shown in Figure 60-2. Plain catheters have a single lumen and are available in French sizes 8F to 18F (Fig. 60-2A). An indwelling catheter has a double lumen and an inflatable balloon distal to the drainage eyes (Fig. 60-2B). It is known as a retention or Foley catheter. The balloon is inflated after insertion and holds the catheter in place within the bladder. Double-lumen Foley catheters are available in French sizes 8F to 10F, with a 3-ml balloon, or sizes 12F to 30F, with a 5- or 30-ml balloon. The usual catheter size used for men is 16F to 18F; for women it is 14F to 16F. For ready identification, the French size is printed on the catheter. A Foley catheter will also have the balloon capacity printed on the balloon lumen. The balloon of a Foley catheter is inflated with a prefilled syringe of normal saline or sterile water that is inserted into an inflation valve on the balloon lumen inlet, either with or without a needle, depending on the brand of catheter.

There are several other styles of catheters, which are usually inserted by the physician. A triple-lumen Foley catheter is used for continuous bladder irrigation as is usually needed after a transurethral resection of the prostate (Fig. 60-2C). A Coudé tip catheter may be used to bypass an enlarged prostate gland that is producing urethral obstruction (Fig. 60-2D). Mushroom and wing-tipped catheters (as are shown in Fig. 35-1, D & E) are normally used for suprapubic drainage.

Indwelling Catheter Drainage Systems

A drainage system for an indwelling catheter consists of a connector, drainage tubing, and a collection bag, such as that shown in Figure 60-3. A wide variety of commercial products is available (Gurevich, 1980).

Drainage tubing is clear semirigid tubing that is similar to suction tubing. Most drainage tubes have a self-sealing latex aspiration port that is used either for removing urine specimens or irrigating the catheter without separating the system. Standard drainage tubing diameter is $9/32$ inch; however, many manufacturers have begun to produce a slightly larger diameter ($11/32$ in) tubing. This larger diameter is too wide to support a standing column of urine and therefore urine drains continuously along the perimeter of the tubing, rather than remaining in the tubing (Gurevich, 1979). This helps decrease the potential for reflux into the bladder if the tubing accidentally is raised above the bladder level. Drainage tubing is attached to the Foley catheter with a connector. A *rubber band* and *safety pin* or *plastic clamp* are used to secure the tubing to the bed linen so as to avoid dependent loops in the tubing and minimize accidental pulling on the catheter.

A *drainage collection bag* is a clear plastic bag, calibrated in 50- to 100-ml increments, with a usual capacity of 2000 ml. When there is a rigid connection between the drainage tubing and the bag, the tube is not likely to kink at that point. Many collection bags have an antireflux valve at the inlet to prevent urine from reentering the tubing if the bag inadvertently is raised above the tubing. No studies have as yet been done to document the effectiveness of these devices. A drainage port with a clamp or a drainage valve is located at the bottom of the bag and is used to empty the collection bag. These ports are usually covered or protected from direct contamination in some way. Drainage bags have handles, hooks, self-adherent straps, or strings with hooks that are used to attach the bag to a bed frame, chair, clothing, or around the client's waist.

A *urine meter* is a smaller urine collection chamber calibrated in 1- to 5- and 10-ml increments, with a capacity up to 200 ml. When used with children, the

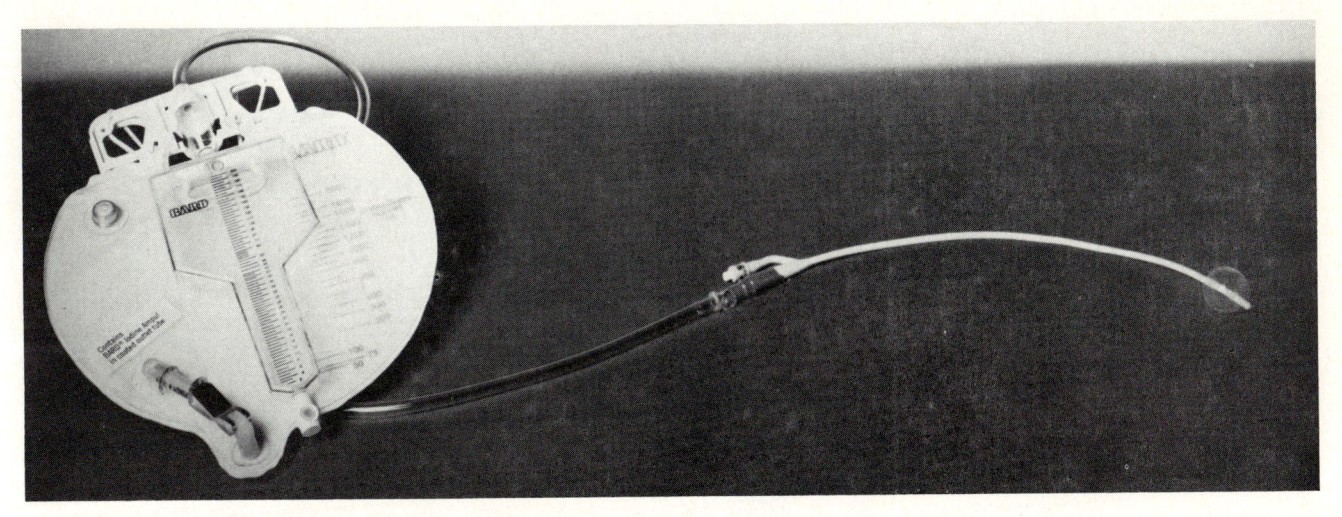

Figure 60-3. Indwelling catheter with tamper-evident drainage collection system: catheter with inflated balloon, sealed connector, tubing, and collection bag with urine meter. Note the valve at the lower end of the urine meter and the drainage port on the collection bag. (Courtesy of Bard Urological Division, C. R. Bard, Inc., Murray Hill, NJ.)

urine meter may be a separate collection chamber; for use in adults, however, it is normally an integral part of a larger drainage bag. Urine meters are usually emptied directly into the larger bag either by turning a valve or tilting the combined collection bag and urine meter. If the urine volume exceeds the urine meter capacity, it simply overflows into the larger collection bag and is emptied at the drainage port. The drainage collection system shown in Figure 60-3 includes a urine meter.

A *calibrated measuring container* called a graduate is used to contain and measure the urine when emptying the drainage bag. Graduates may be made of reusable metal or disposable plastic or waxed cardboard. They are kept in the bathroom and used exclusively for that client. After each use they are rinsed with cool water. Reusable graduates are sterilized between use by clients, and disposable ones are discarded when they deteriorate or when the client is discharged.

A *catheter drainage system kit* contains a sterile drainage collection bag with attached tubing and a covered connector, a sliding clamp, a hangar, safety pin, and rubber band. It is used when the catheterization kit does not contain a preconnected catheter and drainage tubing.

Catheterization Kits

Urinary catheterization kits are sterile and contain all the equipment needed to insert a catheter. The kit also may include the catheter or the catheter may be added to the sterile field after the kit is opened. If a catheter is included in the kit, the size will be identified on the package label, including the balloon capacity if it is a Foley catheterization kit. The equipment is usually arranged in the sequence in which it will be needed, since this makes it easier to use the items without contamination. The contents of a typical plain in-and-out urinary catheterization kit include the following: two plastic-backed drapes, one plain and one fenestrated (having a center opening); one pair of disposable plastic gloves that fit either hand; a small package of water-soluble lubricant; five rayon absorbent balls; one plastic forceps; a specimen container with a label; and a packet of povidone–iodine (Betadine). A kit for inserting a Foley catheter would include all of these items, as well as a prefilled syringe container 10 or 30 ml of sterile water. Most Foley catheterization kits contain a preconnected Foley catheter and complete drainage collection system. An example of a catheterization tray for an indwelling catheter is shown Figure 60-4.

Catheter Irrigation Equipment

The equipment needed for a catheter irrigation depends on whether the irrigation is being done by separating the system or by injecting the solution through the aspiration port or catheter. If done through the aspiration port, a large syringe (25 to 30 ml) with a small-gauge needle (No. 25 or 23) is used. If the system is to be opened, the following sterile equipment is needed: one moisture-resistant barrier drape, bulb (asepto) syringe or large catheter-tipped syringe, calibrated graduate, water for irrigation, alcohol swabs to cleanse the junction before separation, and a sterile pan or tray for containing the returns. Small bottles of sterile water or normal saline are used for an irrigation. The bottle is labeled with the date and time it was opened and discarded after 24 hours.

Sterile catheter irrigation kits may contain only the graduate and syringe, or they may also include a barrier drape, an alcohol swab, and a drainage tube protector to cover the connector while the system is separated. The sterile box containing the equipment serves as a container for the irrigation returns.

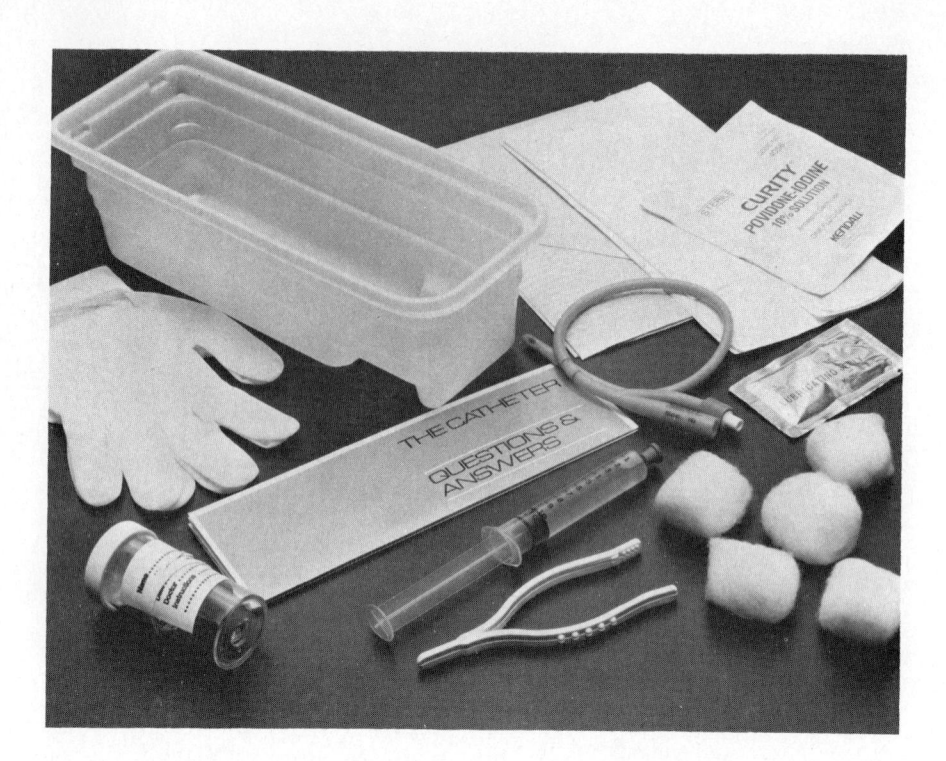

Figure 60-4. Catheterization kit for inserting an indwelling catheter. (Courtesy of The Kendall Co., Boston, MA.)

☐ EXECUTION

CARE OF THE CLIENT WITH AN INDWELLING CATHETER

A variety of nursing interventions will help the client accept and adapt to an indwelling catheter, as well as protect him or her from injury and the hazards of developing a catheter-associated urinary tract infection. In general, clients are more relaxed and cooperative when they understand the reason for having an indwelling catheter, the role it plays in their treatment plan, what to expect while it is in place, and how to care for it.

When a catheter is first inserted, tell the client that the initial constant urge to urinate is normal and that it will diminish as the meatus becomes accustomed to the presence of the catheter. Clients who are groggy from anesthesia or sedation or who are slightly confused will often ask to be put on the bedpan or have a urinal because they feel they need to urinate. Some clients will need repeated explanations that a tube is keeping the bladder empty. You may need to apply mitts or restraints to confused or restless clients to keep them from pulling the catheter out. Use of restraints is discussed in Skill 49.

When clients are in bed, fasten the drainage bag to the stationary bed frame beneath the gatching frame, so as to avoid raising the bag if the foot portion of the bed is elevated.

Since the catheter drainage system can easily become portable, encourage clients to ambulate as permitted by their medical or functional status. Explain that an inflated balloon keeps the catheter in place regardless of the person's position, and that activity is beneficial to general health and helps the flow of urine. If clients are self-conscious about the visibility of the catheter drainage system when they are out of the room, arrange to pin it to the gown inside the robe, or suspend it from the waist or belt with a gauze tie. The drainage bag may also be attached to a rolling intravenous pole, carried like a valise, or, if the client uses a walker, tied to that. Regardless of where the drainage bag is hung, be sure that it is below the level of the bladder and that the tubing has no kinks or dependent loops. When a client is in a wheelchair, the bag can be suspended from the frame in the front or back of the wheelchair. Be sure to position the bag and tubing so they do not get caught in the wheels. The bag is never placed on the floor since that usually occludes the entry tubing into the drainage bag and interferes with gravity flow of urine. In addition, the floor is dirty and the drainage port can become contaminated. Some manufacturers make a supporting frame that stands on the floor and holds the bag upright. A variety of correct ways to position a drainage collection bag and tubing is shown in Figure 60–5.

To reduce the potential for urinary tract infection with an indwelling catheter, maintain a closed system, position the bag and tubing to promote a continuous flow of urine and prevent reflux into the bladder, provide daily perineal care, and maintain an adequate fluid intake and urine output. Place tape around the catheter–tubing junction to prevent accidental separation and to remind personnel not to separate it for convenience. Silk or paper tape is preferred, as they leave less adhesive residue on the catheter than ordi-

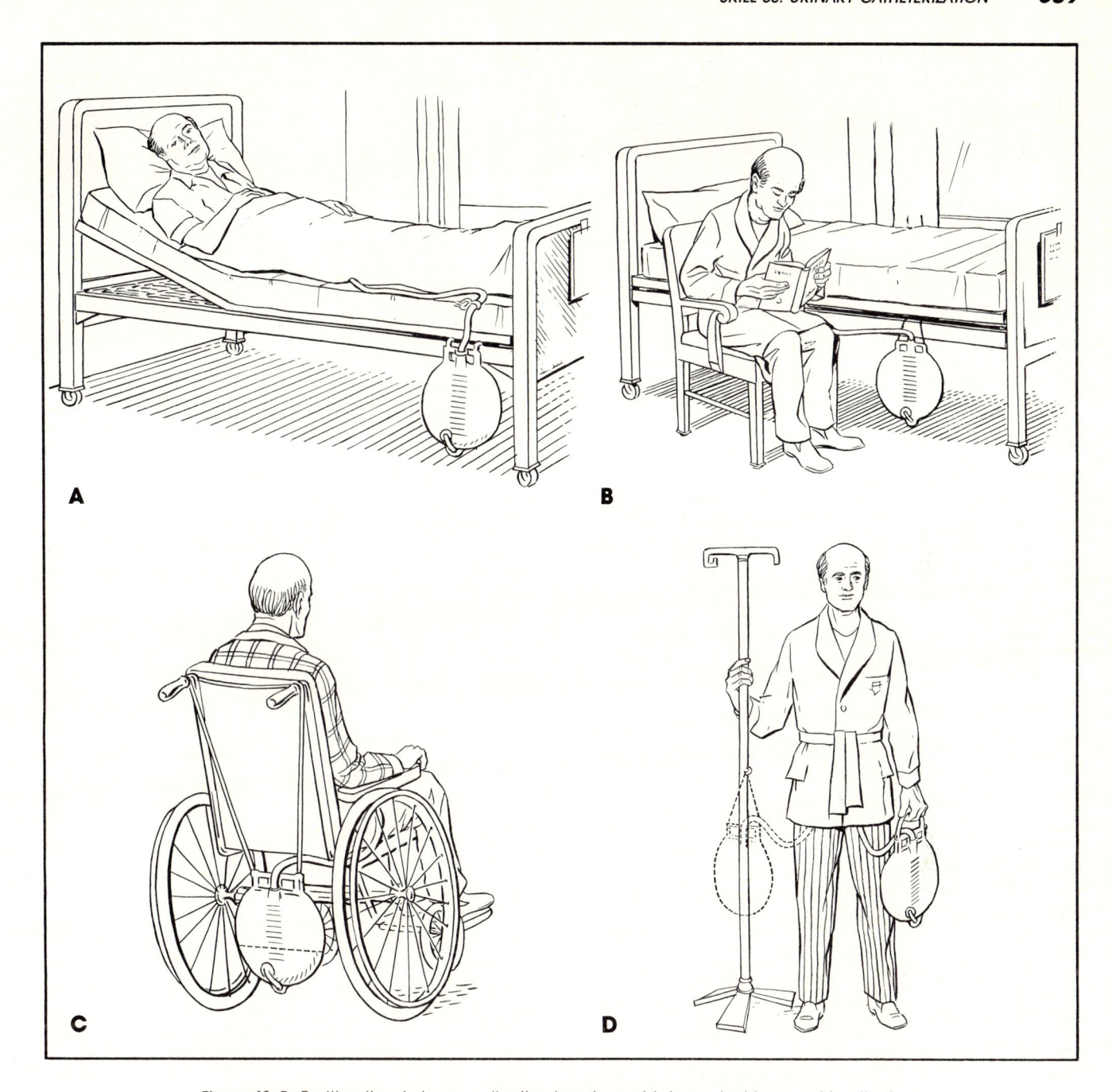

Figure 60–5. Position the drainage collection bag to avoid dependent loops, raising the bag above bladder level, or placing the bag on the floor. **A.** Hang bag from bed frame near foot of bed, with tubing laying on the bed. **B.** Hang bag from bed frame, using string attachment. Bed must be in "low" position when client is up in chair. **C.** Suspend bag from handles in back of wheelchair. **D.** Carry bag in hand or suspend from mobile intravenous pole.

nary adhesive tape. If you must open the system for irrigation, be sure to use surgical aseptic technique as discussed earlier.

It was previously mentioned that urine in the drainage bag becomes contaminated before urine in the bladder does and that the offending organisms are often the same ones. Therefore, it is crucial to avoid urine reflux into the bladder. To do this, avoid tubing kinks and dependent loops that interfere with straight gravity drainage and never raise the drainage bag above the bladder level without first clamping the tubing.

There are a number of ways to prevent urine reflux into the bladder. Place the tubing between the edge of the bed and the siderail, coil the excess tubing, and place it on the bed. Be careful not to catch or pinch the tubing with the siderail. Never place the tubing over the siderail because if the rail is raised it would raise the tubing above the bladder level. If you find dependent loops of urine-filled drainage tubing when checking a client, first pinch off the tubing or catheter *between* the client and the dependent loop. Then raise the tubing to empty the urine into the drainage bag. Release the pinched portion only after you have lowered the tubing. Reposition the tubing to prevent dependent loops.

There is a difference of opinion about whether the drainage tubing is best placed under or over the client's leg. When the tubing goes over the leg, enough urine needs to accumulate in the bladder to push the column of urine up over the thigh, after which a siphon effect occurs. If the bladder needs to be kept totally empty, run the tubing under the leg. On the other hand, constant pressure from lying on the tubing may increase the probability of pressure sores or interfere with circulation, especially in debilitated and malnourished clients. These problems can be minimized by changing the location of the tubing every time the client's position is changed and by not placing it under the popliteal space. If the client is quite inactive, place the tubing between the legs and hang the drainage bag from the foot of the bed. If clients are quite active, however, they are likely to become entangled with the tubing in this position and perhaps cause it to disconnect or become kinked.

Be especially careful about tubing position when ambulating or transferring clients from the bed to a chair or cart and back again. It is unacceptable to place the drainage bag on the client's abdomen during a transfer unless the catheter is clamped. Keeping the bag below the bladder level during transfer takes some preplanning about whether to move the bag or the client first and where to place the bag. In transfer situations where the drainage bag will inevitably and unavoidably be above the bladder level, there are two actions that will protect the client from urine reflux. If you can anticipate the need in advance, clamp the catheter itself before beginning the transfer. If no clamp is available or the need is not anticipated, fold and pinch the catheter *before* lifting the bag above the bladder level and release it only *after* the bag has been returned below the bladder. *Do not separate the tubing.*

As indicated earlier, special antiseptic meatal care is believed to be unnecessary and even harmful. However, careful daily perineal care is an important aspect of preventing extraluminal entry of microorganisms into the bladder. When they are able, encourage clients to continue their usual bathing practices while the indwelling catheter is in place. Clamp the tubing before the client gets into the bathtub for a bath to prevent urine backflow from the tubing to the bladder. There is no need to clamp the tube when the client is showering; the drainage bag may be hung from a towel bar, shower door handle, or propped in the corner of the shower. Instruct the client to wash the perineal area well with soap and water, rinse and dry carefully, and avoiding pulling on the catheter. Replace the catheter taping after bathing as needed. When females have vaginal discharge, bleeding, or other perineal secretions and are unable to take a shower or tub bath, a sitz bath or perineal care on a bedpan are the best alternatives. A bedpan allows the nurse to soap and rinse the perineum as often as needed, with less manipulation of the catheter than when using a washcloth. Use a clean pitcher or graduate to pour warm water over the perineum. Teach male clients to retract the foreskin when bathing and to keep the area as clean as possible.

When a client has an indwelling catheter in place, increase his or her fluid intake to 2000 to 2500 ml per day unless contraindicated for medical reasons such as renal or cardiac disease. This volume will generally produce a urine flow of at least 50 ml per hour. A urine flow rate of at least 25 ml per hour has been found to be helpful in reducing upward mobility of microorganisms through the catheter toward the bladder. In addition, a more concentrated urine tends to cause more odor problems in the drainage system and contributes to bypassing, as indicated earlier. If a catheter drainage seems sluggish, give the client an additional glass or two of water or juice and check the urine flow in 10 to 15 minutes, when an increased rate of flow should be visible in the drainage tubing. Irrigate *only* when repeated obstruction is a problem or when ordered for a specific purpose.

OBTAINING A URINE SPECIMEN

When a urine specimen is needed, collect it from the aspiration port in the drainage tubing, or from the catheter itself. Use surgical aseptic technique as described below and shown in Figure 60-6. Do *not* disconnect the catheter to obtain the specimen. Before collecting the specimen, clamp the tubing for 15 to 20 minutes to allow enough urine to accumulate in the bladder and tubing. Cleanse the aspiration port with an alcohol swab and allow the alcohol to dry. Use a 5- to 30-ml syringe and a small-gauge needle, such as a No. 23 or 25, and insert it into the aspiration port, using surgical aseptic technique. If there is no aspiration port in the drainage tubing, cleanse the catheter distal to the balloon inlet. Insert a small-gauge needle at a 25 degree angle, directing it toward the drainage tubing to avoid entering the balloon inlet lumen. The angle entry will seal more completely than a straight puncture and will decrease the possibility of the needle going through the lumen and exiting on the other side of the catheter.

The urine specimen may be transferred to a sterile container or the needle cover can be replaced and the sample transported to the laboratory in the syringe. Be sure to remove the clamp from the drainage tubing after the specimen is collected.

Collect a 24-hour urine specimen from the collection bag, following agency policies for collection and refrigeration. If a client does not have an indwelling catheter and a sterile catheterized urine specimen is ordered, use a plain catheter with an in-and-out procedure. Most catheterization kits include a sterile specimen container for this purpose. In most instances,

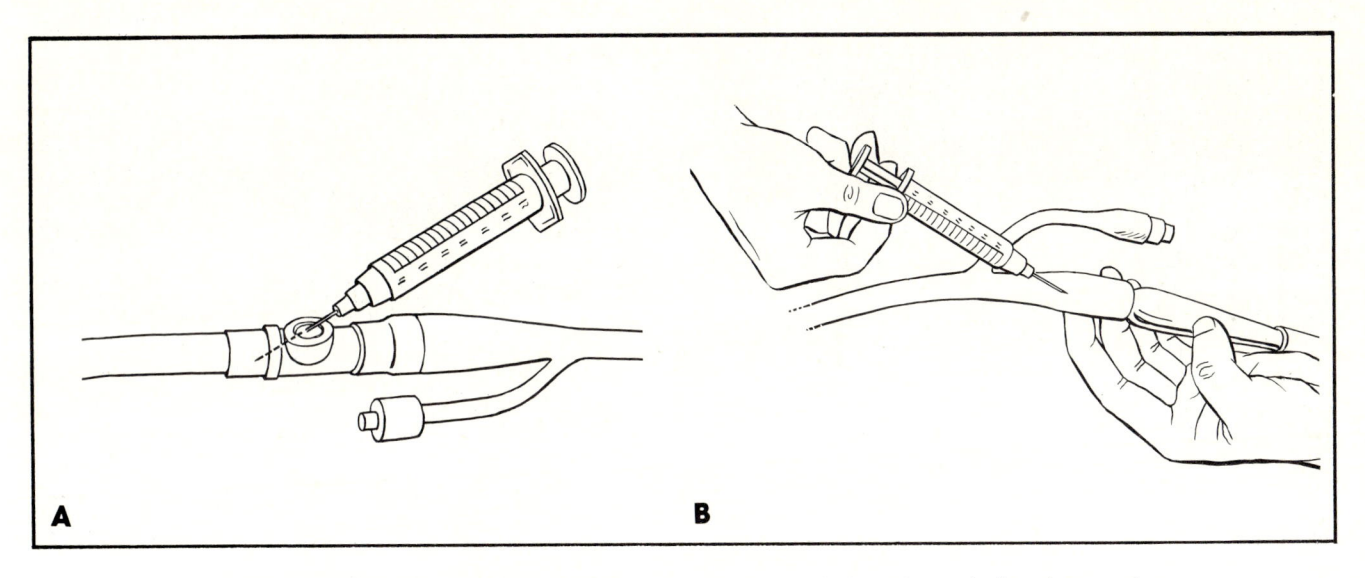

Figure 60–6. Obtain a urine specimen from an indwelling catheter, using a sterile syringe and needle, and aseptic technique. **A.** Cleanse aspiration port with alcohol swab; insert needle at an angle. **B.** If there is no aspiration port, cleanse distal portion of catheter with alcohol swab; insert needle at an angle, distal to the balloon inlet, and directed toward the collection tubing.

however, clean-catch midstream urine specimens are used to obtain a urine specimen for culture purposes, rather than inserting a catheter with its accompanying risks.

INSERTION OF A URINARY CATHETER

It is helpful to have an assistant when inserting a catheter, especially if you are inexperienced, or the client is heavy, weak, acutely ill, confused, uncooperative, or for any reason may have difficulty maintaining the necessary position for the needed length of time. Inspect and cleanse the perineal area to remove soiling before beginning the catheterization procedure. Because of the location of the female urethra, you will need an additional external light source. A gooseneck floor lamp works well since it can easily be adjusted, or a flashlight can be used. If the catheterization kit is packaged in a protective plastic bag, use it for a trash container. Stand it upright in a place that is convenient for discarding used supplies, preferably just beyond the far side of the sterile field. This avoids potential contamination from used supplies such as soiled rayon balls. If no plastic bag comes with the kit, obtain a small, moisture-resistant trash bag for this purpose.

Positioning the Client
Place a female in either a dorsal recumbent or lateral position. For the dorsal recumbent position, have her lie on her back with her knees flexed and spread apart, feet flat on the bed, as shown in Figure 60–7A. If the client is heavy or the bed is soft, elevate the buttocks with a folded towel or bath blanket, which makes it easier to see the meatus. Plan to work from the side of the bed that puts your dominant hand toward the foot of the bed, since that makes it easier to handle the equipment. Have your assistant stand on the opposite side of the bed to support the client's legs, offer comfort and reassurance, and direct the light beam on the meatus. If no assistant is available, adjust the gooseneck lamp or position the flashlight on the bed with a folded towel or washcloth. After positioning, drape the client with a bath blanket for privacy and warmth. Place the catheter kit between the client's legs about 45 cm (18 in) from the perineum so that the sterile equipment is readily accessible. Before opening the sterile catheter kit, use a clean glove to separate the labia and check the visibility of the meatus. Place the light source to focus on the meatus.

For the lateral position, have the client lie on her side with her knees drawn up toward her chest. If you are right-handed, the client lies on her left side, and vice versa. Pull the client's buttocks close to the near side of the bed, and see that her shoulders are closer to the opposite side of the bed, as shown in Figure 60–7B. Have the assistant stand on the far side of the bed where he or she can talk to the client and also hold her knees, either lightly as a reminder or more firmly to help maintain the position. Stand with your dominant hand toward the foot of the bed and place the catheterization kit on the bed near the client's legs.

The lateral position for catheterizing a female offers a number of benefits, although it is not widely used. It is often more comfortable, less embarrassing, and clients tend to be less anxious, which makes insertion of the catheter easier. The nurse is closer to the working area and since there is no leg to reach over, body mechanics are better. There is also less likelihood for contaminating the equipment since the urethra is generally more visible in this position. Since

642 PROFESSIONAL CLINICAL NURSING SKILLS

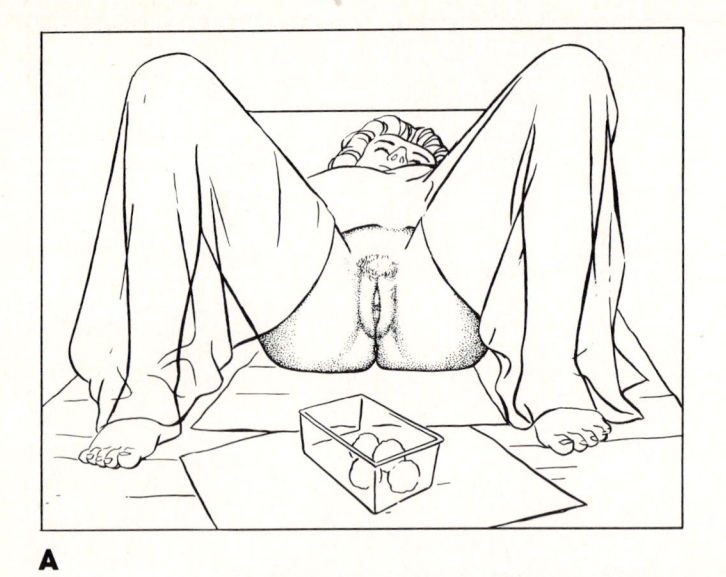

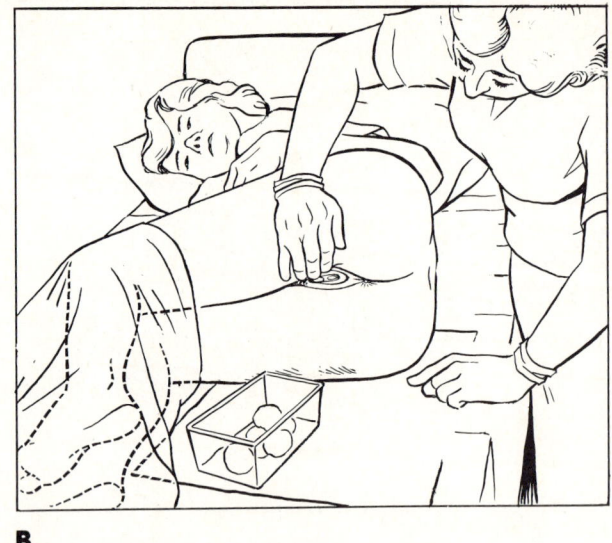

Figure 60–7. Positions for inserting catheter in female client. Note convenient location of catheterization kit. **A.** *Dorsal recumbent position.* **B.** *Lateral position, with a left-handed nurse.*

only one labium needs to be lifted, there is less likelihood of the labia coming together before the catheter is inserted. If the labium is slippery, a gauze square or absorbent ball can be used to hold it securely.

Although it is a comfortable position for many women and an ideal one for clients with leg contractures, the lateral position is not suitable for all clients. For example, some clients need to remain in a supine position, such as after a fractured hip; postpartum clients with an episiotomy may experience pain from having the labium lifted, and visualization of the meatus may be difficult in clients with very heavy buttocks (Dobbins and Gleit, 1971; Rowson, 1970).

To catheterize a male client, place him in a supine position with the legs together or slightly apart. Fold the top linen down to the middle of his thighs and drape him for privacy and warmth. Plan to stand so that your dominant hand is toward the client's feet. Place the catheterization kit on the bed on the near side of his knees or on the overbed table positioned across his knees.

Inserting the Catheter

After the client is in position, place the catheterization kit about 45 cm (15 in) from the perineal area and open it to provide a sterile work area. Position the kit so that it will form a continuous sterile field with the drapes that will be placed under the perineal area. Most catheterization kits are packaged so that the equipment is available in the sequence it will be needed, with sterile gloves on top. If the first drape is on top, pick it up at a corner and allow it to fall open without contaminating. Touch only the corners and place one edge under the female client's buttocks or over the male client's legs just below the penis. The second drape is usually fenestrated; that is, it has a center opening designed to fit over the perineum. The use of this drape is optional since it often does not stay in place over the female perineum and is difficult to position over the penis without contaminating the gloves or drape.

After putting on the sterile gloves, pour the antiseptic on the absorbent balls, open the specimen container, lubricate the catheter, test the balloon inflation, and do any other necessary preparation with two sterile hands. Once the nondominant hand separates the labia or holds the penis, it is contaminated and must not be returned to the sterile area; all sterile equipment must be handled only with the other hand.

Hold the absorbent balls with the forceps to cleanse the labia or penis, since that avoids contamination of the gloved hand. Once the labia have been cleansed, they must not be allowed to close over the meatus until the catheter is inserted. If they do close, separate the labia again and use the remaining saturated sterile absorbent ball to cleanse directly over the meatus again. In the same way, if the foreskin closes over the tip of the penis, retract it and cleanse the meatus again. Since the cleansing agent makes the labia slippery, many nurses keep one sterile absorbent ball dry and use it to help hold the labia apart or to lift the upper labium when the client is in the lateral position. It may also be used to blot the excess cleansing solution from the meatus, making it more clearly visible. Figure 60–8 shows female perineal anatomic landmarks, the thumb and finger positions used to separate the labia for clients in both the dorsal recumbent and lateral positions, the urethral meatus, and the placement of an indwelling catheter within the female bladder.

After cleansing the urethral orifice, insert the well-lubricated catheter slowly and gently. For a fe-

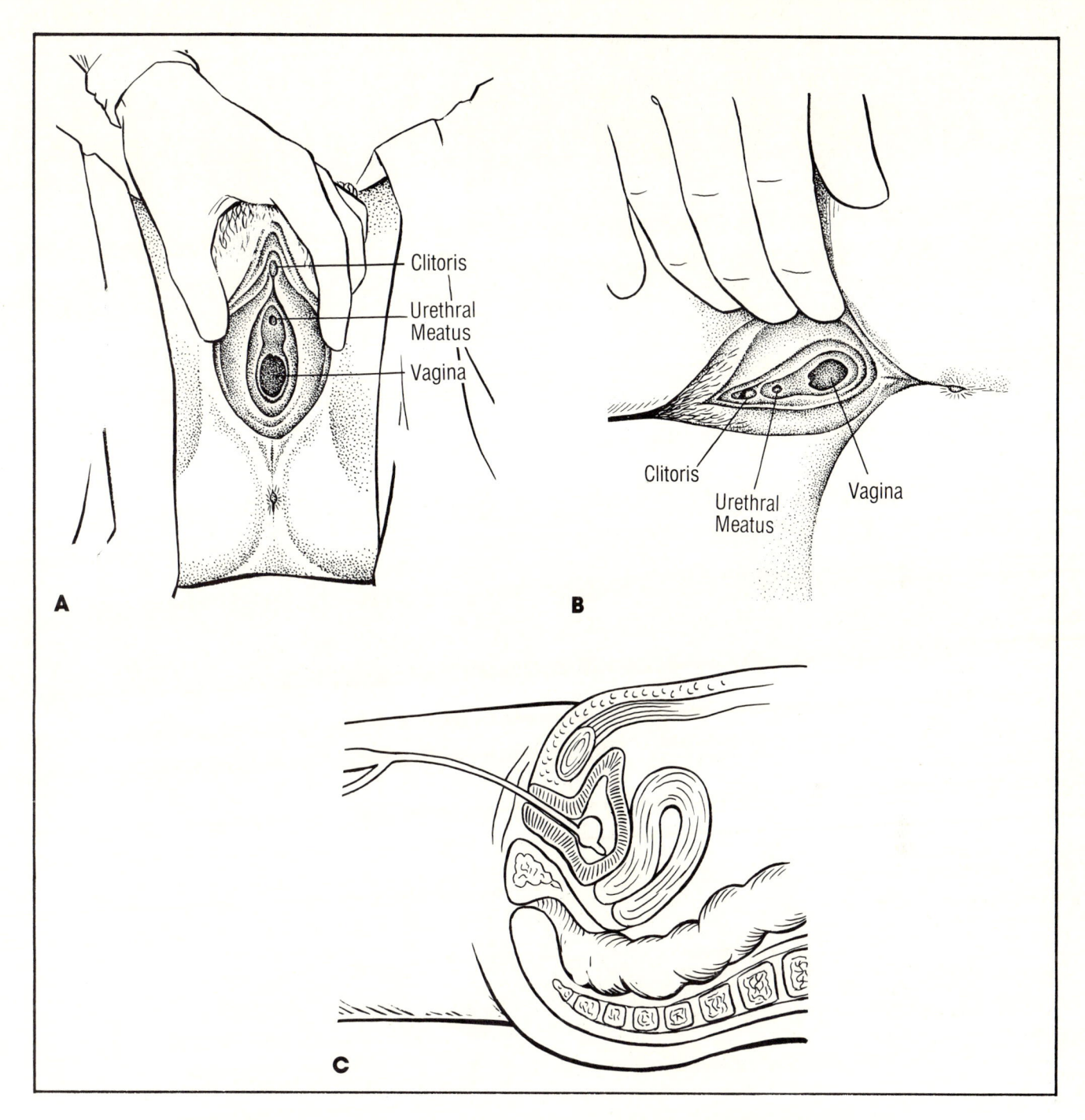

Figure 60-8. Female perineal anatomic landmarks and finger positions for separating the labia. **A.** Dorsal recumbent position. Separate labia with thumb and forefinger. **B.** Lateral position. Lift upper labia with fingers. **C.** Indwelling catheter in place in female bladder.

male, direct the catheter slightly downward to follow the natural curve of the urethra. In the male, stretch the penis upright, at a right angle to the abdomen, and direct the catheter straight downward. Figure 60-9 shows how the penis is held for cleansing and the positions needed for inserting a catheter, as well as the placement of an indwelling catheter within the male bladder. If you encounter resistance, do not force the catheter. Rotate it, wait briefly, and ask the client to take a deep breath, which usually relaxes the urethral sphincters. Resistance is more likely to occur in the male than the female, and occurs primarily when the catheter reaches the external sphincter, just distal to the prostate gland, that is, after about 12.5 to 15 cm (5 to 6 in) of the catheter has been inserted. If the catheter meets resistance at this point, first put a little more upward traction on the penis. If that is not effective, change the angle of the penis and direct it toward

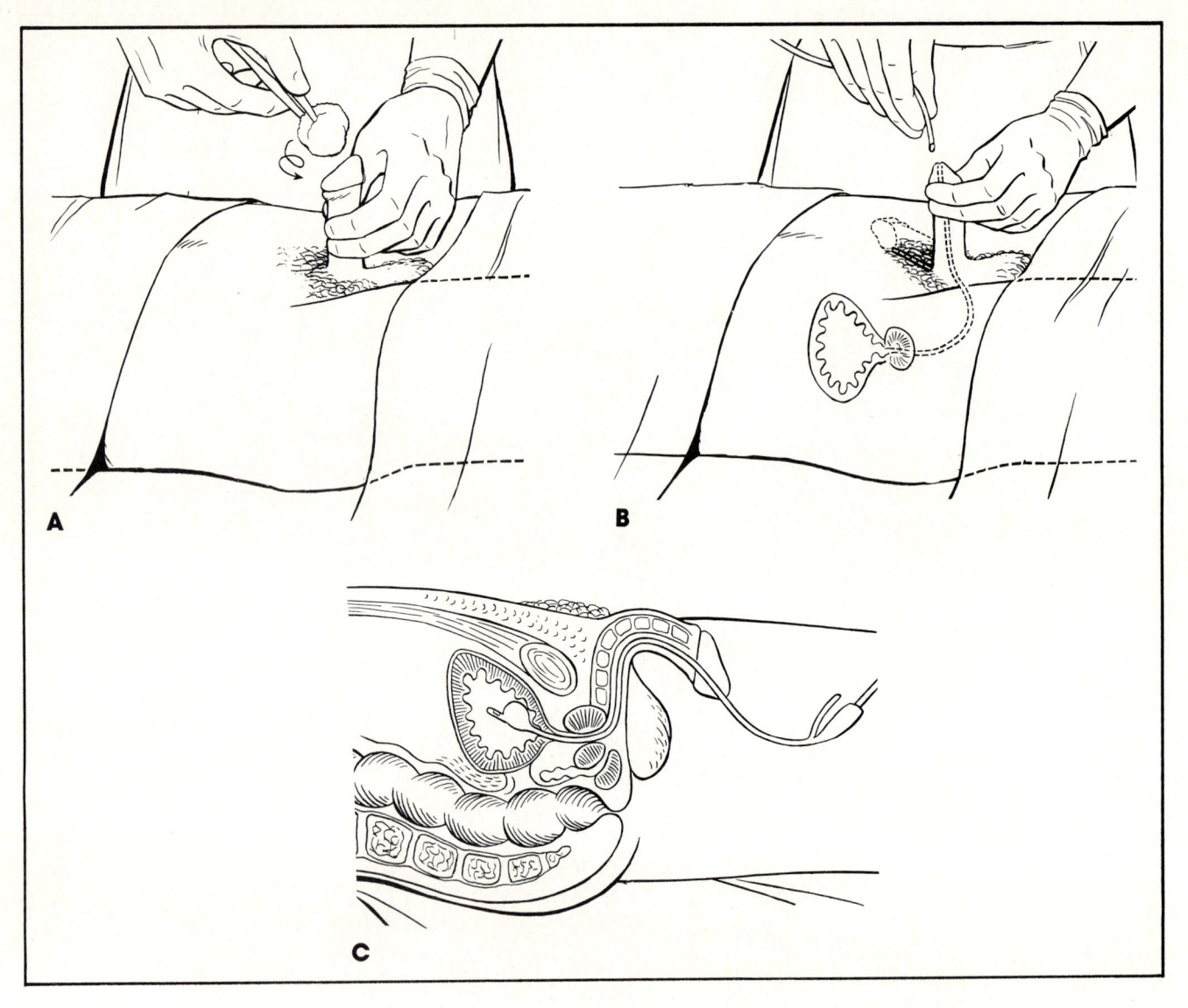

Figure 60-9. Insertion of a catheter in a male. **A.** Cleanse penis in a circular motion from the meatus downward. **B.** Exert firm yet gentle upright tension on the penis to straighten the urethra; pinch head of penis slightly to open the urethral meatus. If resistance is encountered, lower penis toward abdomen. **C.** Indwelling catheter in place in male bladder.

the client's head, while still maintaining tension. These maneuvers will usually direct the catheter around the prostate gland. If resistance continues, do not force the catheter, since it can easily enter the spongy tissue that surrounds the male urethra and produce what are known as blind pouches or passages. Resistance may also occur 1 to 2 cm (½ to ¾ in) from the meatus, because of membranous folds in the glans. Sometimes a smaller-diameter catheter can be inserted more readily. Contact a physician to insert the catheter if necessary.

If you contaminate the catheter at any time during the procedure, obtain a new catheterization kit and begin the procedure over. If the catheter inadvertently enters the vagina, leave it there as an identifying landmark when inserting the next catheter. In some women, the urethral meatus is almost inside the vaginal orifice, making it difficult to locate. Many nurses like to add a sterile applicator to the sterile field and use it to locate and identify the urethra after cleansing the labia.

If you are inserting a plain catheter for one-time use, insert the catheter just a little beyond the point at which urine begins to flow. If you are inserting a Foley catheter, insert it an additional 2.5 to 5 cm (1 to 2 in) to be sure the balloon will be out of the urethra when it is inflated. The client will experience pain if the balloon is inflated within the urethra. Some sources advocate inserting the catheter in a male client nearly to the balloon lumen bifurcation to be certain it is in sufficiently far (Bates, 1981).

The prefilled syringe in the catheterization kit usually contains more solution than the stated balloon capacity. Since the balloon inflation lumen has a capacity of less than 1 ml, it is best to insert only 1 or 2 ml more than the stated balloon capacity and discard

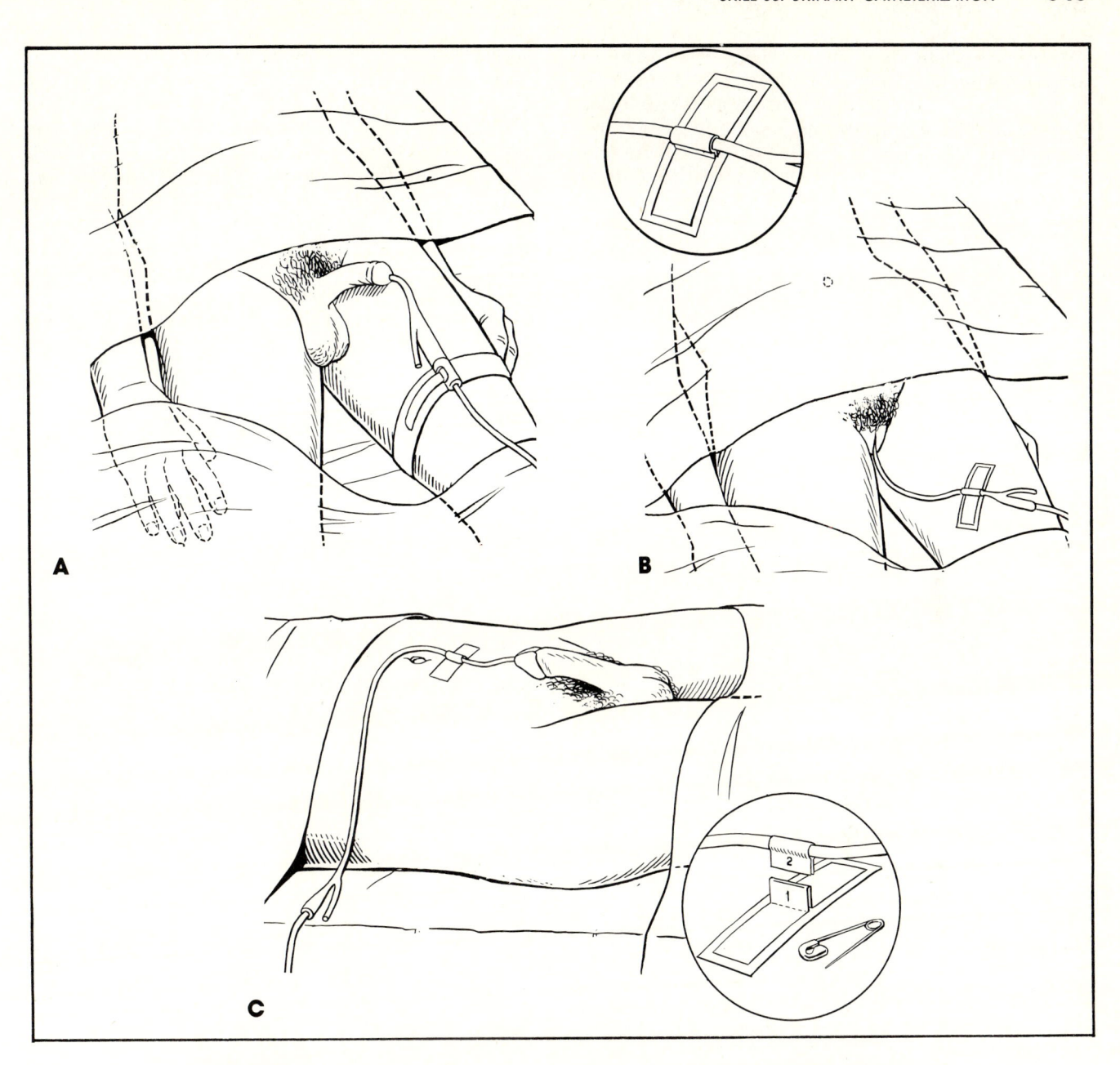

Figure 60-10. Urinary catheters may be attached to the inner thigh or to the abdomen (for long-term use with males). **A.** Catheter secured to thigh with commercial self-adherent catheter strap that loops around catheter. (Note lateral direction of penis and slack that allows for leg abduction.) **B.** Catheter secured with two strips of tape. Inset: Place first strip of tape on thigh (or abdomen). Place center of second strip of tape around catheter. Attach ends of strip to first tape strip. **C.** Catheter secured to abdomen below navel, using three strips of tape. Inset: Place first tape strip on abdomen. Form Tab 1 with second tape strip and attach to first strip. Form Tab 2 around catheter with third tape strip. Pin the two tabs together.

the remaining fluid. After inflating the balloon, tug gently on the catheter to be sure it is in place securely. Attach the drainage tubing connector to the catheter if it is not a preconnected system, being careful to avoid contaminating either opening. Remove the equipment, clean and dry the perineum, and return the client to a comfortable position. Secure the catheter to the leg or abdomen as described below. Tape the catheter-tubing junction if it is not a preconnected system. Coil the excess tubing on the bed, attach a rubber band to the tubing in a clove hitch fashion, and secure it to the bed linen with a safety pin.

Monitor the client's comfort level and urine output at regular intervals for the first few hours after inserting the catheter, particularly if the bladder has been quite distended. Although many sources caution against removing more than 1000 ml of urine at one time because of a potential for hypovolemic shock, there is no documentation in the literature to support this (Sorensen and Luckmann, 1979; Steele, 1983). In clinical practice, large amounts of urine are often removed at one time from clients with acute urinary retention without harm to the client other than an occasional small amount of temporary bleeding from minor injury to the bladder mucosa as the detrusor muscle contracts. Clients with long-term chronic retention and elevated blood urea nitrogen (BUN) and creatinine levels may develop postobstructive diuresis if adequate hydration is not provided as the bladder is emptied (Steele, 1983).

Securing an Indwelling Catheter
Secure an indwelling catheter with sufficient slack to avoid continuous urethral pressure, even during activities, as indicated earlier. For females, secure the catheter to the inner thigh; for males, use either the thigh or the abdomen. The thigh is more confortable for ambulatory males, but for bedfast, paralyzed, or debilitated clients, the abdomen may be preferable because that position straightens the urethra and avoids pressure from the catheter on the penosacral junction. If the thigh is used, be sure the penis is directed laterally toward the thigh with considerable slack. Shave the hair from the thigh or abdomen before applying adhesive tape. Catheters can be secured in several ways. Figure 6-10 shows three methods, each of which avoids repeated removal of tape from the skin. A piece of Op-Site placed on the leg before applying the tape will protect the skin (Fig. 60-10B).

☐ SKILL SEQUENCES

INSERTING A URINARY CATHETER: FEMALE

Step	Rationale
1. Validate physician's order or identify client's need for catheterization.	Ensures appropriate implementation of treatment plan.
2. Wash hands.	Avoids transfer of microorganisms.
3. Prepare equipment and place on overbed table. Plan to stand so that your dominant hand is toward the foot of the bed.	Energy-efficient measure; provides convenient work space. Provides for easier insertion of catheter.
4. Explain procedure.	Enlists client cooperation.
5. Close door or draw curtains.	Provides privacy.
6. Raise bed to comfortable working height and lower side rail if used.	Provides for nurse safety and comfort.

7. Position client in:
  a. Dorsal recumbent position, with knees flexed and apart and feet about 60 cm (2 ft) apart.
  b. Lateral position, with knees drawn up toward chest and hips pulled toward edge of bed.
Drape with bath blanket.
	Provides for adequate visualization of meatus.
	
	May be more comfortable and provide more sense of privacy and better visualization.
	Protects client's privacy, decreases embarrassment and tension, and provides warmth.

8. Position light source to focus on perineum; adjust gooseneck light or position person holding flashlight in appropriate place.	Additional light source is needed to see meatus clearly.
9. If soiled, wash perineal area with soap and water, rinse, and dry.	Decreases likelihood of introducing microorganisms into bladder along with catheter.
10. Remove plastic protector from catheterization kit. Place in convenient place so that it can be used as a trash container without needing to reach across sterile field.	Maintains sterility of contents and provides for disposal of soiled absorbent balls.
11. Place catheterization kit between client's legs (for dorsal recumbent position) or near legs (for lateral position), about 45 cm (1½ ft) from perineal area. (NOTE: If inserting Foley catheter and kit does not contain a preconnected catheter-drainage system, first open separate drainage kit, being careful not to dislodge protective cap on tubing connector. Attach collection bag to bed frame near foot of bed with hook provided. Bring drainage tubing between bed and side rail and place connector in safe and convenient place.)	Provides convenient sterile working area. Maintains sterility of connector and helps prevent intraluminal contamination. Provides for straight downhill drainage. Avoids contamination and keeps tubing readily available.
12. Pick up one corner of moisture-resistant barrier drape, stand back from bed and allow it to fall open with plastic side away from you. Grasp drape at opposite corners of one side and place it under the client's buttocks. Touch only the corners of drape.	Avoids sterile drape becoming contaminated from touching bed or table. Provides sterile area adjacent to perineum. Avoids contaminating sterile drape during placement.
13. Don sterile gloves.	Enables nurse to handle sterile equipment.
14. Discard fenestrated drape at side of sterile field or open to half of full size and place on lower abdomen above symphysis pubis. OR: Place over perineal area with labia visible.	Provides additional sterile area but often does not remain in place over perineum and thus increases likelihood of contamination of catheter.

(continued)

Step	Rationale
15. If urine specimen is desired, remove cap from specimen container and replace it lightly. Place container upright within easy reach. If not needed, discard away from sterile field.	Specimen container opens more easily if nurse uses both hands.

16. For indwelling catheter:
   a. Attach prefilled syringe to balloon outlet on catheter and inflate balloon.
   b. Deflate balloon and leave syringe in place.
	Tests balloon for leaking or bursting.
	
	Balloon can be inflated when nurse has only one hand available.

17. Lubricate distal 4 to 5 cm (1½ to 2 in) of catheter, using water-soluble lubricant. Avoid occluding drainage holes in tip with lubricant. Place in safe place inside catheterization kit container or on sterile field. (If using prelubricated catheter, remove external protector.)	Reduces friction and facilitates catheter insertion. Avoids accidental contamination of catheter.
18. Pour antiseptic cleansing agent over 3 or 4 absorbent balls.	Preparatory for cleansing meatus.

19. Separate labia with nondominant hand, exposing meatus.
   a. Dorsal recumbent position: Place thumb and forefinger or two fingers between labia minora, spread fingers outward and pull upward slightly.
   b. Lateral position: Lift upper labia with two fingers. (NOTE: Do not allow labia to come together until catheter is inserted.)
	Provides visualization of meatus.
	Upward pull smooths out area and increases visibility of meatus and opens it slightly.
	
	Area becomes contaminated if labia are allowed to close after cleansing and before catheter is inserted.

20. Use forceps and moistened absorbent balls to cleanse labia and meatus, firmly but gently. Use each ball one time; wipe from clitoris toward anus; first cleanse far side of labia, then cleanse near side, and finally cleanse directly over meatus. Discard soiled balls in small trash bag.	Maintains sterility of gloved hand. Cleansing direction proceeds from cleaner to dirtier area. Cleansing minimizes entry of microorganisms into bladder. Cleansing motion increases visibility of meatus.
21. Move urine collection container or preconnected drainage bag near perineum. Pick up catheter with gloved dominant hand about 7.5 cm (3 in) from tip, leaving open end of catheter in urine collection container. Ask client to take a deep breath or bear down as if preparing to urinate. Gently insert catheter 5 to 7.5 cm (2 to 3 in) until urine flows freely.	Positions container to receive urine. Maintains open end of catheter as sterile. Relaxes urinary sphincter and allows catheter to enter more easily. Force can injure tissues.
22. Direct catheter slightly downward. If no urine flows, insert catheter 2 cm (¾ in) farther and rotate catheter. (NOTE: For an indwelling catheter, insert an additional 2.5 to 4 cm (1 to 1½ in).)	Follows natural curve of urethra. Catheter drainage eyes may be against bladder wall. Ensures balloon is not in urethra when inflated.
23. Release labia; rest nondominant hand on pubis and hold catheter firmly and steadily with fingers. Keep open end of plain catheter in urine collection container or stabilized in notch on container. Maintain catheter position until bladder is emptied, catheter balloon inflated, or urine specimen obtained.	Steadies catheter and avoids in-and-out movement, which increases probability of microorganisms entering bladder. Avoids dripping or spilling urine.

24. For indwelling catheter:
   a. Inflate balloon with preattached syringe. Tug gently on catheter.
   b. Attach open end of catheter to drainage collection tubing connector without contaminating either opening.
   c. Secure catheter to inner thigh, allowing enough slack to permit adduction of leg.
	Identifies whether balloon is inflated.
	
	Provides sterile closed system and avoids intraluminal contamination.
	
	Avoids pressure on urethral meatus.

25. To obtain specimen: Use dominant hand to remove loosened cap from specimen container and place it on sterile field. Place specimen container on bed near urine collection container. Pinch catheter to stop flow of urine; place open end in specimen container; release fingers to allow 30 to 45 ml (1 to 1½ oz) of urine to drain into container. Pinch catheter and return open end to urine container. Close specimen container.	Avoids contamination of specimen container and spilling urine onto sterile field.
26. When urine flow decreases, remove catheter slowly (1 cm at a time) until urine scarcely drips. Pinch catheter and remove it. Place catheter on sterile field.	Empties bladder completely. Avoids dripping.

(continued)

INSERTING A URINARY CATHETER: FEMALE (Cont.)

Step	Rationale
27. Remove drapes and use them to wipe perineal area. Remove wrapper and all contents and place on foot of bed or chair. Remove gloves. Return client to position of comfort and safety.	Comfort measure. Allows client to return legs to usual position more quickly.
28. Attach collection bag to bed frame as in step 11, avoiding dependent loops or kinks.	Provides for straight downhill drainage.
29. Measure and empty urine; discard disposable equipment; return reusable equipment to central service.	Appropriate care for supplies.
30. Wash hands.	Avoids transfer of microorganisms.
31. Label specimen container and send it to the laboratory or place in refrigerator.	Ensures correct identification and care of specimen.
32. Record time, amount and character of urine removed, client's reaction, and any problems encountered. Record purpose for specimen collection and time specimen was sent to laboratory.	Fulfills nurse accountability and provides ongoing data base.

INSERTING A URINARY CATHETER: MALE

Step	Rationale
1. Repeat Skill Sequence, "Inserting a Urinary Catheter: Female," steps 1 to 6.	Same as Skill Sequence, "Inserting a Urinary Catheter: Female," steps 1 to 6.
2. Position client on back near edge of bed, with legs together. Fold top linen below genitals; place towel or bath blanket over abdomen and chest.	Provides ease in working and gives adequate visualization. Protects client's privacy and provides warmth.
3. If soiled, wash genitals with soap and water, rinse and dry.	Decreases likelihood of introducing microorganisms into bladder along with catheter.
4. Remove plastic protector from catheterization kit. Place in convenient place so it can be used as a trash container without needing to reach across sterile field.	Maintains sterility of contents and provides for disposal of soiled absorbent balls.
5. Place catheterization kit on bed beside client's knees or on overbed table. (NOTE: If catheterization kit does not contain a preconnected catheter-drainage system, open separate drainage kit before opening catheterization kit, being careful not to dislodge protective cap on tubing connector. Attach collection bag to bed frame near the foot of bed with hook provided. Bring drainage tubing between bed and siderail and place connector in safe and convenient place.)	Provides convenient sterile working area. Maintains sterility of connector and helps prevent intraluminal contamination. Provides for straight downhill drainage. Avoids contamination and keeps tubing readily available.
6. Pick up one corner of moisture-resistant barrier drape, stand back from bed and allow it to fall open with plastic side away from you. Grasp drape at opposite corners of one side and place it on client's legs just below penis.	Avoids accidental contamination from bed or overbed table. Provides a sterile area adjacent to perineal area.
7. Don sterile gloves.	Enables nurse to handle sterile equipment.
8. Open fenestrated drape to half of its size and place it on lower abdomen above penis; or discard away from sterile field.	Fenestrated drape is difficult to place over penis without contaminating gloves and drapes.
9. For indwelling catheter, see Skill Sequence, "Inserting a Urinary Catheter: Female," step 16.	Tests balloon for leaking or bursting.
10. Pour antiseptic cleansing agent over three or four absorbent balls.	Preparatory for cleansing meatus.
11. If urine specimen is needed, follow Skill Sequence, "Inserting a Urinary Catheter: Female," step 15.	Specimen container opens more easily if nurse uses both hands.
12. Generously lubricate 15 to 18 cm (6 to 7 in) of catheter with a water-soluble lubricant. Avoid occluding drainage holes in tip with lubricant. Place in safe place on sterile field.	Generous lubrication needed because of bends, turns, and length of male urethra. May prevent drainage of urine. Avoids accidental contamination of catheter.
13. Using nondominant hand, hold penis at a 90 degree angle and retract foreskin and grasp penis gently but firmly just below glans. Using thumb and fingers, pinch glans together slightly, to open meatus. (NOTE: Non-dominant hand is now unsterile.)	A light touch is more likely to stimulate an erection than a more firm touch. (See text for what to do if an erection occurs.) Prepares meatus and glans for cleansing prior to catheter insertion.

(continued)

Step	Rationale
14. Use dominant hand to hold forceps and moistened absorbent balls and cleanse from meatus outward in a circular motion and down over glans to hand holding penis. Repeat twice more, using fresh absorbent ball each time. Discard used balls in small trash bag.	Maintains sterility of gloved hand. Cleansing direction proceeds from cleaner to dirtier area. Cleansing minimizes entry of microorganisms into bladder.
15. Continue to hold penis at a 90 degree angle to the legs, pulling upward slightly. Gently pinch glans between thumb and fingers. Using dominant hand, move urine collection container near base of penis.	Straightens urethra and opens meatus, facilitating catheter entry. Preparatory for collecting urine.
16. With thumb and finger of nondominant hand, pick up catheter about 5 to 7.5 cm (2 to 3 in) from tip. Hold remainder of catheter curled up in palm of hand with other three fingers.	Long, lubricated catheter is difficult to control without contaminating.
17. Ask client to take a deep breath or bear down as if about to urinate. Insert catheter 3 to 5 cm (1½ to 2 in) into urethra, shift hand position and insert catheter 5 to 7 cm (2 to 3 in) into urethra. Repeat to a total depth of 18 to 20 cm (7 to 8 in). When resistance is met, pause briefly to allow external sphincter to relax. Have client take a deep breath, apply a little more traction to penis or change its position, lowering it toward his abdomen. Do not force catheter into urethra. If urine does not flow, rotate the catheter or insert it an additional 2.5 to 5 cm (1 to 2 in).	Relaxes and opens sphincters, facilitating catheter entry. Catheter entry may cause temporary sphincter spasm. Helps move catheter around prostate gland. Force can perforate urethra and cause a blind pouch. Catheter drainage hole may be against bladder wall.
18. Hold catheter in place securely with nondominant hand; lower penis and insert open end of catheter into urine collection container. Rest nondominant hand on pubis.	Avoids in-and-out movement of catheter while urine is draining. (In-and-out movement facilitates entry of microorganisms.) Steadies hand holding catheter.

19. For indwelling catheter:
  a. Insert catheter an additional 5 to 7 cm (2 to 2½ in) or to balloon lumen bifurcation.
  b. Return foreskin to anatomic position after removing catheter or when an indwelling catheter is in place.
	Ensures balloon is not in urethra when inflated.
	
	Avoids constriction of glans.

20. Complete procedure as in Skill Sequence, "Inserting a Urinary Catheter: Female," steps 25 to 32.	See Skill Sequence, "Inserting a Urinary Catheter: Female," steps 25 to 32.

CATHETER AND BLADDER IRRIGATION AND INSTILLATION

A catheter system can be irrigated in three ways, depending on the type of equipment used: (1) manually through the aspiration port without disconnecting the system, (2) manually through the catheter after separating the catheter and tubing, and (3) through a closed three-way catheter with a continuous in-and-out flow of fluid. Regardless of the method used, strict surgical aseptic technique is required to avoid introducing microorganisms into the system.

When a catheter is irrigated manually, small amounts of irrigant solution are used. If handled aseptically, bottles of normal saline may be labeled with the date and time and kept for 24 hours. Follow directions or ask the pharmacist about the length of time an antibiotic solution or other irrigant may be kept safely. For a continuous irrigation through a three-way catheter, large bags or bottles (2000 ml) or a physiological irrigant fluid are used. A quite rapid flow rate should be maintained when there is a lot of bleeding or if clots are present, as is common immediately after surgery for transurethral removal of the prostate gland. The rapid flow rate avoids retention of blood in the bladder and prevents clots from clogging the catheter. Remember to empty the drainage bag frequently and to keep accurate intake and output records.

For home use, clients and their families are usually taught to separate the system for irrigation. Teach them to boil the irrigation set for 20 minutes before each use. (Adjust the time according to the altitude, as in Skill 30.) Water for irrigation is boiled for 20 minutes and stored in a boiled jar with a screw-top lid. Acetic acid solution (0.25 percent) may be made by adding 2 T white vinegar to 1 qt distilled water. Store a sterilized drainage tubing cap in a clean covered jar. Before irrigating the catheter, the family member should wash his or her hands thoroughly and scrub the catheter junction with alcohol before separating it. Sterile gloves are not necessary.

To irrigate a catheter through the aspiration port you will need the following equipment: a 25- or 50-ml syringe with a No. 23 needle, sterile saline or other irrigant as ordered, a sterile basin, and alcohol swabs. To irrigate through the catheter lumen, you will need a sterile catheter irrigation kit or the following equipment: a large sterile asepto or catheter-tipped syringe; sterile saline or other irrigant; a sterile pan to contain the irrigant; a sterile pan for the returns; alcohol swabs; and a protector for the connector, such as a sterile 4×4 gauze pad and a rubber band.

☐ SKILL SEQUENCE

CATHETER IRRIGATION AND INSTILLATION

Step	Rationale
1. Validate physician's order.	Ensures appropriate implementation of treatment plan.
2. Wash hands.	Avoids transfer of microorganisms.
3. Prepare sterile equipment.	Energy-efficient measure.
4. Explain procedure to client.	Enlists client cooperation.
5. Raise bed to comfortable working height.	Provides for nurse safety and comfort.
6. Turn back top linen to expose catheter junction site.	Provides adequate visualization.

7. To irrigate through aspiration port:
  a. Pour irrigating solution into sterile pan, draw it into syringe, and attach a No. 23 needle.
  b. Cleanse aspiration port with an alcohol swab.
  c. Fold over and pinch tubing distal to aspiration port, or close catheter tubing clamp.
  d. Insert needle, touching only upper portion of syringe.
  e. Inject 30 or 50 ml of solution into catheter.
  f. Release tubing.
  g. Observe for return flow of fluid through catheter.
  h. Remove syringe from needle, refill syringe, and reattach to needle. Avoid touching syringe tip. Repeat irrigation as needed to clear catheter of debris or clots.
	Small-gauge needle makes a resealable puncture in latex port.
	Removes microorganisms.
	Directs irrigant toward bladder rather than down tubing.
	
	Maintains syringe tip as sterile to avoid contaminating solution when refilling syringe.
	
	Allows for irrigant to flow out of bladder by gravity.
	Identifies nature of returns and need for further irrigation.
	Avoids contamination of lower portion of syringe.
	
	Promotes catheter patency.

8. To irrigate through catheter lumen:
  a. Pour irrigant into sterile container. Remove tip guard from catheter or asepto syringe and fill syringe. Touch only the part of syringe that will not need to be returned to sterile container for refilling.
  b. Place a sterile collection basin near catheter-tubing junction.
  c. Remove tape seal around catheter-tubing junction, if one is present.
  d. Cleanse catheter-tubing junction with one or two alcohol swabs.
  e. Separate tubing from connector, being careful not to contaminate either end. Hold catheter with thumb and forefinger of nondominant hand and place drainage tubing between second and third fingers with connector upright and not touching catheter opening. Slip catheter protector over connector or wrap it with a sterile gauze pad and secure with rubber band. Place protected connector end of tubing in a safe place on the bed.
  f. Insert 30 to 50 ml of solution into catheter, pinch catheter between fingers, remove syringe, and allow solution to return by gravity into collection basin. If there is no return, use gentle suction with syringe. Do not touch tip or lower end of syringe.
  g. Repeat irrigation two or three or more times until returns are clear.
  h. Hold drainage tubing in nondominant hand as in step 8e.
  i. Hold tubing connector in dominant hand and reconnect catheter to tubing without touching either one.
  j. Retape catheter-tubing junction.
	Prepares sterile irrigant for use.
	
	Convenient location for collecting returns.
	
	Provides access to junction.
	
	Removes microorganisms.
	
	Avoids intraluminal contamination.
	
	Protects connector opening.
	
	Avoids having tubing become contaminated or fall to the floor during procedure.
	
	Avoids contamination of solution when refilling syringe.
	Clearing catheter will decrease frequency with which irrigation is needed.
	Protects sterility of catheter and connector openings.
	
	Avoids contamination.
	
	Discourages unnecessary separation of system.

9. Return client to a position of comfort and safety.	
10. Discard disposable equipment.	Appropriate care for equipment.
11. Wash hands.	Prevents transfer of microorganisms.
12. Record amount and type of irrigant used.	
13. Record method of irrigation, amount and type of irrigant used, amount and character of returns, and any problems associated with procedure. Add amount of nonreturned fluid to both intake and output record. Report unusual findings.	Fulfills nurse accountability and provides ongoing data base. Ensures accurate intake and output measurement.

REMOVING AN INDWELLING CATHETER

Sometimes the physician will order that an indwelling catheter be alternately clamped and released several times before it is removed. A usual routine for this bladder reconditioning is to clamp the catheter for 3 to 6 hours and then release it for 5 to 10 minutes to drain the bladder, leaving the drainage system intact. The cycle is repeated two or more times. This reconditioning is based on the fact that when the bladder is kept empty, the detrusor muscle remains contracted and the bladder tends to lose its capacity both to hold urine and to contract adequately. Some clients who have had an indwelling catheter have temporary dysfunction after it is removed, experiencing urinary retention and residual urine after voiding. This dysfunction tends to diminish with each voiding following removal of the catheter (Sorenson and Luckmann, 1979; Williamson, 1982). In Williamson's (1982) study of eight women, a significant increase in regaining regular micturition was achieved when the bladder was reconditioned for as short a time as three cycles of a 3-hour clamping followed by a 5-minute draining.

To remove an indwelling catheter, you will need a syringe of the same capacity as the balloon capacity, an emesis basin, round pan, or a towel, a trash bag, a flashlight, and cleansing materials for perineal care. Depending on the style of balloon lumen inlet, you may also need a No. 22 needle on the syringe.

Before removing the catheter, explain the procedure to the client, indicating that it is a quick procedure and will not be painful. Also explain that he or she will probably not feel the urge to void for several hours after the catheter is removed, and that urinary output will need to be measured for 24 hours to evaluate the bladder's function.

For this procedure, position the client on his or her back in a supine position. Turn the linens back to expose the genital area and drape the client as needed for warmth and privacy. Have a female client spread her legs apart and place the pan or towel near the perineal area. Place the pan or towel beside or on a male client's legs. Remove the tape or leg band from the leg or abdomen. Attach the syringe to the balloon inlet port or insert the needle into the port, depending on the catheter, and withdraw the inflation fluid. Although the catheter will be discarded, it is best not to deflate the balloon by cutting off the inlet lumen. Sometimes the balloon lumen will have become obstructed, preventing the balloon from deflating. When the inlet port has been cut off, there is no way to apply suction with a syringe. If the balloon cannot be deflated, do not attempt to burst it by inserting additional water because the balloon pieces become foreign bodies and can produce bladder irritation or calculi. Although a physician usually punctures a nondeflated balloon, the nurse may be designated to do this. Mocsny (1980) suggests the following procedure for puncturing a catheter balloon, using surgical aseptic technique and the wire stylet from a long catheter such as that used in subclavian intravenous therapy. If the stylet is shorter than the catheter, cleanse the catheter with an alcohol swab and use a sterile scissors to cut it off about 1 inch from the meatus. Carefully thread the stylet through the balloon lumen until it meets the firm resistance of the balloon. Press the stylet firmly and steadily but gently, until you feel it puncture the balloon and see water flowing from the catheter. If the stylet cannot be removed easily, contact a physician.

After deflating the balloon, ask the client to take a deep breath to relax the sphincters, remove the catheter slowly, and place it in the pan or towel. Inspect the urethral meatus, using a flashlight if needed. Note any redness, edema, or discharge. Wash and dry the perineal area and return the client to a position of comfort and safety. Inspect the catheter to make certain that it is intact, measure and empty the collection bag, and discard all used disposable equipment. Have the client increase his or her fluid intake and monitor fluid intake and output for the next 24 hours to determine whether the bladder is emptying properly. Sometimes the physician will ask that the client be catheterized for residual urine after the catheter is removed. In this case, first have the client void, measure the urine, and then insert a straight catheter as soon as possible after voiding. Measure the urine obtained through the catheter and report and record the amount of residual urine. If the amount of residual urine is greater than the amount determined acceptable by the physician, it may be necessary to reinsert the indwelling catheter. The amount regarded as acceptable will vary depending on the client's diagnosis, bladder status, and physician's directive.

TEACHING CLIENTS INTERMITTENT SELF-CATHETERIZATION

Involve the client and his or her family in the decision about self-catheterization and be sure they understand the goal and procedure for this approach to bladder emptying. The self-catheterization process is relatively simple and most clients learn it quite readily. A family member is usually taught the procedure also, in case the client is unable to do it. The following procedure is based on the work done by Lapides et al. (1976) with clients with dysfunctional bladders.

For each teaching session, the client should have a full bladder and washes his or her hands before beginning. To teach a female client how to catheterize herself, position her on an examining table, seated with her feet on the table and her knees flexed and held apart. Use a mirror to help her identify her perineal anatomy and locate the urinary meatus. Have her hold the catheter 1 cm (½ in) from its tip with her dominant hand and hold the labia apart with the index and fourth fingers of the nondominant hand, pressing against the meatus with the third finger. Next, have her lift the third finger from the meatus and insert the catheter. Have her partially empty the bladder, remove the catheter completely and recatheterize herself with the same catheter for additional practice. If she is able, have her use the bathroom for the next practice session and either sit on the toilet or stand facing it with one leg on the toilet seat. The standing position helps separate the labia. Most women can catheterize themselves without a mirror after a few days. Lubricant is optional for the female client.

Have a male client sit on or stand in front of the toilet, if he is able. Have him hold his penis at a right angle to the abdomen and insert a well-lubricated catheter far enough for the urine to flow. Instruct him to direct the urine flow into the toilet.

Teach clients to empty the bladder completely each time and always to empty the bladder at the scheduled time, even if they are not able to wash their hands or had not washed the catheter after the last use. After the bladder is empty, clients should wash their hands and the catheter with soap and water, then rinse the catheter, shake off the excess water, and store it in a clean plastic bag, toothbrush holder, or compact. If water is not available, commercial wet wipes may be substituted for handwashing. Advise clients to carry an extra catheter or two with them when they are away from home.

RECORDING

After inserting an indwelling catheter, record the size of the catheter, balloon capacity, the amount of water used to inflate the balloon, and the purpose for which the catheter was inserted. If the catheter was inserted to relieve urine retention, record data about bladder distention and urinary output before inserting the catheter, and record the amount of urine that drained from the bladder during the first 30 to 45 minutes after the catheter was inserted. If an in-and-out catheterization was done for residual urine, record the amount of urine voided, the amount of urine obtained through the catheter, and the time interval between voiding and catheterizing.

Record the client's reaction to the procedure, his or her ability to assume and maintain the needed position and willingness to cooperate with the procedure. If the catheter was irrigated, indicate the reason for the irrigation, the type and amount of solution used, whether the aspiration port was used or the system separated, and the characteristics of the returned fluid. Recording also includes whether a urine specimen was sent to the laboratory, the time, the purpose, and whether it was obtained through the aspiration port or directly from the catheter. Always indicate the amount of urine obtained and include a description of the color, appearance, and odor of the urine obtained by catheterization or when emptying the drainage collection bag. Report any unusual findings to the nursing supervisor or the attending physician.

Sample POR Recording
- S—"I don't think my catheter's working right! I feel like I need to go to the bathroom!"
- O—No urine in drainage tubing. Tubing kinked and under client. Catheter drained 300 ml urine in 10 min after tubing repositioned. Urine is clear amber with a few visible mucous shreds.
- A—Positional catheter malfunction.
- P—Relocated drainage bag nearer foot of bed. Reinforced teaching re importance of drainage tubing position. Check position and catheter drainage q 2–3 hr.

Sample Narrative Recording
Experienced strong urge to void. Catheter found kinked under client. Catheter drained 300 ml urine in 10 min after repositioning drainage bag near foot of bed. Teaching reinforced re importance of drainage tubing position. Tubing checked q 2–3 hr during remainder of shift. Urine is clear and amber with a few mucous shreds.

☐ CRITICAL POINTS SUMMARY

1. Catheterization is used selectively for specific purposes rather than as a routine therapeutic measure.
2. Being catheterized and having an indwelling catheter in place is often emotionally distressing and perceived as an invasion of privacy.
3. The primary problem with indwelling catheters is the high incidence of urinary tract infection.
4. Women are at greater risk for developing a catheter-associated urinary tract infection than are men because the female urethra is shorter than the male and the meatus is in closer proximity to the anus.
5. Microorganisms may enter the bladder at the time of insertion, ascend around the catheter (extraluminal contamination), or ascend inside the catheter (intraluminal contamination).
6. Nursing interventions are of crucial importance in preventing urinary tract infections associated with indwelling catheters.
7. Catheter-associated urinary tract infections can be prevented by:
   a. Maintaining a completely closed catheter–drainage tubing–collection bag system.
   b. Providing daily soap and water perineal care.
   c. Positioning the drainage tubing and collection bag so there is a continuous downflow of urine.
   d. Careful handwashing before and after providing any care to any part of the catheter system.
   e. Avoiding touching the drainage port when emptying the collection bag.
   f. Using a separate container to empty each client's collection bag.
8. The risk of infection can be reduced by increasing fluid intake to 2000 to 2500 ml per day unless contraindicated.
9. Change an indwelling catheter when it contains concretions or is too soild to be cleared adequately.
10. Catheter irrigation is done only when specifically ordered, usually for actual or potential obstruc-

tion from mucus, blood, or other debris, but not sediment.
11. Use strict aseptic technique to irrigate a catheter either through the aspiration port or by separating the system.
12. Use strict aseptic technique and a syringe and needle to collect a urine specimen through the aspiration port or from the catheter.
13. Secure an indwelling catheter to the thigh (or abdomen for males) with enough slack to avoid pressure on the meatus.
14. Never raise the urine collection bag above the bladder level unless the catheter or tubing is clamped or pinched before the bag is raised; the clamp is not released until the bag is again below bladder level.
15. Forceful insertion of the catheter can damage the uretha.
16. Intermittent self-catheterization is often a successful alternative to an indwelling catheterization.
17. Intermittent catheterization is done with surgical aseptic technique in an institution and with clean technique at home.

☐ LEARNING ACTIVITIES

1. Examine several different kinds of urinary catheters; note the difference in consistency and composition. Note the French size, the balloon size for an indwelling catheter, and the type of balloon inflation inlet port.
2. Examine a drainage collection system, noting the location of the drainage tube entrance into the bag, the calibrations on the bag, and the manner in which the drainage port functions. Note whether there are any protections against accidental contamination of the drainage port.
3. Look at several kinds of catheterization kits; note the sequence of the equipment; identify the purpose for each item. Identify advantages and disadvantages of each type of kit.
4. Look at catheters that are secured to clients in several different ways and identify the advantages and disadvantages of each.
5. Interview persons who have been catheterized or have had indwelling catheters in place. Inquire about the nature of explanations they were given, how their privacy was protected, and what was for them the most uncomfortable or distressing part of being catheterized or having a catheter in place.
6. Interview several staff nurses and inquire about ways they have found to avoid separating a catheter system when providing care or transferring clients.
7. Interview an infection control nurse and inquire about the incidence of catheter-associated urinary tract infections in that institution and the measures that are currently being used to control those infections.

☐ REVIEW QUESTIONS

1. For what reason(s) is surgical aseptic technique used for inserting a catheter in both the acute- and home-care setting?
2. Why are women with an indwelling catheter more likely than men to develop a urinary tract infection?
3. What proportion of nosocomial infections are related to an indwelling catheter?
4. Give an example of both extraluminal and intraluminal microorganism entry into the bladder.
5. Where long-term use is indicated, what are the advantages of intermittent self-catheterization as opposed to an indwelling catheter?
6. Identify each of the following actions as correct (C) or incorrect (I) when caring for someone with an indwelling catheter. Explain your rationale for each choice.
    a. ____ Avoid showers or tub baths.
    b. ____ Avoid touching the drainage port of the collection bag to the side of the graduate used to empty the bag.
    c. ____ Empty a dependent loop of tubing by lifting it at the most dependent part.
    d. ____ Encourage bed rest.
    e. ____ Increase fluids to 2500 ml per day, unless contraindicated.
    f. ____ Insert a catheter with surgical aseptic technique.
    g. ____ Place the catheter drainage bag on the floor when the client is in a chair.
    h. ____ Place the collection bag on the client's abdomen when transferring him or her from the bed to a stretcher.
    i. ____ Provide perineal care on a bedpan.
    j. ____ Provide daily careful meatal care with an antiseptic solution.
    k. ____ Remove and reinsert a fresh indwelling catheter every 2 weeks.
    l. ____ Secure the catheter to the thigh so as to exert tension on the catheter.
    m. ____ Separate the catheter and drainage tubing to collect a urine specimen or irrigate a catheter.
    n. ____ Use clean technique for intermittent self-catheterization.
    o. ____ Use the same graduate to empty collection bags from several clients.
7. How would you (1) protect a client's privacy and (2) offer emotional support during each of the following activities?
    a. Ambulating in the hallway.
    b. Sitting in a chair.
    c. Emptying a drainage collection bag.
    d. Inserting an indwelling catheter.
    e. Irrigating an indwelling catheter.
    f. Removing an indwelling catheter.
    g. Transporting to another department.

PERFORMANCE CHECKLISTS

OBJECTIVE: To use surgical aseptic technique to insert a urinary catheter in a female client.

CHARACTERISTIC	RANGE OF ACCEPTABILITY	SATISFACTORY	UNSATISFACTORY
1. Validates order.	No deviation		
2. Washes hands.	No deviation		
3. Prepares equipment.	No deviation		
4. Explains procedure.	No deviation		
5. Closes door or draws curtains.	No deviation		
6. Places bed in working position.	No deviation		
7. Positions client in dorsal recumbent or lateral position.	No deviation		
8. Drapes with bath blanket.	No deviation		
9. Positions external light source to focus on perineum.	No deviation		
10. Works from side of bed that places dominant hand toward foot of bed.	No deviation		
11. Washes perineal area with soap and water.	Omit if area is not soiled.		
12. Places and opens catheterization kit about 45 cm (1½ ft) from perineal area.	Open drainage collection kit first if indwelling catheterization kit does not contain a preconnected catheter–drainage tubing system.		
13. If separate drainage system used, positions collection bag and tubing connector safely.	Omit if using preconnected system.		
14. Places edge of first drape under buttocks, touching only the corners.	No deviation		
15. Dons sterile gloves.	No deviation		
16. Discards fenestrated drape.	May place over perineal area or on lower abdomen if desired.		
17. Prepares equipment: a. Pours antiseptic on all but one absorbent ball. b. Opens urine specimen container. c. Tests Foley catheter balloon. d. Lubricates catheter.	No deviation No deviation Omit if using plain catheter. No deviation		
18. Separates labia with fingers of nondominant hand.	No deviation		
19. Uses forceps to cleanse labia and meatus with absorbent balls.	No deviation		
20. Cleanses from anterior to posterior with one stroke per absorbent ball, ending with meatus.	No deviation		
21. Inserts catheter with gloved dominant hand until urine flows (total depth of 5 to 7.5 cm (2 to 3 in)).	Insert additional 2.5 to 4 cm (1 to 1½ in) for indwelling catheter.		
22. Releases labia and holds catheter in place firmly until: a. Bladder is emptied. b. Foley balloon is inflated. c. Urine specimen is obtained.	 No deviation No deviation No deviation		
23. Secures indwelling catheter to inner thigh, allowing slack for movement.	No deviation		
24. Pinches and removes plain in-and-out catheter.	No deviation		

(continued)

CHARACTERISTIC	RANGE OF ACCEPTABILITY	SATISFACTORY	UNSATISFACTORY
25. Removes drapes and equipment.	No deviation		
26. Cleanses and dries perineal area.	No deviation		
27. Returns client to position of comfort and safety.	No deviaion		
28. Positions drainage bag and tubing correctly.	Will have been done earlier, if separate drainage system used.		
29. Measures urine.	Omit if indwelling catheter was inserted.		
30. Disposes of equipment.	No deviation		
31. Washes hands.	No deviation		
32. Reports and records findings.	No deviation		

OBJECTIVE: To use surgical aseptic technique to insert a urinary catheter in a male client.

CHARACTERISTIC	RANGE OF ACCEPTABILITY	SATISFACTORY	UNSATISFACTORY
1. Validates order.	No deviation		
2. Washes hands.	No deviation		
3. Prepares equipment.	No deviation		
4. Explains procedure.	No deviation		
5. Closes door or draws curtains.	No deviation		
6. Places bed in working position.	No deviation		
7. Positions client on back.	No deviation		
8. Drapes with bath blanket.	No deviation		
9. Works from side of bed that places dominant hand toward foot of bed.	No deviation		
10. Washes perineal area with soap and water.	Omit if area is not soiled.		
11. Places and opens catheterization kit on bed beside client's knees or on overbed table.	Open drainage collection kit first if indwelling catheterization kit does not contain a preconnected catheter–drainage tubing system.		
12. If separate drainage system is used, positions collection bag and tubing connector safely.	Omit if using preconnected system.		
13. Places first drape over legs near penis.	May don sterile gloves first, if preferred.		
14. Dons sterile gloves.	No deviation		
15. Places half-opened fenestrated drape on lower abdomen.	Discard drape, if preferred.		
16. Prepares equipment: a. Pours antiseptic on all but one absorbent ball. b. Opens urine specimen container. c. Tests Foley catheter balloon. d. Lubricates catheter.	No deviation No deviation No deviation No deviation		
17. Cleanses head of penis and meatus: a. Uses forceps to hold absorbent balls. b. Uses each ball for one stroke. c. Uses circular strokes from meatus outward.	No deviation No deviation No deviation		
18. Holds penis at right angle to body.	Adjust position downward toward client's abdomen if resistance encountered.		
19. Inserts catheter with gloved dominant hand until urine flows (total depth of 18 to 20 cm (7 to 8 in)).	Insert additional 5 to 7 cm (2 to 2½ in) for indwelling catheter.		

(continued)

PROFESSIONAL CLINICAL NURSING SKILLS

OBJECTIVE: To use surgical aseptic technique to insert a urinary catheter in a male client (cont.).

CHARACTERISTIC	RANGE OF ACCEPTABILITY	SATISFACTORY	UNSATISFACTORY
20. Holds catheter securely in place until: a. Bladder is emptied. b. Foley balloon is inflated. c. Urine specimen is obtained.	No deviation No deviation No deviation		
21. Secures indwelling catheter to inner thigh or abdomen, allowing slack for movement.	No deviation		
22. Pinches and removes a plain in-and-out catheter.	No deviation		
23. Removes drapes and equipment.	No deviation		
24. Cleanses and dries perineal area.	No deviation		
25. Returns client to position of comfort and safety.	No deviation		
26. Positions drainage bag and tubing correctly.	Will have been done earlier, if separate drainage system was used.		
27. Measures urine.	Omit if indwelling catheter was inserted.		
28. Disposes of equipment.	No deviation		
29. Washes hands.	No deviation		
30. Reports and records findings.	No deviation		

OBJECTIVE: To use surgical aseptic technique to irrigate a urinary catheter.

CHARACTERISTIC	RANGE OF ACCEPTABILITY	SATISFACTORY	UNSATISFACTORY
1. Validates physician's order.	No deviation		
2. Washes hands.	No deviation		
3. Prepares equipment.	No deviation		
4. Explains procedure.	No deviation		
5. Raises bed to comfortable working height.	No deviation		
6. Turns back linen to expose catheter junction.	No deviation		
7. To irrigate through aspiration port: a. Prepares solution. b. Clamps catheter tubing. c. Inserts solution with syringe and needle. d. Releases tubing. e. Observes for return gravity flow. f. Repeats procedure as needed or ordered.	No deviation Fold over and pinch tubing after cleansing if no clamp available. No deviation No deviation No deviation No deviation		
8. To irrigate through catheter lumen: a. Prepares solution and fills syringe. b. Places collection basin near junction. c. Removes tape seal at catheter–tubing junction. d. Cleanses junction with alcohol. e. Separates tubing from connector and holds tubing and catheter so as to avoid contaminating either opening. f. Covers connector with sterile protector and places in safe place. g. Inserts solution with catheter syringe. h. Removes syringe and allows fluid to return by gravity. i. Repeats as needed or ordered. j. Reconnects catheter and tubing without contamination. k. Retapes catheter–tubing junction.	May fill syringe just before using it. No deviation Omit if no seal present. No deviation No deviation No deviation No deviation No deviation No deviation No deviation No deviation		

(continued)

CHARACTERISTIC	RANGE OF ACCEPTABILITY	SATISFACTORY	UNSATISFACTORY
9. Returns client to position of comfort and safety.	No deviation		
10. Discards disposable equipment.	No deviation		
11. Washes hands.	No deviation		
12. Reports and records findings.	No deviation		

REFERENCES

Andriole V: Hospital acquired urinary infections and the indwelling catheter. Urology Clinics of North America 2(3):451–469, 1975.

Bates P: A troubleshooter's guide to indwelling catheters. RN 44(3):63–68, 1981.

Blannin JP: Catheter management. Nursing Times 78(11):438–441, 1982.

Burke JP, Garibaldi RA, et al: Prevention of catheter-associated urinary tract infections: Efficacy of daily meatal care regimens. American Journal of Medicine 70(3):665–658, 1981.

Champion VL: Clean technique for intermittent self-catheterization. Nursing Research 25(1):13–18, 1976.

Cunha BA: Nosocomial urinary tract infection. Heart and Lung 11(6):545–551, 1982.

Dobbins J, Gleit C: Experience with the lateral position for catheterization. Nursing Clinics of North America 6(2)373–375, 1971.

Ferrie BG, Glen ES, Hunter B: Long-term urethral catheter drainage. British Medical Journal 2(6197):1046–1047, 1979.

Garibaldi RA, Burke JP, et al: Meatal colonization and catheter-associated bacteriuria. New England Journal of Medicine 303(6):316–318, 1980.

Garibaldi RA, Burke JP, et al: Factors predisposing to bacteriuria during indwelling urethral catheterization. New England Journal of Medicine 291(5):215–219, 1974.

Gurevich I: The new urine meters: A Nursing80 product survey. Nursing80 10(12):47–52, 1980.

Gurevich I: Selection criteria for closed urinary drainage system. Supervisor Nurse 10(2):39–43, 1979.

Haley RW, Schaberg DR, et al: Extra charges and prolongation of stay attributable to nosocomial infections: A prospective interhospital comparison. American Journal of Medicine 70(1):51–57, 1981.

Kinney AB, Blount M, Dowell M: Urethral catheterization: Pros and cons of an invasive but sometimes essential procedure. Geriatric Nursing 1(4):258–263, 1980.

Kunin CM: Detection, Prevention, and Management of Urinary Tract Infections, ed 3. Philadelphia, Lea & Ferbiger, 1979.

Lapides J, Diokno AC, et al: Further observation on self-catheterization. Journal of Urology 116(2):169–171, 1976.

Maki DG, Hennekens CH, Bennett JV: Prevention of catheter-associated urinary tract infection: An additional measure. Journal of the American Medical Association 221(11):1270–1271, 1972.

McGill S: Catheter management: It's the size that's important. Nursing Mirror 154(14):48–49, 1982.

Mocsny N: Puncturing catheter balloons. Nursing80 10(3):88, 1980.

Morel A: Urethral catheters—An ancient device. RN 35(4):41–44, 1972.

Parrott PL, Garibaldi RA, et al: CDC's urinary tract guidelines: What really works? Conversations in Infection Control 3(6):1–12, 1982.

Platt R, Polk BF, et al: Mortality associated with nosocomial urinary-tract infection. New England Journal of Medicine 307(11):637–642, 1982.

Priefer BA, Duthie EH, Gambert SR: Frequency of catheter change and clinical urinary tract infection. Urology XX(2):141–142, 1982.

Product Information. Bard Urological Division, CR Bard, Inc., Murray Hill, NJ, 1982.

Rowson L: The lateral position in catheterization. Nursing Clinics of North America 5(1):189–190, 1970.

Sheckler, WE: Hospital costs of nosocomial infections: A prospective three-month study in a community hospital. Infection Control 1:150–152, 1980.

Sorensen KC, Luckmann J: Basic Nursing: A Psychophysiologic Approach. Philadelphia, WB Saunders, 1979.

Steele RE: Personal communication, Indianapolis, Urologist, December 21, 1983.

Warren JW, Muncie HL, et al: Sequelae and management of urinary infection in the patient requiring chronic catheterization. Journal of Urology 125(1):1–8, 1981.

Williamson ML: Reducing post-catheterization bladder dysfunction by reconditioning. Nursing Research 31(1):28–31, 1982.

Wong ES (with Hooton TM): Guidelines for prevention of catheter-associated urinary tract infections. In Guidelines for the Prevention and Control of Nosocomial Infections. Atlanta, GA, Centers for Disease Control, 1981.

BIBLIOGRAPHY

Altshuler A, Meyer J, Butz MKJ: Even children can learn to do clean self-catheterization. American Journal of Nursing 77(1):97–101, 1977.

Bielski M: Preventing infection in the catheterized patient. Nursing Clinics of North America 15(4):703–713, 1980.

Blannin JP, Hobden J: The catheter of choice. Nursing Times 76(48):2092–2093, 1980.

Clifford CM: Urinary tract infection—A brief selective review. International Journal of Nursing Studies 19(4):213–222, 1982.

Cule J: Forerunners of Foley. Nursing Mirror 150(8)(Suppl):i–vi, 1980.

DeGroot J: Urethral catheterization: Observing "niceties" prevents infections. Nursing76 6(12):51–55, 1976.

DeGroot J, Kunin CM: Indwelling catheters. American Journal of Nursing 75(3):448–449, 1975.

Friedman FB (ed): Why *not* use a Foley? RN 45(11):71–76, 1982.

Garner JS: Urinary catheter care. Nursing74 4(2):54–56, 1974.

Hartman M: Intermittent self-catheterization: Freeing your patient of the Foley. Nursing78 8(11):72–75, 1978.

Kennedy AP: The nursing management of patients with long-term indwelling catheters. Journal of Advanced Nursing 7(5):411–417, 1982.

Kluge RM, Rowan RL, et al: Play it safe with urethral catheters. Patient Care X(18):106–107, 1976.

Kunin CM: Indwelling urinary catheters. Journal of the American Medical Society 237(17):1859–1860, 1977.

Lapides J, Diokno AC, et al: Followup on unsterile intermittent self-catheterization. Journal of Urology 111(2):184–187, 1974.

Pinner RW, Haley RW, et al: High-cost nosocomial infections. Infection Control 3(2):143–149, 1982.

Platt R, Murdock B, et al: Reduction of mortality with nosocomial urinary tract infection. Lancet I(8330):893–897, 1983.

Reid RI, Pead PJ, et al: Comparison of urine bag-changing regimens in elderly catheterized patients. Lancet II(8301):754–756, 1982.

Rutala AA, Kennedy VA, et al: Serratia marcescens nosocomial infections of the urinary tract associated with urine measuring containers and urinometers. American Journal of Medicine 70(3):659–663, 1981.

Turck M, Stamm W: Nosocomial infection of the urinary tract. American Journal of Medicine 70(3):651–654, 1981.

Wentworth A, Cox B: Nursing the patient with a continent ileostomy. American Journal of Nursing 76(9):1424–1428, 1976.

Woodrow M, Wilsey G, Wiley N: Suprapubic catheters. Part I: A direct line to better drainage. Nursing76 6(10):40–45, 1976.

AUDIOVISUAL RESOURCES

Be Aware of the Urinary Catheter
Slide-cassette. (1978, Color, 18 min.)
Available through:
University of Michigan
Medical Center Media Library
Ann Arbor, MI 48109

Bladder Catheterization
Videorecording. (1982, 15 min.)
Available through:
Southern University School of Medicine
Medical Television
Carbondale, IL 62901

Care of the Ostomate
Videocassette. (1984, Color, 29 min.)
Available through:
American Journal of Nursing Company
Educational Services Division
555 West 57th St.
New York, NY 10019

Foley Catheterization of the Female
Videorecording, 1 cassette. (1978, 6 min.)
Available through:
University of Washington
Health Sciences Learning Resources Center
Seattle, WA 98195

Infection Control III: Program 5. Urinary Catheter Procedures
Filmstrip and cassette. (1985, Color, 19 min.)
Available through:
Concept Media

SKILL 61 *Ostomy Care*

PREREQUISITE SKILLS

Skill 19, "Inspection"
Skill 28, "Handwashing"
Skill 57, "Bedpans and Urinals"
Skill 58, "Bowel Elimination Procedures"

☐ STUDENT OJBECTIVES

1. Identify the most common reasons for bowel and urinary diversions.
2. Describe three ways ostomies are constructed.
3. Define ileostomy, colostomy, urostomy, ileal conduit, and vesicostomy.
4. Differentiate between conventional and continent bowel and urinary ostomies.
5. Explain the relationship of a colostomy location to the character of the drainage and the care required.
6. Explain the differences in the care of an ileostomy and a sigmoid colostomy.
7. Identify the purposes of a colostomy irrigation.
8. Identify ways to manage common problems associated with an ostomy.
9. Discuss factors that influence a client's reaction and adaptation to having an ostomy.
10. Identify nursing interventions that enhance self-worth and social acceptance for a client with an ostomy.
11. Explain the importance of successful self-care in long-term management of an ostomy.
12. Identify advantages and disadvantages of disposable versus reusable and one-piece versus two-piece appliance systems.

13. Explain the purposes of various skin products designed for ostomy care.
14. Explain factors that contribute to leakproof ostomy appliance application.
15. Explain factors that contribute to successful and unsuccessful colostomy irrigation.
16. Change an ostomy appliance and pouch, using appropriate medical aseptic technique.
17. Irrigate a colostomy using appropriate medical aseptic technique.

☐ INTRODUCTION

Temporary or permanent bowel and urinary diversions are achieved through a surgical creation of an artificial opening into any portion of the intestinal or urinary tract, with the bowel or urinary tract sutured to the abdominal surface. The opening is called an ostomy and the bowel or urinary tissue forming the opening is called a stoma. An ostomy permits bowel and bladder elimination to take place when the usual anatomic routes are nonfunctional due to pathology, trauma, or birth defects. Ostomy is a general term that includes a colostomy (opening into the colon), ileostomy (opening into the ileum), or urostomy (opening into the urinary tract). The term *ostomate* is sometimes used to refer to a person who has an ostomy.

A colostomy was first used to relieve bowel obstruction in the mid-1700s, and ostomy care has been described in medical and nursing literature since the 1930s. The literature has always included recommendations that persons with ostomies be able to manage independently before leaving the hospital (Jackson and Broadwell, 1982).

The goals of ostomy management are (1) to provide a leakproof, odorproof, and socially acceptable way to contain bowel or urinary drainage and (2) to maintain the peristomal skin (skin around the stoma) in an intact and normal state. Most clients with urostomies, conventional ileostomies (see below), and some clients with colostomies must wear a pouch at all times. Clients with sigmoid colostomies can usually be regulated, primarily with irrigation, and do not need to wear a pouch. Clients with a continent ileostomy (see below) and vesicostomy (bladder opening) also do not need a pouch.

Because of the expanded technology and knowledge in the field of ostomy care, a relatively new nursing specialty has developed: that of enterostomal therapist (ET). In many agencies an enterostomal therapist assumes the primary responsibility for fitting all clients with an appropriate appliance and for teaching the client and a family member how to care for the stoma. It is important, however, that staff nurses know how to use ostomy appliances and provide stomal care, because they have more extended contact with the client and his or her family, and an enterostomal therapist is not always available. Clients also find it reassuring when staff nurses understand and can provide ostomy care (Mikolon, 1982). In one study, 21 percent of 138 hospitalized persons with ostomies specifically commented on the inadequate knowledge of ostomy care that nursing staff demonstrated (Achterberg et al., 1979). There is a high probability that a nurse practicing in any setting will need to provide some type of ostomy care because of the increased numbers of persons who, as a result of modern medical practice, have ostomies. It is not uncommon for infants, children, and handicapped persons to have an ostomy. Because these persons have highly complex needs, their care is usually managed by a nurse who specializes in ostomy care, and is not discussed here.

This skill presents the common aspects of appliance and skin care methods used for all ostomies, as well as differences that depend on the type of ostomy and its anatomic location. Because of continuing new developments in ostomy equipment, a general approach to using ostomy equipment is presented. This background, plus current professional literature and manufacturers' directions, will enable the nurse to adapt to a variety of equipment styles. Although teaching self-care to a client with an ostomy is a crucial aspect of nursing care, that aspect is beyond the scope of this text. The nurse is expected, however, to be aware of and participate in the teaching plan developed by the ostomy therapist.

☐ PREPARATION

The management goal for any client with an ostomy of any kind is to provide leakproof and odorproof containment of ostomy drainage or regulation of a sigmoid colostomy so as to maintain the integrity of the peristomal skin. A variety of ostomy appliances and other equipment is available to help achieve this goal. An ostomy appliance is a disposable or reusable pouch that is attached to a disposable self-adherent wafer or a reusable faceplate. It is designed to fit around the stoma on the peristomal skin (skin around the stoma). The pouch may be closed or open at the bottom to allow drainage of ostomy effluent without removing the pouch.

BOWEL DIVERSIONS

The bowel may be diverted from its usual functional route and connected to the abdomen at any point from the ileum to the sigmoid colon, as shown in Figure 61–1. Depending on the surgical procedure used in creating a bowel diversion, the resulting ostomy is known as an end, double-barreled, or loop ostomy, as shown in Figure 61–2. In an *end ostomy* (Fig. 61–2A), a single stoma is created and the distal portion of the bowel is surgically removed or left in place as a blind pouch. In a *double-barreled ostomy* (Fig. 61–2B), the

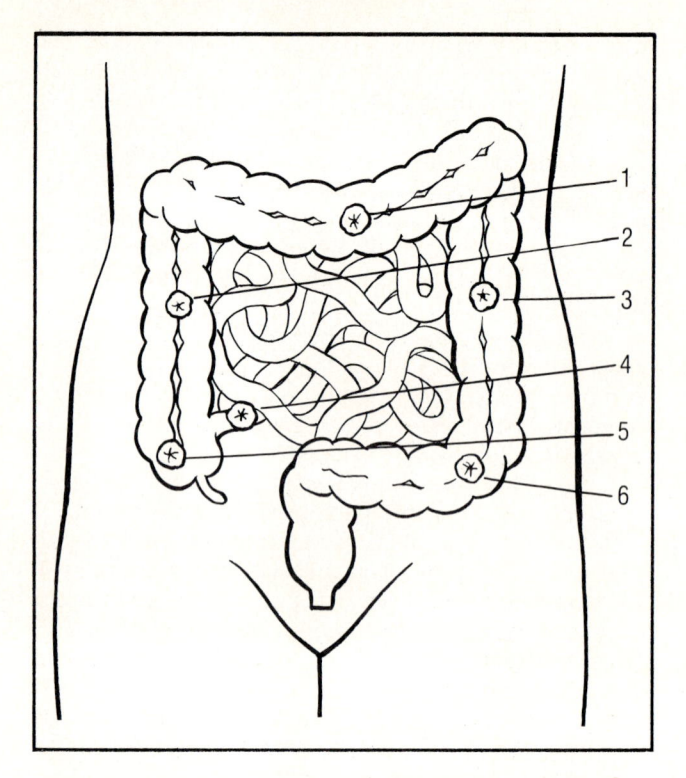

Figure 61-1. Common locations and names of bowel diversions. **1.** Transverse colostomy. **2.** Ascending colostomy. **3.** Descending colostomy. **4.** Ileostomy. **5.** Cecostomy. **6.** Sigmoid colostomy.

bowel is completely severed and two stomas (openings) are created. The proximal or functional stoma drains stool, and the distal or nonfunctioning stoma drains mucus. A *loop ostomy* (Fig. 61-2C) has one stoma that opens into both the proximal and distal bowel segments. Only the anterior portion of the bowel is opened, leaving a connecting wall between the proximal and distal segments. This type of ostomy is usually done as a temporary measure and later is either closed or redone as an end ostomy.

A healthy intestinal stoma is red or pink in color. It may be flush with the skin, inverted, or protruding. Because it is a part of the bowel, the stoma produces mucus and has slight visible peristaltic movements. Since the bowel is a nonsterile organ, the stoma is handled with clean nongloved hands. The stoma has no pain sensations but may bleed if handled carelessly. However, the peristomal skin has pain sensation and is especially tender during the first 8 to 10 days after surgery. A newly created stoma will gradually shrink in size. After about 6 months to 1 year the ideal intestinal stoma rises about 2 cm (¾ in) above the skin level. Because of the peristaltic movements in the stoma, water will not enter the stoma during bathing. For aesthetic and hygienic reasons, however, a stoma cap or pouch should be worn when swimming.

Colostomy

A colostomy is a surgically created opening that connects the colon to the surface of the abdomen and allows feces to exit at that point. A colostomy may be created at any point in the colon from the cecum to the sigmoid colon, as was shown in Figure 61-1.

A *temporary* colostomy is created when the surgeon anticipates being able to restore the bowel to its original state at some future time. The client's condition does not always permit the major surgery involved in colostomy closure, however. A *permanent* colostomy involves complete or partial removal of the colon segment distal to the stoma. When the distal portion of the colon is not removed, that segment continues to secrete mucus, which is expelled either through a stoma known as a mucous fistula or through the rectum. Thus, a client with a colostomy may have the urge to defecate even though no feces is present in the rectum. The mucous fistula is often located in the distal end of the abdominal incision (Fig. 61-2D), but may be placed anywhere on the abdomen. A small dressing is usually worn over a mucous fistula to absorb the mucus that is discharged.

A *sigmoid colostomy* is the most common kind of permanent bowel diversion. It is an end colostomy that is most often performed for cancer of the rectum. Cancer of the rectum or colon often requires a surgical procedure referred to as an abdominoperineal resection. This procedure includes removal of the rectum and anus through a perineal incision.

A *descending colostomy* is an end colostomy created at any point in the descending colon and located somewhere on the left side of the abdomen. Its position may be quite similar to a sigmoid colostomy and often is distinguished only by the physician's report. A descending colostomy may be created when a large pelvic tumor is removed prior to instituting radiation therapy.

A *transverse colostomy* is the most frequently constructed temporary colostomy. In one study, 105 of 257 persons with transverse colostomies eventually had normal bowel function restored (Wara et al., 1981). Transverse colostomies are located at any point in the transverse colon. They are performed to relieve obstruction, inflammation, or to provide a temporary elimination route prior to repairing trauma or birth defects. They may also be done as a palliative measure on terminally ill patients, with no intent for closure. Transverse colostomies are often loop colostomies, in which a loop of bowel is brought to the abdominal surface and held in place with a glass rod or plastic colostomy bridge. The anterior bowel wall is opened, creating both a proximal functional stoma and a distal nonfunctioning or mucous stoma.

An *ascending colostomy* is located in the right lower quadrant of the abdomen. It is the least common type of colostomy, is usually temporary, and is performed in a similar manner to a transverse colostomy. A temporary *cecostomy* is sometimes done to relieve an obstruction. It may drain either through a tube or a stoma.

Since stool becomes more solid as it progresses through the large bowel because of the absorption of water from the fecal mass, the management of a colostomy depends on its anatomic location. The drainage from an ascending colostomy is liquid or semiliquid

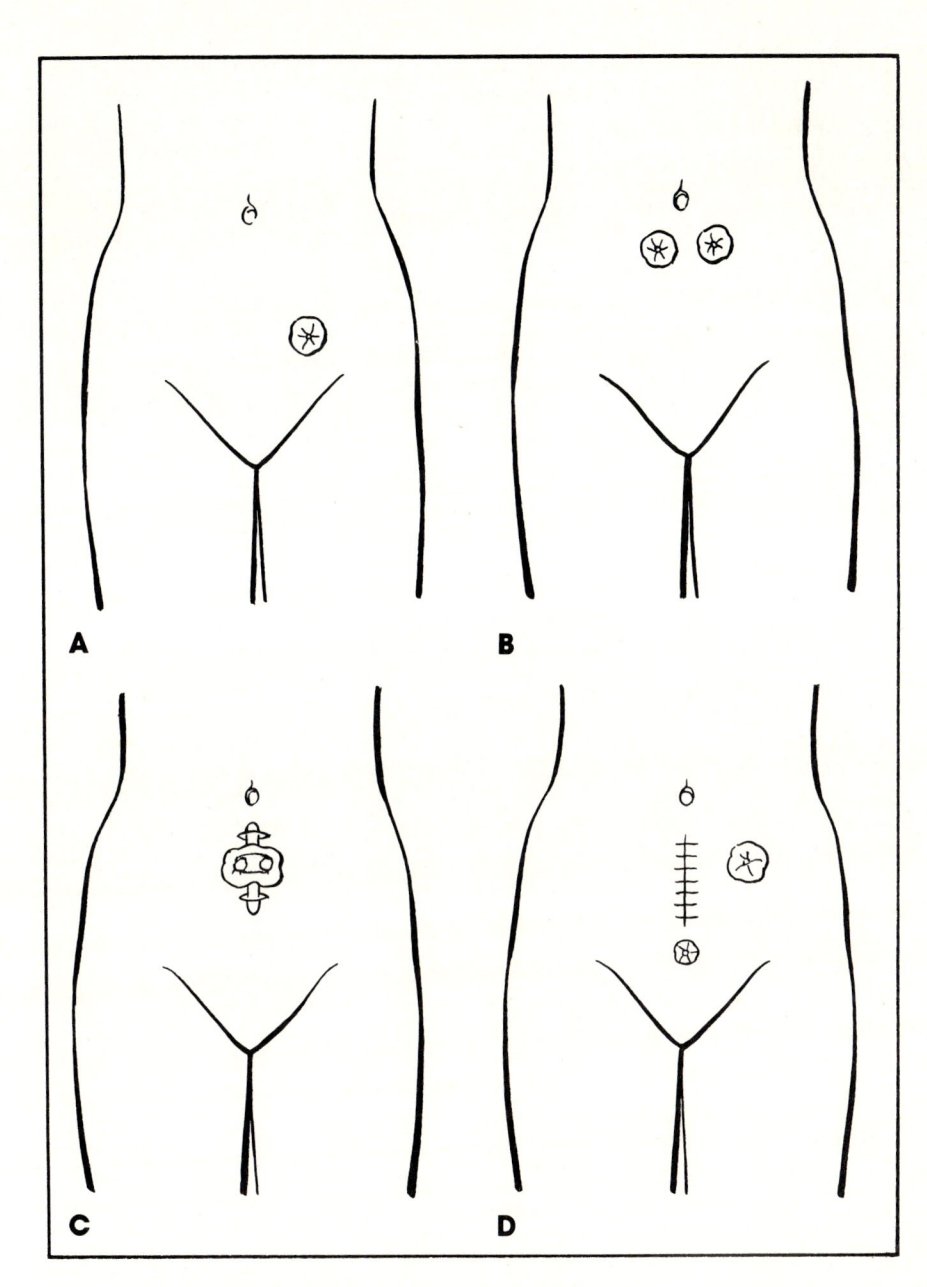

Figure 61-2. Four types of colostomies. A. End sigmoid colostomy, with single proximal stoma. B. Double-barreled transverse colostomy with the proximal stoma on the left and the distal stoma on the right. C. Loop transverse colostomy with an opening in the anterior bowel wall, allowing drainage from both the proximal and distal bowel segments. D. Descending colostomy with mucous fistula in distal end of incision.

and requires that a pouch be worn continuously. Drainage from a transverse colostomy is often quite malodorous and varies from a thick liquid if it is located on the right side to a more pasty consistency if it is on the left side. A transverse colostomy cannot be regulated and a pouch must be worn at all times.

A sigmoid colostomy will discharge loose stools in the initial postoperative period, but in a few days the stools will become formed and firm and regulation of bowel evacuation can be initiated. In the majority of persons with sigmoid colostomies, regulation and control of evacuation is most successfully achieved through irrigations. In general, persons who had regular bowel habits before a colostomy are more likely to be able to regulate their colostomies than those who had irregular bowel habits. A well-regulated colostomy requires only a cap or patch between evacuations. For some people, evacuation of a sigmoid colostomy is more successful when it occurs spontaneously and naturally into a drainable pouch, without irrigation. This is especially true for people who lack the capability of, time for, or interest in irrigating their colostomies, such as people with inadequate hand-to-eye coordination or insufficient strength, or those whose schedules or bathroom facilities make irrigation difficult. The function and care of a descending colostomy is similar to that of a sigmoid colostomy.

Colostomy Irrigations. Irrigation of a new sigmoid colostomy is usually begun 5 to 7 days postoperatively, when bowel sounds have been reestablished and flatus is passed through the colostomy. Irrigations are begun on a daily basis, and if no spillage of stool occurs between irrigations, irrigations on alternate days are tried. Although morning is the usual irrigation time, some people find evening irrigations fit their schedule better. Irrigation after meals generally produces better results because it takes advantage of the gastrocolic reflex and increased peristalsis that occur at that time.

A colostomy irrigation is similar to a tap-water or saline enema in that introduction of fluid into the colon stimulates peristalsis and produces an evacuation of feces. Instead of a rectal tube, an irrigation cone or a soft catheter with a shield is used to administer the solution. A conventional rectal tube may injure the bowel, and the cone or shield holds the solution in the colon since the stoma has no sphincter. An irrigation is used to produce colon evacuation at a time the client finds desirable and convenient and to avoid fecal drainage between evacuations. A colostomy will, however, function adequately without irrigation. Irrigations are done around the same time every day or every other day and take between 45 minutes and 1 hour for the total procedure. When done properly, one irrigation is usually sufficient for adequate evacuation. Like a tap-water enema, a colostomy irrigation is meant to stimulate evacuation of the distal colon, and not completely empty the colon.

Some advantages of irrigations are that the client regains control of his or her own fecal elimination, selects the time for the colostomy to evacuate stool, and may not need to wear a pouch between evacuations. Regular irrigation also seems to decrease the amount of flatus and odor the client experiences, since the number of intestinal bacteria is reduced by irrigations. Also, when there is no fecal drainage between irrigations, peristomal irritation is decreased.

Some disadvantages of irrigation include the fact that it is quite time consuming, bowel evacuations between irrigations may occur if the irrigation is not done correctly and completely or if elimination patterns change, and some people find the procedure repulsive.

Dietary Considerations. After surgery, a liquid diet is used at first, then a low-residue diet, and finally, a progression to a regular diet in a week or so. There are no specific dietary or fluid restrictions for a client with a colostomy. He or she is advised to maintain a well-balanced diet and may want to avoid foods that have previously caused gas, odor, and loose stools.

Ileostomy

A *conventional ileostomy* connects the distal end of the ileum to the abdominal surface. The most common conditions for which an ileostomy is performed are ulcerative colitis and Crohn's disease, both of which occur most often in young adults. An ileostomy may also be done for familial polyposis, cancer of the colon, congenital defects, and trauma to the colon.

With a permanent ileostomy, either a total colectomy and proctectomy (removal of the colon and rectum) or a partial colectomy is done. With a partial colectomy, the colon is removed but the rectal stump is left in the abdomen as a blind pouch or brought to the abdominal surface as a mucous fistula. A temporary ileostomy may be used to bypass or rest the colon, such as after abdominal trauma.

Initially after surgery, an ileostomy drains 2000 ml or more dark green, viscid and generally odorless fluid in a 24-hour period. Over a period of weeks and months, the drainage becomes thicker and changes to a yellow-brown color with a more characteristic fecal odor. This adaptation is the body's response to the absence of a colon where water and electrolytes are usually reabsorbed. A well-functioning adapted ileostomy drains 1000 ml or less in 24 hours (Wentworth, 1982).

A *continent ileostomy* (ileal reservoir) is a newer, somewhat experimental procedure in which an internal reservoir or pouch is created from a section of the terminal ileum and attached to the abdominal wall, as shown in Figure 61-3. A nipple valve formed by intussuscepting the terminal ileum keeps the fecal drainage in the pouch until a catheter is inserted to drain the fluid material. The capacity of this reservoir can be expanded gradually until it reaches about 500 ml

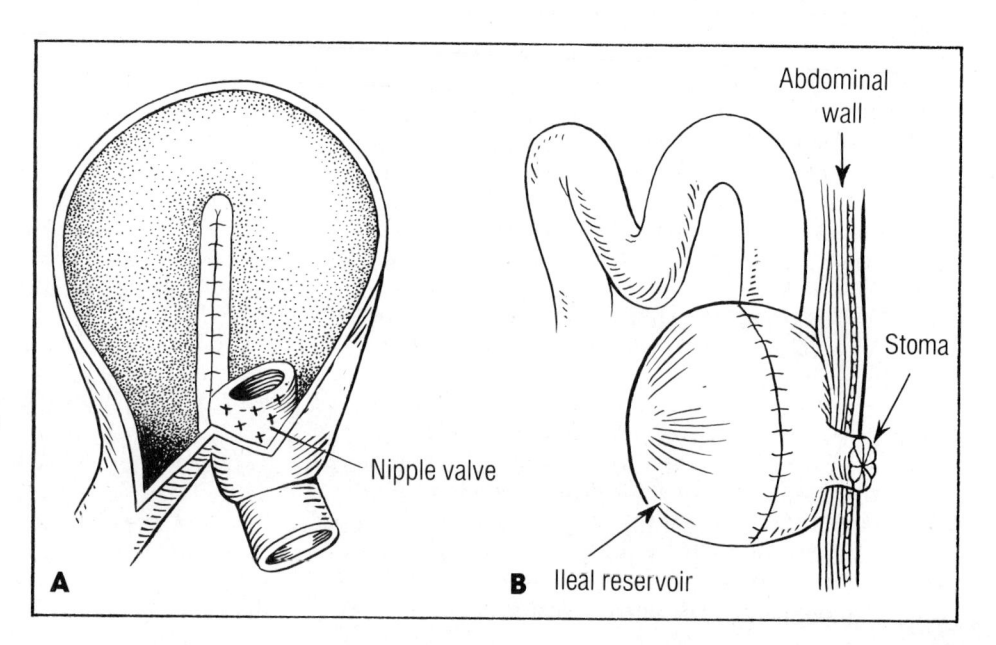

Figure 61-3. Continent ileostomy. *A.* A reservoir (pouch) is created out of a section of ileum, sutured to the abdominal wall, and a flush stoma created. As the reservoir fills, pressure closes the nipple valve at the ileal-reservoir junction until a catheter is inserted for drainage. *B.* The nipple valve is created by intussuscepting the terminal ileum backward into the ileal reservoir about 5 cm (2 in).

(Wentworth, 1982). Instead of a pouch, a patch is worn over the stoma to absorb mucus and protect the peristomal skin.

Because of the initial large volume of fluid losses after an ileostomy has been created, the client's fluid intake is monitored while he or she is in the hospital. The primary differences between the management of a conventional ileostomy and that of a colostomy are that drainage is constant, a pouch is always needed, regulation is not possible, and an ileostomy is not irrigated.

Initially the pouch on a conventional ileostomy is emptied frequently to avoid overfilling and loosening of the appliance. For home care, clients are usually taught to empty the pouch when they urinate or ½ to 1 hour after meals when the pouch is likely to be full and again before bedtime. Appliance changes are best done when the bowel is most quiet, such as before meals, several hours after meals, or at bedtime.

A functioning ileal reservoir must be intubated and drained three or four times in 24 hours. Average drainage time is 5 to 10 minutes, but if the fecal drainage is thickened, it may take up to 30 minutes. Specific management problems for ileostomies are discussed in the section on Common Problems in Ostomy Management.

A client with a conventional ileostomy will sometimes choose to have a continent ileostomy with an ileal reservoir created. He or she then has the freedom of not having to wear a pouch. However, it is sometimes more time consuming to drain an ileal reservoir and keep it patent than to care for a well-functioning conventional ileostomy. Psychological and physiological problems can arise when clients have unrealistic expectations from the surgery (Goldman and Rombeau, 1978).

URINARY DIVERSIONS

Urinary diversion with creation of a *urostomy* is accomplished in several ways. The distal ends of the ureters may be transplanted to the abdominal surface (cutaneous ureterostomy) or into a loop of the bowel, forming either an ileal or a colon conduit. Urine may also be diverted from the bladder directly to the abdominal surface, forming either a cutaneous or continent *vesicostomy*. Urostomies may be performed when part of the urinary tract is absent or malfunctions because of birth defects or is removed for cancer, or when normal voiding is impossible because of a neurogenic bladder. Several types of urinary diversions are shown in Figure 61-4.

A urostomy pouch is emptied about every 3 to 4 hours, depending on fluid intake. This interval can be extended if a leg bag is attached to the pouch. During the night, the pouch is connected to a leg bag or to straight drainage using a catheter drainage collection system (or a plastic jug for home use). The best time to change a urostomy pouch is in the morning or late at night when fluid intake and urine output are decreased. A rolled gauze, tampon, or dental wick can be held *over* the stoma to absorb the urine while the skin is being cleaned, dried, and prepared for a new appliance. Nothing is ever inserted into the stoma. Medical aseptic technique is used to apply a pouch to a urostomy.

Ureterostomy

A *cutaneous ureterostomy* may have one or two stomas located on the flanks or the abdominal wall. They may be permanent or temporary. A ureteral stoma is smaller than an intestinal stoma and when healthy, is slightly purple or flesh colored.

Ileal Conduit

An *ileal conduit* is currently the most popular type of urinary diversion. An ileal segment is resected, leaving the mesentery attached. One end is closed and the other attached to the abdominal surface, creating a stoma. The ureters are detached from the bladder and attached to the ileal segment, which simply serves as a conduit for urine. Urine drains continually from an ileal conduit; thus, a pouch is needed at all times. It is important for both the nurse and the client to understand that an ileal conduit is simply a conduit, not a reservoir or bladder, and cannot be controlled voluntarily.

A healthy ileal conduit stoma is pink or red because it consists of bowel tissue. If the bladder has been removed, an ileal conduit is a permanent procedure. For reasons beyond the scope of this text, the surgeon may elect to use a segment of colon rather than the ileum; however, the nursing care is the same as for an ileal conduit.

Ileal Bladder Conduit

An *ileal bladder conduit* (continent ileal reservoir) is similar in structure and function to a continent ileostomy, except that it contains urine. The ureters are attached to a pouch that is created surgically from a segment of the distal ileum, and a narrow canal connects the pouch to the abdominal surface where a stoma is created. A catheter is used to drain the urine from the ileal reservoir at regular intervals. No pouch is needed; a small dressing may be worn.

Vesicostomy

A *cutaneous vesicostomy* provides direct drainage of urine from the bladder into a pouch through a stoma that is flush with the skin. Used primarily for children, this diversion is usually a temporary one. In recent years, a *continent vesicostomy* has been used for some persons with a neurogenic and completely areflexic bladder. Similarly to a continent ileostomy, a nipple valve is created that allows urine to drain from the bladder only when a catheter is inserted and no pouch is needed (Barrett, 1979). Because of its location, it is difficult to keep a pouch on a vesicostomy.

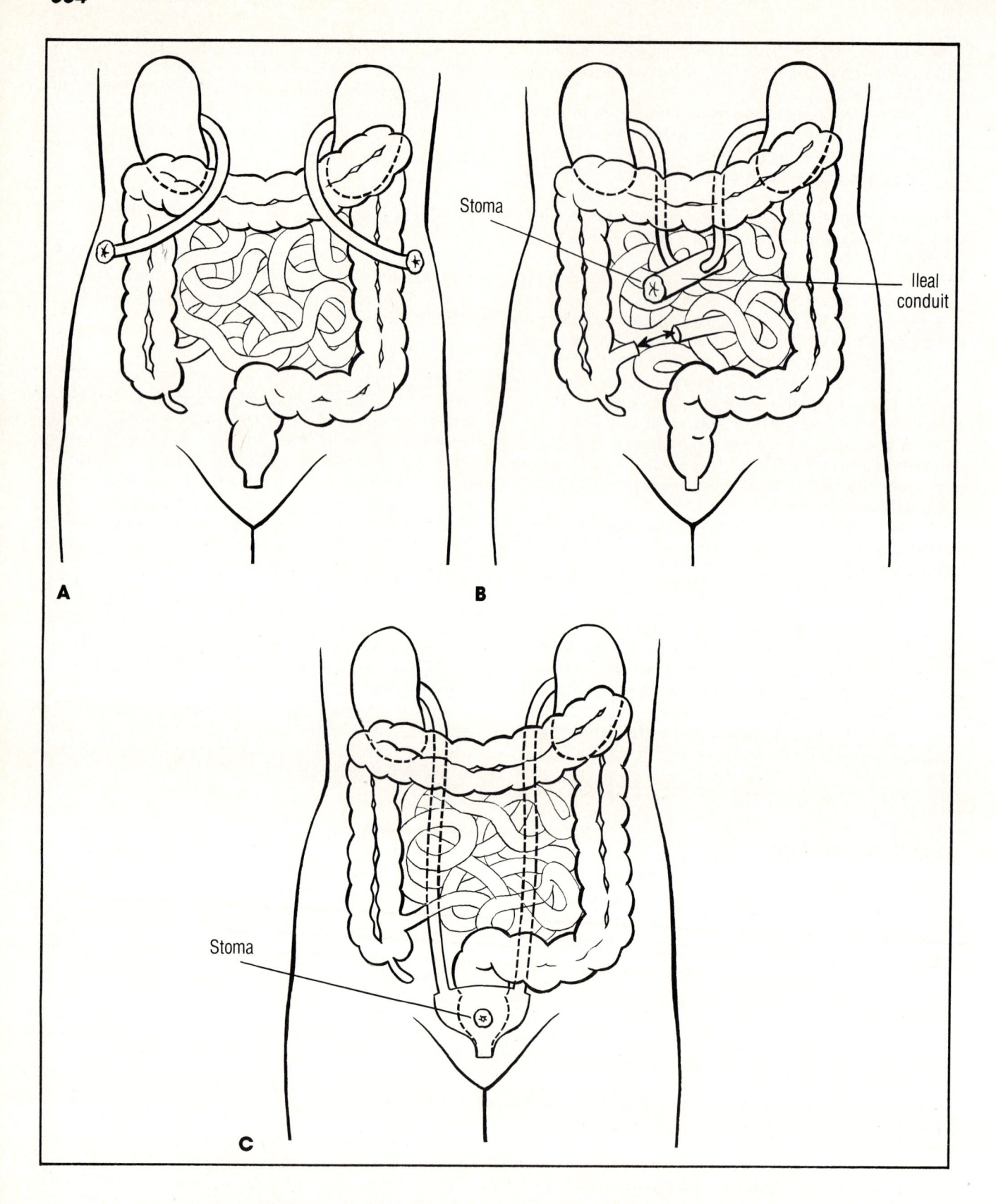

Figure 61–4. **A.** Bilateral cutaneous ureterostomy. Ureters are attached to the abdominal wall. **B.** Ileal conduit. A distal segment of the ileum is resected, leaving the mesentery intact. It is closed at one end and a 1 to 2 cm (½ to 1 in) abdominal stoma created, usually in the RLQ. **C.** Cutaneous vesicostomy. A surgical connection is created between the bladder and the skin surface.

COMMON PROBLEMS IN OSTOMY MANAGEMENT

Regardless of the type of ostomy, most persons with ostomies have problems with appliance leakage, skin irritation, and odor at some time. Persons with any bowel diversion may also have trouble with flatus and diarrhea, those with ileostomies may develop food blockage from excess fiber or residual food particles, and those with urinary diversion have an increased risk of developing urinary tract infection.

Leakage

Major sources of leakage are from pouches that are poorly fitted or poorly applied and are allowed to overfill because the weight of an overfull pouch tends to loosen the seal and allow leakage.

Leakage occurs when the appliance becomes visibly loosened from the skin. It also occurs when drainage seeps under the wafer or faceplate that holds the pouch in place. This is sometimes called "hidden leakage." When it occurs, most clients feel burning or itching in the peristomal area. Although the placement of the stoma affects the ease of pouching, a skilled enterostomal therapist can usually help fit a client with an appliance that has minimal leakage problems.

Skin Irritation

The peristomal skin can become irritated from the ostomy drainage itself or from practices associated with the use of appliances. To avoid irritation and actual erosion, the skin must be protected from the drainage and kept clean and dry and remain intact.

Fecal drainage from an ileostomy is highly irritating because the small bowel contains proteolytic digestive enzymes. Ileostomy drainage can cause skin erythema within several hours. Stool from the ascending and right transverse colon most likely contains some digestive enzymes and can cause similar problems (Watt, 1982).

Stool from a sigmoid colostomy does not contain these enzymes, but stool from any part of the colon is an irritant if left in continued contact with the skin. Urine is highly irritating to the peristomal skin and must be kept from direct contact with the skin or serious excoriation will occur.

Another source of skin irritation is stripping of the stratum corneum from overly rough and frequent removal of adhesive appliances, overly vigorous and excessive use of solvents to remove adhesives, or an overly vigorous drying and rubbing of the peristomal skin. Prevention of irritation and care of irritated skin are discussed in the section on Execution of this skill.

Odor

Odor control is especially important because urine and stool odors are considered socially unacceptable for most people. Regular emptying and careful cleaning of reusable appliances are crucial for odor control. It is helpful to use a pouch made of an odorproof material or one designed to control the odor released, such as those with replaceable charcoal filters. Deodorizers such as Banish (United), Ostomy Deodorant (Sween), or charcoal may be inserted into an ileostomy or colostomy pouch; deodorants such as Peri-wash (Sween) or Skin Care (Bard) can be used to clean the appliance and the peristomal skin if needed. Odors are also avoided when the lower end of a drainable ostomy pouch and the spout of a urostomy pouch are dried with toilet tissue after they have been emptied.

Some foods, such as cheese, fish, onions, and cucumbers produce more odorous feces, while foods such as buttermilk, yogurt, cranberry juice, and parsley decrease fecal odors for some people. Deodorizers such as bismuth subgallate or chlorophyll can be taken orally to control fecal odors. Foods such as asparagus and fish often produce odorous urine and vitamin C helps decrease urine odors for some people. Medications may also cause both feces and urine to become malodorous, as identified in Skill 57.

An alkaline urine and urinary tract infections contribute to urostomy odor. Urine can be acidified through diet or by placing 10 ml of vinegar into the pouch before applying it; urinary tract infections can be treated promptly by the physician.

Flatus

Flatus is an unavoidable source of odor with bowel diversion ostomies, since there is no sphincter control. Ways to decrease flatus are discussed in Skill 58. Gurgling sounds of flatus passing through an ileostomy or colostomy can be muffled by placing the hand gently over the stoma.

When gas accumulates in a pouch, it can be released in the bathroom. Sometimes nurses or clients prick holes in the pouch to release flatus. This practice also releases odors and is to be avoided.

Diarrhea

When diarrhea is caused by food, it can usually be controlled by adjusting the diet and eating less bulk and roughage. Since people with an ileostomy have decreased capacity for reabsorbing water, sodium, and potassium, they are at particular risk of developing fluid and electrolyte imbalance with diarrhea. If dietary adjustment and home remedies are not readily effective, a physician's assistance is required.

Food Blockage

Another common diet-related problem for people with an ileostomy is food blockage near the stoma from accumulation of cellulose. The ileum has limited capacity to expand and becomes obstructed at the stoma more readily than does a colostomy. Blockage can be prevented by eating slowly, chewing food thoroughly, and increasing fluid intake when eating high-fiber and cellulose foods such as popcorn and celery-type vegetables. These foods should be eaten in moderation and with other foods (Lamanske, 1977).

Clients who have continent ileal reservoirs can help keep their drainage liquefied by increasing their total intake and drinking grape or prune juice. If the ostomy does not drain readily, gentle pressure on the abdomen, coughing, or performing Valsalva's maneuver may help. The reservoir may also be irrigated several times with a syringe, catheter, and 30 to 40 ml of normal saline.

Urinary Tract Infections

There is a fairly high incidence of urinary tract infections in persons with ileal conduits. This is generally associated with reflux of urine into the ureters or with a conduit that does not drain properly and contains residual urine. To avoid urinary tract infections, clients are taught to observe their urine for color changes associated with hydration status and to drink 2 to 3 liters of liquid each day to provide adequate urine flow. They are also taught to recognize and report the signs and symptoms of a urinary tract infection: cloudy or foul-smelling urine, fever, chills, hematuria, and flank pain. To help avoid reflux during the night, clients are encouraged to connect the ostomy pouch to a leg bag (see Skill 59) or straight drainage (see Skill 60).

PSYCHOSOCIAL ADJUSTMENT TO AN OSTOMY

Psychosocial support and encouragement are crucial aspects of ostomy care. It is important to help the client accept and feel good about his or her ostomy because the client's feelings are projected to others and will influence how family and friends feel about the ostomy. Broadwell and Jackson (1982) cite several studies that indicate psychosocial adjustment after an ostomy is less successful than physiological functioning. Clients indicated a need for more information, counseling, and psychological and educational preparation before and after surgery.

The nurse's attitude about the ostomy influences the client's reaction. A nurse who is able to care for an ostomy willingly, without appearing disgusted, and in a knowledgeable way conveys the message that an ostomy is acceptable and manageable. Nurses do not wear gloves to handle bedpans and urinals. Wearing gloves while caring for an ostomy is therefore not necessary or recommended. Use of gloves tends to suggest that the ostomy is dirty and unacceptable.

A certified visitor from the local ostomy chapter can have a very positive effect on the client's adjustment, both by providing practical guidance from firsthand experience and by serving as a successful role model. The ostomy chapter tries to match age, sex, and type of stoma to the client. In many hospitals, the physician's consent is needed before such a visit may take place. Encourage clients to join the local and national ostomy chapters since excellent educational material is available, along with information about new products and practices.

Reaction to having an ostomy varies greatly. After having an ostomy, elimination becomes a public event, with nurses assisting in a formerly private function. It is unnatural for urine or feces to exit from the abdomen, clearly visible, unpredictably, and without control. Loss of elimination control is associated with loss of self-control, helplessness, and feelings of being infantile and dirty. Many people with ostomies lead quite normal and varied lives, although caring for a stoma and appliance is time consuming. Regular living habits help a person cope with an ostomy. Adaptation and adjustment will vary with the state of health, preoperative preparation, postoperative education and support, relationships with spouse and family, and attitude toward life in general. Initially, most people experience a sense of loss and go through a grieving process similar to that experienced with any loss. This normal process should be supported and encouraged, but it if persists, counseling before discharge is recommended.

For persons who have had cancer, a colostomy may be a reminder of a successful or unsuccessful bout with death. Regardless of the outcome, lingering fears often remain. People who have an ileostomy created for ulcerative colitis often welcome their ostomy as a life-saving measure that allows them a freedom and a normalcy that they have not experienced for many years. These people are usually young and active, but often physically emaciated and psychologically distressed from years of excessive and repeated bouts with diarrhea. As young adults, their concerns often focus on appearance, sexuality, activity level, profession or occupation, and having a family.

Sexuality is an issue often overlooked by healthcare professionals. Sexual function need not be altered for most women with an ostomy and is usually not impaired for males with an ileostomy when the rectum is excised for benign disease. However, sexual functioning is impaired for up to 50 percent of male patients with colostomies and rectal resection for malignant disease, primarily from damage to pelvic nerves (Kirkpatrick, 1980). References at the end of this skill include additional information about sexuality and the person with an ostomy (Dericks, 1974; Kirkpatrick, 1980; Shipes, 1982; Simmons, 1983; and Young, 1982). Ostomy publications available through the United Ostomy Association deal with sexual function, marriage, and pregnancy. Addresses are included at the end of this skill.

SELF-CARE FOR CLIENTS WITH OSTOMIES

The main focus of the nurse's care for a client with an ostomy is not simply to give care but to help him or her learn self-care and management of elimination, which enhances self-confidence and self-worth. In general, people are able to cope with an ostomy and recover more quickly when they understand their treatment and care and know what they are expected to do. Before a client with a new ostomy is discharged, if at all possible, he or she demonstrates self-care for pouching, irrigation, or both without supervision or assistance. This gives a measure of confidence about being able to cope at home and gives the nurse a chance to identify any problems or misunderstandings. Another family member is also taught how to provide care in case that is needed, but when family members are taught first, clients often continue to be dependent and never learn self-care.

Because there is so much to learn, explanations often need to be repeated and reinforced. A referral to a home-care agency is often helpful because the community nurse can evaluate the home setting and family capabilities and provide follow-up supervision after the client is discharged. To avoid confusion for the client, the community nurse reinforces and supports the plan of care taught at the hospital. In many larger cities, an enterostomal therapist is available as a consultant after the client is discharged.

DATA BASE

In some settings, persons with newly created ostomies are housed in specialty units where nurses develop increased skill in providing ostomy care. Nevertheless, people with ostomies are admitted to the hospital for a wide variety of reasons secondary to their existing ostomies, so it is important for nurses in all types of settings to be familiar with the kind of equipment used in their agency and to know agency policy for cleansing peristomal skin, changing appliances, and irrigating colostomies. Agency policies also specify the role of the enterostomal therapist in managing ostomy care. The enterostomal therapist always works collaboratively with the physician but may also function quite independently and is generally available for both direct care and nurse and client consultation.

Client History and Recorded Data

The client's health record provides information about the date and reason an ostomy was created, its placement on the abdomen (often including diagrams), whether the ostomy is permanent or temporary, and the person's progress and prognosis. This information helps the nurse offer support, provide appropriate explanations, and develop a relevant teaching plan. If there are two colostomy stomas, the physician indicates which stoma is functional and designates whether one or both will be irrigated. The physician's orders also specify any medications needed to prevent or treat peristomal skin problems and indicate the type and frequency of colostomy irrigations. If this information is not available, the physician or the enterostomal therapist is contacted.

When a person with an ostomy is admitted to a health-care agency, whether for purposes related or unrelated to the ostomy, it is important to record the client's home-care practices and an indication of the level of success of that self-care. As much as is possible, these practices are continued during hospitalization, unless the client's history or direct observation reveals serious problems in procedure. A physician's order is generally needed for these practices to be continued in the hospital setting.

Data about the client would include current participation in appliance change, irrigation, or both; the teaching plan and the teaching that has already been done; the activity level and medical or functional limitations that affect the client's ability to use the bathroom; and indicators of how well he or she is coping psychologically with the ostomy.

A data base about the status of the ostomy itself would include a description of the location, size, and color of the stoma; the condition of the peristomal skin; skin preparations used; and the amount and kind of drainage that usually occurs. Data about the appliance include the style of appliance used; the type of adhesives used to attach the appliance; the interval at which the pouch is emptied or changed, including when that was last done; and any problems with leakage, odors, or excessive flatus.

The nursing-care plan or kardex provides much of this information. Because the client's status may change rapidly, however, this information is validated by direct observation and interviews with the client and his or her family.

Physical Appraisal Skills

Inspection. On inspection, a healthy bowel tissue stoma, such as with a colostomy, ileostomy, or ileal conduit, is red or pink. A urinary tissue stoma, such as with a urostomy, is purple–gray or flesh colored. Inspection may reveal problems with the stoma such as edema, ulceration, or a dark red or cyanotic color from lack of adequate blood supply. Peristomal skin problems may also be evident, such as erythema, abrasions, folliculosis, hyperplasia, ulceration, and erosion.

The nurse inspects the appliance for leakage under the pouch to identify if the pouch needs to be emptied or changed, if two-piece systems are attached tightly, and if drainable pouches are closed securely. The wafer or faceplate is inspected to see if the opening is the correct size and is centered over the stoma. The wafer or faceplate should be tightly sealed to the abdomen with no loose areas or leaking.

Palpation. Gentle palpation around the stoma reveals any edema, induration, or excessive tenderness that may need to be called to the physician's attention. When a stoma is dilated with a finger, the sense of touch reveals the tightness of the stoma and the direction of the colon.

Auscultation. Before an order for an initial irrigation to a new colostomy is implemented, auscultation of bowel sounds reveals whether peristalsis has been reestablished.

Sense of Smell. The sense of smell reveals typical odors of urine, feces, or flatus, altered odors from dietary sources or urinary tract infections as discussed earlier, or the unpleasant odors associated with poor appliance care and hygiene.

EQUIPMENT

Ostomy Appliances

An ostomy appliance consists of a wafer or faceplate that fits around the stoma and a pouch to contain the ostomy drainage. Appliances are available in a wide variety of styles and sizes designed to accommodate a variety of needs. An appliance is selected and fitted individually, based on the person's anatomy, size, life style, and amount and type of ostomy drainage. Detailed information about specific brands of appliances can be obtained from package directions or from the manufacturer. An international listing of ostomy appliances and product manufacturers can be found in the references (Manufacturer's, 1982).

Ostomy appliances are of two general types—disposable and permanent. It is important that the nurse be able to distinguish between them. It is not uncommon for a nurse working in the operating room, emergency room, or on a general care unit to discard a client's permanent appliance, mistakenly thinking all ostomy appliances are disposable. Permanent appliances are quite expensive and represent an investment that should be handled with care. They are, however, considerably more economical for long-term usage than disposable appliances.

Permanent Appliances. Several permanent appliances are shown in Figure 61-5. A permanent appliance has a hard or flexible plastic faceplate that fits around the stoma and a reusable pouch made of soft rubber or vinyl. The faceplate is held in place with an adhesive disc with or without an ostomy belt. The pouch collar is stretched over the flange that surrounds the stoma opening in the faceplate. The pouch is held in place with a firm elastic band and bead known as a Bead-O-Ring. After the elastic band is placed around the flange, the bead is pulled into place snugly against the flange, tightening the elastic and holding the pouch collar firmly in place, as shown in Figure 61-6. Sometimes a stiff, hard rubber ring known as an O-ring is used to hold the pouch in place.

Vinyl pouches look and feel more substantial than the disposable pouches described below; they can be reused for 4 to 6 months. An ostomate has at least two permanent appliances so that a clean one is always ready for use. A permanent pouch may be changed daily. It is rinsed with cool water, washed with mild dish detergent and warm water and rinsed. It is then soaked in a bleach solution (60 ml per L, or ¼ c per qt) for 20 minutes and rinsed again. To remove urine crystals from a urostomy pouch, it is soaked in full strength white vinegar for 20 minutes and then rinsed with water. The pouch may be towel-dried or have a frame or towel placed inside it to keep the sides apart while drying.

Permanent reusable pouches are drainable; that is, they are open at the lower end to allow for drainage of the urinary or fecal contents. Pouches used for bowel diversion have a wide flat opening that is closed by folding the end over and fastening it with a snap-lock closure or rubber bands. Pouches used for urinary diversion have a leakproof drainage valve or tap at the bottom for easy drainage of liquid contents.

Disposable Appliances. Several styles of disposable appliances are shown in Figure 61-7. Disposable appliances are available in one- or two-piece styles. A one-piece appliance consists of a pouch with an attached adhesive area around the stomal opening. This adhesive area is placed on a skin barrier that surrounds the stoma.

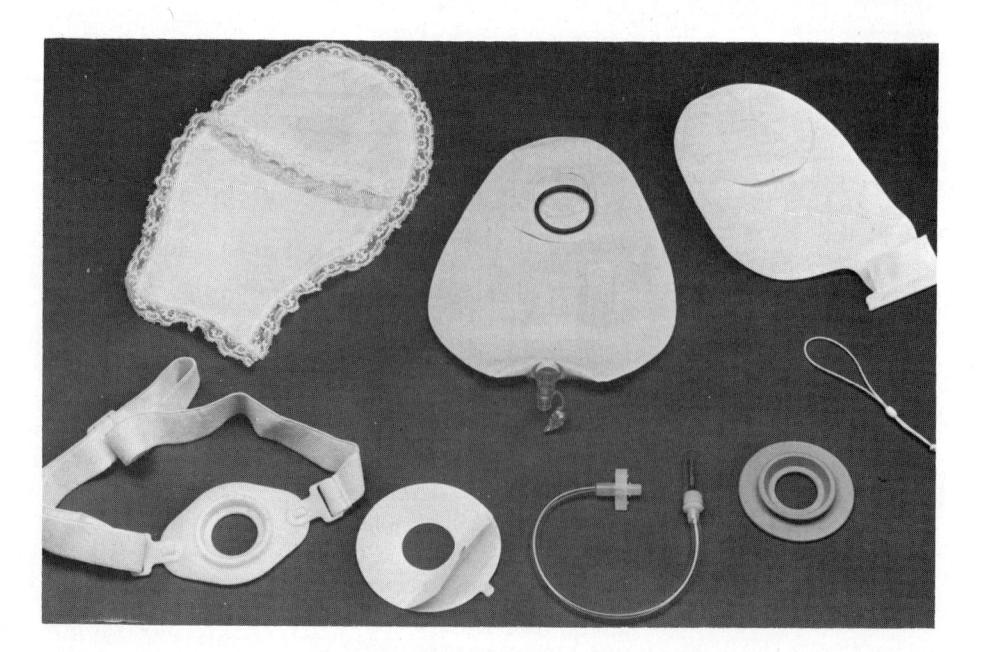

Figure 61-5. Permanent ostomy products. Clockwise, beginning at upper left: washable pouch cover, urostomy bag and an "O" ring, ileostomy bag, Bead-O-Ring, plastic faceplate, adaptor for connecting a urostomy bag to a leg bag, double adhesive disc, and plastic faceplate with adjustable belt.

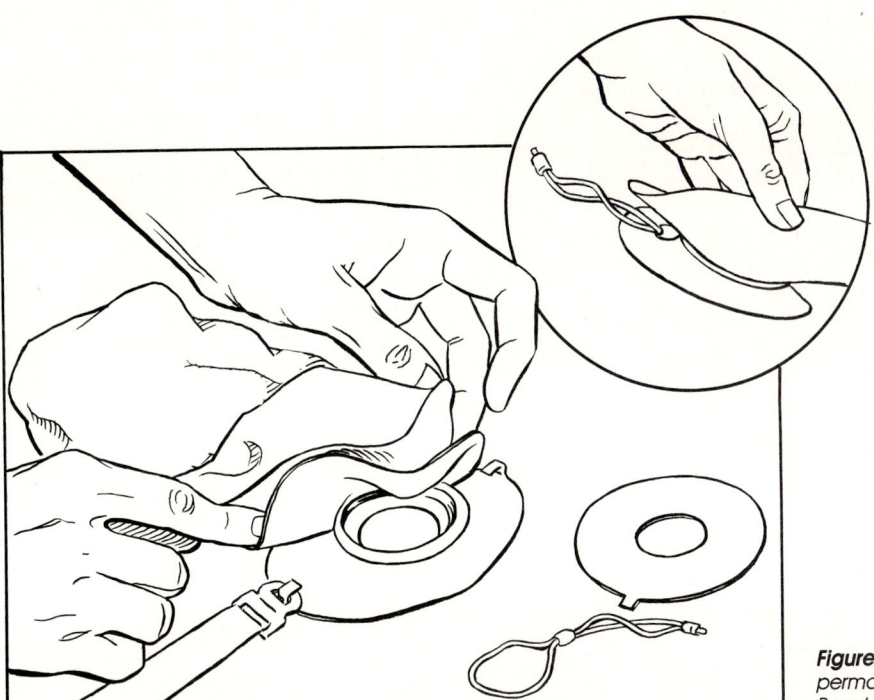

Figure 61–6. Permanent vinyl pouch applied to a permanent plastic faceplate and fastened with a Bead-O-Ring.

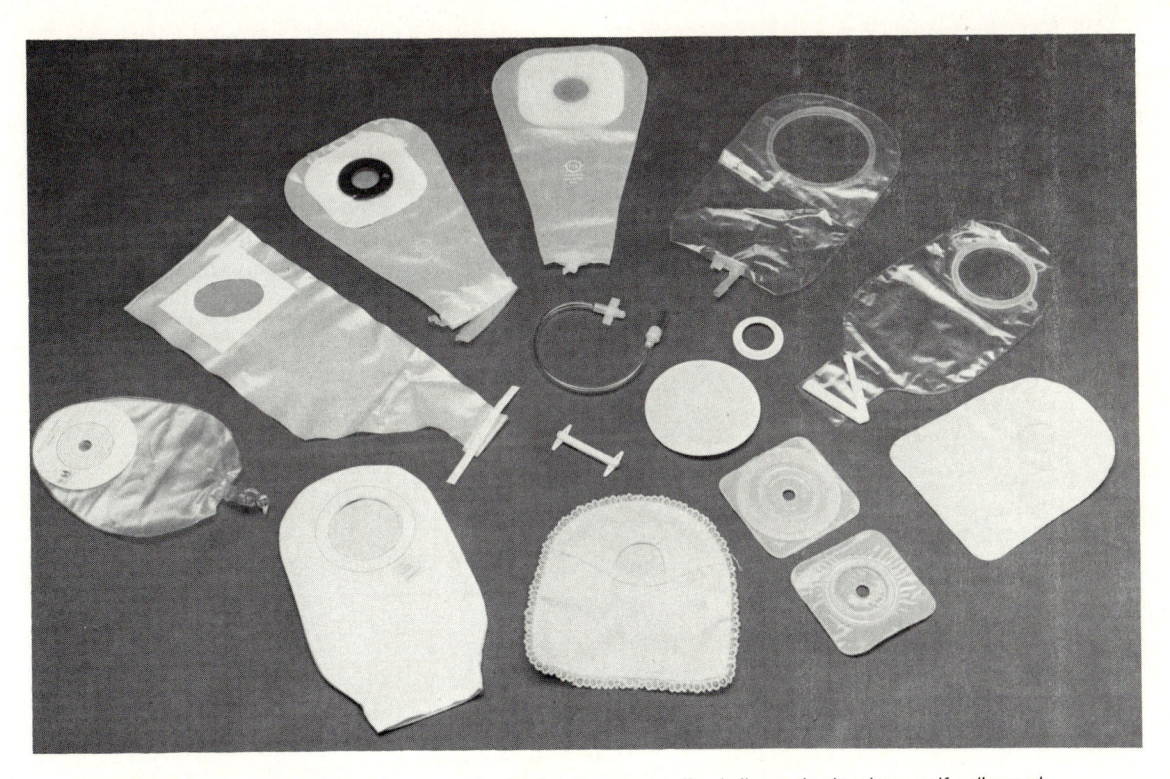

Figure 61–7. Disposable ostomy products. Appliances on the left are single-piece self-adherent pouches; those on the right consist of a two-piece pouch and flange. Note variable types of drains and closures on lower ends of pouches, and the degree of transparency of the pouches.

A two-piece disposable appliance system consists of a skin-barrier wafer with an attached plastic snap-on/snap-off circular flange and a separate disposable pouch. The pouch has a matching plastic ring that snaps securely onto the flange in a manner similar to plastic storage containers. The wafer may or may not have a precut stomal opening. The opening can be cut easily with scissors to fit around the stoma. The skin-barrier wafer can be left in place for up to 1 week, with a fresh pouch snapped into place as needed.

Several newer two-piece systems have a flexible accordion-style or floating flange, such as the Sur-Fit System (Squibb) and the Hollister Two-Piece Ostomy System. The fingers can be placed behind this flange so that the snap-on pressure is directed toward the fingers rather than on the abdomen, which may be tender after surgery (see Fig. 61–8).

Disposable ostomy pouches are made of clear, translucent, or opaque vinyl or plastic. Although they are less substantial than permanent reusable pouches, they can often be emptied, washed, rinsed, and reused several times. Many people find them more convenient than reusable pouches; they are more expensive to use than permanent appliance pouches, however. Clear pouches are normally used in hospitals after surgery so that the stoma and drainage can be monitored. For long-term use, most people prefer translucent or opaque pouches since they are not accustomed to looking at their urine and stool. Many people use a commercial or homemade cloth pouch cover for comfort, appearance, and to prevent a perspiration rash from developing under the pouch, especially in the summer.

A *stoma cap* is a small patch or cap that fits over the stoma. It is designed to give some protection, absorb mucus, and control odors with a built-in charcoal filter. Stoma caps may fit a two-piece snap-on/snap-off system or they may be a separate adhesive-backed patch.

Skin Protection Products

In addition to the appliance itself, a variety of products is often used to protect the peristomal skin, such as skin barriers, skin sealants, pastes, and powders. These products also help provide a more secure and leakproof fit for the appliance.

A *skin barrier* is a disc or wafer that is placed on the peristomal skin before the faceplate is put in place. It may be made of karaya (a natural gum from trees in India) or of a mixture of gelatin and pectin that may or may not contain karaya. Skin barriers are quite flexible, easily cut to fit around the stoma, and will adhere to the skin without an adhesive, simply by being held in place against the warm skin. Skin barriers protect the skin from contact with urinary or fecal drainage. They also help heal irritated skin, improve the wearability of the pouch, and serve as a filler for creases, dips, and scars around the stoma. Examples of nonkaraya skin barriers are Stomahesive (Squibb), HolliHesive (Hollister, Inc.), and Reliaseal (Bard). Tape is usually placed around the edges of the skin barrier to keep the edges from lifting, thus allowing the wafer to loosen.

A *skin sealant* is an alcohol-based solution used to provide a protective film over the skin before an appliance or adhesive tape is put in place. Skin sealants help prevent removal of the stratum corneum of the epidermis when the appliance is removed. They are not needed under a skin barrier. If done carefully, most barriers can be removed without removing superficial skin layers. Skin sealants also increase the adherence of permanent appliances. Examples of skin sealants include Skin Prep (United) and Hollister SkinGel. They are available as sprays, liquids, gels, or wipes. They should be used only on intact skin because of their high alcohol content.

Skin adhesives are available as sprays, latex skin cement, or double-faced discs. They are used to adhere a permanent faceplate or disposable appliance to the skin. Most adhesives can be removed with the pouch or rubbed off gently with the fingers or a dry gauze. Vigorous rubbing can cause skin irritation.

Pastes and *powders* are used to fill in uneven areas on the skin surface or open spaces between the stoma and the skin barrier. They are made of materials similar to those used for skin barriers and adhesives.

Colostomy Irrigation Equipment

The equipment used for a colostomy irrigation is similar to that used for a tap-water enema: warm tap water, container for the water, a cone-tip or a catheter

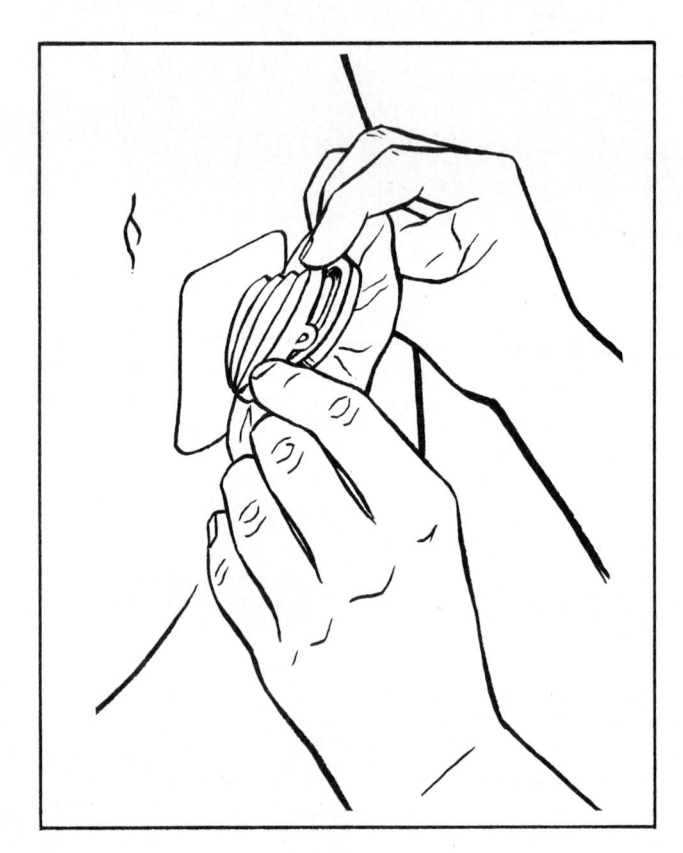

Figure 61–8. Barrier wafer with flexible flange and closed ostomy pouch with snap-on ring. To apply, place fingers beneath the flange and press the ring into place on flange.

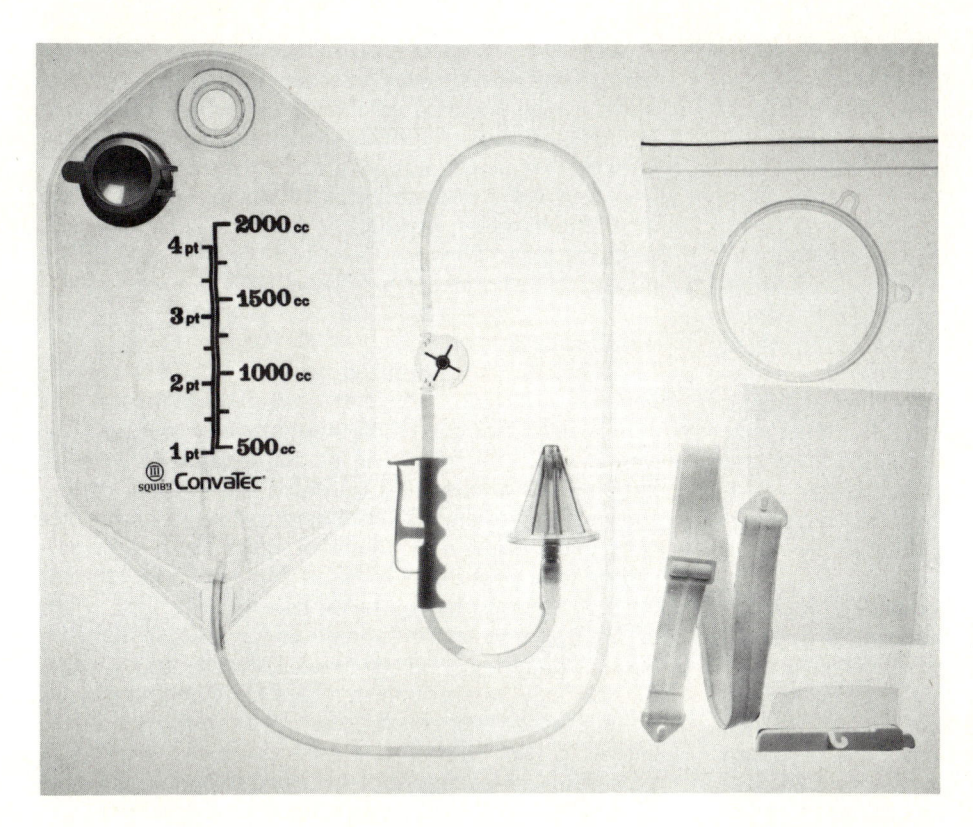

Figure 61-9. Visi-Flow Irrigation System for colostomy irrigations. Note regulator clamp, paddle-wheel flow indicator, irrigation cone, irrigation sleeve, and adjustable belt. (From Convatec, Division of ER Squibb and Sons, Inc., Princeton, NJ, with permission.)

with a shield, water-soluble lubricant, an irrigation sleeve, sleeve clips, and sometimes an ostomy belt (Fig. 61-9).

Tap water at a temperature of 40.5°C (105°F) is usually used for irrigating, although normal saline may be used.

Water containers are usually large plastic bags (1500 to 2000 ml capacity) with an attached connecting tube that has a regulating clamp for adjusting the rate of flow. One company (Squibb Convatec) has added a paddle-wheel flow indicator to the tubing near the thumb control. This device allows the client or nurse to determine whether the fluid is flowing by observing whether the paddle-wheel turns, rather than having to watch the fluid level in the irrigation container.

A *cone-tip* or a straight catheter with a *sliding shield* is used to administer the solution. The cone-tip is preferred over a straight catheter since it prevents backflow of fluid more effectively, gently dilates the stoma, and makes colon perforation almost impossible. A sliding shield is always used on a straight catheter to guide the insertion depth. The shield serves the same purposes as the cone-tip.

A *water-soluble lubricant* is needed for catheter insertion, but it is optional for cone-tip insertion.

An *irrigation sleeve* is used to contain the irrigation returns or direct them into the toilet. A typical sleeve is 75 cm (30 in) long, 20 cm (8 in) wide at the top, and 7.5 cm (3 in) wide at the bottom. A stoma opening is located on one side of the sleeve near the top edge. It may be designed to fit the snap-on/snap-off flange of a two-piece appliance system, be held in place with a belt, or be backed with an adhesive. Irrigation sleeves have either a slide-seal closure or a foldover top that closes with a flexible band or *sleeve clips*. These designs help keep the irrigant returns from splashing out when the cone-tip or catheter is removed from the stoma. An adjustable *ostomy belt* (described below) may be used to hold the sleeve in place if the sleeve is reusable.

Other Ostomy Products

An adjustable *ostomy belt* may be used to hold the irrigating sleeve in place around the stoma or to hold a permanent faceplate in place. A belt is not generally needed with the newer, wafer-style disposable appliances. If the stoma is below the waist, a belt tends to ride up on the hips and dislodge the pouch, sometimes causing injury to the stoma. If the stoma is at the waist, a belt is usually needed. An overly tight belt places undue pressure on the peristomal skin and may cause stomal prolapse or ulcers under the belt. If a belt is worn, it must be loose enough to accommodate two fingers being inserted between the belt and the skin.

Solvents are sometimes used to help dissolve the adhesive that holds the faceplate in place. They are available as sprays, liquids, or wipes and are to be used sparingly, if at all. The skin is washed and rinsed after solvents are used, since they are skin irritants and often cause allergic reactions. Examples of solvents are Uni-Solve Wipes (United) and Hollister Remover.

Other products available for ostomy care include greaseless skin conditioners and special soaps and skin cleansers that leave no residue or film on the peristomal skin. Examples of skin conditioners are Uni-Salve (United), Hollister Skin Conditioning Creme, and Hollister Moisture Barrier Skin Ointment.

☐ EXECUTION

When caring for a person with an ostomy, the technical skills with which the nurse is most often involved relate to preventing or treating peristomal skin irritation, preventing leakage, emptying pouches, changing appliances, or irrigating a colostomy. The nurse may also find that the appliance needs to be modified and can make a referral to the enterostomal therapist. However, for many people, the nurse's role is primarily that of instructing and assisting them in providing self-care.

In the immediate postoperative period, it is important to inspect the stoma frequently. If a bowel tissue stoma loses its red–pink color and becomes pale, cyanotic, purple, or dark red, notify the physician immediately since those changes indicate an interference with the blood supply to the stoma. It is easier to inspect a stoma if a transparent pouch is used so that it is not necessary to remove the pouch so often. If necessary, use a flashlight for adequate visualization of the stoma.

COPING WITH PROBLEMS

Peristomal Skin Irritation

Peristomal skin irritation is a common problem because of the frequent application and removal of adhesive products and from contact with irritating fecal or urinary drainage. Additionally, any ostomy care product is a potential allergen at any time. If the peristomal skin is already irritated, contact the enterostomal therapist or physician.

To prevent erythematous and irritated peristomal skin, wash the area with soap and water, rinse well, and pat dry. Avoid rubbing as it is abrasive to the stratum corneum of the epidermis. Apply a skin barrier such as Stomahesive or HolliHesive to the peristomal skin before attaching the appliance to an ileostomy, urostomy, or a colostomy with liquid and semiliquid fecal drainage. A skin barrier is usually not needed with the formed or semiformed stools of a sigmoid colostomy. Cut the stomal opening in the skin barrier so that it fits closely against the base of the stoma and protects all the peristomal skin without coming into contact with any part of the stoma tissue. Fill in any unprotected area around the stoma with an adhesive paste, protective powder, or karaya paste. Since karaya dissolves in liquids it is not useful with urostomies. A skin sealant protects against irritation because it provides a tighter and more occlusive seal between the skin and the appliance adhesive and minimizes skin stripping when the appliance is removed. If hair in the peristomal area needs to be shaved, use an electric razor—as a safety razor may irritate the skin or cut the stoma. Some skin barriers may be used on irritated skin, such as Stomahesive or HolliHesive, whereas others such as karaya are used only on dry, intact skin as a preventive measure. Various antibiotic and antifungal skin preparations are available in spray, powder, or paste form to help heal irritated skin. They are used only on the advice of a physician or enterostomal therapist.

Appliance Leakage

Leakage can be minimized by judicious use of skin barriers, adhesives, adaptors, and pastes. Be sure the skin is clean and dry before applying any product. Use a mild soap and rinse well, or use alcohol. Do not use bath oils or a soap that contains oils or cold cream, since adhesives and skin barriers will not stick to oily skin. When using a skin-barrier wafer, the weight of a full pouch is less likely to cause leakage under the wafer if it is supported by being framed with four strips of moisture-resistant nonallergenic adhesive tape. Some wafers have an attached adhesive tape frame.

Leakage can often be avoided by changing the appliance before it begins to leak. For example, if a wafer begins to leak on day 4, change it on day 3 the next time. Hidden leakage sometimes occurs when the seal around the stoma or between the barrier and pouch is not tight, and drainage can seep under the barrier or pouch. This hidden leakage may be signaled by burning and itching of the peristomal skin. To avoid this leakage, press the barrier and pouch firmly against the abdomen around the stoma and use a paste to fill in the space between the barrier and stoma.

REPLACING A POUCH

Empty a drainable pouch before removing it, since it is easier to empty while attached, and there is less chance of spilling when removing it. When a client with an ostomy is hospitalized, ostomy drainage is always measured to monitor fluid output. Inspect the stoma carefully while the pouch is removed.

To remove a pouch with a two-piece system, steady the wafer or accordion flange with one hand and loosen the upper part of the snap-on ring. Remove the entire ring, discard or empty the pouch, and then rinse it. To apply a new pouch, place the pouch ring over the faceplate flange, with the pouch at the desired angle. For bedfast clients, position the pouch so that it hangs downward toward the bed; for ambulatory clients, allow it to hang toward the thighs. Beginning at the bottom of the flange and working toward the top, apply gentle pressure around the ring until it clicks into a secure position. Tug gently downward to confirm that it is secure. If the flange is flexible and extends away from the wafer, place your fingers between the wafer and the client and press against your fingers to avoid pressing on the abdomen.

To remove a permanent pouch, remove the O-ring or Bead-O-Ring and place it in a secure place to guard against loss. Stretch the pouch opening slightly and remove it from the faceplate. To apply a fresh pouch, stretch the opening slightly and pull the collar over the faceplate flange until it is secure. Pull the ring over the pouch and flange so that it rests in the groove between the collar and pouch. Adjust the pouch so that there is no bunching or overlapping around the flange. Remove the protective paper from one side of a double adhesive disc and press it onto the faceplate. Prepare the peristomal skin as for a disposable appliance, using sealants, barriers, pastes, or cements as needed. Figure 61–8 shows application of a disposable pouch for a two-piece system and Figure 61–6 shows application of a permanent pouch to a permanent faceplate.

REPLACING AN APPLIANCE

Gather all equipment needed to provide skin care and attach the particular kind of appliance so that the procedure is not interrupted to obtain needed supplies. In general, it is best to use products from only one manufacturer for one client, thus avoiding confusion and possible incompatibility of parts and products. Encourage the client to do as much of the procedure as possible. Before replacing a urostomy appliance, have the client limit his or her fluid intake for 2 hours. This produces a temporary decrease in the amount of urinary drainage from the stoma and makes it easier to change the appliance.

If the client is wearing a belt, first unhook and remove it. To remove a skin-barrier wafer or faceplate, lift one corner and, while pulling gently with one hand, press the skin downward and away from the wafer or faceplate with the other hand until it is completely removed. Do not peel the wafer or faceplate from the skin because that can strip the stratum corneum of the epidermis.

Clean the stoma with warm water and a washcloth to remove mucus and drainage. Place a folded gauze, washcloth, or tampon over an ileostomy, urostomy, or draining colostomy while preparing the skin. If this is not done, drainage will run onto the clean skin and the preparation will need to be repeated. Never insert anything into the stoma.

Inspect and clean the peristomal skin, drying it thoroughly, as discussed earlier. If the skin is irritated, apply any medications or treatments the physician may have ordered. To prepare the skin barrier, cut the opening $1/16$ to $1/8$ inch larger than the stoma. If the pouch does not have an attached skin barrier, cut the opening $1/8$ to $1/4$ inch larger than the stoma so that it does not contact the stoma and cause injury. The opening in the wafer or faceplate must fit closely and snugly around the stoma. However, if it fits too closely, peristaltic movements of the stoma can cause the wafer or faceplate to loosen and leak. If it fits too snugly, the stoma may become edematous.

If the base of the stoma is smaller than the stoma tissue, the opening may be too small to fit over the stoma. If so, split the upper part of the barrier or disc from the opening outward; place it around the stoma so that the cut edges meet or slightly overlap and the barrier fits snugly around the base of the stoma. Fill any space around the stoma with a stoma paste. For additional security and a moisture-resistant seal, tape the four edges of the barrier.

The skin should be as dry as possible when a skin barrier is applied. Stomahesive and HolliHesive will adhere to a weeping skin, while ReliaSeal adheres only to dry skin. If a skin sealant is used, apply it to dry and intact skin and allow it to dry until tacky. Place the dull side of a separate skin barrier on the skin and apply the adhesive-backed pouch to the shiny side.

It is easier to apply any skin barrier or adhesive disc if you remove only half of the protective paper backing initially. Place the barrier or disc around the stoma, pressing the first half into place firmly and smoothly. Remove the paper backing on the second half and smooth it into place. Be sure to press firmly within the flange of a wafer and adjacent to the stoma.

Apply a one-piece system in a similar manner. Because of decreased access to the stoma with a drainable pouch and the absence of access with a closed pouch, apply stoma paste or a karaya ring around the stoma before applying the pouch. When using an opaque pouch, press your forefinger into the pouch opening from the closed side of the pouch to use as a guide for centering the opening over the stoma. Sometimes a dissolvable paper guide strip is placed around the stoma to help center the pouch opening over the stoma.

More specific procedures for using various brands of equipment will accompany that equipment or be found in the agency's procedure manual.

☐ SKILL SEQUENCE

REPLACING AN OSTOMY POUCH

Step	Rationale
1. Validate physician's or enterostomal therapist's orders for stoma care. Determine need for changing pouch.	Ensures appropriate intervention.
2. Wash hands.	Prevents transferring microorganisms.

(continued)

REPLACING AN OSTOMY POUCH (Cont.)

Step	Rationale
3. Assemble needed equipment and familiarize self with type of appliance used by client.	Prevents delays and interruptions during care. Increases nurse's confidence and skill.
4. Determine client's knowledge of procedure and explain as needed.	Involves client in self-care.
5. Raise bed to comfortable working height. Close door or draw curtains.	Promotes nurse safety; ensures client privacy.
6. Position client for maximum visibility of stoma and smooth abdominal contours. Drape and cover with bath blanket or towel to provide minimum exposure.	Provides easier application of leakproof pouch. Protects client's privacy.
7. Inspect pouching for security of seal and fit around stoma. Inquire about problems with pouching.	Enables nurse to follow previous method or modify as needed.
8. Prepare replacement permanent pouch, if used. Be sure faceplate is clean and dry and has had a sealant applied and allowed to dry.	Adhesive disc removes more completely if sealant is used first.
a. Peel protective paper from one side of a double-faced adhesive disc. Align opening in disc with opening in faceplate and smooth disc into place, working from center opening to outside edge of faceplate.	Bubbles or wrinkles may cause leakage.
b. Peel protective paper from other side of disc and set it aside, with adhesive side upward.	Pouch is prepared for application.
c. Close lower end of pouch.	Contains drainage.
9. Empty used drainable pouch into graduated container; note characteristics of contents, measure and record.	Provides ongoing data base.
10. Remove appliance:	
a. Remove belt if one is being worn.	Provides access to appliance.
b. Lift a corner of wafer or faceplate and slowly and gently press skin downward and away from wafer or faceplate. (NOTE: Use small amount of adhesive remover or solvent if needed. After solvent is used, wash skin thoroughly with soap and water, rinse, and pat dry.)	Rapid removal can remove superficial skin layers and cause skin irritation. Helps dissolve adhesives but is a skin irritant.
c. Discard disposable pouch and wafer in moisture-resistant trash bag (or newspapers for home use).	
d. Place a permanent pouch in moisture-resistant bag and set aside for later cleaning.	
11. Provide stoma care:	
a. Observe condition of stoma and peristomal skin.	Provides information for making needed modification in care.
b. Cleanse stoma and peristomal skin with warm water and damp washcloth if needed. Use soap and water if fecal material or urine is on the peristomal skin. Rinse and pat dry. Avoid rubbing.	Removes fecal or urinary deposits. Stoma is not fragile or sterile. Soap film under an appliance can cause skin irritation. Rubbing can cause skin abrasions. Skin must be dry for adhesives and barriers to adhere to skin.
c. Place folded gauze, toilet tissue, tampon, or soft facial tissues over stoma if drainage is constant.	Absorbs drainage and keeps peristomal skin dry during skin preparation and application of appliance.
d. Apply any medications or implement ordered treatment for irritated peristomal skin. Avoid oily or powdery substances.	Prevents excoriation or irritation, erosion, or infection. Appliance will not adhere to oily or powdered substances.
12. Apply skin barrier:	
a. Use measuring guide to cut opening in new skin barrier or barrier wafer so it fits 1/8 to 1/16 inch away from stoma. (NOTE: If using skin sealant, apply and allow to dry before applying skin barrier.)	Protects peristomal skin from irritation from contact with ostomy drainage. Avoids injury to stoma. Promotes tight seal.
b. Place skin barrier or barrier wafer evenly and tightly around stoma; press firmly into place.	Prevents seepage beneath barrier.
c. Use stoma paste to fill in area between stoma and barrier.	Protects skin and prevents seepage under wafer.
13. Close lower end of a drainable pouch with a clamp or rubber band, or close urostomy pouch valve. Place deodorant in pouch as ordered.	Prepares pouch for application. Helps control odors.
14. Apply pouch, keeping it flattened during application.	Keeping air out of pouch helps it lie flat on abdomen without bulging. Provides for tight seal.
a. Disposable pouch, two-piece system: Snap pouch ring of a two-piece system onto wafer flange, beginning at bottom and pressing it around toward top until ring clicks into a secure position. Tug downward gently on pouch.	Identifies if pouch is snapped in place correctly.

(continued)

Step	Rationale
b. Disposable pouch, one-piece system: Remove protective paper backing from adhesive-backed one-piece pouch and press into place with opening centered over stoma. (NOTE: A skin barrier may be applied before the pouch.)	Provides for tight seal.
c. Permanent pouch:	
(1) Position prepared faceplate around stoma. (NOTE: A skin barrier may be applied first. Fill in area between face plate and stoma with stoma paste.)	Necessary to hold a permanent appliance in place. Avoids leakage under faceplate and irritation of peristomal skin.
(2) Stretch pouch opening over flange of faceplate. Begin at bottom of flange and slowly work pouch collar up and over flange. With finger, feel if pouch fits smoothly on flange.	
(3) Slide Bead-O-Ring over pouch and place around flange and between collar and pouch. Pull bead tightly against flange. (NOTE: O-ring also may be used.)	Determines correct pouch placement. Anchors pouch and provides leakproof seal.
15. Frame edges of a skin barrier wafer with moisture-resistant nonallergenic adhesive tape.	Helps support weight of full pouch and avoids leakage of water during bathing.
16. Rinse used permanent pouch; wash with mild soap or detergent and water; rinse with water. Soak in bleach or vinegar solution as needed and rinse. Towel dry or hang to air dry.	Removes fecal contaminants; prevents odors and removes urine crystals.
17. Wash hands.	Avoids cross-contamination.
18. Report unusual findings. Record condition of stoma and peristomal skin; amount and character of drainage; medications used on skin or stoma; type of pouch used; and any skin sealants, barriers, cements, or pastes used in pouching. Record client's reaction to and participation in procedure.	Fulfills nurse accountability. Provides ongoing data base. Maintains continuity of client care.

COLOSTOMY IRRIGATION

When a client is having his or her colostomy irrigated for the first time, explain the procedure before beginning and encourage the person to help you with part of the irrigation, even if he or she plays only a small role. With each irrigation, match the increase in the amount of self-care to the rate at which the client is capable of learning. When clients with colostomies are admitted to a hospital for purposes not related to their colostomies, encourage them to do as much of their own irrigation and ostomy care as they are able. Irrigation time gives the nurse a chance to assess a client's methods and make suggestions for changes that might make care easier and more effective. However, support the client's usual practices and not push for change unless those practices are harmful. For example, in an effort to increase the effectiveness of the irrigation, some persons use several quarts of water and insert the catheter very deeply into the colon. Both of these practices are likely to cause leakage between irrigations, and deep insertion may cause colon perforation (Goode, 1982; Schauder, 1974).

A colostomy irrigation is very similar to a tap-water enema and has similar precautions and hazards about pressure and temperature. However, pressure is usually adjusted with a regulator clamp rather than with the height of the container.

Before irrigations are begun on a new colostomy, the physician often orders digital dilatation of the stoma. To do this, gently insert a heavily lubricated gloved finger into the stoma for a distance of 2 inches and leave it there for 1 minute (Goode, 1982). Although not recommended as a daily practice, dilatation is thought to relax the stoma and prevent stricture. It also helps the client learn the direction of the colon, which is helpful in directing the cone-tip or catheter in the correct direction.

The bathroom is the best place for a colostomy irrigation since that is the usual place for bowel elimination. Also, water is available for rinsing the sleeve and it is easy to dispose of the irrigation returns and control odors by regular flushing of the toilet. However, an irrigation can also be done with the client in bed. Be sure the bottom of the sleeve is clipped securely to prevent leakage in bed. When doing an irrigation in the bathroom, have the client sit on the toilet in the usual manner or on a chair facing the toilet, with the lower end of the sleeve in the toilet. Use a chair with a foam pad for a client with a recent abdominoperineal resection because a toilet seat or rubber ring causes much discomfort and places strain on the perineal sutures. A chair also works better for an obese person. Protect the client's privacy by closing the door or curtains, have him or her wear a short shirt or turn a hospital gown so it opens in the front, and place a towel over the lap to decrease exposure of the genital area.

Assemble all the equipment in the bathroom, including an intravenous pole on which to hang the irrigating fluid. When preparing the equipment, fill the irrigation container with 1500 ml of water so that 500

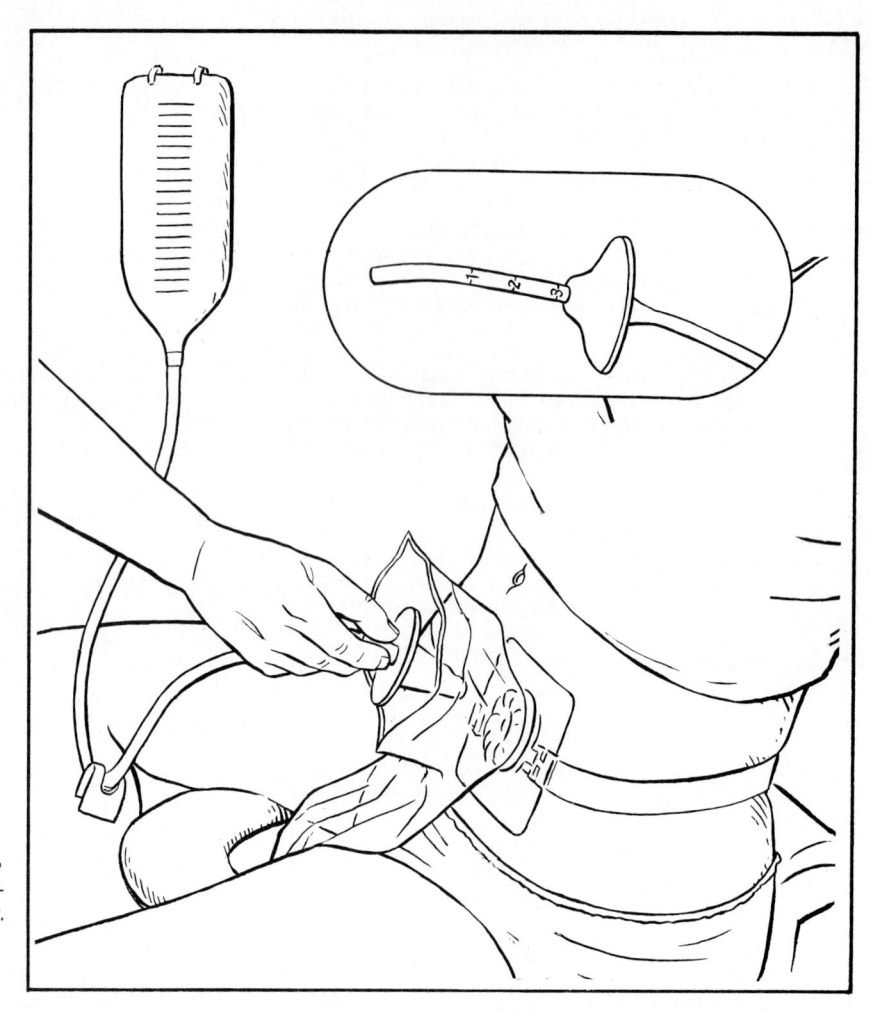

Figure 61-10. Colostomy irrigation using stoma cone and snap-top closure disposable irrigation sleeve. Patient is seated on toilet; irrigating solution is 45 cm (18 in) above stoma. **A.** Insert cone through top of irrigating sleeve. (Insert shows catheter with sliding shield.)

ml is available for rinsing the irrigation sleeve after the initial returns. After everything is assembled, remove the pouch or patch and place an irrigation sleeve over the stoma or snap a sleeve ring onto the flange of a two-piece wafer system. An ostomy belt may be used to hold the irrigation sleeve in place, even when using wafer-style equipment. This is because of the fluid weight the sleeve is required to hold during the irrigation. A wafer will need to be changed more frequently if it is used for irrigation without the additional support of a belt.

As with a tap-water enema, enough water needs to flow into the colon to produce distention and stimulate peristalsis. Since the stoma has no sphincter, a cone-tip or catheter shield is used to seal the stoma so the fluid will be retained in the colon. Slide the shield to a point 5 to 10 cm (2 to 4 in) from the distal tip of a straight soft catheter. If the catheter has no shield, insert it through a baby bottle nipple and use the nipple as a shield. Lubricate the distal 5 cm (2 in) of the straight catheter. Lubrication of the end of a cone-tip is optional, but excessive lubrication is likely to allow the cone to slip from the stoma and make it more difficult to achieve a tight seal in the stoma.

Reach in through the top opening of the sleeve to insert the cone-tip or catheter into the stoma (Fig. 61-10A). Hold the tip or shield firmly from the outside of the sleeve during the irrigation (Fig. 61-10B). Pull the top of the sleeve together around the tubing to avoid having fluid splash out of the sleeve.

Regulate the fluid flow with the regulator clamp or by adjusting the height of the container, as with a large-volume enema. The goal is to insert 1000 ml (500 ml for a first irrigation) over 10 to 15 minutes. If cramping occurs, slow the rate, as when giving a tap water enema. If leakage occurs around the cone-tip, adjust the angle of insertion rather than increasing the pressure exerted. After the desired amount of fluid is instilled, leave the cone-tip in place for a few minutes, since this helps stimulate peristalsis. A cramp similar to ones that accompany a bowel movement often signals that the colon is ready to evacuate (Schauder, 1974).

In most instances, fluid and some stool will return immediately when the cone-tip or catheter is removed. If the fluid does not return readily, have the client massage his or her abdomen, deep breathe, or change position. It is rarely necessary to siphon a colostomy irrigation. Remember that if a client is dehydrated, the colon will absorb water to restore fluid balance and less will be returned than was inserted. To avoid splashing out of the top of the sleeve, close a self-seal top or fold the top over twice and close it with clips.

After initial returns (10 or 15 minutes), rinse the

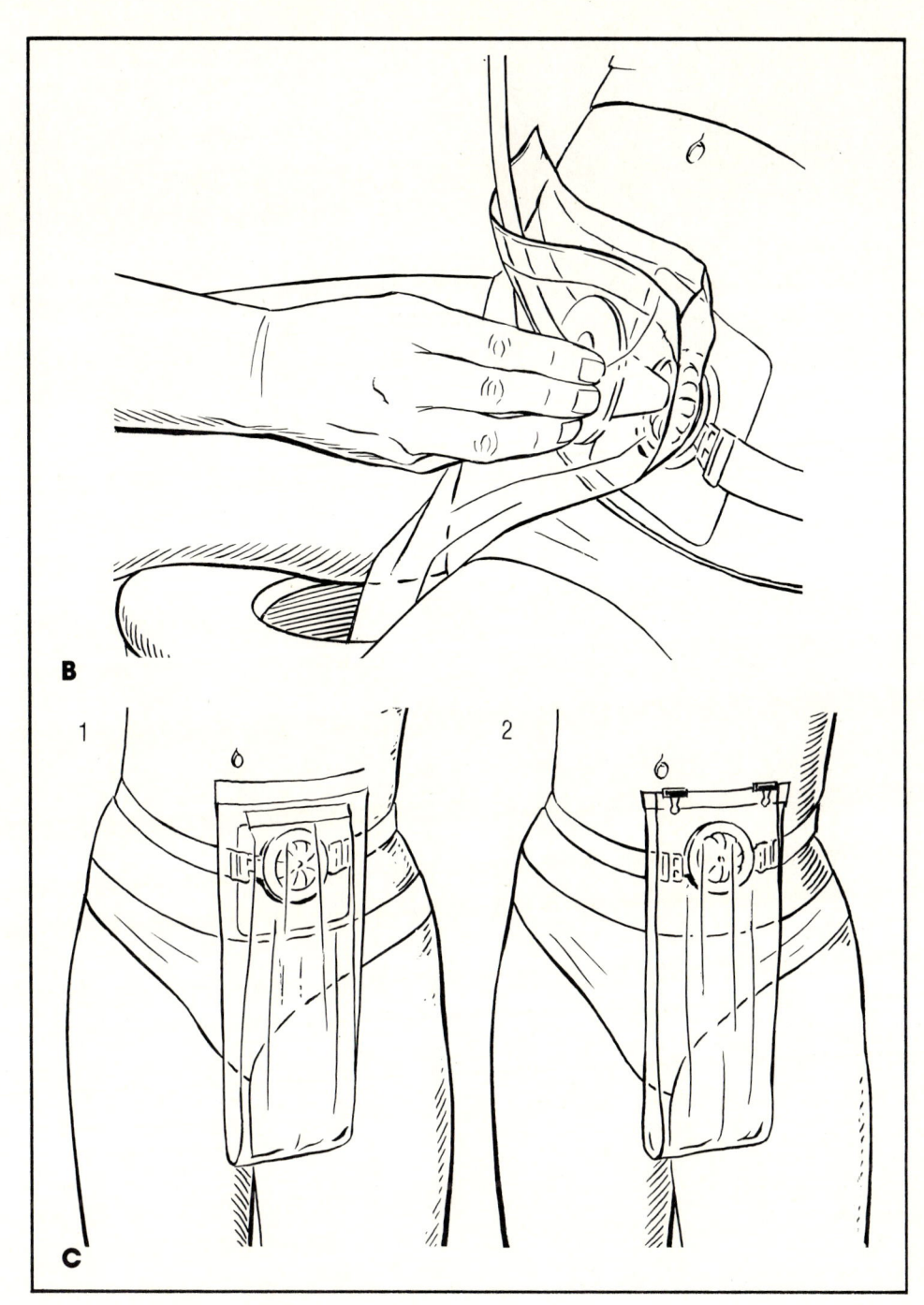

Figure 61-10. B. Hold in place from outside the sleeve. C. After initial returns, fold up lower end of the irrigation sleeve to form a large pouch to contain the later returns. (1) Close clamp clip and hook to snap-on ring or (2) fold lower and upper ends of sleeve together and anchor with clip fasteners.

sleeve with the remaining 500 ml of irrigant, remove the lower end of the sleeve from the toilet, dry it off with toilet tissue, and attach it to the upper part of the sleeve by folding the upper and lower edges over twice and securing them with clips (Fig. 61-10C). This forms a large pouch to contain the remaining water and stool that will be evacuated over the next 20 to 30 minutes. Encourage the client to ambulate during this time, since activity facilitates evacuation. This is also a good time for the person to shave, fix hair, or engage in other personal hygiene activities. If the irrigation is done in bed, initial returns can be emptied into a measuring container or bedpan through the lower end of the sleeve.

After all the fluid and stool have returned, refill the irrigation container, unclamp the large pouch, empty and rinse the sleeve. Hold the catheter or cone-tip against the sides of the sleeve and remove as much drainage as possible (Fig. 61-10D). Remove the sleeve, wash it with soap or detergent and rinse and dry it with towels or hang it in the bathroom to air-dry. This helps control odors and bacteria.

Some clients like to shower or bathe before they care for their stoma. Because of peristaltic action, wa-

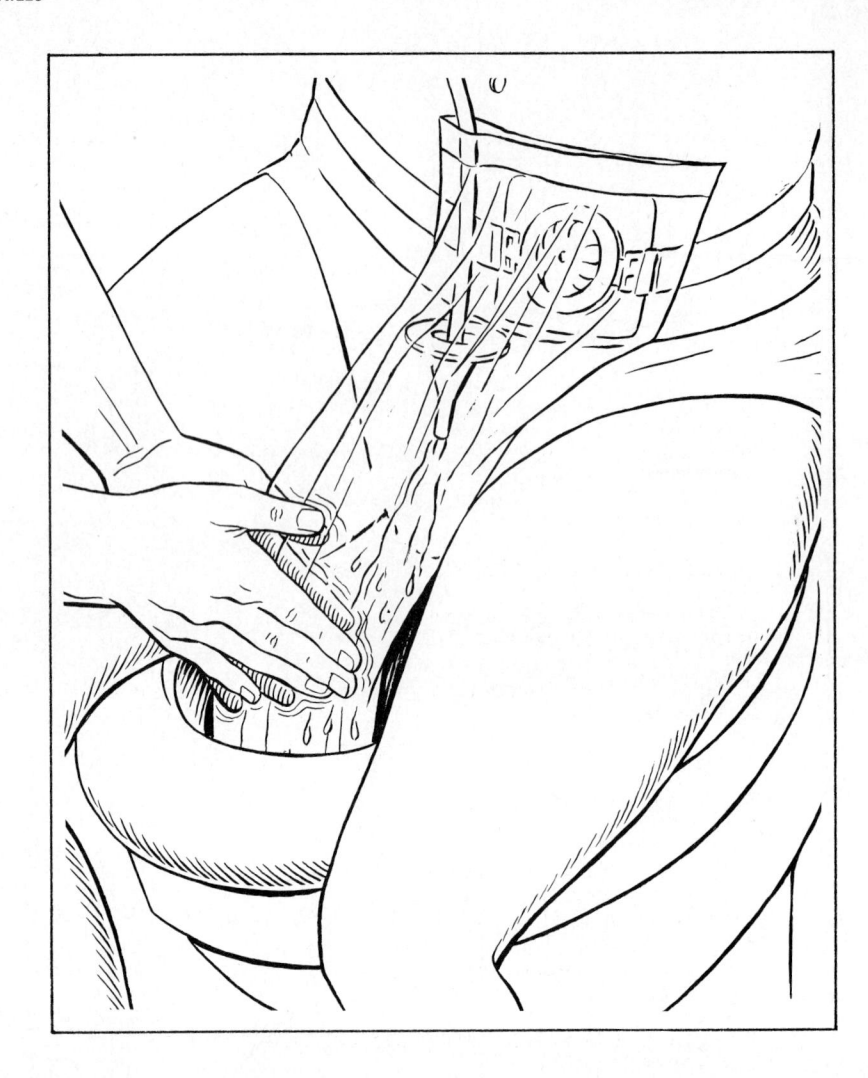

Figure 61-10. D. After emptying later returns, rinse sleeve before removing from toilet.

ter will not enter a stoma made from bowel tissue. The only caution about bathing is to avoid the soaps and oils that decrease appliance adherence. Many ostomates wear only a patch or stoma cap between irrigations, usually one with a charcoal filter for odor control.

☐ SKILL SEQUENCE

COLOSTOMY IRRIGATION

Step	Rationale
1. Validate physician's order for irrigation.	Ensures appropriate intervention.
2. Identify client's knowledge of procedure and ability to assist. Explain as needed.	Aids nurse in explanations and determining participation of client.
3. Wash own hands.	Prevents transfer of microorganisms.
4. Gather and prepare needed equipment:	Prevents delays and interruptions during care.
a. Fill irrigating container with 1500 ml tap water or saline at 40.5° to 43°C (105° to 110°F).	Irrigation procedure is similar to large-volume enema. Additional water is ready for rinsing. Cooler temperatures may cause cramping; higher temperatures can injure bowel mucosa.
b. Attach cone tip or catheter with shield to irrigating tubing. Catheter shield or baby bottle nipple should be placed 5 to 10 cm (2 to 4 in) from the distal tip of the catheter.	Cone or shield seals stoma and prevents leakage and allows correct insertion depth and direction.
c. Lubricate distal 5 cm (2 in) of catheter with water-soluble lubricant. Cone-tip lubrication is optional.	Facilitates insertion of catheter but may cause cone-tip to slip from stoma.
d. Place or hang container at least at client's shoulder level or 30 to 45 cm (12 to 18 in) above stoma.	Provides sufficient pressure for fluid to flow into colon.

(continued)

SKILL 61: OSTOMY CARE   **679**

Step	Rationale
5. Assist client to a seated position on toilet or on chair facing toilet; close door. Place client's gown with opening in front; place towel on lap. (NOTE: Alternate method for bedfast clients: Position patient on back near side of bed. Drape with bath blanket.)	Allows irrigation returns to flow into toilet for easy disposal and odor control. Provides privacy. Using a chair avoids strain on perineal sutures. Avoids unnecessary exposure; allows for gravity drainage.
6. Remove pouch or stoma cap from abdomen. Discard pouch in moisture-resistant bag.	Prevents transfer of microorganisms.
7. Dilate stoma with lubricated and gloved finger if ordered.	May relax stoma and allow fluid to flow more readily; helps determine direction of colon; may prevent stoma stenosis.

8. Attach irrigation sleeve:
  a. Reusable sleeve:
    Hook ostomy belt to one side of plastic ring of irrigation sleeve. Place plastic ring of sleeve over stoma and hook other side of belt to plastic ring.
    Or: Snap ring of a two-piece system onto wafer flange and attach an ostomy belt to flange.
  b. Disposable adhesive-backed sleeve:
    Cleanse and dry area around stoma. Remove protective paper from adhesive backing and apply adhesive opening of sleeve over stoma. Add ostomy belt if equipment permits.
  c. Place long narrow end of sleeve in toilet. For bedfast clients, clip end of sleeve and lay it beside client on bed.
	
	Provides secure attachment.
	
	Secures sleeve and provides additional support.
	
	Ensures that sleeve will adhere to peristomal skin.
	
	Provides additional support.
	
	Allows drainage to enter appropriate receptacle.

9. Administering irrigation fluid:
  a. Hold cone-tip or catheter over toilet; release clamp and fill tubing with warm water. Close clamp.
  b. Insert cone-tip or catheter through top opening of irrigation sleeve and into stoma, using a gentle rotating motion. Insert catheter 5 to 10 cm (2 to 4 in) or as specified. Hold cone-tip or catheter firmly in place from outside of sleeve. Pull top of sleeve around catheter.
  c. Release and adjust regulator clamp and allow fluid to flow into colon over 10 to 15 minutes. (NOTE: If cramping occurs, slow the rate of flow. If pain occurs, close clamp and allow client to rest. Do not remove cone-tip or catheter.)
  d. Close regulator clamp and hold cone-tip or shield in place for several minutes.
	
	Air in tubing can cause cramps and slows rate of flow. Avoids leaking.
	Facilitates insertion and avoids injury to colon. Greater insertion depth with catheter may cause perforation.
	
	Avoids leaking fluid from sleeve and stoma.
	
	Adequate fluid volume is needed to provide effective stimulation of peristalsis and colon evacuation. Slowing or stopping fluid eases pressure and relieves cramping and pain.
	
	Closing clamp avoids leaking when cone is withdrawn.

10. Contain initial returns:
  a. Remove cone-tip or catheter from stoma, pulling upward and out of sleeve and holding top of sleeve close to body.
  b. Fold top of sleeve together twice and clip together or close slide-seal closure.
  c. Have client remain on toilet or in same position in bed for 10 to 15 minutes.
  d. Place nurse call signal within reach. Remain with clients who are fearful, weak, or inexperienced.
	
	Avoids leakage from spurting return fluid.
	
	Allows for initial return of water and stool.
	
	Promotes physical and psychological safety. Gives client the chance to verbalize feelings.

11. Contain later returns:
  a. Open top of sleeve and use cone-tip or catheter to rinse inside of sleeve with remaining water in irrigating container.
  b. Remove lower end of sleeve from toilet, rinse, and dry with toilet tissue. Fasten lower end to top of sleeve with hook, flexible closure, or ostomy clips. Flush toilet. (NOTE: For bedfast clients: drain contents into graduated container; measure and discard.)
  c. Leave sleeve in place for 30 to 45 minutes. Encourage ambulatory clients to move around.
	
	Clears initial returns from sleeve.
	
	Creates large pouch to contain remaining drainage securely.
	
	Appropriate disposal of returns. Provides space for later fluid returns; provides data for evaluating returns.
	
	Allows time for complete return of water and feces. Facilitates colon evacuation.

12. Finish irrigation:
  a. Close regulator clamp and refill irrigation container with water.
  b. Have client sit or stand by toilet, if ambulatory.
  c. Remove clips and place lower edge of sleeve in toilet and allow sleeve to empty.
	
	Preparatory for rinsing irrigation sleeve.

(continued)

COLOSTOMY IRRIGATION (Cont.)

Step	Rationale
d. Place cone-tip or catheter in top opening of sleeve; open regulator clamp and rinse sleeve until clean, holding cone-tip against inside wall of sleeve. Rub sleeve together with hands. For bedfast client, remove sleeve; discard disposable sleeve or clean reusable sleeve in bathroom.	Ensures complete rinsing of fecal contents.
e. Close regulator clamp and remove cone-tip or catheter.	Avoids dripping fluid.
f. Unhook belt. Remove sleeve.	Completes irrigation procedure.
13. Wash peristomal skin with soap and water, rinse, and dry.	Removes irritating fecal drainage.
14. Apply pouch, cap, or patch over stoma as in Skill Sequence, "Replacing an Ostomy Appliance," steps 12 to 14.	Provides needed degree of protection.
15. Wash reusable irrigation sleeve with mild soap or detergent and warm water, rinse and dry with towels or hang to air dry. Store equipment in bathroom or bedside stand with bedpan.	Avoids bacterial overgrowth; decreases odors; prolongs life of sleeve. Equipment is contaminated from contact with fecal drainage and should not be stored with personal hygiene materials.
16. Provide for client handwashing.	Hygienic measure.
17. Wash own hands.	Avoids cross-contamination.
18. Record kind and amount of irrigant used, nature and amount of returns, any problems with irrigation, and length of time needed to complete irrigation. Record condition of stoma and peristomal skin. Record skin care provided and type of pouching or stoma protection used. Record client's reaction and participation.	Fulfills nurse accountability. Provides ongoing data base. Provides continuity of client care.

RECORDING

Record the appearance and condition of the stoma and the ostomy drainage at least daily. When a permanent faceplate or skin-barrier wafer is changed, record the length of time since the last change and the appearance and condition of the peristomal skin. Record the frequency with which a pouch is changed or emptied. Regular recording of these data will help identify problem areas promptly. Record any leakage that occurs between appliance changes. Recording also includes any medications or treatment used on irritated skin and any products used to prepare the skin and appliance.

After giving a colostomy irrigation, record the type and amount of solution used, the nature and amount of the returns, the length of time needed to complete the irrigation, the amount of self-care the client was able to accomplish, the degree of fatigue experienced, and any problems encountered. If the appliance was changed after the irrigation, record findings related to stoma care. In addition to data about the ostomy itself, include information about the client's affect and acceptance of the stoma, such as whether he or she participates in giving care, looks at or touches the stoma, or makes any comments about the stoma or its care.

Sample POR Recording

- S—"I usually get good results from an irrigation. At home it takes me about 45–50 min. to irrigate." "I don't usually leak between irrigations. This wafer has been on 4 days now!"
- O—Did own irrigation in B.R., using 1000 ml tap water. Returned water with formed and semiformed stool. Irrigation time: 50 min. Stoma red-pink with no bleeding. Wearing minipouch after irrigation.
- A—Colostomy successfully regulated with irrigations. No problems with stoma or pouching.
- P—Support client's methods and continue observations.

Sample Narrative Recording

Irrigated own colostomy in B.R. with 1000 ml tap water. Returned water with formed and semi-formed stool. Total irrigation time: 50 min. States "At home it takes about 45–50 min. to get this kind of results." "I don't usually leak between irrigations." Stoma cap attached to wafer which remains tightly adhered to abdomen after 4 days. Stoma red-pink; no bleeding.

☐ CRITICAL POINTS SUMMARY

1. Most people with an ostomy are able to lead fairly normal lives.
2. The nurse's acceptance of the client's ostomy is crucial to its acceptance by the client and his or her family.

3. The main way to prevent peristomal skin irritation is with a properly fitting and leakproof appliance.
4. Odor control is achieved by regular pouch changes, careful cleaning of reusable pouches, use of deodorizers in the pouch, use of internal deodorizers, and dietary adjustments.
5. Except for sigmoid colostomies, conventional ostomies drain constantly and need continual pouching.
6. Continent ostomies are drained with a catheter at regular intervals.
7. Two-piece appliance systems increase the ease with which pouches are changed and decrease skin irritation from frequent faceplate changes.
8. Skin barriers and sealants are used with appliances to protect peristomal skin from ileal drainage and urine.
9. Ostomy belts are used primarily for irrigation purposes.
10. Sigmoid colostomies can usually be regulated with daily irrigations done at the same time each day and by avoiding foods that cause constipation or diarrhea.
11. A cone-tip irrigation system or catheter with sliding shield helps prevent backflow during irrigation and is less likely to injure the colon than a plain straight catheter.
12. The mode of action, procedure, and precautions for a colostomy irrigation are similar to those for a tap-water enema.
13. Initial irrigation returns occur in 15 to 20 minutes; a complete irrigation requires 45 to 60 minutes.
14. Persons with sigmoid colostomies and continent ostomies often wear only a patch or pouch over the stoma.
15. Urostomy pouches are connected to straight drainage at night to help prevent urinary reflux from an overly full pouch.

☐ **LEARNING ACTIVITIES**

1. Examine various types of ostomy appliances available in the central supply department. Identify advantages and disadvantages of the different types and the purposes for which they may be used.
2. Obtain a two-piece disposable appliance with a drainable pouch, closed pouch, irrigation sleeve, and stoma cap from the central supply department. Apply the wafer to the mannequin and practice attaching and removing a pouch and sleeve, as well as opening and closing the clamp on a drainable pouch. Position the pouch for a bedfast and ambulatory client. Note the length of the irrigation sleeve in comparison to the pouches and the mannequin. Repeat procedure, using a two-piece permanent ostomy appliance.
3. Interview an enterostomal therapist or a nurse who works regularly with persons who have ostomies and ask what he or she has found helpful in providing emotional and psychological support for them.
4. Contact your local or national ostomy association and obtain literature available for people with ileostomies, colostomies, and urostomies.
5. Invite a representative from your local association to speak to your professional group about ostomy care, problems faced by people with ostomies, and expectations they have of professionals.

☐ **REVIEW QUESTIONS**

1. Would you expect to find one (1) stoma or two (2) with the following procedures?
   ____ Double-barreled colostomy
   ____ End colostomy with a blind pouch
   ____ End colostomy with a mucous fistula
   ____ Loop colostomy
   ____ Sigmoid colostomy with abdominoperineal resection
2. If you are asked to irrigate a colostomy that has two stomas, how would you determine which one to irrigate?
3. Why might a client with a colostomy experience an urge to defecate?
4. In what ways might the reaction of a person with a recent ileostomy differ from that of a person with a recent sigmoid colostomy, and for what reasons?
5. How is a continent ostomy different from a conventional ostomy?
6. What advantages and disadvantages does a continent ostomy have as compared with a conventional ostomy?
7. What kind of drainage, skin problems, and pouching needs would you expect with an ileostomy; ascending, transverse, or sigmoid colostomy; ileal conduit; ureterostomy; or vesicostomy?
8. For what reasons is a sigmoid colostomy the only colostomy that can usually be regulated?
9. What can a nurse do to promote self-worth and independence for the person with an ostomy?
10. For what purposes are the following ostomy products used? Barriers, sealants, adhesives.
11. What are the advantages of a two-piece appliance system as compared to a one-piece system?
12. What are the best ways to prevent peristomal skin irritation and appliance leakage?
13. In what ways is taping a faceplate to the abdomen preferable to wearing an ostomy belt?
14. How is a colostomy irrigation different from and similar to a tap-water enema?
15. For what reasons is a cone-tip or catheter with a sliding shield preferred over a plain, straight catheter for a colostomy irrigation?

PERFORMANCE CHECKLISTS

OBJECTIVE: To use medical aseptic technique to change an ostomy appliance in a secure manner.

CHARACTERISTIC	RANGE OF ACCEPTABILITY	SATISFACTORY	UNSATISFACTORY
1. Validates order.	No deviation		
2. Washes hands.	No deviation		
3. Assembles equipment.	No deviation		
4. Explains procedure.	No deviation		
5. Closes door or draws curtains.	No deviation		
6. Places bed in working position.	No deviation		
7. Positions and drapes for visibility and privacy.	No deviation		
8. Inspects existing pouch seal.	No deviation		
9. Applies sealant and adhesive to permanent pouch.	Omit if using disposable equipment.		
10. Removes existing appliance from skin without damaging skin.	No deviation		
11. Discards disposable pouch.	Place reusable pouch in moisture-resistant bag and clean when procedure is completed.		
12. Observes stoma condition.	No deviation		
13. Cleanses stoma and peristomal skin without irritation or injury.	No deviation		
14. Implements ordered skin care.	No deviation		
15. Cuts opening in skin barrier wafer to appropriate size.	Omit if not used under a permanent faceplate.		
16. Applies skin barrier wafer around stoma.	No deviation		
17. Fills area around stoma with stoma paste.	No deviation		
18. Applies disposable pouch: a. Snaps ring of two-piece pouch onto flange. b. Places adhesive-backed one-piece pouch around stoma.	No deviation No deviation		
19. Applies reusable pouch: a. Positions faceplate around stoma. b. Attaches pouch. c. Slides O-ring or Bead-O-Ring into place.	No deviation No deviation No deviation		
20. Frames edges of wafer with tape.	Omit if wafer not used.		
21. Washes and rinses reusable equipment.	No deviation		
22. Washes hands.	No deviation		
23. Reports and records findings.	No deviation		

OBJECTIVE: To use medical aseptic technique to irrigate a colostomy in a safe and effective manner.

CHARACTERISTIC	RANGE OF ACCEPTABILITY	SATISFACTORY	UNSATISFACTORY
1. Validates order.	No deviation		
2. Explains procedure.	No deviation		
3. Washes hands.	No deviation		
4. Assembles equipment: a. Fills irrigation container with 1500 ml tap water. b. Lubricates catheter with sliding shield with water-soluble lubricant. c. Positions container at 30 to 45 cm (12 to 18 in) above stoma.	Normal saline may be used. Less volume is used for initial irrigation. Optional to use a small amount of lubricant with cone-tip. No deviation		

(continued)

CHARACTERISTIC	RANGE OF ACCEPTABILITY	SATISFACTORY	UNSATISFACTORY
5. Positions client seated on toilet or chair.	Position on back if bedfast.		
6. Protects privacy.	No deviation		
7. Removes and discards pouch or stoma cap.	No deviation		
8. Dilates stoma with lubricated finger.	Omit if not ordered.		
9. Attaches irrigation sleeve and ostomy belt.	Omit if equipment does not permit.		
10. Places lower end of sleeve in toilet.	For bedfast client, clip end together and place beside client.		

11. Administers irrigant:
  a. Fills tubing with warm water.
  b. Inserts cone-tip or catheter with shield into stoma.
  c. Holds cone-tip or shield firmly in place from outside the sleeve.
  d. Adjusts regulator clamp to allow fluid to flow in over 10 to 15 minutes.
  e. Slows or stops if cramping occurs.
	No deviation
	No deviation
	
	No deviation
	
	No deviation
	
	No deviation		

12. After 2 to 3 minutes, removes cone-tip or catheter while holding top of sleeve together and upward.	No deviation		
13. Waits 10 to 15 minutes for initial returns.	No deviation		
14. Forms large pouch with irrigation sleeve.	For bedfast client, empty sleeve before forming pouch.		
15. Waits 30 to 45 minutes for later returns.	No deviation		
16. Places call signal within reach when leaving the room.	No deviation		
17. Empties irrigation sleeve.	No deviation		
18. Refills container and rinses irrigation sleeve into toilet.	For bedfast client, remove and discard or wash and rinse.		
19. Removes sleeve.	No deviation		
20. Cleanses peristomal skin.	No deviation		
21. Applies stoma pouch, cap, or patch.	No deviation		
22. Cleans reusable equipment.	No deviation		
23. Provides for client handwashing.	Omit if client did not participate.		
24. Washes own hands.	No deviation		
25. Reports and records findings.	No deviation		

REFERENCES

Achterberg J, Lawlis GF, et al: The psychosocial road to recovery. Ostomy Quarterly 16(3):19-20, 1979.

Barrett N: Continent vesicostomy: The dry urinary diversion. American Journal of Nursing 79(1):462-464, 1979.

Dericks VC: The psychological hurdles of new ostomates: Helping them up . . . and over. Nursing74 4(10):52-55, 1974.

Goldman SL, Rambeau JL: The continent ileostomy: A collective review. Diseases of the Colon and Rectum 21(7):594-599, 1978.

Goode PS: Colostomy irrigation. In Broadwell DC, Jackson BS (eds): Principles of Ostomy Care. St Louis, CV Mosby, 1982, pp 369-380.

Jackson BS, Broadwell DC: Philosophy and issues in ostomy care. In Broadwell DC, Jackson BS (eds): Principles of Ostomy Care. St Louis, CV Mosby, 1982, pp 3-7.

Kirkpatrick JR: The stoma patient and his return to society. Frontiers of Radiation Therapy and Oncology. Basel, Switzerland, S Karger, 14:20-25, 1980.

Lamanske J: Helping the ileostomy patient to help himself. Nursing77 7(1):34-39, 1977.

Manufacturers of ostomy aids (Appendix 2). Clinics in Gastroenterology 11(2):422-430, 1982.

Mikolon S: Psychosocial issues in ostomy management. In Broadwell DC, Jackson BS (eds): Principles of Ostomy Care. St Louis, CV Mosby, 1982, pp 438-442.

Schauder MR: Ostomy care: Cone irrigations. American Journal of Nursing 74(8):1424-1427, 1974.

Shipes E: Sexual implications of stoma surgery, Part 2. Clinics in Gastroenterology 11(2):383-391, 1982.

Simmons KN: Sexuality and the female ostomate. American Journal of Nursing 83(3):409-411, 1983.

Wara P, Sorensen K, Berg V: Proximal fecal diversion: Review of 10 years' experience. Diseases of the Colon and Rectum 24(2):114-119, 1981.

Watt RC: Pathophysiology of peristomal skin. In Broadwell DC, Jackson BS (eds): Principles of Ostomy Care. St Louis, CV Mosby, 1982, pp 241-253.

Wentworth A, Cox B: Nursing the patient with a continent ileostomy. American Journal of Nursing 76(9):1424-1428, 1976.

Young CH: Sexual implications of stoma surgery, Part 1. Clinics in Gastroenterology 11(2):383-391, 1982.

BIBLIOGRAPHY

Barer AE: Stoma care in conventional ileostomy. Clinics in Gastroenterology 11(2):274-277, 1982.

Barrett N: Ileal loop and body image. AORN Journal 36(4):712-722, 1982.

Broadwell DC, Jackson BS (eds): Principles of Ostomy Care. St Louis, CV Mosby, 1982

Broadwell DC, Sorrells S: Loop transverse colostomy. American Journal of Nursing 78(6):1029-1031, 1978.

Dericks VC, Donovan CT: The ostomy patient really needs you. Nursing76 6(9):30-33, 1976.

Dunne LK: Ileal bladder conduit. In Broadwell DC, Jackson BS (eds): Principles of Ostomy Care. St Louis, CV Mosby, 1982, pp 783-785.

Gross L: Ileostomy: A Guide. Los Angeles, The United Ostomy Association, 1979.

Gross L, Lenneberg ES: Transverse Colostomy. Los Angeles, The United Ostomy Association, 1983.

Hyman E, Ashenmacher FE, et al: The pouch ileostomy: New nursing applications of time-tested techniques. Nursing77 7(7):44-47, 1977.

Jackson BS: Colostomates' reactions to hospitalization and colostomy surgery. Nursing Clinics of North America 11(3):417-425, 1976.

Jensen V: Better techniques for bagging stomas. Part 1: Urinary ostomies. Nursing74 4(7):60-64, 1974.

Jensen V: Better techniques for bagging stomas. Part 2: Colostomies. Nursing74 4(8):30-35, 1974.

Jensen V: Better techniques for bagging stomas. Part 3: Ileostomies. Nursing74 4(9):60-65, 1974.

Jeter KF: Urinary Ostomies—A Guidebook for Patients, ed 2. Los Angeles, The United Ostomy Association, 1978.

Lennenberg E, Mendelssohn AN: Colostomies: A Guide, ed 2. Los Angeles, The United Ostomy Association, 1974.

MacDowell DE: The special needs of the older colostomy patient. Journal of Gerontological Nursing 9(5):294-296, 1983.

Mahoney JM: What you should know about ostomies. Nursing78 8(5):74-84, 1978.

Mather DG: Ileal conduit surgery: How to help a terrified patient. RN 44(10):29-31, 1981.

Mullen BD, McGinn KA: The Ostomy Book: Living Comfortably with Colostomies, Ileostomies, and Urostomies. Palo Alto, CA, Bull Publishing, 1980.

Nortridge JAS: Helpful hints for assessing the ostomate. Nursing82 (Horsham) 12(4):72-77, 1982.

Ostomy Care at a Glance. United, Division of Howmedica, Largo, FL, 1978.

Palselius I: Stoma care in continent ileostomy. Clinics in Gastroenterology 11(2):278-284, 1982.

Product Data Sheets. Hollister, 2000 Hollister Drive, Libertyville, IL, 1983.

Product Information. Convatec, a division of ER Squibb & Sons, Princeton, NJ, 1983.

Stoma Care. Nursing Times (Community Outlook), July 13, 1983, pp 181-196.

Watson PG, Wood RY, et al: Comprehensive care of the ileostomy patient. Nursing Clinics of North America 11(3):427-444, 1976.

Watt R: Ostomies: Why, how, and where: An overview. Nursing Clinics of North America 11(3):393-404, 1976.

Wentworth A: Internal ileal reservoir (continent ileostomy). In Broadwell DC, Jackson BS (eds): Principles of Ostomy Care. St Louis, CV Mosby, 1982.

SUGGESTED READING

Dericks VC: The psychological hurdles of new ostomates: Helping them up . . . and over. Nursing74 4(10):52-55, 1974.

Mahoney JM: What you should know about ostomies. Nursing78 8(5):74-84, 1978.

Schauder MR: Ostomy care: Cone irrigations. American Journal of Nursing 74(8):1424-1427, 1974.

Simmons KN: Sexuality and the female ostomate. American Journal of Nursing 83(3):409-411, 1983.

To locate the nearest enterostomal therapist:
International Association for Enterostomal Therapy
1701 Lakeview Avenue, Suite 470
Glenview, IL 60025
(312) 724-1910

To obtain ostomy publications:
United Ostomy Association Inc.
2001 West Beverly Boulevard
Los Angeles, CA 90057
(213) 413-5510

AUDIOVISUAL RESOURCES

Care of the Ostomate
Videocassette. (1984, Color, 28 min.)
Available through:
American Journal of Nursing Company
Education Services Division
555 West 57th Street
New York, NY 10019

Caring for the Ostomy Patient
Videorecording. (1977, Color, 75 min.)
Available through:
Greater Cleveland Hospital Association
1226 Huron Road
Cleveland, OH 44124

Enterostomal Therapy
Videorecording. (1978, Color, 46 min.)
Available through
State University of New York
Upstate Medical Center
Division of Educational Communications
750 East Adams Street
Syracuse, NY 13210

Nursing Care of Patients with Colon Stomas
Videorecording. (1977, Color, 22 min.)
Available through:
The American Cancer Society
777 Third Avenue
New York, NY 10017

14 Mobility Assistance

◻ INTRODUCTION

People are in constant motion: walking, eating, sitting, and gesturing. Even in sleep, we turn and reposition our bodies. Generally, illness produces short or long-term changes in a person's mobility and capacity for self-care. When this occurs, the nurse is expected to assist that person in performing activities of daily living as well as to implement or teach measures designed to restore function or prevent complications and further disability, such as range-of-motion exercises. In addition, the person may need to be taught new methods for being mobile if the usual ones are no longer feasible, such as learning to use crutches, canes, or walkers.

It is important to know how to perform these and other direct-care activities in a way that is safe for both the nurse and client. It is not always possible to prevent skin and tissue damage or problems from immobility, particularly in aged, malnourished, immunosuppressed, or severely ill and injured persons. However, it is unacceptable nursing practice for a client's skin to become denuded from improper lifting and turning techniques, to have decubitae develop from improper positioning or insufficient position changes, or to have clients experience preventable negative results of immobility because they were inadequately turned or ambulated.

In the course of daily living, everyone has a need to lift, carry, push and pull objects or people. Because of the nature of direct nursing-care activities, nurses are involved in a great deal of that type of work. And, like workers in heavy industry, that fact is often demonstrated in a negative way—through low back pain and injury (Cust et al., 1972; Troup, 1965). The high incidence of low back pain is reported to be related to activities of turning, lifting, transferring, and moving clients (Raistrick, 1981; Scholey, 1983; Stubbs et al., 1981). British studies indicate that nurses have nearly twice as much sick leave as a result of back pain as the rest of the working population, and an estimated 43 percent of all English and Welsh nurses will suffer back pain at least once a year (Stubbs et al., 1981). Scholey (1983) reports that women take a surprisingly long time to become experienced lifters. For example, in heavy industry, it took women 3 years to reduce their subjective feelings of pain and fatigue associated with repetitive tasks. The problem is compounded for nurses. Most nurses are women, but their tasks during the work day are not repetitive and the type of task varies considerably with the client's weight, strength, ability to assist with activities, and the presence of imbalancing factors such as heavy casts or partial paralysis. In addition, most lifting is done without mechanical assistance, equipment may be heavy and awkward to use, and the level of staffing may preclude adequate help in lifting, transferring, and handling clients.

Back injuries apparently are the result of two major processes: an acute injury or the cumulative effect of minor back trauma. It is crucial that the nurse understand the basic principles of body mechanics and movement, as well as learn to perform daily living activities and direct nursing-care tasks in ways that will decrease the probability of strain and injury for self and the client. Scholey (1983) points out that safe lifting and handling of clients demands a high level of skill and suggests that students practice in the clinical setting with workers who are more experienced. She also proposes that nurses need to understand the causes of back stress, analyze each lifting situation, and plan the lifting task carefully so the least possible stress is induced. If given the opportunity, many clients can participate and cooperate in lifting and moving, thus gaining some beneficial exercise and reducing the work load of the nurse. It is also important to take a few minutes time to adjust the environment to facilitate moving and transferring. For example, it only takes a short time to raise the bed to a proper working height, move a chair to the correct spot, or use a mechanical lifting device. Omitting preparations such as these may save a few minutes, but contribute to development of back pain and injury.

◻ ENTRY TEST

1. Identify the large bones of the upper and lower extremities.

2. What are the three normal curves of the vertebral column?
3. Define the following terms: ligaments, tendons, cartilage, bursae.
4. Identify the parts of a skeletal muscle.
5. Describe the actions of skeletal muscles.
6. Describe characteristics of skeletal muscle contractions.
7. Compare isometric and isotonic muscle contractions.
8. What action on a joint is caused by muscle contraction?
9. Identify normal structures within a freely movable joint.
10. What are intervertebral discs?
11. What are the major muscles used when moving clients?

☐ BODY MECHANICS PRINCIPLES

Body mechanics is the application of scientific knowledge about movement of body parts to the use of the body in daily life activities and to the prevention and correction of problems related to posture (Miller and Keane, 1983). Posture refers to body position or manner of carrying oneself.

A "good" body posture means standing or sitting in a naturally erect and straight, but not rigid, position. Good body alignment is essentially a balanced neutral position, as described in Skill 63. Rather than being a single solid unit, the body consists of a series of segments placed one above the other: the head, upper and lower trunk, and legs. When the body is well aligned, the segments are in line vertically, with the line of gravity (described below) running through the center of gravity of each segment. With good body alignment, muscles are under enough tension to maintain the alignment of the body segments without any undue strain on joints, muscles, tendons, or ligaments.

A well-aligned standing or sitting position helps promote normal organ function, improves one's appearance, increases muscle efficiency and therefore decreases fatigue, and helps prevent injury or strain when moving, lifting, and turning clients. When clients are confined to a bed or chair, it is essential to help them maintain good posture and a normal body alignment. Appropriate posture and alignment contribute to a general feeling of well-being, promote adequate organ function, and help prevent disability and injury to muscles and joints. Maintaining a client's normal body alignment often requires supporting body parts with pillows, blankets, and towels. It also may involve using braces, crutches, or canes. The skills in this chapter describe the correct use of supports and assistive devices.

When the body is in motion, alignment leaves the neutral position. A person will have a more stable balance, be less likely to become fatigued, and will experience less muscle or joint injury if body segments are kept in alignment as much as the movement allows or if the person compensates for the altered alignment. For example, it is safer and easier to maintain the trunk erect when walking or lifting than to twist, slouch, or bend the trunk.

MECHANICAL PRINCIPLES IN BODY MECHANICS

To understand the use of body mechanics for both the nurse and the client, it is important to understand some basic concepts about weight, balance, force, frictional forces, inertia, motion, momentum, and work.

Weight

Weight is a measure of the earth's gravitational attraction for an object. This downward attraction occurs along all parts of an object, but for practical use it can be considered to be concentrated at one point known as the *center of gravity*. In the human body, the center of gravity is located between the umbilicus and the symphysis pubis and is slightly higher for men than for women.

The *base of support* is the total area over which the weight of an object is distributed. When a person is erect, the distance between the feet forms the base of support; in a seated position, the horizontal distance between the feet and the buttocks forms the base of support.

The *line of gravity* refers to an imaginary vertical line passing downward through the center of gravity. In an erect person in good alignment, the line of gravity extends downward from the head through the center of gravity, the knees, and the feet proximal to the great toes.

Balance

When the line of gravity falls within the base of support, an object is said to be in *balance*, or in a state of equilibrium. The closer the line of gravity falls toward the center of the base of support, the better balanced the object. The closer the line of gravity falls toward the edge of the base of support, the less stable and well-balanced the object. For example, if a person leans too far forward without placing one foot forward and a little apart (widening the base of support), he or she will become imbalanced and either fall or take a step forward to establish a wider base of support and avoid falling.

An object or person can be made more stable by lowering the center of gravity as this position will be more likely to bring the line of gravity within the base of support. For example, a brick turned on its long side is more stable and balanced than when it is standing upright on its short end—because its center of gravity is lower and has to be raised higher to make it tip over.

Clinical Application: A bed client who is turned on the side is less stable than one who is lying on the back, because turning on the side raises the center of gravity. (See Skill 64.)

An object can also be made more stable by widening its base of support.

Clinical Application: To move a client upward in bed, place the feet apart, so that the nurse's center of gravity remains above the base of support (between the feet) before, during, and after the movement.

In the human body, maximum stability occurs when the centers of gravity of all the weight-bearing segments lie in a vertical line that is centered over the base of support (Luttgen and Wells, 1982). When one body segment gets out of line, a compensatory disalignment of another segment usually occurs in order to maintain a balanced position of the body as a whole. At every disaligned point, uneven tension is placed on the ligaments and uneven muscle tonus occurs in the opposing muscle group, thus causing fatigue and sometimes actual muscle strain.

Force
Force refers to a push or pull that produces a change in the position or direction of movement of an object. The description of any force must include both the direction and magnitude of that force. A *disrupting force* is one that tends to move an object or the body out of balance and thus make it less stable. A *restoring force* is one that tends to maintain the object or body in balance, thus increasing its stability. Within the human body, force is exerted by muscle tension, which is a pulling force.

Friction
Whenever two or more objects are in contact with each other, *friction* resists the relative motion of those objects against each other. There are several concepts about frictional forces that have implications for how nurses move objects and clients.

1. Friction is directly proportional to the force that is pressing the two objects together. The heavier an object, the greater the frictional force exerted, and the more displacement force required to overcome that frictional force and produce motion.

   Clinical Application: More force is required to slide a heavy chair than a lighter weight one, or to slide a heavy client in bed than to move a lighter weight client.

2. Friction acts parallel to the surfaces that are in contact and in the direction opposite to the force producing or tending to produce motion.

   Clinical Application: When moving a client in bed, a sliding movement of the client's body across the sheet is accompanied by a sliding movement of the client's skin in the opposite direction, called a "shearing force." When skin is thin or fragile, this shearing force can cause damage to the skin and subcutaneous tissues, resulting in abrasion of the epithelium. (See Skill 64.)

3. Friction varies with the composition of the object's surface. Although a surface may look smooth, nearly all surfaces are uneven or have minute projections that mesh together and resist movement of two or more objects together that are adjacent to each other. Some surfaces exert less frictional force than others; for example, teflon or plastic surfaces exert much less frictional force than do cotton, wool, or painted surfaces.

   Clinical Application: When using a drawsheet to slide a client in bed, a plastic sheet beneath the drawsheet decreases frictional forces and therefore less displacement force is required to slide the client. (See Skill 65.)

4. Starting static friction is greater than sliding friction. Starting friction is a force that prevents motion of an object until the displacing force is sufficient to overcome the static friction force. Once in motion, a sliding object requires less force to continue the movement than it did to initiate the movement, that is, less sliding friction is encountered.

   Clinical Application: More force is required to begin sliding a heavy object or client than to continue the movement.

5. Rolling friction requires less displacing force to overcome it than does starting or sliding friction.

   Clinical Application: Less force is required to move a wheelchair or a bed with castors than to slide a conventional chair of equal weight or a bed without castors.

6. Friction is independent of speed. However, although speed does not decrease friction, it does increase momentum (see below), and therefore increased speed can move an object more easily.

   Clinical Application: A more forceful motion can move a client higher in bed more quickly and with less effort. (See Skill 65.)

7. Friction is independent of the total area of contact between the two surfaces.

   Clinical Application: Turning a large carton on its smallest side would decrease the contact surface area, but it would not decrease the amount of friction exerted or the force required to move it, because the weight of the carton remains unchanged and simply is exerted in a smaller area. In addition, turning the carton would raise the center of gravity and make the carton less stable and harder to move without imbalancing.

Inertia
Inertia describes the property that keeps an object at rest or in uniform motion until an outside force acts upon the object.

Motion
Motion refers to the continuous change of an object's location in relation to objects that are regarded as being at rest. Most human body motions are angular or rotary motions (curvilinear, or motion along a curve) rather than rectilinear (motion along a straight line).

Momentum
Momentum refers to the tendency of a moving object to continue in motion until outside forces slow or stop it. Momentum is the result of both the mass (weight) of a body and its velocity (speed in a given direction).

Work
In terms of physics and laws of motion, when a force acts on an object and produces motion, *work* is said to have been accomplished. In direct-care nursing activities, work is accomplished when clients are turned, moved, or lifted, or when objects are lifted, carried, pushed, or pulled. Lifting is the least efficient way to accomplish work, because a lifting force directly opposes gravity. Pulling and pushing are more efficient because they do not oppose the force of gravity. Work is more efficient if force is augmented by applying it at an angle, by using an inclined plane or a lever, or by substituting a rolling motion for a sliding motion.

In body mechanics, angular movement (motion about an axis) results from the action of *levers*. Levers are simple machines used to accomplish work (moving an object which exerts a resistance) when a force is exerted on a *lever arm* supported at some point by a *fulcrum* (a hinge or joint). This action causes the resisting object to move in an *arc* (a partial circle), that is, causes it to rotate. For the most effective rotation, a force is applied as far away from the axis as possible. Any movement of a partial or total extremity involves an angular movement because the extremity is being moved in some or all of a circle around the axis (joint).

Levers can increase force or speed, but not both. The portion of the lever arm from the fulcrum to the point at which the applied force is exerted is called the *effort arm*. The portion of the lever from the fulcrum to the point at which the resistance is exerted is called the *resistance arm*. If the effort arm is longer than the resistance arm, then the lever multiplies force. If the resistance arm is longer than the effort arm, then the lever multiplies speed.

Levers fall into three classes, depending on the relative placement of the effort, fulcrum, and resistance.

Class I levers have the fulcrum between the resistance and the effort. An example of a class I lever is the scissors: the swivel pin is the fulcrum, the effort is exerted at the handles, and the resistance is presented by the item being cut. Because the fulcrum can be anywhere between the effort and the resistance, a class I lever can multiply either force or speed, depending on the precise placement of the fulcrum.

A wheel is a special case of a Class I lever: the fulcrum is the wheel's axle, the force is applied with a hand at the top of the wheel, and the friction between the wheel and the floor is the resistance.

Clinical Application: When a person pushes forward on the top of the wheelchair wheel, a backward force is exerted at the bottom of the wheel through the action of the hand's forward force on the fulcrum (axle). This backward force overcomes the resistance between the wheel and the floor, and the wheelchair moves forward.

Class II levers have the resistance between the fulcrum and the effort. A nutcracker is a lever of this type: the hinge is the fulcrum, the nut is the resistance, and the hand squeezing at the ends of the handles supplies the effort. Because the effort arm is always longer than the resistance arm, class II levers always multiply force.

Clinical Application: Moving a client's arm or leg to do range-of-motion exercises involves using a class II lever. When moving a client's leg, the hip joint is the fulcrum, the resistance is the center of gravity of the leg (at the midthigh point), and the applied force is exerted as the nurse holds and moves the leg.

Clinical Application: Moving a heavy box by pushing first one end and then the other also uses a Class II lever. A pushing force exerted at one corner of the box causes that end of the box to pivot around the far diagonal corner of the box (resistance). To slide heavy objects across the floor, the nurse can repeat this lever action at alternate corners of the box.

Class III levers have the effort between the fulcrum and the resistance. An example of a class III lever is the forearm: the elbow is the fulcrum, the effort is applied by the biceps (which attaches to the forearm at a distance of 5 to 8 cm (2 to 3 in) from the elbow), and the resistance is the forearm itself. Because the resistance arm is always longer than the effort arm, levers of this class always multiply speed. The body contains many third-class levers, thus giving people dexterity and quickness, rather than simple brute force.

A lever and fulcrum produce an angular motion in which a force is exerted against a lever arm. A lever is most efficient (uses less effort to accomplish work) when there is a long distance from the applied force to the fulcrum (a long lever arm) and a short distance between the fulcrum and the object to be moved.

Clinical Application: To place a heavy client on a bedpan, use the upper arm as a lever arm and the elbow as a fulcrum. Rest the elbow on the bed, push downward with the upper arm, and raise the client with the hand and lower arm. This action requires far less effort than lifting straight upward.

An inclined plane can be used to raise or lower a load by sliding or rolling an object up or down the plane rather than by lifting it.

Clinical Application: When a bed and chair or an automobile seat and wheelchair are of uneven heights, a sliding board can be used to connect the two levels. The person then can slide rather than lift from one level to the other. For increased efficiency and decreased potential for tissue injury from shearing forces, the sliding board may have fabric-covered rollers instead of a flat surface. (See Skill 65.)

When an object is on an inclined plane, the force of its weight is directed straight downward (gravitational pull) and also downward along the surface of the incline. To move an object up an inclined plane requires both an upward and forward force.

Clinical Application: When the head of a bed is elevated, body weight will gradually pull the client downward into a slouched position. It is more efficient and requires less work if the head of the bed is lowered before moving the client back up into a correctly aligned position. In the horizontal position, only a forward force is needed, while both an upward and forward force are required to overcome the force of gravity as well as move the client forward.

MUSCLE MOVEMENTS

Body movements are produced as the muscles exert a pulling force against the bones, causing them to move like levers; muscle movement also is used to produce work, such as pushing, pulling, or lifting. Most human body segment motions are angular movements, in which the body part moves in an arc around a fixed line or axis. This arc may be quite small, such as that permitted by the muscles of the back, or it may be the complete circle in which the arm may move around the axis in the shoulder. Several concepts about muscle movement are helpful in understanding how to use one's own body muscles efficiently in moving clients and objects.

During flexion and extension of a joint, the angular motion exerted by the muscles that support and connect a joint serves two simultaneous functions. The function of the primary extensors and flexors is to move the body part as a lever arm and through an arc, as when the arm is moved toward the face to take a drink. Smaller muscles within the joint stabilize the joint by drawing the lever arm (the bone being moved) closer to the fulcrum (joint). These simultaneous actions allow the joint to function without dislocating the two articulating surfaces.

The primary direction of a muscle force is along a straight line from muscle insertion to origin. The point of application of force is at the muscle insertion site. A muscle also exerts a rotary (twisting) force that also helps stabilize the joint. A muscle is capable of producing a greater pulling force when it is at a resting length than when it is in either a more shortened or a more elongated length.

Clinical Application: When moving and turning clients, position the client's arms and legs in an anatomic near-neutral position, rather than hyperextended or sharply flexed.

When a muscle shortens as it contracts (concentric contraction), it exerts a greater force than when it lengthens as it contracts (eccentric contraction).

Clinical Application: Greater quadriceps femoris muscle force is required to step up a stairstep or rising from a chair than to step down a stairstep or sit down in a chair. Stepping up and rising from a chair involve lengthened (eccentric) muscle contractions, while stepping down and sitting involve shortened muscle contractions (concentric).

When muscles are contracted without any appreciable shortening or visible movement, they are said to be under static or isometric contraction, sometimes referred to as "muscle setting." In usual daily activities, muscle setting is fatiguing and should be avoided. However, muscle setting can be helpful when moving clients.

Clinical Application: To pull clients toward the edge of the bed or upward in bed, set the muscles of the arms before beginning to pull. When this is done, the movement produced by the nurse's quadriceps muscles (knee extensors) is transferred directly to the client through the "set" arms and shoulders. The movement of the client is thus produced by the stronger leg muscles, rather than by lifting or pulling with the weaker arm muscles.

BODY MECHANICS USED IN LIFTING

In a lifting action, downward compression on the intervertebral discs comes from several sources: the usual weight of the body, the additional weight being lifted, and contraction of the muscles of the back. This compression is the greatest at the lumbosacral junction. When these pressures are exerted on a healthy spine that is held erect, problems usually do not occur, especially if the person is young and has intact vertebrae and discs. Older persons and those with a history of back injury and pain tolerate this compression less well. If the spinal column is twisted while lifting, or if lifting occurs with the back bent, the downward force becomes a twisting force or a shearing friction force. Intervertebral discs are much more prone to injury from twisting and shearing forces than from compression forces.

Characteristically, at the beginning of a lift, a person will perform Valsalva's maneuver; that is, take a breath, contract the abdominal muscles, close the glottis, and hold the breath while lifting. This action elevates the intraabdominal and intrathoracic pressures and apparently relieves some of the compression on the intervertebral discs that is exerted as the muscles of the back contract, because the increased pressure tends to force the vertebrae apart. The increased pressure also tends to reduce shearing forces when the back is flexed during lifting. Tightening the gluteal muscles also aids in stabilizing the pelvis and spinal column. Setting the abdominal and gluteal muscles is sometimes referred to as "tightening the pelvic girdle."

APPLICATION OF SELECTED PHYSICS CONCEPTS FOR SAFE BODY MOVEMENTS

Generally accepted correct and safe techniques for lifting, pushing, pulling, and sliding objects and people include the following:

1. Hold the trunk nearly erect. In this position, most of the weight of the upper body and the load being lifted is directed straight downward through the vertebral column.
2. Place the feet apart with one behind the other to provide a wide base of support.
3. Face the object to be lifted, to avoid twisting and shearing forces.
4. Flex the knees and assume a crouch position. When possible, begin to lift when the angle between the thigh and lower leg is approximately 120 degrees, as this provides the maximum contraction potential of the quadriceps. If the object is on the floor, obviously this is not possible. When feasible, if heavy objects are to be lifted and moved, they should be stored on elevated shelves.
5. Tense the abdominal and gluteal muscles to support the abdominal organs and brace the pelvic area. This increases the pressure within the abdomen and relieves some compression on the intervertebral discs.
6. Bring the object close to the body and keep it there while lifting it. This action minimizes the shift in the line of gravity toward the object as its weight is added to the body's weight.
7. Lift by contracting the quadriceps and gluteal muscles, thus extending the knees. Keep the trunk almost vertical.
8. Avoid jerking and twisting, as those actions place undue stress on the intervertebral discs.
9. Carry heavy items at the waist level. When carried above the waist, the center of gravity is raised, resulting in decreased stability.
10. To conserve energy and prevent injury, divide heavy loads into several smaller loads if they must be carried; slide heavy objects or tip them from corner to corner; use a mechanical lift for heavy objects or clients; or seek assistance from other nurses.
11. When carrying a heavy object in one hand, broaden the base of support by placing the feet farther apart. Extend the opposite arm to balance the load or tilt the entire body to maintain the line of gravity within the base of support.
12. Use a pulling movement to move clients, because a pull tends to have a slight upward component and therefore reduces sliding friction forces. A pushing movement tends to have a downward component that increases the sliding friction force. In addition, pushing tends to compress tissues and joints in an undesirable manner. A pushing force is, however, quite appropriate for inanimate objects.
13. When pulling clients up in bed, turn the feet and body to face the direction of the pull, thus avoiding twisting and shearing forces.
14. Pull objects or people on a level plane to avoid working against the force of gravity unnecessarily.
15. For a straight pull, position the feet apart, with one behind the other. Set the muscles of the upper extremities and pelvic girdle. Pull by straightening (extending) the forward leg while shifting body weight to the backward leg. The force exerted by shifting body weight adds to the force of the pull. Setting muscles transmits the force exerted by the strong leg muscles and the body weight directly to the client, and avoids excessive pull on the upper extremities.

Overview

This chapter presents skills that are used to assist clients with mobility needs. Those skills include "Assistance with Ambulation" (Skill 62), "Maintenance of Range of Motion" (Skill 63), "Moving, Turning, and Positioning" (Skill 64), and "Transfer Activities" (Skill 65). Clients who require ambulation assistance often are partially or completely bedfast, on either a short-term or long-term basis. Therefore, this chapter also includes "Bedmaking Procedures" (Skill 66).

REFERENCES

Cust G, Mair A: The prevalence of low back pain in nurses. International Nursing Review 19(2):169–178, 1972.

Luttgen K, Wells K: Kinesiology: A Scientific Basis of Human Motion, ed 7. Philadelphia, College Publishers, 1982.

Miller BF, Keane CB: Encyclopedia and Dictionary of Medicine, Nursing, and Allied Health, ed 3. Philadelphia, WB Saunders, 1983.

Raistrick A: Nurses with back pain—can the problem be prevented? Nursing Times 77(20):853–856, 1981.

Scholey M: Back stress: The effects of training nurses to lift patients in a clinical situation. International Journal of Nursing Studies 20(1):1–13, 1983.

Stubbs DA, Rivers PM, et al.: Back pain research. Nursing Times 77(20):857–858, 1981.

Troup J: The relation of lumbar spine disorders in heavy manual workers and manual lifting. Lancet 1(7390):857–861, 1965.

BIBLIOGRAPHY

Duff AW (ed): Physics for Students of Science and Engineering, ed 8. Philadelphia, P. Blakiston's Sons, 1937.

Flitter HH: An Introduction to Physics in Nursing, ed 7. St Louis, CV Mosby, 1976.

Jensen JT: Physics of the Health Professions, ed 3. Philadelphia, JB Lippincott, 1982.

Williams JE, Metcalfe HC, et al.: Modern Physics. New York, Holt, Rinehart and Winston, 1976.

SKILL 62 Assistance with Ambulation

PREREQUISITE SKILLS

Skill 19, "Inspection"
Skill 20, "Palpation"
Skill 28, "Handwashing"

☐ STUDENT OBJECTIVES

1. Identify the types of clients who may require assistance with ambulation.
2. Describe the types of conditioning exercises that can be used to prepare clients for ambulation with assistive devices.
3. Differentiate among the different types of gaits.
4. Indicate the types of assistive devices commonly used for ambulation.
5. Describe how to move the client to the dangle position.
6. Describe how to assist a client to stand at the bedside.
7. Describe how to assist a client to ambulate without assistive devices.
8. Indicate the gaits used with specific assistive devices.
9. Indicate the methods used to measure a client for crutches.
10. Describe how to execute the gaits used with each of the assistive devices.
11. Identify safety hazards when ambulating clients.
12. Demonstrate the ability to assist a client to dangle.
13. Demonstrate the ability to ambulate a client with and without ambulation assistive devices safely.

☐ INTRODUCTION

Ambulation, the act of walking, is an activity most people take for granted. For a client who has had surgery, experienced a stroke, or had a broken leg, the act of walking can be very difficult. A few days of bedrest can reduce a client's activity tolerance rather quickly. When inactivity is combined with some disease process, injury, or pain, the client is most apt to require some assistance with ambulation. The nurse assists with ambulation while maintaining normal body alignment in a safe environment. Some clients may need to relearn how to use muscle groups for balance and ambulation. It also may be necessary for some clients to learn how to use assistive devices such as a cane, walker, or crutches when they are not able to bear their full body weight on their legs. Normally, ambulation retraining and teaching clients how to use assistive devices is done by physical and occupational therapists, but the nurse is informed about how a client uses common assistive devices so that the nurse can either teach clients or supervise them as they learn.

In addition to concern about ambulating clients who obviously require some assistance, it is important to recognize that immobility in itself and without illness or injury, has adverse effects that result in deconditioning. Deconditioning, as defined by Spencer et al. (1965), includes three components: (1) a reduced maximum range of response to physical activity, that is, weakness; (2) a decreased endurance for activity, that is, fatigue; and (3) changes in the normal physiological adjustments which occur in response to changes in activity, that is, light-headedness or faintness which may occur with changes in body position. It is wise to remember that relatively healthy clients who have decreased physical activity while hospitalized may need some assistance with ambulation.

☐ PREPARATION

The components of ambulation include good body alignment, weight shifting, balance, and coordination. Good body alignment during ambulation facilitates the efficient functioning of the body parts involved in ambulation. Coordination adequate enough to provide a stable balance and allow for weight shifting is essential for ambulation. Failure to achieve balance results in an unstable and tiring gait (Kottke, 1982, p. 420). In ambulation, the center of gravity shifts from one side to the other and from front to back. Normal upright body position is maintained by the action of the muscles of the back, abdomen, and lower extremities. When a step is taken forward the center of gravity is moved to a point above the foot that is in contact with the floor. This produces a tendency for the body to rotate forward. As the second foot is moved forward and placed on the ground and the first foot is lifted in preparation for forward movement, the center of gravity again shifts to a point over the second foot, thus causing the body to rotate forward (Flitter, 1976).

THE PHASES OF AMBULATION

There are two phases in ambulation: the weight-bearing phase and the swing phase. Ambulation begins with the weight-bearing phase in the double stance position (both feet on the floor). The swing phase begins with a shift of body weight to one foot as the other foot moves forward. Swinging the arm on the side opposite the moving foot helps to maintain balance. This phase terminates when the moving heel is planted on the floor. As the weight on the newly planted foot is distributed forward to the ball of the foot, the opposite foot prepares to push off for the next step (Rambo and Wood, 1982, pp. 246-247).

CONDITIONING EXERCISES

Exercise develops strength and endurance. The value of the exercise a client obtains while providing as much self-care as possible should not be overlooked. Have the client be actively involved in providing personal care as much as possible. In addition, conditioning exercises may be indicated for specific muscle groups in the shoulders, arms, wrists, and hands prior to ambulation with an assistive device. These exercises include range of motion exercises presented in Skill 63, and resistive, isotonic, and isometric exercises.

Resistive Exercises

Resistive exercises help to increase the size and strength of the muscle; they are done either by pushing against a stationary object or resisting movement. Pushups and pull-ups are resistive exercises. Clients can do modified versions of each of these in bed to help strengthen the arms and the legs. To strengthen the arms pull-ups can be done with a trapeze as shown in Figure 62-1. In this exercise the client pulls the upper body off the mattress. The arm and shoulder muscles can be exercised by using a strap or rope attached to the lower end of the bed to pull up to a sitting position. Pushups can be used to strengthen the arms and the legs. For the arms, the client lies on the abdomen, palms flat against the mattress at shoulder level and pushes the upper body up off the bed. While sitting in a chair the client can push with the hands against either the chair seat or arms to lift the hips up off the chair. For the legs, the client bends the knees and pushes against the bed to move up in the bed or pushes against a foot board. These exercises should be done in repetitions of three to ten for each exercise, two to three times a day.

Isometric Exercises

Isometric exercises, otherwise known as muscle-setting, help to maintain muscle strength. These exercises are done by contracting a group of muscles as hard as possible and holding the contraction for 10 seconds. These exercises are usually done in repetitions of ten for each exercise two to three times a day, using muscle groups such as the quadriceps, abdominals, and gluteals. An advantage of isometric exercise is that it can be done at any time, quickly, and without special equipment. Isometric exercises produce a transient elevation in blood pressure in normal people that is considered to be of no harm to those persons with a healthy cardiovascular system. However, in persons who have vascular or cardiac disease the elevation may initiate a chain of events that result in

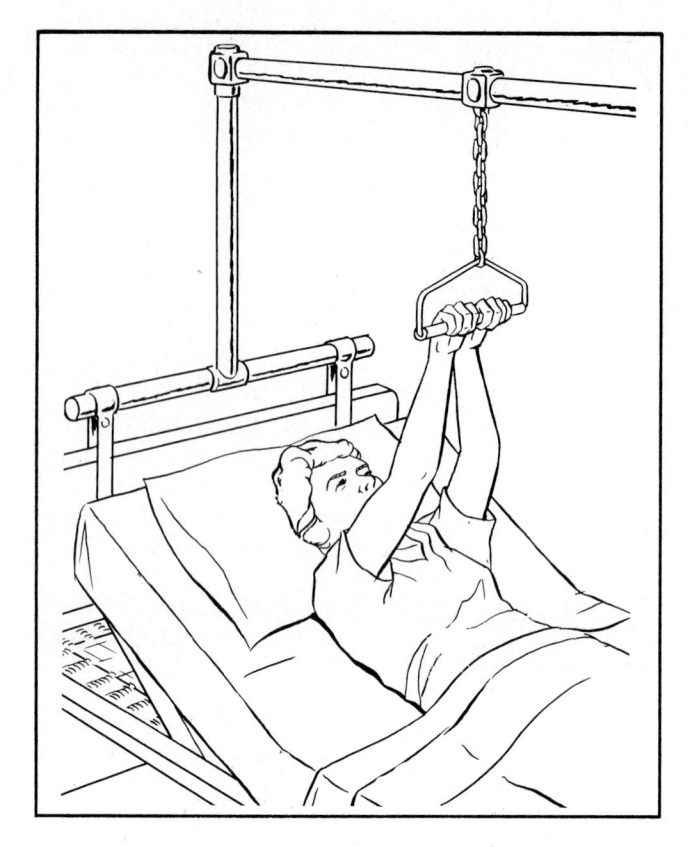

Figure 62-1. Using the trapeze on a balkan frame to do pull-ups.

cardiac problems such as myocardial infarction or heart failure. Therefore, isometric exercises are not to be initiated with clients who have a history of cardiovascular problems without a physician's order (Mitchell and Loustau, 1981). In addition to the concern about elevation in blood pressure, the nurse cautions these clients to avoid executing Valsalva's maneuver during exercise. This maneuver occurs when the breath is held during an isometric contraction or while straining during a bowel movement. It results in an increased intrathoracic pressure which decreases cardiac output and coronary blood circulation because venous return is reduced. Myocardial infarction may be precipitated in persons who have coronary artery disease or diseased heart muscle (Mitchell and Loustau, 1981). It is wise always to instruct clients to try to develop a rhythmic pattern of inhaling and exhaling during exercise and other activities that may involve straining. Although it is usually recommended that exhalation occur during the exertional aspect of the exercise, clients often have problems remembering when to inhale and when to exhale. The most important point for them to remember is to keep breathing and not hold the breath.

Isotonic Exercises

Isotonic exercises maintain and increase muscle strength. They are dynamic exercises in which muscles contract and lengthen to lift, hold, and move objects.

Weight lifting is an example of an isotonic exercise. Exercise programs that include isotonic exercise are most apt to be designed and implemented by a physical therapist.

DANGLING

Dangling is a term commonly used to describe the position of a client sitting on the edge of the bed with the feet resting on the floor or a foot stool. It is frequently used as an alternative to sitting up in bed and clients often find it more convenient for performing some personal hygiene activities such as combing the hair or brushing the teeth since it allows more freedom of arm movement. The dangling position is beneficial because it is an intermediate step between bed rest and ambulating or sitting up in a chair. Initially, a client who has been on bed rest for an extended period of time may not be able to sit or stand up erectly without experiencing some faintness or dizziness because of the effects of deconditioning. Orthostatic (postural) hypotension is a frequent phenomenon of immobility. Before the client is able to sit erectly in the bed and then dangle without faintness, it may be necessary to raise the head of the bed a few degrees at a time and to stop when symptoms are noted. It may take a few days of this gradual increase in the degree of elevation before the client is asymptomatic. Once the client is able to dangle without feeling the effects of orthostatic hypotension, the client is ready for ambulation. Orthostatic hypotension may occur when the client moves from the sitting to the standing position, so it is important that the client be instructed and guided to move slowly, thus permitting the autonomic nervous system to compensate.

GAITS

The term *gait* describes the manner of walking. Special types of gaits are necessary for maintaining body alignment and balance when canes, walkers, or crutches are used. These gaits are described in terms of the number of weight-bearing contacts that the client's feet and the ambulatory device make with the floor during one complete stride; for example, two-, three-, and four-point gaits.

The type of gait selected for a particular client is related to the client's muscle strength, coordination, and ability to use and bear full or partial weight on both feet. Usually, the physician or physical therapist selects the best gait for the client, but in some situations the nurse may be expected to do this after consultation with the physician. Clients who will be using an ambulatory device for an extended period of time may benefit from learning more than one gait so that they can reduce the amount of exertion required, alter the speed with which they move, and adjust to the amount of space available for ambulation.

The *four-point gait* is used when a client cannot support the full body weight on either leg, for example, a client who has loss of strength in the leg muscles from disease or injury or who has loss of balance. There are two types of *three-point gaits*. In one, partial weight bearing on one leg is permitted with full weight bearing on the other. This may occur when a client has a cast on one leg or a new prosthesis on one leg. In the other type, weight bearing is not permitted on one leg when the other leg is able to bear the full weight (Providing Early Mobility, 1981). Additional gaits are those used with crutch walking. These include the *two-point alternate*, the *swing-to*, and the *swing-through gaits*.

DATA BASE

Client History and Recorded Data

A nursing decision to ambulate a client must be in accord with the medical diagnosis, the physician's order for activity, and the client's strength, tolerance, and endurance level. Such information in both the client's health record and nursing kardex provides guidance about the ability to ambulate, the need for help from an assistant, or the use of ambulatory devices. When a client uses an ambulatory device, it is helpful for the nurse to know how long the client has used the device and how skilled the client is in its use.

If the client has experienced a prolonged period of immobility it is beneficial for the nurse to know the extent to which the client might be experiencing the symptoms of deconditioning and how the client has responded to the most recent ambulation. The nurse would also want to know the client's mental status and ability to understand or follow directions. This information is helpful when working with neurologically impaired persons, such as clients who have some residual loss of function following a stroke.

Snyder and Baum (1974) developed a tool for assessing a neurologically impaired client's problems with regard to posture, positioning of the feet (station), and gait. Some of the items on the tool provide information that is useful for the nurse to know about any client. This information includes: any difficulty the client may have in ambulating, pain or discomfort on ambulation, use of assistive devices for ambulation, the need for help in sitting or standing up, the length of time the client is able to stand, the need for support while standing, and the distance that can be ambulated without difficulty. In addition, it is also important to be aware of any concerns the client might have in relation to ambulating. For example, a client who has had recent surgery may be fearful that the incision will rupture or a client who has either fallen or experienced near falls may be fearful of repeated incidents. On the other hand, some clients are apt to overestimate their strength and ability. It is important to know this about them and also to be aware of any instruction given to them about pacing and about gradually increasing their ambulation.

Physical Appraisal Skills

Inspection. In addition to using inspection for determining the client's general appearance, state of rest, and respiration rates prior to and during ambulation, inspection is used to detect differences in the size of the extremities and the ability to move them with coordination. Inspection reveals balance, posture, the width of the base of support used in the stance and gait, the type of gait, the arm swing, and the ability to use ambulatory devices correctly. It is also used to detect signs of fatigue such as pallor, perspiration, and dyspnea.

Palpation. Palpation is used to appraise the client's pulse prior to, during, and after the activity.

EQUIPMENT

Canes, walkers, and crutches can be obtained from pharmacies, health-aid supply stores, voluntary health organizations in the community, and inpatient care facilities. These assistive devices can either be purchased or rented. When it is known that the device will be required for a short period of time, renting may be more desirable. For safety purposes it is extremely important that a rubber tip be in place on the end or ends of the ambulatory device to prevent slipping. The tip is inspected frequently for signs of wear and replaced promptly whenever it is worn.

Canes

The types of canes most commonly used include the four pronged (quad cane), three pronged, bent shaft, and regular cane. These canes are often made of lightweight metal and are either adjustable or sized for the client. The handle of the cane may be curved or straight. Straight handles may have either smooth or contoured hand grips and generally provide a more secure grip since there is more surface for the hand to grasp. The quad cane shown in Figure 62-2A offers the most support as it has the broadest base; it is particularly useful for clients who are unsteady on their feet. The bent-shaft cane also shown in Figure 62-2B permits the force applied by the client on the hand grip to be directed over the cane's vertical axis. The regular straight cane is single-ended and has a semicircular handle.

For a proper fit, the top of the hand grip of the cane should be at the level of the client's hip joint. When bearing weight, the tip of the cane is placed about 10 cm (4 in) laterally to the foot and the arm is bent to a 30 degree angle at the elbow. Canes are appropriate for clients who have minimal weakness of the lower extremities and who have good balance.

Walkers

A walker is a four-point aluminum ambulatory device with bars across the top and sides. Walkers are adjustable or are sized to the client. There are several models of walkers. Some *standard walkers* are designed to be

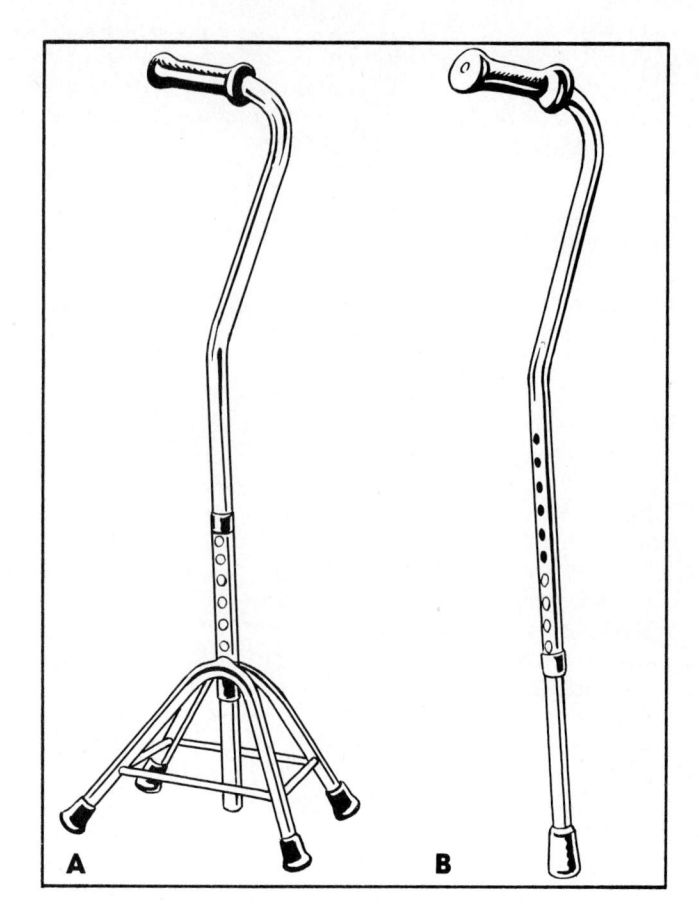

Figure 62-2. **A.** A quad cane. **B.** A bent-shaft cane.

picked up, and other models slide or roll ahead of the client with each step. The standard walker is used with clients who have good arm strength and balance. Another type, referred to as a *reciprocal walker,* is designed to advance alternately from one side to the other as the client moves the legs. This model, shown in Figure 62-3, is considered more stable than the standard walker. It is better for the client with reduced arm strength and impaired balance, and it also encourages a normal walking pattern. Clients who are unable to lift a standard walker might be able to use a model with wheels on the front legs that permit the walker to be rolled ahead of the client.

A proper fit for a walker permits the client to grasp the hand grip while having the elbows flexed at a 30 degree angle when the hand grip is grasped with the wrist extended. Clients who might use a walker include those who are learning how to walk again after a long period of not ambulating, those who are unable to bear full weight on a leg, and those who are preparing for ambulation with a brace or crutches (Rambo and Wood, 1982, p. 270).

Crutches

Types of crutches, as shown in Figure 62-4, include the axillary, the Lofstrand (Canadian), and the platform, all of which are adjustable. *Axillary crutches* may be made of wood or aluminum. The axillary

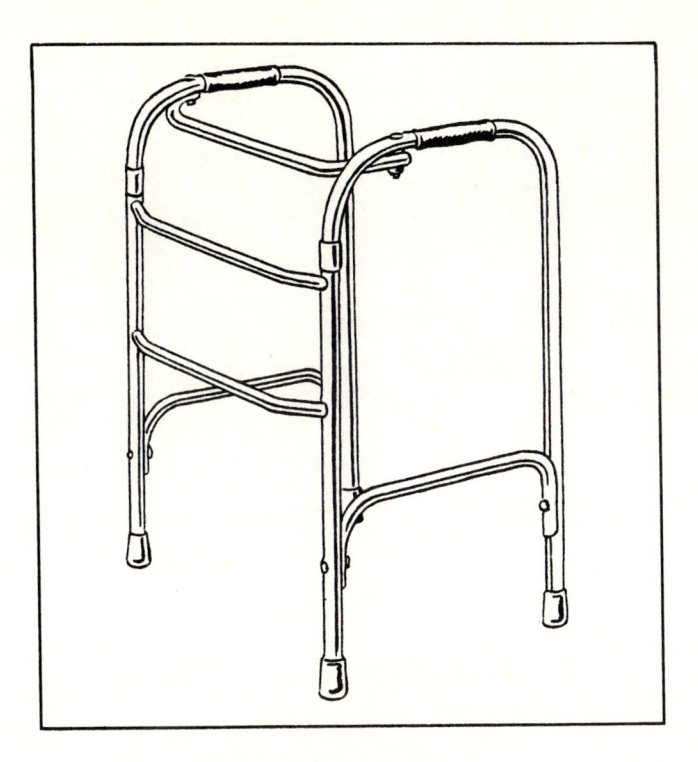

Figure 62–3. Reciprocal walker.

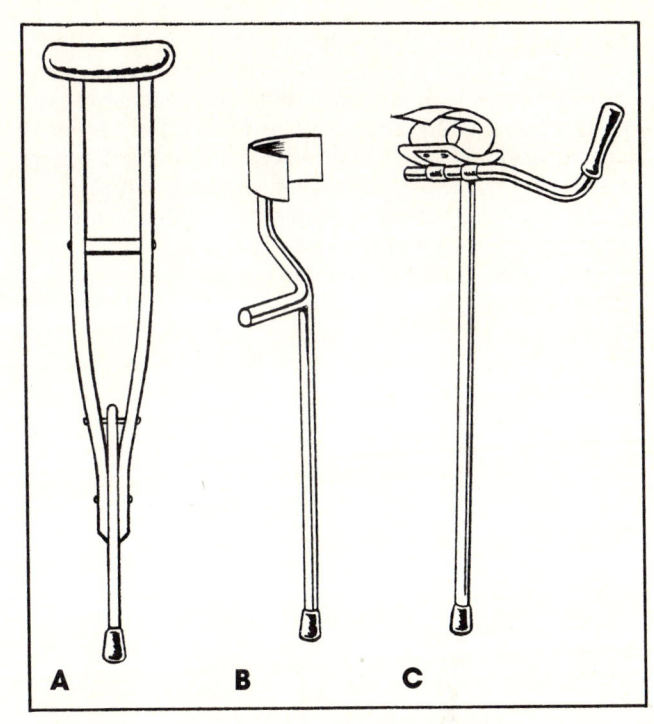

Figure 62–4. Types of crutches. **A.** Axillary crutches. **B.** Lofstrand crutches. **C.** Platform crutches.

crutch has a crossbar at the top that is usually referred to as the axillary bar and a hand bar about midway down the length of the crutch. The crossbar may be padded. These crutches are most often used for short-term conditions. *Lofstrand crutches* do not have the axillary crossbar; instead there is a cuff that encircles the forearm to stabilize the crutch against the arm. The hand bar extends out from the main shaft of the crutch. This crutch enables the client to release one hand grip and to use that hand without losing the crutch. Lofstrand crutches are used by clients who have long-term problems. The axillary and Lofstrand crutches require the body weight to be borne by the hands. The platform crutch is shorter than the other types. It has a platform for the forearm to rest on and a horizontal bar with a hand grip that extends out from the main shaft. This crutch is used by clients who require long-term assistance but are not able to bear their weight on their hands or wrists. The length can be adjusted so that the elbows are bent to a 30 degree angle with the crutch tip placed about 15 to 20 cm (6 to 8 in) lateral to and in front of the foot. The handle bars may be padded.

Gait Belt

A gait belt is a safety device that is placed around a client's waist before ambulating. It is made of a cotton twill or nylon material and is available in different lengths and widths. Some models have hand holds on each side and on the back to permit the helper to maintain a secure grip on the client.

☐ EXECUTION

Prepare the client for ambulation by explaining what is going to be done and how the client can help. If necessary, assist the client in donning the appropriate clothing and make sure well-fitting shoes or house slippers that will provide good support are worn. Arrange the furniture in the room to provide open space to move about in and make sure the floor is dry and free from clutter that the client could trip over. After the client is sitting on the side of the bed apply a gait belt around the waist for additional support and reassurance during ambulation. If the client will be using an assistive device after a procedure or surgery, teach its use before the procedure.

ASSISTING THE CLIENT TO DANGLE

The amount of assistance any client requires to move from the supine position in bed to a dangle position depends on physical abilities and strength, sitting balance, and ability to understand and follow directions. There are two starting positions from which any client can prepare to dangle: Fowler's position or the supine position. Clients who find it easier to start from Fowler's position include those with recent abdominal surgery, those with generalized weakness, those with orthostatic hypotension, and the obese. Many clients are able to move directly from the supine to the sitting position without difficulty. Encourage clients to do as much as possible for themselves because the activity provides exercise and a client often finds it more comfortable to move unassisted. When a client moves unassisted, it is often useful for the nurse to be present to provide help if needed, to monitor the client's technique, and to assess the tolerance for the activity.

Regardless of the starting position, there are three stages in moving to the dangling position. The client moves to a side of the bed, turns on the side and faces the edge of the bed, and moves upright to the sitting position. Stand nearby to protect the client from falling and to provide necessary assistance. Many clients are able to move themselves to the side of the bed in a flat position. This can be done by alternately pushing downward against the mattress with the feet and raising and moving the buttocks and then moving the shoulders and feet. Clients can also use side rails to pull themselves to the side of the bed. Assisting the client who needs help is described in Skill 65. When the client is near the edge of the bed, elevate the head of the bed to a semi-Fowler's position to decrease the distance to the sitting position. Most clients who are able to dangle can turn themselves on the side with minimal assistance. Teach them how to turn by crossing the far leg over the near leg, pulling on the side rail or the edge of the bed, and then placing the feet near or just over the edge of the bed. This allows the feet to move to the floor easily as the client pivots to sit up. Pushing against the bed with the hands while letting the feet fall over the edge of the bed to the floor initiates the force that moves the client upright. The weight of the legs serves as a counterforce and helps to move the client upright. Some clients will need assistance to move to the dangle position, as shown in Figure 62–5.

Clients with one-sided weakness or paralysis require some modification in the dangling procedure. The most secure way for these clients to dangle is to move the impaired side toward the edge of the bed and turn onto that side. Clients generally have better balance and more mobility when the impaired side is turned toward the bed and the unimpaired side is left free to do the moving. If necessary assist the client to move the impaired side toward the edge of the bed because this is more difficult than moving the unimpaired side. If the client moves the unimpaired side to the near edge of the bed and turns on that side, the impaired side is then turned upward. Because the impaired side is dead weight, the client is unable to control it and has more difficulty maintaining balance. If for some reason it is necessary for the client to dangle so that the impaired side of the body is the side that turns, remain close at hand to prevent the client from falling. To maintain sitting balance once in the sitting position, have the client place both hands firmly on the mattress on each side of the buttocks and plant the feet firmly on the floor or stool. If the client experiences symptoms of orthostatic hypotension, have him or her alternately plantar flex and dorsiflex the feet; this provides a pumping action that enhances venous return. The following skill sequence presents the technique for dangling a client with minimal nurse assistance.

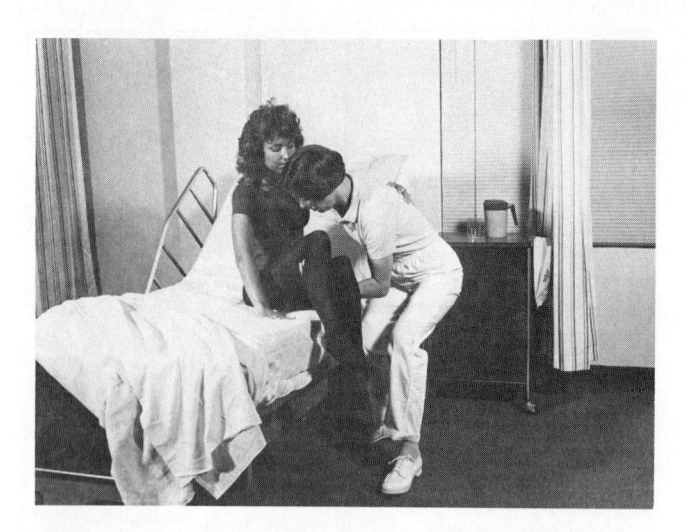

Figure 62–5. A nurse pivoting a client to the dangle position. (Photo by James Haines.)

☐ SKILL SEQUENCE

ASSISTING THE CLIENT TO DANGLE

Step	Rationale
1. Check kardex for medical and nursing orders.	Provides direction for special care needs.
2. Wash hands.	Prevents transfer of microorganisms.
3. Explain procedure to client.	Enlists cooperation and increases involvement in own care.
4. Close door or draw cubicle curtains, assist client to don appropriate clothing.	Provides privacy.
5. Place bed in low position.	Allows client's feet to reach floor while dangling.
6. Fold top linen to foot of bed.	
7. Help client to move to side of bed.	Facilitates swinging legs over edge of bed.

(continued)

Step	Rationale
8. Elevate head of bed 45 to 60 degrees.	Decreases distance to move to sitting position.
9. Stand facing bed near client's hips. Position feet apart, with one behind the other.	Provides broad base of support and allows for weight shifting.

10. To turn a client on the side facing you:
   a. Abduct client's near arm slightly
 	
   b. Cross client's far arm over body to grasp side rail or edge of mattress.
   c. Cross client's far leg over near leg and bring feet to edge of bed.
   d. Place hands on shoulder and hip and assist as client pulls on side rail or mattress and turns on side.
	Avoids trapping near arm under body and places it in position to assist in sitting up.
	Places arm over body's center of gravity and prepares to assist with turn.
	Allows weight of legs to assist with turn.
	
	Encourages self-help.

11. Prepare to move to a dangling position:
   a. Have client use near hand to grasp edge of mattress.
   b. Have client use far hand to grasp your shoulder or side rail, or prepare to push down on mattress with hand.
   c. Position self adjacent to bed, near client's hips, facing far corner of foot of bed. Assume a broad-based stance with foot farthest from bed advanced forward.
   d. Place on arm around client's lower shoulder and the other under both thighs, near knees.
   e. Flex your knees to 120 degree angle and set abdominal and gluteal muscles.
	
	Provides broad base of support and allows for weight shifting.
	
	Increases contraction capability of quadriceps muscles. Prevents strain on intervertebral discs.

12. Assist client to sit up on edge of bed. Simultaneously:
   a. Have client pull on your shoulder or side rail or push with one hand down into mattress.
   b. Have client push elbow of other arm into mattress.
   c. Have client move feet over edge of bed and allow them to fall toward floor.
   d. Pivot on your rear foot and shift your weight to rear leg; lift client's shoulders and pull legs off bed. Provide minimal assistance as indicated.
	Client actively involved in moving self.
	
	Weight of legs and gravity help to pull client upright.
	Allows client to obtain exercise.

13. Hold on to client until sitting balance is established. Tell client to press both hands down into mattress and plant both feet firmly on floor.	Stabilizes client until adjusted to upright position. Aids in maintaining balance.
14. To return to bed, reverse procedure, assisting client as needed.	Client may be fatigued and need more help to return.
15. Document in health record amount of assistance client needed, any adverse responses, length of time client dangled, any changes in blood pressure and pulse, tolerance for activity.	Fulfills nurse accountability and adds to data base.

ASSISTING THE CLIENT TO STAND

When supervising or helping a client to get out of bed, elevate the head of the bed and have the client dangle to attain a sitting balance before attempting to stand. In preparation for standing tell the client to place the feet about 25 cm (10 in) apart to establish a wide base of support. As shown in Figure 62-6, help the client to stand by having him or her place each arm on the top of your shoulders while you grasp the client under the arms and around the back. Having the client lean forward slightly at this time helps to position the trunk within the base of support. Then flex your hips and knees, brace your knees against the client's knees or legs, and have the client push against the floor with the feet as you move yourself and the client up to an erect, standing position. Instruct the client to count and move with you to help to synchronize movements and to avoid unnecessary strain. It is important to

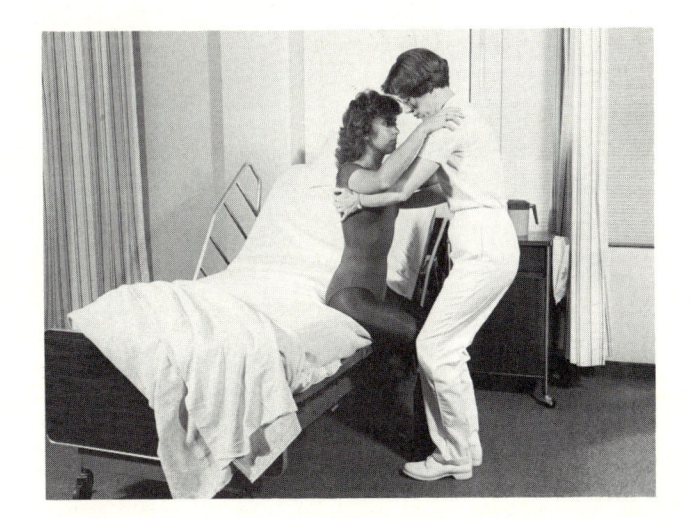

Figure 62-6. Assisting a client to stand at the bedside. (Photo by James Haines.)

hold the client as close to your body as possible to prevent injury from poor body mechanics. Tell the client not to grab you around the neck because this action permits the client to pull you too far forward, which will change your center of gravity and pull you off balance. To help the client establish standing balance place both hands on his or her waist or hold on to the gait belt while standing at the bedside for a few minutes. Observe the client for signs of fainting or weakness while standing at the side of the bed before ambulation begins. If the client feels faint or weak permit him or her to sit down on the bed.

ASSISTING THE CLIENT TO AMBULATE WITHOUT ASSISTIVE DEVICES

Ambulating a client who has no physical impairment or who does not require the use of an assistive device is a common nursing activity. Keep in mind that it is often embarrassing to ask for help, and that when help is offered it may be refused. For some individuals, accepting help creates uncomfortable feelings of inadequacy and dependence. Help the client to accept the idea that using help to ambulate is expected and is intended to prevent injury. An evaluation of a client's physical and emotional status may clearly indicate the need to be supported securely during ambulation, or a need for reassurance that is provided by being held loosely around the waist, by a gait belt, or at the arm during the first few ambulations. One way of ambulating with a client is to walk at the side as shown in Figure 62–7A. Hold on to the client's arm on the side nearest you to help provide balance, stability, and reassurance. If the client has weakness on one side, then stand close on the stronger side and grasp the gait belt securely. Have the client extend the weak leg at the same time you extend your opposite leg, as shown in Figure 62–7B; this helps to maintain stability and a broader base of support for both bodies. If there are two helpers, each helper holds onto one of the client's upper arms.

ASSISTING THE CLIENT TO USE AMBULATORY DEVICES

Much of the instruction and supervision a nurse provides to a client learning how to use an assistive device is duplication and reinforcement of what has already been taught by a physical therapist. The client who is learning to use assistive devices must learn to adjust to a base of support that includes the feet (or one foot) and the device, and learn to shift the line of gravity within that unfamiliar and wider base. Allow adequate time for the client to learn how to use the device safely, and provide for frequent practice opportunities under the direct supervision of a knowledgeable

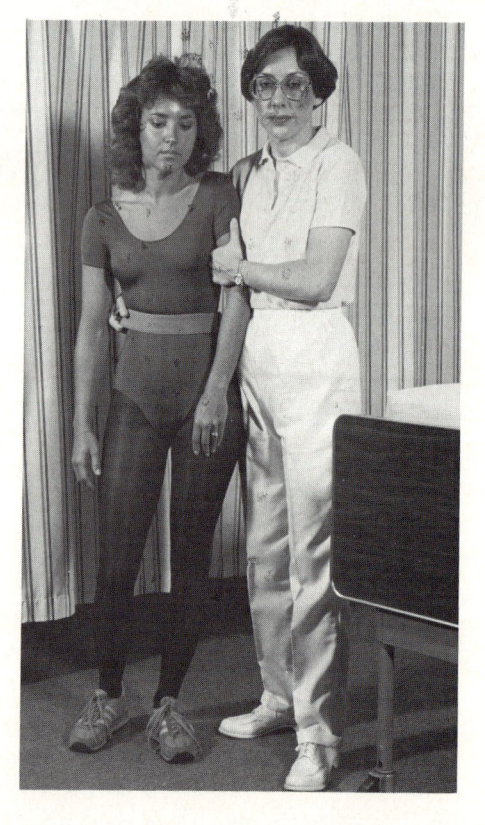

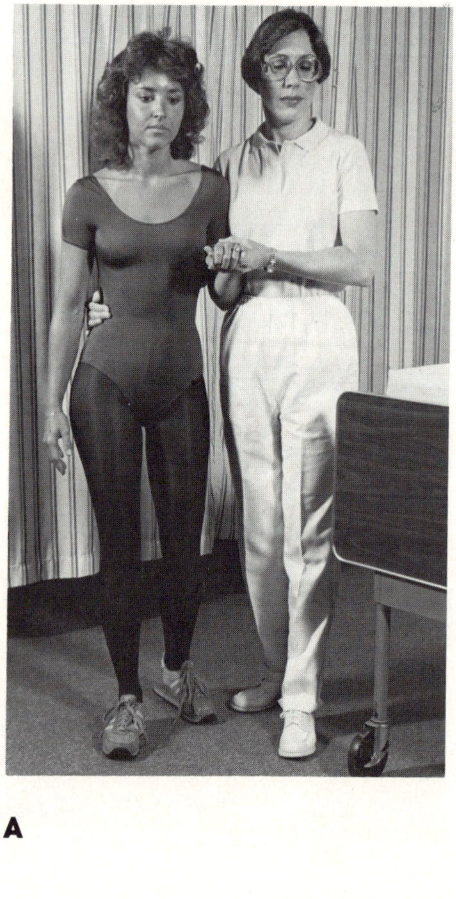

Figure 62–7. Assisting the client to ambulate: **A.** Ambulating a client who needs minimal assistance. **B.** Ambulating a client with right-sided weakness, using a gait belt. (Photo by James Haines.)

A   B

health professional. Such opportunities help the client to correct errors in techniques while being protected from injury and also increase the client's strength, endurance, and skill in using the device. Clients need to be taught about the hazards associated with incorrect use of assistive devices and helped to plan how to accomplish their activities of daily living at the pace permitted by the device. A common problem faced by people who use assistive devices is the difficulty in carrying objects. Workable solutions to this problem include attaching a lightweight tote bag to the walker or using a lightweight back pack.

The following guidelines suggested by Sorensen and Luckman (1979, pp. 1122–1125) include points that are important to observe when assisting and supervising any client using ambulatory devices.

1. Make sure that the client is physically and psychologically prepared and able to use the device.
2. Select comfortable and well-fitting clothes that will permit unrestricted movement and permit you to observe the client's movements.
3. Make sure the client is wearing well-fitted shoes or house slippers that allow a secure stance and gait.
4. Create enough space in the room for the client to move about without obstruction.
5. Check the floor for clutter and wet or slippery areas that could precipitate an accident.
6. Be sure to have the client distribute the body weight evenly between the foot (feet) and the ambulating device (devices).
7. When the client is able to bear partial or full weight on both feet be sure the feet are positioned about 15 to 20 cm (6 to 8 in) apart to establish an adequate base of support.
8. Instruct the client to shift the body weight to the assistive device and the leg remaining in contact with the floor at the same time the other leg is moved forward.
9. Instruct the client to stand erect, keeping the body in good alignment, holding the head up and looking straight ahead.
10. Position yourself behind and slightly to the side of the client; this puts you in a position ready to provide assistance to the client.

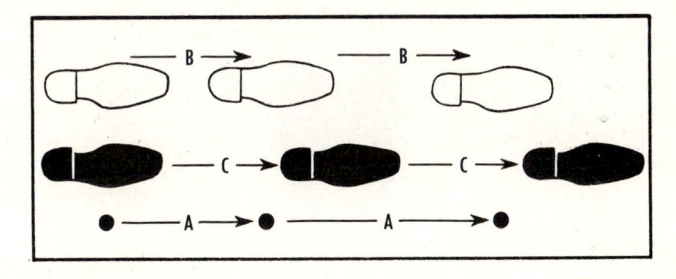

Figure 62–8. To use the cane-first gait, repeat this pattern having the client hold the cane on the strong side: **A.** Advance the cane ahead of the strong leg (solid foot). **B.** Advance the weak leg (open foot) so that it is parallel with the cane. **C.** Advance the strong leg ahead of the weak leg and cane.

Using a Cane

When using a cane, have the client hold the cane in the hand on the strong side of the body with the cane tip placed about 10 cm (4 in) out to the side of the foot. Sine et al. (1981) describe two different gaits that the client may use with a cane: one is the cane first and the other is the cane together. Cane first, shown in Figure 62–8, is used when the client's balance and strength are adequate enough to advance the strong leg ahead of the cane safely. The second type of gait, cane together, is used with clients who are stronger and well coordinated. With this gait the weak leg and the cane are advanced at the same time and the strong leg then is moved forward of the cane.

Using a Walker

Have the client stand in front of the walker with the feet positioned about 20 cm (8 in) apart and the handgrips held firmly. The elbows are flexed about 30 degrees with the wrists extended. Teach the client to advance the walker and walk with it using the appropriate gait.

The reciprocal walker can be used with either a two- or four-point gait. The two-point gait is shown in Figure 62–9. The four-point gait is similar to the crutch four-point gait described below.

To use a standard walker with a three-point gait follow the description below for the three-point crutch gait.

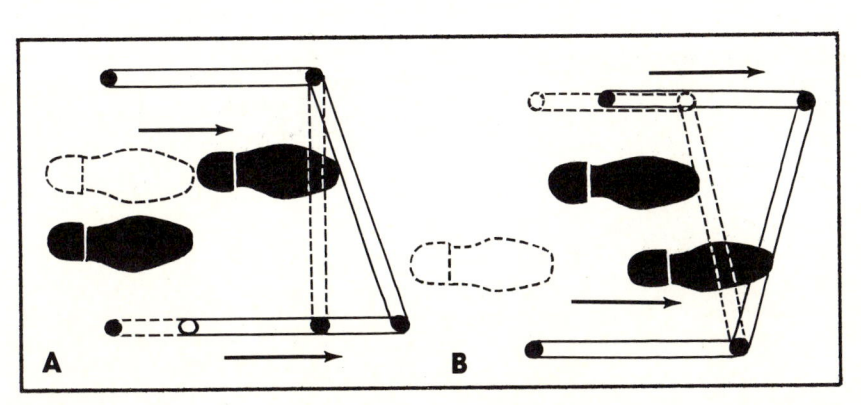

Figure 62–9. To use a reciprocal walker with a two-point gait have the client stand in front of the walker and repeat this pattern: **A.** Move one side of the walker forward and at the same time advance the opposite leg. **B.** Move the other side of the walker and at the same time advance the opposite leg.

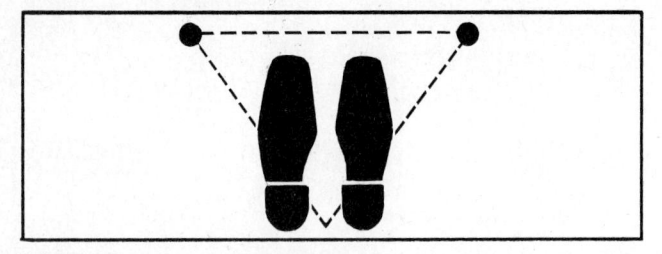

Figure 62-10. The triangular base of support for crutches with the tips of the crutches 15 to 20 cm (6 to 8 in) in front of the feet and out to the sides about 10 to 15 cm (4 to 6 in).

Measuring the Client for Crutches

Nurses are often in a position to assist clients with the proper fit of axillary crutches since these are the most common type used for short-term problems. There are two ways in which a client may be measured for axillary crutches; both are done with the client lying flat in bed wearing shoes. The measurements include an allowance for the axillary bar padding and the rubber crutch tip. To measure a client for crutches either measure the length from the axillary fold to the heel of the foot and add 5 cm (2 in) or measure from the axillary fold to a point 15 to 20 cm (6 to 8 in) out from the client's heel. While the client is standing, adjust the hand bars so the elbows are bent about 30 degrees while the wrist is hyperextended slightly. Since the body weight is born by the hands and not the axillae, a proper fit for the crutches can be determined by having the client stand erect with the crutches in place and inserting two or three fingers between the top of the axillary bar and each axilla.

Using Crutches

As shown in Figure 62-10, the base of support for crutches is the area bounded by the feet and the crutches; this triangular base increases stability. The stance forms the starting position for each of the crutch gaits described below. The base should not be too wide and may be established by placing the crutches either in front of or behind the feet. Keep the legs beneath the pelvis to avoid placing the legs in a slanting position which introduces a horizontal and downward force. Slipping occurs when there is insufficient friction on the supporting surface, as occurs with wet spots on the floor or ice on the ground outside (Luttgen and Wells, 1982). The appropriate technique with axillary crutches is to support the body weight on the arms by pressing the hands against the crutch hand bars. It is not uncommon, however, to observe people with axillary crutches supporting all of the body weight on the axillae. This practice places pressure on the radial nerves and can eventually cause weakness of the arms, wrists, and hands.

When teaching and supervising the client who is learning to use crutches, make sure the client is able to establish and maintain balance and is alert and able to follow instructions. Have the client place the tips of the crutches about 15 to 20 cm (6 to 8 in) in front of the feet and out to the side of the feet about 10 to 15 cm (4 to 6 in). The exact distance that provides both balance and comfort for each client depends on the client's height, so the client may need to do some experimenting to find the best position. Keep in mind that as the client's height increases, the center of gravity rises, so a wider base of support is necessary to maintain balance. Using crutches for ambulation is hard work but it becomes easier if the momentum from one step is used to make the next step. To do this requires that each step be followed quickly by another. Stopping after each step loses momentum and increases the amount of energy expended. When beginning to learn how to use crutches, the client may feel more comfortable and secure taking small steps. The particular gait pattern a client uses with crutches depends upon the client's ability to bear weight on one or both legs and the extent to which the client is able to balance on one or both legs. The various gaits are described below.

The Four-point Gait. The four-point gait shown in Figure 62-11 is the most stable because three points provide support at a time. The client must be able to bear some weight on both legs to use this gait.

The Three-point Gait. The three-point gait shown in Figure 62-12 is used when the client is able to bear full weight on one leg and only partial or no weight on the other leg.

The Two-point Gait. Since the two-point gait provides only two points for support at any one time, the client using this gait must have good balance. The two-point gait permits faster ambulation than the

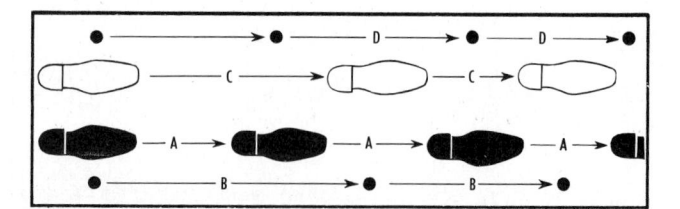

Figure 62-11. To use the four-point gait, first advance the left crutch forward about 20 cm (8 in). Then repeat the following right leg–right crutch, left leg–left crutch pattern: **A.** Advance right leg parallel to left crutch. **B.** Advance right crutch forward about 20 cm (8 in) ahead of right foot. **C.** Advance left leg parallel to right crutch. **D.** Advance left crutch 20 cm (8 in) ahead of left leg.

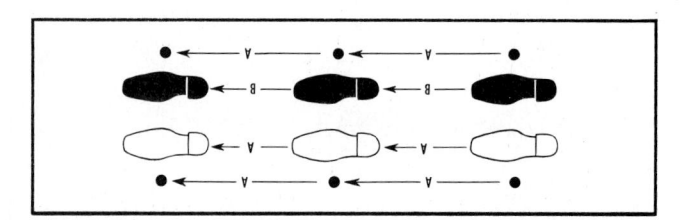

Figure 62-12. To use the three-point crutch gait, repeat this pattern: **A.** Advance both crutches and the non-weight-bearing leg forward about 20 cm (8 in). **B.** Advance the weight-bearing leg forward so it is even with the crutches and the non-weight-bearing leg.

four point. The pattern for this gait is the same one used with the reciprocal walker and is shown in Figure 62-9. One crutch at a time is moved forward simultaneously with the opposite leg.

The Swing-to and Swing-through Crutch Gaits. Both the swing-to and swing-through gaits shown in Figures 62-13 and 62-14 require that the client have good muscle strength in the upper arms to lift the body to pass through the crutches. These are advanced gaits that permit the client to move very quickly and they are usually used by people who have permanent disabilities.

RECORDING

At the end of the dangling or ambulatory activity record the client's physical and emotional tolerance, the pulse and respiration rates, any signs or symptoms of orthostatic hypotension such as pallor, perspiration, weakness, dizziness, or fainting, and the amount of anxiety you perceive the client is experiencing. In addition, indicate the amount of time the client was up and specify the distance ambulated so that this episode can be used as a comparison with previous and future activities. Specify the type of aid used during the activity such as a gait belt or crutches.

Sample POR Recording

- S—"I'm really bushed, using these crutches is harder than it looks. Guess I'm not in very good shape."
- O—Maintained good balance and posture during first ambulation on crutches with gait belt assistance. P 100, R 28, perspiring and face flushed after walking about 20 ft using a three-point gait.
- A—Fatigue related to exertion of crutch walking; able to use proper technique.
- P—Continue pushups and pull-ups to increase strength in arms. Continue ambulation q 4 hr as ordered.

Sample Narrative Recording

Very tired after ambulating about 20 ft on crutches for the first time, wearing gait belt. Able to use three-point gait and maintain good balance and posture. P 100, R 28, perspiring and face flushed. Continues to do pushups and pull-ups to strengthen arms.

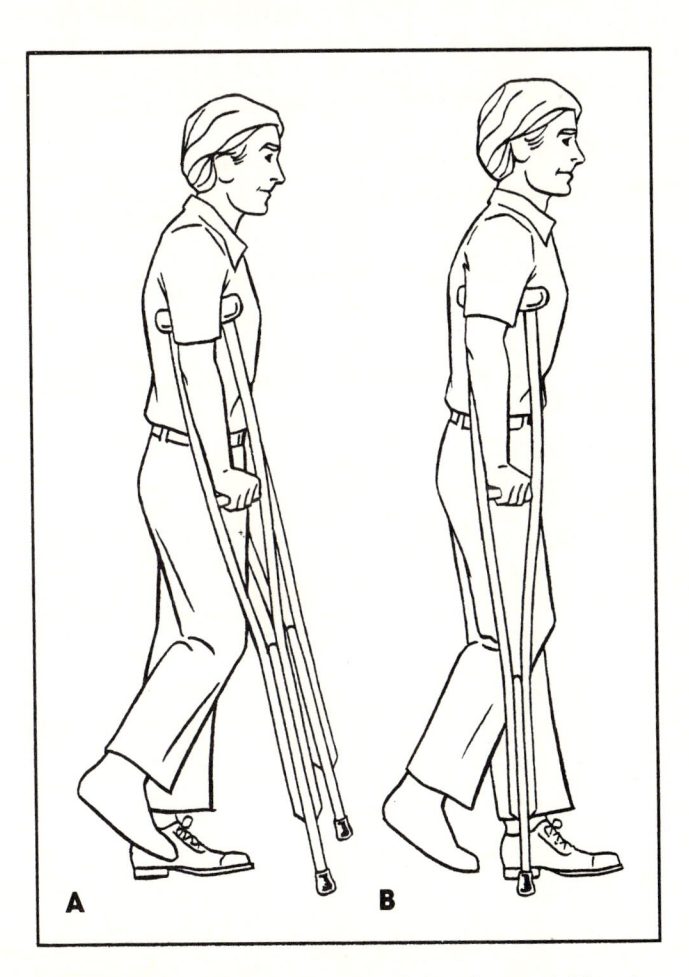

Figure 62-13. *To use the swing-to crutch gait, repeat this pattern:* ***A.*** *Advance the crutches while supporting the body weight on one leg.* ***B.*** *Advance the supporting leg to a point parallel with the crutches.*

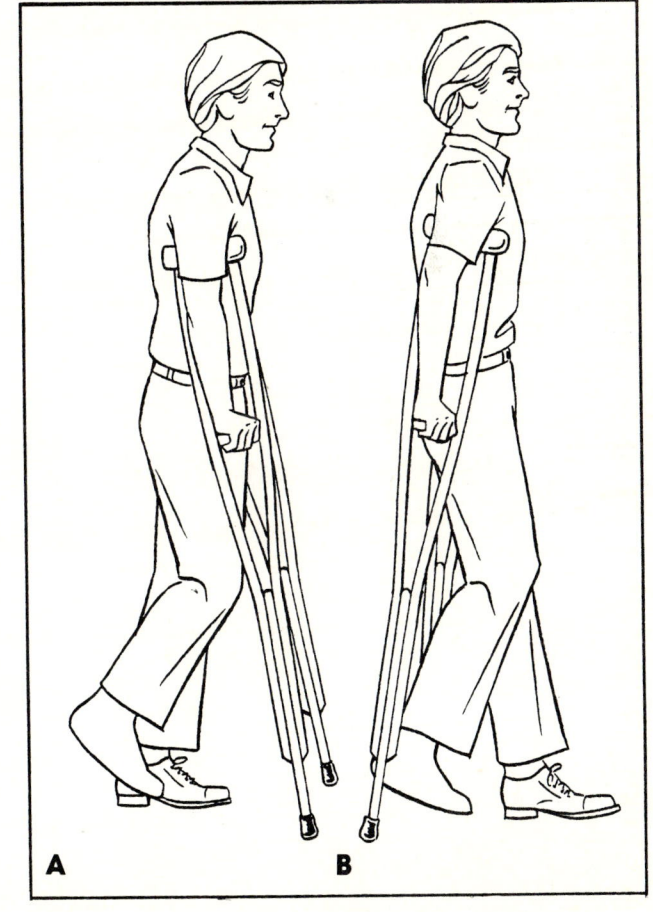

Figure 62-14. *To use the swing-through crutch gait, repeat this pattern:* ***A.*** *Advance both crutches while supporting the body weight on one leg.* ***B.*** *Swing both legs through and ahead of the crutches.*

☐ CRITICAL POINTS SUMMARY

1. Assess the client's physical and emotional ability to ambulate.
2. Teach and supervise the client appropriate conditioning exercises and supervise the activity in preparation for ambulation with assistive devices.
3. Be sure the client is wearing appropriate clothing and well-fitting shoes.
4. Prepare the environment before the client ambulates by removing clutter that could precipitate a fall.
5. Select the appropriate ambulatory device according to the client's physical ability.
6. Use a gait belt for clients who are learning how to ambulate.
7. Remind the client to stand erect and look straight ahead.
8. Remind the client how to shift body weight while moving the legs and ambulatory device.
9. Stand close to side of the client, ready to provide assistance if necessary.
10. Provide frequent encouragement and opportunities for the client to practice ambulation.

☐ LEARNING ACTIVITIES

1. Measure a peer for axillary crutches.
2. Practice resistive and isometric exercises to strengthen the upper body.
3. If possible obtain a pair of axillary crutches and practice the three- and four-point gaits.
4. Visit a pharmacy or medical appliance store and compare the weight and stability of different types of ambulatory devices.
5. Interview a person who uses some type of ambulatory device to find out how long it took to become skilled and comfortable using the device.

☐ REVIEW QUESTIONS

1. What types of clients require help with ambulation?
2. Match the type of conditioning exercise listed in Column I with the example of the exercise listed in Column II.

    COLUMN I
    a. Isotonic
    b. Resistive
    c. Isometric

    COLUMN II
    ___ Pushups
    ___ Holding a contracted muscle
    ___ Lifting weights

3. Describe exercises for the arms that would help prepare a client to use crutches.
4. Name the types of gaits that can be used with different assistive devices.
5. Describe assistive devices used for ambulation.
6. Indicate the steps you would use to provide minimal assistance in dangling.
7. Describe the position you would assume in relation to the client when helping a client to stand at the bedside.
8. Describe two ways you can support a client ambulating without assistive devices.
9. What are some of the safety hazards that must be guarded against when ambulating a client using assistive devices?
10. Describe the procedure you would use to teach and supervise a client using each of the following assistive ambulatory devices and gaits.
    a. A cane with the "cane first" gait.
    b. A reciprocal walker with the two-point gait.
    c. Crutches with the four-point, three-point, swing-to, and swing-through gait.

☐ PERFORMANCE CHECKLIST

OBJECTIVE: To assist a client to dangle safely.

CHARACTERISTIC	RANGE OF ACCEPTABILITY	SATISFACTORY	UNSATISFACTORY
1. Checks kardex for medical and nursing orders.	No deviation		
2. Washes hands.	No deviation		
3. Explains procedure.	No deviation		
4. Closes door or cubicle curtains, helps client to dress, puts bed in low position, folds back linen.	No deviation		
5. Assists client to side of bed, elevates head of bed.	No deviation		

(continued)

CHARACTERISTIC	RANGE OF ACCEPTABILITY	SATISFACTORY	UNSATISFACTORY
6. Stands facing the bed near the client's hips. Positions feet apart, with one behind the other.	No deviation		

7. To turn client to face you:
  a. Abducts client's near arm slightly
  b. Places far arm across body to grasp side rail or edge of bed
  c. Crosses far leg over near leg and brings feet to edge
  d. Places hands on shoulder and hip and assists as client pulls on side rail or edge of bed and turns
	Strong clients may not need to position limbs as described.		

8. Prepares to move to a dangling position:
  a. Has client use near hand to grasp edge of bed and far hand to grasp shoulder, side rail or prepares to push against bed
  b. Stands next to bed at client's hips, faces far corner of foot of bed. Takes a broad-based stance and advances foot farthest from the bed forward
  c. Places one hand around client's shoulder and other over both thighs, near knees, and flexes your knees to about a 120 degree angle to set abdominal and gluteal muscles
	Client may be strong enough to dangle without help.		

9. To assist client to dangle, simultaneously:
  a. Has client:
    (1) Pull on shoulder or side rail, or push into bed
    (2) Push elbow of other arm into bed
    (3) Move feet over edge of bed to floor
  b. Pivot rear foot, shifting weight to rear leg while lifting client's shoulders and pulling legs off bed
	Client may be strong enough to dangle without help.		

10. Holds client in sitting position until balanced. Instructs to support self by pressing hands into mattress and planting feet firmly on floor.	No deviation		
11. To return to bed, reverses procedure, assists client as needed.	No deviation		
12. Records amount of assistance provided, adverse responses, length of time client dangled, any changes in vital signs, tolerance for activity.	No deviation		

REFERENCES

Flitter HH: An Introduction to Physics in Nursing, ed 7. St Louis, CV Mosby, 1976.

Kottke FJ: Therapeutic exercise to maintain mobility. In Kottke FJ, Stillwell GK, et al. (eds): Krusen's Handbook of Physical Medicine and Rehabilitation, ed 3. Philadelphia, WB Saunders, 1982.

Luttgen K, Wells K: Kinesiology: A Scientific Basis of Human Motion, ed 7. Philadelphia, College Publishers, 1982.

Mitchell P, Loustau A: Concepts Basic to Nursing, ed 3. New York, McGraw-Hill, 1981.

Providing early mobility. Nursing Photobook. Horsham, PA, Intermed Communications, 1981.

Rambo BJ, Wood LA (eds): Nursing Skills for Clinical Practice, ed 3. Philadelphia, WB Saunders, 1982, vol 1.

Sine RD, Holcomb JD, et al.: Basic Rehabilitation Techniques: A Self-instructional Guide, ed 2. Rockville, MD, Aspen Systems Corporation, 1981.

Snyder M, Baum R: Assessing station and gait. American Journal of Nursing 74(7):1296–1297, 1974.

Sorensen KC, Luckman J: Basic Nursing: A Psychophysiological Approach. Philadelphia, WB Saunders, 1979.

Spencer WA, Vallbona RE, et al.: Physiologic concepts of immobilization. Archives of Physical Medicine and Rehabilitation 46(1):89–100, 1965.

BIBLIOGRAPHY

Crutches & walkers. Nursing 72 2(12):21–24, 1972.

Jungreis SW: Exercises for expediting mobility (and decreasing disability) in bedridden patients. Nursing 77 7(8):47–51, 1977.

Klabak L: Getting a grip on the transfer belt technique. Nursing 78 8(2):10, 1978.

Kozier B, Erb G: Techniques in Clinical Nursing: A Comprehensive Approach. Menlo Park, CA, Addison-Wesley, 1982.

Programmed instruction. Teaching a patient how to use crutches. American Journal of Nursing 79(6):1111–1126, 1979.

AUDIOVISUAL RESOURCES

Crutch and Cane Measurement
  16mm. (1969, Color, 6 min.)

Independent Ambulation and Elevation Activities of the Hemiplegic Patient
  16mm. (1966, Color, 11 min.)

Orientation to the Use of Crutches
  16 mm. (1965, Color, 6 min.)
    Available through:
    National Medical Audiovisual Center
    Order Section E Q
    Washington, DC 20409

The Use of Canes and Walkers
  Filmstrip with cassette. (1979, Color, 14 min.)

The Use of Crutches: Four, Two, Three Point Gaits
  Filmstrip with cassette. (1979, Color, 16 min.)
    Available through:
    Medcom, Inc.
    PO Box 116
    Garden Grove, CA 92642

SKILL 63 Maintenance of Range of Motion

☐ PREREQUISITE SKILL

Skill 19, "Inspection"
Skill 20, "Palpation"
Skill 28, "Handwashing"

☐ STUDENT OBJECTIVES

1. Indicate the purpose of range of motion (ROM) exercises.
2. Differentiate among the types of range of motion exercises.
3. Define the terms associated with ROM exercises.
4. Demonstrate the ability to execute passive and active assistive range of motion exercises safely.

☐ INTRODUCTION

Range of motion refers to the degree of movement that is possible for a joint. Range of motion (ROM) exercises are used for joint mobility and they consist of moving each joint through its normal range. These exercises are considered an integral part of nursing care for partially or completely immobilized clients and are also an important part of care for those who are not immobilized. ROM exercises are used to maintain joint mobility, increase joint movement, maintain muscle strength, increase activity tolerance, develop coordination, prevent deformities, and stimulate vascular circulation. In addition to these physiological benefits, ROM exercises also provide the client with increased opportunities to interact with the nurse, express concerns, and become aware of improvement in joint flexibility and muscle strength.

☐ PREPARATION

There is some degree of variation in the normal flexibility of each joint, and there also may be variation in the range of movement between a pair of joints. The movements that each person performs each day and the type of work done affects the type and amount of flexibility present in each joint. Although females tend to be more flexible than males, a gradual decrease in flexibility in both sexes begins after birth and continues throughout the life span (Rasch and Burke, 1978).

In addition to the normal decrease in the range of flexibility of any joint, pathologic changes in the neurologic, muscular, and skeletal systems from disease or trauma also reduce mobility. Mitchell and Loustau (1981) describes external factors that influence motor function and cites some therapeutic interventions which are often responsible for curtailing body joint movement (p. 345–346). For example, although bed rest may be prescribed either to prevent damage to a body system or permit a body part to rest, it reduces the opportunities the client has for movement of all the joints through their normal range. Kyphosis of the spine, flexion contractures of the hips, knees, and ankles can result from prolonged bed rest if the normal range of motion for the joints is not maintained by regular exercise (Kottke, 1982, p. 397). Mechanical restrictions on a client's movements result from the use of casts, skeletal traction, intravenous and other types of feeding modalities, and body system monitors as well as physical restraints that are used to control a client's movements. Clients who are capable of full physical activity may curtail their movements voluntarily because of physical or emotional lethargy or because they assume a sick-role behavior in response to the influence of the clinical environment.

Reduction or elimination of joint movement through the full range results in tightness in the joint. This occurs because lack of movement results in an alteration of the normal metabolic processes of connective tissue replacement. There is a continuous replacement of connective tissue in body areas which have repeated movement, such as in joint capsules, subcutaneous tissue, and intramuscular layers. This tissue is a network of fibers that is kept loose by virtue of the movements that occur during the time the fibers are forming. When movement is restricted or absent the connective tissue becomes contracted and dense and lacks the pliability essential for movement. The process by which the connective tissue becomes dense is known as fibrosis. Fibrosis affects the flexibility of joints in two different ways: within the joint and within the muscle. Within the joint, the dense connective tissue makes the joint tight and restricts the arc of motion. Fibrosis in the muscle causes it to shorten, and this pulls the joint to which it is attached into an abnormal position. This results in a contracture, which is a permanently contracted muscle that interferes with mobility and function. Kottke (1982) identifies four factors that promote fibrosis: immobilization, edema, trauma, and impaired circulation. He also cites studies that show that reduced or lost range of motion in normal joints can result after 4 weeks of immobilization. In an injured joint, however, loss of motion can occur in 2 weeks. Range of motion exercises help to ensure that pliable connective tissue will be formed instead of fibrosed tissue. Kottke recommends that ROM exercises be initiated immediately after trauma or surgery, except in the case of necessary immobilization (1982, p. 392).

TYPES OF RANGE OF MOTION

There are four types of range of motion exercises. The type selected depends upon the client's ability to assist with the exercises and the goal of the exercise program. *Passive range of motion exercises* are done completely by someone other than the client. They are used when the client is unable to participate actively in executing the movements. *Active assistive range of motion exercises* are performed collaboratively by the client and another person. *Free active range of motion*

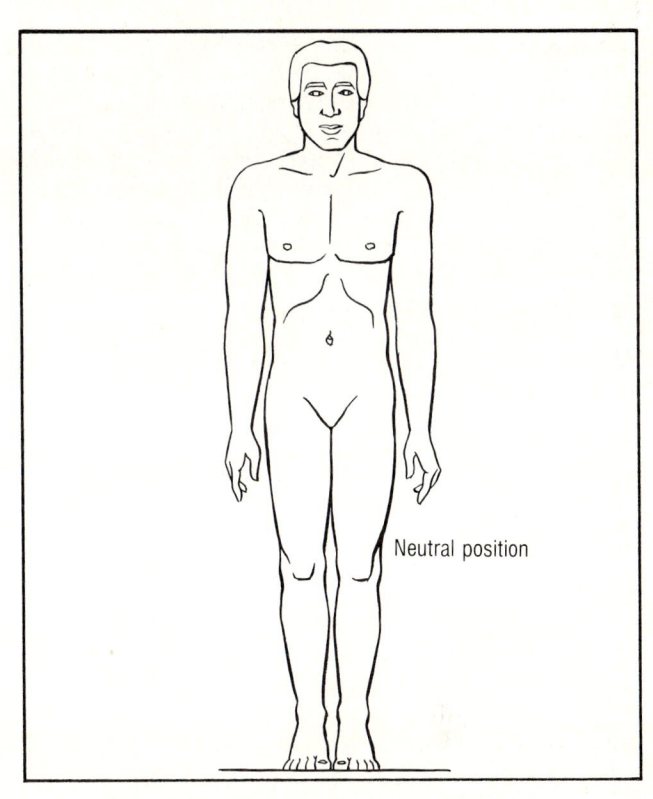

Figure 63–1. The anatomic neutral position.

exercises are performed completely by the client. *Resistive range of motion* exercises are active exercises performed against a resistant force created either by an assistant or some type of equipment.

ROM Movement Terms

The terms used to describe the movements of body parts assume that the part is in the neutral anatomic position, as shown in Figure 63-1. These terms are used to describe both the results of an evaluation of a joint's mobility and the performance of a joint within a specific range.

- *Abduction:* To move a part away from the midline.
- *Adduction:* To move a part toward the midline.
- *Circumduction:* To move a part in a circle.
- *Eversion:* To turn a part outward.
- *Extension:* To move the two ends of any jointed part away from each other, increasing the angle between the two parts.
- *Flexion:* To decrease the angle between two jointed parts.
- *Hyperextension:* To move a part beyond the normal extension.
- *Inversion:* To turn a part inward.
- *Pronation:* To position a part facing downward.
- *Supination:* To position a part facing upward.

TYPES OF JOINTS

A joint is defined as the junction of two bones. Although there are three different classes of joints in the body, because of their movements the class of most interest is the diarthrodial. The joints in this class are freely movable and have synovial fluid in the joint cavity. Joints that fall within this class are the pivot, gliding, ball and socket, hinge, condyloid, and saddle joints. These joints are located in different parts of the body and are the ones that are exercised during ROM exercises. For example, the first and second cervical vertebrae form a pivot joint while other cervical vertebrae are gliding joints, the shoulder and hip are ball and socket joints, the elbow is a hinge, the wrist is a condyloid joint, and the base of the thumb is a saddle joint.

DATA BASE

Client History and Recorded Data

Much of the information pertinent to determining a client's need for and the feasibility of implementing a program of ROM exercises is available on the client's health record and the nursing kardex. Although designing a program of ROM exercises for a client is usually considered an independent nursing function, it is essential that the nurse understand the types of diagnoses and conditions that would prohibit such independent nursing action. It is also wise to find out about the institution's policy regarding independent nursing actions and the use of passive range of motion exercises without a physician's order. A physician's order should be obtained for range of motion exercises for clients with diagnoses that indicate pathologic conditions of the joints such as arthritis or other inflammatory processes. Acute cardiac problems also contraindicate range of motion exercises unless specifically ordered by the physician.

The activity level permitted by the physician provides some indication of the amount and type of exercise the client is able to tolerate. In addition, information available on the admitting nursing history and the medical history should include problems with joint pain, swelling, weakness, paralysis, ambulation, balance, and the level of ability to perform activities of daily living. Clients who have existing disabilities involving the neuromuscular and skeletal systems may have a complete evaluation of function and mobility performed by a physical therapist. The report of such an evaluation in the health record provides another source of data. Talking with and observing the client's movements may reveal limitations in joint mobility which may be otherwise obscured by the way in which the client has consciously or unconsciously learned to adapt. Other important items of data pertinent to ROM exercises include the client's ability to understand, follow directions, and cooperate with the plan of care.

If the client is already receiving ROM exercises, the nursing-care plan or physical therapy record would indicate the type of ROM exercises to be used, the recommended frequency, and the client's ability to assist with the exercises. Current vital signs serve as a baseline for evaluating changes that may occur during ROM exercises.

Physical Appraisal Skills

Inspection. The joints and limbs on each side are inspected to detect similarities and differences in size and contour, atrophy, swelling, masses, and contractures. Inspection is also used to note the range of motion through which each joint is able to move.

Palpation. Swelling, masses, edema, or other deformities are identified by palpation. Abnormalities of a joint may be determined by palpating the joint while it is being moved through its range. Among the abnormalities that may be felt are dislocations in which the bone at a joint is displaced, or a subluxation, which is a slipping or partial dislocation of a bone, or muscle spasms that occur while the part is at rest.

EQUIPMENT

Bath blankets are often used to cover the client in bed to prevent exposure and drafts. Shorts, pajamas, or a towel can be used to drape the genital area while the lower extremities are exercised.

☐ EXECUTION

Prior to implementing any program of ROM exercises, clearly explain to the client what is to be done, how it will be done, and how the joint should feel during the exercise. When implementing active assistive or active exercises, demonstrate what the client is to do. Although the exercises may be done at any time, try to schedule them at a time when the client is rested and will be able to relax. It is important to enlist the client's cooperation and to advise him or her to inform you immediately if any pain or discomfort is felt at any time during the exercises. Keep in mind that normal movements used to perform personal care such as bathing, brushing the teeth, grooming the hair and nails all require a variety of joint movements and that these activities can be used to enhance a client's mobility even if confined to bed or restricted to sitting in a chair. Kottke (1982) recommends that to maintain range of motion each joint should be put through its complete range three times and that this regime be implemented two times a day. The frequency and number of times the exercises are performed each day may need to be increased if the goal is to restore or increase the range of motion and muscle strength.

POSITION OF THE CLIENT

Passive range of motion exercises are usually executed with the client lying on a bed or exercise table. Some joints may be exercised while the client is sitting on the side of the bed or in a chair. Elevate the level of the bed to a height appropriate for you to work without bending over, as this will decrease the back strain that contributes to developing a back injury. Position the client on the side of the bed nearest you for easy access. Whenever possible place the client flat on the back without a pillow. Have the client wear a hospital gown, shorts, pajama bottoms, or use a towel to cover the genital area. Use a bath blanket to provide warmth and privacy and draw the curtains or close the room door to avoid a draft.

IMPLEMENTING THE EXERCISES

Assume a position facing the body part and the direction of the intended movement. Provide secure support for the body part being exercised by holding limbs as close to the joint as possible. This serves several purposes: it stabilizes the joint; guides it through the desired direction; controls the movement of the part; and also provides an opportunity to palpate the joint to detect any abnormal placement of a bone in the joint. The grasp used to hold a part depends on the joint to be moved and the size of the client. Figures 63–2A and B show two different ways to hold and support an extremity during an exercise. Two persons may be required to implement ROM exercises safely with large clients. If possible, keep the client in good body alignment during the exercises. Maintain correct alignment of the limb segments during ROM exercises to avoid undue stress and strain on the joint structures. When doing resistive ROM exercises, support the part in a balanced and aligned position and use your muscles to provide a counterforce to the client's muscular contractions.

When moving the extremities through their range of motion, spread your feet apart to increase your base of support and stability. Set your arm, shoulder, abdominal and gluteal muscles, and shift your weight from one leg to the other as you move the extremity. Using large leg muscles and body weight helps move a heavy extremity more smoothly and with less effort and fatigue than when arm or shoulder muscles alone are used. Use measures that promote relaxation, such as approaching the client with a gentle manner, warming the hands before touching the client, keeping the client warm, and ensuring privacy.

Use smooth, rhythmic, and controlled movements during each of the exercises since painful muscle spasms can be initiated by jerky movements. Move each joint through as complete a range of motion as possible without causing pain or forcing the joint. Stop movement of the joint when the client feels pain or when resistance is met as the joint moves. A joint can be injured if it is moving during a muscle spasm or tremor because movement stretches a contracted muscle or ligament. Begin with and return the part to its neutral position, which is usually, but not always, the same as anatomic neutral. For example, when the shoulder is in a neutral position for ROM exercises, the arm is extended horizontally from the shoulder rather than suspended at the side. Expect the client to have an increase in respiratory and cardiac rates during and immediately following the exercises.

When performing a complete program of passive range of motion exercises, start with the neck and then progress down the body distally to the shoulders and upper extremities and then to the hips and lower extremities. After grasping and securely holding a part, watch the client's facial expression while moving the part. This enables you to detect early signs of pain or discomfort and to gain some sense of the client's endurance for the exercises.

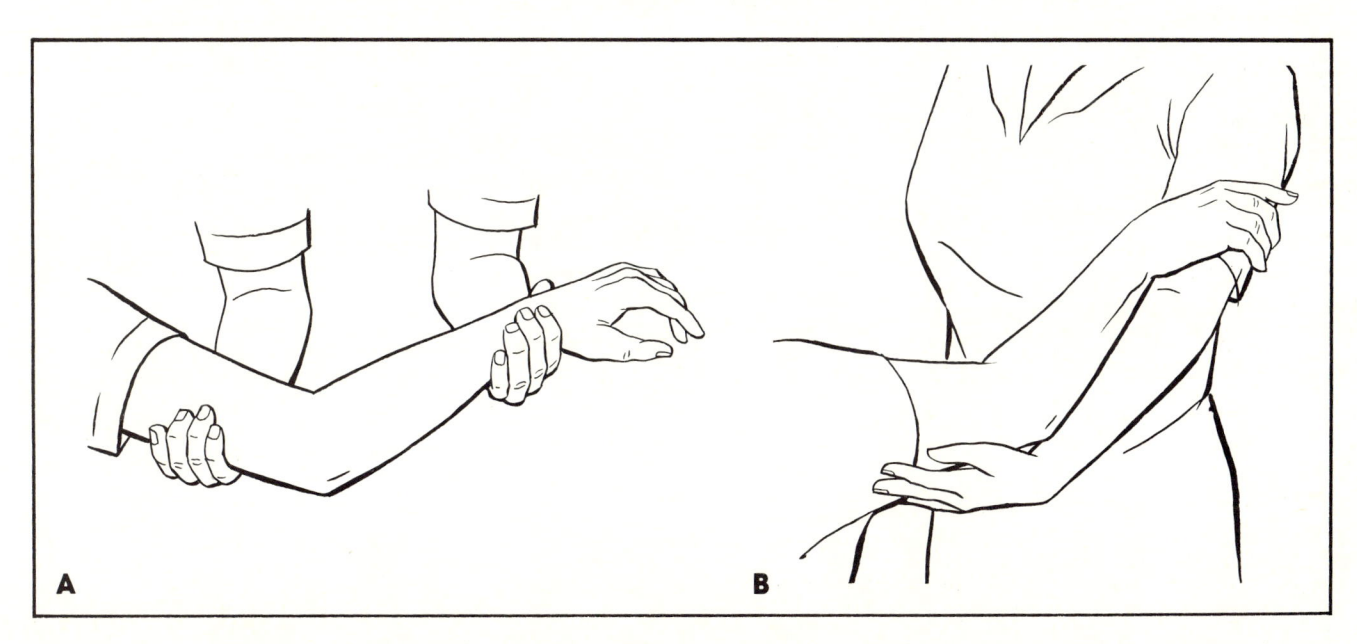

Figure 63–2. Methods of holding and supporting an extremity. **A.** Using cupped hands to support the extremity close to a joint. **B.** Using an arm and hand to support the client's extremity.

RANGE OF MOTION EXERCISES

The movements used for range of motion exercises for each body part are the same for passive, active, assistive, or independent exercises. If the purpose of the exercise is to increase strength through the use of resistive exercise, consult a physician or physical therapist for the amount of resistance to use; if the purpose of the exercise is to increase the range of motion, consult them to find out how far to extend the movement beyond the client's normal range. The movements involved in the exercises for various parts of the body are identified below and the movements are shown in Figures 63–3 through 63–11. Begin with the body part in the neutral position for each specific exercise and return the part to the anatomic neutral position at the end of the exercise. Each movement is repeated on both sides of the body.

Neck Movements
The exercise movements for the neck include *flexion, hyperextension, lateral flexion,* and *rotation.* Support the head between your hands if the client is unable to control the movements.

Shoulder Movements
The exercise movements for the shoulder include *forward flexion, extension, hyperextension, abduction, adduction, circumduction, external rotation, internal rotation, horizontal abduction, horizontal adduction, elevation,* and *depression.*

Elbow Movements
Exercises for the elbow include *flexion, extension, supination,* and *pronation.*

Wrist Movements
Exercises for the wrist include *flexion, extension, hyperextension, adduction,* and *abduction.*

Finger Movements
Exercises for the fingers include *flexion, extension, hyperextension, abduction, adduction,* and *opposition of the thumbs.*

Hip Movements
The movements for the hip include *flexion, extension, hyperextension, abduction, adduction, cross adduction, internal rotation, external rotation,* and *circumduction.*

Knee Movements
The movements for the knee include *flexion* and *extension.*

Ankle Movements
The movements for the ankle include *dorsiflexion, plantar flexion, eversion,* and *inversion.*

Toe Movements
The movements for the toes include *flexion, extension, abduction,* and *adduction.*

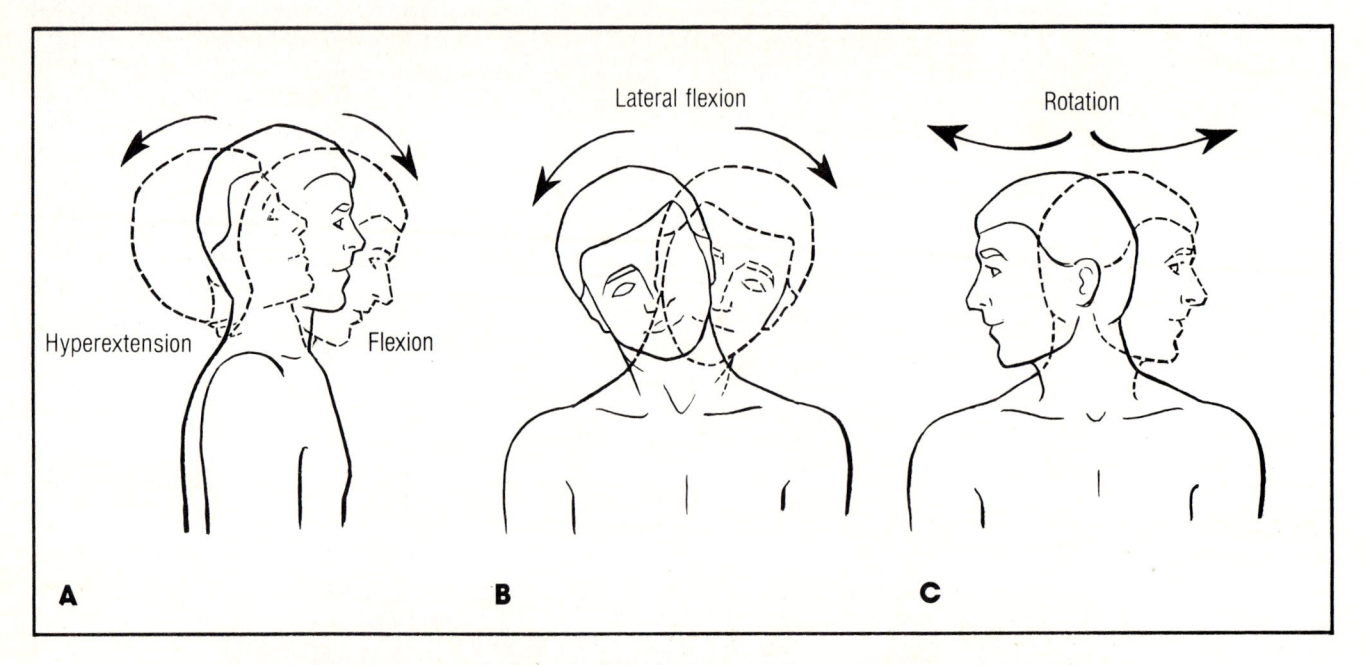

Figure 63–3. Neck movements. **A.** Flexion: *Tilt the head forward until the chin touches the chest.* Hyperextension: *Tilt the head back as far as possible.* **B.** Lateral flexion: *Tilt the head as if to move the ear toward one shoulder and then the other.* **C.** Rotation: *Turn the head so the person is looking over first one shoulder and then the other.*

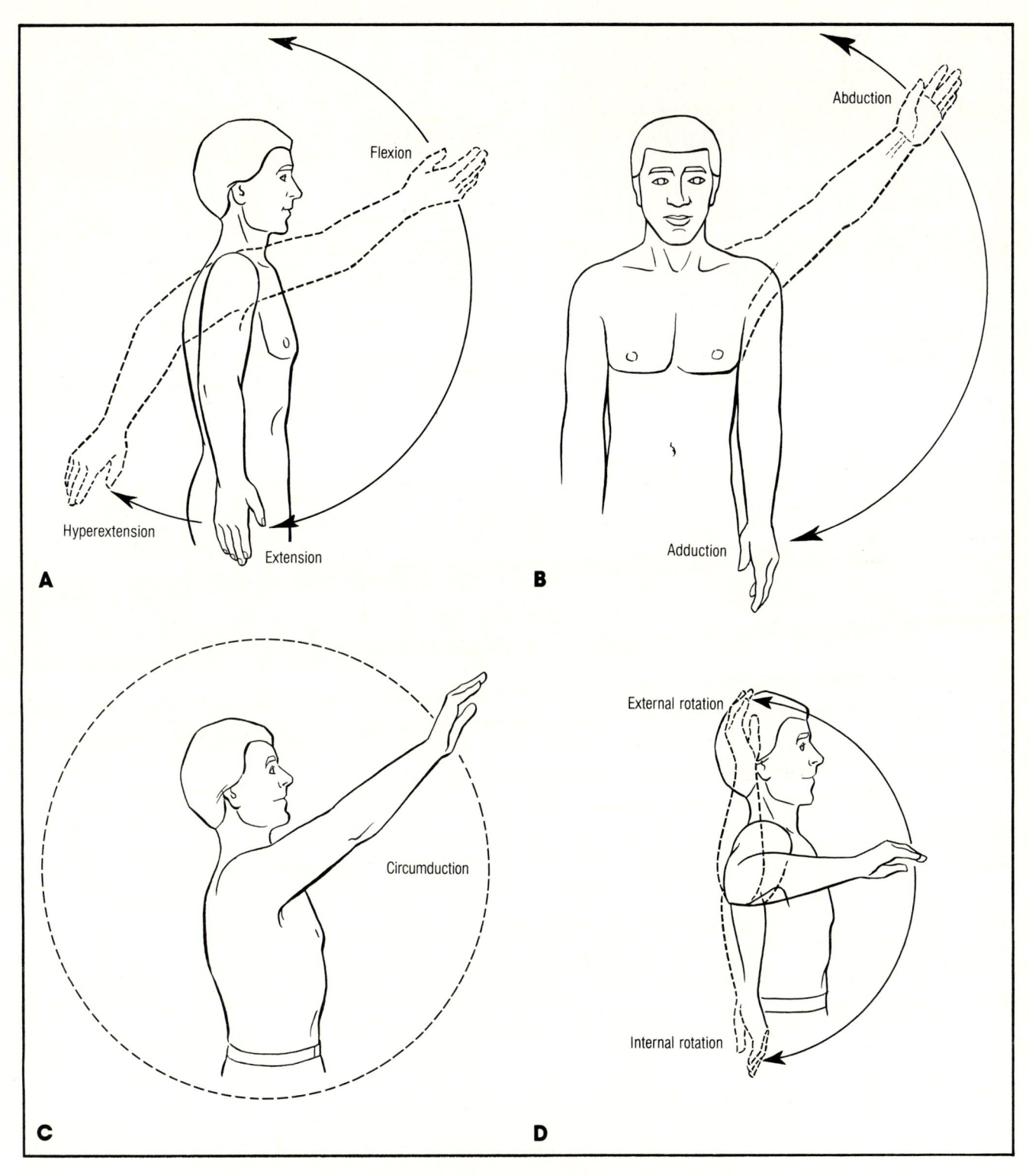

Figure 63–4. Shoulder movements **A.** Forward flexion: *Raise the arm (keeping the elbow straight) forward and upward until it is alongside the head.* Extension: *Lower the arm to the neutral position.* Hyperextension: *Move the arm backward from the neutral position.* **B.** Abduction: *Move the arm laterally away from the body and up above the head.* Adduction: *Return the arm to the neutral position.* **C.** Circumduction: *Move the straight arm in a 360 degree circle in a plane alongside the body.* **D.** External rotation: *Hold the arm at shoulder height with the elbow bent at a 90 degree angle and the palm facing the feet. Rotate the arm until the palm and forearm face forward.* Internal rotation: *Hold the arm at shoulder height with the elbow bent at a 90 degree angle and the palm facing the feet. Rotate the arm until the palm and forearm face backward.*

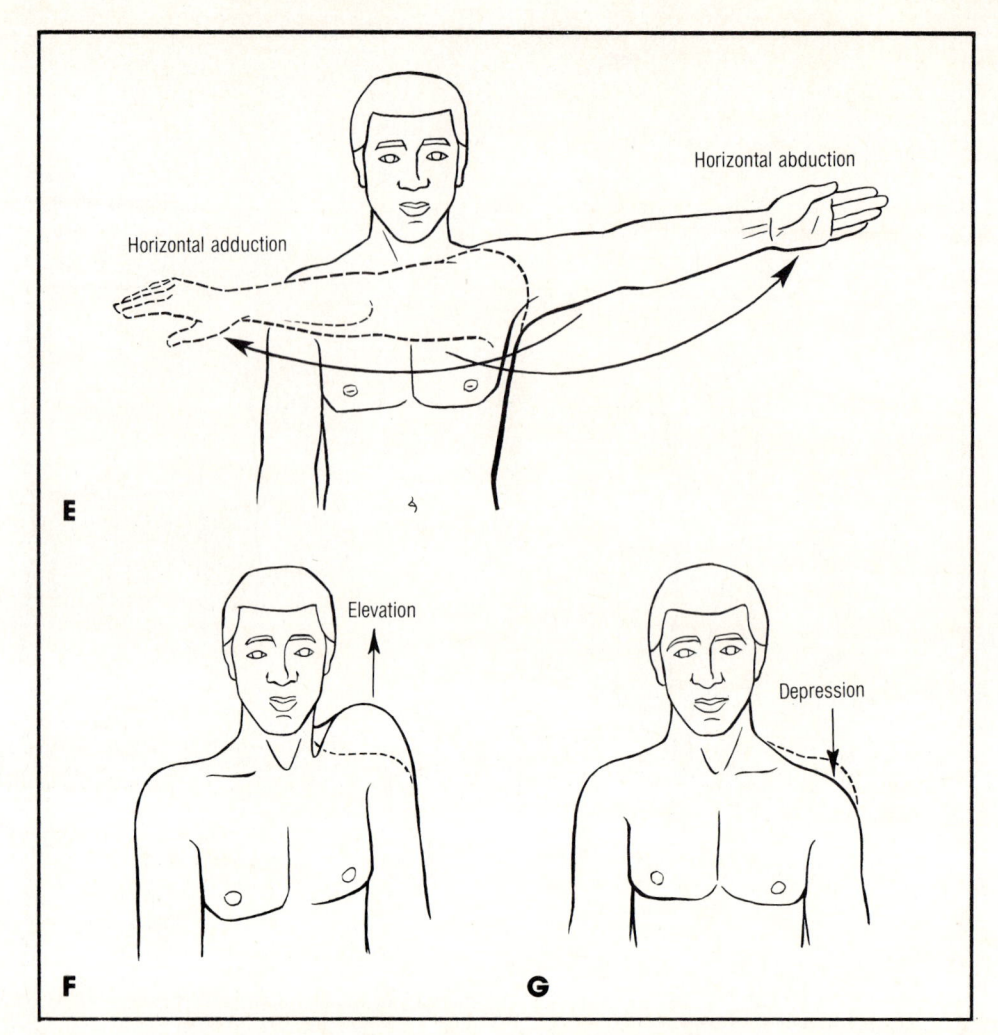

Figure 63-4. E. Horizontal abduction: *Extend the arm laterally at shoulder height and move the arm backward.* Horizontal adduction: *Extend the arm laterally at shoulder height and move the arm across the front of the body toward the opposite shoulder.* **F.** Elevation: *Raise one shoulder up toward the ear.* **G.** Depression: *Lower one shoulder down toward the foot.*

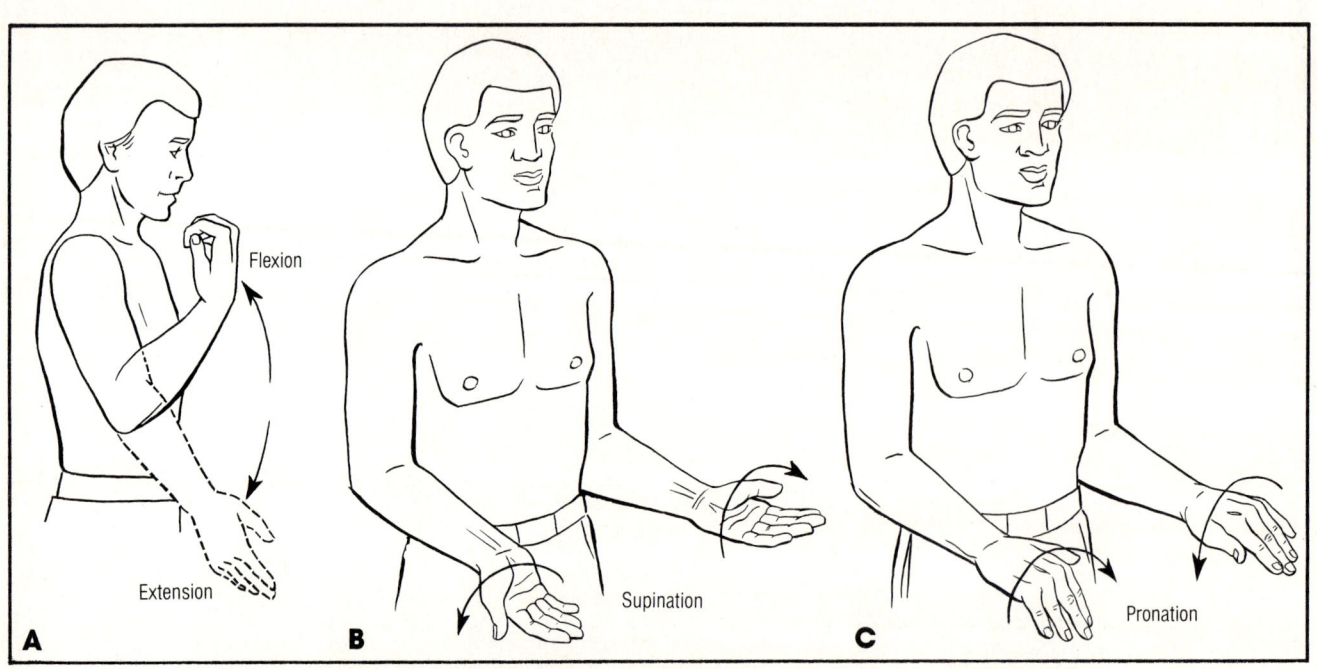

Figure 63-5. Elbow movements. **A.** Flexion: *Bend the elbow and bring the forearm and hand toward the shoulder.* Extension: *Return the forearm and hand to the neutral position.* **B.** Supination: *Stabilize the elbow with the forearm extended in front of the body, rotate the forearm 90 degrees until the palms face upward.* **C.** Pronation: *Stabilize the elbow with the forearm extended in front of the body, rotate the forearm 90 degrees until the palm faces downward.*

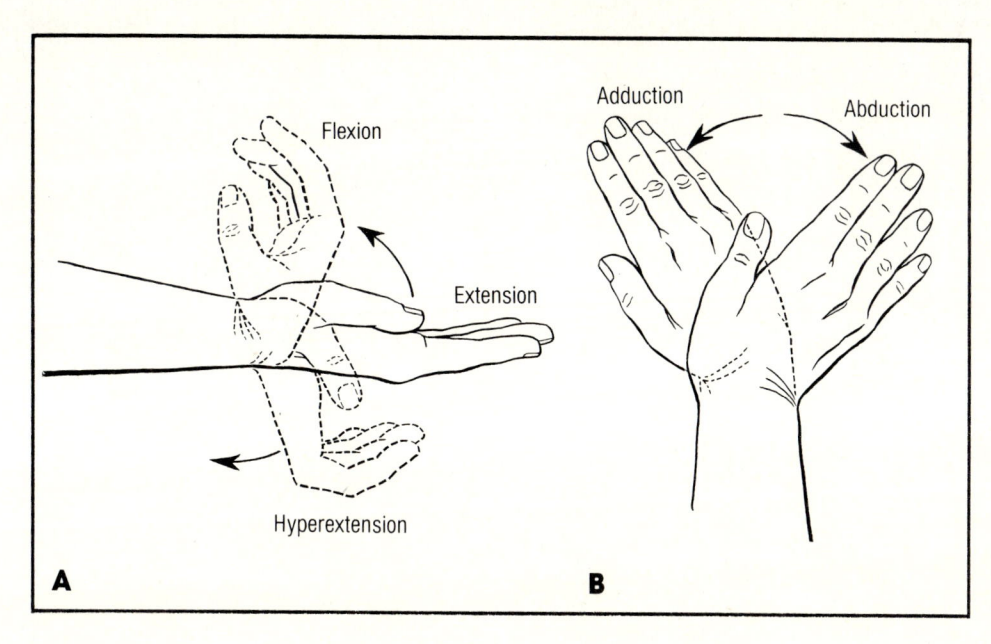

Figure 63-6. Wrist movements. **A.** Flexion: *Bend the wrist so the palm is toward the inner aspect of the forearm.* Extension: *Straighten the wrist to the neutral position.* Hyperextension: *Bend the wrist back toward the forearm.* **B.** Adduction (radial deviation): *Move the hand sideways with the thumb side toward the forearm.* Abduction (ulnar deviation): *Move the hand sideways with the little finger toward the forearm.*

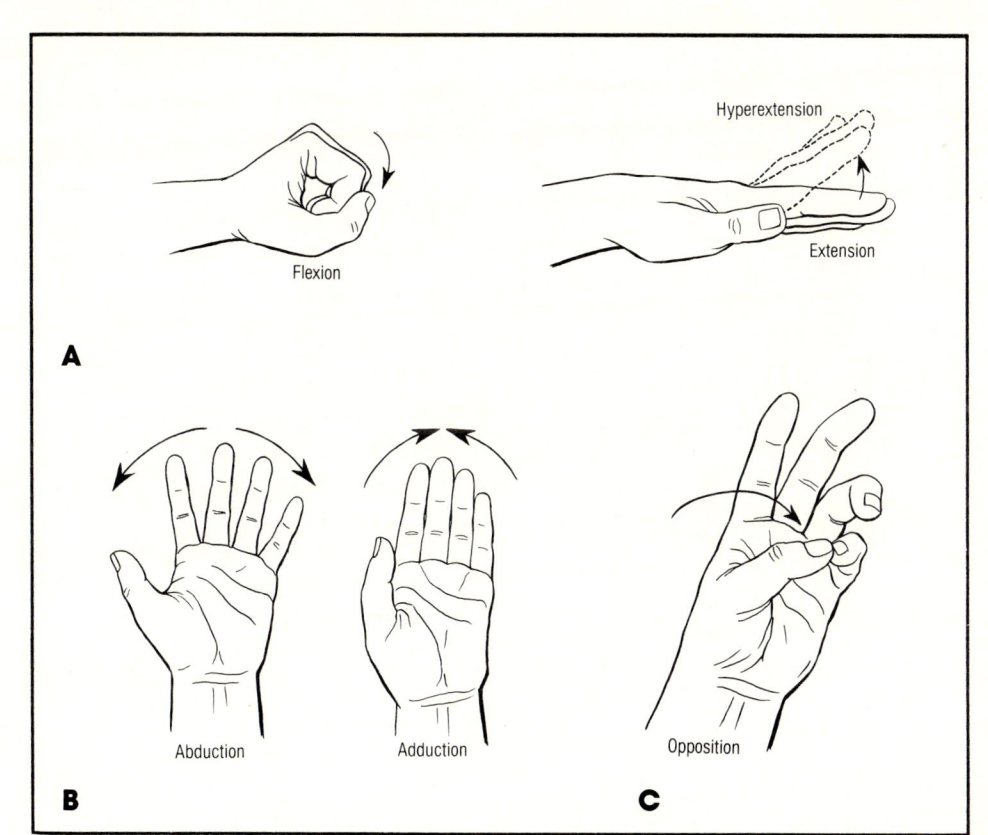

Figure 63-7. Finger movements. **A.** Flexion: *Bend the fingers and thumb toward the palm.* Extension: *Return the fingers to the neutral position.* Hyperextension: *Bend the fingers backward toward the forearm.* **B.** Abduction: *Spread the fingers apart.* Adduction: *Move the fingers toward each other.* **C.** Opposition of thumbs: *Move the thumb to touch the little finger.*

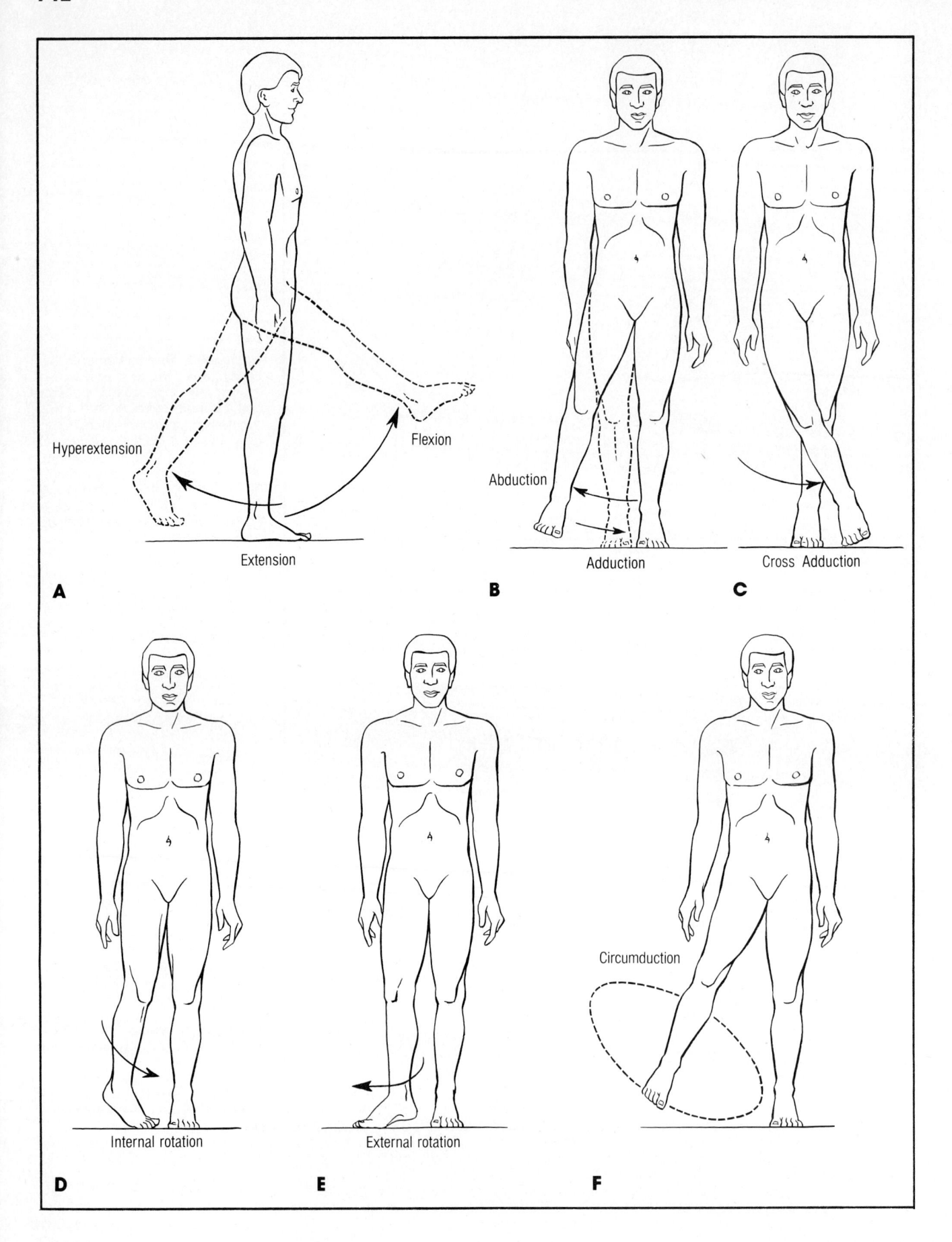

A

Hyperextension · Flexion · Extension

B

Abduction · Adduction

C

Cross Adduction

D

Internal rotation

E

External rotation

F

Circumduction

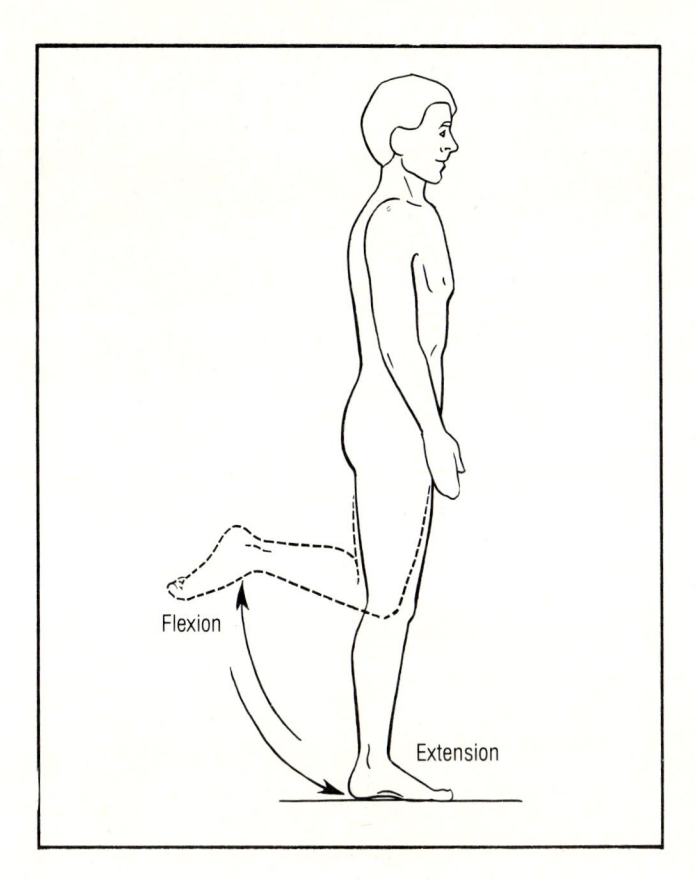

Figure 63-9. Knee movements. Flexion: *Bend the knee and direct the foot backward and upward toward the body, decreasing the angle between the foot and the back of the leg.* Extension: *Return the knee to the neutral position.*

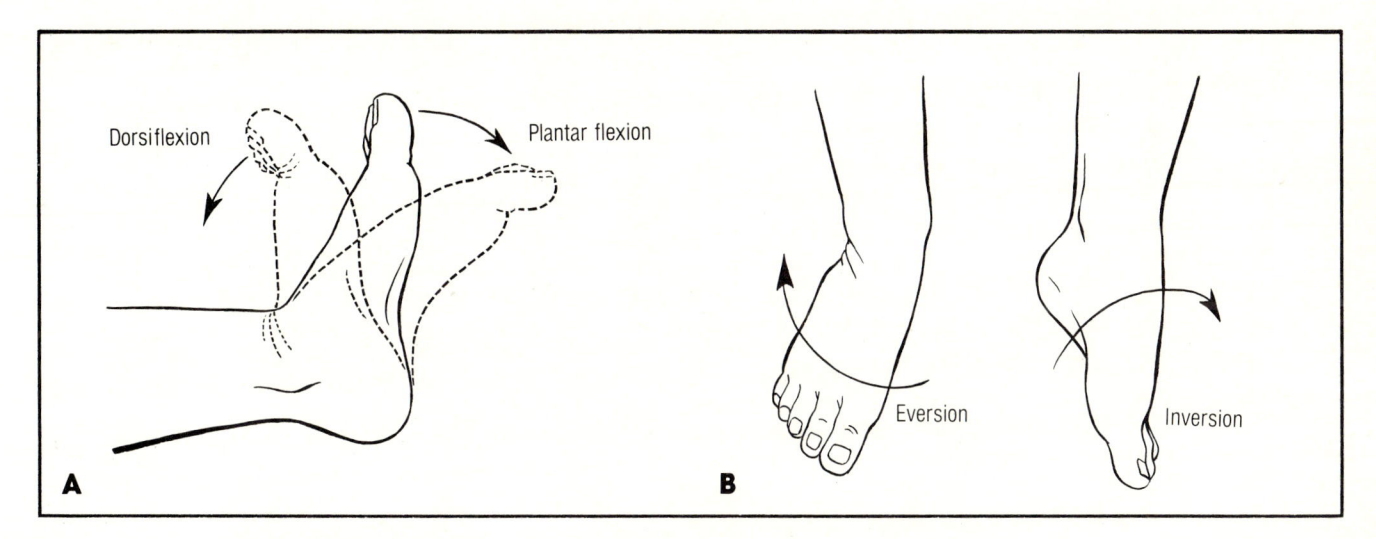

Figure 63-10. Ankle movements. **A.** Dorsiflexion: *Pull the foot up toward the body.* Plantar flexion: *Press the foot downward while pointing the toes.* **B.** Eversion: *Turn the sole of the foot laterally outward.* Inversion: *Turn the sole of the foot inward toward the midline of the body.*

Figure 63-8. Hip movements. **A.** Flexion: *Bend the hip with the leg moving forward and upward.* Extension: *Return the hip to the neutral position.* Hyperextension: *Move the leg backward from the neutral position.* **B.** Abduction: *Move the leg laterally from the side of the body.* Adduction: *Return the leg to the neutral position.* **C.** Cross adduction: *Move the leg across the midline over the opposite leg.* **D.** Internal rotation: *Turn the leg and foot toward the midline.* **E.** External rotation: *Turn the leg and foot outward away from the midline.* **F.** Circumduction: *Hold the leg straight and move it in a 360 degree circle in a plane alongside the body.*

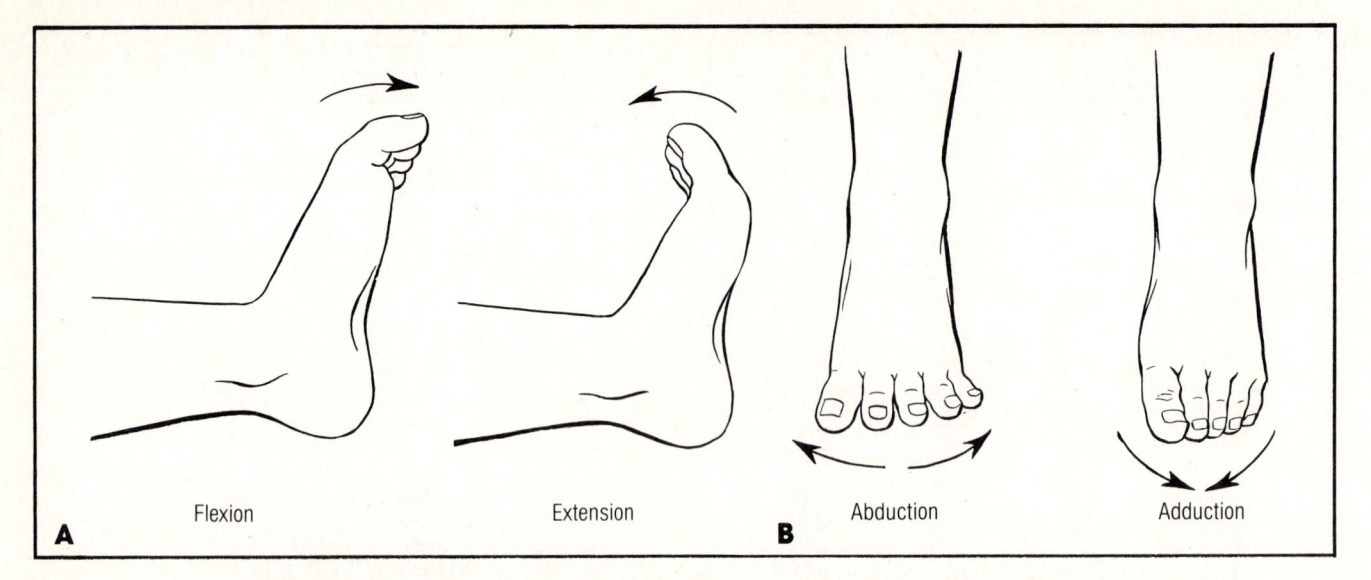

Figure 63-11. Toe movements. **A.** Flexion: *Point the toes downward.* Extension: *Pull the toes upward toward the foot.* **B.** Abduction: *Spread the toes apart.* Adduction: *Move the toes toward each other.*

☐ SKILL SEQUENCE

RANGE OF MOTION EXERCISES

Step	Rationale
1. Wash hands.	Prevents transfer of microorganisms.
2. Explain procedure to client; specify joints to be exercised.	Allays anxiety. Allows client to participate in own care.
3. Adjust bed to appropriate working height.	Prevents back strain from bending, stretching, and lifting.
4. Close room door or draw curtains around bed; cover client with a bath blanket and place a drape over genital area or have client wear shorts.	Keeps client warm and protects privacy.
5. Position client in neutral body alignment on the near side of bed.	Neutral anatomic position provides reference point for movements.
6. Position self to face the body part being exercised and the intended direction of movement. Place feet apart and one in front of the other.	Avoids exerting a twisting or shearing force on spine and increases effectiveness of muscular movements. Broadens base of support and makes weight shifting possible.
7. Expose part to be exercised; place warm hands in position to support body part.	Provides access to the part. Promotes relaxation.
8. Move the part gently in desired direction to the limit of its normal range or until resistance is felt. Repeat at least three times.	Avoids pain and injury to the joint.
9. Document in record joints exercised, number of repetitions, client's reaction and ability to participate, and any unusual findings.	Fulfills nurse accountability and provides ongoing data base.

RECORDING

After ROM exercises are performed, record the type of exercises, that is, passive, active, active assistive, resistive; the joints exercised; the types of movements; and the number of times the exercises were done. Indicate the presence of any discomfort such as pain or spasms during or after the exercises, and note any increase or decrease in the range of movement. Include information about the client's tolerance for the exercises and the ability to cooperate and assist with the exercises.

Sample POR Recording

- S—"I feel stiff lying in bed so much."
- O—Full range of motion in all joints without discomfort during active assistive ROM to all joints.
- A—Joint stiffness related to bed rest.
- P—Continue ROM to all joints; three repetitions, three times per day.

Sample Narrative Recording

Reports joint stiffness in all joints. Active assistive ROM to all joints without discomfort. Will continue with exercises, three repetitions, three times a day.

CRITICAL POINTS SUMMARY

1. Position self and client to prevent stretching and muscle strain.
2. Explain exercises and promote relaxation prior to beginning ROM exercises.
3. Use gentle, smooth, and rhythmic movements.
4. Stop the exercises immediately when the client experiences pain.
5. Move the joint only to the point of resistance or pain.

LEARNING ACTIVITIES

1. Perform a complete set of ROM exercises on yourself. Note the mobility of each joint, the point at which stretch on the muscles is felt, and the point at which discomfort is present.
2. With a partner, execute all four types of ROM exercises. Note the sensations of assisting with and receiving these exercises.

REVIEW QUESTIONS

1. What are the reasons ROM exercises are performed?
2. How would you describe the differences in the four types of ROM exercises?
3. Match each of the terms listed in Column I with its definition listed in Column II

COLUMN I	COLUMN II
1. Supination	___ To move a part inward.
2. Adduction	___ To move a part outward.
3. Abduction	___ To move a part toward the midline.
4. Inversion	___ To position a part facing upward.
5. Eversion	___ To move a part away from the midline.

PERFORMANCE CHECKLIST

OBJECTIVE: To execute range of motion exercises safely.			
CHARACTERISTIC	RANGE OF ACCEPTABILITY	SATISFACTORY	UNSATISFACTORY
1. Washes hands.	No deviation		
2. Explains procedure.	No deviation		
3. Adjusts bed to working height.	No deviation		
4. Provides privacy.	No deviation		
5. Positions client in neutral body position.	No deviation		
6. Positions self to face body part being exercised; faces direction of intended movement; places feet for broad base support.	No deviation		
7. Exposes part to be exercised.	No deviation		
8. Moves body part smoothly and gently to limit of normal range or until resistance is felt. Repeats each movement at least three times.	No deviation		
9. Shifts body weight to help move heavy body parts.	No deviation		
10. Uses this sequence to perform ROM exercises on each side of the body: a. Neck: (1) Flexion (2) Hyperextension (3) Lateral flexion (4) Rotation (right and left)	No deviation		

(continued)

OBJECTIVE: To execute range of motion exercises safely (cont.).			
CHARACTERISTIC	RANGE OF ACCEPTABILITY	SATISFACTORY	UNSATISFACTORY
b. Shoulder: (1) Forward flexion (2) Extension (3) Hyperextension (4) Abduction (5) Adduction (6) Circumduction (7) External rotation (8) Internal rotation (9) Horizontal abduction (10) Horizontal adduction (11) Elevation (12) Depression	No deviation		
c. Elbow: (1) Flexion (2) Extension (3) Supination (4) Pronation	No deviation		
d. Wrist: (1) Flexion (2) Extension (3) Hyperextension (4) Adduction (5) Abduction	No deviation		
e. Fingers: (1) Flexion (2) Extension (3) Hyperextension (4) Abduction (5) Adduction (6) Opposition of thumbs	No deviation		
f. Hip: (1) Flexion (2) Extension (3) Hyperextension (4) Abduction (5) Adduction (6) Cross adduction (7) Internal rotation (8) External rotation (9) Circumduction	No deviation		
g. Knee: (1) Flexion (2) Extension	No deviation		
h. Ankle: (1) Dorsiflexion (2) Plantar flexion (3) Eversion (4) Inversion	No deviation		
i. Toe: (1) Flexion (2) Hyperextension (3) Abduction (4) Adduction	No deviation		
11. Documents the joints exercised, the number of repetitions, the client's reaction and ability to participate, and any unusual findings.	No deviation		

REFERENCES

Kottke FJ: Therapeutic Exercise to Maintain Mobility. In Kottke FJ, Stillwell GK, et al. (eds): Krusen's Handbook of Physical Medicine and Rehabilitation, ed 3. Philadelphia, WB Saunders, 1982.

Mitchell P, Loustau A: Concepts Basic to Nursing, ed 3. New York, McGraw-Hill, 1981.

Rasch PJ, Burke RK: Kinesiology and Applied Anatomy, ed 6. Philadelphia, Lea & Febiger, 1978.

BIBLIOGRAPHY

Ciuca R, Bradish J: Active range-of-motion exercises encore: A handbook. Nursing78 8(8):45–49, 1978.

Ciuca R, Bradish J: Passive range-of-motion exercises encore: A handbook. Nursing78 8(7):59–65, 1978.

Hirschberg GG, Lewis L, et al.: Promoting patient mobility: And other ways to prevent secondary disabilities. Nursing77 7(5):42–46, 1977.

Rambo BJ, Wood LA (eds): Nursing Skills for Clinical Practice, ed 3. Philadelphia, WB Saunders, 1982, vol 1.

Sorensen KC, Luckman J: Basic Nursing: A Psychophysiological Approach. Philadelphia, WB Saunders, 1979.

AUDIOVISUAL RESOURCE

Range of Motion Exercises
Filmstrip with cassette (1984, Color, 17 min.)
Available through:
Medcom, Inc.
PO Box 116
Garden Grove, CA 92642

SKILL 64 Turning, Moving, and Positioning

PREREQUISITE SKILLS

Skill 28, "Handwashing"
Skill 38, "Skin Care"
Chapter 14, "Introduction"
Skill 63, "Maintenance of Range of Motion"

☐ STUDENT OBJECTIVES

1. Indicate the purposes for which clients are placed in the different types of positions.
2. Identify pressure points associated with various body positions.
3. Differentiate among the devices used to support clients in various positions.
4. Differentiate among the various devices and mechanisms used to prevent pressure problems and to increase circulation.
5. Describe correct turning and moving techniques.
6. Describe the appearance of a client who is positioned correctly in the supine, lateral, prone, and Sims positions.
7. Describe the appearance of a bed that has been placed in various Fowler and Trendelenburg positions.
8. Demonstrate the ability to turn, move, and place a client in different therapeutic positions in a safe manner.

☐ INTRODUCTION

Changing the body position is a natural and frequent activity that most people do either unconsciously or consciously. For example, a healthy person with normal innervation shifts body position when pressure and tissue anoxia produce discomfort, or moves from a lying down to a sitting position when experiencing respiratory distress. An important component of nursing practice is moving and changing a client's body position for comfort as well as for therapeutic purposes. There are many types of clients who are unable to make these automatic changes in body position without assistance; those who are weak, ill, or debilitated, and those who have pain, impaired cerebral function, or decreased sensorimotor status. There are also clients who have conditions such as a heart attack, surgery, or fractures that require restricted physical activity to permit a body system or part to rest. There are specific body positions used for therapeutic purposes; for example, Fowler's position is used to facilitate increased expansion of the chest during inspiration and the Trendelenburg position is used in hypovolemic shock to increase the circulation of the available fluid volume to the vital organs as one means of compensating for a deficit in total body fluid volume.

Although a physician may specify turning and positioning activities for a given client, the nurse is expected to identify all of the clients who require such assistance and to implement turning and repositioning as an independent nursing function. Any person who is physically inactive and confined to partial or complete bed rest or is limited to being up in a chair might develop negative consequences in several body systems, merely from the immobility. These consequences are manifested in the altered function of the cardiovascular, respiratory, gastrointestinal, motor, and urinary systems, as well as in metabolic and psychosocial disequilibrium. Further elaboration of these consequences can be found in medical–surgical textbooks.

Clients who are more vulnerable to the consequences of immobility include those whose physical condition is deteriorating rapidly; those with an altered sensorium or decreased mobility; those who are thin, emaciated, malnourished, obese, elderly, in pain, or terminally ill; and those who are restrained for prolonged periods of time or have had recent anesthesia or surgery. Many of the consequences of immobility can either be eliminated or minimized by periodic movement and position change.

The moving, turning, and positioning activities described in this skill are in common use in most acute, chronic, and home-care settings. They may be performed by the nurse, family, or other primary caregiver.

☐ PREPARATION

There are several factors involved in careful positioning. First, it is imperative for the nurse to use correct body mechanics during the pulling, turning, and lifting that are part of positioning. These activities range from mildy strenuous positioning to the more strenuous activity of moving clients up in bed. Because one of two major contributing factors to the development of low back injury is repeated episodes of low to moderate levels of back strain (Scholey, 1983; Stubbs et al., 1981), the nurse will want to protect himself or herself by using techniques that avoid twisting the spine and causing strain on the intervertebral discs.

Second, it is imperative that the client be positioned and supported in a correct body alignment, with joints in a neutral or slightly flexed position, so as to avoid placing strain on joint structures and muscles. Correct alignment and adequate support also increase the client's comfort and promote rest and relaxation.

Third, neither the position itself nor the supportive devices used to maintain the position may place extensive pressure on skin and subcutaneous tissues, particularly at places known as "pressure points." Most of the body's weight is transmitted to a bed or chair at these pressure points, that is, at places where the bones are nearest the skin surface and where the subcutaneous tissue is thin. Pressure points vary with the body position. For example, in a supine position, pressure points are the back of the head, the spines of the scapulae, the elbows, sacrum, and heels, as shown in Figure 38–1. In the lateral position, pressure points shift to the side of the head and ear, acromion process, elbow, ribs, greater trochanter, medial and lateral aspects of the knees, and the malleolus. In the prone position, pressure points are on the cheek and ear, acromion process, breasts (females), genitalia (males), knees, and toes.

Although other factors contribute, the primary causative factor for pressure sores (decubitus ulcers) is pressure. Vascular pressures in the extremities include an arteriolar pressure of 38 mm Hg, venous pressure of 20 mm Hg, and a capillary pressure of 12 mm Hg (Leavitt, 1966). By contrast, in the sitting position, pressure in the area under the ischial tuberosites can be as high as 700 mm Hg. In a lying-down position, many body areas are subjected to pressures that are much greater than that within the circulatory system, particularly in areas over bony prominences. This pressure narrows and obliterates blood vessels, thus reducing or eliminating blood flow to a portion of the body (Linden et al., 1965; Miller and Sachs, 1974). It is also known that greater tissue damage occurs from sustained lower levels of pressure than from shorter periods of higher pressure (Rudd, 1962).

POSITIONING A CLIENT IN BED

The frequency with which clients who are confined to bed need to have their position changed depends on the client's condition and the type of mattress in use. Some clients may need to have their position changed every hour, while every 2 to 4 hours is adequate for others. Client's who are on flotation devices need less frequent position changes than those on conventional mattresses. Using a variety of positions decreases the probability that any one or two body areas are subjected to excessive and prolonged pressure. The degree of joint flexibility, general health status, and illness condition provide some limits to the number of positions that are possible for a given client.

The common positions used for a person in bed are known as supine (back lying), lateral (side-lying), prone (front-lying), and Sims (modified prone) positions. These positions are achieved through specific placement of the body segments and the use of supportive devices such as pillows, towels, and blankets. The bed usually is in level position when these positions are used. An adjustable bed serves as a mechanical facilitator for maintaining a client in some specific positions such as the Fowler's and Trendelenburg positions.

Supine

The most common position for a person in bed is the supine position, that is, lying on the back. When a sacral decubitus is present, this position is used only for the minimal amount of time required for providing basic care or meals.

Prone Position

In the prone position, the person lies on the abdomen, with one or both arms at the side and the head turned toward one side or the other. It is an ideal position for clients who have posterior decubitae that require treatment. In addition, it provides for hip extension and shoulder retraction. It is, however, the least commonly used position. Both nurses and clients often are unfamiliar with it; clients fear being unable to breath or being left alone for long periods of time; and nurses often are unsure of its value and of how to move a client to this position. The prone position is an important alternative that too often is overlooked. It can be tolerated, however, for shorter times than others and is contraindicated for persons who have respiratory distress, heart disease, recent abdominal surgery, or decreased joint flexibility such as occurs with arthritis or contractures.

Lateral Position

Another common position is the lateral or side-lying position, in which the person is on the side with the hips and arms flexed and the uppermost extremities supported with pillows. This position is quite comfortable and provides for increased respiratory excursion.

Sims Position

The Sims position is a semiprone position named for James Marion Sims (1813–1883), an American surgeon and gynecologist (Miller and Keane, 1983). It is useful for clients who find the prone position uncomfortable, and avoids excessive pressure on the male genital area or on large pendulous female breasts.

Fowler's Position

In a Fowler's position, the head of the bed is elevated between 30 and 90 degrees. The position is named for an American surgeon, George R. Fowler (1848–1906) (Thomas, 1981). Depending on the degree of elevation, this position is identified as "low," "semi," and "high" Fowler's position. A Fowler's position reduces pressure on the heart and diaphragm from the abdominal organs, thus decreasing the cardiac work load and allowing increased respiratory excursion and easier breathing. Low Fowler's position (30 degree elevation) is often used for comfort, rest, and relaxation. A semi-Fowler's position (40 to 50 degree elevation) is useful when eating meals in bed or when dyspnea (difficulty breathing) occurs with a lower head elevation. A high Fowler's position (90 degree elevation or upright) primarily is used when clients have orthopnea, which is the ability to breathe easily only in the upright position.

A Fowler's position may or may not include knee flexion, as agency usage of the term varies. Slight knee flexion is helpful in eliminating uncomfortable hyperextension of the knee joint and in decreasing strain on the hamstring tendons in that joint. Knee flexion also helps keep clients from sliding downward toward the foot of the bed, and therefore maintains a correct position for a longer time and decreases the effects of sliding friction, also known as "shearing force."

Knee flexion can be provided safely when the gatch mechanism can be operated independently of elevating the head of the bed, because the degree of flexion can be controlled. Knee flexion can also be provided with small pillows or towels.

Shearing force occurs whenever the head of the bed is elevated above 30 degrees or when a client assumes a slumped sitting position. Shearing force results from a combination of the downward and forward force exerted by the weight of the torso and the static friction produced between the skin and the bed surface. The deep fascia is attached securely to the bony structure, while the deeper portions of the superficial fascia are rather loose and slide easily on the deeper fascia. As the tissue layers slide upon each other, blood vessels become kinked and torn, the tissues tear, and deep injury occurs. Eventually this injury extends to the surface and a decubitus ulcer has formed (Mitchell and Loustau, 1981). Tissues in the sacrum and heel are the most prone to injury because the body weight is concentrated in the pelvic area and the heels provide additional static friction and resistance to sliding. However, shear injuries can occur any place where frictional force is exerted.

Although knee flexion helps prevent the client from sliding down toward the foot of the bed, it can also cause specific problems with the circulatory system. These problems are more apt to occur with the electrical or manual mechanical beds that automatically raise the knee gatch as the head of the bed is elevated. The dependent position of the lower legs combined with pressure on the popliteal area causes dependent edema and venous stasis in the lower legs, with a tendency toward thrombus formation. When both the legs and the torso are elevated, the pelvic area is in a dependent position, again resulting in venous stasis and the possibility of thrombus formation in the deep pelvic veins. Raising the entire lower part of the bed to the level of the knee gatch so that the lower legs and knees are on the horizontal plane relieves the circulatory problems with the legs but not with the pelvic area. Another problem associated with the semi- to high Fowler's positions is that they functionally limit a client's activity, because clients tend to remain in one position and have less spontaneous side-to-side turning.

In both agency and home-caring settings, the Fowler's position usually is created by using an adjustable, mechanical hospital bed. If this type of bed is not available, Fowler's position can be created with a straight chair and multiple pillows. The straight chair is tilted so the back forms an inclined plane. When padded and placed in bed, it provides a firm support to maintain the client in a Fowler's position. The client is supported in the Fowler's position with pillows or folded towels and blankets, as shown in Figure 64-1. A medium-sized pillow supports the head in a neutral or slightly flexed position; a folded pillow supports the arms to prevent dependent edema and shoulder strain; a folded towel, blanket, or small pillow provides slight knee flexion to prevent joint hypertension; and a folded towel decreases pressure on the heels. Heel protectors often are used to provide additional protection from pressure and shearing force.

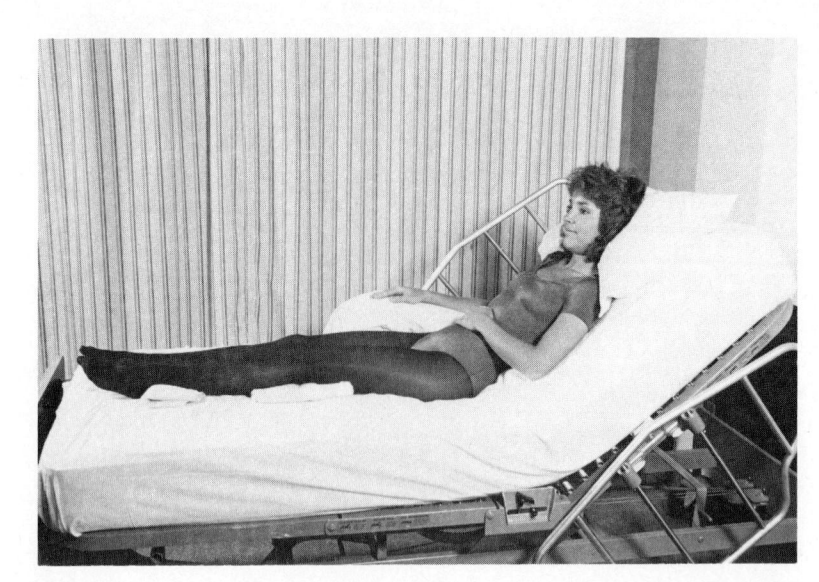

Figure 64–1. Semi-Fowler's position. The pillow has been removed from the left arm to show the relationship between the client's position and the bed elevation. (Photo by James Haines.)

Trendelenburg Positions

The three types of Trendelenburg positions are the regular, modified, and reverse Trendelenburg. In the regular Trendelenburg position, the entire bed is tilted so that the feet are elevated above the head (Fig. 64-2). In the modified Trendelenburg position, the trunk and head are lowered, mildly elevating the legs (Fig. 64-3). In the past, the Trendelenburg position was used to treat shock. Because the position causes increased pressure in the brain and on the heart and lungs, it is now contraindicated for that purpose as well as for clients with heart disease, respiratory distress, or head injuries. Currently, the regular Trendelenburg position sometimes is used to promote drainage of respiratory secretions. The modified Trendelenburg position may be used in hypovolemic shock. In the reverse Trendelenburg position, the entire bed is tilted so the client's head is higher than the feet (Fig. 64-4). This position may be used to increase arterial circulation to the legs or to increase respiratory excursion when a Fowler's position is not possible, such as with back injuries.

The Trendelenburg positions can be obtained by adjusting an automatic bed by inserting metal pins into beds with expandable legs or by placing blocks called "shock blocks" under the legs of the bed. To obtain the modified Trendelenburg position, first lower the bed to a level position; then lower the head of an automatic bed or raise the foot end of a manually operated bed and place its brace into a notch on the bed frame. With the regular Trendelenburg position, a pillow may be placed between the client's head and the headboard to protect against injury if he or she slides down the inclined surface. A bath blanket may be placed over the foot of the bed to protect the feet in the reverse Trendelenburg position.

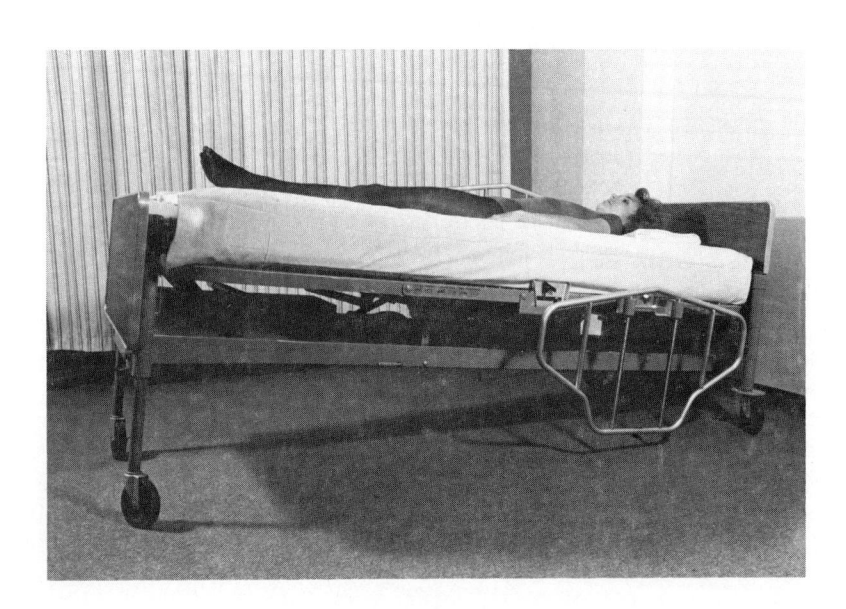

Figure 64–2. Trendelenburg Position. (Photo by James Haines.)

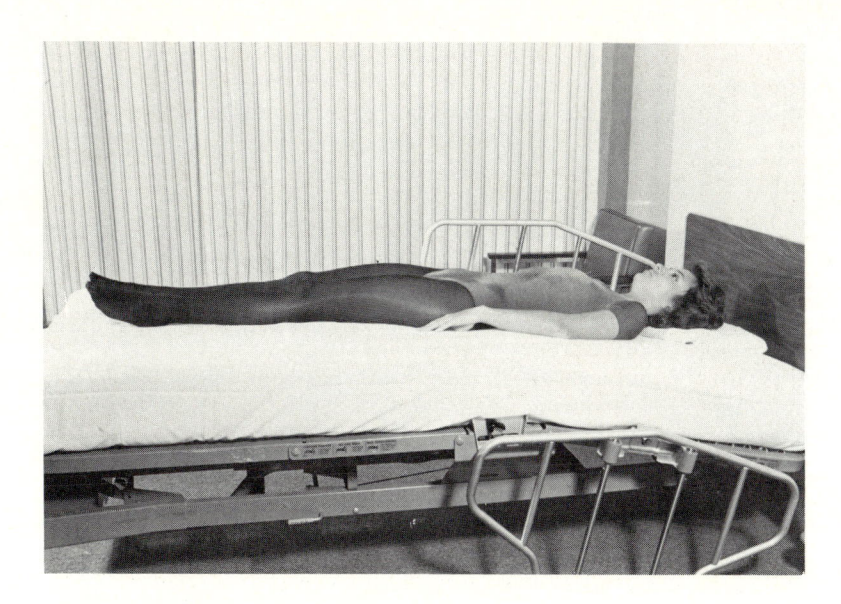

Figure 64-3. Modified Trendelenburg position, with the head and shoulders lower than the legs and hips. (Photo by James Haines.)

DATA BASE

Decisions about the types of positions used and the frequency with which a client is turned and repositioned usually are based on nursing judgment. The physician, however, may specify that certain positions are preferred or contraindicated. The nursing-care plan or kardex and the client's health record contain information that helps the nurse make these decisions. Other information will be obtained through direct observation and conversation with the client or family.

A decision about the *frequency* of turning is influenced by the client's age, size, weight, diagnoses, circulatory and integumentary status, and the probability of developing negative consequences from immobility. The *positions* used are influenced by similar factors, plus the client's respiratory and cardiac status; level of consciousness and mental alertness; degree of joint flexibility; skeletal deformities; presence of surgical incisions, traumatic injuries, existing or potential decubitae, dressing, casts, traction, and tubes of various kinds; and individual preferences and degree of comfort in the various positions. This information also helps determine the number of people needed to accomplish turning and repositioning in ways that are safe for both the client and nurse, as well as the amount and type of supports that are needed to maintain that particular client in correct alignment.

Decisions based on the above information become part of the data base for a specific client. A schedule for turning and repositioning, the positions used, the number of persons required for turning, and the amount and type of supportive devices needed are included in the nursing-care plan or kardex.

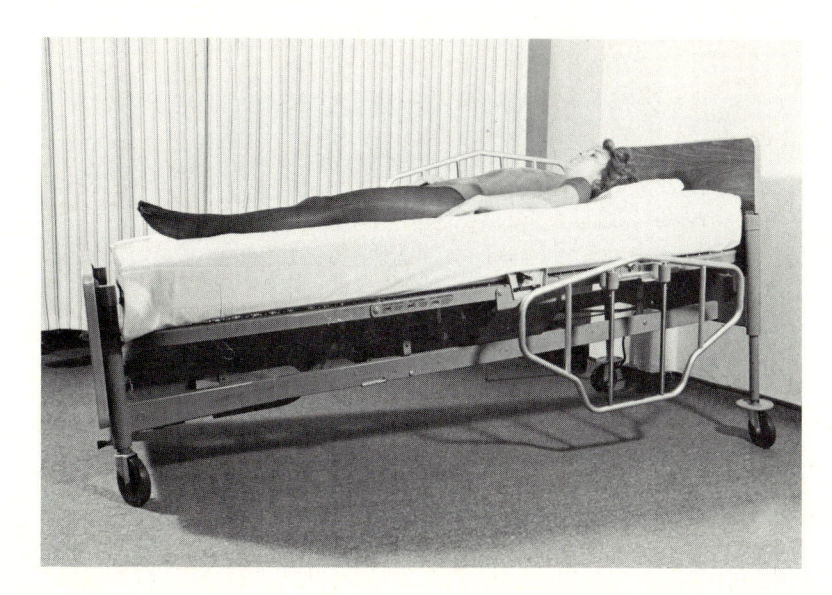

Figure 64-4. Reverse Trendelenburg position. (Photo by James Haines.)

Inspection

Inspection is used to determine whether body alignment is correct after repositioning, as well as to identify the presence of any pressure areas.

EQUIPMENT

The equipment used to turn and position clients varies considerably with the agency and with the client's state of health and illness. Supportive aids are used to maintain a client in correct alignment and position. Protective aids are used to prevent negative effects from excessive or sustained pressure. Turning devices are used when spinal column alignment is crucial or whenever turning is difficult.

Supportive Devices

Clients can be stabilized in the positions described above by using pillows, towels, and bath blankets that are folded and arranged so they provide needed support and slight flexion, avoiding hyperextension of joints. Trochanter rolls and sandbags are used to stabilize joints and prevent external rotation.

Trochanter Rolls. To make and place a trochanter roll, first fold a bath blanket in thirds lengthwise or use several large bath towels. Place one end of this rectangle well under the client's hips. Roll the other end under until a snug roll rests tightly against the body, as shown in Figure 64–5. This action will noticeably correct external rotation of the hip and leg. A wider roll could include the knee, or a second trochanter roll may be used, especially if the client's legs are very heavy. However, a trochanter roll is not placed at the knee in preference to the hip, as that would not support the joint being rotated.

Sandbags. Sandbags are bags of canvas, rubber, or plastic that are filled with sand. They are heavy, yet slightly flexible, weighing from 2.2 to 22 kg (1 to 10 lb) each. Sandbags can be used to prevent external rotation of a joint, support an extremity in correct alignment, or prevent rotation of the head when that movement is contraindicated.

Footboards. Footboards are wooden boards placed at the end of the bed or over the lower mattress for one of two purposes. They can relieve the pressure of the upper linens on the feet and lower legs. They are used to relieve pressure of the upper linens on the feet and legs and to avoid causing plantar flexion from too tight linens. Although footboards are in common use for preventing foot drop (plantar flexion), there is some controversy about their use. Some sources indicate that foot drop can be prevented by resting the feet at a 90 degree angle against a footboard (Sorensen and Luckmann, 1979). There is some thought that a footboard may actually increase the problem of plantar flexion because the pressure against the ball of the foot can produce a reflex plantar flexion and foot drop, especially if there is neuromuscular impairment. Talbot (1978) indicates that the feet should not be placed against a footboard if there is a tight heel cord or spasticity, and that the feet should never be forced against the footboard.

Handrolls, Cones, and Splints. Handrolls are soft or hard devices that are placed in the palms of the hand to prevent flexion contractures of the fingers and wrists. Research suggests that a hard cone-shaped device is more effective than a soft roll in decreasing or preventing flexion spasticity in the hand (Dayhoff, 1975; Jamison and Dayhoff, 1980). Sometimes splints are used to support the wrist and fingers in a slight hyperextension.

Protective Aids to Prevent Sustained Pressure

A variety of techniques and devices are available to relieve excessive pressure at the body's pressure points

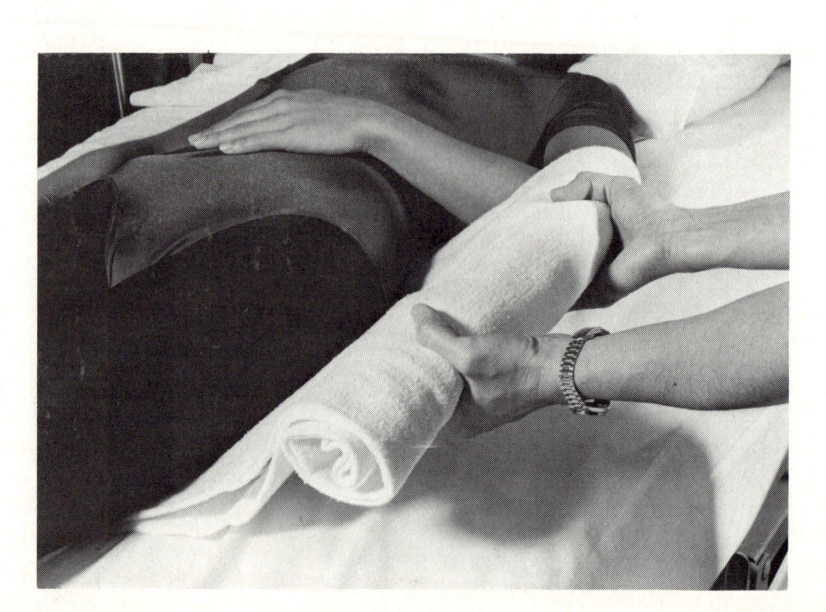

Figure 64–5. Rolling a trochanter roll into place. (Photo by James Haines.)

and provide for broad and equal distribution of weight. Intensified pressure over bony protuberances can be reduced by placing pillow or towel supports in the body contour indentations that occur adjacent to the bony protuberances. Filling out these indentations (such as the waist above the iliac crest when in a lateral position) distributes the body weight over a greater surface area and reduces peak pressures in any given area. Pressure over a bony protuberance can be reduced by supporting the body part on both sides of the joint, using foam pads or pillows. Care must be used to avoid additional pressure on adjacent tissues.

Antidecubitus Pads

Sheepskin Pads. Sheepskin pads have a deep fluffy pile that feels confortable and distributes weight evenly because of the air trapped in the deep pile; they help keep the client dry because they are slightly absorbent. A sheepskin pad is placed next to the skin and should reach from above the hips to below the knees. It is sturdy and can be used to help turn and move the client. Although they are fairly expensive, sheepskins last about a year when cared for properly. Both synthetic and real sheepskins should be washed and dried when wet or soiled, and then shaken gently to fluff them. To avoid the possibility of being a reservoir for infection, sheepskins should be sent to central service for washing rather than be laundered in the clinical area (Jackson, 1983).

Foam Pads. Foam padding about 1.25 to 2.5 cm (½ to 1 in) thick can be used over part or all of the mattress or be cut to fit any size area. Thick foam pads and mattresses that resemble the inside of an egg carton are available commercially. The pad is placed on the mattress with the projections extending upward. The client's weight compresses the projections somewhat, but trapped air in the foam distributes pressure evenly.

Plastic Foam. Plastic foam pads developed through research for the NASA space program will respond to body weight and conform to body contours when at body temperatures, thus distributing the weight over the entire surface of the pad (Culclasure, 1974).

Overbed Cradles. An overbed cradle is a semicircular or square wooden or metal frame that is placed on the mattress near the foot of the bed. The top linens are placed over the cradle, thus avoiding pressure on the feet and legs. Some overbed cradles have a light bulb that can supply dry heat to an area, such as an ulcer, as ordered by the physician.

Heel Protectors. Heel protectors are sheepskin-lined pads that are shaped to fit the heel or elbow. They often fasten with self-adherent straps. In addition to decreasing undue sustained pressure, they decrease the static and sliding friction forces when moving and turning the clients. The client shown in Figure 64–18 is wearing heel protectors.

Donuts. Rolled washcloths or dressings called "donuts" and inflated rubber rings are considered inappropriate devices for relieving pressure except in very selective situations, such as after rectal surgery. Although pressure is decreased in one area, the ring increases pressure in surrounding tissues and may compound the pressure problems.

Flotation Devices

Flotation devices distribute body weight equally throughout substances such as water, air, or a gel. They are used to prevent the negative effects of prolonged pressure. To be effective, only a single sheet must be placed over a flotation device. Heavy pads or thick fabrics interfere with the weight distribution and cause additional pressure on the tissues. It is important to avoid puncturing the surface and causing the flotation device to leak.

Silicone Gel Pads. A silicone gel pad contains a gellike fluid that has the consistency of human fat. The gel is encased in an elastic membrane; it supports weight, keeps its shape, and flows freely with the client, thus avoiding shearing friction force when a client moves. Silicone gel pads can be placed in cutout areas in foam pads, or can be designed to fit the seat of a wheelchair (Grabenstetter, 1968; Mitchell and Loustau, 1981).

Water Beds. Water beds have been used during the past years to equalize the pressure of the body weight over the entire body surface. Although water beds are effective in equalizing pressure, there are problems associated with their use. It is difficult to maintain proper positioning in a floating bed; the pelvic area always remains lower and causes problems with urinary drainage; skin maceration can occur because there is little surface air circulation; and some individuals are unable to tolerate weightlessness and will develop psychotic symptoms (Pfaudler, 1968; Thornhill and Williams, 1968). In addition, the beds are quite heavy and bulky.

Alternating Pressure Air Mattresses. Alternating pressure air beds provide both flotation and pressure changes. The plastic mattress is made of odd and even sections or pockets that are alternately inflated and deflated by a mechanical pumping apparatus. Although a slight shifting motion continually changes the pressure on the body, clients must be turned regularly and positioned carefully. When using an alternating pressure mattress, be careful to avoid kinking the tubing as that would interfere with the inflation.

Air Suspension Beds. A new design in air beds involves multiple, specially designed, air-filled cushions. In the KinAir bed, the cushions are made of a waterproof fabric that allows air and water vapor, but not bacteria, to pass through. The patient support surface is divided into 5 sections (head, back, seat, legs, and feet), each of which has independent pressure controls, thus allowing for selective pressure at various body areas. The KinAir support surface rests on a base designed like a regular adjustable hospital bed; it can be adjusted to provide the same positions as a regular hospital bed. This bed is approximately one-fourth the weight of an air fluidized bed (described below), which makes it easier to transport in the clinical area.

Air Fluidized Beds. An air fluidized bed such as the CLINITRON Unit (Fig. 64-6) is a mobile tank containing approximately 1500 pounds of tiny microspheres (glass beads) and covered with a monofilament polyester filter sheet upon which the individual lies. Warm pressurized air sets the beads in motion and produces a dry fluid medium on which the client floats. Pressure is distributed evenly over the entire body. Clients are supported well below capillary closing levels (11 to 15 mm Hg), allowing unimpeded circulation to all areas. Body fluids and exudates pass through the filter sheet, mix with the beads, and fall to the bottom of the tank. The clumps are sequestered away from the client in an environment hostile to bacterial growth. The filter sheet is changed every 2 weeks while the person is on the unit and the beads are changed between clients (Coker, 1979; Sanchez, et al., 1983; Scheulen and Munster, 1983; Turnock, 1983). Air fluidized beds are leased to the hospital on a per diem basis. This per diem cost might be prohibitive for many clients were it not that most insurance companies cover the cost of these beds.

Air fluidized beds have been found to be very beneficial for persons with multiple injuries, burns, dressings, and the acute pain associated with some terminal illnesses, and for obese and emaciated clients.

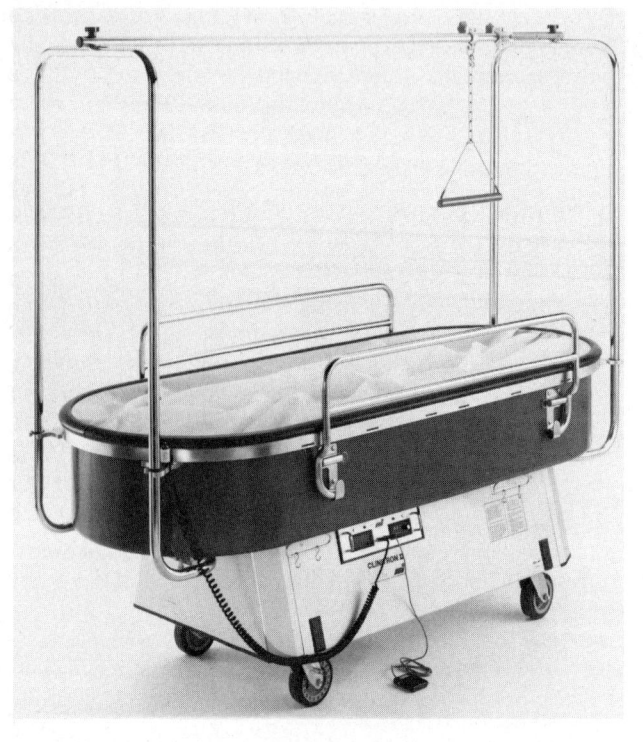

Figure 64-6. CLINITRON II, and Air-Fluidized Support System. (Courtesy, Support Systems International, Inc., Charleston, SC.)

In addition to pressure reduction, clients experience less pain, require less sedation and pain medication, and sleep better. Since less frequent turning is needed to relieve pressure areas, there is more time to focus on other nursing-care needs. However, the need for turning is not eliminated, as position changes continue to be needed for maintenance of adequate pulmonary function.

When giving personal care and performing procedures, the bed is defluidized (the air turned off) to provide a stable surface. Before turning off the bed, the beads can be pushed around so as to support the client or expose body areas as the beads stabilize. The bed will automatically refluidize within 30 minutes if not turned back on earlier. There are some problems associated with the bead bed. Fluid balance should be monitored closely to avoid occurrence of dehydration because of the continuous circulation of warm, dry air. Coughing and deep breathing exercises must be done regularly to avoid pulmonary congestion. In addition, these beds are very heavy to move. Care should be used to avoid back injuries when nurses are required to move the unit from one area to another. Transporting a client in the CLINITRON Air Fluidized Support System is to be avoided whenever possible.

SPECIAL TURNING DEVICES

Special beds or frames designed as turning devices are available for clients who must be immobilized or who are difficult to turn without causing further injury or great discomfort. For example, persons with recent cervical spine injury are kept in continuous traction, but still require turning; new quadriplegics and paraplegics are difficult to care for in regular beds; and turning may be very painful and difficult for persons with massive burns or injuries. The Stryker frame, wedge turning frame, and the CircOlectric bed are the most common types of turning devices. Directions for using these devices often are attached to the frame, and videotaped operating instructions may be included in orientation sessions. When these turning frames are not used regularly, it is important to consult those resources before operating the device, and to work with someone who is familiar with them. The turning frames described below are extremely useful devices, but clients can fall out as the device is being turned if they have not been positioned and secured properly and if the locking mechanisms are not fastened correctly. Families and clients need thorough explanations about the purpose and use of these frames. Because the frames are narrow and the turning unfamiliar, the individual initially may be quite fearful about their use.

Stryker Frames

The Stryker frame was designed by Dr. Homer Stryker in 1938 as a modification of the older Bradford frame (Skinner, 1946). A Stryker frame consists of two narrow lightweight metal frames that are covered

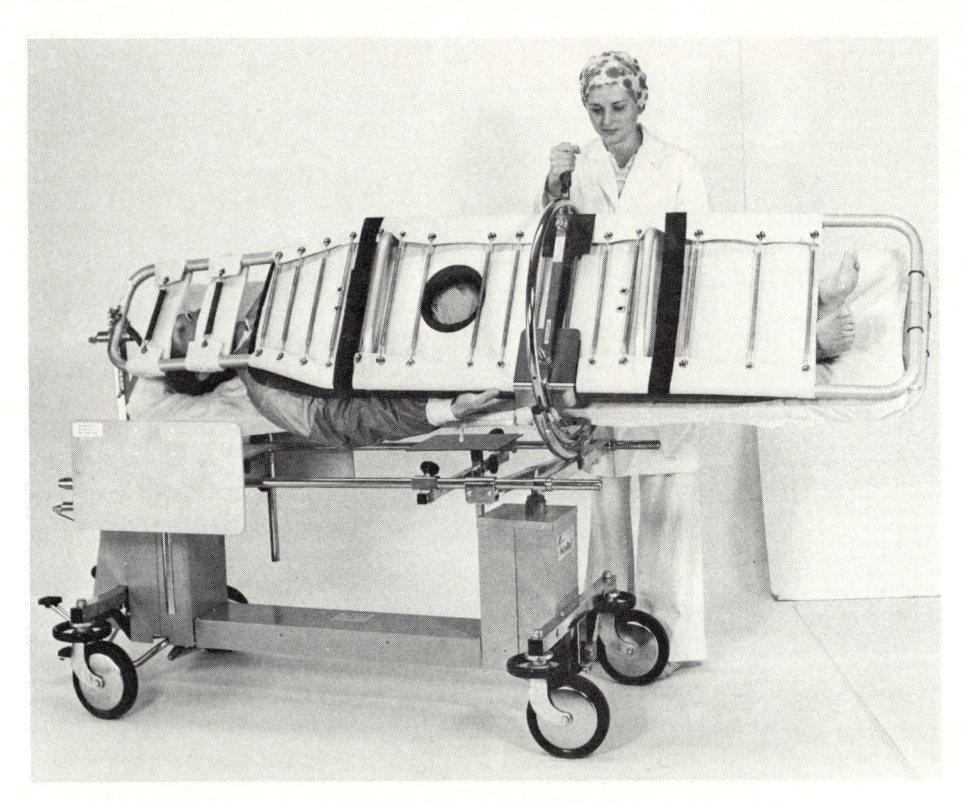

Figure 64–7. Wedge turning frame. (Courtesy, Stryker Corporation, Kalamazoo, MI.)

with heavy canvas and attached to a portable stand in such a way that the frames can be rotated anteriorly to posteriorly. The original Stryker frame was supported at both ends within a rectangular frame. The newer Wedge turning frame is supported at the head and in the center; the center support is a circular two-sectioned ring that serves as a turning ring (See Fig. 64–7).

The canvas cover on the posterior frame is in at least three separate segments; that is, an upper section for supporting the trunk and head, a lower section for the legs, and a 10 to 15 cm (4 to 6 in) middle section to support the buttocks area. The middle section is removable so the person can use the bedpan without being lifted. The canvas on the anterior frame (used for the prone position) may be in one piece with a round opening for elimination purposes, or it may be in segments similar to the posterior frame canvas. The upper portion of the anterior frame cover extends from just below the shoulders to just above the symphysis pubis and from just below the symphysis pubis to the internal malleolus, and the feet extend over the canvas and rest against a canvas foot support. A specially designed mattress is available for the posterior frame, and sheets designed to fit the frames eliminate bulk and decrease wrinkles. It is essential to have the center openings on the anterior and posterior frames match, so the person does not need to be moved for elimination purposes.

The Stryker Wedge frame has various attachments that support the arms or allow the individual to eat, read, and perform some personal care functions. The head end of the stand has a hole through which a traction rope is passed, and the person can be rotated without disturbing the traction.

To turn someone on a Stryker frame, place the second frame on top of the person, sandwiching the person between the two frames. Secure the frame by tightening the knurled nut at the head of the frame and closing the ring until it locks automatically. Place a pillow on the legs to help hold them in place securely during turning. Position drainage tubes, intravenous feedings, and other attachments so they will not be pulled out when the frame is turned. If the client is able, he or she can hold on to the frame while it is turned; if the client is unable to do this, use several safety belts. Turn the client quickly to the right. The turning lock automatically locks when the lower frame is horizontal and level. After turning, remove the top frame and provide necessary care. Always return the knurled nut to its place on the frame.

It is possible for pressure problems to develop, particularly at the edges of the canvas sections, even if the client on a Stryker frame is turned every 2 hours. Check the skin carefully with each turn and provide protective measures as needed. Post a schedule for turning and include the supports needed and the methods the client prefers. Plan adequate time for giving care, because haste sometimes causes care-givers to omit important details.

Circle Beds

The CircOlectric bed, shown in Figure 64–8, is another type of Stryker frame. An electric mechanism turns the frames slowly from head to foot within a portable

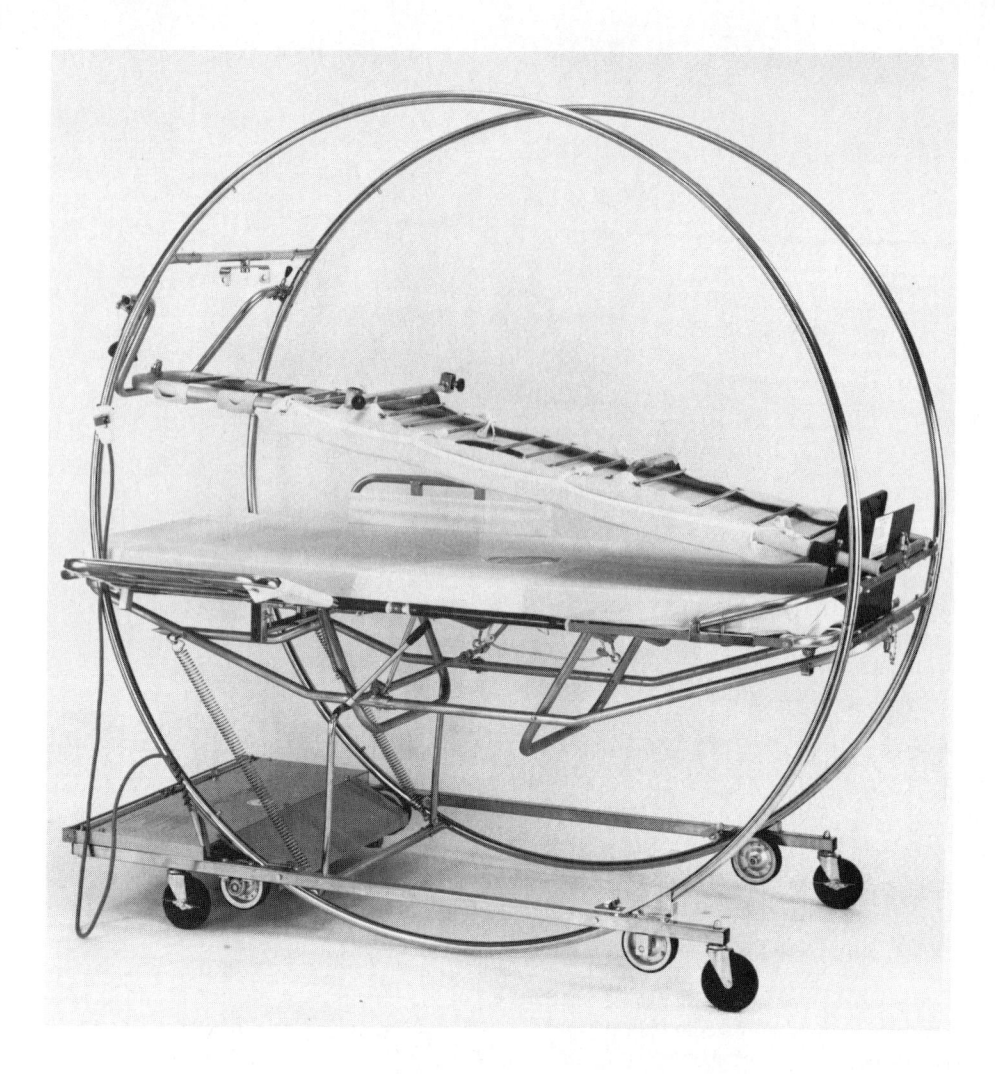

Figure 64-8. CircOlectric frame. (Courtesy, Stryker Corporation, Kalamazoo, MI.)

circular stand, rather than from side to side as in the Wedge turning frame. Because the rotation can be stopped at any point, any position between supine and upright is possible. This gradual tilt is particularly important for paraplegics and quadriplegics who have lost nervous innervation to their blood vessels, as it allows the cardiovascular system to accommodate gradually to a position change and minimizes postural hypotension.

The posterior frame on a CircOlectric bed is wider than that on a Wedge frame and has a foam mattress. A variety of attachments is available to provide for comfort, support, and personal care. Several kinds of traction are possible, and a transfer sling, similar to that used with a portable mechanical patient lift, can be used to transfer a person from the frame to a wheelchair as the frame turns.

When turning someone in a CircOlectric bed, position and secure the upper frame in the same manner as described above. The addition of a footboard prevents the client from sliding. Rotate the bed smoothly, without interruptions. When the client is in the prone position, release the head end of the mattress frame from the stand; a spring attachment raises it upward and it is locked in place on the circular stand.

In the initial phases of using a circle bed, it is important to observe the client for distress, particularly cardiac arrhythmias. As with the Wedge turning frame, the skin needs to be inspected for pressure problems with each turning.

☐ EXECUTION

Correct repositioning involves three components: moving, turning, and positioning. Clients often need to be moved up higher in bed and be repositioned prior to mealtime or using a bedpan. Before being turned to a new position in bed, the client usually must be moved to the side of the bed to provide adequate space to turn safely or be moved lower in bed for turning to the prone position. After being moved up or down in bed, the client must be supported in the new position in correct body alignment. Advance planning and preparation can make these activities efficient and safe. The risk of personal back injury can be minimized by using correct body mechanics during each of these activities.

SKILL 64: TURNING, MOVING, AND POSITIONING   **727**

The following guidelines apply to the processes of moving, turning, and repositioning:

1. Plan to have sufficient help present to accomplish the task promptly.
2. Use two or more nurses for heavy or helpless persons.
3. Have enough supportive devices such as pillows, towels, or bath blankets within easy reach so the person is not left unattended.
4. Always have the side rails raised except when a nurse is next to the bed and adjacent to the individual.
5. Whenever two or more nurses work together to move or turn a client, designate one nurse to be in charge of the move and give a prearranged signal to initiate the move. Usually, this nurse is the one who will be assuming the greatest share of the person's weight.
6. Use a broad-based stance, flex your legs, and shift your body weight from one foot to the other as you exert lifting or pulling forces.
7. Before turning or moving a client, remove supportive pillows or blankets that would interfere with the move and place them within easy reach on the foot of the bed, nearby chairs, or the overbed table.
8. Position the extremities so they will not be injured during the move or turn and so their weight will assist with rather than interfere with the activity.
9. Support and move the extremities in the same way as when performing ROM exercises.
10. Keep all turning, moving, and positioning within the normal range of motion for each joint.
11. Smooth and tighten the lower sheets; remove crumbs or debris.
12. Place the nurse-call signal within easy reach.
13. Monitor the client's tolerance for and ability to maintain the position.

MOVING CLIENTS IN BED

Clients are always moved and turned with a pulling rather than a pushing action because a pushing action requires more effort and also compresses tissues and joints. A safe and effective way for one or more nurses to move someone in bed is with a pull sheet. A pull sheet is an additional sheet made of heavy fabric or a regular sheet folded crosswise. It is placed under the client and on top of the lower bed sheet so that it extends from the shoulders to the midthighs. If the person is helpless, the pull sheet should extend the full length of the body, or additional nurses can support the head and feet during the move. Roll the edge of the pull sheet tightly so the roll is parallel with and adjacent to the person's body. Grasp the rolled edge and move the sheet and person together. Using a pull sheet eliminates most of the static and sliding friction between the client's skin and the bed. Friction between the pull sheet and the bed linen can be further decreased by adding a slight lifting component to the pulling action. A plastic sheet beneath the pull sheet also decreases friction.

Moving a Client to the Side of the Bed

When moving a client to the side of the bed without assistance and using a pull sheet, face the bed directly and use a straight forward pull; use the force exerted by the quadriceps muscles and shifting body weight, as discussed in the Introduction to this chapter. Two nurses can work together to pull the person toward themselves with the pull sheet, or the second nurse can add a lifting component from the opposite side of the bed. To do this, the second nurse assumes a position fairly near the bed, with the body weight resting on the backward leg. As the nurse on the near side of the bed begins to pull, the second nurse lifts by raising the arms and shifting his or her body weight onto the forward leg. This lifting action should not require a

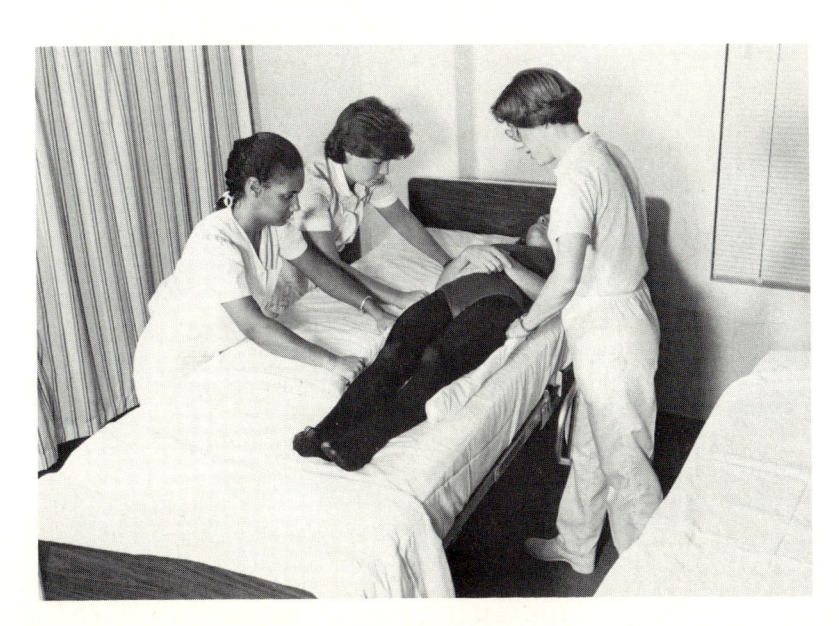

Figure 64-9. Three nurses moving a client from the side of the bed. The two nurses on the far side are prepared to pull; the nurse on the near side will lift. (Photo by James Haines.)

large amount of effort; it simply increases the efficiency of the first nurse's pulling action by decreasing the sliding friction. If necessary, or if sufficient help is available, two or three nurses can share the pulling and lifting from the opposite sides of the bed. Three or more nurses may be required to move large or helpless clients. Figure 64-9 shows three nurses moving a client from the side of the bed back toward the center of the bed.

When moving someone toward you without a pull sheet, place your hands and arms under the client to decrease friction and add a lifting component. Position yourself as described above, but with more knee flexion and with the arms closer to the surface of the bed. Two nurses can pull in unison from the same side of the bed, one supporting the shoulders and head, the other the hips

One nurse can also move a heavy or helpless person to the side of the bed without a pull sheet in a series of segmental movements. First, move the head and thorax, then the abdomen and hips, and finally the legs. If this action is repeated several times from alternate sides of the bed, it can also be used to move a person toward the head of the bed.

☐ SKILL SEQUENCE

MOVING A CLIENT TO THE SIDE OF THE BED

Step	Rationale
1. Wash hands.	Avoids transfer of microorganisms.
2. Explain procedure to client; include position to be used.	Allays anxiety; allows client to participate in own care.
3. Adjust bed to appropriate working height.	Prevents back strain from bending and working against force of gravity.
4. Close room door or draw curtains around bed. Turn back upper bed linen as needed to visualize client during procedure. Cover client with gown or blanket.	Protects client privacy and keeps client warm while providing for adequate visualization.

A. Straight Pull, Using a Pull Sheet

Step	Rationale
(1) Position pull sheet under client so it extends at least from shoulders to hips.	Enables pulling force to be directed toward heaviest parts of body. Provides additional support as needed.
(2) Place client's arms across chest or abdomen; remove pillow from under client's head.	Prevents injury from shear force and decreases static friction force by bringing arms over client's center of gravity. Decreases resistance to pulling action.
(3) Roll the near edges of pull sheet toward client's side. With palms turned downward, grasp the roll near shoulder and hip levels.	Provides for a firm grasp of sheet. Uses muscles of arms most effectively and enables pulling force to be exerted at heaviest body segments.
(4) Face bed directly.	Avoids twisting the spine when pulling; decreases shearing force on nurse's spine and avoids back strain.
(5) Place feet apart, with one behind the other; body weight rests on forward leg.	Provides broad base of support; maintains line of gravity within base of support during weight shift involved in moving.
(6) Flex knees to approximately a 120 degree angle.	Provides for maximum contraction potential of the quadriceps; lowers nurse's center of gravity and increases stability.
(7) Take a breath and set muscles of arms, shoulders, abdomen, and buttocks.	Relieves some of the compression on the intervertebral discs caused by lifting and pulling.
(8) Simultaneously, pull directly toward yourself, push with your forward leg (contract the quadriceps), and shift your body weight to the back leg.	Transmits pulling force from the quadriceps and the shifting body weight directly to client, avoiding excessive strain on upper extremities.
(9) Two nurses: First nurse grasps pull sheet at client's shoulders and head. Second nurse grasps sheet at hips and thighs. Second nurse gives signal to begin move.	Distributes weight between the two nurses and supports client. Nurse pulling the greatest amount of weight directs the move.
(10) Three nurses: Two nurses pull as in step 9; third nurse adds lifting component from opposite side of bed.	Lifting component decreases static and sliding friction, requiring less pulling force.
(11) Turn and position in correct body alignment.	Completes intended procedure.

B. Straight Pull, Without a Pull Sheet

Step	Rationale
(1) Place one arm under client's hips, reaching across to the far trochanter. Place second arm under shoulders, reaching to far shoulder.	Provides support and decreases static and sliding friction between client's skin and the bed linen during the move.
(2) Position client and remove pillow as in step A(2).	Same as step A(2).
(3) Position self and pull as in steps A(4 to 8).	Same as steps A(4 to 8).
(4) Two nurses: First nurse places both arms under client's shoulders (and head, if client is weak or helpless). Second nurse places both arms under buttocks and thighs. Position selves and pull as in steps A(5 to 8).	Distributes weight and decreases friction as in step B(1). Same as in steps A(5 to 8).

Moving a Client Up or Down in Bed

A client can be moved up or down in bed by two or more nurses with or without a pull sheet, or by one nurse without a pull sheet. The techniques described here are for moving someone up in bed. The same techniques are used in reverse for moving a person down toward the foot of the bed.

Moving a person up or down in bed requires that the direction of the pull be toward the head or foot of the bed, as compared to the straight pull toward the side of the bed, discussed in the preceding section. To avoid exerting twisting and shearing forces on your intervertebral discs, modify your stance, turning your feet and trunk toward the direction of the pull.

The client can help with the move by flexing the knees and, if possible, pushing downward. Even if the client is not able to assist actively by pushing, this flexed position decreases resistance from the legs, helps avoid shearing force against the heels, and contributes to the pushing force.

Moving Clients with a Pull Sheet. Two or more nurses can work together to move a client up in bed with a pull sheet. The pull sheet is prepared and placed in the same manner as for moving a client to the side of the bed.

☐ SKILL SEQUENCE

MOVING A CLIENT UP IN BED WITH A PULL SHEET

Step	Rationale
1. Prepare self, client, and environment as in Skill Sequence, "Moving a Client to the Side of the Bed", steps 1 to 4, p. 728. For this move, two or more nurses work on opposite sides of the bed.	Same as in Skill Sequence, "Moving a Client to the Side of the Bed," steps 1 to 4, p. 728. Divides the work between two persons.
2. Place and prepare the pull sheet as in Skill Sequence, "Moving a Client to the Side of the Bed," steps A(1) and A(3), p. 728.	Same as in Skill Sequence, "Moving a Client to the Side of the Bed," steps A(1) and A(3), p. 728.
3. Place the client's arms across the chest or abdomen.	Same as Skill Sequence, "Moving a Client to the Side of the Bed," step A(2), p. 728.
4. Remove pillow from under head and place against head of bed.	Decreases resistance to moving upward. Protects client from accidental injury.
5. Instruct the client to flex the knees and assist with the move by pushing downward into the mattress and toward the foot of the bed. (NOTE: If the client is unable to assist, flex knees and position feet for the client. Have an assistant stabilize the feet if possible.)	Additional force decreases nurse effort. A horizontal pushing force combined with a vertical downward pushing force results in a horizontal move in the opposite direction. Weight of client's legs does not resist pulling action; decreases shear friction on heels. Flexing the knees increases contraction capability of the quadriceps. Stabilizing feet increases static friction of feet against bed.
6. Turn your feet and trunk toward head of bed and assume a broad-based stance; place the foot farthest from the bed in a forward position and turned in the direction of the pull. Body weight rests on the foot nearest the bed (the backward leg).	Broad base increases stability, lowers nurse's center of gravity, and provides a base for shifting the weight with the pull.
7. With palms downward, grasp the rolled sheet near the shoulders and hips.	Uses muscles of arms most effectively and directs pulling force toward the heaviest body segments.
8. Flex your knees and set muscles as in Skill Sequence, "Moving a Client to the Side of the Bed," steps A(6) and A(7), p. 728.	Same as in Skill Sequence, "Moving a Client to the Side of the Bed," steps A(6) and A(7), p. 728.
9. On a prearranged signal by the designated nurse, simultaneously straighten the backward leg, shift your body weight to the forward leg, and pull and lift the pull sheet and client toward the head of the bed. The client pushes his or her feet downward into the mattress and toward the foot of the bed.	Same as in Skill Sequence, "Moving a Client to the Side of the Bed," step A(8), p. 728. Decreases shearing force on heels from dragging on sheet, and decreases force required to move client.
10. Turn and position in correct body alignment.	Completes intended procedure.

Moving Clients without a Pull Sheet. One nurse can move a client up in bed without a pull sheet if the client is able to help, as shown in Figure 64-10. Note that the client's one arm is placed on the abdomen to decrease static friction forces and avoid shearing injury; the other arm assists with the move by pulling on the side rail opposite the nurse. The nurse uses the stance described above and places one arm and hand completely under the client's buttocks; the other hand is placed under the shoulders. These positions enable the nurse to provide a lifting and pulling force at the centers of gravity for the heaviest body segments, thus decreasing shear friction force between the client's skin and the bed linens. The client assists by flexing

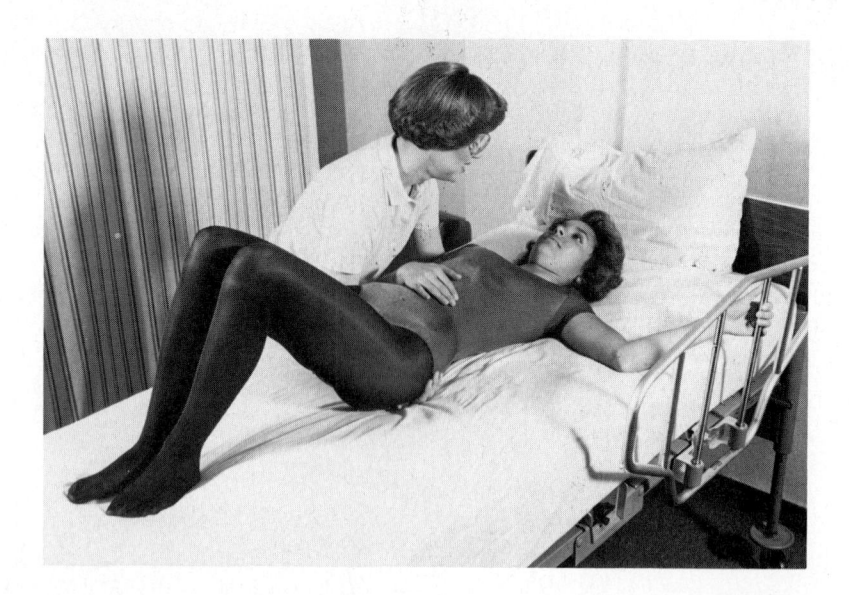

Figure 64-10. One nurse moving a client up in bed without using a pull sheet; client assisting. (Photo by James Haines.)

the knees and pushing downward into the mattress as described above. It is unacceptable practice to move someone up in bed by grasping under the armpit and pulling, as this action causes excessive strain on the shoulder joint and can dislocate a joint that lacks normal muscle stabilization.

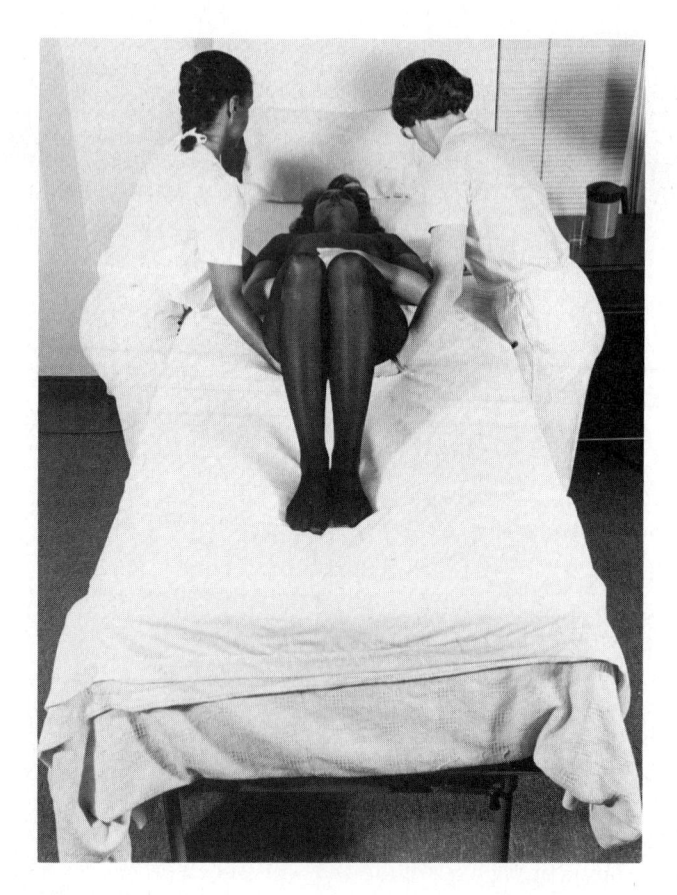

Figure 64-11. Two nurses moving a client up in bed without using a pull sheet. (Photo by James Haines)

If the client is unable to help or is quite heavy, two nurses can use a similar technique, working together from opposite sides of the bed. Each nurse places one hand and arm under the client's buttocks so the hand nearly meets the opposite nurse's hand. Each nurse places the other arm and hand under a shoulder in a similar way, as shown in Figure 64-11.

If the client has strong arms and needs minimal assistance in moving up in bed, leave the side rails in place and assist as shown in Figure 64-12. With this technique, the nurse is able to achieve a stance that allows for only minimal assistance with the move.

TURNING AND POSITIONING CLIENTS IN BED

Before turning and repositioning a client, offer a bedpan or urinal, drink of water or juice, or pain medication (if appropriate). Attention to these basic physiological needs will increase comfort and help the client maintain the position for a longer time.

Decide in advance of turning where you want the client to be located after being turned, and reposition the client in such a way that he or she will be in a safe, appropriate place in the bed after the turn is completed. When possible, have the client assist with turning by crossing the near leg over the far leg and pulling on the far side rail while the nurse assists from the near side of the bed.

To protect yourself and to turn a client toward yourself smoothly and with minimal exertion, use body mechanics that are similar to those used in moving a client straight toward you in bed, as described in Skill Sequence, "Moving a Client to the Side of the Bed," steps A(4) to A(8), p. 728. As the client is turned and positioned, inspect pressure areas and assess skin integrity, circulation, and current potential for skin breakdown, as discussed in Skill 38.

After turning is complete, place the client in one of the positions described below and position so that all body segments and parts are in good alignment and

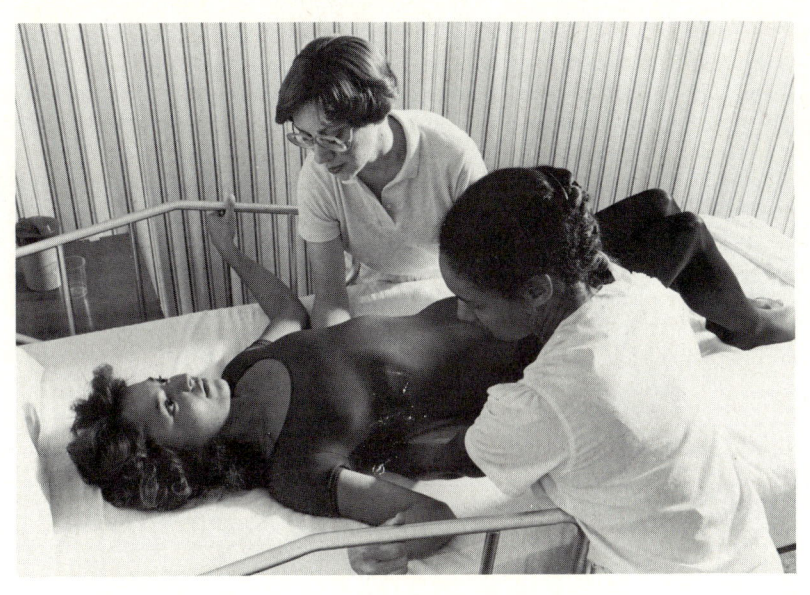

Figure 64-12. Two nurses assisting a client to move up in bed while client assists by pulling on the side rails. (Photo by James Haines.)

the client is balanced and secure. Protect and pad all body areas that are in contact with each other to avoid direct and intensive pressure. Support the extremities in a way that avoids dependent edema and prevents strain on the joints. Positioning can be used to supplement ROM exercises in maintaining joint flexibility and in providing for extension, flexion, or abduction, as identified below. When positioning the hands, place the wrists in either a straight or slightly hyperextended position, thus avoiding a natural tendency toward flexion and increased potential for contractures. If no contractures or reflex clenching of the fists occur, alternate between these two hand positions. A hard roll or cone may be placed in the hand, or the fingers may be extended on the surface of the pillow.

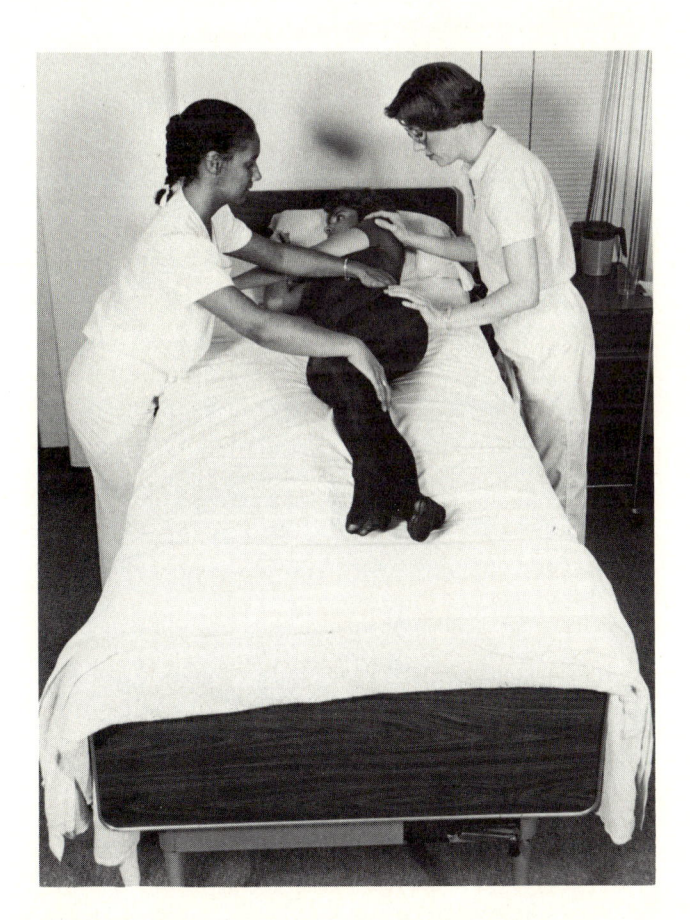

Figure 64-13. Two nurses turning a client to the side. (Photo by James Haines.)

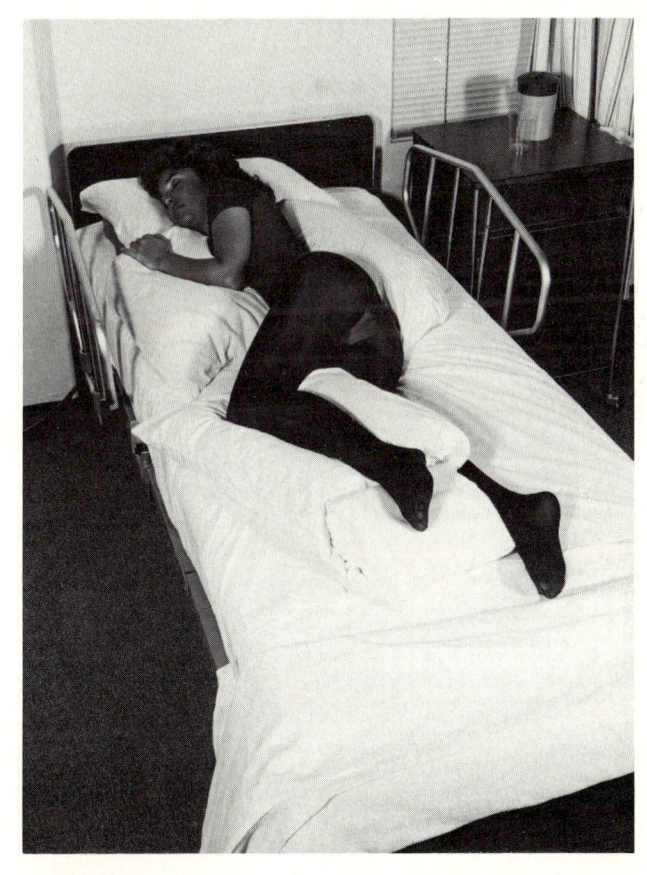

Figure 64-14. Lateral position: Client supported with pillows. (Photo by James Haines.)

Turning to Lateral and Supine Positions

Before turning the client from a supine to a lateral position, move the client toward the side of the bed opposite the side he or she will face after being turned. This action ensures that the client will be located safely in the center of the bed after turning. Position the extremities so they are near the body's center of gravity and serve as an angular force to assist in the turning. Grasp the major body segments such as the shoulder and hip prior to and during a turn, as that action stabilizes the client and controls the movements. Helpless or heavy persons may be turned by two nurses (Fig 64-13), or by pulling the far side of the pull sheet toward yourself. After the turn is completed, position and support the trunk and extremities as described below and shown in Figure 64-14.

To turn the client back to a supine position, stabilize the client with your hand and remove the support pillows. Support the client at the shoulder and hip and allow gravity to slowly return the body to the mattress. Reposition the extremities and return the client to the center of the bed.

☐ SKILL SEQUENCE

TURNING TO LATERAL AND SUPINE POSITIONS

Step	Rationale
1. Prepare self, client, and environment as in Skill Sequence, "Moving a Client to the Side of the Bed," steps 1 to 4, p. 728. Remove supportive pillows and place nearby. Use body mechanics and techniques described in Skill Sequence, "Moving a Client to the Side of the Bed," parts A and B, to move and turn the client.	Same as Skill Sequence, "Moving a Client to the Side of the Bed," steps 1 to 4, p. 728. Facilitates repositioning. Same as Skill Sequence, "Moving a Client to the Side of the Bed," parts A and B.

A. Turning from a Supine to a Lateral Position

Step	Rationale
(1) Move client to side of bed opposite direction client is to face.	Prepares for safe turning and protects client from falling.

(2) Return to near side of bed to position client for turning:
  a. cross far leg over near leg
  b. place far arm on abdomen or chest
  c. abduct near arm slightly
	
	Weight of extremities provides added force to help turn client.
	
	Avoids having client turn onto arm.

(3) Face client directly and place hands on client's shoulder and hips, or reach across client and grasp rolled pull sheet in those areas.	Directs pulling force toward center of gravity of heaviest body segments.
(4) Pull far side of client's body toward yourself, turning client on side.	Uses own body weight to turn client, conserving nurse effort.

(5) Support client in lateral position, using the following guidelines:
  a. Head: place a pillow under head.
  b. Trunk: pull hips toward edge of bed.
     Tuck pillow lengthwise along client's back and roll it under snugly, as shown in Figure 64-15
  c. Legs: flex top leg and bring it forward to rest on one or two pillows, as shown in Figure 64-16.
 	
     Bottom leg may be flexed slightly at hip and knees or kept straight.
  d. Shoulders: pull lower shoulder forward slightly.
  e. Arms: support top arm on one or two pillows, level with shoulder.
     Flex bottom arm more acutely and place hand beside or under head pillow.
	
	Maintains head level with the spine.
	Maintains line of gravity through both trochanters.
	Supports trunk securely.
	
	Supports entire extremity in comfortable and balanced positions. Avoids dependent edema and internal rotation of hip.
	Provides for comfort.
	
	Increases client's comfort and provides balance.
	Same as step A(5)c except avoids internal rotation of shoulder.
	Position of comfort. Avoids hyperextension of elbow joint.

(6) Document type of position used, purpose, length of time client remained in position, client's comfort level, and any problems encountered or special techniques used.	Fulfills nurse accountability, contributes to ongoing data base.

B. Turning from a Lateral to a Supine Position

Step	Rationale
(1) Remove support pillows from beneath top arm and leg. Rest client's arm on abdomen. Uncross top leg from bottom leg.	Positions arm near client's center of gravity. Position and weight of leg facilitates turning.
(2) Stabilize client with your hand and remove support pillow from back. Hold client at shoulder and hip and allow trunk to return slowly to mattress. Do not allow client to drop onto back.	Protects client from physical and emotional discomfort.

(continued)

SKILL 64: TURNING, MOVING, AND POSITIONING   **733**

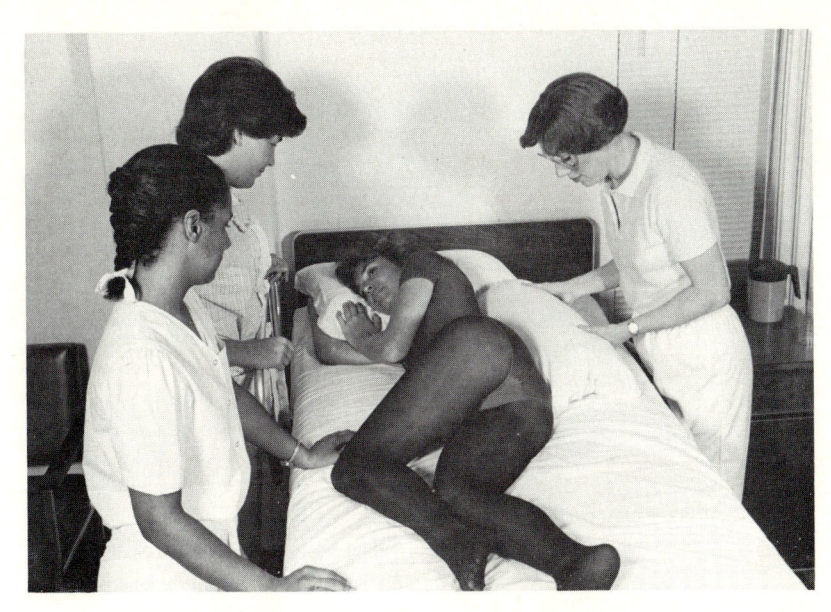

Figure 64–15. Tuck the pillow edge securely under the client's back before rolling it under; this holds the pillow securely in place. (Photo by James Haines.)

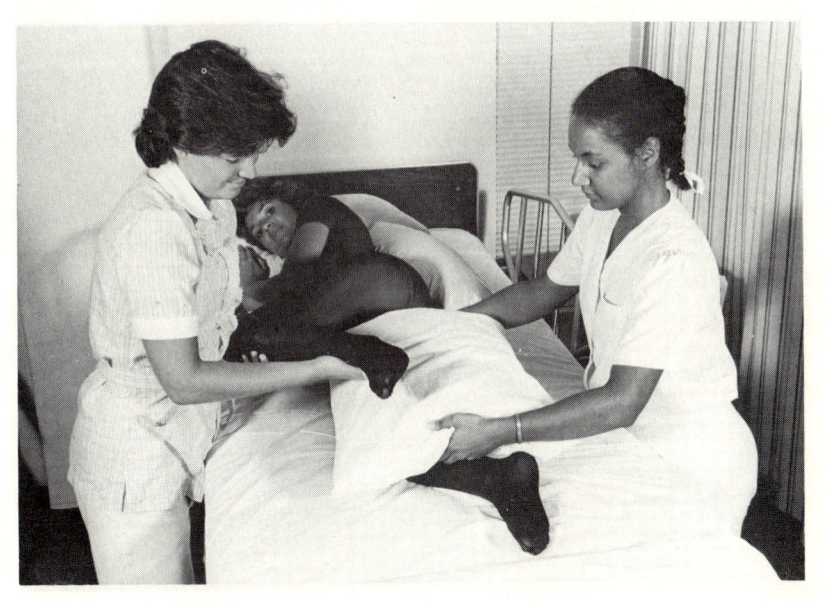

Figure 64–16. One nurse supports the client's leg while a second nurse places the pillow in position. (Photo by James Haines.)

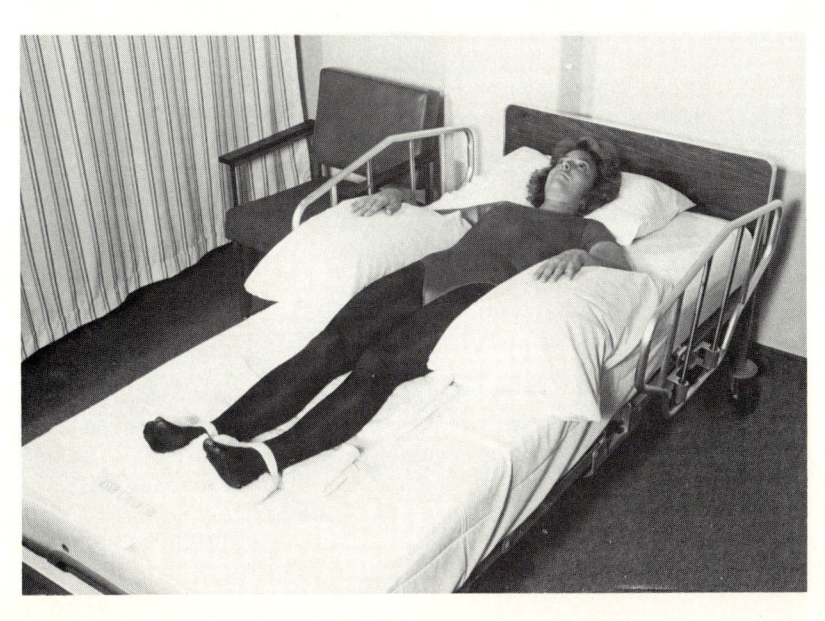

Figure 64–17. Supine position: Client supported with pillows and folded towels, heel protectors, and trochanter roll (beneath pillow). (Photo by James Haines.)

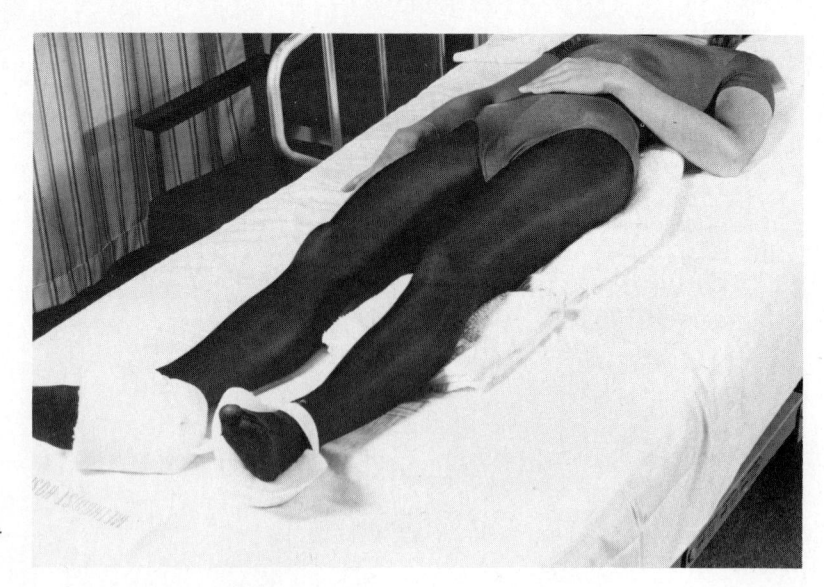

Figure 64-18. *Trochanter roll in place at left hip joint. The right leg is in external rotation because a trochanter roll has not yet been placed on that side. (Photo by James Haines.)*

TURNING TO LATERAL AND SUPINE POSITIONS (Cont.)

Step	Rationale
(3) Move client into center of bed.	Provides for client safety.
(4) Position with pillows and towels in the supine position, as shown in Figure 64-17 and described below.	
a. Head: place a small to medium-sized pillow under the head.	Comfort measure; avoids excessive neck flexion.
b. Back: place a small pillow or folded towel under the small of the back, based on the degree of swayback present and on the client's comfort and preference.	Comfort measure.
c. Knees: provide slight flexion for the knees with a small pillow or folded towel, avoiding excessive pressure on the popliteal area or calves.	Avoids hyperextension of lumbosacral area and avoids excessive pressure on nerves and blood vessels.
d. Heels: place a folded towel under the ankles and apply commercial heel protectors.	Decreases pressure and shearing force on heels.
e. Legs: when clients are weak or have neurologic impairment, place trochanter rolls beside hip joint as shown in Figure 64-18, or beside both the hip joint and knees.	Prevents external rotation and maintains legs in alignment. Weight of a helpless or relaxed body part acts as a lever and causes the part to rotate. Support must be placed at hip joint to prevent external rotation of leg.
f. Arms: support one or both arms on pillows in one of the following ways:	
i. abduct arms slightly; pronate forearms and hands and place them on pillows beside body.	Avoids dependent edema and internal shoulder rotation.
ii. abduct forearms at right angles to the shoulder; pronate forearms and place them on pillows parallel to the body.	Provides for lateral shoulder extension and avoids dependent edemas.
iii. abduct arms slightly, fully extend the elbow; and place beside the body in a supinated position.	Provides for elbow extension.
iv. abduct the forearms at right angles to the shoulder; supinate the forearms and hands and place them beside the head and on a pillow that is placed above the shoulder level.	Provides for external shoulder rotation.
(5) Document as in step A(6).	Same as step A(6)

Turning to Prone and Supine Positions

The technique for turning a client to and from a prone position is similar to turning someone to a lateral position, but with several differences. First, move the client nearer the foot of the bed, so the feet hang over the end of the mattress. Second, place *both* arms fully extended and parallel, directly against the body. This position avoids trapping the arms under the body as the client turns onto the abdomen. Third, turn the client's face away as you pull the client toward yourself. Two nurses can work together by having the first nurse exert a straight forward pull while the second nurse adds a lifting component from the far side of the bed. Support the client as he or she is lowered to the bed; being dropped is frightening and uncomfortable. After the turn, position as described below.

SKILL 64: TURNING, MOVING, AND POSITIONING   735

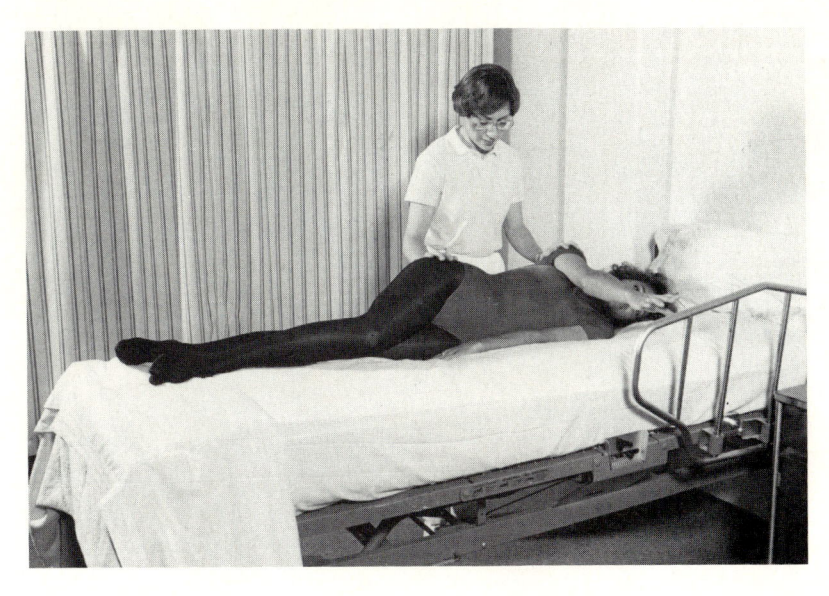

Figure 64–19. The arm is placed very close to the client as the client prepares to turn to a prone position. The nurse is positioned to guide the client steadily down toward the mattress. (Photo by James Haines.)

☐ SKILL SEQUENCE

TURNING TO PRONE AND SUPINE POSITIONS

Step	Rationale
1. Prepare self, client, and environment as in Skill Sequence, "Moving a Client to the Side of the Bed," steps 1 to 4, p. 728.	Same as Skill Sequence, "Moving a Client to the Side of the Bed," steps 1 to 4, p. 728.
2. Use body mechanics and techniques described in Skill Sequence, "Moving a Client to the Side of the Bed," parts A and B, to move and turn the client.	Same as Skill Sequence, "Moving a Client to the Side of the Bed," parts A and B.
3. Remove supporting pillows and place nearby.	Facilitates turning and positioning
A. Turning from Supine to Prone Position	
(1) Move client toward foot of bed so feet will hang over mattress.	Avoids excessive plantar flexion.
(2) Move client to near side of bed.	Ensures client will be in center of bed after turn is completed.
(3) Remove pillow from under client's head or place head near edge of pillow.	Allows face to turn onto mattress rather than pillow.
(4) Cross near leg over far leg.	Weight of leg provides additional turning force.
(5) Place client's arms against body, fully extended; OR have client extend near arm to pull on far side rail, as shown in Figure 64–19.	Avoids trapping arm under body when turning. Able clients can assist by pulling.
(6) Move to far side of bed, turn client on side, and support trunk with a pillow; OR have a second nurse support client.	Stabilizes client prior to completing the turn.
(7) Return to near side of bed, grasp shoulder and hip and support trunk as client turns onto abdomen.	Supports trunk while gravity causes it to return to the mattress. Client's near arm is held in place with nurse's arms.
(8) Position client in prone position as shown in Figure 64–20 and described below:	
a. Head: Turn face toward side with raised arm. Alternate face and arm positions on successive repositionings.	Position of comfort.
b. Shoulders: Place a small pillow or folded towel under each shoulder, if needed.	Avoids shoulder rounding; may or may not increase comfort.
c. Abdomen: Place a bath blanket or towel under abdomen and pubic area. For women with large breasts, place a folded towel or small pillow in the epigastric area.	Decreases swayback and increases comfort. Avoids pressure on male genitalia. Avoids pressure on the breasts.
d. Knees: Place a small pillow, folded blanket, or towel under ankles.	Avoids hyperextension of the knee joint.
e. Feet: Allow feet to hang freely over the foot end of mattress. Place folded towel under ankles.	Feet over end of bed avoids excessive plantar flexion. Towel under ankles avoids knee hyperextension.

(continued)

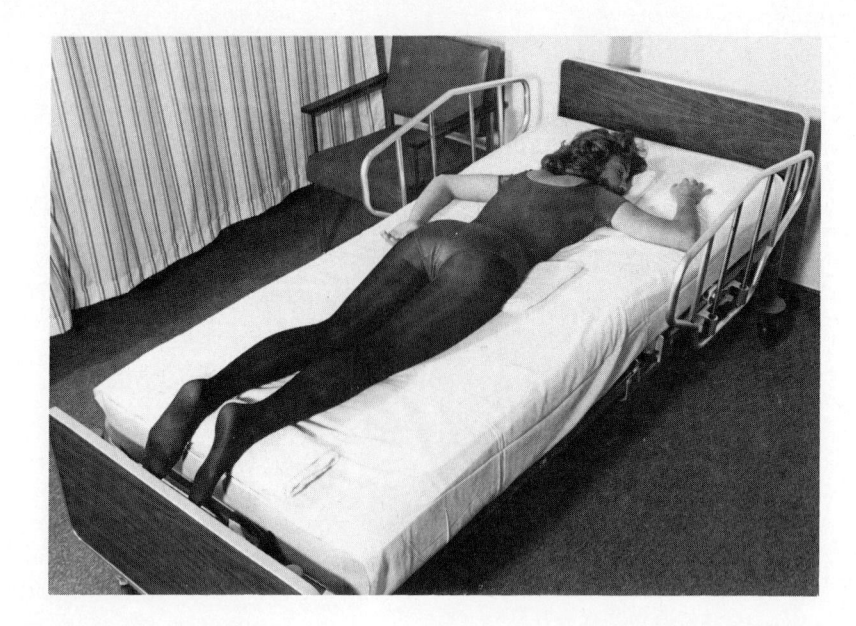

Figure 64-20. Prone position: Client supported with folded towels and bath blankets. (Photo by James Haines.)

TURNING TO LATERAL AND SUPINE POSITIONS (Cont.)

Step	Rationale
f. Arms: Position arms in one of the following ways:	Provide variation for comfort.
i. Abduct both arms laterally from shoulder, bend elbows and place forearms parallel to face.	
ii. Abduct both arms laterally from shoulder, bend elbows and place one forearm parallel with face and second forearm parallel with body.	
iii. Place one arm as described above in (i), abduct second arm slightly and extend it fully so it is pronated and parallel with the body.	
iv. Place both arms prone and fully extended, parallel with the body.	
(9) Document as in Skill Sequence, "Turning to Lateral and Supine Positions," step A(6).	Same as Skill Sequence, "Turning to Lateral and Supine Positions," step A(6).
B. Turning from Prone to Supine Position	
(1) Place client's arms directly adjacent and parallel to the body.	Brings arm weight nearer center of gravity and facilitates turning. Avoids trapping near arm under body.
(2) Turn client's face away from yourself.	Essential for turning without twisting neck.
(3) Cross client's far leg over the near leg.	Weight of leg aids in turning client.
(4) Reach across and grasp far shoulder and hip.	Exerts force at areas of greatest body weight.
(5) Pull toward yourself, turn client on side and support weight of trunk as it is lowered to the mattress. (NOTE: Depending on size of client, it may be easier to do this in two steps as in step A(6) and step A(7).)	Accomplishes turn without discomfort for client.
(6) Move client to center of bed and up in bed to correct position for elevating head of bed.	Provides for comfort and safety.
(7) Support with pillows and towels in the supine position, as in Skill Sequence, "Turning to Lateral and Supine Positions," step 4.	Same as Skill Sequence, "Turning to Lateral and Supine Positions," step 4.
(8) Document as in Skill Sequence, "Turning to Lateral and Supine Positions," step A(6).	

Turning to a Sims Position

A client is turned to and from the Sims position in the same manner as for the prone position. When the client is on the side, however, flex the uppermost hip and knee sharply and rest the knee and foot on the bed, raise the arm on the same side so it is parallel to the head, and allow the client to turn toward the abdomen. The flexed leg forms a triangular prop that keeps both the gluteal and lower abdominal areas raised off the bed on that side. The other leg will rotate internally somewhat at the hip joint and the knee will flex slightly (see Fig. 64-21). A pillow may or may not be

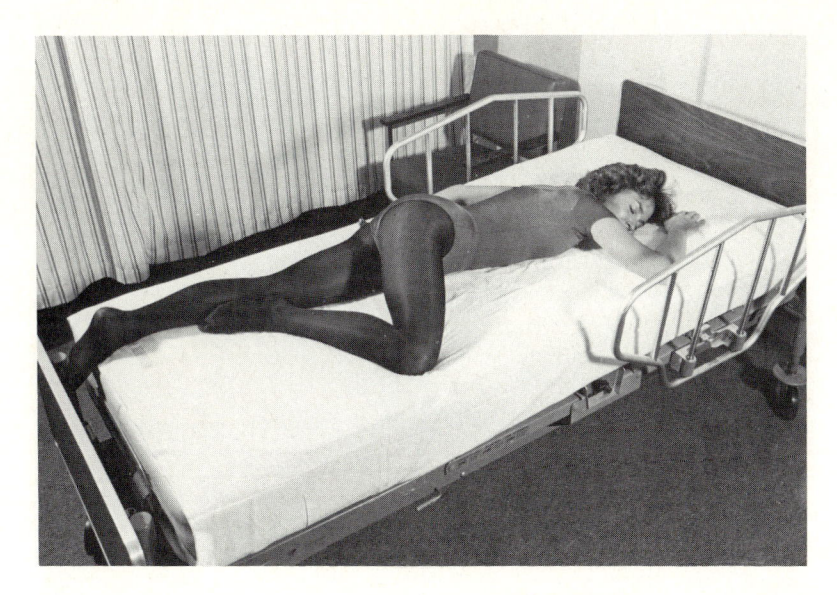

Figure 64-21. Sims position. (Photo by James Haines.)

needed to support the abdomen; this will depend on the contour of the client's abdomen, the client's comfort and personal preference, and the degree of swayback present. Other pillows usually are not necessary. Clients may find this position more comfortable than the completely prone position.

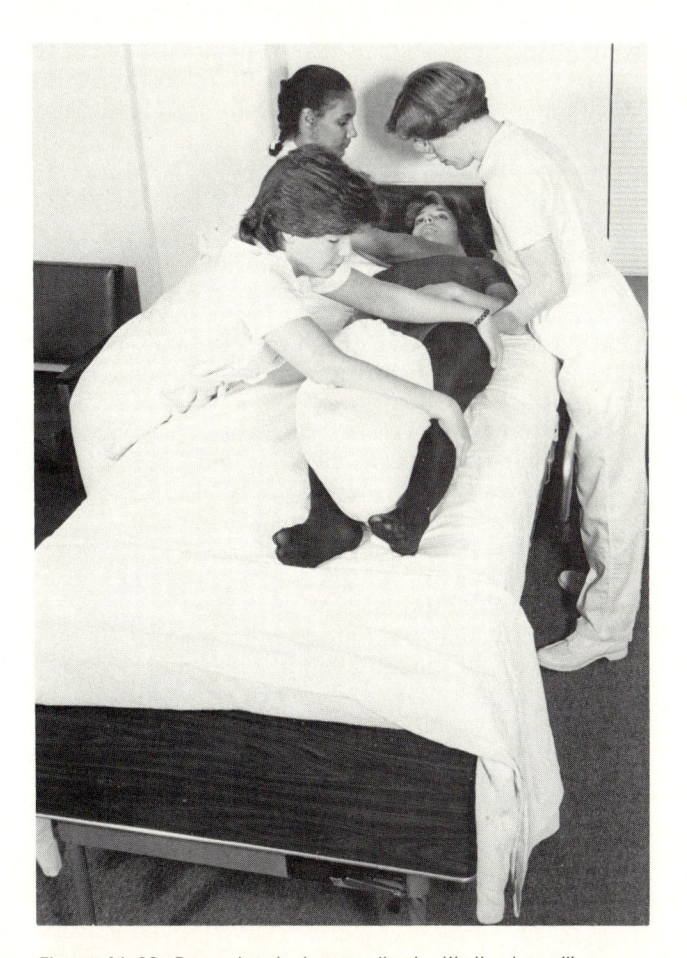

Figure 64-22. Preparing to turn a client with the logrolling technique. (Photo by James Haines.)

Logrolling a Client

After some types of spinal surgery, the client must be turned without twisting the spine or neck. This technique is known as "logrolling" and requires at least three nurses working in synchrony. Figure 64-22 shows a client prepared for logrolling. A pillow is placed between the legs to keep them apart and parallel to each other. Two nurses work from the side toward which the client is to be turned. One nurse prepares to pull the hips and legs toward himself or herself and the other supports and stabilizes the client's head and neck by placing the left hand under the base of the head and neck and the right hand on the far side of the neck. The third nurse on the opposite side of the bed prepares to lift and turn the client's shoulder and waist. The client is turned as a single unit, with all body segments maintained in vertical alignment. The head is not allowed to rotate on the spinal column. Figure 64-23 shows the completed turn, with the nurses' hands still in the positions used for turning. To maintain the client on the side, place pillows in ways that support the head, back, abdomen, and arms. Both legs may be flexed slightly at the hips and knees, with the legs remaining parallel to avoid twisting the spine.

RECORDING

Documentation of turning and positioning includes the type of position used and the purpose for the position; the client's ability to help turn; the degree of comfort in the position; the length of time the client remained in the position; and any special techniques used, such as logrolling. In addition, document any changes in skin condition, actual or potential pressure sores, and any untoward reactions to being turned and repositioned, such as discomfort or cardiovascular and respiratory changes.

Sample POR Recording

- S—NA
- O—Apparently slept for 30 min. when in lateral po-

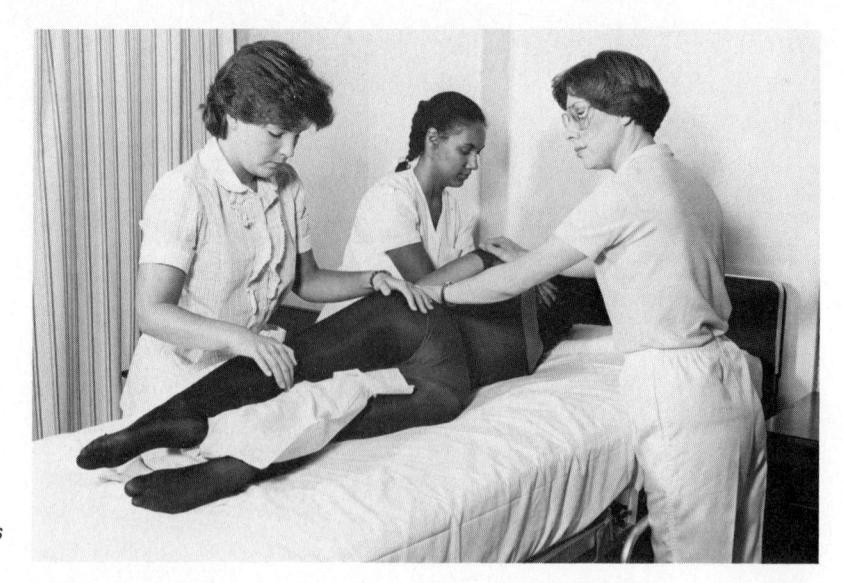

Figure 64–23. Logrolling completed, nurses hands remain in position. (Photo by James Haines.)

sition. Reddened sacral area smaller and less red today.
- A—Regular turning apparently decreasing potential for skin breakdown.
- P—Continue turning and repositioning q 2°, avoiding supine position.

Sample Narrative Recording
Turned to lateral position for 2 hours; decubitus care given. Remains minimally responsive; apparently slept for 30 minutes. Reddened area on sacrum smaller and less red today.

☐ CRITICAL POINTS SUMMARY

1. Regular and frequent turning is a crucial aspect of preventing skin, respiratory, and circulatory problems.
2. Use correct body mechanics to move, turn, and position clients:
    a. Assume a broad-based stance.
    b. Face the direction of a pulling action.
    c. Flex the knees to approximately 120 degree angle with the thigh before beginning to pull.
    d. Use body weight shifts to help pull and turn client.
3. Pull, rather than push, clients to change their position.
4. Support each body part when moving and positioning clients.
5. Position a client in good alignment and balance, with adequate support for each body segment.
6. Use adequate supports to avoid dependent edema and direct contact between body parts.
7. The logrolling technique maintains all body segments in alignment when turning the client.
8. Flotation devices decrease the frequency of, but do not substitute for, regular turning and repositioning.
9. Correct use of turning frames facilitates caring for clients who are difficult to turn.

☐ LEARNING ACTIVITIES

1. In a laboratory setting, turn and position a "client" in supine, lateral, prone, and Sims positions. Use pillows and towels to fit the body contours. Allow the person to remain in one or more positions without moving for at least 30 minutes. Reverse roles. Compare initial and later feelings of comfort and safety.
2. Use the controls on several different types of electric beds to place someone in regular and modified Trendelenburg, reverse Trendelenburg, semi-Fowler's and high-Fowler's positions. Determine how to engage and disengage the gatching mechanism of the bed that is used for Fowler's positions.
3. A. In a laboratory setting, use correct body mechanics to move a "client" upward in bed in the following ways. Work with several peers and a faculty preceptor as needed.
    (1) One nurse: client assits by flexing knees and pushing down toward the mattress and up toward the head of the bed.
    (2) Same as in (1), except client assists by pulling on the far side rail.
    (3) Same as (1), except with two nurses on opposite sides of bed.
    (4) Two nurses, using a pull sheet: client flexes knees but does not assist.
    (5) Same as (4), except client assists as in (1).
   B. Ask an observer to give feedback on your use of body mechanics.
    (1) Ask the "client" to give feedback on perceived safety and the comfort and smoothness of the movements.
    (2) Identify for yourself the muscles you were

aware of using, and whether any back strain was experienced.
        (3) If possible, repeat activity with persons of variable weight and height.
4. A. In a laboratory setting, use correct body mechanics to move a helpless "client" from the center of the bed to the near edge in the following ways. Use assistance as needed.
        (1) One nurse, move client in segments.
        (2) Two nurses, using a pull sheet.
        (3) Two nurses, without a pull sheet.
        (4) One nurse, using a pull sheet.
    B. Obtain the same type of feedback as in 3B.
5. In a Central Service area or a rehabilitation unit:
    A. Look at various types of foam pads, egg crate mattresses, heel protectors, and other devices used to prevent excessive pressure on bony protuberances.
    B. Look at turning frames (Stryker Wedge and CircOlectric) and airfluidized beds. If possible, operate these devices, watch a demonstration, or read the directions for use.
    C. Talk with staff nurses who have cared for a client on the special beds in 5B. Inquire about the benefits and problems associated with each.

☐ REVIEW QUESTIONS

1. Match the description in Column II with the position in Column I.

   COLUMN I
   ___ Fowler's
   ___ Lateral
   ___ Modified Trendelenburg
   ___ Prone
   ___ Reverse Trendelenburg
   ___ Sims
   ___ Supine

   COLUMN II
   A. Bed flat, head higher than foot.
   B. Bed flat, head lower than foot.
   C. Head and shoulders lower than legs and hips.
   D. Head of bed elevated to 30 to 90 degrees.
   E. Lying flat on abdomen.
   F. Lying on abdomen, one leg flexed sharply.
   G. Lying on back.
   H. Lying on side with both legs extended.
   I. Lying on side with one or both hips and knees flexed.

2. Why is it necessary to change a bed client's position regularly and frequently?
3. Why is each of the following practices an essential aspect of correct body mechanics used to position and move clients?
    a. Broaden the base of support
    b. Set the muscles of the arms, abdomen, and buttocks
    c. Face the direction of the pull
    d. Flex the knees to about a 120 degree angle before beginning the pull
    e. To pull, shift body weight from one foot to the other
    f. Pull, rather than push clients to change their position
4. Circle correct response. A pillow placed between the knees of a client in the lateral position will (increase/decrease) the pressure on the knee joints and avoid (inward/outward) rotation of the upper hip joint.
5. Where are the pressure points located for a client in the supine, lateral, and prone positions?
6. What specific techniques can be used to prevent dependent edema formation when positioning clients?
7. Why is it easier to move either helpless or nonhelpless clients up in bed when their knees are flexed?
8. Why is it easier to turn a person to the side when the far leg is crossed over the near leg and the far arm is placed across the chest or abdomen?
9. Why is the near arm placed against the body tightly when preparing to turn someone to a prone position?
10. Why is the near arm abducted slightly from the body when preparing to turn someone to a lateral position?
11. What is "shear force?"
12. How can the effects of shear force be minimized when moving a person up in bed, moving to one side of the bed, and when positioning in the Fowler position?

☐ PERFORMANCE CHECKLISTS

OBJECTIVE: To move a client to the side of the bed in a safe manner.			
CHARACTERISTIC	RANGE OF ACCEPTABILITY	SATISFACTORY	UNSATISFACTORY
1. Washes hands.	No deviation		
2. Explains procedure to client.	No deviation		
3. Adjusts bed to working height.	No deviation		

(continued)

OBJECTIVE: To move a client to the side of the bed in a safe manner (cont.).

CHARACTERISTIC	RANGE OF ACCEPTABILITY	SATISFACTORY	UNSATISFACTORY
4. Provides privacy.	No deviation		
5. Provides adequate visualization of client and procedure.	No deviation		
A. Straight Pull with Pull Sheet			

(1) Positions client on pull sheet:
   a. Includes hips and shoulders.
   b. Places client's arms across the chest or abdomen.
   c. Removes pillow.
	No deviation
	No deviation
	
	No deviation		

(2) Positions self:
   a. Faces bed directly.
   b. Uses wide base of support; rests weight on forward leg.
   c. Grasps rolled pull sheet at client's hips and shoulders; palms downward.
   d. Flexes knees.
   e. Sets muscles of arms, shoulders, abdomen, and buttocks.
	No deviation
	No deviation
	
	No deviation
	
	No deviation
	No deviation		

(3) Pulls directly toward self, shifting weight to back leg.	No deviation		
(4) Two or three nurses use prearranged signal when moving client.	No deviation		
(5) Positions client correctly.	No deviation		
B. Straight Pull without Pull Sheet			
(1) Places one arm completely under client's hips.	No deviation		
(2) Places other arm completely under client's shoulders.	No deviation		
(3) Positions self and pulls directly toward self. (See A(2) a to e and (3).)	No deviation		
(4) Positions client correctly.	No deviation		

OBJECTIVE: To move a client up in bed in a safe manner, using a pull sheet.

CHARACTERISTIC	RANGE OF ACCEPTABILITY	SATISFACTORY	UNSATISFACTORY
1. Washes hands.	No deviation		
2. Explains procedure to client.	No deviation		
3. Adjusts bed to working height.	No deviation		
4. Provides privacy.	No deviation		
5. Provides adequate visualization of client and procedure.	No deviation		

6. Positions client on pull sheet:
   a. Includes hips and shoulders.
   b. Places client's arms across chest or abdomen.
	No deviation
	No deviation		

7. Places client's pillow at head of bed.	No deviation		
8. Instructs client to flex knees.	Flex knees for client and stabilize his or her feet against mattress, as necessary.		

9. Positions self:
   a. Turns feet and trunk toward head of bed.
   b. Uses wide base of support; rests weight on backward leg.
	No deviation
	
	No deviation		

(continued)

CHARACTERISTIC	RANGE OF ACCEPTABILITY	SATISFACTORY	UNSATISFACTORY
c. Grasps rolled pull sheet at client's hips and shoulders, palms downward.	No deviation		
d. Flexes knees.	No deviation		
e. Sets muscles of shoulders, arms, abdomen, and buttocks.	No deviation		
10. Moves client up in bed with help of second nurse on opposite side of bed.	No deviation		
a. Gives prearranged signal.	No deviation		
b. Straightens backward leg.	No deviation		
c. Shifts weights to forward leg.	No deviation		
d. Client pushes feet downward and toward foot of bed.	Omit if client unable to assist.		
11. Positions client correctly.	No deviation		

OBJECTIVES: (1) To turn a client to the lateral and supine positions in a safe manner and (2) to support a client correctly in the lateral and supine positions.

CHARACTERISTIC	RANGE OF ACCEPTABILITY	SATISFACTORY	UNSATISFACTORY
1. Washes hands.	No deviation		
2. Explains procedure to client.	No deviation		
3. Adjusts bed to working height.	No deviation		
4. Provides privacy.	No deviation		
5. Provides adequate visualization of client and procedure.	No deviation		
6. Uses correct body mechanics throughout procedure.	No deviation		
7. Removes supportive pillows and places nearby.	No deviation		
A. Turning: Supine to Lateral Positions			
(1) Moves client to side of bed.	No deviation		
(2) Positions client:			
a. Crosses far leg over near leg.	No deviation		
b. Places far arm on abdomen or chest.	No deviation		
c. Abducts near arm slightly.	No deviation		
(3) Places own hands on client's shoulders and pulls straight toward self. or: Grasps rolled pull sheet on far side of client and pulls straight toward self.	No deviation		
(4) Supports client in lateral position:			
a. Places a pillow under the head.	No deviation		
b. Tucks a pillow along the back.	No deviation		
c. Pulls hips toward edge of bed.	No deviation		
d. Flexes and supports top leg on pillow(s).	No deviation		
e. Pulls bottom shoulder forward slightly.	No deviation		
f. Abducts and flexes bottom arm.	No deviation		
g. Flexes and supports top arm on pillow(s).	No deviation		
B. Turning: Lateral to Supine			
(1) Removes support pillows from arms and legs.	No deviation		
(2) Places top leg beside bottom leg.	No deviation		
(3) Stabilizes client with hand and removes pillow from back.	Omit if client can support self.		
(4) Holds client at shoulders and hips and allows trunk to return to bed slowly.	No deviation		
(5) Moves client to center of bed.	Client assists as able.		

(continued)

OBJECTIVES: (1) To turn a client to the lateral and supine positions in a safe manner and (2) to support a client correctly in the lateral and supine positions (cont.).

CHARACTERISTIC	RANGE OF ACCEPTABILITY	SATISFACTORY	UNSATISFACTORY

(6) Positions in supine position:
  a. Places pillow under head.
  b. Supports small of back with folded towel or small pillow.
  c. Provides slight knee flexion with towel or pillow.
  d. Relieves pressure on heels with towels or blanket under ankles.
  e. Places trochanter roll beside hip joint.
  f. Supports arms with pillows.
	No deviation
	Omit if unnecessary for comfort.
	
	No deviation
	
	No deviation
	
	Omit if client has adequate neuromuscular control.
	No deviation		

(7) Documents positioning in health record.	No deviation		

OBJECTIVES: (1) To turn a client to the prone and supine positions in a safe manner and (2) to support a client correctly in the prone and supine positions.

CHARACTERISTIC	RANGE OF ACCEPTABILITY	SATISFACTORY	UNSATISFACTORY
1. Washes hands.	No deviation		
2. Explains procedure to client.	No deviation		
3. Adjusts bed to working height.	No deviation		
4. Provides privacy.	No deviation		
5. Provides adequate visualization of client and procedure.	No deviation		
6. Uses correct body mechanics throughout procedure.	No deviation		
7. Removes supportive pillows and places nearby.	No deviation		
A. Turning: Supine to Prone			
(1) Moves client to foot of bed so feet will hang over mattress.	No deviation		
(2) Moves client to near side of bed.	No deviation		

(3) Positions client:
  a. Removes pillow.
  b. Crosses near leg over far leg.
  c. Places arms against body, fully extended.
	Place head near edge of pillow.
	No deviation
	Client may use near arm to pull on far side rail and help with turn.		

(4) From far side of bed, turns client on side and supports with pillow.	Second nurse may support client on the side.		
(5) From near side of bed, supports client at shoulder and hip as client turns onto abdomen.	Second nurse may complete the turn.		

(6) Supports client in prone position:
  a. Turns face toward side with raised arm.
  b. Relieves swayback and reduces pressure on genitals (male) and breasts (female) with blankets, towels, or small pillows.
  c. Provides slight flexion with folded blanket or towel under ankles.
  d. Allows feet to hang over end of mattress.
  e. Positions arms beside body or head.
	No deviation
	No deviation
	
	No deviation
	
	No deviation
	
	No deviation		

B. Turning: Prone to Supine			
(1) Places client's arms adjacent to and parallel with body.	No deviation		
(2) Turns client's face away from self.	No deviation		

(continued)

CHARACTERISTIC	RANGE OF ACCEPTABILITY	SATISFACTORY	UNSATISFACTORY
(3) Crosses client's far leg over near leg.	No deviation		
(4) Grasps client's far shoulder and hip, pulls client to side, and supports weight of trunk as it lowers to mattress.	May be done in two steps, first turning client to a lateral position.		
(5) Moves client to center of bed and toward head of bed.	No deviation		
(6) Positions in supine position: a. Places pillow under head. b. Supports small of back with folded towel or small pillow. c. Provides slight knee flexion with towel or pillow. d. Relieves pressure on heels with towels or blanket under ankle. e. Places trochanter roll beside hip joint. f. Supports arms with pillows.	No deviation Omit if unnecessary for comfort. No deviation No deviation Omit if client has adequate neuromuscular control. No deviation		
(7) Documents positioning in health record.	No deviation		

REFERENCES

Coker KE: The intermittent air-fluidized bed and the neurologically impaired patient. Journal of Neurological Nursing 11(1):31-33, 1979.

Culclasure DF: Medical benefits from space research. American Journal of Nursing 74(22):275-278, 1974.

Dayhoff N: Re-thinking stroke: Soft or hard devices to position hands? American Journal of Nursing 75(7):1142-1144, 1975.

Grabenstetter J: Synthetic fat helps prevent pressure sores. American Journal of Nursing 68(7):1521-1522, 1968.

Jackson J: Sheepskins—A potential hazard? Nursing Times 79(18):41-45, 1983.

Jamison SL, Dayhoff NE: A hard hand-positioning device to decrease wrist and finger hypertonicity: A sensorimotor approach for the patient with nonprogressive brain damage. Nursing Research 29(5):285-289, 1980.

Leavitt L: Decubitus ulcers. Hospital Medicine 2(11):76-78, 84-85, 1966.

Linden O, Greenway RM, et al.: Pressure distribution on the surface of the human body: 1. Evaluation in lying and sitting positions using a "bed of springs and nails." Archives of Physical Medicine and Rehabilitation 46(5):378-385, 1965.

Miller BF, Keane CB: Encyclopedia and Dictionary of Medicine, Nursing, and Allied Health, ed 3. Philadelphia, WB Saunders, 1983.

Miller ME, Sachs ML: About Bedsores: What You Need to Know to Help Prevent and Treat Them. Philadelphia, JB Lippincott, 1974.

Mitchell PH, Loustau A: Concepts Basic to Nursing, ed 3. New York, McGraw-Hill, 1981.

Pfaudler M: Flotation, displacement, and decubitus ulcers. American Journal of Nursing 68(11):2351-2355, 1968.

Rudd TN: The pathogenesis of decubitus ulcers. Journal of the American Geriatric Society 10(1):48-53, 1962.

Sanchez DG, Bussey B, et al.: How air-fluidized beds revolutionize skin care. RN 46(6):46-48, 1983.

Scheulen JJ, Munster AM: Clinitron air-fluidized support: An adjunct to burn care. Journal of Burn Care and Rehabilitation 4(4):271-275, 1983.

Scholey M: Back stress: The effects of training nurses to lift patients in a clinical situation. International Journal of Nursing Studies 20(1):1-13, 1983.

Skinner G: Nursing care of a patient on a Stryker frame. American Journal of Nursing 46(5):288-292, 1946.

Sorensen KC, Luckmann J: Basic Nursing: A Psychophysiologic Approach. Philadelphia, WB Saunders, 1979.

Stubbs DA, Rivers PM, et al.: Nursing Times 77(20):857-858, 1981.

Talbot D: Principles of Therapeutic Positioning: A Guide to Nursing Action. Minneapolis, MN: Sister Kenny Institute, 1978.

Thomas CL: Taber's Cyclopedic Medical Dictionary, ed 14. Philadelphia, FA Davis, 1981.

Thornhill HL, Williams ML: Experience with the water mattress in a large city hospital. American Journal of Nursing 68(11):2356-2358, 1968.

Turnock H: Benefits of a bead bed. Nursing Mirror 157(20):32-34, 1983.

BIBLIOGRAPHY

Bilger AJ, Greene EH (eds): Winter's Protective Body Mechanics: A Manual for Nurses. New York, Springer Publishing Co., 1973.

Foss G: The "how to's" of bed positioning. Nursing72 2(8):14-16, 1972.

Harvin JS, Hargest TS: The air-fluidized bed: A new concept in the treatment of decubitus ulcers. Nursing Clinics of North America 5(1):181-187, 1970.

Hrobsky A: The patient on a CircOlectric bed. American Journal of Nursing 71(12):2352-2353, 1971.

Kozier B, Erb G: Techniques in Clinical Nursing. Menlo Park, CA, Addison-Wesley, 1982.

Lewis LW: Fundamental Skills in Patient Care, ed 3. Philadelphia, JB Lippincott, 1984.

Norton D: Breakdown of pressure areas. Nursing Times 20:399-401, 1964.

Nursing74 editorial staff: How to negotiate the ups and downs, ins and outs of body alignment. Nursing74 4(10):46-51, 1974.

Rambo BJ, Woods LA: Nursing Skills for Clinical Practice, ed 3. Philadelphia, WB Saunders, 1982.

Rantz MF, Courtial D: Lifting, Moving, and Transferring Patients: A Manual, ed 2. St Louis, CV Mosby, 1981.

744 PROFESSIONAL CLINICAL NURSING SKILLS

AUDIOVISUAL RESOURCES

Basic Nursing Care: Lifting and Moving the Patient
Slides, filmstrip, videocassette, film. (1982, Color, 18 min.)
Available through:
Medcom, Inc.
P.O. Box 116
Garden Grove, CA 92642

Bed Positioning
20 slides

Moving and Lifting Patients
Film (1969, 25 min.)

Moving in Bed
26 slides
Available through:
Sister Kenny Institute
1800 Chicago Avenue
Minneapolis, MN 55404

Bed Care and Positioning of the Patient with Arthritis
Film (16mm). (1968, Color, 18 min.)

Bed Positioning of the Acute Hemiplegic Patient
Film (16mm). (1966, Color, 8 min.)
Available through:
National Medical Audiovisual Center
Washington, DC 20409

The Hemiplegic Patient: Changing Position in Bed
Film (16mm). (1968, Color, 8 min.)

How to Turn a Patient on a Stryker Frame Bed
8 Slides. (1978, B & W)
Available through:
Health Sciences Consortium
200 Eastowne Drive, Suite 213
Chapel Hill, NC 27514

Moving a Patient in Bed
Videorecording (¾ in). (1972, Color, 16 min.)
Available through:
Comprenetics, Inc.
5805 Uplander Way
Culver City, CA 90230

SKILL 65 Transfer Activities

PREREQUISITE SKILLS

Skill 28, "Handwashing"
Chapter 14, "Introduction"
Skill 62, "Assistance with Ambulation"
Skill 64, "Turning, Moving, and Positioning"

☐ STUDENT OBJECTIVES

1. Identify types of clients who may require assistance in transferring from one place to another.
2. Indicate the types of transfers in common use.
3. Describe safety precautions that must be used to prevent injury during transfer.
4. Describe the appropriate position for clients who are seated in a chair.
5. Describe how to use a mechanical lift for transfers.
6. Demonstrate the ability to implement safe bed-to-stretcher and bed-to-chair transfers and vice versa.

☐ INTRODUCTION

Transferring activities involve moving clients from a bed to a chair, stretcher, treatment table, or another bed. Some persons are able to do this unassisted; others need varying degrees of assistance, depending on their strength, general condition, or the activity restrictions imposed by their illness.

Transfer activities are a common occurrence in any direct-care setting. In some agencies, transportation personnel do most of the bed-to-stretcher transfers, while in other agencies, this task is shared with the nursing staff. As with the activities of moving, turning, and lifting (Skill 64), it is essential that nurses protect themselves from injury by using correct body mechanics. When a transfer is accomplished correctly, the nurse exerts minimal effort and avoids self-injury, and the client is moved with maximum safety and the amount of exercise appropriate for that person.

☐ PREPARATION

Transfer activities are modified to fit the person's strengths and capabilities, as well as the space, equipment, and staff available. Clients should be allowed and encouraged to do as much of the transfer as possible and permissible. Active participation increases a client's independence, sense of control of both self and environment, and often provides needed exercise. In addition, even a small amount of lifting help from a client decreases the resistance of static friction and requires less lifting by the nurse. It is especially important that clients with long-term disability (such as a spinal cord injury or cerebral vascular accident) achieve a maximum degree of independence, as that will increase their ability to cope with chronic weakness or paralysis.

ASSESSMENT OF TRANSFER CAPABILITIES

Before a client is transferred to a chair for the first time, or whenever a nurse is uncertain of the client's ability to transfer, it is important to assess strength, balance, and ability to cooperate and help with the transfer. To assess upper extremity strength, have the person grasp, squeeze, and release both of your hands. Clients with a weak grasp lack the ability to push up in bed or hold on to a chair or bed. Those who are unable to release may have difficulty performing the arm movements associated with balance and support during a pivot transfer. To assess lower extremity strength (primarily the quadriceps muscles), have the client flex the knees while lying on the back; support the leg with one arm, place your hand beneath the sole of the foot, and ask him or her to push against your hand and extend the leg. Clients with weak quadriceps have limited ability to stand and will need more assistance from the nurse. To assess balance, first assist the person to dangle. Next, place one hand about 18 cm (5 in) away from one shoulder to guard against falling, and use the other hand to push the person sideways slightly. If the person regains balance readily, he or she probably will have adequate standing balance. To assess general ability to transfer, evaluate vital signs before and after dangling, observe for postural hypotension, and determine the client's ability to hear, understand, and follow directions (Long and Buergin, 1977).

POSITIONING A CLIENT IN A CHAIR

Correct alignment is as important when sitting in a chair as when lying in bed. When in a sitting position, the three major pressure points are the ischial tuberosities, sacrococcygeal area, and the trochanters (greater, lesser, and intertrochanteric crests) (Peterson and Adkins, 1982). Tissues over the ischial tuberosities are specially adapted to tolerate intensive pressure in the normal upright sitting position. Postural changes, such as slouching or sitting unevenly, affect the distribution of pressure on the different pressure points and cause increased pressure at one or more points, resulting in capillary occlusion and tissue ischemia. A person with normal innervation will change position automatically, and no damage occurs. When people are not aware of pressure sensations or are unable to change their position, tissue necrosis will occur if the pressure remains unrelieved. In addition, a slouched position exerts a shearing force on the deeper tissues and increases the potential for pressure-sore development.

Slouching is most likely to occur when the chair seat depth exceeds the person's upper leg length, so that the trunk tilts backward against the chair back when the knees are flexed over the front of the seat. Norton (1964) suggests that the risk of pressure sores may be greater when clients are in chairs than when in bed, particularly if the chair does not fit them. Position changes are limited in a seated position, and nursing staff tends to reposition a seated client less often than a bed client.

Clients who are at an increased risk for developing pressure sores when sitting include those who have decreased innervation; atrophy of the gluteal or thigh muscles; pathologic conditions of the hip joint that do not allow a normal sitting position, such as arthritis; or clients with an altered sitting position, such as may occur with scoliosis or after some orthopedic surgeries.

A correct sitting position includes the following characteristics:

1. The lower back is against the back of the chair so the spinal column is directly above the ischial tuberosities.
2. Feet are flat on the floor or on a support.
3. Hips are at approximately a right angle to the trunk and the knees are at the same angle to the thighs; body weight is distributed evenly over the buttocks and posterior thighs; the chair edge does not place pressure on the popliteal space.
4. Forearms are supported at elbow level without causing elevation or drooping of the shoulders.

There are several ways to decrease the risk of developing pressure sores when clients are in a sitting position. First, adapt the chair to fit the client by placing cushions or pillows behind the client's back, on either side of the client, on the armrests, on the chair seat, or on the floor under the client's feet. Second, teach clients to raise themselves from the chair for a total of at least 1 minute out of each hour, or tilt on alternate hips. Third, use antidecubitus pads to decrease and redistribute pressure, as discussed in Skill 64. Fourth, never allow clients to sit on a plastic or wooden chair without adequate padding or clothing. In addition to being uncomfortable, moisture cannot evaporate and shearing force associated with slouching is exaggerated because of the increased static and sliding friction between skin and the hard chair surface.

DATA BASE

A decision about the methods used to transfer and transport clients may be made by the physician or physical therapist; however, it often is made by the nurse. This nursing judgment is based on the client's activity orders and medical and nursing diagnoses; personal preference, physical strength and movement capability, age, size, mental alertness and ability to follow directions; the presence of injuries, lesions, incisions or prostheses that require special protection; and the placement of tubings attached to the client, such as intravenous tubing, nasogastric tubes, or urinary catheters. A decision may also be based on the availability of staff persons or special equipment, or on the requirements of the department to which the client is being transported.

746 PROFESSIONAL CLINICAL NURSING SKILLS

The nursing-care plan or kardex will provide information about prescribed transfer methods or about those methods which have been used successfully, as well as the number of people and type of equipment required. When this information is available and used by the nursing staff, clients benefit from the familiarity and security of consistent methods. Because a client's condition may change on a daily basis, it is important to make direct observations at the time of transfer and evaluate whether any changes need to be made in the planned method of transfer.

Physical Appraisal Skills

Inspection. Inspection is used to determine whether transfer equipment such as mechanical lifters, stretchers, and wheelchairs are positioned correctly and securely before the client is actually transferred. Inspection is also used to assess the correct position of the client and nurse before, during, and after transfer.

EQUIPMENT

Wheelchairs

A wheelchair is used to transport clients who are able to support themselves in an upright position. Clients may propel themselves or be pushed by another person, or the wheelchair may be motorized and self-propelled.

A wheelchair consists of a frame and a seat that is suspended between wheels. The large rear wheels have a turning rim used by clients to propel themselves; the smaller front wheels swivel, allowing the wheelchair to turn.

A hand brake can be forced against the rear wheel to keep the wheelchair from moving while getting in and out of the chair. The feet and legs are supported by foot pedals and adjustable leg rests; these items can be folded back or removed while getting in and out of the chair, or to allow the chair to be propelled with the feet. Most wheelchairs have a vinyl seat and back that can be cleaned easily, and most are constructed so they can be folded for storage or transportation. A folding wheelchair is shown in Figure 65–1, along with the mechanical lift described below.

Stretchers

Stretchers are used to transport clients who are seriously ill, limited in movement, unable to sit upright, or who are required to lie flat for some reason. A stretcher is a narrow, lightweight metal bed with large wheels that make it easy to roll. A stretcher has a pad for comfort and side rails or a safety belt to protect the client from falling. Most stretchers used in hospitals are approximately the same height as a bed (in high position) or a treatment table, thus decreasing the amount of lifting required to transfer from one to the other. Some stretchers have adjustable headrests which allow the person to be placed in the Fowler's position, and many have a portable intravenous standard that can be inserted into a bracket.

Roller Bars

A roller bar is used to transfer a client to and from a bed, stretcher, or treatment table without lifting. The roller bar consists of a vinyl-covered metal frame containing rows of metal rollers. When a client is placed on one side of the frame and pulled across it, the cover rolls around the frame and rollers, moving the person

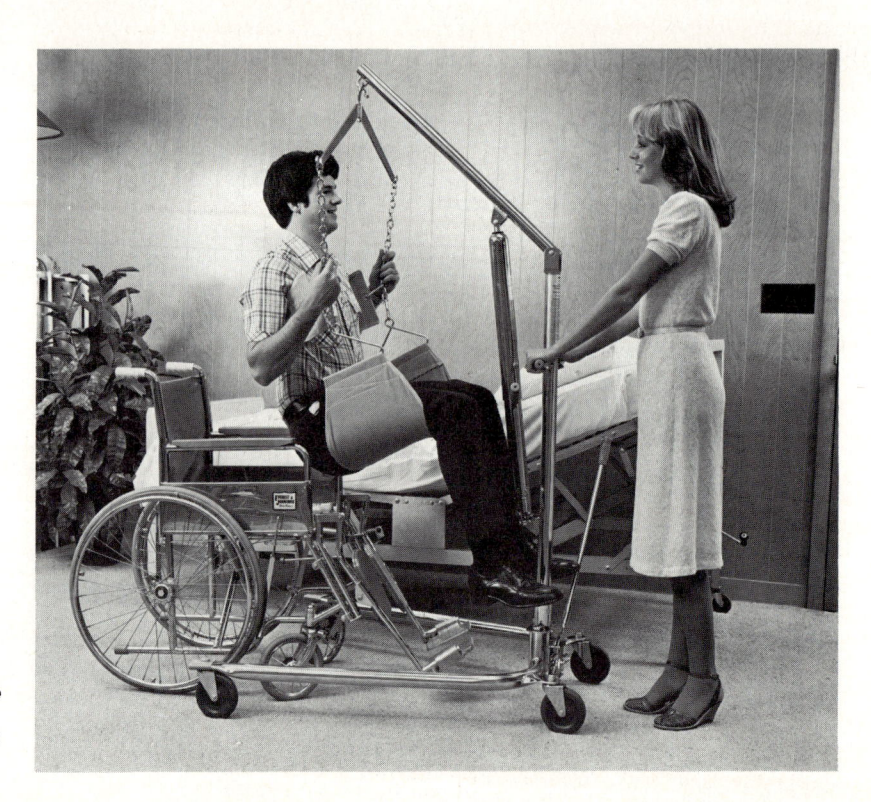

Figure 65–1. Hoyer Patient Lifter with two-piece sling. As the boom lowers, the client will move over the seat of the wheelchair. (Courtesy, Ted Hoyer and Company, Inc. OshKosh, WI.)

along with the cover. This device decreases significantly the resistance to moving that is exerted by static and sliding friction forces.

Mechanical Lifters
A portable mechanical lift, such as the Hoyer Patient Lifter, is used to transfer heavy or helpless clients from a bed to a chair, stretcher, bathtub, or commode. The Hoyer Patient Lifter (Figure 65-1) has an adjustable base that can be widened to 39 inches, thus broadening the base of support and increasing its stability, or it can be narrowed to 24 inches so it can pass through a door or maneuver in tight quarters. Not all lifts have this adjustable base. The lift is designed to be raised and lowered with a hydraulic pump or a mechanical jack, thus adjusting the lift to any height bed or chair.

While being transported by the lift, the client is suspended in a one- or two-piece canvas, fabric, or mesh sling attached with straps or chains to hooks on the swivel bar of the lift. Some one-piece slings are designed with a higher back rest to support the head; some have an opening to accommodate using a commode or toilet; and mesh slings can be used to lift the client into a tub for bathing. A two-piece sling consists of a wide strap that goes under the buttocks and a narrower strap that fits across the back and under the arms. The straps or chains are attached to the sling with S-hooks and to the lift by placing metal rings over the swivel bar hook.

☐ EXECUTION

Most transfers between a bed and a stretcher require that several nurses work together to share the work load. Transfers between a bed and chair may be done with only one nurse; however, it is helpful to have an assistant when a weak, heavy, or partially paralyzed client is transferred between a bed and chair for the first time. Having a second person available to assist with a first-time transfer provides a margin of safety in the event that the client is physically unable to help as much as was anticipated. Once the degree of active client participation in the transfer is determined, a second person may not be necessary.

Advance planning is crucial for a successful transfer. A few minutes spent planning and organizing will save much time, energy, and possible injury at the time of the actual transfer. When others are helping with the transfer, it is especially important to have all supplies and equipment ready, the furnishings in the room or unit arranged properly, and a plan devised that specifies who will do what and how it will be done so as to accomplish the transfer readily and safely.

TRANSFERRING BETWEEN A BED AND A CHAIR

A key factor in transfers between a bed and chair is the placement of the chair in relation to the client and the bed. Chair placement is determined by the client's capabilities, the room arrangement, and the location of any equipment attached to the client, such as intravenous infusions, nasogastric suction, or urinary catheters.

When a client has adequate mobility and needs assistance because of generalized weakness, place the chair on the side of the bed where tubes or equipment are attached. If space is inadequate on that side, relocate the client's tubes and equipment or rearrange the unit so that space, equipment, and chair all are on the same side of the bed. If space permits, choose to have the chair on the client's dominant side and place the bedside table against the wall beside the head of the bed; the chair can then be braced against the table to prevent the chair from moving during the transfer.

When a client has impaired function of the arm or leg or both on one side, position the chair to face either the head or foot of the bed, with the uninvolved arm nearest the chair. For example, if a person with a paralyzed left arm must get out of bed on the left side of the bed because of space limitations, place the chair facing the head of the bed. This position allows the client to reach for the chair arm with the uninvolved strong arm and help with the transfer. It also provides a sense of security and a better balance than when the client leads with a weakened or paralyzed arm. Following this principle usually means that the chair must face one direction to move *from* the bed, and the opposite direction to return *to* the bed. Rearrange tubing, equipment, and space as needed.

Plan the placement of tubings and equipment to avoid becoming tangled in them during the pivot turn. When tubing and equipment are attached to the side of the body nearest the chair, position these items at the far side of the chair before beginning the transfer. When these items are on the side of the client that is farthest from the chair, maintain the tubing and equipment in that relationship.

When a wheelchair is being used, set the brake tightly. If it does not seem secure or if the client is very heavy, have an assistant hold the wheelchair in

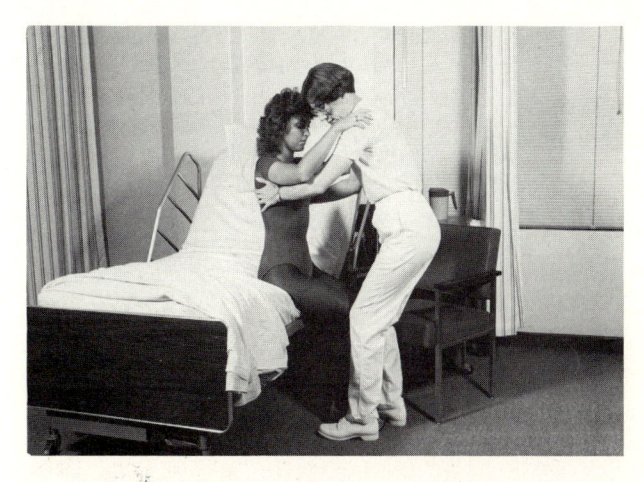

Figure 65-2. Preparing to stand at bedside; nurse's knees and feet brace client's knees and feet. (Photo by James Haines.)

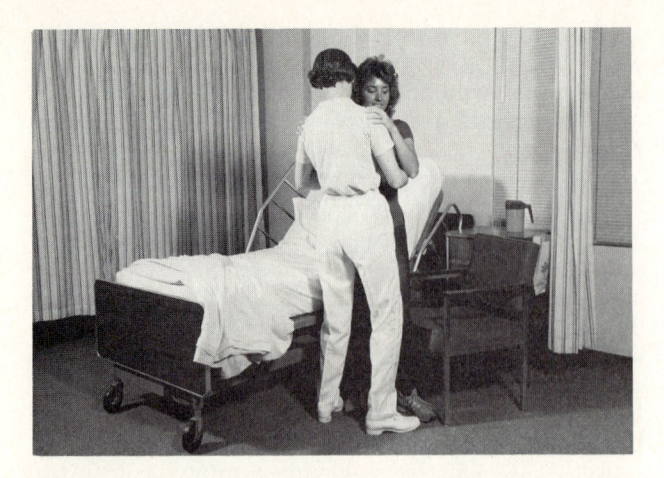

Figure 65-3. Standing and pivoting; bracing continues. (Photo by James Haines.)

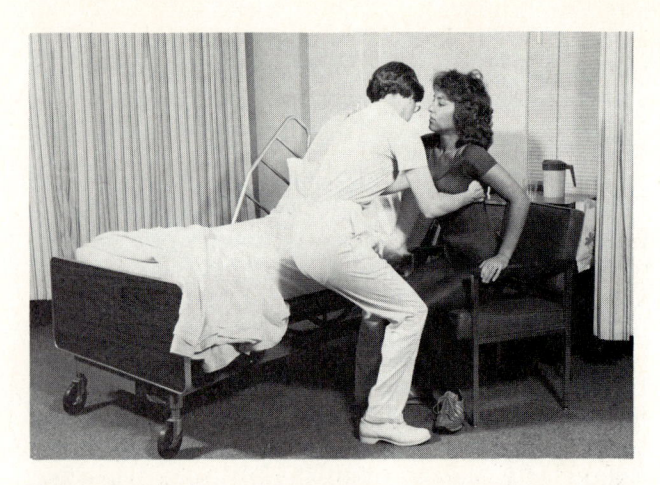

Figure 65-4. Nurse lowers client to chair; client assists in effort. (Photo by James Haines.)

place. Remove the leg supports nearest the bed to allow more space for yourself and the client to pivot your feet. If the client has difficulty standing or is hard to transfer, remove the near arm rest to eliminate any interference from the arm height.

To assist a client to move from a bed to a chair, the nurse faces the person seated on the side of the bed, and then assists him or her to stand, pivot, and sit down in the chair as shown in Figures 65-2, 65-3, and 65-4. These activities are described in the Skill Sequence, "Transfer from Bed to Chair." It is important for both the nurse and the client to use a forward-backward broad-based stance (described in Skill 64), as these positions enable both persons to use shifts of body weight to help the person rise to a standing position. It usually is more effective and requires less effort on the part of both the nurse and the client if the client stands completely upright before pivoting and sitting down. Clients sometimes want to stand only partly upright, turn, and sit quickly in one motion, perhaps out of fear of falling. Before beginning the transfer explain the procedure step by step; during the transfer, coach the client verbally with each step.

☐ SKILL SEQUENCE

TRANSFER FROM BED TO CHAIR

Step	Rationale
1. Wash hands.	Prevents transfer of microorganisms.
2. Check activity orders on care plan, kardex, or health record.	Ensures correct implementation of medical and nursing care plans.
3. Explain procedure to client.	Enlists client's help and cooperation.
4. Close room door or draw curtains around bed.	Provides for privacy.
5. Place bed in low position.	Allows for easier move to the chair.
6. Place chair beside bed at a slight angle, facing head or foot of bed. (See text for determination of chair placement.)	Chair is positioned for client to reach with strong arm; client is able to stand, pivot, and sit without walking.
7. Assist client to don a bathrobe or pajamas, or be certain client is adequately covered with gown.	Provides for privacy and warmth.
8. Position tubings that are attached to client in a way that will not interfere with the transfer.	Avoids accidental dislodging of tubings such as intravenous infusions and bladder catheters.
9. Assist client to move to side of bed, dangle, and stand, as in Skill 62, Skill Sequence, "Assisting the Client to Dangle," p. 696. (See Fig. 65-2.) Be sure client is wearing nonskid shoes or slippers.	Provides support; increases static friction between the feet and the floor, decreasing the potential for slipping and falling.
10. Have client stand in place briefly; continue to brace knees and feet.	Allows client to gain balance in upright position; prepares for careful, planned pivot and seating; uses muscles of both nurse and client more effectively.

(continued)

Step	Rationale
11. Instruct client to turn by pivoting on ball of foot farthest from chair and shifting the other foot toward far side of chair.	Maintains client's balance; avoids twisting action, and positions client directly in front of chair.
12. Simultaneously, nurse turns by pivoting on ball of foot nearest chair and shifting other foot toward chair. Knees remain braced against client's knees as shown in Figure 65-3.	Maintains nurse's balance; avoids twisting action on intervertebral discs and straining the back. Positions nurse to assist with a straight lift. Helps client maintain balance, keeps knees from buckling, and prevents feet from slipping.
13. Instruct client to move back toward chair until legs touch seat of chair.	Places client securely in center of chair seat after sitting down.
14. To assist client to sit down, as shown in Figure 65-4, simultaneously:	
a. Instruct client to grasp far arm of chair; lean forward; flex knees; and lower body weight steadily to chair. Second arm remains on nurse's shoulder.	Client's arm supports part of the body weight. Leaning forward keeps client's center of gravity over base of support. Flexed quadriceps support body weight.
b. Nurse continues to brace client's knees, flexes own knees and hips sharply, and supports client in lowering to chair.	An abrupt drop to the chair can be painful and cause injury.
15. Position client in chair, using pillows, cushions, or blankets to achieve a correct sitting position.	Supports body in correct alignment, avoids shearing force, and reduces fatigue.
16. Place a blanket over client's legs as needed.	Provides for privacy and warmth.
17. Place nurse-call signal within reach.	Provides for safety.
18. Monitor tolerance to position.	Provides for safety and gathers data.
19. Document in health record time spent in chair and client's tolerance for the activity.	Provides ongoing data base. Fulfills nurse accountability and responsibility.

To return the client to the bed, first relocate the chair as needed. Then help the client slide toward the front of the chair so that one leg can be placed backward under the chair and create a broad, forward-backward stance. Use the same procedure and sequence to help the patient stand, pivot, and sit on the edge of the bed (see Fig. 65-5). Return the client to bed as described in Skill 62.

When a client is not able to stand, a mechanical lift may be used, as described below. When no lift is available, two people can lift the client from a bed to a chair and back again. To lift a client from a bed to a chair, first assist the person to a sitting position in the bed. The strongest and tallest nurse then stands behind the head of the bed and grasps the person under the axilla or around the trunk. The second nurse supports the legs, and the person reaches for the arm of the chair and pushes against the bed with the other arm for support. On a prearranged signal, the nurses lift the client to the chair. A transfer from the chair to the bed is done in the same way, with the nurse standing behind the chair. If the client is too heavy to be moved in this way without causing excessive strain on the nurses, the technique is not attempted.

TRANSFERRING BETWEEN A BED AND STRETCHER

Most bed to stretcher transfers are accomplished with the stretcher placed adjacent to the bed and stabilized in that position by setting the brakes on *both* pieces of equipment, or by having two people hold them together at the head and foot ends. This security is crucial to avoid having the client fall to the floor if the bed and stretcher move apart inadvertently. A nurse always stands on the far side of the stretcher to assist the client to move from the bed and to guard against falling off the narrow stretcher. Some clients are able to shift themselves to the edge of the bed and onto the stretcher with minimal or no assistance. When clients are unable to do this, several nurses work together and accomplish the transfer with a pull sheet or roller bar, as shown in Figures 65-6 and 65-7 and described in the Skill Sequence, "Transfer from Bed to Stretcher" (sections A and B).

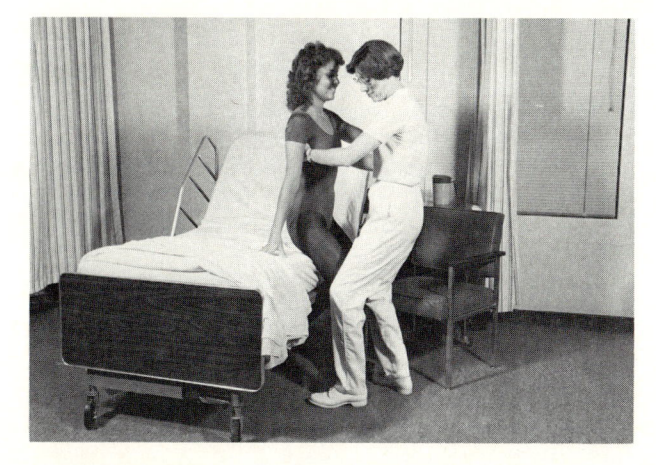

Figure 65-5. Returning to bed; nurse continues to brace client's knees and feet; client assists in effort. (Photo by James Haines.)

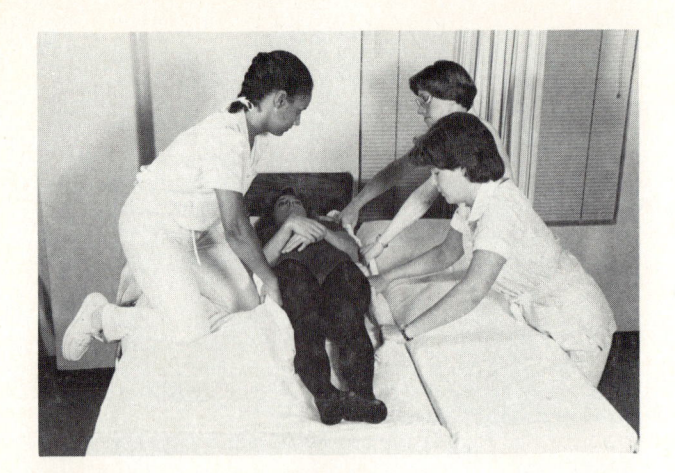

Figure 65-6. Bed-to-stretcher transfer, using pull sheet. Additional nurses may be required to move the client's feet and head. (Photo by James Haines.)

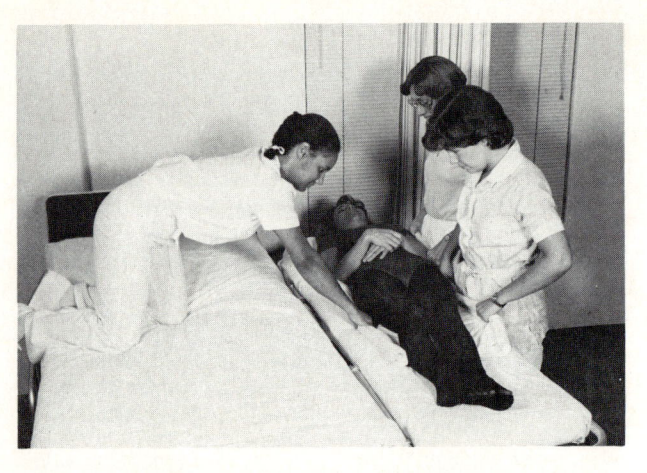

Figure 65-7. Stretcher-to-bed transfer, using pull sheet. The nurse on the bed shifts her body weight backwards and pulls, rather than lifting. (Photo by James Haines.)

When space does not permit the stretcher to be placed adjacent to the bed, it can be positioned at a right angle to the foot or head of the bed and stabilized there. The client then can be carried to the stretcher by at least three nurses, as described in the Skill Sequence, "Transfer from Bed to Stretcher" (section C). The client's weight is shared among the nurses, with the strongest nurse carrying the hip area (for a woman) or the shoulder area (for a man), a taller nurse carrying the head, and the shortest nurse carrying the feet. When this principle is followed, the client is carried in a fairly level fashion.

The following Skill Sequence presents techniques for transferring a client from a bed to a stretcher. The same techniques are used in reverse to transfer from a stretcher to a bed.

☐ SKILL SEQUENCE

TRANSFER FROM BED TO STRETCHER

Step	Rationale
(NOTE: Three persons are required for these transfers.)	
1. Wash hands.	Prevents transfer of microorganisms.
2. Explain procedure to client.	Enlists client's help and cooperation.
3. Draw curtains around bed or close room door.	Provides for privacy.
4. Rearrange furniture in room or unit as needed to accommodate stretcher.	Facilitates transfer.
5. Raise bed to same height as stretcher.	Provides for easy, level transfer.
A. Pull Sheet Transfer	
(1) Place pull sheet under client and move toward side of bed as in Skill 64, Skill Sequence, "Moving a Client to the Side of the Bed," steps A(1) to A(10), p. 728.	Same as Skill 64, Skill Sequence, "Moving a Client to the Side of the Bed," steps A(1) and A(10), p. 728. Decreases distance client must be moved.
(2) Place stretcher parallel to and adjacent to bed. Lock wheels on both bed and stretcher.	Places stretcher in correct position. Protects client from injury.
(3) Place folded blanket or towels between bed and stretcher to bridge the gap between the two surfaces evenly.	Protects from injury and facilitates sliding from one surface to the other.
(4) To move client to the stretcher, as shown in Figure 65-6:	
a. First nurse (leader): kneel on bed at level of client's waist; place knee nearest client's head forward from the other knee. Grasp rolled pull sheet at shoulder and hip levels.	Allows nurse to use quadriceps muscle and shifting body weight to assist in lifting and moving. Applies lifting force at heaviest body segments.
b. Second nurse: stand beside stretcher, reach across, and grasp rolled pull sheet near head and below shoulders.	Prevents injury to head during transfer and supports partial weight of shoulders.
c. Third nurse: stand beside stretcher, reach across and grasp rolled pull sheet above and below the hips.	Applies pulling force heaviest at body segments.

(continued)

Step	Rationale
d. On a prearranged signal given by the leader (first nurse), the first nurse straightens his or her legs and lifts; the second and third nurses pull; moving client in unison to center of the stretcher.	Uses correct body mechanics to pull, lift, and move client. Unison move is experienced by client as smooth and safe. Stretcher is narrow.
(5) Position client for comfort with pillows; cover with blanket or sheet; raise side rails and secure safety strap. (NOTE: Return client to bed in a similar manner, as shown in Figure 65–7.)	Provides for comfort, privacy, and safety.

B. Roller Bar Transfer

Step	Rationale
(1) Place pull sheet under client as in Skill 64, Skill Sequence, "Moving a Client to the Side of the Bed," step A(1). Do not move client to side of bed.	Directs force toward the heaviest parts of the body. Provides additional support as needed. Prevents injury from shear force and decreases static friction force and resistance to pulling action. Facilitates placement of roller bar.
(2) Prepare for transfer:	
a. First nurse: turn client on side, away from side where stretcher is to be placed.	Positions client for placement of roller bar.
b. Second nurse: place roller bar under client so that both the hip and shoulder areas are included (and head if using a long bar).	Provides adequate support; places roller under heaviest body segments.
c. First nurse: allow client to turn onto back onto roller bar.	Stabilizes roller bar in correct placement.
d. Second and third nurses: place stretcher parallel and adjacent to bed. Fill in the gap between bed and stretcher with blankets and towels as needed. Lock wheels on both bed and stretcher.	Places stretcher in correct place. Protects from injury, facilitates sliding from one surface to the other.
e. Roll pull sheet close to client on both sides.	Keeps pull sheet taut and uses pulling force more efficiently.
(3) To move client to the stretcher:	
a. First nurse: stand at far side of bed, reach across and grasp rolled pull sheet at shoulders and hip levels; hold firmly throughout the move.	Applies steady pulling force at heaviest body segments. Taut sheet provides slight lifting motion that protects client from hard rollers and decreases nurse effort.
b. Second nurse (leader): Reach across stretcher, grasp rolled pull sheet and hold sheet taut. For short roller bar; grasp at top and bottom of roller bar. For long roller bar; grasp at shoulder and hip levels.	Applies steady pulling force at heaviest body segments. Adapts pulling action to length of roller bar.
c. Third nurse: reach under pull sheet and support client's head (and shoulders, if using a short roller bar).	Provides for client's comfort and assists with move.
d. On prearranged signal from leader (second nurse), second nurse pulls client toward self; third nurse supports and moves client's head and shoulders; first nurse continues to hold sheet taut; client is moved in unison from bed to center of stretcher by these simultaneous actions.	Uses correct body mechanics to pull, lift, and move client. Unison move is experienced by client as smooth and safe. Stretcher is narrow.
(4) Second nurse turns client toward self slightly while third nurse removes roller bar.	Provides for safe removal of roller bar from narrow stretcher.
(5) Position client on stretcher as in step A(5).	Provides for client comfort, privacy, and safety.

C. Three-Person Transfer

Step	Rationale
(1) Place stretcher or second bed at right angles to foot of bed, or in convenient place.	Provides for convenient transfer and minimizes carrying distance.
(2) Lock wheels. If possible, place stretcher against wall or have fourth nurse hold it in place.	Safety measures.
(3) Plan for strongest nurse to carry heaviest part of client; tallest nurse to carry client's head and shoulders; and shortest, least strong nurse to carry client's legs. (NOTE: Nurse at heaviest portion is leader.)	Distributes weight evenly, shares work load, and provides relatively level position for client.
(4) Move client toward near side of bed.	Brings client near to nurses' centers of gravity, increases efficiency of arm flexors, and decreases lifting force needed.
(5) Assume a forward to backward broad-based stance with knees flexed.	Provides stability and balance, enables nurses to lift by contracting the quadriceps, straightening the knees, and shifting body weight to the backward foot.
(6) Place arms completely under client so hands grasp far side of body, elbows resting on the bed. Arms of first and third nurses should touch the middle nurse's arms.	Places client's weight (resistance) on the forearm level; elbows serve as fulcrum. Provides additional support for heavy body segments.
(7) On leader's call of "Turn" or "One," roll client toward own chests in unison, keeping elbows on bed.	Brings client's weight close to nurse and within nurse's base of support.

(continued)

TRANSFER FROM BED TO STRETCHER (Cont.)

Step	Rationale
(8) On call of "Lift" or "Two," stand upright, straightening legs and pushing upward with large leg muscles. Continue to hold client against chest.	Uses large muscles for major lifting work. Maintains client in secure position and within nurses' line of gravity.
(9) On call of "Pivot" or "Three," nurses step backward from the bed, turn and walk toward the stretcher in unison.	Maintains client in alignment and avoids exerting a twisting force on nurses' intervertebral discs.
(10) On call of "Ready" or "Four," nurses assume broad-based stance, flex knees, and lower elbows to stretcher edge.	Maintains client within nurses' line of gravity and prepares to use large leg muscles to lower client to stretcher.
(11) On call of "Down" or "Five," lower client to stretcher surface by slowly straightening both knees and lowering forearms to stretcher.	Large muscles provide controlled movement toward stretcher.
(12) Position as in step A(5) above.	Provides for client, comfort, privacy, and safety.
(13) Document in health record the time, type of transfer used, client's destination, and any problems encountered.	Fulfills nurse accountability and responsibility.

TRANSFER WITH A MECHANICAL LIFT

Before using a mechanical lift to transfer a client for the first time, demonstrate and explain the procedure to clients and families. Although this usually is an unfamiliar procedure initially, most clients feel safe after the first few transfers are accomplished. To ensure a sense of security for the client, two or three nurses should work together when using the lift. The first nurse maneuvers the lift and operates the jack. A second nurse lifts the client's legs to assist in clearing the bed as the client is moved away from the bed. This nurse continues to hold the legs and steady the client during the move. A third nurse manages the environment as needed, holds the chair or wheelchair in place, and guides the client's trunk into the chair. The first nurse lowers the mechanical jack and stabilizes the lift while the second nurse pushes downward gently on the client's knees to help maintain a correct sitting position and guides the client to the chair.

The following guidelines will help you use a mechanical lift to transfer a client safely.

1. Plan the move carefully and rearrange the client's furniture as needed to accommodate the movement of the lift.
2. Widen the base, if possible, with the adjusting lever and lock it in place when raising and lowering the client.
3. Narrow the base only for transporting in narrow places or for storage.
4. Attach the shortest strap to the shoulder portion of a one-piece sling and the longer straps to the hip area, as shown in Figure 65-8. When using a two-piece sling, attach the chain to the seat section and hook the back section into the first, second, or third link of the chain, thus forming a seat with the two straps as shown in Figure 65-1. If possible, the client's arms should be outside this back section.
5. *Always* insert all hooks with the open end turned away from the client, to avoid injury and the possibility of having the hooks slip out of place during the transfer process.
6. *Always* lock the wheels before raising and lowering a client.
7. To raise the hydraulic jack, pump it steadily, stabilizing the lift by holding the steering handle. Lower it slowly and steadily to avoid sudden jolts and allow time to position the client carefully.
8. As the lift is raised and lowered, observe how the client's position changes in relationship to the mast and boom; protect the client from being injured by the boom or swivel bar.
9. Hold the client's legs or knees to guide and stabilize during the move. A free-swinging movement can be quite frightening and can cause the lift to imbalance.

After the transfer is complete, leave the sling in place under the client when it would be difficult to replace it, such as when a weak, paralyzed, or obese person is sitting in a chair. When left in place, be sure there are no wrinkles to cause undue pressure. Remove the sling when it can be replaced readily, such as when a client has been transferred to a flat surface (bed or stretcher) or when the client has enough strength to lift himself or herself in a chair.

RECORDING

Documentation includes data about the ability of the client to assist with the transfer; the number of people required to accomplish the transfer; any special devices or techniques used, such as a mechanical client lifter or roller bars; and the reaction of the client to the transfer. Documentation of transfers between a bed and stretcher includes information about the area of the hospital or treatment procedure to which a client is going or from which the client is returning. Other recorded data would relate to the specific reason for transferring to and from a stretcher, such as

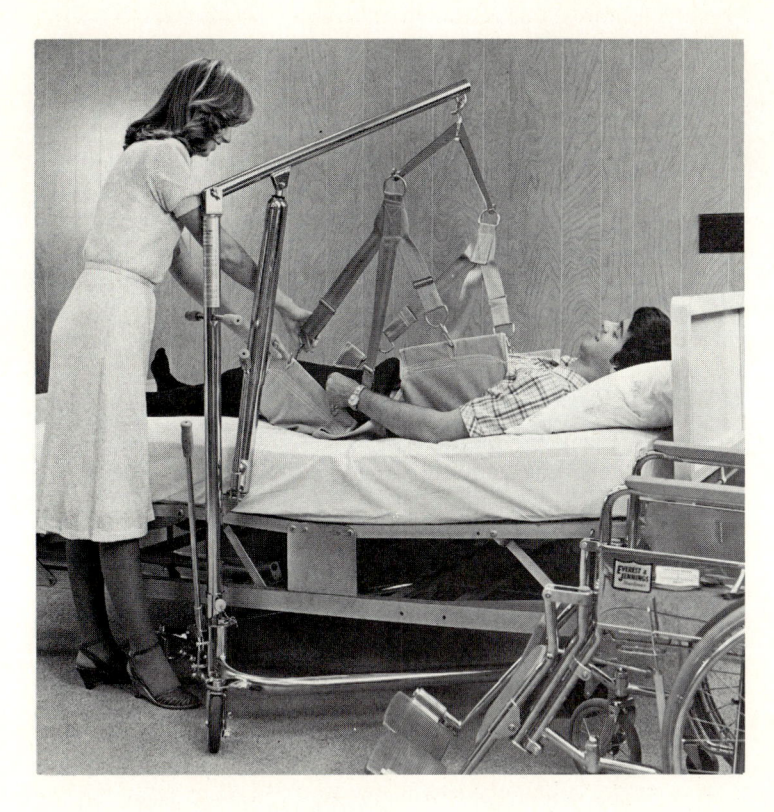

Figure 65-8. Hoyer Patient Lifter with one-piece sling. Note S-hooks turned away from client. (Courtesy, Ted Hoyer and Company, Inc. OshKosh, WI.)

documentation of postoperative status for a client returning from surgery.

Sample POR Recording

- S—"I don't feel scared anymore when you use this lift!"
- O—Relaxed, joking while being transferred to chair via Hoyer Lift. Able to hold onto straps today.
- A—Has adapted well to Hoyer Lift transfer.
- P—Continue use of lift on regular basis.

Sample Narrative Recording

Relaxed and joking when transferred to chair this AM, using Hoyer Lift. Able to hold onto straps today. States "I don't feel scared anymore when you use this lift!" Has adapted well to lift.

☐ CRITICAL POINTS SUMMARY

1. Evaluate a client's ability to assist with a bed-to-chair transfer.
2. Use adequate assistance and plan a transfer in advance to avoid injury to the client and the nurse and to use time and energy more effectively.
3. Arrange the furniture in the room to accommodate needed equipment and personnel.
4. Encourage clients to do as much of the transfer as possible or as is permitted.
5. Stabilize a bed, wheelchair, and stretcher by setting the brakes; or have an assistant hold the equipment in place during the transfer.
6. When transferring a client between a bed and a chair:
   a. Position the chair so the client can assist with the transfer without becoming entangled in any attached tubings.
   b. Have both nurse and client use a broad, forward-backward stance.
   c. Have nurse brace client's knees and feet with own feet.
   d. Coach client with each step.
7. Support a seated client to provide equal distribution of pressure and to avoid slouching.
8. Transfer between a bed and stretcher by pulling and lifting in unison on a prearranged signal.
9. When using the three-person transfer, hold the client close to own chests and use large leg muscles for lifting and lowering the client.
10. During a transfer with a mechanical lift, stabilize the client to avoid a free-swinging motion.

☐ LEARNING ACTIVITIES

1. In a central service area, learning laboratory, or a rehabilitation, orthopedic, or geriatric clinical area, examine a mechanical lift, such as the Hoyer Lift. Identify all working parts. Practice moving a peer from the bed to a chair with the mechanical lifter, using adequate assistance and supervision. Identify own feelings of safety or insecurity with using the mechanical lift or being transferred with this device.

754 PROFESSIONAL CLINICAL NURSING SKILLS

2. In a simulated setting:
   a. Assist someone to move from the bed to a chair and back again. Role play having a weakened right side.
   b. Assist someone to move from the bed to a stretcher and back again, using a pull sheet or a roller bar. Role play having a weakened left side.
   c. Compare experiences and identify teaching points for the person who is being transferred.
3. In a laboratory or clinical setting, examine a wheelchair. Apply and remove the brakes; remove and replace the leg supports and arms (if relevant); and fold and unfold the chair. Practice wheeling yourself in the chair and push a peer in the chair, preferably up and down a ramp. Identify own sense of safety when being pushed, and any concerns you may have about pushing someone else.

REVIEW QUESTIONS

1. What type of clients need assistance with transferring from a bed to a chair or stretcher?
2. How would you determine the number of persons required to help with a transfer?
3. How would you determine a client's ability to assist with a transfer between a bed and chair?
4. Explain the reason for these actions when transferring clients between a bed and chair:
   a. Nurse braces the client's knees and feet.
   b. Both nurse and client use a forward-backward stance.
   c. Nurse coaches client with each step of transfer.
5. Match the type of client situation in Column I to the correct placement of a chair in Column II.

COLUMN I
___ Client with right-sided weakness, transferring from a bed to a chair
___ Client with left-sided weakness, transferring from a chair to a bed

COLUMN II
A. Chair on left side of bed, facing foot of bed
B. Chair on left side of bed, facing head of bed
C. Chair on right side of bed, facing foot of bed
D. Chair on right side of bed, facing head of bed

6. For each of the following circumstances, identify how you would support a client who is seated in a chair. Explain the rationale for each answer.
   a. Chair too low for thighs to rest on the chair seat.
   b. Chair seat too deep for hips to reach the back of the chair.
   c. Elbows do not reach the chair arms.
   d. Feet do not reach the floor.
   e. Client tilts to one side in the chair.
7. Explain the position and task of each nurse during a bed-to-stretcher transfer when using a:
   a. Pull sheet
   b. Roller bar
   c. Three-person transfer
8. Explain the reason for these actions when using a mechanical lift to transfer a client:
   a. Attaching the hooks so they turn away from the client.
   b. Broadening the base of the lift when raising and lowering the client.
   c. Steadying the client by holding his or her legs during the transfer.
9. What are the primary sources of injury for the client and nurse during transfer activities?

PERFORMANCE CHECKLISTS

OBJECTIVE: To transfer a client between a bed and a chair safely.

CHARACTERISTIC	RANGE OF ACCEPTABILITY	SATISFACTORY	UNSATISFACTORY
1. Washes hands.	No deviation		
2. Explains procedure to client.	No deviation		
3. Provides privacy.	No deviation		
4. Places bed in low position.	No deviation		
5. Places chair beside bed at a slight angle.	No deviation		
6. Provides adequate clothing, shoes, or slippers.	No deviation		
7. Positions tubings so they will not interfere.	No deviation		
8. Assists client to dangle and stand.	No deviation		

(continued)

CHARACTERISTIC	RANGE OF ACCEPTABILITY	SATISFACTORY	UNSATISFACTORY
9. Braces client's knees and feet with own knees and feet.	No deviation		
10. Simultaneously: a. Client pivots and turns. b. Nurse pivots and turns. c. Nurse continues to brace client's knees and feet.	No deviation No deviation No deviation		
11. Instructs client to move back to front edge of chair.	No deviation		
12. Assists client to sit down: a. Client grasps chair arm. b. Nurse flexes own knees and hips to lower client to chair.	No deviation No deviation		
13. Positions client in chair to avoid slouching.	No deviation		
14. Covers knees with blanket or sheet.	Omit if not needed for warmth or privacy.		
15. Places call signal within reach.	Omit if remaining in room entire time client is in chair.		
16. Documents in health record.	No deviation		

OBJECTIVE: To transfer a client between a bed and a stretcher, using a pullsheet, roller bar, or a three-person transfer.

CHARACTERISTIC	RANGE OF ACCEPTABILITY	SATISFACTORY	UNSATISFACTORY
1. Washes hand.	No deviation		
2. Explains procedure.	No deviation		
3. Provides privacy.	No deviation		
4. Rearranges furniture to accommodate stretcher.	No deviation		
5. Raises bed to same height as stretcher.	No deviation		
A. Pull Sheet Transfer			
(1) Places pull sheet under client.	No deviation		
(2) Moves client to near side of bed.	No deviation		
(3) Places stretcher parallel to and adjacent to bed.	No deviation		
(4) Fills space between bed and stretcher with folded blanket or towel.	No deviation		
(5) Locks wheels on bed and stretcher.	Use two additional assistants to hold bed and stretcher together.		
(6) First nurse kneels on bed in forward-backward kneeling stance and grasps pull sheet.	No deviation		
(7) Second and third nurses stand beside stretcher and reach across to grasp pull sheet.	No deviation		
(8) Designates nurse on bed as leader.	No deviation		
(9) On prearranged signal, pull and lift client onto stretcher.	No deviation		
(10) Positions client for comfort.	No deviation		
(11) Raises side rails and secures safety strap.	No deviation		

(continued)

OBJECTIVE: To transfer a client between a bed and a stretcher, using a pullsheet, roller bar, or a three-person transfer (cont.).

CHARACTERISTIC	RANGE OF ACCEPTABILITY	SATISFACTORY	UNSATISFACTORY
B. Roller Bar Transfer			
(1) Places pull sheet under client.	No deviation		
(2) First nurse turns client on side away from stretcher placement.	No deviation		
(3) Second nurse positions roller bar under client to include hip and shoulder area.	Include head if using a long roller bar.		
(4) First nurse lowers client onto roller bar.	No deviation		
(5) Second and third nurses place stretcher adjacent and parallel to bed.	No deviation		
(6) Fills space between bed and stretcher with folded towels or blanket.	No deviation		
(7) Locks wheels on bed and stretcher.	Uses two additional assistants to hold bed and stretcher together.		
(8) Designates nurse beside stretcher and at client's hip area as leader.	No deviation		
(9) Holds pull sheet taut and on prearranged signal and in unison, pulls client across roller bar to stretcher.	No deviation		
(10) Removes roller bar.	No deviation		
(11) Positions client for comfort.	No deviation		
(12) Raises side rails and secures safety strap.	No deviation		
C. Three-Person Transfer			
(1) Places stretcher at right angles to bed.	Place in a convenient place away from bed.		
(2) Locks wheels.	Place bed against wall or have fourth nurse hold stretcher in place.		
(3) Positions nurses at bedside: a. Tallest at client's head and shortest at client's feet. b. Strongest at male client's shoulders and head.	No deviation Strongest nurse supports female client's hip area.		
(4) Designates strongest nurse as leader.	No deviation		
(5) Moves client to near side of bed.	No deviation		
(6) Assumes flexed, forward–backward stance.	No deviation		
(7) Inserts arms completely under client's body.	No deviation		
(8) Nurses' arms touch other nurses' arms.	No deviation		
(9) Leader calls "turn"; nurses roll client toward own chests; elbows remain on bed.	Alternate call: "one."		
(10) Leader calls "lift"; nurses stand.	Alternate call: "two."		
(11) Leader calls "pivot"; nurses step back, turn, and walk toward stretcher in unison.	Alternate call: "three."		
(12) Leader calls "ready"; nurses assume a flexed forward–backward stance and lower elbows to stretcher edge.	Alternate call: "four."		
(13) Leader calls "down"; nurses lower client to stretcher by straightening knees and lowering forearms to stretcher.	Alternate call: "five."		
(14) Positions client for comfort.	No deviation		
(15) Raises side rails and secures safety belt.	No deviation		
(16) Documents transfer, destination, and time in health record.	No deviation		

REFERENCES

Long BC, Buergin PS: The pivot transfer. American Journal of Nursing 77(6):980–982, 1977.

Norton D: Breakdown of pressure areas. Nursing Times 20(13):399–401, 1964.

Peterson MJ, Adkins HV: Measurement and redistribution of excessive pressures during wheelchair sitting. Physical Therapy 62(7):990–994, 1982.

BIBLIOGRAPHY

Ford JR, Duckworth B: Moving a dependent patient safely, comfortably: Part 1—Positioning. Nursing76 6(1):27–36, 1976.

Jordan HS, Kavchak MA: Transfer techniques. Nursing73 3(3):19–22, 1973.

Klabak L: Getting a grip on the transfer belt technique. Nursing78 78(2):10; 1978.

Kozier B, Erb G: Techniques in Clinical Nursing. Menlo Park, CA, Addison-Wesley, 1982.

Lewis LuVW: Fundamental Skills in Patient Care, ed 3. Philadelphia, JB Lippincott, 1984.

Nursing74 Staff: How to negotiate the ups and downs, ins and outs of body alignment. Nursing74 4(10):46–51, 1974.

Rambo BJ, Wood LA: Nursing Skills for Clinical Practice. Philadelphia, WB Saunders, 1982.

Rantz MF, Courtial D: Lifting, Moving, and Transferring Patients, ed 2. St Louis, CV Mosby, 1981.

Sorensen KC, Luckmann J: Basic Nursing: A Psychophysiologic Approach. Philadelphia, WB Saunders, 1979.

Talbot D: Techniques of Therapeutic Positioning: A Guide to Nursing Action. Minneapolis, MN, Sister Kenny Institute, 1978.

SUGGESTED READING

Jordan HS, Kavchak MA: Transfer techniques. Nursing73 3(3):19–22, 1973.

Long BC, Buergin PS: The pivot transfer. American Journal of Nursing 77(6):980–982, 1977.

AUDIOVISUAL RESOURCES

Independent Bed Transfer
  Videorecording.
    Available through:
      Dalhousie University
      A-V Division, Faculty of Medicine
      W. K. Kellogg Health Science Library
      Halifax, Nova Scotia, Canada

Independent Transfers and Basic Functional Activities
  Videorecording. (1976, Color, 30 min.)
    Available through:
      AudioVisual Concepts
      1525 East 53rd Street
      Chicago, IL 60615

Moving In and Out of Your Wheelchair
  Film (16 mm). (1969, Color, 5 min.)
    Available through:
      National Audiovisual Center
      Order Section E-Q
      Washington, DC 20409

Transfer Activities and Ambulation
  Filmstrip with cassette. (1978, Color, 23 min.)

The Use of Stretchers
  Filmstrip with cassette. (1979, Color, 14 min.)

The Use of Wheelchairs
  Filmstrip with cassette. (1979, Color, 10 min.)

Use of Patient Lifters
  Filmstrip and cassette.
    Available through:
      Medcom, Inc.
      PO Box 116
      Garden Grove, CA 92642

SKILL 66 Bed Making Procedures

PREREQUISITE SKILL

Skill 28, "Handwashing"
Chapter 14, "Introduction"

☐ STUDENT OBJECTIVES

1. Describe the various ways in which a bed may be made.
2. Indicate the type of bed making required to meet various client needs.
3. Describe the techniques used to handle clean and soiled linen.
4. Describe ways to maintain client and nurse safety during bed making.
5. Demonstrate the ability to make a bed in different ways.

☐ INTRODUCTION

Bed making refers to the application or changing of bed linens. It is a commonly used skill that every nurse is able to execute efficiently and teach and supervise ancillary personnel and family members to perform. Bed making is a skill that is an integral part of nursing care provided in direct-care settings and the home. It is done to ensure that a client's environment in bed is clean and comfortable. A clean, wrinkle-free bed prevents skin problems and infections that might result from wrinkles, lumps, moisture, and debris that accumulate on bed linen. A clean wrinkle-free bed enhances a client's psychological comfort as well as physical comfort and promotes a sense of well-being. There are many different ways of making beds; the method used depends on the type of bed and the particular needs of the client.

☐ PREPARATION

Although clients who are ill spend a great deal of time in bed, most are able to get out of bed at least once a day to have the bed made. This not only reduces the amount of work for the nurse but may conserve the client's energy; it also provides an opportunity to increase the client's activity level. Normally a client has the linen changed once a day after bathing. There are situations in which a client may need to have the bed linen changed either partially or completely more than once a day. In addition, the linen often needs to be tightened to remove wrinkles and lumps and to have accumulated crumbs and lint brushed away to keep the client comfortable.

TYPES OF BEDS

The contemporary standard hospital bed is a modification of the manually operated gatch bed which was designed with cranks and screws to permit elevation of the client's head and knees. Most of the beds in use today are operated electrically and permit lowering and raising the height of the bed in addition to changing the position of the head or knees. The controls are attached to the side of the bed and are operated by either push buttons or a sliding lever; they may be operated by the nurse or the client to select different positions for comfort or therapeutic purposes. Various positions used for comfort and therapeutic purposes are described in Skill 64. The electric controls on some beds may be locked in place to maintain a permanent position or to prevent the bed from being placed in an undesired position. Activation of the electric controls that change the high-low position on most bed models requires direct and constant contact with the control button or lever for movement to occur. Some models have a "walk-away" control that allows the bed to continue to raise or lower itself after the control is activated; this type of bed should not be used with children, senile, heavily sedated, mentally retarded and psychiatric clients. At least three persons have been crushed to death under this type of bed because the down control was activated while they were under the bed. In the event that this type of bed is accidentally used for inappropriate clients, the switch can be changed within a few minutes or the bed can be kept unplugged when someone is not in attendance at the bedside.

Electric beds also have hand cranks for manual control. There usually are three manual hand cranks; one to raise the head of the bed, another for the foot, and a third to raise the height of the bed; these controls are located at the foot of the bed. The hand cranks are pulled out for use and then retracted to prevent people from bumping into them. Operating a bed manually takes physical effort, so the nurse needs to be conscious of maintaining good body alignment and using body mechanics to prevent back strain. Hospital-type beds are often used in the home and may be rented or purchased from health-care supply vendors in most communities. All hospital-type beds have locks on the wheels in the form of levers that are activated by stepping on them. The wheels must be locked at all times when a bed is in use to prevent it from rolling when a client is getting in or out and when the nurse is making it.

Side rails are safety devices attached to the sides of the bed to protect the client and prevent falls. They are available in full or half lengths and are attached to most hospital beds used in health-care facilities. They have special buttons or levers to permit them to be raised or lowered. Side rails are often used by clients to grasp hold of when changing position or getting out of or into bed. In addition to side rails, other attachments commonly used with beds include bed boards, intravenous poles, overbed frames such as the balkan frame and trapeze shown in Figure 62–1, and various types of traction with weights that are used to keep bones in alignment while healing occurs. These devices do not interfere with bed making, but the nurse sometimes needs to modify the way in which the bed is made when they are in use. For example, to avoid adding weight to a leg that is in traction and taking the risk of interfering with the proper alignment of the leg, the top linen may either be tucked under the mattress only on the side not in traction or it may merely be draped over the leg not in traction. A folded sheet may be used to cover the upper part of the client.

Specially designed sheets should always be used with special beds such as the CircOlectric beds and Stryker or Foster turning frames. Sheets designed for the posterior frame or mattress have openings that permit the client to use the bed pan. The standard size hospital sheet often is too large to use on the narrow frames and mattresses of special beds because they are narrower than the hospital bed mattress. The special-sized sheets are preferable to folded standard sheets, as multiple layers of folded linen produce wrinkles that create skin problems and discomfort.

TYPES OF BED MAKING

Several names are used to refer to different ways to make a bed; these names usually describe how the bed appears after it is made as well as the purpose to be achieved by the method used. The way in which a bed is made for a particular client depends on the client's condition and the agency's policy. Beds made without the client in them are referred to as unoccupied beds. This category of bed making includes the open, closed, and anesthesia (surgical) bed. Beds that are made with the client in them are referred to as occupied beds.

Unoccupied Bed
An unoccupied bed may be made *open,* with the top sheet, blanket, and bedspread folded back to the foot of the bed in preparation for the client to enter it easily, or it may be made *closed* with the top linen drawn up to the head of the bed under the pillows in a manner similar to that used in the home. Closed beds are usually made by housekeeping personnel after a client is discharged and the client unit is cleaned and prepared for the next admission. This type of bed also may be used for clients who are in short- or long-term care facilities in which the clients are ambulatory or where the focus is on self-care.

An *anesthesia bed,* also referred to as a surgical, postoperative, or recovery bed, is an open bed made in preparation for the client returning from surgery or a diagnostic procedure for which anesthesia was administered. It is often made for clients on regular clinical units. In addition, it is made routinely in recovery rooms and intensive care units. With this bed, the top linens are folded back to one side to permit easy transfer of the client from a stretcher or another bed.

Occupied Bed
An *occupied* bed is one that is made with the client in it. Making this type of bed often requires that the client move to one side of the bed while the other side is made. However, an occupied bed may be made from the head to the foot instead of from one side to the other.

HANDLING LINENS

Reusable cotton linens are most commonly used in health-care facilities, although disposable tissue fiber-laminate bed linens are available. Reusable linen usually is laundered by a commercial laundry and delivered to the facility. The strong detergents used by these laundries may be irritating to some clients' skin. In each health-care facility clean linen is distributed daily to clinical units on a specially designed large linen cart. During transit from the central linen room the open sides of the linen cart are covered with a clean canopy to prevent contamination from airborne organisms in the environment. Clean linens are always removed from the linen cart with freshly washed hands. In the interests of economizing on the linen inventory and to avoid the ever-present potential for contaminating linens at the client's bedside, only those linens that are to be used at one time are taken to the client's bedside. Once linens are placed in a client's room they cannot be returned to the linen cart because they are considered contaminated.

Soiled linen is handled as little as possible and with a minimum of agitation to prevent contamination of others and of the air in the immediate environment. Contamination occurs from the dispersion of potentially infectious microorganisms shed from the client; these microorganisms are showered upon others and into the air when soiled linen is vigorously removed from the client and the bed. The nurse's uniform also becomes contaminated by transfer of microorganisms when soiled linen is held close to the body.

In a study to evaluate the number of living microorganisms and inanimate particles shed during bed making and stripping in a nursing home facility, Litsky (1971) compared two types of bed linens: reusable cotton and the disposable tissue fiber-laminate. She found making beds with clean reusable linen yielded $2\frac{1}{2}$ times the number of viable bacteria in the air counts than did the disposable linen. Similarly, she found $7\frac{1}{2}$ times the number of viable bacteria during bed stripping of reusable linen than with the disposable linen. The results of this study provide the basis for the author's conclusion that bed making and bed stripping are dirty activities. Litsky presents the following recommendations for bed making (p. 56):

1. Ambulatory clients should leave the room while the bed is stripped and made.
2. Assign a two-person team to bed making: one person wearing a protective gown to prevent contamination of the uniform assumes responsibility for stripping all of the beds; the second person handles the clean linen and makes all of the beds.
3. Carry clean linen into the room immediately before making the bed and do not store it in any place not intended for linen storage.
4. Place soiled linen in a linen bag immediately upon removal from the bed; remove it from the room and place in the appropriate area on the unit for soiled linen.
5. Wash hands immediately before and after making each bed.

In addition to these recommendations, Litsky suggests that it may be appropriate to have personnel and clients wear masks to prevent cross-infection caused by airborne organisms (p. 56). Nurses will find few if any health-care facilities with bed making policies that specifically include implementation of Litsky's recommendations. The results of the study and her recommendations should make all nursing personnel more aware of the importance of using good aseptic techniques while bed making. Safe practices used for the disposal of linen from an isolation unit are presented in Skill 29.

DATA BASE

Client History and Recorded Data

Prior to making a client's bed the nurse needs to know the activity level permitted for the client to determine whether an occupied or unoccupied bed is to be made. This information usually is available on the nursing kardex but the nurse may need to verify that the information is current. In addition, the nurse assesses the client's energy level because a person who is not required to be on bed rest for therapeutic purposes may be either too fatigued or too weak to get out of bed at the time the bed is to be made. The nurse also needs to be aware of any limitations a bed-rest client might have on movement of the total body or a body part in the bed; for example, a client with an immobilized extremity, in traction, must have the leg kept in alignment as well as maintaining the traction and weight on the leg. Or a client with cardiopulmonary disease may be unable to tolerate lying flat in bed. Special precautions often need to be observed during bed making when moving clients who have extensive dressings or burns as well as those who are experiencing a great deal of pain. These precautions may include working with an assistant or handling the extremity with special care. Clients in pain may need an analgesic administered before moving about to have the bed made. Apart from knowing whether an occupied or unoccupied bed is to be made, the nurse also finds out if the client is scheduled for a procedure that would require the preparation of an anesthesia bed.

EQUIPMENT

The equipment used for bed making varies with the type of bed being made and with agency policy. Many facilities use a *mattress pad* that is sized to cover the entire top surface of the mattress. In many direct-care facilities, mattresses are covered with a plastic fabric to protect the mattress. A mattress pad often is placed over the mattress before the sheet is applied. A mattress pad is made of heavy cotton-flannel fabric and may have ties or elastic bands that attach it to the mattress. Pads to protect the mattress are also used with regular beds in the home. Mattress pads are used over a plastic mattress cover to protect the client from discomfort that is apt to result from the body heat radiated to and held by the plastic cover. Heat accumulates because it cannot be dissipated readily from the dorsal side of the client by conduction or radiation and the client begins to perspire in an effort to dissipate the heat. The pad also helps to anchor the bottom sheet in place and reduces some of the wrinkling by providing some friction for the sheet. *Plastic or rubber drawsheets* are usually about 90 cm (36 in) wide and sufficiently long to tuck under each side of the mattress and be anchored in place securely. They are used to protect either the bottom sheet or the mattress from soiling.

Flat *sheets* made of cotton fabric are commonly used in health-care facilities for both the top and bottom sheet, but the use of fitted sheets is becoming more common. Special sheets designed with holes are used for mattresses and frames on special beds such as CircOlectric, Foster, and Stryker frames. *Drawsheets* are about 90 cm (36 in) wide and are used to protect the bottom bed sheet from soiling; they are also used with a plastic mattress cover (in lieu of a mattress pad) to protect the client from the heat retention caused by the plastic cover. Drawsheets may be devised by folding a regular bed sheet in half lengthwise. *Blankets* normally are made of cotton or a synthetic blend. There are generally two types of blankets available in most health-care facilities: the cotton bath blanket which is very lightweight and a heavier type, often of a loosely woven fabric, that helps to trap warm air close to the client. Bath blankets often are used to make the bed of those clients who have difficulty keeping warm. When used for this purpose, one blanket is usually placed directly over the bottom bed sheet and a second is placed under the top sheet so that the blanket is in direct contact with the client. *Pillowcases* also are made of cotton; they are available in different sizes suitable for small, medium, and standard pillows. *Bedspreads* used in health-care facilities are often made of cotton or a synthetic blend; colored spreads are becoming more common.

☐ EXECUTION

A client's bed usually is made after the client bathes; in most health-care facilities bed making, like bathing, is scheduled as part of the morning work. When staffing level or the type of nursing personnel organization permit, bed making may be performed when it is most convenient for the client. Consider the best way to organize the work involved in the nursing care for all aspects of client care to conserve the nurse's energy as well as that of the client. Conserve energy by planning the work sequence in terms of the number of occupied and unoccupied beds that need to be made after evaluating each client's condition, energy level, and ability to help. The use of good body mechanics is essential to prevent back strain. Good body mechanics for bed making include: maintaining a wide-base stance, advancing one foot in front of the other, keeping the back straight and the knees and hips slightly flexed, facing the direction in which one is working, and raising the bed to working height. These maneuvers keep the center of gravity within the base of support established by the wide stance. It is also important to set the abdominal and gluteal muscles and use the large muscles of the leg rather than the small muscles of the arms and shoulders when turning the client and lifting the mattress. This avoids back strain and shear force on the spine and keeps the center of gravity within the base of support established by the wide stance. When folding linen or blankets, hold the upper extremities near the body rather than having them stretched out in front of the body, taking care not to bring the item in contact with the clothing. Outstretched extremities combined with the weight of the item act on the center of rotation at the shoulder joint and increase the torque exerted (Flitter, 1976, p. 44). Contact of the linen with the clothing transfers microorganisms from the item to the clothing or from the clothing to the linen. Establishing a pattern of working smoothly and rhythmically helps to reduce muscle tension and is less fatiguing.

It is possible to individualize each client's care and make the physical aspects of the work less demanding by planning the sequence of activities in collaboration with the client and in accord with the client's physical abilities. For example, the client may be too tired to get out of bed immediately after bathing but may be able to do so after a brief rest. Postponing making the bed until the client has a rest period and is able to get up reduces the amount of time needed to make the bed, and also conserves the nurse's physical energy. In addition, it often requires less energy and stress for a client to get out of bed than to move around in bed and over the rolled or folded linens. Keep in mind that both clients on bed rest and those who are able to get up are frequently debilitated, weak, have little energy, and may also be in pain. Singly or in combination, these conditions can result in a client becoming exhausted easily after bathing. Even with the nurse doing all of the work, the energy required for bed making may exceed the reserve the client has at the time. A rest period after bathing and prior to moving about the bed or getting out of bed may be a welcome relief. Clients with pain may need to have an analgesic administered before they can comfortably tolerate the activity involved in bathing or having their bed made. It is important to monitor the client's comfort, stamina, and tolerance for activity before and during bed making. Bed making also may be postponed after bathing for clients who will leave the room for scheduled diagnostic tests, surgical procedures, or therapeutic services, such as physical therapy.

In addition to using good body mechanics to protect yourself from injury, it is important to provide for client safety through the appropriate use of side rails. Side rails prevent clients from falling out of the bed and also serve as a reminder not to get out of bed without assistance. The policy in most health-care facilities requires that side rails always be raised when the bed is in the elevated position. Sometimes a client's condition is cause for keeping the side rails up even when the bed is in the low position. When making an occupied bed, raise the side rail on the side opposite from which you are working; this provides for client safety and also gives the client something to hold onto when shifting and turning in bed. It is also important to keep the call signal within the client's reach at all times when a nurse is not present at the bedside.

MAKING THE BED

Removing all rings and the wristwatch before making a bed is a safe practice that helps to prevent injuries and scratches that might occur from getting them caught on the bedsprings. If rings and watches are worn while beds are made it is important to lift the mattress high enough for the hand to reach safely under the mattress without getting caught on the springs. Lifting the mattress high enough for safe entry of the hand is not always easy to do, particularly when making a bed with a heavy client in it. Holding the hand with the palm turned downward while tucking the linen under the mattress protects the nails from tears that might result from getting them caught on the bed frame.

In preparation for making the bed, lock the bed wheels to prevent rolling and determine all of the supplies needed. To do this inspect the bed and look for supplies that might be available in the bedside stand. It is also a wise practice to look for and remove personal belongings before stripping the linen to avoid losing the personal possessions in the laundry. Be aware of whether the client is scheduled for surgery, as that would require making an anesthesia bed (described below). Some health-care facilities have a policy that sheets, drawsheets, and pillowcases are changed daily, while others may leave the decision of what linen to change up to the nurse. Linen that is visibly soiled or damp from perspiration must be changed. Linen may be conserved by using the unsoiled top sheet as the bottom sheet or folding it for use as a drawsheet. When this is done fold the linen when you remove it from the bed and place it over the back of a chair so that it is available for later use.

There are basically two ways in which a bed may be made. With one method the foundation, consisting of the bottom sheet and drawsheet, is made by making a mitered corner at the head of the bed and then tucking the sheet and drawsheet under the mattress on one side and then moving to do the same thing on the opposite side of the bed. The top linen is applied in the same manner, moving from one side of the bed to the other before making the mitered corners at the foot with all layers of the linen. This method may be easier for the novice nurse to learn, although it is not the most efficient in terms of energy conservation. An alternative and more efficient method is to make only one side of the foundation and then to apply each layer of the top linen on that same side, fan-folding it lengthwise back to the center of the mattress. Then make the mitered corner with all the layers of linen at the foot of the bed on that side. Then all layers of the second side are made. There is more than one acceptable way to make a mitered corner.

When making an occupied bed, make a pleat with the top layers of linen to allow room for the client to move the feet freely. A toe pleat may be made either vertically or horizontally.

SKILL SEQUENCES

MAKING AN UNOCCUPIED BED

Step	Rationale
1. Wash hands.	Prevents transfer of microorganisms.
2. Obtain clean linen and linen bag or hamper.	Prevents delays and interruptions.
3. Raise bed to working height and lower side rails.	Reduces effort and prevents back strain.
4. Place a chair near foot of bed with back toward bed.	Provides place for folded linen that will be reused.
5. To remove linen:	
a. Place linen bag or hamper at bedside.	Prevents transfer of microorganisms. Reduces unnecessary movement.
b. Start at head of bed and loosen all linen from mattress while moving around bed.	Prepares linen to be folded or rolled and avoids risk of tearing linen. Avoids back strain from reaching across bed.
c. Slide pillows out from pillowcases while pillows are on the bed. Fold or roll pillowcases and place in linen bag or hamper. Place pillows on chair at bedside.	Avoids transfer of microorganisms from linen to chair.
d. Grasp center top edge of spread with both hands and pull it to bottom of bed. Grasp center of folded spread and lift from bed. Place it over the back of chair if it is to be reused. Roll soiled spread and place in linen bag if soiled.	Avoids vigorous movement of linen and dispersion of microorganisms. Prevents linen from falling to floor.
e. Remove blanket, top and bottom sheet in same manner as spread. Place soiled linen in laundry bag or hamper.	Prepares linen for reuse. Prevents linen from falling to floor and prevents dispersion of microorganisms.
6. Grasp lugs on side of mattress or push against foot of mattress to move it up to head of bed.	Mattresses slide down toward foot of bed when head of bed is elevated.
7. Wash hands.	Prevents transfer of microorganisms from soiled to clean linen.
8. Move to side of bed where clean linen is placed.	Conserves energy.
9. Smooth mattress pad (if there is one) with palms of hands to remove wrinkles. Place unfolded bottom sheet on lower half of mattress and determine if sheet is folded lengthwise or crosswise.	Prevents unnecessary wrinkles.
10. Place center fold of sheet on appropriate half of bed and unfold sheet toward head and foot of bed. As shown in Figure 66–1A and B, move sheet so bottom hem is even with lower edge of mattress; do not tuck under mattress.	Provides for adequate amount of sheet to be tucked under the head and secures sheet in place.
11. Use one hand to lift mattress on near side at head of bed, use other hand to tuck excess sheet under head of mattress. Pull sheet taut and smooth out wrinkles.	Anchors sheet in preparation for making a mitered corner.
12. To make a mitered corner, as shown in Figure 66–2 A, B, and C:	A mitered corner provides a more secure anchoring for linen because it conforms to shape of mattress. Use of good body mechanics prevents back strain.
a. Stand facing head of bed; use one hand to lift lower edge of sheet so that it forms a triangle with edge of mattress. Use other hand to tuck lower portion of sheet securely under mattress.	
b. Place free hand at upper edge of mattress and base of triangle to hold sheet against mattress.	Holds sheet in place.
c. Bring triangular portion of sheet down firmly over hand, remove hand and tuck mitered corner under mattress.	
13. Tuck all of remaining sheet under mattress on near side of bed, moving from head to foot of bed. (NOTE: At this point top layers of linen may be placed sequentially on bed so that one side of bed may be completely made at one time. Fan-fold top layers back to center of bed to allow access to bottom sheet on opposite side of bed. Unfold each layer of linen, smooth wrinkles before tucking linen under foot of mattress and before making mitered corner.)	Making one side at a time conserves energy and time.
14. Place center fold of drawsheet at center of midsection of bed, unfold sheet across bed and tuck it under mattress.	Places sheet in proper location under client's hips.
15. Make other side of bed in same manner. Gather excess sheet in both hands and pull it taut before tucking it in as shown in Figure 66–3.	Removes wrinkles.

(continued)

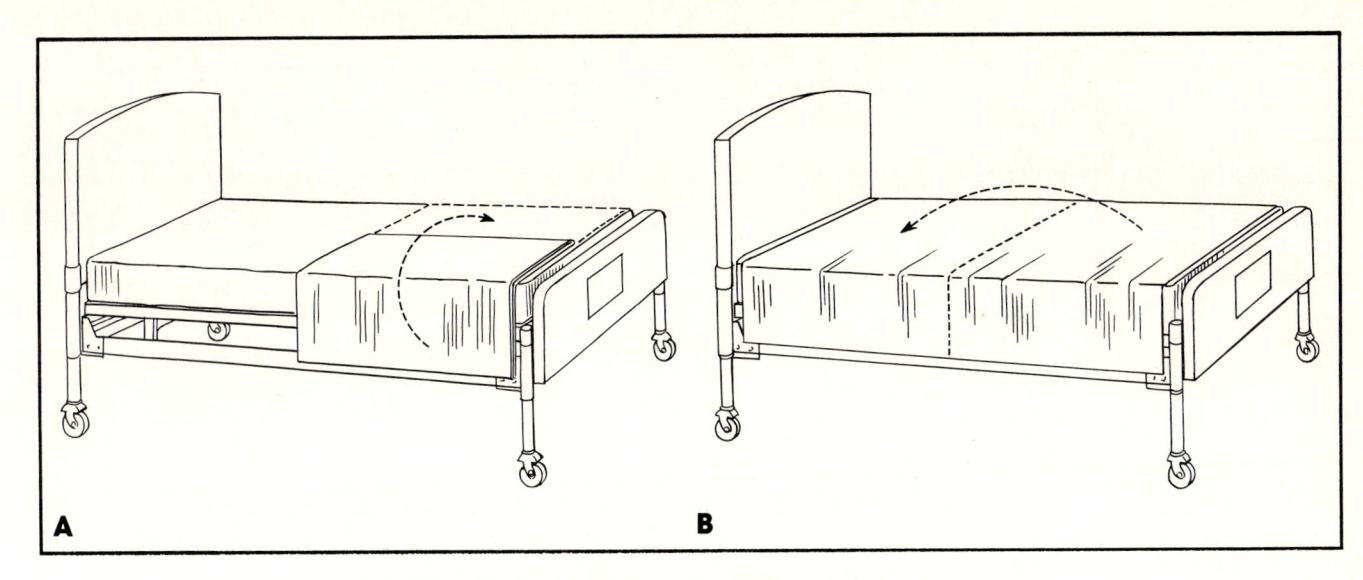

Figure 66–1. A. and **B.** Placing a clean bottom sheet on the mattress

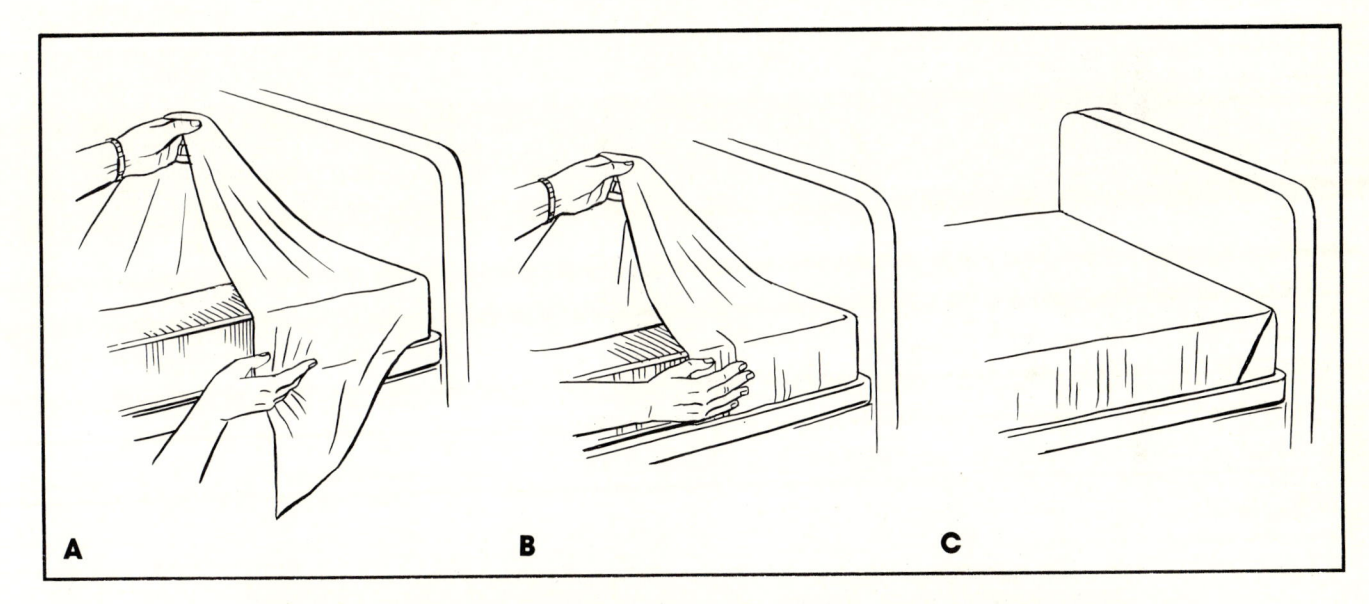

Figure 66–2. A, B, C. Making a mitered corner involves forming a triangle by folding the top portion of the sheet upward toward the bed and then tucking the lower portion under the mattress. The triangle is brought over the edge of the bed and tucked under the mattress.

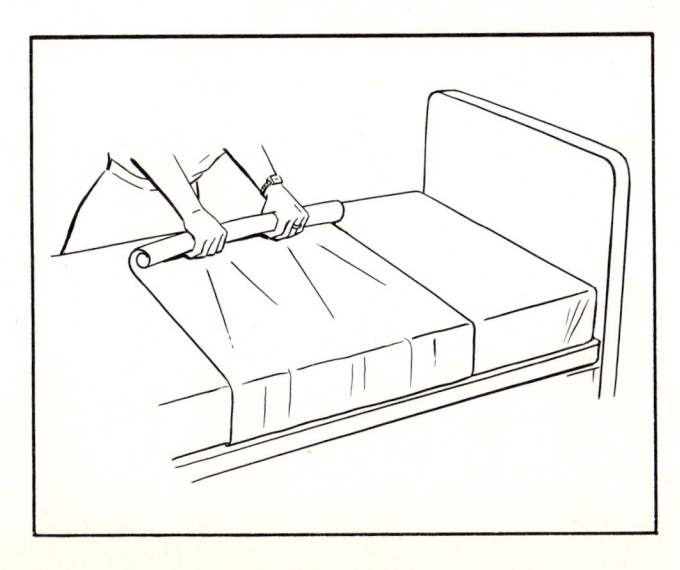

Figure 66–3. Pulling the drawsheet taut after it is anchored on one side of the bed.

MAKING AN UNOCCUPIED BED (Cont.)

Step	Rationale
16. Place top sheet at head of bed with hem at edge of mattress and center fold in middle of bed. Unfold sheet toward foot of bed, then out to sides. Position sheet with top edge at head of bed.	Provides for ample sheet to be available for tucking under foot of mattress.
17. Place blanket and bedspread over top sheet about 5 cm (2 in) below edge of sheet, unfolding it in same manner used in step 16.	Allows sheet to be cuffed over edge of blanket and spread.
18. Tuck all layers of linen under foot of mattress and then make a mitered corner on each side of bed.	Making mitered corner with all layers treated as a single unit permits making toe pleat.
19. To make a toe pleat, as shown in Figure 66-4: a. Stand at foot of bed, reach over foot frame and with both hands grasp all layers of linen as a single unit. Lift layers and fold them back about 10 cm (4 in) to create a pleat.	Allows room for feet to move freely without pressure from top covers.
20. Move to head of bed and fold top sheet back to make a cuff about 5 cm (2 in) wide.	Cuff protects edges of blanket and spread from soiling.
21. Grasp edge of cuff with both hands and fan-fold all of layers down to lower half of bed as shown in Figure 66-5. (NOTE: For a closed bed, top linen is left at head of bed.)	This "opens" bed for easy entry.
22. To dress pillows, as shown in Figure 66-6: a. Open pillow case and lay it flat on bed. b. Pick up pillow and fold it in half lengthwise. c. Use one hand to hold pillow under arm while other hand holds pillow case open. d. Insert pillow into case; flatten it and adjust pillow to fit into corners of case. (NOTE: Tuck a pleat in long side of case when case is too wide for pillow.)	Avoids shaking pillow case and eliminates need to hold case. Smooths out pillow and improves appearance. Helps to hold pillow in place in case and improves appearance.
23. Place pillows at head of bed.	
24. Lower height of bed, place signal light on bed.	Enables client to get into bed more easily.
25. Close linen bag and place it in laundry chute or other designated area.	

MAKING AN OCCUPIED BED

Step	Rationale
1. Explain procedure to client.	Allays anxiety.
2. Wash hands.	Prevents transfer of microorganisms.
3. Obtain clean linen, linen bag or hamper, place linen near client on clean surface.	Reduces unnecessary walking.
4. Close room door or cubicle curtains.	Provides privacy.
5. Position a chair near foot of bed with back toward bed.	Provides place for reusable linen.
6. Raise side rails, then bed to working height.	Provides safety for client. Prevents back strain.
7. Lower side rail on side near linen supply. Place bath blanket over client and top bed linen (or keep the top sheet over client in place of blanket while bed is made).	Provides easy access to bed. Cover client when linen is removed.
8. Reach under blanket and remove spread and top sheet as in Skill Sequence, "Making an Unoccupied Bed," steps 5d and e.	Same as Skill Sequence, "Making an Unoccupied Bed," steps 5d and e.
9. Move mattress to head of bed as in Skill Sequence, "Making an Unoccupied Bed," step 6. (NOTE: If necessary, have a helper work on opposite side or have client assist by pulling upward on head of bed.)	Same as Skill Sequence, "Making an Unoccupied Bed," step 6.
10. Turn client to opposite side of bed and reposition pillow under client's head.	Permits vacant side of bed to be made. Provides for client comfort.
11. Loosen all bottom linen from side and head of bed.	Prepares linen for removal.
12. Roll or fan-fold each layer of soiled linen as close to client's back as possible.	Positions linen for retrieval from opposite side. Forms compact fold or roll of linen for client to roll across.
13. Proceed to make one side of bed as described in Skill Sequence, "Making an Unoccupied Bed," steps 9 to 13.	Same as Skill Sequence, "Making an Unoccupied Bed," steps 9 to 13.

(continued)

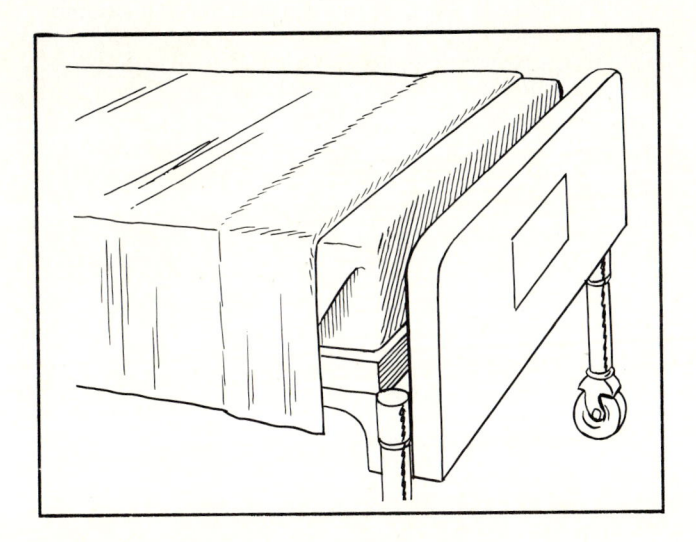

Figure 66-4. The horizontal toe pleat is a fold of all the top layers of linen made near the foot of the bed to allow room for the client to move the feet freely.

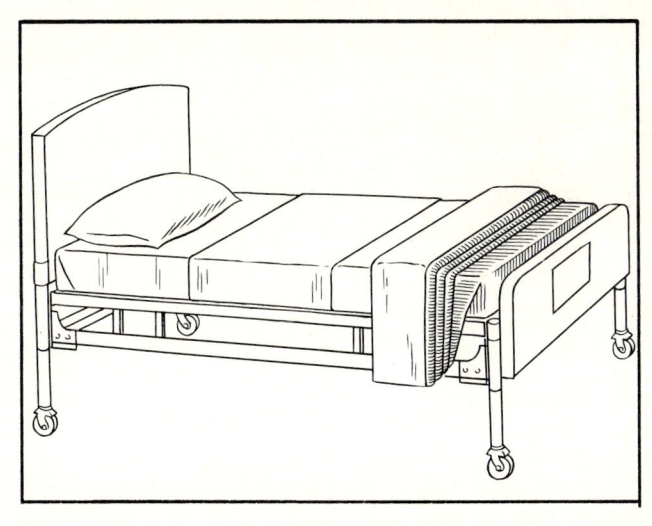

Figure 66-5. For an open bed, the top layers of linen are fanfolded back to the bottom of the bed to permit easy entry for the client.

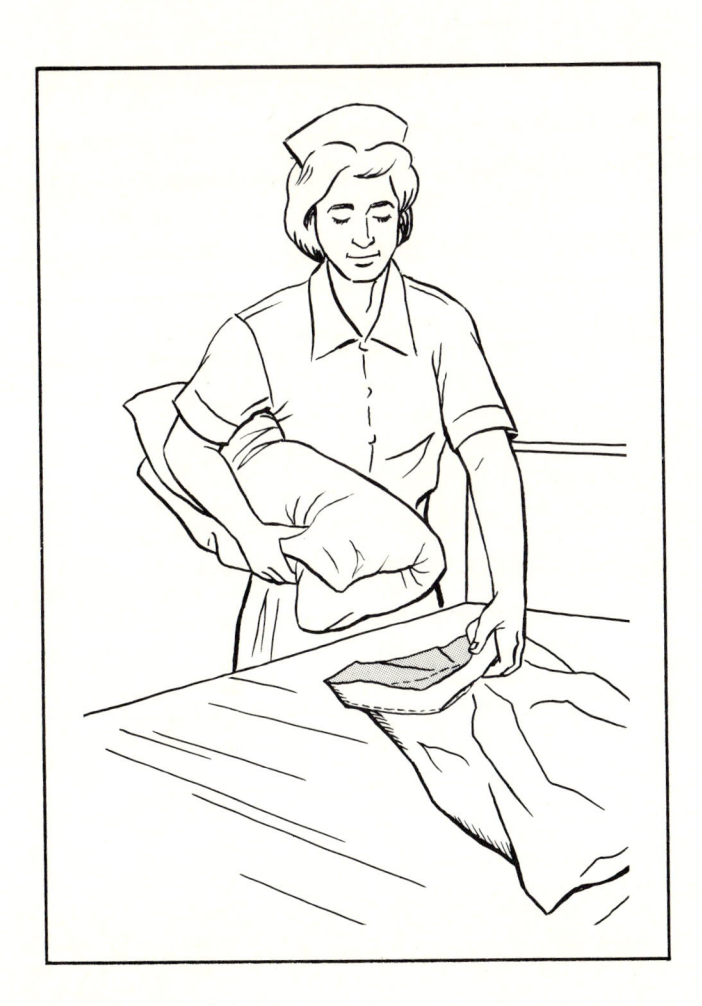

Figure 66-6. Dressing the pillow by folding it in half and inserting it into the case.

MAKING AN UNOCCUPIED BED (Cont.)

Step	Rationale
14. Raise side rail and move to opposite side of bed.	Prevents client from falling. Client can grasp rail to move and change position.
15. Lower side rail and move client over rolled linen to clean side of bed; move pillow to clean side.	Permits easy access to client and bed; permits second side of bed to be made.
16. Loosen linen from side and head of bed.	Prepares linen for removal.
17. Roll layers of soiled linen toward edge of bed, remove and place in linen bag or hamper.	Helps to contain organisms and protects clean linen. Prevents contamination from linen.
18. Smooth mattress pad; unroll clean bottom sheet and draw-sheet, pulling them toward you; smooth bottom sheet then gather it in both hands and pull it taut to remove all wrinkles. Make mitered corner and tuck in remaining sheet. Pull drawsheet taut, and tuck it under mattress.	Wrinkles are uncomfortable and create skin problems. Weight of client on sheets requires additional strength to remove all wrinkles.
19. Dress one pillow at a time as described in Skill Sequence, "Making an Unoccupied Bed," step 22, and place under client's head.	Same as Skill Sequence, "Making an Unoccupied Bed," step 22.
20. Return client to the center of bed or to a position of comfort.	Enhances client's comfort and allows nurse to position client properly and more easily before top linen is applied.
21. Apply top linen as described in Skill Sequence, "Making an Unoccupied Bed," steps 16 and 17.	Same as Skill Sequence, "Making an Unoccupied Bed," steps 16 and 17.
22. Have client hold on to top linen or tuck it around shoulders while you reach under it to remove bath blanket.	Anchors top linen in place.
23. Fold bath blanket, place in bedside stand or linen bag or hamper if soiled.	Makes available for future use or disposes of properly.
24. Tuck all layers of linen under foot of mattress; make mitered corners as in Skill Sequence "Making an Unoccupied Bed," step 18.	Same as Skill Sequence, "Making an Unoccupied Bed," step 18.
25. Make a toe pleat with top linen as in Skill Sequence, "Making an Unoccupied Bed," step 19.	Creates room for feet to move freely.
26. Raise side rail: lower height of bed; place call signal within reach of client.	
27. Tidy bedside unit, obtain clean towels and facecloth if necessary.	Provides clean environment for client.
28. Dispose of linen bag or hamper in appropriate designated area.	

Variations for Making Unoccupied and Occupied Beds

The Anesthesia Bed. The anesthesia bed is one variation of the unoccupied bed. With this bed the top linens are folded back to one side of the bed to permit easy transfer of the client into the bed. Some facilities have a specific procedure for this bed while others leave it to the nurse's discretion.

To make an anesthesia bed, make the foundation of the bed with a drawsheet as for a regular unoccupied bed. One bath blanket may be placed over the foundation and tucked in at the head and sides of the bed and a second used under the top sheet. Bath blankets provide additional warmth and absorb the increased perspiration that clients usually experience during the immediate postoperative hours when recovering from the effects of anesthesia. Place a bed protector, such as a pad, at the head of the bed to prevent the bed linen from getting soiled in the event that the client vomits or has excessive oral secretions. Leave the layers of top linens hanging over the foot and sides of the bed; then fold back the top and bottom edges of all layers to make wide cuffs. There are alternative ways to fold the top linen back to one side of the bed. One way to make the top of an anesthesia bed is to fan-fold the linen lengthwise to one side of the mattress as shown in Figure 66–7. Another way is to form four triangles with the top linen before fan-folding it to one side of the bed. To do this, bring the lower corner of the cuffed edge from both the head and foot of the bed to the horizontal and vertical center of the bed, first on one side and then the other. Fan-fold each side toward the center of the bed and then move the folded linen to one side of the bed.

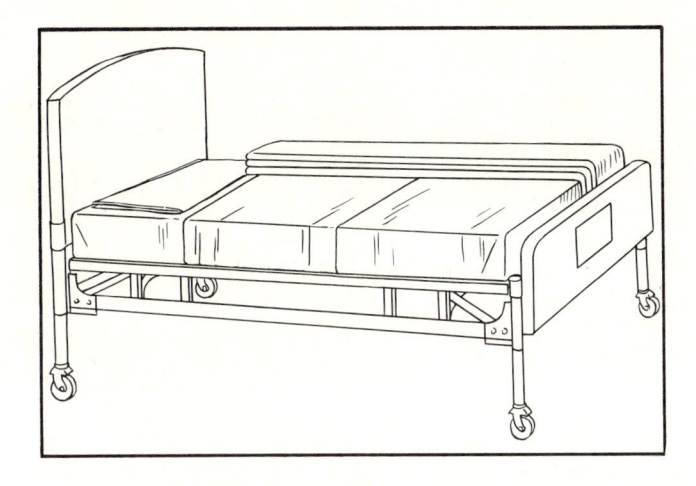

Figure 66–7. An anesthesia bed with the top covers fan-folded back to one side of the bed.

Making the Bed from Head to Foot. An occupied bed may be made by starting at the head of the bed and moving toward the foot. It is sometimes necessary or more desirable to make the bed in this manner when a client must remain in the Fowler position because of cardiopulmonary problems that interfere with respiratory or cardiac function. In addition, clients who have abdominal infections, such as peritonitis, are also required to stay in high Fowler position to promote the localization of the infection. Making a bed in this manner is usually best done with at least two persons, one working on each side of the bed. This helps to get the bed made quickly and conserve the client's energy. There are times when it is necessary for three persons to help in making the bed of a critically ill client, particularly for those who are completely helpless. To conserve the client's energy as well as the nurses', each nurse alternates roles in assisting and supporting the client to lean forward while the nurse on the opposite side is making the head of the bed. When three nurses are working together, one or two may assume the primary role of assisting or lifting the client while the others make the bed.

Begin by preparing the bottom sheet for use by opening it and folding it into quarters crosswise. Instruct the client about how the procedure will be done. Either remove the pillows or move them to one side and then loosen all of the linen. Start at the head of the bed and roll or fold the bottom sheet down from the head of the bed to a point as close to the client's buttocks as possible. Then place the upper edge of the sheet across the head of the mattress, smooth out the wrinkles as much as possible, and tuck the sheet under the top of the mattress on one side of the bed. Exchange roles, anchor the sheet under the head of the mattress on the opposite side, then pull the sheet down over the mattress close to the client's buttocks. Assist the client to turn to the side as much as possible and provide support while the other nurse pulls down and removes the soiled sheet and then pulls the clean sheet from under the buttocks and toward the foot of the bed. Smooth out the wrinkles, tighten the sheet, and make a mitered corner on one side and then the other. Apply a drawsheet or pull sheet and add the top linen to the bed in the same manner as making a standard occupied bed. Permit the client to rest if necessary between any of the bed-making steps.

RECORDING

Normally it is standard practice not to document that a client's bed has been made since it is generally assumed that this is done as often as necessary. Refusal of a client to have the bed made may be documented with the reasons for refusal. It is important to record the client's physical and psychological responses to the physical activity and exertion experienced when an occupied bed is made. This includes vital signs: pulse, respirations, and blood pressure, and the degree of fatigue or discomfort. Information concerning any special precautions required when making the bed are placed on the nursing kardex.

Sample POR Recording

- S—"Don't bother me, I don't know why you insist on changing my sheets, they were changed yesterday. I don't change my sheets every day at home. This bed isn't dirty and I'm not dirty, I washed this morning and straightened the sheets. It seems to me that you are just wasting time and energy. Go away and leave me alone."
- O—Became very agitated when the nurse wanted to change the linen and make the bed. Refused to have linen changed and bed made.
- A—Does not understand the reason why hospital linen is changed daily, feels staff is implying that she is not clean. Not comfortable in having personnel doing things for her.
- P—Change linen when soiled and explain purpose of frequent linen changes in the hospital and personnel's responsibilities in infection control.

Sample Narrative Recording:
Refused to have linen changed and bed made. Feels staff is implying she is not clean and unable to take of herself. Explained purpose of linen changes and its importance in relation to infection control. Will continue to change linen when soiled.

☐ CRITICAL POINTS SUMMARY

1. Handle all linen with aseptic technique.
2. Dispose of soiled linen promptly.
3. Determine the appropriate type of bed to be made for each client.
4. Use good body mechanics while stripping linen and making beds.
5. Determine the client's physical and psychological status prior to beginning bed making.
6. Secure adequate assistance when making occupied beds.
7. Plan activities with the client and other staff to conserve energy.
8. Lock the wheels on the bed prior to making the bed.
9. Keep the side rail raised on the side toward which the client is turned when making an occupied bed.

☐ LEARNING ACTIVITIES

1. Practice making an unoccupied bed with a drawsheet.
2. Practice making an anesthesia bed with bath blankets.
3. Practice making an occupied bed having a peer act as a client; exchange roles to experience how it feels to have a bed made while you are in it.
4. Practice making an occupied bed with a peer, using the head to foot approach. Have a second peer act the role of a totally dependent, acutely ill client who must be kept in high Fowler position at all times. Have the client (peer) share how he or she felt while the bed was being made and then have the bed makers discuss the type of problems encountered during the procedure. Develop alternative ways to make the bed and practice some of these, discussing the difference among the methods from each person's perspective.

☐ REVIEW QUESTIONS

1. Why is a clean, wrinkle-free bed important for a client's physical and psychological well-being?
2. What are the reasons for having so many different ways to make a bed?
3. How would you handle clean and soiled linen?
4. How would you explain to a peer how to make a bed with a client in it?
5. How would you explain to a peer how to make an occupied bed from the head to the foot?
6. What do you need to know about a client's status before planning how the bed will be made?

☐ PERFORMANCE CHECKLISTS

OBJECTIVE: To make an unoccupied bed using aseptic technique and good body mechanics.

CHARACTERISTIC	RANGE OF ACCEPTABILITY	SATISFACTORY	UNSATISFACTORY
1. Washes hands.	No deviation		
2. Obtains clean linen and linen bag or hamper.	No deviation		
3. Raises bed to working height, lowers side rails, places chair near foot of bed.	No deviation		
4. To remove linen: a. Places linen bag or hamper at bedside, loosens linen on all sides of bed. b. Removes pillow cases while pillows are on bed; folds or rolls pillow cases and places in linen bag or hamper. Places pillows on chair. c. Grasps center top edge of spread with both hands; pulls it to bottom of bed. Takes center of folded spread and lifts from bed. Places it over back of chair for reuse; if soiled, places in linen bag or hamper. d. Removes blanket, top and bottom sheet in same manner as spread. Discards soiled linen in laundry bag or hamper.	No deviation		

(continued)

CHARACTERISTIC	RANGE OF ACCEPTABILITY	SATISFACTORY	UNSATISFACTORY
5. Grasps lugs on side of mattress or pushes against foot of mattress to move it up to head of bed.	No deviation		
6. Washes hands.	No deviation		
7. Moves to side of bed where clean linen is placed; smooths mattress pad, places unfolded bottom sheet on lower half of mattress, determines if sheet is folded lengthwise or crosswise.	No deviation		
8. Places center fold of sheet on appropriate half of bed, unfolds sheet toward head and foot of bed, places sheet even with lower edge of mattress; does not tuck it under mattress.	No deviation		
9. Lifts the mattress on near side at head of bed with one hand, uses other hand to tuck excess sheet under head of mattress. Pulls sheet taut and smooths out wrinkles.	No deviation		
10. Makes a mitered corner: a. Stands facing head of bed; with one hand lifts lower edge of sheet to form a triangle with edge of mattress. Tucks lower portion of sheet under mattress with other hand. b. Places free hand at upper edge of mattress at base of triangle to hold sheet in place. c. Brings triangular portion of sheet down firmly over hand, removes hand and tucks mitered corner under mattress.	No deviation		
11. Tucks all of remaining sheet under mattress on this side of bed, moving from head to foot of bed.	No deviation		
12. Places the center fold of drawsheet at center of midsection of bed, unfolds sheet across bed and tucks it under mattress.	No deviation		
13. Makes other side of bed in same manner. Gathers excess sheet in both hands and pulls it taut before tucking it in.	Use alternative method of completing one side of bed at a time.		
14. Places top sheet at head of bed, hem at edge of mattress, and center fold in middle of bed. Unfolds sheet toward the foot of the bed, then out to the sides. Places the sheet at the top edge of the head of the bed.	No deviation		
15. Places the blanket and spread over the top sheet about 5 cm (2 in) below the edge of the sheet, unfolding it in the same manner as in step 14.	No deviation		
16. Tucks all layers of linen under the foot of the mattress, then makes a mitered corner on each side of the bed.	No deviation		
17. To make a toe pleat: Stands at the foot of the bed, reaches over the foot frame and with both hands grasps all layers of linen; lifts and folds them back about 10 cm (4 in) to create at toe pleat.	No deviation		

(continued)

OBJECTIVE: To make an unoccupied bed using aseptic technique and good body mechanics (cont.).

CHARACTERISTIC	RANGE OF ACCEPTABILITY	SATISFACTORY	UNSATISFACTORY
18. Moves to the head of the bed, folds top sheet back to make a cuff about 5 cm (4 in) wide. Uses both hands to grasp cuff, fan-folds linen down to the lower half of the bed.	No deviation Leave linen at head of bed for closed bed.		
19. To dress pillows: a. Opens pillow case, lays it flat on the bed. b. Picks up and folds pillow in half lengthwise; holds pillow under arm with one hand, uses other hand to hold pillow case open. c. Inserts pillow into case; flattens it and adjusts the pillow to fit into the corners.	No deviation		
20. Places pillows at head of bed, lowers height of bed, places signal light on bed.	No deviation		
21. Closes linen bag and places it in laundry chute or other designated area.	No deviation		

OBJECTIVE: To make an occupied bed using aseptic technique and good body mechanics.

CHARACTERISTIC	RANGE OF ACCEPTABILITY	SATISFACTORY	UNSATISFACTORY
1. Explains procedure to client.	No deviation		
2. Washes hands.	No deviation		
3. Obtains clean linen and linen bag or hamper.	No deviation		
4. Closes room door or cubicle curtains.	No deviation		
5. Places chair near foot of bed; raises side rails and bed to working height.	No deviation		
6. Lowers side rail on side near linen; places a bath blanket over client and top linen or keeps the top sheet over the client while bed is made.	No deviation		
7. Reaches under blanket and removes spread and top sheet.	No deviation		
8. Pushes mattress up to head of bed as in Performance Checklist, "Making an Unoccupied Bed," characteristic 5.	No deviation		
9. Turns client to opposite side of bed and repositions pillow under client's head.	No deviation		
10. Loosens all bottom linen from side and head of bed. Rolls each layer of linen close to client's back.	No deviation		
11. Proceeds to make one side of bed as in Performance Checklist, "Making an Unoccupied Bed," characteristics 7 to 11.	No deviation		
12. Places drawsheet as in Performance Checklist, "Making an Unoccupied Bed," characteristic 12, tucking it under one side.	No deviation		
13. Raises side rail and goes to opposite side of bed; lowers side rail, moves client over rolled linen to clean side of bed; shifts pillow to clean side.	No deviation		

(continued)

CHARACTERISTIC	RANGE OF ACCEPTABILITY	SATISFACTORY	UNSATISFACTORY
14. Loosens linen from side and head of bed. Rolls layers of soiled linen toward edge of bed, removes and places in linen bag or hamper.	No deviation		
15. Smoothes mattress pad; makes remaining side of bed, pulling sheets taut to remove all wrinkles.	No deviation		
16. Dresses one pillow at a time as described in Performance Checklist, "Making an Unoccupied Bed," characteristic 19.	No deviation		
17. Returns client to center of bed, positions for comfort.	No deviation		
18. Applies top linen as in Performance Checklist, "Making an Unoccupied Bed," characteristics 14 and 15. Has client hold linen around shoulders or tucks it under to remove bath blanket.	No deviation		
19. Completes making top of bed by following Performance Checklist, "Making an Unoccupied Bed," characteristics 16 and 17. Folds bath blanket, places in bedside stand or linen bag or hamper.	No deviation		
20. Raises side rail, lowers height of bed, places signal light within client's reach.	No deviation		
21. Tidies bedside unit, obtains clean towels and face cloth if necessary; disposes of linen bag or hamper in appropriate place.	No deviation		

REFERENCES

Flitter HH: An Introduction to Physics in Nursing, ed 7. St Louis, CV Mosby, 1976.

Litsky BY: Germs make trouble when nurses make beds. Modern Nursing Home 27(5):52–56, 1971.

BIBLIOGRAPHY

King EM, Weick L, et al.: Illustrated Manual of Nursing Techniques, ed 2. Philadelphia, JB Lippincott, 1981.

Kozier B, Erb G: Techniques in Clinical Nursing. Menlo Park, CA, Addison-Wesley, 1982.

Lewis LuVW: Fundamental Skills in Patient Care, ed 3. Philadelphia, JB Lippincott, 1984.

Rambo BJ, Wood LA (eds): Nursing Skills for Clinical Practice, ed 3. Philadelphia, WB Saunders, 1982, vol 1.

Sorensen KC, Luckmann J: Basic Nursing: A Psychophysiological Approach. Philadelphia, WB Saunders, 1979.

AUDIOVISUAL RESOURCES

Bedmaking
  Slides with cassette. (1976, Color, 18 min.)
    Available through:
    Media Systems Corporation
    757 3rd Avenue
    New York, NY 10017

Fundamental Skills: Making an Occupied Bed
  Videotape (½ in, ¾ in). (1978, Color, 14 min.)
Fundamental Skills: Making an Unoccupied Bed
  Videotape (½ in, ¾ in). (1978, Color, 14 min.)
    Available through:
    Indiana University School of Nursing
    NICER Department
    110 West Michigan Street
    Indianapolis, IN 46223
Hospital Beds: Variable Height
  Videorecording (¾ in). (1976, Color, 15 min.)
Making a Surgical (Postoperative) Bed
  Videorecording (¾ in). (1972, Color, 17 min.)
Making the Unoccupied (Closed) Bed
  Videorecording (¾ in). (1978, Color, 13 min.)
    Available through:
    Comprenetics, Inc.
    5805 Uplander Way
    Culver City, CA 90230
Occupied Bed Making
  Filmstrip with cassette. (1974, Color, 10 min.)
    Available through:
    Medcom, Inc.
    PO Box 116
    Garden Grove, CA 92642

15 Respiratory Care

☐ INTRODUCTION

Since oxygen cannot be stored in the body, respiration is vital to life. Nursing care directed toward the respiratory system function is an integral component of care given to clients in any setting in which the nurse practices. The goals of this care are to ensure that the client has an adequate supply of oxygen to meet the body's metabolic demands and to prevent the occurrence of pulmonary complications. To meet these goals, the nurse uses interventions that *promote, maintain,* or *restore* an individual client's respiratory function to its maximal level.

Nurses promote optimal respiratory function when working with both healthy and ill clients. Healthy people often develop the habit of shallow breathing or have poor posture that does not permit maximum ventilation. The nurse can teach these people how to improve their respiratory function by periodic deep breathing and by holding their body in better erect alignment.

Compromised respiratory function occurs in clients whose primary problems are pulmonary in nature, such as with bronchitis, pneumonia, or chronic obstructive lung disease. It also occurs when the primary problems are in body organs and systems other than the respiratory. For example, decreased physical activity and recumbent immobility lead to decreased strength in the muscles of respiration. In addition, some medications depress the respiratory center, and pain often keeps clients from breathing deeply or moving about adequately.

The nurse is involved in a variety of interventions assigned to assist ill clients with their respiratory functions. For example, the nurse often teaches deep breathing and coughing to clear secretions from the airway. Clients who are immobilized or have decreased physical activity require change in their body position to prevent pooling of pulmonary secretions that can lead to atelectasis. When clients are unable to clear their own airway of secretions effectively, the nurse may be required to suction the airway to ensure its patency. When clients have artificial airways, such as tracheostomies, the nurse is also responsible for ensuring the patency of those airways. When clients are unable to obtain an adequate supply of oxygen from the ambient air they may require a supplemental source of oxygen. It is the nurse's responsibility to administer and monitor the effects of oxygen.

In addition to implementing interventions that are specifically directed toward the respiratory system, the nurse also monitors and promotes the client's nutritional and fluid status. Adequate nutrition and fluids are needed for tissue repair, to provide enough energy for adequate respiratory function, and to minimize a client's vulnerability to infection.

The skills included in this chapter include "Chest Therapy Exercises" (Skill 67), "Oxygen Therapy" (Skill 68), "Tracheostomy Care" (Skill 69), and "Suctioning the Airway" (Skill 70).

☐ ENTRY TEST

Review the entry test for Chapter 7, items 13 to 18.

1. How many lobes are in the right and left lungs?
2. What are the anatomic positions of the right and left main bronchi?
3. What is meant by dead space in the respiratory tract?
4. What are the types of pulmonary tidal volume?
5. What does the term *ventilation* mean?
6. What are the respiratory gases?
7. How is oxygen carried in the blood?
8. What is meant by the partial pressure of oxygen?
9. What relevance does the partial pressure of oxygen with the blood have to a person's oxygenation status?
10. What is surfactant?

SKILL 67 Chest Therapy Exercises

PREREQUISITE SKILLS

Skill 19, "Inspection"
Skill 22, "Auscultation"
Skill 24, "Pulse Appraisal"
Skill 25, "Respiration Appraisal"
Skill 28, "Handwashing"
Skill 51, "Monitoring Fluid Balance"

STUDENT OBJECTIVES

1. Differentiate between the purposes of preventive and restorative respiratory exercises.
2. Describe the benefit to ventilation from periodic deep breaths.
3. Explain the normal processes by which bronchial hygiene is maintained.
4. Describe how retained secretions interfere with ventilation.
5. Indicate the characteristics of sputum.
6. Describe how to collect a sputum specimen.
7. Describe normal and abnormal breath sounds.
8. Specify where normal and abnormal sounds are best heard with a stethoscope.
9. Use the appropriate technique to auscultate for breath sounds.
10. Describe each type of preventive respiratory exercise.
11. Describe each type of restorative respiratory exercise.
12. Specify the data to be collected prior to having a client perform respiratory exercises.
13. Demonstrate the ability to teach clients how to perform preventive and restorative exercises accurately.

INTRODUCTION

The chest therapy exercises that are used to improve bronchial hygiene and prevent pulmonary complications can be classified into preventive and restorative respiratory exercises. Preventive exercises include deep breathing, the use of incentive spirometry, and coughing. Restorative exercises include diaphragmatic breathing, pursed-lip breathing, and postural drainage. Although most institutions have respiratory therapists to teach clients how to perform these exercises, many times the responsibility for reinforcing instruction and supervising the exercises are part of the nurse's role. The nurse may also be expected to provide the preliminary instruction to clients for preventive respiratory exercises. Preventive exercises are taught to clients as an integral part of nursing care and are of particular importance for clients who are immobile and those who are scheduled for abdominal and chest surgery. Restorative exercises are used most often for clients who have a chronic pulmonary disease such as emphysema.

PREPARATION

In normal respiration, inspiration is an active process and expiration a passive one. It is helpful to keep in mind that air that does not go into the lungs cannot come out. In the normal healthy person with eupneic respirations, involuntary sighs act as intermittent deep breaths and occur between five to ten times an hour. These sighs serve to open up alveoli that are not normally opened during eupnea. It is believed that this normal process results in varying tidal volumes and plays an important role in preventing alveolar collapse. When breathing patterns are altered and become shallow (without sighs) there is a gradual collapse of the alveoli within 1 hour (Shapiro et al., 1979). Alveolar collapse inhibits the oxygen and carbon dioxide exchange (alveolar ventilation) and the capillaries return unoxygenated blood to the left side of the heart. This eventually results in hypoxemia, which is a deficiency of oxygen in the arterial blood. Collapsed alveoli, a condition known as atelectasis, are often the result of monotonous shallow breathing which occurs most often in obese, geriatric, inactive, or postoperative clients. The excessive weight of an obese person restricts lung expansion and results in low inspiratory volumes. With aging the small airways begin to close at higher volumes during expiration than in the young. Inactivity, particularly in the supine position, results in shallow breathing and can result in atelectasis in a few hours. Other pulmonary complications that can result from prolonged bedrest or immobility include dependent lung edema and thromboembolitic episodes.

There are other factors that affect the quality of respiration and thus pulmonary gas exchange. Breathing patterns may become altered because of narcotic, sedative, and hypnotic drugs or anesthetics that depress the central nervous system, which in turn depresses the respiratory center. General anesthesia may irritate the mucous membranes, which respond by producing an increased amount of secretions. Oxygen therapy may also irritate or dry the mucous membranes. Anticholinergic drugs such as atropine and belladonna act to decrease the gag and swallow reflexes. This interferes with the control a person has over the normal bronchial secretions by preventing them from being swallowed.

NORMAL BRONCHIAL HYGIENE

For normal pulmonary gas exchange to occur, the tracheobronchial tree must be kept clean. The primary cleansing mechanism is through mucus-covered cilia. The continuous film of viscous and elastic mucus combines with the action of the cilia to move debris and secretions through the bronchioles and bronchi to the trachea and then to the pharynx where it is swallowed. However, a change in the properties of mucus and the cilia can occur as a result of inflammation of the pulmonary epithelium, abnormalities of the mucous and serous glands, and many diseases that involve the tracheobronchial tree. Abnormal mucus can cause the film movement to slow or stop and when the mucus film is interrupted in the large airways, secretions are retained. Any physiological stress can cause changes in the normal ciliary function. The alveoli do not have a mucous film but are lined with a fluid that is believed to become part of the mucus film in the bronchioles and bronchi (Shapiro et al., 1979).

RETAINED SECRETIONS

The potential for retained secretions exists when any physiological stress to the pulmonary system interrupts the normal bronchial cleansing mechanisms, such as the inhalation of irritants like smoke or dust or when an inflammatory process such as pneumonia occurs. Retained secretions are the most common cause of poor pulmonary function in sick people. Some of the common causes of retained secretions are dehydration, acute pulmonary disease, a foreign body in the trachea, tubes placed in the trachea, generalized muscular weakness, and an inability to use the abdominal muscles because of surgery, infection, pain, or paralysis of the lower part of the body. When secretions are retained, the inflammatory response of the pulmonary mucosa causes edema, which results in increased resistance to air flow. Additional resistance is created as the retained secretions partially plug and narrow the bronchial openings. This increased resistance leads to an increase in the work of breathing because it takes more energy to move adequate amounts of air in and out of the lungs.

Since the inflammation and plugging are not evenly distributed in the lung, there are uneven areas of air flow resistance. This results in an uneven distribution of ventilation, which leads to hypoxemia. Either minor or major degrees of retained secretions may cause an increased work of breathing and hypoxemia. Another undesirable effect of retained secretions is stasis pneumonia. When the normal secretions are blocked from movement as described previously, they provide an ideal culture medium for bacterial growth, and stasis pneumonia is a common result of this bacterial growth. It is important to keep in mind that although retained secretions are potentially hazardous for any client, they pose particularly significant hazards for clients who have either cardiopulmonary disease or a disease that limits the effectiveness of the normal processes of bronchial hygiene (Shapiro et al., 1979).

There are four important clinical indicators of retained secretions. One is an increase in the work of breathing which is manifested by subjective complaints of dyspnea and objective signs of the use of accessory muscles for respiration, tachypnea, and the client's preference for sitting up rather than lying down. Another indicator is hypoxemia, which should be suspected if the client has tachycardia, arrhythmia, and an elevated blood pressure. A third indicator is that of frequent weak, ineffective, and nonproductive cough resulting from the client's attempts to improve ventilation. These futile attempts often make the client lethargic, sweaty, and anxious. (To obtain relief from the symptoms resulting from ineffective coughing, it is not uncommon for the nonhospitalized client to use over-the-counter cough suppressant medications or to request such medication from the nurse or physician.) The fourth indicator of retained secretions includes signs of pulmonary infection. The signs for which the nurse is alert consist of any combination of the following: chills, elevated temperature, increased pulse rate, chest pain, and either the absence of breath sounds or the presence of abnormal breath sounds heard on auscultation. The abnormal breath sounds (described later in this skill) include crackles, wheezes, and bronchial breath sounds. When the nurse detects any of these clinical signs it is essential that the physician be informed immediately so that the client can have a complete pulmonary appraisal and the necessary diagnostic tests such as white blood count, chest x-ray and sputum culture. (Shapiro et al., 1979, pp. 161–162, 263–264).

SPUTUM

When retained secretions are coughed up they are then referred to as sputum. Sputum may consist of either mucus or mucopurulent matter. The characteristics and amount of sputum a client expectorates are important indicators of the respiratory status and response to therapy. Saliva can be differentiated from sputum from the lungs by attending to the sounds and actions the client used to produce the expectorant and by inspecting it carefully. Saliva may be thin, ropy, or mucoid. The *consistency* of sputum can be thin or thick, watery or viscous (sticky and adhesive). Its *color* can be either clear, white, yellow, or green depending on the type of organisms present. Blood may be present in the sputum in small amounts which will only tinge the sputum or in large amounts as frank bleeding. It is important to note the amount and the color of blood in the sputum because it can help to identify the source of the bleeding. Bright red blood comes from arteries and dark red from veins. The *volume* of sputum a client coughs up and expectorates varies with the nature of the pulmonary condition and whenever possible, it should be estimated by having the client use a sputum cup to expectorate into instead of tissues. Some clients produce only 1 to 2 tsp a day while others may produce as much as a pint. When clients produce large quantities of sputum, using a covered sputum cup provides safer control of microorganisms. The full, sealed container or soiled tissues are placed in a waterproof paper bag and disposed of with trash that will be incinerated.

Sputum Collection
Sputum specimens are collected for laboratory analysis either to identify organisms producing infections such as pneumonia or tuberculosis or for tissue cell examinations to diagnose malignancies. Therefore, it is important that the specimen be of sputum and not saliva. Normally the best quality specimens are obtained from the first sputum expectorated in the morning because the secretions accumulate during the night while the client sleeps. To collect a specimen, give the client the appropriate collection container and instruct the client to take several deep breaths, cough deeply and forcefully, and expectorate into the container. Once the specimen is obtained, cover it snugly with the lid and place it in a paper bag; then wash your hands. Complete the laboratory requisition with the client's full name, room number, and the specific test to be performed as ordered by the physician. Record a description of the specimen and that it was sent to the laboratory. Sputum specimens must be sent to the laboratory promptly once they are collected since they need to be as fresh as possible. For example, specimens for bacteriologic analysis or cytology are to be sent to the laboratory within 30 minutes of collection.

APPRAISAL OF THE RESPIRATORY SYSTEM

In addition to appraising the characteristics of a client's respiratory rate, rhythm, depth, and pattern, the nurse can auscultate the lungs with a stethoscope. This permits the nurse to obtain data about the air flow through the tracheobronchial tree and the presence of mucus or airway obstruction.

Breath Sounds
Movement of air in the tracheobronchoalveolar system creates vibrations that are perceived as sounds. The absence of normal breath sounds usually represents either obstruction in the airways or an abnormal interference with the respiratory sounds in the pleural cavity. Breath sounds may be increased with any condition that produces consolidation of lung tissue (DeGowin and DeGowin, 1981).

Breath sounds have distinctive qualities that are analyzed according to pitch, intensity, quality, and duration in relation to the inspiratory and expiratory phases. *Normal breath sounds* are classified as vesicular, bronchial, and bronchovesicular. *Vesicular sounds* are normally heard in the entire lung area except beneath the manubrium sterni and the upper interscapular region. They are soft and low-pitched and characterized by a long inspiratory phase and a short expiratory phase without separation between the phases. *Bronchial sounds* are normal only when heard over the anterior midline of the trachea. They are high-pitched, usually louder than vesicular sounds, have a harsh quality, and are characterized by an inspiratory phase that is half the duration of the expiratory phase, with a brief pause between the phases. When bronchial sounds are heard in peripheral lung tissue it is an indication that consolidation or compression of that lung tissue has occurred. These conditions enhance the transmission of sound from the bronchial tree. *Bronchovesicular sounds* are a mixture of vesicular and bronchial sounds. They are normal only when heard over the major bronchi at the sternal border of the first and second intercostal spaces. They are moderate both in pitch and intensity and have inspiratory and expiratory phases of equal duration and without a pause. If bronchovesicular sounds are heard in other parts of the lung, it is an indication that some degree of pulmonary consolidation or tissue compression is causing the sounds to be transmitted there from the bronchial tree. Figure 67–1 shows the lung areas where the normal vesicular, bronchial, and bronchovesicular sounds are heard on the anterior and posterior chest.

Abnormal breath sounds, also referred to as *adventitious sounds,* are indicative of an alteration in normal pulmonary function. There are three types of abnormal sounds: crackles, wheezes, and friction rubs. *Crackles,* known also as rales, are sounds that result either from the movement of fluid or exudate in the airways and alveoli. They are categorized as fine or coarse. *Fine crackles* are high-pitched and coarse crackles are low-pitched. The smaller the size of the affected airway, the higher the pitch of the crackles. Fine crackles are discrete and noncontinuous sounds heard on inspiration that are similar to the sounds of rubbing several strands of hair between the forefinger and thumb. *Coarse crackles* are similar in all respects to fine crackles except that the sounds are louder. Crackles that are heard *early* in the inspiratory phase are found in clients who have obstructed chronic bronchitis, emphysema, and asthma. They are usually few in number, low-pitched, and heard at both the mouth and the lung bases. These crackles are caused by a delayed recoil that allows the airway to close during the previous expiration. Crackles that are heard late in the inspiratory phase are numerous, are usually found at the base of the lungs, and occur in clients who have conditions such as congestive heart failure or fibrotic alveoli. Crackles are not cleared by coughing (DeGowin and DeGowin, 1981).

Wheezes are also known as *rhonchi.* They are produced by air moving through narrowed or partially obstructed airways. Wheezes are continuous sounds caused by airways that are reduced in size by secretions, swelling of the mucosa, foreign bodies, stenosis,

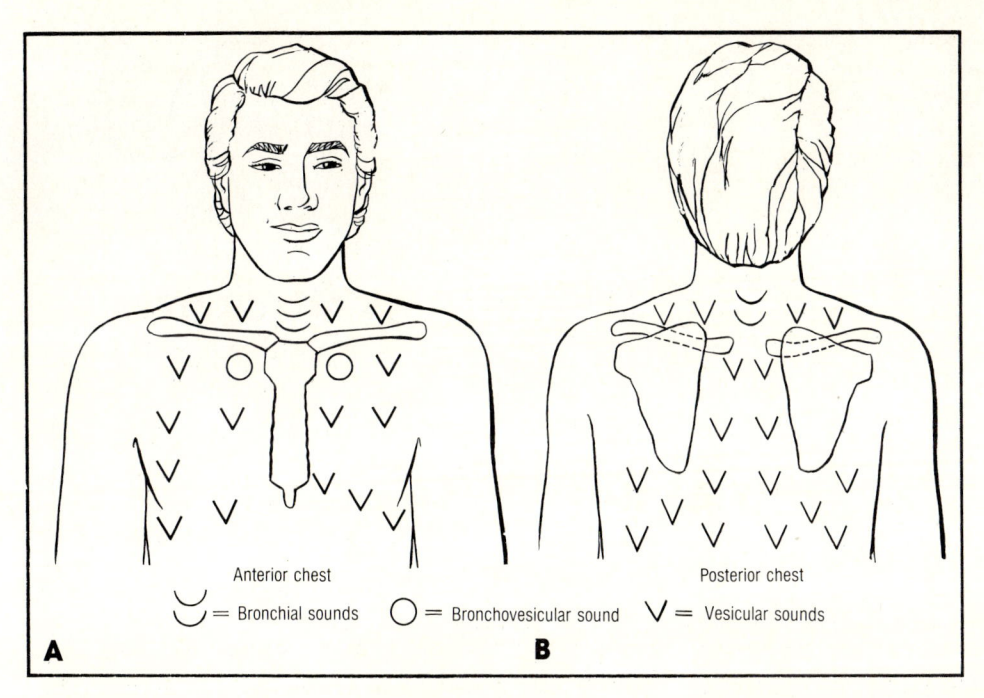

Figure 67-1. Auscultation sites for normal breath sounds. **A.** Anterior chest. **B.** Posterior chest.

a tumor, or spasms. As with crackles, the pitch depends upon the size of the airway that is involved. Wheezes may be heard both during inspiration and expiration but are more dominant on expiration. When wheezes are caused by secretions in the airways they are apt to decrease or disappear after coughing or suctioning.

Friction rubs are caused when inflamed pleural layers rub together. The sounds have a superficial creaking or grating quality that is likened to that of creaking leather. Friction rubs may be heard during both inspiration and expiration but may be limited to only inspiration. The sounds may be constant for a few respiratory cycles and then disappear for a while. They are best heard over the anterolateral chest where the greatest thoracic movement occurs. Friction rubs are not changed by coughing and may be difficult to differentiate from inspiratory crackles.

Auscultation of Breath Sounds

As with appraisal of other aspects of body functioning, practice in listening to normal breath sounds throughout the lungs helps the learner distinguish among the characteristics of normal breath sounds expected in different parts of the chest. It is also helpful to have a more experienced person validate what is heard. These activities increase confidence in listening to breath sounds and help the nurse distinguish between normal and abnormal sounds in the client-care setting.

Before beginning to auscultate for breath sounds, wash your hands, provide a private setting, and ask the person to remove all clothing from the chest area and to assume a comfortable sitting position with the head held erect and in the midline. Clothing interferes with identification of the chest landmarks and can cause adventitious sounds to be heard through the stethoscope. Use the diaphragm of the stethoscope for appraising the lungs because it covers a larger area than the bell and is suited for the frequencies of sound that will be heard.

Warm the stethoscope diaphragm with your hands and ask the person to breathe through the mouth slightly more deeply than normal. In a systematic manner, listen to all areas of the chest. First, place the diaphragm at the anterior midline of the trachea and listen for bronchial sounds. Then lift the diaphragm completely off the chest and move it to the apex of the lungs. Continue to move the stethoscope alternately from one side of the chest to the other so that comparisons can be made of the sounds heard. Figure 67-2 shows the sequence and sites used on the anterior and posterior chest for auscultation.

PREVENTIVE RESPIRATORY EXERCISES

Deep breathing and coughing are two of the most common methods a nurse uses to prevent clients from having pulmonary complications. These interventions are important because they are the least expensive means available and can help clients avoid the increased costs of medical care and extended hospital stay. Incentive spirometry, a mechanical aid that helps clients to take deep breaths, is becoming more commonly used in the clinical setting. However, as with other adjunct services it is an additional expense to the client.

Deep Breathing

During normal inspiration, the upper chest rises slightly as the diaphragm, the principal muscle of inspiration, contracts and descends; the abdomen rises and protrudes slightly and the lower ribs flare outward as the lower thorax expands. During normal ex-

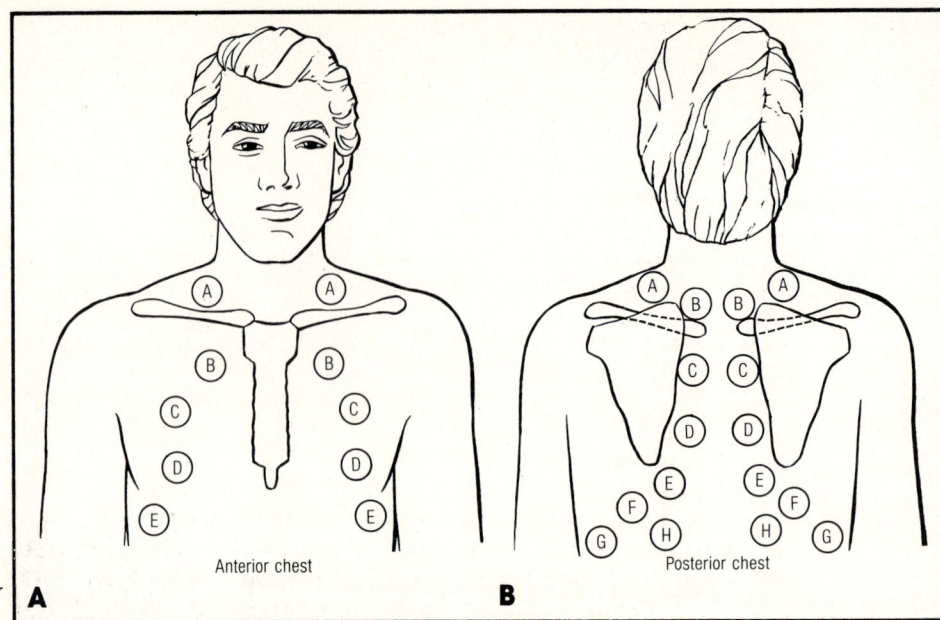

Figure 67-2. Sequence and sites used for auscultation of breath sounds. A. Anterior chest. B. Posterior chest.

piration, the abdomen and ribs move slightly inward as the diaphragm relaxes and ascends.

Deep breathing is a conscious, slow, deliberate inspiration that requires full chest expansion. For a deep breath to be effective in prevention of atelectasis, the inspiratory phase must be sustained for three seconds. Deep breathing has many benefits; it enhances maximum alveolar inflation, helps to maintain normal lung capacity, loosens secretions prior to coughing, improves venous return to the heart, facilitates muscle relaxation, and helps to control anxiety that occurs with shortness of breath. It is also believed that deep breathing helps to stimulate the production of surfactant, a "detergentlike" substance that reduces the surface tension of the fluid that lines the alveolar epithelium. Without a continuous production and secretion of surfactant, normal alveolar function is significantly impaired.

Incentive Spirometry

When a client is unable to sustain deep inspirations effectively enough to prevent the pulmonary complications that result from shallow respirations, the physician may order that the client use an incentive spirometer. This device encourages the client to take sustained maximal inspirations by presenting some type of visible goal for him or her to achieve when inspiring through the device. Incentive spirometry produces increased lung volume by generating a high pressure within the lung tissue that would be attained by the client if he or she were able to take a sustained deep breath voluntarily.

Coughing

Coughing is an important protective mechanism for the lungs because it is a natural method of removing substances from the lower respiratory tract. A cough is a reflex that may be initiated voluntarily or activated by irritation of the respiratory tract either by secretions or inhaled foreign elements such as smoke, fluid, or food. A cough consists of a series of five coordinated sequential movements. It begins with a deep inspiration which is followed by a pause and then the epiglottis and vocal cords close, trapping the air in the lungs. Intraabdominal pressure increases, pushing the diaphragm up and decreasing the volume of the thoracic cavity. As the diaphragm is forced upward, the intercostal muscles simultaneously resist the chest wall expansion and as a result the intrathoracic pressure increases. The trapped air in a nonexpanding cavity causes an increase in the alveolar pressure and the epiglottis opens to release a high velocity air flow from the lungs. For a cough to be effective, secretions must be mobilized by a high velocity air flow (Shapiro et al., 1979, pp. 158–159). Since coughing compresses and deflates the alveoli, reduces lung volume, increases the pleural pressure, and reduces the venous return to the heart it is encouraged only when the client has noisy respirations that suggest retention of secretions (Harper, 1981).

RESTORATIVE BREATHING EXERCISES

Diaphragmatic Breathing

Although diaphragmatic breathing is the normal manner of breathing, clients who have chronic obstructive lung disease (COLD) overuse the muscles in the upper chest and pull in the abdomen during inspiration, thus making it difficult for the diaphragm to descend. The reduction of elasticity in the lung that is associated with COLD prolongs expiration and the terminal and respiratory bronchioles tend to collapse and trap air within them. When a great deal of air is trapped, the diaphragm becomes flattened and less effective in increasing the vertical dimension of the thorax.

Clients with obstructive lung disease need to be taught how to improve the efficiency of their breathing by increasing their use of the diaphragm and decreasing the use of the accessory muscles of respiration. Diaphragmatic breathing increases ventilation of the lower lobes by reexpanding the alveoli, preventing abnormal alveolar closure and reducing alveolar overinflation. Diaphragmatic breathing also assists in the removal of secretions by preventing the secretions from pooling within the alveoli. It improves the efficiency of breathing by distributing ventilation more evenly throughout the lung tissue, reduces the work of breathing, and coordinates the breathing patterns by reducing the use of the accessory muscles. Diaphragmatic breathing improves a client's tolerance for physical activity. It also enables him or her to exert some control of breathing when dyspnea occurs and this helps to reduce anxiety and panic (Harper, 1981).

Pursed Lip Breathing
Pursed lip breathing is actually a method used to control expiration. With pursed lip expiration, the lips are partially closed, as with a whistle, to create a resistance for the outflow of air. This helps delay closure of the airway by keeping the bronchial pressure increased, which in turn increases the tidal volume. The airways remain open longer, resulting in less air trapped in the alveoli. Prolonged expiration also slows the respiratory rate and helps to distribute air in the lungs more evenly. Pursed lip expiration makes a soft blowing sound. Clients with chronic obstructive lung disease are taught how to breathe in this manner because the diseased airways tend to collapse and trap air during expiration.

Postural Drainage
Postural drainage is used to reduce airway resistance and minimize the client's potential for developing infection from retained secretions and obstruction of the airways. This type of treatment is often necessary because coughing alone may be ineffective; it is most frequently used in combination with coughing. During a treatment, twelve different body positions, with the client facing upwards and downwards, are used to treat all segments of both lungs. This is necessary because various parts of the lung are directed anteriorly, laterally, and posteriorly. The specific positions used for any one client depend on the lung areas that need to be drained. The physician usually prescribes the lung areas that require treatment.

Postural drainage should be done *only* by skilled personnel; in most institutions it is performed either by a respiratory or physical therapist. Situations in which the nurse may be required to perform postural drainage include pediatric clients or adult clients who are in intensive care units. When learning postural drainage techniques, it is important that the nurse be taught by a skilled clinician and be properly supervised while gaining the necessary skill. Even when not performing postural drainage, the nurse must be aware of the following important points when clients are receiving this form of treatment: (a) Postural drainage is done at least 1½ to 2 hours after meals to avoid nausea and vomiting. (b) A complete treatment in which all segments of the lungs are treated takes about 1 hour. This can be very fatiguing to the client and may inhibit the ability to cough or be physically active after therapy. (c) Sputum production may be delayed from ½ to 1 hour following the treatment. This occurs because it is theorized that postural drainage, percussion, and vibration move secretions from the small to the large airways where they can then be coughed up and expectorated (Traver, 1982, p. 125). Physical activity following a treatment facilitates continued movement of the secretions and enhances sputum production. (d) Clients who become excessively fatigued from a complete treatment may need to have shorter sessions in which different parts of the lungs are treated at one time so that they will be able to move about after the treatment and realize the maximum benefits of the therapy. (e) In addition to monitoring the client's fatigue level, the nurse is also responsible for monitoring changes in the client's condition over time to determine positive or adverse responses to therapy.

Percussion and Vibration. During the time a client is in each of the positions used for postural drainage, the physical therapy techniques of percussion and vibration are frequently used over the lung area that requires treatment so as to aid in dislodging the secretions. *Percussion* is a series of rapid rhythmic gentle blows to the client's skin that is performed with cupped hands. The hands create an air pocket that transmits vibrations to the lung tissue being treated. *Vibration* is a more gentle maneuver than percussion and is used over each area immediately following percussion, but only during exhalation. Vibration is believed to increase the velocity and movement of exhaled air, thereby helping to move secretions.

DATA BASE

Client History and Recorded Data
There are several types of data that the nurse collects in preparation for providing chest therapy to a client so that an appropriate goal of care can be established. It is important to know if the client has either a previous history of, or an existing acute or chronic pulmonary disease such as pneumonia, bronchitis, asthma, or emphysema, and to know if the client has a nonproductive or productive cough, and the nature of any sputum. Diseases or conditions such as muscular weakness, paralysis, and pain further compromise the respiratory function because they interfere with the movement of muscles used in respiration. Any medications a client receives that alter the normal processes of respiration must also be considered in relation to the client's current respiratory function. It is also im-

portant to know if a client is scheduled for surgery or has had surgery in the recent past because of the effect that anesthesia and immobility have on respiratory function. Other factors to consider include the client's age, weight, and level of consciousness; these factors affect the quality of respirations in well people and are even more significant in illness.

The nurse also reviews the health record to determine if the client has any symptoms of retained secretions such as an increase in temperature, pulse, respiratory rate, and blood pressure; for example, an elevated temperature may be indicative of a pulmonary infection. The health record also includes results of the physician's examination of the lungs and reveals the presence or absence of retained secretions or obstruction.

Physical Appraisal Skills

Inspection. The client's respiratory rate, rhythm, depth, and pattern, and the use of accessory muscles are inspected at rest. Note any changes related to activity as well as any evidence of inadequate gas exchange such as an anxious facial expression, a decrease in the level of mental alertness, and the presence of cyanosis around the mouth, lips, nose, and in the ear lobes. It is significant to note if the client prefers a sitting position to facilitate respiration. Since dehydration increases the potential for retained secretions, the nurse looks for the signs indicative of dehydration such as decreased urinary output, dry mucous membranes, loss of skin turgor, and thirst. Inspection is used to detect the characteristics of any expectorated secretions.

Auscultation. The quality of breath sounds during inspiration and expiration may be listened to with and without the use of a stethoscope. A stethoscope should be used whenever there is a suspicion of retained secretions or an obstruction in the airway. Systematic auscultation of all of the lung areas permits the nurse to detect the presence or absence of normal breath sounds. This information provides the nurse with some basis for evaluating the effects of either preventive or restorative breathing exercises. When abnormal sounds are heard, they should be reevaluated by auscultating after the client coughs to determine if they are eliminated by coughing; this helps to identify the type of abnormal sounds.

EQUIPMENT

The equipment required for chest therapy depends on the type of treatment the client is receiving. All clients need to have a supply of tissues at the bedside and a paper bag taped to the bedside table for the proper disposal of sputum.

Incentive Spirometers

Incentive spirometers are designed on the basis of normal physiological principles of respiratory function and generally provide an inspiratory volume between 500 to 2500 ml. There are two main types of incentive spirometers; those that measure the amount of client effort in flow and those that measure it in volume. Some models are lightweight and can be hand held while others must be placed on the bedside table. Many are inexpensive and disposable. Those that are not completely disposable have disposable parts that can be discarded to prevent cross-contamination between clients and the other parts can be sterilized. Other features of incentive spirometers that are found on some models and not others include an adjustable flow/volume rate, a locking device that prevents the client from changing the preset goal, a setting that allows for application of resistance during expiration to keep the alveoli inflated during expiration, and complete portability without a need for an electrical power source. Figure 67-3 shows one type of incentive spirometer.

Pillows

Pillows are used to support the client in a position that facilitates respiration, deep breathing, and coughing.

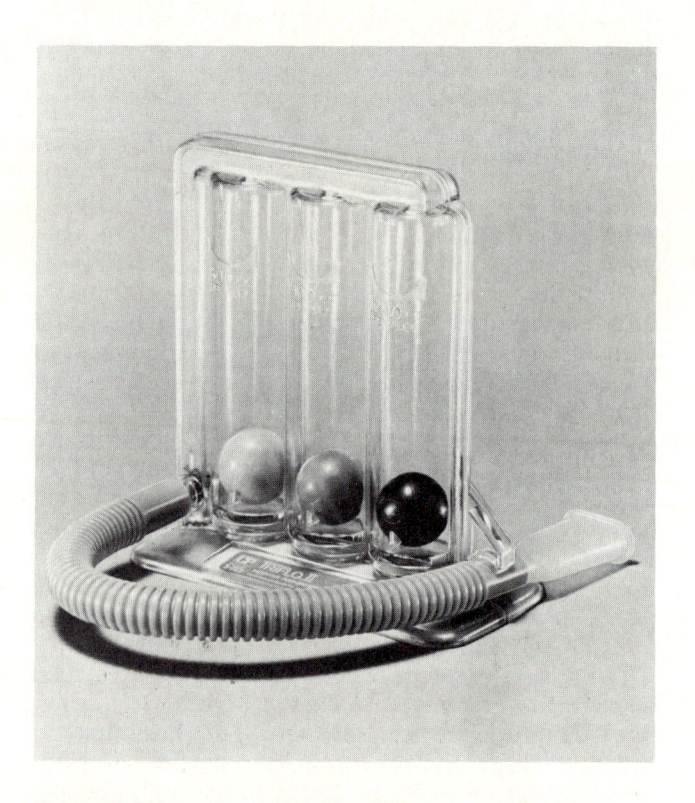

Figure 67-3. Incentive Spirometer. This device allows the client to perform sustained maximum inspiration and provides a visible goal through the use of light-weight balls that rise in response to the client's inspiration. (Courtesy of Cheseborough-Pond's, Inc. Greenwich, CT 06830.)

☐ EXECUTION

Since respiratory exercises can only be done by the client, it is essential to establish a good rapport with that client prior to teaching or supervising the exercises. A sense of confidence in the competence of the nurse helps the client perform the exercises. Confidence is promoted by explanations of the goals that are to be achieved and by helping the client to understand why the exercises are important to recovery or improvement. Doing the exercise with the client helps him or her to see what is expected.

Avoid doing chest therapy exercises during or near mealtimes because they may precipitate nausea or vomiting. Whenever possible, remove all uncomfortable or restrictive clothing to prevent interference with the movement of the thorax and abdomen. Ideally, a client is first instructed in how to perform preventive breathing exercises before the onset of pulmonary complications or surgery in order to be able to perform them at a maximum level without interference from drugs or pain. This permits the nurse to establish a baseline of data about the client's ability which can then be used later to evaluate performance after surgery. When a client is in pain, administer analgesic medication sufficiently in advance of the exercise so that pain does not prevent the client from deep breathing or coughing in an effective manner. Pain from a surgical incision can also be minimized during breathing or coughing by placing one or both hands gently but firmly over the surgical dressing or by having the client support the incision with both hands or hold a pillow in place over the incision.

DEEP BREATHING

To instruct a client in how to deep breathe effectively, place the client in a comfortable sitting position whenever possible since this promotes full expansion of the chest. First, have the client cough to clear the airway of any secretions. Then place your flat hand over the lower border of the sternum and have the client take a slow, controlled, deep inspiration and note the elevation of your hand as the chest expands. Have the client hold the breath while you count off three seconds; one-one thousand, two-one thousand, three-one thousand. Then have the client exhale slowly. Have the client place his or her own hand over the lower border of the sternum and repeat the exercise so the client can observe and feel the difference between deep breathing and normal breathing. The physician may prescribe five to ten deep breaths for each exercise session or the number may be left to the nurse's descretion. The client's pulmonary condition and fatigue level at the time of each session will help determine the number of deep breaths taken. Deep breathing exercise sessions are usually performed between two and four times a day; in the morning, before meals, and at bedtime. However, postoperative clients should perform the exercises at least every hour for the first 24 hours after surgery. During the second 24-hour period the exercises may be performed every 2 hours unless the client's respiratory status is compromised, in which case the hourly exercises must be continued.

INCENTIVE SPIROMETRY

In hospitals with respiratory therapists it is usually the therapist that sets the goal for the client (based on the physician's order) and evaluates the client's respiratory function. The nurse may be responsible for reinforcing the therapist's teaching and for supervising the client's use of the spirometer. Prior to instructing a client in the use of the spirometer, find out if the client is to use the device for inspiration alone or for both inspiration and expiration and familiarize yourself with the model to be used.

To use the device for inspiration, instruct the client to exhale slowly and completely, place the lips tightly over the mouthpiece, inhale only through the mouth and mouthpiece, and hold the inspiration as long as needed to gain the reward provided by the spirometer. Remove the mouthpiece and have the client exhale into the room. Instruct the client to take about five normal breaths between each use of the spirometer, then repeat the exercise. Limit the use of the spirometer to four to five breaths per minute to prevent hyperventilation. The spirometer may need to be used as often as 10 to 15 times per hour around the clock for 1 to 3 days postsurgery. Validate the frequency of use with the physician or therapist. After the first few days, the frequency of use may be decreased. Make sure that the client understands how often it is to be used.

The parts of the spirometer that come in contact with the client need to be sterilized or changed at least every 48 hours to prevent growth of organisms and other parts should be kept dust free with a plastic cover (Rarey, 1981, p. 147).

COUGHING

The effectiveness of a cough depends upon the amount of air inhaled, a tight closure of the epiglottis, and a rapid forceful expulsion of air. The effectiveness can be judged by a cough's sound; an effective cough is deep and hollow and produces sputum if any is present, while an ineffective cough is weak and high-pitched and does not result in expectoration (Harper, 1981). It is important to teach a client how to cough effectively. Although it seems simple, it is an intervention that too often is slighted. Body position, comfort, timing, and muscle contraction are critical components of an effective cough. High velocity air flow is essential for a maximal forced expiratory cough. A client should be requested and assisted to cough when there is evidence that retained secretions are present. It may be necessary to have the client cough as often as every 1 to 2 hours.

SKILL SEQUENCE

COUGHING

Step	Rationale
1. Explain procedure to client.	Enlists cooperation.
2. Close door and cubicle curtains.	Provides privacy.
3. Position client on side of bed with legs dangling and arms supported, or elevate bed-rest client to a semi-Fowler's position with head flexed, supported with a pillow, arms and knees slightly flexed. Have client rotate shoulders slightly inward. (NOTE: Place a pillow over abdominal incision.)	Allows full expansion of the chest. Promotes relaxation. Provides support during cough.
4. Instruct client to take 2 to 3 slow slightly deep breaths; then to take an additional breath with the mouth partially open, holding the breath for a count of one.	Lungs should feel half full of air.
5. Have client lean forward to contract the abdominal, thigh, and buttock muscles for a count of two.	Increases abdominal pressure.
6. Have client cough forcefully twice.	First cough raises secretions and second expels them.
7. Have client expectorate into tissue.	Controls dispersion of microorganisms.
8. Let client relax for a few minutes before attempting to cough again.	Helps client to remobilize efforts for effective cough.
9. Dispose of tissue in paper bag.	Controls dispersion of microorganisms.
10. Return client to a comfortable position.	Facilitates rest after coughing.
11. Wash hands.	Prevents cross-contamination.
12. Record client's ability to cough effectively, degree of assistance required, fatigue level after coughing, and a description of the sputum.	Adds to data base, promotes accountability.

PURSED LIP BREATHING

Place the client in a semi-Fowler's position with the knees slightly flexed to relax the abdominal muscles. Instruct the client to exhale through the mouth with the lips in a whistling or kissing position. It is sometimes helpful to have the client whistle or to imagine blowing out a candle when learning the shape for the lips. Once a client learns how to use pursed lip breathing, it should be used all of the time.

DIAPHRAGMATIC BREATHING

Since diaphragmatic breathing is used most often for clients who have chronic pulmonary disease and have developed the habit of using the accessory muscles during respiration, it is important that clients learn how to relax these accessory muscles while retraining their breathing pattern. During the exercises, observe the client for forced and prolonged expiration and encourage the client to avoid those actions because they cause shortness of breath and gasping. Help the client to concentrate on breathing slowly without the use of accessory muscles because this inhibits the downward movement of the diaphragm and limits the effectiveness of the exercises.

Begin by placing the client on bed rest in a semi-Fowler's position with the knees slightly flexed and in good body alignment. The ambulatory client can sit in a high-backed armless chair. First, demonstrate the technique so that the client has some idea of what is expected. Then place both of your hands over the costophrenic margins as shown in Figure 67-4 and have the client inspire slowly, keeping the upper chest and shoulders relaxed. During expiration, gently squeeze down and outward. This helps to stretch the costophrenic angle. Have the client take the next inspiration while the hands continue to exert gentle pressure. After several respiratory cycles, begin to squeeze more

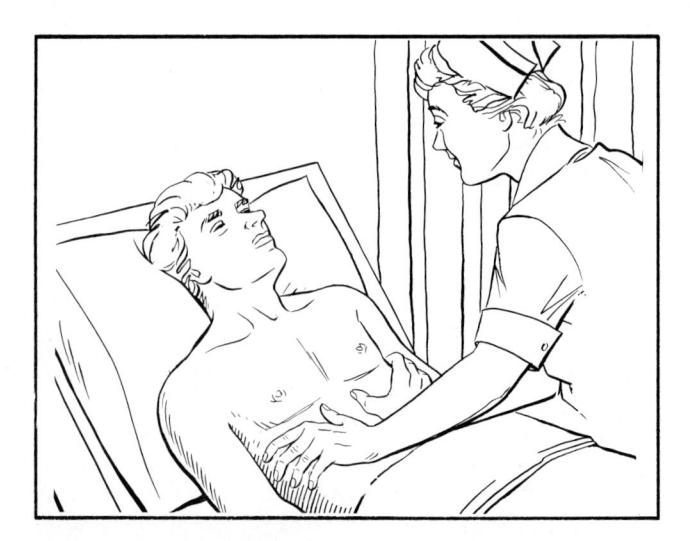

Figure 67-4. Diaphragmatic breathing. The client is in semi-Fowler's position and the nurse's hands are placed over the costophrenic margins.

firmly during exhalation. This stretching helps to enhance the normal muscular response. When the client has performed several cycles of this maneuver, find out if he or she feels the difference in this new breathing pattern over the old method. Once a client can feel this proper way of breathing, have him or her try it alone. Once a client has learned diaphragmatic breathing in the supine position, have him or her practice it while standing, walking, and during other activities such as lifting and carrying so that the maximum benefit can be obtained from the retraining.

RECORDING

In addition to the characteristics of a client's respirations the nurse records the type, frequency, and effectiveness of chest therapy exercises. The volume and characteristics of sputum are noted as well as information pertinent to the collection of specimens sent to the laboratory. The client's ability to execute a cough, the degree of assistance required, and tolerance of and extent of fatigue are all important aspects that are included in the recording.

Sample POR Recording

- S—"The stuff I'm coughing up is so thick that I can barely spit it out."
- O—Coughing up small amounts of thick viscous yellow sputum.
- A—Cough effective, needs increased fluid intake.
- P—Increase fluid intake to 200 ml/hr, continue to have client cough q 1–2 hr.

Sample Narrative Recording

Effective cough, producing small amounts of thick yellow viscous sputum. Will increase fluid intake to 200 ml/hr and continue to have client cough q 1 to 2 hr.

□ CRITICAL POINTS SUMMARY

1. Deep breathing helps to prevent alveolar collapse.
2. Retained secretions are a common cause of poor pulmonary function.
3. The color, consistency, and volume of sputum are important indicators of a client's respiratory status.
4. The best quality sputum specimen is collected in the morning.
5. Since a client's posture affects lung volume, position the client properly before each exercise.
6. Effective deep breaths require full chest expansion.
7. Diaphragmatic breathing improves the efficiency of breathing.
8. Appraisal of the client's respiratory status includes respiratory rate, rhythm, depth, pattern, and the sounds heard by auscultation.

9. Avoid doing respiratory exercises during or just prior to mealtime.
10. Administer an analgesic to a client in pain before beginning respiratory exercises.
11. Demonstrate each respiratory exercise before having the client execute it.

□ LEARNING ACTIVITIES

1. Observe a respiratory or physical therapist teaching a client how to perform deep breathing, coughing, and diaphragmatic breathing exercises and pursed lip breathing exercises.
2. Practice demonstrating and teaching each of these exercises with a peer.
3. Review the health records of several different clients who have either pulmonary disease or respiratory complications and note the type of medications and treatment used to improve the respiratory status. Follow the sequence of interventions and note the positive and negative effects on the clients' progress toward improvement.

□ REVIEW QUESTIONS

1. How do preventive respiratory exercises differ from restorative exercises?
2. How do periodic deep breaths benefit ventilation?
3. How do retained secretions interfere with ventilation?
4. What are the characteristics of sputum?
5. How would you collect a sputum specimen?
6. Match the normal type of breath sound listed in Column I with its qualities of breath sounds listed in Column II.

COLUMN I	COLUMN II
A. Vesicular	___ High-pitched, harsh
B. Bronchial	___ Soft, low-pitched
C. Bronchovesicular	___ Inspiratory phase half as long as expiratory phase
	___ Long inspiratory phase, short expiratory phase
	___ Inspiratory and expiratory phases equal
	___ Moderate pitch

7. At what location on the chest would you listen for vesicular, bronchial, and bronchovesicular sounds?
8. What are the three types of abnormal breath sounds?
9. Describe how you would tell a peer to auscultate a person's chest to hear normal breath sounds.
10. What are the three preventive respiratory exer-

cises used most often by nurses? How are they performed?
11. What are three restorative respiratory exercises? How would you teach two of them to a client with chronic obstructive lung disease?
12. What data does a nurse need to collect from the health record and the client before providing chest therapy?
13. What data are collected by inspection and auscultation?

PERFORMANCE CHECKLIST

OBJECTIVE: To teach clients how to cough effectively.

CHARACTERISTIC	RANGE OF ACCEPTABILITY	SATISFACTORY	UNSATISFACTORY
1. Explains procedure to client.	No deviation		
2. Closes door and cubicle curtains.			
3. Places client in a relaxed position on side of bed or in semi-Fowler's position. Has client rotate shoulders slightly inward.	No deviation		
4. Instructs client to take 2 to 3 slow deep breaths, followed by another with the mouth partially open, holding it for a count of one.	No deviation		
5. Has client lean forward and contract the abdominal, thigh, and buttock muscles for a count of two.	No deviation		
6. Has client cough forcefully twice and expectorate into tissue.	No deviation		
7. Lets client relax before repeating cough.	No deviation		
8. Disposes of tissue in paper bag and returns client to a comfortable position.	No deviation		
9. Washes hands.	No deviation		
10. Records results and client's response.	No deviation		

REFERENCES

DeGowin EL, DeGowin RL: Bedside Diagnostic Examination, ed 4. New York, Macmillan, 1981.

Harper RW: A Guide to Respiratory Care: Physiology and Clinical Applications. Philadelphia, JB Lippincott, 1981.

Rarey KP, Youtsey JW: Respiratory Patient Care. Englewood Cliffs, NJ, Prentice-Hall, 1981.

Shapiro BA, Harrison RA, et al.: Clinical Application of Respiratory Care, ed 2. Chicago, Year Book Medical Publishers, 1979.

BIBLIOGRAPHY

Frownfelter DL: Chest Physical Therapy and Pulmonary Rehabilitation. Chicago, Year Book Medical Publishers, 1978.

Glover DW, Glover M: Respiratory Therapy. St Louis, CV Mosby, 1978.

Malasanos L, Barkauskas V, et al.: Health Assessment, ed 2. St Louis, CV Mosby, 1981.

Spearman CB, Sheldon RL, et al.: Egan's Fundamentals of Respiratory Therapy, ed 4. St Louis, CV Mosby, 1982.

Stanley L: You can really teach COPD patients to breathe better. RN 41(4):43–49, 1978.

Traver GA (ed): Respiratory Nursing: The Science and Art. New York, John Wiley & Sons, 1982.

Wade JF: Comprehensive Respiratory Care: Physiology and Technique. St Louis, CV Mosby, 1982.

SUGGESTED READING

Acee S: Helping patients breathe more easily. Geriatric Nursing 5(6):230–233, 1984.

Tyler ML: The respiratory effects of body positioning and immobilization. Respiratory Care 29(5):472–483, 1984.

Wesatra B: When your patient says "I Can't Breathe". Nursing84 (Horsham) 14(5):34–39, 1984.

AUDIOVISUAL RESOURCES

Abnormal Breath Sounds
Filmstrip and cassette. (1979, Color, 23 min.)

Adventitious Breath Sounds
Filmstrip and cassette. (1979), Color, 16 min.)

Introduction to Breath Sounds
  Audiocassette.
  Available through:
    American College of Chest Physicians
    911 Busse Hwy
    Park Ridge, IL 60068
Introduction to Incentive Spirometry
  Filmstrip and cassette. (Color, 12 min.)
Normal Breath Sounds
  Filmstrip and cassette. (1977, Color, 19 min.)
Physical Assessment: The Chest
  Filmstrip and cassette. (1977, Color, 26 min.)

Available through:
  Medcom, Inc.
  P.O. Box 116
  Garden Grove, CA 92642

A Simplified Introduction to Lung Sounds
  Audiocassette.
  Available through:
    Raymond L.H. Murphy, Jr., M.D.
    Stethophonics
    Box 122
    Wellesley Hills, MA 02181

SKILL 68 Oxygen Therapy

□ PREREQUISITE SKILLS

Skill 19, "Inspection"
Skill 20, "Palpation"
Skill 22, "Auscultation"
Skill 24, "Pulse Appraisal"
Skill 25, "Respiration Appraisal"
Skill 26, "Blood Pressure Appraisal"
Skill 28, "Handwashing"

□ STUDENT OBJECTIVES

1. Identify the purposes for which oxygen therapy is administered.
2. Differentiate between the signs and symptoms presented in acute and chronic hypoxia.
3. Specify the precautions used to administer oxygen safely.
4. Indicate the various types of physiological hazards associated with oxygen therapy.
5. Explain why low concentrations of oxygen are essential for clients who have chronic obstructive lung disease.
6. Indicate the reasons why oxygen must be humidified.
7. Identify the data which the nurse collects prior to and during oxygen therapy.
8. Describe the types of equipment used in oxygen supply systems.
9. Describe the types of equipment used for low and high flow oxygen delivery systems.
10. Describe the procedures used to administer oxygen with each type of delivery system.
11. Specify the nursing interventions required by any client receiving oxygen therapy.
12. Administer oxygen therapy safely.

□ INTRODUCTION

Oxygen is a transparent, colorless, and odorless gas that is used as a drug. A concentration of 100 percent oxygen under pressure is administered for the purposes of restoring a sufficient level of oxygen to the tissues for metabolic function and to prevent the activation of physiological responses that stress the circulatory and respiratory systems. Oxygen therapy is administered when the arterial oxygen level is lower than that needed for these purposes and to prevent irreversible brain damage. Using oxygen therapy, however, does not necessarily guarantee relief of a reduced level of arterial oxygen, since this depends on the client's hemoglobin concentration, the adequacy of cardiac function, and the distribution of blood through the pulmonary and systemic circulation. Clients who require oxygen therapy include those who have pulmonary conditions such as pneumonia, chronic obstructive lung disease, or chest trauma that interferes with alveolar ventilation, or cardiac disease such as congestive heart failure or impaired circulation of blood to the lungs.

Most institutions employ respiratory therapists who evaluate a client's need for oxygen therapy, set up the necessary equipment, and monitor the client's response to therapy. However, it is the nurse who is responsible for the subsequent administration of oxygen and for monitoring both the function of the equipment and the client's response to therapy. In the event of an emergency, it is the nurse who initiates the oxygen therapy and thus must be knowledgeable about the basic types of therapy and when and how they are used.

□ PREPARATION

For the normal healthy adult inspiring the 21 percent oxygen present in the atmospheric air at sea level, the normal partial pressure of oxygen (oxygen tension) present in the arterial blood (PaO$_2$) ranges between 80 to 100 mm Hg. A decreased oxygen tension is associated with a variety of illness conditions.

HYPOXEMIA AND HYPOXIA

Hypoxemia, which is a low level of oxygen tension in the arterial blood, is considered to be present when the PaO$_2$ is below 50 mm Hg, assuming that the client has a normal concentration of hemoglobin (Luckmann and Sorensen, 1980). Blood gas analyses are used to determine the specific amount of gases present in the blood and they provide the most accurate data to the physician to identify when a client has hypoxemia. *Hypoxia* is the term used when the amount of oxygen delivered to the tissues is inadequate to meet the metabolic needs. Hypoxia follows hypoxemia and is responsible for the signs and symptoms a client manifests when the oxygen tension is inadequate.

Cyanosis, which is a common sign of hypoxia, is not a reliable indicator of the level of oxygen tension in the arterial blood. This is true for several reasons. Cyanotic skin color occurs when there are about 5 g of hemoglobin per 100 ml of blood without oxygen in addition to inadequate perfusion of the skin capillaries. The perception of cyanosis is dependent not only upon the appraiser's skill but it is also influenced by the client's skin color and the environmental light. Since the rate of circulation differs in various parts of the body, an area with a slow rate of blood flow, such as a hand or foot, may be cyanotic even though the actual PaO$_2$ is adequate. On the other hand, a client may be cyanotic without having 5 g of hemoglobin without oxygen. This can occur in clients who have a low level of hemoglobin, as with severe anemia, and a decreased level of oxygen tension. The opposite of this situation occurs with clients who are cyanotic but have an increased number of red blood cells (polycythemia) and an increased level of hemoglobin with an adequate level of PaO$_2$ (Traver, 1982, pp 63–64).

The four basic causes of hypoxemia are:

1. A decreased amount of inspired oxygen tension as may occur when a person is at an elevation above sea level where the amount of oxygen present in the air is less.
2. An increase in the amount of carbon dioxide in the blood, hypercapnia (PaCO$_2$), which results in a decrease in the alveolar oxygen tension. This occurs when there is hypoventilation.
3. Anatomic shunting of blood in which some blood does not come in contact with oxygen because it bypasses some component of the pulmonary circulation such as the pulmonary artery or the capillaries in the lung tissue.
4. Abnormal matching of the oxygen flow into the alveoli and the blood flow through the pulmonary capillaries as many occur in pulmonary conditions such as asthma or pneumonia.

The presenting signs and symptoms of hypoxemia may be apparent only when the client is already hypoxic. It is important for the nurse to be alert to the earliest signs and symptoms of tissue hypoxia. These signs and symptoms depend on four factors: where the process of respiration is interrupted; the extent of the interruption; the rapidity of the onset; and the client's ability to compensate for the interruption. Hypoxia may be either acute or chronic and the signs and symptoms vary with each type.

Acute Hypoxia

Acute hypoxia occurs because of a rapid reduction in either the supply or distribution of oxygen and is seen in conditions such as asphyxia, airway obstruction, or sudden cardiorespiratory failure. The earliest signs and symptoms of acute hypoxia have been likened to those of alcohol intoxication because the initial clinical manifestations result from the effect of oxygen deprivation on the nervous system. These manifestations may include any one or a combination of the following: impaired mental judgment, confusion, headache, double vision, restlessness, anxiety, and irritability. As the level of hypoxia increases, depression, apathy, and drowsiness occur and muscular weakness results in loss of muscular coordination. There are also some cardiovascular system signs that are activated by the sympathetic branch of the autonomic nervous system in compensation for the reduced level of oxygen in the arterial blood. Heart rate, cardiac output, and vasoconstriction are increased, resulting in an increase in pulmonary vascular resistance which causes an increase in the arterial blood pressure. Cyanosis is a late sign. The client may also demonstrate an increase in the respiratory rate, experience dyspnea, and have Cheyne-Stokes respirations. A client who has a partially obstructed airway may have noisy, gasping respirations (Harper, 1981).

Chronic Hypoxia

When hypoxia develops slowly or is present for a prolonged period of time, the body adjusts to a reduced level of oxygen to the tissues and attempts to compensate and provide adequate oxygen to the tissues. The primary compensatory response is circulatory, in that pulmonary vasoconstriction occurs. This increases the work of the right ventricle and can result in hypertrophy of the right ventricle. Hypoxia stimulates the bone marrow to increase production of red blood cells so that more hemoglobin is present to carry the available oxygen. This is demonstrated by elevated red blood cell, hemoglobin, and hematocrit levels. Some of the conditions that cause chronic hypoxia include chronic obstructive lung disease and certain types of cardiovascular disease such as cyanotic heart defects (Harper, 1981).

OXYGEN AS A THERAPY

When considering the use of oxygen as a therapeutic intervention, it is important to be aware that except in an emergency, it is the physician who prescribes oxygen therapy. The medical order should include the method of administration and the amount of oxygen to be given, specified either by liters per minute or the percent of oxygen concentration desired. Since oxygen is a drug, the nurse administers it as a medication and is responsible for checking both the accuracy of the dose and the route of administration. The nurse also monitors and evaluates the client's response to the therapy and reports adverse reactions to the physician.

To administer oxygen safely, the nurse is knowledgeable about the potential hazards inherent in the use of oxygen, the need for humidification of the oxygen, and the value of blood gas analysis in monitoring the client's response to the therapy.

Hazards

The hazards associated with the use of oxygen as a therapeutic intervention are classified as physical and physiological.

Physical Hazards. Oxygen is heavier than air and exerts a partial pressure of 150 mm Hg in the atmospheric air at sea level. It is not flammable but supports combustion. As the concentration of oxygen in an environment increases, the combustion point of materials in that environment decreases. In an enriched oxygen environment a small spark or burning object such as a cigarette can rapidly become a large fire. When oxygen is under pressure, as occurs in hyperbaric chambers or with portable oxygen cylinders, the hazard increases significantly. Grease, oil, or other flammable substances must not be permitted to come in contact with an oxygen source or the equipment used to deliver oxygen to a client. When oxygen is in use, no smoking rules must be enforced rigidly, and all highly combustible materials or spark-producing appliances such as electric razors and transistor radios are removed from the immediate environment. Some institutions require that the nurse-call signal be disconnected. Static-producing materials such as wool or synthetics are not used around clients receiving oxygen (Rarey, 1980).

Physiological Hazards

Absorption Atelectasis. Alveolar collapse can occur with the inspiration of high concentrations of oxygen. Nitrogen is the major gas present in the alveoli since it normally comprises about 78 percent of room air. When the inspired high concentration of oxygen is diffused from the alveoli into the blood stream more rapidly than the nitrogen is replaced, the alveoli collapse. This is apt to occur in clients who are either very relaxed or well-sedated and who have a low tidal volume with a tendency to retain secretions that partially block the alveoli (Rarey, 1981).

Retrolental Fibroplasia. Blindness in newborn infants can be caused by high concentrations of oxygen that maintain the PaO_2 at abnormally high levels for a prolonged period of time. The blindness is caused by retinal arterial vasoconstriction and tissue scarring. It is important to monitor the arterial oxygen to keep it within the normal physiologic range (Rarey, 1981).

Oxygen-induced Hypoventilation. Oxygen-induced hypoventilation is also known as oxygen-induced carbon dioxide narcosis. Normally, the stimulus to breathe comes from the carbon dioxide level in the arterial blood. With adequate alveolar ventilation the carbon dioxide level is maintained at 40 mm Hg by the elimination of about 200 ml of carbon dioxide per minute. This is usually about the same amount produced by the tissues. However, when the alveolar ventilation is inadequate to maintain this balance, the carbon dioxide level increases. In clients who have chronic obstructive lung disease with chronic hypoventilation, increased carbon dioxide retention, and hypoxemia, the drive to breathe comes from a compensatory response that is activated as the hypoxemia stimulates carotid and aortic chemoreceptors. The respiratory center also becomes insensitive to the increased levels of carbon dioxide and no longer responds by increasing the respiratory rate. Inhaled high concentrations of oxygen remove the stimulus to breathe and the respiratory rate decreases, which raises the carbon dioxide level. The carbon dioxide can reach a narcotic level causing mental confusion that can progress to a loss of consciousness, coma, and then death. Since these physiological changes may occur either rapidly or slowly enough to go unnoticed, the nurse must be alert for warning signs of marked increases in carbon dioxide retention in a client with chronic obstructive lung disease who is receiving oxygen therapy. Depending on the level of carbon dioxide to which the client has become adapted, the early signs may include the inability to concentrate, mental confusion and irritability, headache, and an inability to sleep. The normal night sleep patterns may be reversed. However, it is dangerous to give these clients a sedative because this further depresses the respiratory center and increases the SaO_2 (Rarey, 1981).

Oxygen Toxicity. Lung tissue damage can occur with oxygen therapy since there are limits to the ability of lung tissue to tolerate and adapt to concentrations above the normal 21 percent present in air. The common signs and symptoms that may be observed when the amount of oxygen inspired exceeds the client's adaptive limits include substernal pain, headache, and shortness of breath. The lungs become congested and inflamed; poor function of the cells lining the bronchial tree leads to a decreased production of surfactant and the development of atelectasis and pulmonary edema (Harper, 1981).

Humidification

Normally the inspired oxygen in air that reaches the lungs is warmed and humidified as it passes over the mucous blanket in the nasopharynx, pharynx, and trachea. Since oxygen is a dry gas, when it is administered therapeutically it must be humidified with a sufficient quantity of water or other prescribed fluid so that it becomes saturated. This is particularly important if the route of administration bypasses the nasal cavity. Inadequately humidified oxygen causes the mucous membranes to become dry and respiratory secretions to become thickened. Lack of adequate humidity can also contribute to a client's dehydration because the dry oxygen absorbs moisture from the body.

Blood Gases

Arterial blood gases measure the partial pressure of oxygen (PaO_2), oxygen saturation (SaO_2), carbon dioxide ($PaCO_2$), actual bicarbonate (HCO_3), and the arterial pH. These measurements are used by the physician or advanced nurse clinician to determine either the client's respiratory status or acid-base balance or both. A complete discussion about the meaning and interpretation of blood gases can be found in a medical-surgical nursing text. The nurse administering oxygen therapy needs to be aware that the physician may order blood gases because they provide the most accurate data about the respiratory status of a client. Any interpretation of blood gas results must be done in terms of their relationship to a specific client's other physiological mechanisms and the changes and patterns that occur in a given client over time. The clinical management of a hypoxic client is not done on the basis of one isolated blood gas analysis.

DATA BASE

Client History and Recorded Data

To be able to monitor oxygen therapy, it is necessary to have information about the reason why the oxygen is being given, the desired goal of the therapy, and how it relates to the client's current respiratory status. Information pertinent to the client's previous respiratory history and current respiratory status is available on the health record. The nurse reviews the health record for results of appraisals of the respiratory system, and blood pressure and pulse measurements. Although subtle changes in the client's mental-emotional status indicative of the early signs of hypoxia may be revealed on the medical or nursing notes, these data are supplemented or validated by direct observation and interaction with the client. It is important for the nurse to know if the client has received oxygen therapy in the past, the type of response and how well the client was able to tolerate and cooperate with the therapy. This information should be included in the nursing history.

Knowledge of the client's medical diagnosis helps to direct the nurse to note conditions that are apt to promote or result in hypoxemia and with this information the nurse can be alert for the early signs and symptoms of acute or chronic hypoxia. The nurse also identifies the presence of factors that increase the demand for oxygen such as infection, pain, and anxiety. These stressors can rapidly change a stable client's respiratory status and result in a need for supplemental oxygen to meet metabolic needs.

Physical Appraisal Skills

Inspection. Early detection of a client's hypoxic state and changes in a client's response to oxygen therapy are dependent upon the nurse's use of inspection skills. The skills are used to make observations of an altered mental and emotional status; detect changes in the respiratory pattern; look for indications of cyanosis in the nail beds, ear lobes, and mucous membranes; notice any signs of pressure on the skin due to the equipment used in the delivery system; and observe the nature of respiratory secretions and signs of dehydration.

Palpation. The client's need for or response to therapy is evaluated, in part, by palpation of the client's pulse. Palpation is also used to appraise skin turgor to determine the client's state of hydration.

Auscultation. To evaluate respiratory status, the adequacy of breath sounds in different parts of the lungs is detected by auscultation with a stethoscope as presented in Skill 67. Auscultation is also required for blood pressure measurement.

EQUIPMENT

There are two different categories of equipment used to provide oxygen therapy to a patient: equipment used with oxygen supply systems and equipment used with oxygen delivery systems.

Oxygen Supply Systems

A *wall system* supply of oxygen provides a central source of oxygen under 50 to 60 pounds of pressure per square inch (psi) and is delivered to outlets near the client's bed by a pipeline. The oxygen at each outlet has the same amount of pressure as in the pipeline. The system of pipelines has zone valves that control the flow of gas and can be closed by nurses or other responsible personnel in the event of a fire in an area. Alarms installed at different locations throughout the facility serve as a safety feature to alert the staff of a pressure failure in the pipeline. In the event of a pressure failure, emergency oxygen cylinders are kept in client-care areas so that a supply of oxygen is available at all times. The wall oxygen system is the most economical and safest method for use in a large health-care facility (McPherson, 1981).

To reduce the pressure and regulate the flow of oxygen which is measured in liters per minute (L/m) a *flow meter* is attached to the wall outlet. Flow meters are available in different sizes and designs and are either screwed on or plugged into the outlet. It is important to learn how to connect the design used in the

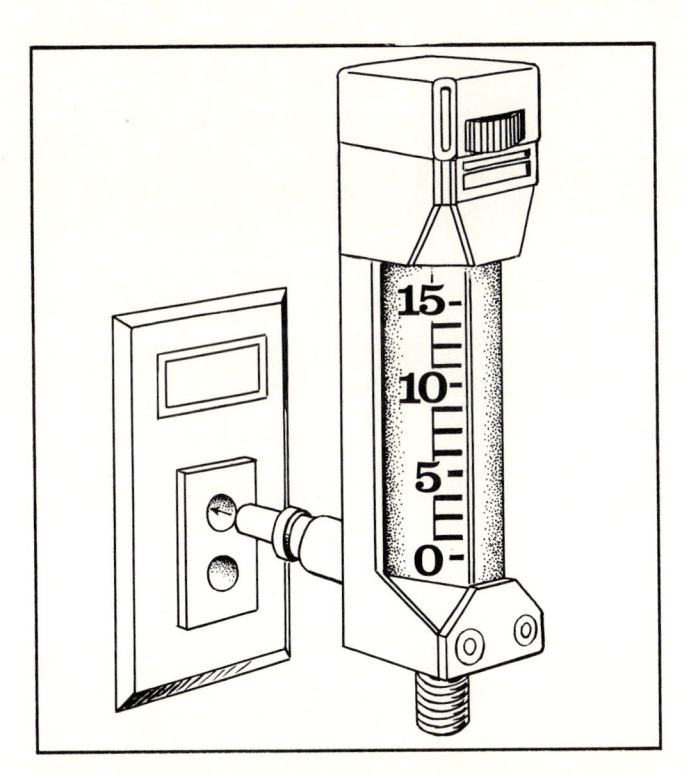

Figure 68-1. Wall outlet flowmeter measures oxygen flow in liters per minute.

facility in which the nurse is practicing. Figure 68-1 shows one type of wall outlet.

Portable steel cylinders containing pressurized oxygen are used when wall system oxygen is not available. Since similar shaped steel cylinders are used for several different medical gases, they are differentiated by a color code system. In the United States, the cylinders used for oxygen are green. In addition to the color code, each tank is labeled with the name of the gas it contains. Cylinders of oxygen are available in large and small sizes and are used both in health-care facilities and homes. Large cylinders are transported on a self-supporting cart with wheels and casters; they are secured on the cart by either a strap or chain. Once in place at the client's bedside, they must be kept on the cart or chained to the wall to prevent them from falling as this could cause violent decompression of the cylinder, greatly increasing existing fire hazards. Smaller cylinders of oxygen are available and may be either attached to wheelchairs or stretchers or wheeled on a small cart when it is necessary to transport an oxygen-dependent client to other areas of the facility. These small cylinders are also used by noninstitutionalized persons who require supplemental oxygen. The storage area for all gas cylinders must meet local fire department regulations to prevent explosions and keep the potential for fire at a minimum. A protective cap is kept over the cylinder outlet when the cylinder is not in use to prevent accidental damage to the outlet that would permit the escape of gas. Since a fully standardized cylinder of oxygen is under more than 2000 psi, a partially opened outlet is extremely dangerous and can cause the cylinder to jettison like a rocket (McPherson, 1981).

A pressure flow regulator is used to regulate the pressure of oxygen from a cylinder. A hand wheel controls the flow of oxygen from the tank into the pressure regulator. The regulator reduces the oxygen pressure as it flows from the cylinder, permitting the oxygen to be adjusted at a flow rate in liters per minute. The regulator is attached to the cylinder outlet with a large nut. A wrench is used to tighten the nut securely. The regulator is equipped with two gauges; one measures the contents of the cylinder, and the other indicates the oxygen flow rate. An adaptor on the regulator is used to attach oxygen tubing or a humidity bottle. A large oxygen cylinder must be changed when the regulator pressure shows 500 psi. Figure 68-2 shows a large oxygen cylinder with a pressure flow regulator attached (McPherson, 1981).

Small oxygen cylinders complete with flow meter and delivery equipment are kept in client-care areas and are used for either emergencies or as a temporary supply of oxygen for clients.

Humidifiers are devices that moisturize the oxygen. They are attached either to the flow meter or the tubing that delivers the oxygen to the client. *Simple humidifiers* that attach to the flow meter have a bottle that is filled to a designated level with either sterile distilled water, normal saline, or a medicated solution. Simple humidifiers are designed to provide enough moisture to the oxygen to make the therapy more comfortable for the client. With this model, known as a bubble humidifier, oxygen flows below the fluid sur-

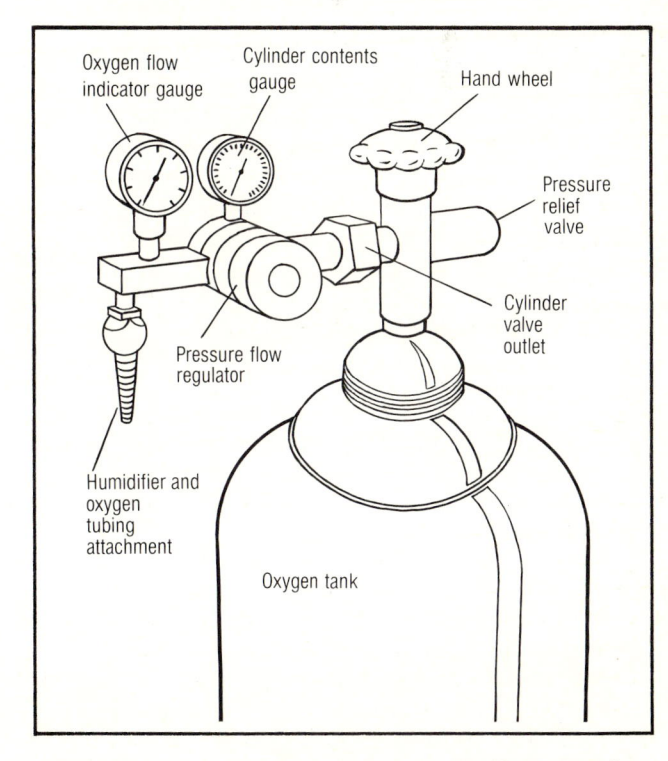

Figure 68-2. Large portable oxygen cylinder with pressure flow regulator.

face and then bubbles back up to the top of the bottle where it then flows through the connecting tube to the client. This type of humidifier is most commonly used with nasal cannulas, nasal catheters, and face masks because it is intended to supplement the normal humidification that occurs in the nasopharynx (Harper, 1981).

The humidification of a gas is influenced by the duration of contact between the gas and water, the surface area of the gas and water, and the temperature of the gas and water. Increasing the temperature of the gas and water increases the capacity of the gas to hold water vapor. *Heated humidifiers* produce a relative humidity of 100 percent at body temperature and are used when the oxygen delivery route bypasses the client's nose such as occurs with clients who have either a tracheostomy or endotracheal tube. When a heated humidifier is used, the tubing carrying the oxygen to the client must be placed downward away from the client without any low spots to prevent an accumulation of water and blockage of the tubing. When water does accumulate in the tubing, the tubing can be disconnected from the humidifier so that it can be emptied into a receptacle (Harper, 1981).

Oxygen Delivery Systems

The equipment systems that are used to deliver oxygen directly to the client produce either a low or high flow of oxygen.

Low flow systems provide a variable concentration of oxygen and are used most commonly for clients who are clinically stable. These systems do not provide all of the oxygen needed for each breath, and the remaining oxygen the client uses comes from room air. Consequently, in this system the oxygen delivered to the client is diluted. Low flow systems are easy to administer, economical, and more comfortable for the client to wear. A major disadvantage of the low flow system is that the concentration of oxygen the client receives varies with the breathing pattern. The equipment used with low flow systems includes nasal cannula, nasal catheter, simple mask, partial rebreathing mask, and tent (Rarey, 1981).

High flow systems provide all of the oxygen that the client inspires and are used with clients who are critically ill and have variations in the depth and rate of respiration and require carefully controlled oxygen concentration. The equipment used with high flow systems that are presented in this text are the nonrebreathing mask and the venturi mask (Rarey, 1984).

Low Flow Oxygen Systems. A *nasal cannula* is a plastic small-bore tube with two prongs approximately ½ inch long that are shaped to fit into the client's nares, as shown in Figure 68–3. The cannula is held in place either by an adjustable sliding ring on the tubing that passes over the client's ears and under the chin or by an elastic band that wraps around the back of the head. It is used for general oxygen therapy or for short-term emergencies. The oxygen flow rate is set between 1 and 6 L/min and provides the client

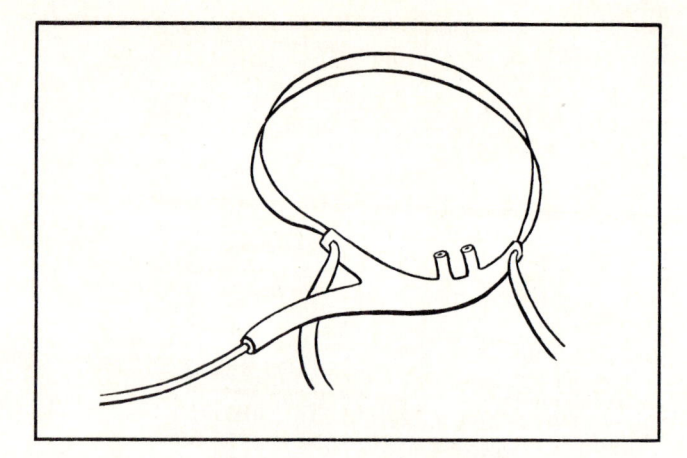

Figure 68–3. Nasal cannula.

with an oxygen concentration of 24 to 44 percent. The advantages of the cannula are that it is disposable, easy to put on, comfortable for the client to wear, and can be left in place while drinking and eating. The disadvantages include a lack of control of the concentration of oxygen because of air inspired around the cannula, easy displacement of the prongs from the nares, drying and irritation of the nares and nasal mucosa from the oxygen and the prongs, and less oxygen delivery to the client who has any obstruction in the nasal cavity such as excessive nasal secretions, edema of the mucous membranes, or a severely deviated nasal septum (Frownfelter, 1978).

A *nasal catheter* is a plastic small-bore tubing with perforations at the distal end. It is inserted through a naris and nasal cavity into the oropharynx until it lies behind the uvula, as shown in Figure 68–4, and is held in place by a strip of nonallergenic adhesive tape over the client's nose or forehead. It is used when it is not possible to keep a nasal cannula in place and with clients who have facial trauma. It is contraindicated for clients who have nasal bleeding or an obstructed nasal cavity. The catheter is lubricated with a water-soluble lubricant before insertion. The nasal catheter is used for short-term emergencies and with the same flow rates provides the same oxygen concentration as the cannula. The advantages of the catheter are that it permits the client to breathe through the nose or mouth and it is disposable. Its disadvantages are that it is uncomfortable for the client to wear and may cause drying of the oropharyngeal mucous membranes, which can result in having the catheter become lodged in the nasal cavity. The catheter can also cause thickening of secretions because the oxygen does not absorb humidity from the nose. Because of the location of the catheter, the oxygen flow may become misdirected into the stomach and result in abdominal distention (Rarey, 1981).

The *simple oxygen mask* shown in Figure 68–5 is a plastic dome-shaped device that fits over the client's nose and mouth and is held in place by an elastic strap that wraps around the back of the head. A flexible steel metal strip in the nose area of the mask can be molded to conform to the client's nose. The mask has

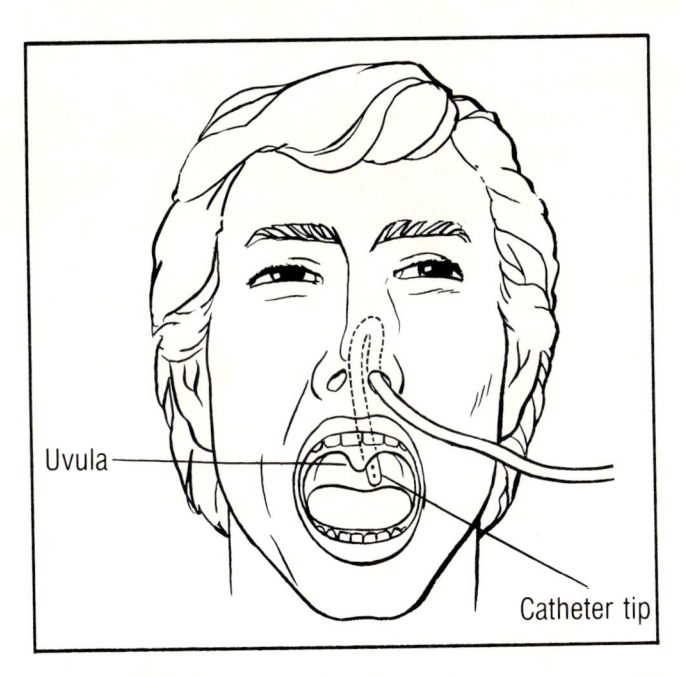

Figure 68-4. Nasal catheter in proper position.

a series of small holes on each side that serve as exhalation vents. It is used when clients need an increased oxygen concentration for less than 12 hours. The simple mask is used less often than other types of masks because the concentration of inspired oxygen is so variable. The simple mask can deliver a concentration of oxygen between 44 and 68 percent at a flow rate between 6 and 10 L/min. Depending on the shape of the mask, an additional 70 to 100 ml of oxygen is held around the nose and mouth. The advantage of the simple mask is that it is lightweight and disposable. Its disadvantages are that it is difficult to obtain a good fit over the client's face and the plastic and elastic strap can cause skin irritation. It cannot be used if the client has any type of facial trauma or a nasogastric tube in place. It must be removed when the client eats or drinks and can be particularly hazardous if worn by clients when vomiting occurs because it prevents the vomitus from clearing the mouth and may result in aspiration of vomitus. Room air can be inspired through the vent holes in the mask and this reduces the oxygen concentration. The flow rate must be at least 5 L/min so that the exhaled carbon dioxide can be flushed through the vents in the mask; otherwise the client may rebreathe the exhaled gas. As with all masks, clients dislike it because they feel smothered (Rarey, 1981).

A *partial rebreathing mask* is similar to a simple mask; however, it has a transparent plastic reservoir bag attached (Fig. 68-6) which permits the client to inspire a reserve of oxygen from the bag. It is called a rebreathing mask because the first third of the air exhaled by a client returns to the bag and the remaining air is exhaled through the vents in the mask. The air returned to the bag is essentially the same oxygen that the client inhaled because it comes from the dead spaces in the respiratory tract, that is, the trachea and bronchi where little or no gas exchange occurs. The partial rebreather mask is used with clients who are acutely ill or who have cardiac disease. Therapy with this mask relieves moderate to severe hypoxia. This mask can deliver an oxygen concentration of about 60 to 91 percent when the flow rate is set at 10 or more L per minute. The advantages of the mask are that it is lightweight and disposable and can provide high concentrations of oxygen. Some of the disadvantages are the same as with the simple mask in terms of fit, skin irritation, and client tolerance. In addition, the mask

Figure 68-5. Simple face mask.

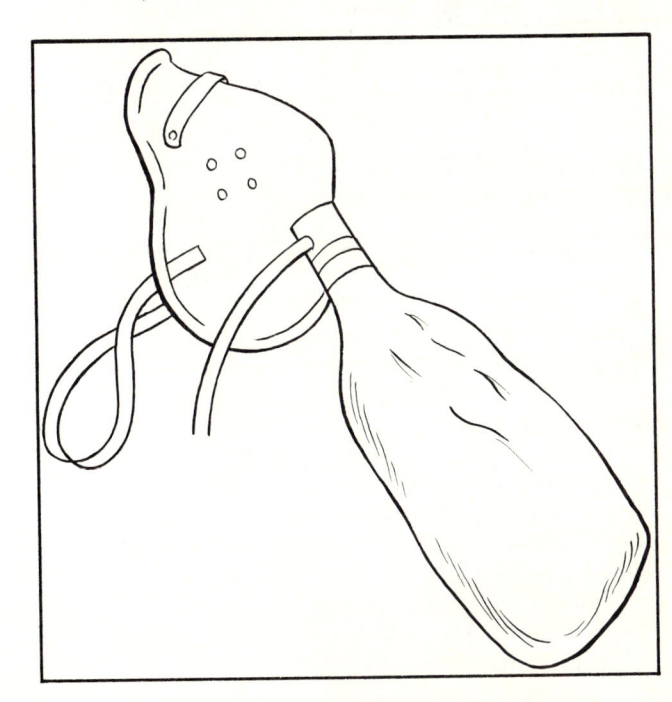

Figure 68-6. Partial rebreathing mask.

must be kept in a position that does not allow the bag to become kinked for this would prevent air from being inhaled from the reservoir and thus reduce the mask to a simple model (Rarey, 1981).

An oxygen *tent* is a large plastic canopy that encloses the client in a controlled environment. It has a motor-driven unit with a thermostat that helps to circulate and cool the air. The canopy supported by a frame fits over the top of the bed and has side openings to permit access for nursing care. When used for adults usually only the head and upper chest are enclosed, but with children the entire body is contained within the tent. Tents are not often used for adults. They are used primarily for children who have a fever with pulmonary congestion and need a cool, highly humidified environment plus oxygen therapy. Oxygen is heavier than air, so for a tent to be effective the lower border of the canopy is tucked securely under the mattress to prevent leaks and to allow the oxygen concentration to build up to between 30 and 35 percent. The oxygen flow rate must be set at a minimum of 10 L/min to prevent an accumulation of carbon dioxide within the tent. The advantages of the tent are particularly realized with children because it allows the client unrestricted movement while providing a cool moist oxygenated environment. It is also beneficial for other clients who require oxygen and have extensive areas of the body traumatized such as occurs with burns. The disadvantages of the tent are: There is a loss of oxygen concentration each time the tent is opened; the noise from the motorized unit can be very annoying to the client; and there is an increased potential for fire because of the lowered combustion point of the plastic in the presence of oxygen (Rarey, 1981).

High Flow Oxygen Systems. The *nonrebreathing mask* is a variation of the simple mask. It has an attached reservoir bag that contains a one-way valve that is placed between the mask and the bag to prevent exhaled gas from flowing into the bag. A second set of valves located on the mask's vents prevents the client from inspiring any room air, thus controlling the concentration of oxygen the client inhales. This mask is useful for short periods of time when the client needs high concentrations of oxygen. The flow rate is set between 6 and 15 L/min at the point at which the reservoir bag remains one-third full during inspiration. It can deliver an oxygen concentration between 60 and 90 percent. The advantages of this mask are that it controls the oxygen concentration as the client inhales and permits the highest possible concentration for a client who is able to breathe spontaneously. Its disadvantages are: The mask must fit so snugly over the client's face for proper function that the client is able to tolerate it for only a few hours; the exact concentration of oxygen the client receives depends upon the bag not totally collapsing when the client inspires; and kinks or separation of the oxygen tubing will reduce the client's oxygen supply to what little can be obtained from the room air through a small hole in the mask (Fuchs, 1980; Rarey, 1981).

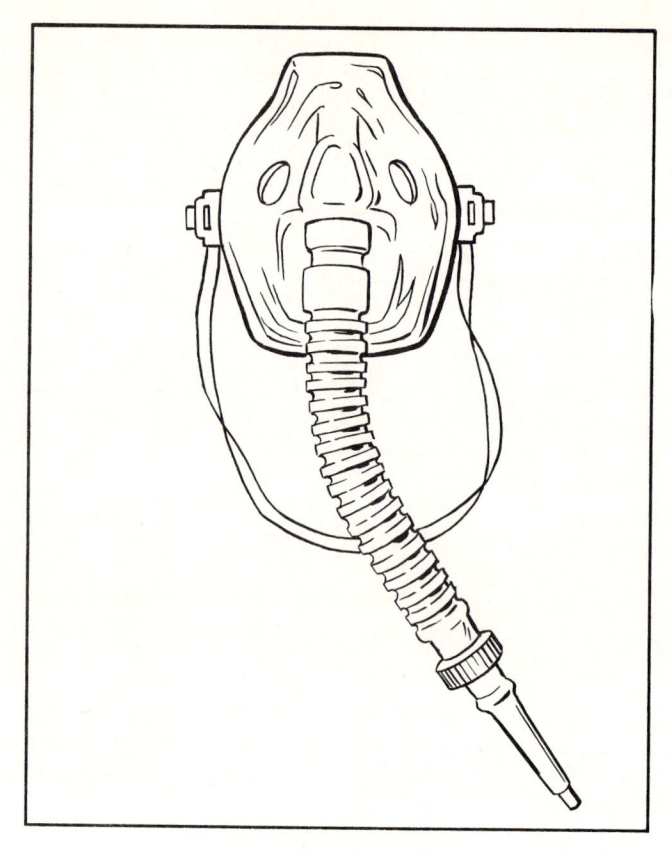

Figure 68–7. Venturi mask.

Venturi mask is the name given to several different types of masks that permit a specific amount of room air to be mixed (entrained) with a specific concentration of oxygen before it is delivered to a client's airways. One type of venturi mask is shown in Figure 68–7. The venturi-type mask is considered a high flow system because the mixture of room air and the oxygen provides a high flow of gas to the client. The components of a venturi type mask include: a venturi device, which is a restricted orifice through which oxygen flows with a high velocity; air entrainment ports that allow specific amounts of room air to enter the system, and a mixing chamber through which the combined oxygen and room air then flows before it reaches the mask and the client. The face mask has vents that prevent the client from rebreathing the exhaled air. Venturi-type masks are available for various concentrations of oxygen and each type requires that a specific flow rate of oxygen be used. The masks are often color coded according to the percent of oxygen and the related flow rate. The most commonly available models are for concentrations of 24 percent, 28 percent, 35 percent, and 40 percent and the flow rate range is from 4 to 10 L/min, depending on the design of the mask used. Masks delivering a concentration of less than 30 percent do not require humidification but those with greater concentration do. With the lesser oxygen concentration, humidification will restrict the room air flow and result in a higher than desired oxygen concentration being delivered.

The venturi-type mask was designed primarily for chronic obstructive lung disease clients because of their need for carefully controlled concentrations of oxygen but the mask can be used for any client when a known required concentration of oxygen is essential. The advantage of the venturi-type mask is its ability to control the specific concentration of oxygen. The disadvantages of the mask are that the large vents on the entrainment component can be blocked by the client's body position, clothing, or bed linen. When this occurs, the inspired oxygen concentration is raised. The mask is also uncomfortable and can cause skin irritation. Clients cannot drink or eat with the mask in place and there is a risk of aspiration when vomiting occurs. There is also a problem of dehydration and thickened secretions if the humidification is inadequate (Rarey, 1981).

Table 68-1 summarizes flow rates and percent of concentration attainable for each type of delivery system.

Additional Items. *Connecting tubing* made of transparent flexible plastic at least 180 cm (6 ft) long is used to transport the oxygen from the flow meter to the delivery system. The length allows some degree of mobility for the client at the bedside and reduces the need to use a temporary supply of oxygen. The excess length of tubing can be coiled and pinned to the bed to prevent it from falling on the floor or becoming kinked. Connecting tubing is available in small and large diameters. Small diameter tubing is used mostly with low-flow delivery systems. Tubing with a lumen diameter of at least 1½ cm should be used to deliver oxygen with high humidity masks. This size tubing reduces the amount of condensation that collects on the inner wall and allows the oxygen to flow without obstruction (Administering, 1980).

Water-soluble lubricant is used to insert a nasal catheter. Oil-based lubricant is not used because of its potential to be inhaled into the lungs where it could cause pulmonary complications.

A *nonallergenic adhesive tape* strip is used to anchor a nasal catheter to the client and *rubber bands* and *safety pins* are used to anchor the connecting tubing to the bed linen.

TABLE 68-1. Oxygen Delivery Systems, Flow Rate, and Concentrations

System	Oxygen Flow Rate (L/min)	Oxygen Concentrations (%)
Nasal cannula	1 to 6	24 to 44
Nasal catheter	1 to 6	24 to 44
Simple mask	6 to 10	44 to 68
Partial rebreathing mask	10 or more	60 to 91
Tent	10 or more	30 to 35
Nonrebreathing mask	6 to 15	60 to 90
Venturi-type mask	4 to 10	24 to 40

EXECUTION

PREPARING THE CLIENT FOR OXYGEN THERAPY

Once it has been determined that a client requires oxygen therapy, the nurse directs his or her attention to preparing the client and the environment. Keep in mind that oxygen therapy may be an anxiety-producing experience for both the client and family because of the common belief that it is used only for critically ill people. There may also be some fears related to the dangers of fire and explosion. The nurse can allay these concerns by taking the time to give careful explanations about why the oxygen therapy is necessary, how it will be administered, and how the client and family can help to make it more effective. They also need to know what safeguards are used to prevent accidents from occurring. It is appropriate to link these explanations with no-smoking policies and the reasons for removing all materials that have a potential for creating static electricity. Some institutions require that the electric signal light be disconnected (if it is not grounded) and be replaced by a clapper bell. In the event that the client is in a semiprivate room, the same explanations regarding safety are made to others in the room so that the environment is safe. Place the no-smoking sign on the door so that all entering are aware of the need for safety.

Whenever possible, place the client in a semi-Fowler's position so that respirations can be executed with a maximum of efficiency. Use pillows to support the client's head, shoulders, and arms as necessary. Change the client's position at least every 2 hours and have the client take periodic deep breaths and cough to clear secretions from the lungs to facilitate gas exchange at the alveolar level. Even with the use of a humidification system, a client breathing some room air may have some drying effects of the oxygen on the mucous membranes. Inspect the mucous membranes and appraise the hydration status of the client by keeping a careful eye on the intake and output record and by appraising the skin. Hydration can be improved by increasing oral intake of liquids unless contraindicated by the client's condition or by the physician's order. An additional room humidifier may be required to increase the ambient humidity if the drying effects persist in spite of good nursing care.

Handle all equipment used for oxygen delivery to the client with medically aseptic technique. Contaminated equipment can cause infections of the respiratory system. The parts of the system that become wet, such as the humidifier and connecting tubing, and items placed on the client such as the cannula need to be replaced at least every 8 hours to prevent the growth of microorganisms.

Prior to attaching the oxygen delivery device to the client, turn on the oxygen and allow it to flow through and fill the system. Permit the client to feel the oxygen flow, because this provides some reassurance that oxygen is indeed flowing. Position the connecting tubing so that the client will not lie on it and so that it cannot become kinked. Wrap the excess connecting tubing in a coil and secure it to the bed linen with a rubber band and safety pin, taking care not to puncture the tubing.

Keep in mind that a client's oxygen requirements change in relation to the respiratory pattern, which varies with rest, sleep, and activity. The amount of oxygen prescribed by the physician is usually based on the client's needs at rest and, because oxygen is administered only as prescribed, it may be necessary to have a second order for a different flow rate when the client is active. The adequacy of the flow rate and concentration may be determined by careful observation of the client for signs of hypoxia as activity levels change.

PREPARING OXYGEN SYSTEMS

Wall Systems
When using a wall oxygen system, attach a flow meter to the wall outlet and fill the humidifier bottle to the designated level with sterile distilled water or normal saline. Attach the connecting tube to the nozzle on the flow meter and the appropriate oxygen delivery device. Open the flow meter valve before slowly opening the wall system outlet and then adjust the flow to the desired rate. Observe the bubbles in the humidifier to ensure that the oxygen is flowing through the solution.

Oxygen Cylinders
Whenever possible, prepare an oxygen cylinder in some area other than at the client's bedside because it is a noisy procedure that may alarm the client. The cylinder must be "cracked" before attaching the pressure flow regulator to remove dust and debris from the valve outlet that might clog the pressure flow regulator. Cracking makes a loud hissing sound. Remove the protective cap and point the cylinder valve outlet away from yourself and others in the area. Place both hands on the hand wheel and open it slightly by turning it counterclockwise, then close it quickly. Close the pressure flow regulator before attaching it to the cylinder. To attach the regulator, hold it level so that the nut is aligned with the cylinder valve outlet. Begin by turning the nut clockwise to start it on the threads of the valve outlet and then use the correct size wrench to tighten it securely. Take care not to cross the threads and do not force the nut. Once the regulator is in place, transport the cylinder to the bedside and position it so that it is not in the way and in danger of being overturned. Secure it to the wall or leave it on the carrier. To administer the oxygen to the client, attach the connecting tubing to the nozzle on the regulator, attach the oxygen delivery device before opening the cylinder valve completely, and then turn it back a quarter or half turn. Open the flow regulator and adjust the flow to the desired rate. Check the oxygen flow through the device. Attach and fill the prescribed humidifier. After all of these activities are completed, position the delivery system device on the client.

ADMINISTERING OXYGEN

Nasal Cannula and Catheter Administration
There are specific problems associated with the use of both the cannula and the catheter that good nursing care can either help to prevent or minimize. Prior to inserting either device, and routinely during the course of the therapy, inspect the nasal cavity by raising the tip of the nose and using a flashlight to detect the condition of the mucous membranes and the presence of any secretions or obstructions due to a deviated septum. Have the client blow his or her nose if possible to clear the airways or carefully remove secretions and crusted material with cotton-tipped applicators moistened with water or half-strength hydrogen peroxide. Inspect the condition of the oral mucous membranes and provide oral hygiene if the client is unable to do so independently. Wash and dry the client's face to remove accumulated perspiration and oil. Apply a thin film of either water-soluble lubricant or vaseline to the aspect of the naris or nares over which the cannula or catheter rests to prevent friction of the plastic tube from irritating the tissues. If the prongs of the cannula are too long to fit comfortably within the nares, trim off the excess carefully with scissors. This helps to remove undue pressure against the nares. Keep alert for early signs of pressure over the ears and at the back of the head where the elastic band on the cannula contacts the skin. Place small pieces of absorbent cotton or a gauze pad between the skin and elastic to prevent pressure areas and change the position of the padding periodically (Fuchs, 1980).

When inserting a nasal catheter, estimate the length of the catheter to be inserted in the client's nasopharynx by using the catheter to measure from the tip or bridge of the nose to the tip of the ear lobe. Mark this spot on the catheter with a narrow piece of tape. Use this length only for a guide because the actual distance from the tip of the nose to the tip of the uvula may be greater or lesser than this. Apply a thin film of water-soluble lubricant on the tip of the catheter to facilitate its entry. Do not force the tube into the cavity but gently slide it along the floor of the nose. Insertion is usually easier if the client holds the head in a normally erect position. Clients who have received nasal catheter oxygen frequently may prefer assisting with inserting the catheter. Find out if the client has a preference for the naris to be used or determine if one side of the nasal cavity is obstructed.

After inserting the catheter, inspect the position of the tip of the catheter by using a flashlight and tongue depressor. The catheter is to be located behind and at the same level as the uvula. If it is above this level the oxygen is less apt to enter the respiratory tract and will increase the dryness of the mucosa; if it is below this level it will enter the esophagus and distend the stomach as well as cause irritation of the oropharynx.

To anchor a nasal catheter in place, place a nonallergenic adhesive tape strip around the catheter and on the client's cheek or mandible with enough slack and in such a position that it will not apply pressure on the external naris. When changing the catheter, remove the old tape residue from the skin, using adhesive tape remover if necessary. Alternate the anchoring sites as much as possible to prevent skin irritation.

Mask Administration

A client who receives oxygen by mask requires the same type of care to the nasopharynx as one receiving it by cannula or catheter. However, one of the differences in the use of the mask is that the client has a sense of being smothered by the snug mask. The mask also becomes warm and increases the amount of moisture on the skin. When this is combined with the pressure of the mask against the skin there is great potential for irritation or breakdown of the skin, especially in clients who are malnourished or debilitated. To prevent or reduce these effects, remove the mask at least every 8 hours and preferably every 2 hours; bathe and dry the face and apply a thin film of absorbent powder, being careful not to create a cloud of dust that the client will inhale. Use a damp wash-cloth to clean the inside of the mask and dry it thoroughly before replacing it. Clients who require continuous oxygen and are using a mask must have either a cannula or catheter available at the bedside so that oxygen can be administered when the mask is removed for bathing, eating, and drinking.

Clients who are edentulous or have a small, large, or irregularly shaped face may not have a good fit with the mask. To prevent loss of oxygen, insert small gauze pads to fill in the gaps. Pads can also be used to relieve some of the pressure from the snug mask.

When a client has a reservoir bag or venturi component, take care to prevent the bag or component from kinking or becoming covered with clothing or bed linen. It is also important to check the connecting tubing frequently for dependent loops in which condensation is apt to accumulate. Disconnect the tubing and empty the condensation to permit the oxygen to flow without obstruction. Explain the importance of these actions to the client and the family so that they can be involved in assisting to ensure good oxygen therapy (Fuchs, 1980).

☐ SKILL SEQUENCE

ADMINISTERING OXYGEN BY NASAL CANNULA, CATHETER, AND MASK

Step	Rationale
1. Check physician's order or nursing kardex.	Ensures accurate flow rate and correct delivery system.
2. Wash hands.	Prevents transferring microorganisms.
3. Prepare equipment and supplies.	Prevents delays and interruptions.
4. Explain procedure to client.	Allays anxiety and lets client know how to cooperate.
5. Place client in semi-Fowler's position.	Facilitates efficient respiration.
6. Fill humidifier with sterile distilled water. (NOTE: Omit if venturi mask <30 percent concentration is used.)	Water vapor humidifies dry oxygen and reduces drying of mucous membranes.
7. Attach flow meter to wall outlet, connect tubing and delivery system. Check delivery system for O₂ flow. (NOTE: Prepare cylinder away from bedside.)	Ensures proper gas flow. Avoids creating unnecessary noise at bedside.
8. Instruct client to breathe normally when delivery system is applied.	Prevents hyperventilation or hypoventilation.
9. Apply delivery system:	
a. Nasal cannula	
(1) Insert prongs into both nares with concave surface against nares. (NOTE: Trim prongs that are too long with scissors.)	Conforms to normal shape and directs flow up into nasopharynx. Prevents pressure on nasal mucosa.
(2) Arrange tubing over ears and adjust ring under chin or apply elastic band around head.	Holds cannula in place.
(3) Secure tubing to clothing or bed linen. (NOTE: Inspect condition of nares every 3 to 4 hours and change cannula at least every 8 hours.)	Prevents pulling on cannula.
b. Nasal catheter	
(1) Measure distance from bridge or tip of nose to tip of ear lobe with catheter and mark with tape.	Provides gauge for length of catheter to be inserted into nasopharynx.
(2) Place a thin film of water-soluble jelly on tip of catheter, avoid plugging holes in distal end of tube.	Facilitates catheter insertion.

(continued)

ADMINISTERING OXYGEN BY NASAL CANNULA, CATHETER, AND MASK (Cont.)

Step	Rationale
(3) Hold catheter so natural curve corresponds with normal curvature of nasal cavity. Use nondominant hand to raise tip of nose while inserting catheter into nares along floor of nose until desired length is reached.	Facilitates catheter insertion.
(4) Hold catheter in place and have client open mouth; depress tongue with tongue blade. Use a flashlight to locate tip of catheter at level of uvula; adjust by withdrawing or inserting farther.	Catheter tip should be just out of sight behind the tip of the uvula to prevent drying and irritation of nasopharynx or inflation of stomach with oxygen.
(5) Secure catheter with a narrow strip of nonallergenic tape to bridge of nose or mandible area of face.	Prevents catheter from dislodging.
(6) Secure connecting tube to client's gown or to bed linen.	Prevents pulling on cannula.
(NOTE: Inspect condition of nares every 3 to 4 hours and change cannula at least every 8 hours.	Reduces irritation of mucous membranes.
Alternate nostrils at least every 8 hours if possible. Use moist applicators to cleanse nasal cavity.)	Removes secretions.
c. Face mask	
(1) Hold mask close to client's face for a few seconds before applying.	Feeling flow of oxygen allays client's anxiety.
(2) Place mask over client's nose and mouth, then wrap elastic band around back of head.	
(3) Adjust mask to fit facial shape. Use small gauze pads if necessary to fill in gaps between mask and skin.	Snug fit required to prevent loss of oxygen.
(4) Secure tubing to client's gown or bed linen.	Prevents pulling on cannula.
(NOTE: Remove mask and cleanse client's face and nostrils; use damp cloth to clean mask at least every 8 hours.)	Removes accumulated perspiration and prevents skin irritation.
When using mask with reservoir bag or venturi-type mask: position client, clothing, and linen so that function of bag or venturi component is not hampered.	Kinks in the bag or occlusion of the venturi ports, or blocking the connecting tube with water, prevent the client from inspiring the prescribed O_2 concentration.
Position connecting tubing to avoid dependent loops in which condensation from the humidifier is apt to accumulate.	Permits full flow of oxygen.
10. Record time, type of delivery system and flow rate, effects of therapy on health record.	Provides data for nursing care and demonstrates accountability for nursing actions.

Tent Administration

Placing a client in an oxygen tent can be done most efficiently by two persons. First, prepare the bed by placing a cotton bath blanket over the plastic mattress cover to prevent the potential for static electricity caused by the movement of the linen over the plastic. Cover the blanket with a regular sheet and place an additional bath blanket over the sheet. The second blanket helps to absorb perspiration if the client is febrile and keeps the client more comfortable. To prepare the tent, position it near the head of the bed, plug it into the electrical outlet, and connect the oxygen. Turn the oxygen on at maximum flow and reach inside the tent to check the patency of the oxygen and exhaust outlets and then set the thermostat control to the desired temperature setting. Close all of the side openings, gather the lower border of the canopy together, tie it with a cord and allow the canopy to fill with oxygen for about 5 minutes. Open the canopy and place it over the client and begin to tuck the edge of the canopy under the mattress first at the head of the bed, then the sides, and finally the foot (if it is to cover the entire client). Be sure to tuck in as much tent as possible to prevent leaks. When an adult is to be enclosed only from the waist up, place a lengthwise folded sheet across the client's hip or thigh area and place the edge of the canopy within the fold. Fold the sheet and canopy upon itself and tuck the ends under the mattress. This helps to seal off the lower border of the canopy. Reduce the oxygen flow to the prescribed rate and check the client to ensure that there are no drafts blowing directly on the head or shoulders. During the first hour of therapy, check the client and the temperature inside the canopy at frequent intervals to be sure that the desired temperature is achieved and that the client is comfortable. Some clients may want a blanket or towel around the shoulders and chest for additional warmth. As with other methods of oxygen therapy, the flow rate and equipment and the client's status need to be carefully monitored at least every 3 to 4 hours (Rarey, 1980).

Provide the client with a clapper bell in lieu of the electric signal light. Noncritically ill clients may enjoy having some personal items in the tent with them to provide some distraction from the isolation. Children may feel more secure with a favorite toy and adults may enjoy reading material or playing cards. Do not permit the client to have items that have a potential for producing static electricity. Plan nursing care for a client in an oxygen tent carefully so it can be carried out in an efficient manner, preventing unnecessary loss of oxygen from the tent. When changing bed linen, it is easier to keep the tent tucked around the client if two people work together from the opposite sides of the bed.

Clients who are confined in a tent may eat their meals while remaining in the tent. If clients require feeding, they may be fed or assisted through the side openings. Sometimes, however, a therapeutic oxygen level is more easily maintained by removing the tent and using a nasal cannula during meals.

RECORDING

All aspects of oxygen therapy are fully documented on the client's health record. This includes the time and type of therapy, the rate of flow or concentration, and the client's positive or negative responses to the therapy. If arterial blood gas analyses are performed, the results may be recorded on a flow sheet that also has space for the oxygen flow rate or concentration used at the time the blood sample was obtained. Since these records permit the physician to evaluate the effects of the therapy and the client's response to specific oxygen concentrations, it is important that they are kept accurately and include the date and specific time of each entry. The flow sheet may also make provision for including brief notes about the client's response to therapy.

Sample POR Recording

- S—"I don't like this tube in my nose, but I can breathe easier now."
- O—More relaxed and less dyspneic; respirations 24, pulse 120 with O_2 by nasal catheter at 3 L per minute.
- A—Responding well to oxygen.
- P—Continue to monitor response.

Sample Narrative Recording

Doesn't like nasal catheter but admits to some relief of dyspnea with oxygen flow at 3 L per minute. More relaxed, less dyspneic, R-44, P-120. Will continue to monitor response.

☐ CRITICAL POINTS SUMMARY

1. The earliest signs of acute hypoxia are revealed by changes in the client's mental–emotional status.
2. Cyanosis is an unreliable sign of hypoxia.
3. A safe environment for oxygen therapy requires the elimination of all fire hazards and items that have potential for producing sparks.
4. Adequate humidification and fluid intake are needed to prevent dehydration during oxygen therapy.
5. Oxygen has the potential for causing absorption atelectasis, hypoventilation, damage to lung tissue, and blindness in infants when administered at concentrations higher than the client can safely tolerate.
6. Prepare oxygen cylinders with caution to prevent accidents and damage to the valve outlet.
7. Low flow oxygen systems provide a variable concentration of oxygen.
8. High flow oxygen systems provide a fixed oxygen concentration.
9. Whenever possible, place clients receiving oxygen therapy in a semi-Fowler's position.
10. Periodic deep breathing, coughing, and position change facilitate alveolar gas exchange and prevent respiratory complications.
11. Use medically aseptic technique when handling all oxygen delivery equipment.
12. Change wet components of the delivery system at least every 8 hours.
13. Prevent skin irritation and excessive dryness of the mucous membranes by providing frequent care.
14. Use padding under snug masks and elastic bands to prevent pressure areas on the skin.

☐ LEARNING ACTIVITIES

1. Visit the Respiratory Therapy department or central supply department and look at the different types of equipment used to administer oxygen therapy.
2. Observe a respiratory therapist who is setting up oxygen therapy and instructing a client on its use.
3. Interview clients who have had different types of oxygen therapy to learn about their positive and negative experiences.
4. Find out from the nursing or the engineering staff where the zone area shut-offs for the central oxygen system are located on the clinical unit.

☐ REVIEW QUESTIONS

1. For what reasons is oxygen therapy administered?
2. Match the type of hypoxia listed in Column I with the correct signs and symptoms listed in Column II.

COLUMN I	COLUMN II
A. Acute hypoxia	____ Increased hemoglobin level
B. Chronic hypoxia	____ Headache
	____ Restlessness
	____ Drowsiness
	____ Right ventricular hypertrophy

3. What are some of the static electricity-producing items that you would remove when using oxygen so as to ensure a safe environment?
4. Name three of the physiological hazards to which a client is exposed when oxygen is administered.
5. Why does a client with chronic obstructive lung disease need to have a low concentration of oxygen delivery?
6. What information does a nurse collect from the client's health record before administering oxygen?
7. What data does a nurse collect by using physical appraisal skills prior to and during the use of oxygen?
8. Why does oxygen need to be humidified before it enters the client's respiratory system?
9. What are some of the advantages and disadvantages of each of the following oxygen delivery systems? Nasal cannula, nasal catheter, face mask, and tent.
10. What precautions do you need to observe when administering oxygen with a nonbreathing and a venturi-type mask?
11. How would you prepare a client to receive oxygen?
12. What would you do to prepare both a wall and cylinder oxygen supply system for administering oxygen?
13. How can you be sure that oxygen is flowing through a delivery device before applying the device to the client?
14. How would you describe to a peer the way to insert a nasal catheter?
15. What can you do to prevent skin irritation from pressure applied by a nasal cannula, catheter, and face mask?
16. How would you describe to a peer the way to place a client in an oxygen tent?

☐ PERFORMANCE CHECKLIST

OBJECTIVE: To use the appropriate method to administer oxygen safely.

CHARACTERISTIC	RANGE OF ACCEPTABILITY	SATISFACTORY	UNSATISFACTORY
1. Checks physician's order or nursing kardex.	No deviation		
2. Washes hands.	No deviation		
3. Prepares equipment.	No deviation		
4. Explains procedure and places client in semi-Fowler's position.	Omit if contraindicated.		
5. Fills humidifier.	No deviation		
6. Attaches flow meter, connects tubing and delivery system, and checks for O_2 flow.	No deviation		
7a. To apply nasal cannula: (1) Inserts cannula into the nares with concave surface against nares.	No deviation		
(2) Arranges tubing over ears and adjusts ring under chin or applies elastic band around head.	No deviation		
(3) Secures tubing to client's gown or bed linen.	No deviation		
7b. To apply nasal catheter: (1) Measures distance and marks catheter.	No deviation		
(2) Lubricates catheter with thin film of water-soluble lubricant.	No deviation		
(3) Inserts catheter by raising tip of nose following natural curves until desired length is reached.	No deviation		
(4) Checks for position at level of uvula using tongue depressor and flashlight. Adjusts if necessary.	No deviation		

(continued)

CHARACTERISTIC	RANGE OF ACCEPTABILITY	SATISFACTORY	UNSATISFACTORY
(5) Secures catheter to face or nose with tape.	No deviation		
(6) Secures tubing to client's gown or bed linen.	No deviation		
7c. To apply face mask: (1) Holds mask over client's face before applying over nose and mouth; wraps elastic band around head.	No deviation		
(2) Adjusts and fits mask with gauze pads if necessary.	No deviation		
(3) Positions connecting tubing to prevent dependent loops.	No deviation		
8. Records time, type of delivery system, flow rate, and effects of therapy on health record.	No deviation		

REFERENCES

Administering oxygen safely: When, why, how. Nursing80 (Horsham) 10(10):54–56, 1980.

Frownfelter DL: Chest Physical Therapy and Pulmonary Rehabilitation. Chicago, Year Book Medical Publishers, 1978.

Fuchs PL: Getting the best out of the oxygen delivery systems. Nursing80 10(12):34–43, 1980.

Harper RW: A Guide to Respiratory Care: Physiology and Clinical Applications. Philadelphia, JB Lippincott, 1981.

Luckmann J, Sorensen K: Medical–Surgical Nursing: A Psychophysiological Approach, ed 2. Philadelphia, WB Saunders, 1980.

McPherson S: Respiratory Therapy Equipment, ed 2. St Louis, CV Mosby, 1981.

Rarey KP, Youtsey JM: Respiratory Patient Care. Englewood Cliffs, NJ, Prentice-Hall, 1981.

Traver GA (ed): Respiratory Nursing: The Science and Art. New York, John Wiley & Sons, 1982.

BIBLIOGRAPHY

Glover DW, Glover M: Respiratory Therapy. St Louis, CV Mosby, 1978.

Shapiro BA, Harrison RA, et al.: Clinical Application of Respiratory Care, ed 2. Chicago, Year Book Medical Publishers, 1979.

Stanley L: You can really teach COPD patients to breathe better. RN 41(4):43–49, 1978.

Wade JF: Comprehensive Respiratory Care: Physiology and Technique. St Louis, CV Mosby, 1982.

AUDIOVISUAL RESOURCE

Oxygen Administration
Filmstrip and cassette. (1976, Color, 20 min.)
Available through:
Medcom, Inc.
P.O. Box 116
Garden Grove, CA 92642

SKILL 69 Tracheostomy Care

PREREQUISITE SKILLS

Skill 19, "Inspection"
Skill 20, "Palpation"
Skill 22, "Auscultation"
Skill 28, "Handwashing"
Skill 30, "Sterile Supplies"
Skill 31, "Donning Sterile Gloves"
Skill 32, "Dressings and Wound Care"
Skill 40, "Oral Care"
Skill 67, "Chest Therapy Exercises"

☐ STUDENT OBJECTIVES

1. Describe a tracheostomy.
2. Describe reasons why a tracheostomy is performed.
3. Indicate the disadvantages of a tracheostomy.
4. Differentiate among the signs and symptoms associated with each type of complication that can result from a tracheostomy.
5. Specify the components of the physiological aspects of care for a client with a tracheostomy.

6. Specify the components of the psychological aspects of care for a client with a tracheostomy.
7. Describe data the nurse collects from the health record prior to giving care to a client with a tracheostomy.
8. Indicate the data the nurse obtains with physical appraisal skills.
9. Differentiate among the different types of tracheostomy tubes.
10. Specify the equipment that must be kept available at the bedside at all times when a client has a tracheostomy.
11. Describe the precautions that need to be observed when removing, cleaning, and reinserting an inner cannula of a tracheostomy tube.
12. Describe the precautions that must be observed when providing wound care and changing tracheostomy neck ties.
13. Demonstrate the ability to provide tracheostomy care safely.
14. Demonstrate the ability to change a permanent tracheostomy tube.

INTRODUCTION

Tracheostomy care is required by clients who have a surgically created opening in the trachea (tracheotomy) into which a tracheostomy tube is inserted to maintain a patent airway. The complete care of a tracheostomy includes keeping the airway patent by suctioning to remove secretions, cleansing the tube, preventing complications of the respiratory tract, and wound care to the incision and stoma. Since suctioning the airway is an intervention that is also used with clients other than those with a tracheostomy, it is presented as a separate entity in Skill 70.

Many aspects of the care and the observations required for the client with a new tracheostomy are the same as those that are used after the immediate postoperative period. The focus of this skill, however, is on the care provided to a client on the regular clinical unit, since a client with a new tracheostomy requires continuous monitoring and is usually kept in an intensive care unit for the first 24 to 48 hours after surgery.

A tracheostomy is one method used to maintain an artificial patent airway. The other method is endotracheal intubation, in which a tube is inserted through the nose or mouth into the trachea. A tracheostomy is used when an artificial airway is used for a prolonged period of time; if an endotracheal tube is contraindicated either because of trauma to the tissues, as may occur with burns, or because of a laryngeal obstruction such as a tumor or edema; or when a conscious client is unable to tolerate an endotracheal tube. Although there is a higher risk of infection with a tracheostomy, it is often selected as a method for maintaining a patent airway over the option of an endotracheal tube because it is more comfortable, allows the client to take food and fluids by mouth, and permits the client to communicate verbally to some extent.

The specific reasons for a tracheostomy are to:

1. Relieve upper airway obstructions in the respiratory tract that are due to conditions such as tumors, edema, or burns.
2. Provide an open airway for clients who require an artificial airway for a prolonged period of time.
3. Provide an alternate route to remove secretions from the trachea and bronchi when chest therapy exercises or intubation are not effective.
4. Prevent aspiration of secretions such as food or vomitus from the pharynx into the lower respiratory tract.
5. Provide a route for mechanical ventilation.

A tracheostomy may be performed either as an emergency or elective procedure. It is done as an emergency procedure when an insurmountable obstruction prevents adequate gas exchange. As an elective procedure, it may be done for the client's comfort, to facilitate nutritional intake, or to reduce the dead space in the respiratory tract and to lessen the work of breathing as well as to facilitate the removal of secretions. Depending on the purpose and the condition of the client, the tracheostomy may be either temporary or permanent. A temporary tracheostomy is closed after the client has been taught how to resume breathing through the upper respiratory tract. A permanent tracheostomy is commonly used with clients who have had a laryngectomy performed for removal of a carcinoma of the larynx. These clients must be taught how to care for the artificial airway before discharge from the hospital.

PREPARATION

To understand some of the problems that can occur with a tracheostomy and have a basis on which to relate aspects of care, the nurse should have some knowledge of how a tracheostomy is performed.

THE TRACHEOSTOMY PROCEDURE

A tracheostomy is performed with the patient in a high semi-Fowler's position and the neck hyperextended to provide good access to the trachea. An incision is made in the midline of the trachea below the larynx and through the second and third tracheal rings, unless an obstruction dictates a lower site. An oval window of tracheal tissue is removed and a tracheostomy tube is inserted. If the tracheostomy is to be permanent, the margins of the tracheal opening are sutured to the skin so that a permanent stoma is formed. Otherwise the skin is loosely sutured together around the tube. A small dressing is applied between the tube and the skin to prevent irritation of the skin

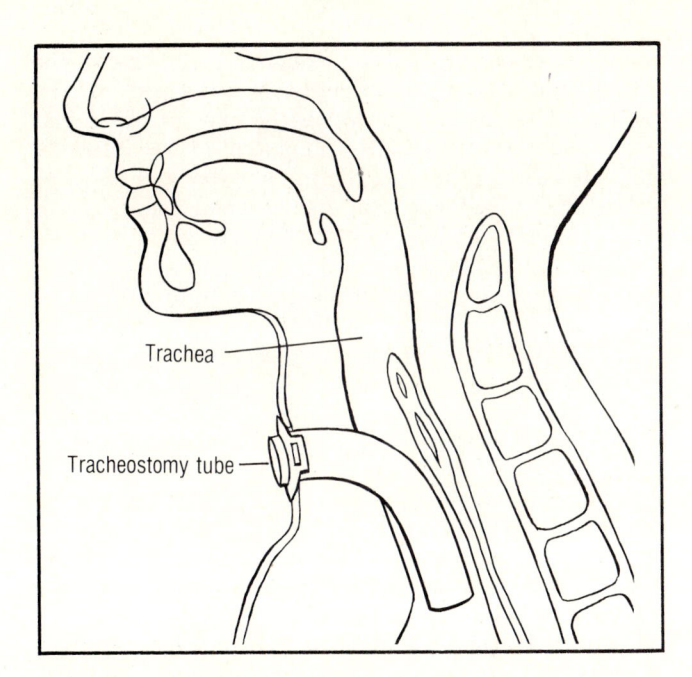

Figure 69-1. Correct placement of the tracheostomy tube.

from the tube and to protect the fresh incision. The tube is held in place by a pair of ties attached to each side of the tracheostomy tube flange and tied around the client's neck.

The selection of the tracheostomy tube size is an important consideration. The tube must not only have a diameter that permits ventilation, but it must be of proper length so that it lies above the bifurcation of the bronchi and it must have a curvature that approximates that of the normal contour of the client's trachea and neck as shown in Figure 69-1. Tubes that do not fit properly interfere with adequate ventilation and can cause serious tissue damage to the trachea. Tracheostomy tubes are available in both metal or synthetic materials and consist of single or double cannula. Double-cannula tubes permit the removal of the inner tube for cleaning. Some tracheostomy tubes are also designed with a balloon cuff that can be inflated in the trachea to provide a closed system within the lungs when mechanical ventilation is necessary. A more in-depth description of tracheostomy tubes is presented in the equipment section.

ADVERSE EFFECTS OF A TRACHEOSTOMY

Disadvantages of a Tracheostomy

There are three inherent disadvantages with the use of a tracheostomy that the nurse needs to be aware of because of the implications they have for affecting a client's normal function. First, the normal protective cough mechanism is impaired because of the inability to close the glottis tightly; this prevents the necessary increase in intrathoracic pressure essential for an effective cough. The loss of this ability makes it difficult for the client to clear foreign particles and material from the lungs. Second, inspired air bypasses the upper airway structures of the nose and pharynx, thus removing the filtering, warming, and humidification of inspired air. Third, the client also loses the ability to speak normally because the tracheostomy lies below the pharynx and there is inadequate air pressure within the larynx to permit the vocal cords to function properly.

Complications of a Tracheostomy

There are several complications that require direct intervention or prompt notification of the physician.

Emphysema (air in the tissues) can occur in the subcutaneous or mediastinal tissues either because of an accidental laceration of the pleural domes during the surgery or because the sutures in the incision are too numerous or too tight. These conditions cause a negative intrathoracic pressure that forces air from the lungs into the tissues. Crepitus, which is air in the subcutaneous tissues, may be detected by palpating around the tube to feel the gas bubbles in the tissues and by listening for the fine crackling sound of those bubbles during palpation. The gas bubbles feel like small nodules that move freely when the tissue is pressed (DeGowin and DeGowin, 1981). When the cause of the emphysema is due to sutures, it is corrected when the surgeon removes or loosens the sutures. Figure 69-2 shows subcutaneous emphysema.

Hemorrhage at the incisional site or from within the tracheobronchial tree is an additional concern. Moderate serosanguinous drainage from the incision is to be expected for the first 2 to 3 postoperative days. However, frank blood or persistent serosanguinous drainage is abnormal because it may be from a small blood vessel that has been opened by vigorous cough-

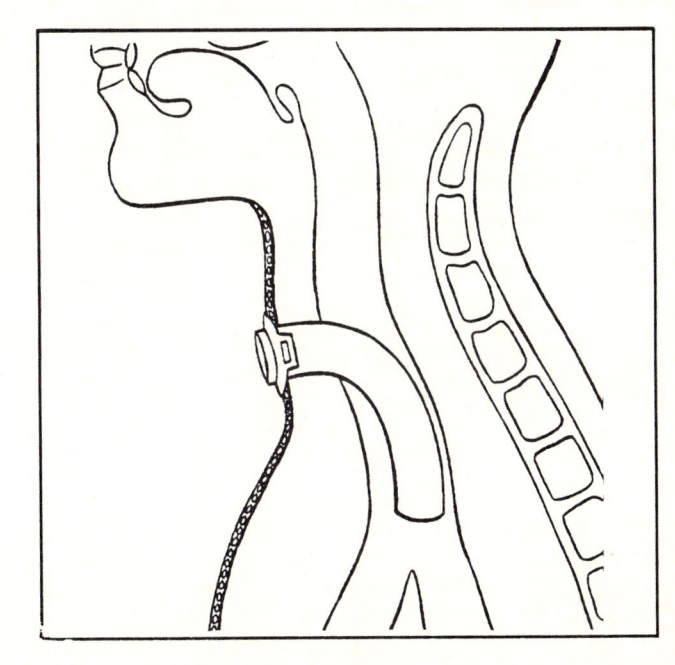

Figure 69-2. Subcutaneous emphysema in the tissues above and below the tracheostomy tube.

ing. Blood mixed with the secretions that come from the tracheostomy tube is normal during the first 8 hours following surgery. However, blood appearing after this period is abnormal and may be due to erosion through the anterior wall of the trachea to the innominate artery, caused by an improperly positioned tube. Any abnormal bleeding must be reported to the physician immediately.

Respiratory insufficiency can result from obstructions in the airway, either within the tracheostomy tube or below it. Accumulated secretions in the tube can partially or completely block the tube, and edema of the mucous membrane lining of the tracheobronchial tree, foreign bodies, or excessive secretions can occlude the airway below the tube. The signs that are indicative of respiratory insufficiency are unequal movement of both sides of the chest during respiration, marked effort during inspiration, and retraction of the accessory muscles in the supraclavicular, intercostal, and substernal areas during inspiration.

Partial or complete *expulsion of the tube* can occur accidentally. This is not a common occurrence but can happen if the ties are not secured with a square knot which cannot slip, if the ties are too loose around the neck, or if adequate precautions are not observed when the ties are changed. Even partial expulsion of the tube is considered an emergency because the airway may become completely occluded. The client with a partial occlusion can manifest the same signs of respiratory insufficiency described above. The client with complete obstruction will be apneic and become cyanotic rapidly.

A *tracheoesophageal fistula* can be caused by erosion of the posterior wall of the trachea to the esophagus by a tube that is not the proper length or curvature. This problem is manifested by coughing or choking while eating or drinking or by leaking or aspiration of food or liquids from the tracheostomy.

Inflammation or infection of the incision can occur from contamination of the wound by tracheobronchial secretions. The warm moist environment that may be present around the wound is conducive to the growth of organisms. Frequent inspection of the wound is essential to detect early signs of inflammation. Measures to reduce the potential for infection include keeping the wound clean and dry and frequent dressing changes with the use of good aseptic technique. Clients are also vulnerable to pulmonary infections and atelectasis because the loss or weakening of an effective cough enhances the accumulation and pooling of secretions in the lungs.

The *placement of the tracheostomy tube* is important for proper ventilation and the prevention of complications. As mentioned above, the tracheostomy tube size must be of an appropriate length and curvature. Correct placement of the distal tip of the tube is 5 cm (2 in) above the carina (ridge) that separates the right and left main bronchi at their junction with the trachea (Traver, 1982). X-ray can be used to determine the specific location of the tube. If the tube becomes displaced into a bronchus, the lung served by that bronchus can collapse due to mucus plugging and pneumonia can result. There are clues that the nurse can be alert for that indicate incorrect placement of the tube. These include: depressed or absent breath sounds in either the left lung or the upper right lobe or both; decreased excursion of the left chest during inspiration; and the inability to pass a suction catheter beyond the tip of the tracheostomy tube, which can mean that the tip of the tube is on or just above the carina. Figures 69–3A and B show some examples of tube displacement.

NURSING CARE FOR THE CLIENT WITH A TRACHEOSTOMY

A tracheostomy is a client's lifeline. It is therefore important that the nurse realize that in addition to using a number of technical skills, a great deal of clinical judgment is required. Nursing care must address both physiological and psychological needs of the client.

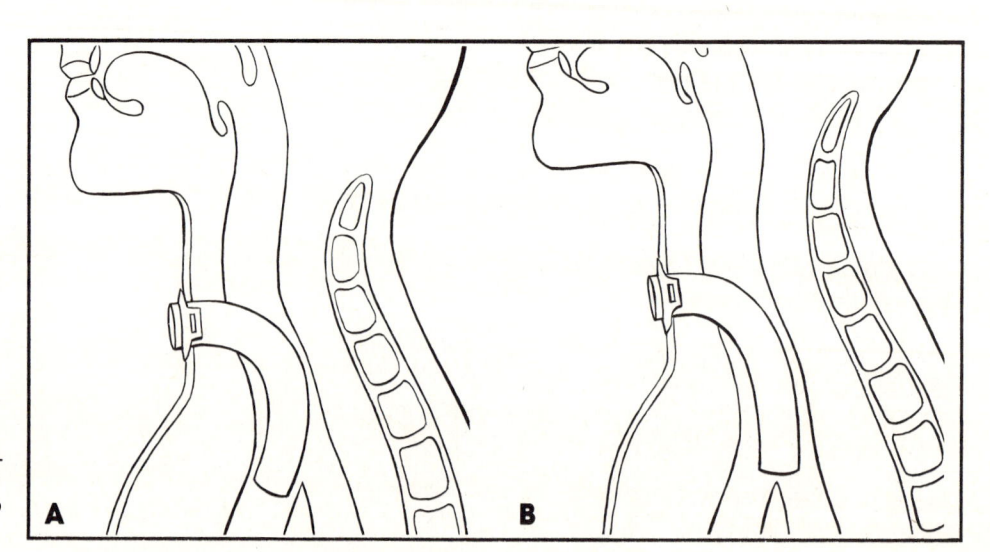

Figure 69–3. Tracheostomy tube displacement. **A.** Cannula in the right mainstem bronchus. **B.** Cannula too close to the carina.

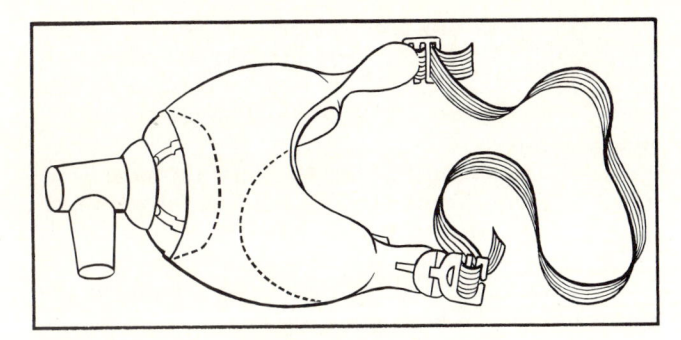

Figure 69-4. A tracheostomy mask used for humidification.

Physiological Aspects of Care

Humidification of inspired air is essential to prevent damage to the tracheal mucous blanket and drying of the tracheal secretions. Heated humidifiers can provide 100 percent of the needed humidity and enough hydration to prevent drying and crusting of the secretions (Traver, 1982). Humidity is provided either through a mask (Fig. 69-4) which is placed over the tracheostomy or through oxygen therapy if the client requires it. In the event that no humidity is prescribed by the physician, the nurse can provide humidity by keeping a gauze square moistened with sterile distilled water or saline over the tracheostomy.

A daily *fluid intake* of 3000 to 4000 ml will keep the pulmonary secretions liquid enough for removal either by coughing or suctioning. To achieve this volume, increase the fluids offered at and between meals. Clients who are unable to ingest orally an adequate fluid volume often require intravenous fluids. Careful monitoring of the client's intake and output is done at least once every 8 hours.

The amount of *nutrients and calories* provided must be adequate to meet the requirements for proper cellular function, tissue repair, and energy. This can be a real problem for the client because some dysfunction of the swallowing mechanisms may occur as a result of the presence of the tracheostomy tube. There is a danger that orally ingested food and fluids may be aspirated into the lungs. When a client takes oral nutrition and fluids it is important that the client be observed carefully for evidence of aspiration. This may be noted by the client coughing or choking while eating or by the appearance of the food or liquids through the tracheostomy. Often a client is able to swallow solid food easier than liquids. However, when there is a doubt about the ability to swallow effectively, the physician may order that the client drink a dilute solution of methylene blue dye before each meal and that the nurse observe for the appearance of the dye through the tracheal secretions (Harper, 1981). Clients who are unable to take fluids and nourishment by mouth may be fed either through a nasogastric or gastrostomy tube (Skill 54).

In addition to the potential for contamination of the lower respiratory tract from fluids or food, there are other sources of contamination. Personnel and equipment that come in contact with the tracheostomy can harbor organisms that produce nosocomial infections. Since clients with a tracheostomy are particularly vulnerable to respiratory infection, it is extremely important that strict aseptic technique is used at all times. *Handwashing* and the *use of either medical or surgical aseptic technique* when directly contacting the tracheostomy tube and dressing are essential.

Dry oral mucous membranes provide another source of infection. Frequent *oral care* is necessary to prevent infections and halitosis. Clients who are unable to take oral nourishment are particularly vulnerable to oral-cavity problems.

As with any other type of respiratory system problem, the client's *position must be changed* frequently to prevent pooling of secretions in the lungs. To permit full lung expansion, place the client in the semi-Fowler's position at frequent intervals and assist him or her to perform *chest therapy exercises* such as deep breathing and coughing as often as required to keep respiratory function at its maximum. To cough effectively, it may be necessary to occlude the opening in the tracheostomy immediately prior to the expiratory phase of the cough so that adequate intrathoracic pressure can be attained.

Psychological Aspects of Care

A client with a tracheostomy is apt to be *apprehensive* about the ability to breathe and fearful of choking. It is therefore important that the nurse be sensitive to the client's concerns and provide frequent reassurance. Careful explanations of procedures before they are executed help the client know what to expect. Working in a careful and competent manner also helps the client to feel secure in knowing that he or she will be taken care of properly. Having equipment ready at all times and anticipating the client's needs are integral parts of nursing care. A major difficulty that the client has is an *inability to communicate verbally* to make needs known. This occurs because expired air bypasses the larynx and vocal cords and the client is unable to speak or whisper. Whenever possible, plan for alternate means of communication before the client has surgery. Some of the methods that are used include a magic slate or pad and pencil for writing out messages, an alphabet board can be used so that the client can spell out words in the event that writing is not possible, or some form of sign language communication. When these methods are not suitable the nurse can request that the client nod or blink the eyes to give yes or no responses to questions. After having adapted somewhat to the tracheostomy, a client is able to speak a few words by placing a finger over the airway during expiration. This permits air pressure to increase within the larynx so that sound can be created.

Analgesics, sedatives, and tranquilizers must be used with extreme caution because they depress the respiratory center. Since there is very little pain normally felt with a tracheostomy, frequent use of analgesics is usually not necessary. A nurse can help reduce a client's anxiety and minimize the need for drugs by making frequent contact, providing reassurance, keeping the call signal readily available, and by anticipating and responding quickly to the client's needs.

DATA BASE

Client History and Recorded Data

Prior to caring for a client with a tracheostomy, the nurse needs to know the medical diagnosis, why and when the procedure was performed, whether it was an emergency or elective procedure, and if it is temporary or permanent. The nurse also needs to know the type and size of the tube that is in place. If the tube has a cuff, the method and amount of inflation should be specified on the record. Single-cannulated tubes are normally changed by the physician, and the date and time of changes are recorded on the health record. In addition, it is important to know how the client is coping with having a tracheostomy, the frequency of care required for the tube and the wound, if humidification and oxygen therapy are prescribed, and if so, the types and amounts to be administered. Orders for medications and oral intake and the client's response to the treatment regime must also be reviewed. The pattern of recorded temperature, pulse, and respirations provides important data about a client's respiratory status and can alert the nurse to early indications of an infection. Since the respiratory status of a client with a tracheostomy can change rapidly, it is essential that the nurse not rely only on the recorded data but conduct frequent evaluations.

Physical Appraisal Skills

Inspection. The condition of the wound and dressing, the presence and character of secretions and crustations in and around the tube, and signs of respiratory distress or hypoxia are appraised by inspection. Inspection is equally important in the appraisal of the client's coping ability and responses to all interventions. Expressions of concern or anxiety may be manifest only by nonverbal communication since the client is unable to speak normally.

Palpation. Light palpation of the tissues around the tracheostomy is used to detect the presence of crepitus.

Auscultation. The quality of breath sounds is determined by auscultation with or without the use of a stethoscope.

EQUIPMENT

Tracheostomy tubes are made of either a metal or synthetic material such as nylon, silicone, or polyvinyl chloride. They are available in different lengths, diameters, and curvatures. *Metal tubes* are made of silver because this metal is nontoxic and does not react with tissue. Silver tubes are often used for permanent tracheostomies; however, they cannot be used with clients who are receiving radiation therapy. Since silver is a soft metal, it must be handled carefully to prevent it from denting. Dents may interfere with insertion or proper fit and sharp edges can injure the trachea. *Synthetic tubes* are disposable and lighter weight than metal tubes. They tend to soften at body temperature and conform to the normal contour of the trachea.

Tracheostomy tubes are designed with both a single or double cannula. Double-cannulated tubes consist of an inner and an outer set of tubes which permit the removal of the inner cannula for cleaning. Double-cannulated tubes may have a duplicate inner cannula that can be inserted as a replacement for the one that has been removed for cleaning. Metal tubes are double-cannulated. Synthetic tubes are available in both single- and double-cannulated models and may include an inflatable cuff.

An *obturator* fits inside and extends beyond the tip of the outer cannula. It occludes the outer cannula and is used to guide the tube through the tracheostomy when it is inserted. The obturator is then removed and is replaced by the inner cannula when a double-cannula tube is used. The inner cannula is held securely in place by a locking device and is removed only for cleaning or suctioning. Once the obturator has been used during surgery for insertion of the outer cannula, it is cleaned and sterilized and kept at the client's bedside for immediate use in the event that the tracheostomy tube is expulsed and must be reinserted. Since the parts of a tracheostomy set are not interchangeable with other sets, it is vital that parts be clearly labeled and kept together.

Figure 69–5 shows examples of metal and synthetic tracheostomy tubes. *Cuffed tubes* have an elastic balloon sleeve that encircles the distal part of the outer cannula. A small-caliber elastic tube runs from the center of the cuff along the outer cannula to the outside of the client's tracheostomy. A small test balloon located on the tubing serves as a guide for proper inflation. A cuff is inflated to prevent air from escaping from or entering the upper respiratory tract. The cuff is inflated with a *syringe* containing a prescribed amount of air or fluid and then clamped with a rubber-covered *hemostat*. The rubber protects the cuff tubing from damage. Cuffed tubes are used to prevent an unconscious client from aspirating secretions, to exert pressure on bleeding points in clients who have had surgery on the neck or throat, and to maintain the closed system that is required for clients who are mechanically ventilated. Discussion of mechanical ventilation is beyond the scope of this text.

Umbilical tape is a lightweight ¾-inch cotton twill tape. It is attached to both sides of the flange on the outer cannula and then tied around the client's neck to hold the tracheostomy tube in place.

Tracheostomy care equipment is available in

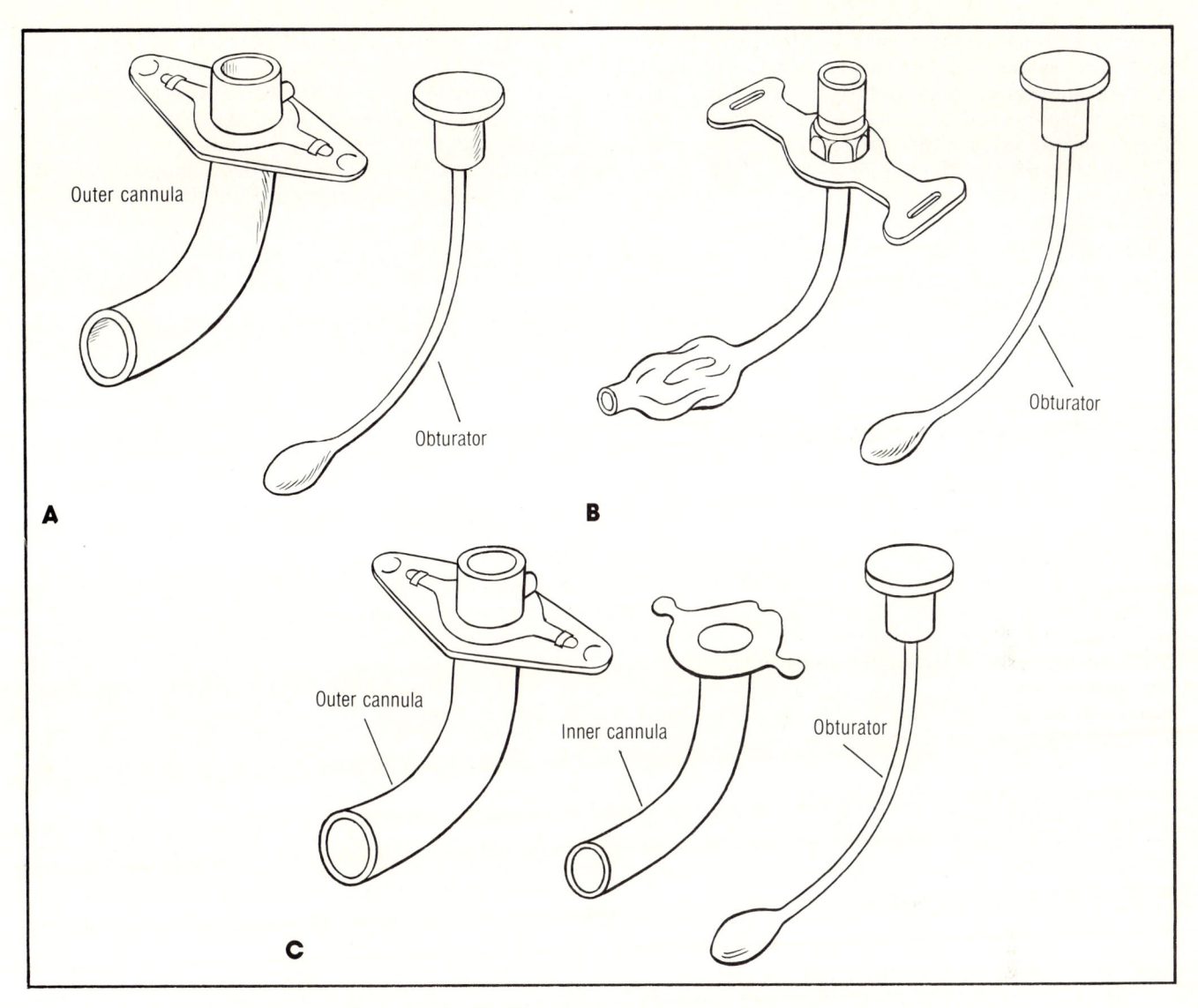

Figure 69-5. Tracheostomy tube sets. **A.** Single-cannula tube and obturator. **B.** Single-cannula cuffed tube and obturator. **C.** Double-cannula tube, inner cannula, and obturator.

commercially prepared disposable single-use kits or it may be assembled from items obtained from central supply. *Pipe cleaners* and a *small test-tube brush* are used to clean the inner cannula. *Sterile disposable gloves* are worn when implementing surgical aseptic technique. *Hydrogen peroxide* or a *liquid detergent* solution is used to cleanse the inner cannula and *sterile distilled water* or *normal saline* is used for rinsing the cannula and cleansing the wound. *Isopropyl alcohol (70 percent)* may be used if it is necessary to sterilize the inner cannula before it is replaced in the client. Another option for sterilizing the cannula is to immerse it in boiling water for 3 to 5 minutes. *Three bowls or basins* are used to hold the cleaning and rinsing solutions. *Sterile unfilled gauze 4 × 4 squares* are used to hold the inner cannula and to dress the wound. When surgical aseptic technique is used, sterile scissors are used to cut the wound dressing halfway down the center. In commercially prepared kits the gauze square for the wound dressing may be already split halfway down the middle and have the edges sewn to prevent raveled threads from adhering to the wound or falling into the trachea. *Scissors* with blunt tips must be kept at the bedside at all times to cut the umbilical tapes in the event that they become too tight, as well as to prepare them for changing. A *small sterile forceps* is required to handle the sterile gauze squares and to retrieve the sterilized inner cannula from the alcohol or boiling water. A *sterile drape* is used for a sterile field on which to lay out the equipment and supplies. *Silver polish* may be used occasionally to polish a silver tube after it is cleaned and before it is sterilized.

The equipment used to suction the tracheostomy is described in Skill 70.

Additional sterile instruments that need to be kept at the bedside for emergency use as well as for scheduled tube changes include a *tracheal dilator*, which is a smooth curved forceps with blunt rounded tips; and two tracheal hooks that are, as the name implies, instruments with a hook on the tip. These instruments are used to open a collapsed trachea and to gain access to it for tube insertion.

Most institutions have a policy that an extra tracheostomy kit of the same size the client has in place be kept at the bedside at all times in addition to the equipment and supplies needed for routine tracheostomy care.

☐ EXECUTION

Even though the tracheostomy tube and the client's airway are not sterile, the use of either surgical or medical aseptic technique is essential to prevent nosocomial infections. The selection of surgical versus medical aseptic technique depends upon how new the tracheostomy is; whether the tracheostomy is temporary or permanent; the nature of the microorganisms in the immediate environment; and the vulnerability of the client to nosocomial infections. Most institutions have a policy that surgical aseptic technique be used for all clients for at least the first 72 hours after surgery. To maintain sterile aseptic technique when providing complete tracheostomy care, it may be necessary to change sterile gloves several times if they become contaminated. Medical aseptic technique is implemented with sterile equipment and supplies to eliminate the potential of transferring organisms from the environment to the client's respiratory tract. Medical aseptic technique is used most often with clients who have a permanent tracheostomy because these clients are going to be living in a normal environment and it is believed that they are able to adapt to the organisms present in that environment without acquiring a nosocomial infection.

Whether you are implementing surgical or medical aseptic technique, label the bottles of sterile distilled water or normal saline with the date and time they are opened so they can be discarded at the end of a 24-hour period. This is important even when using medical asepsis, because the solution provides a medium for the growth of microorganisms. Discard solutions that are known to be contaminated. There are two reasons why tap water is usually not recommended for cleansing the tracheostomy tube. Tap water often has a high bacterial count with a potential for harboring pathogenic microorganisms and it may have a high concentration of minerals. It is difficult to remove secretions from the inner cannula with hard water (water with a high mineral content). Since minerals become concentrated when the water is boiled, they can accumulate on the equipment.

At all times, a complete set of equipment for cleansing the tube, suctioning the airway, providing wound care, and changing the tapes must be available at the bedside.

CLEANING THE TRACHEOSTOMY TUBE

Clean a tracheostomy tube at least every 8 hours. It may be necessary to clean the inner cannula of a double-cannulated tube as often as every hour to prevent it from obstruction. Determine the cleaning frequency for each individual depending on the amount and character of pulmonary secretions. Think through the type of care needed and prepare all of the equipment and supplies before beginning. This is particularly important when the client has a double-cannulated tube because the inner cannula can be left out for only a few minutes and it is essential that you work as quickly as possible to prevent the outer cannula from becoming obstructed with secretions. In the event that the client has the type of tube which has a duplicate inner cannula, use it to replace the one that is removed for cleaning. This ensures patency of the airway.

When cleaning a silver tracheostomy tube, it is preferable to use a liquid detergent rather than hydrogen peroxide to reduce the discoloration and tarnishing that occurs from peroxide. A silver tube can be polished occasionally with silver polish to keep the tube smooth for easier insertion. However, this takes more time and leaves the client without the protection of the inner cannula.

Prior to removing an inner cannula, suction the tracheostomy as described in Skill 70 to remove accumulated secretions, if there is an indication that they are present. Use one hand to hold the flange of the outer cannula while unlocking the inner cannula. This prevents unnecessary movement of the tube in the trachea, which causes irritation and is likely to stimulate coughing. Remove the inner cannula by pulling it forward. Do not force the removal of the cannula. If it resists removal, check to see if dried crustations around the outside of the flange are the cause. Cleanse this area with cotton-tipped applicators moistened with either a half-strength solution of hydrogen peroxide or sterile distilled water and try again. If the tube still resists removal, seek help from a staff nurse who is more experienced than you. The tracheostomy tube may need to be changed if the inner cannula cannot be removed.

After removing the inner cannula, take the time to note carefully the amount and characteristics of the secretions inside the cannula before immersing it in the cleansing solution. This enables you to determine how often the tube requires cleaning and provides an indication of the adequacy of the humidity the client is receiving. Thick or crusted secretions usually mean that the client is not receiving adequate hydration.

While the inner cannula is soaking, clease around the flange surface of the outer tube with applicators or gauze squares that are slightly moistened with half-strength hydrogen peroxide or sterile distilled water or saline. When the inner cannula is thoroughly cleaned and rinsed and sterilized if necessary, shake it to remove any residual fluid before reinserting it. If the client shows evidence of having accumulated secretions, suction the outer cannula before inserting the inner cannula.

WOUND CARE

Care of a tracheostomy wound includes cleansing the wound and changing the dressing. Normally the surgical dressing is not changed during the first 24 hours. After that it is changed whenever it becomes soiled or at least every 8 hours.

It is often difficult to provide care to a tracheostomy incision because it is small and lies beneath the flange of the tracheostomy tube. After the dressing is removed, the wound can be partially inspected by gently retracting the skin around the incision. Remove any wound drainage with either sterile applicators or a gauze square slightly moistened with sterile saline or half-strength hydrogen peroxide. Do not use full-strength hydrogen peroxide because the foam created may flow into the trachea and irritate the tracheal mucosa. Dry the area with clean applicators or gauze squares. Some serosanguinous wound drainage is normal for the first 2 to 3 days, but persistent drainage after this period is abnormal and should be reported immediately to the physician. The physician may prescribe a broad-spectrum antibiotic ointment such as baciguent (Bacitracin) or an antiseptic ointment such as povidone-iodine (Betadine) for the wound until it is healed. Apply this to the cleaned wound in a thin film to prevent it from leaking into the trachea.

A surgical dressing is used to protect a fresh incision from pathogenic organisms present in the environment and also to prevent irritation of the skin from the flange on the tracheostomy tube. The dressing must fit around the tube. There are two different ways in which this can be done. One way is to use an unfilled 4 × 4 gauze square that is split halfway down the center and the other is to open and refold a gauze square so that it is mitered into a U-shape which can then be placed on both sides of the wound. An important point to keep in mind is that cutting a gauze square results in frayed edges and poses the hazard of aspirating loose threads. Gauze squares available in commercially prepared tracheostomy-care kits have the split edges sewn closed to prevent this from occurring. To prepare a mitered gauze square, unfold the square so that it is an open rectangle and then fold it upon itself lengthwise. Fold it again in half crosswise and then make a 45 degree angle fold on each side of this center fold, as shown in Figure 69-6. To apply the dressing, have the client raise the chin slightly to provide better access to the wound. Place the dressing by approaching the wound from the top of the tracheostomy site and gently insert the gauze between the flange of the tube and the skin, as shown in Figure 69-7.

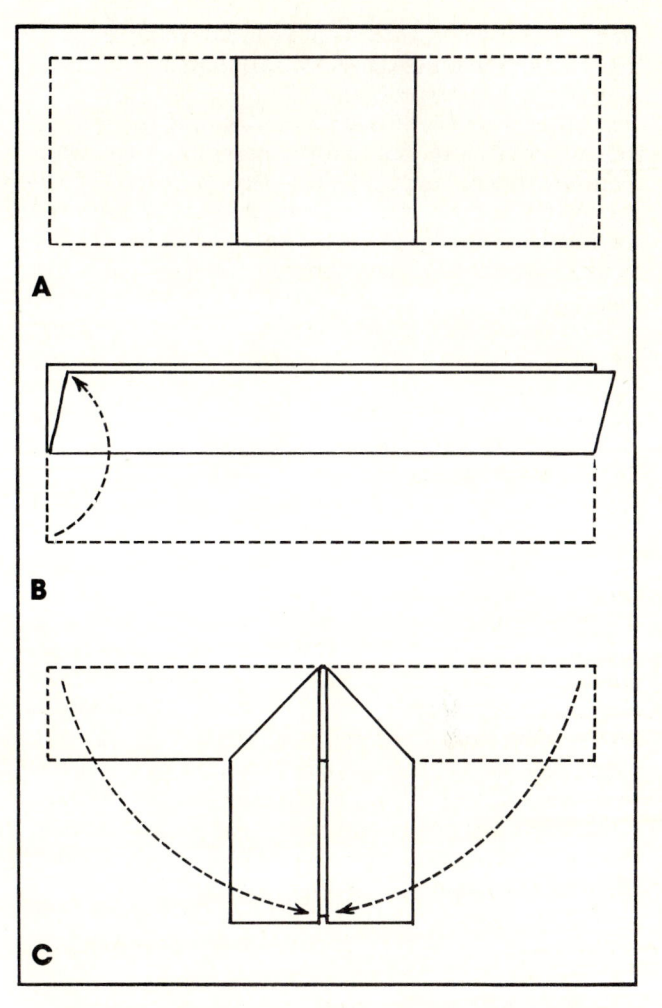

Figure 69-6. Preparing a tracheostomy dressing. **A.** Unfolding the gauze square. **B.** Folding the open gauze square lengthwise. **C.** Making 45 degree angle folds on each side of the center of the square.

CHANGING THE TRACHEOSTOMY TUBE TIES

The ties are changed whenever they become soiled. This procedure requires the assistance of a second person to eliminate the hazard of an accidental expulsion of the tube when the soiled ties are cut. Because of the danger of having the tube expulsed, many institutions

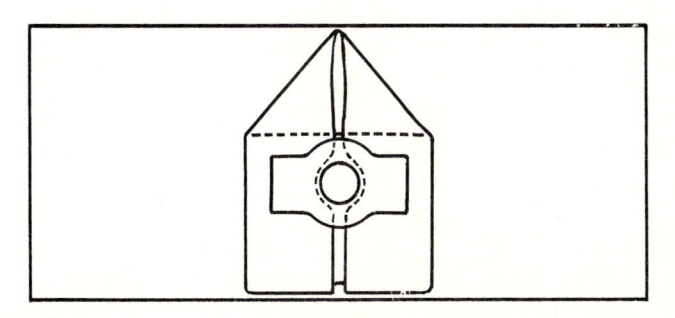

Figure 69-7. A mitered gauze square tracheostomy dressing in place.

have a policy that prohibits anyone from changing the ties on children unless specifically ordered by the physician.

There are two different methods that can be used to secure the clean ties to a tracheostomy tube. Both require two lengths of umbilical tape at least 37.5 cm (15 in) long. With one method, the ties are secured with square knots at the flange; with the other method the tie is slipped through a slit that is cut in the twill tape. Prepare the ties in advance.

Have an assistant wash his or her hands and don a sterile glove before placing a hand with the fingers on the flange to hold it securely in place. Cut the ties on the side of the neck and remove them from the flange. To use the *square-knot method,* grasp the end of the tie and insert it through the underside of the flange and into the slot, pull it through and make a square knot on the top side of the flange. Repeat this on the other side. Have the assistant use his or her free hand to raise the client's head as you bring one of the ties around the back of the neck. Tie the ends together on the side of the neck in a square knot, leaving enough slack so that one finger can be slipped under the ties. The knot placement avoids pressure on the back of the neck when the client is supine, and the slight amount of slack avoids pressure on the blood vessels in the neck. To use the *slit method,* prepare the tapes by folding a 2.5 cm (1 in) end of the tape on itself and cut a lengthwise slit about 1 cm (½ in) long through the center of the fold. Repeat this with the second tie. Have the assistant assume the same role as

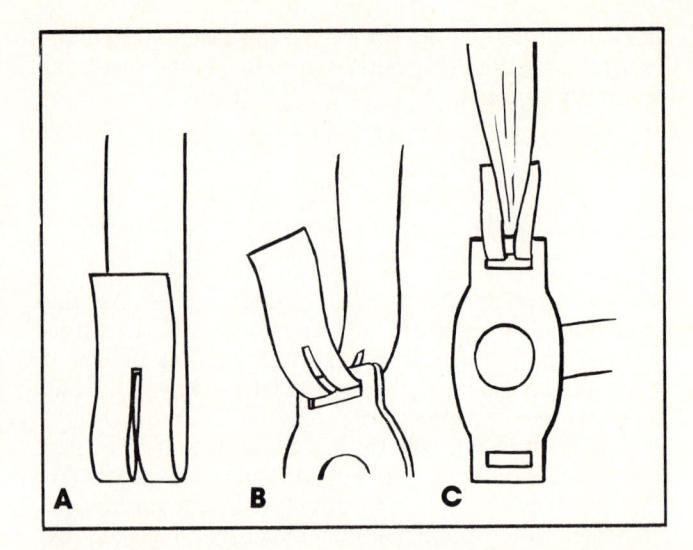

Figure 69–8. Preparing the neck tapes using the slit method. **A.** Cutting the slit. **B.** Attaching the tape to the flange. **C.** Pulling the tape through the slit.

described above before cutting the ties on the side of the neck. Hold the end of the tie with the slit and insert it from the underside through the slot, pull it through about 5 cm (2 in) and then insert the opposite end of the tie through the slit. Pull the tape all the way through the slit until the tape is snugly secured. Figure 69–8 shows how to prepare and attach the ties. Repeat on the opposite side. Tie the tape around the client's neck as described in the first method.

☐ SKILL SEQUENCE

ROUTINE TRACHEOSTOMY CARE

Step	Rationale
1. Check physician's orders or nursing kardex.	Provides direction for special care needs.
2. Wash hands.	Prevents cross-contamination.
3. Explain procedure to client and place client in low semi-Fowler's position.	Allays anxiety. Facilitates access to neck.
4. Assemble necessary equipment.	Prevents delays.
5. Close door and cubicle curtains.	Ensures privacy.
6. To cleanse a double-cannula tube:	
a. Open kit, prepare sterile field and organize equipment and supplies. Pour solutions into containers.	Prepares equipment for use.
b. Don sterile gloves.	
c. Hold flange securely with one hand and use other to unlock and remove inner cannula in an upward and outward arc.	
d. Observe inside of cannula for crustations; place in hydrogen peroxide or detergent solution.	Amount and character of secretions helps to provide guide for frequency of cleansing. Soaking loosens secretions. Accumulated secretions can interfere with proper fit and locking of inner cannula.
e. Cleanse flange of outer cannula with sterile cotton-tipped applicators moistened with half-strength hydrogen peroxide or sterile distilled water or normal saline and rinse.	
f. Use brush or pipe cleaners to remove all secretions from inside of inner cannula.	Prevents cross-contamination.

(continued)

Step	Rationale
g. Rinse clean cannula by pouring sterile distilled water or normal saline over inside and outside. Shake off residual fluid.	Removes residual cleansing agent to prevent tissue irritation. Avoids inserting fluid into trachea.
h. Insert inner cannula and lock it in place. Remove gloves.	Prevents cross-contamination.
7. Wound care:	
a. Remove soiled dressing by pulling it gently up from under flange; discard in waterproof paper bag.	Prevents cross-contamination.
b. Wash hands.	
c. Inspect condition of wound. Moisten applicators or gauze squares with sterile distilled water or normal saline and gently remove all exudate and dry. Discard soiled applicators/gauze squares in bag.	Determines condition of wound. Promotes wound healing; prevents exudate from falling into trachea.
d. Don sterile gloves.	Prevents cross-contamination.
e. Prepare and apply sterile dressing by approaching wound from top. Gently insert gauze between flange of tube and skin. Remove gloves.	Prevents contaminating dressing. Gauze must interface tube and skin.
8. To change neck ties:	
a. Wash hands.	Prevents cross-contamination.
b. Use clean scissors to cut 2 lengths of umbilical tape 37.5 cm (15 in) long. Cut slit if desired.	
c. Have assistant wash hands and don a sterile glove before holding tube in place.	Prevents cross-contamination. Tube must be held in place when ties are cut to prevent accidental expulsion.
d. Cut tape on both sides of neck and remove from flanges.	Prepares flange for clean tapes.
e. Insert end of clean tape through slot; secure through slit or with a square knot tied on outside. Repeat on opposite side.	Ties must be secure to prevent tube expulsion.
f. Tie tapes on side of neck with square knot leaving enough slack to permit insertion of one finger under tape.	Same as above; avoids pressure on back of neck. Prevents pressure on skin and blood vessels.
9. Place client in comfortable position.	Facilitates relaxation.
10. Discard supplies and clean and return equipment to appropriate area.	
11. Wash hands.	
12. Inventory equipment and supplies.	Assures readiness for subsequent care.
13. Record procedure, character, and amount of secretions, condition of wound, and client's responses on health record.	Provides data for continuity of care and nurse accountability.

CLEANSING A PERMANENT TRACHEOSTOMY

Clients with a permanent tracheostomy or laryngectomy may or may not have a tube in place. Once the incision of the tracheostomy or laryngectomy is healed, the remaining opening in the trachea is referred to as a stoma. With or without the presence of a tube, dried secretions around the stoma must be removed to prevent them from occluding the airway. To remove the secretions, place the client in a supine position for better access and visibility. Use a flashlight to visualize the stoma and use forceps to remove the crustations around the stoma. If the client is unable to cough out mucus plugs that lie within the trachea, remove these with forceps and then cleanse around the stoma with a warm moist washcloth or gauze square. The physician may prescribe an ointment for use around the stoma to prevent it from becoming dry. Apply a thin film with cotton-tipped applicators, avoiding the inner aspect of the stoma so that the ointment is not inhaled into the trachea.

CUFF INFLATION

When the physician inserts a cuffed tube, it is normally inflated at that time. Thereafter, it is the nurse's responsibility to maintain the correct inflation to achieve the desired purpose. Some cuffs need to be deflated periodically to relieve pressure on the tracheal mucosa; others do not require this. There are numerous types of cuffs and different procedures used to inflate them. Know the type of cuff being used, the physician's orders for inflating and deflating the cuff, and the amount of air required to keep the cuff inflated. The information presented here is intended as a general guide.

Inflate a cuff slowly. Depending on the size of the cuff, 1 to 6 ml of air may be needed to provide an adequate seal. It is frequently recommended that a slight leak of air from the lungs be permitted around the cuff to prevent undue pressure on the tracheal wall. To inflate the cuff, withdraw the plunger of a 5 to 10 ml syringe to permit the desired amount of air to fill the syringe. Insert the tip of the syringe into the end of the cuff tubing and slowly inject the air. The air inflates both the cuff and the test balloon at the same time. When they are filled to the desired capacity, clamp the rubber-tipped hemostat on the tubing distal to the test balloon and leave it in place to prevent the air from escaping. The test balloon serves as an indicator of the degree of the cuff inflation. Deflation of the test balloon means that the cuff has deflated. Notify the physician of any difficulty you have when inflating the cuff or if the cuff deflates spontaneously.

EMERGENCY AIRWAY MAINTENANCE

Nurses are not usually expected to reinsert a temporary tracheostomy tube because of the potential for improper placement. Since the margins of the trachea are not sutured to the skin as they are with a permanent tracheostomy, there is a potential for inserting the tube under the skin instead of in the trachea. In an emergency the nurse does need to know how to prevent a client from asphyxiation when a tube is expelled accidentally. When a tube is expelled accidentally, either partially or completely, it is imperative to take immediate action to maintain a patent airway. If the tube is partially expelled, do not attempt to force it back into the trachea. Cut the ties and remove the tube so that it does not occlude the airway or damage the tissues. Open the sterile package with the tracheal dilator forceps, insert the forceps into the trachea, and open them to dilate the trachea to prevent its collapse and asphyxiation. Call for help. A temporary tracheostomy tube should be reinserted by a qualified person.

CHANGING A PERMANENT TRACHEOSTOMY TUBE

Nurses are expected to know how to insert a permanent tracheostomy tube and be able to teach the client and family how to care for the tube and the stoma. Insertion of a permanent tube is easier and safer because the margins of the tracheal opening are sutured to the skin. When the wound is healed, a permanent stoma is formed thus eliminating the potential for incorrect placement of the tube.

Prepare for insertion of the clean replacement tube by first checking to make sure all of the parts fit properly. First, insert the obturator into the outer cannula, check the fit and then remove it. Insert the inner cannula, check its fit, then remove it and reinsert the obturator. Attach clean ties to the tube. Immerse the outer cannula in sterile distilled water or normal saline, because wetting the tube reduces the friction against the tracheal mucosa and facilitates insertion. The alert, cooperative client may be able to assist with the tube change by holding the clean tube in place while the ties are secured.

☐ SKILL SEQUENCE

CHANGING A PERMANENT TRACHEOSTOMY TUBE

Step	Rationale
1. Check physician's order or nursing kardex.	Validates order for procedure.
2. Wash hands.	Prevents delays.
3. Assemble necessary equipment.	Prevents cross-contamination.
4. Check all parts of tracheostomy set for fit and proper size.	Parts are not interchangeable.
5. Close door and cubicle curtains.	Ensures privacy.
6. Attach clean ties to tube. (NOTE: Suction airway if necessary.)	Avoids delay in completing procedure.
7. Wet outer cannula with sterile distilled water or normal saline; shake off excess.	Reduces friction against tracheal mucosa.
8. Insert obturator in outer cannula.	Prevents damage to tracheal mucosa and facilitates insertion.
9. Cut ties on client's neck.	Permits removal of tube.
10. Remove old tube, withdrawing it in an upward and an outward arc; remove and discard dressing.	Permits removal of tube. Follows normal contour of trachea.
11. Insert clean tube into stoma in a downward and inward arc. Hold tube in place at flange with one hand while removing obturator with the other hand.	Follows normal contour of trachea. Prevents expulsion of tube; obturator must be removed immediately to permit respiration.
12. Hold tube in place with one hand. Use other hand to bring one tie around neck to meet other tie.	Prevents expulsion.
13. Grasp both ties in one hand securely and pull them together snugly on side of neck.	Prevents expulsion. Too much slack in ties can allow tube displacement.

(continued)

Step	Rationale
14. Remove hand holding tube and tie the tapes in a square knot on the side of the neck. (NOTE: Suction airway if necessary.)	Irritation of airway may stimulate coughing.
15. Insert and lock inner cannula.	Essential to prevent accumulation of secretions in outer cannula.
16. Cleanse stoma and apply clean dressing.	
17. Clean and discard equipment and supplies appropriately.	
18. Obtain a replacement tracheostomy tube of same size or cleanse and sterilize the set removed from client; wrap it in a clean towel. Keep at bedside.	Prepares for next tube change.
19. Record date and time of change, nature of secretions on outer cannula, and client's response to procedure.	Provides data for continuity of care and helps to determine frequency of tube changes.

TEACHING THE CLIENT SELF-CARE

The client and family are taught how to use clean technique to care for a permanent artificial airway in the home. Begin teaching at least 7 days before discharge so that the client feels confident in the ability to provide adequate self-care. Some institutions have a procedure covering all aspects of care as well as a list of equipment and supplies that can be given to the client.

Teach the client and family how to wash their hands, giving careful attention to the areas around the fingernails. Provide the client with a mirror so the client can see to remove and insert the cannulas and care for the stoma. Provide instruction about checking all of the parts of the clean tracheostomy tube set to ensure that they fit properly since the parts are not interchangeable with another set. Show the client how to prepare the replacement tube with the ties attached and how to remove and insert the inner and outer cannulas. Make sure the client knows how to clean the tubes and how to handle silver tubes to prevent denting the soft metal.

Small bowls or glass jars can be used as receptacles to hold the cleansing and rinsing solutions. The client may need to purchase distilled water to prevent minerals in hard water from building up on the equipment. Telfa dressings are often recommended for use in the home because they do not adhere to the wound or fray when cut. Instruct the client and family to wash the receptacles and small brush with soap and water, rinse them thoroughly, and boil them in distilled water for 10 minutes at least once a day to disinfect them. When not in use supplies are to be kept covered with a clean towel as described in Skill 30. When a soiled tube set is removed, it is thoroughly washed, rinsed, then boiled and wrapped in a clean towel. In addition, instruct the client about suctioning the tracheostomy and caring for suction equipment, as described in Skill 70.

Clients with permanent artificial airways need to be cautioned about the hazards of getting foreign materials in the trachea. Some may elect to wear a small covering over the stoma to prevent inhalation of the foreign substances while others may chose to wear a high-neck shirt or dress. There is also a danger of water dripping into the trachea during a bath, shower, or shampoo unless the stoma is protected by a permeable shield such as a thin towel.

RECORDING

Data pertinent to both the physiological and psychological status of the client need to be entered on the health record. Document the frequency of tracheostomy care, the nature of the secretions, any signs and symptoms of complications caused by the tracheostomy, respiratory characteristics, condition of the wound, hydration status, any change in a client's level of apprehension, and the client's response to care.

Sample POR Recording

- S—Writes "I can't cough or breathe good."
- O—Anxious expression. Frequent cough weak and ineffective. Tracheal secretions thick and tenacious, difficult to remove from inner cannula. Wound clean, no drainage on dressing.
- A—Decreased air exchange due to thick secretions and inability to cough effectively. Inadequate hydration.
- P—1. Explain reasons why cough weak and demonstrate effective cough technique.
  2. Offer 200 ml of fluids q 2 hr.
  3. Maintain current level of humidity.
  4. Clean trach tube q 2 hr.

Sample Narrative Recording

Writing notes to communicate concern about weak cough. Reason for weak cough explained and taught how to cough more effectively. Tracheal secretions thick and tenacious, difficult to remove from inner cannula. Offer 200 ml of fluids q 2 hr, maintain current humidity and schedule trach care q 2 hr. Wound clean, no drainage on dressing.

☐ CRITICAL POINTS SUMMARY

1. Use strict aseptic technique when providing tracheostomy care.

2. Be alert for the signs and symptoms indicative of complications related to the tracheostomy.
3. Adequate humidity and hydration keep pulmonary secretions thin and facilitate their removal.
4. Frequent oral care helps to prevent infection and enhances client comfort.
5. Frequent position changes, deep breathing, and coughing improve respiratory function.
6. Use analgesics, sedatives, and tranquilizers cautiously because they depress the respiratory center.
7. Keep each part of the tracheostomy set together to avoid mismatches.
8. Handle silver tubes carefully to prevent denting.
9. Keep all the necessary equipment and supplies needed for routine tracheostomy care and emergencies at the bedside at all times.
10. Label bottles of sterile distilled water or normal saline with the date and time they are opened.
11. Use a square knot to secure the neck ties on the tracheostomy tube.
12. Begin teaching self-care to a client with a permanent tracheostomy at least 7 days before discharge.

☐ LEARNING ACTIVITIES

1. Visit the central supply department and look at the different types of single- and double-cannulated tracheostomy tubes, tracheal dilators, tracheal hooks, and tracheostomy-care kits.
2. If possible, visit a client who has a tracheostomy and observe how tracheostomy care is given.
3. Talk with a person who has a permanent tracheostomy tube and find out how that person takes care of it and what types of problems are encountered in living with it.

☐ REVIEW QUESTIONS

1. What is a tracheostomy?
2. Give five reasons why a tracheostomy is performed.
3. Why may a client with a tracheostomy have an ineffective cough?
4. What prevents a client with a tracheostomy from speaking normally?

5. Match the type of complications listed in Column I with the signs and symptoms with which they are associated, listed in Column II.

COLUMN I
A. Hemorrhage
B. Tracheoesophageal fistula
C. Tube displacement
D. Emphysema
E. Respiratory insufficiency
F. Tube expulsion

COLUMN II
____ Bubbles in the subcutaneous tissues
____ Choking while eating or drinking
____ Absent breath sounds in any part of either lung
____ Unequal movement of both sides of the chest during respiration
____ Apnea and cyanosis
____ Frank bleeding from within the trachea
____ Food returning through the tracheostomy

6. How can the pulmonary secretions be kept thin enough to be easily removed by coughing or suctioning?
7. What are the reasons for using strict aseptic technique?
8. Why is frequent oral care important?
9. What effects do position change, deep breathing, and coughing have on respiratory function?
10. What can the nurse do to help reduce apprehension for a client with a tracheostomy?
11. What data does the nurse collect from the client's health record?
12. What data does the nurse collect by using physical appraisal skills?
13. What are the differences between a single-cannulated and a double-cannulated tracheostomy tube?
14. What equipment and supplies must be kept at the bedside at all times?
15. How would you explain to a peer how to remove, clean, and reinsert an inner cannula?
16. How would you explain to a peer how to give wound care and change the neck ties?

☐ PERFORMANCE CHECKLISTS

OBJECTIVE: To use the correct procedure to give routine tracheostomy care safely.

CHARACTERISTIC	RANGE OF ACCEPTABILITY	SATISFACTORY	UNSATISFACTORY
1. Checks physician orders or nursing kardex.	No deviation		
2. Washes hands.	No deviation		

(continued)

CHARACTERISTIC	RANGE OF ACCEPTABILITY	SATISFACTORY	UNSATISFACTORY
3. Explains procedure and places client in low semi-Fowler's position.	Modify position according to client's respiratory status.		
4. Assembles necessary equipment.	No deviation		
5. Closes door and cubicle curtains.	No deviation		

6. To cleanse a double-cannula tube:
  a. Opens kit, prepares sterile field, organizes equipment and supplies, and pours solutions.
  b. Dons sterile gloves.
  c. Holds flange, unlocks and removes inner cannula in an upward and outward arc.
  d. Observes inside of inner cannula for crustations before placing it in cleansing solution.
  e. Cleanses flange.
  f. Uses brush or pipe cleaners to cleanse inner cannula. Rinses cannula by pouring sterile distilled water or normal saline over it. Shakes off residual liquid.
  g. Inserts cannula and locks it in place. Removes gloves.
	No deviation
	
	No deviation
	No deviation
	
	No deviation
	
	No deviation
	No deviation
	
	No deviation		

7. Wound care:
  a. Removes soiled dressing.
  b. Washes hands.
  c. Inspects condition of incision and skin. Cleanses wound.
  d. Dons sterile gloves.
  e. Prepares and applies sterile dressing. Removes gloves.
	No deviation
	No deviation
	No deviation
	
	Omit if using medical aseptic technique.
	No deviation		

8. To change neck ties:
  a. Washes hands.
  b. Uses clean scissors to cut 2 lengths of cotton twill tape 37.5 cm (15 in) long. Cuts slit in tape if desired.
  c. Has assistant don a sterile glove before holding tube in place.
  d. Cuts ties on both sides of neck and removes from flanges.
  e. Inserts end of clean tape through slot and secures. Repeats on opposite side.
  f. Ties tapes at the side of the neck using a square knot. Leaves enough slack to permit insertion of one finger under tape.
	No deviation
	No deviation
	
	No deviation
	
	No deviation
	
	No deviation
	
	No deviation		

9. Positions client comfortably.	No deviation		
10. Discards used supplies. Cleans and returns equipment to appropriate area.	No deviation		
11. Washes hands.	No deviation		
12. Records procedure.	No deviation		

OBJECTIVE: To use the correct procedure to change a permanent artificial airway tube safely.

CHARACTERISTIC	RANGE OF ACCEPTABILITY	SATISFACTORY	UNSATISFACTORY
1. Checks physician's order or nursing kardex.	No deviation		
2. Washes hands.	No deviation		

(continued)

OBJECTIVE: To use the correct procedure to change a permanent artificial airway tube safely (cont.).

CHARACTERISTIC	RANGE OF ACCEPTABILITY	SATISFACTORY	UNSATISFACTORY
3. Assembles necessary equipment and checks size and fit of all tracheostomy set parts.	No deviation		
4. Closes door and cubicle curtains.	No deviation		
5. Attaches clean ties to tube.	No deviation		
6. Suctions airway if necessary.	No deviation		
7. Inserts obturator in outer cannula and wets outer cannula with sterile distilled water or normal saline; shakes off excess.	No deviation		
8. Cuts ties on client's neck and withdraws old tube in an upward and outward arc. Removes old dressing.	No deviation		
9. Inserts a clean tube into stoma in a downward and inward arc. Holds it in place with one hand and removes obturator with the other.	No deviation		
10. Holds tube in place while bringing ties together at one side of neck.	No deviation		
11. Grasps both ties securely in one hand pulling them together snugly.	No deviation		
12. Ties tapes with a square knot.	No deviation		
13. Inserts and locks inner cannula.	No deviation		
14. Cleanses stoma and applies a clean dressing.	No deviation		
15. Cleans and discards equipment appropriately.	No deviation		
16. Obtains a replacement tube set of the same size or cleanses and sterilizes same set removed from client and wraps it in a clean towel.	No deviation		
17. Records date and time of tube change.	No deviation		

REFERENCES

DeGowin EL, DeGowin RL: Bedside Diagnostic Examination, ed 4. New York, Macmillan, 1981.

Harper RW: A Guide to Respiratory Care: Physiology and Clinical Applications. Philadelphia, JB Lippincott, 1981.

Traver GA (ed): Respiratory Nursing: The Science and Art. New York, John Wiley & Sons, 1982.

BIBLIOGRAPHY

Conner GH, Hughes D, et al.: Tracheostomy: Post-operative care. American Journal of Nursing 72(1):72–74, 1972.

LeMaitre G, Finnegan J: The Patient in Surgery: A Guide for Nurses, ed 4. Philadelphia, WB Saunders, 1980.

Luckmann J, Sorensen K: Medical–Surgical Nursing: A Psychophysiologic Approach, ed 2. Philadelphia, WB Saunders, 1980.

Rarey KP, Youtsey JW: Respiratory Patient Care. Englewood Cliffs, NJ, Prentice-Hall, 1981.

Wade JF: Comprehensive Respiratory Care: Physiology and Technique. St Louis, CV Mosby, 1982.

AUDIOVISUAL RESOURCES

Elements in Tracheostomy Care
  Filmstrip and cassette. (1982, Color, 18 min.)
  Available through:
    Medcom, Inc.
    P.O. Box 116
    Garden Grove, CA 92642

Infection Control: Tracheostomy Care
  Filmstrip and cassette. (1974, Color, 20 min.)
  Available through:
    Concept Media
    P.O. Box 19542
    Irvine, CA 93714

SKILL 70 Suctioning the Airway

PREREQUISITE SKILLS

Skill 19, "Inspection"
Skill 22, "Auscultation"
Skill 28, "Handwashing"
Skill 30, "Sterile Supplies"
Skill 31, "Donning Sterile Gloves"
Skill 67, "Chest Therapy Exercises"

STUDENT OBJECTIVES

1. Indicate the purpose for suctioning the airway.
2. Differentiate among the routes used to suction the airway.
3. Indicate when each route is used.
4. Describe the adverse effects of suctioning.
5. Indicate how a nurse can minimize the adverse effects of suctioning.
6. Indicate the type of aseptic technique used to suction the upper and lower airways.
7. Describe the data a nurse collects prior to and after suctioning a client's airway.
8. Indicate the safe ranges for the force of suction used for infants, children, and adults.
9. Describe the items used for suctioning a client by each route.
10. Describe how you would prepare for and implement a suctioning procedure for each route.
11. Suction a client by each route in a safe manner.

INTRODUCTION

An airway is suctioned to remove accumulated secretions from the respiratory tract to ensure a patent airway. It is done with a catheter connected to a vacuum source. Clients who require suctioning are those who are not able to clear the airway adequately by coughing. These include clients with neurologic conditions, such as myasthenia gravis; pulmonary disease, such as chronic obstructive lung disease; and those who have artificial airways or are weak and debilitated. Because anesthesia and pain decrease pulmonary ventilation, postoperative clients may also need to be suctioned. Suction is used only when there is evidence that accumulated secretions are present that cannot be removed by coughing.

PREPARATION

The respiratory tract can be divided into the upper and lower airway. The upper airway extends to the larynx and includes the nose, mouth, and pharynx while the trachea and right and left main bronchi are part of the lower airway. Clients with accumulated secretions may require suctioning of the upper or lower airway or both. Suctioning an upper airway is usually considered to be an independent nursing judgment and most institutions permit it to be initiated by a nursing order. A nurse, however, needs to know the policies of the institution in which he or she is practicing. Lower airway suctioning of the tracheobronchial tree may be routinely permitted only for clients with an artificial airway; even then there may be a policy limiting the depth to which the nurse may insert the catheter in the tracheobronchial tree.

ROUTES FOR SUCTIONING

Upper Airway

The *oropharyngeal route* of suctioning is probably the most familiar to anyone who has had dental care, since suction is often used to remove saliva from the oral cavity during dental procedures. With this route, the catheter is inserted into the oral cavity and back toward the pharynx. This route is commonly used with clients who have difficulty swallowing saliva, fluid, or food and is intended to prevent aspiration of material into the lungs. Clients who are at risk for aspiration need to have suction equipment kept at the bedside in a state of readiness. Suction may also be used in combination with oral hygiene to remove cleansing agents from the mouth when the client is unable to expectorate voluntarily. Suction through the oropharyngeal route may also be used to stimulate a client to cough.

The *nasopharyngeal route* is used to remove secretions from the nose and pharynx and therefore the catheter is inserted through one of the nostrils. It can be used as an alternate route for access to the upper airway when it is not possible to insert a catheter into the oral cavity.

Lower Airway

The *nasotracheal route* is used to remove secretions from the trachea or the bronchi or both. It is used with clients who are unable to cough effectively. Although this route is normally used by physicians, with proper preparation nurses can use it.

The *tracheostomy or laryngectomy routes* provide direct access to the trachea and through it to the bronchi. Suctioning an artificial airway is an integral part of client care. However, there may be a restriction on the depth for inserting the catheter. Some institutions or physicians may not permit a nurse to routinely insert the catheter more than 12.5 cm (5 in) without a specific order because the catheter would be entering a bronchus.

SPUTUM SPECIMEN COLLECTION

Since clients who require suctioning to maintain a patent airway are vulnerable to pulmonary infections, specimens are often collected during the suctioning procedure. If they are not collected and handled properly, sputum specimens obtained by suction have a high probability of being contaminated.

ADVERSE EFFECTS OF SUCTIONING

Although suctioning is a therapeutic intervention, it does have adverse effects when not used properly. Suctioning can induce hypoxemia because it removes oxygen from the respiratory tract. To prevent or minimize suction-induced hypoxemia, suction is applied for no more than a maximum of 15 seconds for each attempt and there needs to be an interval of 3 minutes between each attempt (Traver, 1982, p. 274). Some clients may require oxygenation prior to suction to prevent hypoxemia. The amount of oxygen and the method used to deliver the oxygen depends on the cardiopulmonary status of the client and the type of oxygen therapy the client may be already receiving. As with any administration of oxygen, a physician's order is required.

Excessive suctioning can cause *alveolar collapse* either by removing nitrogen from the alveoli or by blocking a lung segment. *Bradycardia* followed by *hypotension* can occur from stimulation of the vagus nerve which is the major nerve supplying the tracheobronchial tree. When a vagal response is combined with hypoxemia, cardiac arrhythmias can develop. Monitoring the client's pulse before and after suctioning enables the nurse to detect this adverse effect.

The presence of the catheter and the action of the suction on the mucosal tissue has an irritating effect that interferes with the protective cilia and mucous blanket and results in increased tracheobronchial secretions. *Traumatized tissue* can become edematous or erode. Gentle insertion and manipulation of the catheter will minimize these effects.

Clients who require suctioning to maintain a patent airway often have compromised pulmonary function and are particularly vulnerable to infection. Suctioning is performed with strict aseptic technique to prevent nosocomial infections. Suction catheters used to suction one route are not used to suction another airway route because of the potential for transferring microorganisms from one location to another. While it may appear to be cost-effective to reuse the same catheter for oropharyngeal suction as was used for tracheobronchial suctioning, this practice is not acceptable.

DATA BASE

Client History and Recorded Data
Prior to suctioning a client, it is important to know the medical diagnosis and understand why the client is unable to expectorate or cough out the accumulated secretions. It is important to know of any impairment of the cardiopulmonary system that may require special precautions in the use of suction or if the client needs supplemental oxygen prior to suctioning to prevent hypoxemia. Oxygen therapy is prescribed by a physician.

Clients find suctioning to be an unpleasant and uncomfortable procedure, so the nurse finds out what experience they have had with airway suctioning and how they have responded. Since suctioning removes even minimal secretions that are not actually obstructing the airway, the nurse may find some apprehensive clients wish to be suctioned more often than necessary. It is important to determine if the client knows how to deep breathe and cough, since these exercises help to prevent the accumulation of secretions, decrease the need for frequent suctioning, and often make necessary suctioning attempts more successful. The nursing-care plan should include clear documentation about the frequency with which a client needs to be suctioned, the nature of the secretions, collection of sputum specimens, and the schedule for deep breathing and coughing. In addition, the nurse remains alert to those clients who have a potential need for upper and lower airway suctioning because of their inability to swallow, deep breathe, or cough properly. The pattern of temperature, pulse, respiration, and blood pressure measurements may reveal the presence of an infection or indicate adverse reactions to suctioning.

The decision to suction a client must be made on the basis of evidence that the client has accumulated secretions obstructing the airway and that the client is unable to remove with effective coughing. The nurse uses physical appraisal skills to validate the need for suctioning.

Physical Appraisal Skills

Inspection. Changes in a client's respiratory states that indicate a need for suctioning include an increased rate and labored breathing. Inspection is also used to determine the characteristics of the secretions obtained by suctioning.

Auscultation. Abnormal breath sounds indicating the presence of retained secretions and a need for suction may be detected with the use of a stethoscope. Although noisy, moist respiratory sounds can often be heard with the naked ear, it is best to develop the habit of listening with a stethoscope before and after each suctioning. The breath sounds that are indicative of an obstructed airway are crackles and wheezes. A complete description of these sounds, where they can be heard, and how to listen for them is presented in Skill 67.

EQUIPMENT

Suction Source
The negative pressure required to create a partial vacuum necessary for suction is provided either by a cen-

tral pipeline source throughout the institution or by a mobile suction machine. The suction that is used for removing secretions from the respiratory tract is similar to that which is used for gastrointestinal purposes discussed in Skill 56. It is not, however, applied continuously. When suctioning the airway, the nurse applies and controls the suction by manually covering and releasing a vent in the suction tube. This action prevents inducing hypoxemia from excessive suctioning. *Pipeline systems* are accessible at outlets in the wall near the client's bed. These are often located in the same compartment as the outlet for pipeline oxygen. A *mobile suction unit,* as shown in Figure 70–1, is plugged into standard grounded electrical outlets and placed at the bedside. Both suction systems produce a continual flow of negative pressure and require a pressure regulator to adjust and limit the maximum amount of negative pressure to a safe therapeutic range. Safe suction force ranges for secretion removal vary among clients and it is important to use the appropriate range to prevent tissue damage. The safe ranges are: adults, 120 to 150 mm Hg; children, 80 to 120 mm Hg; and infants, 60 to 80 mm Hg (Rarey, 1981, p. 196).

The *collection reservoirs* for the secretions are made of glass or plastic and are marked with milliliter calibrations. Depending upon the type of suction system, one or two containers are used. With two containers, one serves as an overflow collector to prevent secretions from flowing into the pressure regulator and vacuum system. Plastic disposable containers may have a device that blocks and prevents overflow from moving into the regulator and vacuum system; with these models, a second container is not used. Since the size of the container affects the amount of time required for the desired negative pressure to build up, it is recommended that the size not exceed two liters (Rarey, 1981, p. 204).

Suction Catheters

Catheters are hollow cylindrical tubes made of rubber or polyvinyl chloride (PVC); they have a series of openings at the distal end. Suction catheters are available with a wide variety of tip styles, some of which are shown in Figure 70–2. The tip may be blunt, beveled, or bent at an angle (O'Malley, 1979). Catheters with a bent tip are called Coudé and are often used when it is necessary to enter and suction the left bronchus. Polyvinyl chloride tubes are transparent, less expensive than rubber, and easier to insert and cause less tissue reaction. Catheters range in diameter from 5 to 18 F and come in different lengths. To avoid obstructing the airway, the size selected for use should not be more than half the inside diameter of the airway into which it is inserted. It also needs to be long enough to reach the distal area to be suctioned. Some

Figure 70–1. Mobile suction unit. (Courtesy of GOMCO, Division of Allied Healthcare Products Inc., St Louis, MO 63110.)

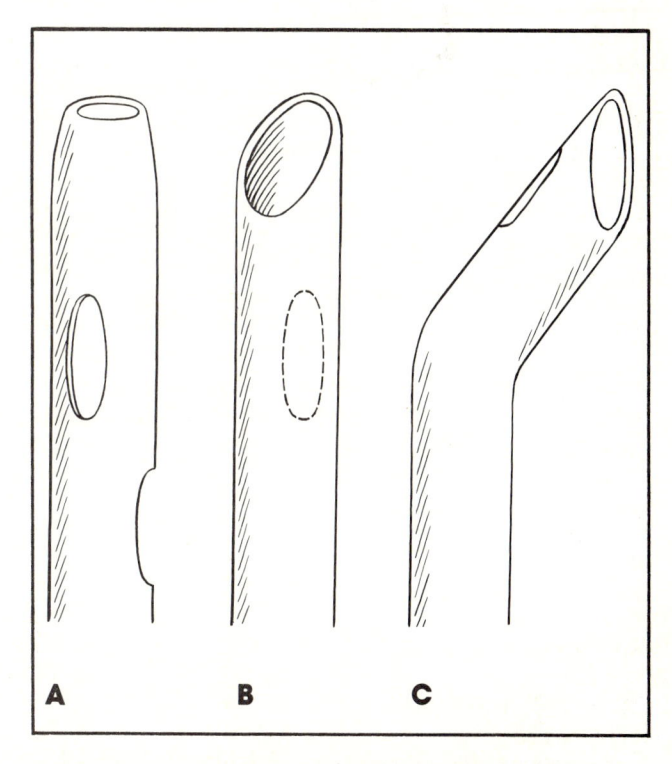

Figure 70–2. Suction catheter tips. **A.** Blunt tip. **B.** Beveled tip. **C.** Coudé tip.

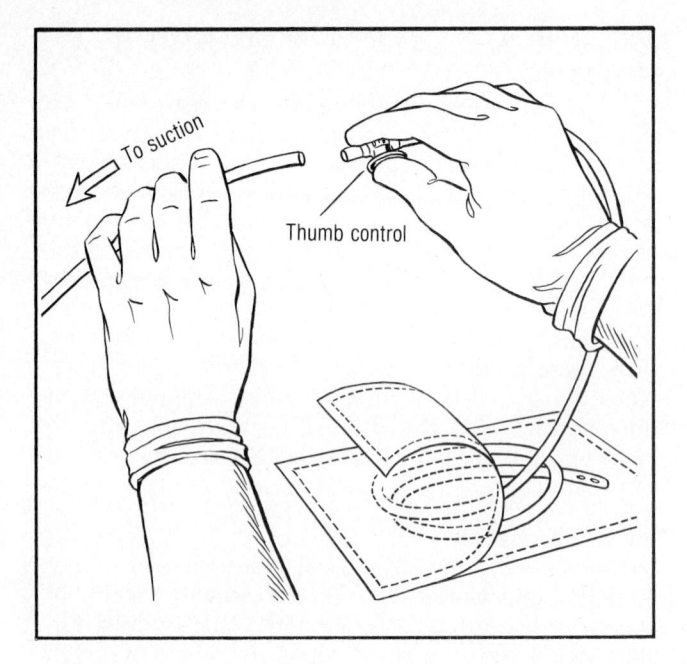

Figure 70-3. Thumb occluding a side-arm vent on suction catheter.

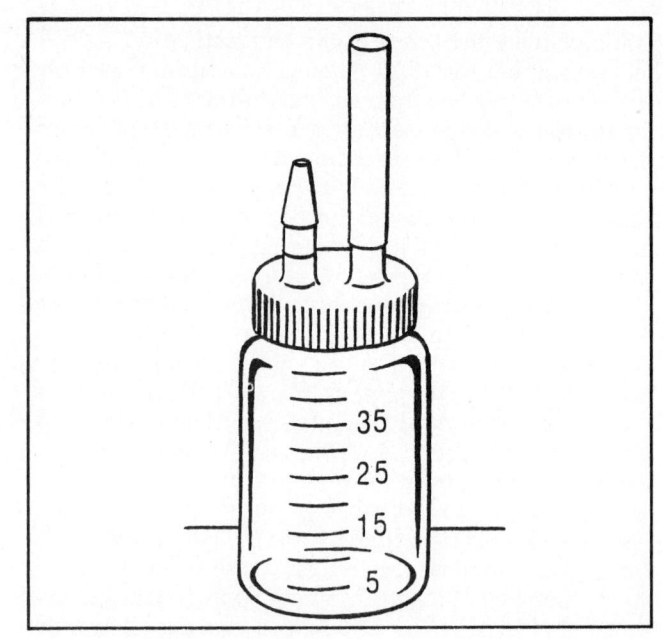

Figure 70-4. Entrapment type of sputum specimen container.

disposable catheters have a raised side-arm vent (as shown in Figure 70-3) that permits the nurse to create suction easily by occluding the vent with the thumb or finger. Elevation of the vent prevents contact with the secretions as they flow through the catheter.

Additional Items

A *connecting tubing* of durable plastic that will not collapse with negative pressure is attached to the container and used to link the suction catheter to the suction source.

A *"Y" or "T" connector* is required as a vent if the suction catheter does not have a side-arm vent. The connector is inserted between the connecting tubing and the catheter.

Regardless of whether medical or surgical aseptic technique is used, sterile items are normally required in institutions. These include *disposable gloves* to wear while handling the sterile catheter, *normal saline* to wet the catheter to facilitate entry into the airway and flush the secretions into the collection container, a *basin* to hold the saline, and a *sterile drape* on which to place the catheter between successive suctioning attempts to prevent contamination from the environment.

Specimen collection containers are sterile plastic containers. Some are designed so that they can be inserted between the catheter and the connector tubing. These containers have two separate outlets; one that connects to the suction catheter and another to the connecting tubing. This permits the entrapment of the specimen without the need to transfer it to and from the catheter to the container. Figure 70-4 shows one type of specimen collection container.

When a suction catheter is inserted through the mouth or nose, *tongue blades* and *4 × 4 gauze squares* may be used to depress the tongue or hold it extended to facilitate entry and visualization of the oral cavity.

Commercially available catheter kits include all of the items needed for a single suctioning procedure.

☐ EXECUTION

Since suctioning has inherent adverse effects, the decision to suction a client must be made on the basis of clear evidence that secretions need to be removed. With many clients, the frequency of suctioning may be decreased by the effective use of deep breathing and coughing exercises, because these exercises can prevent pooling of secretions and facilitate their removal. Suctioning the lower airway should be done only after auscultation of the lungs verifies the presence of secretions.

PREPARING THE CLIENT

Having the airway suctioned is not a comfortable procedure. Be sure to explain what needs to be done in a way that the client can understand. Let the client know that he or she can cooperate by breathing as you instruct and by not pulling on the catheter. A cooperative client helps to prevent some of the adverse effects and enables you to get the suctioning done in the most efficient and effective manner. If you have reason to believe that the client is unable or unwilling to cooperate, have a second person available if it becomes necessary to control the client's movements. Some clients may attempt to pull the suction catheter away during the procedure, thus posing a potential for traumatizing the mucous membranes and contaminating sterile equipment. Position the bed at an appropriate height for you to have easy access to the client and work from the side which is easiest for you to reach all of the necessary items. Whenever possible, place the client in a semi-Fowler's position with the head erect and in the midline, using pillows to support the head and shoulders as necessary.

PREPARING THE EQUIPMENT

Inventory the available equipment and supplies to make sure that they are adequate for more than one suctioning attempt. This prevents delays in implementing the procedure and allows for proper discarding of contaminated items. Set up the sterile field so that all of the items are readily available and accessible and place it in a location where it will not get contaminated by yourself or the client. Check the collection container to be sure that it is not too full; empty it if necessary before beginning. Select catheters that are sufficiently long and of the proper diameter for the entry route. Turn on and check the suction equipment to ensure proper function and adjust the pressure regulator to the desired level before attaching the sterile catheter.

SUCTIONING TECHNIQUES

The decision to use either medical or surgical aseptic technique is usually made on the basis of what part of the airway requires suctioning. In general, use medical aseptic technique to suction the upper airway through the oral or nasal route. Permanent artificial airways are also suctioned with medical aseptic technique after the first 72 hours after surgery when there is no evidence of pulmonary infection. When using medical aseptic technique, wear a clean or sterile glove on the hand that will be used to manipulate the catheter. Handle all items used during the suction in such a way to prevent introduction of organisms from the environment. Surgical aseptic technique is used to suction the trachea and bronchi through the nasal route and also for an artificial airway for at least the first 72 hours after surgery. When using surgical aseptic technique, don sterile gloves on both hands and use only sterile equipment and supplies for each suction attempt.

To lubricate the catheter, insert the tip into the basin of sterile saline, briefly occlude the vent, and aspirate a small amount of saline. This wetness helps the secretions flow through the tube more easily. Regardless of the route used for suctioning, always insert the catheter into the airway without occluding the vent and never force the catheter. Applying suction during the insertion prolongs the period when oxygen is removed and adds to the trauma to the mucous membranes. If the catheter's insertion is blocked by a mucus plug, apply suction and withdraw it. Once the catheter is in place in the airway, apply the suction intermittently as you withdraw the catheter to minimize the undesired effects. While withdrawing the catheter, rotate it between the thumb and forefinger to facilitate removal of the secretions through the holes in the catheter tip. The practice of moving the catheter up and down in the airway is not an effective technique and strips the epithelium and cilia thus traumatizing the tissues. Keep in mind that the suction is applied intermittently for no more than a maximum of 15 seconds for each attempt and that there needs to be a 3 minute interval between suctioning attempts to permit the client to breathe and be reoxygenated. To apply suction, cover the vent on the catheter or the "Y" connector with a thumb or finger. Alternate closing and opening the vent so that the suction is not continuous.

When a client requires suction by more than one route, use a separate catheter and glove for each route. When both the upper and lower airway require suctioning, suction the lower airway first, unless otherwise directed. An air sucking sound can be heard at the distal tip of the catheter during effective suctioning. When the sound is absent, it may indicate that the catheter either is blocked with secretions or is against a tissue wall. If this occurs, open the vent, withdraw the catheter slightly, and apply suction again.

Oropharyngeal Route
The specific placement of the catheter tip in the oropharynx depends on the location of the secretions. Depress the tongue with a tongue blade so that the secretions can be seen, insert the tip between the gum line and the buccal mucosa, and then slide it along the floor of the mouth to the pharynx.

Nasal Route
When using the nasal route as an entry for either upper or lower airway suctioning, ask the client if he or she has a preference for which nostril is to be used. It is also wise to inspect both nostrils with a flashlight to determine if one is obstructed because of a deviated septum. If one nostril is obstructed, use the unobstructed one; otherwise, alternate nostrils to prevent trauma to one nostril from repeated catheter insertions.

Use the nasal route for nasopharyngeal suctioning when it is not possible to enter by the mouth because of trauma or the client is unable to open the mouth. To ensure proper placement of the catheter in the nasopharynx, measure the distance from the tip of the nose to the earlobe with the catheter before insertion.

To reach the trachea for nasotracheal suctioning, measure the distance from the tip of the nose to the earlobe and down the side of the neck to the thyroid cartilage ("Adam's apple") and make a mental note of this location on the catheter. Have the client hyper-

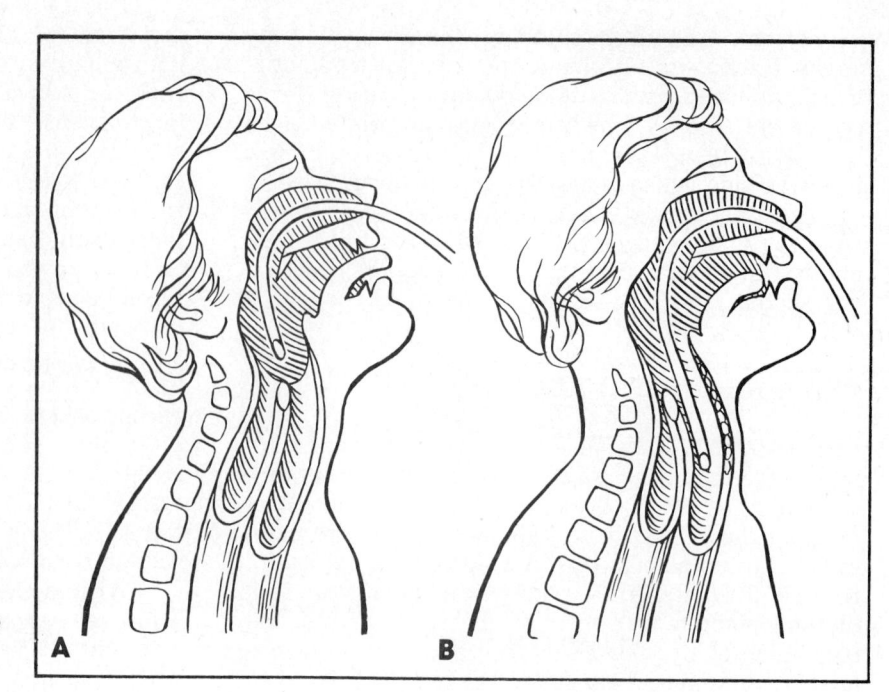

Figure 70-5. Nasotracheal suctioning. **A.** Inserting the catheter into the nasopharynx with the tongue extended and the head hyperextended. **B.** The tongue can be retracted and the head lowered slightly once the catheter has passed through the vocal cords and into the trachea.

extend the head and extend the tongue with the mouth wide open as shown in Figure 70-5. This displaces the glottis forward, in line with the trachea, preventing entry into the esophagus and allowing the catheter to pass through the vocal cords into the trachea. It may be necessary to have a second person hold the tongue with a gauze square if the client is unable to do this voluntarily. Some clients are able to take slow deep breaths during the insertion procedure while others may need to breathe in a panting fashion. Insertion during inspiration facilitates passing the catheter. Advance the catheter slowly and gently until the trachea is reached. At this point air will flow through the catheter and the client will be unable to speak. In the event that the client begins to cough, withdraw the catheter immediately to prevent damage to the mucosa which occurs because the catheter partially occludes the larynx and causes negative pressure within the trachea.

There are times when secretions in the bronchi must be removed by suctioning. To facilitate entry of the catheter into a bronchi, place the client in different positions. For the right bronchus, turn the client slightly on the right side with the head turned to the far left and for the left bronchus turn the client slightly to the left side with the head turned to the far

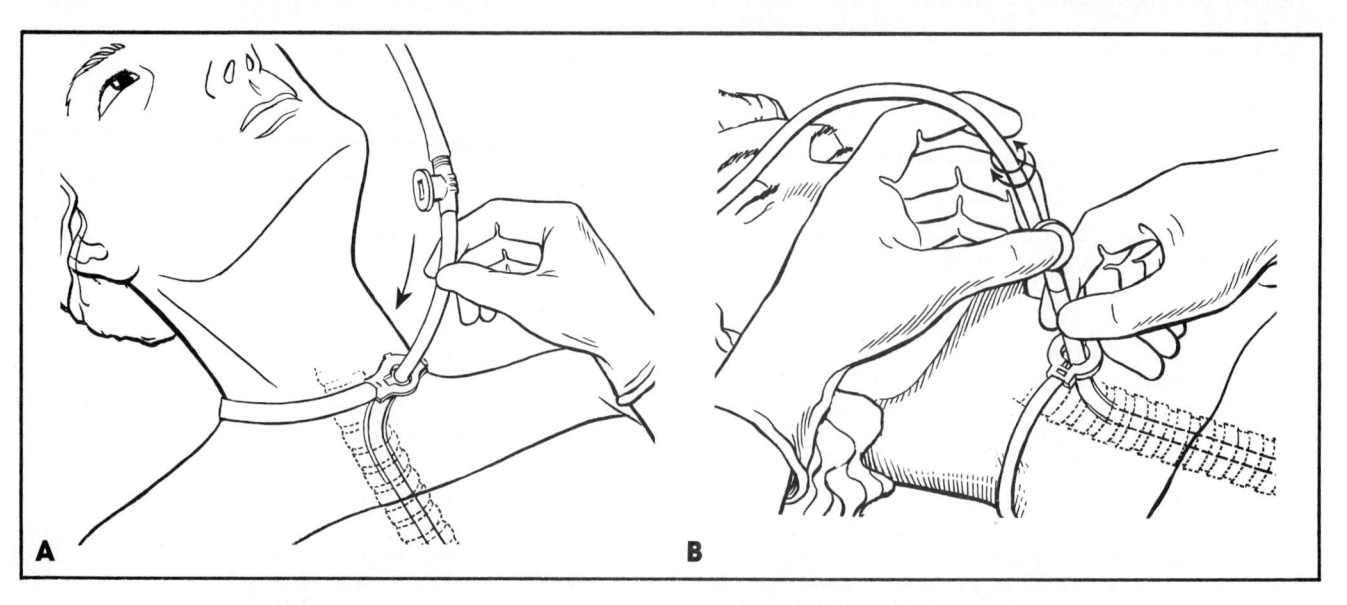

Figure 70-6. Suctioning a tracheostomy. **A.** Inserting the catheter into the tracheostomy tube. **B.** Applying suction by occluding the vent while simultaneously rotating the catheter and withdrawing it from the tracheostomy tube.

right. Because the normal position of the left bronchus is more horizontal than vertical, the catheter will most often enter the right bronchus unless a Coudé-tipped catheter is used (Rarey, 1981, p. 204).

In addition to the routine suctioning required to clear the artificial airway of secretions, the tracheostomy is usually suctioned before the inner cannula is removed for cleaning and before it is reinserted. Both of these suctioning procedures are done only if there is evidence that the client is unable to expel the secretions voluntarily by coughing. The catheter is usually inserted only 12.5 cm (5 in) to avoid entering the bronchi unless otherwise specified. Figure 70–6 shows suctioning a tracheostomy.

Prior to suctioning a tracheostomy, isotonic normal saline may be instilled into the tracheostomy as a way of mobilizing and liquefying secretions. Use this practice only if institutional policy or the physician's order indicates that it is an acceptable practice for nurses. To do this procedure, use a sterile 5 ml syringe and needle to aspirate 3 to 5 ml of sterile isotonic saline from a 30-ml vial as in Skill 73. Remove the needle and instill the liquid into the tracheostomy immediately before suctioning.

☐ SKILL SEQUENCE

SUCTIONING THE AIRWAY

Step	Rationale
1. Check physician's order or nursing kardex.	Verifies order and indicates restrictions.
2. Explain procedure and instruct client on how to cooperate.	Allays anxiety, facilitates cooperation.
3. Wash hands.	Prevents cross-contamination.
4. Assemble necessary equipment.	Prevents delays.
5. Close door and cubicle curtains.	Ensures privacy.
6. Open and prepare clean or sterile field, pour sterile normal saline into basin.	Maintains sterile field and avoids delays in procedure.
7. Place client in high semi-Fowler's position if possible, with head erect and in midline. Support head with pillows if necessary.	Facilitates entry into airway and enhances client's ventilation.
8. Turn on, check, and adjust suction pressure.	Ensures proper function and appropriate level of pressure.
9. Open one end of package with sterile suction catheter package, leaving catheter in package.	Prepares catheter for removal from package.
10. Attach catheter to connecting tubing on suction source while holding catheter in wrapper. (NOTE: Omit this step for nasotracheal suctioning.)	Wrapper maintains sterility.
11. Hold wrapper at the distal end and remove catheter, then place catheter on the field.	Maintains sterility of catheter.
12. Don clean or sterile gloves as indicated for aseptic technique used.	Prepares for handling catheter.
13. Pick up catheter with gloved hand, insert tip in saline while using opposite hand to occlude vent. Aspirate small amount of saline then open vent and remove catheter from saline.	Wets catheter for lubrication while maintaining sterility.
14. Oropharyngeal route:	
a. Have client open mouth and instruct client to breathe normally.	Reduces potential for client gagging.
b. Hold tongue blade in non-sterile gloved hand and insert in mouth to depress tongue.	Provides access to oropharynx.
c. Hold catheter with gloved hand and insert into oropharynx.	
d. Alternately occlude vent and rotate catheter between thumb and forefinger while simultaneously withdrawing catheter from oropharynx.	Reduces time suction is applied.
e. Immerse catheter tip in saline, occlude vent to aspirate fluid, then open vent.	Flushes secretions from catheter.
f. Wait 2 to 3 minutes before next suction attempt.	Rest period necessary to permit client to inspire.
15. Nasopharyngeal route: (NOTE: Do not attach catheter to suction connecting tubing until catheter is in the trachea. Immerse sterile catheter in saline for lubrication. Place connecting tubing across chest for accessibility.)	Facilitates catheter insertion.

(continued)

SUCTIONING THE AIRWAY (Cont.)

Step	Rationale
a. Use gloved hands to hold catheter near but not touching skin. Measure distance from tip of nose to earlobe and down side of neck to thyroid cartilage. Make a mental note of length of catheter to be inserted to reach trachea.	Provides gauge for length of catheter to be inserted into nasopharynx.
b. Instruct client to hyperextend neck, open the mouth wide, and extend the tongue.	Facilitates catheter insertion.
c. Have assistant grasp tongue with gauze square.	Facilitates catheter insertion.
d. Instruct client to pant through mouth.	Reduces potential for gag reflex.
e. Insert catheter through nostril, nasopharynx, and into trachea. Note air flow through catheter.	Verifies position of catheter in trachea.
f. Have assistant release tongue and ask client to breathe normally.	Helps client to relax.
g. Hold catheter securely in trachea with gloved hand; use other hand to pick up and attach connecting tube.	Prevents catheter from slipping farther down into airway.
h. Alternately close and open the catheter vent while rotating catheter between thumb and forefinger and slowly withdrawing catheter.	Suction is present only when vent is occluded. Rotating catheter provides access to more secretions.
i. Flush catheter with normal saline.	
j. Repeat steps 12 b to i if necessary.	
16. Tracheostomy route: (NOTE: Administer oxygen therapy before suctioning if ordered.)	Prevents hypoxemia.
a. Insert catheter into inner cannula 12.5 cm (5 in).	
b. Apply alternating suction and rotate catheter between thumb and forefinger while slowly withdrawing catheter.	Suction is present only when vent is occluded. Rotating catheter reduces potential for trauma to the tissues.
c. Flush catheter with normal saline. If necessary, repeat suctioning after a 3-minute rest period. (NOTE: Remove, cleanse, and reinsert inner cannula if necessary and provide wound care. Repeat steps 15 a to c using a new sterile catheter.)	Flushes secretions from catheter. Rest interval prevents hypoxemia inducement. Inner cannula does not always require cleaning with each suctioning. Additional suctioning may be required after inner cannula reinserted.
17. Clean reusable and discard disposable equipment.	Prevents transfer of microorganisms.
18. Place client in a comfortable position.	Procedure fatiguing to client.
19. Record amount and characteristics of secretions, client's response to suctioning, and respiratory status during and following suction.	Provides data for continuity of care.

Sputum Specimen Collection

Handle the sterile collection container in a way that does not contaminate the interior because this causes inaccurate test results. When using containers that are inserted between the catheter and the connecting tubing, read the directions to ensure that the catheter and the connector tubing are attached to the proper outlets. Hold the container upright during the suctioning procedure to prevent losing the specimen to the suction system. Label the specimen with the client's name, room number, and date.

TEACHING SUCTIONING TO THE CLIENT WITH A TRACHEOSTOMY TUBE

Clients with permanent artificial airways need to learn how to suction before they are discharged. Begin teaching at least 7 days prior to discharge so the client and family feel competent to keep the airway patent. As with routine care of an artificial airway, some institutions have a procedure that covers all aspects required for suctioning as well as a list of the equipment and supplies needed.

As with the other artificial airway care procedures used in the home, teach the client and family how to wash their hands, giving careful attention to the areas around the fingernails. Provide the client with a mirror so that he or she can see to insert the catheter into the airway. Teach the same technique you have been using. To help the client acquire the manual skills needed to maneuver the catheter in the tracheostomy and occlude the Y-vent, provide opportunities to handle the equipment, and allow simulated practice sessions if necessary. To prevent the danger of oversuctioning, instruct the client to limit each suction attempt to 5 to 6 seconds with a 3-minute rest period between attempts. Help the client to understand the danger of oversuctioning and the importance of deep breathing and coughing effectively to clear the airway.

The client will need a mobile suction unit for use in the home, as well as having some understanding of how it operates. If a wall system is in use in the hospital, provide an opportunity to see and become familiar with the parts of a mobile unit before going home. Although the unit used at home will have specific directions for its care and use, it is helpful to see a mobile unit before discharge.

Small bowls or *glass jars* can be used in the home to hold the solution used to flush the catheter. *Tap water* is usually used in the home to flush the suction catheter. Instruct the client to use soap and water to clean the reusable suction catheters, Y-connector, connecting tubing, and bowls and to rinse them thoroughly. To disinfect these items by boiling, cover them with enough water so that there is at least 1 inch over them. See Skill 30 for information about disinfecting supplies. Wrap the disinfected items in a clean towel. The collection container on the suction unit needs to be emptied, washed, and rinsed at least once a day.

RECORDING

The amount and characteristics of the aspirated secretions and the client's tolerance of the suctioning are recorded. Include the frequency of suctioning and how well the client is able to deep breathe and cough out secretions voluntarily.

Sample POR Recording

- S—NA
- O—Difficult to arouse client; respirations 28 and noisy; occasional weak, ineffective cough; coarse wheezes heard in both lungs.
- A—Unable to clear airway for adequate ventilation.
- P—Maintain in semi-Fowler's position, suction nasopharynx p.r.n. Notify physician of congested lungs and request order for nasotracheal suctioning.

Sample Narrative Recording

Difficult to arouse, respirations 28 and noisy. Cough weak and ineffective, coarse wheezes heard in both lungs. Placed in semi-Fowler's position; nasopharynx suctioned. Notified physician of lung congestion and obtained order for nasotracheal suctioning.

☐ CRITICAL POINTS SUMMARY

1. Suctioning the upper airway is usually an independent nursing function.
2. Medical aseptic technique is generally used to suction the upper airway, whereas surgical aseptic technique is used for the lower airway.
3. Avoid contaminating sputum specimens.

4. Suctioning can induce hypoxemia and alveolar collapse.
5. The time interval during which suction is applied while the catheter is in the airway should not exceed 15 seconds during a 3-minute period.
6. The mucous membranes in the respiratory tract become irritated from suctioning and by the presence of the catheter.
7. There are specified safe ranges for the force of suction for adults, children, and infants.
8. The diameter of the suction catheter should not exceed one-half the diameter of the airway.
9. Suction an airway only when there is evidence of the presence of secretions to be removed.
10. Inspect the nostrils for occlusion before inserting a catheter.
11. Measure the length of the catheter to be inserted into the trachea.
12. Before insertion, lubricate the catheter by immersing it in normal saline.
13. Do not apply suction while inserting the catheter into the airway.
14. Rotate the catheter and apply intermittent suction only when withdrawing the catheter from the airway.
15. Use a fresh catheter for suctioning through another route.
16. Release the suction when there are no air-sucking sounds coming from the distal tip of the catheter.

☐ LEARNING ACTIVITIES

1. Visit the central supply department and look at different types of suction catheters, mobile suction units, and sputum collection containers. Find out which types are used most often.
2. Look at the bacteriologic reports on sputum specimens obtained by suctioning. Note if the report indicates that the specimen was contaminated.
3. Interview clients who have been suctioned to find out how it feels and what difference they detect in their breathing as a result of being suctioned.

☐ REVIEW QUESTIONS

1. Why would a client require airway suctioning?
2. What routes can be used to suction an airway?
3. When would each route be used?
4. Match the adverse effect of suctioning listed in Column I with the preventive nursing intervention in Column II. Each adverse effect may be used once, more than once, or not at all.

COLUMN I
A. Hypoxemia
B. Edematous mucous membranes
C. Alveolar collapse
D. Bradycardia
E. Hypotension
F. Infection
G. Increased secretions

COLUMN II
___ Suction client only when evidence indicates it is necessary
___ Limit suction time to 15 seconds
___ Use aseptic technique
___ Use gentle insertion and manipulation of the suction catheter
___ Change the suction catheter for each different route
___ Keep the vent open when inserting the catheter in the airway

5. What information does the nurse need to collect before suctioning a client?
6. Give the safe ranges of the force of suction for each of the following groups of clients:
   - Children = _____ mm Hg
   - Adults   = _____ mm Hg
   - Infants   = _____ mm Hg
7. What equipment would you need to suction a client through the oropharyngeal and nasotracheal routes?
8. How can you know when a catheter is in the trachea?
9. How would you describe to a peer the way to suction a client using the oropharyngeal, nasotracheal, and tracheostomy routes?

☐ PERFORMANCE CHECKLIST

OBJECTIVE: To use the correct procedure to suction an airway safely.

CHARACTERISTIC	RANGE OF ACCEPTABILITY	SATISFACTORY	UNSATISFACTORY
1. Checks physician's order or kardex.	No deviation		
2. Explains procedure and instructs client on how to cooperate.	No deviation		
3. Washes hands.	No deviation		
4. Assembles equipment.			
5. Closes door and cubicle curtains.			
6. Opens and prepares clean or sterile field, pours sterile normal saline into basin.	No deviation		
7. Places client in high-Fowler's position if possible with head erect and in midline. Supports head with pillows if necessary.	No deviation		
8. Turns on, checks, and adjusts suction pressure.	No deviation		
9. Opens package with sterile suction catheter and attaches catheter to suction source.	Omit if suctioning by nasotracheal route.		
10. Removes wrapping from catheter and places catheter on sterile field.	No deviation		
11. Dons clean or sterile gloves according to aseptic technique used.	No deviation		
12. Picks up catheter with gloved hand, flushes it with saline.	No deviation		
13. Oropharyngeal route: a. Instructs client to open mouth and breathe normally. b. Uses tongue depressor to depress tongue. c. Inserts catheter tip into oropharynx with gloved hand.	No deviation No deviation No deviation		

(continued)

CHARACTERISTIC	RANGE OF ACCEPTABILITY	SATISFACTORY	UNSATISFACTORY
d. Alternates occluding vent and rotates catheter while simultaneously withdrawing catheter from oropharynx. e. Flushes catheter with saline. f. Waits 2 to 3 minutes before next attempt.	No deviation No deviation No deviation		
14. Nasopharyngeal route: a. Uses gloved hands to hold catheter near face to measure distance from tip of nose to earlobes and thyroid cartilage. Notes length of catheter to be inserted. b. Has client hyperextend neck, open the mouth wide, and extend the tongue. c. Has assistant grasp tongue with gauze square and has client pant through mouth. d. Inserts catheter through nostril, nasopharynx, and into trachea. Notes air flow through catheter. e. Has assistant release tongue and asks client to breathe normally. f. Holds catheter securely in trachea and uses other hand to attach connecting tubing. g. Alternately applies suction while rotating catheter and slowly withdrawing catheter. h. Flushes catheter with normal saline. i. Repeats steps 14 b to i if necessary.	No deviation No deviation No deviation No deviation No deviation No deviation No deviation No deviation No deviation		
15. Tracheostomy route: a. Inserts catheter into inner cannula 12.5 cm (5 in). b. Applies alternate suction and rotates catheter while slowly withdrawing catheter. c. Flushes catheter with normal saline. d. Repeats steps 15 a to c if necessary after a 3-minute rest period. (NOTE: Cleanses inner cannula and provides wound care if necessary. Repeats suctioning if necessary using a new sterile catheter.)	No deviation No deviation No deviation No deviation		
16. Cleans reusable and discards disposable equipment.	No deviation		
17. Places client in a comfortable position.	No deviation		
18. Records relevant data on health record.	No deviation		

REFERENCES

O'Malley P, Zankofski MA: Disposable suction catheters: Nursing79 product survey. Nursing79 9(5):70–75, 1979.

Rarey KP, Youtsey JW: Respiratory Patient Care. Englewood Cliffs, NJ, Prentice-Hall, 1981.

Traver GA (ed): Respiratory Nursing: The Science and Art. New York, John Wiley & Sons, 1982.

BIBLIOGRAPHY

Fuchs PL: Streamlining your suctioning techniques, Part I: Nasotracheal suctioning. Nursing84 (Horsham) 14(4):55–61, 1984.

Fuchs PL: Streamlining your suctioning techniques, Part III: Tracheostomy suctioning. Nursing84 14(7):39–43, 1984.

Harper RW: A Guide to Respiratory Care: Physiology and Clinical Applications. Philadelphia, JB Lippincott, 1981.

Luckmann J, Sorensen KC: Medical–Surgical Nursing: A Psychophysiological Approach. Philadelphia, WB Saunders, 1980.

Perkins JJ: Principles and Methods of Sterilization in Health Sciences, ed 2. Springfield, IL, Charles C Thomas, 1969.

Skelley BF, Deeren SM, et al.: The effectiveness of two pre-oxygenation methods to prevent endotracheal suction-induced hypoxemia. Heart and Lung 9(2):316–323, 1980.

Sorensen KC, Luckmann J: Basic Nursing: A Psychophysiologic Approach. Philadelphia, WB Saunders, 1979.

SUGGESTED READING

Fuchs PL: Streamlining your suctioning techniques, Part I: Nasotracheal suctioning. Nursing84 14(5):55–61, 1984.

Fuchs PL: Streamlining your suctioning techniques, Part II: Endotracheal suctioning. Nursing84 14(6):46–51, 1984.

Fuchs PL: Streamlining your suctioning techniques, Part III: Tracheostomy suctioning. Nursing84 14(7):39–43, 1984.

AUDIOVISUAL RESOURCES

Pharyngeal Suctioning
   Filmstrip and cassette. (1982, Color, 14 min.)

Tracheobronchial Suctioning in the Intubated Patient
   Filmstrip and cassette. (1982, Color, 17 min.)
   Available through:
      Medcom, Inc.
      P.O. Box 116
      Garden Grove, CA 92642

16 Medication Administration

☐ ENTRY TEST

1. What are the metric units of weight and measures of volume and length?
2. What is the basis of the relationship among units in the metric system?
3. How are smaller metric units converted to larger units, and vice versa?
4. What is the relationship between metric weight and fluid volume measures?
5. What are the units of weight and measures of volume and length in the U.S. household system?
6. What are commonly known equivalents between the metric system and the U.S. household system?
7. Write the Roman numerals from one to twenty, using lowercase letters.
8. Express the following values as a ratio, decimal fraction, or common fraction:

RATIO	DECIMAL FRACTION	COMMON FRACTION
1 : 2	____	____
____	____	$\frac{1}{3}$
____	0.75	____

9. Solve the following equations:

   a. $\frac{2}{3} \times \frac{3}{4} = x$

   b. $\frac{1}{2} + \frac{2}{5} = x$

   c. $\frac{3}{4} + \frac{5}{8} = x$

   d. $\frac{3}{4} - \frac{5}{8} = x$

   e. $\frac{3}{4} \div 2 = x$

   f. $\frac{3}{4} \times 2 = x$

   g. $0.25 \times 3.5 = x$

   h. $8.5 \div 2.5 = x$

   i. $1\frac{5}{8} - \frac{3}{4} = x$

   (express answer as decimal)

   j. $3x + 5 = 20$

   k. $6x - 12 = 4x$

   l. $10 \times \frac{3}{21} \times \frac{8}{3} \times \frac{14}{30} = x$

10. What characteristics of mucous membranes make it possible for substances to be absorbed into the body through these tissues?
11. Describe the structures and functions of the external nose, nasal cavity, and accessory sinuses.
12. Describe the structures and secretions of the external ear.
13. Describe the structures and functions of the external eye cavity.
14. For location of the anal sphincters, review Chapter 13, Entry Test, items 1 and 2, p. 562.
15. For structure and function of the female genitalia and vagina, review Chapter 10, Entry Test, items 5 and 7 to 9, p. 357.
16. Identify the absorptive surface of the lungs.
17. Compare the vascularity and nerve supply of the epidermis, dermis, subcutaneous, and skeletal muscle tissues.
18. Where are the major muscle masses of the body located?
19. Describe the three layers in the strucutre of a vein.
20. Identify the purpose and location of valves in the venous system.

PREREQUISITE SKILLS

Skill 17, "Using the Health Record"
Skill 18, "Nursing Records"

INTRODUCTION

Drugs are chemicals that produce biologic effects in living organisms. Medications are drugs that are used for therapeutic, diagnostic, or preventive purposes in human beings. The term *dosage* refers to the amount of pure drug available in a given amount or quantity of medication, such as the number of milligrams of drug in one tablet. It also refers to the amount of drug ordered to be given at one time. The term *dose* generally means the number of tablets, milliliters, or other quantity needed to administer a specified dosage (amount of drug).

Medications are received into the body through the oral (by mouth or nasogastric tube), topical (applied to skin or mucous membranes), or parenteral (other than the gastrointestinal tract) routes. Medications are usually quite beneficial, but they also have the potential for undesirable or even harmful effects. Correct administration of medications increases their therapeutic effectiveness and can decrease some of the negative side effects. For example, the effectiveness of some antibiotics is decreased if taken within 1 to 2 hours of the ingestion of food, milk, or antacids, while giving aspirin with food or milk decreases the potential for gastric irritation from that drug.

Nurses administer medications in acute, long-term, and ambulatory settings, monitor clients' self-administration of medication in the clinic and home, and teach clients and families safe medication administration in any of these settings. To be able to fulfill these functions, the nurse must know how to prepare a wide variety of medications, be able to administer them correctly through the appropriate route, and possess enough knowledge about both the client and the drug so that the procedure is both safe and therapeutic.

Safe medication administration is often summarized as the "Five Rights": the right *drug,* the right *dosage,* the right *client,* the right *route,* and the right *time.* To be able to administer medications safely, the nurse must know the terms, abbreviations, symbols, and systems of weights and measures used with medications; how to calculate dosages and equivalent weights and measures; the processes used to obtain, administer, and record medications in an inpatient setting; and how to gather information about the medications he or she administers. Because this information is necessary for administering medications through any route, it is presented in the introduction to this chapter. The specific skills within the chapter include the techniques for administering medications through the various routes and dosage calculation problems specific for those routes. These skills include "Oral Medication Administration" (Skill 71), "Topical Medication Administration" (Skill 72), "Injectable Medication Administration" (Skill 73), and "Intravenous Fluid and Medication Administration" (Skill 74).

LEARNING TO ADMINISTER MEDICATIONS

With the increased use of prepackaged and prelabeled (unit-dose) medications and the increasingly common use of the metric system of weights and measures, nurses currently spend much less time preparing medications, that is, less time calculating dosages, measuring and pouring liquids and tablets, and preparing injectable medications. These changes, however, do not diminish the importance of developing and using safe habits of preparing and administering medications. As drugs become more potent and complex, there is an even greater risk of untoward effects when errors in administration occur. Hopefully, the reduced time required for preparing medications will enable the nurse to use the time for observations that detect the effectiveness of the drug and any problems associated with the drug therapy, as well as to teach clients and families about the drugs.

In most agencies, it is still necessary to do some dosage calculations. The computational skills needed for these calculations are not difficult and were initially learned by most people prior to entering high school. These calculations include the use of decimal and common fractions and a basic proportion equation. As with all skills that are not used frequently, the student may need some refreshing and additional practice with these math skills. The pretest questions can help the student determine the need for this review and practice. If additional assistance is needed, it is recommended that the student use a basic math review book.

For safe medication administration, the nurse also must learn to interpret a variety of abbreviations and symbols used in ordering, preparing, and administering medications. Common abbreviations and symbols are included in this skill; however, agency variations exist.

Medication administration is one of the functions in nursing practice where precise habits must be developed to the point of becoming automatic and ritualistic. It is absolutely imperative that the student do three things: (1) memorize the formulas for calculating equivalents and dosages so they become as familiar as the basic multiplication and division tables; (2) use these formulas to determine correct weights and measures and calculate correct dosages; and (3) follow specific procedures, checks, and safeguards when selecting medications from the supply source and giving them to the client. These automatic sets of behaviors are essential to avoid errors in medication administration, particularly when the nurse is in a hurry, under pressure, or working in unfamiliar circumstances. A parallel example is that of driving a car, in which the learned automatic habits and behaviors of turning, braking, steering, alertness, and cautious driving produce safe driving in a variety of circumstances.

Unfortunately, medication errors and the inability to figure drug doses are common enough that they are a major concern of nurses who work in orientation and inservice programs. For example, when 95 nurses in a pediatric center were tested for their ability to correctly implement medication orders, it was found that their computation scores ranged from 40 to 100 percent correct, with a mean score of 86.2 percent correct answers, with very little difference between experienced and inexperienced nurses. An answer was considered incorrect only when it would have resulted in an administered dose at least 10 times greater or less than the ordered dose. Nurses were also asked to judge the appropriateness of the ordered dosage. Nurses with more than three years experience admitted to less uncertainty about dosages and had a significantly higher error rate than inexperienced nurses (17 percent as compared with 14 percent). The most common source of computational error was misplaced decimal points, often related to the nurse's careless and unclear writing. Experienced nurses admitted to writing answers (usually wrong) based on their experience, without doing any calculations (Perlstein et al., 1979).

Medication errors are discussed in more detail later in this Introduction.

WEIGHTS AND MEASURES IN MEDICATION ADMINISTRATION

Although most drugs are ordered and available in the metric system of weights and measures (volume and length), there are two other systems used with medications: the familiar U.S. household system, and the older apothecary system, currently used only in pharmacy practice. From the perspective of the nurse administering medications, these different systems become a problem only when a drug is *ordered* using weights and measures of one system and the drug is *available* labeled in weight and measurement terms of another system. An example of this problem is the common preoperative medication order of atropine, gr 1/150 (apothecary system term). Atropine is an injectable liquid available in ampules or vials labeled 0.4 mg of atropine per ml solution (metric terms). To know what volume of atropine solution to administer so as to give gr 1/150, the nurse must convert the apothecary dosage to the metric system and then determine the correct volume of atropine to use for the ordered dose. In the home setting, teaspoons and other household measures are often used to measure medications. Therefore, the nurse must be able to work with all three measurement systems and exchange values between them. Each of the systems is described briefly here to help the student understand the meaning and value of the terms used in each system.

Some drugs are measured in units or milliequivalents instead of weight or liquid volume. A milliequivalent (mEq) is a unit of chemical activity or combining power equivalent to the activity of one milligram of hydrogen. Electrolytes such as potassium are measured in mEq. A unit is a measure of the biologic activity of a substance. Drugs such as penicillin and insulin are measured in units.

The Metric System

The metric system is about 300 years old and is the system of weights and measures used throughout most of the world. Although the Metric Conversion Act of 1975 has promoted increased use of the metric system, the United States remains the only industrialized nonmetric nation.

The *meter* is the basic unit of the metric system. It originally was defined as one ten-millionth of the distance from the equator to the North Pole along the meridian that passes through Paris. Since 1960, the meter is defined as the length equal to 1,650,763.73 wave-lengths of the orange-red light of the Krypton-86 isotope (Remington's Pharmaceutical Sciences, 1985). A bar of platinum of this length is kept at the International Bureau of Weights and Measures near Paris, with duplicates in various nations around the world, including the United States, Britain, and Canada. The metric units and abbreviations that are most often used with medications are as follows:

- Weight: kilograms (kg), grams (g), milligrams (mg), micrograms (mcg)
- Volume: liter (L) and milliliter (ml)
- Length: centimeters (cm) and millimeters (mm)

Arabic numerals are always used with the metric system and precede the abbreviation; for example, 250 mg, 60 ml, or 1 g. In this text, gram is abbreviated as "g" (following the recommended usage in the United States Pharmacopeia). Although "gm" is often used as an abbreviation, it can be confused with "gr" when handwritten carelessly. To avoid errors, a zero is always used before the decimal point when writing a fractional part of a metric unit; for example, 0.5 or 0.4 ml. A misplaced decimal can mean a serious overdose or underdose of medication. Quantities between 1 milligram and 1 gram are usually referred to as milligrams; quantities less than 1 milligram are expressed as micrograms; and quantities larger than 1000 grams are expressed as kilograms (Remington's Pharmaceutical Sciences, 1975; United States Pharmacopeia, 1980).

Activity 16-A: Metric Weights

Complete the following table of metric weights:

$$3 \text{ mg} = \underline{} \text{ g}$$
$$50 \text{ mg} = \underline{} \text{ g}$$
$$250 \text{ mg} = \underline{} \text{ g}$$
$$\underline{} \text{ mg} = 6 \text{ g}$$
$$\underline{} \text{ mg} = 0.4 \text{ g}$$
$$\underline{} \text{ mg} = 0.005 \text{ g}$$

(See Appendix II, p. 1013 for answers.)

The Apothecary System

The apothecary system is a very old system of weights and measures. It was used in England at the time the United States was colonized, but at the present time it is used only in pharmacy practice and measuring wine. The basic and smallest unit of weight in the apothecary system is the *grain,* which initially referred to the weight of a grain of wheat. The basic and smallest unit of liquid measure is the *minim.* It is approximately the volume of water that would weigh a grain. There is no unit of length in the apothecaries' system, and the apothecary pound does not have the same value as the common United States household (avoirdupois) pound.

The most common unit of weight used in administering medications is the grain, and the most common liquid measures are the minim, fluidram, and fluidounce. The dram and ounce are rarely used as units of weight. When there is no doubt that the medication is a liquid, "fluid" may be omitted. When dram, ounce, or their abbreviations and symbols are used alone in a medication order or dosage problem, it is assumed to be fluid measure. Table 1 shows the relationship of units of weight and volume in the apothecary system, indicating abbreviations and symbols. Fluid and weight units are distinguished in this table.

Guidelines for hand-writing amounts of medications in the apothecary system are as follows:

1. With symbols, use lowercase Roman letters *after* the symbol. Draw a line over these lowercase letters to help distinguish them from Arabic numerals. The symbol $\overline{ss}$ is used for one-half.
2. With abbreviations, use Arabic numerals *before* the abbreviations. Use common fractions for partial units.

Examples of written apothecary abbreviations and symbols:

SPOKEN AS:	ABBREVIATIONS	SYMBOLS
Seven and one-half grains	7½ gr	gr $\overline{viiss}$
Two minims	2 m	m $\overline{ii}$
Two and one-half fluidounces	2½ foz or 2½ oz	f℥ $\overline{iiss}$ or ℥ $\overline{iiss}$
One dram	1 fdr or 1 dr	f℥ $\overline{i}$ or ℥ $\overline{i}$

TABLE 1. Apothecary Weights and Fluid Measures

WEIGHT		
60 grains	= 1 dram (dr) ( )	ℨ
480 grains or 8 drams	= 1 ounce (oz) ( )	
12 ounces	= 1 pound (lb) = 5760 grains (gr)	℥

VOLUME		
60 minims	= 1 fluidram (fdr) ( )	f℈
8 fluidrams or 480 minims	= 1 fluidounce (foz) ( )	f℥
16 fluidounces	= 1 pint (pt)(O) = 7680 minims (m)	
2 pints	= 1 quart (qt)	
4 quarts	= 1 gallon (gal); (Cong = 1 wine gallon)	

Activity 16-B: Abbreviations and Symbols

1. Write the following amounts, using abbreviations and symbols:

	ABBREVIATION	SYMBOL
twelve minims	_____	_____
two fluidrams	_____	_____
four fluidounces	_____	_____
two and one-half grains	_____	_____
1/60 grain	_____	_____

2. Using the values given in Table 1, determine the following units of volume measure:

$\overline{ss}$ = _____
$\overline{ss}$ = _____
$\overline{ii}$ = _____
$\overline{ii}$ = _____
$\overline{xvi}$ = _____
90 m = _____

(NOTE: Answers to these problems can be found in Appendix II, p. 1013.)

The Household System

The household system of measurement is used in the home setting when other measures are not available. These measures are not considered accurate and should be avoided whenever possible, because there is no standardization in droppers or in teaspoons and tablespoons used for eating. For example, a teaspoon has often been regarded as containing a fluidram or 4 ml, but the average present-day teaspoon is more likely to contain 5 ml. Kitchen measuring spoons are fairly accurate measurement devices, but modern teacups, tablespoons, dessertspoons, and teaspoons have been found to average 25 percent greater capacity than the quantities commonly listed in equivalent tables (Remington's Pharmaceutical Sciences, 1985). Drops and minims have also been regarded as equivalent. The volume of a drop, however, will vary with the viscosity of the liquid, the diameter of the dropper, and the angle at which it is held. Standardized medicine spoons, droppers, or cups are available quite inexpensively in most drug stores, and families should be encouraged to purchase these items.

Exchanging between Systems

The metric and apothecary systems have different size units and subdivisions which are incompatible with each other. Any exchanging between the systems results in approximate equivalents, and a 10 percent margin of difference greater or less than the desired dose is considered acceptable for administering medications. The most common reason a nurse would need to calculate equivalent dosages is when a medication order is written in the apothecary system and the pharmacy only stocks the drug in metric units. In these situations, change the ordered apothecary dosage to a metric unit, since metric is the more accurate system.

TABLE 2. Approximate Equivalent Weights and Measures

WEIGHT		
Metric	Apothecary	Household
1 mg	1/60, 1/64, 1/65 gr	
60, 64, or 65 mg	1 gr	
1 g	15 or 16 gr	
30 or 32 g	1 oz or 8 dr	2 tablespoonfuls (tbsp) or 6 teaspoonfuls (tsp)
1 kg		2.2 lb (avoirdupois)
FLUID VOLUME		
1 ml	15 or 16 m	15 or 16 drops (gtts)
4 ml	1 fdr	—
5 ml	—	1 tsp
12 ml	—	1 dessertspoonful (dssp)
30 or 32 ml	1 foz	2 tbsp
240 or 250 ml	8 foz	1 cup (c)
500 ml	16 foz	1 c or 1 pint (pt)
1000 ml (1 L)	32 foz	4 c or 1 quart (qt)
4000 ml (1 L)	1 gallon (gal)	1 gallon

Although conversion tables are often found in a medicine room or on a medicine cart, this does not always occur, so the nurse cannot plan to rely on tables alone. Memorize the most commonly used metric, apothecary, and household equivalents, as given in Table 2. Many of these values are likely to be familiar, because they are used every day as well as in basic science courses.

When an apothecary-metric conversion is needed, select the conversion ratio (equivalent) that divides out most evenly with the ordered dosage and available dose. Generally, using this equivalent will yield an answer (dose) that is easily given at the bedside, such as whole tablets or capsules, rather than fractions of tablets or capsules that cannot be measured. This method will also yield an answer that is within the 10 percent acceptable margin of difference.

CALCULATION OF DRUG DOSAGES

Drug dosage calculations are used to determine the amount of medication to administer in order to implement the physician's order for a given amount of pure drug. In all dosage problems, there are at least two known values: (1) the ordered (desired) dose to give the client, and (2) the strength of the medication on hand from which to give this dose (the available dosage).

There are two ways to calculate dosage problems: the factor-label method and the proportion equation method. Both are presented here, since students and faculty will find one or the other more compatible with their own mathematics background. Both methods involve multiplying and dividing common fractions and both begin by identifying the *ordered* (desired, or known) dose and an *unknown* dosage (amount) to be given. They are different in that the factor-label equation has the advantage of including all needed calculations in one equation, regardless of the number of conversions needed. With this method, both unit labels and numbers are divided out when solving the equation. With the proportion equation, several equations are used to solve problems involving conversions, and labels are disregarded when dividing and solving the equation.

Most of the skills in this chapter contain examples and practice problems that use both the factor-label and the proportion method. If the student has any difficulty with those problems, he or she is advised to seek additional help or consultation.

Factor-Label Method

The conceptual formula for a factor-label dosage calculation equation is as follows:

Factor-Label Equation:

$$\text{Ordered Dosage} \times \substack{\text{Conversion Factor(s)} \\ \text{or} \\ \text{Known Relationships}} = \substack{\text{Unknown Dose} \\ \text{to be given}}$$

The factor-label method is based on the mathematical concept that multiplying the ordered dosage by known relationship or conversion factor ratios that have a value of 1 yields a dose of medication that can be given at the bedside. Ratios with a value equal to 1 describe a relationship between two different unit labels for the same entity. An example of a ratio equivalent to 1 is $\frac{30 \text{ ml}}{1 \text{ oz}}$. That this ratio equals 1 can be demonstrated mathematically as follows:

1. Write an equation stating the relationship between the two units: 30 ml = 1 oz.
2. Because the two sides of the equation are equal, each side of the equation can be divided by the same amount without changing the equality:

   $$\frac{30 \text{ ml}}{1 \text{ oz}} = \frac{1 \text{ oz}}{1 \text{ oz}}$$

3. Because anything divided by itself is equal to 1, the equation in (2) is equivalent to $\frac{30 \text{ ml}}{1 \text{ oz}} = 1$.

Any known relationship can be expressed in the form of a ratio equivalent to 1. When calculating dosage problems, the ratios equivalent to 1 include: (a) dosage strength, such as mg/tablet, mg/ml; (b) fixed conversion factors between different units of measure, such as 15 gr/1 g, 60 mg/1 gr; or (c) conversion factors within the metric system, such as 1000 mg/1 g. Using one or more ratios equal to 1 in the equation does not alter the value of the ordered dose; it simply changes the dose into an equivalent unit that can be administered at the bedside. For example, to give an ordered dose of 200 mg of the drug Nembutal, you need to determine the number of capsules (dosage) that are needed to administer that dose. The "bridge" between the ordered dose and the dosage to be given is the ratio of 100 mg/1 capsule.

There are three steps involved in setting up the factor-label equation:

1. Identify the *ordered dosage*. That is, determine the exact amount of drug that is to be given to the client at one time or in a specific amount of time. This known amount is always expressed in terms of the pure drug to be given. For example: Give 5 mg, gr x̄, or 30 ml of a drug at 8 AM or every 4 hours; or give 1000 ml of an intravenous fluid over 6 hours of time.
2. Identify the *label or unit of the unknown dose* (amount) of available medication needed to administer the ordered dosage. This unknown amount to be given is always expressed in units that may be administered at the bedside; for example, number of tablets, capsules, milliliters, drops per minute, or milliliters per hour.
3. Identify the necessary *known relationships or conversion factors* that will convert the unit label of the ordered dosage to the unit label of the amount of available medication needed and form a "bridge" between the two values. For example, if the ordered dosage is expressed in different units from the available dosage, insert the necessary relationship ratios in the equation to form "bridges" between the ordered dosage label and the label of the dose to be given at the bedside. That is, when the ordered dosage is written in grains and the available medication is labeled in grams, it is necessary to insert a known relationship ratio about grains and grams, such as $\frac{15 \text{ gr}}{1 \text{ g}}$. These unit label conversions may include a conversion between metric and apothecary units, a conversion within the metric system, a conversion between units of time, all three, or any two of the three.
4. *Set up the equation*. Place the unknown amount (dose) to be given to the client on the right side of the equal sign, and place all other values on the left, in the following sequence:
   a. Place the unknown dose to be given to the right of the equal sign.
   b. Place the ordered dosage on the far left.
   c. Insert the needed conversion or known relationship ratios in the equation.
5. Solve the problem by dividing out both the unit labels and the numerals. Arrange the values within the ratios and place the ratios in the equation in a sequence that allows all unit labels to be divided out *except the unit label that is identical to the unit label of the desired dose to be given at the bedside.*

The following examples illustrate this sequence and further explain the arrangement of the values within the ratio as well as the placement of the ratios within the equation. The first example requires only a dosage strength ratio to calculate the problem.

Example A: You are asked to administer 650 mg of an oral drug. You have tablets containing 325 mg per tablet. How many tablets will you administer? (Although the answer of 2 tablets is readily apparent, the following process of using the factor-label equation would be the same for more complex problems.)

1. Identify the ordered *dosage: 650 mg*
2. Identify the unknown *dose: x tablets*
3. Place the *ordered* dosage on the far left and the *unknown* dose on the right side of the equal sign.

$$650 \text{ mg} = x \text{ tablets}$$

4. Insert the *dosage strength ratio* (325 *mg/tablet*) into the equation. Place the values in the numerator or denominator position in a way that one unit label can be divided out with the unit label of the ordered dose.

$$650 \text{ mg} \times \frac{1 \text{ tablet}}{325 \text{ mg}} = x \text{ (tablets)}$$

Divide out the unit labels, leaving only the label identical to the unit label of the desired dose to be given at the bedside.

$$650 \cancel{\text{mg}} \times \frac{1 \text{ tablet}}{325 \cancel{\text{mg}}} = x$$

5. Solve the equation.

$$\frac{\overset{2}{\cancel{650}} \times 1 \text{ tablet}}{\underset{1}{\cancel{325}}} = x$$

$$x = 2 \text{ tablets}$$

This equation will always work if it is set up so that unit labels will divide out evenly (except for the unit label that corresponds with the unit label of the unknown dose to be given). If the equation is set up incorrectly, it will not be possible to divide out unit labels. Therefore, *it is crucial to label all terms in the equation.* For example, the equation could not be solved if the known relationship between milligrams and tablets were set up in the reverse sequence, as shown in the following INCORRECT equation:

$$650 \text{ mg} \times \frac{325 \text{ mg}}{1 \text{ tablet}} = x \text{ (tablets)}$$

In this equation, there is no way to divide out the milligram labels and have only the tablet labels left.

NOTE: If the ordered dosage in the previous example is written as 0.65 g, a metric conversion is needed. To do this, change the ordered 0.65 g dosage to milligrams by moving the decimal point three places to the right (650 mg), or change the available 325 mg dosage to grams by moving the decimal point three places to the left (0.325 g). Either of these actions yields an ordered dosage and an available dosage with the same unit label. Or, insert the metric conversion ratio of 1000 mg/1 g into the equation, as shown below.

Example B: Ordered dosage: Seconal gr iii
Available dosage: Seconal 100 mg (capsules)

In this problem, a metric-apothecary conversion is needed. The conversion ratio "15 gr/1 g" will be used because it can be divided evenly by the ordered dosage of 3 gr. Because the dosage is labeled in milligrams, the 1 g in the conversion ratio must be changed to milligrams. This can be done by moving the decimal point as indicated earlier or by inserting a conversion ratio for grams and milligrams into the equation as shown below.

1. Place the ordered dosage on the far left and the unknown dosage on the right side of the equal sign.

   $$3 \text{ gr} = x \text{ (capsules)}$$

2. Insert the conversion ratio for grains and grams immediately after the ordered dosage, arranging the values so the grains labels will divide out.

   $$3 \text{ gr} \times \frac{1 \text{ g}}{15 \text{ gr}} = x \text{ (capsules)}$$

3. Insert the conversion ratio for grams and milligrams after the apothecary-metric conversion ratio. Arrange the values so the unit labels will divide out with the grain :: gram ratio.

   $$3 \text{ gr} \times \frac{1 \text{ g}}{15 \text{ gr}} \times \frac{1000 \text{ mg}}{1 \text{ g}} = x \text{ (capsules)}$$

4. Insert the available dosage strength ratio after the grams :: milligrams ratio.

   $$3 \text{ gr} \times \frac{1 \text{ g}}{15 \text{ gr}} \times \frac{1000 \text{ mg}}{1 \text{ g}} \times \frac{1 \text{ capsule}}{100 \text{ mg}} = x \text{ (capsules)}$$

5. Divide out the unit labels.

   $$\frac{1}{\cancel{3} \cancel{\text{gr}}} \times \frac{1 \cancel{\text{g}}}{\cancel{15} \cancel{\text{gr}}} \times \frac{\cancel{1000}^{10} \cancel{\text{mg}}}{1 \cancel{\text{g}}} \times \frac{1 \text{ capsule}}{\cancel{100} \cancel{\text{mg}}} = x \text{ (capsules)}$$

6. Solve the equation.

   $$\frac{1 \times 1 \times 10 \times 1 \text{ capsule}}{5 \times 1 \times 1} = x \text{ (capsules)}$$

   $$\frac{10 \text{ capsules}}{5} = x$$

   $$x = 2 \text{ capsules}$$

Proportion Equation Method

Dosage Calculations. A known values DOSAGE FORMULA is used to calculate drug dosage problems, using the following conceptual formula.

Dosage Formula:

$$\frac{\text{Known Dosage}}{\text{Known Amount}} = \frac{\text{Ordered Dosage}}{\text{Unknown Amount}}$$

Example : You are asked to give Equanil, 100 mg at bedtime, p.r.n. (as needed). You have available scored tablets labeled Equanil, 200 mg. How many tablets will you administer?

Although the answer to this problem would be readily evident without doing any calculation, it illustrates the use of the proportion equation. The ratio on the left represents the dosage available for use and has a *known dosage* in a *known amount;* that is 200 mg in 1 tablet. The ratio on the right represents the ordered medication and has an *ordered dosage* in an *unknown amount;* that is, 100 mg in an undetermined number of tablets. In this equation, the term *amount* refers to number of oral tablets, but it may mean any other unit or quantity; that is, capsules, milliliters, minims, milligrams, fluidrams, teaspoons, or liters. *Dosage* refers to any measured amount of drug, expressed as grams, milligrams, grains, milliequivalents, or units. Solve the problem as follows:

$$\frac{\text{Known Dosage}}{\text{Known Amount}} = \frac{\text{Ordered Dosage}}{\text{Unknown Amount}}$$

$$\frac{200 \text{ mg}}{1 \text{ tablet}} = \frac{100 \text{ mg}}{x \text{ tablets}}$$

$$100 = 200x$$

$$x = \frac{100}{200}$$

ANSWER: $x = \frac{1}{2}$ *tablet*

The Equanil example illustrates the following guidelines for using this proportion equation to calculate drug dosages. Use these guidelines to solve proportion equations correctly.

1. Use the same units in each of the two ratios. There may be *no more* than two units of weight or measure in any one equation.
2. Place the terms in the same sequence on both sides of the equation.
3. Label *every* term when setting up the equation.
4. Cross-multiply to solve the equation.
5. Label the unknown quantity, x, with the appropriate unit of weight or measure.

Conversion Calculations. A known values CONVERSION FORMULA is used to determine equivalent values between two systems of weights and measures. This proportion equation has a known ratio of equivalent values on one side of the equation and the value needing to be converted on the other side of the equation. The conceptual formula is as follows.

Conversion Formula:

Known Equivalents = Unknown Equivalents

Example : Ordered Dosage: Nembutal, gr iii, at bedtime
Available Dosage: Nembutal, 100 mg capsules

To solve this dosage problem, you will need to convert the apothecary gr iii to a metric equivalent before you can calculate the number of capsules to give the client.

To set up a conversion equation, first write the side of the equation that contains the *unknown value* you want to determine, labeling both terms. Next, select a set of *known equivalent values* for those two terms and put it on the other side of the equation. Change grams to milligrams as needed to set up the equation. Choose an equivalent that divides evenly with the ordered dosage.

Known Equivalent = Unknown Equivalent

$$\frac{1000 \text{ mg}}{15 \text{ gr}} = \frac{x \text{ mg}}{3 \text{ gr}}$$

$$15x = 3000$$

$$x = 200 \text{ mg}$$

ANSWER: 3 gr = 200 mg

Notice that the conversion calculations in the Nembutal example came out even, with no fractions, and that the answer of 200 mg is directly comparable to the available dosage of 100 mg. It is evident that you would need to administer two capsules of Nembutal 100 mg in order to give a dose of 200 mg. This relationship is not always so evident, and the DOSAGE FORMULA is then used to calculate the needed amount of medication. Choosing an equivalent that produces an even answer directly comparable to the available dosage makes it much easier to determine the desired dose of medication.

Children's Dosage Calculations

Dosage calculations for infants and children are done in the same way as for adult dosages. Because the amounts of the drug and the volume are smaller, the nurse must be particularly careful when doing the calculations, must know the usual dosages, and must validate unusual or unfamiliar orders. Infant and children's dosage calculation formulas (Young's, Clark's, and Fried's rules) are not included in this text because those calculations are done by the physician when determining the prescribed dosage, and nurses rarely need to use them. Most pediatric textbooks contain the nomograms and formulas used for calculating dosage on the basis of body surface area (BSA). The nurse might need to use this formula to evaluate whether an ordered dose is within the safe range for that particular child or infant. Whenever the nurse is uncertain about a pediatric dosage, it is important to consult with the physician, a pharmacist, or a printed guide or formula available in the clinical unit.

THE MEDICATION ORDER

Most people are familiar with the prescription method used for ordering medications and have taken a prescription to a pharmacy to purchase the medication as dispensed by a pharmacist. Another way to obtain medications is through clinics or outpatient departments where medications are distributed under the supervision of physicians or pharmacists. In each of these settings, the individual receiving the drug will administer it to himself, herself, or a family member.

The process of receiving a medication is quite different in an inpatient setting than in a clinic or home setting. That is, rather than giving a prescription directly to the client or family, the physician gives a medication order to a nurse, pharmacist, or computer. Clients generally remain in a room or a unit within the agency and nurses are responsible for administering the medications to the clients. In some agencies, pharmacy personnel are beginning to assume this function. As of yet, there is no data to reflect the success of this approach.

Health-care agencies use a variety of systems to ensure that the ordered medications are given to the right person at the right time and in the right manner. These systems vary somewhat with the specific agency.

Initiating the Medication Order

Medications are prescribed or ordered by a licensed medical physician (MD), osteopathic physician (DO), dentist (DDS), an optometrist (OD), or a podiatrist (DPM). In some states, physician's assistants, nurse practitioners, or clinical pharmacists are legally authorized to prescribe certain drugs. For a medication order to be implemented, it must be complete. This means it must include the following information: date (and sometimes time of day), name of the drug, desired dose, route of administration, time of day or frequency of administration, expiration date (if relevant for that drug), any special instructions for administration, and the signature of the physician or other professional authorized to prescribe medications. Abbreviations and terms commonly used in medication orders and administration of medications are given in Table 3.

TABLE 3. Abbreviations and Terms Used in Medication Orders

ABBREVIATION	LATIN DERIVATION	MEANING
aq.	aqua	water
aa.	ana	of each
c̄	cum	with
s̄	sine	without
os	os	mouth
p.o.	per os	orally, by mouth
o.d.	oculus dexter	right eye
o.s.	oculus sinister	left eye
o.l.	oculus laerus	left eye
o.u.	oculo utro	both eyes
Sig	signa	write on the label
IM		intramuscular
SQ, SubQ		subcutaneous
IV		intravenous
ID		intradermal
q.s.	quantum sufficit	as much as is required; a sufficient amount
no.	numerus	number
d.c. or d/c	discontinua	discontinue

TABLE 4. Medication Administration Schedule

ABBREVIATION	LATIN DERIVATION	MEANING	EXAMPLE OF ADMINISTRATION TIME
ad lib	ad libita	as desired, freely	
a.a.	ana	of each	
a.c.	ante cibos	before meals	7:30–11:30–4:30
p.c.	post cibos	after meals	8:30–12:30–5:30
q.d.	quaque die	every day	9:00 AM
o.h.	omni hora	every hour	1–2–3, etc.
q.h.	quaque hora	every hour	1–2–3, etc.
q.i.d.	quater in die	4 times each day	8–12–4–8 or 6–12–6–12 or 9–3–9–3
t.i.d.	ter in die	3 times each day	10–2–6 or 10–6–2
b.i.d.	bis in die	twice each day	9–9
p.r.n.	pro re nata	as needed; when required	
q. 2 h.	quaque 2 hora	every 2 hours	8–10–12, etc.
q. 3 h.	quaque 3 hora	every 3 hours	9–12–3–6 9–12–3–6
q. 4 h.	quaque 4 hora	every 4 hours	8–12–4–8 12–4
q. 6 h.	quaque 6 hora	every 6 hours	6–12–6–12
q. 8 h.	quaque 8 hora	every 8 hours	6–2–10
q. a.m.	quaque ante meridiem	every morning	9:00 AM
q.o.d.	quaque altero die	every other day	1–5, 1–7, 1–9
h.s.	hora somni	hour of sleep; bedtime	10:00 PM
q. h.s.	quaque hora somni	at every bedtime	10:00 PM

Medications are administered at different times of the day to achieve a variety of therapeutic effects or to minimize side effects. For example, cimetidine (Tagamet) is always taken with or immediately after meals to prolong its action and counteract drug-induced gastric acid secretion. Some drugs, such as antibiotics, need to be given every 4 to 6 hours throughout a 24-hour day so as to maintain therapeutic blood levels, while other drugs, such as antacids, may be given only during waking hours. Abbreviations used to designate varied administration times are shown in Table 4.

Types of Medication Orders

All medication orders must be in writing to be valid. There are some circumstances in which a client may need the medication before this written order is possible. For example, in emergencies *verbal orders* (VO) are used when there is not enough time to write the orders or when a physician cannot stop a procedure to write the orders. In other circumstances, the physician may not be available in person, and a *telephone order* (TO or PO) is given over the telephone to the nurse or pharmacist. The practice of having unit clerks or secretaries receive telephone orders is not considered safe because of their level of understanding about drugs. When taking a verbal or telephone order, the nurse promptly writes it in the health record as a complete order, indicates it is a verbal or telephone order, includes the time the order was given, and signs his or her own name as well as that of the physician giving the order. As soon as circumstances permit, the physician then countersigns the order.

Another kind of medication order is the *standing order*. Standing orders are written physician directives or protocols that are available for nurses to implement according to agency policy and nursing judgment. They are most often used where care for many clients is similar, such as in maternity units, coronary care units, or for routine pre- and postoperative care in specialty areas where the physician has many clients with similar kinds of surgeries.

Each type of medication order described above may be *one-time, stat, standard,* or *p.r.n.* orders. *One-time* orders are for medications that are to be given only once, such as for a preoperative medication. A *stat* order indicates that the medication is to be given immediately and only once, such as for relieving the current distress of pain or nausea. A *standard* order is one that may be given for a specified number of days, such as a postoperative pain medication or antibiotic; or it may be given indefinitely, such as with vitamins. In many agencies, policy dictates that standard orders are automatically discontinued after a specified number of days and must be reordered by the physician in writing if the medication is to be continued. Other

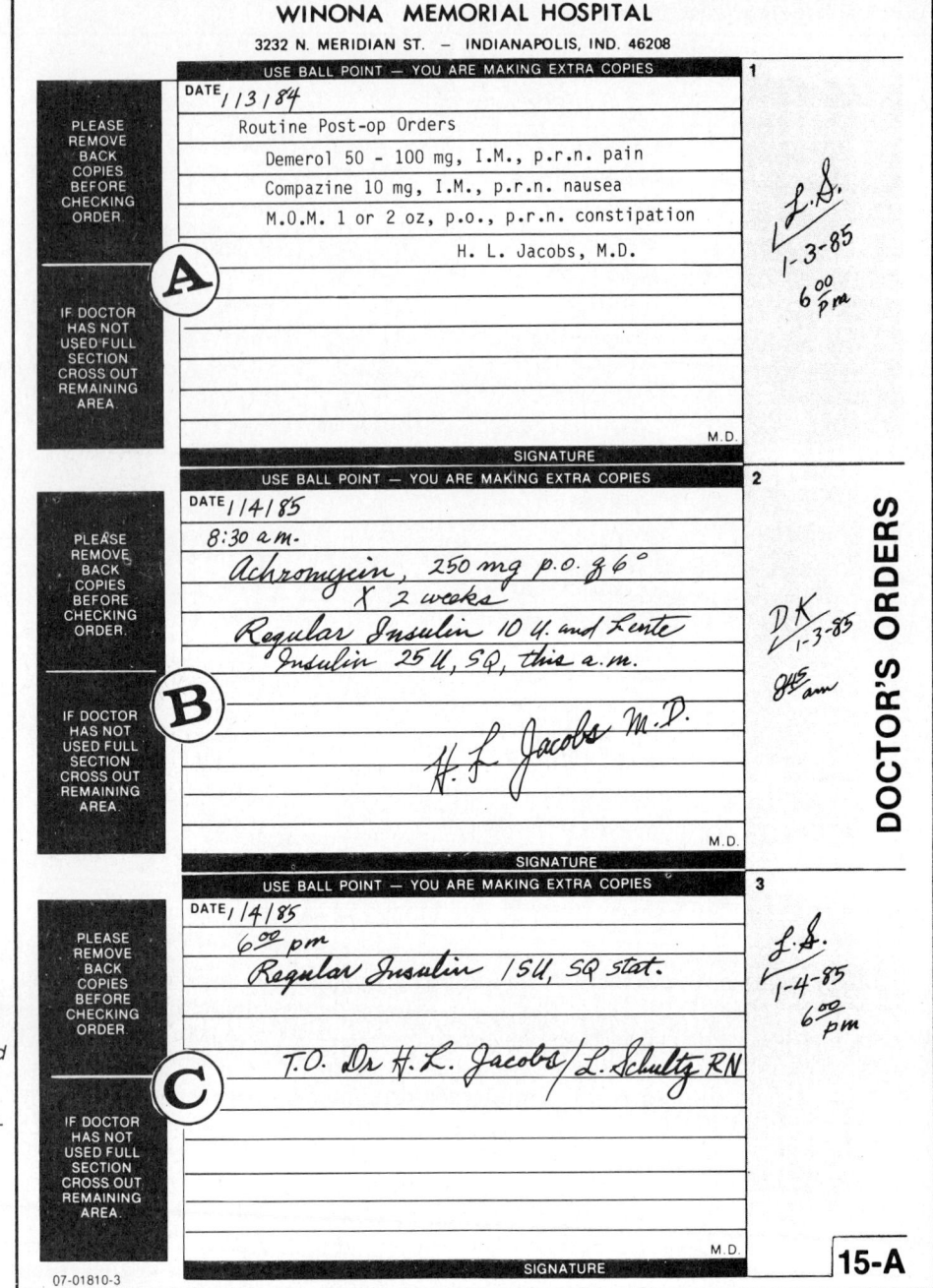

Figure 1. Physician's written medication orders. **A.** Standing orders printed or typed on the physician's order form. Note the checkmark, nurse's initials, and date that indicate the orders were activated and entered into the system for this client. **B.** Standard, routine order for antibiotic, with expiration date indicated; and a onetime order for insulin. Both orders were written and signed by the attending physician. **C.** Stat one-time telephone order for insulin. This order has not yet been countersigned by the physician.

agencies may implement such a policy primarily for antibiotics and controlled substances (sedatives, tranquilizers, and narcotics). Agency policy usually dictates that all medication orders are automatically canceled when a client goes to surgery unless the physician specifies otherwise. These policies and practices are designed to promote safe administration and avoid developing drug toxicity, tolerance, or addiction. P.r.n. medications are given at the discretion of the nurse for the purpose indicated by the physician when writing the order; for example, analgesics are often ordered to be given when the client has pain.

The medication orders discussed here are shown in Figure 1. These orders are either typed or written on a physician order page.

Transmitting the Order to the Pharmacist

After a medication order is written, there are several different ways it can be sent to the pharmacy department. In some agencies, the physician's order form in the health record is a multiple page form, such as that shown in Figure 1. With this system, a duplicate of the written order is sent to the pharmacist to interpret and dispense the ordered medications, while the original order remains in the health record. A third copy is sent to the financial department for billing purposes. In some agencies, the written physician order is inserted into a computer system by a unit clerk or staff nurse. In other agencies, the medication order is transcribed by hand from the physician's order form in the health record onto a requisition form, which is sent to the pharmacy department. Because of the potential for transcription error, this system is not in common use.

The pharmacist's role is to dispense the medication. In some situations this may mean mixing, preparing, and labeling the drug, but more commonly includes correctly measuring and labeling the drug with the correct name, client's name, and instructions for administering the drug. The pharmacy department uses one of several different ways to deliver the medications to clinical units, as discussed below.

Medication Delivery Systems

The three primary systems used to deliver medications to clinical units are the *unit-dose, individual,* or *stock* supply systems. Modifications or combinations of these systems are often used, according to agency preference.

Unit-dose System. In the unit-dose system, the drug is packaged in separate doses that are labeled with the drug name (generic or proprietary or both), dosage, expiration date (if appropriate), and warnings, storage recommendations, or administration directions, as needed. Any type of medication may be packaged in this way, including tablets, capsules, vaginal inserts, oral liquids, or injectable medications. Some medication are always packaged in multiple-dose containers, such as insulin. Several unit-dose and multiple-dose package styles are shown in Figure 2.

In a typical unit-dose system, a carbon copy of the medication order or a computer message is sent to the pharmacy department. The pharmacist keeps a record of the drugs each client receives and checks new orders for compatibility or antagonistic actions with the drugs the client is already receiving. Unit-dose packages of all the medications needed for an 8-, 12-, or 24-hour period are placed in individual drawers for each client and then taken to the clinical unit. A module containing these individual drawers is placed in a portable medicine cart or in a medicine room, replacing the module already there. Figure 3 shows a portable medicine cart. To administer medications to a group of clients, the nurse takes the cart to or into each client's room in sequence and then selects from the drawer the medications to be given to that client at that time. With this system, the nurse works with only one client's medications at a time, thus decreasing the potential for administration errors.

Advantages of the unit-dose system include: substantial savings in nurse's time spent in preparing medication; less chance for errors in preparation and administration of medications; decreased medication costs because medications can be returned to the client's drawer and clients are billed only for the medica-

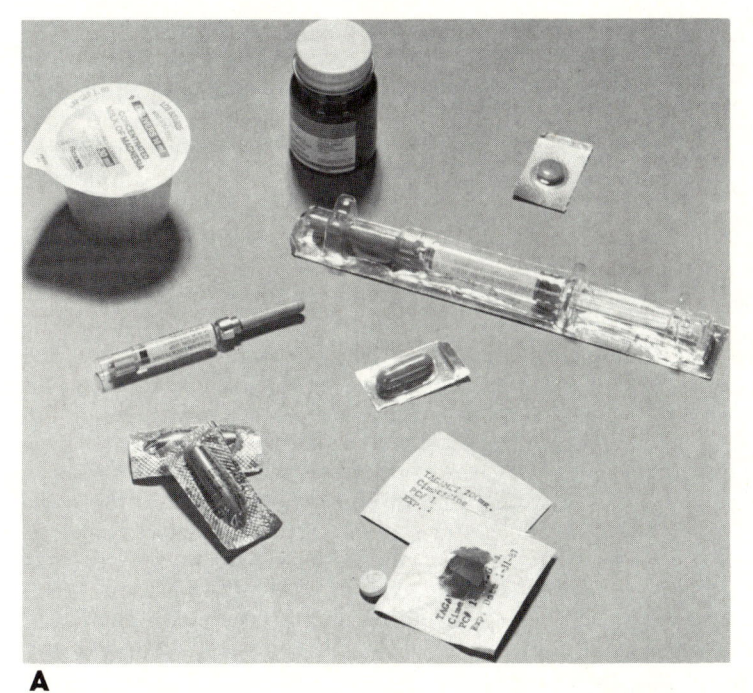

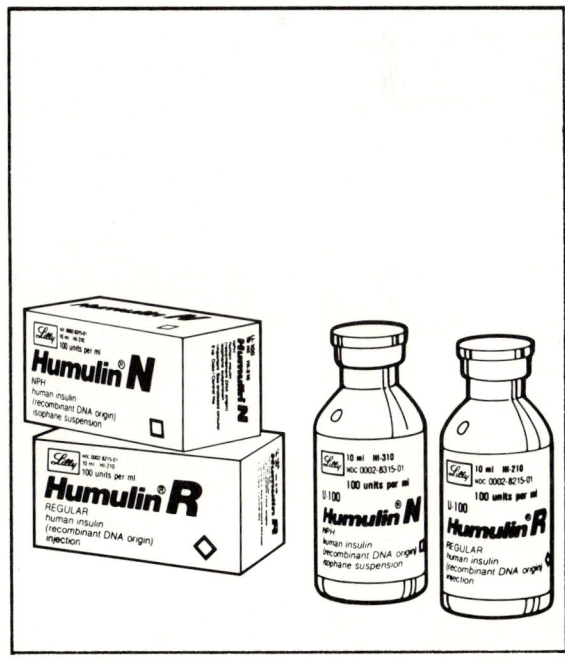

Figure 2. A. Unit-dose packaging: Oral liquids, tablets, capsules, suppositories, prefilled syringe, and cartridge-needle unit. (Photo by James Haines.) B. Multiple-dose vial of Humulin, regular and NPH. (Courtesy of Eli Lilly and Company, Indianapolis, IN.)

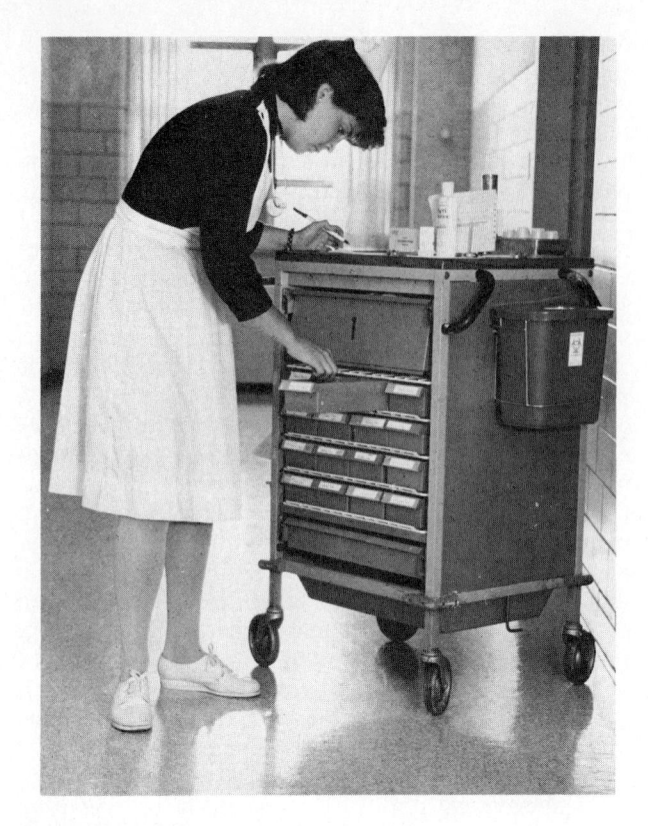

Figure 3. Portable medication cart, with individual drawers for each client's medications. (Photo by James Haines.)

tions they actually receive; improved control and monitoring of drug administration within an agency; and reduction of the amounts of stock drugs that need to be kept on each unit (Buccerl and Baker, 1978). Recent guidelines from the American Society of Hospital Pharmacists and current standards of the Joint Commission on Accreditation of Hospitals recommend using the unit-dose system of drug distribution (Davis and Cohen, 1981). The primary disadvantage of this system involves time delays for newly ordered medications to reach the clinical unit, or delays in replacing drugs that have been contaminated or damaged during attempted administration. Decentralized clinical pharmacy services generally help resolve these problems (Jackson et al., 1978).

Individual Supply System. In the individual supply system, each client has a separate drawer in a portable cart or a cubicle in a medicine room that contains about a five-day supply of the medications ordered for that client. These medications may be in multiple-dose containers or individual unit-dose packages. When a medication is discontinued, it may be returned to the pharmacy either at that time or when the client is discharged. The nurse may need to select the correct medication from among other, currently unused, medications. To give a medication with this system, the nurse selects the correct medications for that particular time and prepares the correct amount of the prescribed drug. If using a medicine cart, the nurse would prepare one client's medications at a time and give them to that client immediately. If no cart is used, the nurse prepares a large number of clients' medications while in the medicine room, places them in plastic or paper containers, and then delivers them to the clients in some logical sequence. Medicine cards must be used with this system so that each client's medications are clearly identified. Medicine cards are described below.

Stock Supply System. In the stock supply system, a wide variety of medications is stored in bulk in the medicine room on the clinical unit. The nurse uses a medicine card system as a guide for selecting the correct medicine from the bulk supply at the right time for each client. This system eliminates the need for requisitions to the pharmacy, allows the medication regime to be changed without waiting for new medications to be delivered from the pharmacy, and eliminates the need to return unused medications to the pharmacy. This system is used infrequently because it has more sources for error in that the nurse has to select the correct medication from among a large variety of medications that often are similar in name and dosage. It also requires that many medications be constantly available on each clinical unit and usually requires that the nurse do more dosage calculation, as every dosage form cannot be available on the clinical unit. Other disadvantages include the risk of contamination through incorrect handling being greater with a bulk drug supply than with smaller amounts of drug, and the large amount of time required for the nurse to inventory the stock and reorder the drugs.

ADMINISTERING THE MEDICATION

Transmitting the Order to the Nursing Staff

Several different systems are used to transmit the medication order from the health record to a medicine record used by the nurse who will actually administer the medications. Regardless of the system used, each one has built-in safeguards and checks that help avoid the potential for human error in the transmission process.

Computer Systems. In a computerized system, the computer prints out a list of regularly scheduled and p.r.n. medications for a given work shift for all the clients on that unit. New medications or order changes are inserted into the computer system and printed out automatically. Medications are recorded in the computer system after they are given, as described below. A printed record of medications given on the previous day is placed in the health record. In addition, information about the medications given to a particular client is retrievable from the computer system at any time. When medications are discontinued, they are deleted from the system. Figure 4 shows a computer printout for regularly scheduled medications, a computer screen for recording medications, and a computer terminal.

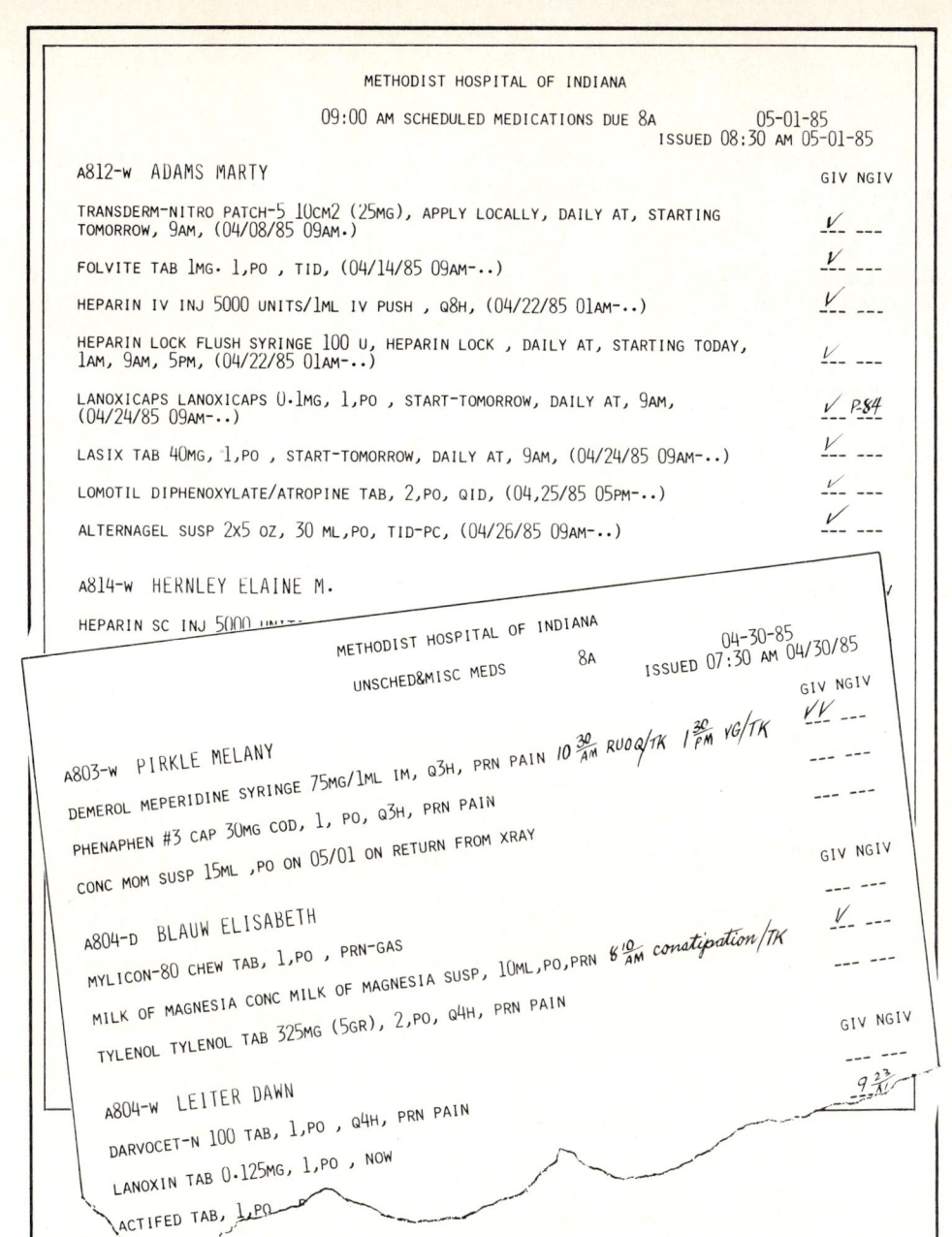

Figure 4. Computer system for transmitting medication orders and recording medication administration: **A.** Computer printout used at the medication cart. Note the "given" and "not given" columns for recording at the time of administration. Scheduled medications, given at regular intervals (top). Unscheduled and miscellaneous medications, given p.r.n., one time only, or as a stat medication (bottom). (Courtesy of Methodist Hospital of Indiana, Inc., Indianapolis, IN.) **B.** Computer screen for recording medications with a light pen and entering that information into the system. **C.** Computer terminal. The nurse is using a light pen to record medication administration on the computer screen. He will then enter that information into the system. (Courtesy of Methodist Hospital of Indiana, Inc., Indianapolis, IN. Photos by James Haines.)

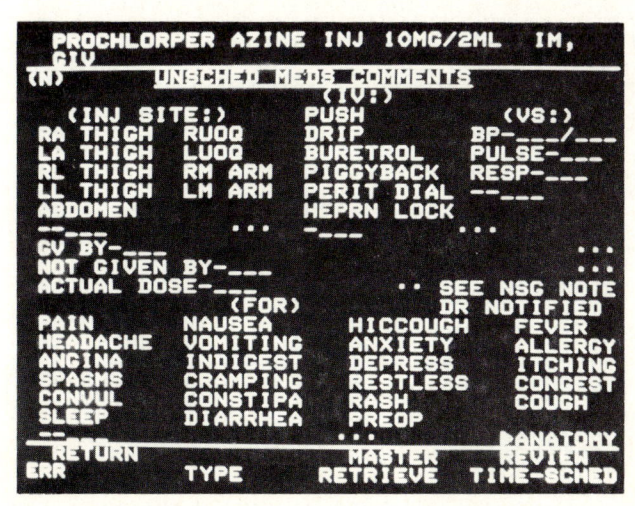

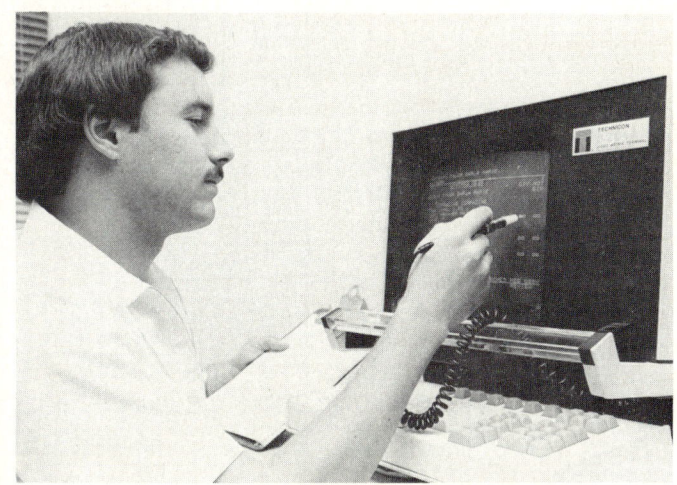

840 PROFESSIONAL CLINICAL NURSING SKILLS

Manual Systems. In a manual or noncomputerized system, the medication order is transcribed onto a medication record page or kardex form that lists all regularly scheduled, p.r.n., or stat medications. A medication record page is a multiple page form with four or five copies, as shown in Figure 5. The medication pages for a group of clients are kept in a loose-leaf notebook on the portable medicine cart. After each client's medications are given, the nurse records that administration on that client's medication page. A line is drawn through discontinued medications. At the end of each 24 hours, the bottom copy is removed and placed in the health record, replacing the previous day's copy. When all columns on the original page are completed, it is placed in the record and becomes a part of the permanent record. This system provides documentation in the health record of the medications given on the previous day, as with the computerized printout system.

In another kind of manual system, the medication order is transcribed onto a medication kardex which is kept on a portable medicine cart. The nurse uses the kardex as the source of information for administering medications, and prepares one client's medications at a time, just prior to giving them to the client. The medication order is usually deleted with a yellow marker when it is discontinued. In a modification of this system, the medication order is transcribed onto a medicine kardex and a medication card is made out for each medication. These cards are usually color-coded to help identify the different time intervals for administering medications. The cards are stored in the medicine room or on the medicine cart in a rack with compartments for each hourly time inter-

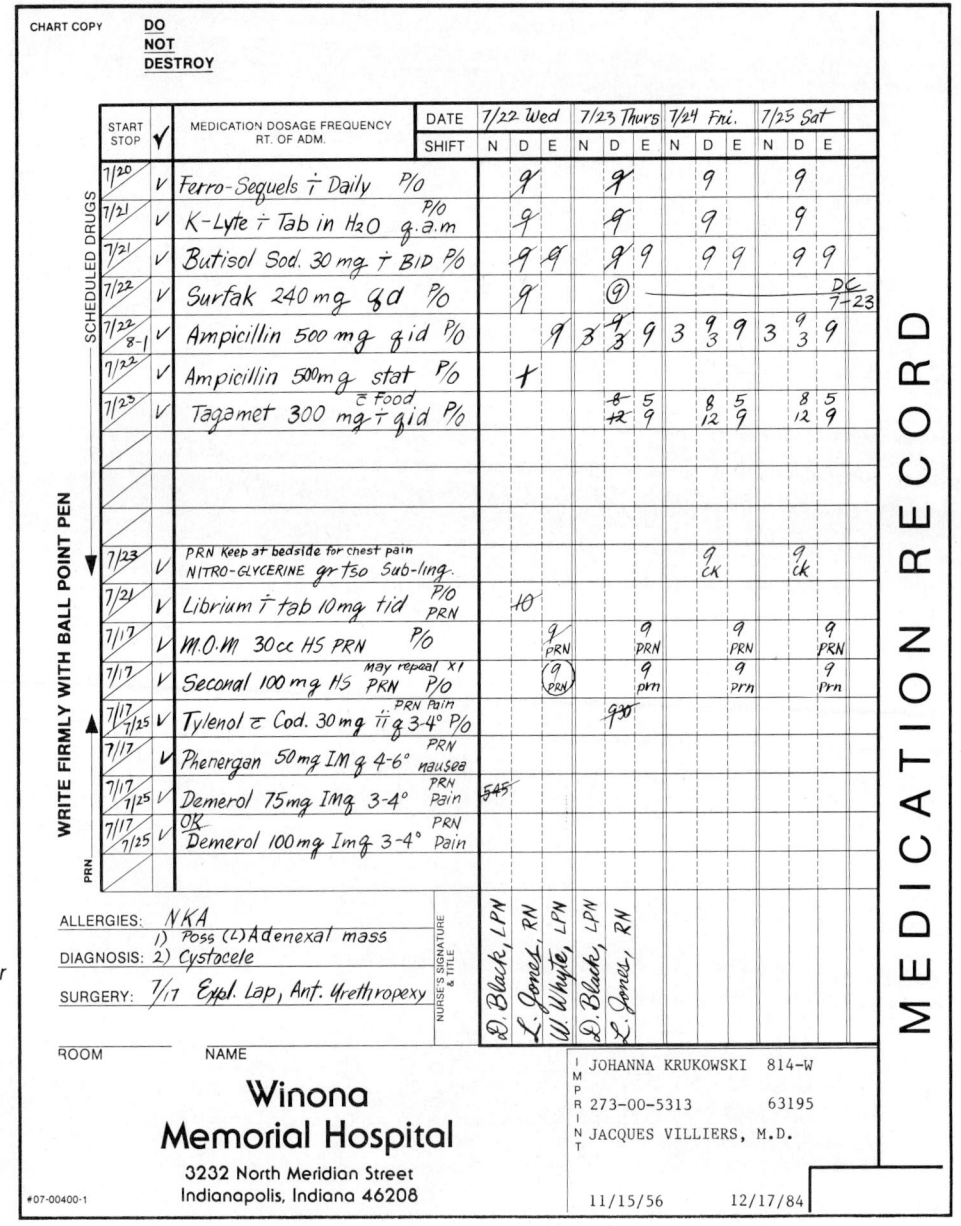

Figure 5. Medication record form, with three duplicate sheets. The scheduled administration times are written when the order is transcribed onto the sheet. The nurse draws a line through the correct time and signs his or her name after the medication is given. Note that regularly scheduled medications are separated from p.r.n. medications to avoid accidentally giving them at scheduled times. Note the discontinued medication, the starting date, and the automatic stop date for some medications. (Courtesy of Winona Memorial Hospital, Indianapolis, IN.)

MEDICATION ADMINISTRATION 841

```
NAME
  Neal, Becky
ROOM
  428-W
DRUG
  Achromycin-Q
DOSE
  250 mg, p.o.
TIME
  9-3-9-3
```

Figure 6. A. *Medication card with all needed information.*

val. A medication card *must* contain the following information: client's first and last name, room and bed number, name of drug, dosage, route, times to be given, and any special directions for administration such as "give with milk or juice" or "check pulse." The starting and expiration dates and the initials of the nurse who prepared the card may be written on the back of the card. When medication cards are used, there is *always* a permanent listing of medications to be given to each client in case individual cards are misplaced or lost. Figure 6 shows a completed medication card and a tray designed to hold cups of prepared medications and medication cards for a large number of clients. A small tray is used for medications for one client. With this system, in addition to transcribing the medication order onto a kardex and medication card, the order also needs to be transcribed onto a medication record sheet that is kept in the health record and is used to document medication administration.

Regardless of the system used, at regular intervals during the day, the medication record (computer printout, medication page, or kardex and medication card) is checked for accuracy with the original written

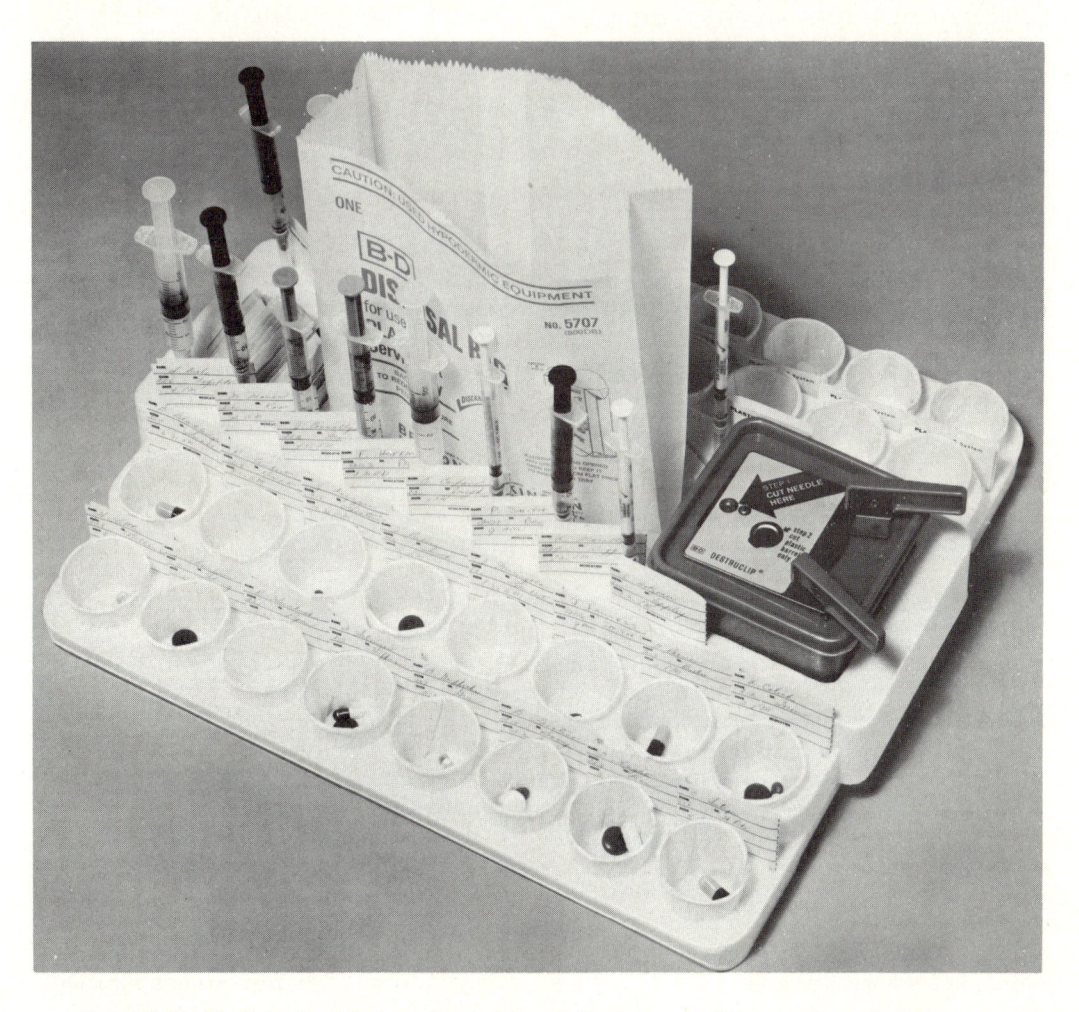

Figure 6. B. *Medicine tray designed to hold medicine cups, medicine cards, and syringes. (Courtesy of Becton-Dickinson Company, Rutherford, NJ.)*

medication order. This checking may be done on every shift, on a daily basis, or on any other schedule as determined by agency policy; it is done by two nurses or by a nurse and the unit clerk.

Preparing and Administering Medications

Preparing and administering medications is presented in specific detail within the context of each of the skills in this chapter, with some general comments included here.

It is not always possible to administer medications at the exact time specified, particularly when giving medications to more than a few clients or when other activities are occurring. A general rule of thumb has been that medications may be given 30 minutes before or after the specified time without being regarded as an error. However, there are times when a 30-minute delay may have a negative effect on a diagnostic or therapeutic plan, such as when clients are given preoperative sedatives just as they are leaving for surgery instead of 30 minutes earlier, which would have allowed time for relaxation. On the other hand, a variation of several hours for a daily vitamin would not cause harm to a client. These examples are not meant to negate in any way the importance of administering medications on time; they are given to emphasize the need for knowledgeable rather than rote administration of medications. Francis (1980) suggests reconsidering the definition of medication error so as not to include a specific 30-minute rule, since professional nursing judgment may result in a nurse placing a higher priority on attending to urgent client needs in preference to giving a routine medication exactly as scheduled.

When administering medications to more than one person, plan to give the medications first to those clients who are able to take them readily, and then to clients who need assistance. This sequence enables you to give more medications at or near the specified time and allows more unhurried time with those who need assistance. A key factor in giving medications to groups of clients is to work sequentially and in an orderly manner, both when preparing and when administering the medications.

Recording Medications

Record medications immediately after they are administered. When this is not done, there is a potential for a duplicate dose to be given. For example, a client with pain may ask for and receive pain medication from one nurse. Before the medication takes effect, the client may report the pain to another nurse. If the second nurse finds no record of recent administration of pain medication, that nurse may also give the client pain medication, resulting in a double dose. This duplication can also occur with stat drug orders or regularly scheduled medications.

Never record medications before they are administered. This practice is unethical and creates the potential for needing to alter a legal document. Clients have been known to refuse medications; they may leave the unit for a test or a treatment and need to omit the medication or take it later; their condition may change so that the medication is no longer needed; they may die; or the nurse may be called to an emergency before the medication is actually given. Recording medications prior to administering them can result in missed doses or a need to alter the health record unnecessarily.

When using a medication record page, the nurse records the medications on that page as each client's medications are given. With a computer system, the nurse marks the printout columns labeled "given" or "not given" at the time the medication is administered and then later enters all the medications into the computer system at the same time. When bedside computer terminals are used, medications can be recorded in the computer as soon as they are administered. With the medication card system, the nurse records medications in all client's health records after giving all the medication for that particular time period, such as all the 10:00 AM medications for a group of clients.

MEDICATION ERRORS

The system for administering medications in an inpatient setting is complex, often involves many persons, and is vulnerable to human and mechanical error. Davis and Cohen (1981) define a medication error as being one or more of the following: a client receives a medication intended for another client; a client receives the wrong dose or an extra dose of medication; a medication is given by the wrong route; the client receives a wrong medication; a medication is omitted; an outdated medication is given; the medication is given at the wrong time. These authors comment that giving a medication at a wrong time is relative, and whether it is regarded as a medication error is determined by the ordering physician. They cite a hospital protocol that requires scheduled medications given one hour before or after the scheduled time to be reported to the physician.

Use of the unit-dose system significantly reduces medication error rates. In their summary of medication errors, Davis and Cohen (1981) cite an overall error range of 5.3 to 20.6 percent with an average of 11.67 percent for eight hospitals with nonunit-dose medication systems. The three hospitals using unit-dose had error rates of 3.5 percent, 1.7 percent, and 0.64 percent. Wrong-time medication errors were not counted in either system.

A study involving 309 nurses in an acute-care setting revealed the following self-reported types of medication errors and the approximate percentage of the total errors: medication not recorded, 11 percent; omitted dose, 6 percent; wrong dose, 5.6 percent; wrong drug, 3.5 percent; wrong patient, 0.7 percent; and wrong route, 0.6 percent. The largest category of self-reported errors was "wrong time" (72.7 percent), but that category comprised only 0.8 percent of the errors reported on incident reports. In this study the total self-reported medication error rate was 2.7 per 1000 doses of medications given (including "wrong time" errors), most of which did not result in harm to the client (Francis, 1980).

Research for developing the State Board Test Pool Examination (SBTPE) included a study of 13,963 critical incidents (effective and ineffective actions and "close calls") reported by 2700 nurses in 67 hospitals and community agencies. The study was done for the National League for Nursing (NLN) by the Council of State Boards of Nursing of the American Nurses' Association (ANA). With two exceptions, all of the negative incidents reported involved medication errors related to a nonadherence to the administration schedule or administering medications by an incorrect route, rate, or mode. In this study, incorrect scheduling included treatments and tests as well as medications. However, there were 77 reports of errors such as giving medication by a different route than ordered and using the wrong orifice or site. The two exceptions were errors in reading or interpreting physician's orders and failure to use monitoring equipment when needed (Jacobs et al., 1978).

Medication errors can and do occur at any point from the time the medication order was written to the time it was recorded after it was given. Sources of medication errors include: poorly written and incorrectly interpreted physician orders; incomplete medication orders; confusion of drug names; inappropriate abbreviations; confusing labels on drug containers; incorrect reading of labels; incorrect dispensing of the medication by the pharmacist; inadequate knowledge of drugs by nurses or pharmacy technicians; incorrect client identification; clients not questioning changes in drug administration; or dosage calculation errors. It is crucial that extreme care be exercised in all aspects of the complex system and multiple steps between ordering and receiving a medication in the average inpatient setting.

Davis and Cohen (1981) point out that while many medication errors have no clinical significance and do not have an adverse effect on the client, they do affect the client's confidence in the quality of the health-care system and its personnel. Some errors, however, have very serious and even fatal consequences, as these and other sources indicate (Creighton, 1975; Davis and Cohen, 1981; Fink, 1983; Perlstein et al., 1979).

If a medication error does occur, it is imperative that the nurse assume the responsibility for acknowledging and reporting the error so that any needed corrective action can be taken. All agencies have an established policy for completing incident reports. The person with the most knowledge about the error should complete the written incident report, including the facts associated with the error and the corrective action taken at that time. Medication error reports are used to analyze the source of the error and take constructive action with the system or personnel as needed. They are to be kept confidential and not used to berate or criticize an individual or department.

MEDICATION ADMINISTRATION AND THE LAW

As indicated earlier in this text, the health record is a legal document; therefore, recording the administration of medications in the record is a legal activity. In addition, most state nurse practice acts identify the persons legally entitled to administer medications: usually registered nurses, student nurses under supervision, or licensed practical nurses who have been prepared to do this.

As with other nursing skills, the nurse can be found to be legally negligent in administering medications incorrectly, such as by giving an incorrect dosage or injecting a medication in an inappropriate site, thus causing harm to the client. Failure to report a known medication error so that corrective action can be taken would also constitute negligence.

Administration of controlled substances (narcotics, sedatives, and tranquilizers) is governed by law, and there are special regulations for manufacturing, transporting, storing, prescribing, dispensing, and administering these drugs. Agencies develop their own practices and procedures for implementing these regulations. For example, controlled substances are kept locked and the key is kept by the person responsible for their administration. All drugs must be accounted for at the end of each shift, usually through a counting process done by two nurses at the end of each work shift. When administering a controlled substance to a client, the nurse must enter the following information in a pharmacy record: date and time of administration, client's name, prescribed drug, name of the physician who prescribed the medication, and the signature of the nurse who is giving the drug. Additional records are kept by the pharmacy department. Controlled substances are packaged by the pharmacy department and delivered to the clinical unit in various ways that facilitate counting and recording the individual doses of medication, as shown in Figure 7. Figure 8 shows a controlled substance record used in one agency. Each time a nurse uses a controlled substance, he or she counts the remaining drugs and signs the controlled substance record before removing the drug from the container. The nurse who gives the medication must be the one who signs the controlled substance record. In addition, at the end of each work shift, an oncoming nurse and an offgoing nurse count the remaining drugs together and record the totals on a form designed for that purpose.

There is a legal basis for drug names. Drugs have both a proprietary name (trade name, protected by a trademark) and a nonproprietary or generic name that reflects the drug's chemical structure. Drugs are

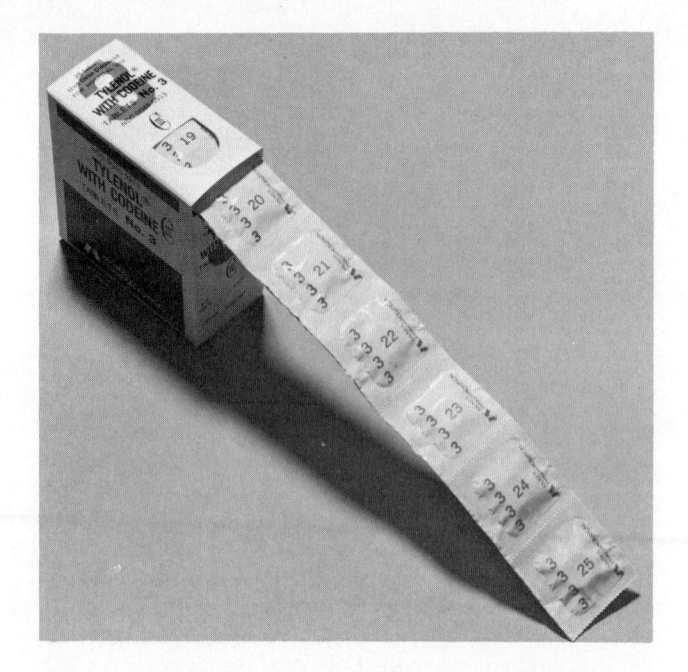

Figure 7. Controlled substances prepared for use on the client-care unit. These methods allow medication to be counted and removed from the containers without being touched. **A.** Perforated strips of sequentially numbered medications. (Photo by James Haines.)

often produced by several different manufacturing companies, each of whom places its own trade name on the drug it produces. Proprietary drug names are always capitalized, and generic names begin with a lower-case letter. Many health-care agencies have policies that require or permit use of an equivalent generic labeled drug for the proprietary drug named in the medication order. In some states, the law allows pharmacists to substitute an equivalent generic labeled drug for the proprietary drug specified in the prescription. The primary reasons for these substitutions are space and money. Fewer drugs need to be available in the pharmacy department if prescriptions and medication orders can be filled with generic labeled drugs and generic drugs are generally less costly.

When generic drugs are used, the nurse may receive a drug from the pharmacy that has a different name than appears in the medication order. When this happens, the pharmacist usually labels the drug "same as . . . (trade name of drug)" or includes a note to that effect. Sometimes a list of commonly used generic and trade name equivalents is posted in the medicine room. If this information is not readily available, contact the pharmacist for the needed information and request inclusion of equivalent names in routine pharmacy labeling. In addition, equivalent names can be validated in one of the types of drug reference sources described below. Do not assume that the generic drug sent by the pharmacy is the equivalent of the proprietary drug name without validation. Pharmacists sometimes make errors too! (Cohen, 1981).

KNOWLEDGE BASE FOR SAFE MEDICATION ADMINISTRATION

It is expected that the student will use a pharmacology textbook to learn about general drug classifications, drug actions and interactions, as well as specific information about individual drugs, such as usual dose, route of administration, actions, uses, side effects, toxicity, specific techniques of administration, nursing observations, and teaching implications. In addition, the nurse must know the client's diagnosis and how the drug fits the diagnostic or therapeutic plan.

There are various sources for obtaining needed information about drugs. *The American Hospital Formulary Service Drug Information (current year's date)* (McEvoy and McQuarrie, 1985) describes and gives rationale for most therapeutic agents. It is kept current with quarterly bound supplements and a revised master volume that is issued each January. This reference replaced the earlier loose-leaf format in 1984. It is available in most clinical areas. Another reference, *Facts and Comparisons,* (Kastrup and Boyd, 1984), is similar to a formulary, except that drug information is arranged in therapeutic categories. This loose-leaf drug information service is updated monthly. Many agencies also publish an *individual hospital formulary* that includes the drugs most commonly used at that agency. Other valuable references are *nursing-oriented drug references* that include information about

Figure 7. B. Round plastic container with 25 numbered compartments, covered with a rotating clear top. The top is rotated counterclockwise so the small opening is over the compartment with the next numbered dose. The container is then inverted over a medicine cup and the capsule or tablet drops out. **C.** Plastic box with numbered compartments and sliding clear plastic lid. The lid is moved toward the smaller numbers, exposing one compartment at a time and allowing that medication to be dropped into the medicine cup.

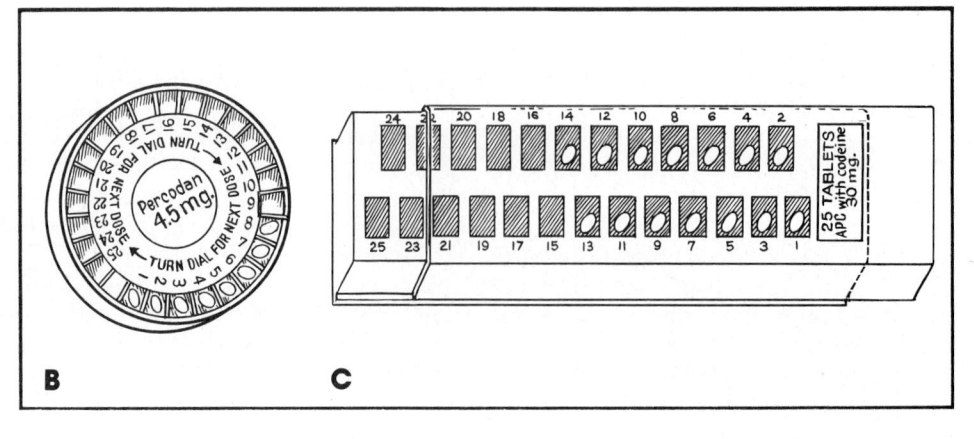

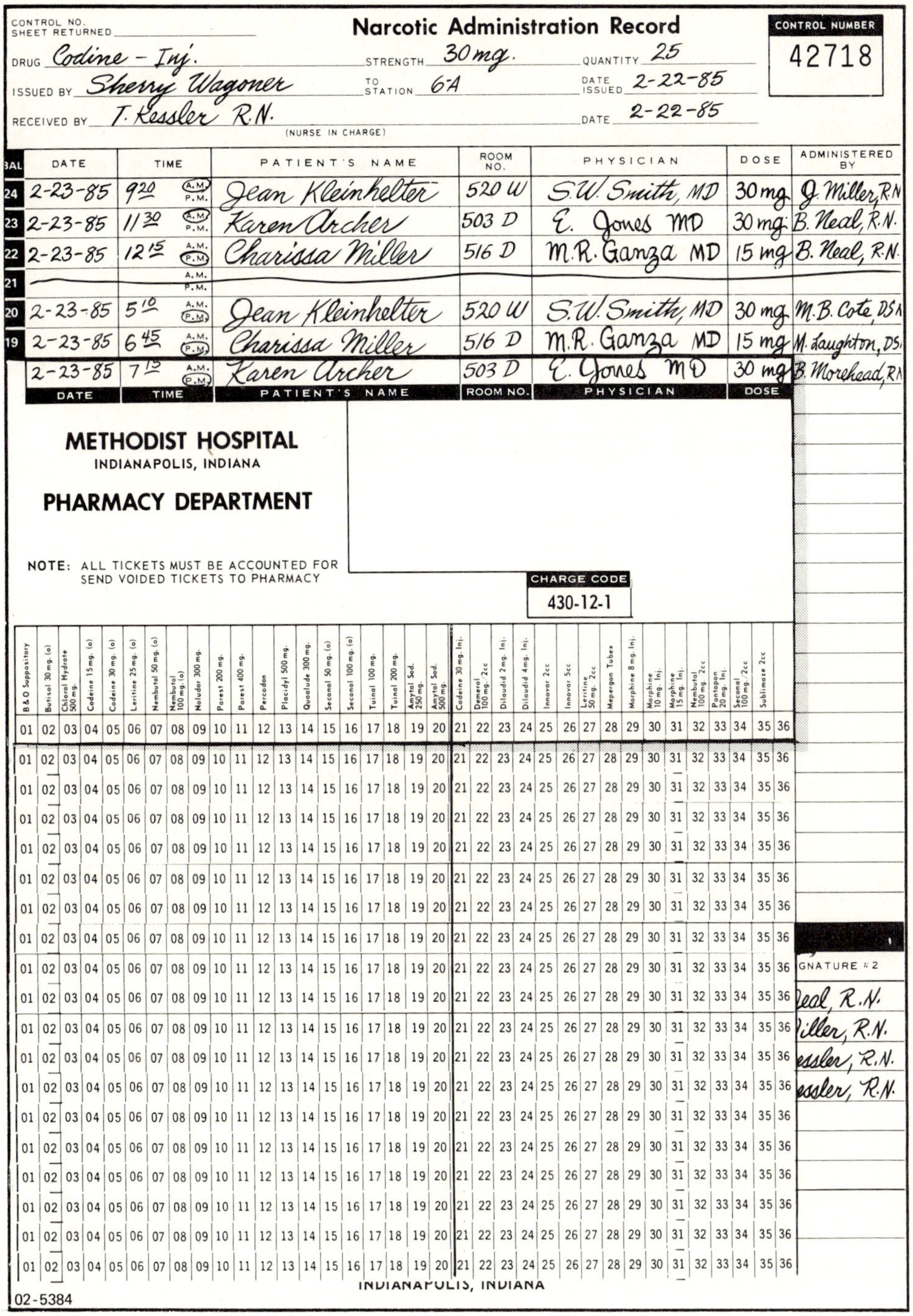

Figure 8. Sign-out sheet for one dosage strength of one controlled substance, injectable codeine, 30 mg. The nurse administering the medication fills in the identifying data and signs his or her name on the self-carboning charge ticket, removes the ticket, and stamps it with the client's charge plate. The charge ticket is used for billing purposes and the master record of the controlled substance use is returned to pharmacy when all doses are given. The section at the bottom is used when a second nurse must countersign for the medication, such as when part of the unit-dose is destroyed, a medication is wasted, or when students administer a controlled substance drug. (Courtesy of Methodist Hospital of Indiana, Inc., Indianapolis, IN.)

usual dosages, expected actions, teaching needs, and nursing responsibilities in administration, making observations about side effects and toxicity (Govoni and Hayes, 1985; Malseed, 1983; Scherer, 1985).

Nursing journals, such as the *American Journal of Nursing, Nursing (Horsham),* and *RN* have regular monthly updates on medications. Product inserts from manufacturers are usually available in boxes used to package medications. The pharmacist often has package inserts when they are not available on the clinical unit. One of the best, most up-to-date resources for information about medications is the agency pharmacist. Consult the pharmacy department whenever you are unable to locate information about any medication. Another common reference is the *Physicians' Desk Reference (PDR),* 1985. The PDR is an annual publication that compiles information about medications from drug manufacturers. The colored illustrations of numerous medications are a valuable reference for helping identify medications visually, which may be necessary when clients bring unlabeled drugs to a clinic, physician's office, or emergency room. Because it is not directed toward nurse administration of drugs and does not always include information the

```
                                         Student Name _____
                                         References Used _____
NAME: Furosemide, U.S.P. (Lasix)         _____
CLASSIFICATION: Diuretic
ACTION: Potent sulfonamide "loop" diuretic. Depresses sodium and chloride reabsorption
    and enhances excretion of potassium.
    Oral administration: effect begins 30-60 min., peeks 1-2 hrs., and lasts 6-8 hrs.
    IV administration: effect begins 5 min.(somewhat later afterIM), peaks 20-60 min.,
    and lasts 2 hrs.
USE: Reduces edema in congestive heart failure, cirrhosis of liver, and renal disease.
    Reduces blood pressure in treatment of hypertension; may be used alone as first step
    in treating hypertension or in combination with other antihypertensives.
USUAL ADULT DOSE: Oral: diuresis - 20 - 80 mg. daily or b.i.d.
                        hypertension - 40 mg. daily or b.i.d.
                  IV:   diuresis - 20 - 40 mg. per dose (give 4 mg./min.)
ADMINISTRATION ROUTE: oral tablet, oral solution, IM or IV
NURSING IMPLICATIONS: Schedule daily and b.i.d. doses to avoid nocturia (i.e., 8 am daily
    or 8 am and 2 pm b.i.d.). Weigh patient daily for diuretic effect. Monitor I&O for
    diuretic effect. Monitor BP for diuretic effect and treatment of hypertension.
    Electrolytes should be checked at beginning of therapy for imbalances in K, Na, and
    Cl. Monitor blood glucose; Lasix may cause hyperglycemia.
SIDE EFFECTS: Frequent urination, postural hypotension when combined with antihyperten-
    sives, glycosuria.
TOXIC EFFECTS: Mild intoxication: weakness, fatigue, lightheaded, dizzy, confusion,
    vomiting, muscle cramps, hyponatremia, hypokalemia, hypochloremia, acute gout.
              Marked intoxication: same plus hearing loss, fullness in ears, tinnitus.
PATIENT TEACHING: Encourage intake of potassium rich foods; physician may need to
    prescribe potassium supplement if dietary measures are inadequate. Schedule home
    intake of medication around daily routine to accommodate peak and duration of
    action. If used in hypertension, encourage periodic BP checks. Alert to signs of
    fluid and electrolyte imbalance.
```

Figure 9. Sample drug card prepared prior to administering the medication and used for reference purposes.

nurse needs to know, it is not an adequate reference by itself.

Drug Cards

A drug card is a useful tool for recording information about drugs in a way that is readily accessible. Figure 9 shows a format for recording information on a 4" × 6" or 5" × 8" card. Students are often required to prepare cards such as these for the medications they will be giving to clients. Commercially prepared drug cards are also available. The cards can be kept in a pocket while on the clinical unit and stored in a personal file until needed for another client. It is helpful to use a second card or the back of the first card to keep an account of the various circumstances in which the medication was used. This process helps the student note drug effectiveness and make comparisons of various clients' responses to the drug.

Overview

The skills in this chapter include "Oral Medication Administration" (Skill 71), "Topical Medication Administration" (Skill 72), "Injectable Medication Administration" (Skill 73), and "Intravenous Fluid and Medication Administration" (Skill 74).

REFERENCES

Buccerl P, Baker JA: Management strategy for the diffusion of innovation: Unit dose distribution. American Journal of Hospital Pharmacy 35(2):168–173, 1978.

Cohen MR: Medication errors: If a drug doesn't look right, check with the pharmacist. Nursing81 (Horsham) 11(10):81, 1981.

Creighton HC: Law Every Nurse Should Know, ed 3. Philadelphia, WB Saunders, 1975.

Davis NM, Cohen MR: Medication errors: Causes and Prevention. Philadelphia, George F Stickley, 1981.

Fink JL III: Preventing lawsuits: Medication errors to avoid. NursingLife 3(2):26–29, 1983.

Francis GM: Nurses' medication "errors": A new perspective? Supervisor Nurse 11(8):11–13, 1980.

Gennaro AR: Remington's Pharmaceutical Sciences, ed 17. Martin AN (ed): Part 2, Pharmaceutics. Easton, PA, Mack Publishing, 1985.

Govoni LE, Hayes JE: Drugs and Nursing Implications, ed 5. Norwalk, CT, Appleton-Century-Crofts, 1985.

Jackson JC, Anderson RK, et al.: Decentralized pharmacist concept solves unit dose problems. Hospitals 52(4):107–108, 1978.

Jacobs AM, Fivars G, et al: Critical Requirements for Safe/Effective Nursing Practice. Kansas City, MO, American Nurses' Association, 1978.

Kastrup EK, Boyd JR(eds): Facts and Comparisons. Philadelphia, JB Lippincott, 1984.

McEvoy GK, McQuarrie GM: American Hospital Formulary Service: Drug Information '85. Bethesda, MD, American Society of Hospital Pharmacists, 1985.

Malseed RT: Quick Reference to Drug Therapy and Nursing Considerations. Philadelphia, JB Lippincott, 1983.

Perlstein PH, Callison C, et al.: Errors in drug computations during newborn intensive care. American Journal of Diseases of Children 1(3):376–379, 1979.

Physicians' Desk Reference, ed 39. Jack E. Angel (Publisher). Medical Economics Company, Inc., Oradell, NJ, 1985.

Scherer JC (ed): Lippincott's Nurse's Drug Manual. Philadelphia, JB Lippincott, 1985.

United States Pharmacopeia, ed 20. Rockville, MD, United States Pharmacopeial Convention, 1980.

BIBLIOGRAPHY

Bergersen BS, in consultation, Goth A: Pharmacology in Nursing, ed 14. St Louis, CV Mosby, 1979.

Blume DM, Cornett EF: Dosages and Solutions, ed 4. Philadelphia, FA Davis, 1984.

Cohen MR: Medication errors: Look up an unfamiliar drug before administering it. Nursing83 (Horsham) 13(3):74, 1983.

Cohen MR: Medication errors: Don't forget to check the administration route. Nursing83 (Horsham) 13(2):116, 1983.

Cohen MR: Consultation: Liability for unit-dose injectables. Nursing79 9(10):80, 1979.

Dexter P, Applegate M: How to solve a math problem. Journal of Nursing Education 19(2):49–53, 1980.

Kozier B, Erb G: Techniques in Clinical Nursing. Menlo Park, CA, Addison-Wesley, 1982.

Lewis LVW: Fundamental Skills in Patient Care, ed 3. Philadelphia, JB Lippincott, 1984.

Ptasynski EM, Silver SMcD: Experience in posology. Journal of Nursing Education 20(8):41–46, 1981.

Rodman MJ, Smith DW: Pharmacology and Drug Therapy in Nursing, ed 2. Philadelphia, JB Lippincott, 1979.

Scherer JC: Lippincott's Nurses' Drug Manual. Philadelphia, JB Lippincott, 1985.

Sheridan E, Patterson HR, et al.: Falconer's The Drug, the Nurse, the Patient, ed 7. Philadelphia, WB Saunders, 1982.

Smith MJ, Smith DW: Pharmacology and Drug Therapy in Nursing, ed 2. Philadelphia, JB Lippincott, 1979.

Smoot RC, Price J, et al.: Chemistry: A Modern Course (teacher's annotated ed). Columbus, OH, Chas. E. Merrill, 1979.

Sorensen KC, Luckmann, J: Basic Nursing: A Psychophysiological Approach. Philadelphia, WB Saunders, 1979.

Stewart DY, Kelly J, et al.: Unit-dose medication: A nursing perspective. American Journal of Nursing 76(8):1308–1310, 1976.

Wilson BA, Shannon MT: A Unified Approach to Dosage Calculations. New Orleans, Gifford Test Preparation Services, 1983.

SUGGESTED READING

Davis NM, Cohen MR: Learning from mistakes: 20 tips for avoiding medication errors. Nursing82 (Horsham) 12(3):65–72, 1982.

Fink JL III: Preventing lawsuits: Medication errors to avoid. NursingLife 3(2):26–29, 1983.

Levine ME: Breaking through the medication mystique. American Journal of Nursing 70(4):799–803, 1970.

Newton DW, Newton M: Guidelines for preventing drug errors. Nursing77 7(9):62–68, 1977.

AUDIOVISUAL RESOURCES

Apothecary Measurements
 Filmstrip. (1973, Color, 25 min.)
Fractions and Decimals
 Filmstrip. (1973, Color, 17 min.)
Household Measurements
 Filmstrip. (1973, Color, 23 min.)
The Metric System
 Filmstrip. (1973, Color, 17 min.)
 Available through:
 Medcom, Inc.
 P.O. Box 116
 Garden Grove, CA 92642

SKILL 71 Oral Medication Administration

PREREQUISITE SKILLS

Skill 19, "Inspection"
Skill 28, "Handwashing"
Skill 53, "Assistance with Eating"
Skill 56, "Insertion and Care of Gastrointestinal Tubes"
Chapter 16, "Introduction"

☐ STUDENT OBJECTIVES

1. Identify the benefits and disadvantages of the oral route of medication administration.
2. Describe guidelines for safe preparation and administration of oral medications.
3. Describe the three safety checks designed to ensure accurate preparation of medications in the unit-dose, individual client, or stock supply system.
4. Describe the safety checks designed to identify the correct client before administering medications.
5. Explain the rationale for opening unit-dose medications at the client's bedside.
6. Describe ways to assist clients who have difficulty swallowing oral medications.
7. Describe safe administration of enteric-coated and time-release tablets and capsules.
8. Describe the correct procedure for pouring liquid and solid oral medications from individual or stock supplies.
9. Determine the prescribed amount of oral medication from the dosage available.
10. Administer oral medications in a safe manner.

INTRODUCTION

Oral medications are those medications that are taken into the gastrointestinal tract, primarily through swallowing. Since most medications taken orally are absorbed from the small intestines, they may also be inserted through nasogastric feeding tubes directly into the stomach. The oral route for administering medications is the simplest, safest, most economical, and most convenient route for giving medications. It is, therefore, the preferred way to give medications unless contraindicated or if another route produces a greater therapeutic action. For example, the oral route is not used when clients are nauseated, vomiting, when a more rapid action is desired, or when a drug might be inactivated by gastrointestinal secretions or might be too irritating for that system. In general, drug action by the oral route has a slower onset and less potent effect than a parenteral route. The duration of action by the oral route varies with a variety of factors, such as the presence or absence of food in the stomach, gastric pH, and rate of gastrointestinal emptying. Some disadvantages associated with the use of the oral route include its slower onset of action, possible inactivation by digestive enzymes, sometimes incomplete absorption, and the possibility of gastrointestinal irritation with anorexia, nausea, and vomiting, or irritation and ulceration of the gastric mucosa.

PREPARATION

PREPARATIONS OF ORAL MEDICATIONS

Oral medications are of two basic forms: solids and liquids. A solid preparation contains a specified amount of pure drug combined with other ingredients (such as binders, lubricants, diluents, and coatings) to produce a stable and easily swallowed tablet or capsule. The type of ingredient and coating used is determined by the drug and its therapeutic intent. Tablets and capsules are labeled with the amount of pure drug contained in one tablet or capsule, sometimes referred to as its *strength*. For example, "Lanoxin, 0.125 mg" means that each tablet contains 0.125 mg of the pure drug Digoxin. Some tablets are scored; that is, they have a grooved line across the center of the tablet and, therefore, can be split evenly with a sharp knife. Likewise, a liquid preparation is a specified amount of drug diluted in a given volume of a liquid that is an appropriate vehicle for that drug and its intended therapeutic purpose. Liquids are labeled with the amount of drug contained in one or more milliliters, minims, fluidrams, or ounces, sometimes referred to as the *concentration* of a liquid. For example, "Kaon elixir (potassium gluconate), 20 mEq/15 ml" means that 15 milliliters of Kaon elixir contains 20 mEq of the pure drug potassium gluconate.

Types of Oral Medications

Common types of oral solid and liquid preparations are defined and illustrated in Table 71-1. The terms used here are included on a drug label, and the nurse is expected to know what the terms mean in order to administer the drug correctly. For example, the nurse will choose other ways of administering a medication to a client than crushing or emptying enteric-coated tablets or capsules when he or she knows that doing so would release the drug into the stomach where it can produce gastric irritation or be destroyed by gastric secretions rather than being released in the intestines as intended.

Food and Oral Medications

The presence of food influences gastrointestinal motility, gastric emptying time, and the rate of blood flow to the gastrointestinal tract. Increased gastric secretion and bile production can alter the rate of drug breakdown. Since these factors affect the amount of drug actually received by the client, it is necessary to know whether a drug is best given with food or on an empty stomach. For example, food may delay the absorption of some drugs but not interfere with their overall effectiveness, such as digoxin (Lanoxin) and acetaminophen (Tylenol). Food will decrease the absorption of some drugs, such as cloxacillin (Tegopen) or erythromycin (EES). Other drugs are given with food to avoid gastrointestinal irritation, even though the food delays the absorption of the drug, such as with aspirin and furosemide (Lasix). The presence of food in the stomach will also minimize the nausea and vomiting that may accompany administration of estrogens such as Premarin or corticosteroids such as dexamethasone (Decadron). However, some drugs must be given on an empty stomach to avoid interference with absorption, such as the tetracyclines (Terramycin, Panamycin); or delayed absorption, such as the sulfonamides (Gantrisin) (Giovannitti and Schwinghammer, 1981; Govoni and Hayes, 1985; Rosenberg and Sangkachand, 1981, volumes 5 and 6).

If uncertain whether a drug should be given with or without food, check various references as described in the Introduction to this chapter or references at the end of this skill.

CALCULATION OF ORAL MEDICATION DOSAGES

The physician's medication order usually specifies the amount of pure drug to be given, rather than the volume of liquid or the number of tablets or capsules needed to administer the ordered dosage. The most common calculations used in administering oral medications are for the purpose of determining the quantity of tablets or capsules or the volume of liquid needed to provide the ordered dosage. Scored tablets can be split evenly to provide a dosage of one-half tablet; nonscored tablets cannot be accurately divided. Highly potent oral drugs with a potential

TABLE 71-1. Oral Dosage Forms

DOSAGE FORM	DESCRIPTION	ADMINISTRATION GUIDELINES
Solids		
Capsules	Hard or soft one- or two-piece gelatinous shell containing powdered, granular, oily, or liquid drugs.	Do not chew.
Tablets	Powdered drugs compressed or molded into small discs; combined with other ingredients to aid in swallowing and dissolution. May be coated to protect the drug from air, light, disguise an unpleasant taste, or add a distinctive color.	Do not chew coated tablets.
Enteric-coated tablets and capsules	Coating resists the action of gastric secretions and dissolves in the small intestines.	Do not crush tablets or empty capsules.
Time-release	Capsules contain small particles of drug that are coated with materials that dissolve at varying times. Examples: *Spansules, Sequels*. Tablets are layered or constructed so the drug is released at several different times. Examples: *Repetabs, Extentabs*.[a]	Do not crush or chew.
Liquids		
Solution	Homogenous liquid preparation of a soluble substance.	Does not need shaking. Do not give if there is sediment in the bottom.
Syrup	Somewhat viscous, sugared or fruit-based solution containing a drug. Examples: *Cough syrup, pediatric or infant medications*.	Check label to see if it can be diluted.
Saturated solution	A solution that contains all of the solute that can be held by the solvent. Example: *SSKI (saturated solution of potassium iodide)*.	Often diluted.
Suspension	Preparation of finely divided, undissolved substances dispersed in a liquid vehicle. Settles out when standing.	Shake prior to each administration.
Gels and magmas	Thick, milky suspensions.	Shake prior to each administration.
Emulsion	Suspension of fine oil or fat droplets in water.	Shake prior to each administration.
Elixir	Nonviscous hydroalcoholic liquid with flavoring and sugar added. Example: *Elixir of terpin hydrate (cough medication)*.	May be diluted.
Tincture	Alcoholic or hydroalcoholic solution without added sugar. Example: *Tincture of belladonna (smooth muscle relaxant)*.	May be diluted.
Fluid-extract	Bitter solution of vegetable drugs; highly concentrated and unpleasant tasting.	

[a]When attached to a drug name, these terms and abbreviations indicate a sustained-release drug form: -bid ,SA, Plateau Cap, Dur- , SR, and Span- (Wordell, 1982).

for toxicity (such as digitalis products and anticoagulants) cannot be split accurately, as there is no guarantee that the drug is dispersed evenly in all parts of the tablet.

Oral dosage problems can readily be solved with either the factor-label method or the known values dosage formula (proportion method), as shown in the following examples.

Example A: Ordered Dose: Kaon elixir, 15 mEq, q.i.d.
Available Dosage: Kaon elixir (potassium gluconate), 20 mEq/15 ml

Factor-Label Method:

Ordered Dose × Known Relationship = $\dfrac{\text{Ordered}}{\text{Dosage}}$

$$15 \text{ mEq} \times \dfrac{15 \text{ ml}}{20 \text{ mEq}} = x \text{ (ml)}$$

$$\dfrac{3 \times 15 \text{ ml}}{4} = x$$

$$\dfrac{45 \text{ ml}}{4} = x$$

$$x = 11 \text{ ml (approx.)}$$

Proportion Equation—Dosage Formula:

$$\dfrac{\text{Known Dosage}}{\text{Known Amount}} = \dfrac{\text{Ordered Dosage}}{\text{Unknown Amount}}$$

$$\dfrac{20 \text{ mEq}}{15 \text{ ml}} = \dfrac{15 \text{ mEq}}{x \text{ ml}}$$

$$20x = 225 \text{ ml}$$

$$x = 11 \text{ ml (approx.)}$$

ANSWER: Give 11 ml Kaon elixir orally, four times a day.

Example B: Ordered Dose: Codeine, gr $\overline{ss}$, orally, stat
Available Dosage: Codeine Phosphate, USP, 0.015 g (tablets)

To solve this problem, you need to convert the ordered dose from the apothecary to the metric system in which it is available. Because the answer will be in the metric system, change the common fraction ½ to the decimal fraction 0.5 when setting up the equation. Change the 0.015 g to 15 mg to avoid working with more fractions.

Factor-Label Method:

To use the *factor-label* method, first identify the ordered dose and the dosage to be given; second, insert the appropriate conversion factor in the equation after the ordered dose. Use a label in the denominator that will divide out with the ordered dose label. Third, insert the known relationship ratio between the drug and the quantity, as shown here.

$\dfrac{\text{Ordered}}{\text{Dose}} \times \dfrac{\text{Conversion}}{\text{Factor}} \times \dfrac{\text{Known}}{\text{Relationship}} = \dfrac{\text{Ordered}}{\text{Dosage}}$

$$0.5 \text{ gr} \times \dfrac{60 \text{ mg}}{1 \text{ gr}} \times \dfrac{1 \text{ tablet}}{15 \text{ mg}} = x \text{ (tablet)}$$

$$0.5 \times 4 \times 1 \text{ tablet} = x$$

$$x = 2 \text{ tablets}$$

Proportion Equation:

To use a proportion equation, first use the conversion formula to convert the apothecary unit to a metric unit.

Known Equivalents = Unknown Equivalent

$$\dfrac{60 \text{ mg}}{1 \text{ gr}} = \dfrac{x \text{ mg}}{0.5 \text{ gr}}$$

$$x = 60 \times 0.5$$

$$x = 30 \text{ mg}$$

Second, use the dosage formula to calculate the number of tablets to use.

Known Dosage : Known Amount =
Ordered Dosage : Unknown Amount

$$\dfrac{15 \text{ mg}}{1 \text{ tablet}} = \dfrac{30 \text{ mg}}{x \text{ tablets}}$$

$$15x = 30 \times 1$$
$$x = 2 \text{ tablets}$$

ANSWER: Give 2 tablets Codeine Phosphate, orally, now.

Activity 71-A:
Practice Problems for Preparing Oral Medications

Solve the following oral dosage problems. Remember that the answer must be a measurable *amount* of liquid or a *number* of tablets or capsules. In some of the problems, you will need to convert to the metric system as well as determine the dosage to be administered. Write the complete answer, including drug, amount, route, and time of day.

1. Ordered dose: Isordil, 160 mg
   Available dosage: Isosorbide dinitrate (Isordil Tembids), 40 mg (bottle of capsules)
   Administer: _____
2. Ordered dose: Ilotycin Suspension, 400 mg q 6 h.
   Available: Erythromycin (Ilotycin) oral suspension, 0.2 g/5 ml
   Administer: _____
3. Ordered dose: Sudafed, gr $\overline{iss}$, q 6° p.r.n.
   Available dosage: Pseudoephedrine hydrochloride (Sudafed), 30 mg (tablets)
   Administer: _____
4. Ordered dose: Ephedrine liquid, gr 1/20, q 4 h.
   Available dosage: Ephedrine sulfate, 8 mg/5 ml
   Administer: _____

(NOTE: Answers to these problems can be found in Appendix II, p. 1013.)

DATA BASE

Before giving any medication, the nurse must know its expected action, side effects, and toxicity so he or she can observe for therapeutic effectiveness, potential or actual problems, and provide information to the client. Most agencies encourage clients to know about their medications since informed and knowledgeable clients tend to be more actively involved in their own health care. Occasionally, agency or physician policy may differ from this stance.

The nurse must also know whether the dosage is within normal limits, if the ordered route is appropriate for this drug, and what special precautions are needed to administer it correctly and safely.

Client History and Recorded Data

To be able to interpret a medication regime to the client and to make knowledgeable observations and judgments, the nurse must know the client's diagnosis and how the medication fits into the therapeutic and diagnostic plans. The health record includes any indications of potential problems with swallowing, such as may occur with lesions of the esophagus or mouth, oral surgery, neurologic impairment, n.p.o. status, presence of nausea and vomiting, level of consciousness, and mental status. The health record also includes known allergies and documentation of the need for p.r.n. and stat medications.

The kardex or nursing-care plan contains information about allergies and special problems affecting medication administration. For example, this information might include the client's level of consciousness; mental capability; difficulty in swallowing; inability to use the hands and arms due to weakness, restraints, or casts; positional restrictions such as needing to remain flat in bed; willingness to take medications; hearing or visual impairment; or a spoken language different from that of the nurse.

In addition to knowing these data, the nurse also observes for many of these factors at the time the medication is administered, since client status can change quickly.

While it is not possible to have extensive information about large numbers of clients, most agency systems have essential information readily available on the medication record page or kardex, in a kardex, on a computer care plan printout, and through the regular report process between work shifts. It is crucial that the nurse administering medications assume the responsibility of adding to these sources the information gained while administering medications.

Physical Appraisal Skills

Inspection. The nurse uses inspection to observe the client swallowing the medication and sometimes to determine if tablets or capsules remain in the client's mouth.

EQUIPMENT

The type of equipment used to administer oral medications varies with the agency and the system of medication administration used. Portable medicine carts, medication record pages and kardexes, computer printouts, medication cards, and the specially designed trays used with medication cards have been described earlier. Although less measuring equipment is needed with the unit-dose prepackaged system, some medications will most likely always need measuring and special preparation. The equipment described below and shown in Figure 71-1 is routinely available on most clinical units.

Medicine cups are used to measure oral liquid volumes ranging from 5 ml to 30 or 32 ml. They are made of disposable clear plastic, translucent waxed paper, or reusable glass. Since they are calibrated in milliliters, drams, ounces, teaspoonfuls, dessertspoonfuls, and tablespoonfuls, they can be used with several different measurement systems.

There are several ways to measure amounts less than 5 ml. One way is to use a regular *syringe* of appropriate size without a needle, or use an oral syringe that is calibrated in milliliters and teaspoons and may have a short piece of attached rubber tubing. Some liquid drugs have a *calibrated eye dropper* attached to the bottle cap; they are calibrated only for use with the particular drug in that bottle. Small volumes of liquids can also be measured with a reusable glass *minim glass* (1 dram capacity), *minim pipette,* or small *glass graduates* calibrated in milliliters. *Medication spoons* calibrated in teaspoonfuls and tablespoonfuls can be purchased in most drug stores.

Paper souffle cups or *medicine cups* are used to transport nonpackaged oral tablets and capsules from a medicine room or cart to the client's bedside.

Two clean *spoons* or a *mortar and pestle* may be used to crush some tablets when clients have difficulty swallowing them.

When using reusable measuring containers, the dosage is always transferred to a medicine cup for transporting and administering the medication to the client. If the drug can be diluted, a small amount of water can be used to rinse the reusable container. All reusable equipment used to measure or prepare medication must be washed and rinsed after each use to prevent leaving residual traces of the drug that could contaminate the next drug being measured or prepared.

☐ EXECUTION

KNOWLEDGE BASE FOR ADMINISTERING MEDICATIONS

Before administering a medication, review its general actions and know whether the dosage and route are appropriate both for that drug and for the client for

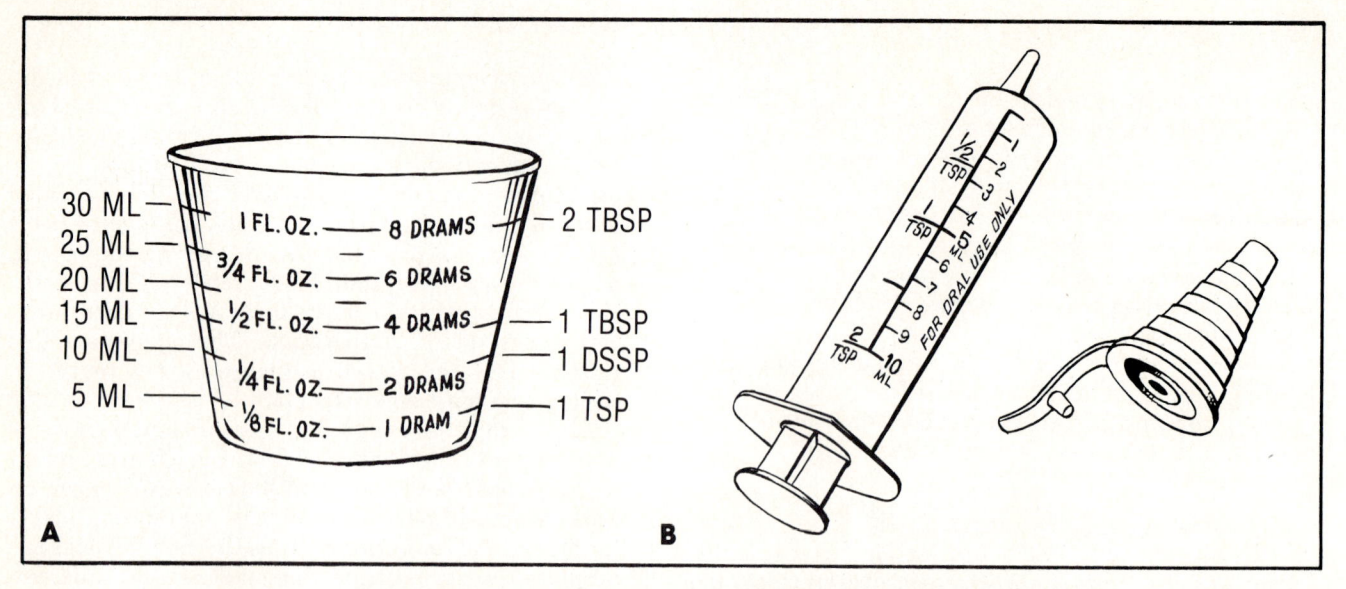

Figure 71-1. Containers used for measuring and preparing oral medications. **A.** Medicine cup, 30 ml capacity. Note calibrations for milliliters, tablespoonfuls, ounces, and drams. **B.** Oral liquid dispenser, calibrated in milliliters and teaspoonfuls. Note bottle adaptor insert.

whom it is intended. Medication given by a route other than intended can be hazardous, cause damage, or be inactivated by gastric enzymes if not intended for oral use. Remind yourself mentally that any drug that is potent enough to be therapeutic is also potent enough to harm, or even kill.

GUIDELINES FOR SAFE PREPARATION OF MEDICATIONS

There are some practices that can safeguard against making errors when preparing medications. Except for the specific references to the oral route, these safe practices apply to preparation of drugs for all routes.

1. *Avoid distractions.* Work in a quiet place and refuse to become involved in conversations with someone else.
2. *Prepare one medication at a time.* This avoids confusing different drugs and dosages.
3. *Check the medication order and the selected dosage three times: Three SAFETY CHECKS.* That is, compare the medication order with the drug and the amount of drug you are planning to give at *three separate times.* To do this, hold the medication unit-dose package or multiple-dose container adjacent to the medication order. Place a finger at the proper place on the medication record, or hold the medication card in your hand and mentally read word-for-word the medication order and the client's name, drug name, dosage, and route indicated on the medication package or container. Be particularly careful with look-alike drug and client names. *If there is any discrepancy in the client's name, drug name, or route, do not give the medication.* Investigate the problem and take

whatever corrective action is needed, such as obtaining a different drug from the pharmacy, obtaining a new medication order, or locating the correct medication record form.

The three safety checks are performed at different times when the unit-dose system is used as compared with individual or stock supply systems.

a. Unit-dose medications:

SAFETY CHECK 1 is done when removing the unit-dose package from the client's individual medicine drawer.

SAFETY CHECK 2 is done after deciding the number of unit-dose packages needed for this dosage and before placing them on the medicine cart near the medication order or in a medicine cup.

SAFETY CHECK 3 is done *at the bedside,* before opening the medication package and handing it to the client. *Do not open a unit-dose package and transfer it to a medicine or souffle cup before arriving at the bedside.*

b. Individual or stock supply medications:

SAFETY CHECK 1 is done when removing the container from the client's medicine drawer or stock supply shelf.

SAFETY CHECK 2 is done after pouring the required number of tablets or capsules into a souffle cup or after measuring the correct amount of liquid in a measuring cup.

SAFETY CHECK 3 is done before returning the container to the drawer or shelf.

With the individual or stock supply system, there is no way to identify the drug after you have poured it into the cup except by its shape, size,

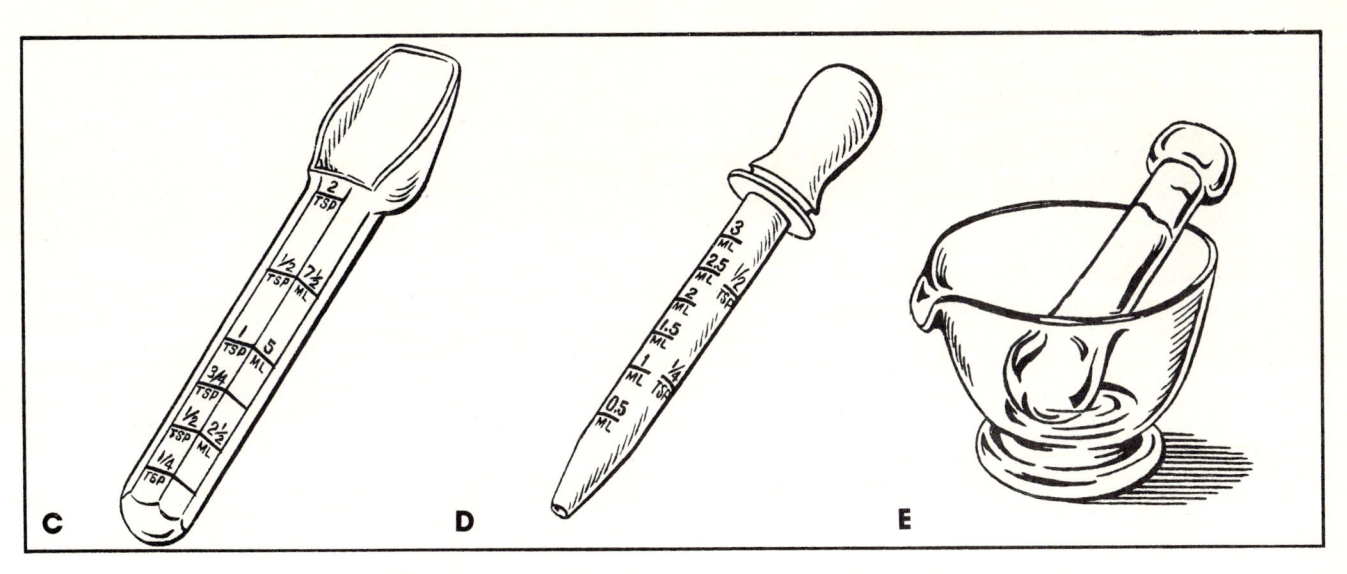

Figure 71-1. C. Calibrated measuring spoon, used in the home setting. **D.** Calibrated medicine dropper. **E.** Mortar and pestle for crushing some tablets.

color, or aroma. Since none of these characteristics is an accurate way to identify drugs, be *very* careful to keep the medication card or medication order record form near the prepared drugs until you have reached the client's bedside.

4. *Have a complete medication order.* The only exception is that when the route is not specified, the oral route is assumed. Find out if your agency policy differs from this.
5. *Question unusual medication orders.* When a drug, dosage, or route seems inappropriate for the client, contact the pharmacist or physician for clarification of the order. *You are legally accountable for the medications you give,* regardless of the order, and can be found legally negligent in a court of law for following an incorrect medication order.
6. *Check the expiration date for the medication order* for drugs such as controlled substances and antibiotics. These drugs will need to be reordered at regular intervals or after a specified number of doses. For narcotics, this may be as frequently as every 72 hours.
7. *Validate a generic drug substitution for a proprietary medication order.* If the pharmacy department has not indicated that the generic drug is equivalent to the ordered proprietary drug name, check a posted list of equivalent drugs if one is available, look in a drug reference book, or call the pharmacist. In addition, request that the pharmacy department provide this information routinely.
8. *Note any orders, tests, or procedures that might mean omitting a medication.* Each agency has some method of noting when medications are discontinued for procedures such as surgery, or when they are to be omitted temporarily, such as for some diagnostic tests or when on n.p.o. status.
9. *Calculate equivalent values and dosages as needed.* If you are in doubt about your answer, validate it with another staff person who is licensed to administer medications. If the identified number of tablets or amount of liquid does not fit within the usual range of dosage, contact the pharmacist or supervisor, and the physician as needed. If more than three unit-dose packages are needed to provide the correct dose, there probably is something wrong with the calculations or the medication provided by the pharmacy. Contact the pharmacist for assistance and clarification.
10. *Check the drug expiration date: DO NOT administer outdated drugs.* Discard them or return them to the pharmacy. Age causes drugs to deteriorate and lose their potency, or to change their composition and have an effect other than intended.
11. *Read the directions for preparation and administration.* Read carefully and follow the directions on the label or package insert. For example, a label may read "For oral use only; dilute in at least 100 ml"; "Chew tablets, follow with water"; "Give diluted with fruit juice or water"; "Sprinkle on glass of water and mix well just before drinking." Obtain the juice, milk, or food you will need to administer your medications. Coordinate medications with meal schedules so that drugs will be given with or without food as directed.
12. *Reconcile and sign the controlled substance record before removing the drug from the supply.* The number of drugs in the supply must balance with the number of drugs that have been signed out *each time a drug is removed* and again at the close of each work shift. Compare the supply with the record *before and after* you remove the controlled substance drug. If the client refuses to take the drug or if it is not administered for any reason, non–unit-dose packaged controlled substances

must be discarded by flushing them down a drain while a co-worker licensed to give medications witnesses this action. Both persons then must sign the controlled substance record, indicating the drug was wasted or destroyed.

13. *Do not open or break enteric-coated oral capsules.* Removing the enteric coating releases the medication into the stomach rather than the intestines and eliminates the protection designed to prevent gastric irritation or destruction by gastric enzymes.
14. *Do not crush time-release oral tablets or capsules.* Crushing alters the structure of the tablet and releases the drug all at one time rather than at intervals, which may lead to an overdose. Time-release capsules may be opened and added to soft foods or inserted through a nasogastric tube, as long as the capsule is not enteric-coated or the client does not chew the tiny granules of medication contained in the capsule. Chewing would have the same result as crushing.
15. *Do not return unused or excess medication to the supply container.* This practice applies both to individual and stock supply medications. Federal law prohibits dispensing prescription medications except by authorized persons, such as pharmacists, and most state pharmacy practice acts maintain that medications may be dispensed only by a pharmacist. Returning unused or excess medication to a stock or individual client supply is legally regarded as dispensing medications. In addition, when a medication is placed in a medicine cup and then returned to the supply, there is a potential for contamination of the supply from the cup or the environment and a potential for that contamination to alter the composition of the drug. When drugs have been taken to the client's room, there is no way to know for certain if an unlabeled drug is being returned to the correct container.
16. *Store drugs in the specified manner.* Read and follow the label or package insert and store as directed; for example, "Refrigerate after opening"; "Avoid exposure to sunlight or air"; or "Store at room temperature."
17. *Clean up after yourself!* When you finish preparing medications for one client or for a group of clients at the medicine cart or in the medicine room, clean the area so it is ready for someone else to use while you are administering your medications. This includes washing all equipment used to prepare and measure the medication, disposing of single-use supplies, and wiping work surfaces as needed. Cohen (1982) reports an incident of a client having a near-fatal anaphylactic reaction as a result of residual penicillin dust when a mortar and pestle were not cleaned after preparing a previous client's medication.

PREPARING ORAL MEDICATIONS

Safe preparation of oral medications is based on the preceding guidelines and includes selecting the correct number of unit-dose packages, pouring the correct number of tablets or capsules from a stock container, or pouring the correct volume of a liquid from a stock container. It is crucial to follow an orderly routine to prepare medications and to use the three safety checks to avoid errors.

☐ SKILL SEQUENCE

PREPARING ORAL MEDICATIONS

Step	Rationale
1. Check medication orders on medication page, kardex, computer printouts, or medication cards, according to agency policy.	System of checks helps detect human errors in ordering and transcribing medication orders.
2. Review own knowledge of drugs, using drug cards or other drug reference source.	Reinforces knowledge about the drugs.
3. Wash hands.	Helps avoid cross-contamination.
4. Prepare equipment. (NOTE: When using a portable medicine cart, prepare the medications in the hall outside each client's room or in the room, according to agency policy. When no portable medicine cart is used, prepare medications in the medicine room, place them in sequence on a tray and transport them to clients' rooms after all medications are prepared.)	Time-efficient action.
5. Read one medication order and select the correct medication container or unit-dose package from client's individual supply or from unit stock supplies. Prepare only one medication at a time, following steps 6 and 7 and then step 8 or 9.	Avoids confusion between different medications.

(continued)

Step	Rationale
6. SAFETY CHECK 1: Compare drug label and client's name with written or printed medication order.	Guards against errors.
7. Calculate dosage as necessary; that is, determine the number of tablets, capsules, milliliters, fluidrams, fluidounces, or minims of medication needed for the ordered dose.	Ensures correct dosage is administered.
If medication is a controlled substance, follow agency policy to sign for and obtain medication.	Fulfills legal accountability with controlled substances.
8. Unit-dose medications: a. Select the number of unit-dose packages needed for the ordered dosage.	Ensures correct dosage is administered.
b. Place medication package on medicine cart near medication page, printout, kardex, or medication card. **Do not open package and remove medication.**	Labeled package provides for final safety check at bedside.
c. SAFETY CHECK 2: Compare prepared dosage and label on unit-dose packages with medication order. (NOTE: Safety check 3 is performed at the bedside.)	Guards against errors. Provides final check before administering the medication.
9. Multiple-dose tablet or capsule containers: a. Remove cap and hold cap and container together with cap beneath opening.	Avoids dropping the medication.
b. Shake desired number of tablets or capsules into container cap, returning extra tablets or capsules to container without touching them, as shown in Figure 71-2. (NOTE: Use a slight rolling motion while pouring the medications from the container.)	Medications have touched only the inside of the container and can be returned without contamination. Often helps medications come out of the bottle one at a time.
c. Pour tablets and capsules into medicine cup or souffle cup.	Preparatory for giving medications to client.
d. SAFETY CHECK 2: Before placing medicine or souffle cup on the medicine tray or cart near the medication order, compare the prepared tablet or liquid dosage and container label with the medication order.	Guards against errors.
e. Place on medicine tray or on medicine cart near medication order.	
f. SAFETY CHECK 3: Before returning the container to the individual or stock supply, compare the container label with the medication order. (NOTE: Medication can now be identified only by color and shape. Keep medication order with medication at all times.)	Guards against error. Guards against confusing medications with each other and causing errors.
10. Multiple-dose liquid medications: a. Read and follow directions on label, such as "shake well"; obtain food or milk as needed for administration.	Ensures correct administration.
b. Remove cap and place it upside down on cart or countertop.	Protects edge and inside of cap from contamination.
c. Place thumb nail at desired level on medicine cup.	Gives visual identification and reminder of amount of liquid to pour.
d. Hold bottle and medicine cup at eye level, with bottle label facing you.	Direct line of vision required for accurate measurement. Label is visible while pouring. Avoids illegible labels from medication dripping on label when bottle is upright.
e. Pour slowly into medicine cup to desired level, measuring at the bottom of the meniscus as shown in Figure 71-3. (NOTE: As you finish pouring, use a slight rolling motion to raise the bottle.)	Avoids pouring excess medication. Bottom of meniscus is true fluid level. Avoids dripping.
f. Pour excess medication into sink or trash container. Do not return to bottle.	Avoids potential contamination of bottle contents from contact with environment.
g. Do SAFETY CHECK 2 as in step 9d.	
h. Wipe off bottle and screw neck with damp paper towel.	Avoids illegible labels and caps that stick or do not close well.
i. Replace cap securely.	Avoids leakage.
j. Do SAFETY CHECK 3 as in step 9f.	
11. Prepare additional medications for one or more clients, following steps 5 to 10.	

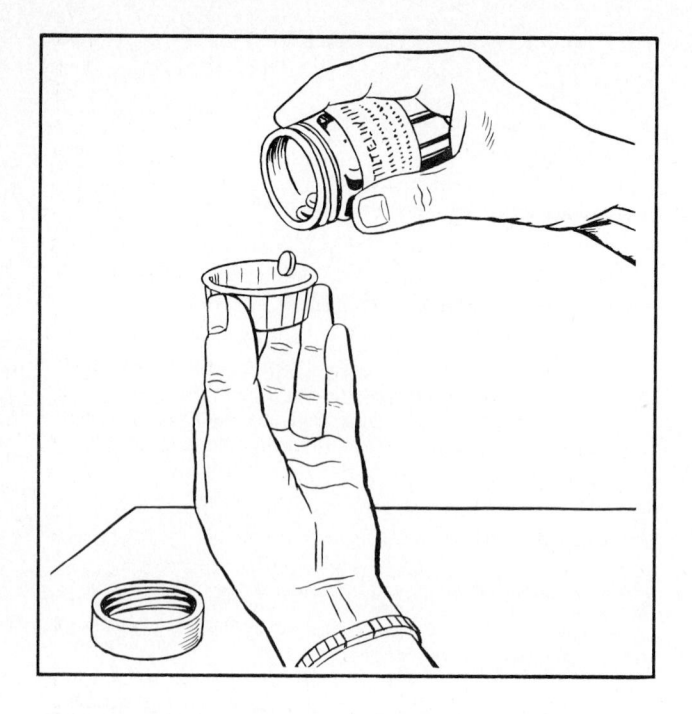

Figure 71-2. Pouring oral tablets or capsules from a multiple-dose container.

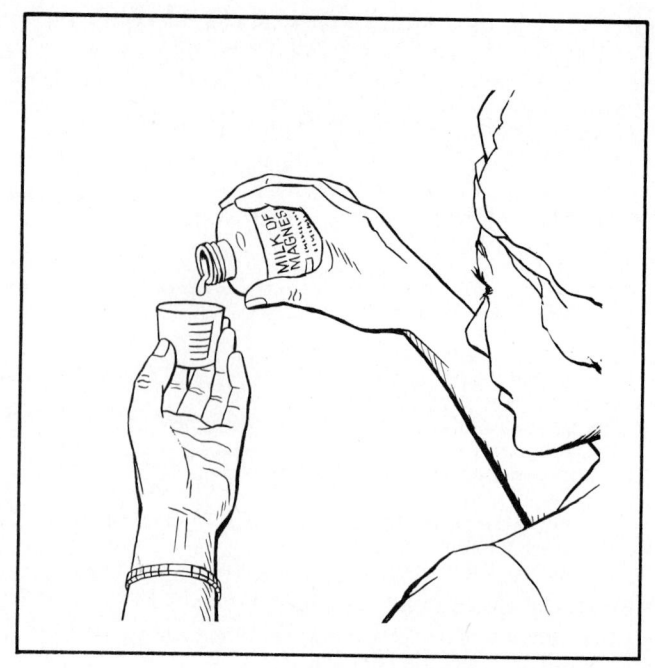

Figure 71-3. Pouring oral liquid medications from a multiple-dose container.

ADMINISTERING ORAL MEDICATION

In most agencies, the nurse takes the portable medicine cart into the room to administer medications. Students giving medications to one or two clients may or may not work from the cart, depending on agency and unit policy. Regardless of the system, the student must have possession of a valid medication order and form for recording medication when administering any medications to clients.

Most clients find it easier to swallow medications in an upright position, or as nearly upright as their condition permits. Since most people cannot draw enough water through a straw to swallow medications, offer a fresh glass of water without the straw. Some people prefer to take one medication at a time; others prefer to take them all at once to get it over with. If the person has a dry mouth or difficulty swallowing medications, offer a drink of water or juice before the medication to moisten the mouth and throat. Have the client place the medications on the back of the tongue, take a drink of water, flex the neck slightly, and swallow. The common practice of tilting the head backward and hyperextending the neck narrows the oropharynx and makes swallowing more difficult. Capsules are sometimes easier to swallow when they are placed in the front of the tongue and allowed to float back with the drink of water. Unless fluid intake is restricted, encourage drinking a full 8-oz glass of water with oral medications. Water helps dissolve the drug, and if only a few sips of water are taken, it is possible for the drug to adhere to the esophagus, contributing to development of esophagitis.

If a client is unable to take the medications unassisted, pour the medications into the client's mouth from the cup or place them on the tongue with clean fingers. To prevent cross-contamination of microorganisms to other clients, remember to wash your hands promptly after touching the client's mouth or the rim of the medicine cup or water glass where the client's lips touched them. When a client has neuromuscular impairment involving tongue displacement, such as with a cerebrovascular accident (stroke), place the tablet or capsule on the side of the tongue toward the displacement, since the displaced side is the most functional.

There are several other interventions that are often helpful for clients who have difficulty swallowing medications. If the tablet can be crushed or the capsule opened without interfering with its intended action, medication may be added to soft foods such as ice cream, applesauce, custard, or mashed potatoes. Tell the client the medication is in the food, since some medications will change the food's taste. Stroking the neck on both sides of the thyroid cartilage and manually closing the mouth while flexing the client's neck will often assist in swallowing, as will other swallowing facilitation techniques described in Skill 53.

Liquid oral medications can be given with a regular syringe of an appropriate size. To do this, pour the correct amount of medication into a medicine cup and withdraw the medication into the syringe, or attach a large-gauge sterile needle and withdraw the medication directly from the medication bottle into the syringe, and then discard the needle. To avoid contaminating the medication in the bottle, do not insert a syringe directly into the bottle (unless you can do so without touching any part of the syringe that enters the bottle neck) and do not return excess medication to the bottle. For easier administration to the client, add a 5 cm (2 in) length of latex tubing to the syringe so you can insert the medication slowly into the client's mouth between the cheek and the teeth. The syringe may be rinsed, kept at the bedside, and reused for the next medication administration.

Because the size of a drop is so variable, droppers are not used to measure medications in an inpatient setting, unless they are calibrated and attached to the medication bottle cap. Since the dropper attached to a medication bottle is calibrated for that bottle of medication *only*, do not use it to measure medication from another bottle. When measuring drops with a dropper in the home setting, hold the dropper at a 45 degree angle and at eye level where the drops can be counted readily.

Although most medications have flavorings added to increase their palatability, some medications are quite unpleasant, such as castor oil, or bitter, such as potassium products. Since cold numbs the taste buds, bitter medications are more palatable if they are chilled, given with ice water, or if the client sucks ice chips before taking them. Chilling also decreases the aroma of oily odorous medications such as castor oil, making them easier to tolerate. Medications which discolor the teeth if they are swallowed in the usual way (such as iron preparations) should be diluted and given with a straw, followed with a glass of water.

GUIDELINES FOR SAFE ADMINISTRATION OF MEDICATIONS

As with preparation of medications, there are practices that can safeguard against errors while administering the drug to clients. Except for the information specific to the oral route, these safe practices apply to administration through any route.

1. *Know the client.* Most medication record pages or kardexes contain brief vital data about that client, such as age, sex, date of admission, diagnosis, type of surgery and the date (if relevant), some diagnostic tests, allergies, and the physician's name. As you administer medications, *think* about the relationship of the medication to that particular client and his or her condition.
2. *Identify the client clearly.* To do this, compare the name and room number on the medication order with the actual room and client in four ways:
   a. Before you enter the client's room, *check the room number.*
   b. After you are in the room, *check the bed number or letter,* unless it is a private room. Know your agency's policy about whether Bed 1 is near the door or the window.
   c. *Check the identification band* for the client's name and compare it with the medication record.
   d. *Address the client by name or ask the client to state his or her name.* This can be done in a variety of ways, depending on the personalities and circumstances involved. For example, "Mr. John Smith? I have your morning medications," or "Are you Mr. John Smith? Let me see your identification band, please." To avoid confusion between clients with similar names, the name should always be written and stated with the complete first and last names, not just first initial and last name. If the name is one that is used for both sexes, such as Marian/Marion, Carol/Carroll, or Francis/Frances, include a title that indicates gender.

   It is imperative that none of these checks is omitted, even though you may know the client well. These safeguards are a crucial part of the rigid habits that will help you avoid making a medication error. If you are uncertain about the identity of the client after these checks, consult with another staff member who knows the client. Clients have been known to answer to names other than their own or crawl into someone else's bed, either from confusion or as a joke. *Do not give a medication if you are in doubt about the client's identity.*
3. *Open unit-dose medications at the bedside.* As indicated previously, major benefits of the unit-dose system include being able to identify the medication at the time it is given to the client and being able to return unused or refused medications to the client's supply rather than destroying them. Before opening the unit-dose packages, do the final SAFETY CHECK 3 with the medication order. As you open each package and give the medication to the client, use the time to talk with the client about the medication's therapeutic action or significant side effects. For example, when giving a diuretic, you might ask about frequency of urination, presence of edema, or fluid intake. Many clients will find it easier to take the medication if you pour it into a souffle cup before handing it to them. As an additional safety check, before discarding the empty package, compare it with the medication order on the medication record form.
4. *Make needed assessments before giving the medication.* You are accountable for making appropriate judgments about medication administration, based on specific knowledge of the drugs you are working with. For example, digitalis products are nearly always omitted if the pulse is below 60; some antiarrhythmics are omitted if the blood pressure is too low for that client; and narcotics are sometimes delayed if the respiratory rate is too low. You are also responsible for investigating whether medications are having any untoward effects. For example, it is not uncommon for a client to have mild diarrhea and continue to have a stool softener administered on a regular basis without anyone determining whether the stool softener was still needed.
5. *Listen to the client.* If clients tell you they are allergic to a medication or that the physician has changed the order—*listen* to what they are saying.

Check the health record, validate the order, or check with the physician. The history of allergy may have been accidentally omitted from the medication record form, nursing-care kardex, or the health record; or the information may never have been obtained from the client. *Never* give a medication if someone tells you he or she is allergic to it. Serious harm and even death have been known to occur when people have received medication to which they were allergic.

6. *Observe the client take the medication.* To do this, observe for swallowing. Sometimes it is necessary to inspect the inside of the client's mouth to see if the medication is still there. Clients do not swallow medications for a variety of reasons, such as a refusal to take medication, an intent to hoard medication for later overdose, from mental confusion or incapacity, or from physiological difficulty in swallowing.

7. *Do not leave medications at the bedside.* If a client is eating, is in the bathroom, or not able or willing to take the medication while you are in the room, wait or negotiate a time to return. Do not leave the medications for the client to take later. When you record a medication is given, you are assuming the responsibility that it actually was taken by the client. There are a few medications that are exceptions to this rule of not leaving medications at the bedside. For example, nitroglycerin and hourly antacids are almost always left at the bedside, either by agency policy or physician order. If you are working in an agency where clients give their own medications, follow those policies.

8. *Do not leave medications unattended.* If you are interrupted for any reason while giving medications and need to do something else, such as answer the telephone, return the medicine cart or tray to the medicine room. You may leave them briefly under the watchful eye of a trusted co-worker, but never leave prepared medications where clients or the public have access to them.

9. *Check bedside medications.* At least one time each day, ask the client about the need for and use of drugs that are kept at the bedside, check the supply, and replenish as needed. There should be at least a 24-hour supply of medication available.

10. *Record medications promptly, after they are given.* As you record the medication as having been given, compare the empty unit-dose package with the medication order as it appears on the medication record form. Medication errors related to not recording medications at the time of administration are among the most commonly reported errors (Davis and Cohen, 1981).

11. *Record water on intake-output record as needed.* When intake and output is being measured, be sure to record the water used to give oral medications. When intake is restricted, plan the liquid allotment to include medication administration. One study indicated that the average intake with medications exceeded 30 percent of the total daily intake for 30 percent of the clients studied, and that those persons on fluid restriction took the largest volume of liquid with medications (Holmes et al., 1965). To decrease the amount of fluid needed for medication administration, give medications with meals when feasible, disguise the taste so less water is needed after the medication, offer small glasses of water, and negotiate the allocation with the client.

☐ SKILL SEQUENCE

ADMINISTERING ORAL MEDICATIONS

Step	Rationale
1. Prepare medications as in Skill Sequence, "Preparing Oral Medications," p. 854.	Ensures administration of correct drug.
2. Take portable medicine cart or tray of medications to client's room.	Follows agency policy.
3. Identify the client. Check the following and compare with the written medication order:	Ensures identification of correct client.
a. Room number on door.	Identifies correct room.
b. Bed number or letter.	Identifies correct bed.
c. Name on identification band. Replace band if missing.	Most accurate identification.
d. Address client by complete name or ask client to state his or her name. (CAUTION: Some clients will respond automatically without listening, or will exchange beds because of confusion or as a joke.)	Identifies correct person. Involves client in identification process.
4. Introduce self by name and inform client about medications he or she is to receive, according to agency policy.	Provides information about own identity. Provides information about therapeutic and diagnostic plan.
5. Perform preliminary assessments as needed; for example, pulse, blood pressure, or the need for a laxative.	Ensures appropriateness of administration of medication at this time.

(continued)

Step	Rationale
6. Assist client to as near an upright position as condition will permit.	Upright position facilitates swallowing.
7. Unit-dose SAFETY CHECK 3: Compare label and prepared dosage with medication order.	Guards against error.
8. To administer tablets or capsules:	
a. Unit-dose package: At the bedside, open packages one at a time directly into client's hand or into a souffle cup and hand it to the client.	Avoids handling medication. Provides time to discuss need for, effectiveness of, or problems with the medication.
b. Multiple-dose medications: Hand prepared souffle cup with medication to client or pour medications into client's hand.	Avoids handling medication.
c. If assistance is needed, place souffle cup to client's lips and pour medication into mouth. (NOTE: ORAL medications may be given one at a time, or several at the same time.)	Appropriate action when client unable to handle own medications. Client preference varies.
d. Offer glass of water to client without using straw. Hold glass and assist as necessary.	Volume of water drawn through a straw is usually not enough to swallow a medication.
e. Have client flex neck slightly and swallow medication. (NOTE: See text for suggested actions when client has difficulty swallowing medication.)	Position facilitates swallowing.
f. Observe client for swallowing.	Identifies if client actually receives the medication.
9. To administer oral liquids:	
a. Follow directions on unit-dose label; remove sealed top.	Provides for correct administration.
b. Dissolve or dilute unit-dose or stock supply medication as needed.	Provides for correct administration.
c. Hand unit-dose container or medication cup to client, or hold container to client's lips as needed.	No need to transfer unit-dose liquid to medicine cup. Appropriate assistance if client unable to handle own medication.
d. Observe client for swallowing.	Identifies inability to take medication, and validates that client actually receives the medication.
10. Observe initial reaction to medication.	Identifies any initial untoward reactions.
11. Return to position of comfort and safety.	Provides for client comfort and safety.
12. Record medications on medication page or kardex, make notation on computer printout or record in computer, or turn medicine cards upside down in separate area. Compare the empty unit-dose package with the medication order on the medication record form.	Fulfills nurse accountability for recording or noting that medication was given, according to system used. Serves as final check for accuracy of medication administration.
13. Discard disposable containers in trash container. Return reusable glasses or medicine cups to separate area on medicine cart or tray.	Follows principles of medical asepsis in caring for used equipment.
14. Record fluid intake of client on intake-output measurement.	Promotes accurate intake-output measurement.
15. Continue to next client and repeat procedure for each person.	Ensures correct administration of medications to group of clients.
16. Replace supplies on medicine cart or in medicine room. Leave the medicine cart, medicine trays, and medicine room clean and tidy.	Prepares equipment for the next nurse.
17. Record medications in client's record or in the computer system, unless a multiple-page medication record or kardex system is used. Recording to include: date, time, drug, dosage, route, and initials or signature.	Provides permanent record of medication administration.

GIVING MEDICATIONS THROUGH A NASOGASTRIC TUBE

A nasogastric tube is not inserted for the purpose of giving medications. When a feeding tube is in place, oral medications can be inserted through the tube. Since the action of an oral medication is the same when given through a tube as when swallowed, administration guidelines about crushing tablets, emptying capsules, and giving medication with or without food remain unchanged. Many medications are available in liquid form as well as tablets and capsules. Before you decide to crush and dissolve a tablet or empty a capsule, contact the pharmacist to see if that particular medication is available as a liquid.

If the medication can or should be administered with food, it may be given when an intermittent enteral feeding is given. It should not be mixed with the formula, but given as a single dose. If the client is not tolerating the tube feeding very well or if there is delayed absorption, give the medication at a time other than with the feeding. This is particularly important if gastric contents are aspirated soon after the feeding to relieve distress. When continuous enteral feedings are being given, disconnect the tubing from the nasogastric tube to administer the medication.

To give a medication through a nasogastric tube, the following equipment is required: a tubing clamp or hemostat, a large bulb or plunger syringe, a glass of water, and the liquid medication. Follow these steps to administer the medication:

1. Prepare and check the medication and identify the client in the usual ways.
2. Position the client in as nearly upright a position as possible to avoid gastric reflux.
3. Protect the bed linen with a towel or protective pad.
4. Unclamp the tube and check its placement to determine whether it is in the stomach as described in Skill 56. Be sure to check residual gastric contents.
5. Remove the squeeze bulb or plunger from the syringe, attach it to the tube, pour the medication into the syringe, and allow it to flow in by gravity.
6. Rinse the syringe and tube with 30 to 50 ml of water to clear the tube of medication so the medication does not cling to the sides of the tube or clog the inlet port and so that the client receives the entire dosage.
7. Clamp the tube and leave the client in a semi-Fowler's position for about 30 minutes.
8. Record the volume of water in the intake and output record.

GIVING INSTRUCTIONS ABOUT MEDICATION ADMINISTRATION

As you give medications to clients, include any special instructions for administration. For example, if a cough syrup has local soothing action, the client should take it *after* other medications, but if the cough syrup has a systemic action (as many do), then it is all right to drink water afterward. Other examples of special instructions are reminding clients to drink 8 to 10 glasses of water per day when taking sulfa drug preparations, drinking minimal water immediately after taking an antacid, and not chewing or swallowing tablets intended for sublingual or buccal administration. Unless agency policy dictates otherwise, tell clients what medications they are receiving. For example, you might say "Mr. Smith, here is your antibiotic (or sulfa or erythromycin)." Not only does this provide information about the therapeutic or diagnostic plan, it also gives the client an opportunity to report previous allergies or idiosyncratic reactions to the drug.

When clients are to take medications at home, be sure they know how often to take each drug, whether to take it with food or on an empty stomach, as well as possible side effects that should be reported to the physician. Review with clients any over-the-counter (OTC) medications that may interact unfavorably with the prescribed medication, or suggest they check with the physician or pharmacist about those drugs. Explain the need for taking all of a prescribed medication as ordered rather than discontinuing it when the symptoms subside, unless otherwise directed. Advise clients not to take medications prescribed for another family member and to check the expiration date on medications that are used infrequently.

Some clients have difficulty remembering to take their medications as scheduled, particularly if they take quite a number of medications or if they are somewhat confused or forgetful. A written schedule of the medications to be taken at specific clock times provides a guide for these clients and a referral to a community-based nurse is usually quite helpful.

RECORDING

Record medications immediately after administering them, following the agency system. On the medication flow sheet, record the drug name and dosage, the frequency, route of administration, the date and time given, and the initials or signature of the nurse who gave the medication. In the nurses' notes, record any relevant information you may have obtained while administering medications; for example, data about the therapeutic effectiveness of the drug, untoward reactions, problems encountered in administration, and the client's reaction to the medications. In most agencies, specific drugs are recorded in the nurses' notes only when it is a stat, p.r.n., or unusual medication. It is then included within the context of the SOAP or narrative recording. When these types of drugs are given, it is important to record the effectiveness or ineffectiveness of the drug and any delayed problems. Periodically, as a part of ongoing charting, record those same kinds of data about all regularly scheduled medications the client receives, since responsible charting includes recording the client's response to the therapeutic plan.

For a sample medication flow sheet recording, see Chapter 16, Introduction, Figure 5, p. 840.

☐ CRITICAL POINTS SUMMARY

1. Store, prepare, and administer medications according to directions on the label or package insert.
2. Read labels and medication orders carefully.
3. Think about the relevance and appropriateness of the medications you are preparing and administering.
4. Avoid distractions while preparing and administering medications.
5. Prepare one medication at a time.

6. Use the factor-label method or a known values proportion equation (conversion formula and dosage formula) to calculate medication dosages correctly.
7. Check the medication order and the selected dosage *three times:*
    a. Unit-dose system:
       SAFETY CHECK 1: When removing the unit-dose package from the medicine drawer.
       SAFETY CHECK 2: After deciding the number of unit-dose packages needed for the correct dosage.
       SAFETY CHECK 3: At the bedside, before opening the packages.
    b. Individual or stock supply system:
       SAFETY CHECK 1: When removing the medication container from the medicine drawer or the supply shelf.
       SAFETY CHECK 2: After pouring the desired number of tablets or capsules or the amount of liquid needed for the correct dosage.
       SAFETY CHECK 3: When returning the container to the drawer or shelf.
8. Always open unit-dose medication packages at the bedside.
9. Do not return unused medications to a stock or individual supply.
10. Identify the correct client by room number, bed number, identification band, and verbal use of his or her name.
11. Make appropriate drug-related assessments before administering the medication.
12. Observe the client actually swallow the medication.
13. Assist the client to swallow oral medications as needed.
14. Do not leave prepared medications unattended.
15. Do not leave medications at the bedside, except as indicated by physician order or agency policy.
16. Record water used to administer medications on the intake–output record.
17. Give liquid or dissolved medications through a nasogastric tube as a single dose and rinse the tube afterward.

☐ LEARNING ACTIVITIES

1. Examine unit-dose packages as prepared by a drug manufacturer and a hospital pharmacy. Note similarities and differences in the style and information contained on the label.
2. Observe one or more systems of medication administration (unit-dose, individual, or stock supply) and talk with nurses who use or have used those systems. What benefits and problems do you or they identify with each system?
3. For your agency, identify the methods by which the physician's medication order reaches the pharmacy; the medication order system used by the nurses to administer medications; the method by which medications are recorded after administration; the process by which the medication order used by the nurse to administer the medication is validated as being the same as the one the physician wrote; and the process by which clients are charged for the drugs they receive.
4. Interview nurses who work in various kinds of client-care areas, such as general medical–surgical, intensive care, or pediatric units. Ask what kind of oral medication dosage calculations they encounter in their areas of work, and the kind of conversions between the metric and apothecary system they need to use. Practice calculating those kinds of problems.
5. Interview a visiting or public health nurse and inquire about the ways clients measure medications in the home setting and what kinds of aids they have used to help clients remember to take their medications.
6. Examine enteric-coated and non–enteric-coated tablets and capsules. What differences do you note in their appearance and composition?
7. Examine time-release capsules and tablets. Note the different colored granules in the capsule and the layers in the tablet.
8. Obtain a medication cup calibrated in three systems, a beaker calibrated in milliliters, and a minim glass. Measure the volume contained in several teaspoons, tablespoons, and soupspoons. Obtain several eye droppers and measure 15 drops into a minim glass or milliliter beaker. Compare the volume obtained by holding each one at the same angle and the same dropper at different angles. Measure 15 drops of concentrated sugar syrup and compare that volume with the water volume. What do these volume measurements tell you about accuracy of measuring with the household system? (NOTE: If a milliliter beaker or minim glass is unavailable, measure the drops into a medicine cup and withdraw the water into a tuberculin syringe to measure in milliliters. Tuberculin syringes are calibrated in tenths of a milliliter.)
9. Examine a liquid medication that needs to be shaken before it is administered and one that does not need to be shaken. What differences do you note between the two liquids? Shake both medications and note what happens. Would shaking contribute to a more or less accurate measurement of these medications?

862 PROFESSIONAL CLINICAL NURSING SKILLS

10. Investigate the statements about medication administration that are contained in the Nurse Practice Act in your state.

☐ REVIEW QUESTIONS

1. In what ways is the oral route of administering medications preferable over the parenteral route?
2. What are some disadvantages of the oral route?
3. In what ways are the SAFETY CHECKS used in preparing medications *alike* and *different* for the unit-dose versus the individual or stock supply system?
4. What four ways must be used to identify the client before administering medications?
5. What problems might be encountered if you rely only on verbal identification of a client?
6. What are the reasons it is important to know the drugs being administered and the client to whom they are being administered?
7. What are the reasons for developing rigid automatic habits for safe medication administration?
8. Give the rationale for the following guidelines of medication administration:
    a. Avoid distractions while preparing and administering medications.
    b. Prepare one medication at a time.
    c. Do not return unused medications to a stock or individual supply.
    d. Observe the client actually swallow the medication.
    e. Do not leave prepared medications unattended.
    f. Do not leave medications at the bedside, except as indicated by agency policy or physician order.
9. Why are unit-dose medication packages opened at the bedside rather than in a medicine room or in the hallway?
10. Why are enteric-coated capsules never emptied and added to food to facilitate swallowing the medication?
11. Why should enteric-coated and time-release tablets never be crushed?
12. How can a medication's unpleasant taste be disguised?
13. What interventions will usually help clients swallow medications when they are having difficulty?
14. Describe the process for giving oral medications through a nasogastric tube.
15. What problem sometimes occurs when medications are given through a nasogastric tube at the same time as the tube feeding?
16. Solve the following dosage calculation problems, converting to the metric system as needed. Use the factor-label or known values proportion equation method.

    a. Ordered dose: Cortisone 0.025 g, p.o. q.i.d. Available dosage: Cortisone Acetate, 10 mg (scored tablets).
    b. Ordered dose: Lanoxin gr 1/300 p.o. daily. Available dosage: Lanoxin, 0.1 mg (tablets).
    c. Ordered dose: Phenobarbitol, 12 mg b.i.d. Available dosage: Elixir of Phenobarbitol, 30 mg/5 ml.

☐ PERFORMANCE CHECKLISTS

OBJECTIVE: To prepare oral medications safely, using safety checks and correct calculations.

CHARACTERISTIC	RANGE OF ACCEPTABILITY	SATISFACTORY	UNSATISFACTORY
1. Checks medication order for accuracy.	No deviation		
2. Reviews knowledge of drug.	No deviation		
3. Washes hands.	No deviation		
4. Prepares one medication at a time.	No deviation		
5. Signs for controlled substances as needed.	No deviation		
6. Selects correct medication.	No deviation		
7. Does SAFETY CHECK 1: Compares drug label and client's name with the medication order.	No deviation		
8. Calculates the correct dosage (amount needed).	No deviation		

(continued)

CHARACTERISTIC	RANGE OF ACCEPTABILITY	SATISFACTORY	UNSATISFACTORY
9. Unit-dose medication: 　a. Selects the correct number of unit-dose packages. 　b. Places medication near medication order and does SAFETY CHECK 2: Compares drug label and client's name with the medication order. 　c. Leaves medication packages unopened.	No deviation No deviation Opens only if medication is to be crushed or inserted into a nosaogastric tube.		
10. Multiple-dose tablets or capsules: 　a. Shakes desired number into container cap without touching contents. 　b. Pours medication into souffle or medicine cup. 　c. Does SAFETY CHECK 2 as in 9b. 　d. Places medication near medication order or on medicine tray. 　e. Does SAFETY CHECK 3: Compares drug label and prepared dosage with medication order before returning container to individual or stock supply.	No deviation No deviation No deviation No deviation No deviation		
11. Multiple-dose liquid medications: 　a. Reads and follows directions for shaking, dilution, or giving with food. 　b. Removes cap and places it upside down in safe place. 　c. Places thumbnail at desired level on medicine cup and holds bottle and medicine cup at eye level, with bottle label facing self. 　d. Pours correct amount, measured at meniscus. 　e. Does SAFETY CHECK 2 as in 9b. 　f. Wipes off bottle and neck and replaces cap. 　g. Does SAFETY CHECK 3 as in 10e.	No deviation No deviation No deviation No deviation No deviation No deviation No deviation		

OBJECTIVE: To administer oral medications safely.			
CHARACTERISTIC	RANGE OF ACCEPTABILITY	SATISFACTORY	UNSATISFACTORY
1. Takes medicine cart or tray to client's room.	No deviation		
2. Identifies the client: 　a. Compares medication order with client's 　　(1) Room number 　　(2) Bed number 　　(3) Identification band 　b. Addresses the client by name.	 No deviation No deviation No deviation No deviation		
3. Informs client about medication being given.	Modify according to client's capability or agency and physician policy.		
4. Performs needed preliminary assessments.	No deviation		
5. Assists client to a near-upright position.	No deviation		
6. Does unit-dose SAFETY CHECK 3: Compares label and dosage with medication order before handing it to the client.	No deviation		

(continued)

OBJECTIVE: To administer oral medications safely (cont.).

CHARACTERISTIC	RANGE OF ACCEPTABILITY	SATISFACTORY	UNSATISFACTORY
7. To administer tablets or capsules: a. At the bedside, opens unit-dose package and pours medication into client's hand or souffle or medication cup. b. For multiple-dose medications, hands prepared cup to client. c. Offers glass of water without straw.	No deviation May need to place medication in client's mouth. May need to hold glass for some clients.		
8. To administer oral liquids: a. Removes sealed top from unit-dose package. b. Dilutes or prepares medication as needed. c. Hands unit-dose container or medication cup to client.	No deviation No deviation Hold container for client as needed.		
9. Observes for swallowing.	Facilitate as needed.		
10. Observes initial reaction.	No deviation		
11. Repositions for comfort and safety.	No deviation		
12. Records medication on medication record page, kardex, or in bedside computer.	Mark computer printout or stack medicine cards for later recording.		
13. Discards disposable containers.	No deviation		
14. Returns reusable containers to separate place on tray or cart.	No deviation		
15. Records fluid intake.	Omit if not on intake-output measurement.		
16. Records medication on permanent form in health record or computer.	Omit if already done.		

REFERENCES

Cohen MR: Medication errors: Always clean the mortar and pestle after crushing tablets. Nursing82 (Horsham) 12(12):25, 1982.

Davis NM, Cohen MR: Medication errors: Causes and prevention. Philadelphia, George F Stickley, 1981.

Giovannitti C, Schwinghammer T: Food and drugs: Managing the right mix for your patient. Nursing81 (Horsham) 11(7):26-31, 1981.

Govani LE, Hayes JE: Drugs and Nursing Implications, ed 5. East Norwalk, CT, Appleton-Century-Crofts, 1985.

Holmes JH, Sitprija V, et al.: Fluid intake with medication. Archives of Internal Medicine 116(6):813-818, 1965.

Rosenberg JM, Sangkachand P: "Take with meals" . . . or not? Part I. RN 44(6):60-65, 1981.

Rosenberg JM, Sangkachand P: "Take with meals" . . . or not? Part I. RN 44(5):47-52, 1981.

Wordell DC: Should you crush that tablet? Nursing82 (Horsham) 12(9):78, 1982.

BIBLIOGRAPHY

Kozier B, Erb E: Techniques in Clinical Nursing. Menlo Park, CA, Addison-Wesley, 1982.

Lewis LuVW: Fundamental Skills in Patient Care, ed 3. Philadelphia, JB Lippincott, 1984.

Nursing80 Photobook. Giving medications. Horsham, PA, Intermed Communications, 1980.

Palmer HA, Fraser GL: Crushing tablets, opening capsules: When is it safe? RN 41(8):53-59, 1978.

Sorensen KC, Luckmann J: Basic Nursing: A Psychophysiologic Approach. Philadelphia, WB Saunders, 1979.

Wood LA: Nursing Skills for Allied Health Services, vol 3. Philadelphia, WB Saunders, 1975.

SUGGESTED READING

Giovannitti C, Schwinghammer T: Food and drugs: Managing the right mix for your patient. Nursing81 (Horsham) 11(7):26-31, 1981.

Rosenberg JM, Sangkachand P: "Take with meals" . . . or not? Part II. RN 44(6):60-65, 1981.

Rosenberg JM, Sangkachand P: "Take with meals" . . . or not? Part I. RN 44(5):47-53, 1981.

Sandroff R: Booby-trapped orders. RN 44(11):24-31, 1981.

Wordell DC: Should you crush that tablet? Nursing82 (Horsham) 12(9):78, 1982.

AUDIOVISUAL RESOURCES

Medicating the Patient: Administering Oral, Topical, Suppository and Inhalant Medications
Filmstrip, video. (1982, Color, 21 min.)

Medicating the Patient: Preparing Medications
Filmstrip, video. (1982, Color, 19 min.)
Available through:
Medcom, Inc.
P.O. Box 116
Garden Grove, CA 92642

Preparation and Administration of Oral Medications
Videorecording. (1981, 8 min.)
Available through:
Robert J. Brady Company
Route 197
Bowie, MD 20715

SKILL 72 Topical Medication Administration

PREREQUISITE SKILLS

Skill 19, "Inspection"
Skill 28, "Handwashing"
Skill 32, "Dressings and Wound Care"
Skill 36, "Wet Sterile Dressings"
Skill 39, "Perineal Care"
Skill 40, "Oral Care"
Skill 43, "Vaginal Irrigation"
Skill 58, "Bowel Elimination Procedures"
Skill 60, "Urinary Catheterization"
Chapter 16, "Introduction"
Skill 71, "Oral Medication Administration"

STUDENT OBJECTIVES

1. Distinguish between local and systemic effects of locally applied medications.
2. Indicate the various anatomic sites to which topical medications may be applied.
3. Identify the advantages and disadvantages of topical application of medications to the skin and mucous membranes.
4. Describe the relationship of the application site to the absorption and effectiveness of locally applied medications.
5. Define common terms used to identify various types of topical medications.
6. Describe the correct positioning and procedures for instilling eye drops and ointments, ear drops, nose drops and sprays, and for irrigating the eye and ear.
7. Describe the correct positioning and procedures for inserting rectal, vaginal, and urethral suppositories and inserts.
8. Describe the correct methods of applying powders, lotions, creams, ointments, and pastes to skin surfaces.
9. Administer topical medications in a safe manner.
10. Describe the correct method for administering sublingual and buccal tablets.
11. Describe the correct method for using mouth and throat sprays and throat lozenges.
12. Compare transdermal application of systemic-acting topical medications with dermal application of local acting drugs.

INTRODUCTION

Topical administration of medication refers to local application of drugs to the skin and mucous membranes. Topical medications are prepared in various dosage forms ranging from powders and liquids to pastes and suppositories. Topical application of medication to mucous membranes includes inserting medication into the eyes, nose, mouth, lungs, rectum, vagina, and occasionally, the urethra. Topical application to the skin includes the skin anywhere on the body, including the external ear and auditory canal, as both are lined with epithelial tissue.

Topical medications applied to mucous membranes may have either local or systemic action. For example, sublingual and buccal tablets are rapidly absorbed through the thin epithelium and rich capillary network under the tongue and in the cheek, resulting in rapid drug action such as occurs when nitroglycerin given sublingually relieves the chest pain of angina pectoris within 1 or 2 minutes. Drugs given through these two routes are rapid acting and potent because they enter the systemic circulation directly, without first traversing the portal circulation. Because of this characteristic, these routes are useful for drugs that would be deactivated or destroyed by gastric enzymes or hepatic processes.

Topical medications applied to the skin are almost always intended for local action. With the exception of nitroglycerin, cytotoxic drugs, and some toxic chemicals encountered in industry, most drugs are not readily absorbed into the circulation through intact skin. Itching and burning of the skin generally is relieved more promptly with a topical dermal drug application than with a systemic drug given orally, subcutaneously, or intramuscularly. In general, there are fewer side effects and less severe allergic reactions to topical drugs as compared to drugs given by other routes. Topical drugs are also easy to administer, can often be applied by the client, and their visible connection with the problem is of psychological benefit.

Disadvantages of topical dermal medications include difficulty in delivering precise dosages; possible staining of clothing, skin, or linens; often time-consuming application; and potential client embarrassment if the medication is applied to the total body surface or body areas considered private.

This skill presents the methods for administering sublingual and buccal medications and mouth and throat preparations; instilling eye drops and ointments, ear drops, nasal drops or sprays; inserting rectal and urethral suppositories and vaginal inserts, suppositories, or cream; and applying various powders, liquids, and semisolid preparations to the skin. In addition, eye irrigations are included here, since this procedure is used to apply medication to or mechanically cleanse the mucous membranes of the eye.

☐ PREPARATION

Topical medications are applied for a variety of purposes, usually specific to the route being used. Each client's specific illness condition or health problem will determine the medication needed and therefore the purpose for which it is intended. There are, however, some general purposes for using each topical medication route. While drugs are well-absorbed across mucosal surfaces, the mucous membranes are highly selective in their absorption and differ in their sensitivity to drugs. For example, topical eye medications are one-fourth to one-half as concentrated as nasal medications. With a few notable exceptions as indicated in the following discussion, application of topical medications is considered a clean, medical aseptic technique.

ROUTES AND PURPOSES FOR TOPICAL MEDICATIONS

Mouth and Throat
Drugs given in the mouth and throat are for either systemic or local action.

Sublingual and Buccal Tablets. Medications given by the sublingual and buccal routes are designed for systemic action. Sublingual tablets are usually small in size. They are placed under the tongue and quickly absorbed into the circulation. The most common sublingual drug is nitroglycerin, which begins to give relief from the chest pains of angina pectoris within 1 minute. Buccal tablets are larger in size and are held in the cheek pouch adjacent to the upper molars until they are absorbed. For example, oxytocin is sometimes administered buccally to stimulate uterine contractions.

Mouth and Throat Drugs. Topical medications may be sprayed onto the mucous membrane of the mouth and throat to produce local effects, using a spray pump or atomizer. They may also be applied as a mouthwash or gargle. These medications include antiseptics, such as chloraseptic, to inhibit growth of microorganisms; anesthetics, such as xylocaine viscous, to diminish sensations, and astringents for local constriction and relief of inflammation. Since topical anesthetics applied to the throat and mouth can be absorbed systemically, it is essential that the nurse record the volume and dosage used during a procedure to avoid overdosage and untoward systemic effects.

Nasal Administration
Many nose drops and nasal sprays are intended for local action within the nasal cavity or sinus passages; for example, decongestant vasoconstrictive drops and sprays, such as oxymetazoline (Afrin, Duration), are used to open blocked nasal passages and reduce nasal hyperemia. Adverse cardiovascular and central nervous system effects can occur if nose drops are given incorrectly and pass down the throat without producing local action. Some nasal sprays, however, are designed for systemic absorption of drugs that would be digested if taken by mouth, such as the hormone vasopressin used in the treatment of diabetes insipidus.

Nasal preparations are aqueous, isotonic, slightly acidic, and nonirritating. Most are not oily because oils would inhibit ciliary cleansing action and increase the risk of respiratory infections such as a lipid pneumonia if they are inhaled.

Ear Administration
Ear drops and ear ointments, referred to as 'otic' medications, are used for local action on or within the external auditory canal or the tympanic membrane. For example, ear drops such as Debrox may be used to soften cerumen for later removal; antibiotic drops are used to treat infections; itching may be relieved with 70 percent alcohol. When ear wax is impacted, the physician will usually remove it with an irrigation or teach and supervise this activity.

Instillation of ear drops, insertion of ear ointment, and ear irrigations are performed with either aseptic or clean technique, depending on the reason for the treatment. The technique would be determined either by the physician or the client's condition; for example, if open denuded areas are present or if the tympanic membrane is not intact, aseptic equipment and technique should be used.

Eye Administration
Eye drops and ointments, referred to as 'ophthalmic' medications, are used for local action, such as to apply antibiotics to the conjunctiva, anesthetize the cornea prior to corneal surgery or for a tonometry measurement for glaucoma; to dilate the pupil for eye examinations; to constrict the pupil for treatment of glaucoma; or to soothe irritated tissues. Eye medications are usually a dilute solution in a strength less than 1 percent strength, and are made with a nonirritating base suited for sensitive eye tissues. Eye irrigations

with sterile saline are used to flush foreign bodies or contaminants from the eye.

Rectal Administration
Medications are administered rectally in suppository form for either local or systemic effects. A suppository is a drug form that contains a pure drug mixed with a firm base such as cocoa butter, lanolin, glycerin, carbowax, or gelatin, and then molded into a shape suitable for inserting into a body orifice or organ. Suppositories are in a solid state at room temperature or when refrigerated, but they melt at body temperature. Rectal suppositories are usually about 3.5 to 4 cm (1½ to 1¾ in) long, slightly larger in diameter than a lead pencil, and have a tapered tip for easier insertion. Some are self-lubricated and others require additional lubrication for insertion. Examples of local acting suppositories are glycerin (humectant and bulk-producing actions) and bisacodyl, USP (Dulcolox), a stimulant laxative. Examples of systemic acting suppositories are Belladona and Opium (B & O), an antispasmodic used to treat bladder spasms; ergotamine and caffeine (Cafergot), used to treat migraines; and trimethobenzamide (Ticon, Tigan), an antiemetic.

Vaginal Administration
Topical medications for vaginal use may be in the form of conical, globular, or cylindrical shaped inserts made similarly to rectal suppositories. They may also be in cream, jelly, or foam form, dispensed by squeezing the medication from a tube into a tubular applicator that has a plunger which is used to insert the medication high into the vaginal vault. Topical vaginal preparations may be used for local treatment of vaginal infections; for example, a fungicide such as miconazole nitrate (MicaTin or Monistat) is used to treat a *Candida albicans* infection. Topical hormones such as conjugated estrogens, U.S.P. (Estroate, Premarin) are used to treat atrophic changes in the vaginal mucosa.

Dermal Administration
Topical medications are applied to the skin for purposes such as to protect skin integrity, treat skin infections, apply antiseptics or disinfectants, or to relieve the itching and burning associated with many skin conditions and with the side effects of medications or diagnostic tests. The therapeutic effectiveness of a topical dermal medication is related not only to the drugs it contains but also to the form in which it is available and how it is applied to the skin. Table 72-1 shows common forms of topical dermal medications, the general purpose of the form itself, how it is applied, and common examples. Depending on the consistency of the medication, it will be available in jars, tubes, bottles, or sprays.

Transdermal Administration
Some topical medications are intended for systemic action and are absorbed into the circulation through the skin, called the transdermal route. Topical application and transdermal absorption of drugs such as nitroglycerin and scopolomine provide a sustained release in any easy to use form.

Respiratory Administration
The mucous membranes of the respiratory tract provide a quick, rapid, and easily accessible route for administering medications by inhalation of volatile or nonvolatile preparations. The vast expanse of alveolar surface with its adjoining rich capillary network provides for rapid absorption of drugs. Only the intravenous route will achieve a higher blood level of a drug more quickly than will the respiratory route. Respiratory inhalants are given for purposes such as to open the airway with bronchodilators and decongestants; dissolve and mobilize secretions with mucolytics; and prevent or treat allergic reactions.

Volatile inhalants may be administered for a systemic effect, such as when aromatic spirits of ammonia are used to revive a fainting person. Nonvolatile preparations can be inhaled primarily for a local action on the tracheobronchial tree through a medium that is readily inhaled, as occurs with an aerosol or the steam produced by humidifiers and vaporizers. These methods are used primarily to apply medications for local action on the tracheobronchial tree.

An aerosol is a suspension of fine particles of a liquid or powder carried in a stream of gas (usually air). For particles to enter the alveolar spaces, they must be no more than 1 to 3 microns in size. Particles between 3 and 10 microns reach the bronchi, and larger particles only reach the mouth, throat, and upper trachea before they are deposited (Nursing80 Photobook, 1980; Sorensen and Luckmann, 1979).

A nebulizer produces uniformly sized aerosol particles through a system of baffles or blades. Hand-held nebulizers are operated by manual compression or through the force exerted by inhaled air. Clients can carry them conveniently in a purse or pocket and use them quite easily to provide quick relief or prevention of allergic or asthmatic reactions.

DATA BASE

As with any medication, prior to giving a topical drug, it is important to determine that the medication order is complete, the ordered dosage form and amount appropriate for the specific person, and the available dosage form compatible with that order. A valid medication order for topical medications includes the strength of the medication, its dosage form (such as ointment, lotion, or suppository), the route by which it is to be applied, and some indication of the amount to be given. The amount may be expressed as drops of liquid, milliliters or inches of ointment, the grams of cream to be applied with a calibrated inserter, or a recommendation such as apply liberally, apply sparingly, or apply as needed to control itching. Unless otherwise specified, an order to apply eye ointment

TABLE 72-1. Common Forms of Dermal Topical Medications

DOSAGE FORM	DESCRIPTION AND PURPOSE	ADMINISTRATION GUIDELINES
Powder	Finely divided solid inert substance; reduces maceration and moisture. Examples: Talcum powder, cornstarch, neosporin powder.	Have client turn head away. To apply near or on face, have client cover nostrils and exhale while applying. Do not apply to raw, denuded areas as powders can foster bacterial and fungal growth.
Lotion	Liquid suspension or dispersion of drugs; leaves a layer of powder that protects the skin. Examples: Calamine lotion, U.S.P.; flurandrenolide (Cordran) lotion.	Shake bottle vigorously prior to each use. Apply by patting, since rubbing can cause further irritation.
Cream	Emulsion of oil and water in a semisolid form; lubricates and prevents water loss. Examples: Flurandrenolide (Cordran) cream; betamethasone (Valisone) cream; fluocinonide (Lidex) cream.	Apply even, thin layer and rub in well.
Ointment	Mixture of drug with a semisolid base such as petrolatum and lanolin in a soft spreadable consistency; provides prolonged contact of the medication. Examples: Zinc oxide ointment, U.S.P.; triamcinolone acetonide (Kenalog) ointment, Desitin ointment.	Apply thin film and rub in well. Avoid applying to hairy areas, as ointments can clog hair follicles and cause folliculitis. Little or no rubbing is required, since in most cases the ointment itself is not significantly absorbed into the skin.
Paste	Thick, stiff mixture of ointment and powdered drugs that do not melt at body temperature. Repels moisture, absorbs secretions, and retains drugs in prolonged direct contact with the skin. Less greasy than ointments. Example: Zinc oxide paste, U.S.P.	Spread even coat with tongue depressor or gloved fingers. Cover with a cloth to protect the clothing or with plastic to retain the paste on the skin.
Gel	Semisolid gelatinous colloidal aqueous suspension of drug. Used where an occlusive effect is not desired. Example: Lidocaine (Xylocaine) gel	Apply even coating. Appropriate for hairy areas. May be drying to the skin.
Sprays and Aerosols	Liquid drug preparation dispersed in droplet form as it is applied to the skin or mucous membranes through the use of compressed gas or air. Very finely divided particles are known as an aerosol, which gives a more uniform application. Examples: Benzocaine (Americaine, Dermoplast spray); betamethasone (Diprosone) spray; Chloraseptic throat spray.	Read instructions on can to determine if product needs to be shaken before application and to determine the proper distance to use so as to get the right level of application, usually 6 to 12 inches. Hold container upright and direct toward the area. When spraying near the face, have the client turn the head away, hold the nose shut, or exhale.

generally means placing a ribbon of ointment along most of the conjunctiva inside the lower lid.

Client History and Recorded Data

The physician's order and the nursing-care plan indicate whether clean or aseptic technique is to be used to apply the medication. If this information is not available, the nurse makes that decision based on his or her own knowledge of the area to be treated, the medication being applied, and the potential for introducing contaminants to the area. The client's diagnosis, therapeutic plan, progress, and prognosis provide information for explanations and for evaluating the condition of the area to which the medication is being applied. The health record contains a description of the color, odor, and other characteristics of the exudate, secretions, or discharges from the body orifice or surface being medicated. These data provide a basis from which to evaluate the therapeutic effectiveness of the medication or any untoward reactions.

In addition to recorded data, the nurse also elicits data directly from the client and family; for example, subjective reports of discomfort such as itching, burning, pain, or nasal congestion, as well as objective observations of behaviors such as blinking, squinting, frowning, pulling the ears, rubbing, or scratching. These data are collected as a baseline prior to beginning topical therapy and again at regular intervals during the treatment process to evaluate effectiveness.

Physical Appraisal Skills

Inspection. Whenever topical medications are to be applied to skin or mucous membranes, the area is always inspected for redness, swelling, irritated areas, open lesions, and the presence of any unusual discharge, exudate, or drainage.

Ear. Inspection is used to determine the status of the pinna and the lining of the external auditory canal, and the color and amount of cerumen in the canal. Observations of the client may reveal he or she is rubbing or tugging at the ear because of discomfort and itching.

Eye. Inspection will determine the status of the conjunctiva, sclera, or eyelids. Observations of the client may reveal rubbing of the eyes because of itching, or frowning, squinting, and blinking because of irritation, altered vision, or photophobia.

Nose. Inspection reveals the status of the external nose. A flashlight is used to inspect the external nares for crusts, clots, discharge, or obstruction of any kind. Observations of the client may reveal mouth-breathing, sniffing, or blowing of the nose.

Mouth. The nurse uses inspection to examine the tongue and cheeks for cleanliness and freedom from debris prior to inserting buccal or sublingual tablets.

Anal Area. The nurse inspects the anal area for the presence of external hemorrhoids or fissures that may cause pain when a suppository is inserted, or for incontinent feces that must be cleansed before insertion of the suppository.

Vaginal Area. The nurse inspects the vaginal and perineal area for the presence of redness, irritation, or discharge prior to inserting any vaginal creams or tablets.

Skin. Inspection reveals whether the skin is intact, broken, irritated, inflamed, or edematous; whether there are open, draining lesions; and the nature of any drainage or secretions.

Auscultation. The nurse uses the sense of hearing to detect nasal congestion.

Palpation. Palpation detects the edema and warmth that may occur with an infection or inflammation involving the eyelids, external ear, or other body parts.

Sense of Smell. The sense of smell will detect the presence of fecal incontinence and of some vaginal and ear discharges or suppurative (pus-forming) skin conditions.

Equipment

Topical medications are applied to the skin with *ungloved hands* or with *clean or sterile gloves,* depending on the medication and the status of the body part being treated. Pastes, because of their stiff consistency, are often applied with *tongue blades.* *Swabs* or *sponges* may be used with some medications but can be wasteful if they absorb excessive amounts of medications. *Eye droppers* and dropper bottles are used for eye and ear drops; *squeeze bottles, nebulizers,* and *spray devices* are used with mouth products and inhalation medications; a variety of *applicators* is used with vaginal and rectal suppositories and creams; and *finger cots* are used to insert rectal suppositories. Illustrations of this equipment are included later in this skill.

☐ EXECUTION

When preparing and administering topical medications, follow the guidelines for safe medication preparation and administration as discussed in Skill 71, modifying the preparation as needed for each specific topical dosage form. The method for applying topical medications varies with the site to which the medication is being applied. In general, skin surfaces should be clean and dry before applying medication. That often means removing secretions, debris, and old medication by cleansing the area with sterile saline, water, soap and water, or other agents as specified by the physician, indicated on the package label or insert, or determined by the body area being treated. Use hydrogen peroxide for cleansing only if specifically ordered by the physician. Store topical medications as indicated on the package; for example, some suppositories need to be refrigerated.

When applying topical medications, it is unacceptable practice to return the applicator to the container if it touches the client's skin because this contaminates the contents and may result in colonization of microorganisms within the container. This means the dropper should not touch the eye, ear, or nose while instilling drops; tubes of ointment or atomizer and spray tips should not be allowed to touch the orifice in which they are used; and tongue depressors or applicators used to remove pastes, creams, or liquids should not be returned to the container if they touch the client. If a dropper attached to the bottle cap inadvertently touches the client, use several alcohol swabs to cleanse the dropper, wiping toward the tip. Allow the dropper to dry before returning it to the bottle.

Although the eye, ear, nose, and throat are not private body areas, it is a courtesy to close the client's door or draw the curtains to administer medications into those orifices. Privacy is mandatory for inserting rectal and vaginal medications and for applying medication to private parts of the body.

When clients are taught how to continue using a topical medication at home, plan a return demonstration by the person who will be applying, inserting, or instilling the medication. In addition, it is advisable to teach clients correct procedures for administering medications in the eye, ear, nose, throat, and to the skin because many over-the-counter (OTC) drugs are used in these areas. For example, people often use OTC eye drops to soothe irritated eyes, nose drops or sprays to relieve congestion, ear drops to soften ear wax, and throat sprays or gargles to relieve sore throats.

ADMINISTERING TOPICAL MEDICATIONS

Administration in the Mouth

Sublingual and Buccal Tablets. Place sublingual tablets directly under the tongue and buccal tablets in

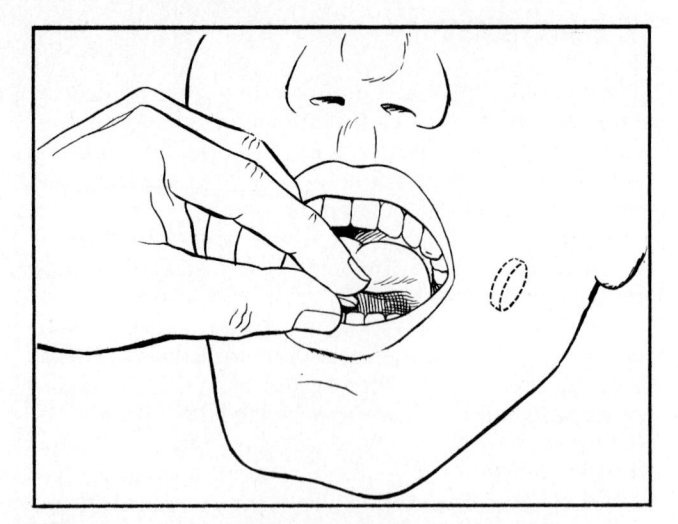

Figure 72-1. Place a sublingual tablet under the tongue. Place a buccal tablet in the cheek.

the cheek pouch adjacent to the upper molars, as shown in Figure 72-1. Ask the person to hold the tablet in place until it is absorbed and caution not to swallow or chew the medication since that would alter its effect and effectiveness. Lozenges or troches for local action on irritated throat tissues are allowed to dissolve, swallowing the medication and saliva as needed.

Sprays. When using mouth and throat sprays, place the client in a semi-Fowler's or near upright position to help prevent aspiration of the medication and for increased ease of administration. Offer a drink before administering the spray, because water is often contraindicated after throat sprays, especially anesthetic sprays that depress the gag reflex. Ask the client to open the mouth wide and say "ah." Use a flashlight and a tongue depressor to inspect the condition of the area to be treated. Clients may prefer to hold the tongue depressor themselves.

To use a spray pump, hold the nozzle just outside the client's mouth and direct the spray toward the throat; to use an atomizer, insert the tip just inside the mouth and direct it toward the back of the throat, as shown in Figure 72-2. Press the spray pump nozzle or squeeze the atomizer bulb quickly, firmly, and with enough pressure to propel the spray to the inflamed areas. Before applying the spray, instruct the client not to swallow immediately afterward so that the medication can run down the throat and coat the mucous membranes. Remain with the client until you are certain he or she will not aspirate the medication.

Mouthwashes and Gargles. To assist someone with a mouthwash or gargle, you will need the following equipment: the ordered solution, a drinking glass, emesis basin, and tissues. Warm the solution to room temperature or slightly warmer and assist the client to an upright seated or standing position. Have the client take about 30 ml (1 oz) of solution into the mouth and swish it around the mouth, over the gums, and between the teeth. Instruct the client to spit the solution into the emesis basin and repeat this procedure several times. Use tissues for wiping the mouth as needed.

Gargling is done in a similar way, except that the client tilts the head back slightly and allows the solution to run into the throat. Simultaneously, he or she exhales slowly through the mouth, creating a gargling action. Instruct the client to spit the solution into the emesis basin, unless ordered otherwise. For example, a lidocaine gargle sometimes is swallowed so it can decrease pain sensations deeper in the throat and esophagus and thus increase swallowing ease.

Some mouth and throat medications are known as swish and swallow drugs. With these drugs, the client is instructed to rinse the mouth with the medicated solution, hold it in the mouth as long as possible, and then swallow it. Examples of these drugs are the antifungal nystatin (Candex, Mycostatin) used to treat oral thrush, and viscous xylocaine, used to relieve oral discomfort. Because xylocaine interferes with swallowing, do not give food for an hour after this medication.

Administration through the Nasal Route

When inserting drops into the nose, the degree of head tilt will determine whether the medication will remain in the nasal cavity, enter the sinuses, or run wastefully

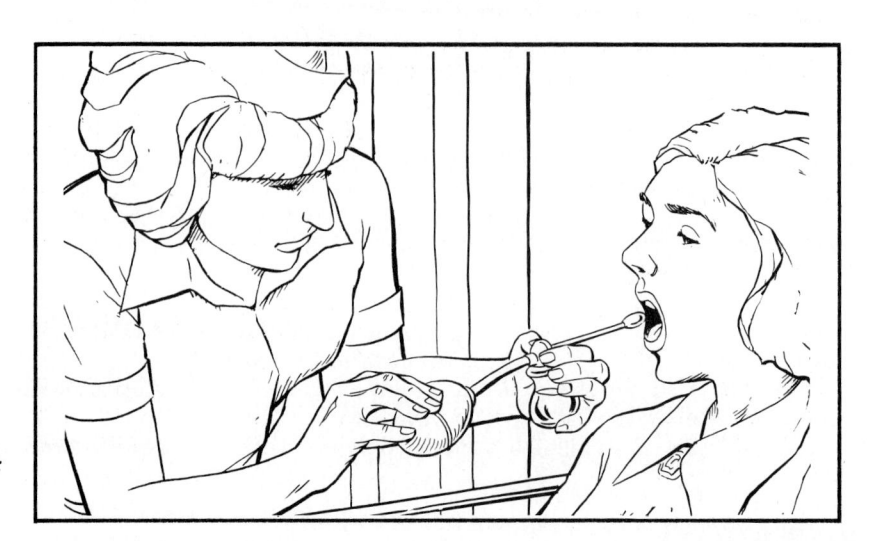

Figure 72-2. Topical application to the throat: place the atomizer tip just inside the client's mouth.

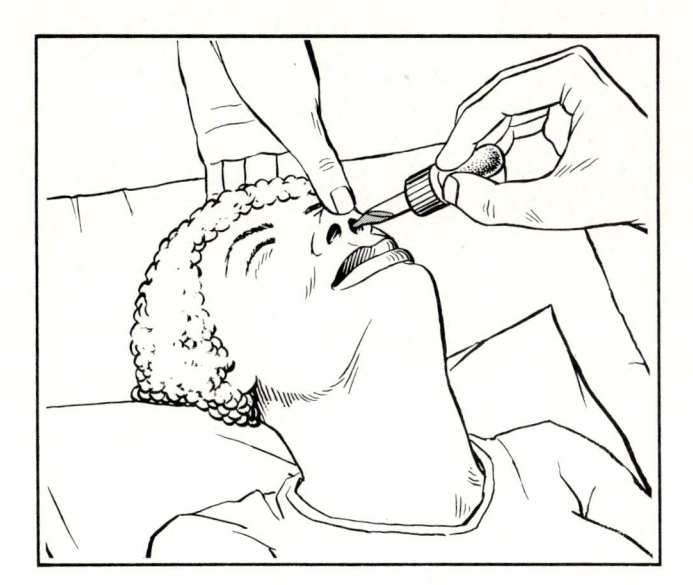

Figure 72-3. Administer drops into the nasal cavity. Position the client so the drops can flow toward the posterior nasal turbinates.

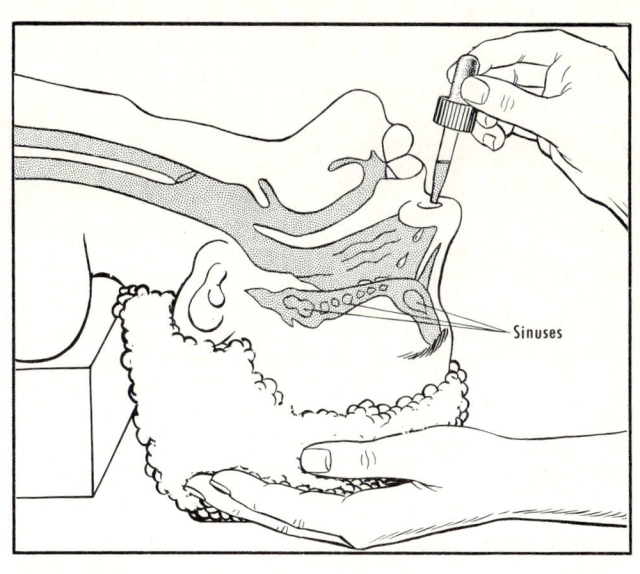

Figure 72-4. Administer drops into the sinuses. Position the client so the drops flow downward into the sphenoid and ethmoid sinuses.

down the throat, as occurs if the appropriate positions are not used.

To administer nose drops to an adult with ordinary nasal congestion, place him or her in a nearly upright position with a pillow behind the shoulders and neck to tilt the head backward until the columella nasi (anterior and external portion of the nasal septum) is as nearly vertical as possible, as shown in Figure 72-3. If the client cannot assume this position, place a pillow or folded bath blanket under the shoulders to achieve the same nasal angle. Draw enough medication into the dropper for one administration to both nostrils, to avoid returning the dropper to the bottle for more medication for the second nostril. Inform clients that they may taste the medication after it is instilled and ask them to mouth breathe while you instill the drops. This action helps suppress the urge to sniff and propel the medication up into the sinuses. For increased visibility of the nasal openings, raise the tip of the nose with the thumb of your nondominant hand. Direct the drops toward the center or upper part of the nasal cavity, rather than toward the nasal floor, as that helps avoid medication running down the throat.

Generally, it is helpful to insert 3 or 4 drops in each nostril and wait 2 to 4 minutes while the client remains in position so that the medication can begin to clear the anterior nasal turbinates. Then insert 3 or 4 more drops in each nostril to reach the posterior portions of the turbinates. It is not usually necessary to keep the head tilted backward to keep the drops in this portion of the nose, but you should suggest that the client not blow the nose for about 10 minutes to allow the medication to remain in contact with the nasal tissues.

To administer medicated drops to the sinuses, position the client with the neck hyperextended over the edge of the bed so that the columella nasi is horizontal, as shown in Figure 72-4. Support the head with one hand and instill 3 to 4 drops into each nostril, wait 2 or 3 minutes if the client is able to tolerate the position, and then instill 3 or 4 more drops. Elderly persons may not be able to maintain this position long enough to wait for the second administration.

To administer a nasal spray medication with a nasal atomizer, tilt the client's head back as for instilling nose drops. Insert the atomizer tip 1 cm (3/8 in) into the naris and squeeze quickly and firmly one time, using enough force to coat the inside of the nostrils with a spray. Too much force will cause the medication to enter the sinuses and cause headaches. Keep the head tilted back for 5 minutes and avoid blowing the nose, as for nose drops. Repeat 1 time after 3 or 4 minutes, as needed.

☐ SKILL SEQUENCE

INSTILLING NASAL DROPS

Step	Rationale
1. Check medication orders on medication page, kardex, computer printout, or medicine card, according to agency policy.	System of checks helps detect human errors in ordering and transcribing medication orders.

(continued)

INSTILLING NASAL DROPS (Cont.)

Step	Rationale
2. Review own knowledge of drug, using drug cards and other drug reference sources.	Reinforces knowledge about the drugs.
3. Wash hands.	Avoids transfer of microorganisms.
4. Select correct unit-dose package or medication container, compare label with medication order (SAFETY CHECK 1), and determine appropriate amount to be given. (Determine that medication is labeled for nasal use.)	Guards against errors in administration. Ensures correct dosage form is administered.
5. Place medication on medicine cart or tray with client's other medications and again compare dosage and label with medication order (SAFETY CHECK 2).	Guards against errors in administration.
6. Gather additional equipment as needed.	Time-efficient nursing action.
7. Identify client by comparing room, bed number, and client's name (identification band and verbal response) with medication order.	Guards against errors in administration.
8. At client's bedside, compare container or unit-dose package with medication order before administering medication (SAFETY CHECK 3).	Guards against errors in administration.
9. Explain procedure to client.	Increases ability to cooperate and assist with procedure and decreases apprehension.
10. Close door or draw curtains.	Provides privacy.
11. Raise bed to comfortable working height.	Allows for correct body mechanics and promotes nurse safety.
12. Unless contraindicated, ask client to blow the nose; cleanse crusts from external nares with tissues or applicators as needed.	Usually removes old crusts, debris, secretions.
13. To administer drops into nasal cavity: a. Position client in near-upright or semi-Fowler's position, with a pillow behind shoulders, allowing neck to hyperextend so columella nasi are nearly vertical. (NOTE: if this position is contraindicated, place a pillow under the shoulders while client is flat, and allow the head to tilt backward at a similar angle.)	Allows medication to flow against upper surface of nasal cavity; avoids swallowing medication or having it enter sinuses.
b. Withdraw enough medication into dropper for both nostrils.	Avoids having to return dropper to bottle during administration of drops.
c. Ask client to breathe through the mouth.	Avoids having client sniff medication into sinuses.
d. Elevate tip of client's nose with your thumb and insert dropper 1 cm (1/3 in) inside naris without touching it.	Opens the nostril for easier insertion of dropper. Touching nares contaminates dropper and medication when dropper is returned to medication.
e. Hold dropper on a horizontal plane and direct flow of medication toward upper center back of nasal cavity; insert 3 or 4 drops, or amount ordered.	Directs medication toward nasal conchae, rather than down client's throat. Provides adequate amount for decongestion effect on anterior tissues.
f. Ask client to remain in position for 2 to 4 minutes if condition permits; instill 3 to 4 more drops, and allow client to assume a position of comfort. Provide tissues.	Allows time for medication to shrink anterior nasal tissues so additional medication can reach posterior tissues. Nasal drainage often occurs.
14. To insert drops into sinuses: a. Withdraw enough medication into dropper for both nostrils.	Avoids having to return dropper to bottle during administration of drops.
b. Position client with the neck hyperextended over edge of the bed, supporting the head with your nondominant hand.	Allows medication to reach sinuses through gravity. Support makes position more tolerable.
c. Insert 3 or 4 drops; wait 2 or 3 minutes; insert 3 or 4 more drops.	Allows for more complete entry of medication into sinuses.
d. Return client to position of comfort and safety.	Promotes comfort and safety.
15. Document administration of nose drops on medication record form, in health record, or in computer. Record character of nasal discharge, degree of nasal congestion, and client's reaction to procedure in nurses' notes.	Fulfills nurse accountability and provides ongoing data base.

Administration into the Ear

Administration of ear medication is considered a clean procedure unless the health record indicates the tympanic membrane is damaged or torn. If there is an opening between the outer and middle ear, aseptic technique must be used to prevent entry of contaminants into the middle and inner ear. If there is any question about whether the tympanic membrane is intact, use sterile solutions and aseptic technique. Warm ear drops to body temperature prior to instilling them into the ear, since cold drops can stimulate the inner ear vestibular apparatus and cause discomfort and

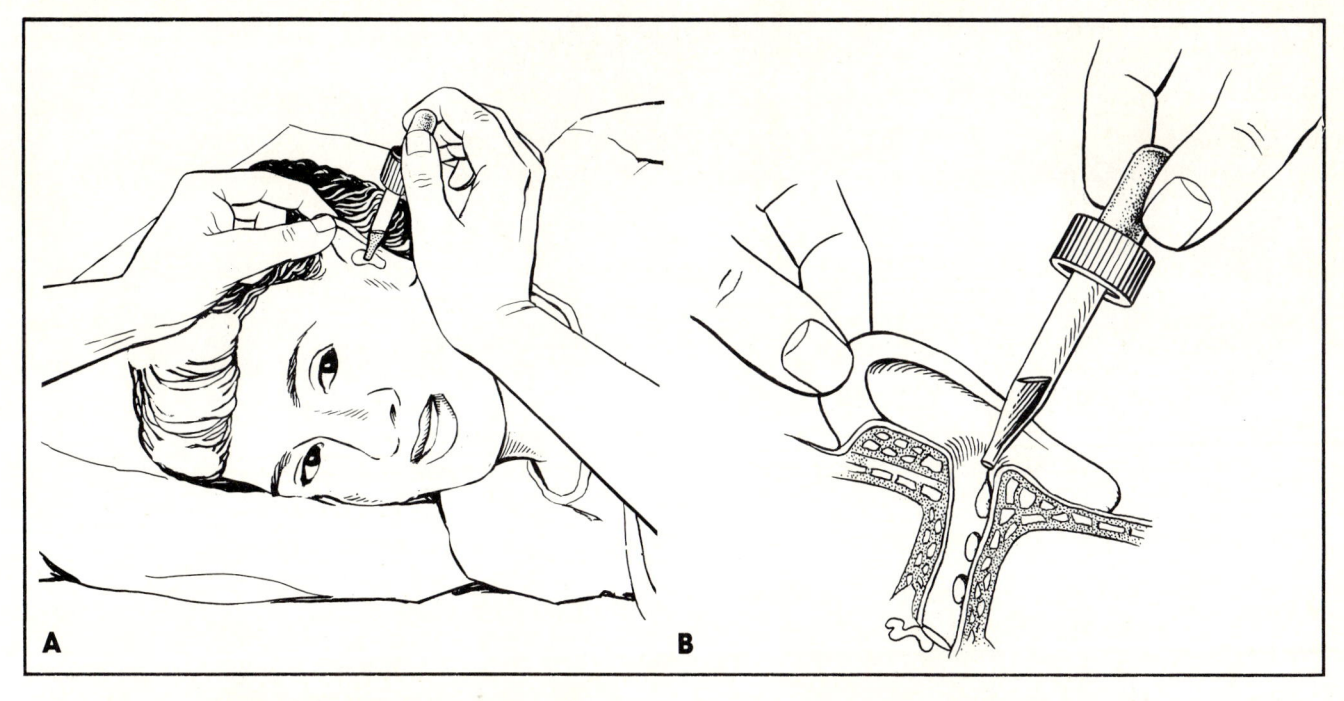

Figure 72–5. Instill drops into the external ear canal. **A** Rest both hands on the client's head to stabilize it. Pull the adult ear upward and backward to straighten the external auditory canal. **B.** Insert drops toward the side of the canal.

vertigo. Warm the drops by holding or rolling the bottle in your hands for a few minutes.

Position the client in a side-lying position on a pillow, so that the ear to be treated is exposed. Stand so your dominant hand is toward the client's chin, since this position makes it possible to instill medication in both ears without repositioning yourself. After drawing up the desired amount of medication, rest your nondominant hand on the head near the client's ear and rest the side of your dominant hand on the jaw. These positions stabilize both the client's head and your hands, thus avoiding injury or contamination of the dropper in the event that the client moves unexpectedly or your hand is unsteady. Straighten the external auditory canal by pulling on the pinna with the nondominant hand. For adults, pull the pinna upward and backward, as shown in Figure 72–5A; for a child under three, pull downward and backward. Direct the medication toward the ear canal (Fig. 72–5B) since direct application on the tympanic membrane can cause discomfort.

After instilling the medication, press on the tragus three or four times with a gentle pumping action to help disperse the medication throughout the canal and toward the tympanic membrane. Conscious clients will be able to tell you when the medication reaches the membrane. Allow the person to remain in position for about 3 minutes before repositioning and instillation of drops in the second ear, if that is needed. If desired, a small dry absorbent ball may be placed loosely in the canal opening for about 30 minutes to absorb excess drainage.

Remember that an ear infection often causes the pinna and tragus to be extremely painful, even if it is not visibly swollen or inflamed. Be very gentle when manipulating the ear.

☐ SKILL SEQUENCE

ADMINISTERING EAR MEDICATIONS

Step	Rationale
1. Repeat Skill Sequence, "Instilling Nasal Drops," steps 1 to 11. Determine that medication is labeled "otic," "oto-," or for use in the ear.	Ensures correct dosage form is administered.
2. Warm medication to body temperature by holding bottle in your hand for 2 minutes.	Cold ear drops can cause discomfort and vertigo.
3. Cleanse debris, secretions, and old medication from pinna and external auditory canal opening.	Preparatory to applying new medication.

(continued)

ADMINISTERING EAR MEDICATIONS

Step	Rationale
4. Wash hands.	Avoids transfer of microorganisms.
5. Position client in flat, side-lying position with the head on a pillow, exposing ear being treated.	Provides easy access to ear.
6. Withdraw desired amount of medication into dropper and hold it in dominant hand.	Provides correct dosage.
7. Position yourself so your dominant hand is toward client's feet.	
8. Rest your nondominant hand on client's head and grasp upper 2/3 of pinna and pull upward and backward. (For children under 3, pull downward and backward.) Rest the side of dominant hand on client's lower jaw.	Stabilizes client's head. Straightens adult external auditory canal. Straightens child's external auditory canal. Stabilizes nurse's hand and client's head, avoiding accidental injury or contamination of dropper.
9. Instill desired number of drops; hold ear in position and press gently on tragus 3 or 4 times in a pumping action until client reports feeling ear drops on tympanic membrane.	Promotes adequate distribution of medication throughout external auditory canal.
10. Encourage client to remain on side for 3 or 4 minutes. If desired, place a small dry absorbent ball in opening of external auditory canal for 30 minutes.	Retains medication in ear. Helps absorb excess medication or drainage.
11. Reposition client and repeat procedure with other ear as indicated.	Completes administration process.
12. Return client to position of comfort and safety.	Promotes client comfort and safety.
13. Document medication administration on medication record form, in health record, or in computer. Record status of ear, nature and extent of discharge, and client's reaction to medication procedure in nurses' notes.	Fulfills nurse accountability and provides ongoing data base.

Administration into the Eye

Always use sterile equipment and surgical aseptic technique to administer medications into the eyes because eye tissues are quite sensitive and eyesight is too valuable to risk unnecessary infection. Many ophthalmologists require that a separate tube of ointment or bottle of drops be used for each eye, thus avoiding any possibility of cross-contamination such as a transfer of microorganisms from an infected to an uninfected eye. Wash your hands very thoroughly before beginning the procedure. Use sterile saline and absorbent balls or gauze squares to cleanse secretions and residual medication from the eyelids and lashes. To avoid any possible problems, always use separate equipment, medica-

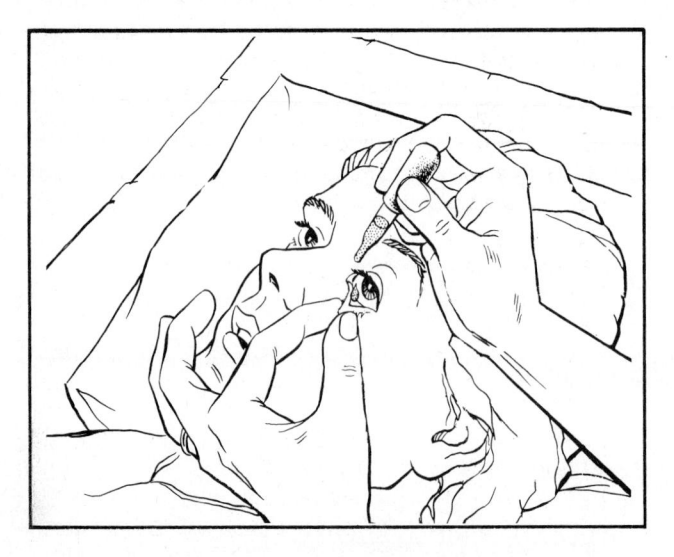

Figure 72-6. Instill eye drops into the small pouch created by pinching the tissues beneath the eye and pulling them outward.

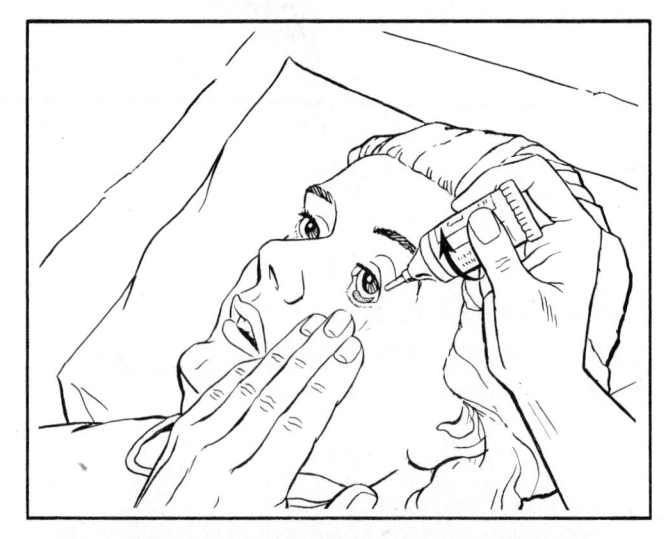

Figure 72-7. Insert eye ointment along the conjunctival surface from the inner canthus outward. Twist tube toward head and upward to disconnect ointment strip.

tion, and tissues for each eye, and discard used items promptly. As with ear drops, warm the bottle of ophthalmic drops or tube of ointment to body temperature. Explain to the client that his or her vision will be blurred temporarily by the ointment, but that it will clear spontaneously.

To instill eye drops, position the client comfortably in a semi-Fowler's position, with the head turned slightly so the eye being treated is somewhat lower than the other eye. Ask the client to look upward. Use the nondominant hand to pinch the skin gently below the lower lid and pull it outward to create a small pouch. Hold the hand and dropper off to one side of the eye, as this action decreases the client's blink reaction. Place one or two drops of medication into the center of the pouch, as shown in Figure 72-6. More than that amount is wasteful because it will overflow when the eye is closed. Hold the lower lid in place for a few seconds while the drop settles, raise the lower lid up toward the eye, and then release it. Next, have the client close the eye slowly, without blinking or squeezing; apply gentle pressure over the inner canthus for two minutes. This action increases contact time of the medication with the ocular tissues and delays the drug's overflow into the lacrimal duct, thus increasing the drug's effectiveness and decreasing the potential for systemic absorption and occurrence of side effects.

Wipe the excess medication away with a clean tissue, moving from the inner canthus outward; discard tissues promptly.

To administer an eye ointment, position the client as above and have the client look upward. Remove the cap from the tube of eye ointment, hold it upside down vertically, and squeeze a small amount of ointment onto a sterile gauze square or into a trash bag without touching the edges of the bag, thus insuring that the ointment present at the tube opening is sterile.

Place two or three fingers of the nondominant hand on the skin beneath the eyelid and pull downward, gently and firmly with the fingers; expose the conjunctival surface inside the lower eyelid. Begin at the inner canthus and squeeze a ribbon of ointment into the conjunctival space inside the lid, as you direct the ointment across the exposed conjunctival surface. As you approach the outer canthus, stop squeezing the tube and simultaneously rotate the tube inward toward the eye and lift the tube upward, as shown in Figure 72-7. This action will usually disconnect the ribbon of ointment from the tube. After inserting the ointment, release the eyelid and ask the client to close the eye gently to avoid squeezing the medication out of the eye. Wipe the excess medication from the lids and lashes in the same way as for eye drops.

☐ SKILL SEQUENCE

ADMINISTERING EYE MEDICATIONS

Step	Rationale
1. Repeat Skill Sequence, "Instilling Nasal Drops," steps 1 to 11. (Determine that medication is labeled "ophthalmic" or for use in the eyes.)	Ensures correct dosage form is administered.
2. Warm eye drops or ointment to body temperature by holding in your hand for 2 minutes.	Decreases sensitivity of eye to medication.
3. Cleanse eyelids with sterile saline and absorbent balls or gauze squares to remove secretions and old medications, wiping from inner canthus outward.	Prepares eye for administration of current medication. Avoids introducing debris and microorganisms into lacrimal duct at inner canthus.
4. Wash hands.	Avoids transfer of microorganisms.
5. Position client on the back so that eye being treated is slightly lower than other eye.	Prevents transfer of microorganisms to other eye.
6. Withdraw correct amount of medication into dropper.	Ensures correct dosage.
7. Hold tube vertically and discard first drop of ointment.	Ensures sterility of ointment at tube opening.
8. Position yourself so your dominant hand is toward top of client's head.	Convenient position for inserting medication.
9. Rest the side of your dominant hand on client's forehead and hold dropper, squeeze bottle or ointment tube held vertically between thumb and index finger.	Stabilizes nurse's hand and client's head, avoiding accidental injury or contamination.
10. Ask client to look upward.	Helps open the eye and expose conjunctival sac; helps avoid accidentally dropping medication directly on cornea.

11. To administer eye drops:
  a. With nondominant hand, gently pinch skin beneath eyes and pull outward, forming a small pouch.
  b. Instill only desired number of drops.
	Creates a space in which to drop the medication.
	
	Avoids wasting medication by overflowing.

(continued)

ADMINISTERING EYE MEDICATIONS (Cont.)

Step	Rationale

12. To administer eye ointment:
   a. Place three fingers of nondominant hand beneath eyelid and pull downward gently but firmly.
   b. Hold tube vertically and discard first drop of ointment.
   c. Beginning at inner canthus, place a ribbon of ointment along conjunctiva. As you near outer canthus, rotate tube toward the head and simultaneously lift it upward.
	Exposes entire length of lower conjunctival sac.
	
	Ensures sterility of ointment being inserted.
	Follows principle of working outward from inner canthus. Disconnects ointment ribbon from tube.

13. Ask client to close eye gently and avoid squeezing eyes shut tightly. Allow eyes to remain closed for 2 to 3 minutes. Wipe excess medication with absorbent ball, gauze sponge, or tissues, and discard promptly in an impervious trash container.	Avoids squeezing medication out of eye. Allows medication to spread over entire eye. Comfort and hygienic measure; decreases amount of later crusting. Safe disposal of contaminated items.
14. Repeat procedure for other eye as needed. Use a separate tube or bottle of medication for each eye.	Completes administration procedure. Avoids accidental transfer of microorganisms from one eye to the other.
15. Return client to position of comfort and safety.	Promotes client comfort and safety.
16. Record medication administration on medication record form, in health record, or in computer. Record status of eye and eyelids, character of drainage, and client's reaction in nurses' notes.	Fulfills nurse accountability and provides ongoing data base.

Eye Irrigations. To irrigate the eye, use sterile saline or an ordered medicated solution and a sterile irrigation set such as is used to irrigate urinary catheters (Skill 60). Warm the solution to body temperature by placing a 250-ml solution container in a pan of hot tap water for 10 to 15 minutes. If large amounts of solution are needed, a sterile intravenous infusion container and equipment can be used.

Position the client on his or her side with the head near the edge of the pillow. Turn the head so the eye being irrigated is nearest the bed. Use a moisture-resistant drape or bath towel to protect clothing, pillow, and linen and place an emesis basin so it will contain the returns. Use the thumb and forefinger of the nondominant hand to hold the eyelids open, as shown in Figure 72-8. Direct the stream of liquid downward across the eye from the inner canthus toward the outer canthus, rather than directly toward the cornea. Avoid contaminating the syringe or tubing tip during the procedure. When finished with the irrigation, dry the excess fluid from around the eye with absorbent balls, gauze squares, or tissues.

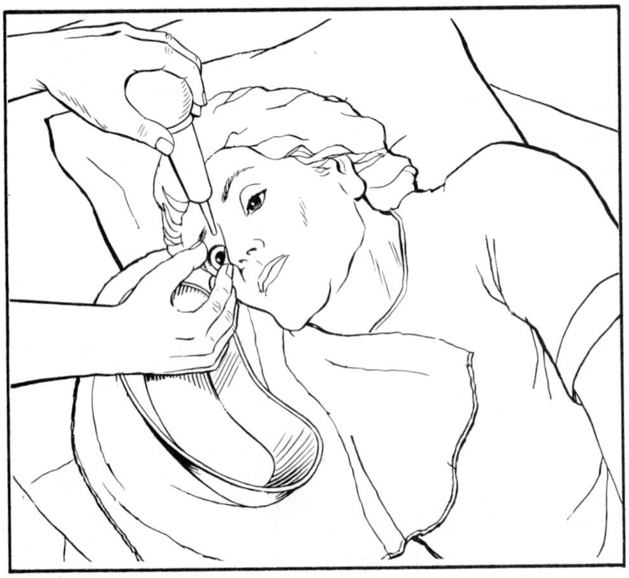

Patching the Eye. Sometimes the physician orders an eye patch to be applied after instilling ophthalmic drops or ointment, or after an irrigation. Use specially designed sterile oval eye pads for this purpose. After washing your hands, ask the client to close the eye. Place a sufficient number of oval pads over the eye to fill the orbital cavity and keep the eyelid from opening (Fig. 72-9A). Anchor the pads in place with two or three strips of nonallergenic silk or paper tape as shown in Figure 72-9B. For added protection, sometimes a lightweight oval plastic or metal shield (Fig. 72-9C) is placed over the pads before anchoring with tape, or a black eye patch is added over the tape.

Vaginal Administration

You will need the following equipment to instill vaginal medications: the specified vaginal medication, a sterile or clean applicator (if available with the medication), sterile gloves, water-soluble lubricant, a gauze sponge or clean paper towel, a bed-protector pad, cleansing materials for perineal care, and a bedpan as needed for perineal care.

Position the client in a dorsal recumbent position as for a urinary catheterization and drape with a sheet or bath blanket to provide privacy (Skill 60). Before

Figure 72-8. Eye irrigation (left-handed nurse). Position client on side. Direct irrigant downward and across the eye.

877

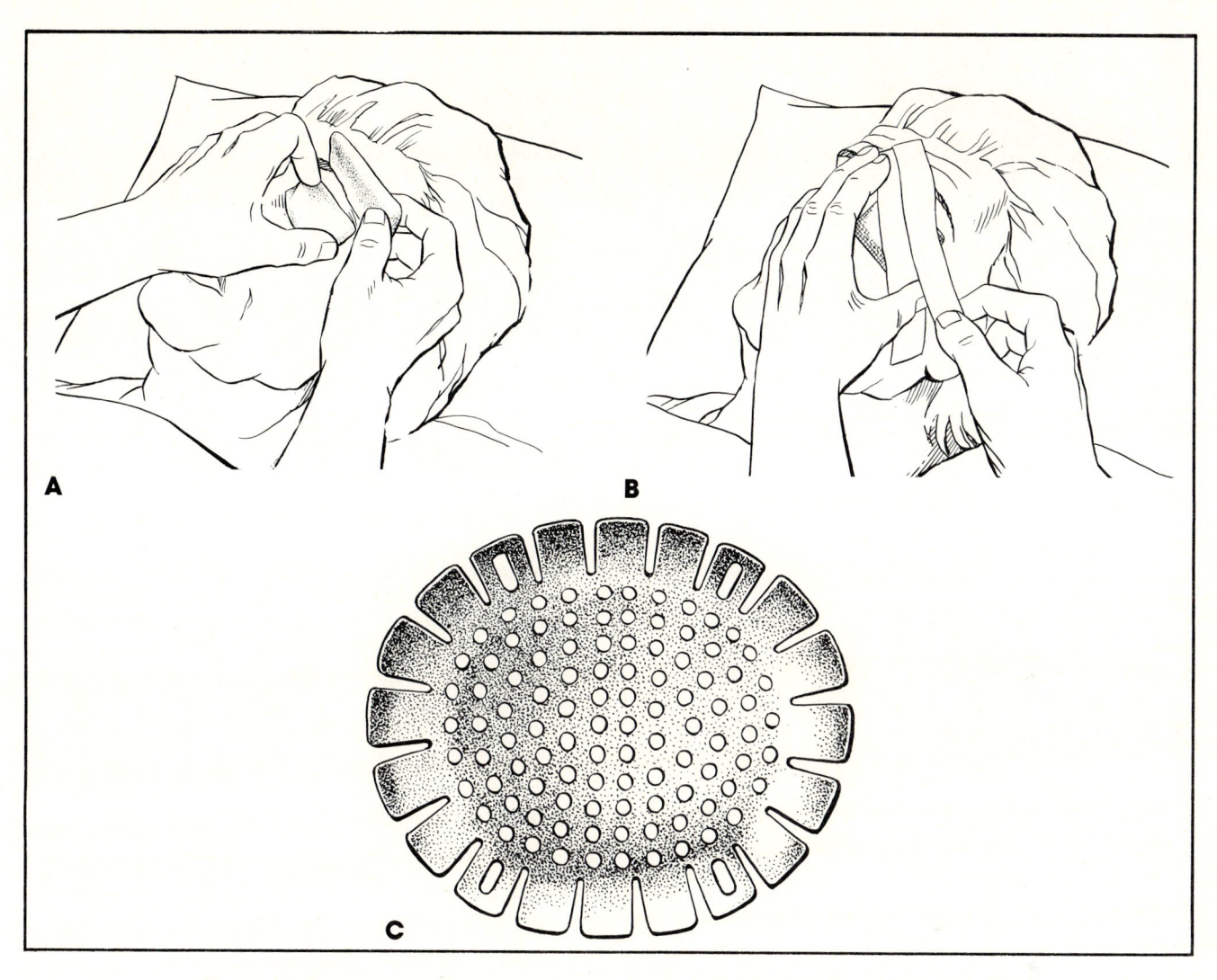

Figure 72–9. **A.** Applying an eye patch. Place gauze pads over the eye to fill the orbital cavity. **B.** Secure with nonallergenic tape. Place tape at an angle from the forehead to the jaw. **C.** Metal eye shield, used to provide increased protection.

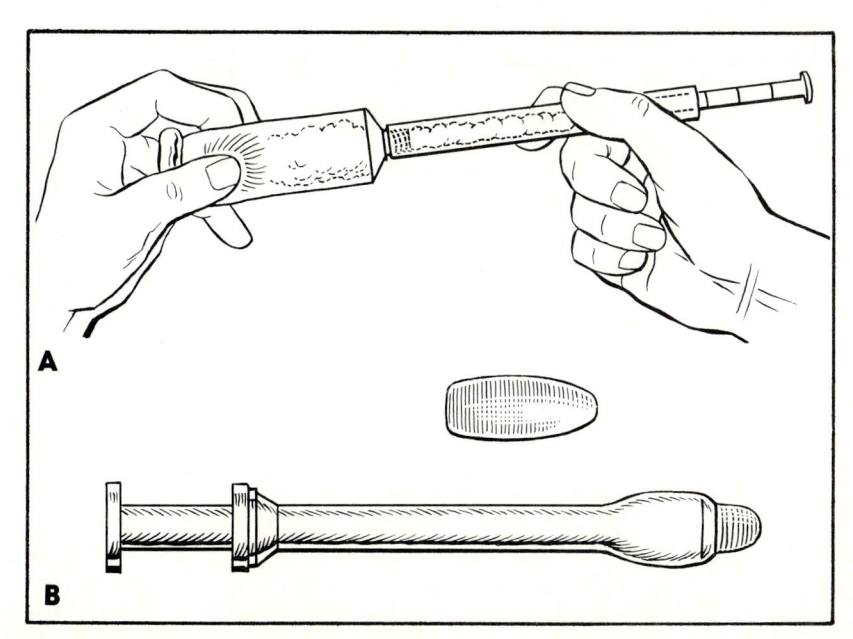

Figure 72–10. Inserting vaginal medications. **A.** Squeeze ointment from the tube into calibrated applicator, or **B.** Place vaginal tablet in applicator.

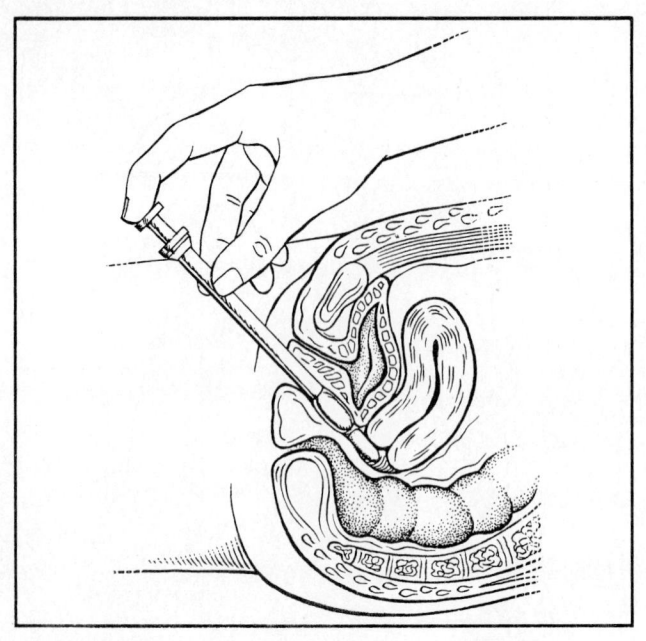

Figure 72-10. C. Insert applicator 5 to 7.5 cm (2 to 3 in) into the vagina. Depress applicator plunger to release tablet or ointment into the vaginal vault.

inserting the medication, cleanse the perineal area to remove secretions, drainage, or old medication. When possible, plan to insert vaginal medications after the client completes her personal hygiene care, as this will decrease the need for perineal care prior to inserting the medication. If this is done, be sure to make observations of the perineal area and its drainage at other times.

Ointments, gels, and creams must be inserted with an applicator. Tablets and suppositories can be inserted with specially designed inserters or with a lubricated and gloved finger tip. Although the vagina is not a sterile area and in health is self-cleansing, use sterile gloves to avoid introducing any environmental contaminants. Since the vagina has no sphincter, ask the client to remain flat for at least 30 minutes to allow the medication to disperse throughout the vagina. Suggest that she wear some type of sanitary protection to avoid staining her clothing or the bed linen. Some clients may prefer to insert the medication in the vagina themselves, which may be appropriate, providing they are taught to and can follow instructions. Figure 72-10 shows insertion of vaginal medications.

☐ SKILL SEQUENCE

ADMINISTERING VAGINAL MEDICATIONS

Step	Rationale
1. Repeat Skill Sequence, "Instilling Nasal Drops," steps 1 to 11. (Determine that medication is labeled for vaginal use.)	Ensures correct dosage form is administered.
2. Position client in a dorsal recumbent position as for urinary catheterization (Skill 60).	Provides access to vaginal area and protects client's privacy.
3. Drape with a bath blanket or sheet for privacy.	
4. Place protective bed pad under client's buttocks.	Protects bed linen.
5. Inspect and cleanse perineal area, using bedpan as needed.	Gathers baseline data; removes secretions, drainage, and old medication.
6. Don sterile gloves.	Minimizes risk of introducing contaminants.
7. Place water-soluble lubricant on gauze sponge or clean paper towel and lubricate applicator tip (if one is to be used).	Allows easier insertion.
8. Use nondominant hand to separate labia.	Provides access to vaginal orifice.
9. Using dominant hand, insert the applicator about 5 to 7.5 cm (2 to 3 in) into vagina, directing it toward sacrum. Push plunger in all the way. (NOTE: If no applicator is available with medication, place tablet or suppository on tip of a lubricated gloved index finger. Curl other fingers into the palm of the hand and insert medication as far as you can comfortably reach.)	Follows anatomic direction of vagina. Releases the suppository or insert; instills the cream, gel, or ointment into vaginal vault.
10. Remove applicator; discard if disposable; if reusable, wash with soap and warm water, rinse and return to container.	Appropriate care of equipment.
11. Remove gloves and discard them in a trash container.	Contains any contamination.
12. Request that client remain in a lying-down position for 30 minutes. Apply a perineal pad or small adhesive-backed underwear liner.	Since vagina has no sphincter, pad absorbs medication drainage and protects clothing from staining.

(continued)

Step	Rationale
13. Wash hands.	Avoids transfer of microorganisms.
14. Return client to a position of comfort and safety.	Promotes comfort and safety.
15. Record medication administration on medication record form, in health record, or in computer. Record character of vaginal drainage, status of perineal area, and client's reaction in nurses' notes.	Fulfills nurse accountability; provides ongoing data base.

Rectal Administration

You will need the following equipment to insert a suppository into the rectum: the rectal suppository, a clean examination glove or finger cot, water-soluble lubricant, and a protective bed pad. If the suppository is warm and soft, it will be difficult to insert and may adhere to the wrapper. It can be firmed up quite readily by holding it under cold running water or placing it in the refrigerator for a few minutes. If the suppository is not self-lubricated or if the client has external hemorrhoids, fissures, or has had recent rectal surgery, lubricate the tapered tip with a water-soluble lubricant. Never cut a suppository to administer a partial dose, such as to use an adult suppository for a child's dosage. There is no guarantee that the dosage is distributed evenly throughout the suppository, and an inaccurate dosage can result.

Position the client as for a large-volume cleansing enema (Skill 58), wear a clean examination glove or finger cot, and insert the suppository about 7.5 cm (3 in) into the anal canal, until it is past the internal sphincter, as shown in Figure 72–11. Assist the client to relax in a similar way as for an enema. Since the insertion procedure stimulates the defecation reflex, apply pressure after you remove your finger by pressing the buttocks together or compressing the anus with a pad of gauze or tissues. Ask the client to remain lying down for about 20 minutes so the suppository can be absorbed systemically or achieve its local action. Explaining the purpose for the suppository helps clients accept this limitation. Place a protective bed pad under the client's buttocks if the suppository is given to stimulate bowel evacuation or if there is a history of rectal incontinence. If the client is able and prefers to do so, allow him or her to insert the suppository after giving instructions about the procedure.

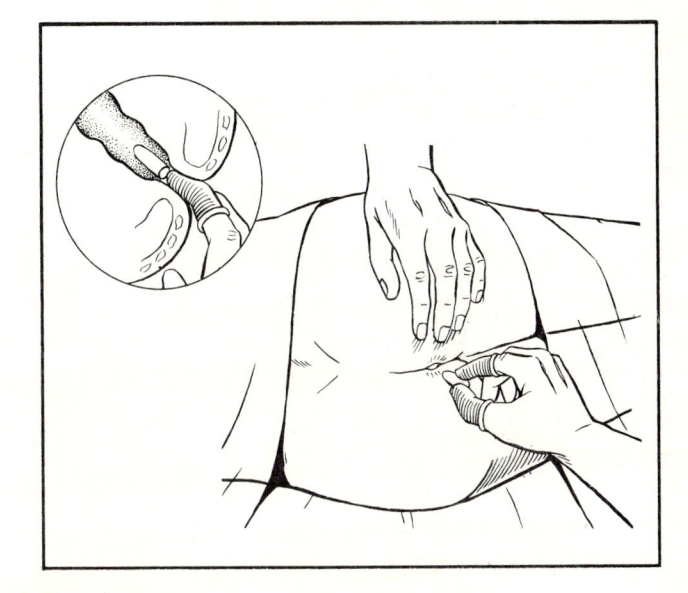

Figure 72–11. With a gloved finger or finger cot, insert a suppository into the rectum until it is past the internal sphincter.

☐ SKILL SEQUENCE

INSERTING A RECTAL SUPPOSITORY

Step	Rationale
1. Repeat Skill Sequence, "Instilling Nasal Drops," steps 1 to 11. (Determine that medication is labeled for rectal use.)	Ensures correct dosage form of medication is administered.
2. Position client on right or left side with upper leg drawn up, as for a large-volume cleansing enema (Skill 58). Drape with sheet or bath blanket.	Preparatory for inserting a suppository. Provides for privacy and increases psychological comfort.
3. Don a clean examination glove on dominant hand, or place a finger cot on that index finger.	Protects hand from direct contact with rectum.

(continued)

INSERTING A RECTAL SUPPOSITORY (Cont.)

Step	Rationale
4. Lubricate tapered end of suppository with a water-soluble lubricant as needed.	Provides for easier insertion and decreases client discomfort.
5. Use nondominant hand to separate buttocks and expose anus.	Avoids discomfort or pain associated with blind entry, especially if client has rectal problems.
6. Have client take a deep breath, touch anus lightly with suppository, and wait briefly.	Relaxes external anal sphincter. Reflex sphincter contraction from being touched is followed by relaxation.
7. Insert suppository and direct it along posterior rectal wall toward umbilicus, as with an enema tube. Insert suppository about 7.5 cm (3 in), until it passes the internal sphincter. Do not insert into a fecal mass.	Follows anatomic direction of anal canal. Aids in retaining suppository. Retards absorption and delays drug action.
8. Press buttocks together with hands or hold a pad of gauze or tissues over the anus for a few minutes.	Counteracts reflex defecation impulse caused by insertion procedure.
9. Clean excess lubricant from anal area; ask client to retain suppository for at least 20 minutes.	Comfort and hygienic measure. Allows time for systemic absorption or local action.
10. Remove and discard glove or finger cot.	Contains contamination.
11. Wash hands.	Avoids transfer of microorganisms.
12. Document medication administration on medication record form, in health record, or in computer. Record data about status of anal area and client's reaction to the procedure in nurses's notes. If suppository was for laxative purposes, record its effectiveness.	Fulfills nurse accountability. Provides ongoing data base.

Administering Medication to the Skin

In most agencies, it is acceptable practice to allow clients to apply dermal medications themselves if they prefer. The nurse, however, is responsible for teaching and supervising correct application.

When using medication from a jar, use a tongue depressor to remove the required amount and place it on a gauze sponge or clean paper towel. If the tongue depressor is used to apply the ointment or paste, use a second, clean one to remove additional medication from the jar.

When medication is to be applied to the scalp, determine from the physician's order or package insert directions whether the hair needs to be shampooed before each application of medication, on a daily basis, or as needed for comfort and cleanliness. It is important that the medication be applied to the scalp itself, rather than to the hair. This is best accomplished by successively parting the hair at 1.5 cm (5/8 in) intervals and applying the medication to the visible scalp at each parting. Follow package directions about whether to massage the medication into the scalp.

When applying topical medication to the face, avoid applying it near the eyes since dermal medications are not intended for ophthalmic use and the aroma alone can be irritating to the eyes. Apply medication sparingly around the mouth and under the nose to avoid inadvertent entry into the mouth, and because some dermal medications have an unpleasant odor or may be quite aromatic.

Apply medication to the body in a cephalocaudal direction, working with the direction of the hair growth since that is more comfortable and less irritating.

A decision about using bare hands or wearing gloves to apply dermal medications is based on factors specific to each situation. For example, instructions on the package may indicate gloves are to be used. Gloves are worn if the nurse has breaks in his or her own skin, if the medication would be irritating to the nurse's skin, if the nurse has sensitive skin, if the client has an infectious skin condition, or if the medication can be absorbed through the nurse's skin and thus deliver some medication to the nurse also. If there is any question about introducing microorganisms that would exacerbate the client's condition, wear sterile gloves to apply the medication. With some exceptions, drugs applied to the skin are not readily absorbed through the skin of the nurse's hand during application to the client's skin, and therefore gloves are not needed for routine dermal application. If gloves are worn, use surgeon's sterile gloves because of their close fit. Clean exmination gloves fit too loosely to be worn for this purpose. If wearing gloves, explain to the client that you are wearing gloves for the client's protection and to avoid introducing any microorganisms from your hands. Explanations are especially important when clients have unsightly skin conditions about which they may already be quite sensitive.

Transdermal Administration of Medications

Topical nitroglycerin ointment provides a sustained vasodilation that helps prevent anginal attacks. Nitroglycerin ointment (Nitro-bid, Nitrol) is prescribed

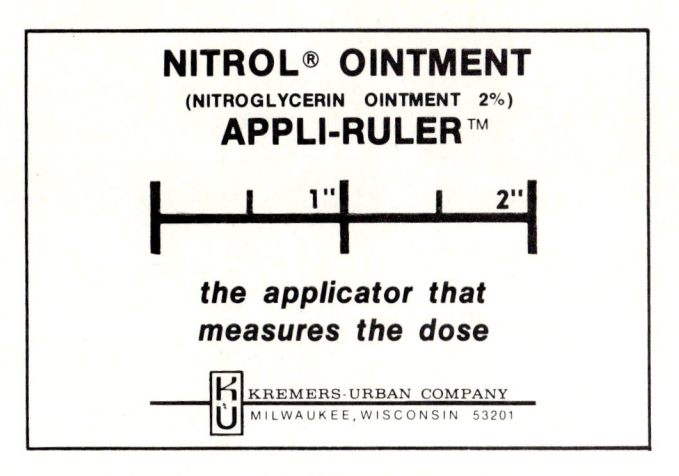

Figure 72-12. Applicator paper for measuring dosages of nitroglycerin ointment. (Courtesy of Kremers-Urban Company, Milwaukee, WI.)

in centimeters or inches, rather than milligrams or milliliters, with a usual dosage strength of 15 mg/inch. It is squeezed from a tube onto a specially designed firm plastic or paper applicator with inch markings on it, as shown in Figure 72-12. Use the applicator or a rubber glove to spread a thin uniform film of the prescribed amount over an area of nonhairy skin the size of the applicator; that area has been found to be sufficient to achieve desired clinical effects and blood levels (Iafrate et al., 1983; Product Information, 1984). Nitroglycerin ointment is never applied with an ungloved hand, because some of the medication can be absorbed through ungloved fingers. The ointment is not massaged or rubbed into the skin as this would increase the rate of absorption and interfere with its sustained action. After spreading the ointment, the applicator may be removed or left in place. Cover the area with a transparent plastic kitchen wrap and fasten it with tape on all sides. Covering the area increases skin temperature and hydration at the site, which is known to increase percutaneous absorption. It also keeps the medication in contact with the skin and protects the clothing from the ointment (Hansen and Woods, 1980). Rotate sites to avoid skin irritation and remove all of the previous dose of ointment before applying a new dose. A newer modification of the applicator paper has an adhesive patch attached to the applicator paper, such as NITROL *T*ape *S*urrounded *A*ppli-*R*uler, or TSAR (Kremers-Urban Company). Topical nitroglycerin also is available as premeasured adhesive patches with dosage strengths ranging from 2.5 mg to 15.0 mg; for example, Transderm-Nitro (Ciba). Before applying one of these easy-to-use patches, remove the old patch and cleanse any residual adhesive and medication from the skin. Apply to body areas as described above, rotating application sites.

Transdermal scopolomine (such as Transderm-V) can be used to prevent motion sickness associated with traveling. In this form, the drug has fewer negative side effects than when administered orally or parenterally. Transdermal scopolomine discs are applied behind the ear (Gever, 1982). It is important to instruct the client to wash hands thoroughly after applying this medication. Transfer of scopolomine from

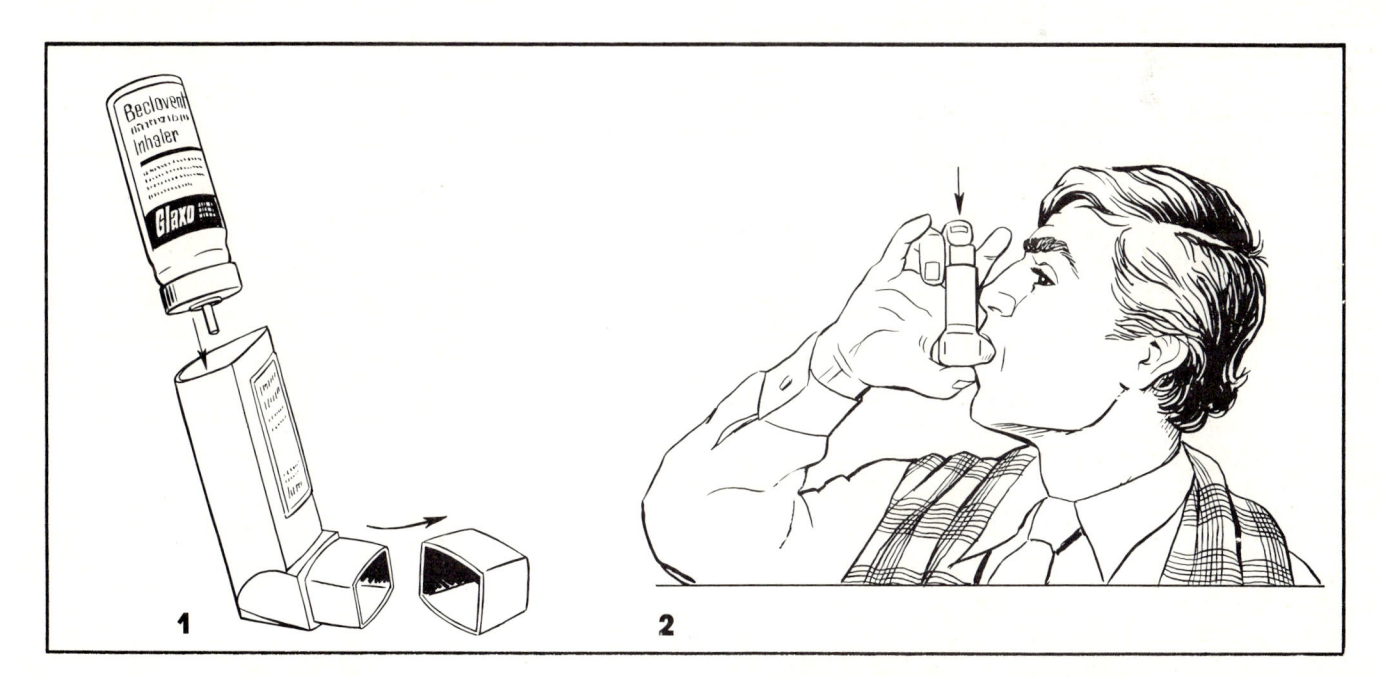

Figure 72-13. Inhalant medications. **A.** Using a metered-dose nebulizer: (1) Insert the medication bottle securely into the plastic holder; remove the mouthpiece; (2) Exhale. Hold the nebulizer upside down, with lips closed loosely around the mouthpiece. Inhale slowly. While inhaling, push the bottle into the holder one time firmly. This releases one dose of medication. Remove mouthpiece and exhale slowly, through pursed lips. Repeat only as directed. Rinse mouthpiece with warm water.

882 PROFESSIONAL CLINICAL NURSING SKILLS

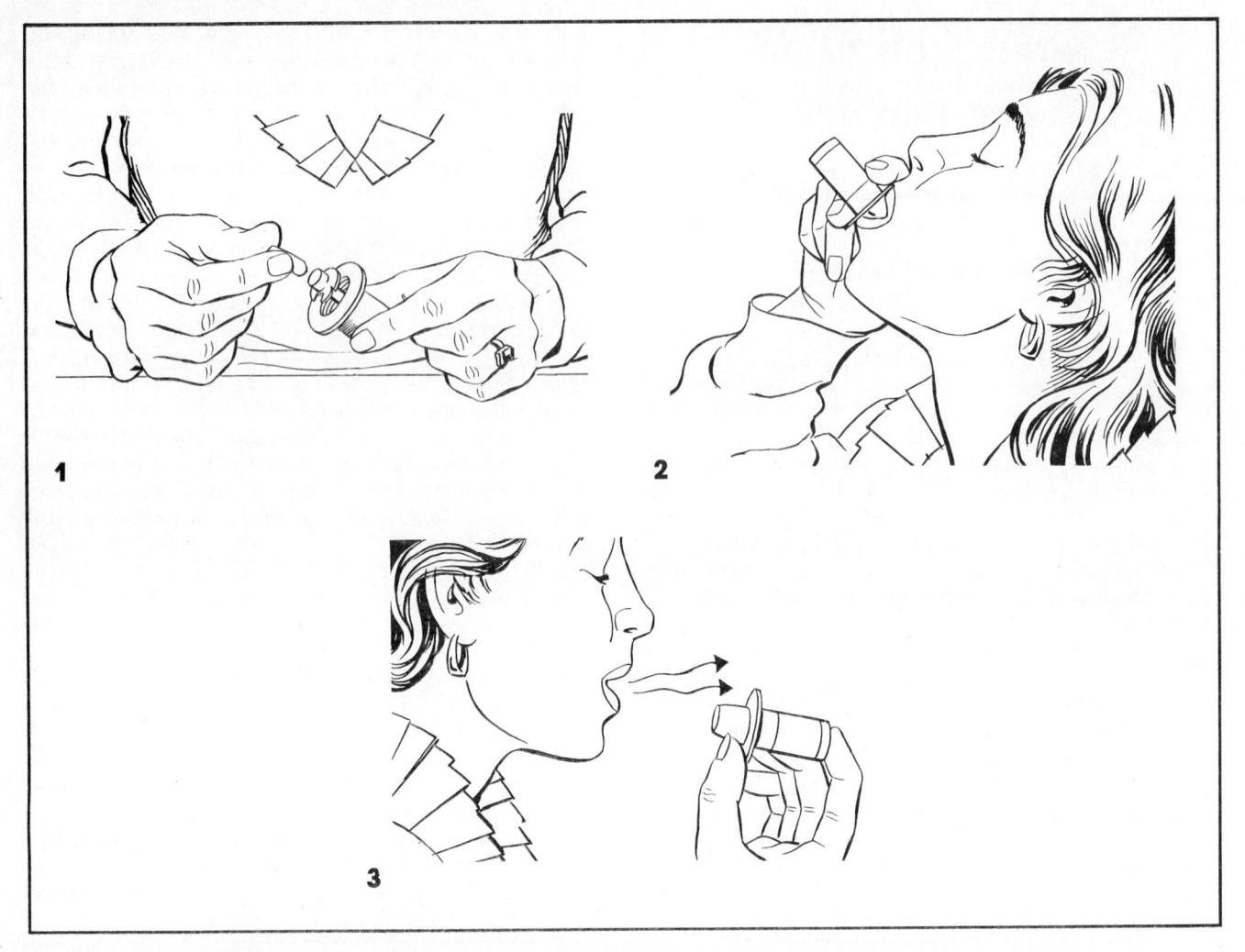

Figure 72–13. B. Using a turbo-inhaler device: (1) Place capsule of medication in turbo-inhaler; (2) Exhale as much air as possible; place mouthpiece in mouth and close the lips around it; tilt head backward and inhale once, deeply and quickly, to fill the lungs; (3) Hold the breath for several seconds; remove the device from the mouth; exhale as deeply as possible. Repeat these two steps several times, until medication is gone. Rinse mouthpiece with warm water.

the hands to or near the eye can result in pupil dilatation that may take several days to subside.

Administering Medications through Inhalation

Inhalant medications are usually self-administered with a nebulizer or inhaler and are accompanied by specific instructions on how to operate them most effectively. Instruct clients to inhale as deeply as possible to achieve the maximum benefit from the medication and to avoid swallowing aerosolized medication. However, they are not to exhale through the device. With some equipment, this action delivers medication to the surrounding air. As with all medication, nebulizers and inhalers are used only as often as directed by the physician or as cautioned on the package insert.

Some respiratory nebulizers and inhalers are disposable and may contain one dose of medication or a series of metered doses. Others are reusable and the client places a capsule of powdered medication in the device for each dose. Some devices come apart for washing. Figure 72–13A shows the use of a metered-dose nebulizer and Figure 72–13B shows a turbo-inhaler.

To use a mesh-covered crushable ampule of volatile spirits of ammonia for a person who has fainted, break the ampule in your fingers and hold it under the person's nose.

RECORDING

Record the administration of the medication in the computer or on the medication record form that is a part of the client's permanent health record. In the nurses' notes, record information about the therapeutic effectiveness of the medication and any untoward effects. Include the status of the area prior to applying the medication and any changes noted from the previous application. For example, note the color and appearance of the area, breaks in the skin, presence of edema and inflammation, and the amount and character of any crusts, secretions, or drainage from the area being treated. Include the client's reaction to the application; for example, if burning, redness, or discomfort occurs at that time or later. A sample medication record flow sheet with recorded medications is shown in Chapter 16, Introduction, Figure 5.

Sample POR Recording

- S—"I really itched after my shower this morning! I itch so bad before it's time for my medication—it's hard to keep from scratching! I do scratch some times!"
- O—Fine red macular rash on torso and extremities. Skin intact. Observed rubbing and scratching arms and abdomen about 45 minutes before medication applied.
- A—Incomplete relief from itching, possibly from prolonged interval between applications of medication.
- P—1. Corticosteroid ointment applied to arms, back, abdomen, and legs × 3 between 8 AM and 3 PM.
  2. Contact physician regarding incomplete relief.
  3. Continue to apply corticosteroid ointment.
  4. Plan diversional activities during hour before medication is due.

Sample Narrative Recording

Corticosteroid ointment applied to abdomen, back, arms, and legs × 3 between 8 AM and 3 PM. Observed scratching and rubbing arms and abdomen about 45 minutes before medication applied. States ointment gives temporary relief and helps her forget about the rash; also states that she was particularly itchy after her shower this AM. Fine red macular rash on torso and extremities. Skin intact with some redness on abdomen and forearms from rubbing and scratching. Physician notified about incomplete relief from symptoms.

☐ CRITICAL POINTS SUMMARY

1. Observe the status of the area being treated prior to administering a topical medication.
2. If an applicator touches the skin or mucous membranes, it is not returned to the medication container, since that would contaminate the medication.
3. Observe the client's initial and later response to application of topical medications.
4. To administer drops into the nasal cavity, tilt the head so the columella nasi is vertical and direct the drops toward the upper part of the nasal cavity.
5. To administer drops into the sinuses, hyperextend the neck over the side of the bed so the columella nasi is horizontal.
6. While administering eye and ear medications, rest the dominant hand on the client's head to avoid accidental contamination or injury.
7. Warm ear drops to body temperature to avoid discomfort and potential vertigo.
8. To administer ear drops, straighten the adult external auditory canal by pulling upward and backward; direct the drops toward the canal and pump the tragus gently. Straighten a child's auditory canal by pulling downward and backward.
9. Warm eye drops and ointment to body temperature to avoid discomfort.
10. Work from the inner toward the outer canthus to cleanse the eye, insert ophthalmic ointment, or wipe excess medication from the lids.
11. To administer eye drops, grasp the skin gently beneath the lower eyelid, pull it outward, and instill one or two drops.
12. To administer eye ointment, pull the lower lid downward and lay a ribbon of ointment along the conjunctival surface.
13. Use an applicator, inserter, or gloved finger to insert medications into the vaginal vault.
14. Use a glove or finger cot to insert a rectal suppository beyond the internal rectal sphincter.
15. Most topical medications are poorly absorbed through the skin.
16. Wear gloves to apply topical medications to the skin if the medication or the skin condition might adversely affect the nurse or if the condition is infectious.
17. Instruct clients to deep breathe when inhaling respiratory inhalant medications.

☐ LEARNING ACTIVITIES

1. With a peer, practice the positions and hand placements used to instill ear drops, eye drops and eye ointment, and nose drops for use in both the nasal cavity and the sinuses. Do not insert any medication into these orifices unless it is prescribed by a physician for that person or is an OTC product *used by that person only,* such as contact lens wetting drops, drops used to soothe irritated eye tissues, or to soften ear wax. Reverse roles and repeat positions. Compare your perspectives of the comfort or discomfort of each position.
2. Use a flashlight to inspect a peer's external nasal cavity. Note the color of the mucous membranes, patency of nostrils, and any crusts and secretions. Reverse roles and repeat.
3. Inspect a peer's external ear and note its color and appearance. Pull the pinna backward and upward and note any visible changes. Reverse roles and repeat.

4. Using a flashlight and tongue depressor, inspect a peer's mouth. Look at the vascularity of the area under the tongue and on the cheeks. Note where you would place sublingual and buccal medications.
5. In a central service department or simulation laboratory, familiarize yourself with mechanical atomizers, nebulizers, and sprays. Determine the amount of pressure you need to use to disperse a fine spray.
6. In a pharmacy or simulation laboratory, examine various forms of medications for topical use such as rectal suppositories; vaginal inserts and applicators; liquids, creams, ointments, pastes; sublingual and buccal tablets; and medications for the eye, ear, and nose. Read the labels carefully to determine how the administration route is indicated. Read directions for application on the label or the package insert. Note any relationships between the route and method of application and the desired effect of the medication.

☐ REVIEW QUESTIONS

1. Why are sublingual and buccal routes useful for medication that would be deactivated or destroyed by the liver?
2. Why does administration of medication through the mucous membranes of the respiratory tract and mouth result in rapid drug action?
3. Why should an applicator or dropper not be returned to the medication supply container if it has touched the client?
4. Explain the reasons for the following recommended actions:
    a. Instilling ear drops
        (1) Warm the drops prior to insertion.
        (2) Rest your dominant hand on the client's jaw.
        (3) Pull the pinna upward and backward.
        (4) Pull the pinna downward and backward.
        (5) Direct the drops toward the side of the canal.
        (6) Press the tragus in a pumping manner.
    b. Instilling eye drops and ointment
        (1) Warm drops and ointment prior to insertion.
        (2) Rest your dominant hand on the client's forehead.
        (3) Grasp the skin gently beneath the lower eyelid and pull it outward to instill eye drops.
        (4) Pull the lower eyelid downward with two or three fingers to insert eye ointment.
        (5) Work from the inner canthus outward.
    c. Instilling nasal drops
        (1) For nasal action, tilt the head so the columella nasi is vertical.
        (2) For sinus treatment, hyperextend the neck so the columella nasi is horizontal.
        (3) Raise the tip of the nose with the thumb for added visibility.
        (4) Insert drops in two stages, waiting between stages.
5. How does insertion of vaginal tablets and inserts differ from insertion of vaginal creams and gels?
6. Explain the position and procedure for inserting a rectal suppository.
7. Why is it often safe to apply topical medications to the skin with ungloved hands?
8. What factors would you consider when deciding whether to apply a topical medication to the skin with gloved or ungloved hands?
9. How is applying a nitroglycerin ointment different from applying other topical medications to the skin?
10. Why would you instruct a client to inhale very deeply when using respiratory inhalant medications?

☐ PERFORMANCE CHECKLISTS

OBJECTIVE: To use appropriate medical aseptic technique to insert drops into the nasal cavity and the sinuses.			
CHARACTERISTIC	RANGE OF ACCEPTABILITY	SATISFACTORY	UNSATISFACTORY
1. Checks medication order for accuracy.	No deviation		
2. Reviews knowledge of drug.	No deviation		
3. Washes hands.	No deviation		
4. Selects correct medication, labeled for nasal use.	No deviation		
5. Does SAFETY CHECK 1: Compares drug label and client's name with medication order.	No deviation		

(continued)

CHARACTERISTIC	RANGE OF ACCEPTABILITY	SATISFACTORY	UNSATISFACTORY
6. Places medication near medication order and does SAFETY CHECK 2.	No deviation		

7. Identifies the client:
   a. Compares medication order with:
      (1) Room number
      (2) Bed number
      (3) Identification band
   b. Addresses client by name.
	No deviation
	
	No deviation		

8. Does SAFETY CHECK 3.	No deviation		
9. Informs client about medication being given.	No deviation		
10. Closes door or draws curtains	No deviation		
11. Raises bed to working height.	No deviation		
12. Performs needed preliminary assessment and cleansing.	No deviation		
13. For nasal cavity, positions client with columella nasi nearly vertical.	For sinuses, position client with columella nasi nearly horizontal.		
14. Withdraws medication into dropper.	No deviation		
15. Elevates tip of nose with thumb.	No deviation		
16. Inserts 3 or 4 drops without touching dropper to nasal tissue.	Other amount may be specified.		
17. Waits 2 to 4 minutes.	Client's condition may not allow this.		
18. Inserts 3 or 4 additional drops.	Other amount may be specified.		
19. Observes client's initial reaction.	No deviation		
20. Repositions for comfort and safety.	No deviation		
21. Records medication on medication record form.	Mark computer printout or stack medicine cards for later recording.		
22. Records medication on permanent form in health record.	Omit if already done.		

OBJECTIVE: To use appropriate medical aseptic technique to instill drops into the ear correctly.

CHARACTERISTIC	RANGE OF ACCEPTABILITY	SATISFACTORY	UNSATISFACTORY
1. Checks medication order for accuracy.	No deviation		
2. Reviews knowledge of drug.	No deviation		
3. Washes hands.	No deviation		
4. Selects correct medication, labeled for use in the ears.	No deviation		
5. Does SAFETY CHECK 1: Compares drug label and client's name with medication order.	No deviation		
6. Places medication near medication order and does SAFETY CHECK 2.	No deviation		

7. Identifies the client:
   a. Compares medication order with:
      (1) Room number
      (2) Bed number
      (3) Identification band
   b. Addresses client by name.
	No deviation		

8. Does SAFETY CHECK 3.	No deviation		
9. Informs client about medication being given.	No deviation		

(continued)

OBJECTIVE: To use appropriate medical aseptic technique to instill drops into the ear correctly (cont.).

CHARACTERISTIC	RANGE OF ACCEPTABILITY	SATISFACTORY	UNSATISFACTORY
10. Warms ear drops in hands.	No deviation		
11. Closes door or draws curtains.	No deviation		
12. Raises bed to working height.	No deviation		
13. Performs needed preliminary assessment and cleansing.	No deviation		
14. Positions client in flat, side-lying position, head on pillow, exposing ear to be treated.	No deviation		
15. Withdraws medication into dropper.	No deviation		
16. Positions self with dominant hand toward client's foot.	No deviation		
17. Rests nondominant hand on client's head.	No deviation		
18. Pulls pinna upward and backward.	For children: pull pinna downward and backward.		
19. Instills drops; holds ear in position and presses tragus gently several times.	No deviation		
20. Instructs client to remain in position 3 to 4 minutes.	No deviation		
21. Repositions for comfort and safety.	No deviation		
22. Records medication on medication record form or in bedside computer.	Mark computer printout or stack medicine cards for later recording.		
23. Records medication on permanent form in health record.	Omit if already done.		

OBJECTIVE: To use appropriate sterile equipment and medical aseptic technique to instill drops and ointment into the eye correctly.

CHARACTERISTIC	RANGE OF ACCEPTABILITY	SATISFACTORY	UNSATISFACTORY
1. Checks medication order for accuracy.	No deviation		
2. Reviews knowledge of drug.	No deviation		
3. Washes hands.	No deviation		
4. Selects correct medication, labeled for use in the eyes.	No deviation		
5. Does SAFETY CHECK 1: Compares drug label and client's name with medication order.	No deviation		
6. Places medication near medication order and does SAFETY CHECK 2.	No deviation		
7. Identifies the client: a. Compares medication order with: (1) Room number (2) Bed number (3) Identification band b. Addresses client by name.	No deviation		
8. Does SAFETY CHECK 3.	No deviation		
9. Informs client about medication being given.	No deviation		
10. Warms eye drop container in hands.	No deviation		
11. Closes door or draws curtains.	No deviation		
12. Raises bed to working height.	No deviation		

(continued)

SKILL 72: TOPICAL MEDICATION ADMINISTRATION

CHARACTERISTIC	RANGE OF ACCEPTABILITY	SATISFACTORY	UNSATISFACTORY
13. Performs needed preliminary assessment and cleansing.	No deviation		
14. Cleanses from inner canthus outward.	No deviation		

15. Eye drops:
   a. Withdraws medication into dropper.
   b. Positions self with dominant hand toward top of client's head.
   c. Rests dominant hand on client's forehead.
   d. Asks client to look upward.
   e. Pinches skin beneath eye with non-dominant hand to create pouch.
   f. Instills drops.
	Omit if medication is in a sqeeze bottle.
	No deviation
	
	No deviation
	
	No deviation
	No deviation
	
	No deviation		

16. Eye ointment:
   a. Holds tube upright vertically and discards first drop of ointment.
   b. Positions self with dominant hand toward top of client's head.
   c. Rests dominant hand on client's forehead.
   d. Asks client to look upward.
   e. Pulls tissues below the eye downward.
   f. Holds tube upright vertically and places ribbon of ointment in canthus.
   g. Works from inner canthus outward.
	No deviation
	
	No deviation
	
	No deviation
	
	No deviation
	No deviation
	No deviation
	
	No deviation		

17. Asks client to close eye gently and remain closed 2 to 3 minutes.	No deviation		
18. Use separate medication, equipment, and tissues on each eye.	No deviation		
19. Records medication on medication record form or in bedside computer.	Mark computer printout or stack medicine cards for later recording.		
20. Records medication on permanent form in health record.	Omit if already done.		

OBJECTIVE: To use appropriate medical aseptic technique to insert medication into the vagina.

CHARACTERISTIC	RANGE OF ACCEPTABILITY	SATISFACTORY	UNSATISFACTORY
1. Checks medication order for accuracy.	No deviation		
2. Reviews knowledge of drug.	No deviation		
3. Washes hands.	No deviation		
4. Selects correct medication, labeled for vaginal use.	No deviation		
5. Does SAFETY CHECK 1: Compares drug label and client's name with medication order.	No deviation		
6. Places medication near medication order and does SAFETY CHECK 2.	No deviation		
7. Obtains inserter or applicator, sterile gloves, and water-soluble lubricant.	Tablets and inserts may be inserted manually.		

8. Identifies the client:
   a. Compares medication order with
     (1) Room number
     (2) Bed number
     (3) Identification band
   b. Addresses client by name.
	No deviation		

9. Does SAFETY CHECK 3.	No deviation		
10. Informs client about medication being given.	No deviation		

(continued)

OBJECTIVE: To use appropriate medical aseptic technique to insert medication into the vagina (cont.).

CHARACTERISTIC	RANGE OF ACCEPTABILITY	SATISFACTORY	UNSATISFACTORY
11. Closes door and draws curtains.	No deviation		
12. Raises bed to working height.	No deviation		
13. Positions client in dorsal recumbent position with legs apart and knees flexed.	No deviation		
14. Drapes for privacy.	No deviation		
15. Places protective pad under hips.	No deviation		
16. Inspects and cleanses perineal area as needed.	No deviation		
17. Dons sterile gloves.	No deviation		
18. Lubricates applicator tip.	No deviation		
19. Separates labia with nondominant hand.	No deviation		
20. Inserts applicator or inserter 5.0 to 7.5 cm (2 to 3 in) into vagina and releases tablet.	Insert tablet a similar distance with gloved finger.		
21. Discards disposable applicator.	Wash reusable applicator with soap and warm water.		
22. Applies protective pad.	No deviation		
23. Requests that client remain in lying-down position for 30 minutes.	No deviation		
24. Removes and discards gloves.	No deviation		
25. Repositions for comfort and safety.	No deviation		
26. Washes hands.	No deviation		
27. Records medication on medication record form or in bedside computer.	Mark computer printout or stack medicine cards for later recording.		
28. Records medication on permanent form in health record.	Omit if already done.		

OBJECTIVE: To use appropriate medical aseptic technique to insert rectal suppositories.

CHARACTERISTIC	RANGE OF ACCEPTABILITY	SATISFACTORY	UNSATISFACTORY
1. Checks medication order for accuracy.	No deviation		
2. Reviews knowledge of drug.	No deviation		
3. Washes hands.	No deviation		
4. Selects correct suppository, labeled for rectal use.	No deviation		
5. Does SAFETY CHECK 1: Compares drug label and client's name with medication order.	No deviation		
6. Firms suppository in refrigerator or ice water as needed.	No deviation		
7. Places medication near medication order and does SAFETY CHECK 2.	No deviation		
8. Obtains clean gloves or finger cots and water-soluble lubricant.	No deviation		
9. Identifies the client: a. Compares medication order with: (1) Room number (2) Bed number (3) Identification band. b. Addresses client by name.	No deviation		

(continued)

CHARACTERISTIC	RANGE OF ACCEPTABILITY	SATISFACTORY	UNSATISFACTORY
10. Does SAFETY CHECK 3.	No deviation		
11. Informs client about medication being given.	No deviation		
12. Closes door and draws curtain.	No deviation		
13. Raises bed to working height.	No deviation		
14. Positions client on side with upper leg drawn up.	No deviation		
15. Drapes for privacy.	No deviation		
16. Dons clean gloves or two finger cots.	No deviation		
17. Lubricates suppository.	Omit if prelubricated and client has no hemorrhoids or rectal problems.		
18. Separates buttocks and exposes anus.	No deviation		
19. Has client take deep breath and touches anus with suppository.	No deviation		
20. Inserts suppository 7.5 cm (3 in).	No deviation		
21. Presses buttocks together.	Alternate action: Compress anus with pad of tissues or gauze.		
22. Asks client to retain suppository for 20 minutes.	Ability to retain varies with individual and type of suppository.		
23. Removes gloves or finger cots and discards.	No deviation		
24. Repositions for comfort and safety.	No deviation		
25. Washes hands.	No deviation		
26. Records medication on medication record form or in bedside computer.	Mark computer printout or stacks medicine cards for later recording.		
27. Records medication on permanent form in health record.	Omit if already done.		

REFERENCES

Gever LN: Administering drugs through the skin. Nursing82 (Horsham) 12(3):88, 1982.

Hansen MS, Woods SL: Nitroglycerin ointment—Where and how to apply it. American Journal of Nursing 80(6):1122–1124, 1982.

Iafrate RP, et al: Effect of dose and ointment application technique on nitroglycerin plasma concentrations. Pharmacotherapy 3(2):118–124, 1983.

Nursing80 Photobook. Giving Medications. Horsham, PA, Intermed Communications, 1980.

Product Information. Kremers-Urban Company, Milwaukee, WI, 1984.

Sorensen KC, Luckmann J: Basic Nursing: A Psychophysiologic Approach. Philadelphia, WB Saunders, 1979.

BIBLIOGRAPHY

Kirilloff LH, Tibbals SC: Drugs for asthma: A complete guide. American Journal of Nursing 83(1):55–61, 1983.

Kozier B, Erb G: Techniques in Clinical Nursing. Menlo Park, CA, Addison-Wesley, 1982.

Lewis LuVW: Fundamental Skills in Patient Care, ed 3. Philadelphia, JB Lippincott, 1984.

Nurses' drug alert: Instilling eyedrops correctly. American Journal of Nursing 83(7):1061 (NDA p 51), 1983.

Shiery S: Insight into the delicate art of eye care. Nursing75 5(6):50–55, 1975.

Wood LA: Nursing Skills for Allied Health Services. Philadelphia, WB Saunders, 1975, vol 3.

SUGGESTED READING

Matus NR (consultant): Topical therapy: Choosing and using the proper vehicle. Nursing77 7(11):8–10, 1977.

AUDIOVISUAL RESOURCE

Medicating the Patient: Administering Oral, Topical, Suppository and Inhalant Medications
Filmstrip, video. (1982, Color, 21 min.)
Available through:
Medcom, Inc.
P.O. Box 116
Garden Grove, CA 92642

SKILL 73 Injectable Medication Administration

PREREQUISITE SKILLS

Skill 19, "Inspection"
Skill 20, "Palpation"
Skill 28, "Handwashing"
Skill 30, "Sterile Supplies"
Chapter 16, "Introduction"
Skill 71, "Oral Medication Administration"

☐ STUDENT OBJECTIVES

1. Identify the purposes for administering medications through the intradermal, subcutaneous, and intramuscular routes.
2. Identify the volume and types of medication given through each injection route.
3. Identify the anatomic landmarks for the common injection sites of each injection route.
4. Describe the client's body position for administering medication in each injection site.
5. Differentiate the palpation findings for intradermal, subcutaneous, and muscle tissue.
6. Identify potential hazards associated with administering injectable medications.
7. Differentiate the angle and depth of needle entry into the tissues for each injection route.
8. Identify the various parts of a syringe and needle.
9. Describe methods used to stabilize and stretch the skin while giving an injection through the different routes and sites.
10. Explain special precautions needed to administer insulin and heparin subcutaneously.
11. Describe the purpose and technique for the Z-track method of giving an intramuscular injection.
12. Determine the correct volume of injectable medication to administer so as to give the prescribed dosage.
13. Describe correct procedures for withdrawing medication from vials and ampules.
14. Describe correct procedures for combining the contents of two vials or a vial and ampule in one syringe.
15. Describe correct procedures for administering injectable medications through each route.
16. Use aseptic technique to prepare and administer intradermal, subcutaneous, and intramuscular medications in a safe manner.

☐ INTRODUCTION

The injectable medication routes presented in this skill are the intradermal, subcutaneous, and intramuscular routes. The intravenous route is presented in Skill 74.

The intradermal route is used for administering small doses (0.1 ml or less) of antigens as diagnostic skin tests for histoplasmosis or tuberculosis and for giving test doses of drugs that have a potential for producing anaphylactic shock, such as tetanus toxoid or penicillin. It may also be used to administer immunotherapy for cancer with drugs such as bacille Calumette-Guérin (BCG) or for allergy testing in preference to a patch test.

The subcutaneous route is useful when clients cannot take medications orally; when the drug would be inactivated or destroyed by the gastrointestinal system; when a more rapid drug action is desired than is possible with the oral route; or when the drug is too toxic or irritating for oral administration. This route is useful for small amounts (up to 1.5 ml) of nonirritating water-soluble drugs that are absorbed readily into the circulation.

The intramuscular route is used when a more rapid or more potent action is desired; when the drug is an oil preparation; or when the volume to be injected is greater than 1.5 ml and no more than 3 ml at each site.

The physician determines the most appropriate administration route for an injectable drug, based on the physical properties of the drug, its rate of absorption, and its solubility. Any change in administration route is done only after consultation with the physician.

Injectable drugs are packaged in sterile vials and ampules and the nurse uses surgical aseptic technique to prepare and administer them with sterile syringes and needles. Injectable drugs often are available in dosage forms suitable for several different routes. For example, heparin and insulin can be given through the subcutaneous or intravenous route but not the intramuscular route, while Vitamin B_{12} can be given only intramuscularly. Fat-soluble vitamins can be given by the oral or intramuscular route; vaccines and tetanus toxoid, by either the subcutaneous or intramuscular route; and some narcotics by the subcutaneous, intramuscular, or intravenous routes. Some antibiotics and anticoagulants are given by the oral, intramuscular, and intravenous routes, and other drugs such as morphine can be given by all four routes. It is essential to be alert to drug labeling and to use a dosage form designed for the route being used because many drugs prepared for parenteral use would be irritating, toxic, or destroyed if used orally; because infections can occur if nonsterile oral preparations are used for injections; and because a drug intended for subcutaneous use can act too rapidly if given intramuscularly.

This skill presents the techniques for administering intradermal, subcutaneous, and intramuscular medications in a safe way.

☐ PREPARATION

The activities and assessment practices associated with administering injectable medications are designed to ensure that the medication is injected into the designated body tissue, that is, into the skin, subcutaneous, or muscle tissue. To do this requires that the nurse be able to select the most appropriate site for a particular medication and specific person; know the variables that affect drug absorption from various injection sites; and be able to inject the medication in a safe manner that minimizes untoward effects of the injection procedure. In addition, safe injection technique requires being able to distinguish between healthy and unhealthy tissue and between subcutaneous and muscle tissue, and to determine the length of needle and injection technique that will deliver the medication to the desired tissue. Figure 73-1 shows the skin, subcutaneous, and muscle tissues and the depth and angle at which the needle is inserted to reach each of those sites.

MEDICATION INJECTION SITES

Selecting an appropriate site for an injection requires that the nurse be able to distinguish between subcutaneous and muscle tissue; to recognize when medications can be injected safely into skin, subcutaneous, and muscle tissues; and to identify and select from a variety of injection sites. Clients will experience less discomfort and fewer complications at the injection site when the nurse is able to use a variety of sites and rotates use of the most appropriate ones.

To identify the precise injection site, inspect and palpate specific landmarks as described in the following section. Be sure to remove enough clothing and bed linen to be able to see and palpate those landmarks as well as the intended injection site. It is unacceptable practice to expose only a portion of the gluteus, side, or thigh and give a blind injection in a false attempt to maintain privacy. Likewise, it is an unacceptable practice to give an injection in the arm with the sleeve pushed up tightly so as to distort or hide anatomic landmarks, or to give an injection to an ambulatory client who is leaning over a table with the trousers only partially pulled down from the waist or the undergarments lifted from below. Although an intramuscular injection site may have a fairly sizable muscle mass, the medication must be injected only into specific portions of those muscles because of their proximity to major bones, blood vessels, and nerves. The goal is to insert the medication into the belly of the muscle, since that area can accommodate the fluid more readily.

Healthy skin tissue is clear, without breaks, irritation, inflammation, or induration. On palpation, it feels smooth and resilient. Healthy subcutaneous tissue is vascular and contains substantial amounts of interstitial fluid; in obese people it is less vascular because of increased numbers of fat cells. On palpation, subcutaneous tissue feels full, smooth, soft, and resilient and has no indurated or tender areas. When grasped between the thumb and fingers preparatory to giving an injection, this tissue feels firm and fairly solid. When clients are severely dehydrated, subcutaneous tissue feels softer and less full, because of decreased fluid volume.

Healthy muscle tissue is more vascular than subcutaneous tissue. On palpation, this tissue feels firm, solid, and dense in contrast to the softer subcutaneous tissues, although the degree of density varies with the client's level of exercise and nutritional status. Muscle tissue feels softer when it is relaxed, firm when tensed, and has no hard masses or painful areas. If uncertain as to whether muscle or subcutaneous tissue is being palpated, ask the client to tense and then relax the underlying muscle.

Intradermal Injection Sites

The most common site used for administering diagnostic skin tests and giving test doses of medications is the volar surface of the forearm. For the average adult, the forearm site is located 2 to 4 inches below the antecubital space in the nonhairy fleshy area of the forearm. The scapular area may also be used for allergy testing. The back or the medial aspects of the thigh may also be used if the forearms are unavailable

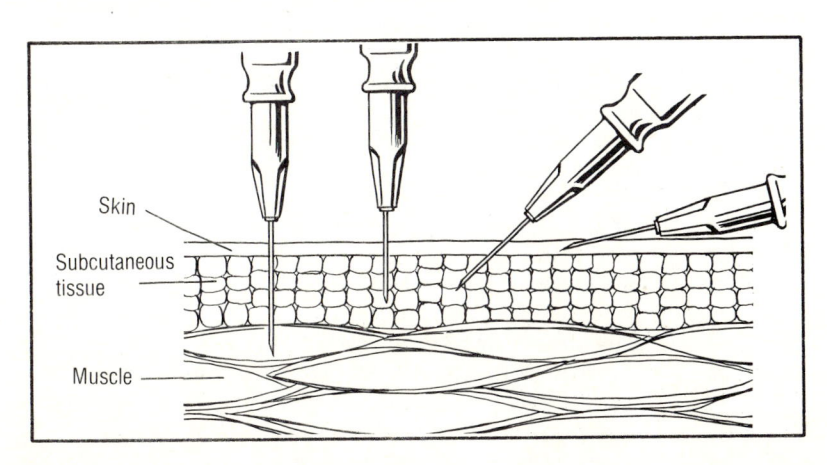

Figure 73-1. Tissues penetrated by injections. Note needle entry angle and depth used for injection into each type of tissue.

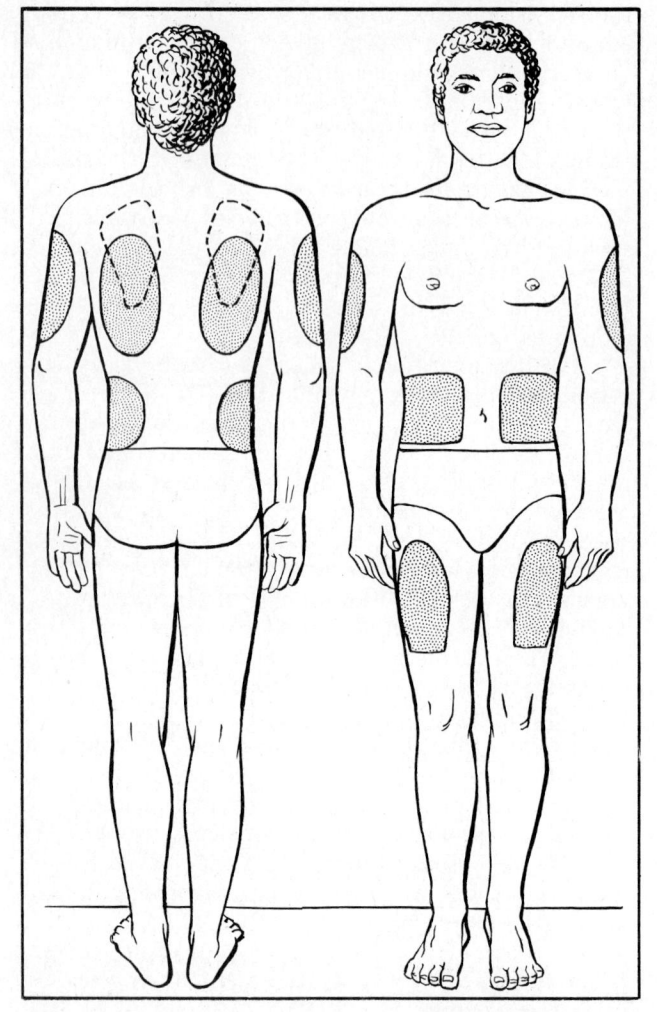

Figure 73-2. Common body areas used for subcutaneous injections.

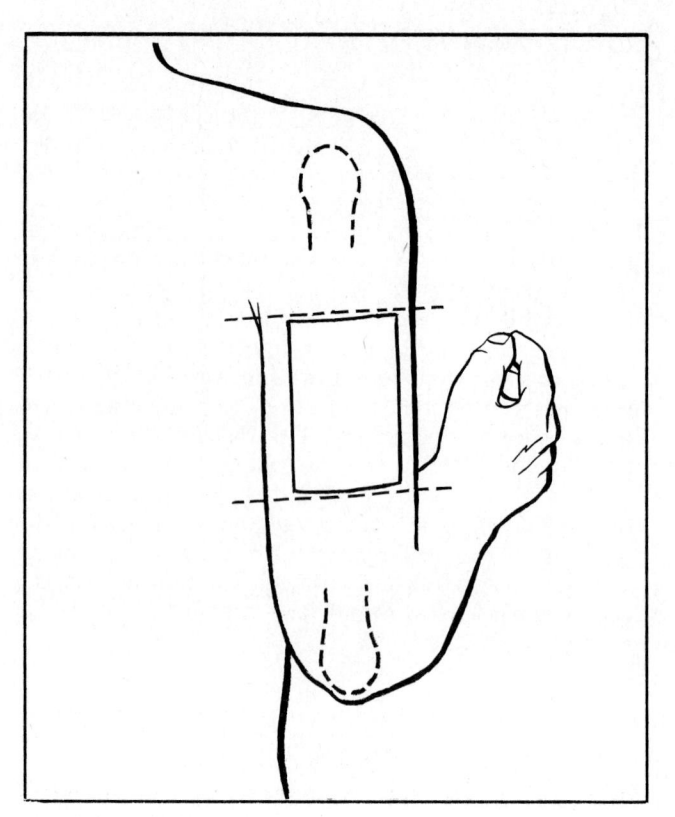

Figure 73-3. Subcutaneous injection site: upper arm area.

or if a rash in present. Intradermal injections for immunotherapy may be administered at the tumor site or elsewhere on the body, as determined by the physician.

Subcutaneous Injection Sites

The most commonly used sites for administering subcutaneous injections to adults are the outer aspects of the upper arms, the anterior aspects of the thighs, and the abdomen. Other areas that usually have an adequate amount of subcutaneous tissue are the scapular and buttocks areas. These areas are shown in Figure 73-2.

Upper Arm Area. Place the client's arm at the side of the body in a relaxed position. Identify the center third of the lateral aspect of the upper arm in a line from the olecranon (bony protuberance of the elbow) to the acromion process (point of the shoulder), as shown in Figure 73-3.

Anterior Thigh Area. Place the client in a seated, semi-Fowler's, or supine position with the leg relaxed. Identify the center third of the anterior thigh by placing one hand above the knee and the other hand just below the groin, as shown in Figure 73-4.

Abdomen. Place the client in a semirecumbent position. Visualize horizontal lines between the right and left anterior superior iliac spines and between the tenth ribs. The anterior abdominal area between these two lines is considered appropriate for subcutaneous injections, excluding the midline and the belt area. The midline apparently has more pain receptors than other abdominal tissues, and pressure from belts or waistbands can cause discomfort at the injection site and may contribute to bruising with heparin injections.

Scapular Area. Place the client on the side, prone, or in a seated position. To locate this site, identify the fleshy area covering the lower half of the midscapula and extending a similar distance below the scapula. Avoid the midline where there is little subcutaneous tissue over the spine.

Buttocks Area. Place the client in a prone position or on the side. Inject the medication in the upper outer fleshy aspects of either buttock.

Intramuscular Injection Sites

Common intramuscular injection sites include the deltoid (upper arm below the acromion process), vastus lateralis (anterior lateral midthigh), ventrogluteal area (between the greater trochanter and the anterior

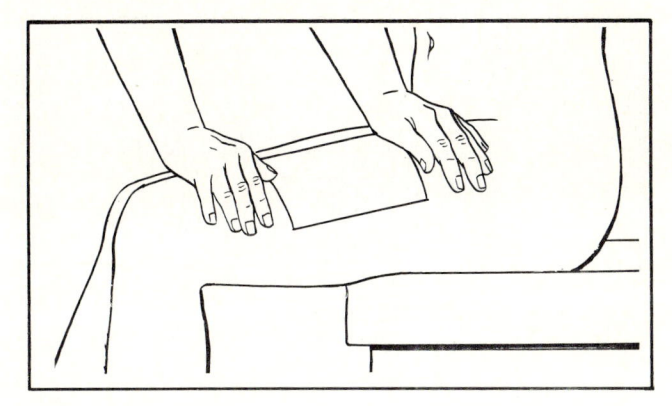

Figure 73-4. Subcutaneous injection site: anterior thigh area.

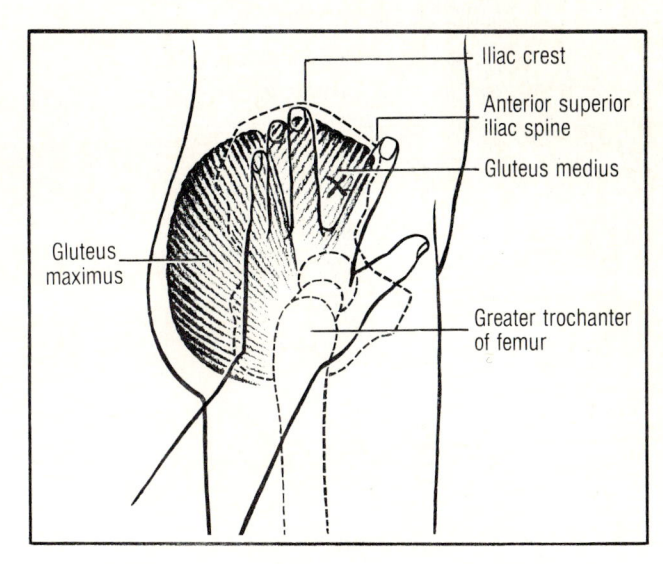

Figure 73-5. Intramuscular injection site: ventrogluteal muscle.

superior iliac spine), and the posterior or dorsal gluteal area (gluteus medius and gluteus maximus). In infants and children, the rectus femoris (anterior midthigh) is commonly used, but the posterior gluteal area is never used for children who weigh less than 9 kg (20 lb), *or* who have walked less than 1 year, since this muscle mass develops through the exercise of walking and is related to total body size.

The particular muscle mass selected for an injection depends upon the volume of drug to be injected and the desired rate of absorption as well as the size, physical condition, and age of the client. The various muscle sites are described here in a sequence of preferred use.

Ventrogluteal Site. The ventrogluteal site uses the gluteus medius muscle. Its lack of widespread use is most likely caused by lack of familiarity with this site. Although it is not as large as the vastus lateralis, it is an excellent injection site because there are no major nerves or blood vessels in the area, there is less adipose tissue than over the buttocks, and it can be used for both adults and children. In addition, there is much less postinjection discomfort with walking, sitting, and lying down than with the more commonly used posterior gluteal site.

To use this site, position the client on the side, on the back, or prone, and expose the side from the gluteal fold to the waist. For the right ventrogluteal site, rest the palm of your left hand on the client's right greater trochanter. Place the index finger on the anterior superior iliac spine and spread the middle finger posteriorly away from the index finger and along the superior iliac crest as far as possible, forming a V-shaped area. The desired injection site is in the center of that V space, as shown in Figure 73-5. Identify the left ventrogluteal site with the right hand. Always remember to *direct your thumb anteriorly* on the client's body. Palpate the selected site; spread the skin taut; and insert the needle directed slightly upward toward the crest of the ilium.

Vastus Lateralis Site. The vastus lateralis muscle usually is thick and well-developed in most adults and children. It has no major blood vessels or nerves in the area, is easily accessible, and an injection in this site causes little discomfort for bedfast persons. Its primary disadvantage is that the client can readily see the injection. Encourage looking away or closing the eyes during the injection.

Position the client either on the back or in a seated position. Expose the entire leg from the greater trochanter to the knee. Palpate the trochanter and visualize the center third of the distance between it and the knee. The injection area is in that third, and includes the midanterior and midlateral thigh, as shown in Figure 73-6. If the muscle mass is fairly large, spread the skin taut at the injection site; if it is small, grasp the muscle mass in your hand. Insert the needle at a 90 degree angle.

Deltoid Muscle. The deltoid muscle is a readily accessible muscle that is satisfactory for nonirritating medications of volumes less than 1.5 ml. However, in some women and in emaciated persons, this muscle is not well enough developed to accommodate even this small volume. Irritating medications or volumes larger than 1.5 ml should be injected into other, larger muscle masses.

To use this site, the client can assume a seated, standing, supine, or prone position. To identify the site, first raise the sleeve of a loose-fitting gown or shirt, or ask the client to remove a tight sleeve. Constriction from tight sleeves distorts the muscle contour, making site selection difficult. Palpate the acromion process with the flat fingers or palm of one hand and with the fingertips of the other hand locate the tip of the deltoid, usually at the axillary crease. The desired injection site is in the center of the inverted triangle thus formed, and about 5 cm (2 in) below the acromion process, as shown in Figure 73-7. Recall that the brachial artery and vein and radial nerve are very close to the deltoid. For this site, grasp the muscle between the thumb and fingers and direct the needle slightly toward the acromion process as an added safety precaution against striking nerves and vessels.

894 PROFESSIONAL CLINICAL NURSING SKILLS

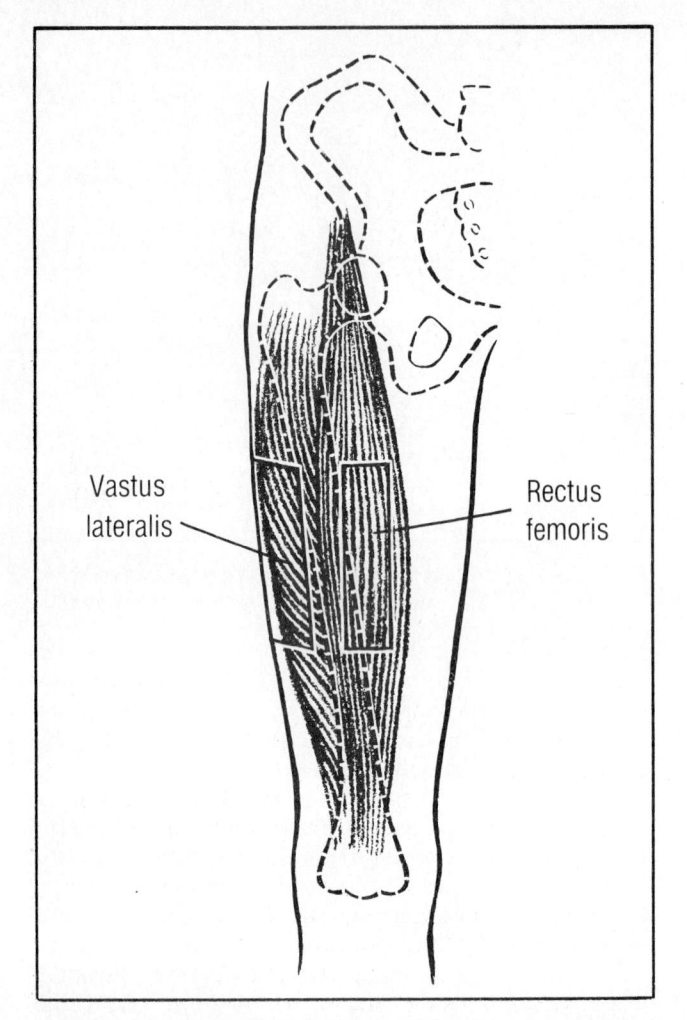

Figure 73-6. Intramuscular injection sites: vastus lateralis and rectus femoris muscles.

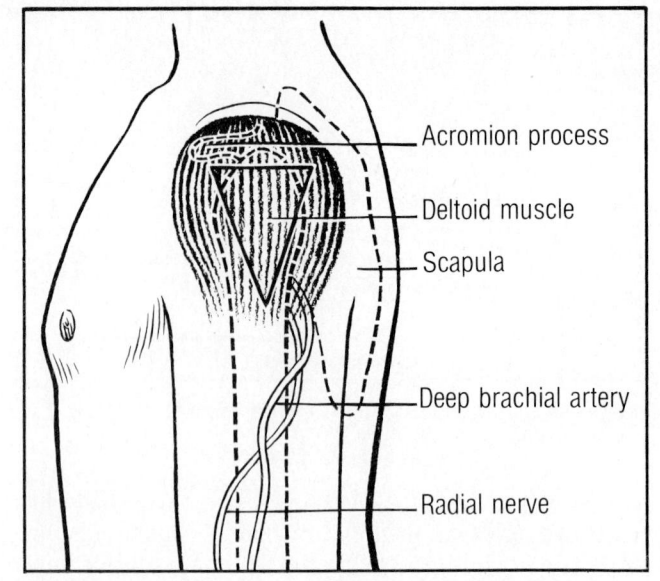

Figure 73-7. Intramuscular injection site: deltoid muscle.

Posterior or Dorsal Gluteal Area. This site uses the gluteus medius muscle and the upper edge of the gluteus maximus muscle. Although it is often the most commonly used site, it is also the one with the most potential for injury from incorrectly placed injections. The amount of adipose tissue in that area often makes it difficult to identify correct landmarks. If landmarks are not identified carefully, it is easy to inject the medication into the subcutaneous tissues lateral to the gluteus muscle or below it into the portion of the gluteus maximus where the superior gluteal artery and sciatic nerve are located.

Since an anxious person can easily tense the gluteus muscle, position the client so the femur rotates internally, which relaxes the muscle. Kruszewski et al., (1979) found that internal rotation of the femur with the client in the prone position and the toes pointing inward resulted in significantly less discomfort with injections of a narcotic and a tranquilizer. Internal rotation of the femur can also be accomplished by having the client in a side-lying position, with the knee and hip joints of the upper extremity flexed and placed anterior to the lower leg. This position is sometimes called the lateral position; it is similar to that used for a large-volume enema.

To identify the site, remove clothing or bed linen to expose the complete buttocks on one side of the body, including the medial and gluteal folds. There are two different ways to identify the posterior gluteal site. One is to palpate the *posterior superior iliac spine* and the *greater trochanter.* Visualize a diagonal line between these points, which is parallel and lateral to the sciatic nerve. The desired injection site is at the midpoint and 2.5 to 4.0 cm (1 to 1½ in) superior to this line, as shown in Figure 73-8A.

A second way to identify this site is to divide the buttock visually into four quadrants of a square, as shown in Figure 73-8B. The upper horizontal side of this square is at the iliac crest; the lateral vertical side is at the greater trochanter, not the client's side. The medial and gluteal folds form the other two sides of the imaginary square. (The medial fold refers to the crease between the buttocks; the gluteal fold is the crease below the buttocks.) The central horizontal line bisecting the square extends from the beginning of the medial fold to slightly above the trochanter. The vertical bisecting line is halfway between the trochanter and medial fold. The desired injection site is the upper outer quadrant of this imaginary square, excluding a triangular portion in that quadrant where the sciatic nerve and superior gluteal artery are located, as shown in Figure 73-8B.

To give an injection at this site, spread the overlying skin taut and insert the needle at a 90 degree angle.

Rectus Femoris Site. The rectus femoris muscle is located adjacent and medial to the vastus lateralis, and is identified with the same landmarks as shown in Figure 73-6. It is used primarily with infants and children.

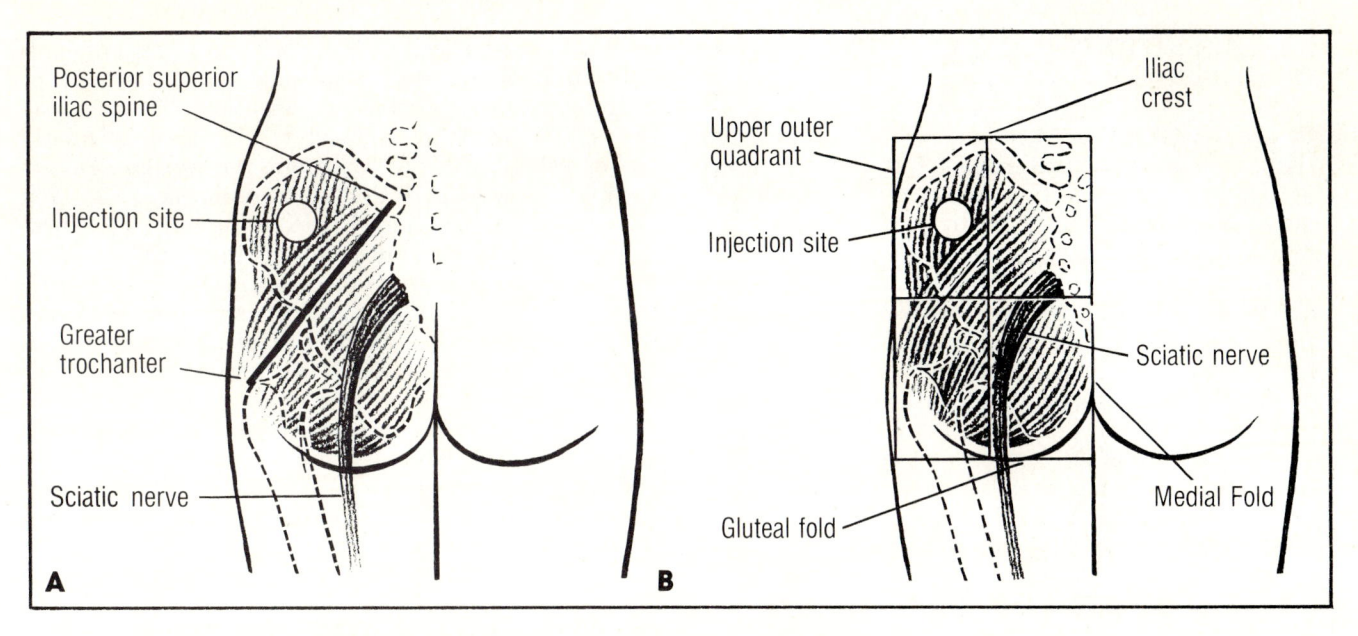

Figure 73–8. Intramuscular injection site: dorsal gluteal area. **A.** Diagonal line location method. **B.** Quadrant location method.

DRUG ABSORPTION FROM VARIOUS INJECTION SITES

An *intradermal medication* is injected between the epidermal and dermal layers of the skin. Most intradermal medications are used to produce a local reaction, are not absorbed into the general circulation, and do not have systemic effects. The volume of solution injected is very small; for example, a standard antigen dosage is 0.1 ml.

Medication that is injected into the *subcutaneous* or *muscle* tissue enters the interstitial spaces (extracellular fluid compartment) within those tissues and then is absorbed through the capillary network, dispersed throughout the body via the cardiovascular system to the target tissues, metabolized by the liver, and excreted through the kidneys. Absorption is more rapid from highly vascular muscle tissue than from the less vascular subcutaneous tissue. Therefore, a drug injected intramuscularly is expected to produce a more rapid action, while subcutaneous injection is expected to provide a slower and more sustained effect.

In addition to tissue vascularity, a variety of factors influences drug absorption from the injection site. Muscle movement and exercise increase the rate of absorption because blood flow to skeletal muscles increases during exercise. Massaging the site after injection tends to help disperse the medication mechanically. Some drugs, such as heparin, are not massaged. The nurse is responsible for knowing when massage is appropriate. Absorption of medication is decreased when there is inadequate circulation at the injection site, in the extremity used for the injection, or in the total cardiovascular system. Medications are not injected into indurated or edematous tissues, and the intravenous route is often substituted for the subcutaneous or intramuscular route when decreased tissue perfusion and decreased cardiac output exist, such as in shock.

Administering an injectable medication to a client with decreased tissue perfusion results in an insufficient dosage at the time of the injection, but can later produce an unexpected overdose if the peripheral circulation improves. Medications are also not given in open, irritated, or inflamed tissues because of altered tissue vascularity, potentially increased tissue irritation, and additional discomfort for the client. Insulin is never injected in areas of lipodystrophy or hypertrophy, as described later.

Other significant factors influencing drug absorption relate to the drug itself, its concentration, the type of solution in which it is dispersed, the solubility of the drug in the surrounding tissues, and the specific muscle in which it is injected. Drug absorption is more rapid after injection into the deltoid than into the vastus lateralis muscle, and slowest (especially in females) after injection into the gluteus maximus (Greenblatt and Koch-Weser, 1976).

Recent studies show that the amount of drug actually available for therapeutic action after intramuscular injections is sometimes inconsistent, incomplete, or slow and sometimes does not equal that obtained through oral or intravenous administration. For example, intramuscular injection of digoxin and phenytoin (Dilantin) is not recommended because of their incomplete availability and erratic absorption (Greenblatt and Koch-Weser, 1976). Increasingly, antibiotics and other medications formerly given by the intramuscular route are being given through the intravenous route quite successfully.

MINIMIZING UNTOWARD EFFECTS OF INJECTIONS

It is essential that medications be injected into the tissues for which they are intended. If a subcutaneous or intramuscular injection is inadvertently injected into a blood vessel, it will act too rapidly or have too potent an action, and when medications intended for the subcutaneous route are injected into a muscle, the action may be incomplete or erratic. Some medications intended for intramuscular use are quite irritating to the subcutaneous tissues and can cause bruising or actual tissue damage. Greenblatt and Koch-Weser (1976) indicate that although there is little definitive information about the frequency of adverse reactions to intramuscular injections, serious complications are probably uncommon. Like Hanson (1963), they believe most injection injuries can be avoided by using correct techniques, although there are some apparently inevitable untoward effects associated with injections.

Some *local pain or discomfort* almost always occurs because the needle entry stimulates the numerous pain receptors located in the skin and subcutaneous tissues. Although skeletal muscle is poorly innervated by pain receptors, distention of the tissue from the medication solution can be very painful. This is especially true for large volumes of fluid, irritating solutions, or solutions with a pH or tonicity far from physiological. When given correctly, subcutaneous injections are generally less uncomfortable than intramuscular injections, although the volume or fluid composition can cause discomfort.

Although perception of discomfort with injections is subjective and varies with the individual, a variety of practices will minimize pain and discomfort with injections. These techniques include: (1) using a sharp needle of the smallest gauge (bore or diameter) that can deliver the medication to the desired location in the tissues; (2) inserting the needle quickly through taut skin; (3) exerting counterpressure as the needle is withdrawn; and (4) gently massaging the injection site to help disperse the medication, unless contraindicated. Pain and discomfort can also be reduced by correct site selection and by helping the client relax. General relaxation decreases perception of pain, and relaxation of a muscle allows the needle to enter the tissues more easily and helps the medication to disperse more readily. To minimize the psychological discomfort associated with injections, explain the purpose of the injection or the particular site and method being used, protect the client's privacy, and suggest that he or she avert the eyes during the actual injection. The nature of the medication makes some intramuscular injections more painful than others; ice or ethyl chloride may be used to chill the tissues locally and thus reduce perception of pain sensations. Sometimes 1 ml of ½ percent lidocaine is mixed with antibiotics to decrease pain.

The *trauma* of any intramuscular injection releases the enzyme creatinine phosphokinase (CPK) from muscle cells and causes some elevation of serum CPK levels, particularly with frequent injections. This elevation can interfere with some diagnostic tests for cardiac and liver problems. *Other complications* may occur from incorrect injection techniques, particularly when using the common posterior gluteal site. For example, abscess and cyst formation, necrosis, skin sloughing, and continued pain can occur from subcutaneous injection of medications intended for intramuscular administration; bone bruising or periostitis can occur when a bone is struck; and peripheral nerve damage (including paresthesia and paralysis) can occur when the sciatic nerve is struck (Hanson, 1963).

Correct selection of the injection site and choosing a sufficiently long needle will ensure that the medication actually enters the desired muscle or subcutaneous tissue, thus avoiding many complications. Needle length selection is discussed later, with injection techniques.

INJECTABLE MEDICATION DOSAGE FORMS

Injectable medications are available as drugs already dissolved in water or oil, or as powdered drugs needing to be reconstituted, that is, needing to be dissolved in a diluent to form a solution. As with oral medications, injectable medications are labeled with the amount of pure drug (expressed in grams, milligrams, grains, milliequivalents, or units) in a given volume (expressed in milliliters or minims) of solution. Injectable medications are sterile, labeled for subcutaneous or intramuscular use, and are usually administered in smaller volumes than oral medications.

Powdered drugs are labeled with the volume and type of diluent needed to reconstitute the drug as well as the strength of the resulting solution. Because of the displacement created by the powdered drug, the diluent volume is usually less than the reconstituted volume. For example, when cephalothin sodium (Keflin) is reconstituted by adding 4 ml of sterile water for injection to each gram of drug, the resulting solution has a strength of 500 mg/2.2 ml and a total volume of 4.4 ml.

Sometimes a vial label will list varying amounts of diluent to use to produce varying concentrations. For example, a vial of penicillin containing 5,000,000 units is labeled:

ADD DILUENT	CONCENTRATION OF SOLUTION
23 ml	200,000 U/ml
18 ml	250,000 U/ml
8 ml	500,000 U/ml
3 ml	1,000,000 U/ml

In this example, the correct amount of diluent is the one that produces a concentration comparable to the desired dosage. For example, if the ordered dosage is 2,000,000 units, the nurse prepares the most concentrated solution listed, and uses the concentration of 1,000,000 U/ml in setting up the dosage calculation equation.

Another kind of instruction may accompany a ready-to-mix combination vial. The label may read: "Turn top clockwise and push downward. Shake well to dissolve. Withdraw entire contents to provide a 1 g dose. Provides an approximate volume of 3 ml (330 mg/ml)." If less than the total 1 g contained in the vial is needed, the concentration of 330 mg/ml is used to calculate the dosage.

Sometimes the directions specify only a minimum volume of diluent and give no indication of the displacement involved. In this situation, the minimum amount of diluent is used to dissolve the drug and the entire volume of reconstituted solution is withdrawn into the syringe to measure it. Dosage calculations are based on that volume and the total amount of drug (mg or g) in the vial or ampule. An exception to this rule occurs when a very small portion of the drug in a vial is to be given. In that situation, a larger than minimum volume of diluent would yield a larger and more easily calculated dosage volume.

CALCULATION OF INJECTABLE MEDICATION DOSAGES

With a few exceptions, injectable medication dosages are calculated like oral liquid medications, and similar apothecary–metric conversions may be needed. Insulin dosages are not calculated, but are simply measured in a syringe calibrated in units of insulin. No other syringe is ever used to measure insulin, and an insulin syringe is never used with any other medication. When calculating dosages of reconstituted drugs, remember to *use the reconstituted volume and concentration* rather than the amount of diluent.

The following problems are examples of common types of injectable medication calculations.

1. *Drugs already in solution*
   PROBLEM: You are asked to give 50 mg of meperidine hydrochloride (Demerol), IM. You have on hand a vial containing 75 mg/ml. What volume of medication will you give?
   a. *Factor-label method*

   $$\overset{2}{\cancel{50}} \, \cancel{mg} \times \frac{1 \text{ ml}}{\underset{3}{\cancel{75}} \, \cancel{mg}} = x \text{ (ml)}$$

   $$\frac{2 \times 1 \text{ ml}}{3} = x$$

   $$x = 0.66 \text{ ml or } 0.7 \text{ ml}$$

   b. *Proportion equation method*

   $$\frac{75 \text{ mg}}{1 \text{ ml}} = \frac{50 \text{ mg}}{x \text{ ml}}$$

   $$75 \, x = 50$$

   $$x = \frac{50}{75} = \frac{2}{3} = 0.66 \text{ or } 0.7 \text{ ml}$$

   ANSWER: Give 0.7 ml of meperidine hydrochloride (Demerol), IM.

2. *Dosage calculation requiring apothecary–metric conversion*
   PROBLEM: You are asked to give 0.25 g of Aminophylline, IM. You have on hand a vial labeled "Aminophylline, gr 7½ in 2 ml." How much medication will you give?
   a. *Factor-label method*

   $$0.25 \, \cancel{g} \times \frac{\overset{2}{\cancel{15}} \, \text{gr}}{1 \, \cancel{g}} \times \frac{2 \text{ ml}}{\underset{1}{\cancel{7.5}} \, \cancel{gr}} = x \text{ (ml)}$$

   $$0.25 \times 2 \times 2 \text{ ml} = x$$
   $$x = 1 \text{ ml}$$

   b. *Proportion equation method*

CONVERSION	DOSAGE CALCULATION
$\dfrac{15 \text{ gr}}{1 \text{ g}} = \dfrac{7\frac{1}{2} \text{ gr}}{x \text{ g}}$	$\dfrac{0.5 \text{ g}}{2 \text{ ml}} = \dfrac{0.25 \text{ g}}{\text{ml}}$
$15 \, x = 7.5$	$0.5 \, x = 2 \times 0.25$
$x = 7.5 \div 15$	$0.5 \, x = 0.5$
$x = 0.5 \text{ g}$	$x = 1 \text{ ml}$

   ANSWER: Give 1 ml Aminophylline, IM.

3. *Displacement with reconstituted drugs*
   PROBLEM: You are asked to give Penicillin G Potassium, 300,000 U, IM. You have available a vial containing 1,000,000 units of powdered Penicillin G Potassium. The label reads: "Adding 4.6 ml of Sterile Water for Injection yields 200,000 U/ml." How much medication would you give?
   a. *Factor-label method*

   $$\overset{3}{\cancel{300{,}000}} \, \cancel{U} \times \frac{1 \text{ ml}}{\underset{2}{\cancel{200{,}000}} \, \cancel{U}} = x \text{ (ml)}$$

   $$\frac{3 \text{ ml}}{2} = x$$

   $$x = 1.5 \text{ ml}$$

   b. *Proportion equation method*

   $$\frac{300{,}000 \text{ U}}{x \text{ ml}} = \frac{200{,}000 \text{ U}}{1 \text{ ml}}$$

   $$200{,}000 \, x = 300{,}000$$
   $$x = 3 \div 2$$
   $$x = 1.5 \text{ ml}$$

   ANSWER: Add 4.6 ml Sterile Water for Injection and give 1.5 ml of the resulting solution.

Activity 73-A: Practice Problems for Preparing Injectable Medications

Determine the correct volume of medication to administer.

1. Ordered dose: Demerol, 75 mg, IM p.r.n. q 3 hr. for pain

Available dosage: Meperidine hydrochloride (Demerol) 50 mg/ml
2. Ordered dose: 15,000 U Heparin, SQ, now
Available dosage: Heparin sodium, 20,000 U/ml
3. Ordered dose: Morphine, gr 1/8, SQ q. 3 hr p.r.n.
Available dosage: Morphine sulfate, USP, 16 mg/ml
4. Ordered dose: Prostaphlin, 300 mg IM q 6 h
Available dosage: A 10-ml vial of sodium oxacillin (Prostaphlin), 1 g (powdered drug). Directions on the vial read: "Adding 5.7 ml D_5W results in 250 mg/1.5 ml"

(NOTE: Answers to these problems can be found in Appendix II, pp. 1013-1016.)

DATA BASE

As with oral and topical medications, safe administration of parenteral medications requires a knowledge of the drug and its intended actions and potential side effects, as well as knowing whether the ordered drug and the dosage form are appropriate for the route designated.

Client History and Recorded Data

The health record contains a variety of data that help determine where to administer an injection and what length and gauge needle to use. For example, it contains the client's age, weight, height, diagnosis of client's condition, general state of health, circulatory status, and factors that might interfere with site availability, such as casts, traction, local infections, injuries, or rashes.

The record, kardex, or nursing-care plan reflect the client's mobility, level of consciousness, ability to cooperate, and level of involvement in own care. These factors influence whether an assistant is needed for turning or positioning the client. Knowledge of basic facts about the medication and how it fits into the diagnostic and therapeutic plans provides a basis for explanations or instructions to the client. In addition, the nurse considers the client's level of consciousness, alertness, language skills, understanding of the medical plan and the medication, and the length of time the client has already taken the medication. Although the nursing or medical history indicates the client's mental status and ability to cooperate, those factors change rapidly and are validated by direct observation at the time of the injection.

The record also indicates where previous injections have been given and identifies any problems with past injections, such as hematomas or tender areas. It may also include a prohibition against giving an injection in a particular body part; for example, injections are not given in the arm on the side where a complete mastectomy was performed because of inadequate circulation. Information about needle length or special injection technique may be included on the kardex or the medication record form. Allergy information is always included in the health record and kardex. It is essential that a client's allergy history be known when administering antibiotics or serums (toxoids or diagnostic allergens) because of the potential for anaphylactic reactions. Allergy information is always elicited from or validated with the client. If the client's report contradicts the record, that report must be investigated before administering the drug.

Physical Appraisal Skills

Inspection. Inspection is used to identify anatomic landmarks needed to locate the desired injection site. Adequate visibility is dependent on having a good light source and exposing the entire area. Inspection also reveals any bruises, edema, or open areas at the intended site, which would eliminate the use of that site.

Palpation. Palpation is used to identify the anatomic landmarks pertinent to each injection site. Palpation identifies bony protuberances and the difference between subcutaneous and muscle tissues, as well as the presence of any edema, induration, or tenderness at the intended site, which would eliminate the use of that site.

EQUIPMENT

Syringes

Although there are many different syringe styles and sizes, all syringes have three parts, as shown in Figure 73-9: a barrel with printed calibrations, a plunger which fits inside the barrel, and a tip for attaching a needle. The syringe may have a plain or Luer (spiral threaded) tip. Disposable syringes are made of plastic or glass; reusable syringes are made only of glass. Most agencies use disposable syringes and needles, primarily for convenience and cost. Sterility is guaranteed by the manufacturer, and the cost is less than that for cleaning, resterilizing, and replacing reusable syringes and needles.

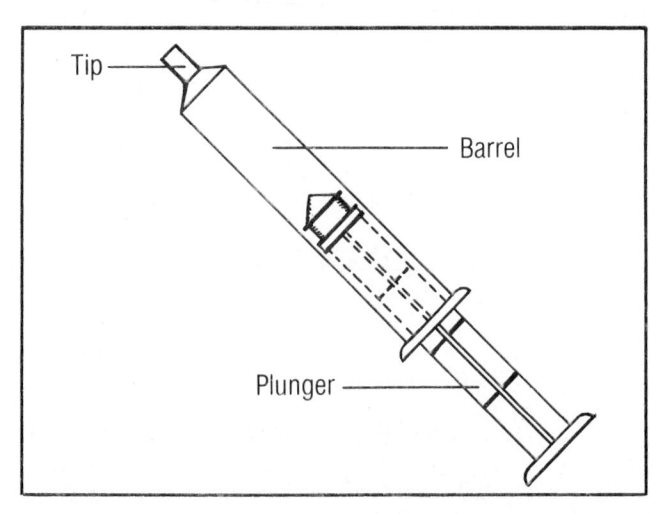

Figure 73-9. Three parts of a syringe: barrel, plunger, and tip for attaching needle.

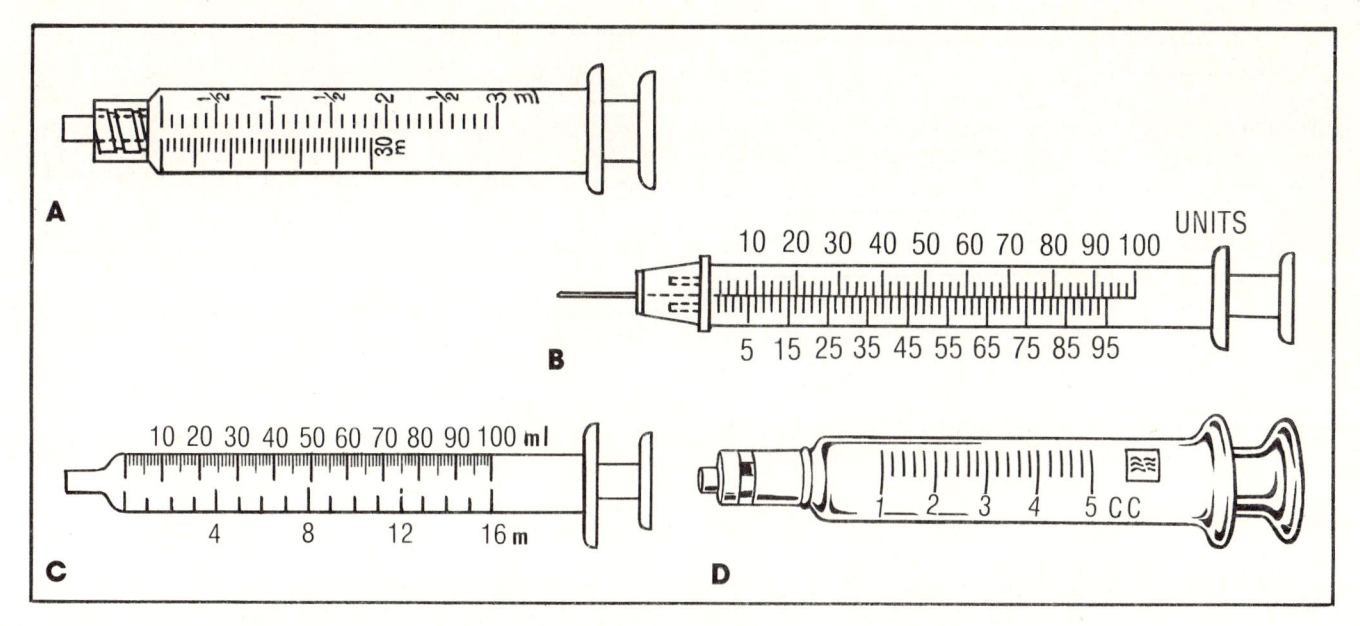

Figure 73-10. Four common types of syringes: **A.** Hypodermic syringe with 3 ml capacity and Luer-Lok tip. **B.** Insulin syringe with preattached needle designed to eliminate dead space. **C.** Tuberculin syringe with conventional tip. **D.** Glass multifit syringe with Luer-Lok tip.

Disposable syringes are packaged individually in a paper or plastic heat-sealed wrapper or rigid plastic container. They may or may not have an attached needle. Needles are also packaged individually, giving a wide variety of available combinations of syringe and needle sizes. The wrapper or container cap is always labeled with the syringe capacity and the needle size, and is usually color-coded to aid in easy selection of the desired syringe and needle.

Many syringes are constructed so there is a small amount of *dead space* in the syringe tip; that is, fluid contained in the tip is part of the measured volume in the syringe but is not emptied when the medication is injected—unless a small amount of air is added to the syringe *after measuring the correct volume*. This air rises to the top of the syringe when it is held vertically and clears the medication from the needle when the plunger is pushed down all the way. The amount of dead space in a 2.5 ml or larger syringe is quite small in relationship to the volume and dosage of medication, and whether the needle is cleared is not a significant factor in determining the accuracy of the dosage. Dead space, however, *can* be a significant factor when measuring potent drugs such as insulin or heparin in narrow diameter, small-volume syringes, as discussed below.

The three most common types of syringes used for medication administration are the common hypodermic, insulin, and tuberculin syringes, as shown in Figure 73-10, along with two types of packaging.

Hypodermic Syringes. Hypodermic syringes are available in 2, 2.5, 3, and 5 ml sizes. Smaller sizes are calibrated in both minim and milliliter scales and larger ones only in milliliters. Larger syringes with a 10, 20, 30, or 50 ml capacity are made similar to hypodermic syringes and used for purposes other than giving medications directly to clients, such as for adding sterile solutions to intravenous infusions or adding medication to a special procedure tray.

Insulin Syringes. Insulin syringes are longer and more slender than a 3 ml hypodermic syringe and have a maximum capacity of 1 ml. The small diameter makes it possible to measure small amounts of the drug insulin accurately. Insulin syringes are made of either glass or plastic; most are calibrated with a 100-unit scale designed only for U-100 insulin. Because U-40 insulin still is available, some syringes are calibrated with a 40-unit scale designed only for U-40 insulin. Some insulin syringes are designed to eliminate or substantially decrease the amount of dead space in the syringe; these syringes have either a preattached nonremovable #28 needle or a specially designed syringe tip and removable needle with the shaft extending into the hub.

Tuberculin Syringes. A tuberculin syringe also has a maximum capacity of 1 ml and is similar in size and shape to an insulin syringe. It is calibrated in tenths and hundredths of milliliters and usually in 16ths of minims up to 1 minim. Although it is designed to administer tuberculin antigen, it can be used whenever small or precise measurement of any medication is needed, such as with heparin or pediatric dosages. Tuberculin syringes have either a removable or nonremovable preattached needle.

Reusable Glass Syringes. Glass syringes are available in sizes similar to disposable syringes and with either plain or luer tips. Many glass syringes are made with an interchangeable (multifit) plunger that fits any barrel, as shown in Figure 73-10D. Glass syringes with a more precise fit are made so that one plunger fits only one barrel, with both the plunger and the barrel numbered so they can be matched after cleaning and resterilizing. Glass syringes can be sterilized along with other equipment in treatment sets prepared by the agency. They are also used to draw arterial blood gas samples, since the gases would diffuse out through a plastic syringe. Disposable commercially prefilled syringes are often made of glass because of the possibility of interaction with plastic during long storage. Glass syringes are used in some physicians' offices and some clinics. The nurse is usually responsible for cleaning and sterilizing the syringes and needles. It is important to follow appropriate cleaning procedures and correct sterilization procedures to prevent transmitting microorganisms from one client to another (see Skill 30). Syringes should be completely disassembled and sterilized without a needle attached.

Prefilled Syringes. Some medications are available in commercially manufactured prefilled plastic or glass unit-dose syringes, labeled and ready for immediate use. In some hospitals the unit-dose system includes prefilling syringes with injectable medications in the pharmacy rather than sending vials or ampules to the clinical unit. In addition to the benefits of the unit-dose system, pharmacy prefilled syringes have the advantages of being prepared under a laminar flow hood using aseptic technique and by persons who are experienced in choosing diluents and calculating dosages.

Needles

The three parts of a needle are the *hub,* which attaches to the syringe tip, the *shaft* or cannula, which is attached to the hub, and a *beveled tip,* which is the slanted opening at the tip of the shaft (see Fig. 73-11A). Needles are made of stainless steel; reusable needles have a stainless steel hub and disposable needles have a plastic hub. Needles are packaged either as part of a syringe-needle unit, or separately, so the needle can be changed to meet the needs of the client, the requirements of the medication, or to provide sterility if the first needle is contaminated. Like syringes, needle packages are also color-coded. Some insulin and prefilled syringes have a nonremovable attached needle. Special care must be taken to avoid contaminating these needles during preparation or administration, since the needle cannot be replaced.

There are three variables that affect selection of a needle for a given purpose or site: gauge, length, and bevel angle. The most commonly used needle *shaft lengths* vary from ⅜ inch to 2½ inches, but lengths from 3 to 6 inches are available for special purposes such as spinal anesthesia or intracardiac and intrathoracic use.

Gauge refers to the diameter of the shaft lumen. Gauge sizes range from 14 to 28, in an inverse relation-

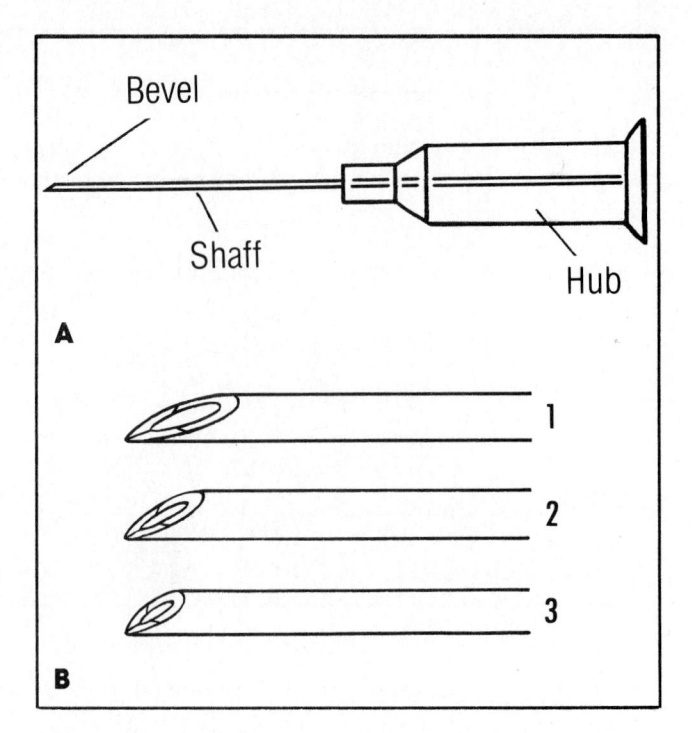

Figure 73-11. Needles for injection purposes. **A.** Three parts of a needle: hub, shaft, and beveled tip. **B.** Three types of beveled tips: (1) long, (2) regular, and (3) short or intradermal.

ship of number to size; that is, the larger the number, the smaller the gauge.

Bevel refers to the narrow slanted tip of the shaft, containing the opening to the shaft, as shown in Figure 73-11B. A long or regular bevel is used for subcutaneous and intramuscular injections because the longer, sharper, and more distinct point enters the skin and tissues more easily. A short (also called intradermal) bevel is used for intradermal injections, because the short bevel more easily enters and remains within the intradermal space.

Vials and Ampules

Both powdered and liquid medications for injection are available in single or multiple-use glass vials or ampules, as shown in Figure 73-12A, B. Vials have a rubber diaphragm that is protected with a lightweight metal cap, lift-up tab, or both. Some ready-mix vials have dual compartments for the powdered drug and its special diluent, separated by a rubber stopper or plug. Compressing the stopper on the upper compartment releases the diluent directly into the powder and reconstitutes the drug. The drug can then be withdrawn with a syringe and needle in the usual manner. Most glass ampules have a prescored neck so the top snaps off easily. Scoring refers to a fine etching line that surrounds the narrowest part of the ampule neck. This etching line enables the glass to break evenly. Manufacturers sometimes indicate prescoring with a colored band around the neck at that point. In the event an ampule is not prescored, use a metal ampule file to etch a line on one side of the ampule neck. To open the ampule, place the thumbs at the etching

SKILL 73: INJECTABLE MEDICATION ADMINISTRATION 901

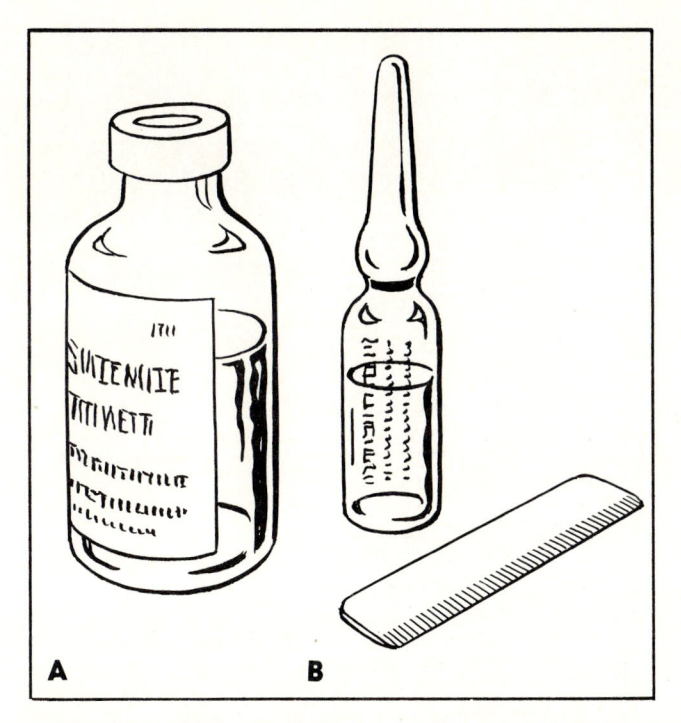

Figure 73-12. Injectable medication containers. **A.** *Vial with rubber diaphragm.* **B.** *Ampule with band indicating prescoring; metal file is used to score unscored ampules.*

mark and snap off the top, as described below. Another option is to use a commercial ampule breaker, as designed by some drug companies.

Prefilled Cartridges
Many injectable drugs are available in prefilled, labeled, disposable glass cartridge-needle units. Instead of a plunger, the cartridge has a piston with a threaded shaft, as shown later in this skill. The cartridges are inserted into a metal device called a Tubex (Wyeth) or a plastic holder such as Carpuject (Winthrop) cartridge holder and administered in the same way as a conventional syringe. Tubex cartridge-needle units are single closed-system sealed units, while Carpuject cartridges are designed so the needle portion penetrates a rubber diaphragm on the cartridge as it is anchored into the holder.

Diluents for Powdered Drugs
The most common diluents used are Sterile Water for Injection, USP or Normal Saline, USP, both of which are available in single or multiple-dose ampules and vials. Some drugs require a special diluent supplied with the drug by the manufacturer, as indicated on the drug label.

Alcohol Swabs
Alcohol swabs are used to cleanse a vial diaphragm before inserting the needle, to cleanse an ampule neck before opening it, and to cleanse the skin before inserting the needle. Most agencies use individually packaged alcohol-saturated cotton wipes for these purposes.

SYRINGE AND NEEDLE DESTRUCTION

Syringes and needles must be disposed of in a way that protects the nurse from accidental needle punctures and makes the used equipment unavailable for illegal drug traffic. The most recent Centers for Disease Control (CDC) recommendations are that personnel use caution when handling all used syringes and needles because it is not always known when blood is contaminated with hepatitis virus or other microorganisms (Garner, 1983). The CDC recommends that needles neither be recapped after use nor be purposely bent or broken by hand because of the potential for accidental needle punctures. No recommendation is made about needle-cutting devices because of incomplete data about their role in needle-transmission of infections from spattered blood. The CDC also recommends placing uncapped needles in a prominently labeled, puncture-resistant container specifically designated for this purpose.

Commercially manufactured boxes are available for discarding syringes with attached needles. The practice of using a disposable plastic gallon jug is unacceptable because needles can readily puncture the thin-walled container. Containers of used syringes and needles may be placed in the general trash for transport to the hospital incinerator where high temperatures completely destroy them. Nurses who work in clinics and physicians' offices will want to find safe methods for disposing of syringes and needles to eliminate the practice of placing intact syringes and needles into the trash for general collection. Many clinics use a syringe and needle destruction device for this purpose, as shown in Figure 73-13. This device severs the needle and damages the syringe, making both unusable for later use with illegal street drugs. There is also a relatively new process available that involves pulverizing syringes and needles and treating them with a chemical that renders them inert.

☐ EXECUTION

The amount of subcutaneous tissue and muscle mass varies with each individual; therefore, the preparation and administration of injectable medications will also vary with the individual. Careful attention to a wide variety of details helps minimize discomfort and promotes absorption of the medication.

PREPARING INJECTABLE MEDICATIONS

Preparation of injectable medications is similar to preparing oral and topical medications in that it is necessary to know the drug's expected action, possible side effects, its role in the therapeutic or diagnostic plan for a particular person, and how to calculate the correct dose to be given. In addition, preparation of injectable medications involves choosing an appropriate

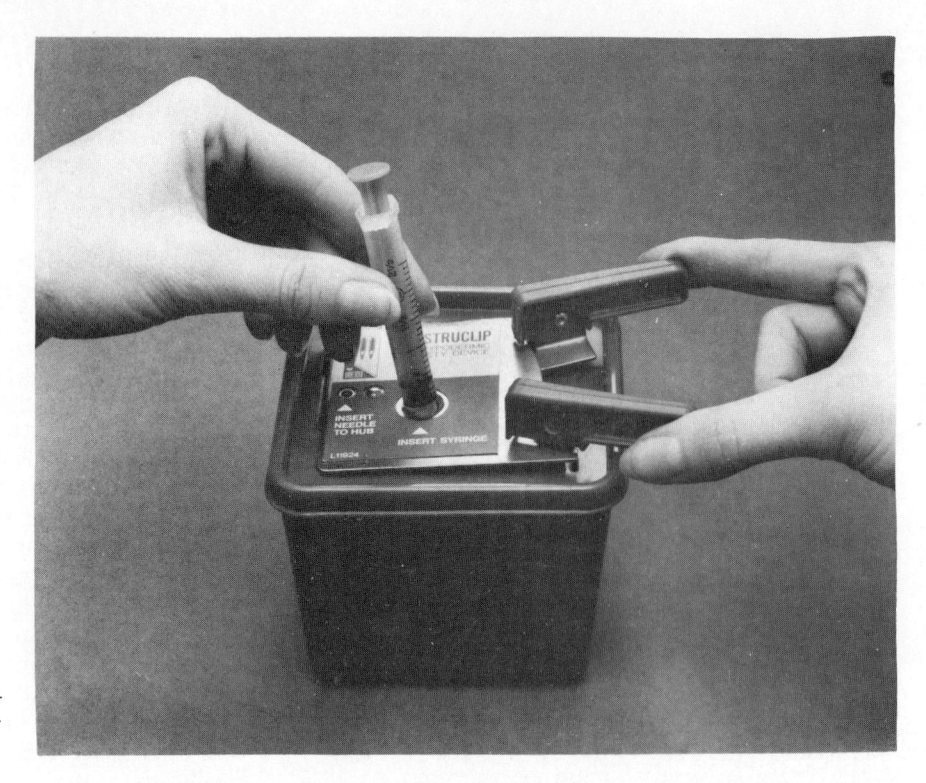

Figure 73-13. Needle and syringe destruction device. (Courtesy of Becton-Dickinson Company, Rutherford, NJ.)

size syringe and needle and being able to use surgical aseptic technique to manipulate syringes, needles, vials, and ampules while withdrawing the medication.

Selecting and Handling Syringes and Needles

Selection of the appropriate syringe and needle sizes is based on the type of injection, type and volume of medication, size of the client, and the site selected. Thick, viscous medications will require large gauge needles. Otherwise, select the smallest gauge needle in the desired length, as smaller gauge needles are less painful. The needle must be long enough to reach the intended site, leaving 0.6 to 1.25 cm (¼ to ½ in) of the needle exposed. On rare occasions, a needle breaks off and it can be lost into the tissues if it was inserted completely to the hub. Criteria for determining needle length are included later, with administration of intradermal, subcutaneous, and intramuscular medications. Common sizes of syringes and needles for various types of injections are shown in Table 73-1.

TABLE 73-1. Common Sizes of Syringes and Needles Used for Injections

TYPE OF INJECTION	SYRINGE SIZE	NEEDLE SIZE
Subcutaneous	2, 2.5, 3 ml	25, 26 gauge ½, ⅝ inch
Insulin	1 ml insulin (calibrated in 100 or 40 units/ml)	25, 26, 27, 28 gauge ½, ⅝ inch
Intramuscular	2, 2.5, 3, 5 ml	20, 22, 23, gauge 1, 1½, 2, 2½ inch
Intradermal	1 ml tuberculin syringe	26, 27 gauge ½, ⅝ inch

Remove the syringe and needle from the package without contaminating the needle. Remove the protective sheath by pulling it straight off, since a twisting motion often dislodges the needle. Always replace the needle sheath after withdrawing the medication or giving an injection. To avoid accidental contamination while withdrawing the medication, stabilize the ampule or vial with the syringe and needle by holding them together in one hand or by resting one hand against the other, as described in the Skill Sequence, "Preparing Injectable Medications."

When pulling back on the plunger to withdraw air or medication, handle only the tip of the plunger, not the plunger itself. The plunger becomes contaminated when it is touched and then the inside of the barrel becomes contaminated as the plunger is pushed back into the syringe to insert air into a vial.

Withdrawing Medication from Vials and Ampules

Vials. Remove the metal cap or cover on the top of a vial. Use an alcohol wipe to cleanse the rubber diaphragm on newly opened single-use vials and multiple-dose vials that are being reused. If there is a round metal perforated tab over the center of the vial, remove it with your scissors or a metal file to avoid injury to your nails or fingers. Withdraw a volume of air into the syringe that is equal to the volume of fluid you plan to withdraw from the vial. Inject that air into the vial. If that volume of air is not inserted, a partial vacuum is created as the medication is withdrawn, making it difficult to measure accurately. Insertion of too much air makes it difficult to control the withdrawal, since the increased pressure forces the

SKILL 73: INJECTABLE MEDICATION ADMINISTRATION **903**

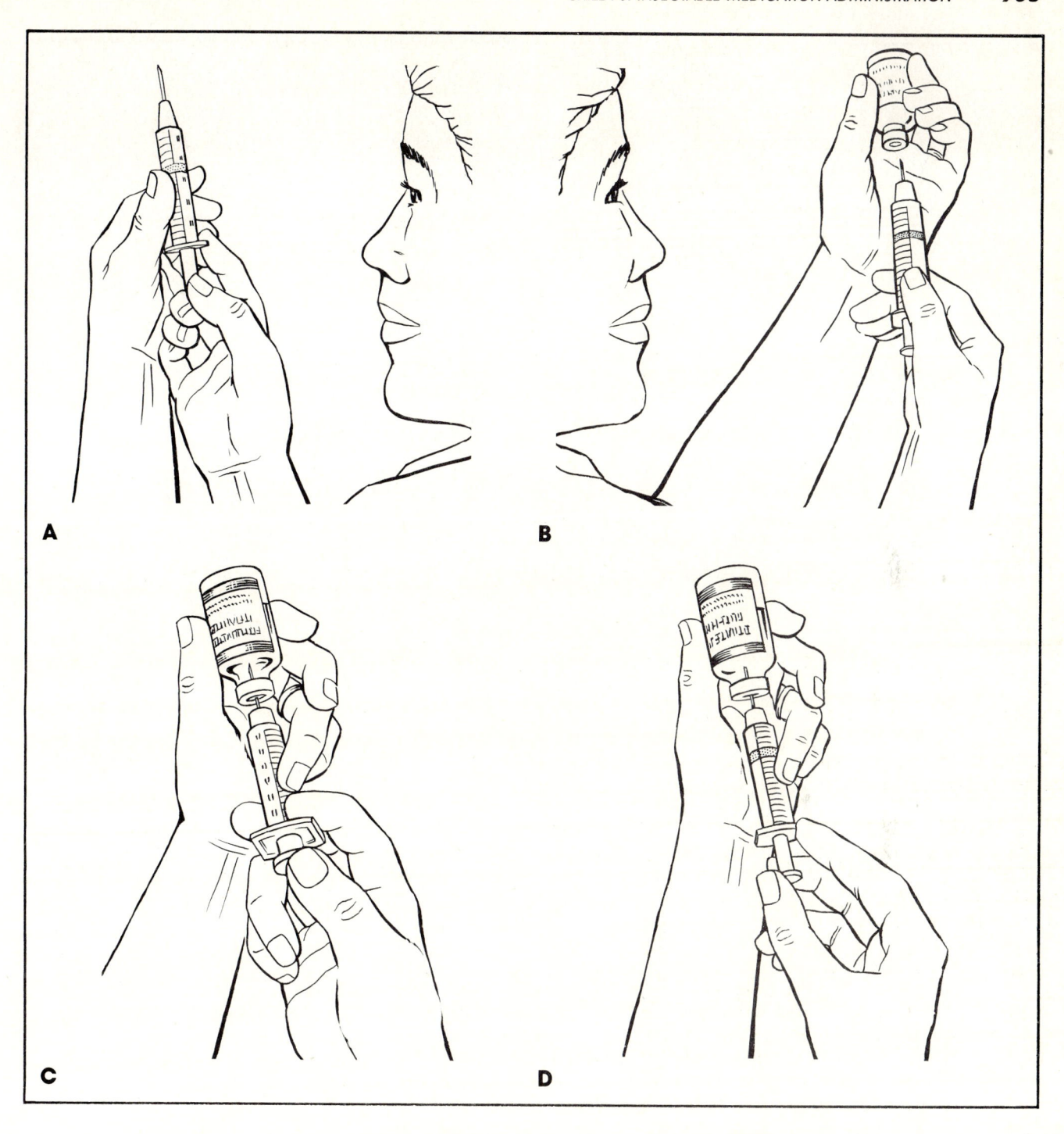

Figure 73–14. Sequence for withdrawing medication from vials. Touch only the plunger tip in each step. **A.** Withdraw volume of air equal to volume of medication to be withdrawn; hold syringe at eye level for accurate measurement. **B.** Hold the inverted vial between nondominant thumb and finger; rest syringe on the hand to stabilize it; and insert needle through the diaphragm. **C.** Inject premeasured air; apply pressure on tip of plunger with thumb. **D.** Withdraw desired volume of medication; use the index finger to provide leverage for withdrawing the plunger.

plunger backward, sometimes quite rapidly. Inject the air into the airspace within the vial to avoid creating bubbles and possibly an inaccurate dosage.

There are several ways to manipulate the syringe and needle to insert the measured amount of air into a vial and withdraw the corresponding volume of medication, as described in the Skill Sequence, "Preparing Injectable Medications," and shown in Figures 73-14 and 73-15. Note that each method stabilizes the syringe, needle, and vial in the nondominant hand, leaving the dominant hand free to manipulate the plunger without any possibility of the needle being withdrawn

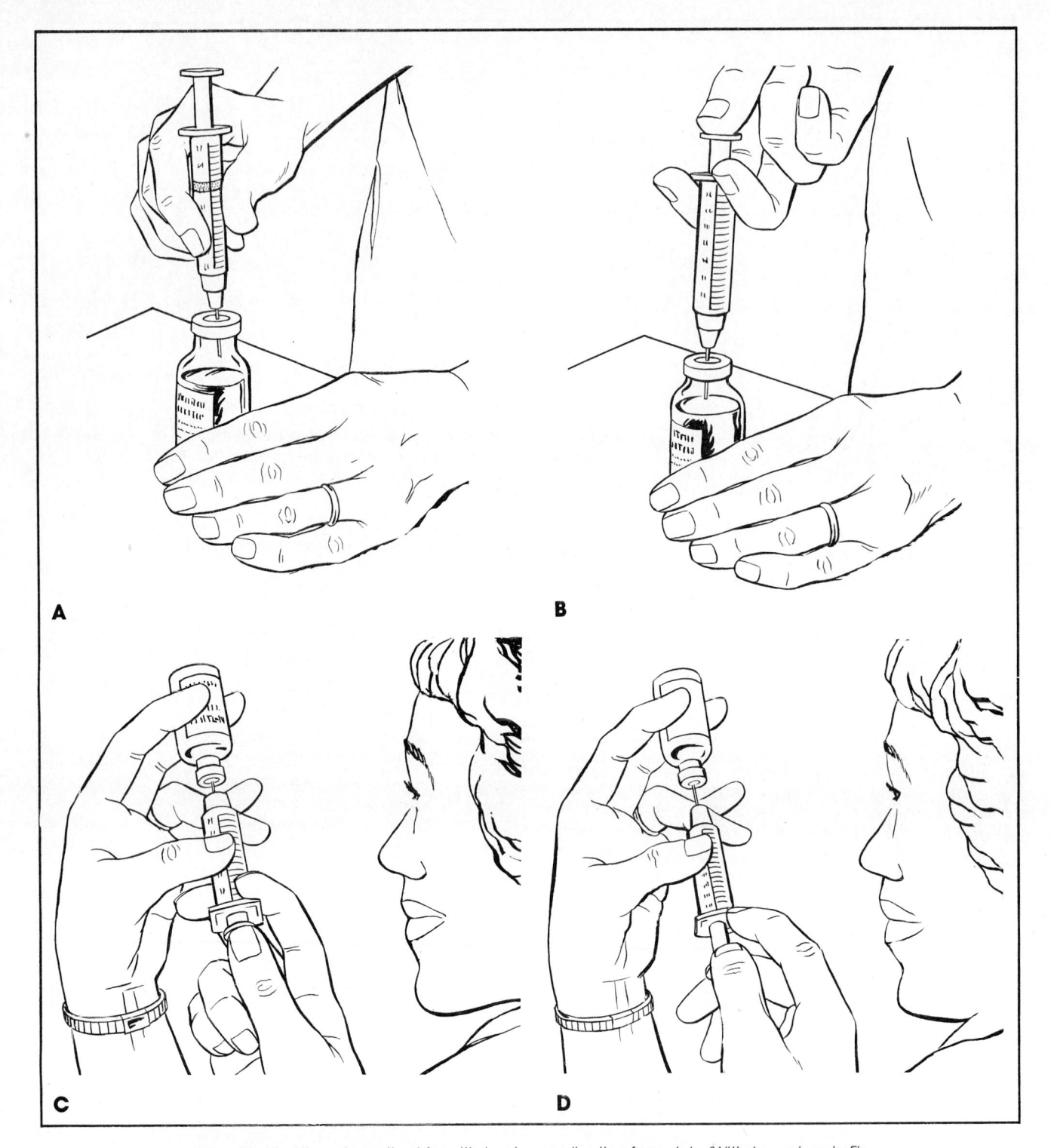

Figure 73-15. Alternate method for withdrawing medication from vials. (Withdraw air as in Figure 73-14A.) **A.** Stabilize upright vial on a solid surface and insert needle through diaphragm but not into the solution. **B.** Inject premeasured air with vial remaining on work surface. OR: **C.** Invert vial and syringe. Hold vial between nondominant index and middle fingers. Hold syringe with thumb and third finger of same hand. Inject air with dominant hand. **D.** Withdraw correct volume of medication.

inadvertently from the vial and becoming contaminated. The vial is always placed upright (as shown in Fig. 73-15B) when inserting the first air for mixing the contents of two vials in one syringe, as described later. If air is inserted with the vial inverted (as in Fig. 73-14C), insert it slowly to avoid causing bubbles.

When air inadvertently enters the syringe while withdrawing the medication, return the air bubble to

SKILL 73: INJECTABLE MEDICATION ADMINISTRATION **905**

plunger tip to expel excess air because the plunger sometimes moves abruptly and quickly, causing inadvertent loss of medication through the needle.

Ampules. Before opening an ampule, be sure that all the medication is in the lower portion of the ampule. If not, hold it in your hand like a thermometer and shake it hard or snap the top with your finger, as shown in Figure 73–17A. Cleanse the ampule neck with an alcohol swab and leave it in place around the neck while you open the ampule, to protect your fingers from injury. Place your thumbs and fingers as shown in Figure 73–17B and simultaneously push away with your thumbs and pull toward you with your fingers to snap off the top easily and evenly. Direct the opening force away from other people to avoid injury in the unlikely event that splintering occurs.

Withdraw medication from an ampule as described in the Skill Sequence, "Preparing Injectable Medications," and shown in Figure 73–18. As you insert the needle into the opened ampule, avoid touching the needle against the open edges of the ampule to prevent contamination. Do not insert air into an ampule before withdrawing the medication, as it is open to the air and has no pressure differential. If air enters the syringe, remove it as described in the Skill Sequence, "Preparing Injectable Medications." If the entire contents of an ampule are not used for one injection, discard the remaining contents, since there is no way to keep it sterile for another, later injection. Discard the ampule in a trash container for glass items.

Mixing Medication in One Syringe
Some medications are mixed and administered in the same syringe to avoid giving two injections; for example, regular and long-acting insulins, as discussed later, and preoperative medications such as meperi-

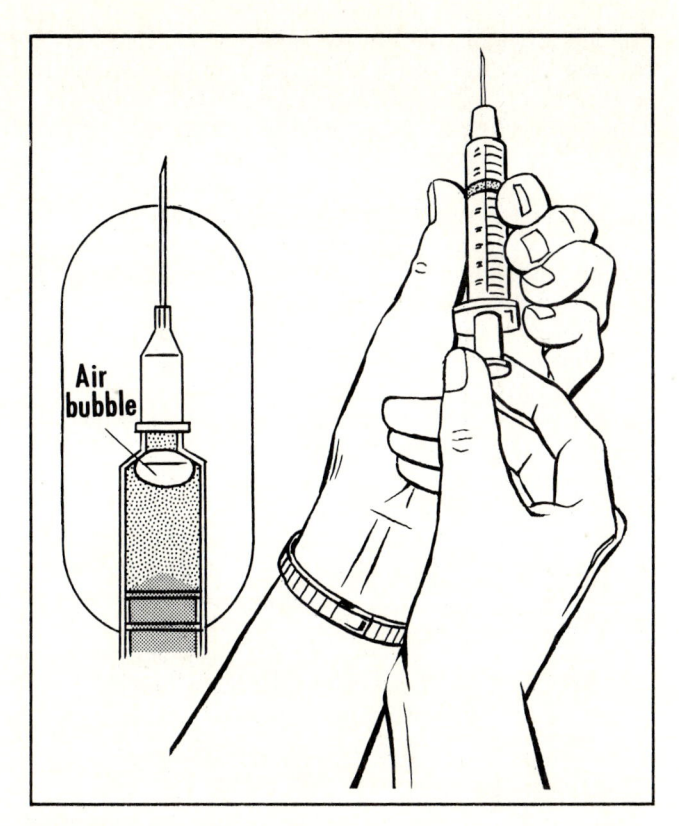

Figure 73–16. To remove air from a syringe, hold it upright and stabilize your hands against each other to avoid inadvertent loss of medication. In this position, the air bubble rises to top of solution, ready to be expelled.

the vial without removing the needle from the vial. If all the medication is withdrawn and excess air is in the syringe, hold it upright and remove the air, as shown in Figure 73–16. Avoid using your thumb on the

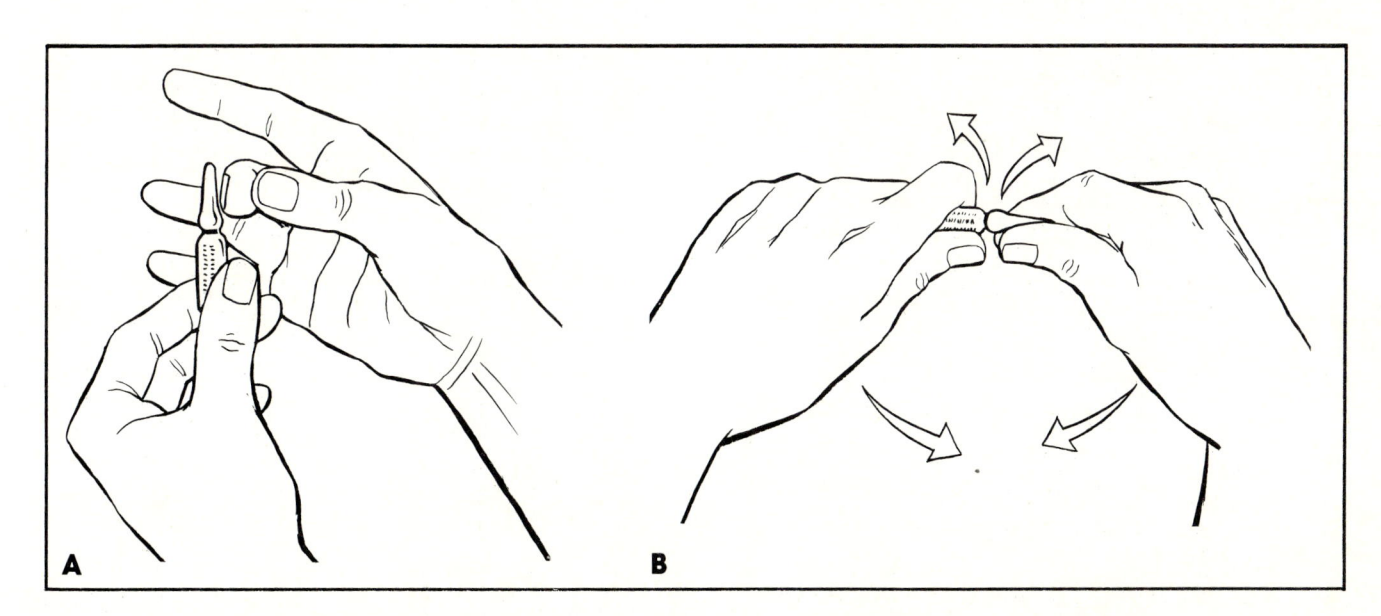

Figure 73–17. Opening an ampule of medication. **A.** Remove solution from the upper portion of an ampule by snapping it with a finger. **B.** Hold ampule with thumbs facing each other. Simultaneously, push away with thumbs and pull back with fingers to snap ampule top off evenly.

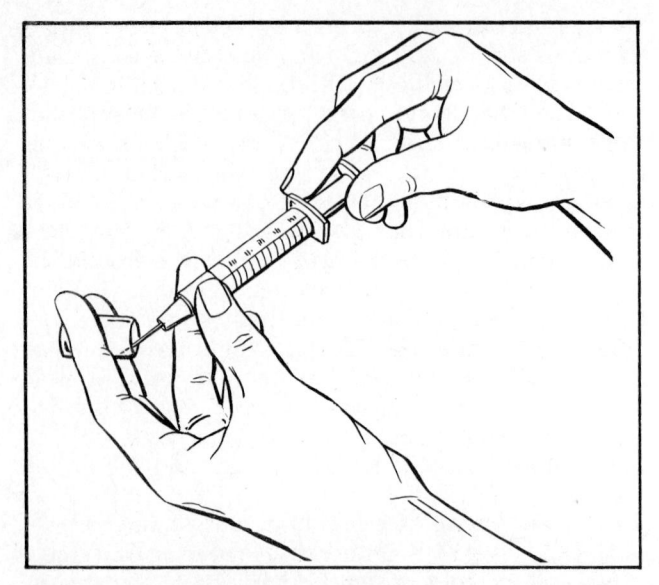

Figure 73-18. Withdrawing medication from an ampule. Stabilize syringe and needle with the ampule in the nondominant hand, leaving dominant hand free to manipulate plunger. Insert needle just inside the opening and tilt ampule gradually to keep bevel within the solution.

dine hydrochloride (Demerol) and atropine. Before mixing two drugs in one syringe, check the compatibility of the two drugs and calculate the total volume that would need to be given. Most clinical units have a list of noncompatible drugs. When in doubt, consult the pharmacist. Incompatible drugs will generally turn cloudy or develop a precipitate when mixed (Kozma and Newton, 1975). If this happens, discard the mixture and give the drugs separately. If the total volume is more than 3 ml, it is usually preferable to give two injections, although clients with large muscles can accommodate up to 5 ml, if injected slowly.

When mixing drugs in one syringe, determine the sequence of inserting air and withdrawing the two drugs that will be the most efficient, the least likely to contaminate a multiple-dose vial, and will most easily obtain the correct amounts of each drug. Always insert air in both vials before withdrawing any medication. Decide which vial you want to withdraw first, and insert air into the other one. Then insert air into and withdraw the medication from the first vial. This makes it possible to insert air in both vials without the possibility of introducing fragments of medication from the syringe or needle into the second vial. *Always insert the air into the first vial with the vial upright on a work surface.* To do this, insert the needle just inside the diaphragm to avoid having it enter the medication. This action avoids the possibility of medication being transferred from one vial to the other either in or on the needle. Use the following guidelines to determine the sequence for mixing medication from two vials in one syringe:

1. If you are using all of the contents of one vial and only part of the contents of another vial, *withdraw the partial volume first.*
2. If you are using a single-dose and a multiple-dose vial, *withdraw the contents of the multiple-dose vial first.*
3. If you are using medication from both a vial and an ampule, *withdraw the contents of the vial before the ampule.*

☐ SKILL SEQUENCE

PREPARING INJECTABLE MEDICATIONS

Step	Rationale
1. Wash hands.	Avoids transfer of microorganisms.
2. Select appropriate medication.	Ensures correct implementation of physician's order.
3. Compare medication order with injectable medication label (SAFETY CHECK 1).	Guards against errors in administration.
4. Calculate correct volume to be given.	Ensures administration of correct amount of medication.
5. Select correct size syringe for volume of medication needed; select needle gauge and length appropriate for client's size, site to be used, and type of medication. Obtain diluent, Tubex, or cartridge holder as needed.	Preparatory for safe administration.
6. Open syringe package without contaminating syringe hub or needle. Add or change needle as needed for site or medication.	Maintains sterility of equipment. Correct length needed to reach site; viscous medications need a larger gauge needle.
7. To withdraw medication from a vial: a. Remove metal cap, center tab, or both. b. Cleanse rubber diaphragm with fresh alcohol swab. c. Remove needle sheath and place it in a safe, clean place. d. Hold syringe at eye level in nondominant hand and withdraw a volume of air equal to desired volume of medication. Touch only syringe barrel and plunger tip. (See Fig. 73-14A)	Provides access to rubber stopper. Removes transient microorganisms that may be present. Protects sheath from contamination. Injecting air equalizes pressure within vial when medication is withdrawn. Avoids contamination of plunger and interior of barrel.

(continued)

Step	Rationale
e. Inject premeasured air into vial (Fig. 73-14 B and C; Fig. 73-15, A, B, C) and withdraw plunger to obtain desired volume (Figs. 73-14D and 73-15D). (NOTE: To avoid causing bubbles in medication, insert air slowly or into air space within vial. Also, if air enters syringe, hold syringe and vial upright vertically, return air to vial, and then withdraw desired volume.)	Injecting insufficient air into vial will create a partial vacuum and make it difficult to withdraw the solution. Excessive air forces solution into syringe, making it difficult to control withdrawal accurately. Bubbles can cause inaccurate measurement. Provides for accurate measurement.
f. Remove needle from vial. If excess air is in syringe, hold syringe vertically upright and expel air carefully. Stabilize hands against each other, as shown in Figure 73-16.	Ensures accurate measurement without inadvertent loss of medication.
g. Replace needle sheath.	Protects sterility of needle.
h. Compare volume and drug label with medication order (SAFETY CHECK 2).	Guards against errors in administration.
8. To reconstitute powdered drugs in vials:	
a. Obtain appropriate diluent.	
b. Follow steps 7a to g to remove diluent from vial.	
c. Follow steps 7a to e to insert diluent into vial of powdered medication. Withdraw needle and replace sheath.	Produces sterile solution for injection. Protects sterility of needle.
d. Rotate, invert, or roll vial between hands to aid in mixing. Avoid shaking, if at all possible.	Thorough mixing without foaming is needed for accurate measurement.
e. Cleanse rubber diaphragm with alcohol swab, reinsert needle, and withdraw needed volume of medication. Remove air as in step 7f. Remove and resheath needle, do SAFETY CHECK 2 as in step 7h, and replace needle sheath.	Ensures correct dosage of medication; protects sterility of needle.
9. To withdraw solution from an ampule:	
a. Move solution from ampule stem to bottom portion: Tap or snap ampule stem with finger (Fig. 73-17A); or hold in hand with stem upward and shake as for a thermometer.	Vibration and centrifugal force aid in moving solution from stem.
b. Cleanse ampule neck with alcohol swab.	Removes transient microorganisms.
c. Place alcohol swab around ampule neck; hold ampule with one thumb on stem and one on bottom of vial; snap off stem by pushing thumbs away from yourself (and not toward other people), as shown in Figure 73-17B. (NOTE: If ampule neck is not scored, use a metal ampule file to etch the glass on the opposite side of the neck from where it will be broken.)	Protects hands from potential injury. Removes stem readily. Avoids possibility of injury from glass fragments. Many ampules are scored for ease in opening. Scratching helps the glass break evenly.
d. Hold ampule between index and middle fingers of nondominant hand and steady syringe with thumb and other fingers. Insert needle without touching open edge of ampule.	Stabilizes ampule and syringe and avoids contamination. Pressure against broken glass edge could dislodge tiny glass fragments.
e. Use thumb and forefinger of dominant hand to withdraw medication from ampule. Keep needle bevel against side of ampule as you withdraw, tilting ampule as needed to keep bevel under level of medication. Keep needle hub out of neck opening of ampule. (See Figure 73-18.)	Allows for easy manipulation of plunger. Avoids having air enter the syringe. Needle hub is regarded as nonsterile, because it is often touched during syringe preparation.
f. If air inadvertently enters syringe, remove air after withdrawing all medication. If syringe capacity cannot accommodate both medication and air, withdraw needle, hold syringe upright vertically, expel air with plunger, reinsert needle and withdraw remaining medication.	Air rises to the top of the medication in the plunger and cannot be expelled when needle is dependent. If air is expelled into an inverted, partially filled ampule, air pressure will force fluid out of ampule.
g. Compare volume in syringe and label on drug with medication order (SAFETY CHECK 2).	Guards against error in administration.
h. Replace needle sheath and place prepared syringe beside medication order, on medicine tray, or take it to client's room to administer it.	Medication is now ready for administration.
i. If medication is in powdered form and needs to be reconstituted, withdraw appropriate diluent from vial or ampule and instill diluent into opened ampule of powdered drug. Check if powder has dissolved and withdraw desired volume. Administer promptly. Check package insert for stability of drug when in solution.	Special diluent may be required. Reconstituted drugs are often unstable in solution.

(continued)

PREPARING INJECTABLE MEDICATIONS (Cont.)

Step	Rationale
10. Combining several medications in one syringe: a. Check compatibility of drugs to be mixed.	Avoids untoward side effects for client or wasting drug if precipitate forms in the syringe.
b. Calculate total volume of medication needed, and obtain appropriate size syringe, up to a maximum of 3 ml (5 ml for a very large muscle mass).	Determines correct dosage and correct size syringe. Maximum volume depends on size of muscle mass.
c. Decide which medication to withdraw first. (See text for decision factors.)	Determines action sequence.
d. Vials: Cleanse both rubber diaphragms. Withdraw air in syringe to equal total volume of medication. With both vials upright, insert air into second vial. Remove needle and insert it into first vial. Instill air and withdraw medication. Insert needle into second vial and withdraw correct amount of medication. Do NOT again add air to first vial.	Provides for adequate displacement of air in both vials. Upright position avoids needle contact with medication and potential contamination of next vial.
e. Ampules: Cleanse and open both ampules. Withdraw medication from first ampule, expel excess air, and withdraw from second vial.	Air displacement is not involved in using ampules.
11. Remove excess air bubbles as needed to obtain accurate measurement.	Ensures correct measurement of dosage.
12. Compare medication order with vial or ampule and volume in syringe. (SAFETY CHECK 2)	Guards against errors in administration.
13. Write date, time, and dosage strength on multiple-dose vials. (NOTE: Medication is now ready for administration to client.)	Appropriate care of equipment. Identifies medication for use at a later time.

Using Prefilled Cartridges

Prefilled glass cartridge-needle units require no preparation; simply select the cartridge unit with the correct drug and dosage, insert it into the holder, and administer it with the same technique as for a regular syringe and needle, as described later. Instructions for loading and unloading a glass cartridge into the metal Tubex are found in Figure 73-19, and Figure 73-20 presents the instructions for the plastic Carpuject. Metal Tubex syringes are available in 1 and 2 ml sizes. A 2-ml Tubex can be adapted for use with a 1-ml cartridge, as explained in Figure 73-19.

Cartridge-needle units designed for each brand can be used interchangeably. A unit designed for a Tubex will fit a Carpuject. To insert a Carpuject unit into a Tubex, first hold the unit in both hands and push the cartridge and needle together to insert the needle into the cartridge stopper, causing a slight popping sound. This action shortens the cartridge-needle unit enough to fit the Tubex.

Leave the needle sheath in place until ready to inject the medication. When you remove the rubber sheath from a Tubex cartridge-needle unit at the client's bedside, you should hear a popping sound if the seal was secure. If your agency policy is to recap used needles prior to discarding them, replace the needle sheath by holding the Tubex upright and dropping the sheath onto the needle. Shake the syringe gently to help the sheath drop into place and then pull it on securely. This method avoids accidental finger sticks from the needle perforating the rubber sheath.

ADMINISTERING INJECTABLE MEDICATIONS

Always use aseptic technique to administer all injections. The techniques used to administer subcutaneous and intramuscular medications are fairly similar, while intradermal technique is quite different, as described below.

Intradermal Injection Techniques

Use a tuberculin syringe to measure and administer the very small volume of medication used for an intradermal injection. Identify the site and place the client in a comfortable, relaxed position with the site exposed; drape for privacy as needed when the back or thigh is used. Cleanse the site first with acetone to remove oil from the skin and then with alcohol to remove transient bacteria. To use the forearm site, support the client's forearm in the nondominant hand, while grasping and stretching the skin taut as shown in Figure 73-21A and described in the Skill Sequence, "Administering Intradermal Medications." Stretch the skin between the thumb and fingers for the other sites.

Hold the syringe so that the needle is almost parallel (15 degree angle) to the skin, with the bevel side of the needle upward. Insert the needle point just under the skin surface, between the epidermis and dermis, until the lumen and bevel are within the skin—*but the outline is still visible.* A good light will help you see this outline or ridge in the skin. If in doubt,

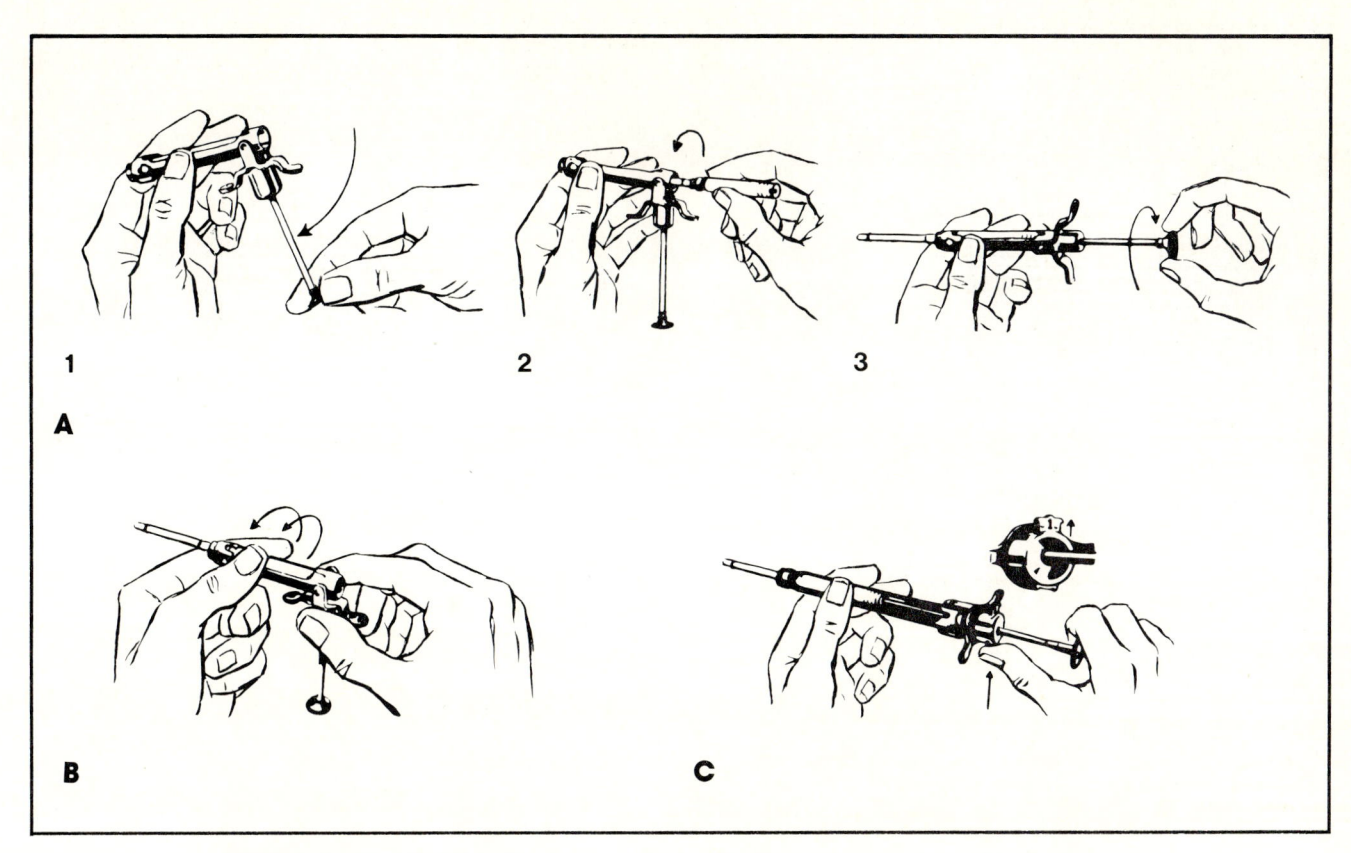

Figure 73-19. Using a Tubex (Wyeth) and glass cartridge-needle unit. **A.** Loading the Tubex syringe: (1) Grasp barrel of Tubex in nondominant hand. With dominant hand, pull back firmly on plunger and swing handle-section downward so that it locks at a right angle to the barrel; (2) Insert prefilled cartridge-needle unit into barrel, needle end first. Rotate unit clockwise until it threads at the front end of the syringe; (3) Swing plunger back into place and attach end to threaded shaft of piston. Hold syringe barrel with one hand and rotate plunger until both ends of cartridge-needle unit are fully, but lightly, engaged. This is indicated by a clicking sound. Do not overtighten, as this makes it difficult to disengage. **B.** Removing the glass cartridge-needle unit: Disengage plunger from piston by rotating it counterclockwise. Pull back plunger rod and swing handle section downward. <u>Do not pull plunger back before disengaging, or syringe will jam.</u> Rotate cartridge-needle unit counterclockwise to disengage it from the front end of syringe. Turn syringe upside down and allow cartridge-needle unit to drop out. **C.** To adapt a 2-ml Tubex syringe for a 1-ml cartridge: engage both ends of cartridge-needle unit and push the slide through so the number "1" appears. After use, syringe resets itself automatically for a 2-ml cartridge. (Courtesy of Wyeth Laboratories, Philadelphia, PA.)

gentle palpation should identify the ridge. If the needle point is freely movable and no outline or ridge is visible or palpable, you have inserted the bevel too deeply. Withdraw it slightly and reinsert it more superficially.

As you begin to inject the medication slowly and gently, you should immediately notice a pale raised wheal (bleb or blister) beginning to form, as shown in Figure 73-21B. In darker-skinned people, the wheal is raised, but remains dark. If a wheal does not form, the needle point is too deep and needs to be repositioned.

After injecting the medication and withdrawing the needle, wipe the site gently with an alcohol swab. Do not massage the site, since that would disperse the medication, rather than allowing it to remain locally. The bleb will gradually disappear or a local allergic reaction will develop within 24 to 72 hours if the person is sensitive to the injected material or if the diagnostic test is positive. After the designated time interval, measure the diameter of the local reaction. Herrmann (1983) gives specific directions for measuring and evaluating the erythema and induration associated with positive reactions.

The following skill sequence gives steps for administering an intradermal injection in the forearm. Alternate sites would be identified and used as needed, depending on the client's status or the physician's directive.

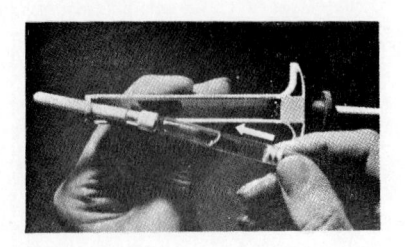

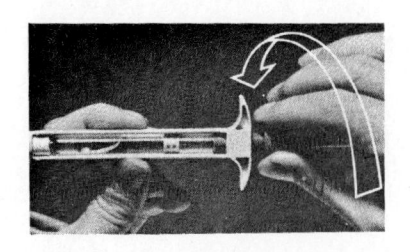

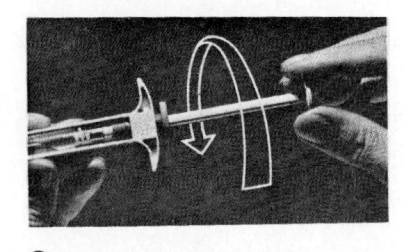

Figure 73-20. Using a Carpuject (Winthrop-Breon) holder and glass cartridge-needle unit. **A.** Insert CARPUJECT Sterile Cartridge-Needle Unit, needle end first, into open side of holder. **B.** Advance and engage blue locking screw and turn clockwise beyond initial resistance until it will no longer rotate. **C.** Advance plunger rod and screw clockwise onto threaded insert in rubber plunger. (NOTE: Reverse procedure to remove cartridge.) (Courtesy of Winthrop-Breon Laboratories, Division of Sterling Drugs, Inc., NY. Carpuject is a registered trademark of Cook-Waite Laboratories, Inc., NY.)

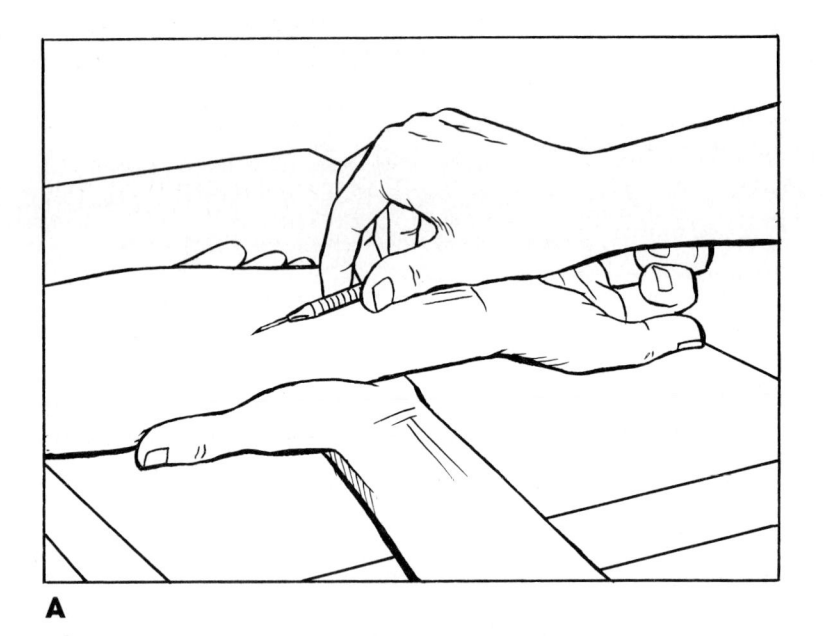

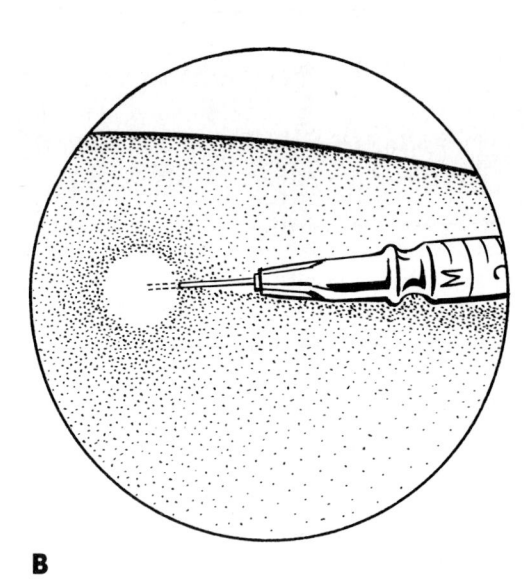

Figure 73-21. Intradermal injection in forearm site. **A.** Cleanse site with acetone and alcohol (not shown). Support and grasp forearm from the under side, stretching skin very taut. Hold the syringe between thumb and four fingers and place needle bevel side up against the skin. Push needle into the skin. Do not aspirate. **B.** Insert solution slowly, beneath epidermis, to create a raised, blanched wheal. Wipe needle entry site; do not massage.

☐ SKILL SEQUENCE

ADMINISTERING INTRADERMAL MEDICATIONS

Step	Rationale
1. Prepare medication as in Skill Sequence, "Preparing Injectable Medications," using a tuberculin syringe.	
2. Identify correct client by comparing the medication order with: a. Room and bed number b. Client's name on identification band c. Client's verbal response to name	Ensures right client will receive medication.
3. Replace needle with a new 27-gauge needle.	Piercing rubber diaphragm on vial dulls small needles on tuberculin syringes. Sharp needle enters the skin more readily. A 27-gauge needle causes less pain and minimizes leakage from needle entry site.
4. Compare medication order with drug label and volume in syringe. (SAFETY CHECK 3).	Guards against errors in administration.
5. Explain procedure and site selection.	Provides information; increases client cooperation.
6. Close door and draw curtains as appropriate for site selected.	Protects client's privacy.
7. Raise bed to comfortable working height.	Promotes nurse safety.
8. Remove clothing or turn back bed linen as needed for complete visualization of site.	Complete visibility is essential for accurate site identification.
9. Identify landmarks and locate site.	Ensures correct anatomic location.
10. Palpate skin for induration or tenderness.	Injection would be more painful at such sites.
11. Instruct client about having site inspected in 24 to 72 hours.	Enlists client cooperation.
12. Cleanse forearm site with acetone, followed by alcohol. Allow to dry.	Acetone defats the skin. Alcohol has antiseptic action. Allowing alcohol to dry prevents stinging with needle entry.
13. Grasp forearm with nondominant hand to hold volar surface skin taut.	Needle entry is easier through taut skin.
14. Hold syringe nearly parallel to the skin (15 degree angle), with bevel upward.	Helps needle enter the skin rather than subcutaneous tissue.
15. Insert needle point into skin until lumen and bevel are within the skin. Outline of needle point is clearly visible in good light.	Needle point needs to be between epidermis and dermis. If needle outline is not visible in good light or distinctly palpable, needle point is inserted too deeply.
16. Inject medication slowly and gently to create a raised wheal immediately.	Medication remains within epidermis, causing distention.
17. Withdraw needle and wipe site gently with alcohol swab. Do not massage site.	If no wheal develops, needle point is inserted too deeply. Massage could disperse medication.
18. Return client to a position of comfort and safety.	Promotes comfort and safety.
19. Provide after-care for equipment: a. Discard empty vial or ampule in designated container. b. Place intact syringes and needles and cartridge-needle units in designated container for later destruction, according to agency policy. Leave needle protector in place over needle. OR c. Sever needle shaft and syringe tip in commercial destruction device. OR d. Rinse glass syringes and reusable needles and return to central service department for cleaning and resterilizing.	Appropriate disposal of glass items. High-temperature incineration completely destroys disposable syringes and needles. Renders syringe and needle unusable for further use. Appropriate care for reusable equipment.
20. Document administration of intradermal medication on medication record form, in nurses' notes, or in computer. Include a description and drawing of location of wheal.	Fulfills nurse accountability. Provides data for later evaluation of response to testing.

General Principles for Subcutaneous and Intramuscular Injections

The following principles and techniques apply to administering medications through both the subcutaneous and intramuscular routes.

1. Palpate bony protuberances used as landmarks. Visual identification alone is inadequate to do this, because the variable amounts of adipose tissue produce visual distortion, unless the person is *very* lean or emaciated. Likewise, it is crucial to *palpate the*

intended site to distinguish between muscle, subcutaneous tissue, and bones. Failure to palpate can result in medication given by an incorrect route and cause harm to the client.

2. Before injecting the medication, add 0.1 to 0.2 ml of air (0.5 ml for iron and other irritating medications, as described later). This air bubble rises to the top of the syringe when it is held vertically, and clears the needle of medication before removing it from the tissues. This action decreases subcutaneous irritation from residual intramuscular medications, helps prevent leakage from the needle entry site, and completely empties the syringe, leaving no dead space filled with medication. Some subcutaneous injections are given with the syringe in a horizontal rather than vertical position, and additional air is not necessary since it will not rise to the top of the syringe (Wong, 1982).
3. Cleanse the skin with alcohol before inserting the needle and allow the alcohol to dry to complete its antibacterial action. Although not widely practiced, there is some indication that skin cleansing may be unnecessary and may actually destroy normal skin flora (Dann, 1966; Koivosto and Felig, 1978; Pitel, 1971).
4. To help the needle enter the skin more easily, stabilize the skin and tissues by stretching the skin taut or by grasping or pinching the tissues between the thumb and fingers.
5. Use a quick darting technique to insert the needle. Slow insertion causes the tissues to "drag" after the needle, stimulates pressure receptors, and causes additional discomfort for the client.
6. Before injecting the medication, aspirate (withdraw the plunger slightly to determine if the needle is in a blood vessel) for all subcutaneous and intramuscular medications, except heparin, as discussed below. It is uncommon to enter a blood vessel during an injection, and if it does happen, blood enters the syringe readily and mixes with the medication quite noticeably. If this happens, discard the medication and syringe and prepare new medication. If only a very slight tinge of red appears at the syringe tip, withdraw the needle and replace it and then administer the medication.
7. Stabilize the syringe and needle while injecting the medication by holding the syringe with the nondominant hand *while that hand remains in contact with the client's body.* This action prevents the needle from moving sideways or in-and-out, which can cause discomfort and tissue injury.
8. Exert slight counterpressure against the needle entry site with an alcohol wipe while removing the needle quickly and in the same direction in which it was inserted. This action again avoids tissue drag, unnecessary tissue trauma, and client discomfort.
9. Massage the injection site to help disperse the medication throughout the tissues, except as noted below.

Techniques that are different for the subcutaneous and intramuscular routes are described in the following sections. They include the method used to hold the skin taut for easy needle entry, the angle at which the needle is inserted, and the way the syringe is held. The needle length varies with the site and the depth of the subcutaneous tissues. In addition, some medications need to be administered with special techniques to avoid hazards or promote optimal absorption, for example, heparin and insulin.

Subcutaneous Injection Techniques

Recommendations and opinions differ about the angle at which a subcutaneous needle is inserted and whether to grasp the subcutaneous tissues between the thumb and fingers or spread the skin at the injection site. For children and most adults, grasping is preferable to spreading, especially if the client is thin, dehydrated, or emaciated. Spreading the skin is satisfactory when there is a sufficient amount of subcutaneous tissue so the end of the needle remains in that tissue, such as in the buttocks area of many females and heavy persons. The decision will depend on the length of the needle and the amount of subcutaneous tissue. A shorter needle (1/2 in) is usually inserted at a 90 degree angle, while a 45 degree angle is used for a longer needle (5/8 in). However, a longer needle could be inserted into a heavy client at a 90 degree angle and a 45 degree angle might be used with a 1/2 inch needle on a very thin adult or a child.

Another acceptable method is to grasp and pick up a layer of skin and subcutaneous tissue and insert a 1/2, 5/8, or 7/8 inch needle at a 20 degree to 45 degree angle at the base of the fold. Learn to use all three methods of inserting a subcutaneous needle and select the method most likely to adequately reach the subcutaneous tissues for the site and that particular client.

Hold the syringe like a dart or hold it between the thumb and four fingers. Various methods of holding the tissues and the syringe are shown in Figure 73-22A-E, subcutaneous injection techniques are shown in Figure 73-23A-C, and both are described in the Skill Sequence, "Administering Subcutaneous Medications."

Heparin Injection. Heparin is an anticoagulant that interferes with clotting time and is used to inhibit clot formation. It is injected deep into the subcutaneous tissues in the abdominal area where the absorption rate is the slowest, thus providing a long-lasting depot of medication. In addition, intramuscular injection may produce a hematoma. Because of the anticoagulant properties of heparin, the following techniques must be used to promote appropriate absorption and avoid causing trauma or bleeding at the site that could result in a hematoma, bruising, and discomfort.

1. Use the dosage strength that yields the smallest volume for the desired dose.

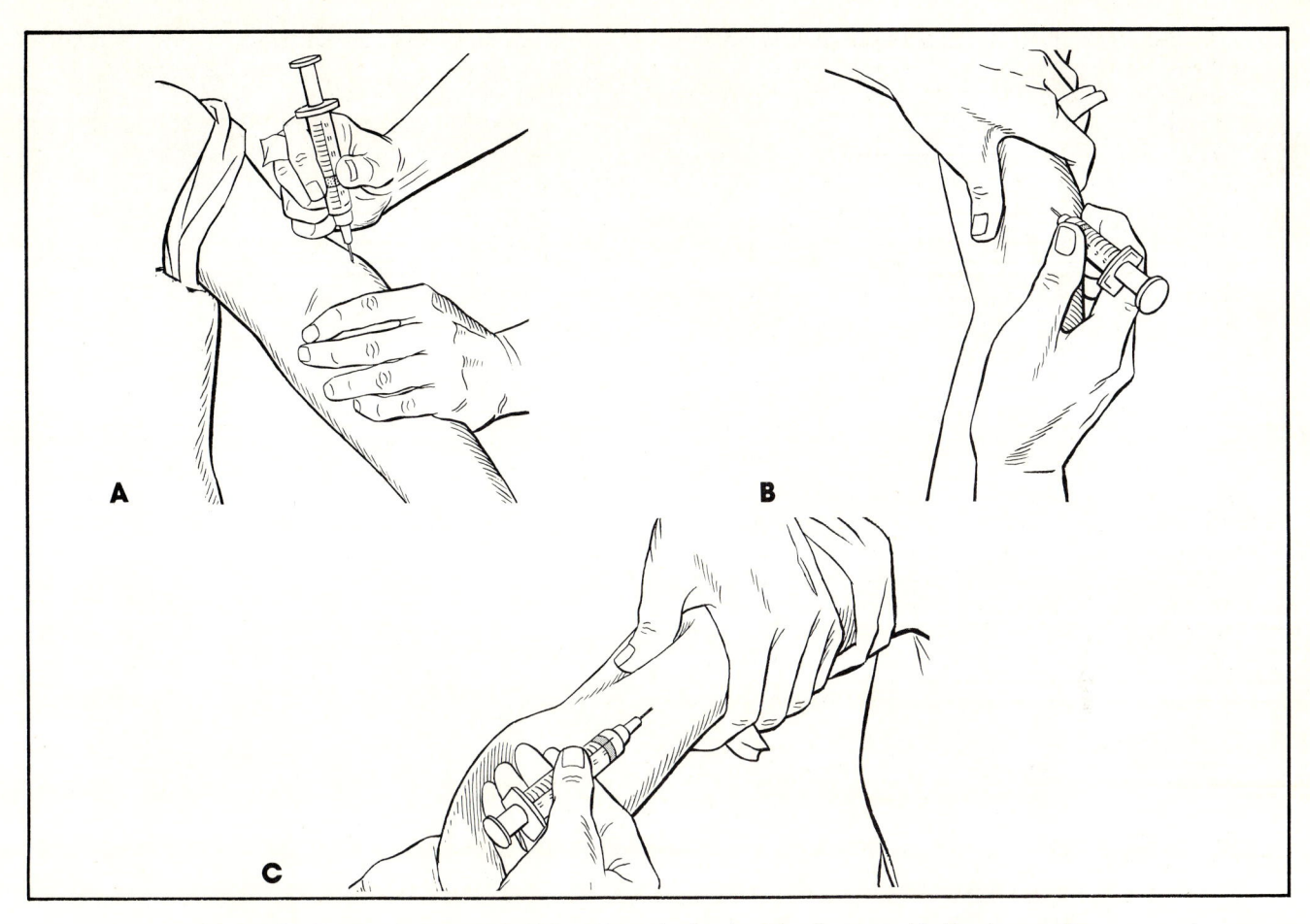

Figure 73–22. *Several ways to hold the skin and subcutaneous tissues and to insert a needle for a subcutaneous injection. Note alcohol swab held between the fingers.* **A** *and* **B.** *Grasp the tissues between thumb and fingers. Hold syringe like a dart. Insert it at a right angle.* **C.** *Grasp the tissues between thumb and fingers. Hold syringe between thumb and four fingers. Insert needle at a 45 degree angle.*

2. Replace the needle used to withdraw the heparin from the vial with a fresh 25-, 26-, or 27-gauge needle.
3. Add 0.05 to 0.1 ml of air to the syringe, to clear the needle after injection.
4. Wipe the selected area gently, rather than massaging it.
5. Stabilize the skin by bunching the tissues gently between the thumb and fingers; by spreading the skin between the thumb and fingers; or with a Z-track technique (described later); the method used will depend on the amount of adipose tissue and agency policy.
6. Avoid injecting heparin within 2 inches of a bruise or scar.
7. *Do not aspirate before injection.*
8. Apply gentle pressure for 1 minute after withdrawing the needle, but *do not massage the area.*
9. Rotate injection sites.

Insulin Injection. Insulin is a potent hypoglycemic (lowers the blood sugar) used in the treatment of diabetes mellitus. Subcutaneous administration provides a depot for gradual absorption. Many diabetic persons take two kinds of insulin, a short-acting regular insulin and a longer-acting modified insulin such as NPH or PZI. Regular insulin is clear, while many long-acting insulins are cloudy in appearance.

Insulin is measured in units of biologic activity, rather than in a weighed volume, and is available in three dosage strengths: U-100 (100 U/ml), U-500 (500 U/ml), and U-40 (40 U/ml). U-100 insulin is the most common insulin. U-500 insulin is available only as regular insulin; it is used for persons with high insulin tolerance and dosage requirements. U-40 insulin is rarely used, but still manufactured. An older insulin strength, U-80, was decertified by the FDA in 1975 and is no longer manufactured.

Insulin is always given with an insulin syringe,

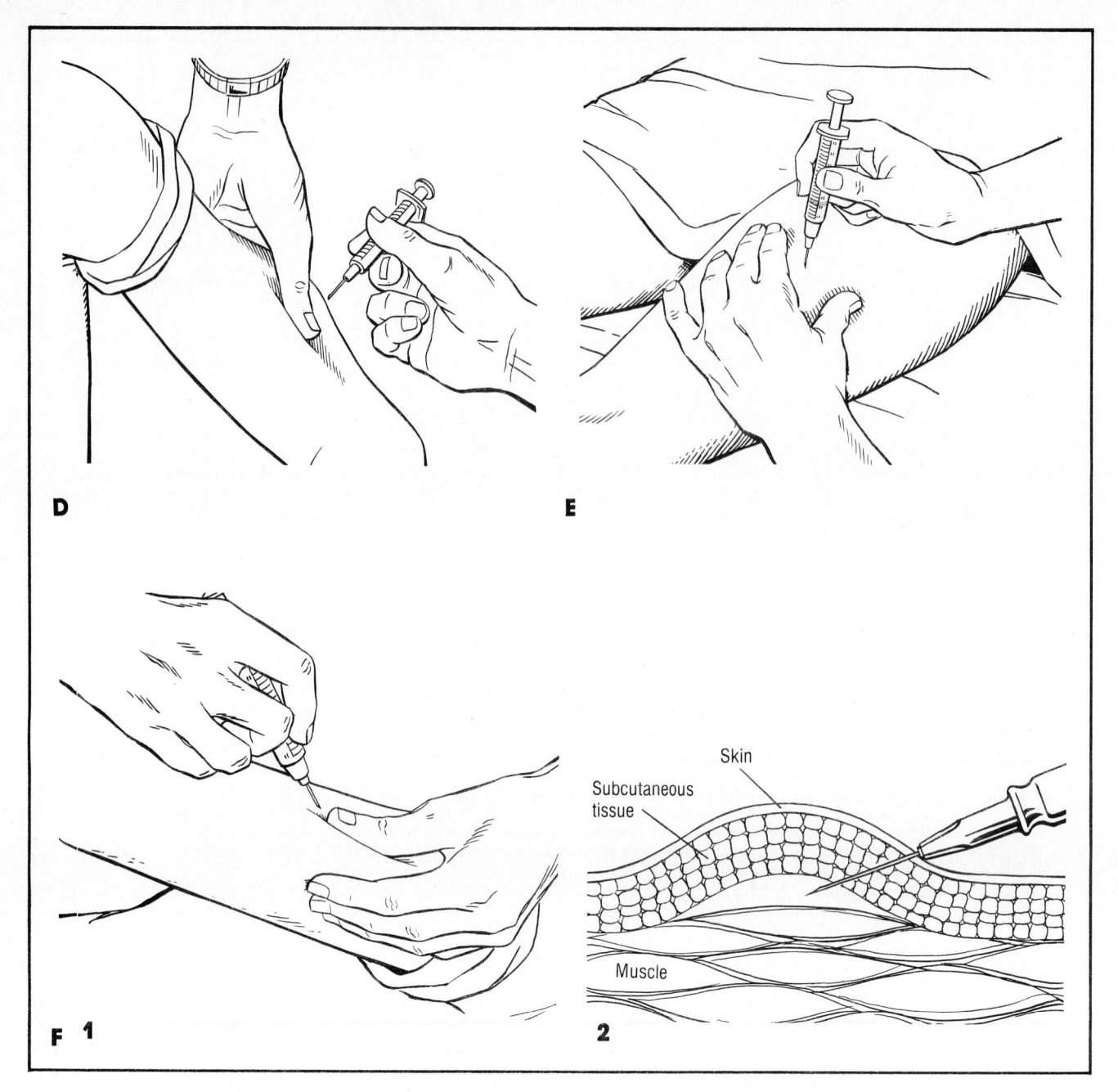

Figure 73-22. *D. Pinch the tissues between thumb and fingers. Hold syringe like a dart. Insert needle at a 90 deree or 45 degree angle. E. Spread the skin between thumb and fingers. Hold syringe like a dart. Insert needle at a 90 degree or 45 degree angle. F. (1) Pinch a fold of tissue between thumb and fingers. Hold syringe between thumb and fingers. Insert needle at base of the fold at a 15 degree to 25 degree angle. (2) Medication is deposited in a "pocket" between subcutaneous and muscle tissues.*

and no other medication is administered with an insulin syringe. Always use a U-100 syringe to measure and administer U-100 insulin, and a U-40 syringe for U-40 insulin. Substituting a syringe with the opposite calibrations would produce a widely different and inaccurate dosage than intended. To administer U-500 insulin, use a U-100 syringe and multiply each calibration by five.

The following techniques are used to administer insulin safely.

1. Rotate vials of modified insulin between the hands to disperse the suspension evenly.
2. Aspirate before injection, since intravenous administration provides a more rapid action than is desired.

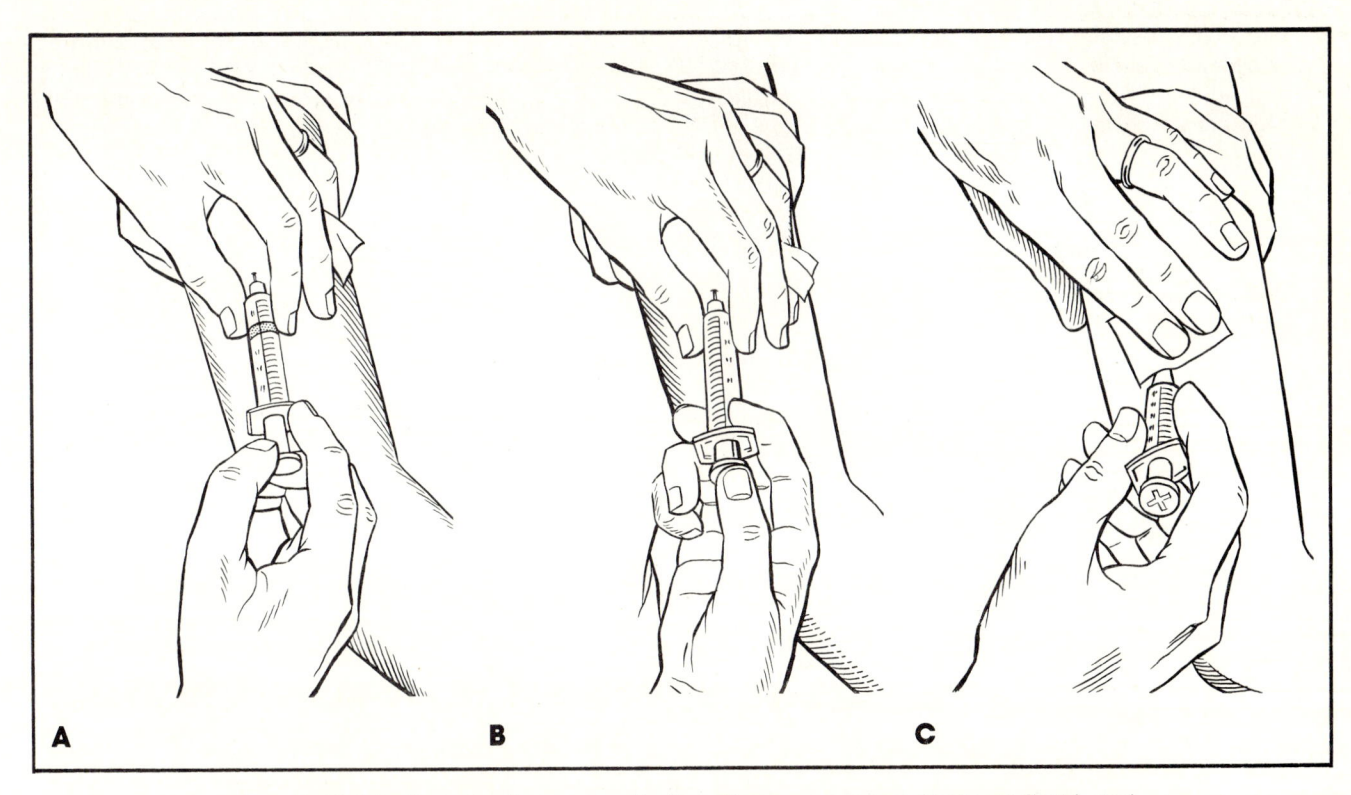

Figure 73-23. Injecting subcutaneous medication. (Tissues were grasped between thumb and fingers and needle inserted at a 45 degree angle, as in Figure 73-22C.) **A.** Stabilize syringe with nondominant hand and aspirate with dominant hand. Index finger on barrel helps stabilize syringe while thumb and middle finger pull back on plunger. Note alcohol swab between fingers. **B.** Place thumb on plunger tip and inject medication slowly. **C.** Place alcohol swab against needle entry site and press gently and firmly while removing needle in the same direction it entered. Massage site gently, unless contraindicated.

3. After withdrawing the needle, apply light pressure without massaging, since massage would hasten absorption.
4. When mixing two kinds of insulin in the same syringe, follow agency policy to determine which one to withdraw first. Syringes with dead space can increase the dosage of the first insulin drawn into the syringe by as much as 8 units, and after mixing in the syringe, the dead space contains an unknown mixture of the two insulins (Wong, 1982). Use the same type of syringe each time and withdraw the two insulins in the same sequence, thus providing the most consistent dosage. In past years the pH of the various types of insulin differed, and there was some concern that inadvertent addition of regular insulin to a vial of long-acting modified insulin could change the pH of the vial over time. All types of insulin now have a neutral pH, so that is no longer a factor. An advantage of withdrawing the longer-acting insulin first is that any contamination of the clear regular insulin is readily visible, because longer-acting insulins usually are cloudy in appearance (Wentworth, 1984). Some sources indicate concern that contamination of the vial of regular insulin with a long-acting insulin can ultimately alter the onset and duration of the regular insulin (Katcher et al., 1983). The problem of mixing two different types of insulin is decreased when each client has his or her own vials. In the home, follow the client's usual mixing sequence to avoid changing the composition of the resulting in-syringe mixture.
5. Rotate injection sites and space the injections about 1 inch apart to avoid lipodystrophy (dimpling or atrophy of adipose tissue) and hypertrophy (thickening of subcutaneous tissues) at the injection site. Avoid reusing a site in less than 6 weeks, if at all possible. Consult medical-surgical nursing textbooks for further information about site rotation, including rotation charts.
6. Follow agency policy about adding air to clear the needle, since consistent use of dead space helps provide consistent dosages.
7. For home use, people with diabetes may soak a glass syringe in 70 percent ethyl alcohol or 90 percent isopropyl alcohol for at least 5 minutes, or boil the syringe for 10 minutes prior to each use. In a recent study, 14 diabetic clients reused their disposable syringe-needle units for 3 successive days over a period of 5 months with no complications and

with considerable cost savings. The needle was wiped with a clean alcohol swab before being recapped, and the syringe-needle unit was refrigerated between uses (Hodge et al., 1980).

8. Store insulin at room temperature, away from excessive heat or cold, as cold insulin contributes to development of lipodystrophy. Refrigerate extra bottles of insulin.

☐ SKILL SEQUENCE

ADMINISTERING SUBCUTANEOUS INJECTIONS

Step	Rationale
1. Prepare medication as in Skill Sequence, "Preparing Injectable Medications."	Ensures correct preparation of medication.
2. Prepare and identify client as in Skill Sequence, "Administering Intradermal Medications," steps 2, and 4 to 8.	
3. Identify landmarks for site. Palpate bony protuberances as needed.	Ensures correct anatomic location.
4. Palpate skin and tissues at selected site. Avoid hardened, inflamed, tender, edematous, or broken skin areas.	Absorption is delayed and injection is more painful at such sites.
5. Cleanse identified site with a fresh alcohol swab, using friction in a circular manner and working from center outward. Hold swab between fingers or place it nearby on client's skin or on bedclothes.	Removes soil and transient microorganisms. Slight local hyperemia helps identify selected site. Alcohol needs to dry for antimicrobial action to occur. Swab is readily available to use when withdrawing needle.
6. Remove needle sheath and withdraw 0.1 to 0.2 ml of air if syringe is to be held vertically or to clear an insulin syringe that has dead space.	Clears needle after injection and helps avoid leakage from needle entry site. Ineffective when syringe is horizontal.
7. Grasp a substantial portion of skin and subcutaneous tissues between thumb and fingers of nondominant hand. OR: Spread skin taut between fingers and thumb, or grasp a fold of tissue between thumb and fingers. (See Fig. 73-22A-F.)	Firms subcutaneous tissue and tightens skin for easier needle entry. Method of holding varies with the site and client.
8. Remove needle sheath and place it in a safe place on the overbed table or hold it between the fingers.	Avoids losing sheath.
9. Hold syringe in dominant hand like a dart in palm of hand, or between thumb and four fingers.	Method of holding syringe varies with the site, insertion angle, or nurse's preference.
10. Insert needle quickly at a 90 or 45 degree angle.	Angle varies with amount of subcutaneous tissue and site.
11. Release pinched or stretched skin, but keep nondominant hand in contact with client and grasp syringe with that thumb and finger. Use dominant hand to aspirate (pull back slightly on the plunger) and observe for blood in syringe. (See Fig. 73-23A.)	Stabilizes syringe and needle during aspiration and injection of medication. Aspiration identifies whether needle is in blood vessel.
12. Inject medication slowly, at a rate of 3 to 4 second/ml. (See Fig. 73-23B.)	Rapid injection causes temporary tissue distention and discomfort from that pressure.
13. With nondominant hand, place alcohol swab on skin adjacent to needle and apply firm but gentle counterpressure as you withdraw needle. Remove needle quickly. (See Fig. 73-23C.)	Helps seal medication in subcutaneous tissue, avoids leakage, and decreases drag of tissues from needle withdrawal.
14. Massage site gently. (Omit massage for heparin and insulin injections.)	Massage increases potential for hematoma at site of heparin injection; increases rate of insulin absorption inappropriately.
15. Observe for superficial bleeding at site and apply bandaid as needed. Replace needle sheath.	Needle may pierce superficial capillaries and cause temporary bleeding. Protects self from accidental needle sticks.
16. Return client to a position of comfort and safety.	
17. Provide after-care for equipment, as in Skill Sequence, "Administering Intradermal Medications," step 19.	Promotes comfort and safety.
18. Document administration of medication on medication record, in nurses' notes, or in computer, according to agency policy. Include site used and any untoward reactions. Record therapeutic action of drug as appropriate.	Fulfills nurse accountability and provides ongoing data base.

Intramuscular Injection Techniques

Estimate the length of the needle you will need to reach through the subcutaneous tissues into the muscle belly and replace the needle on the syringe with one of an appropriate length, if necessary. Avoid the habit of using the same length needle for every person.

Lenz (1983) suggests determining the appropriate needle length for an intramuscular injection by assessing three factors: the muscle mass at the site, the amount of subcutaneous tissue over the site, and the client's overall size. Muscle mass can be estimated for the deltoid and vastus lateralis sites quite easily. To do this, grasp the muscle between the thumb and first two fingers. One-half the distance between the thumb and fingers is the approximate length of needle required to *penetrate* into that muscle. To assess the amount of subcutaneous tissue overlying the muscle, gently pick up the subcutaneous tissue between the thumb and index finger. One-half of the distance between the thumb and finger represents the length of needle required to penetrate the subcutaneous tissue and *reach* the muscle. Adding these two estimated distances to the exposed shaft distance (0.6 to 1.3 cm, or ¼ to ½ in) yields the needle length needed to reach into the muscle belly. Since the ventrogluteal and dorsal gluteal muscles cannot be grasped easily, it is possible only to estimate the depth of the subcutaneous tissue as described above. Estimate the additional needle length required to penetrate the muscle itself on the basis of the client's overall size. For a slender or frail person, a one-inch needle may be required; for a well-developed adult male, perhaps two to three inches; and for an obese person, possibly a four- to six-inch needle. When a very long needle is required, explain its purpose to the client. For consistency of care, record the correct needle length on the kardex or medication record form.

Stabilize the skin and tissues by spreading the site between the thumb and forefinger or by grasping and bunching the muscle between the thumb and fingers. Spreading is preferred when there is a large amount of subcutaneous tissue and fat overlying the muscle, or when the ventrogluteal and dorsal gluteal sites are used, where it would be difficult to grasp the muscle. The action of grasping and bunching small muscles and the muscles in children or thin, frail adults temporarily increases the depth of the muscle and helps insure that the needle point remains in the muscle belly rather than passing through it and striking a bone. To insert the needle into the tissues, hold the syringe like a dart and thrust the needle in quickly and at a right angle to the tissues, as described in the Skill Sequence, "Administering Intramuscular Medications" and shown in Figure 73–24A–E.

Z-track Intramuscular Injection Technique. Some medications, such as iron dextran (Imferon) and chlorpromazine (Thorazine) are so irritating to the subcutaneous tissues that a special Z-track injection technique is used to avoid any leakage into the skin and subcutaneous tissues. In addition to being irritating, iron will cause brown staining in the skin and subcutaneous tissues that lasts for 1 to 2 years.

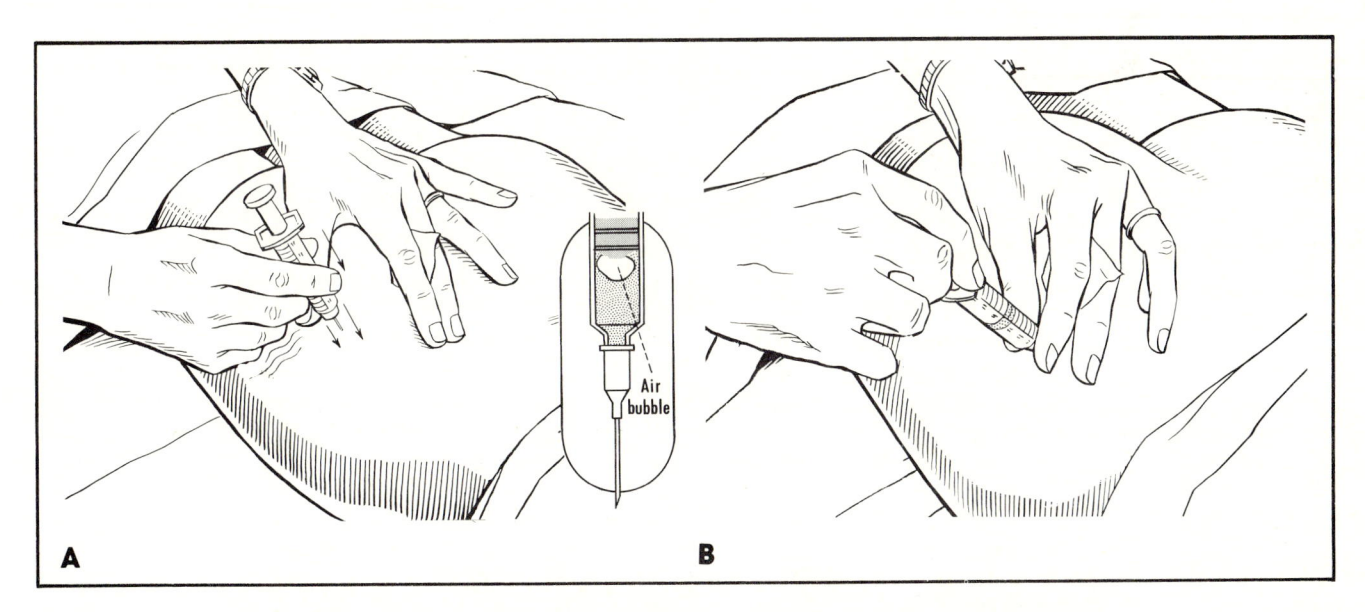

Figure 73–24. *Intramuscular injection sequence, using dorsal gluteal site.* **A.** *Stretch the skin taut between nondominant thumb and fingers. Hold syringe like a dart in dominant hand. Insert needle quickly at a right angle (90 degrees to the skin.) Note alcohol swab between the fingers. Air bubble rises to surface of medication in syringe.* **B.** *Stabilize syringe with nondominant hand* while it remains in contact with client's skin. *Aspirate with thumb and middle finger of dominant hand, placing index finger on the barrel to help stabilize syringe.*

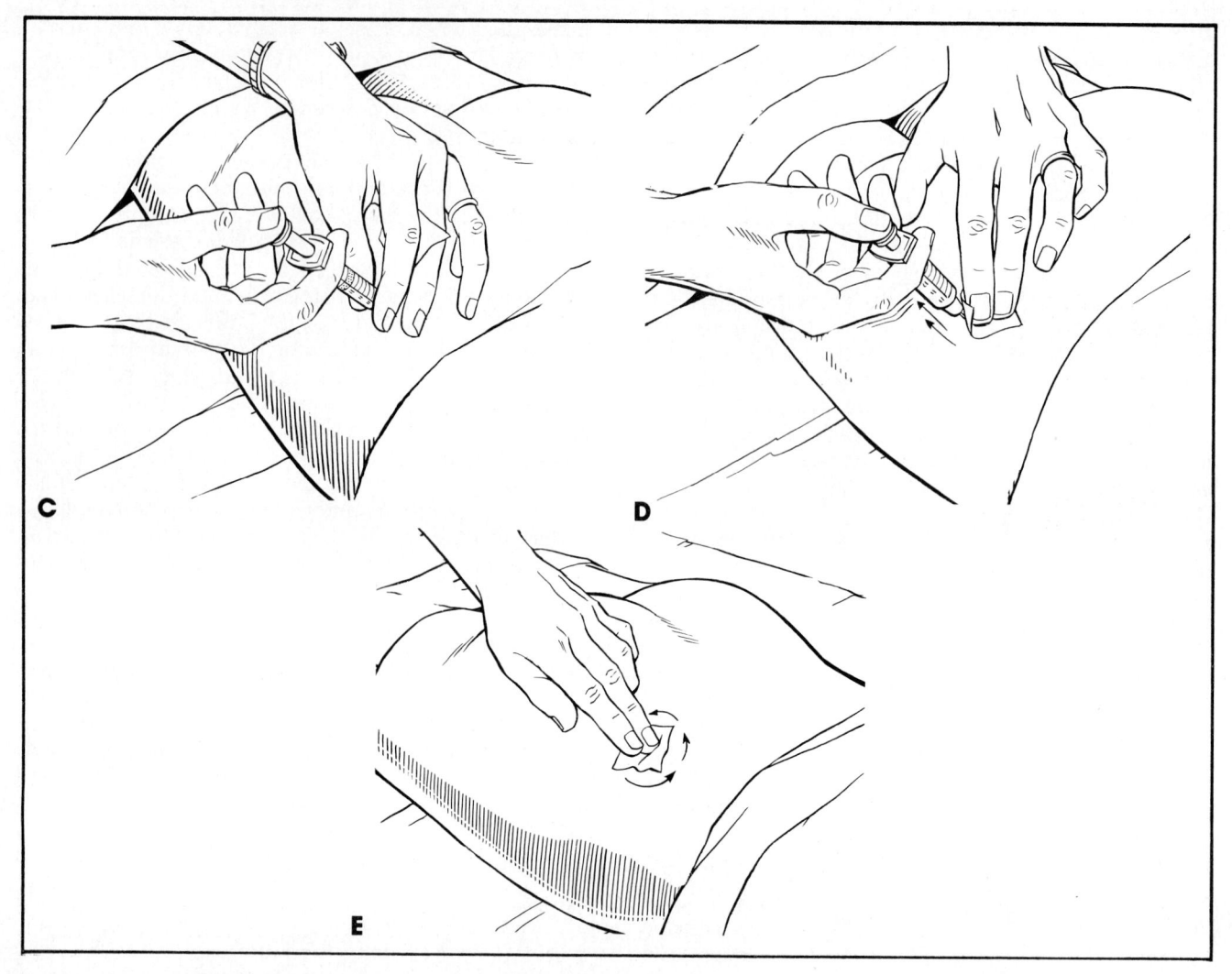

Figure 73-24. C. Continue to stabilize syringe and inject medication slowly. **D.** Place alcohol swab over needle entry site and press gently and firmly while removing needle in same direction it entered. **E.** Massage site gently and firmly.

The Z-track technique uses a clean needle and a lateral displacement of skin and superficial tissues to avoid introducing any medication into the subcutaneous tissues. To implement this technique, first replace the needle used to withdraw the medication with a fresh 19- or 20-gauge needle long enough to penetrate the muscle (2 or 3 inches or longer, depending on body size). Add 0.5 ml of air to the syringe so as to clear it completely after injecting the medication. Use the large dorsal gluteal muscle mass for this technique and identify the site with great care so as to inject the medication into the actual muscle. *Before inserting the needle,* use the side of the hand to displace the skin and subcutaneous tissues laterally *and maintain that displacement* until the medication has been injected. Note that only the skin and overlying tissues have moved laterally, while the muscle tissue remains in position. Insert the needle, therefore, in the identified muscle site, not the laterally displaced skin site. To confirm the presence of muscle tissue after displacement, again palpate the intended site. After injecting the medication, withdraw the needle and release the lateral displacement *simultaneously,* without applying pressure at the injection site. As the tissues are released, a direct needle track from the muscle to the skin surface is eliminated. In addition, the clean needle avoids introducing any medication into the subcutaneous tissues as the needle is inserted and the larger volume of air locks the medication into the muscle.

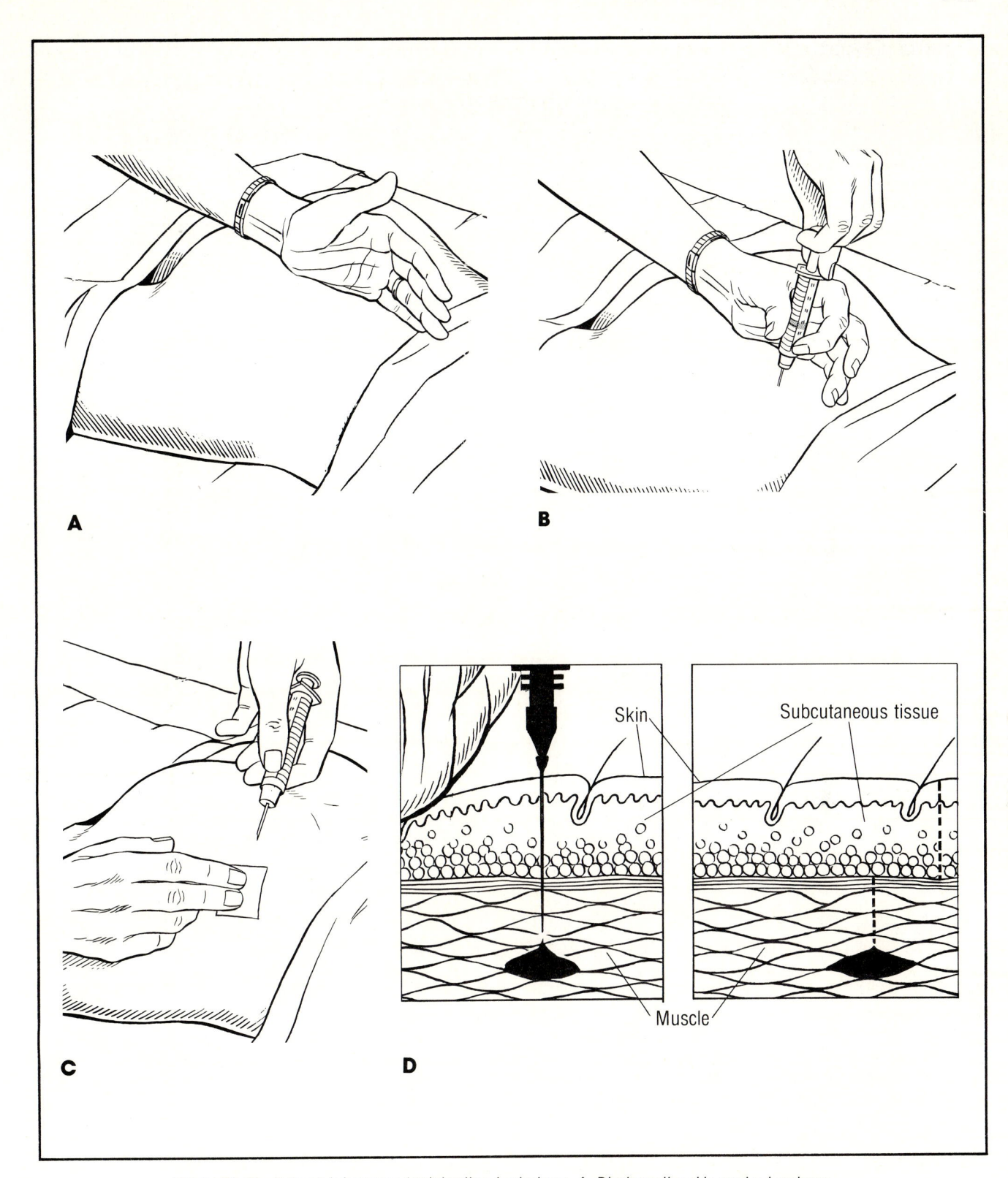

Figure 73-25. Z-track intramuscular injection technique. **A.** Displace the skin and subcutaneous tissues laterally with side of nondominant hand. Insert needle quickly. **B.** Maintain lateral displacement with nondominant hand and use thumb and forefinger to stabilize syringe. Aspirate and inject as for a regular injection. **C.** Remove needle and release tissues simultaneously. Hold alcohol swab lightly on needle entry site. Do not massage muscle injection site. **D.** Diagram shows: (1) Lateral tissue displacement during insertion of needle and medication, (2) Interrupted needle track that seals medication in muscle tissue.

☐ SKILL SEQUENCE

ADMINISTERING INTRAMUSCULAR MEDICATIONS

Step	Rationale
1. Prepare medication as in Skill Sequence, "Preparing Injectable Medications."	
2. Prepare and identify client as in Skill Sequence, "Administering Intradermal Medications," steps 2 to 8.	
3. Identify landmarks and select site, as in Skill Sequence, "Administering Subcutaneous Medications," steps 3 to 5.	
4. Remove needle sheath and withdraw 0.1 to 0.2 ml of air (0.5 ml for iron or other irritating medications).	Clears needle after injection, avoids dead space; helps retain medication in muscle tissue and avoids leakage into subcutaneous tissues with irritation.
5. Spread skin taut between thumb and fingers of nondominant hand; rest side of hand on client's body. (NOTE: For Z-track injection, use side of hand to displace skin and subcutaneous tissues laterally. Keep hand firmly in position until medication has been injected.) (Fig. 73-25A-B.)	Stabilizes tissues and eases needle entry. Provides free thumb and finger to stabilize syringe during injection.
6. Insert needle at 90 degree angle with quick, darting motion. (See Fig. 73-24A.)	Rapid entry decreases tissue drag after needle, thus decreasing discomfort due to pressure sensations.
7. Continue to rest nondominant hand on client's body, release skin and hold syringe with thumb and finger. (Fig. 74-24B.) (NOTE: Modification for Z-track injection: Release tension on skin simultaneously with needle withdrawal in step 10.)	Stabilizes syringe in relationship to client's body. Seals medication in muscle and eliminates direct needle pathway to skin surface.
8. Aspirate with dominant hand (pull back slightly on plunger); observe for blood in syringe. (Fig. 74-24B.)	Identifies whether needle is in blood vessel.
9. Inject medication slowly, at a rate of 1 ml in 3 to 4 seconds. (Fig. 74-24C.)	Rapid injection causes temporary tissue distention and discomfort from that pressure. Also can force medication into subcutaneous tissues.
10. With dominant hand, place alcohol swab on the skin adjacent to needle, apply firm but gentle counterpressure, and withdraw needle. Remove needle quickly. (Fig. 74-24D.)	Helps seal medication in tissues, avoids leakage, and decreases drag of tissues from needle withdrawal.
11. Massage site gently. (Fig. 74-24E.) (NOTE: Modification for Z-track injection: Apply light steady pressure at needle entry site, which is about 1 inch lateral to medication depot; see Fig. 73-25C, D.)	Helps disperse medication. Massage or pressure on medication depot could force medication into subcutaneous tissues.
12. Observe for superficial bleeding; apply bandage as needed.	Needle may pierce superficial capillaries and cause temporary bleeding.
13. Resheath needle or discard it in container or medicine cart, according to agency policy.	Avoids accidental needle stick injuries.
14. Return client to a position of comfort and safety.	Promotes comfort and safety.
15. Provide after-care for equipment, as in Skill Sequence, "Administering Intradermal Medications," step 19.	
16. Document administration as in Skill Sequence, "Administering Subcutaneous Medications," step 18.	

RECORDING

Record the administration of the injection on the medication record form that is part of the permanent health record. In the nurses' notes, record information about the therapeutic effectiveness of the medication and any untoward effects noted. Agency policy varies as to which medications are recorded in nurses' notes as well as in the medication record page or in the computer. In general, p.r.n., stat, intradermal, or experimental drugs are often recorded in the nurses' notes in narrative form or incorporated into POR notes. A sample medication record flow sheet with recorded medications is shown in Figure 5, Chapter 16, Introduction.

Sample POR Recording

- S—"My incision is getting pretty sore! I'd like to have another pain shot now!" "Yes, I have passed some gas today."
- O—Grimacing, holding abdomen. Dressing clean, dry & intact. Abdomen soft; bowel sounds present in LRQ. BP 130/86/80, P 88, R 16.
- A—Post-op incisional pain.
- P—Demerol, 75 mg given IM in Rt. ventrogluteal site for pain @ 5:30 p.m. Continue p.r.n. pain med.; evaluate pain status and medication needs.

Sample Narrative Recording

5:30 PM Reports mod. severe abdominal incisional pain. Dressing clean, dry, & intact. Bowel sounds present in LRQ; abd. soft, states has passed some flatus today. BP 130/86/80, P 88, R 16. Demerol, 75 mg given IM in Rt. ventrogluteal site for incisional pain.

☐ CRITICAL POINTS SUMMARY

1. The subcutaneous route is used for nonirritating drugs in volumes less than 1.5 ml and for sustained slow action.
2. The intramuscular route is used for medication volumes of between 1.5 and 3 ml and for a more rapid absorption.
3. The intradermal route is used primarily for diagnostic testing with minute volumes of drug, such as 0.1 ml.
4. Common subcutaneous sites include the lateral upper arm, the abdomen, lateral thigh, and the scapular and buttocks areas.
5. Common adult intramuscular sites include the deltoid, vastus lateralis, ventrogluteal, and dorsal gluteal areas; the rectus femoris is often used for infants and children.
6. Common intradermal sites are the forearm, upper back, or lateral thigh.
7. Muscle tissue is more solid and firm than the overlying subcutaneous tissues.
8. Stabilize and stretch skin and tissues by grasping, bunching, pinching, or spreading between the thumb and fingers.
9. When both the person and the muscle are relaxed, the needle enters more easily, the medication disperses more readily, and there is less perceived pain.
10. Use surgical aseptic technique to prepare and administer subcutaneous, intramuscular, and intradermal medications.
11. Stabilize the vial or ampule and the syringe and needle in one hand while inserting air or withdrawing medication with the other hand.
12. Dead space is a significant factor in some syringes used to measure small doses of medicine, such as insulin or heparin.
13. Select a needle length and angle of entry that will deliver the medication to the desired location in the subcutaneous or muscle tissue.
14. Stabilize the syringe with a hand that is in contact with the client while aspirating and injecting the medication.
15. Injection of a medication intended for intramuscular use into the subcutaneous tissue can cause tissue destruction.
16. Insert an intradermal needle just under the epidermis so that the needle outline remains visible and palpable.
17. Aspirate before injecting insulin, but do not massage the injection site.
18. To give an injection of heparin, replace the needle used to withdraw the heparin with a fresh needle and do not aspirate or massage the site.
19. A Z-track intramuscular injection displaces the needle track laterally and seals the medication within the muscle.
20. Adding air to the syringe before injecting a medication clears the needle of medication before removing the needle.
21. Accidental needle-sticks can transmit viral infections such as hepatitis from the client to the nurse.

☐ LEARNING ACTIVITIES

1. In a learning laboratory, pharmacy, or central service, examine various sizes and shapes of ampules and vials, including single-dose, multiple-dose, and ready-to-mix vials. Note the scoring on the ampules and the protector for the vial diaphragm. Determine how you would open or prepare each one. Read the instructions for reconstituting powdered drugs, and note whether the label indicates the displacement volume.
2. Work in groups of three: nurse, client, and observer.
    a. Nurse: Locate each subcutaneous, intramuscular, and intradermal injection site on the client, using appropriate anatomic landmarks. Remove enough clothing for adequate visualization of the site and landmarks.
    b. Observer and client: Validate the landmarks and sites identified by the nurse.
    c. Palpate the sites and note the characteristics of the tissues. Ask the client to tense the underlying muscles.
    d. Reverse roles and repeat until each person has played each role.
3. In a practice setting, use unsterile but clean syringes and needles to withdraw fluid from unsterile practice vials and ampules. Inject the fluid into a simulation injection pad, orange, or grapefruit. Empty vials and ampules that originally contained medication may be used for this purpose. Practice

problems appropriate for those vials and ampules of medication can be used to determine the amount of fluid to withdraw. *For simulation purposes, handle the equipment as though it is sterile.* Repeat the activity until you feel comfortable handling the equipment and can calculate correct dosages and withdraw fluid without contamination. Ask for validation of your technique from a lab teacher, peer, or use video-recording if available. Discard fruit that has been used for injection practice.

4. Work with a peer in a practice setting supervised by an experienced person:
   a. Select an appropriate size *sterile syringe and needle.*
   b. *Use aseptic technique* to withdraw Sterile Water for Injection, U.S.P. or Normal Saline, U.S.P. from a vial.
   c. Use correct aseptic technique to inject into the peer:
      (1) 0.5 ml in a subcutaneous site
      (2) 1 ml in an intramuscular site
      (3) 0.1 ml in the forearm intradermal site
   d. Reverse roles and repeat activity.
   e. Compare feelings and perceptions about the experiences of giving and receiving an injection.

☐ REVIEW QUESTIONS

1. In what four body areas are subcutaneous injections most often given?
2. Match the intramuscular injection site in the left column with the anatomic locations in the right column. Items in both columns may be used more than one time.

   INJECTION SITE
   ___ Deltoid
   ___ Dorsal gluteal
   ___ Rectus femoris
   ___ Vastus lateralis
   ___ Ventrogluteal

   ANATOMIC LOCATION
   A. Anterior superior iliac crests and tenth ribs form rectangle.
   B. Center of triangle between acromion process and muscle tip.
   C. Central third of anterior lateral thigh.
   D. Greater trochanter and anterior superior iliac spine form a V.
   E. Greater trochanter and medial and gluteal folds form quadrants.
   F. Greater trochanter and posterior iliac crest form a diagonal line.

3. In what body areas are intradermal injections usually given?
4. Match the site description in Column I with the technique used to stabilize and stretch the skin (Column II).

   COLUMN I
   I. Intramuscular sites:
      ___ Deltoid in an average-sized person.
      ___ Ventrogluteal site in a heavy-set person.
      ___ Dorsal gluteus in a thin person.
      ___ Vastus lateralis in a heavy-set person.
   II. Subcutaneous sites:
      ___ Anterior lateral thigh on a thin person.
      ___ Upper arm site on an obese person.
      ___ Abdominal area on a very thin person.

   COLUMN II
   A. Spread the skin between thumb and fingers.
   B. Grasp tissues between thumb and fingers.
   C. Grasp and bunch muscle tissues.
   D. Pinch tissues between thumb and fingers.

   What factors would be involved in deciding which method to use to stabilize the skin and tissues prior to giving an injection?

5. Match the injection route in Column I with the purpose for that route in Column II.

   COLUMN I
   A. Intradermal
   B. Intramuscular
   C. Subcutaneous

   COLUMN II
   ___ Administer volumes between 1.5 and 3 ml.
   ___ Administer diagnostic tests.
   ___ Provide a depot for slow absorption of medication.
   ___ Provide rapid absorption of medication.
   ___ Provide for local tissue reaction.

6. How would you determine the appropriate needle length and gauge for subcutaneous and intramuscular injections?
7. How would you determine the angle at which to insert a needle for a subcutaneous or intramuscular injection?
8. How do you determine when the needle is inserted correctly for an intradermal injection?
9. How does the Z-track technique avoid subcutaneous tissue irritation and leakage from the needle entry site?

10. Place an "I" (insulin), an "H" (heparin), or an "N" (neither) in front of the appropriate injection technique.
    ____ Aspirate before injecting.
    ____ Massage after injecting.
    ____ Press site gently.
    ____ Use fresh needle for injection.
11. How can you minimize the effect of dead space on insulin dosage if you had insulin syringes with a standard tip?
12. Explain the reasons for each of the following components of preparing injectable medications:
    a. Inserting air into a vial before withdrawing the medication.
    b. Inserting exactly the same volume of air as the desired dosage volume.
    c. Not inserting air into an ampule before withdrawing medication.
    d. Placing an alcohol swab around an ampule neck to break it.
    e. Stabilizing the vial or ampule and the syringe and needle in one hand, leaving one hand free to manipulate the plunger.
    f. Touching only the plunger tip when drawing air into the syringe.
    g. Removing air when measuring the volume in the syringe.
    h. Holding the syringe at eye level to check the volume.
13. Explain the reasons for the following actions involved in giving an injection:
    a. Cleansing the skin with an alcohol swab.
    b. Stabilizing the skin and tissues during needle entry.
    c. Using a quick, darting needle entry.
    d. Stabilizing the syringe during both aspiration and injection with a hand that remains in contact with the person's body.
    e. Aspirating before injecting.
    f. Injecting the medication slowly.
    g. Applying counterpressure as you withdraw the needle.
14. You are asked to give meperidine (Demerol) 75 mg and atropine, 0.2 mg, IM. You have available an ampule of Demerol labeled 100 mg/2 ml and a vial of Atropine labeled 0.2 mg/ml. Answer the following questions.
    a. What volume of Demerol would you give? What volume of atropine?
    b. Why can these two medications be given in the same syringe?
    c. In which vial would you first insert air? Why?
    d. Which vial would you withdraw first? Why?
15. Solve the following dosage calculation problems, using either the factor label or proportion method. Consult an instructor or a peer for assistance as needed.
    a. *Ordered dosage:* Codeine, gr $\bar{ss}$ SQ.
       Available dosage: Codeine sulfate, 60 mg/ml (ampule)
       Answer:
    b. *Ordered dosage:* Atropine, gr 1/300 SQ.
       Available dosage: Atropine sulfate, 0.4 mg/ml (vial)
       Answer:
    c. *Ordered dosage:* Aminophylline 0.5 g, IM.
       Available dosage: Aminophylline 500 mg (7½ gr) in a 2 ml ampule.
       Answer:
    d. *Ordered dosage:* Prostaphlin 750 mg IM.
       Available dosage: Oxacillin sodium (Prostaphlin), 1 g (powdered drug in vial). Directions read: Adding 5.7 ml diluent produces a concentration of 250 mg/1.5 ml.
       Answer:
       (Would you give this volume in one or two injections?)
    e. *Ordered dosage:* Penicillin G 300,000 U, IM.
       Available dosage: Crystalline penicillin G sodium (Penicillin G). Vial contains 5,000,000 U powdered penicillin. Directions:

ADD DILUENT	CONCENTRATION OF SOLUTION
23 ml	200,000 U/ml
18 ml	250,000 U/ml
8 ml	500,000 U/ml
3 ml	1,000,000 U/ml

       Which volume of diluent would you use? What volume would you inject?
       Answer:

☐ PERFORMANCE CHECKLISTS

OBJECTIVE: To use surgical aseptic technique to prepare an injectable medication.			
CHARACTERISTIC	RANGE OF ACCEPTABILITY	SATISFACTORY	UNSATISFACTORY
1. Washes hands.	No deviation		
2. Selects appropriate medication.	No deviation		

(continued)

OBJECTIVE: To use surgical aseptic technique to prepare an injectable medication (cont.).

CHARACTERISTIC	RANGE OF ACCEPTABILITY	SATISFACTORY	UNSATISFACTORY
3. Performs SAFETY CHECK 1.	No deviation		
4. Calculates dosage correctly.	No deviation		
5. Selects syringe and needle appropriate for medication.	No deviation		
6. Opens syringe without contamination.	No deviation		

7. To withdraw medication from vial:
  a. Cleanses diaphragm with alcohol.
  b. Injects volume of air equivalent to dosage into vial.
  c. Withdraws medication into syringe.
  d. Removes excess air.
  e. Replaces needle sheath.
  f. Maintains sterility of needle and syringe plunger (except for plunger tip) throughout procedure.
	No deviation
	No deviation
	
	No deviation
	No deviation
	No deviation
	No deviation		

8. Performs SAFETY CHECK 2.	No deviation		

9. To reconstitute powdered medications:
  a. Injects desired amount of diluent.
  b. Withdraws correct volume.
	No deviation
	No deviation		

10. To withdraw medication from a vial:
  a. Moves solution to lower portion of ampule.
  b. Cleanses ampule neck with alcohol swab.
  c. Snaps off ampule stem away from self.
  d. Inserts needle without touching open edge.
  e. Withdraws desired volume.
  f. Removes excess air.
  g. Replaces needle sheath.
  h. Maintains sterility of syringe plunger (other than tip) throughout procedure.
	Omit if no fluid is in ampule neck.
	
	Score ampule neck first, if not prescored.
	
	No deviation
	No deviation
	
	No deviation
	No deviation
	No deviation
	No deviation		

11. Combining two medications in one syringe:
  a. Calculates total volume.
  b. Obtains correct size syringe.
  c. Inserts air into second vial.
  d. Inserts air into first vial.
  e. Leaves needle in first vial and withdraws medication.
  f. Removes excess air.
  g. Replaces needle sheath.
  h. Maintains sterility of needle and syringe plunger (except the tip) throughout the procedure.
	No deviation
	No deviation
	No deviation
	No deviation
	No deviation
	
	No deviation
	No deviation
	No deviation		

12. Writes date, time, and initials on multiple-dose vials.	No deviation		

OBJECTIVE: To use correct technique to administer an intradermal injection in an appropriate site.

CHARACTERISTIC	RANGE OF ACCEPTABILITY	SATISFACTORY	UNSATISFACTORY
1. Washes hands.	No deviation		
2. Prepares medication. (See first Performance Checklist.)	No deviation		
3. Replaces needle with new 27-gauge needle.	No deviation		
4. Identifies correct client with three checks.	Some clients may be incapable of verbal response to name.		

(continued)

CHARACTERISTIC	RANGE OF ACCEPTABILITY	SATISFACTORY	UNSATISFACTORY
5. Performs SAFETY CHECK 3.	No deviation		
6. Explains procedure to client.	No deviation		
7. Provides privacy.	No deviation		
8. Raises bed to working height.	No deviation		
9. Selects appropriate injection site.	No deviation		
10. Cleanses site with acetone, then alcohol, and allows to dry.	No deviation		
11. Holds skin surface taut.	No deviation		
12. Holds syringe nearly parallel to skin, bevel upward.	No deviation		
13. Inserts needle point into skin only.	No deviation		
14. Injects medication to raise a wheal.	No deviation		
15. Withdraws needle and wipes site with alcohol.	No deviation		
16. Observes client reaction.	No deviation		
17. Returns client to position of comfort and safety.	No deviation		
18. Discards syringe and needle.	Follow agency policy.		
19. Documents in health record.	No deviation		

OBJECTIVE: To use correct technique to administer a subcutaneous injection in an appropriate site.

CHARACTERISTIC	RANGE OF ACCEPTABILITY	SATISFACTORY	UNSATISFACTORY
1. Washes hands.	No deviation		
2. Prepares medication. (See first Performance Checklist, above.)	No deviation		
3. Identifies correct client with three checks.	Some clients may be incapable of verbal response to name.		
4. Performs SAFETY CHECK 3.	No deviation		
5. Explains procedure to client.	No deviation		
6. Provides privacy.	No deviation		
7. Raises bed to working height.	No deviation		
8. Selects appropriate injection site: a. Positions client. b. Exposes area. c. Identifies landmarks. d. Palpates site.	No deviation No deviation No deviation No deviation		
9. Cleanses site with alcohol swab.	No deviation		
10. Adds 0.1 to 0.2 ml air to syringe.	Omit if syringe is to be held horizontally.		
11. Stabilizes skin and tissues with nondominant hand.	No deviation		
12. Inserts needle quickly at a 45 or 90 degree angle, with dominant hand.	No deviation		
13. Stabilizes syringe with nondominant hand.	No deviation		
14. Aspirates.	Omit for heparin administration.		
15. Injects medication slowly.	No deviation		
16. Withdraws needle in same direction as insertion.	No deviation		
17. Applies firm gentle counterpressure as needle is withdrawn.	No deviation		

(continued)

926 PROFESSIONAL CLINICAL NURSING SKILLS

OBJECTIVE: To use correct technique to administer a subcutaneous injection in an appropriate site (cont.).

CHARACTERISTIC	RANGE OF ACCEPTABILITY	SATISFACTORY	UNSATISFACTORY
18. Massages injection site gently.	Omit for heparin and insulin administration.		
19. Observes site and client reaction.	No deviation		
20. Returns client to position of comfort and safety.	No deviation		
21. Discards syringe and needle and medication container.	Follow agency policy.		
22. Documents in health record.	No deviation		

OBJECTIVE: To use correct technique to administer an intramuscular injection in an appropriate site.

CHARACTERISTIC	RANGE OF ACCEPTABILITY	SATISFACTORY	UNSATISFACTORY
1. Washes hands.	No deviation		
2. Prepares medication. (See first Performance Checklist above.)	No deviation		
3. Identifies correct client with three checks.	Some clients may be incapable of verbal response to name.		
4. Performs SAFETY CHECK 3.	No deviation		
5. Explains procedure to client.	No deviation		
6. Provides privacy.	No deviation		
7. Raises bed to working height.	No deviation		
8. Selects appropriate injection site: a. Positions client. b. Exposes area. c. Identifies landmarks. d. Palpates site.	No deviation No deviation No deviation No deviation		
9. Cleanses site with alcohol swab.	No deviation		
10. Adds 0.1 to 0.2 ml air to syringe.	Use 0.5 ml for irritating medications.		
11. Stabilizes skin and tissues with nondominant hand.	Displace superficial tissues laterally for Z-track method.		
12. Inserts needle quickly at a 90 degree angle, with dominant hand.	No deviation		
13. Stabilizes syringe with nondominant hand.	No deviation		
14. Aspirates.	No deviation		
15. Injects medication slowly.	No deviation		
16. Withdraws needle in same direction as insertion.	No deviation		
17. Applies firm gentle counterpressure as needle is withdrawn.	Omit for Z-track method.		
18. Massages injection site gently.	Apply light steady pressure at needle entry site for Z-track method.		
19. Observes site and initial client reaction.	No deviation		
20. Returns client to position of comfort and safety.	No deviation		
21. Discards syringe and needle and medication container.	Follow agency policy.		
22. Documents in health record.	No deviation		

REFERENCES

Dann TC: Routine skin preparation before injection—is it necessary? Nursing Times 62(34):1121–1122, 1966.

Garner JS, Simmons BP: Guidelines for isolation precautions in hospitals. Infection Control 4(4):255, 1983.

Greenblatt DJ, Koch-Weser J: Intramuscular injection of drugs. New England Journal of Medicine 295(10):542–545, 1976.

Hanson DJ: Intramuscular injection injuries and complications. American Journal of Nursing 63(4):99–101, 1963.

Herrmann CS: Performing intradermal skin tests the right way. Nursing83 (Horsham) 13(10):50–53, 1983.

Hodge RH, Krongaard L, et al.: Multiple use of disposable insulin syringe-needle units. JAMA 244(3):266–267, 1980.

Katcher BS, Young LY, et al. (eds): Applied Therapeutics: The Clinical Use of Drugs, ed 3. Spokane, WA, Applied Therapeutics, 1983.

Koivosto VA, Felig P: Is skin preparation necessary before insulin injection? Lancet 1(8073):1072–1075, 1978.

Kozma MT, Newton DW: Nursing guidelines for in-syringe mixtures. Supervisor Nurse 6(8):26–33, 1975.

Kruszewski AZ, Lang SH, et al.: Effect of positioning on discomfort from intramuscular injections in the dorsogluteal site. Nursing Research 28(2):103–105, 1979.

Lenz CL: Make your needle selection right to the point. Nursing83 (Horsham) 13(2):50–51, 1983.

Pitel M: The subcutaneous injection. American Journal of Nursing 71(1):76–79, 1971.

Wong DL: Significance of dead space in syringes. American Journal of Nursing 82(8):1237, 1982.

Wentworth S (Diabetologist): Personal communication. Indianapolis, IN, March 1984.

BIBLIOGRAPHY

All about Tubex. New York, Wyeth Laboratories, 1978.

Blume DM, Cornett EF: Dosages and Solutions, ed 4. Philadelphia, FA Davis, 1984.

Burke EL: Insulin injection: The site and the technique. American Journal of Nursing 72(12):2194–2196, 1972.

Cohen L, Morgan J: The enzymatic and immunologic detection of myocardial injury. Medical Clinics of North America 57(1):105–110, 1973.

Govoni LE, Hayes JE: Drugs and Nursing Implications, ed 5. Norwalk, CT, Appleton-Century-Crofts, 1985.

Intramuscular injections. Philadelphia, Wyeth Laboratories, 1977.

Kozier B, Erb G: Techniques in Clinical Nursing. Menlo Park, CA, Addison-Wesley, 1982.

Lewis LuVW: Fundamental Skills in Patient Care, ed 3. Philadelphia, JB Lippincott, 1984.

Lowenthal W: Factors affecting drug absorption . . . Programmed instruction. American Journal of Nursing 73(8):1391–1408, 1973.

Malseed R: Drug Therapy and Nursing Considerations. Philadelphia, JB Lippincott, 1983.

Newton DW, Newton M: Route, site, and technique: Three key decisions in giving parenteral medication. Nursing79 9(7):18–25, 1979.

Nursing80 Photobook: Giving Medications. Horsham, PA, Intermed Communications, 1980.

Product Information. Winthrop-Breon Laboratories, New York, NY.

Sorensen KC, Luckmann J: Basic Nursing: A Psychophysiologic Approach. Philadelphia, WB Saunders, 1979.

SUGGESTED READING

Hanson DJ: Intramuscular injection injuries and complications. American Journal of Nursing 63(4):99–101, 1963.

Herrmann CS: Performing intradermal skin tests the right way. Nursing83 (Horsham) 13(10):50–53, 1983.

AUDIOVISUAL RESOURCES

Administration of an Intramuscular Injection
  Slides and two cassettes. (1978, Color, 17 min. each.)
  Available through:
    Michigan State University
    Instructional Media Center
    East Lansing, MI 48824

Administration of Medications: Dorsal Gluteal

Administration of Medications: Subcutaneous

Administration of Medications: Vastus Lateralis

Administration of Medications: Ventrogluteal

Administration of Medications: Z-track
  Videorecordings. (1979, Color, 3 min. each.)
  Available through:
    Indiana University
    Nursing Instructional Communications and Educational Resources
    1100 West Michigan Street
    Indianapolis, IN 46223

Location of Sites for Subcutaneous and Intramuscular Injections
  Filmstrip. (1972, Color, 25 min.)
  Available through:
    Henry Ford Community College
    Medical Electronic Educational Services
    954 West Grant Road
    Tucson, AZ 85705

Medicating the Patient: Administering Intramuscular, Intradermal and Subcutaneous Injections
  Filmstrip, video. (1982, Color, 21 min.)
  Available through:
    Medcom, Inc.
    P.O. Box 116
    Garden Grove, CA 92642

SKILL 74 Intravenous Fluid and Medication Administration

PREREQUISITE SKILLS

Skill 19, "Inspection"
Skill 20, "Palpation"
Skill 28, "Handwashing"
Skill 32, "Dressings and Wound Care"
Chapter 16, "Introduction"
Skill 73, "Injectable Medication Administration"

STUDENT OBJECTIVES

1. Identify the primary purposes for which intravenous (IV) therapy is used.
2. Explain principles and practices designed to minimize the risk of intravenous infusion–related infections.
3. Describe the components and purposes of the various fluids available for intravenous infusion.
4. Compare the procedures and rationale for administering medications through a slow infusion, as an IVPB, and as IV push.
5. Specify safeguards needed with intravenous administration of medications.
6. Describe the primary complications associated with intravenous therapy.
7. Explain principles and practices designed to minimize the risk of intravenous infusion–related infections.
8. Describe the signs and symptoms of infiltration and phlebitis at the intravenous infusion site.
9. Identify aspects of intravenous infusion therapy that are left primarily to nursing judgment.
10. Describe special precautions and practices associated with administration of blood and blood products.
11. Describe appropriate physical and psychosocial care required by the client with an intravenous infusion.
12. Specify the components included in a routine hourly assessment of a client with an intravenous infusion.
13. Determine correct flow rates for infusing intravenous fluids by gravity flow or through an infusion control device.
14. Explain the procedures required to change an IV fluid container, administration set, and an infusion site dressing.
15. Describe the procedure required for performing a venipuncture for starting an intravenous infusion and for drawing a blood sample.
16. Demonstrate the ability to perform a safe venipuncture.
17. Demonstrate the ability to prepare an intravenous infusion, add intravenous fluids to an existing infusion, give intravenous medications, and change IV-related equipment.

INTRODUCTION

Intravenous therapy, the administration of fluids, nutrients, or medications into a vein, is an important aspect of the health care received by more than 10 million persons each year. Approximately 30 to 50 percent of all hospitalized clients receive intravenous (IV) therapy (Simmons, 1981). This therapy may be used in acute-care institutions, long-term care facilities, and in the home setting. The intravenous route is being used more frequently than in the past, increasing the nurse's responsibility for safe administration and prevention of complications.

Although administration of fluids by the intravenous route has become widely used only during the past 35 years, the idea has been experimented with for centuries. Initial attempts involved primarily blood transfusions, with the first successful one being performed in Paris in 1667. The enthusiasm surrounding this event led to numerous additional attempts, among them transfusing blood from animals to humans. Not surprisingly, the resulting high fatality rate forced a discontinuation of serious work with transfusions for the following 150 years (Plumer, 1982).

In the early 1900s, at about the time that rapid progress was beginning to be made with blood transfusions, interest in intravenous infusion of other fluids began to develop. Work ensued to make solutions more safe, their variety extensive, and the process of administering an intravenous infusion a less major and more commonly performed procedure.

Currently, over 200 commercially prepared solutions are available for intravenous infusions and a wide variety of administration equipment is in use. Intravenous therapy has become recognized as a highly specialized field, and, in many hospitals, IV therapy teams perform venipunctures and start infusions. This team is composed of highly trained technicians and nurses. In some agencies, these procedures are performed by medical students. Current agency cost-cutting measures, however, may result in these tasks being delegated to the nursing staff in each clinical unit.

Intravenous therapy may be administered by way of a continuous or intermittent infusion of fluid and medication, or by injecting medications directly into the vein. Although this therapy usually is highly successful, it is not without problems, particularly from infections and infiltration. Nurses generally are responsible for overall safe and therapeutic administration of intravenous fluids and medications. This requires a broad knowledge base that is constantly being updated. Nursing interventions and observations are directed toward preventing infection by the use of strict aseptic technique and toward maintaining patency of the cannula by avoiding infiltration and obstruction whenever possible. This skill presents information about intravenous fluids, equipment, and techniques that enable the nurse to assume these responsibilities safely.

☐ PREPARATION

In order to assume competently the responsibility for safe and therapeutic administration of IV therapy, it is imperative that the nurse understand the basic principles of safe fluid administration, become familiar with common parenteral fluids, have a thorough working knowledge of the equipment used, and know how to help the client and family best cope with receiving IV therapy.

THE PHYSICIAN'S ORDER FOR IV THERAPY

The physician's order for intravenous therapy must contain the type of solution to be infused and the rate at which it is to flow. When medications are to be infused, the physician's order includes the specific medication, the dose, and the frequency of administration, exactly as is done for any other medication. When a medication is ordered by the intravenous route, however, the physician must also specify what method of intravenous administration to use. This is not a nursing judgment, and it is not sufficient for the physician simply to indicate that the medication is to be given intravenously. Further clarification, such as "give IVPB" or "give IV push" must also be given.

Typical orders for IV fluid administration might be as follows:

1. IV: 1000 ml D_5W over 10 hr, continuous until D/C'd.
2. IV: 1000 ml NS @ 125/hr.

Typical orders for IV medication administration could be:

1. Tagamet 300 mg IVPB q 6 hr.
2. Lasix 40 mg IV push—now.

Note that the above orders do *not* contain some pieces of information important to successful administration of intravenous therapy. For example, the *IV fluid orders do not specify:*

1. Where the IV is to be started
2. The gauge or type of needle to use
3. The type of equipment to use; for example, bags vs. bottles of fluids and the type of administration set to use
4. The number of drops of solution to infuse per minute

The *medication orders do not indicate:*

1. The type of solution in which to dissolve the IVPB medication
2. The length of time the piggyback should infuse
3. The number of minutes to use to inject the Lasix

These and other aspects of intravenous therapy are decided by nurses each time an intravenous fluid or medication is administered.

PSYCHOLOGICAL REACTIONS TO INTRAVENOUS THERAPY

It is well to remember that although intravenous therapy is a routine procedure for the health team, it is not so for the client and the family, who are likely to view it with fear and concern. Many people assume that intravenous therapy, because of the continued presence of the needle in the vein, will be very painful and therefore need to be reassured that the discomfort is expected to cease once the needle is in place. Clients and families often associate intravenous therapy only with serious illness and are inordinately concerned when told that an IV must be started. This anxiety can be alleviated by explaining the rationale for the therapy and allowing time for questions and concerns before bringing any equipment into the room.

SELECTING AN APPROPRIATE VENIPUNCTURE SITE

A venipuncture (needle entry into a vein) may be performed either to begin an intravenous infusion or to withdraw a blood sample for laboratory analysis. Choosing an appropriate location for a venipuncture plays a large role in the success of both of these procedures, and is one of the most important decisions made in initiating an intravenous infusion. Even in settings where nurses do not start infusions, their input often helps the technician choose a more appropriate site than otherwise might be done. When clients receive long-term intravenous therapy, they are more comfortable when the site is chosen carefully, the venipuncture device anchored securely, and the site protected from trauma.

Selection of an appropriate venipuncture site is based on consideration of the purpose and duration of the venipuncture, the condition of the veins, and the client's safety, mobility, and comfort needs.

When a blood sample is needed for laboratory analysis in either children or adults, one of the large veins in the antecubital fossa is usually an excellent site. With this site, it is important to distinguish between the veins and the superficial arteries in that area. Arteries can be detected by their pulsations and their firm consistency. Suspect an artery puncture when the blood sample is a brighter red than the dusky red color that typifies venous blood. If an artery is punctured accidentally, it is recommended that firm pressure be applied continuously for 10 minutes (longer if the client is receiving anticoagulant therapy), and that the site be observed carefully afterward. Because the pressure within the arterial system is higher than that within the venous system, severe bleeding can result from a single needle stick.

Selecting a venipuncture site for an intravenous infusion is a more complex matter. When large volumes of fluid are to be infused over a relatively short period of time, a larger-bore needle (such as a No. 18 or 20 gauge) is used, and therefore a larger vein is selected. A large vein is also required when administering fluids that are irritating to veins, such as hypertonic solutions or potassium chloride; highly viscous fluids, such as blood or blood products; or when administering chemotherapeutic agents.

When infusions are planned continuously for more than 2 or 3 days, the most distal venipuncture site is selected initially, leaving more proximal sites for subsequent venipunctures. In this way, a vein that has been injured from an infiltration or phlebitis may be reused by going above (proximal to) the injured area. This is especially important during long-term intravenous therapy, because venipuncture sites are changed every 48 to 72 hours, requiring repeated venipunctures.

Palpating the vein prior to performing a venipuncture is an important way to determine whether the vein is healthy enough to receive an intravenous infusion. Veins to avoid are those that feel hard and cordlike (sclerotic) or bumpy (thrombosed or very valvular). A healthy vein feels smooth, pliable, and resilient; this is the preferred type of venipuncture site (Masoorlie, 1981).

Venipuncture site selection is also influenced by the client's medical problems or mobility status. For example, when a client uses crutches or a walker to ambulate, IV sites in either wrist are avoided because of wrist flexion. IV sites in and near joints also are to be avoided because an arm board must be used to prevent joint flexion and there is the potential for the needle to puncture or traumatize the vein.

Intravenous Infusion Sites

Upper Extremities. Most intravenous infusion sites are located somewhere on the upper extremities. The sites on the hands and arms are readily visible, easily accessible, and are the safest and most comfortable for the majority of patients. The veins of the upper extremity and hand are shown in Figure 74–1.

The veins in the *hand* are used when prolonged intravenous therapy is initiated, leaving many proximal venipuncture sites for subsequent use. The most commonly used hand veins are the metacarpal veins, although the digital veins may be large enough to be useful. A short, small-gauge winged needle (described later) is the best choice for venipunctures in the hand. The hand veins are more prone to infiltration; they will not accommodate large needles or irritating fluids, however, and they collapse more quickly when a client is in shock than do more proximal veins.

The size and location of *forearm* veins make them ideal and popular infusion sites. These veins readily receive large needles and irritating fluids and require no joint restriction.

Veins in the *antecubital fossa,* also being large, accommodate large needles, large volumes of fluids, and all but the most irritating of solutions. There are distinct disadvantages associated with the use of these veins for infusions, however. Intravenous infusions in this location require immobilization of the elbow, as damage to antecubital veins would preclude the use of distal sites in that extremity. Another disadvantage is the possibility of accidental entry into an artery. Peck (1985a) indicates that the median antecubital vein is not used to start an infusion as it is too near both the radial vein and artery.

Scalp Veins. The scalp veins are used for intravenous infusion only in the infant and toddler. In these age groups, the scalp veins provide the best site for intravenous therapy due to the abundant supply of superficial veins that are easily located and whose use requires minimal restriction of movement (Plumer, 1982).

Central Veins. The central veins are those in the neck and trunk, such as the external jugular, the cephalic, and the subclavian. The process of infusing fluids into these central veins is a relatively new and rapidly expanding type of intravenous therapy. When a central infusion is started, the nurse's role is that of assisting the physician.

Lower Extremities. The lower extremities are used only as a last resort. Not only are veins in the lower extremities relatively inaccessible, but their use can be quite dangerous. In the lower extremities, superficial veins have frequent connections with the deep veins, and a thrombus that develops in a superficial vein can easily extend into a deep vein, where it can break off and result in pulmonary embolism (Plumer, 1982). The mortality rate for this complication is approximately 38 percent (Luckmann and Sorensen, 1980). Therefore, the risks involved in using the lower extremities are far too great to make them a likely site for intravenous therapy.

INTRAVENOUS FLUIDS

With the multitude of intravenous fluids in current use, it is not surprising that many nurses know little about the composition or effects of the infusions they

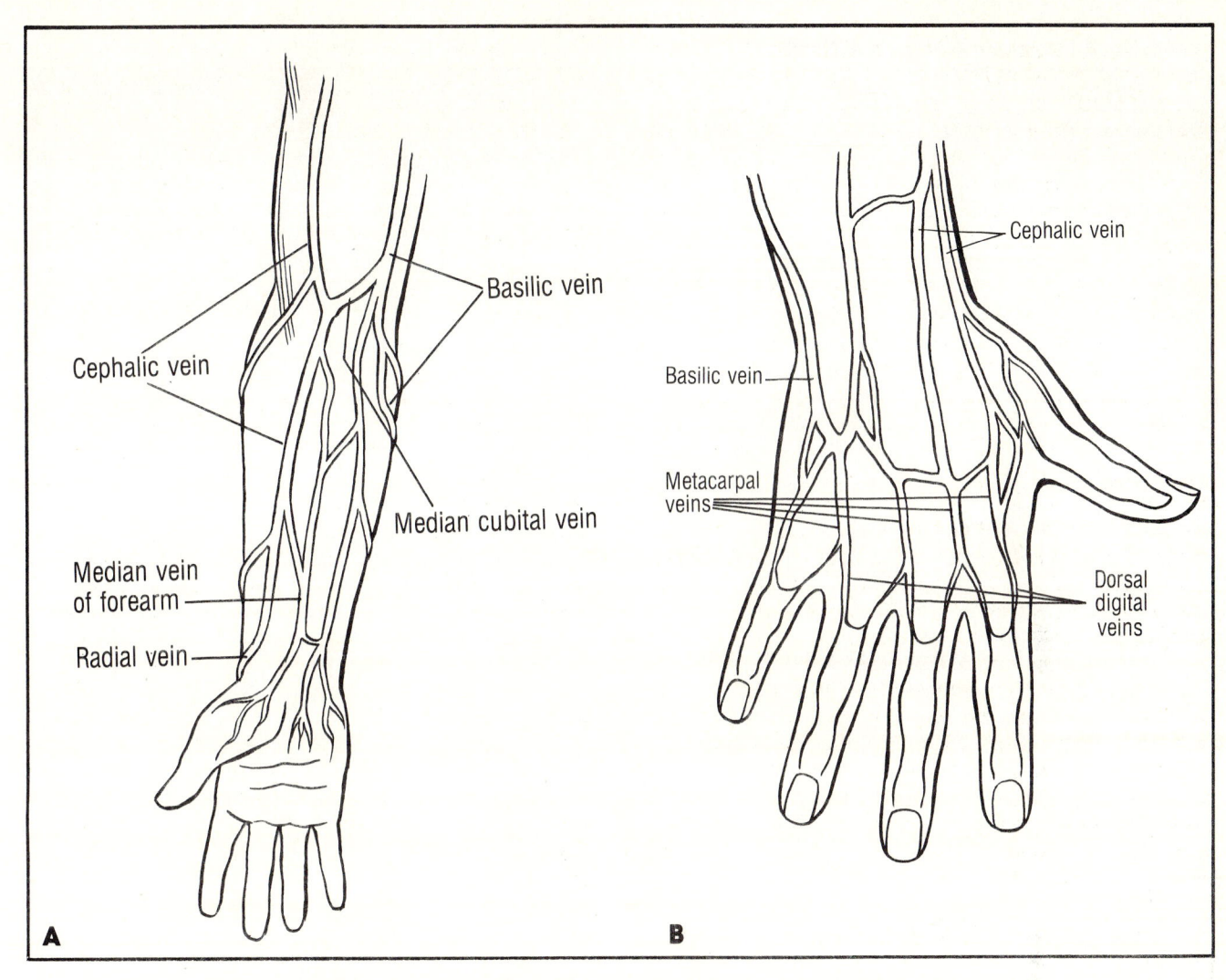

Figure 74–1. Veins of the forearm and hand in common use for venipunctures.

administer. Legally and ethically, however, it is crucial for nurses to know certain basic facts about common intravenous fluids. For example, it is important to know the purpose and tonicity of intravenous fluids, as well as potential hazards for which to observe.

The osmolality of normal blood plasma is 290 mOsm/L; fluids with approximately that osmolality are considered *isotonic*. Fluids with a greater osmolality are considered *hypertonic*, and those with a lower osmolality, *hypotonic*.

Hypertonic fluids increase the osmotic pressure of plasma and draw fluid from cells and interstitial spaces into the intravascular space. Administering excessive amounts of hypertonic solutions can cause both cellular dehydration and circulatory overload. Conversely, hypotonic fluids lower the osmotic pressure of the blood plasma, thereby causing fluid to shift into the cells and the interstitial spaces. Excessive administration of hypotonic fluids can cause water intoxication. Isotonic fluids cause no change in the osmotic pressure of plasma. They function to increase the extracellular fluid volume. If given in excessive amounts, they can cause circulatory overload (Keithley and Fraulini, 1982).

Specific Types of Intravenous Fluids

Many details are available in current literature about intravenous fluids. The most common IV fluids are discussed here briefly. Table 74–1 presents additional information about IV fluids.

Dextrose in Water Solutions. Dextrose solutions are given mainly for their caloric and water content and as a vehicle for administering medications. They are available in four different concentrations; 5, 10, 20, and 50 percent. Five percent dextrose (D_5W) is isotonic only in the fluid container, as the body metabolizes the dextrose quickly, leaving just the water. The other concentrations are hypertonic.

Dextrose for intravenous infusion yields 3.4 calories per gram, rather than the 4.0 calories per gram found in dietary carbohydrates. One liter of D_5W contains 50 g dextrose and yields 170 calories. Three li-

TABLE 74-1. Common Intravenous Fluids

SOLUTION	TONICITY	USE	POTENTIAL HAZARDS	NURSING IMPLICATIONS
Dextrose and Water Solutions				
D_5W	Isotonic in bottle. Hypotonic when administered.	Administration of IV medications. Provides CHO and water.	Hyponatremia (all dextrose solutions) Hypokalemia (all dextrose solutions) Water intoxication	Change solutions every 12 to 24 hours to prevent growth of microorganisms (all dextrose solutions).
$D_{10}W$	Hypertonic (505 mOsm/L)	Provides CHO.	Hypertonic solutions irritate the veins and can cause increased body water loss by osmotic diuresis.	Assess diabetic patients receiving any amount of intravenous dextrose for elevated blood sugar levels.
$D_{20}W$	Hypertonic (1010 mOsm/L)			
$D_{50}W$	Hypertonic (2525 mOsm/L)		Hyperinsulinism	All patients receiving intravenous fluids should have input-output monitored.
Dextrose and Saline Solutions				
$D_5W/0.2$ NaCl	Isotonic (320 mOsm/L)	Promotes diuresis in dehydrated patients. Hydration purposes	Hypokalemia	Do not administer with blood transfusions, as it causes hemolysis of red blood cells.
$D_5W/0.45$ NaCl	Hypertonic (406 mOsm/L)			
$D_5W/0.9$ NaCl	Hypertonic (559 mOsm/L)	Provides calories, water, Na, and Cl.	Same as for normal saline.	
$D_{10}W/0.9$ NaCl	Hypertonic (812 mOsm/L)	For temporary treatment of hypovolemic shock.	Administer only through a large vein.	
Saline Solutions				
0.45 NaCl	Hypotonic (154 mOsm/L)	Supplies normal sodium and water requirements.		
0.9 NaCl	Isotonic (308 mOsm/L)		Hypernatremia Metabolic acidosis Circulatory overload Hypokalemia	
3% NaCl	Hypertonic (1026 mOsm/L)	Corrects severe sodium deficit.	Pulmonary edema	Administer slowly in small volumes.
Multiple Electrolyte Solutions[a]				
Ringer's solution	Isotonic (309 mOsm/L)	Replaces Na, K, Ca, and Cl.		Always ascertain that the client has an adequate urinary output before giving any fluid containing potassium.
Lactated Ringer's (RL)	Isotonic (273 mOsm/L) Electrolyte concentration closely resembles ECF.	Replaces fluid loss from burns, diarrhea, or as bile. Useful in mild acidosis.	Contraindicated in patients with liver disease.	
D_5W/RL	Hypertonic (524 mOsm/L)	Replaces ECF deficits from vomiting or GI suction.	As above	Monitor sodium levels as normal levels can elevate quickly.
$D_{10}W/RL$	Hypertonic (776 mOsm/L)	Provides calories from extra dextrose.	As above	Monitor potassium levels closely, as an excess or deficit can be fatal.

[a] Composition of Multiple Electrolyte Solutions (mEq/L)

	Na	K	Ca	Cl	Lactate
Ringer's solution	147	4	4.5	155.5	—
Lactated Ringer's	130	4	3	109	28
D_5W/RL	130	4	3	109	28
$D_{10}W/RL$	130	4	3	109	27

ters, an amount typically administered in a 24-hour period, only provides 510 calories per day. Obviously, D_5W is not sufficient alone to sustain someone receiving prolonged intravenous therapy (Plumer, 1982).

A main disadvantage of dextrose solutions is that they do not replace electrolyte losses, and over a prolonged period of time, electrolyte-free solutions cause sodium and potassium depletion. Unlike low concentrations of dextrose, higher concentrations, such as $D_{50}W$, can be used to meet most energy requirements. Such hypertonic solutions, however, must be administered through a central vein to avoid irritating a peripheral vein.

Dextrose in Saline Solutions. Solutions of 5 or 10 percent *dextrose in normal saline* (D_5NS, $D_{10}NS$) provide enough calories and electrolytes to prevent catabolism as well as replacing sodium and chlorides (Keithley and Fraulini, 1982).

Saline Solutions. *Normal saline* (0.9 percent) is probably the most frequently administered saline solution. It is used to replenish sodium, replace extracellular fluid, correct metabolic acidosis, and precede and follow blood transfusions. Normal saline is nearly isotonic, as it contains 154 mEq/L each of sodium and chloride; plasma contains 142 mEq/L of sodium and 103 mEq/L of chloride. Normal saline does not contain other electrolytes found in plasma, and therefore its tonicity is entirely dependent on sodium and chloride (Keithley and Fraulini, 1982).

Hypotonic saline (0.45 percent), containing 77 mEq/L each of sodium and chloride, is used to supply normal sodium and water requirements. As it contains less sodium and chloride than normal plasma, it is not a likely choice when deficits need to be replaced. *Hypertonic saline* (3 percent), which contains 513 mEq/L of sodium, is used only to correct severe sodium deficits. It is administered only in small total volumes, and the client must be watched continuously (Keithley and Fraulini, 1982).

Multiple Electrolyte Solutions. Multiple *electrolyte solutions* are used for maintenance therapy and to replace fluid and electrolyte losses. They differ somewhat in their components, as shown in Table 74-1. Electrolyte solutions with dextrose are used when calories as well as electrolytes are required (Keithley and Fraulini, 1982).

Blood and Blood Products. *Whole blood* is given to treat blood volume deficiencies, as occurs in acute hemorrhage. One unit of whole blood contains approximately 500 ml. Preservatives used to prepare whole blood contain sodium citrate and dextrose. Dextrose lengthens the life of red blood cells; sodium citrate combines with ionized calcium, inhibiting clotting and preventing coagulation of the stored blood. Whole blood has a shelf life of 35 days and is stored at carefully controlled temperatures of 1° to 6° C (32° to 42.8°F). It is allowed to reach room temperature only during administration. After a period of time, even with appropriate preparation and storage, whole blood has a decreased capacity to transport and release oxygen and a decrease in coagulation effectiveness. For these reasons, fresh blood may be required during massive transfusions (Plumer, 1982).

Packed red blood cells have the same storage life as whole blood; they consist of a unit of whole blood from which 200 to 225 ml of plasma has been removed. Packed red cells are administered when the blood volume is adequate but the red cell mass is not. They are beneficial in preventing circulatory overload when renal or cardiac disease is present.

Frozen blood is prepared by extracting plasma from whole blood, adding chemicals to protect the red blood cells from damage, and then freezing at −85°C (−121°F). This process allows frozen blood to be stored for 3 years or more; it is quite expensive, however, and therefore used only under unusual circumstances. Both frozen blood and packed cells have a hematocrit level of about 80 percent (Plumer, 1982).

Plasma, the liquid remaining after red blood cells have been removed from whole blood, is used to expand blood volume when the plasma volume is decreased but the red cell mass is adequate, as in acute dehydration or burns. Plasma is also given to replace coagulation factors lacking in certain bleeding disorders (Brunner and Suddarth, 1984). Its shelf life is from 1 to 5 years, depending on how it has been prepared.

Albumin, a plasma protein, provides volume and colloids in the treatment of burns and increases albumin levels in persons with hypoalbuminemia. The risk of transmitting serum hepatitis, always a possibility when administering blood products, does not exist with albumin because the heat used in its processing destroys the hepatitis virus. Because albumin is highly osmotic, it is administered with enough fluids to prevent cellular dehydration, and the client must be observed closely for development of circulatory overload (Plumer, 1982).

Platelets (thrombocytes) are harvested from whole blood and administered as a platelet-rich plasma preparation. Platelets may be stored for no more than 72 hours under FDA regulations and are most effective if infused within 6 hours of donation. Although platelets may be administered without a full compatibility test, Rh matching is preferable and the best platelet donor for any person is a member of his or her own family (Plumer, 1982).

Plasma Substitutes. Various synthetic *plasma volume expanders* are on the market; they are used primarily in the treatment of hypovolemic shock. One such product, Dextran, increases the intravascular osmotic pressure, thereby drawing interstitial fluid into the vessels and increasing the blood volume. Because of the frequency of allergic reactions, Dextran is initially administered very slowly, and the client is observed closely during the first 30 minutes for signs and symptoms similar to a transfusion reaction (described later). Because of the danger of circulatory overload, plasma volume expanders are administered at a carefully controlled rate, particularly for clients with renal or cardiac disease. Advantages of synthetic plasma volume expanders are that they pose no storage problem, there is no danger of transmitting hepatitis (Plumer, 1982), and they usually are acceptable to persons who refuse whole blood transfusions for religious reasons.

INTRAVENOUS MEDICATIONS

Administering medications by the IV route provides more rapid onset of action, more consistent blood levels, more complete absorption, and less discomfort than the other parenteral routes. Because there are hazards associated with its use, the IV route traditionally was used by nurses only in emergency or critical care settings. Currently, intravenous therapy is common in nonacute clinical units in both hospitals and extended-care facilities, as well as in the home setting. For example, antibiotics are often administered by this route in preference to the intramuscular route, and pain medication is often given intravenously for persons with acute pain.

Methods of administering IV medications differ not only in the type of equipment used, but more importantly in the speed with which the medication reaches the bloodstream. Medications may be added to a large-volume IV fluid container and administered by slow infusion. They may also be diluted in a small-volume fluid container and administered as a secondary infusion through a primary IV or through a heparin lock, or they may be injected rapidly and directly into the vein (IV push).

Slow Infusion of Medications
Parenteral electrolytes and vitamins are administered by adding them to the main IV fluid container and infusing them slowly over 8 to 10 hours.

Secondary Infusion of Medication
Secondary infusions of medications dissolved in small volume containers are commonly referred to as intravenous "piggyback" (IVPB) medications because they often are added to the main IV tubing at one of the secondary ports. They also may be given through a heparin lock (described later). Major nursing responsibilities in administering IVPB medications are knowing the period of time for safe infusion and being able to regulate the flow accurately so that they are infused at the correct rate. The danger in giving medications too rapidly is that they can be caustic to the lining of the vein, causing much pain, predisposing the client to thrombosis, and potentially causing serious damage to the vein, making it unusable for infusions until it heals. Pharmacology texts, drug handbooks, or the agency pharmacist may be consulted about correct infusion flow rates, and many nursing units post the infusion rates for commonly administered medications.

IV Push Medications
This method of intravenous medication administration carries the highest potential risk. Medications injected into a peripheral vein reach the heart and are pumped to the brain in only 15 seconds (Geolot and McKinney, 1975). Because of this virtually instant absorption, the client receives almost instant benefits from the drug; if administered too rapidly, however, the plasma drug concentration can reach toxic proportions and cause cardiac arrest. The physician's order for an IV push medication often does not include the infusion time; the actual time is usually determined by agency or unit policy or by the nurse administering the medication. Most IV push medications can be administered safely over a period of 3 to 5 minutes, never in less than 1 minute. If policies or physicians' directives do not indicate safe infusion times or the amount and type of dilution to use, it is imperative to consult current pharmacology literature or the agency pharmacist for this information.

Compatibility of Intravenous Medications
Before administering intravenous medications, it is important to be aware of the potential risk that exists for inadvertent mixing of two incompatible drugs in the same IV tubing. This could result from two or more medications infusing concurrently through the same line, as might occur if an IVPB were being administered through a main IV line at the same time an IV push medication was given. Drug incompatibility may be very obvious, as when precipitation occurs within the tubing; however, incompatible drugs may become less therapeutically active without any visible signs developing (Plumer, 1982). The agency pharmacist is a valuable resource for determining incompatibility, as current literature does not always provide definitive information about drug incompatibilities because of differences in drug formulations from one manufacturer to another (Geolot and McKinney, 1975).

The safest way to prevent an incompatibility is to avoid combining drugs in the same tubing unless they have been absolutely proven to be compatible. Even seemingly harmless multiple vitamin preparations have been known to diminish the potency of antibiotics and therefore are not given through the same tubing. If any doubt exists as to the compatibility of two drugs, the IV tubing must be cleared with a medication-free fluid before and after the medication is infused (Geolot and McKinney, 1975).

COMPLICATIONS OF INTRAVENOUS THERAPY

Intravenous therapy carries with it the potential for several complications, any one of which could be serious, some of which could be fatal. It is important to know how to prevent these complications, identify the signs and symptoms that herald their onset, and be able to intervene appropriately should they develop.

Infiltration

Infiltration is one of the most common complications of intravenous therapy. Infiltration refers to the accumulation of intravenous fluid in the interstitial tissues; it occurs when the venipuncture device becomes dislodged from the vein or punctures the vein wall. Its severity depends upon the type and amount of fluid that accumulates in the tissues.

Signs and symptoms of a developing infiltration occur locally and include swelling, tenderness, coolness, and blanching. Although swelling is usually the first sign noted, if the solution is an irritating one, the client may report pain before the swelling is noticeable. If in doubt as to whether the area is infiltrated, compare it with the same area on the other extremity for difference in diameter, temperature, and appearance.

If little fluid has escaped into the extravascular space, or if the fluid is isotonic, no damage results from infiltration. Reassure the client and family that the surrounding tissues will absorb the fluid in a matter of hours. If, however, large amounts of fluid are allowed to escape into the tissues, or if the infiltrated fluid is hypertonic or otherwise toxic to the extravascular tissues, extensive damage may be done. Examples of fluids that are hazardous if infiltrated include chemotherapeutic agents, concentrated electrolyte solutions, or highly hypertonic solutions. The tissue damage that results from infiltration may be severe enough to require reconstructive surgery (Aisenstein, 1981).

If an IV has infiltrated, it must be discontinued immediately and restarted in another location. An infiltrated IV may be discontinued and restarted without a physician's order. If the swelling is severe or if there is concern about tissue damage, an incident report is filled out and the physician contacted immediately. The swelling from an infiltration may be alleviated more quickly if the part is elevated and warm, moist soaks are applied to the area.

Infiltration can be prevented by some very simple measures, all designed to keep the venipuncture device within the vein. Tape the venipuncture device securely at the insertion site to prevent it from becoming dislodged. If an IV is started near or over a joint, the joint must be immobilized with an armboard to prevent the needle or catheter from puncturing the vein wall during normal joint movement. If the client is very young, disoriented, or restless, the IV site may be protected by taping part of a styrofoam cup over it. Half a medication cup can also be used, after taping its edges for comfort (Gillis, 1983). When moving and turning clients, use care to avoid pulling on the tubing or placing pressure on the insertion site.

Infection

An infection at the venipuncture site can be identified by local warmth, tenderness, redness, and some swelling, as well as by an elevation in body temperature. In spite of impressive advances in the lifesaving capabilities of intravenous therapy, intravenous-associated infections continue to occur, causing prolonged hospitalization, increased hospital costs, and even death. Errors in aseptic technique are the primary cause of this complication; most infections are cannula related, with the gram-positive *Staphylococcus aureus* being the most frequently cultured organism. The Centers for Disease Control (CDC) reports some studies associate steel needles with a lower infection rate than plastic cannulas, and that other studies show no difference; they conclude that plastic cannulas are safe for routine hospital use (Simmons, 1981).

Many infection control measures recommended by the CDC are directed toward preventing contamination at the venipuncture site. These measures include careful handwashing by staff before inserting the cannula and caring for the insertion site, preparation of the venipuncture site with an antiseptic, and application of an antibiotic or antiseptic ointment to the cannula wound at the time of insertion. Placing a sterile dressing over the site helps avoid direct contact with contaminated hands and objects. Securing the infusion device may avoid microorganisms being pushed into the wound. The practice of placing tape over the actual insertion site is to be avoided unless the tape is sterile. Transparent, semipermeable polyurethane dressings such as Op-Site or Tegaderm offer the advantage of direct visualization of the site for the redness associated with infection.

Other CDC recommendations include removing the IV cannula and restarting the IV in a new location every 48 to 72 hours, including heparin lock devices; changing the infusion site dressing every 48 to 72 hours, changing administration sets every 48 hours; and discarding in-use solutions after 24 hours (unrefrigerated solutions show a dramatic increase in bacterial growth beyond that point) (Simmons, 1981). When possible, change the site and the dressing at the same time to avoid interrupting the site unnecessarily. Some believe that administration sets require daily changing, but data so far do not indicate that daily changes further lower infection rates, and the current concern over the high cost of health care discourages unnecessary changing of any equipment. However, some sources do recommend changing administration sets immediately after administering blood, blood products, or lipid preparations (Simmons, 1981).

Additional ways to prevent infection are thorough handwashing before handling of IV equipment and maintenance of strict aseptic technique, including swabbing entry ports with alcohol each time a needle is inserted.

Phlebitis and Thrombophlebitis

Phlebitis, inflammation of the vein wall, occurs as a result of chemical or mechanical trauma caused by the infusion of irritating solutions or by irritation from the infusion device. If the tunica intima is sufficiently damaged, a blood clot may develop from platelets adhering to its roughened surface. This condition is then called thrombophlebitis; it is more serious than phlebitis because the clot can break off and cause an embolism elsewhere in the body. It is not possible to detect the presence of a blood clot within a vein, but its presence is always suspected when signs of phlebitis develop.

The signs of phlebitis are redness, warmth, and induration (hardness) along the course of the vein. The client may complain of burning pain and some swelling may be noted at the site. It is important to palpate the infusion site gently once each shift to assess for the tenderness that accompanies both phlebitis and thrombophlebitis.

When phlebitis is present, restart the infusion in another location. Warm, moist soaks can be applied to the area to help relieve the discomfort associated with this complication.

Although it is not always possible to prevent phlebitis, it is possible to minimize its occurrence. Because large-bore needles and catheters increase the incidence of phlebitis due to mechanical irritation, use them only when necessary. Dilute piggyback medications appropriately and infuse hypertonic solutions as slowly as possible or through as large a vein as is feasible. Maintain stability of the venipuncture device as described above, thus decreasing mechanical trauma to the vein wall, and change sites as recommended (Aisenstein, 1981).

Circulatory Overload
This complication develops when the circulatory system contains more fluid than normal. An adult normally has about 6 liters of blood in circulation; a significant increase in this volume could precipitate pulmonary edema and cardiac failure. The main cause of circulatory overload is overly rapid infusion of IV fluids, as might occur when the infusion has been timed improperly and more than the prescribed amount of fluid has infused, or when the client's physical condition is such that the prescribed amount cannot be tolerated. The latter is especially likely to occur in elderly persons and those with impaired renal or cardiac function (Plumer, 1982).

Signs associated with cardiac failure include dyspnea, rapid and weak pulse, rapid and shallow respirations, reduced urinary output, and edema. Pulmonary edema is identified by dyspnea, cough, and rales heard at lung bases.

It is imperative to prevent infusion of fluid at greater than the prescribed rate. To do this, calculate the flow rate carefully and evaluate it routinely for accuracy. During the course of intravenous therapy, be alert for signs and symptoms of circulatory overload. If an intravenous order requires an excessive amount of fluid administration, question the order and validate its correctness prior to implementing it.

Speed Shock
Speed shock is the result of overly rapid infusion of a drug into the circulatory system, which permits its concentration in the plasma to reach toxic proportions. Syncope, shock, and cardiac arrest may occur. It is prevented by injecting IV push medications slowly, over a 3- to 5-minute time period, and never in less than 1 minute, and by careful timing of adequately diluted piggyback medications so that they infuse over an appropriate time interval.

Bleeding at the IV Site
Bleeding at the IV site is primarily a complication occurring after the site has been discontinued and the needle removed from the vein. Pressure is always applied to the site after removing the needle, and particular attention must be paid to clients who bleed easily or who are on anticoagulant therapy. It is good practice to assess the site 10 or 15 minutes later, as bleeding sometimes begins after it has once stopped.

Air Embolism
An air embolism is the presence of air in the circulatory system. If large enough, an air embolism can interfere with the supply of blood to any body part and cause serious damage. The results can be fatal if the air embolism blocks the pulmonary circulation (Gillis, 1983).

Under normal circumstances, it is unlikely that air would be able to enter the vein. Nevertheless, it is possible, especially when negative pressure exists in the vein and an IV container with an air vent is allowed to empty. (Plastic bags collapse as they empty and air never enters the bag.) Negative pressure may exist in a peripheral vein if the extremity is elevated higher than heart level. Central veins always have a negative venous pressure; precautions for working with central venous infusions are discussed in Skill 55.

Much uncertainty exists regarding the volume of air required to cause a fatal air embolus, but most authorities agree that 10 ml can be a hazard. Although the average administration set has a 5 ml-volume capacity, it is unacceptable practice to permit any air to remain in the tubing and enter the client's bloodstream. In addition, most people know it is unsafe to have air enter the veins and seeing air in the tubing is very alarming (Gillis, 1983).

Air embolism can be prevented by ensuring that all connections of an infusion set are tight, priming the entire length of the tubing properly prior to beginning an infusion, managing central venous catheters as discussed earlier, and removing air promptly from an administration set as described later.

Signs of an air embolism are cyanosis, weak and rapid pulse, lowered blood pressure, raised central venous pressure, and loss of consciousness. If an air embolus is suspected, turn the client on the left side with the head down. This will cause the air to rise in the right atrium and prevent it from entering the pulmonary artery. Administer oxygen and notify the physician promptly (Plumer, 1982).

Errors in IV Solutions or Tubings
There is a potential for making an error when administering medication by any route, but unfortunately, when administering IV therapy, the margin between an error that causes no ill effects and one that proves fatal is very narrow. A mistake is possible in the selection of the drug or solution, the calculation of the dose

or infusion rate, the technique used for administration, or the timing.

All of the safety checks appropriate to safe administration of any medication are used when administering IV solutions and medications. Question any order that seems incorrect and ask a second nurse to verify the dose of any drug before infusing it as a direct IV push.

CALCULATING AND TIMING INTRAVENOUS FLOW RATES

The physician orders the volume of fluid to be administered within a given time period. The nurse determines the correct flow rate and regulates the equipment accordingly.

Calculating Infusion Flow Rates

Flow rates are calculated in either milliliters per hour or drops per minute. A *milliliters per hour* rate is used when administering fluids through an infusion control device (ICD) or when making a time tape to monitor fluid flow. (An ICD is an electronic device that is calibrated to deliver a given volume of fluid, measured in milliliters per hour.) *Drops per minute* are used when administering fluids by gravity flow because gravity infusions are regulated by a manual adjustment of the drop rate that is visible in the drip chamber of the administration set. The flow rate is influenced by the *drop factor* of the equipment being used, that is, the number of drops in 1 ml. The drop factor varies with the manufacturer. For example, as indicated on the package, Travenol macrodrip administration sets deliver 10 drops/ml and Abbott sets deliver 15 drops/ml.

Milliliters per Hour. A *milliliters per hour* flow rate is determined by dividing the total number of milliliters to be infused by the total number of hours over which that volume is to be infused. The drop factor of the administration set has *no* influence on the calculation of a ml/hr rate.

PROBLEM: You are to infuse 3000 ml NS over a 24-hour period of time. What flow rate will you use for setting the ICD and marking the time tape?

$$\frac{3000 \text{ ml}}{24 \text{ hr}} = x \text{ (ml/hr)}$$

$$x = 125 \text{ ml/hr}$$

Drops per Minute. A *drops per minute* flow rate for gravity infusion is calculated by using either the factor-label method or a traditional formula that is quite similar to the factor-label method.

PROBLEM: You are to infuse 3000 ml D$_5$W over 24 hours time, using the gravity flow method and an administration set that has a drop factor of 10 drops/ml. What drops per minute rate is required?

Factor-label method

- Step 1. Set up the equation with the unknown dose to be given (flow rate in drops per minute) on the right side of the equation and the ordered dosage (volume and time period) on the left.

$$\frac{3000 \text{ ml}}{24 \text{ hr}} = x \text{ (drops/min)}$$

- Step 2. Add the known equivalent ratios that are needed to convert hours to minutes and will state the drop factor.

$$\frac{3000 \text{ ml}}{24 \text{ hr}} \times \frac{1 \text{ hr}}{60 \text{ min}} \times \frac{10 \text{ drops}}{1 \text{ ml}} = x \text{ (drops/min)}$$

- Step 3. Divide out the unit labels and solve the equation.

$$\frac{\cancel{3000}^{50} \cancel{\text{ml}}}{\cancel{24}_{8} \cancel{\text{hr}}} \times \frac{1 \cancel{\text{hr}}}{\cancel{60}_{1} \text{ min}} \times \frac{\cancel{10}^{5} \text{ drops}}{1 \cancel{\text{ml}}} = x \text{ (drops/min)}$$

$$\frac{50 \times 5 \text{ drops}}{8 \times 1 \text{ min}} = \frac{250 \text{ drops}}{8 \text{ min}} = x$$

$$x = 31.25 = 31 \text{ drops/min}$$
(approx.)

The drops per minute rate would be divided by 4 to be able to count a 15-second interval easily. This would be approximately 8 drops/15 seconds.

Traditional formula methods

Use the following formula to calculate a drops per minute rate for gravity flow infusions. This formula is in common use by nurses in many settings. The same problem is used to illustrate this method.

$$\frac{\text{volume (ml)}}{\text{time (minutes)}} \times \text{drop factor} = x \text{ drops/min}$$

$$\frac{3000 \text{ ml}}{24 \text{ hr} \times 60 \text{ min}} \times \frac{15 \text{ drops}}{1 \text{ ml}} = x \text{ drops/min}$$

$$\frac{3000 \times 15}{1440 \times 1} = x \text{ drops/min}$$

$$\frac{45,000}{1440} = x$$

$$x = 31.25 = 31 \text{ drops/min}$$
(approx.)

When a choice is possible, select an administration set for a gravity-flow infusion that will produce an easily counted drop rate in the drop chamber, because very rapid rates (such as over 200) or very slow rates (such as under 20) are difficult to count. For example, if calculations based on a drop factor of 60 drops/ml (microdrip set) produce a rate that is too rapid to count accurately, substituting a macrodrip set with a drop factor 10, 12, or 15 drops will produce a rate that can be counted easily. Likewise, a microdrip set can be used when a macrodrip set produces a rate that is too slow to count. Although an infusion control device will deliver a set flow rate regardless of the drop factor, using a macrodrip set facilitates fluid flow from the fluid container.

Activity 74-A:
Practice Problems for Administering Medications

Determine the flow rate required to administer the following intravenous fluids, using either the factor-label or traditional formula method.

1. Infuse 1000 ml of D_5W in 8 hours by gravity flow, using equipment with a drop factor of 15 drops/ml.
2. Infuse 1000 ml of D_5W in 8 hours, using an infusion control device. (Recall that no drop factor is needed for this calculation.)
3. Infuse 1000 ml of Ringer's lactate in 6 hours by gravity flow, using equipment with a drop factor of 12 drops/ml.
4. Infuse 1000 ml of $D_5/0.45$ NaCl in 10 hours by gravity flow, using equipment with a drop factor of 60 drops/ml.

(NOTE: Answers to these problems can be found in Appendix II, p. 1013.)

Timing IV Infusion Flow Rates

A gravity-flow rate is timed by adjusting the manual clamp on the IV tubing until the correct drop rate appears in the drip chamber. To do this, divide the desired number of drops per minute by four and count the falling drops for a 15-second interval. Then count the drops for a full minute to ensure accuracy. It is important to hold your watch beside the drip chamber so that the falling drops may be counted without taking your eye off the second hand.

An IV being infused through an infusion control device is regulated by setting the machine to the desired milliliter-per-hour setting.

A time tape is usually added to a main IV fluid container. If commercial time tapes are not available, a time tape can be made from a strip of adhesive tape, as described in Skill 54 and shown in Figure 54-8. The time tape provides an approximate but quick comparison of the volume of fluid actually infused with the volume scheduled to be infused by a given time. Time tapes are meant to supplement, not substitute for, careful timing and adequate monitoring of an IV infusion.

Calculating IV Medication Flow Rates

Infusion time for IVPB medications is not usually included in the medication order but is determined by agency or unit policy, pharmacy recommendation, or consultation with a drug reference book.

When an infusion control device (ICD) is being used to administer IV fluids, an IVPB medication may be administered by attaching the secondary infusion set to the main IV tubing above the ICD and infusing the medication by readjusting the controls for the desired flow rate. When this is done, it is crucial to reset the machine after the medication is infused, as the rate for the medication is usually more rapid than for the main infusion. Failure to reset the machine can result in grossly incorrect flow rates for the main IV and a potential for fluid overload.

An IVPB medication can also be attached to the main tubing below the ICD and infused by gravity flow. With this method, the ICD setting is unchanged and the flow rate is calculated as described above.

Milliliters per Hour. To calculate a flow rate for IV medications in milliliters per hour when using an ICD, use the formulas given above.

PROBLEM: You are to infuse 75 ml of D_5W containing 30 mEq of KCl as an IVPB through an ICD. An appropriate infusion time is 90 minutes. The available equipment has a drop factor of 60 drops/ml. What flow rate is required?

Factor-label method
Set up the equation as described above. Place the unknown flow rate on the right side of the equation and the ordered volume and time on the left side, insert the minutes/hour conversion and solve the equation. (NOTE: The drop factor is NOT used to calculate the flow rate because an ICD is being used. In addition, the drug dosage (30 mEq KCl) is NOT used to calculate the flow rate because flow rate is based on fluid *volume* rather than *concentration*.)

$$\frac{75 \text{ ml}}{\overset{}{\underset{3}{\cancel{90} \text{ min}}}} \times \frac{\overset{2}{\cancel{60} \text{ min}}}{1 \text{ hr}} = x \text{ (ml/hr)}$$

$$\frac{75 \text{ ml} \times 2}{3 \times 1 \text{ hr}} = x$$

$$x = \frac{150 \text{ ml}}{3 \text{ hr}} = 50 \text{ ml/hr}$$

Traditional formula method
Divide the volume to be infused by the *time in hours*. (90 minutes = 1.5 hours)

$$\frac{75 \text{ ml}}{1.5 \text{ hr}} = x \text{ ml/hr}$$

$$x = 50 \text{ ml/hr}$$

Drops per Minute. A *drops per minute* rate for gravity infusion of IV medications is calculated as described earlier for IV infusions.

PROBLEM: You are to infuse 100 ml of D_5W containing 30 KCl as an IVPB by gravity flow. An appropriate infusion time is 90 minutes. The available equipment has a drop factor of 60 drops/ml. What flow rate is required? For this problem, the factor-label method and the traditional formula method are identical. The *factor-label method* uses the equation described on p. 937, with the unknown flow rate and the drop factor on the right side of the equation and the ordered volume and time on the left side. The *traditional formula method* uses the formula described on p. 937, with the volume divided by the time in minutes and multiplied by the drop factor. (NOTE: The drug dosage is NOT used to calculate the flow rate as described above.)

$$\frac{100 \cancel{ml}^{}}{\cancel{90}_{3} \text{ min}} \times \frac{\cancel{60}^{2} \text{ drops}}{1 \cancel{ml}} = x \text{ (drops/min)}$$

$$\frac{100 \times 2 \text{ drops}}{3 \text{ min}} = x$$

$$x = \frac{200 \text{ drops}}{3 \text{ min}} = 67 \text{ drops/min} \text{ (approx.)}$$

After the flow rate is calculated, the drops per minute rate of 67 would be divided by 4 to count the drops for a 15-second interval. This would be approximately 17 drops per 15 seconds. Although the drug dosage was not used to calculate the flow rate in the above example, it did influence the selection of an infusion time and the choice of an administration set. Potassium chloride is an irritating drug and therefore administered slowly; a microdrip set with a drop factor of 60 to 64 drops/ml is required to administer a relatively small volume over a relatively long period of time.

Activity 74-B
Practice Problems for Administering Intravenous Medications

Determine the flow rate required to administer the following IVPB or heparin lock medications.

1. Infuse 100 ml of D_5W containing 300 mg cimetidine (Tagamet) using gravity flow and an administration set with a drop factor of 15 drops/ml. (Appropriate infusion time: 20 min.)
2. Infuse 75 ml of D_5W containing 1 g cephalothin (Keflin) using gravity flow and an administration set with a drop factor of 12 drops/ml. (Appropriate infusion time: 20 min.)
3. Infuse 50 ml of D_5W containing 3 mEq potassium (KCl) using gravity flow and an administration set with a drop factor of 60 drops/ml. (Appropriate infusion time: 60 min.)
4. Infuse 100 ml of 0.45 percent NS containing 5 million units penicillin through an ICD. (Appropriate infusion time: 30 min.)

(NOTE: Answers to these problems can be found in Appendix II, p. 1013.)

TEACHING HOSPITALIZED CLIENTS ABOUT IV INFUSIONS

Alert and cooperative clients are often willing participants in the care and maintenance of an IV infusion. Generally, the more well informed clients are about their infusions, the more compliant they will be about the therapy and the less anxiety they will experience. Judgment must always be used in determining what to teach because too much information can be overwhelming. Clients should never be made to feel that they, rather than the nursing staff, shoulder the primary responsibility for maintaining an IV infusion.

The following are specific points to be included in a plan for a client who has an IV infusion:

1. Contact the nurse if you experience pain or notice swelling in the arm receiving the IV infusion.
2. If you notice that fluid is not dripping in the fluid chamber, contact the nurse, who will try to get the fluid to flow once more. While waiting for the nurse to arrive, try repositioning your arm and see if that causes the flow to resume. Also check that you are not lying on any part of the IV tubing or that it is not kinked.
3. Avoid touching the IV dressing and never remove it on your own.
4. You may notice when you get out of bed that blood backs up into the IV tubing. If this occurs, try lowering your arm, which should cause the solution to flow and flush the blood from the tubing. Blood in the tubing is only a concern when it is not quickly flushed out again.
5. Other than avoiding vigorous movement of the arm receiving the infusion, having an IV should not limit your movement or activities in any way. The nurses will provide you with a rolling IV pole on which to hang your IV container while you walk or move about.
6. It is very important that you never attempt to readjust the flow rate of your IV in any way. The flow rate has been carefully determined by your physician and set by your nurse and must not be changed.
7. If your IV is running through a pump, please do not touch any of its controls. If the alarm sounds, do not try to silence it, as you might hit the wrong button. Use your nurse call light so that the nurse can come and determine the cause of the problem.
8. Discuss any concerns or questions you have about your IV with your nurse or physician.
9. Having an IV should not be a concern or worry to you. Other than following these guidelines, you should be able to forget it is even there!

INTRAVENOUS THERAPY IN THE HOME

Increasingly, clients with chronic illnesses are being taught to administer their own IV therapy in the home. This may be the method of choice for clients who must receive prolonged antibiotic therapy and is virtually imperative for those persons who must remain on total parenteral nutrition (TPN) for the remainder of their lives. Chemotherapy may also be administered at home as part of a cancer treatment regime.

In the home setting, antibiotics or chemotherapeutic agents are often administered through heparin locks, which are ideal devices for such situations because a continuous infusion is not needed. A group of Canadian investigators found that with properly selected clients, intravenous antibiotic therapy could be given as safely and effectively in the home as in the hospital, and at one-fourth to one-third of the cost! (IV Therapy, 1983). Similar success has been reported with administration of TPN and chemotherapy (Blackburn, 1984; Vogel and McSwimming, 1983).

With the current emphasis on reducing health-care costs, it can be expected that increasing numbers of clients will be taught to administer intravenous therapy in the home. Its key to success is careful selection of clients, superb preparation of clients and families prior to discharge, and follow-up through home and clinic visits. Nurses will continue to play an important role in this type of intravenous therapy.

DATA BASE

As with medication administration by any route, the intravenous infusion of fluids, nutrients, and medications requires knowledge about these substances and their intended actions and potential side effects. It is also important to know whether the amount of solution to be infused is appropriate for that client, and whether the dosage of an ordered medication is appropriate for the intravenous route. Knowledge about the possible complications of intravenous therapy is necessary to the maintenance of scrupulous technique.

Patient History and Recorded Data

The client's overall health status gives some indication of the physiological ability to tolerate an IV infusion. For example, increasing age and the presence of renal and cardiac disease decrease a person's ability to tolerate IV fluids.

Data concerning the client's level of consciousness, ability to cooperate, and willingness to become involved in personal care aid in preventing complications, selecting an appropriate IV infusion site, maintaining an intact infusion, and developing a teaching plan about the infusion. Identifying the client's previous experiences with IVs helps determine what approach is best to provide information to the client and family. Data from the health record indicate the purpose for the intravenous therapy. This information may be helpful in estimating how long intravenous therapy will last, a question that clients and families often ask.

Data from the medical or nursing history provide information that aids in site selection, such as the presence of a shunt or mastectomy, damaged veins, or other factors that prohibit use of an extremity for venipuncture. Past experiences with infusions may also aid in venipuncture site selection, as clients may report the locations of "good" or "poor" veins.

Direct observations and interview are used to confirm data from the health record, as physical and mental condition may change rapidly.

Physical Appraisal Skills

Inspection. Inspection is used to visualize the venous pattern of the arm and to locate superficial, easily cannulated veins. Inspection is also used in the routine assessments crucial to IV maintenance in which early identification of complications is the goal. The swelling associated with infiltration and the redness of phlebitis are also determined by inspection.

Palpation. Palpation is useful in site location and the assessment of the patient for complications of intravenous therapy. The index and middle finger are used to palpate the vein; consistent use of the same fingers is recommended because it increases their sensitivity. Although complications such as infiltration and phlebitis may first be detected by using the skill of inspection, they are confirmed by palpating the area for temperature changes, induration, or swelling.

EQUIPMENT

Fluid Containers

Calibrated IV fluid containers, holding 1000, 500, or 250 ml are available as either evacuated glass bottles or collapsible plastic bags or bottles (Fig. 74–2).

Glass Bottles. Glass bottles with rubber diaphragms were the first fluid containers on the market for intravenous purposes, and although they have largely been replaced by plastic bags in most agencies, they are still in use in some areas. The top of a glass bottle has a rubber diaphragm protected by a metal or plastic cap, similar to injectable medication vials. Markings and labels on the diaphragm indicate the correct spot to insert the administration set spike (described below) or to inject medications.

For fluid to infuse out of a rigid container such as a glass bottle, air must be able to enter the bottle, either through a closed or open system. An open infusion system uses vented glass bottles with a long vent tube in the diaphragm that extends nearly to the bottom of the bottle. After the latex seal is removed from the bottle top, this vent allows room air to enter the bottle as the fluid infuses into the patient, thus equalizing the pressure inside the bottle. A loud hissing sound always occurs when a properly sealed vented bottle is first opened. If this sound is not heard, discard the solution promptly. Because it is open to the air, a vented bottle that has had the seal removed will leak if it is inverted before the administration spike is inserted.

The closed glass bottle infusion system uses a nonvented bottle that requires a vented administration set. This set allows air to enter the bottle through a microporous filter, equalizing the pressure.

Plastic Containers. Plastic containers are popular, as they offer several advantages over glass containers. Plastic bags and plastic bottles collapse as they empty, making air venting unnecessary and thereby reducing the risk of an air embolus and airborne contamination. Plastic containers are easily transported with a minimal risk of damage and are disposed of readily. However, plastic bags are susceptible to punctures, which are difficult to detect unless the bag is squeezed before use. A puncture provides a port of entry for microorganisms; any punctured bag must be discarded.

Plastic IV fluid bags are encased in a protective plastic wrapper that is removed prior to use. The bags have two tab-covered entry ports, one into which the administration set spike is inserted and one for introducing electrolytes, vitamins, medications, or other additives. The administration port has a seal about 1.25 cm (½ in) from the entrance, which prevents fluid from pouring out if the sterile tab is removed while the bag is inverted. However, once the sterile spike from the administration set has pierced this seal, the contents of the container will pour out if the administration set is removed while the bag is inverted. The port for additives has a resealable rubber diaphragm through which a needle can be inserted any number of times, as long as aseptic technique is used. If possible, large-gauge needles (No. 18 and No. 20) should be avoided because they may cause the diaphragm to leak with repeated use.

Volume-Control Containers

Volume-control containers are used to administer a specific small volume of fluid, such as the amount of fluid needed to administer an IVPB or heparin lock medication. Volume control containers include mini-bottles or mini-bags, and burette devices such as that shown in Figure 74-3. Mini-bottles or mini-bags contain 50 to 100 ml of a dextrose or saline solution and are designed with an administration port and a medication port similar to the large plastic bags used for large volume infusions. They can be used with gravity flow or with an infusion control device. These containers may or may not arrive from the pharmacy with the medication already in solution in the container.

A burette, such as a Buretrol, Soluset, Volutrol, or Pediatrol, is a calibrated cylinder with a capacity of 100 to 200 ml. It can either be an integral part of the main IV infusion, or it may be attached to a separate fluid container and added to (piggybacked) the main IV tubing. Burettes have an air filter and a medication port with a rubber diaphragm at the top of the bottle. If the burette is a part of the main IV, only medications that are compatible with the main IV can be administered in this manner.

Administration Sets

An administration set consists of a spike that pierces the fluid container, a drip chamber, tubing that extends down to the venipuncture device or to a filter, several tubing clamps that are used to regulate the rate of flow, one or more Y-type injection ports for infusing piggyback medications, and a rubber flashball

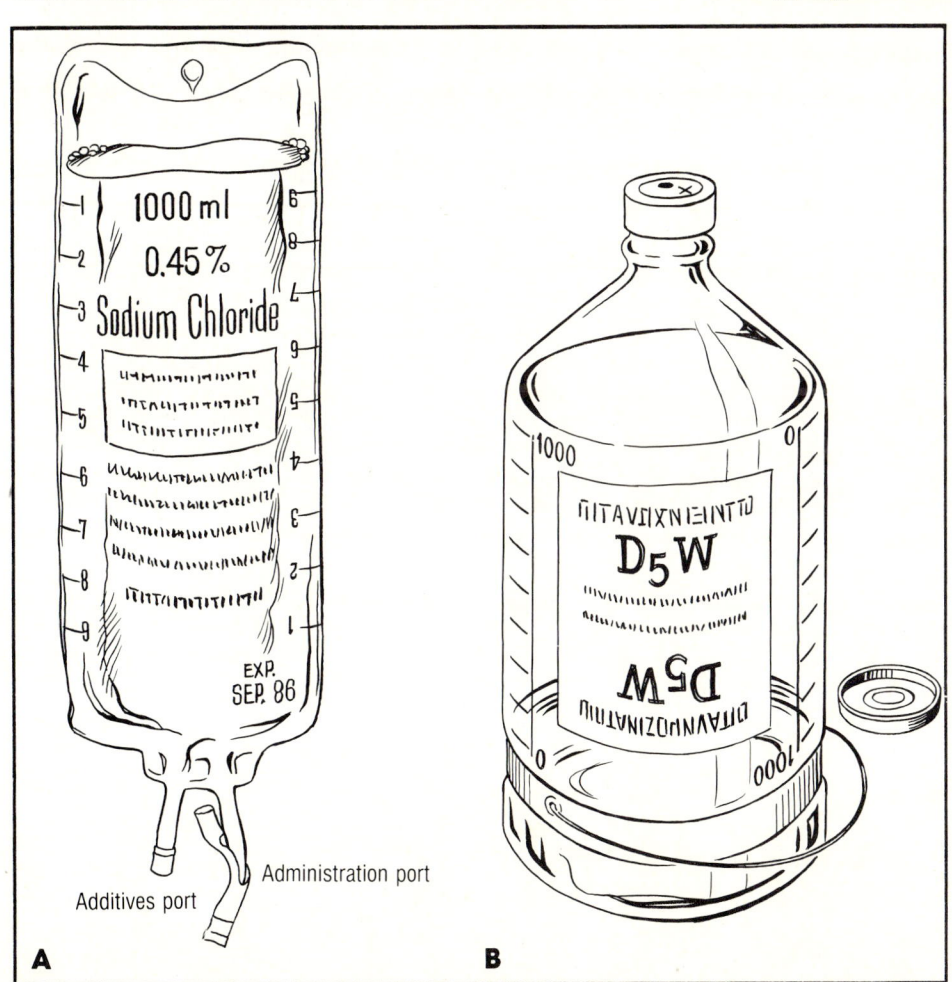

Figure 74-2. Intravenous fluid containers. **A.** Large plastic bag. **B.** Unvented glass bottle. Note that fluid level markings can be read in both the upright and inverted positions. Note entry ports for administration set spike and medications.

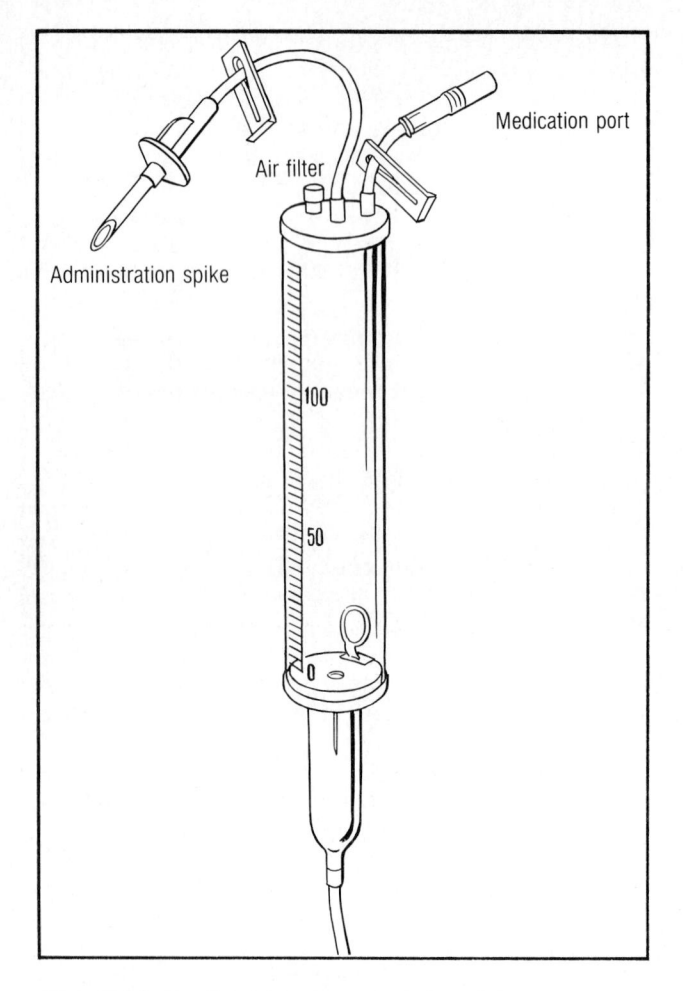

Figure 74-3. Burette style volume-control container.

piece of information used in timing intravenous infusions. The reduced drop size of the microdrip sets allows a constant intravenous flow to be maintained with a minimal amount of fluid. Although they were originally designed for use with infants and children, they also provide safer infusion for adults, unless a rapid flow rate is needed. Adaptors are available that can change the flow rate of a macrodrip set to a microdrip rate; they are easily removed if an increased flow rate is needed.

Administration sets for infusion control devices (electronic equipment that either controls or pumps intravenous infusions) are available in a wide selection, depending on the type of infusion control device being used. Some devices operate using standard administration sets and some require specialty tubing with an in-line pump chamber or cassette that will fit the pumping device.

Filters

Filters are designed to limit the access of bacteria, fungus, and particulate matter to the bloodstream. Filter pores range from 0.22 to 5 microns. They generally are located between the administration set and the veni-

for checking IV tubing patency and administering IV push medications. Many sets include an antireflux valve to prevent backflow into the main IV line from a secondary "piggyback" fluid container. A sample administration set is shown in Figure 74-4. Common tubing lengths are 1.8 m (72 in), 2.1 m (84 in), and 2.7 m (105 in). Shorter secondary administration sets (86 cm, or 34 in.) are used to connect a volume-control container to the main IV tubing. This is done by attaching a needle to the secondary tubing and inserting it through one of the injection ports in the main tubing. Administration sets are prepackaged in sterile packages. However, the only parts of the set that must remain sterile after opening the package are the spike (which is inserted into the fluid container) and the tip of the tubing (which is inserted into the filter or venipuncture device). These parts are covered with protective plastic caps that are removed immediately prior to insertion into the fluid container, filter, or venipuncture device.

Gravity-flow administration sets vary in the rate of flow they are gauged to produce, delivering 10, 15, or 20 drops/ml for a *macrodrip* device, and 50 or 60 drops/ml for a *microdrip* or *minidrip* device. This drop factor is printed on the package and is a vital

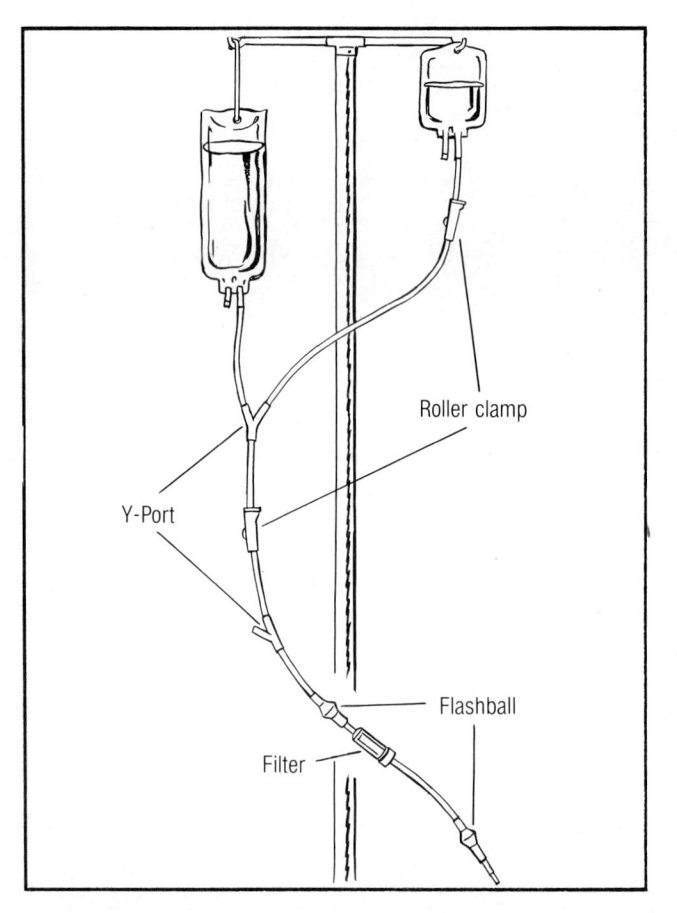

Figure 74-4. Intravenous infusion administration set with secondary "piggyback" tubing attached at one Y-port. A separate filter has been added to the tubing. The volume control container is elevated above the main IV container so the "piggyback" fluid infuses in preference to the main IV fluid.

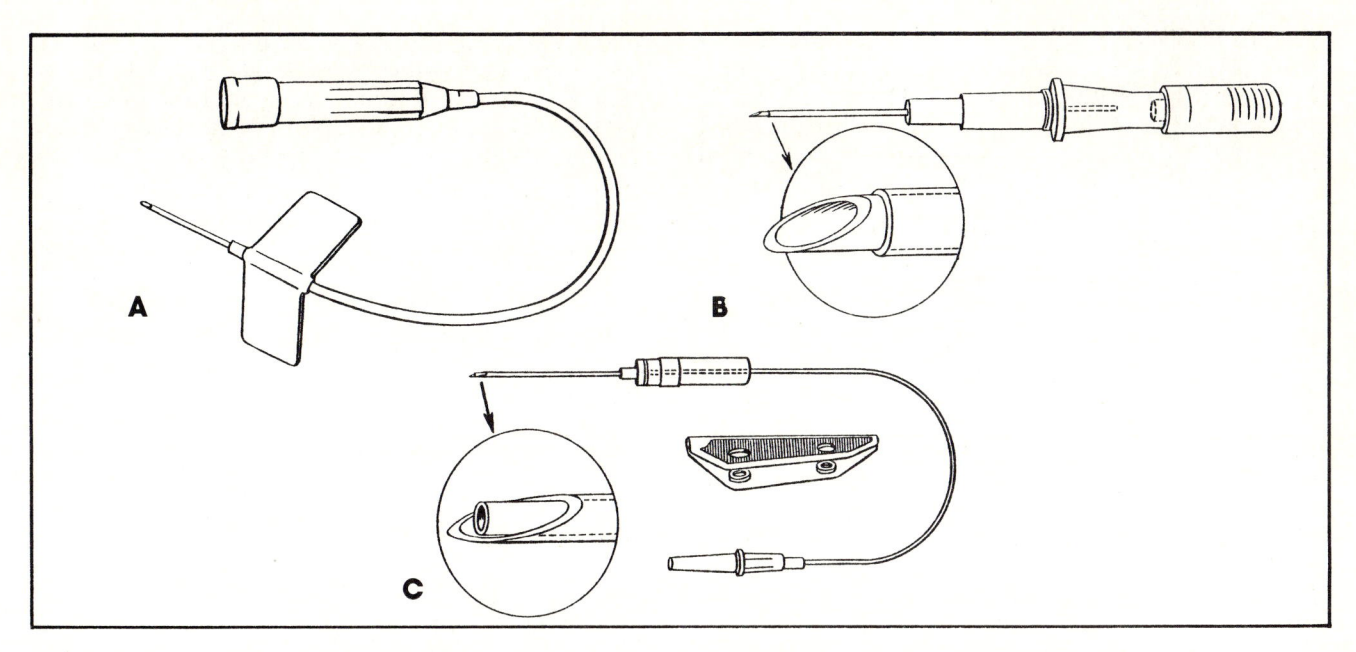

Figure 74-5. Venipuncture devices. **A.** Winged cannula with heparin lock tubing and port. **B.** Over-the-needle catheter. **C.** Through-the-needle catheter.

puncture device, although some administration sets have integral (in-line) filters. Filters are manufactured in a variety of forms, sizes, and materials. They are effective only to the extent that they are used properly. The package should indicate the best position for filling the filter and whether or not the filter prevents air from entering the bloodstream. Special filters are required for administering blood or lipids. Some medications, such as amphotericin-B, are not filtered and are infused distal to the filter (Plumer, 1982).

Filter needles (5-micron pore size) are often used when introducing medications or other additives to IV infusions. Although this is most often done in the pharmacy department, it may be done on some clinical units.

Venipuncture Devices

Venipuncture devices (cannulas) consist of either a steel needle or a plastic catheter from which a needle is removed after venipuncture is completed. Types, lengths, and gauges of venipuncture devices vary; their selection depends on the size of the vein being cannulated, the viscosity of fluid being infused, and the rate of flow required. Several types are shown in Figure 74-5. A No. 20 or No. 22 gauge, short-length needle with a short sharp bevel is used most often for adults. The short sharp bevel pierces the skin more readily, thus causing less discomfort. It is also thought to be less likely to puncture the opposite wall of the vein and cause extravasation, or to become lodged against the vein wall and obstruct the fluid flow. *Winged needles,* often called butterfly needles (Abbot), are small steel cannulas used for unstable veins, difficult insertions, and for children (Fig. 74-5A). The name derives from the winglike plastic projections just above the needle that fold up to form a handle, making it easier to manipulate the needle while inserting it. A plastic catheter needle is flexible and less likely to puncture the vein than is a metal needle. However, the plastic catheter sometimes produces an allergic reaction and a greater risk of infection exists when the plastic catheter is left in place longer than recommended.

An *over-the-needle catheter* (such as an angiocath) is a plastic catheter, 3 to 5 cm (1 to 2 in.) long, containing a steel needle (Fig. 74-5B). Following venipuncture, the needle is withdrawn, leaving the plastic catheter in the vein.

A *through-the-needle catheter* is a large-bore needle with a long plastic catheter inside it (Fig. 74-5C). The catheters are of varying lengths. Following venipuncture, the catheter is threaded into the vein; the steel needle is removed but left in place over the catheter. A plastic protective sheath is snapped over the needle to guard against injury from the needle point.

Heparin Locks

A *heparin lock* is a small device that consists of a winged needle connected to a short tubing as shown in Figure 74-5A. The tubing ends in a self-sealing diaphragm through which medication is injected. The needle remains in the vein continuously and the tubing is taped to the arm. The device is called a heparin lock because a small volume of heparin solution is injected into it to avoid clotting and to maintain its patency. Many agencies use a heparin solution of 100 units/ml of saline, usually in a prepackaged cartridge administered with a Tubex or Carpuject syringe. The only part of a heparin lock that must remain sterile is the needle.

An IV infusion may be converted to a heparin lock by using a small device called an adaptor, which consists of a small piece of plastic tubing. One end of the tubing is designed to be inserted into the venipuncture device already in place after the IV tubing is disconnected, and the other end consists of a resealable rubber diaphragm similar to that in a heparin lock.

Infusion Control Devices

Infusion control devices (ICDs) are electronic machines used to regulate the flow of intravenous infusions. Their use is associated with greatly increased accuracy of IV infusion administration, and they may also be helpful in early detection of some complications associated with IV infusions.

The two main types of ICDs are gravity controllers (rate regulators) and infusion pumps. *Gravity controllers* are the most common type of ICD. They exert no pressure and use only the force of gravity to infuse fluid into the vein. These devices count drops with an electronic sensor or extrude volumes of fluid mechanically or electronically (Turco, 1979). They have no moving components and so are less complex and usually less expensive than the infusion pumps described below. A gravity controller regulates the rate of flow automatically rather than manually, thus bypassing the manual regulator clamps, which have been found to vary considerably in their volume delivery (Turco, 1982). Controllers have audible and visible alarms that are triggered by such occurrences as air in the system, an empty fluid container, or a slowed flow rate, such as may happen with an infiltration or an obstructed tubing. As a slowed rate may occur late in the course of an infiltration, this alarm feature does not eliminate the need for hourly assessment of the infusion. A drawback of controllers is that an accurate drop rate does not necessarily mean that an accurate volume is being delivered (Turco, 1979).

Infusion pumps exert positive pressure to infuse fluid into a client's veins and therefore may also be used for intraarterial infusions. Infusion pumps are classified according to the mechanism that produces the positive pressure, that is, syringe, peristaltic, and cassette pumps. *Syringe pumps,* in which a motor pushes in the plunger of a syringe, are only used to administer small volumes of fluid, because the syringe must be refilled manually. *Peristaltic pumps* work by compressing and releasing a flexible tubing, thereby propelling a small bolus of fluid forward. *Cassette pumps* require use of a special tubing whose cassette (fluid reservoir) fills and is then emptied by pressure from the pump. Of the three types, cassette pumps are the most expensive to operate because of the specially designed administration sets they require.

Both gravity controllers and infusion pumps are available in volumetric and nonvolumetric models. A *volumetric* ICD is the most accurate type; it ensures delivery of fluid at a constant volume. A *nonvolumetric* device delivers fluids at a constant drop rate. Volumetric devices are used when a certain fluid volume must be delivered over a long period of time, as, for example, when administering total parenteral nutrition. Nonvolumetric ICDs are used when short-term accuracy is required, such as when administering certain rapid-acting medications. Most infusion pumps are volumetric, and the fluid delivery rate is measured in milliliters per hour rather than drops per minute.

Blood Sample Devices

Blood samples are often drawn with a specially designed disposable blood collecting mechanism, such as the Vacutainer and Jelco devices. As shown in Figure 74–6, blood collecting devices have a double needle that threads into a plastic needle holder. The longer needle (1 to 1½ in.; No. 20, No. 21, or No. 22 gauge) is covered with a rigid plastic protective cap, similar to other needles used for injection. The smaller and shorter needle is covered with a flexible latex protector. To prepare and use one of these devices, first thread the needle into the holder, leaving the protector in place on both needles; the longer needle then extends from the smaller end of the holder and the shorter needle is inside the holder. After the needle is in the vein, the evacuator blood collecting tube is pushed into the holder and the shorter needle pierces both its own latex protector *and* the sterile rubber diaphragm on the evacuator tube. At that time the negative pressure in the tube draws blood into the tube quite rapidly. When the tube is full and is withdrawn from the needle holder, the latex needle protector reseals itself, thus avoiding blood loss through the venipuncture needle remaining in the vein. Since the shorter needle inside the holder remains sterile, subsequent evacuated blood collecting tubes can be inserted into the needle holder and filled through the same process. With this device, up to 20 evacuator tubes can be filled with blood from one venipuncture.

Additional Infusion Equipment

Armboards. Used to immobilize a joint when an IV has been started over or near it, *armboards* generally consist of a piece of cardboard wrapped in foam rubber with a plastic cover. The upper extremity is taped to it so as to immobilize the elbow, wrist, or fingers. Armboards may be covered with a paper or cloth protector or covering. They may be wiped clean between uses.

Tourniquets. *Tourniquets* are stretchable rubber bands or flexible elastic straps with self-adherent clo-

Figure 74–6. Blood collecting device and evacuated laboratory tube. Note long needle for the venipuncture. The short needle to be inserted into the holder is designed to penetrate the tube diaphragm.

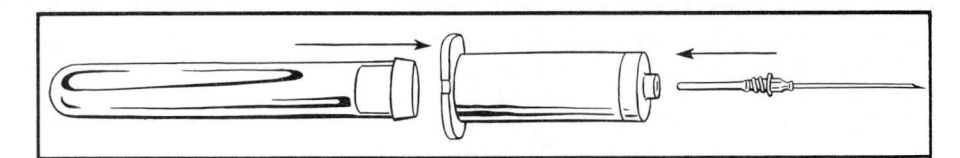

sures. They are placed around the extremity between the intended venipuncture site and the heart, snugly enough to delay venous return and distend the vein distal to the tourniquet during a venipuncture.

Intravenous Poles. *IV poles* (also called IV standards or IV rods) are used for hanging the IV container during administration of an infusion. Some poles are attached to hospital beds, some stand on the floor, some have casters and can be readily moved around, and others consist of chains or rods suspended from the ceiling.

Time Tapes. *Time tapes* are strips of adhesive-backed paper that are calibrated in milliliters to correspond with the volume markings on IV fluid containers. The nurse calculates the number of milliliters to be infused per hour and marks hourly intervals at the appropriate place on the milliliter calibration scale as was described in Skill 54. Time tapes provided by some manufacturers are color coded to assist in this marking. Time tapes also provide space for the nurse to provide identifying client data, the flow rate for the infusion, additives, and the name of the nurse who prepared and hung the infusion.

Intravenous Trays. Most agencies provide intravenous trays that contain the supplies needed to start an IV infusion or perform a venipuncture. The contents of the tray usually include sterile alcohol swabs, antiseptic solution and ointment such as povidone–iodine (Betadine), an antibiotic ointment such as neomycin, adhesive tape, tourniquets, a selection of venipuncture devices, and IV dressing supplies. IV dressings consist of either dry sterile gauze squares or transparent polyurethane material such as Op-Site or Tegaderm.

Equipment for Administration of Blood

Special administration sets are used to transfuse blood. These sets contain a filter inside the drip chamber that is designed to trap bacteria and debris that are present in all blood products, even those stored for only a short time. The filter (and therefore the entire set) should be changed after 2 to 4 units of blood have infused, as continued use allows bacterial contamination and hemolysis (Plumer, 1982).

Blood Administration Sets. *Blood administration sets* are often Y-type sets containing two spikes above the drip chamber. This design permits saline to be hung at the same time as the blood, and infused just prior to, alternately, or simultaneously with the blood.

Blood Warmers. *Blood warmers* are used to warm blood when large or rapid transfusions of cold blood would predispose a client to general hypothermia and cardiac arrest, when doing exchange transfusions of newborns, or when transfusing clients with cold agglutinins. Blood warmers function by a variety of methods. One type involves the placement of blood warming coils in warm water baths, and another uses dry heat to warm blood as it flows through a disposable plastic bag. The directions accompanying the warmer must be read carefully and understood before attempting to use it. It is important that warming devices be submitted to routine quality control procedures to ensure that the blood is being warmed only to the required temperature; this monitoring is usually done by the agency's medical engineering department.

A *pressure cuff* is a device that provides for rapid infusion of blood. The cuff consists of a thin mesh layer stitched to an inflatable bag into which air is pumped manually with a bulb resembling that on a blood pressure cuff. The unit of blood is suspended between the mesh and the inflatable bag, and as air is pumped into the bag, the pressure applied to the unit of blood increases its rate of flow. Connected to the cuff is a pressure gauge calibrated in millimeters of mercury pressure. If allowed to infuse by gravity alone, 1 unit of blood can take up to 2 hours to infuse; with a pressure cuff, 1 unit can be infused in 30 minutes. Rapid administration of blood is often needed in hypovolemic shock.

☐ EXECUTION

Agency policy varies as to whether staff nurses or specially trained teams of nurses or technicians perform venipunctures and start IV infusions. However, all nurses are expected to be able to add subsequent fluids to an existing IV infusion, as well as monitor and discontinue those infusions. Agency policy also determines whether the pharmacy or the staff nurses insert additives into IV fluid containers. Therefore, the practices described in this section may vary depending on the actual clinical situation.

Strict aseptic technique is required when working with IV infusions. This means that all connections are kept capped until they are used, the protective caps are placed in a safe place if they will need to be replaced, and the connections are allowed to touch nothing except each other. It also means that no outdated equipment or tampered packages are used, and that strict aseptic technique is used to instill any additives into the IV fluid container. If any part of the IV infusion setup is contaminated accidentally, discard that item promptly and replace it with a sterile item. The short-term additional cost of new equipment is far less important than the risk of an IV-related infection and its associated personal and economic costs.

PREPARING AN IV INFUSION

To avoid unnecessary anxiety on the part of the client and family, as much as is possible, prepare the infusion in the medicine or clean utility room, away from the bedside.

Collecting Supplies

Check the client's health record for the physician's order to determine the type and amount of solution needed and the time framework for administration. Inspect the *fluid* for clarity and to ascertain that it is free from particulate matter and read the label to ensure that it is the ordered fluid. Select the appropriate *administration set* based on the desired flow rate for the infusion and whether the infusion will be administered with an ICD or by gravity flow. For example, choose a microdrip set when the infusion is to be given very slowly or to a child. Selection of an *IV pole* is limited by what has been purchased by the agency, but, when possible, should be based on the client's mobility. If the client is to be allowed out of bed during the time that the infusion is to be administered, use a sturdy rolling IV pole. If the fluid is to be infused by gravity, check the adjustable mechanism on the IV pole to be certain it is working properly. If an ICD is to be used, ensure that it is functioning properly. Most ICDs are attached to a rolling IV pole or can be bolted onto the pole selected. Inspect the IV tray to be certain that all needed supplies are present.

Setting Up the Infusion

Close the clamp completely on the administration tubing before inserting the spike into the container. This is extremely important because if the clamp is left open, fluid enters the tubing unevenly and allows large air bubbles to form, whereas correct priming (described below) prevents most bubbles.

To prepare plastic bags, first remove the wrapping from around the bag and check to be sure that the administration port is covered with its protective cap. Squeeze the bag gently to check for punctures or leaks. The bag may feel damp when removed from its outer wrapper, but this does not necessarily mean that a leak has developed. Remove the protective cap from the administration port and from the spike on the administration set. Grasp the port firmly near the bag, as this is where the inner seal is located, rather than near the entrance to the port. Use a slightly twisting motion to insert the spike into the port, carefully but firmly.

To prepare a closed system bottle, remove the metal disc and use an alcohol swab to cleanse the rubber diaphragm. With the bottle upright, remove the cap from the tubing and insert the spike firmly through the rubber diaphragm at the point designated "fluids" or "inlet." To prepare an open system bottle with an indwelling air vent, remove the metal disc and the rubber diaphragm beneath it and listen for the hissing sound that indicates that the container was sealed properly. Insert the spike into the larger of the two holes on the rubber diaphragm (the one without the vent).

At this point, the IV fluid container is ready to be hung on an IV pole or on a hook in the medicine room. To prime the tubing (fill it with fluid, thus expelling the air) on a standard administration set, squeeze the drip chamber gently, allowing it to fill half full. The half-full level is quite important. It is difficult for either the nurse or an electronic sensor to count the drips when the drip chamber level is too high. When the level is too low, the fluid splashes and those splashes can be counted by the sensor, giving an inaccurate count. Remove the protective cap from the end of the tubing and hold the tubing over a basin, sink, or cup. Open the clamp slowly and allow fluid to run through the tubing until all air is removed, and then close the clamp.

Occasionally, air bubbles become trapped in the tubing. Minute air bubbles do not constitute a problem. Remove other visible air bubbles, as it is considered unsafe practice to allow air to remain in the tubing as discussed earlier.

To remove air bubbles trapped near the distal end of the tubing, hold that end higher than the rest of the tubing and allow more fluid to flow slowly, so that the air will rise and be expelled. When bubbles are trapped in the tubing near the drip chamber, tapping the tubing will usually coax those bubbles trapped in the middle of the tubing or to remove those bubbles that do not move when tapped, cleanse the medication port distal to the air bubble and insert a sterile needle that is long enough to reach into the lumen of the tubing. Allow the fluid to flow slowly through the tubing until the air passes the site of the needle, at which time the air will escape through the needle, producing a slight hissing sound. Close the clamp, remove the needle, and continue to the next air bubble. Some intravenous filters are designed to remove air; if so, attach the filter, fill it, and observe whether the air bubbles disappear.

Tubing designed for an ICD is primed in a similar way but may require some additional care. For example, some cassette-style tubings require that the chamber be held in a certain way so as to expel all air properly as it is filled. With some sets, failure to expel all air from the cassette chamber causes the entire system to be inoperative.

If a filter is to be used, attach it to the tubing and fill it with fluid so as to expel all air, following the manufacturer's instructions. For example, some filters must be inverted in order to allow air to escape.

Calculate the number of milliliters to be infused per hour when using an ICD, and the number of drops per milliliter when using a gravity flow infusion (based on the drop factor of the administration set). Mark the rate of flow per hour on the bag or bottle with a time tape according to agency policy.

Follow the manufacturer's directions as to how to insert the tubing into the ICD and set the controls properly. Many infusion devices indicate the number of milliliters that have infused from the IV fluid container, and by referring to the time the IV was started, it is easy to determine whether or not the machine is infusing the fluid at the proper rate. It is very important, however, that machines not be trusted blindly, as a malfunction can occur that would prove dangerous or disastrous to the client if watchful nurses did not catch the problem.

☐ SKILL SEQUENCE

PREPARING AN INTRAVENOUS INFUSION

Step	Rationale
1. Validate physician order for intravenous fluids.	Ensures correct implementation of physician's order.
2. Wash hands.	Avoids transfer of microorganisms.
3. Select appropriate IV fluid.	Guards against errors in administration.
4. Inspect fluid for clarity.	Visual check for sterility; a cloudy solution may have been contaminated or sterilized improperly.
5. Read expiration date on fluid container label. Discard if expiration date has passed.	Expired fluid may no longer be sterile, may have become less therapeutic, or both.
6. Compare physician's order with label on fluid container.	Guards against errors in administration.
7. Select appropriate venipuncture cannula.	Provides for correct administration of fluid.
8. Select appropriate infusion control device, if its use is indicated.	Provides for correct administration of fluid.
9. Select correct administration set and type of IV pole.	Promotes correct infusion.
10. Check all packages for intactness.	Contents of an opened package may be unsterile or have been tampered.
11. Maintain surgical asepsis throughout steps 12 to 19.	Avoids contamination and prevents microorganisms from gaining access to the infusion system.
12. Open administration set and close tubing clamp; leave protective caps in place.	Prevents air from entering tubing as it is being filled; prevents contamination of tubing tips.
13. If fluid container is a plastic bag: 　a. Remove wrapping from around bag and check to be sure administration port is protected with a plastic cap. 　b. Squeeze bag gently and inspect for leaks. 　c. Remove protective caps from administration port and spike on administration set; discard caps. 　d. Insert spike into port until it pierces inner seal.	Maintains sterility of equipment. A leak would provide a pathway for entry of microorganisms. Contamination of spike and port would admit microorganisms to IV fluid. Allows fluid to enter drip chamber when it is compressed.
14. If fluid container is a closed-system glass bottle: 　a. Remove metal disc and cleanse the rubber diaphragm with an alcohol swab. 　b. Remove cap from spike on administration set and discard it. 　c. Insert spike firmly through administration port on rubber diaphragm (often marked "fluids").	Avoids transfer of microorganisms. Allows fluid to enter drip chamber when chamber is compressed.
15. If fluid container is an open-system glass bottle: 　a. Remove metal disc and rubber diaphragm beneath it. 　b. Insert spike into larger of two holes in rubber stopper (the one without vent). 　(NOTE: Discard bottle and administration set if a hissing sound is not heard as spike enters bottle.)	 Air vent must remain open so air can enter bottle during infusion. Fluid will be unable to leave bottle if air does not enter to replace it. When properly sealed, open-system bottles contain a vacuum. Improperly sealed bottles must be regarded as contaminated.
16. To prime a standard administration set: 　a. Squeeze drip chamber gently, allowing it to fill half-way. 　b. Remove protective cap from distal end of tubing and hold tubing over a cup, basin, or sink. 　c. Open clamp and allow fluid to fill tubing, thus expelling all air. 　d. Replace protective cap or attach venipuncture device to tubing.	 Fluid in drip chamber prevents air from entering tubing and facilitates counting flow rate. If fluid level is too high or too low, counting is difficult and may be inaccurate. Avoids spilling fluid on floor, which would cause accidents. Prevents air embolism. Avoids inadvertent contamination of tubing tip.
17. To prime an ICD administration set: 　a. Read and follow manufacturer's directions on package, paying special attention to proper filling of cassette or chamber, if present. 　b. Repeat steps 16c and 16d, removing all air from tubing.	Improper filling can lead to total malfunction of system.
18. Remove all visible air trapped in tubing: 　a. Hold distal end of tubing upward, being careful to avoid contaminating tip. 　b. Gently tap or flick tubing with your fingers. 　c. If air bubble is near drip chamber, flick tubing below bubble.	Prevents possible air embolus and allays client's anxiety. Allows air to rise and be expelled more easily. This action sets the bubbles in motion. Moves air up to drip chamber.

(continued)

PREPARING AN INTRAVENOUS INFUSION (Cont.)

Step	Rationale
d. To remove air trapped in middle of tubing, insert a sterile needle into a medication port distal to air bubble, first cleansing port with alcohol.	Provides a sterile pathway for air to exit from tubing.
Open tubing clamp slightly, and allow fluid and air to flow slowly past needle; listen for slight hissing sound as air escapes.	Air will leave tubing through needle.
e. Replace cap on end of tubing.	Maintains sterility of tubing tip.
19. To use a filter:	
a. Following manufacturer's instructions, attach filter to tubing and fill it with IV fluid, being careful to expel all air.	Avoids introducing air into veins.
b. When filter has been filled properly, stop the fluid flow and replace cap on distal end of filter.	Maintains sterility of tubing tip.
20. Calculate number of milliliters to be infused per hour.	Helps monitor administration of correct amount of fluid.
21. Prepare a time tape to attach to bottle or bag that indicates fluid volume to infuse each hour.	Simplifies hourly checks during which proper rate of infusion must be verified. Assists in ascertaining when container will need to be changed.
22. If infusion is to be administered with an ICD, follow manufacturer's instructions for inserting tubing into device and setting controls for desired number of milliliters per hour.	Ensures correct administration of fluid and correct use of ICD.
23. If infusion is to be administered by gravity flow, calculate flow rate in drops per minute, based on drop factor of administration set being used.	Ensures correct rate of administration.

PERFORMING A VENIPUNCTURE

The process of inserting a needle or other type of intravenous cannula into a vein is known as a venipuncture. Venipunctures are usually performed through the skin (percutaneous), but in emergency situations where this is not possible, the physician may make a small surgical incision and insert the cannula. This procedure is done by the physician and is known as a cutdown.

Venipunctures are performed (1) to start an IV infusion to administer fluids, nutrients, or blood, (2) to withdraw blood for laboratory examination, and (3) to administer IV push medications.

Starting an IV Infusion

To perform a venipuncture to start an IV infusion, prepare the IV fluid container as described above, using the correct administration set. You will also need the following equipment: alcohol swabs or an antiseptic solution to cleanse the skin prior to the venipuncture; a tourniquet to slow or halt venous return from the extremity; a clean towel or disposable, moisture-resistant pad to avoid soiling the linen and clothing in case of accidental blood spills; an appropriate venipuncture device; adhesive tape to secure the cannula and dressing; antibiotic ointment to apply to the venipuncture site, along with a sterile applicator (according to agency policy); and sterile gauze squares (4 × 4 in.) or a transparent polyurethane dressing.

Selection of a venipuncture device is based on many factors. Larger-gauge cannulas (such as No. 20 or No. 21) are used to infuse viscous fluids or when rapid infusion is desired (greater than 150 ml/hr). Larger-gauge needles can cause trauma in small veins and thus should be inserted only in large veins. Smaller-gauge cannulas (such as No. 23 or No. 25) are used in small veins and for children. Over-the-needle catheters are probably used more frequently than other types of plastic cannulas. In most agencies, through-the-needle catheters are inserted only by a physician or a specially trained IV therapist.

A winged cannula or straight steel needle is usually attached to the IV tubing prior to the venipuncture. When the needle enters the vein, a "flashback" of blood is seen in the IV tubing at the hub–tubing connection (Plumer, 1982). This method avoids some leakage of blood and decreases the potential for contamination of the IV tubing when attaching it to the needle hub. It is not possible to do this when using an over-the-needle or through-the-needle catheter, however, as the needle must be removed before the IV tubing can be attached.

As you approach the client to perform a venipuncture, be calm and display confidence in your ability to collect the sample quickly. Displaying concern about the procedure will unduly increase the client's anxiety, thus decreasing the chances of a successful venipuncture. Explain the purpose of the venipuncture to the client and also mention that the procedure takes little time, as that information is usually quite reassuring. Ask the visitors or family to step outside the room and close the door or draw the curtain for privacy. Use judgment about this, as it may be unnecessary in some instances. Clients who are unable to cooperate must be restrained, as serious damage could result if movement occurs during the procedure. Highly anxious clients sometimes benefit from having someone hold the uninvolved hand or engage them in diversional conversation.

Select an appropriate site, as discussed earlier. Site selection for starting an IV infusion must be done quite carefully, because the venipuncture device will remain in place for 48 to 72 hours, unless complications develop. Position the client comfortably and inspect the site closely. Use an additional light source if necessary. When previous venipunctures have been difficult and the client is known or suspected to have "poor veins," the chances for a successful venipuncture can be increased by several methods. For example, lower the extremity below the level of the heart for several minutes before attempting the venipuncture. If the client is cold, apply blankets, as superficial veins often constrict under such circumstances. In addition, applying warm moist soaks to the lowered extremity often causes the veins to distend.

Apply the tourniquet between the chosen site and the client's heart. Stretch a rubber tourniquet around the arm and insert a loop under the tourniquet and next to the client's skin to hold it securely. Stretch a flexible elastic band tourniquet around the arm and close the self-adherent closure. If a standard tourniquet is unavailable, a blood pressure cuff inflated just enough to impede venous return provides an ideal tourniquet. Palpate the vein even if it is visible quite clearly, so as to ensure that it is not an artery and to determine that it is healthy enough for a venipuncture and is free from valves. Slapping the area gently may make the vein more prominent. Loosen the tourniquet after identifying the vein. Leaving the tourniquet in place while cleansing the site simply causes discomfort and does not increase the visibility of the vein. Use a circular motion to scrub the area with an alcohol swab or antiseptic solution. Do not touch the insertion site once it has been cleansed.

To stabilize the skin and vein, place the nondominant thumb slightly lateral to and approximately 2.5 cm (1 in) distal to the intended insertion site. This placement avoids having the thumb interfere with inserting the needle. Place the needle at a 25 to 45 degree angle, bevel side up, slightly to one side and parallel to the vein. However, if the vein is small, turning the bevel downward may help prevent extravasation as the needle enters the vein. Steady the dominant hand as it holds the needle by placing the hand or several fingers on the skin, and penetrate the skin with the needle at a point about 1.25 cm (½ in) distal to the planned site of entry into the vein, as shown in Figure 74–7. After the needle has penetrated the skin, relocate the vein with the nondominant hand, lower the needle to a 10 degree angle (nearly flush with the skin), and insert the needle at a gentle angle into the vein. When veins are sclerosed and tend to "roll" away from the needle (as often is true for elderly persons), insertion from above the vein often will be more successful. To do this, place the needle directly above the vein and penetrate the skin and vein simultaneously, with one downward motion.

Experience will help your fingers become sensitive to the resistance encountered as the needle meets the vein wall, and then the snap or pop that is felt as the needle enters the vein. A blood return in the IV tubing or from the venipuncture device will indicate that the cannula is in the vein. When you are certain the needle is in the vein, stabilize the vein with the nondominant hand and thread the cannula carefully into the vein, up to the hub so as to stabilize the cannula (Plumer, 1982). To prevent contamination of the cannula, avoid dragging it across the skin as you insert it. Some nurses place a sterile gauze square distal to the planned insertion site to protect the cannula during its insertion. When inserting an over-the-needle or through-the-needle catheter, it is helpful for an assistant to have the tubing uncapped and ready to insert in the catheter as soon as the needle is removed, thus minimizing blood leakage. Another way to decrease this leakage is to put digital pressure on the vein just proximal to the tip of the catheter while removing the needle and attaching the tubing tip.

As soon as the tubing is attached, open the clamp slowly and observe the site for possible infiltration. If none occurs, secure the infusion device to the client's skin with adhesive tape or a transparent polyurethane dressing. Correct anchoring of the infusion device meets the following criteria: (1) the actual cannual insertion site is free from tape, unless sterile tape is used; (2) the hub–tubing connection is free from tape to facilitate later tubing changes; and (3) the device is secured so that the needle or catheter does not move in and out or from side to side (Hirsch and Hannock,

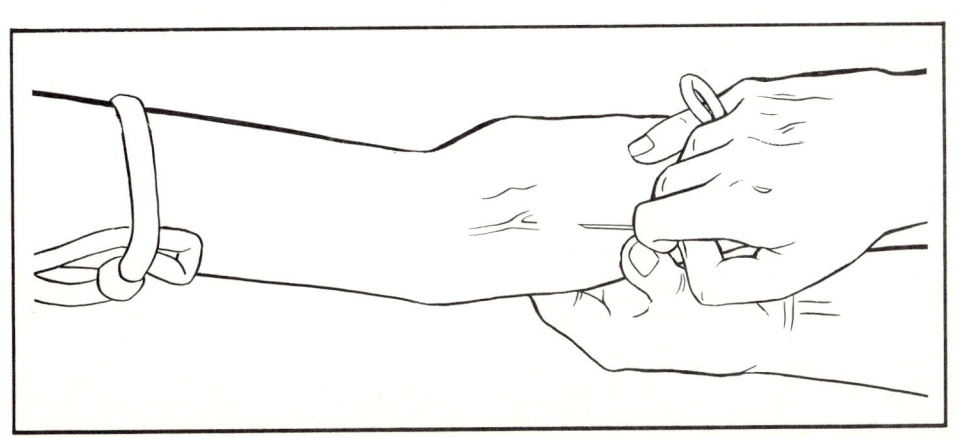

Figure 74–7. Basic venipuncture. Infusion tubing is kinked between ring and little finger. Left thumb keeps skin taut and anchors vein. The needle is held in line with the vein and at an angle.

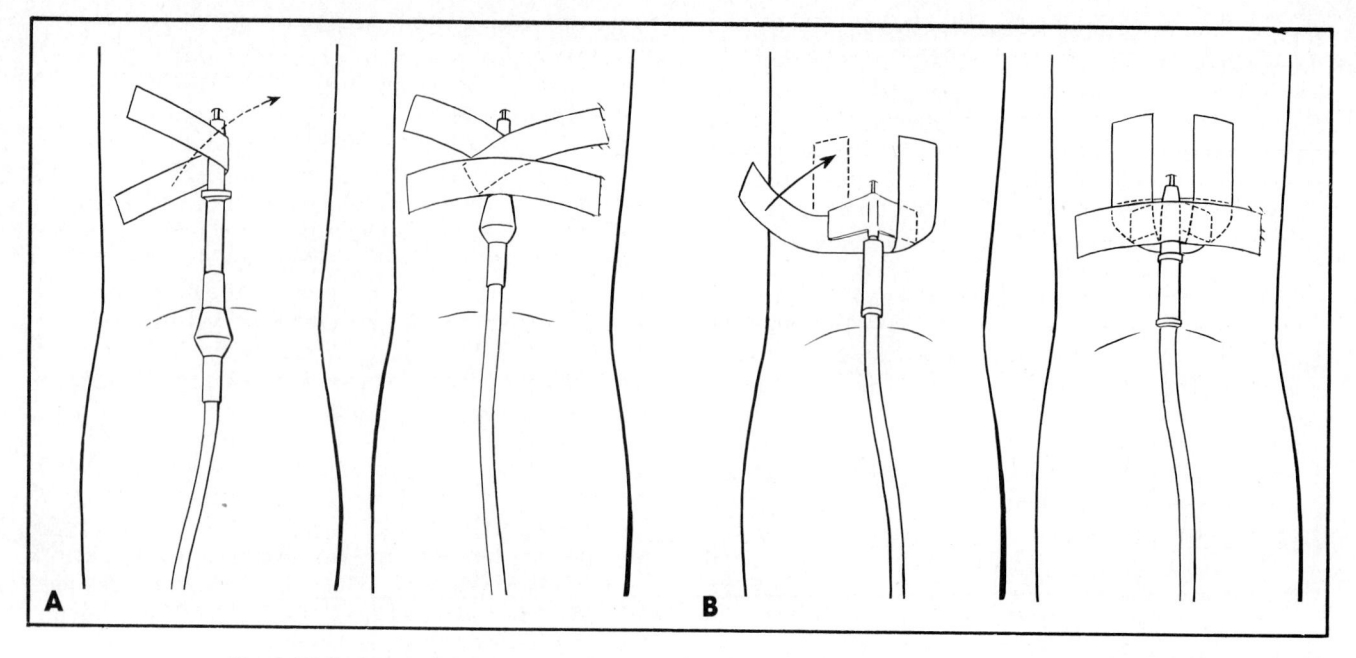

Figure 74–8. Securing an infusion cannula with adhesive tape, leaving both the insertion site and the hub–tubing connections free from tape. **A.** Chevron technique for straight cannulas and steel needles. **B.** Winged needles or cannulas.

1981). Movement of the catheter in and out of the vein admits microorganisms to the vein, and movement of the catheter back and forth traumatizes the tunica intima and predisposes the vein to thrombus formation.

Several common methods used to secure an infusion device with adhesive tape are shown in Figure 74–8. To secure a straight cannula or steel needle with the chevron technique (Fig. 74–8A), place a narrow strip of adhesive tape (adhesive side up) under the hub of the device. Bring the tape up and over the hub and secure it to the client's skin on the opposite side of the hub. Repeat with the other end of the tape. To secure a winged needle (Fig. 74–8B), place two strips of tape across the wings, parallel to the needle. Alternatively, place one strip of tape (adhesive side up) under the winged hub, bring the ends of the tape over the wings, and secure them parallel to the needle. Apply a second strip of tape directly over the hub.

Use great care to maintain strict aseptic technique when working with the venipuncture site, remembering that most IV-related infections are the result of contamination of the insertion site. Before placing a dry sterile gauze dressing over the insertion site, use a sterile applicator to apply a small amount of sterile antibiotic ointment to the cannula insertion site, unless this practice is contraindicated by agency policy. Place a sterile 4 × 4 gauze square over the site and secure it with adhesive tape. Mark on the tape the date, size, and type of venipuncture device used, and your initials. This information assists others to determine when the dressing should next be changed, whether the cannula is large enough to infuse fluids rapidly or to infuse blood should the client's condition warrant, as well as indicating who inserted the cannula. Secure the tubing to the client's skin at an additional spot, or loop it over the dressing and tape it a second time. This action avoids dislodging the cannula accidentally if excessive tension is placed on the tubing. Figure 74–9 shows a dry gauze infusion site dressing.

To use a transparent polyurethane dressing, peel off the protective backing and place the film directly

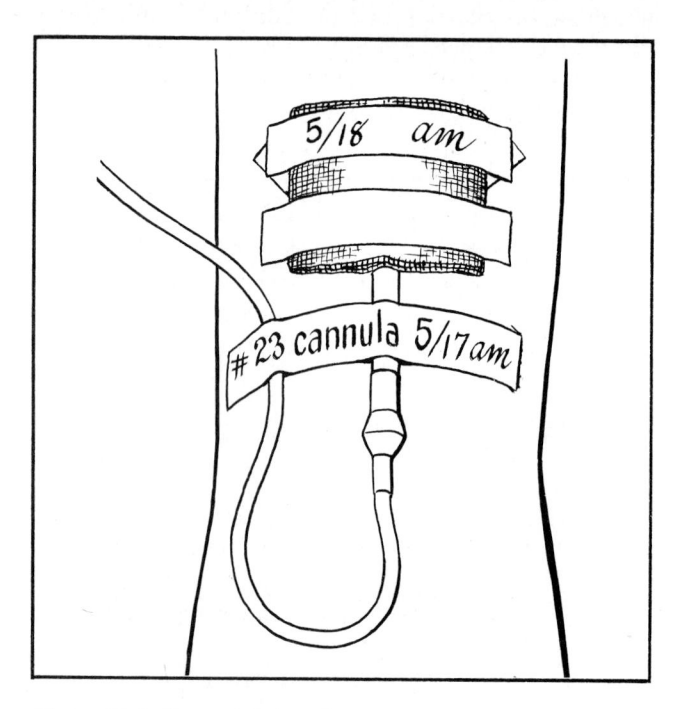

Figure 74–9. Gauze infusion site dressing. Tubing is secured to the client's arm and the dressing is labeled.

over the cannula insertion site. If antibiotic ointment is used, apply only a small dot of ointment, as body heat liquefies the ointment and causes it to spread and loosen the transparent film (Jones, Briggs, and Norton, 1982). The cannula hub is not taped in place, as the dressing secures the cannula as well as sealing the wound. The hub–tubing connection is not covered with the film, thus making tubing changes possible without disturbing the dressing. Do not apply adhesive tape to a transparent dressing; if the tape needs to be removed before the dressing does, the dressing will be destroyed. However, a small tape label may be placed in one corner of the dressing. After the venipuncture device and tubing are secured, regulate the infusion at the proper flow rate. Hold your watch directly beside the drip chamber so you can count the drops per minute without taking your eyes off the second hand. Count the number of drops that fall in a 15-second interval to adjust the flow rate and then count the drop rate for a full minute to ensure accuracy. If the infusion is to be administered with an ICD, set the controls according to the manufacturer's directions, usually in milliliters to be infused in one hour. Before leaving the client's room, again inspect the site for infiltration and to ascertain that the IV is not causing discomfort.

☐ SKILL SEQUENCE

PERFORMING A VENIPUNCTURE AND STARTING AN IV INFUSION

Step	Rationale
1. Validate physician's order for venipuncture or infusion.	Ensures correct implementation of physician order.
2. Prepare IV infusion as in the Skill Sequence, "Preparing an Intravenous Infusion." Attach the venipuncture cannula unless it is an over-the-needle or through-the-needle catheter.	Necessary preparatory step. Needle must be removed from a needle-catheter device after it is inserted into vein, and before infusion tubing is attached.
3. Wash hands.	Prevents transfer of microorganisms.
4. Identify client and self as in Skill 71, Skill Sequence, "Administering Oral Medication," steps 3 and 4.	Ensures that procedure is implemented for correct client.
5. Explain procedure to client. (NOTE: Obtain help to restrain an uncooperative client.)	Allays anxiety and gains cooperation. Prevents injury during venipuncture.
6. Provide privacy and ask visitors to leave the room.	Prevents distraction, allays client and visitor anxiety.
7. Select appropriate location for venipuncture, position client comfortably, and obtain additional lighting as needed. Place a protective pad under extremity.	Promotes successful venipuncture procedure. Avoids accidental soiling of linen and clothing.

8. If client has veins that are difficult to cannulate, try the following steps for 5 to 10 minutes prior to the venipuncture.
  a. Lower arm below heart level.
  b. Put warm blankets on client.
  c. Apply warm, moist soaks to the extremity.
	Helps distend veins, making cannulation easier.

9. Inspect selected site for integrity and bruises.	Avoids using bruised or damaged site.
10. Apply tourniquet between chosen site and client's heart.	Distends veins maximally by retarding or stopping venous return from the extremity.
11. Palpate vein, noting resilience, pliability, and presence or absence of valves. Slap area gently if vein does not seem distended adequately.	Identifies presence of a healthy vein. Makes vein more prominent.
12. Release tourniquet.	Decreases client's discomfort.
13. Cleanse insertion site in a circular manner, using either alcohol swabs or antiseptic solution, according to agency policy.	Removes transient and resident skin bacteria and prevents microorganisms from entering venipuncture site.
14. Reapply tourniquet.	Distends veins maximally by retarding or stopping venous return from the extremity.

15. Insert venipuncture:
  a. Pull skin taut over insertion site with nondominant hand.
  b. Use dominant hand to place cannula parallel to and slightly beside vein, bevel side up and at a 45 degree angle. (NOTE: For above-vein entry, use a 15-degree angle.)
  c. Penetrate skin with cannula, lower needle to 10 degree angle, and penetrate vein at a slight lateral angle.
  d. Observe for blood return.
  e. Thread cannula into vein up to hub.
	Helps immobilize vein and skin.
	Facilitates cannula entry into healthy vein.
	
	Facilitates cannula entry into vein.
	
	Indicates that the device is in the vein and that the infusion may be administered safely.
	Stabilizes cannula in vein.

(continued)

PERFORMING A VENIPUNCTURE AND STARTING AN IV INFUSION (Cont.)

Step	Rationale
16. Release the tourniquet.	Prevents unnecessary discomfort and minimizes blood flow from the venipuncture device.
17. After inserting an over-the-needle catheter, remove the needle inside the catheter, leaving only the plastic catheter inside the vein. Discard the needle according to agency policy.	Avoids accidental needle-stick injuries with a potentially contaminated needle.
18. Insert the tip of the primed administration set tubing into the cannula hub, if not done earlier.	Attaches infusion to cannula without introducing microorganisms directly into the bloodstream.
19. Open the clamp and allow the infusion to flow slowly, observing the site for infiltration. NOTE: If infiltration occurs, remove cannula and attempt another venipuncture at another site.	Infiltration indicates that cannula is not in the vein.
20. Secure cannula so that it does not move laterally or in and out of vein. Leave hub–tubing connection free from tape. NOTE: Do not secure the cannula with tape if a transparent dressing is used.	Secures cannula and avoids accidental removal. Transparent dressing secures cannula.
21. Use a sterile applicator to apply a drop of antibiotic ointment over IV insertion site, according to agency policy. NOTE: If transparent dressing is used, apply a very small dot of ointment.	Recommended by the CDC to help prevent IV-related infections. Body heat liquefies ointment and can loosen transparent dressing.
22. Apply sterile dressing to insertion site. a. Dry gauze dressing: secure a sterile 4 × 4-in. pad over insertion site; label tape with date, time, and initials. b. Transparent polyurethane dressing: peel off protective backing and apply over insertion site; leave hub–tubing connection free. Place label in corner of or adjacent to dressing and identify as in step 22a.	Provides barrier against contact with contaminated items. Provides data for determining subsequent dressing changes. Secures cannula and seals insertion wound. Enables nurse to change tubing without disturbing transparent dressing. Tape label loosens transparent dressing if it is removed.
23. Secure tubing to client's arm and to dressing. (NOTE: Do not apply tape to any part of a polyurethane dressing.)	Avoids dislodging device accidentally. Removing tape destroys polyurethane dressings.
24. Write date, size, and type of insertion device and your initials on tape.	Provides for nurse accountability. Provides data for determining later insertion site care.
25. Set correct gravity infusion flow rate in drops per minute: a. Hold your watch beside drip chamber. b. Count number of drops that fall in 15 seconds and adjust tubing clamp accordingly. c. When rate is correct for a 15-second period, count drops for 1 minute.	Allows for counting drops while simultaneously watching second hand on watch. Quick, easy way to adjust flow rate. Ensures infusion of fluid at intended rate.
26. If infusion is to be administered through an ICD, set controls for desired rate (usually in milliliters per minute), according to manufacturer's directions.	Correct setting ensures infusion of fluid at intended rate. Considerable variation exists among different types of ICDs.
27. Inspect the site again for signs of infiltration and inquire about discomfort at the site.	Ensures that cannula is in client's vein.
28. Discard disposable equipment according to agency policy.	Correct care of equipment.
29. Wash hands.	Prevents transfer of microorganisms.
30. Document procedure in client's health record. Include time, site, purpose, type of cannula, and any problems encountered.	Fulfills nurse accountability. Provides ongoing data base.

Collecting a Blood Sample

The procedure for performing a venipuncture to collect a blood sample is quite similar to that used to start an IV infusion. To withdraw a blood sample for laboratory analysis, you will need a blood collecting device and evacuated blood collecting tubes, or a conventional glass syringe and laboratory tubes. Use a No. 20 or No. 21 gauge needle to withdraw blood, as smaller-gauge needles may cause hemolysis of red blood cells and also prolong the time needed to withdraw the sample; larger-gauge needles are unnecessarily painful. Gather the following additional equipment: a tourniquet; antiseptic solution and protective pad as described earlier; sterile gauze squares or cottonballs for applying pressure to the area during and after the needle is withdrawn; and a band-aid to place over the site after the bleeding has stopped.

Select, inspect, and prepare the venipuncture site as described earlier. As this venipuncture is of short duration, sites at or over joints are acceptable. Some clients automatically clench and unclench their hand after the tourniquet is applied. This practice should be strongly discouraged. Although exercise of the muscle distal to the tourniquet does help distend the vein, this muscle activity can alter the values of some electrolye levels (Metheny and Snively, 1983). Insert the blood collecting device needle into the skin and vein as described earlier and then push the evacuated blood collecting tube into the holder toward the needle so that the short inner needle pierces the rubber diaphragm of the tube. If the needle is in the vein, blood will flow into the tube quite rapidly. When enough blood tubes have been filled to obtain the desired sample, remove or release the tourniquet.

It should be noted that blood collecting devices and evacuated tubes are not recommended for fragile veins or for a person with low blood pressure, as the negative pressure is sufficiently great to collapse the vein. Lesser and more controlled pressure can be applied with a large syringe, such as a 10- or 20-ml syringe. Because of the smaller diameter, a smaller syringe exerts a greater negative pressure than a large one and therefore is more likely to cause a vein to collapse.

To prevent extravasation into the tissues, apply pressure to the site with a sterile gauze square as the needle is being removed and for up to 5 minutes afterward and elevate the arm higher than the heart. Apply a band-aid to protect the wound until it seals over in about 24 hours. Even though venous bleeding is less serious than arterial bleeding, do NOT leave the room until the bleeding has stopped completely. If bleeding seems prolonged or excessive, check the site within 10 to 15 minutes to be sure that the bleeding has not resumed. Bleeding from a venipuncture site can produce unsightly discoloration in subcutaneous tissues, causing the client unnecessary distress and discomfort. Bleeding is likely to be prolonged in persons with blood dyscrasias, clotting disorders, or those who are receiving anticoagulant medications.

CARE OF THE CLIENT WITH AN INTRAVENOUS INFUSION

Caring for a client with an IV requires organization and skill in making routine, accurate assessments. The nurse is responsible for maintaining a continuous flow at the proper rate, making the observations needed to prevent complications or detect them early, and infusing medications at the correct time and rate. The infusion must flow continuously or venous pressure will cause blood to flow back into the cannula, which will then clot and occlude the device. An occluded cannula must be removed and the infusion started in a new site, which causes additional trauma and expense for the client. Never irrigate (inject fluid into) an occluded cannula, as that process sends fibrinous material into the vein, which can result in the development of a thrombus.

☐ SKILL SEQUENCE

PERFORMING A VENIPUNCTURE TO COLLECT A BLOOD SAMPLE

Step	Rationale
1. Validate physician's order according to agency policy.	Ensures correct implementation of physician's order.
2. Follow Skill Sequence, p. 951, steps 3 to 14, "Performing a Venipuncture and Starting an IV Infusion." Note: Do not allow client to clench and unclench the hand.	Alters values of some electrolyte levels.
3. Pull skin taut over insertion site. Insert blood collecting device needle, bevel side up, into skin and vein at a 15 to 45 degree angle, using dominant hand.	Provides for ready entry into skin and vein.
4. Stabilize blood collecting device with nondominant hand. Insert vacuum tube with dominant hand and push tube firmly toward insertion site, so that short needle pierces rubber diaphragm. Observe for prompt blood return into tube.	The vacuum inside tube will draw blood into tube.
5. Leave venipuncture needle in place in vein and remove vacuum tube when full; repeat process until all needed tubes are full. (Note: If blood does not flow into tube, try another tube; if second tube does not fill with blood, assume that needle is not in vein and attempt venipuncture at another site.)	Obtains needed specimen volume. Vacuum tube may have lost its negative pressure.
6. After needed volume of blood has been obtained, release tourniquet.	Helps prevent extravasation into tissues when needle is withdrawn.
7. Withdraw needle while applying pressure at site with a dry sterile gauze square or cottonball. Do not use alcohol swabs for this purpose.	Prevents bleeding at the site. Alcohol stings when applied to a fresh venipuncture site.

(continued)

PERFORMING A VENIPUNCTURE TO COLLECT A BLOOD SAMPLE (Cont.)

Step	Rationale
8. Elevate client's arm higher than heart level while waiting for bleeding to stop. Continue to apply pressure over gauze pad with fingers. Avoid bending client's elbow if antecubital site was used.	Elevation reduces venous pressure and pressure helps seal wound. Bending elbow tends to reopen puncture wound.
9. Apply a band-aid to the site after bleeding has stopped.	Protects insertion site from entry of microorganism.
10. Discard equipment according to agency policy.	Correct care of equipment.
11. Label specimen and send to laboratory promptly.	Ensures correct client receives appropriate diagnostic information.
12. Wash hands.	Prevents transfer of microorganisms.
13. Document procedure in health record. Include date and time specimen was obtained, time it was sent to laboratory, purpose of specimen, and client's reaction to procedure.	Fulfills nurse accountability and provides ongoing data base.

Monitoring the Client with an Intravenous Infusion

Monitor the client who is receiving an IV infusion at least hourly, and more often when potentially hazardous medications are being infused or when the client's condition is not stable. Additionally, every time any nurse comes to the bedside of any person receiving an intravenous infusion, he or she is expected to monitor the infusion. With very little practice, hourly assessments can be made in less than 30 seconds and will greatly increase the safety and effectiveness of IV therapy.

Assessment Sequence. It is important to establish a routine for regular assessments, so that no aspect is omitted. A recommended way to do this is to begin with the fluid container and progress toward the infusion site, using the following sequence, making the following observations, and taking remedial action as indicated.

1. *Fluid container*. Identify if the correct solution is being infused, whether it is infusing on schedule, how much fluid remains in the container, and when it is due to empty. Add a new container as needed. If the fluid will be completely infused within 2 hours or less, it is imperative to ascertain that the next container has been prepared or has arrived from the pharmacy.
2. *Drip chamber*. Note whether drops are falling steadily. If the infusion is on schedule, it is not necessary to count or time the drops, but this should be done if the volume of infused solution is ahead or behind schedule, with adjustments made as needed. If drops are not observed to be falling steadily, or if the IV is behind schedule, investigate and remedy the cause as described below.
3. *Tubing:* Look at the clamp and be sure it is open; check for kinking.
4. *Infusion control device:* Determine that the hourly infusion rate is set correctly and that the indicator lights are functioning.
5. *The client's extremity:* If the IV site is near or over a joint, look for joint flexion that may interfere with the infusion flow. Check the alignment of the extremity for comfort.
6. *Insertion site:* Inspect the infusion site for signs of phlebitis or infiltration as described earlier. If an infiltration is present, discontinue the infusion promptly; do not attempt to clear the needle.

    When an infusion is functioning properly, a gauze dressing is dry and no leakage is present under or around a transparent dressing. A wet or leaking dressing signals that the infusion is leaking either at the hub-tubing connection or at the insertion site itself. Tightening the connection stops that leakage; however, leaking from the insertion site itself usually means that the infusion needs to be restarted in a new site. When a gauze dressing is used, palpate the site gently every 24 hours, as a gauze dressing can hide the signs of infiltration and infection. Because the site is visible when a transparent dressing is used, inspect the site closely, but avoid the unnecessary trauma of palpation unless redness exists.
7. *The client:* Remember that a *person* is receiving the IV infusion! Assess the client for general comfort and discomfort, investigate any complaints of tenderness, pain, or discomfort at the infusion site, and provide additional information as needed. An intravenous infusion causes no pain if it is functioning properly. Observe for signs and symptoms of circulatory overload and monitor intake and output at least every 8 hours. Assess the client for signs of an infection by evaluating body temperature patterns; an elevation may indicate an infusion-related infection, which would necessitate restarting the infusion in another site.

Problems with Flow Rate. Sometimes the IV infusion does not flow at all or at the proper rate, even though no infiltration is evident and all factors have been assessed or corrected as described above. In such circumstances, the following actions may cause the flow to restart. If it does not, the infusion must be discontinued and restarted in another site.

1. Adjust the position of the client's extremity. A flexed joint can obstruct the flow when the needle is at or near the joint. The problem apparently results from the needle bevel being lodged against the vein wall. Move the arm or cannula hub slightly, as some IVs seem to be "positional," that is, a movement or position change can stop or start the flow. Try to determine the position of maximal flow and retape the needle in that position if necessary.
2. Check the tubing for kinks and be sure that the client is not lying on it, as that will slow or stop the flow. Unless too long a time has elapsed, the fluid will begin to flow properly once the tubing has been freed.
3. If the fluid container is a glass bottle, determine whether the air vent is open and functioning properly.
4. Fold the tubing near the venipuncture site and pinch it closed. Squeeze the rubber flashball or tubing distal to the pinched area. If the bevel of the needle or cannula is against the vein wall, this action will move it away and allow the fluid to flow. If, however, the needle has become clotted with backed-up blood, resistance will be felt when the tubing or flashball is squeezed, as squeezing does not produce enough pressure to release the clot and cause a potential embolus.
5. When an infusion is flowing by gravity, raise the height of the IV pole, as the increased pressure may restart the infusion flow.
6. When an ICD is being used, check to be sure it is plugged in, turned on, and that the indicator lights are working. Sometimes machines are turned off inadvertently and then operate on time-limited battery power.

Personal Care
It is important to keep the insertion site dry at all times, as this helps avoid entry of microorganisms. Modify the bathing procedure as needed to accomplish this. *Never separate and reconnect the tubing as a convenience for the nurse.* This practice is considered unacceptable due to the possibility of contaminating the tubing connections and allowing microorganisms to enter the bloodstream (Kozier and Erb, 1982; Simmons, 1981).

Changing the Gown. Some agencies provide special gowns for clients who are receiving IV therapy; these gowns are open not only down the back, but also completely across the shoulders from the neck down through the hem of the sleeve. The openings are closed with snaps, ties, or self-adherent closures. When these gowns are not available, the nurse must know how to get a client and his or her IV into and out of a gown without dislodging the needle, disrupting the flow of the infusion, or disconnecting the tubing.

To change a client's gown, follow the following steps:

1. Remove the soiled gown from the arm that does not have the infusion.
2. Slip the gown down the arm that has the infusion and onto the IV tubing, covering a female's chest with a sheet, bath blanket, or a towel. Unless the gown is wet or badly soiled, allow it to lie on the bed around the IV tubing while you complete the bath or morning care.
3. Place the opened, clean gown near the soiled one.
4. Remove the IV fluid container from the pole and remove the tubing from the ICD, if one is in use. Before removing the tubing, adjust the flow rate manually to a keep-open rate of 20 to 40 drops per minute, as removing the tubing from the ICD may cause the fluid to stop completely or flow at a wide-open rate. A wide-open rate is unacceptable, even for the short time required to change a gown.
5. Hold the fluid container as high as possible, slide the soiled gown up and over the container, and lay the soiled gown on the bed near the client.
6. Pick up the clean gown and insert the fluid container through the sleeve from the inside of the gown, as if it were the client's arm. Allow the clean gown to lay on the bed near the client, with the tubing through the gown sleeve.
7. Rehang the fluid container on the IV pole and check to be sure that the rate of gravity flow has remained unchanged, or replace the IV tubing in the ICD and open the tubing clamp.
8. Assist the client to don the gown, first inserting the arm with the IV site.

The gown can also be removed and replaced in two separate actions if necessary; for example, if the gown is badly soiled or wet, remove it completely before providing care. However, it is easier to remove the soiled gown and replace it with a clean one at the same time, rather than at two separate times. In addition, less manipulation of the IV container and ICD is required.

Ambulation. An ongoing IV infusion should never interfere with the client's need for ambulation, even when there are infusions in several different sites, as is sometimes necessary. The most important principle to follow is to keep the fluid container high enough at all times so that a constant flow is maintained. Use a sturdy portable IV pole for this purpose; the pole can be navigated either by the client or the nurse. A client known to one of the authors walked several times a day in the halls with his IV pole, referring to it as his "dancing partner!"

ROUTINE EQUIPMENT CHANGES

As indicated earlier, IV fluid containers, administration sets, and dressings are changed every 48 to 72 hours, or at more frequent intervals if problems develop. When an administration set is changed at the same time a new IV fluid container is hung, the procedure is the same as preparing an initial IV, except that the venipuncture device is not replaced. However, fluid containers must be changed much more often than administration sets, and sometimes the administration set is changed when the fluid container is not changed.

Changing the IV Fluid Container

The fluid container usually is changed only when it empties, at intervals ranging from 6 to 24 hours. It may also be changed in response to a new order from the physician. New containers of fluid are prepared away from the client's bedside, as described earlier, including a new time tape.

The following sequence of activities is used to change the IV fluid container when the administration set is not being changed. Use aseptic technique and methods similar to those used when preparing an IV infusion, as described earlier.

1. Wash hands.
2. Close the clamp on the administration set or turn off the ICD to stop the fluid flow temporarily and avoid the entry of air into the tubing.
3. Remove the protective cap from the administration port on the new fluid container (cleanse the entry port on a glass bottle with an alcohol swab).
4. Take the old container down from the IV pole.
5. Remove the spike from the old container and insert it into the new container.
6. Hang the new container from the IV pole.
7. Open the clamp and reset a gravity flow rate or restart an ICD.
8. Observe the drip chamber for a few moments to be sure the system is working properly.
9. Discard used items correctly.
10. Wash hands.
11. Document on the IV fluid record.

Changing the IV Administration Set

Although it is easier to change an administration set when a new fluid container is hung, an agency may have a policy that mandates routine tubing changes on certain shifts on certain days of the week. This policy ensures that all tubing is changed at the recommended intervals, even though it may sometimes result in a tubing change after less than 48 hours, for example, if a client's IV was started the day prior to a scheduled tubing change.

The administration set may be prepared at the bedside, in the medicine room, or in a clean utility room. The primary difference between replacing an administration set and preparing an administration set for initial infusion is that a rapid transition between the old and new administration set is needed, as the infusion must be interrupted no longer than is absolutely necessary, so as to avoid clotting in the cannula. This means that you will need to prime the tubing quickly and place the new tubing in the cannula promptly.

The following sequence of activities is used to change the administration set when you are not changing the IV fluid container. Use aseptic technique and methods similar to those used when preparing an IV infusion, as described earlier.

1. Wash hands.
2. Place protective pad under the infusion site to catch any blood lost accidentally when the tubing is separated.
3. Close the tubing clamp on the new administration set and attach a filter (if one is being used), leaving the protective caps on the spike and distal filter tip.
4. Attach a piece of adhesive tape to the tubing and label it with the date and time of the tubing change. This indicates to others when the tubing will again need changing.
5. Remove the IV insertion site dressing to gain access to the cannula insertion site. Loosen the tape that secures the old tubing to the arm.
6. Stabilize the cannula with one hand and grasp the old tubing with the other. Use a twisting motion to loosen the hub-tubing connection, but do not disconnect the tubing. A small hemostat may be used to grasp and stabilize the cannula hub to reduce cannula movement and trauma to the tissue intima. Reattach the loosened tape strip (or use a new short strip of tape) to stabilize the old IV tubing while preparing the new tubing, thus avoiding trauma to the vein.
7. Decrease the fluid flow to a keep-open rate (20–40 drops/min) to maintain cannula patency and avoid blood backup in the tubing.
8. Remove the fluid container from the IV pole and hold the container with the insertion port uppermost.
9. Remove the administration spike from the fluid container and place the used administration set near the head of the bed (for a client in semi-Fowler's position) or hang it from the IV pole or the ICD to allow for a continued gravity fluid flow that will maintain cannula patency and avoid blood backup.
10. Remove the protective cap from the spike on the new administration set and insert it into the fluid container.
11. Rehang the fluid container on the IV pole.
12. Prime the new tubing quickly, close the tubing clamp, and replace the protective cap.
13. Remove the protective cap from the new tubing and hold the tubing between the fingers of one hand. While stabilizing the cannula with the opposite hand, quickly remove the old tubing and insert the new tubing into the cannula. Speed is essential, as disconnecting the old tubing causes blood to flow from the cannula.
14. Open the clamp and restart the infusion flow at a slow rate, to maintain patency of the cannula.
15. Apply a new sterile dressing to the infusion site and secure the tubing to the dressing or extremity.

16. Adjust the flow rate correctly or reset the ICD.
17. Discard used equipment correctly.
18. Wash hands.

Changing the Insertion Site Dressing

The insertion site dressing is changed every 48 to 72 hours when the administration set is changed or whenever a dry gauze dressing becomes wet or soiled or a transparent dressing loosens or leaks.

Remove the old dressing by pulling the tape toward the venipuncture site to prevent accidental dislodging of the needle, and discard the dressing properly. Assess the site for signs of inflammation and infection and relocate the infusion to another site if necessary.

Agency policy may include cleansing the insertion site with an antiseptic such as povidone–iodine (Betadine) and application of an antibiotic ointment such as Neosporin. If so, follow carefully the principles for cleansing wounds described in Skill 32. Cleanse the cannula insertion site with a circular motion, starting at the site and moving outward; repeat twice with a fresh sterile gauze pad. To apply antibiotic ointment, first discard 0.3 cm (⅛ in.) of ointment on a sterile pad. Then squeeze 1.25 cm (½ in.) of ointment on a fresh sterile pad and apply the ointment to the cannula insertion site with a sterile applicator. Apply a fresh sterile gauze pad to the insertion site and tape it in place securely. Write the date of the dressing change on the tape, so that the time for subsequent dressing is readily determined.

If a transparent polyurethane dressing is used, blot the cannula wound dry with a fresh sterile gauze pad and apply the film directly over the insertion site, using the same technique described earlier. When a transparent dressing becomes soiled, wipe it clean with a damp washcloth or gauze square.

Document in the health record the date and time that the dressing change was done. Include the type of antibiotic ointment used, a description of the appearance of the infusion site, noting any abnormalities, and any IV-related complaints expressed by the client.

DISCONTINUING AN INTRAVENOUS INFUSION

Before discontinuing an IV infusion, validate the physician's order and inform the client about the plan. To discontinue an IV infusion, you will need sterile gauze squares and a band-aid. Clamp the infusion tubing and remove the dressing by pulling the tape toward the venipuncture site to prevent inadvertent removal of the cannula. Remove the dressing and discard it in an impervious trash container. Carefully loosen all tape holding the tubing or cannula in place. If the client's arm is hairy, this can be a very painful procedure. Pull the tape quickly, while stabilizing the skin underneath to reduce the pain. After all tape has been loosened, apply gentle pressure directly over the venipuncture site with a sterile gauze square or cotton ball as you remove the cannula gently and steadily. After the cannula is out of the vein, hold firm pressure over the site for 3 to 5 minutes or until bleeding stops, and elevate the arm above the level of the heart. Apply the band-aid after the bleeding has stopped. Instruct the client to keep the site dry for 24 hours, which will allow the wound to seal, thus preventing microorganisms from entering the venipuncture site.

Document in the health record the date, time, and amount of fluid infused. Complete the IV fluid flow sheet or intake record. Total fluid intake and output monitoring is usually continued for at least 24 hours, or as needed, to evaluate the client's ability to ingest oral fluids.

ADMINISTERING IV MEDICATIONS

Medications may be added to the main IV, given as an IV piggyback, or injected directly into the vein. Although any infiltration is a problem, an infiltration with a medication solution produces additional problems resulting from a drug being given by an incorrect route. Patency of the cannula is perhaps most important when injecting medications directly into the vein through a herparin lock or as an IV push medication because the medication is more concentrated than when diluted in an IVPB or the main IV. Therefore, assess the infusion site carefully prior to giving medications directly into the vein.

As with injectable medications, it is crucial that the dosage for IV medications is calculated correctly and that aseptic technique is used to prepare and administer IV medications.

Administering IV Piggyback Medications

In institutions that use the unit-dose system for dispensing medications, piggyback medications are delivered to the clinical unit premixed, labeled properly, and ready to be administered or refrigerated. The medication will have been diluted in the proper amount of D_5W or NS and will be packaged in small volume-control containers. In some institutions, however, the nurse who administers the drug must prepare the piggyback medication solution by adding the designated medication to a small plastic infusion bag or to the buretrol.

Preparing IVPB Medications in Plastic Bags. Prepare IVPB medications away from the bedside. Inject the medication into the small plastic infusion bag through the medication port, using a sterile syringe and needle. When a powdered drug needs to be reconstituted, agency policy may indicate that the diluent is drawn from the small infusion bag. To do this, use a 10-ml syringe and a large-gauge needle (No. 18 or No. 20) to speed the process. Use aseptic technique to withdraw fluid through the medication port and reconstitute the medication as described in Skill 73. After injecting the medication into the medication port, invert the bag, squeeze the port, and invert several more times to mix the medication. After adding the medication, label the bag properly with the client's name, the name and dosage of the medication, the date and time, and your name and title.

Next, select an administration set with a tubing long enough to reach from the IV pole to a medication port on the main IV tubing. This can often be the shorter 86 cm (34 in.) tubing. Insert the tubing spike into the bag and prime it, exactly as when preparing a larger IV infusion, and as described earlier. Be careful to avoid excessive fluid loss during the priming process, so the dosage is not altered. Attach a No. 23 or No. 21 needle to the tubing, leaving the protective cap in place. (A larger needle would make unnecessarily large holes in the medication port.) The medication solution is now ready to be administered in one of several ways, as described below.

Infusing IVPB Medications through the Main IV.
IVPB medications may be administered through the main IV tubing by gravity flow or through an ICD.

For *gravity-flow* administration, calculate the correct flow rate (drops per minute) of the fluid being administered and the length of time over which the IVPB medication will be infused, as discussed earlier. At the bedside, hang the IVPB container on the IV pole and then locate an appropriate medication port on the main tubing—either a Y-type port or the rubber flashball near the venipuncture site. Cleanse the port carefully with an alcohol swab and insert the needle, being very careful to avoid going through the other side of the tubing, as only the flashball or port is self-sealing. If it is institutional policy to run all IVPB solutions through a filter, select a medication port proximal to the filter. Insert the needle all the way into the tubing so that it will not move in and out of the port, thus causing contamination. Tape the needle in place securely to prevent it from becoming dislodged during administration. Open the administration clamp and set the rate as calculated.

For the IVPB to infuse, it must be hung at a higher level than the main IV container. The main IV tubing is not clamped, although sometimes this infusion will stop flowing while the IVPB is running. If the main IV has not been clamped, it will resume its flow when the IVPB empties. The administration set shown earlier in Figure 74-6 includes a secondary "piggyback" solution setup. Note that the secondary container hangs at a higher level than the main IV infusion. The higher level provides a greater pressure, allowing the secondary fluid to flow in by gravity, preferentially over the main IV infusion. The antireflux valve prevents backflow of secondary fluid into the main IV container.

When the main IV is being infused through an infusion control device, the IVPB medication may be infused either through the ICD or inserted into a medication port distal to the ICD and run by gravity flow. To infuse the medication through the ICD, insert the piggyback tubing into a medication port proximal to the ICD, clamp off the main IV tubing proximal to the piggyback insertion site, and reset the ICD controls to deliver the solution at the required flow rate. The alarm on the ICD will sound when the IVPB container is empty, at which time the main IV infusion must be restarted by opening the tubing clamp. If the client is receiving many IVPB medications, this method may pose problems in keeping the main infusion on schedule. However, if the medication is incompatible with the main infusion fluid, the two may not run concurrently.

When a *burette* is used to administer IVPB medications through the main IV, the burette tubing is attached to the main IV as described above. Solution from the main IV fluid container is added to the burette first, followed by the medication, thus diluting the medication. The following sequence of activities is used to administer an IVPB medication with a burette. Use aseptic technique throughout.

1. Determine that the clamp on the burette tubing is closed.
2. Allow 50 to 100 ml of fluid to flow into the burette from the main IV fluid container.
3. Inject the prepared medication into the rubber medication port on top of the burette and agitate gently to mix the medication.
4. Close the clamp on the main administration tubing proximal to the burette tubing insertion.
5. Open the clamp on the burette tubing and adjust the flow rate as needed for the amount of medication and duration of administration.
6. Return to the bedside prior to the time the burette is empty. A delay would allow air to enter the burette tubing and could cause the infusion cannula to become clotted.
7. Allow 15 to 20 ml of additional fluid to flow into the burette from the main IV fluid container and allow this fluid to infuse to clear the medication from the tubing.
8. Close the burette tubing clamp before air enters the burette tubing and open the main IV tubing clamp, adjusting the rate correctly. (*Note:* If the burette is an integral part of the client's main IV tubing, rather than an IVPB, allow at least enough fluid for one hour's infusion to enter the burette from the main IV container.)

Infusing Medications through a Heparin Lock
The patency of a heparin lock is maintained by inserting a dilute heparin solution into the lock at the completion of each infusion. Various heparin solutions are used for this purpose, containing from 10 to 1000 USP units of heparin per milliliter of saline, with 100 units/ml being the most common strength. The heparin lock is always flushed with 1 ml of this solution, even though the capacity of the lock is only 0.2 to 0.4 ml. Using the entire milliliter ensures that the catheter or needle is filled completely with heparin solution, thereby preventing blood from clotting within the lock (Hanson, 1976). To avoid clotting from occurring, the nurse must be sure to have the heparin solution

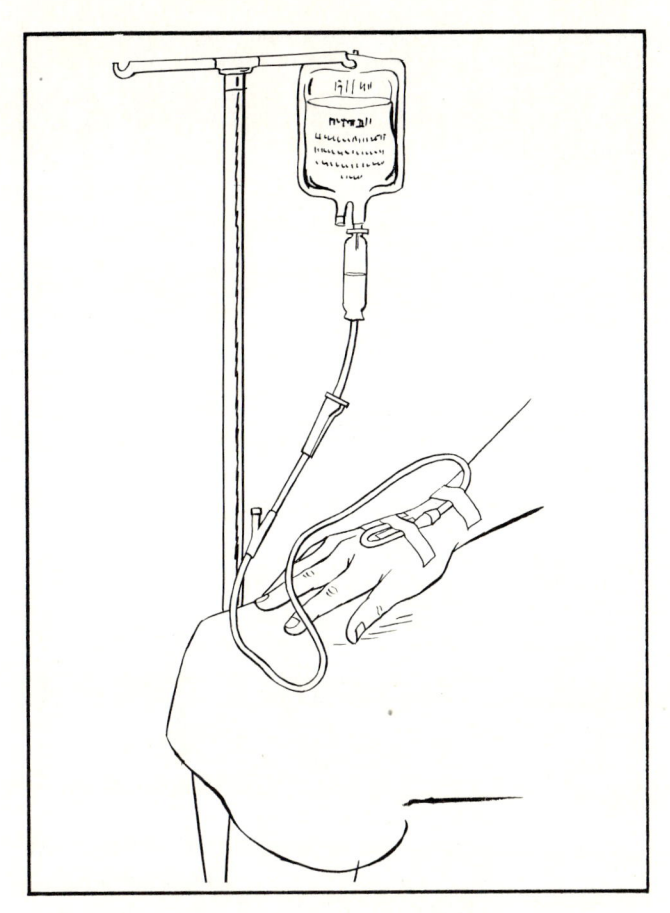

Figure 74-10. Intravenous medication in volume-control container infusing through a heparin lock device.

ready to infuse immediately after each infusion is completed. Figure 74-10 shows an IV medication being infused through a heparin lock.

Medications are prepared for infusion through a heparin lock in the same way as for IVPB medications. However, use a longer administration set, such as a 244-cm (98-in.) tubing. The tubing should allow the small fluid container to be elevated high enough above the infusion site to infuse properly, and yet not restrict the client's movement any more than necessary. Attach a No. 21 or No. 23 needle to the tubing, as a larger gauge would make unnecessarily large holes in the resealable rubber diaphragm of the heparin lock. You will also need to obtain a syringe or cartridge-needle unit containing 1 ml of heparin solution and if agency policy includes the use of saline you will need two cartridge-needle units of saline or a syringe with 2 ml of saline and an extra needle and several alcohol swabs.

The following sequence of activities is used to administer medication through a heparin lock. Use aseptic technique throughout, and cleanse the rubber diaphragm *prior to each needle entry*.

1. Hang the medication container on the IV pole.
2. Inject 1 ml of sterile saline into the heparin lock.
3. Insert the needle on the administration set tubing into the rubber diaphragm, being careful to avoid piercing the other side of the tubing.
4. Tape the needle to the heparin lock securely to prevent it from becoming dislodged during administration of the medication.
5. Adjust the rate of flow correctly.
6. *Return to the bedside prior to the time the small fluid container is empty*. This step is crucial, as the heparin lock can become clotted readily if no fluid is flowing and the heparin solution has not yet been instilled.
7. Clamp the tubing before the drip chamber empties, to avoid the need to reprime the tubing when used with subsequent small fluid containers.
8. Remove the needle from the heparin lock, replace the protective cap, and loop the tubing over the IV pole.
9. Inject 1 ml of saline into the heparin lock.
10. Inject 1 ml of heparin solution into the lock.

When the client no longer needs IV fluids, but still needs IV medications, an IV infusion can be converted to a heparin lock with an adaptor designed for this purpose. One end of the adaptor fits into the infusion cannula, and the other end is sealed with a rubber diaphragm similar to that on a heparin lock. To make the transition from an IV infusion to a heparin lock, clamp the main IV tubing, remove it from the cannula, and insert the adaptor tip quickly to avoid having blood return from the cannula. Inject 1 ml of heparin solution into the adaptor and tape it in place securely.

Adding Medications to the Main IV Fluid Container

When adding medications to the main IV fluid container, use careful aseptic technique and label the bottle as when preparing IVPB medications. With large plastic IV fluid containers, use the same process as for adding medications to the small IVPB bags. With glass bottles, remove the metal cap and rubber disc (if the bottle is vented) and locate the injection port, identified with a triangular indentation on the rubber diaphragm or marked by the word "add." Do not inject the medication through the administration port or through the air vent, as that action can cause the system to malfunction. Agitate the fluid container gently to mix the drug thoroughly with the solution.

Giving IV Push Medications

IV push medications can be given in one of three ways—into the flashball or a Y-port of the main IV tubing, into a heparin lock, or directly into the vein through a venipuncture. With each of these methods, the drug enters the bloodstream rapidly, which is why the IV push route is the most rapid as well as the most potentially dangerous method of administering IV medications. Because of the potential danger, calculate the dosage carefully and validate the prepared dosage with another person licensed to give medications before administering it. When giving an IV push medication into the main IV tubing or a heparin lock, it is crucial to assess the infusion site for potential infiltration; if the cannula is not patent, the medication will not reach the bloodstream. Use careful aseptic technique and inject the medication at the proper rate for the particular medication, as indicated by agency or unit policy, pharmacy guidelines, or drug reference manuals. Observe the infusion site for infiltration as you inject the medication. Stop immediately if the client complains of burning or if you observe swelling at the site. Plan to remain with the client for a few minutes after the medication is given, to observe for immediate effects and any problems. As with the administration of any medication, return later to note its effectiveness.

When administering IV push medications *through the main tubing,* it is necessary to direct the medication toward the vein and minimize its dilution in the tubing. To do this, select the medication port closest to the venipuncture site (preferably the rubber flashball near the cannula hub) and stop the infusion temporarily by folding and pinching the tubing between your fingers. Inject the medication at the proper rate, withdraw the needle, release the tubing, and determine that the infusion is flowing properly.

When administering IV push medications *through a heparin lock,* you will need heparin and saline solutions, as when administering an IVPB medication through a heparin lock. When agency policy includes the use of saline, use the following sequence of actions to administer an IV push medication, cleansing the rubber diaphragm with alcohol before each needle entry:

1. Inject 1 ml saline.
2. Inject the medication at the proper rate.
3. Inject 1 ml saline.
4. Inject 1 ml heparin.

Figure 74–11 shows administration of an IV push medication through the main IV tubing.

To administer an IV push medication through a *direct venipuncture,* insert the needle into the vein as described above, aspirate slightly, and observe the return blood flow into the syringe. Inject the medication at the correct rate, withdraw the needle, and apply pressure to stop the bleeding.

ADMINISTRATION OF BLOOD

There are three main objectives of blood transfusion therapy:

1. Restore blood volume following severe hemorrhage.
2. Restore oxygen-carrying capacity of the blood by supplying red blood cells.
3. Restore coagulation properties by supplying the clotting factors found in platelets and plasma (Kozier and Erb, 1983; Plumer, 1982).

There are several types of preparations that can be administered when transfusion therapy is indicated; examples of these were described earlier. Safe

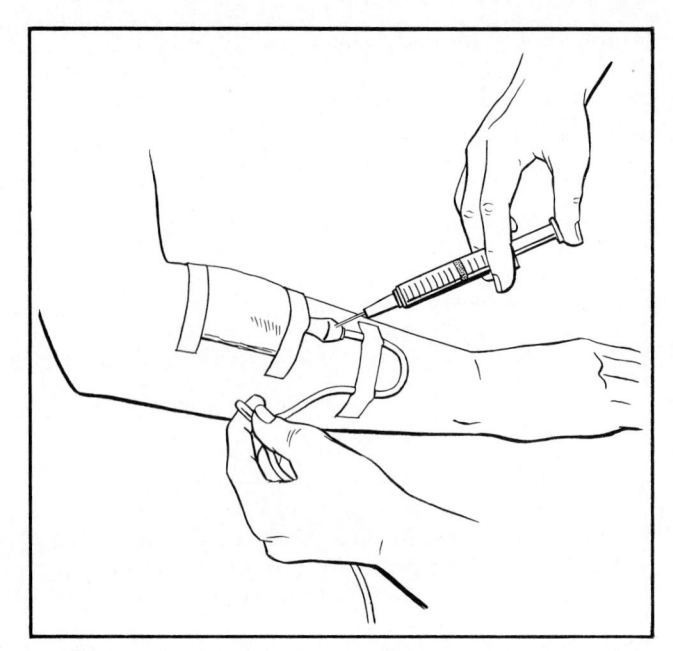

Figure 74–11. *Intravenous medication injected into the main IV tubing through the flashball as "IV push." Tubing is folded and pinched to direct medication toward patient.*

administration of blood and blood products entails being familiar with the various preparations of blood, the purposes for administering them, and possible complications that may develop with each one.

The administration of blood and its components, although an integral part of the care of hospitalized clients, can result in serious problems and complications that can lead to death, permanent disability, and litigation. Untoward responses to blood transfusions include allergic, hemolytic, pyrogenic, and nonhemolytic febrile reactions. The nurse administering blood shares responsibility with the blood bank for the prevention of these unexpected outcomes, or for their earliest possible detection so that serious damage can be avoided.

Selecting and preparing the blood for a particular client is the sole responsibility of the blood bank, whose highly trained personnel type and cross match each unit in an attempt to ensure its compatibility with the person receiving it. It is the responsibility of the nurse on the clinical unit, in conjunction with the transfusion therapist, to make absolute and positive identification of the donor blood and the client receiving it.

Because of the possibility of serious reactions to blood transfusions, hospitals generally have very strict procedures that must be followed when administering blood. The following points should be included in the procedure.

1. Begin infusing blood immediately upon its arrival on the unit, within 30 minutes from the time it is removed from refrigeration. Rapid deterioration occurs once blood has been exposed to room temperature for more than 2 hours. It is not accept-

able practice to store blood in a refrigerator on the clinical unit, as this refrigeration is not controlled.
2. Administer the right blood to the right client.
  a. *With the tranfusion therapist,* check the requisition form against the unit of blood for essential data:
     Client's name and ID number
     Blood group and type (ABO and Rh)
     Blood unit number
     Donor number
     Expiration date
  b. *With the transfusion therapist or another RN,* check the requisition form against the client's identification band, matching the name and identification number.
3. Check the client's temperature prior to infusion as a baseline for future temperature comparisons. Because temperature elevation is one of the signs of a reaction to blood, monitor temperature status at intervals throughout the transfusion and following its completion.
4. Inspect the blood for discoloration or gas bubbles, which indicate probable contamination and necessitate returning the blood to the blood bank.
5. Use only a blood administration set to give blood. It contains a filter specially designed to remove the particulate matter formed during storage, without damaging the blood cells.
6. Use only normal (isotonic) saline to start blood. A 250-ml bag of normal saline is hung with the blood, often through a Y-type administration set. The saline is turned on to keep the line open if the blood is discontinued due to a reaction, or between units of blood if more than 1 unit is being infused consecutively. Additionally, the blood may infuse more readily if infused concurrently with the saline. Using a solution other than saline may cause hemolysis or clotting of the blood.
7. It may be necessary to warm blood during massive transfusions, as rapid administration of cold blood predisposes to cardiac arrest. A mechanical warmer can be used for this purpose, or a length of the tubing can be submerged in a basin of 37°C water. Never attempt to warm the entire unit of blood by placing it in hot water.
8. Never add medication to blood and never infuse blood simultaneously through an administration set being used to administer medications, as there may be a pharmacological incompatibility between the drug and the chemicals used in processing the blood.
9. Administer the first 50 ml of blood slowly and observe the client closely for any adverse reactions. Following this, the rate may be increased as ordered. Continue to observe and monitor the client closely throughout the transfusion and for several hours thereafter.
10. For clients with a normal blood volume, infuse blood at a fairly slow rate to prevent circulatory overload, usually over a 2-hour period. When cardiac, renal, or liver disease is present, however, infuse the blood at a much slower rate. The maximum rate for infusing blood is 500 ml (2 units) every 30 minutes. When the maximum rate must be used to infuse blood, as in severe hypovolemia, a pressure sleeve may be applied to the plastic blood container. By exerting force on the flexible container, blood can be administered at a faster rate than could be attained by gravity flow alone.
11. Include the volume of blood and isotonic saline when calculating the client's daily fluid intake. In some institutions, units of blood are labeled only by weight, and the number of grams in the unit is given, with 1 g the equivalent of 1 ml.

RECORDING AND REPORTING

Intravenous fluids are usually recorded on intake and output flow sheets especially designed for that purpose. All persons receiving intravenous therapy must have intake and output *from all routes* monitored carefully, as described in Skill 51. When intake and output are totaled at the end of a specified time period (often at the end of a shift), read the fluid level on the fluid container with the container remaining inverted and hanging from the IV pole. To be able to read the fluid level on a collapsible plastic bag, grasp and pull the bag from both sides at the fluid level line, thus creating a single line that can be read easily.

Although intake and output flow sheets vary among institutions, the same type of information is always recorded. Record all infused fluids, including the volume of IVPB and heparin lock solutions on the intake-output record, along with the time each was started and ended. A sample IV flow sheet is shown in Figure 74-12.

Record all procedures related to initiating or maintaining IV infusions, either in the narrative notes or on flow sheets designed for that purpose. This recording provides a record of the type and size of infusion devices used, the type, volume, and rate of fluids administered, the name, dosage, and route of all IV medications, and any type of equipment change or modification.

In addition to careful recording of relevant data in the health record, adequate exchange of information at the *change of shift report* helps prevent misunderstandings and errors. This information includes identification of the clients that have an IV infusion or IV medications, the solutions that are being infused and their flow rates, the additives contained in each solution, the remaining volume in each fluid container, the time the next container will be needed, the type of fluid to follow the one being infused, and whether that fluid is on the unit or has yet to arrive from the pharmacy. Any problems or complications are relayed, including questions about whether the IV site was changed that day and where the old site was located. For clients with heparin locks, report the location of the lock and whether it is patent.

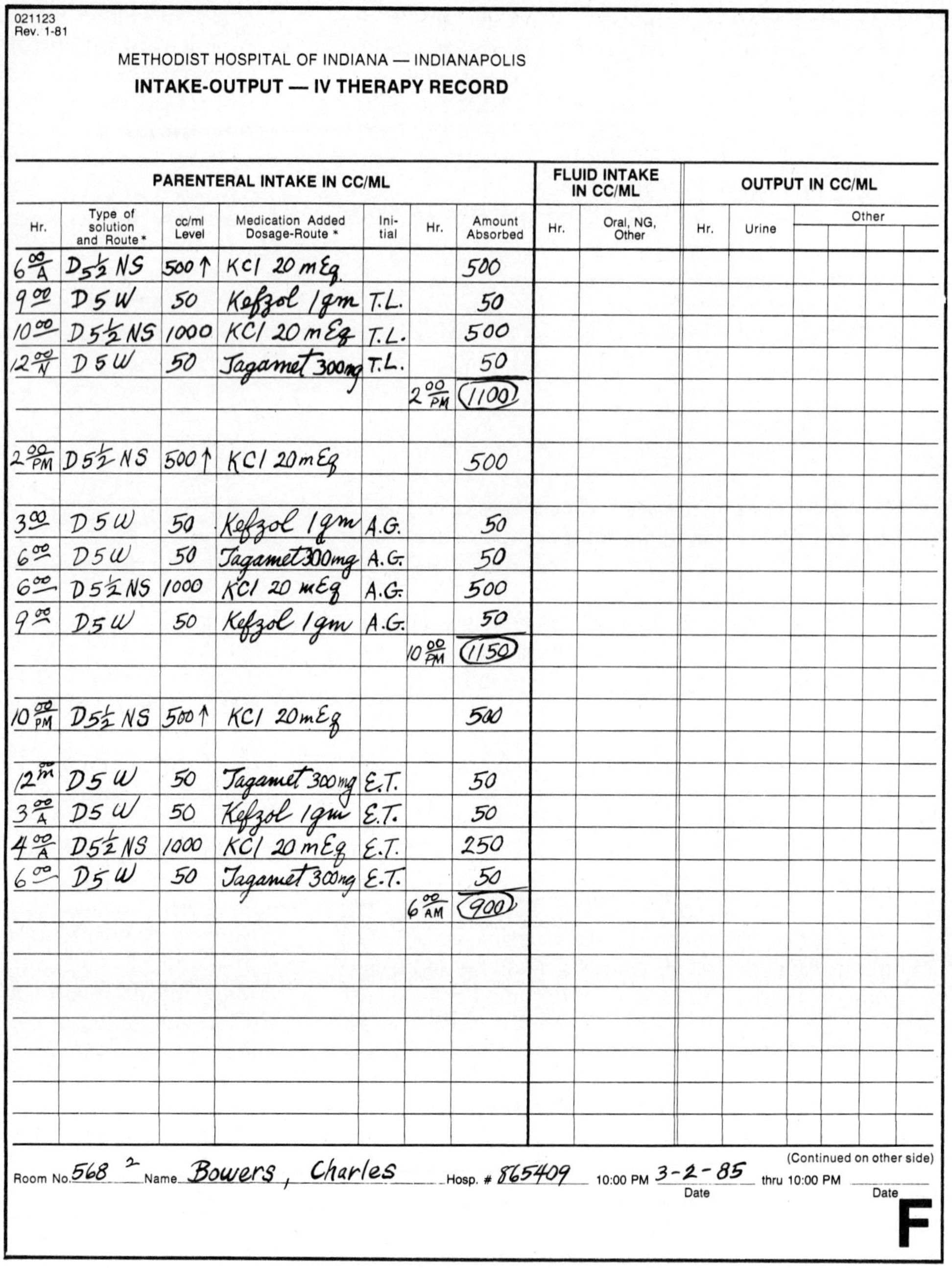

021123
Rev. 1-81

METHODIST HOSPITAL OF INDIANA — INDIANAPOLIS

INTAKE-OUTPUT — IV THERAPY RECORD

PARENTERAL INTAKE IN CC/ML							FLUID INTAKE IN CC/ML		OUTPUT IN CC/ML		
Hr.	Type of solution and Route*	cc/ml Level	Medication Added Dosage-Route*	Initial	Hr.	Amount Absorbed	Hr.	Oral, NG, Other	Hr.	Urine	Other
6 00 A	D5½ NS	500 ↑	KCl 20 mEq			500					
9 00	D5W	50	Kefzol 1gm	T.L.		50					
10 00	D5½ NS	1000	KCl 20 mEq	T.L.		500					
12 00 N	D5W	50	Tagamet 300mg	T.L.		50					
					2 00 PM	(1100)					
2 00 PM	D5½ NS	500 ↑	KCl 20mEq			500					
3 00	D5W	50	Kefzol 1gm	A.G.		50					
6 00	D5W	50	Tagamet 300mg	A.G.		50					
6 00	D5½ NS	1000	KCl 20 mEq	A.G.		500					
9 00	D5W	50	Kefzol 1gm	A.G.		50					
					10 00 PM	(1150)					
10 00 PM	D5½ NS	500 ↑	KCl 20mEq			500					
12 00 m	D5W	50	Tagamet 300mg	E.T.		50					
3 00 A	D5W	50	Kefzol 1gm	E.T.		50					
4 00 A	D5½ NS	1000	KCl 20 mEq	E.T.		250					
6 00	D5W	50	Tagamet 300mg	E.T.		50					
					6 00 AM	(900)					

Room No. 568 2 Name Bowers, Charles Hosp. # 865409 10:00 PM 3-2-85 (Date) thru 10:00 PM ______ (Date) (Continued on other side)

F

Figure 74–12. IV therapy intake–output record. As indicated in the first three columns, at 6:00 A.M. 500 ml fluid remained in the IV fluid container. At 10:00 A.M. that 500 ml had been absorbed (see "Amount Absorbed" column) and a new 1000–ml IV fluid container was added. When the next shift began at 2:00 P.M., 500 ml of fluid remained in that container and 500 ml had been absorbed. In addition to the two 500–ml volumes from two IV fluid containers, two 50–ml IVPB containers with medications had also been infused, totalling 1100 ml for that 8–hour shift.

☐ CRITICAL POINTS SUMMARY

1. The intravenous route is used for fluid replacement, to meet daily fluid and nutrient requirements, and to administer medications.
2. The most common IV infusion sites used for adults are in the forearm and hand.
3. Composition of IV fluids influences nursing observations when IV fluids are being infused.
4. Calculate IV fluid flow rate in drops per minute to regulate a gravity-flow infusion, and in milliliters per hour to set an infusion control device.
5. A time tape helps monitor overall infusion time.
6. Prime an administration set carefully to prevent air from entering the tubing.
7. Select an infusion site appropriate for the type and duration of the infusion, considering client comfort, safety, and mobility.
8. Secure the venipuncture device with adhesive tape so as to leave the insertion site and hub–tubing connections free from tape.
9. After performing a venipuncture for drawing a blood sample, be sure all bleeding has stopped before leaving the client.
10. Infiltration is evidenced by edema, tenderness, coolness, and blanching.

11. Discontinue an infiltrated infusion promptly, without irrigating.
12. Minimize IV-related infections by
    a. Using careful handwashing and aseptic technique when handling equipment
    b. Applying a protective dressing to the insertion site
    c. Changing infusion site dressings and administration sets every 48 to 72 hours
    d. Restarting all infusions every 48 to 72 hours
    e. Discarding in-use IV solutions after 24 hours
13. Phlebitis is evidenced by redness, warmth, and induration along the course of the vein.
14. Minimize the risk of phlebitis by careful venipuncture and administration of medications.
15. On an hourly basis, assess the client with an IV for:
    a. Fluid flow rate
    b. Cannula patency
    c. Equipment function
    d. Signs of infiltration, phlebitis, or leakage at the infusion site
    e. General comfort level
16. Informed clients can help monitor an IV infusion.
17. Monitor fluid intake and output on all clients receiving IV therapy.
18. Do not disconnect the IV tubing to provide personal care.
19. IV medications are given in three ways:
    a. By slow infusion in the main IV
    b. In a small volume through an IVPB
    c. Directly into the vein, in 3 to 5 minutes
20. Administer IV piggyback medications by gravity flow or through an infusion control device.
21. To avoid clotting within a heparin lock, always instill heparin solution immediately after the IV fluid or medication is infused.
22. Follow designated special precautions when administering blood and blood products.

☐ LEARNING ACTIVITIES

1. In a learning laboratory, pharmacy, or central supply department, locate items used to administer IV infusions and perform venipunctures; examine those items to determine the following information:
    a. Fluid containers, including bags and both vented and nonvented bottles: Note air vents and entry ports for the administration spike and additives. Read the label for the contents, volume, indicators of sterility, expiration date, any precautions indicated, and manufacturer's name.
    b. Administration sets of several varieties: For each type, note the drop factor and whether it is a macrodrip or microdrip set. Note the protected spike, the length of the tubing, the number and location of Y-ports, any in-line filters, manual controller, and flashball. If used with an ICD, note any special filling instructions. For what purpose might each type of administration set be used?
    c. Venipuncture devices, including a winged-steel needle, heparin lock device, and both over-the-needle and through-the-needle catheters: Note the gauge and construction of each type. Identify how each type would be secured to the client and for what purpose each might be used.
    d. Filters: Note the micron size and any special filling instructions.
    e. IV tray: List the items on the tray and identify the purpose for which each is used.
    f. IVPB medication equipment, such as volume-control plastic bags and burettes: Note air vents and entry ports for the administration spike and additives. Note type and volume of fluid, medication and its dosage, indicators of sterility, and expiration date.
    g. Infusion control devices: Compare a controller and an infusion pump. Note the flow rate settings, alarms, battery capability, type of administration set required, and any special instructions or cautions for use.
2. In a laboratory setting, using outdated equipment, practice the following techniques. *For simulation purposes, handle the equipment as if it were sterile.* Use the performance checklist for preparing an intravenous infusion to monitor your own or a peer's technique.
    a. Attach an administration set to an IV fluid container, preferably to both a glass bottle and a plastic bag.
    b. Prime the administration set, removing all air bubbles.
    c. Attach and prime a filter, unless it was an integral part of the tubing.
    d. Attach a venipuncture device.
    e. Regulate the flow rate for 45 drops/min (with a macrodrip set) or 90 drops/min (with a microdrip set). Allow the fluid to flow into a basin or waste baskets.
    f. If an ICD is available, insert the tubing or cassette into the device and set the flow rate for 125 ml/hr.
3. Spend time observing nurses perform a venipuncture, change fluid containers, tubing, and site dressings, and provide care for clients with IV infusions. Suggested locations for this activity are a clinical unit or with the IV therapy team in your institution.

☐ REVIEW QUESTIONS

1. For what purposes are intravenous fluids administered?

2. What factors influence the selection of a venipuncture site for an IV infusion versus drawing a blood sample?
3. Why are the veins in the lower extremities seldom used for an IV infusion?
4. Match the IV fluid in Column I with the clinical use in Column II. (Items in Column I may be used more than one time.)

   COLUMN I
   1. D$_5$NS
   2. D$_5$W
   3. D$_5$/0.45 NS
   4. Normal saline (0.9%)
   5. Ringer's lactate solution

   COLUMN II
   ____ Calorie and fluid maintenance or replacement.
   ____ Electrolyte replacement.
   ____ Sodium and fluid maintenance.
   ____ Sodium and fluid replacement.

5. What are the recommended intervals for changing the following components of an IV infusion system?
   _____ administration sets
   _____ discarding in-use solutions
   _____ infusion site dressing
   _____ insertion cannula and infusion site
6. In addition to the practices in the previous question, what other practices are designed to minimize IV-related infections?
7. Place an "I" before the signs associated with infiltration at the infusion site, and a "P" before those associated with phlebitis.
   ____ blanching
   ____ coolness
   ____ hardness along the vein
   ____ redness
   ____ swelling around the insertion site
   ____ tenderness
   ____ warmth
8. Why is an infiltrated IV always discontinued promptly?
9. Which of the following decisions would generally be determined by nursing judgment?
   ____ flow rate for gravity flow IV infusions
   ____ length of time for an IV infusion to infuse
   ____ length of time for an IVPB medication to infuse
   ____ type of administration equipment
   ____ type of IV fluid to be administered
   ____ type of venipuncture device
10. Explain the rationale for the following actions involved in performing a venipuncture:
    a. Applying a tourniquet prior to the venipuncture.
    b. Stretching the skin taut over the site prior to inserting the needle.
    c. Inserting the needle with the bevel turned uppermost.
    d. Loosening the tourniquet immediately after the needle enters the vein when starting an IV infusion.
    e. Keeping the tourniquet in place while withdrawing a blood sample.
11. What interventions are used to stop bleeding after a venipuncture for withdrawing a blood sample?
12. Explain the rationale for the following actions involved in preparing an intravenous infusion and securing a venipuncture device:
    a. Closing the tubing clamp prior to inverting the IV fluid container when priming the administration set.
    b. Removing all air bubbles from the IV tubing.
    c. Not placing adhesive tape over the insertion site.
    d. Not placing adhesive tape on the cannula–tubing junction.
    e. Securing the cannula with adhesive tape before applying a dry sterile dressing.
    f. Omitting tape from the cannula when using a transparent polyurethane dressing over the insertion site.
    g. Securing a loop of IV tubing to the body with adhesive tape.
13. List the factors included in hourly assessments of a client with an IV infusion. Explain the reason for each component.
14. What steps can be taken if a gravity-flow infusion is not flowing at the correct rate?
15. In which units are the flow rate for a gravity-flow infusion calculated and regulated: drops per minute or milliliters per hour?
16. Explain the rationale for using a time-tape when monitoring IV infusions.
17. List the points to include when teaching someone how to help care for and function with an IV infusion.
18. Explain the rationale for using the following injection sequence to administer medications through a heparin lock:
    saline → medication → saline → heparin
19. Match the blood product in Column I with the clinical use in Column II.

    COLUMN I
    1. Albumin
    2. Packed red blood cells
    3. Plasma
    4. Plasma expanders
    5. Platelets

    COLUMN II
    ____ adequate blood volume with inadequate red blood cell mass
    ____ blood volume deficits
    ____ blood volume and protein deficits
    ____ decreased blood volume with adequate red blood cell mass
    ____ hemorrhagic disease

20. Explain the necessity for two people checking the identifying data on blood products prior to transfusing them.

☐ PERFORMANCE CHECKLISTS

OBJECTIVE: To use aseptic technique to prepare an intravenous infusion correctly.

CHARACTERISTIC	RANGE OF ACCEPTABILITY	SATISFACTORY	UNSATISFACTORY
1. Validates physician's order.	No deviation		
2. Washes hands.	No deviation		
3. Selects appropriate IV fluid.	No deviation		
4. Inspects fluid for clarity and expiration date.	No deviation		
5. Validates order with fluid label.	No deviation		

6. Selects and inspects appropriate equipment:
  a. Infusion control device.
  b. Administration set.
  c. Venipuncture cannula.
  d. IV pole.
	
	May not be needed.
	No deviation
	No deviation
	No deviation		

7. Checks all packages for intactness.	No deviation		
8. Closes administration tubing clamp.	No deviation		
9. Checks plastic bags for leaks.	No deviation		
10. Removes protective caps or seals on fluid container and inserts administration spike.	No deviation		

11. Primes tubing:
  a. Fills drip chamber half full.
  b. Fills tubing.
  c. Removes all except minute air bubbles from tubing.
  d. For an ICD, follows manufacturer's directions.
	
	No deviation
	No deviation
	No deviation
	
	No deviation		

12. Attaches and primes a filter, removing all air.	Omit if contraindicated or unnecessary.		
13. Replaces protective cap on end of tubing.	Attach cannula.		
14. Maintains aseptic technique in steps 10 to 13.	No deviation		
15. Calculates the number of milliliters per hour to be administered.	No deviation		
16. Prepares a time-tape and attaches it to IV fluid container.	Not deviation		
17. Inserts tubing into ICD according to manufacturer's directions.	Not relevant for gravity-flow infusions.		
18. Calculates drops per minute flow rate.	Not relevant for ICD infusions.		

OBJECTIVE: To use aseptic technique to start an IV infusion correctly.

CHARACTERISTIC	RANGE OF ACCEPTABILITY	SATISFACTORY	UNSATISFACTORY
1. Validates physician's order.	No deviation		
2. Prepares IV infusion correctly and attaches cannula to IV tubing.	No deviation Omit if using an over-the-needle or through-the-needle catheter.		
3. Washes hands.	No deviation		
4. Identifies client correctly.	No deviation		
5. Explains procedure to client.	Modify explanation according to client's physical, mental, and emotional status.		

(continued)

OBJECTIVE: To use aseptic technique to start an IV infusion correctly (cont).

CHARACTERISTIC	RANGE OF ACCEPTABILITY	SATISFACTORY	UNSATISFACTORY
6. Provides privacy.	Use judgment about family and visitors.		
7. Selects appropriate venipuncture site.	No deviation		
8. Positions client for visibility and comfort.	No deviation		
9. Augments vein visibility as needed.	May not be necessary.		
10. Inspects site carefully.	No deviation		
11. Applies tourniquet correctly.	No deviation		
12. Palpates vein.	No deviation		
13. Loosens tourniquet.	No deviation		
14. Cleanses insertion site in circular manner.	No deviation		
15. Reapplies tourniquet.	No deviation		

16. Inserts cannula:
  a. Stabilizes skin and vein with nondominant hand.
  b. Places cannula parallel to vein, bevel side up.
  c. Holds cannula at 45 degree angle to penetrate skin.
  d. Lowers cannula to 10 degree angle and enters vein at slight lateral angle.
  e. Observes for blood return.
  f. Threads cannula into vein, up to hub.
	No deviation
	
	In some situations, hold cannula to and above the vein, bevel side down.
	Use 15 degree angle when inserting cannula directly above vein.
	Inappropriate for above-vein entry.
	
	No deviation
	No deviation		

17. Releases tourniquet after noting blood return in the cannula or tubing.	No deviation		
18. For an over-the-needle catheter, removes and discards the needle inside the cannula.	No deviation		
19. Inserts tip of primed administration set tubing into the cannula hub.	Omit if done earlier.		
20. Opens tubing clamp to allow fluid to infuse slowly.	No deviation		

21. Secures cannula to skin; avoiding tape on
  a. Insertion site.
  b. Hub–tubing connections.
	Omit if using transparent site dressing.
	
	No deviation
	No deviation		

22. Applies drop of sterile antibiotic ointment over insertion site.	Omit if contrary to agency policy. Optional with transparent dressings.		
23. Applies dry sterile dressing or transparent polyurethane dressing.	No deviation		
24. Labels dressing with date, time, and initials.	No deviation		
25. Secures tubing to client near site.	Do not use adhesive tape on transparent dressings.		

26. Adjusts flow rate:
  a. Gravity flow infusion: counts drops per minute.
  b. ICD: sets desired flow rate in milliliters per hour.
	
	No deviation
	
	Omit with gravity flow infusion.		

27. Inspects site for infiltration.	No deviation		
28. Inquires regarding client's comfort level.	No deviation		
29. Disposes of equipment properly.	No deviation		
30. Washes hands.	No deviation		
31. Documents procedure in health record.	No deviation		

OBJECTIVE: To use aseptic technique to perform a venipuncture for withdrawing a blood sample correctly.			
CHARACTERISTIC	RANGE OF ACCEPTABILITY	SATISFACTORY	UNSATISFACTORY
1. Validates order.	No deviation		
2. Washes hands.	No deviation		
3. Identifies client correctly.	No deviation		
4. Explains procedure to the client.	Modify explanation according to client's physical, mental, and emotional status.		
5. Provides privacy.	Use judgment about family and visitors.		
6. Selects appropriate venipuncture site.	No deviation		
7. Positions client for visibility and comfort.	No deviation		
8. Augments vein visibility as needed.	May not be necessary.		
9. Inspects site carefully.	No deviation		
10. Applies tourniquet.	No deviation		
11. Palpates vein.	No deviation		
12. Cleanses insertion site in a circular manner.	No deviation		
13. Pulls skin taut over insertion site.	No deviation		
14. Inserts blood collecting device needle into the skin and vein a. Bevel side up. b. Parallel to the vein. c. At 45 degree angle.	No deviation May enter vein from top. May use 15 degree angle for above-vein entry.		
15. Stabilizes blood collecting device with nondominant hand.	No deviation		
16. Pushes vacuum tube onto short needle, toward insertion site.	No deviation		
17. Removes vacuum tube when it is full; replaces until required blood samples are obtained.	No deviation		
18. Releases tourniquet.	No deviation		
19. Applies pressure with dry sterile gauze at site while withdrawing needle.	No deviation		
20. Controls bleeding: a. Elevates arm higher than heart. b. Maintains firm pressure with fingers. c. Does not flex a joint, if venipuncture is at joint. d. Inspects carefully.	No deviation No deviation No deviation No deviation		
21. Applies band-aid.	No deviation		
22. Disposes of equipment.	No deviation		
23. Washes hands.	No deviation		
24. Labels specimen and sends to laboratory.	No deviation		
25. Washes hands.	No deviation		
26. Documents in health record.	No deviation		

REFERENCES

Aisenstein TJ: Toward impeccable IV technique: Those all-too-common IV complications. RN 44(3):38–41, 1981.

Blackburn GL: Home TPN: State of the art. American Journal of IV Therapy and Clinical Nutrition 11(2):20–21+, 1984.

Brunner LS, Suddarth DS: Textbook of Medical–Surgical Nursing, ed 5. Philadelphia, J. B. Lippincott, 1984.

Geolot DH, McKinney NP: Administering parenteral drugs. American Journal of Nursing 75(5):788–793, 1975.

Gillis A: Hazards and complications of IV therapy. Dimensions in Health Services 60(5):9,12,13, 1983.

Hirsch J, Hannock L: Mosby's Manual of Clinical Nursing Procedures. St Louis, CV Mosby, 1981.

I.V. therapy in the home...Antibiotic therapy. Emergency Medicine 15(4):82-84, 86, 1983.

Jones BC, Briggs CD, Norton DA: This new type of IV dressing can save you time. Nursing82 (Horsham) 12(12):70-73, 1982.

Keithley JK, Fraulini KE: What's behind that IV line? Nursing82 (Horsham) 12(3):33-42, 1982.

Kozier B, Erb G: Techniques in Clinical Nursing. Menlo Park, CA, Addison-Wesley, 1982.

Kozier B, Erb G: Fundamentals of Nursing, ed 2. Menlo Park, CA, Addison-Wesley, 1983.

Luckmann J, Sorensen KC: Medical-Surgical Nursing: A Psychophysiologic Approach, ed 2. Philadelphia, WB Saunders, 1980.

Masoorlie ST: Toward impeccable IV technique: Trouble-free IV starts. RN 44(2):21-27, 1981.

Metheny NM, Snively WD: Nurses' Handbook of Fluid Balance, ed 4. Philadelphia, J. B. Lippincott, 1983.

Plumer AL: Principles and Practice of Intravenous Therapy, ed 3. Boston, Little, Brown, 1982.

Simmons BP: Guidelines for prevention of intravenous infections (In consultation with Hooten, TM, Wong, ES, Allen JR): In Guidelines for the Prevention and Control of Nosocomial Infections. Atlanta, Centers for Disease Control, 1981.

Turco, SJ: Infusion pumps and controllers: In Modern IV Practices. Chicago, Medical Directions, 1979.

Turco SJ: Mechanical and electronic equipment for parenteral and enteral use: An update. The American Journal of Intravenous Therapy and Clinical Nutrition 9(7):9-15+, 1982.

Vogel TC, McSwimming SA: Teaching parents to give indwelling CV catheter care. Nursing83 (Horsham 13(1):55-56, 1983.

BIBLIOGRAPHY

Dawson HL: Basic Human Anatomy, ed 2. Norwalk, CT, Appleton-Century-Crofts, 1974.

Fineman V, Fleming K: Toward impeccable IV technique: The right things to do about IV's. RN 44(8)29-30, 1981.

Foley R: Administration of intravenous therapy: Nursing policies, procedures, and techniques. (In consultation with D. Godfrey) In Modern IV Practices. Chicago, Medical Directions, 1979.

Giving Medications (Nursing80 Photobook): Horsham, PA: Intermed Communications, 1980.

Hurst JW, Logue RB, et al (eds): The Heart, Arteries, and Veins, ed 5. New York, McGraw-Hill, 1982.

Koszuta LE: Choosing the right infusion control device for your patient. Nursing84 (Horsham) 14(3): 55-56, 1984.

Miller BF, Keene CB: Encyclopedia and Dictionary of Medicine, Nursing, and Allied Health, ed 3. Philadelphia, W. B. Saunders, 1983.

Smith S, Duell D: Nursing Skills and Evaluation: A Nursing Process Approach. Los Altos, CA, National Nursing Review, 1982.

Sorensen KC, Luckmann, J: Basic Nursing: A Psychophysiologic Approach. Philadelphia, J. B. Lippincott, 1979.

Stedman's Medical Dictionary, ed 21. Baltimore, Williams & Wilkins, 1966.

Zenowich D: IV flow control. NITA 7(1):21-25, 1984.

SUGGESTED READINGS

Aisenstein TJ: Toward impeccable IV technique. Those all-too-common IV complications. RN 44(3):38-41, 1981.

Koszuta LE: Choosing the right infusion control device for your patient. Nursing84 (Horsham) 14(3):55-56, 1984.

Masoorlie ST: Toward impeccable IV technique. Trouble-free IV starts. RN 44(2):21-27, 1981.

Peck M: Perfecting your I.V. therapy techniques. Part I. Nursing85 (Horsham) 15(5):38-43, 1985.

Peck M: Perfecting your I.V. therapy techniques. Part II. Nursing85 (Horsham) 15(6):48-51, 1985.

AUDIOVISUAL RESOURCES

Intravenous Therapy
  Videorecording, 3 cassettes. (1974, 90 min.)
  Available through:
    Fairview General Hospital
    Department of Audio-Visual Communication
    18101 Lorraine Ave.
    Cleveland, OH 44111

Intravenous Therapy: Basic Concepts
  Film or videocassette. (1977, color, 28 min.)

Intravenous Therapy: Monitoring and Problem Solving
  Film or videocassette. (1977, Color, 30 min.)
  Available through:
    American Journal of Nursing Company
    Educational Services Division
    555 West 57th St.
    New York, NY 10019

Starting an IV in Children
  Videorecording. (1977, 6 min.)
  Available through:
    Medical College of Virginia
    Learning Resource Center
    McVee Station, Box 510
    1200 E. Broad St.
    Richmond, VA 23298

IV Therapy
  Films, cassettes, slides, filmstrips. (1983, Color.)

Monitoring the Patient, Documenting Nursing Care, Managing Complications (24 min.)

Performing Venipuncture (19 min.)

Preparing Admixtures, Preparing the Administration Set (25 min.)

Preparing the Patient, Selecting the Intravascular Cannula, Selecting the Infusion Site (25 min.)

Principles of Intravenous Therapy (23 min.)

Protecting the Infusion Site (18 min.)

Using the Heparin Lock, Using Central Venous Catheters (21 min.)
  Availble through:
    Medcom, Inc.
    P.O. Box 116
    Garden Grove, CA 92642

17 Emergency Techniques

☐ **INTRODUCTION**

Cardiopulmonary resuscitation (CPR) has been used clinically for only 2 decades. Yet, efforts to restore life have been recorded since before the time of Christ. An ancient miracle performed by the prophet Elisha, and recorded in the second book of Kings, is described in a fashion that resembles mouth-to-mouth resuscitation. Down through the centuries many techniques have been tried. In 1530 Paracelsus used fireside bellows in attempting to revive apparently dead persons. Adaptations of this method were used for 300 years. In the early 1800s victims of near-drowning were placed over the back of a horse. It was hoped that bouncing on the trotting horse would force water out and allow air in. The Schafer Prone Pressure gained acceptance in 1903. Pressure was applied to the back of a face-down victim to induce expiration while release of pressure allowed inspiration (American Heart Association, 1974). In the same year, G. W. Crile of Cleveland reported successful external cardiac compression on three persons (DeBard, 1980). Unfortunately, the heart was viewed as untouchable by the medical community, so his work was not accepted. The effectiveness of closed cardiac massage was demonstrated by Kouwenhoven and his colleagues in the mid-1950s (Kouwenhoven, 1960). At about the same time, Safar, Escarraga, and Elam developed mouth-to-mouth resuscitation (Safar et al., 1958). The two techniques were combined in the early sixties and cardiopulmonary resuscitation as we know it today was discovered. These two techniques were accepted as standards for medical practice in 1966 by the National Academy of Sciences—National Research Council on CPR (Ad Hoc Committee on Cardiopulmonary Resuscitation of the Division of Medical Sciences, National Academy of Sciences—National Research Council, 1966). Performance standards for CPR were developed by the American Heart Association (AHA) and have been most recently revised in 1980.

The 1973 National Conference of Cardiopulmonary Resuscitation (CPR) and Emergency Cardiac Care (ECC) determined that the AHA and the American Red Cross (ARC) would be the primary providers of CPR instruction. Since 60 to 70 percent of sudden deaths due to cardiac arrest occur prior to hospitalization, the AHA recognizes the lay person as an important component in the provision of emergency cardiac care. The goal of the AHA is to train the public in the delivery of CPR because it is very likely that lay people will be available to the victim of cardiac arrest in the community.

The AHA and ARC provide courses in CPR basic life support to the community. Basic life support provides the victim of cardiopulmonary arrest with circulatory and ventilatory support without the use of adjunctive equipment or drugs. Basic life support can be provided by a nurse who enters a client's room and finds him or her unresponsive. The nurse would provide this basic life support until additional help and equipment became available. Basic Life Support (BLS) courses are taught by instructors who have successfully passed the AHA or ARC instructor training program in Basic Life Support. These persons usually are nurses, paramedics, physicians, firemen, or others who may encounter sudden death in the course of their day-to-day work. BLS courses provide practice experience on specially designed mannikins. This is an important learning experience because CPR is never practiced on a conscious person because of the risk of injury associated with the procedure. The Basic Life Support course taught by the AHA includes information about prevention of heart disease. Interested individuals may contact either agency and enroll in scheduled courses, and community groups may call either agency and request that such a course be provided for their groups.

Advanced Cardiac Life Support (ACLS) involves more complex techniques such as defibrillation, drug and intravenous fluid administration, and postresuscitation care, and is delivered only by nurses, physicians, or paramedics. Advanced life support courses are taught by the AHA, often in conjunction with local hospitals.

Certification for Basic Cardiac Life Support is available from both the AHA and ARC. Advanced Cardiac Life Support certification is available from the AHA. Certification in either basic or advanced life support means only that an individual has successfully met the cognitive and performance requirements. Licensure is not implied and future performance of CPR is not guaranteed. Annual recertification for CPR is required because CPR is a psychomotor skill that must be practiced so that the skill will be maintained.

There is evidence (Kelly, 1980) that lay people and rescue personnel are better trained in basic CPR than many health professionals. A possible reason for this may be that the nurse is more often involved in performing advanced life support skills while lay people do only the basic CPR. In a study evaluating the performance of CPR by 35 physicians (Webb and Lambrew, 1978), only eight could properly execute the procedure. Since nurses in the hospital setting are often the first to discover victims of cardiopulmonary arrest, it is essential that they be skilled in performing CPR.

Many communities have developed an organized system for responding to emergencies; these are called emergency medical services (EMS) system. The system includes the local fire department, an ambulance service, and hospital emergency rooms. Trained emergency medical technicians with advanced life support training respond to emergencies in vehicles equipped with advanced life support equipment. They are able to stabilize a victim at the scene and provide safe transport to a hospital with emergency facilities. In many communities this system is activated by calling the emergency telephone number 911. It is important to know the emergency telephone number in your own community.

In a hospital, medical advanced life support for emergencies is obtained by calling the hospital telephone operator who pages a specific emergency code to alert the emergency medical team of the need for their services.

Most states have Good Samaritan Laws which protect both health professionals and lay people who deliver basic or advanced life support either inside or outside the hospital environment. Such a law protects the nurse who unsuccessfully administers CPR to a victim of cardiopulmonary arrest the nurse encounters on the street. A distraught family might assume that because the victim died, CPR was not properly administered and, therefore, sue the nurse. According to the 1980 "Standards and Guidelines for Cardiopulmonary Resuscitation (CPR) and Emergency Cardiac Care (ECC)" (hereafter referred to as the "Standards"), no successful legal action has ever been brought against any person who delivered CPR in a reasonable manner. Nurses have an obligation to perform CPR according to accepted professional standards of care, which are the 1980 AHA standards (American Heart Association, 1980). A nurse's responsibilities include performing those functions for which the nurse has been prepared by education and experience, performing those functions competently, and taking appropriate measures as indicated by observation of the client (Paulson, 1977).

The skills in this chapter include "Cardiopulmonary Resuscitation" (Skill 75), and "Removal of Airway Obstruction" (Skill 76).*

☐ ENTRY TEST

1. What are the two factors that determine cardiac output?
2. What is the difference between ventilation and respiration?
3. What are the points in the cardiac cycle at which each valve in the heart opens and closes?
4. At what point in ventricular contraction do the coronary arteries fill?
5. What is meant by tidal volume?
6. How does air move in and out of the lungs with inspiration and expiration?

REFERENCES

American Heart Association: Standards for cardiopulmonary resuscitation (CPR) and emergency cardiac care (ECC). Journal of the American Medical Association 227(7)(suppl):834–868, 1974.

American Heart Association: Standards for cardiopulmonary resuscitation (CPR) and emergency cardiac care (ECC). Journal of the American Medical Association 244(5):453–509, 1980.

American Heart Association: Instructors Manual for Basic Life Support. Dallas, American Heart Association, 1985.

Debard ML: The history of cardiopulmonary resuscitation. Annals of Emergency Medicine 9(5):273–275, 1980.

Kelly K: CPR: To certify or not to certify. Supervisor Nurse 11(1):41–42, 1980.

Kouwenhoven WB, Jude JR, et al.: Closed cardiac massage. Journal of the American Medical Association 173(10):1064–1067, 1960.

Kouwenhoven WB, Langworthy OR: Cardiopulmonary resuscitation: An account of forty-five years of research. Johns Hopkins Medical Journal 132(3):186–193, 1973.

National Academy of Sciences-National Research Council. Cardiopulmonary resuscitation: Statement by the Ad Hoc Committee on cardiopulmonary resuscitation of the Division of Medical Sciences. Journal of the American Medical Association 198(4):372–379, 1966.

Paulson VS: Legal responsibilities of the nurse in a critical care unit. In Hudak CM, Lohr T, et al. (eds): Critical Care Nursing, ed 2. Philadelphia, JB Lippincott, 1977.

Safar P, Escarraga LA, et al.: A comparison of the mouth-to-mouth and mouth-to-airway methods of artificial respiration with the chest-pressure arm-lift methods. New England Journal of Medicine 258(14):671–677, 1952.

Webb DD, Lambrew C: Evaluation of physician skills in cardiopulmonary resuscitation. Journal of the American College of Emergency Physicians 7(11):387–389, 1978.

---

*The content for both of these skills is adapted from the Supplement to Journal of the American Medical Association, August 1, 1980, the American Medical Association. Reprinted with permission from the American Heart Association. ©The American Heart Association's 1985 Instructors Manual for Life Support has also been used to provide the most current procedures used in both skills.

SKILL 75 Cardiopulmonary Resuscitation

PREREQUISITE SKILLS

Skill 19, "Inspection"
Skill 20, "Palpation"
Skill 22, "Auscultation"
Skill 24, "Pulse Appraisal"
Skill 25, "Respiration Appraisal"

☐ STUDENT OBJECTIVES

1. Explain the purpose of cardiopulmonary resuscitation (CPR).
2. Differentiate between clinical and biologic death.
3. Identify the pathophysiological mechanisms of cardiac arrest.
4. Identify the pathophysiological mechanisms of pulmonary arrest.
5. Compare the technique used for adult and infant CPR.
6. Compare the three methods of opening the airway in the adult victim.
7. Explain the rationale for locating and maintaining the correct compression hand position.
8. Explain the rationale for maintaining the correct compression rate and rhythm when performing CPR.
9. Identify five common errors made when performing CPR and the potential consequence of each error.
10. Correctly demonstrate one-rescuer CPR, two-rescuer CPR, and infant CPR.

☐ INTRODUCTION

Cardiopulmonary resuscitation (CPR) means artificially maintained systemic circulation by manual external compression on the chest and providing oxygen through mouth-to-mouth (mouth-to-nose or mouth-to-stoma) respirations. CPR is basically a means of transporting oxygen to the tissues. It is for this reason that oxygen must be provided prior to and in sequence with external chest compression. CPR is begun when clinical death (cessation of circulation and ventilation) occurs. If successful, it will prevent biologic death (irreversible damage to the vital organs, especially the brain). Statistics reflect success rates of 40 percent to 60 percent for CPR delivered by lay people, paraprofessionals, and health professionals. Cardiopulmonary arrest can be the result of cardiac arrest such as occurs after myocardial infarction or pulmonary arrest such as may result from barbiturate overdose.

CPR can be delivered by one person alone but with adult victims, ideally it is delivered by two people. When two people deliver CPR, it is easier to maintain adequate blood pressure and oxygen levels because there is no need for the rescuer to stop chest compression in order to give artificial ventilation. Infant CPR is performed by only one person because of the small size of the victim. Although the basic principles of CPR are the same for all age groups, children present specific problems that require special attention. These are related to size and anatomic differences and will be discussed later. For the purpose of standardization, the age definitions provided by the American Heart Association will be used in this text: an infant is less than 1 year old and a child is 1 to 8 years old. Adult techniques are used on children over 8 years. However, these are intended only as guidelines since a child's age may be difficult to estimate, and size varies considerably among children of similar age. According to Singer (1977), 20 percent of all arrests occur in the first decade of life; this is more than in any other period of life. The vast majority of these occur in the first year. While children are more vulnerable to arrests than adults, they seem to tolerate them better with higher survival rates and fewer complications, including less central nervous system involvement.

There are two categories of people who receive CPR—those who arrest suddenly and unexpectedly, and those in whom the arrest was anticipated (McCarthy, 1975). The AHA Standards clearly state that "the purpose of CPR is the prevention of sudden, unexpected death. CPR is not indicated in certain situations, such as terminal, irreversible illness where death is expected" (American Heart Association, 1980). The Standards specify that if a decision is made not to resuscitate a hospitalized client in whom death is anticipated, the order should be clearly written on the physician's order sheet and the rationale explained in the progress notes. Such an order is commonly referred to as a "No Code" order and means "Do not resuscitate." The term "Code" is derived from Code Red, Code 99, or other hospital communication signals often used to indicate the need for immediate assistance in resuscitation from specially trained hospital personnel. A "No Code" order is a legitimate medical option, although physicians may be reluctant to write the order, fearing that it implies abandonment of the client and leaves them legally vulnerable. Ideally, the decision of "No Code" is made in cooperation with the family. However, for the protection of the nurse, there should be a hospital policy requiring that "No Code" orders must be written by the attending physician and that verbal "No Code" orders will not be implemented by nursing personnel. If a nurse follows a verbal "No Code" order, the nurse assumes the same risk as with any other type of verbal order; that is, the order could have been misunderstood or the physician might later deny ever having given it (Cushing, 1981).

It is accepted and expected nursing practice to initiate CPR without a written or verbal medical order. It is not accepted practice to stop CPR except under the following circumstances as outlined in the AHA Standards:

1. When effective and spontaneous circulation and ventilation have been restored.
2. When resuscitation efforts have been transferred to another responsible person who knows CPR.
3. When a physician or physician-directed team assumes responsibility for the victim.
4. When the victim is transferred to properly trained personnel charged with responsibilities for emergency medical services.
5. When the rescuer is exhausted and unable to continue resuscitation.

☐ PREPARATION

PHYSIOLOGICAL CHANGES IN CARDIOPULMONARY ARREST

Cardiopulmonary arrest refers to both the absence of circulation and the absence of ventilation. The cessation of either can be the primary event; however, one can quickly lead to the other. In other words, if a cardiac arrest is the primary event, the victim will quickly stop breathing and if a pulmonary arrest is the primary event, the heart will soon cease to contract. In the adult victim, either cardiac arrest or pulmonary arrest is likely to be the primary event. Most pediatric arrests are pulmonary, the exception usually being a child with a primary cardiac defect (Melker, 1978).

Cardiac Arrest

Cardiac arrest refers to the absence of spontaneous cardiac contractions which results in the cessation of all blood flow. The three general causes of cardiac arrest, as described by Ellis and Billings (1980), are: (1) interference with the contractile force of the heart which may result from heart failure or cardiac tamponade; (2) interference with formation and conduction of electrical impulses which may be caused by potassium imbalance, acidosis, or myocardial infarction; or (3) interference with blood flow such as with pulmonary embolus or air embolus.

Pulmonary Arrest

Pulmonary arrest is commonly referred to as a respiratory arrest. When a pulmonary arrest occurs, oxygen and carbon dioxide exchange ceases because ventilation has stopped and air no longer is moving in and out of the lungs. While artificial breathing provides ventilation, the rescuer has no control over whether oxygen–carbon dioxide exchange occurs.

The three general causes of pulmonary arrest (Ellis and Billings, 1980) are: (1) depression of the respiratory center, which can be caused by head trauma or an overdose of barbiturates; (2) interference with ventilation or respiration resulting in interference in oxygen and carbon dioxide exchange, as with airway obstruction or respiratory distress syndrome; and (3) interference with neuromuscular transmission to the ventilatory muscles as may occur in a disease such as myasthenia gravis.

Cardiopulmonary Arrest

The cessation of circulation and ventilation (clinical death) prevents the exchange of oxygen and carbon dioxide not only at the alveolar level, but at the cellular level. Without the delivery of oxygen, tissue metabolism becomes anaerobic; lactic acid is produced, and acidosis develops. This acidotic state evolves quickly, and unless it is corrected, the outcome of the arrest will be death. The reversal of this acidotic state is a primary goal of both basic and advanced life support techniques. Therefore, CPR must be instituted without delay and a sense of urgency must predominate until the decision to stop resuscitative efforts has been made. Biologic death will occur if CPR is not initiated within 4 to 6 minutes. Although there is good evidence that brain damage is not necessarily inevitable if resuscitation is not started within 4 to 6 minutes (Safar, 1978), it is still generally accepted that this is a likely outcome.

PHYSIOLOGY OF CPR

Theories of Blood Flow Mechanisms

Since Kouwenhoven's accidental discovery of external cardiac compression, it has been thought that artificially induced blood flow results from a direct squeezing of the heart between the sternum and the spine. Current research is producing evidence that blood flow may result from one or both of two mechanisms: direct ventricular compression, a global increase in intrathoracic pressure, or both (Babbs, 1980). There is further evidence that simultaneous chest compression and ventilation, that is, inflating the lungs during the downstroke of external cardiac compression, actually increases arterial pressure and carotid blood flow during CPR. This has been described as the "New CPR." However, the effects of this method on the adequacy of ventilation are not yet determined (Chandra et al., 1978). From the practical standpoint of administering basic CPR, the functional result is the same, regardless of the mechanism that produces blood flow. There is no indication that any modification of basic CPR techniques is needed.

Babbs (1980) describes the traditionally accepted theory of blood flow during CPR as the *cardiac pump mechanism,* and the new theory as the *thoracic pump mechanism.* One, if not both, of these mechanisms may be operative during CPR.

Cardiac Pump Mechanism. The cardiac pump mechanism assumes that blood flow during CPR results from compression directly over the heart that squeezes the heart between the sternum and spine, artificially causing it to empty, as depicted in Figure 75-1A. This action is thought to produce an artificial

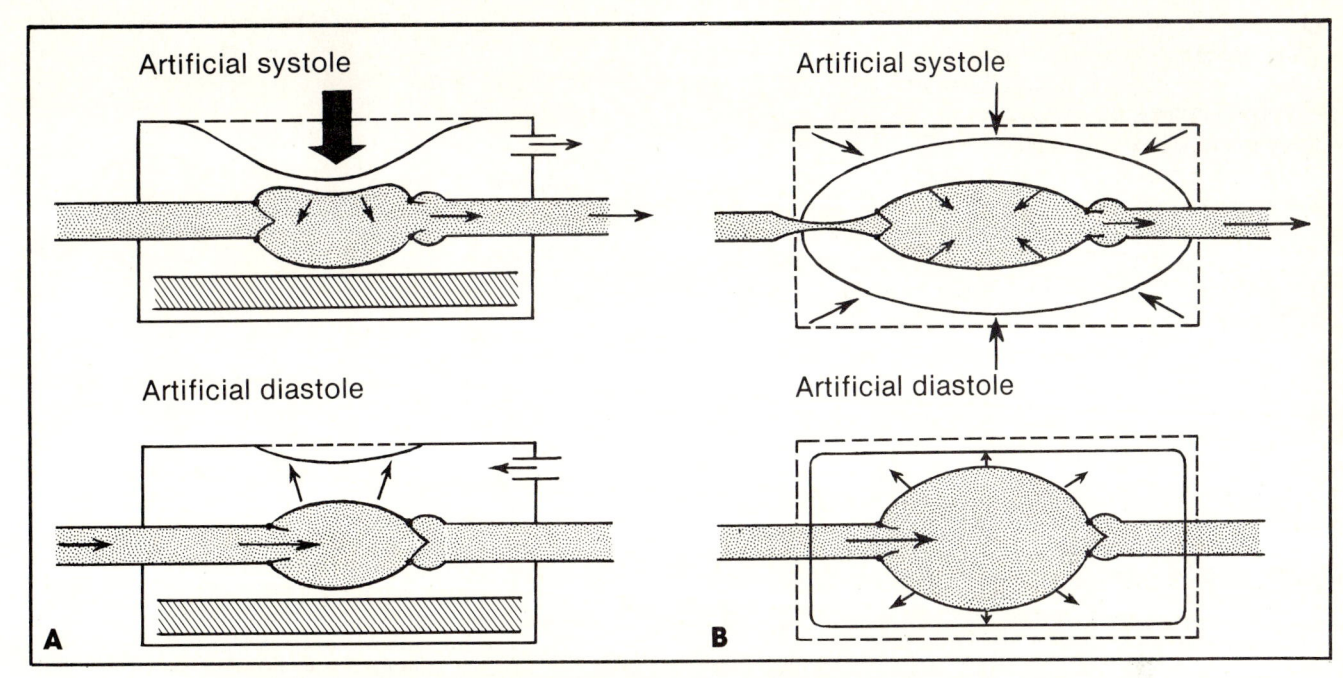

Figure 75-1. Blood flow during CPR: **A.** Cardiac pump mechanism. During artificial systole, central chest compression squeezes the heart against the spine, forcing blood out. Air is vented from the thorax via the trachea (top right). During artificial diastole chest resiliency creates negative pressure for filling. The site of application of force (broad arrow) is critical. For simplicity only one pumping chamber is shown. **B.** The thoracic pump mechanism. During artificial systole, thoracic compression or cough generates intrathoracic pressure which is vented by arterial outflow to peripheral tissues. During artificial diastole, release of intrathoracic pressure allows for filling. Site of application of force is not important. (From Babbs CF: New versus old theories of blood flow during CPR. Critical Care Medicine 8(3):191–195, 1980. Used with permission.)

systole with higher pressures in the ventricles (the compression chamber) than elsewhere in the thorax. The mitral and tricuspid valves are closed, while the semilunar valves are open, forcing blood into the aorta and pulmonary artery. When compression is released, an artificial diastole occurs. Intracardiac pressure drops, the mitral and tricuspid valves open, and the heart passively fills from the peripheral and pulmonary venous circulation. Negative pressure from chest recoil aids ventricular filling. Artificial breathing is delivered during the upstroke of compression (when manual pressure to the chest is released) so as not to hinder cardiac compression and ventricular emptying. If direct compression of the ventricles generates the blood flow, hand position on the sternum is crucial.

Thoracic Pump Mechanism. The thoracic pump mechanism assumes that blood flow during CPR results from an intermittent increase in total intrathoracic pressure, as depicted in Figure 75-1B. The increased pressure (artificial systole) is believed to squeeze blood from the ventricles, pulmonary vasculature, and left atrium, sending it into the systemic and pulmonary circulation. With this mechanism the heart acts essentially like a conduit. Lower pressure outside the thorax aids in blood flow. The release of external thoracic pressure produces an artificial diastole in a manner similar to the cardiac pump mechanism. The global intrathoracic pressure can be enhanced with simultaneous chest compression and ventilation. In other words, artificial breathing is delivered during the downstroke of chest compression. If this theory is operative, hand position for chest compression is not crucial.

Effects of Compression on Blood Flow

The American Heart Association has determined the most effective rate of compression to be 60 beats per minute (BPM) for adults, 80 BPM for children, and 100 BPM for infants. With the adult, this necessitates a rate of 80 BPM when there is only one rescuer to account for time lost giving artificial ventilation. These rates approximate those of healthy adults, children, and infants. They are rapid enough to allow systolic emptying and slow enough to allow diastolic filling, as well as filling of the coronary arteries. Cardiac output is equal to the heart rate times the stroke volume. Because stroke volume is influenced by the volume of blood in the ventricles at the end of diastole, it is important to allow sufficient time for the ventricles to fill.

Compression is applied at a depth of 3.8 to 5.1 cm (1½ to 2 in) for adults, 2.5 to 3.8 cm (1 to 1½ in) for children, and 1.25 to 2.5 cm (½ to 1 in) for infants. These depths are about as far as the sternum can comfortably be compressed for each age group. Compression must be applied evenly and smoothly. The downstroke should consist of 50 percent of the cycle and the upstroke 50 percent. One study (Rudikoff et al., 1976) showed that the effectiveness of external cardiac compression was related to the duration rather than the rate of compression. This finding lends credibility to the widely accepted practice of delivering firm and even compressions. Quick, jabbing compressions do not produce adequate blood pressure or blood flow.

The Mechanics of Ventilation
In the not-too-distant past, it was believed that ventilation by mouth-to-mouth resuscitation was ineffective. The rationale was that expired air contained an inadequate amount of oxygen to sustain life, but it is now known that the amount of oxygen in expired air can maintain life. Normal inspired air contains 20.84 percent oxygen and 0.4 percent carbon dioxide while normal expired air contains 15.7 percent oxygen and 3.6 percent carbon dioxide. The carbon dioxide level in expired air is not detrimental to a victim of cardiopulmonary arrest since a level of 10 percent can be tolerated by most people. In an adult male, normal tidal volume is approximately 500 ml. In giving artificial ventilation to an adult victim, the rescuer delivers about 1000 ml of air, or twice the normal tidal volume.

TECHNIQUES FOR OPENING THE AIRWAY

When breathing is absent for any reason, a person quickly loses consciousness. In the unconscious person, the mandible recedes, the flaccid tongue falls back against the posterior wall, and the flexion of the cervical vertebrae narrows the airway. The result is that the tongue obstructs the airway, which is the most common cause of airway obstruction in the unconscious victim. The American Heart Association (1985) describes four different maneuvers that may be used to open the airway. The first and most important method is the *head tilt*. This method requires that the victim have enough tone in the muscles attached to the jaw to move the lower jaw forward. When the tone is adequate, tilting the head lifts the tongue away from the posterior pharynx and thereby opens the airway. When the head tilt is inadequate to maintain an effective open airway, it may be necessary to combine the head tilt with a second maneuver, the *chin lift,* or a third maneuver, the *jaw thrust.* Either one of these actions actively pulls the lower jaw and tongue forward. A fourth maneuver that has been commonly used combines the head tilt with a *neck lift*. With this movement, the head is extended at the junction of the head and neck; it is not an exaggerated hyperextension of the cervical spine. This method does not provide enough support for the lower jaw, although it is effective in opening the airway. The head tilt-neck lift method should not be used when the victim has or is suspected of having a cervical spine injury because some hyperextension of the cervical spine results when the head is tilted. This movement may either cause or contribute to spinal cord injury. To avoid the potential for spinal cord injury, Donegan (1982) recommends the jaw thrust maneuver *without* head tilt as the preferred method for opening the airway of these victims.

In addition, it is important to remember that because the neck of an infant or small child is pliable, an exaggerated head tilt that may be used safely with adults may actually obstruct an infant or small child's airway. While some degree of head extension is necessary, it is less exaggerated. In children over 4 years, the degree of head extension permitted increases as the child grows.

Guildner (1976) reported a study comparing the effectiveness of the neck-lift, chin-lift, and jaw thrust maneuvers combined with the head tilt. The study indicated that in the unconscious nonbreathing victim and the unconscious breathing victim, the head tilt-chin lift and jaw thrust methods were superior to the neck lift in opening the airway. In addition, it was found that both the neck lift and the jaw thrust methods were consistently more tiring to the rescuer. Since the head tilt-chin lift method also brings the teeth close together, it helps to maintain loose dentures in proper position; otherwise they could serve as an additional obstruction to the airway. Keeping the dentures in proper position also helps the rescuer to obtain a tight mouth-to-mouth seal.

The American Heart Association (1985) currently recommends both the head tilt-chin lift and head tilt-neck lift as appropriate methods, although it emphasizes preferred use of the head tilt-chin lift method because it has some advantages over the head tilt-neck lift.

COMPLICATIONS RESULTING FROM CPR

Under the most ideal circumstances, CPR is not without its hazards, because complications can occur even when the correct technique is used.

Enarson and Gracey (1976) classify complications of CPR as traumatic, circulatory, and aspiration. *Traumatic* complications are the most numerous. The most frequent traumatic injury is rib fracture, which can lead to hemothorax or pneumothorax. Other complications include liver and spleen injuries, flail chest, and gastric rupture. Catastrophic consequences are cardiac tamponade and ruptured heart. *Circulatory* complications occur less frequently than traumatic complications and may result in central nervous system deficits such as hemiplegia, aphasia, or coma. Emboli (blood clots moving in the blood stream) or mural thrombi (small stationary clots) may also result. *Aspiration* may result from regurgitation of stomach contents, expecially when excessive inflation pressures are used, because this can easily cause gastric distention. *Gastric distention* not only leads to regurgitation but decreases lung volume by elevating the diaphragm. Artificial ventilation volume should be limited to that needed to make the chest rise. Excessive ventilation volume can cause hypopharyngeal pressure to exceed 25 cm of water and this can open the gastroesophageal sphincter (McIntyre et al., 1978, p. 1133). Distention may also occur if the victim's airway is partially or completely obstructed. Keeping the airway open by maintaining the head and neck in proper position helps to minimize the problem. Attempts at relieving gastric distention with manual pressure should be avoided due to the risk of aspiration of gastric contents. Aspiration is a very serious complication that significantly decreases chances of a successful resuscitation effort. The American Heart Association (1985, p. 81) recommends that manual relief of distention be attempted *only* if the distention is severe enough to cause inadequate ventilation that cannot be improved by repositioning the airway. To relieve the distention turn the victim on the side to permit air expulsion and prevent aspiration and then apply pressure over the epigastrium (middle upper portion of the abdomen). Continous pressure on the abdomen to prevent distention is not recommended.

McIntyre et al. (1978, p. 1132) refer to victim–rescuer mismatch and caution rescuers to avoid excessive force by taking into account differences in size and age. For example, a young athlete would probably not use his or her full body strength to perform CPR on a frail elderly woman.

DATA BASE

Client History and Recorded Data

When a cardiopulmonary arrest occurs, the nurse quickly, but systematically, assesses the physical state of the victim. The nurse looks for signs of spontaneous respiration and circulation using the physical appraisal skills of inspection, auscultation, and palpation. A hospital-based nurse must know the location of the emergency cart (commonly known as the crash cart) and the cardiac arrest board. The nurse must also know the code status of the clients on the clinical unit. "No Code" orders should be noted in the kardex for clients when cardiopulmonary arrest is anticipated.

Physical Appraisal Skills

Inspection. *Inspection* is used to determine the level of consciousness, respiratory status, pupil response, skin condition, and any obvious cause of cardiopulmonary arrest.

When approaching a suspected arrest victim, it is necessary to establish level of consciousness and differentiate between sleeping, fainting, or cardiac arrest. Since CPR is never done on a conscious person, the adult victim must be stimulated by shaking the shoulder and asking loudly if he or she is okay. An infant is stimulated by tapping the feet, gently attempting to make the infant cry. Rough stimuli could compound injuries that may be present. Adequate time (4 to 10 seconds according to the AHA Standards) should be allowed to make this initial assessment of level of consciousness.

After the nurse has established unresponsiveness, the presence or absence of breathing must then be determined. Place the victim in a supine position and kneel beside the victim, facing the chest. Open the airway and observe the rise and fall of the chest. If no breathing is observed, the nurse assumes that pulmonary arrest is present. If breathing is present, the rate, rhythm, depth, and character are noted.

While positioning the victim, the nurse can simultaneously check for the presence of a tracheal stoma which would be present if the victim had a laryngectomy. Additional observations can be made simultaneously with observations of respiratory status. Indicators of compromised respiratory status are pale, dusky, mottled, or cyanotic skin. Seizures (convulsions) occasionally precede cardiopulmonary arrest. Bladder or bowel incontinence may occur. In addition to inspection of the victim, it is useful to note any obvious environmental cause of cardiopulmonary arrest, such as live electrical wires.

Inspection of pupil reaction to light is best done intermittently during the course of CPR, but only if an extra person with the knowledge base to make this assessment is available. (The one or two rescuers delivering CPR should not stop CPR to make this assessment.) Pupillary response to light is a neurologic indicator of cerebral oxygenation and autonomic nervous system activity. The pupil becomes fully dilated about 1 minute after cardiopulmonary arrest. To inspect the pupils, gently open the eyelids by using the thumb and forefinger to raise the upper lid and depress the lower lid. As the eyelids open, note whether the pupils are dilated or constricted, equal or unequal, and whether they constrict in response to light. While response to light may be an indication of CPR effectiveness, there may be other causes for pupillary changes that may invalidate this assessment. For example, barbiturates and amphetamines can cause the pupils to dilate and narcotics can cause constriction. Until recently, it was accepted that dilated pupils meant irreversible brain damage, but there are now documented cases where this has not always occurred.

Palpation. *Palpation* is used to identify pulses. With adults, central pulses, which are large arteries nearest the aorta, should be used, such as the carotid or femoral arteries. The carotid artery is preferred because it is easily accessible and does not require that clothing be removed. Pulses in the extremities are not used because they may be weak, if not absent, in the event of vascular collapse.

With infants, the AHA currently recommends that the brachial pulse be used to assess circulation. The AHA 1974 Standards recommended placing the hand over the infant's heart to palpate the apical beat. The 1980 AHA Standards, revised recommendation to use the brachial pulse with infants, was made on the basis of a study that compared palpation of the apical and brachial pulse (Cavallaro and Melker, 1983). The study revealed that in healthy infants from 3 weeks to 12 months of age with normal heart function, the apical beat is frequently unreliable and undetectable. After being taught how to palpate both the apical and brachial pulse, 44 percent of the infants' parents could palpate the apical impulse within 10 seconds, but 84 percent could palpate the brachial pulse. In addition, only 27 percent of the parents who were able to palpate the apical beat could count it accurately, while 48 percent of those who could palpate the brachial pulse could do so. A rescuer could mistakenly conclude that circulation was absent if he or she did not feel apical activity (Chameides, 1982). In addition, palpating the carotid pulse on infants is not recommended because the short, chubby neck of an infant makes it difficult to locate and palpate that pulse. Using the brachial pulse site provides the most reasonable alternative to the carotid site; even though it is a peripheral artery, the brachial artery is close to the core of the body.

In the adult, slight hyperextension of the neck makes the larynx, and therefore the carotid pulse, easier to identify. While maintaining the chin lift or head tilt for the open airway with one hand, use the finger tips of the other hand to locate the larynx. Then gently slide the fingers into the groove between the trachea and the sternocleidomastoid muscle, taking care not to compress the pulse. It is important that the pulse be palpated on the side *nearest* the nurse rather than on the side away from the nurse for three reasons: (1) there is a tendency for the fingers to rest on the trachea, so the pulse is not palpated adequately; (2) there is a tendency to use too much pressure, impairing patency of the airway and altering head position; and (3) there is a tendency to feel with both the fingers on the far side and the thumb on the near side. Simultaneous pressure on both the right and left carotid pulses could occlude cerebral blood flow (AHA, 1980). Avoid palpating the carotid artery near the angle of the jaw because stimulation of the carotid sinus located there could result in a severe bradycardia in an already compromised victim.

The brachial pulse of an infant is found on the inner aspect of the upper arm halfway between the shoulder and the elbow. Place the thumb on the outer aspect of the arm and press the tips of the index and middle fingers lightly toward the bone on the inner arm until a pulse is palpated. While the brachial pulse of a healthy infant can be difficult to palpate, a study done with a number of lay adults concluded that this technique can be learned with practice (Chameides, 1982).

Establishing the presence or absence of a pulse should take 3 to 5 seconds.

Auscultation. *Auscultation* is also used to determine the presence or absence of breathing. After opening the airway, remain beside the victim, facing the chest, place an ear over the victim's mouth, and listen for movement of air during exhalation. While listening, simultaneously observe the chest to see if it rises and falls, and wait to feel the expired air move against the cheek. This look, listen, and feel sequence should take 3 to 5 seconds. Listening with the unaided ear is all that is required or recommended. Although the use of a stethoscope would permit finer sound discriminations, valuable time should not be lost obtaining a stethoscope or making these discriminations.

EQUIPMENT

The only equipment needed for basic life support is a firm surface. Hospital emergency carts, commonly referred to as crash carts, include a cardiac arrest board designed specifically for this purpose. Some hospital beds have a removable head or footboard that can be used. If a board is not available, a serving tray or the floor provides an adequate alternative. Outside the hospital, a victim should be placed on the floor or ground, rather than on a bed or a couch.

☐ EXECUTION

CPR TECHNIQUES—ADULT

Cardiopulmonary resuscitation involves three basic skills, referred to by the AHA as the ABC's of CPR: opening the airway, breathing, and maintaining circulation. An adult victim may be given CPR by one or two rescuers.

Begin by placing the victim in a supine, horizontal position for assessment and performance of CPR. The head must be on the same plane as the trunk to facilitate cerebral blood flow; elevating the legs is also recommended by some authorities to aid venous return and cardiac output. If there is reason to suspect trauma, especially to the neck and spinal cord, the victim should be turned as a unit with the head and body in alignment to avoid flexion of the neck.

The airway is then opened and respiratory status is assessed. The presence of a tracheal stoma can be quickly determined at this time.

Establishing an Open Airway

As described above, there are four different methods for opening the adult airway: (1) the head tilt; (2) the head tilt-chin lift; (3) the jaw thrust; and (4) the head tilt-neck lift.

To perform the *head tilt* place a hand on the victim's forehead as shown in Figure 75–2A, kneel at the victim's side, and apply firm, backward pressure with the palm. This moves the lower jaw forward and lifts the tongue away from the posterior pharynx. For victims who have become unconscious because of fainting

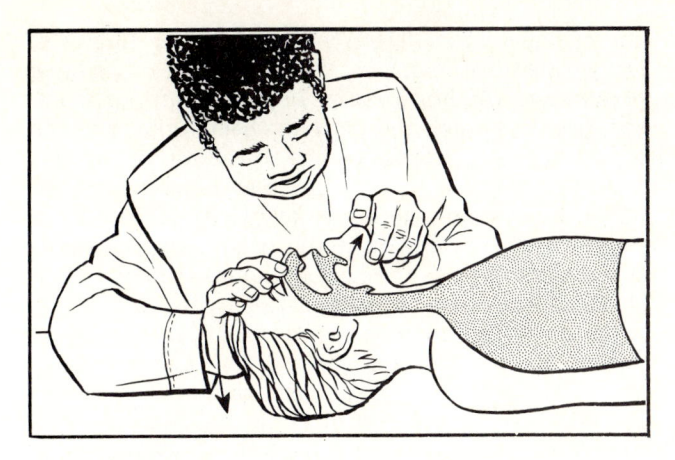

Figure 75-2. Establishing the airway. **A.** Head tilt-chin lift.

or heat prostration, this maneuver may be all that is required to open the airway.

To perform the *head tilt-chin lift* as shown in Figure 75-2A, kneel at the victim's side; first tilt the head backward with one hand, and then place the fingers of the opposite hand under the bony portion of the lower jaw near the chin and raise the chin forward. This brings the teeth nearly together but the mouth should not be closed completely. The thumb may be used to depress the lower lip but not to raise the chin. To deliver mouth-to-nose ventilation, use a modification of the head tilt-chin lift method. Placing the fingers on the soft tissues under the chin is not acceptable because this may obstruct the airway.

To perform the *head tilt-jaw thrust* as shown in Figure 75-2B, kneel at the victim's head and use both hands to grasp the angles of the jaw to displace the mandible forward and upward. This action simultaneously tilts the head backward. The thumbs can be used to pull back the lower lip if the lips close completely. To deliver mouth-to-mouth ventilation, place your cheek tightly against the nostrils to close them. Use the head tilt-jaw thrust for any victim with a suspected or actual neck injury and carefully support the head to prevent it from tilting backward or turning from side to side.

To perform the *head tilt-neck lift* as shown in Figure 75-2C, kneel at the victim's side and place one hand on the forehead and the other under the neck at the base of the head, with both the hands facing away from yourself. Positioning the hand at the base of the head rather than under a lower segment of the neck minimizes hyperextension of the cervical spine. Then apply pressure with the hand on the forehead to tilt the head backward while simultaneously lifting the neck.

After opening the airway, place your ear over the victim's nose and mouth, and look at the chest to listen and feel for the escape of air and observe the rise of the chest.

Ventilation

If, after opening the airway, the victim does not begin to breathe spontaneously, artificial ventilation is given. Artificial ventilation can be given by forcefully breathing into the victim's mouth, nose, or stoma.

To provide *mouth-to-mouth* ventilation, use either the head tilt-chin lift or head tilt-neck lift to maintain an open airway. Pinch the nostrils closed with the hand that is on the forehead to prevent the escape of air through the nostrils during ventilation.

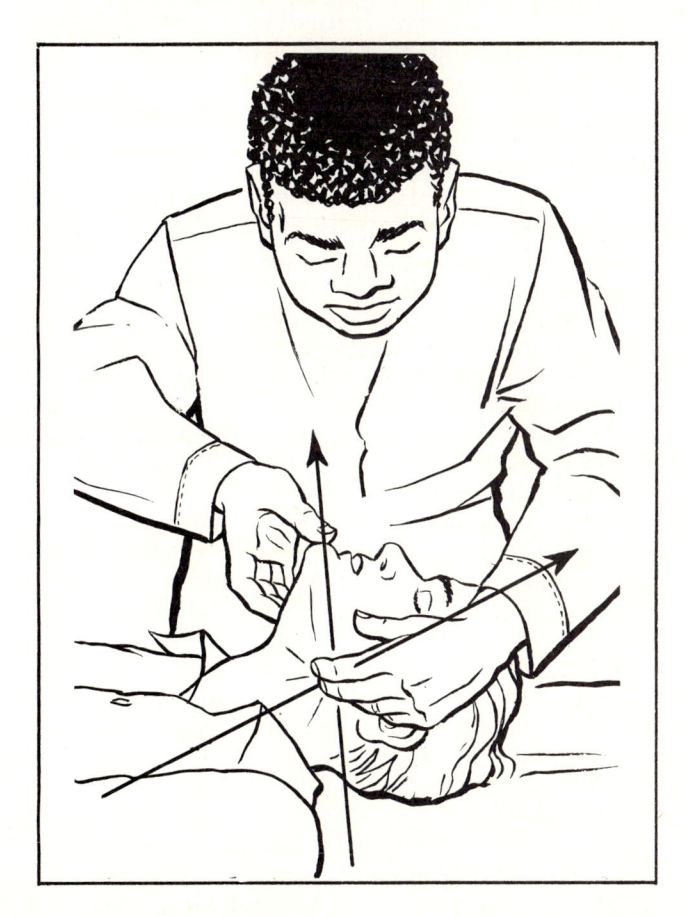

Figure 75-2. B. Head tilt-jaw thrust.

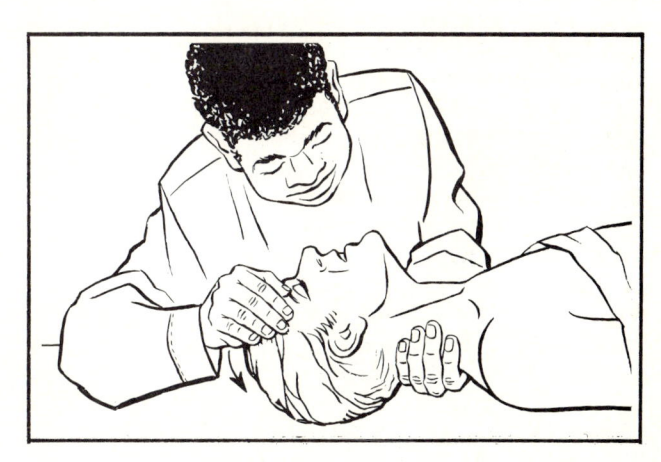

Figure 75-2. C. Head tilt-neck lift.

Open your mouth widely, take a deep breath, and place your mouth over the victim's mouth, creating a seal. Blow forcefully into the victim's mouth.

Initially, four full rapid ventilations are given, allowing no time for the victim's lungs to deflate between ventilations. This increases end expiratory pressure and opens small air sacs which may have collapsed. While giving these four initial ventilations, watch out of the corner of the eye for the chest to rise. If artificial ventilation efforts are ineffective, evaluate your technique and reattempt ventilations. The most common causes of ineffective ventilations are improper head tilt, inadequate mouth seal, and failure to pinch off the nostrils.

If there is mouth trauma and the mouth cannot be opened or a tight seal cannot be maintained, *mouth-to-nose* ventilation may be preferable. With this maneuver, inhale deeply, seal your lips around the victim's nose, and blow forcefully. Greater force may be needed because narrow nasal passages offer more resistance than the wider oral passages. Ventilatory effectiveness is assessed as described above for mouth-to-mouth ventilation. It may be necessary to open the victim's mouth to permit exhalation if the victim is unable to exhale through the nose. This moves the soft palate away from the nasopharyngeal passage, preventing obstruction.

Ventilate victims with tracheal stomas or tracheostomy tubes directly with *mouth-to-stoma* ventilation. Because the oropharyngeal structures are bypassed, it is not necessary to hyperextend the neck. If a tracheostomy tube has an inflatable cuff, it may be helpful to inflate it, if possible, to prevent air from escaping around the tube. Seal the victim's nose and mouth with the hand so air will not be blown out through the nose and mouth, then inhale deeply, seal the mouth around the stoma, and blow directly into the stoma. If the tracheostomy tube is inflated and the lips seal adequately around the tube itself, you may blow directly into the tracheostomy tube.

After administering the initial ventilations, determine the presence or absence of a central pulse and obtain help by calling a code or activating the emergency medical system.

If a pulse is present, deliver 1 breath every 5 seconds or 12 breaths per minute. Since respiratory arrest can be expected to lead to cardiac arrest, continue to assess central pulses every minute. If the pulse is absent, begin cardiac compression immediately after delivering initial ventilations.

Cardiac Compression

Cardiac compression is delivered on the midline of the lower half of the sternum. The correct hand position is determined in two ways. One way is to use the hand nearest to the victim's legs to locate the lower margin of the rib cage with the middle and index fingers (Fig. 75-3A). Run the fingers along the rib cage to the xiphisternal junction, which is the notch where the ribs and sternum meet (Fig. 75-3B). Hold the fingers in this position while placing the heel of the other hand proximal to the fingers (Fig. 75-3C). Remove the fingers from the notch and place the heel of that hand on top of the hand already on the sternum (Fig. 75-3D). (An alternative method, which may be useful for the obese or pregnant victim, is to palpate the xyphoid process with the fingers of the hand nearest the victim's legs and place the heel of the other hand on the sternum.) Place your hands parallel with each other, with the fingers directed toward the far side of the victim. It is imperative to keep the fingers off the chest to minimize the risk of rib fracture. To do this, extend your fingers, or interlace them as shown in Figures 75-3D and 75-4. It is impossible to identify landmarks and use correct hand placement without exposing the victim's chest. This may require tearing or cutting clothing away, since time must not be wasted. When compressions are applied over clothing, the hands tend to slide out of position between compressions, thus increasing the likelihood of causing injury.

The CPR rescuer can lessen the risk of injury to a victim by using the correct technique for the age and size of the victim. For that reason, *locating* correct hand position through correct identification of landmarks is essential. Compression must be midsternal above the xyphoid process. Compression of the xyphoid process can lacerate the liver or other abdominal organs. In *maintaining* correct hand position, it is important that: (a) the rescuer be positioned so the compression is delivered in a vertical, downward motion, and (b) the rescuer does not lose the hand position by allowing the hands to leave the chest wall. Poorly directed force and migration of hands from the midline can lead to lung trauma and fractured ribs, as can failure to keep the fingers raised off the chest wall during compression.

Deliver cardiac compression vertically, that is, with the arms at a 90 degree angle to the victim's chest, and use body weight rather than the arms alone to deliver the force. This technique delivers the maximum compression and minimizes effort expended. To accomplish this, kneel beside the victim if he or she is on the floor or use a stool or kneel on the bed if the victim is in bed. Keep the shoulders directly over the sternum with the elbows locked, and apply enough force to depress the sternum 3.8 to 5.1 cm (1½ to 2 in). This can best be accomplished by rocking forward from the hips and using body weight to deliver the compression. Correct body position and movement are shown in Figure 75-4. A common error is for rescuers to bend their elbows, using only their forearms. This is tiring and most people do not have enough strength to depress the sternum adequately in this manner.

Deliver the compressions regularly, smoothly, and without bouncing.

The compression duration should be equal to, if not slightly greater than, the relaxation between compressions; that is, approximately 0.5 seconds on the

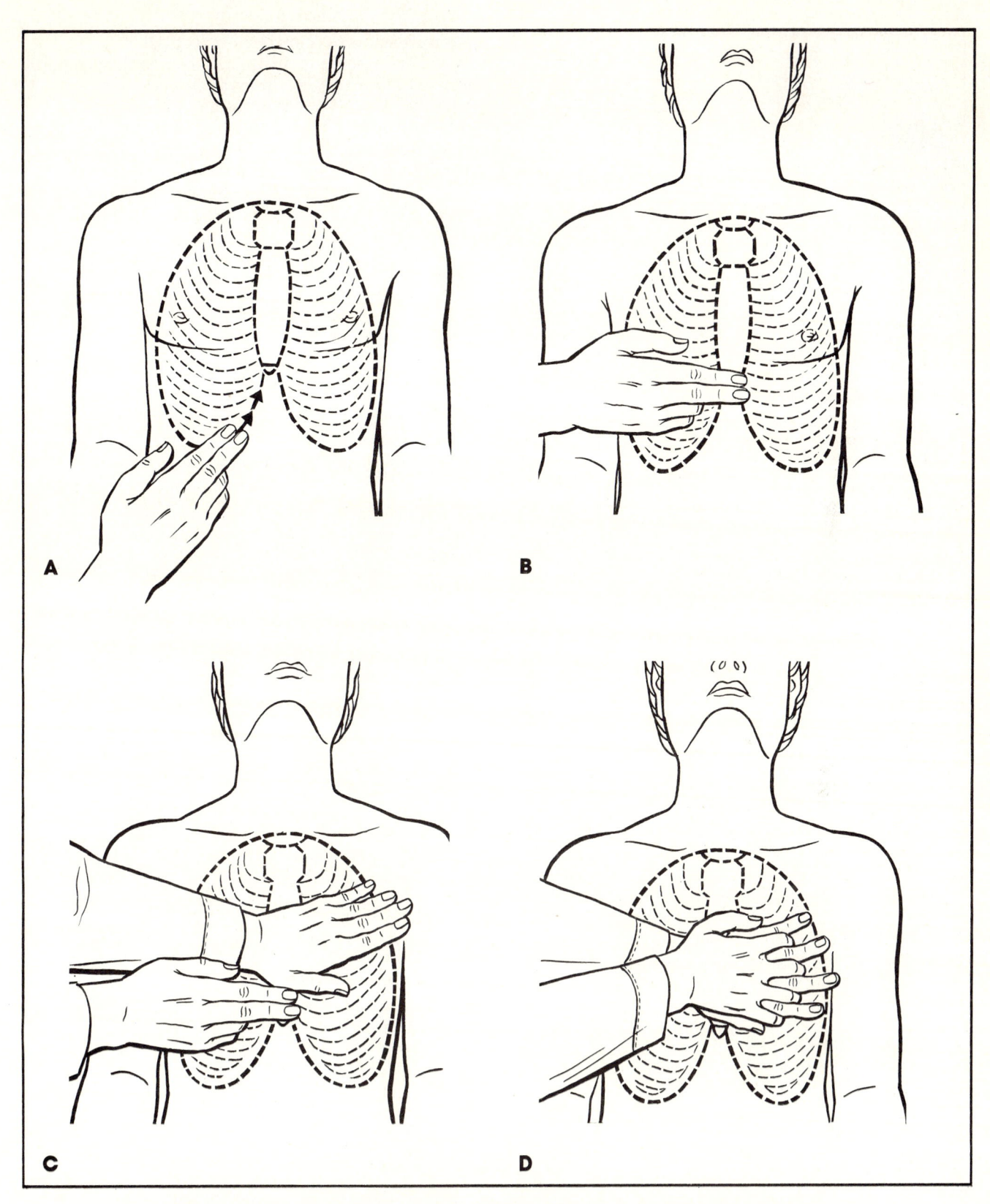

Figure 75–3. Locating correct hand placement: **A.** Locate lower rib margin and run two fingers along rib cage. **B.** Xiphisternal junction. **C.** Keep fingers in this position and place the heel of the other hand on the sternum adjacent to the fingers. **D.** Remove the fingers from the xiphisternal junction and place that hand on top of the other hand, with fingers interlaced and directed away from the rescuer.

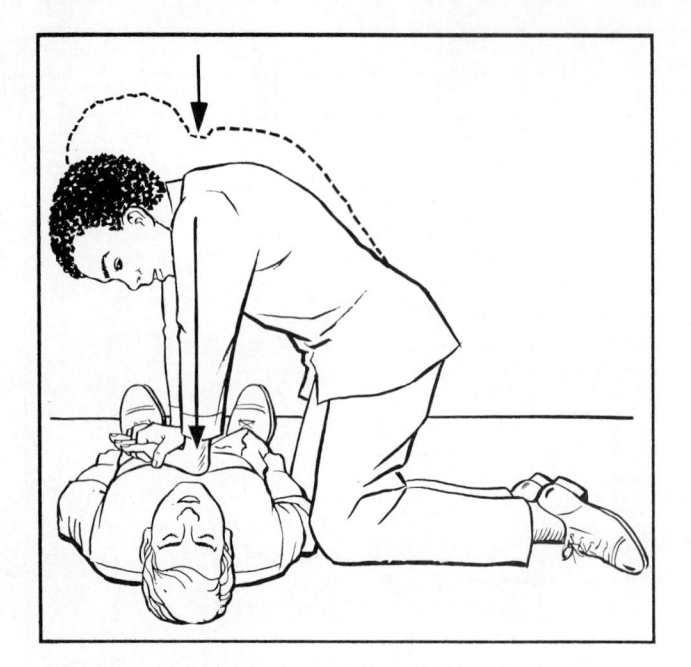

Figure 75-4. Correct body placement and movement for external cardiac compression: Kneel beside victim; keep shoulders directly over the sternum with arms straight and elbows locked. Using body weight and rocking forward from the hips, compress the sternum to a depth of 3.8 to 5.1 cm (1½ to 2 in). Fingers are held away from the chest wall and the hands remain on the chest during both compression and relaxation.

downstroke and 0.5 seconds on the upstroke. This is crucial to achieve an adequate stroke volume and cardiac output and also allows for adequate cardiac filling time. Inadequate cardiac filling can occur if compression is not released completely during the upstroke. When CPR is administered for a long period of time there is a tendency to keep some pressure on the chest at the upstroke because the hands remain in contact with the chest. Another common error is spiking or quick, jerky compression, which significantly diminishes cardiac output.

Ideally, compressions should not be interrupted because systolic pressure drops from a peak of 100 mm Hg to zero when compressions are stopped. George (1978) reports that it takes about five compressions to return the systolic blood pressure to 80 mm Hg. A disadvantage with one-rescuer CPR is that compressions must be interrupted to provide ventilations. With two-rescuer CPR at a rate of 60 BPM, there is sufficient time to interpose a breath on the upstroke of the fifth compression without breaking the smooth, regular rhythm. Ordinarily CPR should not be interrupted for more than 5 seconds. It may be interrupted briefly after the first minute to check for the return of the carotid pulse, and then rechecked a few minutes later. If endotracheal intubation or transporting the victim is required, 30 seconds may be allowed but not more (AHA, 1980).

Compression to Ventilation Ratios

When one rescuer is present, deliver cardiac compressions at a rate of 80 per minute, interspersed with ventilations at a 15:2 compression to ventilation ratio. The rate of 80 provides an effective minute rate of 60, as it compensates for the time lost ventilating the victim. When two rescuers are present, use a compression rate of 60 per minute, with one ventilation interspersed after each fifth compression, a 5:1 compression to ventilation ratio.

To maintain the appropriate compression rates, use an audible mnemonic. For a rate of 80, use "1- and 2- and 3- and- . . . 10- and -1 and -2 and . . . 15- and. For a rate of 60, use "1-1000, 2-1000, . . . 5-1000". These signals help the rescuer maintain the correct rate and rhythm, and communicate the point in the CPR sequence to additional rescuers who become available.

TWO-PERSON RESCUE

When a second rescuer becomes available, that person should communicate that he or she knows CPR and intends to help. This rescuer then kneels next to the victim on the side opposite the first rescuer, and palpates the carotid pulse. If no pulse is felt, the first rescuer's compression technique must be reevaluated and corrected. If a pulse is palpable, the second rescuer says, "good pulse," thus indicating successful technique at that time. Either at that time or at the end of the 15:2 compression–ventilation sequence, the second rescuer says "stop compression" and checks for the return of a spontaneous pulse. If no pulse is felt within 5 seconds, the second rescuer calls, "Continue CPR" and gives a ventilation. CPR is then resumed at the slower rate of 60 BPM and a 5:1 compression to ventilation ratio. When two rescuers deliver CPR, one manages the artificial ventilation and the other manages the cardiac compression. The rescuer managing ventilation interposes a breath during the upstroke of the fifth compression. This avoids the resistance that would be encountered on the downstroke, permitting more effective ventilation and cardiac compression. Failure to interpose ventilation on the upstroke of compression is a common cause of inadequate ventilation in two-rescuer CPR.

When the first rescuer becomes fatigued and wants to change positions, this is communicated to the second rescuer. Rather than the numbered mnemonic, the fatigued rescuer uses the mnemonic "Change-1000, 2-1000. . . ." After the fifth compression, the second rescuer delivers one ventilation and moves into position for compression. Simultaneously, the first rescuer moves to the victim's head and checks the carotid pulse. If no pulse is felt the first rescuer gives one ventilation and says, "Continue CPR." CPR resumes and the rescuers can change positions whenever necessary.

☐ SKILL SEQUENCE

CPR—ONE AND TWO RESCUER

Step	Rationale
1. Kneel at victim's side near the head and shoulders. Shake shoulder. Ask if victim is okay. Place victim in supine position. If no response, call "Help!" (4 to 10 seconds).	Need to assess level of consciousness. Victim can be positioned simultaneously.
2. Open airway. Use head-tilt, head tilt-chin lift, jaw thrust, or head tilt-neck lift. Assess respiratory status. Check for stoma (3 to 5 seconds).	Opening airway may be all that is needed to facilitate breathing. Presence of stoma can be quickly and conveniently determined at this point.
3. If no spontaneous respirations, deliver 4 full, rapid ventilations, allowing no time for deflation between breaths. Observe for rise of chest (3 to 5 seconds).	Oxygenates blood. Increases end expiratory pressure and opens small air sacs. Indicates effectiveness of ventilatory efforts.
4. If unable to ventilate, reposition head and again attempt to ventilate. (NOTE: If unable to ventilate, proceed as for an obstructed airway, Skill 76, before continuing to step 5.)	
5. Assess carotid pulse, placing fingers on near side of trachea (5 to 10 seconds).	Central pulses more likely to be present than peripheral pulses. Carotid usually most convenient.
6. Activate emergency medical system if no spontaneous respirations or pulse present.	Establish arrested state to confirm need for EMS. Have relevant information to give to appropriate person.
7. If pulse is present, ventilate victim once every 5 seconds. Reassess pulse every minute.	Respiratory arrest is likely to deteriorate to cardiac arrest.
8. If pulse is not present, begin external cardiac compression at rate of 80 BPM, alternating with ventilations at a 15:2 compression–ventilation ratio and a compression depth of 3.8 to 5.1 cm (1½ to 2 in). (Mnemonic is 1-and-2-and-3-and-4 . . . 10-and-1-and-2-and . . . 15-and.)	Provides effective minute rate of 60 BPM to compensate for time lost delivering ventilations. Compression depth necessary for artificial blood flow to occur. Mnemonic helps maintain correct rate and rhythm.
9. Assess pulse and respiratory status after first minute. If no response, resume CPR.	Assess for possible return of pulse and breathing.
10. When second rescuer approaches, states that he or she knows CPR and will assist.	Communicates to first rescuer that knowledgeable help is available and he or she must plan to change rate to 60 BPM.
11. Second rescuer kneels at side of victim opposite nurse.	Facilitates changing positions.
12. Second rescuer palpates carotid pulse during cardiac compression and informs rescuer if pulse is present. If pulse is present, second rescuer says, "Stop compressions," and again palpates pulse and checks for breathing.	Evaluates effectiveness of cardiac compression. If no pulse is palpated during cardiac compression, technique must be reevaluated and corrected.
13. If no pulse is palpated, second rescuer calls "No pulse—continue CPR" and delivers one ventilation.	Provides oxygenated air so cardiac compression will be effective when resumed.
14. First rescuer resumes cardiac compression at a rate of 60 BPM and a 5:1 compression–ventilation ratio. Second rescuer delivers ventilation. (Mnemonic is one-1000, two-1000, three-1000, four-1000, five-1000.)	Rate of 60 effectively supports victim hemodynamically and provides sufficient time for second rescuer to ventilate victim without interrupting cardiac compression. Mnemonic helps maintain correct rate and rhythm.
15. When first rescuer is fatigued and desires to change positions he or she uses "Change-1000, 2-1000, 3-1000 . . ." instead of the usual mnemonic.	Communicates to second rescuer to prepare to change positions.
16. On the fifth compression, second rescuer delivers one breath and moves into position for compression.	Oxygenates victim prior to stopping CPR to check pulse.
17. After giving the fifth compression, first rescuer moves to victim's head and palpates carotid pulse and checks for breathing.	Position change provides logical time to reassess victim.
18. If no pulse is felt, first rescuer calls, "Continue CPR" and delivers one breath.	Provides oxygenated air so cardiac compression will be effective when resumed.
19. Resume CPR at same rate of 60 BPM and a 5:1 compression–ventilation ratio.	Rate of 60 effectively supports victim hemodynamically and provides sufficient time for second rescuer to ventilate victim without interrupting cardiac compression.

CPR TECHNIQUES—INFANT AND CHILD

As with the adult, the infant or child is placed in a supine position for assessment and performance of CPR. Some experts suggest that an alternative position for a small infant is to hold it on the nondominant arm. With this method, the infant's head is supported in the antecubital fossa and the legs and torso are supported by the forearm and hand, leaving the other arm free for cardiac compression. Artificial ventilation can also be given in this position but some rescuers find this position rather awkward and have difficulty assessing and maintaining the airway. As the infant or child is being positioned, assess the level of consciousness by gently attempting to rouse him or her.

Establishing an Open Airway

As with adults, open the airway and assess respiratory status. Several authors emphasize initial checking for and clearing secretions. In many instances of pediatric resuscitation, opening the airway may be all that is needed. It is important to remember that because the neck of an infant or small child is pliable, the exaggerated head tilt that may be used with adults flattens the trachea and may actually obstruct an infant's breathing. While neck flexion and head extension are necessary, they are less exaggerated. In children over 4 years of age, the degree of flexion permitted increases as the child grows. The American Heart Association recommends the head tilt-chin lift or the head tilt-neck lift. With the head tilt-chin lift, the tips of the fingers of one hand lift the bony portion of the chin while the other hand slightly presses downward on the forehead, as shown in Figure 75–5A. The head tilt-neck lift is accomplished by lifting the neck slightly with one hand or with the number of fingers that fit easily under the neck and slightly pressing downward on the forehead with the other hand as shown in Figure 75–5B. The mouth should not be completely closed.

It bears repeating that most pediatric arrests are respiratory. Head positioning may be all that is needed, so technique should be critically evaluated on an ongoing basis. Because most arrests are respiratory, strict attention must be given to the airway. Many pediatric experts believe that the airway should be cleared of secretions before beginning CPR (Procter, 1979; Orlowski, 1980; Warren et al., 1977). The current AHA Standards indicate that the rescuer should assess patency of the airway only if the rescuer is unable to deliver the initial breaths. The airway is then cleared of secretions (or any other obstruction) at that point. Continuous evaluation of the airway must be made while performing CPR.

Ventilation

If the absence of breathing is established, deliver four gentle, rapid ventilations. To ventilate the infant or small child, cover both the mouth and the nose. For the larger child, cover only the mouth, pinching the nostrils closed as with the adult. The pediatric victim's air passages are smaller, creating more resistance to air flow, but smaller volumes of air are required. For the infant or small child, puffs from the mouth rather than deep breaths from the lungs should be adequate. Evaluate the adequacy of ventilations by observing the rise and fall of the chest. It is important to avoid excessive volumes of air to decrease the risk of gastric distention, which is more likely to occur in the child than the adult victim. If gastric distention should occur, it should only be corrected if ventilation becomes ineffective. Then the infant or child is turned to its side and pressure is applied to the abdomen.

After delivering the initial ventilations, assess circulation by checking the brachial pulse and seek help as was described for the adult victim. If a pulse is present, ventilate the infant once every 3 seconds (20 times a minute) and a child once every 4 seconds (15 times a minute). These rates approximate normal respiratory rates for healthy infants and children.

If a pulse is not present, begin cardiac compression immediately.

Cardiac Compression

According to most authorities, the heart lies higher in an infant's chest than it does in an adult's. For this reason, cardiac compression should be performed at

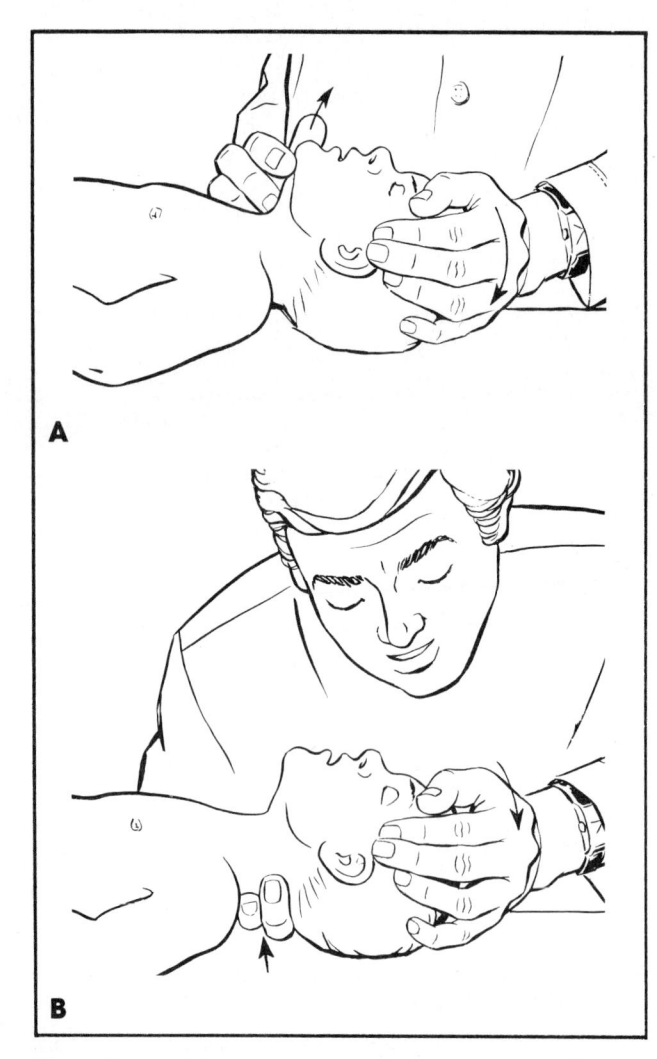

*Figure 75–5. Establishing the infant airway: **A.** Head tilt-chin lift; **B.** Head tilt-neck lift.*

midsternum rather than over the lower half. This avoids injury to the liver or spleen, which lie directly under the lower portion of the sternum. The midsternum can easily be located by visualizing an imaginary horizontal line between the nipples. The sternum is then compressed 1.25 to 2.5 cm (0.5 to 1 in). Two methods can be used for infant cardiac compression. With the first method, the index and middle fingers of the free hand compress the midsternum, as shown in Figure 75-6A. This method is used when there is only one rescuer. The alternative method involves placing the infant on a flat surface, encircling the chest of the infant with both hands, and compressing the midsternum with both thumbs, as shown in Figure 75-6B. There is evidence indicating that better pressures and pulses are obtained with this method (Todres and Rogers, 1975). It is best reserved for when there are two rescuers because it is difficult for a single rescuer to ventilate the infant from this position.

More compression force is required in children than infants; therefore, use the heel of one hand on a child instead of fingers and thumbs, as on an infant, and the sternum should be compressed 2.5 to 3.8 cm (1 to 1½ in). The heart moves down in the thoracic cavity as a child grows; therefore, cardiac compression should be performed on children at the junction of the middle and lower thirds of the sternum, which is slightly higher than for adults and lower than for infants. This point can be determined by mentally dividing the chest into thirds between the suprasternal notch and the xyphoid process.

As with adults, compression duration should be at least 50 percent of the cycle time to maintain sufficient cardiac output. One rescuer may be preferable to two because with these small victims, it is less awkward and the rescuer can easily ventilate and perform cardiac compression without having to change position.

Compression to Ventilation Ratios

For an infant, deliver cardiac compressions at a rate of 100 per minute, interspersed with ventilations at a 5:1 compression to ventilation ratio. For a child, deliver cardiac compressions at a rate of 80 per minute, interspersed with ventilations at a 5:1 compression to ventilation ratio. These rates approximate the higher heart rates of infants and children. Adult ratios can be used as the child approaches adult size. With one rescuer, pause after the fifth compression to give one ventilation. When two rescuers are present give one ventilation on the upstroke of the fifth compression.

To maintain the appropriate compression rates, use an audible mnemonic. For a rate of 100, use "one-two-three-four-five". For a rate of 80, use "1-and 2-and 3-and 4- and 5- and . . ." .

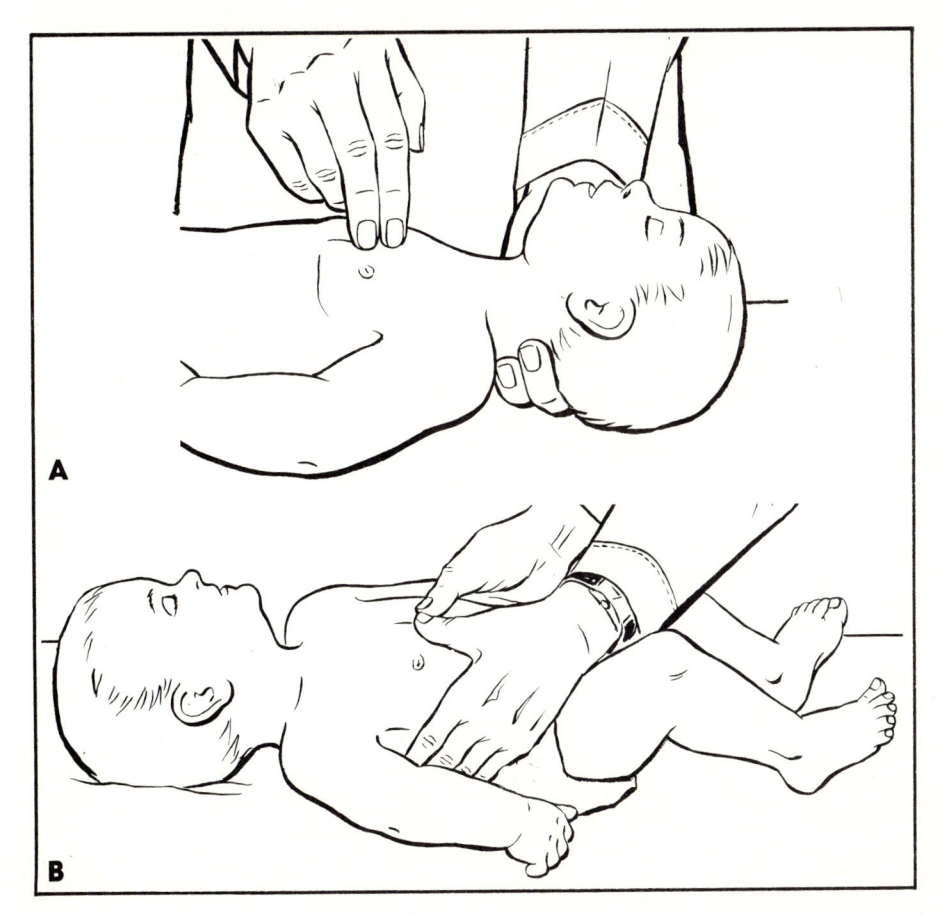

Figure 75-6. Infant cardiac compression, using **A.** index and middle fingers, and **B.** thumbs, with hands encircling the chest.

SKILL SEQUENCE

CPR—INFANT AND CHILD

Step	Rationale
1. Gently attempt to rouse infant or child. Place in supine position (4 to 10 seconds).	Need to assess level of consciousness. Victim can be positioned simultaneously.
2. If no response, call for help. Open airway, avoiding hyperextension of neck. Place ear over mouth to listen for breath sounds and look for chest to rise. Clear secretions if necessary (3 to 5 seconds).	Opening airway, especially in children, may be all that is necessary. Secretions are often present.
3. Deliver 4 gentle, rapid ventilations allowing no time for deflation between breaths. Limit volume to amount needed for chest to rise (3 to 5 seconds).	Oxygenates blood. Increases end expiratory pressure and opens small air sacs. Volume of air required is less than that for adults. Excessive volume can lead to gastric distention.
4. Check for presence of brachial pulse in infant; use carotid artery in older child.	Need to assess circulatory status.
5. Activate emergency medical system if no spontaneous respirations or pulse.	Establish arrested state to confirm need for EMS. Have relevant information to give to appropriate person.
6. If pulse is present, ventilate infant once every 3 seconds (20 times per minute); ventilate child once every 4 seconds (15 times per minute). Reassess pulse every minute.	Breathing rates of infants and children are more rapid than adults. Respiratory arrest is likely to deteriorate to cardiac arrest.
7. If pulse is not present, begin external cardiac compression. Infants: rate of 100 BPM with a compression depth of 1.25 to 2.5 cm (½ to 1 in) and a 5:1 compression to ventilation ratio. (Mnemonic is 1-2-3-4-5 with one ventilation interspersed, without a pause.) Children: rate of 80 BPM with a compression depth of 2.5 to 3.8 cm (1 to 1½ in) and a 5:1 ratio. (Mnemonic is 1-and-2-and-3-and-4-and-5-and . . . .)	Heart rates for infants and children are faster than those of adults.

RECORDING

The time and description of all events are documented for both the cardiopulmonary arrest and the CPR activities. These include: the time the arrest occurred or was discovered; the location; the activities of the client at the time of the arrest; who initiated CPR and the time; any complications that occurred during CPR, such as vomiting; the time the code was called and the time the CPR team responded; the length of time it took for the client to respond; and the time CPR was discontinued either because of rescuer fatigue or lack of client response.

Sample POR Recording

- S—None
- O—Found on floor, unresponsive to stimuli, apneic, & c̄ no palpable carotid pulse. Skin warm but dusky. Responded within 1 minute after CPR initiated by staff nurse. Responded to verbal stimuli, respirations 24/min. & shallow, pulse 114 irregular & thready, BP 96/52, skin pale & warm. Code team responded within 2 minutes after call.
- A—Successful resuscitation from apparent cardiac arrest; condition relatively stable.
- P—Continue careful observations & monitoring vital signs. Notify attending physician.

Sample Narrative Recording

Found on floor, unresponsive to stimuli, apneic, and with no palpable carotid pulse. Skin warm but dusky. CPR initiated by staff nurse. Code 99 called and responded within 2 minutes. Responded within 1 minute to CPR—responding to verbal stimuli, respirations 24/min. & shallow, pulse 114 irregular & thready, BP 96/52, skin pale but warm.

CRITICAL POINTS SUMMARY

1. Assess level of consciousness, absence of breathing, and absence of pulse before initiating CPR.
2. Create an open airway with the appropriate maneuver.
3. Evaluate patency of the airway carefully.
4. Seal the mouth, nose, or stoma tightly when ventilating.
5. Use correct hand placement and body position for the age and size of the victim.
6. Use a compression-to-ventilation ratio of:
   15:2 with one-person rescue for adults
   5:1 with two-person rescue for adults
   5:1 with one- or two-person rescue for children and infants
7. Adjust compression depth according to the age and size of the victim:
   Adults: 3.8 to 5.1 cm (1½ to 2 in)
   Children: 2.5 to 3.8 cm (1 to 1½ in)
   Infants: 1.25 to 2.5 cm (½ to 1 in)
8. Compression rates must be adapted to the age and size of the victim:

Adults: 80 per minute for one rescuer
60 per minute for two-person rescue
Children: 80 per minute for one- and two-person rescue
Infants: 100 per minute
9. Say the correct mnemonic aloud.
10. Do not remove hands from the sternum between compressions.
11. Keep the fingers off the chest at all times during compression.
12. Avoid compression over the xyphoid process.
13. Do not attempt to relieve gastric distention unless unable to ventilate.

☐ LEARNING ACTIVITIES

1. Enroll in an AHA or ARC sponsored Basic Life Support course.
2. Practice locating and palpating the carotid pulse on an adult and the brachial pulse on an infant.
3. Practice identifying chest compression landmarks and the three head tilt maneuvers on an adult and a child.
4. Practice adult and infant CPR on specially designed mannikins such as Resusci-Anni, or Recorder-Anni.
5. Find out how to contact the emergency medical system within your community; within your hospital setting.

☐ REVIEW QUESTIONS

1. What are the causes of cardiac arrest?
2. What are the causes of pulmonary arrest?
3. How would you determine if a person has had a cardiopulmonary arrest?
4. How do you locate the carotid pulse? The brachial pulse?
5. What are the three methods of opening the airway in the adult victim? The infant victim?
6. Why is careful evaluation of the infant airway particularly important?
7. What can you do to minimize the risk of gastric distention?
8. When and how should gastric distention be relieved?
9. What are the two mechanisms believed to be operable in generating artificial circulation?
10. What is the correct hand position for chest compression on the adult? Infant? Child?
11. What are two ways to determine correct hand position for an adult victim?
12. What is the correct position for the rescuer to assume while executing chest compressions on an adult victim?
13. What is the correct rate and rhythm of cardiac compression for the adult? Infant? Child? One rescuer? Two rescuers?
14. What are some of the common errors that occur in the performance of CPR? What are their consequences?
15. Give two reasons mnemonics should be said aloud.

☐ PERFORMANCE CHECKLISTS

OBJECTIVE: To demonstrate one-rescuer and two-rescuer CPR correctly.			
CHARACTERISTIC	RANGE OF ACCEPTABILITY	SATISFACTORY	UNSATISFACTORY
1. Attempts to rouse victim and positions appropriately.	No deviation		
2. Calls for help.	No deviation		
3. Opens airway. Assesses respiratory status. Checks for presence of stoma.	No deviation		
4. Delivers 4 rapid ventilations and observes chest rise.	No deviation		
5. Assesses central pulse.	No deviation		
6. Activates emergency medical system.	No deviation		
7. If pulse present, ventilates victim once every 5 seconds. Reassesses pulse every minute.	May omit and proceed to 8.		
8. If pulse not present, begins cardiac compression at rate of 80 and 15:2 ratio. Says mnemonic audibly.	No deviation		
9. Assesses pulse after first minute, then every 5 minutes.	Assess pulse after first minute.		

(continued)

OBJECTIVE: To demonstrate one-rescuer and two-rescuer CPR correctly (cont.).

CHARACTERISTIC	RANGE OF ACCEPTABILITY	SATISFACTORY	UNSATISFACTORY
10. Resumes CPR.	No deviation		
11. Second rescuer states he or she knows CPR and will assist.	No deviation		
12. Second rescuer kneels at victim's side opposite first rescuer.	No deviation		
13. Second rescuer palpates carotid pulse during cardiac compression. If pulse is present, second rescuer tells first rescuer to stop CPR and again palpates pulse and checks for breathing.	No deviation		
14. If no pulse is present, second rescuer calls, "Continue CPR" and delivers one breath.	No deviation		
15. Both rescuers begin CPR at rate of 60 and 5:1 ratio. Says mnemonic audibly.	No deviation		
16. First rescuer communicates desire to change positions.	No deviation		
17. After fifth compression, second rescuer delivers breath and moves into position for compression.	No deviation		
18. After fifth compression, first rescuer moves to victim's head and palpates carotid pulse.	No deviation		
19. If no pulse is felt, first rescuer calls, "Continue CPR" and delivers one breath.	No deviation		
20. Resumes CPR at rate of 60 and a 5:1 ratio. Says mnemonic audibly.	No deviation		
21. Demonstrates position change.	At least once or until change is demonstrated correctly.		

OBJECTIVE: To demonstrate infant CPR correctly.

CHARACTERISTIC	RANGE OF ACCEPTABILITY	SATISFACTORY	UNSATISFACTORY
1. Attempts to rouse victim and positions appropriately.	No deviation		
2. Calls for help.	No deviation		
3. Opens airway. Assesses respiratory status by listening and looking at chest. Clears secretions if necessary.	No deviation		
4. Delivers 4 gentle rapid ventilations. Observes chest rise.	No deviation		
5. Assesses brachial pulse in infant; uses carotid artery in older child.	No deviation		
6. Activates emergency medical system.	No deviation		
7. If pulse present, ventilates infant once every 3 seconds, child every 4 seconds.	May omit and proceed to characteristic 8.		
8. If pulse is not present, begins cardiac compression at a rate of 100 for infants, 80 for children with 5:1 circulation to ventilation ratio. Says mnemonic audibly.	Correct demonstration of infant CPR.		

REFERENCES

American Heart Association: Standards for cardiopulmonary resuscitation (CPR) and emergency cardiac care (ECC). Journal of the American Medical Association 227(7)(suppl): 834–868, 1974.

American Heart Association: Standards for cardiopulmonary resuscitation (CPR) and emergency cardiac care (ECC). Journal of the American Medical Association 244(5):453–509, 1980.

American Heart Association: Instructors Manual for Basic Life Support. Dallas, American Heart Association, 1985.

Babbs CF: New versus old theories of blood flow during CPR. Critical Care Medicine 8(3):191–195, 1980.

Cavallaro DL, Melker RJ: Comparison of two techniques for detecting cardiac activity in infants. Critical Care Medicine 11(3):189–190, 1983.

Chameides L, Director of Pediatric Cardiology, Clinical Professor, Department of Pediatrics, University of Connecticut. Letter, July 8, 1982.

Chandra N, Rudikoff M, et al.: Simultaneous chest compression and ventilation at high airway pressure during cardiopulmonary resuscitation. Lancet 1(8161):175–178, 1980.

Cushing M: Verbal no-code orders. American Journal of Nursing 81(6):1215–1216, 1981.

Donegan JH: Basic life support for the adult victim: Physiologic principles and practical application. In Donegan JH (ed): Cardiopulmonary Resuscitation: Physiology, Pharmacology, and Practical Application. Springfield, IL, Charles C Thomas, 1982, chap 3, pp 25–66.

Ellis PD, Billings DM: Cardiopulmonary Resuscitation: Procedures for Basic and Advanced Life Support. St Louis, CV Mosby, 1980.

Enarson DA, Gracey DR: Complications of cardiopulmonary resuscitation. Heart and Lung 5(5):805–807, 1976.

George OG: Anatomy and physiology of CPR. AORN 27(5):992–998, 1978.

Guildner CW: Resuscitation—Opening the airway: A comparative study of technique. Journal of the American College of Emergency Physicians 5(8):588–590, 1976.

McCarthy D: The use and abuse of cardiopulmonary resuscitation. Hospital Progress 56(4):64–68, 1975.

McIntyre KM, Parisi CF, et al.: Pathophysiologic syndromes of cardiopulmonary resuscitation. Archives of Internal Medicine 138(7):1130–1133, 1978.

Melker R: CPR in neonates, infants, and children. Critical Care Quarterly 1(1):49–65, 1978.

Orlowski JP: Cardiopulmonary resuscitation in children. Pediatric Clinics of North America 27(3):495–512, 1980.

Proctor A: Pediatric arrest: Scaling down CPR. RN 42(9):58–64, 1979.

Rudikoff M, Tucker M, et al.: Importance of compression rate during external cardiac massage in man. Circulation 54(4)(suppl 2):225, 1976.

Safar P: On the evolution of brain resuscitation. Critical Care Medicine 6(4):199–202, 1978.

Singer J: Cardiac arrests in children. Journal of the American College of Emergency Physicians 6(5):198–205, 1977.

Todres ID, Rogers MC: Methods of external cardiac massage in the newborn infant. Journal of Pediatrics 86(5):781–782, 1975.

Warren RH, Solis LL, et al.: Pediatric review guidelines for cardiopulmonary resuscitation in children. Journal of the Arkansas Medical Society 77(6):231–234, 1980.

BIBLIOGRAPHY

Criley JM, Blaufuss AH, et al.: Cough-induced cardiac compression: Self-administered form of cardiopulmonary resuscitation. Journal of the American Medical Association 236(11):1246–1250, 1976.

Criley JM, Niemann JT, et al.: The heart is a conduit in CPR. Critical Care Medicine 9(5):373–374, 1981.

Guyton AC: Textbook of Medical Physiology, ed 6. Philadelphia, WB Saunders, 1981.

Hart R: A review of CPR for adults. Nursing79 9(2):54–59, 1979.

Kouwenhoven WB, Jude JR, et al.: Closed cardiac massage. Journal of the American Medical Association 173(10):1064–1067, 1960.

Redding JS: Cardiopulmonary resuscitation: An algorithm and some common pitfalls. American Heart Journal 98(6):788–797, 1979a.

AUDIOVISUAL RESOURCES

Cardiopulmonary Resuscitation
  Videorecording (½ and ¾ in). (1982, Color, 20 min.)
Introduction to CPR
  Videorecording (½ and ¾ in). (1982, Color, 12 min.)
  Available through:
    Indiana University School of Nursing
    NICER
    610 Barnhill Drive
    Indianapolis, IN 46223
Cardiopulmonary Resuscitation
  Filmstrip and cassette. (1979, Color, 10 min.)
Cardiopulmonary Resuscitation: Techniques for One Rescuer
  Filmstrip and cassette. (1979, Color, 24 min.)
Cardiopulmonary Resuscitation: Techniques for Two Rescuers
  Filmstrip and cassette. (1979, Color, 18 min.)
Cardiopulmonary Resuscitation: Techniques for Infants and Children
  Filmstrip and cassette. (1979, Color, 17 min.)
  Available through:
    Medcom, Inc.
    P.O. Box 116
    Garden Grove, CA 92642
New Pulse of Life
  Film (16 mm). (1977, Color, 30 min.)
  Available through:
    American Heart Association
    Film Library
    7320 Greenville Avenue
    Dallas, TX 75231
One-Rescuer CPR
  Videocassette (¾ in). (1980, Color, 14 min.)
Two-Rescuer CPR
  Videorecording (¾ in). (1980, Color, 9 min.)
  Available through:
    Health Science Consortium
    200 Eastowne Drive, Suite 213
    Chapel Hill, NC 27514

SKILL 76 Removal of Airway Obstruction

PREREQUISITE SKILLS

Skill 19, "Inspection"
Skill 22, "Auscultation"
Skill 24, "Pulse Appraisal"
Skill 25, "Respiration Appraisal"
Skill 75, "Cardiopulmonary Resuscitation"

☐ STUDENT OBJECTIVES

1. Differentiate between adequate and inadequate air exchange.
2. Differentiate between an airway obstruction caused by a foreign object and an airway obstruction caused by a preexisting disease state.
3. Identify two advantages of chest thrusts over abdominal thrusts.
4. Describe the physiological effects of manual thrusts and back blows.
5. Identify the hazard of performing finger probes.
6. Correctly demonstrate the techniques used to remove a foreign object from a conscious adult.
7. Correctly demonstrate the techniques used to remove a foreign object from an unconscious adult.
8. Correctly demonstrate the techniques used to remove a foreign object from an infant.

☐ INTRODUCTION

Adequate ventilation is impossible without a patent airway. If something other than the tongue obstructs the airway, head positioning by itself will not clear the airway. The additional measures needed before ventilation is possible are a combination of manual thrusts and back blows, which are intended to expel the foreign object from the airway, and finger probes of the mouth, which allow the rescuer to remove the offending object when it becomes accessible in the back of the throat.

R. K. Haugen, a Florida Medical Examiner, is credited with bringing the deaths resulting from food obstruction to the attention of the medical community in 1963. He coined the term "cafe coronary" to distinguish these deaths from those resulting from coronary occlusions (Haugen, 1963).

In 1974 the standards established by the American Heart Association (AHA) gave only cursory attention to foreign object removal techniques. Back blows and finger probes were suggested, but if these maneuvers were unsuccessful, an emergency tracheostomy (a surgical opening of the airway through the throat) was recommended. Clearly, a first aid technique which could be performed by the average person was needed.

Dr. Henry J. Heimlich seemed to answer this need when he first reported his now famous Heimlich Maneuver in 1974. He noted that aspiration (sucking of foreign matter into the lungs) occurs during inspiration while the lungs are expanded. The application of sudden manual abdominal pressure explosively forces air out through the trachea, thereby expelling the foreign object (Heimlich, 1974).

This lifesaving abdominal thrust maneuver was quickly picked up by the news media and widely reported. While Heimlich's technique was recognized by his colleagues as having merit worthy of investigation, there was great concern that the excitement generated by the news media was premature (Redding, 1979). Many scientists believed that back blows were often successful and that neither technique had been adequately researched.

It is now generally accepted that back blows work in some situations and that manual (abdominal or chest) thrusts also work in some situations, but neither is successful all the time. There is also evidence that these maneuvers when used together may be more successful than either used alone (Guildner et al., 1976; Ruben and McNaughton, 1978; Redding, 1979). Therefore, the American Heart Association (AHA) recommends a combination of the two; that is, a series of four back blows alternated with four manual abdominal or chest thrusts, either of which may be executed first. Foreign object removal techniques were developed and integrated into the American Heart Association 1980 Standards and Guidelines for Cardiopulmonary Resuscitation (CPR) and Emergency Cardiac Care (ECC), hereafter referred to as the Standards. This same procedure is taught by the American Red Cross (ARC) and is referred to as the choking technique. The Heimlich maneuver consists only of abdominal thrusts. Posters illustrating these two approaches to relief of airway obstruction may be seen in restaurant dining rooms, kitchens, and restrooms.

☐ PREPARATION

The effect of manual thrusts has been likened to popping a cork on a champagne bottle. Delivering a sharp inward and upward subdiaphragmatic (abdominal) thrust or a sharp, inward, midsternal (chest) thrust compresses the expanded lungs. This sudden increase in intrathoracic pressure increases tracheobronchial pressure, increases the expiratory air flow suddenly, and ejects the bolus. In effect, a powerful artificial cough is created.

Back blows also increase airway pressure and air flow and may also loosen the foreign body. Back blows consist of sharp blows delivered with the heel of the hand over the spine between the shoulders. Both back blows and manual thrusts are delivered in a series of four uniform, forceful blows. To be effective, they must be delivered sharply; that is, each blow in the series should be delivered with the intent of being effective by itself. If possible, the victim's head should be lower than the chest to enlist the aid of gravity.

With unconscious adults, a finger probe or sweep of the back of the throat is performed after the series of back blows and manual thrusts is completed. This maneuver is used in an effort to grasp and remove the foreign object with the finger. If the object has been partially expelled from the lungs, it may be accessible. However, care must be exercised to avoid pushing the object deeper into the airway. With children, a blind finger probe should not be done because the risk of impacting it in the small airway is too great. If the object is visible, it may be removed with a finger.

It is important to consider that airway obstruction can be caused by edema as well as by foreign objects. This possibility is particularly likely in children and it is important to determine if this is the cause before assuming a foreign object is causing the obstruction. This will prevent time being wasted on foreign object removal techniques if other causes, as described below, are responsible.

COMPLICATIONS RESULTING FROM FOREIGN OBJECT REMOVAL TECHNIQUES

When performed properly, manual thrusts are usually safe. However, serious life-threatening consequences can result, so it is a procedure that poses some risks for the client. The two major possible complications of manual thrusts include fractured ribs from chest thrusts and regurgitation from abdominal thrusts. Regurgitation could result in aspiration of more foreign material in the lungs. There have also been reports of abdominal tenderness, ruptured stomach, liver and spleen damage, esophageal laceration, pharyngeal abrasion, and retinal detachment (Redding, 1979; Visintine and Baick, 1975).

DATA BASE

Client History and Recorded Data
If airway obstruction is suspected, it is important to determine whether the obstruction is caused by a foreign object or a preexisting disease state. There are many disease processes which may result in airway obstructions, such as infections, anaphylactic shock, laryngospasm, or tumors. If there is evidence that obstruction is caused by aspiration of a foreign object, foreign object removal techniques should be initiated immediately. If, for example, a restaurant patron who has been laughing, talking with a full mouth, and ingesting alcoholic beverages suddenly becomes unable to breathe, it is quite likely the patron has aspirated a bolus of food. Contributing factors for these cafe coronaries are rapid eating, large bites of food, inadequate chewing, ingestion of alcohol, increasing age, and wearing an upper denture plate. Children and adults who are mentally retarded tend to eat rapidly and chew inadequately, making them prime candidates for mealtime obstruction. Small children tend to place many objects in their mouths, including small pieces from toys and household items that are easily aspirated.

If a person is known to have an illness that has the potential for causing airway obstruction such as croup, and if there is no evidence of aspiration of a foreign object, the nurse must not waste time attempting foreign object removal techniques. Instead, efforts should be made to transport the victim to a hospital, call local emergency services, or otherwise obtain advanced life support. For instance, a child who has been ill with croup and becomes obstructed should be transported immediately to the nearest advanced life support facility.

Physical Appraisal Skills
When assessing the person who is suspected of having an airway obstruction, the nurse must differentiate between adequate and inadequate air exchange. If air exchange is adequate, the victim should be allowed to attempt to expel the foreign object without interference. If, however, air exchange is inadequate or nonexistent, the nurse needs to begin foreign object removal techniques. It must always be remembered that adequate air exchange can deteriorate to inadequate air exchange so it is important to keep a watchful eye on the victim's respiratory status and not leave him or her unattended. There have been reports of choking victims going to the restroom apparently to avoid embarrassment and then later being found dead from asphyxiation. Both inspection and auscultation are used to assess airway obstruction.

Inspection. *Inspection* is used to note the victim's effort to communicate that he or she is choking and to observe the ability to move air in and out of the lungs. The widely publicized, universal distress sign for choking is the hand clutching the throat. The instinctive use of this distress signal may be the first indication that a person is choking.

If air exchange is adequate, note whether the chest is expanding with inhalation efforts. If air exchange is inadequate, there will be exaggerated respiratory efforts, but no air movement. Nasal flaring, a dusky red color, and cyanosis may also be observed as the duration of the obstruction continues unrelieved.

Auscultation. *Auscultation* is used to determine whether the victim can speak or if an infant can cry and to evaluate the quality of breath sounds.

If a victim is communicating distress by using the universal sign for choking or for other reasons seems to be choking, ask the adult victim to speak. If able to speak, the victim is able to move air through the larynx and air exchange is adequate. If unable to speak, air exchange is inadequate and immediate assistance is required. If a baby or small child appears to be choking, attempt to make him or her cry. If the victim is able to cry, air is being adequately exchanged. If the victim is unable to cry, immediate assistance is needed.

If air exchange is adequate, the victim will be able to cough forcefully. The victim may be wheezing between coughs, but the cough will be effective. Poor air exchange can be identified by an ineffective cough and high-pitched crowing noises on inspiration.

☐ EXECUTION

FOREIGN OBJECT REMOVAL—CONSCIOUS ADULT

Back Blows
When the air exchange is inadequate, deliver four back blows alternated with four chest or abdominal thrusts. For delivering back blows to a standing or seated victim, stand beside and slightly behind the victim as shown in Figure 76–1. Direct one foot forward and place the other well behind the victim. This position gives a wide base of support and enables you to support the victim. If the victim loses consciousness, he or she can be allowed to slide down the rescuer's leg to the floor without injury.

If the victim is not too large physically, place him or her in a position leaning over your arm with the head downward to take advantage of gravity as the blows are delivered. One team of investigators (Ruben and MacNaughton, 1978) reported that the greater the size of the obstruction, the greater the effect of shaking and gravity.

Manual Thrusts
If back blows do not dislodge the obstruction, four manual thrusts are delivered, either to the chest or abdomen. Chest thrusts are more effective than abdominal thrusts for obese people and pregnant women. Using abdominal thrusts instead of chest thrusts for an older victim may avoid fracture of brittle ribs. There are not substantial differences in airway flow pressure and volume between chest and abdominal thrusts, although there is a risk of regurgitation with abdominal thrusts (American Heart Association, 1980).

To apply a chest thrust to a conscious victim who is sitting or standing, stand behind the victim and wrap both arms around to the front of the chest, as shown in Figure 76–2A. Form a fist with one hand, having the thumb side of the fist placed against the middle of the sternum, avoiding the xyphoid process and rib margins. Grasp the fist with the opposite hand, keep wrists rigid, and give four quick inward thrusts.

To apply an abdominal thrust, stand behind the victim and wrap both arms around the victim's waist. Form a fist and place the thumb side on the upper abdomen in the area between the ribs and the waist, as shown in Figure 76–2B. Again, avoid the xyphoid process and rib margins. Use the opposite hand to grasp the fist and press it four times into the abdomen with quick inward and upward thrusts. It is important that the abdominal thrust be given inward and upward to exert pressure on the diaphragm, thus increasing intrathoracic pressure. Correct hand placement for both chest thrusts and abdominal thrusts is shown in Figure 76–2C.

The sequence of back blows and manual thrusts may be given in either order and is repeated until the victim expels the obstruction. Remember that each back blow or manual thrust must be given with sufficient force as if to dislodge the obstruction by itself.

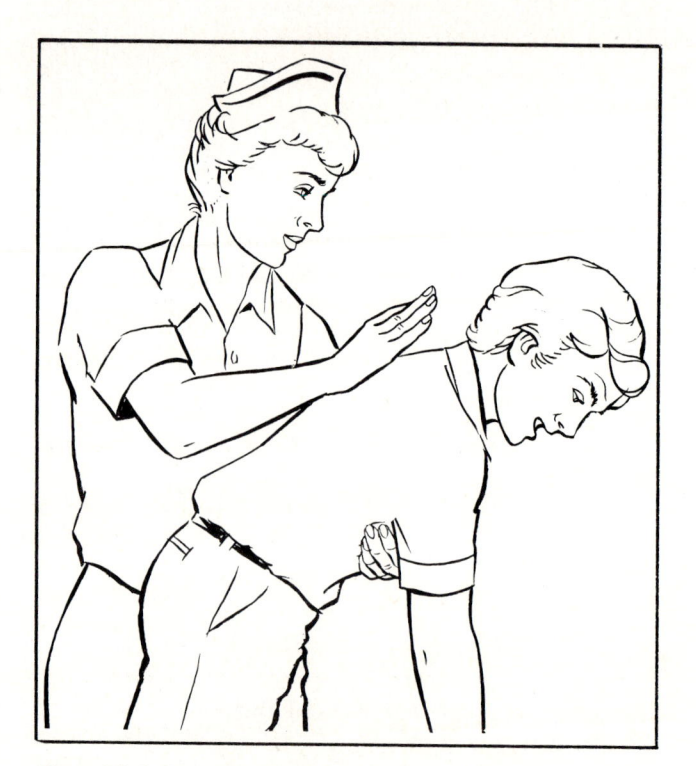

Figure 76–1. Back Blows: conscious adult. Stand beside and slightly behind the victim; deliver four sharp blows with the heel of the hand, over the spine and between the shoulders.

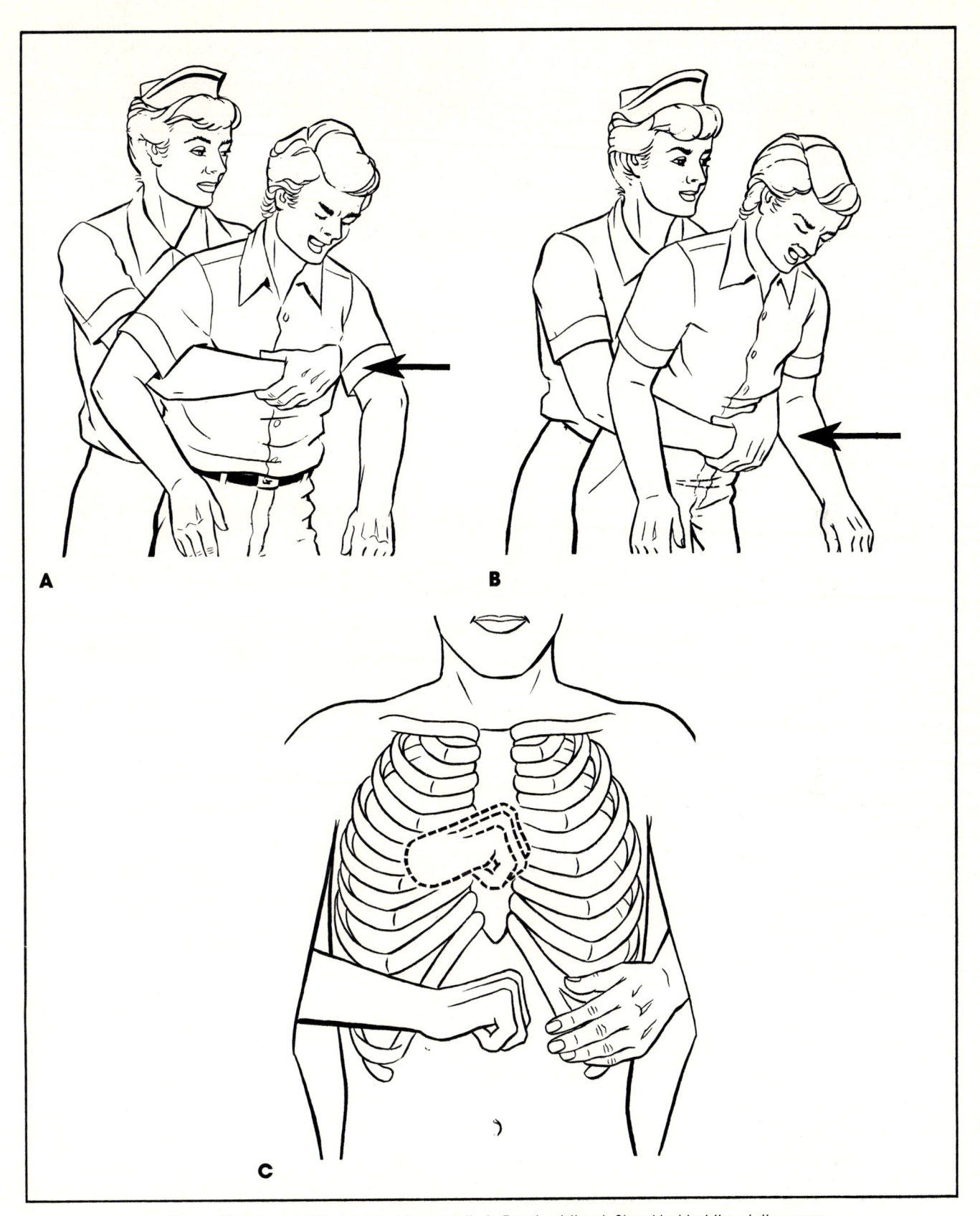

Figure 76–2. Manual Thrust: conscious adult. **A.** For chest thrust: Stand behind the victim, wrap arms around chest and apply sharp inward pressure over the midsternum. **B.** For abdominal thrust: Wrap arms around waist and apply sharp inward and upward pressure over the upper abdomen. **C.** Correct hand placement: One fist is placed with the thumb toward the body, placed in the upper abdomen or over the midsternum and grasped firmly with the other hand.

SKILL SEQUENCE

FOREIGN OBJECT REMOVAL: CONSCIOUS ADULT

Step	Rationale
1. Ask if victim can speak. Evaluate breathing effort (2 to 3 seconds).	If victim is completely obstructed or has inadequate air exchange, he or she will be unable to speak because air cannot pass through the vocal cords. If air exchange is reasonably adequate, victim should be permitted to expel object on his or her own. If air exchange is inadequate treat victim as if a complete airway obstruction exists.
2. Position self beside and slightly behind victim with one arm around chest, supporting victim; place one leg beside other leg behind victim.	
3. With other hand, deliver four back blows (3 to 5 seconds).	Sudden increase in airway pressure may expel obstruction.
4. Deliver four manual (chest or abdominal) thrusts (4 to 5 seconds).	Sudden increase in airway pressure may expel obstruction.
5. Repeat sequence of back blows and manual thrusts until effective or victim collapses.	
6. If victim collapses, allow him or her to slide to the floor and proceed as in Skill Sequence, "Foreign Object Removal: Unconscious Adult," step 5.	Prevents additional injuries from falling.
7. If obstruction is expelled, check for spontaneous respirations.	
8. If obstruction is expelled but there are no spontaneous respirations, initiate CPR, Skill 75.	Implements appropriate actions based on assessment of victim.

FOREIGN OBJECT REMOVAL—UNCONSCIOUS ADULT

If an adult is unconscious, follow the initial steps of CPR; that is, establish unresponsiveness, open the airway, and attempt to deliver the four full rapid ventilations. If ventilation efforts are unsuccessful, reevaluate the ventilation technique and reposition the head. If no chest expansion occurs and ventilation is unsuccessful, assume that an airway obstruction exists. The obstruction must be relieved before any attempt is made to assess and treat circulatory arrest because otherwise there would be no way to oxygenate the blood.

While remaining in the kneeling position for CPR, raise the victim's near arm above the head, and cross the far leg over the near leg. The extended arm supports the victim's head when turned, and the crossed leg uses body weight to help effect the turn. Roll the victim toward you, using your thighs to support the victim. Give four hard back blows with the heel of the hand between the scapulae. Then turn the victim to the back for delivery of the manual thrusts. Two positions are available to the nurse, each offering its own advantage. The nurse can kneel, straddling the victim. With this central position, the thrust is less likely to be misdirected. Or, the nurse may kneel alongside the victim's hips with the shoulders positioned over the victim. This position avoids climbing on and off the victim and provides greater maneuverability. From this position, it is easier to move to the victim's head to do finger probes, remove vomitus, or reattempt ventilation.

To apply the chest thrusts, place the heel of one hand on top of the other on the lower half of the sternum, in essentially the same position as that used for cardiac compression. Give four quick, downward thrusts. To apply the abdominal thrusts, place the heel of one hand on top of the other between the umbilicus and the xyphoid process, with the fingers pointing toward the head, and give four quick, inward and upward thrusts. The victim's head may be turned to the side for abdominal thrusts since regurgitation may occur duing this maneuver. As with the conscious victim, the xyphoid process and rib margins must be avoided when using either of these techniques.

After completing the series of four back blows and four manual thrusts, move to the victim's head to perform a finger probe or sweep. With the victim supine (face up), lift the jaw by grasping the tongue and lower jaw with one hand, as shown in Figure 76–3A. This action pulls the tongue away from the posterior pharynx and may partially relieve the obstruction. Next, insert the index finger of the opposite hand down along the inside of the cheek deeply into the throat to the posterior pharynx. Use a hooking action with the finger to dislodge the object and bring it forward into the mouth.

If the victim's mouth is difficult to open, the crossed finger technique is a useful alternate method. To perform this maneuver, cross the index finger over the thumb and force them into the front of the victim's mouth, as shown in Figure 76–3B.

Twist the finger and thumb open, thereby opening the mouth. Perform the finger probe with the other hand. If the victim's teeth are tightly clenched,

SKILL 76: REMOVAL OF AIRWAY OBSTRUCTION

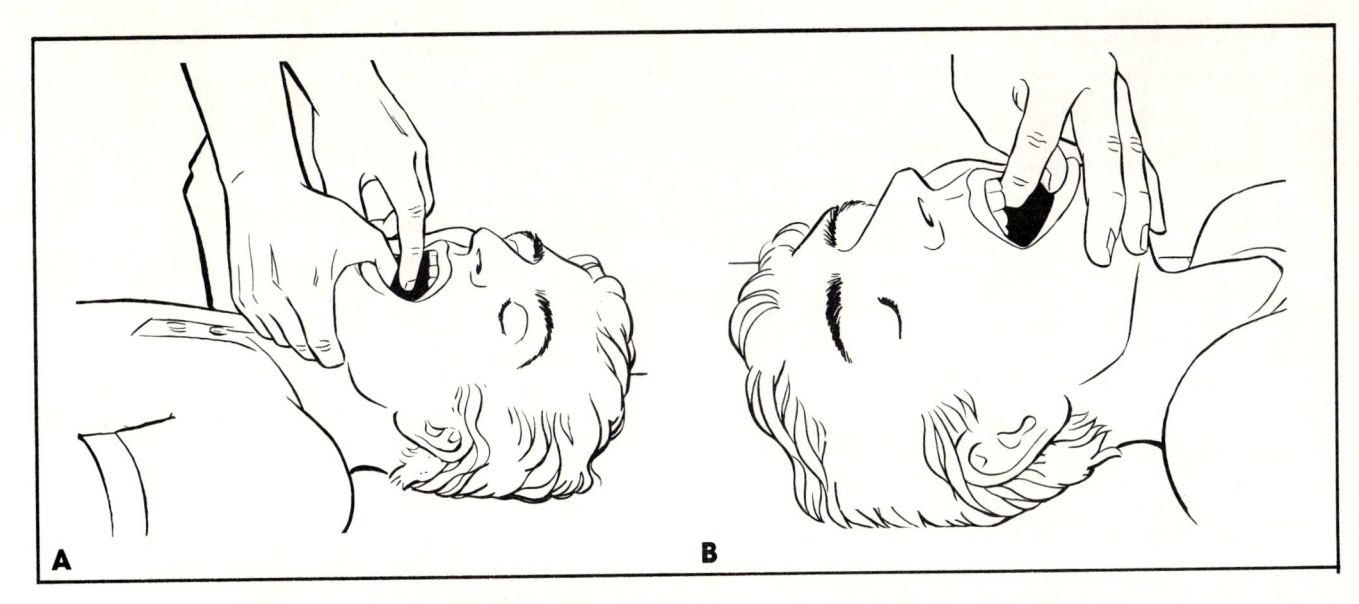

Figure 76-3. Removal of foreign object: unconscious adult. **A.** Open the mouth by lifting the jaw and use the index finger of the other hand to attempt to remove foreign object from the back of the throat. **B.** The crossed finger technique to open the mouth. Use the index finger of the other hand to attempt removal of the foreign object.

you may need to wedge the index finger behind the last molars and twist to open the mouth by rotating the wrist (Ellis and Billings, 1980).

Extreme care must be taken to avoid pushing the foreign object further into the trachea, especially if it cannot be seen, since it can become impacted below the epiglottis. It may be helpful to try to push the object to the opposite side of the throat before attempting to raise it up into the mouth to remove it.

When the foreign object is removed, reevaluate the victim's respiratory status and proceed with CPR if it is indicated. If the victim remains obstructed, make an attempt to ventilate him or her. The tongue-jaw lift maneuver may provide a sufficient airway for some air exchange to occur and as the victim becomes more anoxic the muscles in the throat may relax. If this occurs, slow and deep ventilations along with cardiac compressions may provide adequate oxygen, bypassing the obstruction (Guildner, 1976).

If it is not possible to ventilate the victim because of persistent obstruction, the sequence of back blows, manual thrusts, and attempted ventilations is repeated as often as necessary.

☐ SKILL SEQUENCE

FOREIGN OBJECT REMOVAL: UNCONSCIOUS ADULT

Step	Rationale
1. Same as steps 1 to 4 for Skill Sequence, "CPR—One and Two Rescuer," p. 981.	Time should not be wasted looking for a foreign object unless there is reason to believe one is there.
2. Repeat attempt to ventilate by repositioning head using alternative method to open airway.	Technique should be reevaluated. Inability to expand lungs at this point confirms airway obstruction.
3. In kneeling position, roll victim toward you, using your thighs for support. Position victim's near arm above head before turning. Deliver four hard quick back blows (4 to 6 seconds).	Rapid increase in airway pressure may dislodge the foreign object. Raised arm provides support for head.
4. Roll victim on the back. Deliver four manual thrusts (5 to 6 seconds).	Rapid increase in airway pressure may dislodge the foreign object.
5. Perform finger probe inside mouth (6 to 8 seconds).	Foreign object may be accessible in back of mouth.

(continued)

FOREIGN OBJECT REMOVAL: UNCONSCIOUS ADULT (Cont.)	
Step	Rationale
6. Reattempt to ventilate victim if spontaneous breathing does not begin (3 to 5 seconds).	As muscles relax or if foreign object becomes partially dislodged, it may be possible to ventilate victim, bypassing the obstruction.
7. If unable to ventilate repeat steps 5 to 8 until obstruction is removed.	No effort should be made to assess circulatory status or proceed with cardiac compression until oxygen can be provided.
8. After obstruction removed, continue CPR if there are no spontaneous respirations, as in Skill Sequence "CPR—One and Two Rescuer," steps 5 to 19, p. 981.	

FOREIGN OBJECT REMOVAL—INFANT

If an infant is unconscious, follow the initial steps of CPR; that is, establish unresponsiveness, open the airway, and deliver four rapid breaths. Since an infant's neck muscles are pliable, the airway patency must be evaluated critically.

With a small infant, straddle the body over the forearm in a prone position with the hand supporting the jaw and chest. Keep the head lower than the trunk to take advantage of the force of gravity, as shown in Figure 76-4. If necessary, place the forearm on the thigh for support. If the infant or child is too large to position in this manner, kneel on the floor and drape the child across your thighs with the head lower than the trunk. Ellis and Billings (1980) and the American Heart Association (1985) caution against use of this gravity-dependent position if the obstruction is partial because a foreign object could become lodged under the vocal cords, resulting in complete obstruction.

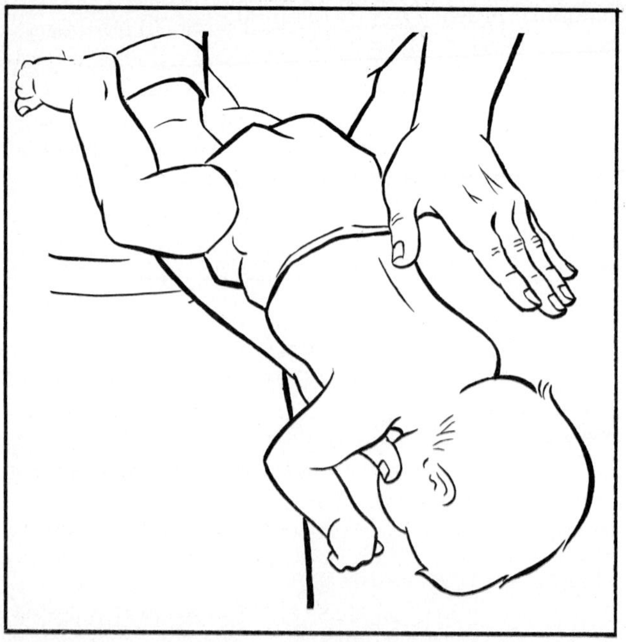

While supporting the infant with the forearm, give four back blows between the scapulae with the heel of the other hand. As with the adult, render each blow forcibly with the intent of dislodging the foreign body, but use less force than is required for the adult.

After the back blows, turn the infant face up. To do this, place the free hand on the infant's back and occiput so that the infant is sandwiched between the forearms, with the head and torso well supported. Rotate both arms to turn the infant face up. Keep the head lower than the trunk. If a larger infant or small child has been draped across the rescuer's knees, roll the child over on the back.

Give four quick chest thrusts by using the middle and index fingers to compress the midsternum. The position and technique are the same as those used for infant cardiac compression. These thrusts will rapidly increase airway pressure and air flow. Abdominal thrusts are not recommended for infants and children because of risk of injury to abdominal organs.

After the chest thrusts have been applied, inspect the inside of the mouth, lifting the tongue and lower jaw forward. To do this, place the thumb over the infant's tongue and grasp underneath the chin with the fingers. If the foreign object can be seen, remove it. Blind finger probes in children are not recommended because a foreign object can too easily be wedged more deeply in the airway.

If the foreign object cannot be removed, reattempt to ventilate the infant. As with the adult, this may be possible if the obstruction has become partially dislodged or the throat muscles have relaxed from anoxia. If it is still impossible to ventilate the infant, the sequence of back blows, chest thrusts, visualizing the airway, and attempts to ventilate is repeated.

Figure 76-4. Back blows: infant. Straddle the infant over the forearm, supporting the jaw and chest with hand. Deliver four back blows between the scapulae with the heel of the hand.

SKILL SEQUENCE

FOREIGN OBJECT REMOVAL: INFANT

Step	Rationale
A. Conscious Infant–Child: 1. Evaluate breathing effort and ability to cry. If air exchange is inadequate, initiate steps 2 to 9, described below for unconscious infant.	If air exchange is adequate, infant will be able to cry and no intervention is needed. If air exchange is poor, infant will be unable to cry and must be treated.
B. Unconscious Infant–Child: 1. Same as in Skill Sequence, "CPR—Infant and Child," steps 1 to 4, p. 984. 2. Reattempt to ventilate after repositioning head and neck, checking for secretions, clearing if necessary. Avoid hyperextending the neck. 3. Sandwich infant face down between forearms with head lower than trunk. (Drape larger infant or small child over thighs with head lower than trunk.) 4. Deliver four back blows. 5. Turn infant face up by sandwiching infant between forearms. Back and head should be supported. Head should be lower than trunk. (Larger infant or small child is rolled to back, keeping head lower than trunk.) 6. Deliver four chest thrusts with middle and index fingers of one hand for infants and heel of one hand for a child. 7. Inspect mouth. Remove foreign object <u>only</u> if it can be seen. 8. Reattempt to ventilate infant. 9. In unable to ventilate, repeat steps 4 to 8 until effective.	Time should not be wasted looking for a foreign object unless there is reason to believe one is present. Airway of infants must be carefully evaluated due to neck pliability. Gravity may help expel foreign object. Rapid increase in airway pressure may dislodge foreign object. Adequate support is provided. Gravity may help expel foreign object. Rapid increase in airway pressure could dislodge foreign object. Abdominal thrusts may injure abdominal organs. Blind finger sweeps are likely to wedge foreign objects more deeply in airway. May be possible to ventilate infant if foreign object becomes partially dislodged or throat muscles relax. No effort should be made to assess circulatory status or proceed with cardiac compression until oxygen can be provided.

RECORDING

The time and a description of the precipitating events, victim's condition, rescuer activities, and the client's response are documented in the health record. It is important to note if airway obstruction preceded cardiac arrest.

Sample POR Recording

- S—"I don't know how that happened, but it was sure scary!"
- O—Found clutching throat and unable to speak while eating. Exaggerated respiratory effort present with no apparent air exchange. Making high-pitched crowing sounds. Large piece of partially chewed food expelled after chest thrusts and back blows were applied, followed by rapid, deep, and unlabored resp. @ a rate of 30/min.
- A—Stable and resting after removal of airway obstruction.
- P—Continue observations of resp. exchange; evaluate eating patterns and habits to determine possible interventions to prevent recurrence of choking and obstruction.

Sample Narrative Recording

Found clutching throat and unable to speak while eating. Respiratory effort exaggerated but did not appear to be moving air. Making high-pitched crowing noises. Chest thrusts and back blows applied. Large piece of partially chewed food immediately expelled. Respirations now rapid and deep but unlabored at a rate of 30 per minute. Stable and resting after airway obstruction removed. Will monitor respirations and air exchange and evaluate eating patterns to identify ways to prevent future airway obstruction.

CRITICAL POINTS SUMMARY

1. Use a combination of alternate back blows and manual thrusts to attempt to remove an obstruction.
2. The force of manual thrusts is delivered with the fists; it is not a bearhug.
3. Chest thrusts are considered safer than abdominal thrusts for infants, pregnant women, and obese people.
4. Abdominal thrusts are safer than chest thrusts for older people.
5. Avoid forcing the foreign object farther into the airway with the finger probe.

6. Blind finger sweeps are not used to attempt removal of a foreign object from the airway of an infant or child.

LEARNING ACTIVITIES

1. Enroll in AHA- or ARC-sponsored Basic Life Support course.
2. Interview nurses who work with mothers of young children to find out what aspects of toy and play safety these nurses include in their teaching that could prevent accidental airway obstruction.
3. When you are in a restaurant, look for posters that illustrate the technique used to remove a foreign body from the airway. Interview a waiter or waitress to find out if or how often they have used this emergency procedure.

REVIEW QUESTIONS

1. What is the correct hand position for chest and abdominal thrusts for a conscious adult and an unconscious adult?
2. What is the significance of differentiating between airway obstruction caused by a foreign object and that caused by a preexisting disease state?
3. How would you decide if air exchange is adequate or inadequate?
4. If airway obstruction is partial but air exchange is adequate, what must you do?
5. If airway obstruction is partial but air exchange is inadequate, what must you do?
6. What is the most important precaution to take when performing a finger probe?
7. What precautions can be taken to avoid choking on a food bolus or other foreign object?

PERFORMANCE CHECKLISTS

OBJECTIVE: To demonstrate foreign object removal technique for a conscious adult correctly.

CHARACTERISTIC	RANGE OF ACCEPTABILITY	SATISFACTORY	UNSATISFACTORY
1. Asks victim if he or she can speak. Evaluates breathing effort.	No deviation		
2. Positions self beside and slightly behind victim. Supports victim correctly.	No deviation		
3. Delivers four back blows.	May deliver manual thrusts first.		
4. Delivers four manual thrusts.	May deliver back blows second.		
5. Repeats sequence of back blows and manual thrusts until effective or victim collapses.	Repeat until evaluator is satisfied.		

OBJECTIVE: To demonstrate foreign object removal technique for an unconscious adult correctly.

CHARACTERISTIC	RANGE OF ACCEPTABILITY	SATISFACTORY	UNSATISFACTORY
1. Attempts to arouse victim and positions appropriately.	No deviation		
2. Calls for help.	No deviation		
3. Opens airway. Assesses respiratory status. Checks for presence of stoma.	No deviation		
4. Delivers 4 rapid ventilations and observes for chest rise.	No deviation		
5. Reattempts ventilation after altering technique.	No deviation		
6. Delivers four back blows.	May deliver manual thrusts first.		
7. Delivers four manual thrusts.	May deliver back blows second.		
8. Performs finger probe.	No deviation		
9. Reattempts to ventilate victim.	No deviation		
10. Repeats sequence of back blows, thrusts, finger probe, and attempted ventilations until effective.	Repeat until evaluator is satisfied.		

OBJECTIVE: To demonstrate foreign object removal techniques for an infant correctly.

CHARACTERISTIC	RANGE OF ACCEPTABILITY	SATISFACTORY	UNSATISFACTORY
A. Conscious Infant–Child:			
1. Evaluates breathing effort and ability to cry. If air exchange inadequate, proceeds to Unconscious Infant–Child, step 2.	No deviation		
B. Unconscious Infant–Child:			
1. Attempts to arouse infant or child. Places in supine position.	No deviation		
2. Calls for help.	No deviation		
3. Opens airway. Listens to and looks at chest.	No deviation		
4. Delivers 4 gentle rapid ventilations and observes for chest rise.	No deviation		
5. Repositions head and attempts to ventilate.	May omit.		
6. Straddles infant face down over forearm.	No deviation		
7. Delivers four back blows.	May deliver chest thrusts first.		
8. Turns infant face up, sandwiching between forearms.	No deviation		
9. Delivers four chest thrusts.	May deliver back blows second.		
10. Visualizes mouth. Removes foreign object if it can be seen.	No deviation		
11. Reattempts to ventilate.	No deviation		
12. Repeats sequence of back blows, chest thrusts, mouth visualization, and attempted ventilations until effective.	Repeat until evaluator is satisfied.		

REFERENCES

American Heart Association: Standards for cardiopulmonary resuscitation (CPR) and emergency cardiac care (ECC). Journal of the American Medical Association 227(7)(suppl):834–868, 1974.

American Heart Association: Standards for cardiopulmonary resuscitation (CPR) and emergency cardiac care (ECC). Journal of the American Medical Association 244(5):453–509, 1980.

American Heart Association: Instructors Manual for Basic Life Support. Dallas, American Heart Association, 1985.

Ellis PD, Billings DM: Cardiopulmonary Resuscitation: Procedures for Basic and Advanced Life Support. St Louis, CV Mosby, 1980.

Guildner CW: Resuscitation—Opening the airway: A comparative study of techniques. Journal of the American College of Emergency Physicians 5(8):588–590, 1976.

Guildner CW, Williams D, et al.: Airway obstructed by foreign material: The Heimlich maneuver. Journal of the American College of Emergency Physicians 5(9):675–677, 1976.

Haugen RK: The cafe coronary: Sudden death in restaurants. Journal of the American Medical Association 186(2):142–143, 1963.

Heimlich HJ: Pop goes the cafe coronary. Emergency Medicine 6(6):154–155, 1974.

Redding JS: The choking controversy: Critique of evidence on the Heimlich maneuver. Critical Care Medicine 7(10):475–479, 1979b.

Ruben H, MacNaughton FI: The treatment of food-choking. The Practitioner 221(1325):725–729, 1978.

Visintine RE, Baick CH: Ruptured stomach after Heimlich maneuver. Journal of the American Medical Association 234(4):415, 1975.

AUDIOVISUAL RESOURCES

Cardiopulmonary Resuscitation: Clearing the Obstructed Airway
Filmstrip and cassette. (1979, Color, 18 min.)
Available through:
Medcom, Inc.
P.O. Box 116
Garden Grove, CA 92642

Obstructed Airway Management
Videorecording (½ and ¾ in). (1982, Color, 17 min.)
Available through:
Indiana University School of Nursing
NICER
610 Barnhill Drive
Indianapolis, IN 46223

Appendix I
Keys to Chapter Entry Tests

☐ CHAPTER 7

1. Body temperature is controlled by a temperature regulating center in the hypothalamus. It operates by means of temperature detectors that identify when the body temperature is too hot or too cold. The detectors respond to a feedback system from temperature receptors in the anterior hypothalamus that receive impulses from cold-sensitive neurons in other parts of the hypothalamus septum and midbrain. Warm and cold skin temperature receptors also send impulses to the spinal cord and hypothalamus to help control body temperature.
2. The seven factors affecting body temperature are: age, circadian rhythm, stress, sleep, hormones, exercise, and internal temperature.
3. The body produces heat by basal metabolism, muscular activity of shivering, thyroxin effect on cells, epinephrine effect on cells, and temperature effect on cells.
4. Heat is lost from the body by radiation, evaporation, and conduction.
5. The major structures that make up the cardiovascular system include the heart, arteries, veins, and blood.
6. The arteries have strong pulsating walls composed of several layers. The arterial system originates from the aorta and its branches, except for the pulmonary artery which originates from the right atrium. Arteries do not have valves. The smallest arteries are called arterioles. Veins have larger lumens and thinner walls than arteries. They are capable of storing blood and are therefore expandable. When veins are empty of blood they collapse. Valves are not present in the veins in the brain, spinal cord, meninges, or superior and inferior vena cavae. However, they are common in the veins of the extremities and serve to support the column of blood, help to direct the flow toward the heart, and prevent back flow. Veins do not pulsate; the blood is moved by action of the muscles on the veins and by changes in pressure in the thoracic and abdominal vessels. Veins are usually under less pressure than the arteries. The smallest veins are called venules. Capillaries are microscopic vessels that connect arterioles with venules.
7. Blood from the superior and inferior vena cavae enters the right atrium, flows through the tricuspid (A-V) valve to the right ventricle, then to the pulmonary artery for oxygenation; the pulmonary veins return the blood to the left atrium through the bicuspid (mitral) valve to the left ventricle. The blood is ejected through the aortic valve into the systemic circulation.
8. The basic functions of the circulatory system are to deliver oxygen and nutrition to the tissues and to remove waste products.
9. The hypothalamus and the cerebral cortex are both capable of exciting or inhibiting the vasomotor center, which controls the degree of vascular constriction and regulates the heart rate.
10. The circulatory factors that influence arterial blood pressure are: circulating blood volume, viscosity of the blood, vascular resistance, stroke volume, and heart rate.
11. The three circulatory reflexes that play major roles in the regulation of the arterial blood pressure are:
    a. Baroreceptors (pressoreceptors) are located in the walls of most of the great arteries in the upper body, especially in the carotid sinuses and the aortic arch. These control mechanisms are nerve receptors that are stimulated by stretching the arterial walls. The baroreceptor system is activated primarily when arterial pressure begins to rise above normal. Baroreceptor impulses inhibit the vasomotor center in the medulla and stimulate the vagal center. These actions decrease sympathetic nervous system stimulation of the cardiovascular system, producing peripheral vasodilation and a decreased rate and strength of cardiac contraction, and therefore, a decrease in arterial blood pressure. Conversely, when arterial pressure drops below normal, the stretch receptors are relaxed and permit the vasomotor center to become more active, thereby causing the arterial pressure to rise back toward normal.

b. Chemoreceptors located in the aortic and carotid bodies are sensory receptors that detect the oxygen level in the arterial blood. When the arterial pressure drops below 100 millimeters of mercury (mm Hg) because the blood flow is depressed, the receptors transmit signals to the vasomotor center to return the pressure to normal.
c. Central nervous system ischemic mechanism is activated when the blood flow is insufficient to maintain normal metabolic function. This is usually when the arterial pressure is below 50 mm Hg. An extremely active and widespread response from the sympathetic nervous system induces vasoconstriction to increase the heart rate and blood flow, resulting in an increase in arterial blood pressure.
12. The kidney regulates blood pressure by responding to a decrease in blood pressure with retention of sodium and fluids. This occurs because of the release of antidiuretic hormone and the production of aldosterone. When the pressure increases, the reverse process occurs.
13. The respiratory tract begins with the nose and includes the nasopharynx, larynx, trachea, bronchus, bronchioles, and alveoli. The trachea is continuous with the main bronchus, which branches left and right to each lung. Bronchioles branch off from each of the main bronchi; these evolve into respiratory bronchioles to which an alveolar duct is attached, leading to the alveolar sacs.
14. Gas exchange occurs at the alveolar level.
15. The capillaries and cells exchange oxygen and carbon dioxide.
16. The respiratory center is located in the medulla oblongata in the brainstem.
17. The primary stimuli for respiration are the blood levels of carbon dioxide and hydrogen ions. Second in importance is a decrease in the level of oxygen concentration in the blood, which stimulates chemoreceptors in the aortic and carotid arteries. The third main stimuli for respiration are the Hering-Bruer reflexes, which are the activation of the stretch receptors in the bronchioles and lung tissues during inspiration and expiration.
18. During inspiration, the diaphragm and the external intercostal muscles act with small muscles in the neck to pull the front of the thoracic cage upward, and the diaphragm moves downward, elongating the thoracic cage. During expiration, the abdominal muscles act to pull the chest cage down to decrease the size of the cavity. They also serve to force the abdominal contents up toward the diaphragm, which decreases the length of the cavity. The internal intercostal muscles help by pulling the ribs downward to decrease further the size of the thoracic cavity.
19. A kilocalorie is a unit of measure that reflects the amount of energy necessary to raise 1 kilogram of water 1 degree Celsius.
20. One gram of protein has 4 kilocalories, as does 1 gram of carbohydrate; 1 gram of fat has 9 kilocalories.
21. Protein is a part of every body cell and it maintains healthy cells and supports their growth. Carbohydrate supplies energy so that protein is available for cell growth and maintenance. Fat is also part of every cell. It also provides the most concentrated energy source for the body.
22. Daily caloric and nutrient requirements are determined by age, state of health or illness, activity level, environmental temperature, and basal metabolic rate.
23. Metabolism consists of three processes:
    a. Assimilating and converting nutrients into living tissue
    b. Breaking down nutrients and body tissues to release energy
    c. Absorption of the nutrients by body tissue

☐ CHAPTER 8

1. A host is a person or any living animal that supports a parasite that lives at the host's expense. The host may serve as a potential course of reinfection and as a means of sustaining the parasite.

   A reservoir may be a host or an environment that supports the survival and multiplication of pathogenic microorganisms. The environment may include soil, air, food, water, milk, or any inanimate substance that provides opportunities for the transmission of microorganisms to a new susceptible host. Living reservoirs include humans, animals, and insects. However, humans are the most frequent reservoir for agents that are infectious to humans.

   A carrier is a person who has an infectious agent in his or her system but does not have any obvious signs of an infection and who serves as a potential reservoir or source of infection for humans.

   Fomites are inanimate substances, such as clothing and rings, that are capable of absorbing and transmitting the infectious agent.

   A contaminant refers to the presence of an infectious agent on an inanimate substance, material, or body surface.

   A vector is any living carrier that transports a pathogenic microorganism from one host to another.
2. The main routes by which microorganisms are transmitted are contact, vehicle, airborne, and vectorborne.
3. The contact route may be divided into three types:
   a. Direct contact involves the direct physical transfer of microorganisms between an infected person and a susceptible host. Personnel and clients may serve in either role.

b. Indirect contact involves personal contact of the susceptible host with inanimate materials that have become contaminated. The materials include such things as clothing, linen, dressings, and instruments.
c. Droplet contact refers to contact with the mouth, nose, or conjunctivae of a susceptible host by an infectious agent through droplets dispersed from talking, coughing, or sneezing by an infected person. The infected person may have the clinical disease or be a carrier.

The vehicle route refers to a substance that serves as an intermediary for the transport of an infectious agent from a reservoir into a susceptible host by ingestion, inoculation, or deposit on the skin or mucous membranes. Food, water, drugs, intravenous fluids, and blood can serve as vehicles.

The airborne route of transmission refers to dust particles or droplet residue that contain an infectious agent in the air. When the microorganisms are disseminated, a susceptible host may inhale them or have the microorganisms deposited on him or her.

The vectorborne route of transmission requires a living microorganism that transports an infectious agent from an infectious person or the wastes of that person to a susceptible host, its food, or its immediate surroundings. Although not a common concern in hospitals, vectors such as rats, bats, and mosquitoes can transmit disease in communities.
4. Infectious agents may enter or leave the body through the respiratory tract, the gastrointestinal tract, the skin or mucous membranes, or directly into the tissues or bloodstream.
5. The skin and mucous membranes are the primary barriers to preventing entry of infectious agents. Blood components, such as plasma, leukocytes, antigens, and antibodies, act to prevent the infectious agent from causing an infection once entry has been gained.
6. The resident flora normally present on the human body are as follows:

LOCATION	MICROORGANISM
Skin	*Staphylococcus epidermidis* and *S. aureus*
	Streptococci—veridans, nonhemolytic and enterococci
	Corynebacteria, diptheroid bacilli
	Gram-negative enteric bacilli, *Escherichia* and *Enterobacter* species
	Mycobacteria, acid-fast bacilli
	Yeasts and fungi
Conjunctiva	*Staphylococcus epidermidis*
	Streptococci—veridans and nonhemolytic
	Branhomella catarrhalis
	Neisseria species
	Corynebacteria, diptheroid bacilli
	Microaerophilic gram-negative bacilli
Nose and throat	*Staphylococcus epidermidis* and *S. aureus*
	Streptococci—veridans, nonhemolytic and enterococcus
	Streptococcus pneumoniae
	Branhomella catarrhalis
	Neisseria species
	Corynebacteria, diptheroid bacilli *Haemophilus* species
	Anaerobes
Mouth	*Staphylococcus epidermidis* and *S. aureus*
	Streptococci—veridans, nonhemolytic, enterococci
	Lactobacillus species
	Spirochetes
	Actinomyces species
	Yeasts
Intestines (adults)	Anaerobic bacilli
	Anaerobic streptococci
	Gram-negative enteric bacilli, *Escherichia, Enterobacter, Proteus, Pseudomonas*
	Streptococci, enterococci
	Yeasts
	Protozoa
Genital Tract	*Staphylococcus epidermidis* and *S. aureus*
	Streptococci, enterococci, nonhemolytic
	Lactobacilli
	Gram-negative enteric bacilli, *Escherichia, Enterobacter, Proteus, Pseudomonas*
	Anaerobic bacilli, *Clostridium* species
	Mycobacteria, acid-fast bacilli
	Spirochetes
	Yeasts
	Protozoa

7. The body area containing the largest number of organisms is the intestines.
8. An antiseptic slows or prevents the growth of organisms; they are used on the body. A disinfectant destroys the pathogenic organisms; they are used on inanimate objects.

CHAPTER 9

1. See Key for Chapter 8 Entry Test, pp. 1000–1001.
2. Pathogenic bacteria are capable of producing disease, whereas nonpathogenic bacteria do not cause disease. Bacteria that are nonpathogenic in one area of the body may become pathogenic when introduced into other body cavities; for example, *Escherichia coli* is a normal flora of the large bowel, but produces infection if present in a wound or the abdominal cavity. A given bacterium may be nonpathogenic for the average person, but for a person with lowered resistance, it may be pathogenic.
3. Medical asepsis refers to the absence of infectious disease-producing microorganisms, while surgical asepsis refers to the absence of all microorganisms. Medical aseptic techniques are designed to confine the spread of pathogens, while surgical aseptic techniques are designed to prevent the entry of all microorganisms to a given area.
4. Spore-forming bacteria are capable of producing forms that are highly resistant to adverse conditions such as heat, cold, disinfection, and drying. Nonspore-forming bacteria have no such mechanisms for survival under adverse conditions.
5. Vegetative forms of bacteria are normal living bacterial forms that are capable of growth and reproduction and have no specialized survival features. Under normal conditions, spore-forming bacteria produce both vegetative forms and bacterial spores that are capable of surviving if adverse conditions such as heat or cold occur.

    Bacterial spores are a resting phase, and neither growth nor reproduction occurs until the spores are stimulated to return to a vegetative form. Under normal conditions, bacterial spores are simply present and inactive. Trauma, such as heat shock or cold shock, causes the bacterial spore to break out of its spore form, become a vegetative form, and then begin to grow.
6. Aerobic bacteria require oxygen in their environment in order to grow and thrive, while anaerobic bacteria require an oxygen-free environment for growth and survival.
7. Facultative anaerobic bacteria are organisms that require an anaerobic environment for optimal growth, but they can survive in an aerobic environment.

CHAPTER 10

1. The functions of the skin are to:
    a. Protect the internal organs from heat, cold, water, trauma, friction, and pressure
    b. Regulate body temperature
    c. Inhibit the growth of microorganisms
    d. Mediate sensations
2. The functions of the three major layers of the skin are:
    a. The epidermis slows the exchange of fluids from either side.
    b. The dermis stores a significant amount of the body's water and provides support for the epidermis, glands, and hair.
    c. The subcutaneous layer serves as an insulator and shock absorber.
3. Sebaceous glands are located on all of the body areas except for the palms, soles, and dorsa of the feet. Although the function of the sebaceous glands is not clearly established, it is believed that sebum provides lubrication to the skin and keeps it supple. Sebum may also have some antibacterial action and antifungal properties. Sebaceous glands function because of stimulation by androgen hormones.

    Aprocrine glands are located in the axillae, areolae, periumbilical, perianal, and genital areas. They continuously excrete an odorless, cloudy fluid. The odor associated with sweat is a result of bacterial growth and decomposition of the bacteria on the body and in the sweat. Apocrine glands are not important for fluid regulation or temperature control. They become active at puberty and atrophy later in life.

    Eccrine sweat glands are found all over the body. There are two types: one type is found on the palms, soles, and axillae. The other type is found in the axillae and on all other parts of the body and responds to thermal and emotional stimuli. Eccrine sweat is clear and odorless. Eccrine glands begin functioning at infancy. Although their output is continuous, these glands increase their secretions in response to emotional stimuli.
4. Melanocytes are special cells in the basal layer of the epidermis. They produce pigment granules called melanosomes that give most of the color to the skin. The pigment is constantly produced and passed to the epithelial cells.
5. The structures included in the external female genitalia are:
    a. The mons pubis, which lies anterior to the pubic symphysis, is a prominent fatty cushion covered with skin. This becomes covered with coarse and somewhat curly hair during puberty.
    b. The labia majora are two thick, rounded folds of skin that are supported by loose areolar and adipose tissue. This tissue is continuous with the mons pubis and extends posterior to the anus. Its thickness decreases toward the posterior aspect. The lateral surfaces are pigmented and after puberty are covered with coarse hair similar to that on the mons pubis.
    c. The labia minora are two small skin folds without hair or fat that lie medial to the large folds of the labia majora and enclose the vestibule where the urethra, the vagina, and the ducts of

the greater vestibular glands open to the surface. The skin is smooth and moist.

d. The clitoris is a small, rounded elevation that is enclosed by the anterior aspects of the folds of the labia minora. It is a dense, fibrous membrane consisting of erectile tissue and is well supplied with sensory nerve endings.

6. The following glands lubricate the female genital area: sebaceous and apocrine sweat glands located in the labia majora and minora; Skene's glands, which are located within the urethral orifice; and Bartholin's glands, which are located on each inner aspect of the labia minora at five and seven o'clock.

7. The urethral orifice is a mucous membrane-lined tube that opens on the vestibule. It lies anterior to the vagina and below the clitoris. The vaginal orifice is located between the labia minora and lies posterior to the urethral orifice and anterior to the distal aspect of the labia majora.

8. The vagina is located in the lower part of the pelvic cavity posterior to the bladder and anterior to the rectum. It extends downward and forward and opens into the vaginal orifice between the labia.

9. Structurally, the vagina is lined with squamous epithelial tissue that becomes several layers thick under the influence of estrogen. The vaginal mucosa has deep furrows known as rugae. There are no glands in the vagina; mucus from the cervix bathes the vagina.

10. Female breast tissue develops at puberty because of the stimulation from estrogens and progesterone.

11. Female breast tissue consists of about 25 separate milk-secreting tubular glands called lobes. The lobes are arranged in a radius, and each lobe is separated by fibrous tissue that extends from the dermis to the underlying pectoralis fascia. Each of the lobes consists of multiple lobules that are surrounded by dense connective tissue. Each gland drains into its own duct that discharges into a separate opening in the breast nipple.

12. The largest area of breast tissue is in the upper outer quadrant and extends along the serratus anterior muscle. The lateral extension of tissue is called the axillary tail.

13. Breast tissue is supported by multiple fibrous bands that run through the breast tissue and attach the tissue to the dermis and muscle fascia; these are known as Cooper's ligaments.

14. The areolar area is a circular surface of pigmented skin around the base of the nipple. Tiny elevations on the areola are produced by glands. The nipple is the pigmented cone-shaped prominence in the center of the areola. It has small openings in its peak that are the orifices of the gland ducts. The skin on the nipple is normally wrinkled.

15. The function of the female breasts is to secrete milk during pregnancy and lactation. These normal secretions may be watery or milky.

16. Lymph nodes are part of the lymphatic system that includes a network of lymph capillaries and vessels and ducts that carry lymph throughout the body. Eventually the lymph drains into the bloodstream. Lymph nodes are round or bean-shaped organs that vary in size and number. Lymph nodes serve an important function by filtering out bacteria and foreign material carried by the lymph that drains from a body area. When the nodes filter lymph from an infected or diseased body area, they become swollen and may be painful. The increase in size or pain may be the first sign of disease.

17. Lymph nodes are distributed throughout the body and are commonly arranged in groups.

18. The external structures of the male genitalia are as follows:

a. The scrotum is a saclike pendant structure of skin that contains the testes and the epididymides. It hangs from the inferior surface of the perineum immediately behind the penis and a short distance anterior to the anus.

b. The penis is an elongated, cylindrically shaped organ that is attached to the front and sides of the pubic arch. The shaft of the penis is covered with dark skin. The foreskin (prepuce) is a circular fold of skin that passes forward over the tip of the organ, known as the glans. The foreskin is retractable and is often surgically removed by circumcision.

c. The urethral orifice opens on the glans.

19. A child developes 20 deciduous teeth equally divided between the upper and lower jaw. A full complement of permanent adult teeth number 32.

20. There are three pairs of salivary glands: the parotids, the submaxillaries, and the sublinguals. The parotid glands lie beneath the skin on the lateral aspects of the face, below and in front of the ear. They produce a serous, watery saliva that contains enzymes. Stensen's duct opens into the mouth opposite the second upper molar teeth. The submaxillary glands lie in front of the parotid glands but below the mandibular angle. They produce a mucous and serous saliva. Wharton's ducts open into the floor of the mouth on each side of the frenulum of the tongue. The sublingual glands lie under the mucous membrane of the mouth under the tongue. They produce a mucous saliva through multiple small ducts.

☐ CHAPTER 11

1. The blood vessels of the skin are found in the epidermal, dermal, and subcutaneous layers.

2. Extensive venous plexus in the subcutaneous tissues hold large quantities of blood. Located in the dermis are capillaries, arteries, veins, and arteriovenous anastomoses. Minute capillaries extend into the papillae of the epidermis.

3. At the back of the neck, the trapezius muscle originates at the occipital bone, the spine of the seventh cervical vertebrae, and the twelve spines of the thoracic vertebrae. The muscle fibers of the upper portion of this muscle run diagonally to the lateral third of the clavicle; the middle portion across the acromion process and the superior border of the scapula; and the lower portion upward and laterally to attach to the medial aspect of the scapula. Over the shoulder, the deltoid muscle has some fibers that begin at the lateral third of the clavicle. Other fibers originate from the side of the acromion process and from the lower edge of the scapula. All of these fibers converge and run vertically to insert onto the middle part of the anterior surface of the humerus.

Over the back, the latissimus dorsi muscle has fibers that originate at the posterior part of the iliac crest, the six lower thoracic vertebrae, all of the lumbar and the upper sacral vertebrae, and the lower four ribs. The fibers run upward and laterally to insert in a groove in the upper aspect of the humerus.

Over the buttocks, the gluteus maximus muscle originates at the outer surface of the ilium and the posterior surface of the sacrum and coccyx. The muscle fibers run downward and laterally with most of them attaching to the lateral aspect of the iliotibial tract. The gluteus medius muscle originates at the outer surface of the ilium and the fibers run downward and laterally to attach to the lateral surface of the greater trochanter.

☐ CHAPTER 12

1. In the healthy adult, the intracellular fluid (ICF) compartment contains 70 percent of the total body water. The major electrolytes in ICF are potassium ($^+$) and phosphates ($^-$). The extracellular fluid (ECF) compartment contains 30 percent of the total body water, with 6 percent in the plasma and 24 percent in the interstitial spaces. The major electrolytes in the ECF are sodium ($^+$) and chloride ($^-$).
2. Water and solutes (including sodium and chloride) move from the bloodstream into the kidney tubules by hydrostatic pressure. To maintain a normal body composition of electrolytes, solutes are reabsorbed into the body through active transport. Normal body fluid concentration is maintained as water passively moves by diffusion and osmosis across the semipermeable tubular membrane to areas of increased solutes.

    When decreased fluid intake or increased fluid loss occurs, the kidneys reabsorb (conserve) more sodium in the proximal tubules. Since sodium is largely responsible for osmotic pressure, water accompanies sodium movement, and therefore water is also retained and conserved. Decreased glomerular filtration accompanying fluid deficit also aids in sodium conservation. When sodium intake increases, there is a corresponding increase in sodium excretion (from a decreased reabsorption from the proximal tubules), increase in glomerular filtrate, and excretion of water. Water and sodium reabsorption are also influenced by antidiuretic hormone (ADH) (alters permeability of the distal tubules and collecting ducts), aldosterone (increases sodium retention), and a complex feedback mechanism known as the countercurrent mechanism.
3. A kilocalorie (kcal) is the amount of heat required to raise the temperature of 1 kg of water at room temperature 1°C. In the body, it represents the energy produced when a specific amount of food is oxidized.
4. One g of carbohydrate metabolizes to produce 4 kcal of energy; 1 g of protein also produces 4 kcal, and 1 g of fat produces 7 kcal.
5. *The milk group* is composed of milk and dairy products, including cheese, yogurt, and ice cream. Adults need two servings per day, children need three, and teenagers and pregnant and lactating women need four.

    The meat group includes meat, poultry, fish, eggs, and legumes. Two or more servings per day are recommended.

    The grain group consists of breads and cereal grains. Four servings per day are recommended.

    The fruit-vegetable group is composed of any fruits and vegetables, and should include a daily source of vitamin C (citrus fruit or juice, tomatoes, cabbage) and a vitamin A source (dark-green or deep-yellow vegetables) three to four times per week. Four servings per day are recommended.
6. RDAs (Recommended Dietary Allowance) are the levels of essential nutrients considered to be adequate to meet the nutritional needs of practically all healthy persons. Recommended levels include a margin of safety for individual differences and normal stresses of living. RDA levels are established by the Food and Nutrition Board of the National Research Council.

    The U.S. RDAs (U.S. Recommended Daily Allowance) are a set of standards developed by the Food and Drug Administration (FDA) to replace the older Minimum Daily Requirements (MDR) for nutrient labeling of foods. Although based on the Recommended Dietary Allowances, U.S. RDAs reflect very broad categories, with values that are fairly standard for all persons over 4 years of age.
7. Anabolism refers to the constructive metabolic processes that build up body substances, a synthesis in living organisms of more complex substances from simpler ones. Anabolism *uses* available energy.

Catabolism refers to the destructive phase of metabolism and includes all processes in which complex substances are progressively broken down into simpler ones. Catabolism involves the *release* of energy. When proteins are broken down for energy, both nitrogenous and nonnitrogenous compounds are formed. When the catabolism of tissue proteins exceeds their anabolism, a negative nitrogen balance is said to exist. This occurs after injury, with illness, and during bed rest of more than 5 to 6 days.

8. The lips, cheeks, tongue, hard and soft palate, glossopharyngeal arches, pharynx (nasopharynx, oropharynx, and hypopharynx), and esophagus are directly involved in swallowing. Related structures include the teeth, mandible, salivary glands (parotid, submaxillary, and sublingual glands), the hyoid bone, thyroid and cricoid cartilages, and the epiglottis. Normal innervation of swallowing is from cranial nerves V, VII, IX, X, and XII.

9. The teeth grind and masticate food, mechanically breaking it down and mixing it with saliva. The starch-splitting enzyme ptyalin found in saliva (secreted by the parotid, sublingual, and submaxillary glands) begins the digestion of starches and other carbohydrates. It also serves as a lubricant for swallowing.

10. The tongue moves the food around in the mouth during chewing and propels the bolus of food backward into the pharynx for swallowing.

11. The pharynx is a funnel-shaped tube with its proximal opening at the mouth and nose, and the distal opening at the esophagus and trachea. It serves as a dual passageway for food and fluids to enter the esophagus through the pharyngoesophageal sphincter, and for air to enter and leave the trachea through the larynx. The esophagus is a musculomembranous passageway between the pharynx and the stomach. The larynx is a cartilagenous structure located between the trachea and the pharynx. It contains the vocal cords and allows air to pass into the trachea. The trachea lies anteriorly to the esophagus within the neck and thorax and serves as the air passageway between the larynx and the main bronchi.

12. The main function of the stomach is the storage, mixing, and liquefaction of food into chyme, which is discharged slowly into the duodenum. Protein digestion begins in the stomach and starch digestion continues from the mouth. Digestion of fats is minimal and very little absorption occurs in the stomach, other than that of alcohol.

13. The small intestine completes the digestion of foodstuffs, absorbs the products of digestion, and moves the waste residue into the colon, where water is reabsorbed.

14. When the digestive functions of the stomach and small intestine are completed, the end products are ready for absorption through the walls of the small intestine in these forms:

- *Carbohydrates* have been transformed into monosaccharides (glucose, fructose, and galactose) and a few disaccharides (maltose and sucrose).
- *Proteins* have been transformed into amino acids and small amounts of dipeptides.
- *Fats* have been transformed into fatty acids, monoglycerides, diglycerides, and glycerol.

15. Gastric fluid is yellow and is composed of mucus, digestive enzymes, hydrochloric acid (hydrogen and chlorides), and potassium and sodium. Its normal pH ranges from 1 to 3.5, which is more acidic than intestinal secretions. Normal daily volume secreted is approximately 2500 ml, much of which is reabsorbed.

16. Blood flows from the lower arms through the brachial vein to the axillary vein to the subclavian vein to the brachiocephalic (innominate) vein to the superior vena cava to the right atrium to the right ventricle to the lungs. Blood flows from the lower arms through the cephalic vein into the axillary vein and through the heart as with the brachial vein. Blood flows from the head through the internal and external jugular veins to a junction with the subclavian vein, forming the brachiocephalic (innominate) vein, which empties into the superior vena cava and then to the right atrium to the right ventricle to the lungs. Blood flows from the legs through the femoral vein to the external iliac vein to the common iliac vein to the inferior vena cava to the right atrium to the right ventricle to the lungs.

17. Enlarging the chest cavity with the muscles of respiration creates a pressure gradient (pressure difference) that causes air to flow into the lungs (inspiration) until the pressure between the atmosphere and the air in the lungs is equal. Expiration is generally quiet and passive, as the thorax recoils and returns to its resting position, compressing the air and causing it to flow out of the lungs to the area of lesser pressure (the atmosphere) until pressures are again equal.

☐ CHAPTER 13

1. Food passes from the mouth through the pharynx and esophagus to the stomach; it enters through the cardiac orifice and passes through the body and antrum of the stomach, leaving through the pyloric sphincter. It then passes through the small intestines (duodenum, jejunum, and ileum) through the ileocecal valve to the large intestines (ascending, transverse, descending, and sigmoid colon) to the rectum and through the anus.

LENGTH OF THE VARIOUS SECTIONS OF THE SMALL AND LARGE INTESTINES:

Duodenum	25 to 30 cm (10 to 12 in)
Jejunum	2.5 meters (about 8 ft)
Ileum	3.7 meters (about 12 ft)

Total small intestine length:
Approximately 6.5 meters (20 to 22 ft)
Ascending colon   12.5 cm (5 in)
Transverse colon   38 cm (15 in)
Descending colon   25 cm (10 in)
Sigmoid colon   25 to 38 cm (10 to 15 in)
Rectum   13 cm (5 in)
Anus   4 cm (1½ in)
Total large intestine length:
Approximately 1.5 meters (4 ft)

2. The internal rectal sphincter is located at the proximal or upper end of the anus and the external sphincter is at the distal or lower end of the anus.

3. In the stomach, mixing and peristaltic waves mix the food with gastric secretions, forming chyme. Strong peristaltic waves in the antral distal portion of the stomach empty small amounts of chyme into the duodenum with each wave; this action is called the pyloric pump. Gastric distention with food and the antral hormone gastrin promote gastric emptying. Reflexes and hormones from the duodenum control gastric emptying by slowing the rate of emptying when too much chyme is already in the small intestine or when the chyme is excessively acid, irritating, hypotonic, or contains too much protein or fat.

   Mixing (segmental) contractions and propulsive (peristaltic) waves move the chyme through the small intestines from the pylorus to the ileocecal valve over an average time of 3 to 5 hours. Gastric distention initiates gastroenteric reflexes that increase the motility of the small intestines. About 800 ml of chyme empties into the cecum each day. Distention in the cecum will cause the ileocecal valve to contract and delay the emptying of chyme into the cecum.

   Chyme moves through the colon by mixing movements (haustrations). A few times each day, propulsive or mass movements propel the fecal contents toward the anus. These contractions are most abundant for about 15 minutes during the first hour after eating breakfast.

4. The stomach stores food, mixes it with gastric secretions to form the semiliquid chyme, and discharges the liquid gradually into the duodenum at a rate at which it can be digested and absorbed. Protein digestion begins in the stomach and starch digestion continues. Little absorption other than of alcohol occurs in the stomach. Finger-like projections in the small intestine, called villi, provide a very large surface for absorption of carbohydrates, proteins, and fats. The small bowel mixes the chyme with digestive secretions and hormones. Normally, all foodstuffs are absorbed from the chyme before it enters the colon.

   The primary function of the proximal half of the colon is to absorb water and electrolytes from the chyme, while the distal half stores fecal matter until it can be expelled. The volume of the chyme is reduced so that approximately 100 ml of water per day is expelled through the feces.

5. Normally, the rectum is empty most of the time as a result of structures that serve as a weak functional sphincter at the rectosigmoid junction. When feces enter the rectum, receptors in the rectal walls are stimulated and initiate the defecation reflex, sending sensory signals to the sacral area of the spinal cord. Reflex parasympathetic stimulation produces strong peristaltic waves and relaxation of the internal smooth muscle sphincter. Stretch receptors also initiate Valsalva's maneuver, which puts downward pressure on the feces and simultaneously causes the pelvic floor to pull outward and upward on the anus to expel the feces. The cerebral cortex controls the voluntary external sphincter muscle, inhibits its contractions, and allows defecation if the time and place are correct. Voluntary contractions of the levator ani muscle reinforce and strengthen voluntary anal sphincter contractions. If the external sphincter is kept contracted, the defecation reflex dies out in a few minutes and usually does not return until additional feces enter the rectum, perhaps hours later.

6. In both the male and the female, the external urinary sphincter is located in the urogenital diaphragm within the levator ani muscle sheath. The sphincter is composed of striated muscle and provides voluntary control over micturition. It is located slightly distal to the prostate gland in the male and about midway between the meatus and the bladder neck in the female.

   In both sexes, the bladder neck is composed of smooth detrusor muscle combined with elastic tissue. Often referred to as the internal sphincter, its natural smooth muscle tone prevents emptying of the bladder until pressure within the bladder rises above a critical threshold.

7. Micturition is also called voiding and urination. As the bladder fills with urine, stretch receptors in the detrusor (bladder) muscle are stimulated and initiate the micturition reflex, sending sensory signals to the sacral area of the spinal cord. Reflex parasympathetic stimulation causes the smooth muscle of the bladder neck to relax and open from the pressure of the urine. Bladder muscle contractions shorten the urethra and pull the bladder downward toward the pubis, at which point micturition occurs, unless the reflex is inhibited by voluntary cerebral cortex control. When a socially acceptable and desired time and place occurs, cerebral cortical control inhibits the external sphincter, allowing it to relax and let urine pass. The cortex also facilitates the micturition reflex and can initiate it when necessary. Voluntary contraction of the abdominal muscles exerts additional pressure on the bladder and aids emptying. Relaxation of the perineal muscles is necessary for voiding, and contraction of these muscles helps the external sphincter retain urine in the bladder. After

voiding, the normal female urethra empties by gravity, while the male urethra requires several contractions of the bulbocavernous muscle to empty it.

8. The female urethra is 3 to 5 cm (1¼ to 2 in) long. It curves downward and forward from the bladder neck to the meatus, which is located on the perineum between the vaginal orifice and the clitoris. Although the meatus is usually located about 2.5 cm (1 in) below the clitoris, it is sometimes located almost within the vaginal orifice.

    The male urethra is 20 to 21 cm (8 to 8¼ in) long. It leaves the bladder in a downward direction, turning anteriorly after it passes through the prostatic gland and the urogenital diaphragm. When the penis is flaccid and hanging in a dependent position, the urethra is S-shaped; when the penis is erect or positioned at a right angle to the body, the urethra becomes J-shaped. The urethral meatus normally is 8 mm in diameter and occurs as a vertical slit in the glans penis.

9. The male urethra extends from the bladder neck to the external urethral meatus, a distance of about 21 cm (8¼ in). It is divided into two main parts: the anterior (distal) and posterior (proximal) urethra. The anterior urethra extends from the urethral meatus at the tip of the glans penis to the external sphincter at the urogenital diaphragm. Within the glans penis, a mucous membrane fold extends into the urethra about 1 to 2 cm (½ to ¾ in) from the meatus. The posterior urethra contains the membranous urethra and the prostatic urethra. The membranous urethra extends through the urogenital diaphragm. It is the shortest and narrowest portion of the urethra and is about 1.5 to 2 cm (⅝ to ¾ in) long. The prostatic urethra extends through the prostate gland for a distance of about 2.5 cm (1 in), and to the bladder neck. It is the widest part of the urethra.

10. The urethral orifice is at the apex of the triangular area at the posterior base of the bladder known as the trigone. The ureters enter the bladder near the other points of the triangle. In contrast to the rest of the bladder, the mucous membrane in the trigone is fixed tightly to the underlying muscle and remains smooth at all times. (The mucous membrane lining of the bladder is attached loosely to the detrusor muscle and is wrinkled when the bladder is empty and smooth when it is full.) The ureters enter the bladder at an oblique angle, through constricted slitlike orifices. This entry helps prevent urine reflux into the ureters and kidney unless the bladder is grossly distended.

☐ CHAPTER 14

1. The large bones of the extremities are:
   a. Upper arm: humerus
   b. Lower arm: ulna and radius
   c. Upper leg: femur
   d. Lower leg: tibia and fibula

2. a. Cervical curve: Cervical vertebrae form an anteriorly convex curve, rounded toward the front of the body.
   b. Thoracic curve: Thoracic vertebrae form a posteriorly convex curve, rounded toward a person's back.
   c. Lumbar curve: Lumbar vertebrae form an anteriorly convex curve.
   d. Sacral curve: Sacral and coccygeal vertebrae form a posteriorly convex curve.

3. a. Ligaments: Broad fibrous bands that hold two or more bones or cartilages together to support and strengthen a joint. They allow some degree of stretch. Ligaments also connect and support other body parts such as organs and muscles.
   b. Tendons: Collagenous fiber cords that attach muscles to bones. They have great tensile strength and do not stretch.
   c. Cartilage: An avascular solid substance found between bones such as the vertebrae.
   d. Bursae: Small closed sacs lined by synovial membrane and containing small amounts of synovial fluid. They serve to decrease friction between adjacent structures such as muscles and bones or tendons and ligaments.

4. The parts of a skeletal muscle are the belly (the central, meaty, contractile portion) and the two tendinous extremities that attach the muscle to the bones, known as the muscle's origin and insertion. The point-of-origin tendon has a more fixed point of attachment, while the point-of-insertion tendon is attached to the bone being moved.

5. Skeletal muscles are classified according to their action as:
   a. Prime movers or agonists: One or two muscles primarily responsible for producing a particular motion.
   b. Synergists: Muscles that assist or supplement a prime mover.
   c. Antagonists: Muscles that oppose a movement produced by another muscle.
   d. Fixators: Muscles that stabilize a joint or joints so as to augment the prime mover's effectiveness.

6. Skeletal muscle contractions are characterized by the following:
   a. A skeletal muscle contracts and pulls toward its center, exerting a pulling force on its attachments.
   b. Skeletal muscles are usually in a state of slight tension or tonus.
   c. Skeletal muscles have their maximum contractile capability when they are at their resting length and are neither shortened nor contracted.
   d. Skeletal muscle fibers contract individually in response to sensory and motor nerve stimulation in an all-or-none manner.

1008   APPENDIX I

    e. Skeletal muscles contract in groups, rather than as individual muscles.
    f. The combination of agonist, antagonist, synergist, and fixator muscle actions provides smoothly correlated and controlled body movements.
7. An isotonic muscle contraction shortens the muscle during contraction and maintains constant tension. An isometric muscle contraction does not shorten the muscle during contraction. Most body movement involves a mixture of isometric and isotonic muscle contractions.
8. Muscle contraction causes joint flexion, that is, it decreases the joint angle and brings the two bones closer together.
9. The *articular surfaces* of adjacent bones are covered with a thin layer of hyaline cartilage. *Ligaments* hold the bones together and create a fibrous *articular capsule* around the articular ends of the bones. The articular capsule is lined with a *synovial membrane* that secretes a lubricating fluid called synovia. Some joints have an *articular disc* or *meniscus* that divides the joint cavity completely or partially. These structures also are covered with synovial membrane.
10. Intervertebral discs are collagenous and fibrous rings that surround a semigelatinous mass. They serve to separate and connect the vertebrae and absorb compression forces on the spine.
11. Major muscles used when moving clients include:
    a. Muscles that move the upper extremity:
      Biceps brachii and brachialis: Flex the elbow joint.
      Triceps: Extends the elbow joint.
      Brachioradialis: Flexes the elbow joint and rotates forearm.
      Deltoid: Abducts the upper arm.
      Pectoralis major: Abducts and rotates arm medially.
      Latissimus dorsi: Extends, abducts, and medially rotates the arm.
    b. Muscles that move the lower extremity:
      Gluteus maximus, medius, and minimus: Extend, rotate, and abduct the thigh.
      Quadriceps femoris: Flexes the thigh and extends the knee joint.
      Biceps femoris: Flexes and laterally rotates the knee joint and leg.
      Gastrocnemius: Plantar flexes foot at ankle and flexes knee joint.
    c. Muscles of the abdomen:
      External and internal oblique, transversus, and rectus abdominis: Flex and rotate the trunk, support the abdominal viscera, and compress the abdomen.
    d. Muscles of the pelvis:
      Levator ani and coccygeus: Support the floor of the pelvic cavity.
    e. Deep muscles of the back:
      Erector spinae (Sacrospinalis): A complex muscle group that extends from the sacral area to the cranium. Its action is to extend the vertebral column and the head. This muscle relaxes when the spine is in an extremely flexed position.

☐ CHAPTER 15

1. The right lung is slightly larger than the left and has three lobes: the superior, the middle, and the inferior. The left lung has only two lobes: the superior and the inferior.
2. The right main bronchus is almost a direct vertical continuation of the trachea, while the left main bronchus is positioned more horizontally.
3. There are two different types of dead air space in the respiratory tract; anatomic and physiological. Air that is inspired with each breath must first fill the anatomic dead space areas in the nasal cavity, pharynx, trachea, and bronchi before it reaches the alveoli. During expiration all of the air in the dead space areas is expired first, before any of the air in the alveoli is expelled into the environment. In a healthy young adult, there is about 150 ml of air in the anatomic dead space. Physiological dead space occurs in persons who have alveoli that are not functional because they do not have blood flow through the adjacent pulmonary blood vessels. In the normal healthy person, the anatomic and physiological dead spaces are about equal. In illness or with respiratory problems the physiological dead space can be as much as ten times the anatomic dead space.
4. There are four different types of pulmonary lung volumes. The *tidal volume* is the volume of air inspired and expired with each normal breath. It is generally about 500 ml in the normal young male adult. The *inspiratory reserve volume* is the additional amount of air that can be inspired above the normal tidal volume; it can be as much as 3000 ml. The *expiratory reserve volume* is the amount of air that can be forcefully expired after the end of a normal tidal expiration; it can be as much as 1100 ml. The residual volume is the amount of air that remains in the lungs after the most forceful expiration occurs; it averages about 1200 ml. When these four volumes are added together, they equal the maximum volume to which the lungs can be expanded: total pulmonary volume.
5. Ventilation is a term that is commonly used in three different ways. It is often used as a synonym for respiration and in this context refers to the tidal exchange of air between the lungs and the atmosphere that occurs during inspiration and expiration. Pulmonary ventilation refers to the total volume of gas exchanged by inspiration and expiration per minute. It is expressed in liters per minute and includes the exchange of gas in the dead spaces. Alveolar ventilation refers to the total volume of new air that is exchanged in the alveoli.

6. The respiratory gases are nitrogen, oxygen, carbon dioxide, and water vapor.
7. At sea level, in a healthy person with normal functioning hemoglobin, the blood has an oxygen content of approximately 20 volumes percent (20 ml of oxygen per 100 ml of blood). Most of the oxygen in the blood is carried in the form of oxyhemoglobin (19.7 volumes percent). Dissolved oxygen (PaO$_2$) represents a very small proportion (0.3 volumes percent) of the total amount of oxygen within the arterial blood.
8. Partial pressure refers to the pressure of any one gas within a mixture of gases and represents the quantity of that gas within the mixture. Since oxygen is one gas within the mixture known as air, partial pressure of oxygen (PaO$_2$) refers to the pressure and therefore the quantity of oxygen dissolved in arterial blood.
9. The PaO$_2$ serves as the driving force for the chemical combination of hemoglobin and oxygen, resulting in the formation of oxyhemoglobin. Oxyhemoglobin is the primary way in which oxygen is carried in the blood. The amount of oxygen carried by oxyhemoglobin is expressed as a percent of saturation of oxygen (SaO$_2$). In adults, the normal partial pressure of oxygen is sufficient to maintain a normal oxygen saturation of 96 to 98 percent in arterial blood. The PaO$_2$ can drop from 100 mm Hg to 50 mm Hg before the oxygen saturation begins to drop below 80 percent. Below 50 mm Hg, the drop in saturation is greatly accelerated and rapidly results in hypoxemia.
10. Surfactant is a lipoprotein substance secreted by cells in the alveolar epithelium. It decreases the surface tension of the fluids that line the alveoli. Surfactant facilitates lung expansion by maintaining the size of the alveoli and by reducing the tendency of the alveoli to collapse.

☐ CHAPTER 16

1. The basic unit of metric weight is the gram (g). The basic unit of metric volume measure is the liter (L). The basic unit of metric length measure is the meter (m).
2. The metric system is a decimal system. The basic unit can be multiplied or divided by 10 or multiples of 10 to form secondary units that differ from each other by 10 or multiples of 10. Subdivisions of the basic units are identified with Latin prefixes and multiples are identified with Greek prefixes. These prefixes and the relationships among the multiples and subdivisions are shown here for the gram. The same prefixes and relationships are used with the liter and the meter. For example, 1 milliliter = 0.001 L and 1 millimeter = 0.001 m.

1 milligram (mg)	=	0.001 g
1 centigram (cg)	=	0.01 g
1 decigram (dg)	=	0.1 g
1 gram (g)	=	1.0 g
1 dekagram (Dg)	=	10.0 g
1 hectogram (hg)	=	100.0 g
1 kilogram (kg)	=	1000.0 g

3. To change from a smaller metric unit to a larger unit, divide the smaller unit by 10 or the appropriate multiple of 10. To change from a larger metric unit to a smaller one, multiply by 10 or the appropriate multiple of 10. An easy way to do this: to divide by 10, move the decimal point one digit to the left; to multiply by 10, move the decimal point one digit to the right. To multiply or divide by hundreds, move the decimal point two places to the right, and so forth. For example, to change milligrams to grams, divide by 1000, since a milligram is one thousandth of a gram. To do this, move the decimal point three places to the left. To change grams to milligrams, multiply by 1000; that is, move the decimal point three places to the right.
4. The relationship between metric weight and fluid volume is that one milliliter (1 ml) of water at 4°C weighs one gram (1 g). The term milliliter (ml) is preferred over cubic centimeter (cc), although they are sometimes used interchangeably. One liter of water at 4°C weighs 1 kilogram (kg).
5. Units of household weights and measures of volume and length:

VOLUME

60 drops (gtts)	=	1 teaspoonful (tsp)
3 teaspoonfuls	=	1 tablespoonful (tbsp)
2 tablespoonfuls	=	1 fluidounce
16 tablespoonfuls or 8 fluidounces	=	1 glassful or 1 measuring cupful (c)
6 fluidounces	=	1 teacupful
2 cupfuls	=	1 pint (pt)
2 pints	=	1 quart (qt)
4 quarts	=	1 gallon (gal)

LENGTH

12 inches (in)	=	1 foot (ft)
3 feet	=	1 yard (yd)
1760 yards or 5280 feet	=	1 mile (mi)

WEIGHT

16 ounces (oz)	=	1 pound (lb)
2000 pounds	=	1 ton (t)

6. Common metric and household equivalent values:

METRIC SYSTEM	U.S. HOUSEHOLD SYSTEM
1 meter	39.37 inches or 1.1 yard

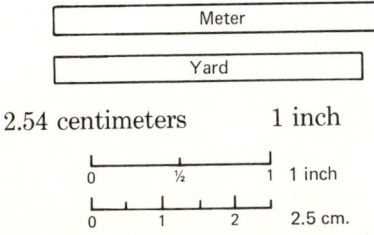

Meter

Yard

2.54 centimeters   1 inch

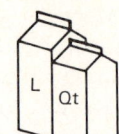

1 kilometer   0.6 miles

1 liter   1.06 qt.

7. 1 = i   6 = vi   11 = xi   16 = xvi
   2 = ii   7 = vii   12 = xii   17 = xvii
   3 = iii   8 = viii   13 = xiii   18 = xviii
   4 = iv   9 = ix   14 = xiv   19 = xix
   5 = v   10 = x   15 = xv   20 = xx

8. | RATIO | DECIMAL FRACTION | COMMON FRACTION |
   |---|---|---|
   | 1 : 2 | 0.5 | ½ |
   | 1 : 3 | 0.33 | ⅓ |
   | 3 : 4 | 0.75 | ¾ |

9.

a. $\frac{2}{3} \times \frac{3}{4} = x$

$\frac{2 \times 3}{3 \times 4} = \frac{6}{12} = \frac{1}{2}$

b. $\frac{1}{2} + \frac{2}{5} = x$

$\left(\frac{1}{2} \times \frac{5}{5}\right) + \left(\frac{2}{5} \times \frac{2}{2}\right) = \frac{5}{10} + \frac{4}{10} = \frac{9}{10}$

c. $\frac{3}{4} + \frac{5}{8} = x$

$\left(\frac{3}{4} \times \frac{2}{2}\right) + \frac{5}{8} = \frac{6}{8} + \frac{5}{8} = \frac{11}{8} = 1\frac{3}{8}$

d. $\frac{3}{4} - \frac{5}{8} = x$

$\left(\frac{3}{4} \times \frac{2}{2}\right) - \frac{5}{8} = \frac{6}{8} - \frac{5}{8} = \frac{1}{8}$

e. $\frac{3}{4} \div 2 = x$

$\frac{3}{4} \div \frac{2}{1} = \frac{3}{4} \times \frac{1}{2} = \frac{3}{8}$

f. $\frac{3}{4} \times 2 = x$

$\frac{3}{4} \times \frac{2}{1} = \frac{6}{4} = \frac{3}{2} = 1\frac{1}{2}$

g. $0.25 \times 3.5 = x$

$x = 0.875$

```
  0.25
 ×3.5
  125
  75
0.875
```

h. $8.5 \div 2.5 = x$

$x = 3.4$

```
      3.4
2.5)8.5
    7.5
    1.0
    1.0
      0
```

i. $1\frac{5}{8} - \frac{3}{4} = x$

$\left(\frac{8}{8} + \frac{5}{8}\right) - \left(\frac{3}{4} \times \frac{2}{2}\right) = x$

$\frac{13}{8} - \frac{6}{8} = \frac{7}{8} = x$

$x = 0.875$

```
    .875
8)7.000
  6.4
   .600
   .56
   .040
   .040
      0
```

j. $3x + 5 = 20$

$3x = 15$

$x = \frac{15}{3} = 5$

k. $6x - 12 = 4x$

$6x - 4x - 12 = 0$

$6x - 4x = 12$

$2x = 12$

$x = \frac{12}{2} = 6$

l. $10 \times \frac{3}{21} \times \frac{8}{3} \times \frac{14}{30} = x$

$\overset{2}{10} \times \frac{\cancel{3}^{1}}{\cancel{21}_{3}} \times \frac{\cancel{8}^{4}}{\cancel{3}_{1}} \times \frac{\cancel{14}^{2}}{\cancel{30}_{6_{3}}} = x$

$\frac{8 \times 2}{3 \times 3} = \frac{16}{9} = x$

$x = 1.64$

10. Mucous membranes consist of a layer of epithelium supported by a layer of connective tissue, designed for secretion of mucus or for absorption of substances through the membrane into the body.

11. The external nose is a triangular cartilaginous pyramid that rests against the bony face. It has two orifices called the nostrils or nares which are separated externally by the columella nasi. The

nasal septum divides the nasal cavity into two halves, called fossae. The lateral walls of the nasal cavity contain three conchae (projections or turbinates). Along with the sphenoethnoid fossae, the conchi warm and filter inspired air. Four pair of paranasal sinuses are named for the bones in which they are located: maxillary, frontal, sphenoid, and ethmoid sinuses. They lighten the weight of the skull and serve as resonance chambers. The sinus cavities are connected with the nasal fossae through small openings, and their mucous membranes are continuous with that of the fossae. The internal auditory (eustachian) tube from the middle ear opens into the nasopharynx just posterior to the nasal conchae.

In a healthy individual, the nasal mucosa is moist, pink, and shiny.

12. The external ear consists of the external auditory canal (external acoustic meatus) that extends from the tympanic membrane to the auricle (external visible portion of the ear). The cartilaginous external ear outside the head is called the pinna, or auricle. The tragus is the cartilaginous projection of the external ear that is anterior to the external meatus of the ear.

The adult external auditory canal is an oval-shaped, tubular, somewhat S-shaped structure about 2.5 cm (1 in) long. In a child under three years it is directed upward inside the head. The canal is lined with skin, and hairs grow in the outer third portion. Sebaceous and apocrine sweat glands in the canal produce cerumen, which lubricates the canal and protects against entry of foreign bodies. Its acid pH inhibits the growth of fungi and bacteria. Cerumen is brown to black in dark-skinned people, yellow in people with light skin, and becomes darker when it is old.

In a healthy individual, the external auditory canal is pink, without lesions.

13. The eyeballs are contained within the bony cavities known as the orbits. The orbital opening is protected by the eyelids, and the elliptical opening between the eyelids is known as the palpebral fissure. The external eye cavity is lined with mucous membrane which forms two conjunctival sacs under the upper and lower eyelids. The cornea is a transparent structure on the anterior portion of the eyeball which covers the pupil and iris and joins the sclera or white portion of the eyeball. The cornea is very sensitive and easily injured.

Lacrimal glands in the upper outer portion of the eye constantly produce tears which continually bathe the eye. The fluid empties into the lacrimal ducts near the inner canthus (angular junction of the eyelids at either corner of the eye) and drains through the lacrimal sac and nasolacrimal duct into the nose.

Healthy conjunctiva is moist and pink in light-skinned persons and darker in dark-skinned persons. Some dark-skinned persons have a slightly brownish sclera.

14. See Keys to Entry Tests, Chapter 12, items 1 and 2, p. 1004

15. See Keys to Entry Tests, Chapter 10, items 5, 7, and 11, pp. 1002 and 1003.

16. Each alveolus is surrounded by a dense capillary network which lies in close contact with the alveolar wall, thus providing a vast surface area for exchange of oxygen and carbon dioxide and absorption of inhalant substances.

17. The epidermis is avascular and has no nerve fibers. The dermis contains a capillary plexus and many nerve endings. Subcutaneous tissue is a mixture of loose areolar connective and adipose tissue, with a capillary network and numerous nerve endings. Skeletal muscle tissue is highly vascular with specialized sensory nerve endings that are stimulated by muscle tension and pressure.

18. The vastas lateralis muscle is one of the four muscles comprising the quadriceps femoris. The vastas lateralis has its origin in the intertrochanteric line and inserts into the tibial tuberosity by the common quadriceps tendon. It works over one joint, that being the knee.

The rectus femoris is also part of the quadriceps femoris muscle. It has its origin in the inferior iliac spine and the ileum above the acetabulum. It works over two joints: the knee and hip.

The gluteus maximus is a thick, coarsely grained muscle that has its origins on the posterolateral iliac blade, sacrum, and coccyx; it inserts into the iliotibial fascia. The gluteus medius has its origin on the lateral surface of the iliac blade, and inserts into the lateral surface of the great trochanter. The gluteus minimus has its origins on the lateral surface of the ilium and its insertion into the anterior surface of the greater trochanter.

The deltoid muscle has its point of origin in the anterior border of the clavicle, lateral border of the acromion process, and the lower border of the scapular spine. Its convergent fibers insert into the deltoid tuberosity on the lateral humerus.

19. The *tunica adventitia,* the outer layer, is comprised of connective tissue that surrounds and supports the vein. The *tunica media,* the middle layer, contains nerve fibers and muscle and elastic tissues. The *tunica intima,* the smooth inner lining of the vein, is comprised of endothelial tissue.

20. Venous system valves are semilunar folds of the tunica intima layer. Their purpose is to keep the blood flowing toward the heart. Valves are detectable in individuals of all ages, but are found more easily in older people. Generally located at places where veins branch, valves feel like small lumps when palpated.

☐ CHAPTER 17

1. Cardiac output is determined by stroke volume and heart rate.

2. Ventilation is the movement of air in and out of the lungs. Respiration is the exchange of both oxygen and carbon dioxide at the alveolar and cellular level.
3. During atrial contraction, the tricuspid and mitral valves open as blood is pumped into the ventricles. The pulmonary and aortic valves are closed at this point. Next, the ventricles contract, opening the pulmonary and aortic valves. Blood is pumped into the pulmonary and systemic circulation. The tricuspid and mitral valves close to prevent backflow into the atria.
4. The coronary arteries fill during ventricular diastole.
5. Tidal volume is the amount of air that is exchanged during normal inspiration and expiration. A healthy male adult has a tidal volume of approximately 500 ml.
6. Inspiration is an active process. In response to impulses in the respiratory center, the chest cavity enlarges as the diaphragm contracts and the ribs elevate, creating a negative pressure within the intrapleural space and the alveoli. The pressure within the alveoli is then lower than the atmosphere, which causes air to enter the lungs until the pressures are equalized.

Expiration is normally a passive process in which air is expelled as the thorax recoils to its resting position. As the chest and lung capacity decreases, air within the lungs is compressed and flows toward the area of lesser pressure, which now is the atmosphere, until the pressures are again equalized.

Appendix II
Keys to Learning Activities

☐ LEARNING ACTIVITY A, CHAPTER 16 INTRODUCTION

$$3 \text{ mg} = 0.003 \text{ g}$$
$$50 \text{ mg} = 0.05 \text{ g}$$
$$250 \text{ mg} = 0.25 \text{ g}$$
$$6000 \text{ mg} = 6 \text{ g}$$
$$400 \text{ mg} = 0.4 \text{ g}$$
$$5 \text{ mg} = 0.005 \text{ g}$$

☐ LEARNING ACTIVITY B, CHAPTER 16 INTRODUCTION

	Abbreviation	Symbol
twelve minims	12 m	m̃ x̄īī
two fluidounces	2 foz	f℥ īī
four fluidrams	4 fdr	f℥ īv
two and one-half grains	2½ gr	gr īīss
1/60 grain	1/60 gr	

☐ LEARNING ACTIVITY 71-A

FACTOR-LABEL METHOD:

1. $160 \text{ mg} \times \dfrac{1 \text{ capsule}}{40 \text{ mg}} = x \text{ (capsules)}$

   $\cancel{160}^{4} \text{ m\cancel{g}} \times \dfrac{1 \text{ capsule}}{\cancel{40}_{1} \text{ m\cancel{g}}} = x \text{ (capsules)}$

   $\dfrac{4 \times 1 \text{ capsule}}{1} = x$

   $x = 4 \text{ capsules}$

2. $400 \text{ mg} \times \dfrac{1 \text{ g}}{1000 \text{ mg}} \times \dfrac{5 \text{ ml}}{0.2 \text{ g}} = x \text{ (ml)}$

   $\cancel{400}^{2} \text{ m\cancel{g}} \times \dfrac{1 \text{ \cancel{g}}}{\cancel{1000}_{200} \text{ m\cancel{g}}} \times \dfrac{\cancel{5}^{1} \text{ ml}}{0.2 \text{ \cancel{g}}} = x \text{ (ml)}$

   $\dfrac{2 \times 1 \text{ ml}}{0.2} = x$

   $x = 10 \text{ ml}$

3. (NOTE: $1\frac{1}{2} = \frac{3}{2}$)

   $\dfrac{3}{2} \text{ gr} \times \dfrac{60 \text{ mg}}{1 \text{ gr}} \times \dfrac{1 \text{ tablet}}{30 \text{ mg}} = x \text{ (tablets)}$

   $\dfrac{3}{\cancel{2}_{1}} \text{ \cancel{gr}} \times \dfrac{\cancel{60}^{2} \text{ m\cancel{g}}}{1 \text{ \cancel{gr}}} \times \dfrac{1 \text{ tablet}}{\cancel{30}_{1} \text{ m\cancel{g}}} = x \text{ (tablets)}$

   $\dfrac{3 \times 1 \text{ tablet}}{1} = x$

   $x = 3 \text{ tablets}$

4. $\dfrac{1}{20} \text{ gr} \times \dfrac{64 \text{ mg}}{1 \text{ gr}} \times \dfrac{5 \text{ ml}}{8 \text{ mg}} = x \text{ (ml)}$

   $\dfrac{1}{\cancel{20}_{4}} \text{ \cancel{gr}} \times \dfrac{\cancel{64}^{8} \text{ m\cancel{g}}}{1 \text{ \cancel{gr}}} \times \dfrac{\cancel{5}^{1} \text{ ml}}{\cancel{8}_{1} \text{ m\cancel{g}}} = x \text{ (ml)}$

   $\dfrac{2 \times 1 \text{ ml}}{1} = x$

   $x = 2 \text{ ml}$

PROPORTION EQUATION METHOD:

1. $\dfrac{160 \text{ mg}}{x \text{ capsules}} = \dfrac{40 \text{ mg}}{1 \text{ capsule}}$

   $40 x = 160$

   $x = 4 \text{ capsules}$

1013

2. (NOTE: 0.2 g = 200 mg)

$$\frac{400 \text{ mg}}{x \text{ ml}} = \frac{200 \text{ mg}}{5 \text{ ml}}$$

$$200x = 2000$$

$$x = 10 \text{ ml}$$

3. CONVERSION:

(NOTE: $1\frac{1}{2} = \frac{3}{2}$)

$$\frac{\frac{3}{2} \text{ gr}}{x \text{ mg}} = \frac{1 \text{ gr}}{60 \text{ mg}}$$

$$\frac{3}{2} \times 60 = x$$

$$x = 90 \text{ mg (equivalent to gr } 1\frac{1}{2})$$

DOSAGE CALCULATION:

$$\frac{90 \text{ mg}}{x \text{ tablets}} = \frac{30 \text{ mg}}{1 \text{ tablet}}$$

$$30x = 90$$

$$x = 3 \text{ tablets}$$

4. CONVERSION:

$$\frac{\frac{1}{20} \text{ gr}}{x \text{ mg}} = \frac{1 \text{ gr}}{60 \text{ mg}}$$

$$x = \frac{1}{20} \times 60$$

$$x = 3 \text{ mg (equivalent to gr } 1/20)$$

DOSAGE CALCULATION:

$$\frac{3 \text{ mg}}{x \text{ ml}} = \frac{8 \text{ mg}}{5 \text{ ml}}$$

$$8x = 15$$

$$x = 1\frac{7}{8} = 2 \text{ ml (approx)}$$

☐ LEARNING ACTIVITY 73-A

FACTOR-LABEL METHOD:

1. $75 \text{ mg} \times \dfrac{1 \text{ ml}}{50 \text{ mg}} = x \text{ (ml)}$

$$\overset{3}{\cancel{75}} \text{ mg} \times \frac{1 \text{ ml}}{\underset{2}{\cancel{50}} \text{ mg}} = x \text{ (ml)}$$

$$x = \frac{3}{2} = 1.5 \text{ ml}$$

2. $15{,}000 \text{ U} \times \dfrac{1 \text{ ml}}{20{,}000 \text{ U}} = x \text{ (ml)}$

$$\overset{3}{\cancel{15{,}000}} \text{ U} \times \frac{1 \text{ ml}}{\underset{4}{\cancel{20{,}000}} \text{ U}} = x \text{ (ml)}$$

$$\frac{3 \times 1 \text{ ml}}{4} = x$$

$$\frac{3 \text{ ml}}{4} = x$$

$$x = 0.75 \text{ ml}$$

(NOTE: 0.75 ml × 16 minims/ml = 12 minims)

3. $\dfrac{1}{8} \text{ gr} \times \dfrac{64 \text{ mg}}{1 \text{ gr}} \times \dfrac{1 \text{ ml}}{16 \text{ mg}} = x \text{ (ml)}$

$$\underset{1}{\cancel{\tfrac{1}{8}}} \text{ gr} \times \frac{\overset{8}{\cancel{64}} \text{ mg}}{1 \text{ gr}} \times \frac{1 \text{ ml}}{\underset{2}{\cancel{16}} \text{ mg}} = x \text{ (ml)}$$

$$\frac{1 \times 1 \text{ ml}}{2} = x$$

$$x = 0.5 \text{ ml}$$

4. $300 \text{ mg} \times \dfrac{1.5 \text{ ml}}{250 \text{ mg}} = x \text{ (ml)}$

$$\overset{6}{\cancel{300}} \text{ mg} \times \frac{\overset{0.3}{\cancel{1.5}} \text{ ml}}{\underset{1}{\cancel{250}} \text{ mg}} = x \text{ (ml)}$$

$$6 \times 0.3 \text{ ml} = x \text{ (ml)}$$

$$x = 1.8 \text{ ml}$$

PROPORTION EQUATION METHOD:

1. $\dfrac{75 \text{ mg}}{x \text{ ml}} = \dfrac{50 \text{ mg}}{1 \text{ ml}}$

$$50x = 75$$

$$x = 1.5 \text{ ml}$$

2. $\dfrac{15{,}000 \text{ U}}{x \text{ ml}} = \dfrac{20{,}000 \text{ U}}{1 \text{ ml}}$

$$20{,}000x = 15{,}000$$

$$x = 0.75 \text{ ml}$$

(NOTE: 0.75 ml × 16 minims/ml = 12 minims)

APPENDIX II **1015**

3. CONVERSION:

$$\frac{\frac{1}{8} \text{ gr}}{x \text{ mg}} = \frac{1 \text{ gr}}{64 \text{ mg}}$$

$$x = \frac{1}{8} \times 64$$

$$x = 8 \text{ mg (equivalent to 1/8 grain)}$$

DOSAGE CALCULATION:

$$\frac{8 \text{ mg}}{x \text{ ml}} = \frac{16 \text{ mg}}{1 \text{ ml}}$$

$$16x = 8$$

$$x = 0.5 \text{ ml}$$

4. $\dfrac{300 \text{ mg}}{x \text{ ml}} = \dfrac{250 \text{ mg}}{1.5 \text{ ml}}$

$$250x = 450$$

$$x = 1.8 \text{ ml}$$

▢ LEARNING ACTIVITY 74-A

FACTOR-LABEL METHOD:

1. $\dfrac{1000 \text{ ml}}{8 \text{ hr}} \times \dfrac{1 \text{ hr}}{60 \text{ min}} \times \dfrac{15 \text{ drops}}{1 \text{ ml}} = x$ (drops/min)

$$\dfrac{\overset{125}{\cancel{1000} \text{ ml}}}{\underset{4}{\cancel{8} \text{ hr}}} \times \dfrac{1 \text{ hr}}{\underset{4}{\cancel{60} \text{ min}}} \times \dfrac{\overset{1}{\cancel{15} \text{ drops}}}{\underset{1}{\cancel{1} \text{ ml}}} = x \text{ (drops/min)}$$

$$\dfrac{125 \times 1 \text{ drop}}{4 \text{ min}} = x$$

$$x = 31.25 = 32 \text{ drops/min (approx)}$$

2. $\dfrac{1000 \text{ ml}}{8 \text{ hr}} = x$ (ml/hr)

$$x = 125 \text{ ml/hr}$$

3. $\dfrac{1000 \text{ ml}}{6 \text{ hr}} \times \dfrac{1 \text{ hr}}{60 \text{ min}} \times \dfrac{12 \text{ drops}}{1 \text{ ml}} = x$ (drops/min)

$$\dfrac{\overset{100}{\overset{200}{\cancel{1000} \text{ ml}}}}{\underset{3}{\cancel{6} \text{ hr}}} \times \dfrac{1 \text{ hr}}{\underset{5}{\cancel{60} \text{ min}}} \times \dfrac{\overset{1}{\cancel{12} \text{ drops}}}{\underset{1}{\cancel{1} \text{ ml}}} = x \text{ (drops/min)}$$

$$\dfrac{100 \times 1 \text{ drop}}{3 \times 1 \text{ min}} = x$$

$$\dfrac{100 \text{ drops}}{3 \text{ min}} = x$$

$$x = 33.33 = 34 \text{ drops/min (approx)}$$

4. $\dfrac{1000 \text{ ml}}{10 \text{ hr}} \times \dfrac{1 \text{ hr}}{60 \text{ min}} \times \dfrac{60 \text{ drops}}{1 \text{ ml}} = x$ (drops/min)

$$\dfrac{\overset{100}{\cancel{1000} \text{ ml}}}{\underset{1}{\cancel{10} \text{ hr}}} \times \dfrac{1 \text{ hr}}{\underset{1}{\cancel{60} \text{ min}}} \times \dfrac{\overset{1}{\cancel{60} \text{ drops}}}{\underset{1}{\cancel{1} \text{ ml}}} = x \text{ (drops/min)}$$

$$\dfrac{100 \times 1 \text{ drop}}{1 \text{ min}} = x$$

$$x = 100 \text{ drops/min}$$

TRADITIONAL METHOD:

1. $\dfrac{1000 \text{ ml}}{8 \text{ hr} \times 60 \text{ min}} \times \dfrac{15 \text{ drops}}{1 \text{ ml}} = x$ (drops/min)

$$\dfrac{15{,}000}{480} = x$$

$$x = 31.25 = 32 \text{ drops/min (approx)}$$

2. $\dfrac{1000 \text{ ml}}{8 \text{ hr}} = 125$ ml/hr

3. $\dfrac{1000 \text{ ml}}{6 \text{ hr} \times 60 \text{ min}} \times \dfrac{12 \text{ drops}}{1 \text{ ml}} = x$ (drops/min)

$$\dfrac{12{,}000}{360} = x$$

$$x = 33.33 = 34 \text{ drops/min (approx)}$$

4. $\dfrac{1000 \text{ ml}}{10 \text{ hr} \times 60 \text{ min}} \times \dfrac{60 \text{ drops}}{1 \text{ ml}} = x$ (drops/min)

$$\dfrac{60{,}000}{600} = x$$

$$x = 100 \text{ drops/min}$$

▢ LEARNING ACTIVITY 74-B

1. $\dfrac{100 \text{ ml}}{20 \text{ min}} \times \dfrac{15 \text{ drops}}{1 \text{ ml}} = x$ (drops/min)

$$\dfrac{\overset{25}{\cancel{100} \text{ ml}}}{\underset{4}{\cancel{20} \text{ min}}} \times \dfrac{\overset{3}{\cancel{15} \text{ drops}}}{\underset{1}{\cancel{1} \text{ ml}}} = x \text{ (drops/min)}$$

$$\dfrac{25 \times 3 \text{ drops}}{1 \text{ min}} = x$$

$$x = 75 \text{ drops/min}$$

2. $\dfrac{75 \text{ ml}}{20 \text{ min}} \times \dfrac{12 \text{ drops}}{1 \text{ ml}} = x \text{ (drops/min)}$

$\dfrac{\overset{15}{\cancel{75}} \cancel{\text{ml}}}{\underset{\cancel{5}}{\cancel{20} \text{ min}}} \times \dfrac{\overset{3}{\cancel{12}} \text{ drops}}{1 \cancel{\text{ml}}} = x \text{ (drops/min)}$

$\dfrac{15 \times 3 \text{ drops}}{1 \text{ min}} = x$

$x = 45 \text{ drops/min}$

3. $\dfrac{50 \text{ ml}}{60 \text{ min}} \times \dfrac{60 \text{ drops}}{1 \text{ ml}} = x \text{ drops/min}$

$\dfrac{50 \cancel{\text{ml}}}{\underset{1}{\cancel{60} \text{ min}}} \times \dfrac{\overset{1}{\cancel{60}} \text{ drops}}{1 \cancel{\text{ml}}} = x \text{ (drops/min)}$

$\dfrac{50 \times 1 \text{ drop}}{1 \text{ min}} = x$

$x = 50 \text{ drops/min}$

4. **FACTOR-LABEL METHOD:**

$\dfrac{100 \text{ ml}}{30 \text{ min}} \times \dfrac{60 \text{ min}}{1 \text{ hr}} = x \text{ (ml/hr)}$

$\dfrac{100 \text{ ml}}{\underset{1}{\cancel{30} \text{ min}}} \times \dfrac{\overset{2}{\cancel{60} \text{ min}}}{1 \text{ hr}} = x \text{ (ml/hr)}$

$\dfrac{100 \text{ ml} \times 2}{1 \text{ hr}} = x$

$x = 200 \text{ ml/hr}$

TRADITIONAL CALCULATION:
(NOTE: 30 min = 0.5 hr)

$\dfrac{100 \text{ ml}}{0.5 \text{ hr}} = \dfrac{x \text{ ml}}{1 \text{ hr}}$

$0.5x = 100$

$x = 200 \text{ ml/hr}$

INDEX

Letters after page numbers represent figures (F) and tables (T).

Abdomen
 appraisal of, 561, 565–568F
 auscultation, 567
 inspection, 566
 palpation of, 172F, 567–568
 percussion, 567
 binder, 456, 459F
 distension of, 568
 injection in, 892
Abdominal thrust, in conscious adult, 990, 991F
Abduction, 705
Abortion, values and, 35
Acceptance
 definition of, 10
 experiencing activity, 11
 helping relationship and, 10–11
 nurse's attitude of, 42
Accountability
 legal, nursing records and, 158
 record keeping and, 141
Acetic acid, in wet-to-dry dressing, 351–355
Acidosis, cardiopulmonary arrest and, 972
Actions
 self-awareness and, 20F
 values and activity on, 33
Activity, food history and, 505
Adduction, 705
Adhesive skin closure, 312F
Adhesive tape
 cotton cloth-backed, 300
 in cast care, 477
 in oxygen administration, 793
 in wet-to-dry dressing, 345
 in wound repair, 299–301F
 IV infusion and, 950F
 paper, 300
 rayon taffeta, 300
 removal, 300
 strapping, 300
 tearing, 330F
 total parenteral nutrition and, 552
Adipose tissue, 224
Administration set
 in IV therapy 941–942, 942F
 changing of, 955–956
Admitting nursing, assessment, 109F
Advanced Cardiac Life Support, 969
Advice
 experiences with activity, 103
 giving of, 103

open questions and, 92
 unsolicited, 103
Aerobic culture tube, wound specimen collection and, 322F
Aerosol, 867, 868T
Affect, 47
Affection, psychological needs and, 25
After meal care, 512
Age
 defecation and, 590
 fluids and, 483
 self-disclosure and, 36
Aging
 atelectasis and, 774
 skin and, 362
Air, in tracheobronchoalveolar system, 776
Air bubble, in IV infusion, 946
Air embolism
 IV therapy and, 936
 total parenteral nutrition and, 550
Air leak, in sphygmomanometer, 215F
Airway
 artificial patent. *See* Tracheostomy
 emergency maintenance of, 810
 obstruction. *See* Obstructed airway, removal of
 opening of
  in children, 982
  in CPR, 974
  technique, 976–977, 977F
 suctioning. *See* Airway suctioning
Airway obstruction, removal of. *See* Obstructed airway, removal of
Airway resistance, postural drainage and, 779
Airway suctioning
 adverse effects of, 816
 auscultation in, 816
 catheters for, 817F
 client preparation, 818–819
 collection reservoirs, 817
 critical points summary, 823
 data base, 816
 equipment, 817F
  preparation, 819
 execution, 818–823
 inspection in, 816
 introduction, 815
 laryngectomy and, 815
 learning activities, 823
 lower, 815
 moble unit for, 817F

nasopharyngeal route, 815, 819
 oropharyngeal route, 815, 819
 performance checklist, 824–825
 physical appraisal skills, 816
 pipeline systems, 817
 preparation, 815–818
 recording
  sample narrative, 823
  sample POR, 823
 review questions, 823–824
 routes for, 815
 self-, 822–823
 skill sequence, 821–822
 source for, 817
 specimen collection containers, 818F
 sputum specimen collection and, 816
 student objectives, 815
 T-connectors, 818
 teaching self-, 822–823
 techniques, 819–822, 820F
  skill sequence, 821–822
 tracheostomy and, 815, 820F, 821
 tracheostomy tube and, 822–823
 upper, 815
 Y-connectors, 818
Albumin
 in nutritional assessment, 506T, 507
 IV, 933
Alcohol
 handwashing and, 242
 in thermal applications, 440
 in thermometer cleaning, 186
Alcohol swab, injection and, 901
Algor mortis, 425
Allergic reaction, to adhesive tape, 301
Alopecia, 399
Alveoli
 airway suctioning and, 816
 collapse, 774, 816
Ambulation. *See also* Crutches
 canes, 694F, 699
 client assistance with, 698–701
 client history and, 693
 clinical history of, 693
 conditioning exercises and, 692–693
 critical points summary, 702
 crutches, 694–695, 695F, 700–701
 dangling, 693
 dangling assistance, 696–697
 data base for, 693–694
 equipment for, 694–695F
 execution, 695–701
 gait and, 693, 699F, 700F, 701F

Ambulation (cont.)
  gait belt, 695, 698F
  inspection of, 695
  introduction, 691
  isometric exercises, 692
  isotonic exercises, 692–693
  IV infusion and, 955
  learning activities, 702
  palpation in, 695
  performance checklist, 702–703
  phases of, 691–692
  physical appraisal skills in, 694
  preparation, 691–695
  recorded data and, 693
  recording, 701
  resistive exercises, 692
  review questions, 702
  skill sequence, 696–697
  standing, 697F
  student objectives, 691
  swing phase, 691–692
  walkers, 694, 695F, 699
  weight-bearing phase in, 691
  with devices, 698F
  without devices, 698F
American Hospital Formulary Service Drug Information, 844
American Journal of Nursing, 845
American Nurses' Association
  medication errors and, 843
  patient values and, 30
Amniotic membrane, in wound repair, 299
Ampule
  inhalation medication, 882F
  injection, 900, 901F
  medication removal from, 902, 905–908F
Anal area, inspection of, 869
Analgesic, tracheostomy and, 803
Ancillary support system, 142
Aneroid manometer, 214F, 216–217, 217F
Ankle
  dorsiflexion, 713F
  eversion, 713F
  ROM exercises for, 708, 713F
  performance checklist, 716
Anorexia, 501
Antecubital fossa, IV infusion in, 930
Antibiotic, wound infection and, 321
Anticholinergic agents, reflex inhibition and, 774
Antidecubitus pads
  donuts, 723
  foam, 723
  heel protectors, 723
  overhead cradles, 723
  plastic, 723
  sheepskin, 723
Antiembolism stockings, 456
Antihelminthic enema, 608
Antiseptic
  dermal administration of, 867
  handwashing and, 242–243
Anxiety
  personal space and, 62
  teaching-learning, 129
  urinary catheterization and, 634
Apical pulse, 197, 199F
  measurement of, 201
Apical-radial pulse, measurement of, 202
Apnea, 206

Apothecary system, 830
  abbreviations and symbols, 830
  activity, 830
  weights and measures, 830T
Appearance, nonverbal communication and, 47
Appetite, 500–501
  food consumption and, 502
Apprehension, of tracheostomy, 803
Approval, reflection of feelings and, 88
Aquathermia pad, 438F
Aqueous benzalkonium chloride, handwashing and, 242
Arm
  injection in, 892F
  muscle circumference, 507
  nutritional assessment and, 507
Armboard, in IV therapy, 944
Armpit
  temperature measurement via, 184, 185F
  techniques, 189
Ascites, 487
Asepsis
  definition of, 239
  medical
    definition of, 239
    entry test, 240–241
    handwashing and, 241–248
    introduction, 239
    isolation technique, 248–266
  surgical
    definition of, 267
    drains and, 328–342
    dressing and, 292–311
    gloves and, 286–292
    injectable medication and, 923–924
    introduction, 267–268
    irrigations and, 328–342
    sterile supplies, 268–285
    suture removal and, 311–318
    wet sterile dressings, 343–351
    wet-to-dry dressings, 351–355
    wound care and, 292–311
    wound culture collection and, 318–328
Aseptic technique
  definition of, 267
  ear drop administration and, 885–886
  eye drop administration and, 886–887
  guidelines for, 275–276
  in dressing change, 302–303
  nose drop administration and, 884–885
  rectal suppositories and, 888–889
  topical administration and, 884–889
  tracheostomy and, 803
  vaginal medication and, 887–888
Asepto syringe
  in oral care, 390
  in wound irrigation, 331–332, 333F
Aspiration
  CPR and, 974
  swallowing and, 517
Aspiration pneumonia, enteral feeding and, 533
Assessment
  admitting history, 109F
  definition of, 107
  in nursing records, 150–151
  nursing history, 110F
Assessment interview, definition of, 107
Assistance
  activities

  assisting with decision making, 104
  experiences with giving advice, 103
  experiencing reassurance, 104
  genuine and false reassurance, 101
  simulation of reassurance, 104
advice as, 103
critical points summary, 104–105
decision making, 101–103
direct physical, 98–99, 105
execution, 103–104
experiences activity, 103
in decision making, 101–103
in problem solving, 101–102
in providing information, 102
introduction, 97–98
need for, 97
offering of, 97–105
performance checklist, 105
preparation, 98–103
problem solving, 101–102
providing information, 102
reassurance, 99–101
  false, 100–101
  genuine, 99–100
referrals as, 102
review questions, 105
self-disclosure as, 102
student objectives, 97
Asthma, hypoxemia and, 786
Atelectasis, 774
  absorption, 787
Atomizer, 870F
Atrial fibrillation, 195
Attending behavior
  activities
    experiencing and using, 73
    observing in others, 72
    simulations of, 73
  components of, 71–72
  counterproductive, 71, 73
  critical points summary, 73
  definition of, 69
  execution, 72–73
  experiencing and using activity, 73
  gestures and, 72
  introduction, 71
  observing activity, 72
  performance checklist, 74
  posture and, 71
  preparation, 71–72
  productive, 71, 73
  review questions, 73–74
  simulation activity, 73
  student objectives, 70–71
  verbal encouragement and, 72
Attentive listening. *See* Listening, attentive
Attitude
  helping relationship and, 11
  teaching-learning, 128
Audit, nursing, 149
Audit process, in record-keeping, 142–144, 143F
Auditory status, assessment of, 113F
Auscultation, 177–180
  critical points summary, 179
  equipment for, 178–179
  execution, 179
  in airway obstruction, 990
  in airway suctioning, 816
  in CPR, 976
  in eating assistance, 522
  in intubation, 567
  in nutritional assessment, 508T

INDEX 1019

in oxygen therapy, 788
in pulse measurement, 200F
in respiration appraisal, 208
in topical medication administration, 869
in wound culture specimen collection, 322
in wound drainage, 330–331
introduction, 177–178
learning activities, 180
of abdomen, 567
of blood pressure, 212F, 214
of breath sounds, 777–778F
of elimination, 595
of fluid balance, 492
of respiration, 780
of tracheostomy, 804
preparation, 178–179
review questions, 180
student objectives, 177
Auscultatory gap, in blood pressure measurement, 212F
Authority, external, helping relationship and, 10
Autonomy esteem and, 26
Awareness, self-understanding and, 22–23
Axilla
in breast examination, 419–420
temperature measurement via, 184, 185F
technique, 189

Back
injuries, 685
lower, pain, 685
massage
skill sequence, 450–451
technique, 449–451
strain, positioning and, 718
Back blow, 989
in conscious adult, 990F
in infant, 994F
in unconscious adult, 992
Back rub, creative use of, 64
Bacteria
in hand cream, 243
medical asepsis and 239
on thermometers, 186
resident, 241
total parenteral nutrition and, 549, 553
transient, 241–242
wound infection and, 319
Bacterial infection, of vagina, 412
Bag
drainage collection, 636
in IV therapy, 940F, 941
isolation precautions and, 260
rubber, in thermal application, 438
trash, dressing changes and, 302
Baking soda, in oral care, 389
Balance
body mechanics and, 686–687
clinical application of, 686–687
definition of, 686
standing and, 697
Baldness, 399
Balkan frame, 692F
Bandage
application. See Bandages and binders, applying

cotton flannel, 455
cotton gauze, 455
elastic, 456
gauze, 455
muslin, 455
stockinet, 456
Bandages and binders, applying
anchoring, 462
body alignment and, 454
care of, 462
circular turn in, 456–457, 457F
client history and, 455
client teaching, 462
clip in, 462
critical points summary, 463
data base, 455
definition, 454
equipment, 455–456
execution, 456–458, 457–458F
extensibility and, 454
factors affecting, 454–455
figure-of-eight turn in, 458F
flexibility and, 454
inspection in, 455
introduction, 454
learning activities, 463
palpation in, 455
performance checklist, 463–464
physical appraisal skills, 455
pin in, 462
porosity and, 454
preparation, 454–456
recorded data and, 455
recording
sample narrative, 462
sample POR, 462
recurrent turn in, 458F
reverse spiral turn in, 457F
review questions, 463
skill sequence, 461–462
skin protection and, 454–455
spica turn in, 458F
spiral turn in, 457F
student objectives, 453
tape in, 462
turns
circular, 456–457, 457F
figure-of-eight, 458F
recurrent, 458
reverse spiral, 457–458
spica, 458
spiral, 457
Barrier drape
in wet-to-dry dressing, 345
sterile field and, 279
Base of support, 686
clinical application of, 687
Basic care sheet, 152
Basic needs
activities
behavior in conflict, 27
behavior in success, 28
looking at basic needs, 25, 26F
and behavior in conflict, 27–28
awareness development, 28
concept of, 25–26
development level and, 26
development of, 25
growth, 25
identification, 24–30
critical points summary, 29
execution, 28–29
introduction, 25
preparation, 25–28

review questions, 29–30
student objectives, 24
looking at activity, 25, 26F
physiological, 25
psychological, 25
reciprocal relatedness of, 18
satisfaction of, 26–27
illness and, 28
self-concept and, 22, 27
values and, 27–28
special, interviewing and, 115–116
values and, 27–28, 31
Basin
emesis, 390, 573
in wet-to-dry dressing, 345
sterile, in wound irrigation, 332
Bath
blanket, 365, 720
cornstarch, 363
in thermal application, 441
medicated, 363
oatmeal, 363
sodium bicarbonate, 363
sponge, 441
whirlpool, 440
Bathing. See also Skin care
bed, 367
body temperature and, 183
execution, 366–369
performance checklist, 370–371
principles of, 362
skill sequence, 368–369
therapeutic, 362–363
Bathtub, skin care and, 365
Beard, grooming, 402
Bed
air fluidized, 724
air suspension, 723–724
alternating pressure air mattress, 723
anesthesia, 766–767, 767F
circle, 725–726, 726F
CircOlectric, 725–726, 726F
client positioning in, 718–720
CLINITRON, 724F
eating in, 511F
footboards, 723
Fowler's position in, 719
head-to-foot, making of, 767
KinAir, 723
lateral position in, 719
logrolling in, 737, 738F
making procedures. See Bed making
moving clients in, 727–730
skill sequence, 728–729
moving to side of, 728
occupied
making up, 759
performance checklist, 770–771
skill sequence, 765–766
positioning in, 730–737
prone position in, 718–719
semi-Fowler's in, 720F
shampooing in, 400F, 402, 403–404
Sims position in 719
supine position in, 718
Trendelenburg position in, 720F
reverse, 720F
turning client in, 730–737
unoccupied
making up, 759
performance checklist, 768–770
skill sequence, 762–765
water, 723
Bed bath, execution, 367–369

Bed linen, isolation precautions and, 252
Bed making
  anesthesia bed, 766–767, 767F
  client history and, 760
  critical points summary, 768
  data base, 760
  equipment, 760
  execution, 760–768
  handling linens in, 759
  head to foot, 767
  introduction, 757–758
  learning activities, 768
  occupied bed, 759
    performance checklist, 770–771
    skill sequence, 764–766
  performance checklist, 768–771
  preparation, 758–760
  recorded data and, 760
  recording, 767–768
    sample narrative, 768
    sample POR, 767
  review questions, 768
  skill sequence
    occupied bed, 764–766
    unoccupied bed, 762–764
  student objectives, 757
  types of, 758–759
  types of beds and, 758
  unoccupied bed, 759
    performance checklist, 768–770
    skill sequence, 762–764
Bedpans and urinals, 588–605, 595–596F
  assistance with, 597–598F, 600–601
  auscultation and, 595
  bowel elimination, 590
  cleaning, 595
  client history, 594
  covers, 595
  critical points summary, 601–602
  data base, 594–595
  definition of, 595, 596
  diarrhea, 593
  equipment, 595–596
  execution, 596–600
  feces appraisal, 591–592
  flushers, 595–596, 596F
  inspection, 594–595
  introduction 589
  learning activities, 602
  maintenance of, 595
  palpation, 595
  percussion, 595
  performance checklist, 602–604
  physical appraisal skills, 594–595
  physiological factors and, 589–590
  preparation, 589–596
  psychosocial factors and, 590–591
  recorded data and, 594
  recording
    sample narrative, 601
    sample POR, 601
  review questions, 602
  sense of smell and, 595
  skill sequence, 599–601
    assisting with bedpan, 599–600
    offering urinal, 600–601
  specimen testing and collection, 593–594
  student objectives, 587–588, 588–589
  urinary retention, 593
  urine appraisal, 591
  voiding difficulty, 592

  voiding inducement measures, 492–493
Bedspread, 760
Behavior
  attending. See Attending behavior
  definition of, 7, 19
  feelings and, 19
  limit setting for, 100
  -needs conflict, activity for, 27–28
  nonverbal. See Nonverbal communication
  paralinguistic, 48
  past experience and, 23
  reciprocal relatedness of, 18F
  "things I love to do" activity and, 32F
  trustworthiness and, 11–12
  values and, 32–33
Being-values, 25
Belonging, psychological needs and, 25
Belt
  gait, 695, 698F
  safety, 466–467
Benign disease, of breast, 419
Benzalkoniumchloride, aqueous handwashing and, 242
Bias, empathy and, 13–14
Bigeminy, of pulse, 195F
Binder
  abdominal, 456, 459F
  antiembolism stockings, 456
  application. See Bandages and binders, applying
  breast, 456, 459
  elastic stockings, 456, 460–467
  elasticized, 459
  scultetus, 459F
  sling, 456, 459–460
  T-, 456, 459
Binding
  of cast edges, 478F
  skill sequence, 478
Bite block, in oral care, 390
Bladder
  instillation of, 633
    execution, 649
    skill sequence, 650
  irrigation of, 633
    execution, 649
    performance checklist, 656–657
    skill sequence, 650
  training, 622
Blame, reflection of feelings and, 88
Blaming, 40
Blanching hyperemia, 360
Blanket, 760
  bathing, 365, 720
  enema and, 611
Bleeding
  IV therapy and, 936
  urinalysis and, 591
  wound repair and, 295
Blindness, neonatal, 787
Blood
  administration of, 960–961
  administration set, 945
  anatomic shunting of, 786
  collection of, 952–953
    skill sequence, 953
  frozen, 933
  in nutritional assessment, 506T, 507
  isolation precautions and, 258T, 259
  IV, 933
  occult. See Occult blood
  sample device, 944F

  warmer, 945
  whole, 933
Blood flow
  cardiac pump and, 973F
  compression and, 973–974
  mechanics of, 972–973, 973F
  thoracic pump and, 973F
Blood gas analysis, 786
Blood gases, 788
Blood pressure appraisal, 210–222
  assessment of, 114F
  auscultation in, 211–213, 212F, 219
  auscultatory gap, 212
  client history, 213–214
  critical points summary, 220–221
  data base for, 213–214
  diastolic, 212
  equipment for, 214–216F
  errors, 217–218
  execution, 217F, 218F
  fluid balance and, 486
  flush method of, 213
  introduction, 210–211
  isometric exercises and, 692
  Korotkoff sounds and, 211–212, 212F
  learning activities, 221
  palpation in, 213
  performance checklist, 221–222
  preparation, 211–217
  recorded data, 213–214
  recording of, 220F
  review questions, 221
  skill sequence, 219–220, 220F
  student objectives, 210
  systolic, 211–212
  thigh, 219
Blood urea nitrogen, fluid balance and, 489
Blood vessel, pulse and, 194
Blood volume, pulse and, 195–196
Body
  surface area of, dosage based on, 834
  topical medication administration to, 880
Body composition, 224
  water and, 483
Body fat, norms, 234T
Body height. See Height and weight
Body language, nonverbal communication and, 48
Body mechanics
  angular movement and, 688
  arc and, 688
  balance and, 686–687
  definition of, 686
  effort arm and, 688
  force and, 687
  friction and, 687
  fulcrum and, 688
  inertia and, 687
  levers and, 688
  momentum and, 687–688
  motion and, 687
  muscle movements and, 689
  principles of, 686–690
  resistance arm and, 688
  standing assistance and, 698
  weight and, 686
  work and, 688–689
Body, movement, physics concepts in, 690
Body odor, nonverbal communication and, 49
Body placement, in CPR, 978, 980F

Body position. *See* Turning, moving, and positioning
Body temperature. *See* Temperature
Body territory, 62
Body weight. *See* Height and weight
Boiling water disinfection, 271–272, 272T
Bottle, in IV therapy, 940F
Bounding pulse, 195–196
Bowel
  auscultation of, 567
  sounds of, 567
Bowel elimination procedures, 605–620. *See also* Enema
  auscultation in, 609
  client history and, 609
  common problems of, 606–607
  constipation, 606
  critical points summary, 617–618
  data base, 609
  enemas, 607–608
    execution, 612–614
    types of, 607–608
  equipment for, 609–611, 610–611F
  execution, 612–617, 613–615F
  fecal disimpaction, 615
  fecal incontinence, 607
  fecal impaction, 606
  flatulence, 606–607
  incontinence protection, 611F
  inspection in, 609
  introduction, 605–606
  learning activities, 618
  palpation in, 609
  percussion in, 609
  performance checklist, 618–619
  physical appraisal skills, 609
  preparation, 606–611
  recorded data, 609
  recording
    sample narrative, 617
    sample POR, 617
  rectal tube insertion, 614–615
  rectal tubes, 611
  review questions, 618
  sense of smell in, 609
  skill sequence, 616–617
  student objectives, 605
Bowel movement. *See* Defecation
Bowles chestpiece, 178F
Brachial pulse, 197, 198F
  measurement of, 202
Bradycardia, 195
  airway suctioning and, 816
Bradypnea, 206
Braiding, hair, 401
Breast
  benign disease of, 419
  binder, 456, 459
  cancer of, 417–424
  examination of. *See* Breast examination
  lesion of, 418–419
    mobility of, 418
  male, 418, 419
  masses, characteristics of, 418–419
  normal, characteristics of, 418
  pregnancy and, 418
  quadrants of, 418F
Breast examination
  bimanual technique, 421F
  breast cancer and, 417
  critical points summary, 423
  data base, 419
  equipment, 419
  execution 420F, 421F
  in males, 421
  inspection in, 419
  instruction, 421
  introduction, 417–418
  learning activities, 423
  palpation in, 419, 421
  performance checklist, 423–424
  physical appraisal skills, 419
  preparation, 418–419
  recording, 422–423
    sample narrative, 423
    sample POR, 422–423
  review questions, 423
  self-, teaching, 421–422
  skill sequence, 422
  student objectives, 417
Breath sounds, 207
  adventitious, 776
  auscultation of, 777F
  bronchial, 776
  bronchovesicular, 776
  crackles, 775, 776
  friction rub, 777
  rales, 776
  rhonchi, 776–777
  vesicular, 776
  wheezes, 775, 776–777
Breathing
  deep, 781
    execution of, 781
  diaphragmatic, 782F
  patterns, 774
  pursed lip, 782
    execution, 782
Bristle, toothbrush, 387
Bronchiole, normal hygiene of, 775
Bronchovesicular sounds, 776
Bronchus
  breath sounds, 775, 776
  normal hygiene of, 775
Brush, in nail care, 408
Bubble, in IV infusion, 946
Bulb syringe
  in oral care, 390
  in wound irrigation, 331–332, 333F
Burette
  in IV therapy, 941F
  in piggyback administration, 958
Burn dressing, 298
Butterfly closure, 312, 313F
Butterfly needle, 942–943, 943F
Buttock, injection in, 892

Calculation. *See* Dosage, drug, calculations
Calculus, dental, 386
Caliper, 228
  in skinfold measurement, 231, 232F, 233–234
Calories, tracheostomy and, 803
Candida albicans infection, 867
Candidiasis, of vagina, 412
Cane
  bent shaft, 694F
  -first gait, 699
  quad, 694F
  types of, 694
Cannula
  in IV therapy, 942–943, 943F
  nasal, 790F

Cantor tube, 570F, 571
Cap, isolation, 260
Cardiac arrest, physiology of, 972
Cardiac pump, 972–973, 973F
Cardiopulmonary arrest, physiology of, 972
Cardiopulmonary resuscitation
  adult techniques, 976–980
    cardiac compression in, 978–980
    compression to ventilation ratios, 980
    establishing open airway, 976–977
    skill sequence, 980
    ventilation and, 977–978
  airway opening, 974
  auscultation in, 976
  blood flow mechanisms, 972
  cardiac arrest, 972
  cardiac pump mechanisms, 972–973
  cardiopulmonary arrest and, 972
  client history and, 975
  complications of, 974–975
  compression and, 973–974
  courses in, 969
  critical points summary, 984–985
  data base, 975–976
  definition of, 971–972
  equipment, 976
  execution, 976–984
  in adult, 976–980, 977F, 979F, 980F
  in infants and children, 981–984, 980F, 983F
    cardiac compression in, 982–983
    compression to ventilation ratios, 983
    establishing open airway, 982
    performance checklist, 986
    skill sequence, 984
    ventilation, 982
  inspection in, 975
  introduction, 970–971
  learning activities, 985
  one-person rescue, 980, 985–986
  palpation in, 976
  performance checklist, 985–986
  physical appraisal skills, 975–976
  physiology of, 972–974, 973F
  preparation, 972–976
  pulmonary arrest, 972
  recorded data and, 975
  recording
    sample narrative, 994
    sample POR, 994
  review questions, 985
  skill sequence, 981, 984
    infant and child, 984
    one and two rescuer, 981
  student objectives, 971
  thoracic pump mechanisms, 973
  two-person rescue, 980
    performance checklist, 985–986
    skill sequence, 981
  ventilation mechanics, 974
  when to stop, 972
Cardiovascular system
  malnutrition and, 508T
  positioning and, 717
Caries, dental, 386
Caring
  definition, 14
  experiencing activity, 14
  helping relationship and, 14–15, 15F
  nurse's attitude of, 42
Carminative enema, 608

Carotid pulse, 197, 198F
Carpuject syringe, 908, 910F
Cart
  insulated meal, 509F
  medication, 838
Cartridge
  injection, 901, 908
  prefilled, 908
Cassette pump, in IV therapy, 944
Casts, care of
  application of, 474–475
  client and, 475
  client history and, 477
  client instructions, 475
  critical points summary, 479
  data base, 477
  drying plaster cast, 475
  equipment, 477
  execution, 477–479, 478F
  finishing edge of, 478F
  inspection, 477
  introduction, 474
  learning activity, 479
  mobility and, 476
  neurovascular status and, 475
  palpation, 477
  percussion, 477
  performance checklist, 480
  physical appraisal skills, 477
  physical problems, 475–476
  plaster, drying the, 475
  preparation, 474–477
  properties of, 474
  recorded data and, 477
  recording
    sample narrative, 479
    sample POR, 479
  removal, 476–477
  review questions, 479
  skill sequence, 478
  skin care and, 476
  stains due to, 476
  student objectives, 473–474
  types of, 474F
Catgut suture, 311
Catheter
  balloon, 633, 636F
  external, 622–624F
    performance checklist, 628
    skill sequence
      application of external catheter, 626
  Foley, 630
    Tamper-Evident Seal, 633
  hydrophilic BN–74 coating on, 633
  in IV therapy, 943F
  nasal, 790, 791F
  over-the-needle, 943F
  suction, 817F
  suprapubic, 630
  through-the-needle, 943F
  urinary. See Urinary catheterization
Catheter drainage system kit, 637, 638F
Catheterization, urinary. See Urinary catheterization
Celsius temperature, 182–183
Center for Disease Control, isolation guidelines of, 255–256F, 257–258T
Center of gravity, 686
Central vein, infusion in, 930
Cerebrovascular accident, oral medication and, 856
Cerumen, removal of, 361
Cervical vertebrae, pivot joint, 706

Challenge, teaching-learning, 128
Chart holder, 145F
Charting. See Record, preparation
Chemical pack, in thermal application, 439
Chemical probe thermometer, 187F
  technique, 190–191, 191F
Chemical reaction, to adhesive tape, 301
Chemical sterilization, liquid, 271
Chemotherapy, hair growth and, 298
Chest
  anatomy of, 199F
  percussion of, 175F
  restraint, 467, 468F
Chest compression
  blood flow and, 973–974
  in adults, 978–980
  in children, 982–983, 983F
  in CPR, 978
Chest therapy exercises
  auscultation and, 780
  breath sounds and, 776–777
    auscultation of, 777
  breathing
    deep, 781
    diaphragmatic, 782F
    pursed lip, 782
  bronchial hygiene and, 775
  client history and, 779–780
  coughing, 781
    performance checklist, 784
    skill sequence, 782
  critical points summary, 783
  data base, 779–780
  deep breathing, 777–778, 781
  diaphragmatic breathing, 782F
  equipment, 780F
  execution, 781–783
  incentive spirometry, 781
  inspection and, 780
  introduction, 774
  learning activities, 783
  percussion and, 779
  performance checklist, 784
  physical appraisal skills and, 780
  postural drainage, 779
  preparation, 774–781
  preventive respiratory exercises, 777–778
  pursed lip breathing, 782
  recorded data and, 779–780
  recording
    sample narrative, 783
    sample POR, 783
  respiratory exercises
    preventive, 777–778
    restorative, 778–779
  respiratory system appraisal and, 776–777
  restorative respiratory exercises, 778–779
  retained secretions and, 775, 776
  review questions, 783–784
  skill sequence, 782
  sputum and, 775–776
  student objectives, 774
  tracheostomy and, 803
  vibration and, 779
Chest thrust
  in conscious adult, 990, 991F
  in infant, 994
  in unconscious adult, 992
Chestpiece
  Bowles, 178F

  of stethoscope, 178F
  open bell, 178F
Chewing
  evaluation of, 518
  facilitating use of, 520F, 521F
Cheyne-Stokes respiration, 206, 207F
Childbirth, urinary catheterization and, 630
Children
  airway obstruction removal in, 994F
  CPR in, 981–984, 982F, 983F
  dosage calculations for, 834
  self-worth development in, 21
  space and, 61
  touch and, 63
  urinary catheterization in, 632
  urine meter for, 636–637
  ventilation in, 982
Chin lift, in CPR, 974, 976–977, 977F
Chin strap, on corpse, 427F
Chronic obstructive lung disease, diaphragmatic breathing and, 778
Circulation
  assessment of, 114F
  CPR complications and, 974
  fibrosis and, 705
  massage and, 446–447
  pulse and, 194
  topical medication and, 866
  Trendelenberg position and, 720
Circulatory overload, IV therapy and, 936
Circumduction, 705
Clarification, open questions and, 92
Clean activity, definition of, 243–244
Cleaning
  concurrent, 253
  of wound, 303–304, 304F
  terminal, 253
Cleanliness, definition of, 267
Clear liquid diet, 504
Cliche's, reassurance and, 100
Client
  capability of, 129–130
  cast instructions for, 475
  combative, 470
  energy of, 129
  motivation for teaching-learning, 128–129
  psychiatric, 470
  restrained, 470
Client history. See Medical history
Clinical nursing, introduction, 165–167
Clip, in bandaging and binding, 462
Clipper, in nail care, 408
Cloth, sterile, 273
Clothing
  isolation, 250, 253
  nonverbal communication and, 47
Clubbing, nail, 407F
Code of nurses, on patient values, 30
Cold
  clinical uses of, 437
  contraindications, 436
  physiological effects of, 435
  systemic effects of, 436
Cold sterilization, 271
Collagen, function of, 359
Collection chamber
  in Gomco Thermotic pump, 572
  in pipeline suction, 571, 572F
Colon, irrigation of, 609
Colostomy. See also Ostomy care
  irrigation, 675–678, 676–678F
    performance checklist, 682–683

skill sequence, 678–680
Combative client, mechanical restraint in, 470
Comfort
  assessment of, 114F, 115
  bedpans and, 597
  teaching-learning and, 129
Commitment
  caring and, 14
  in teaching-learning, 134
Communication
  blaming and, 40
  computing and, 40
  definition of, 2
  distraction and, 40
  in clinical nursing, 165
  interpersonal model of, 3F
  interviewing and, 117F
  intrapersonal model of, 2, 3F
  leveling in, 40
  metal-, 3
  nonverbal. See Nonverbal communication
  nursing and, 1–3
  patterns of, 41
  placating and, 40
  process, 2–3, 3F
  self-disclosure activity on, 41
  self-disclosure and, 40–41
  verbal
    -nonverbal congruence, 51
    tracheostomy and, 803
  written, 141–163
    characteristics of, 141
    health record use, 141–148
    nursing records, 148–163
Communication skills,
  facilitative, 69–105
  introduction, 1
  learning, 3–4
Communication system, purpose of, 142
Community-acquired infection, definition of, 239
Competence, technical, 100
Compress,
  in thermal application, 439, 440–441
  in wet-to-dry dressing, 345
Compression
  chest. See Chest compression
  in massage, 447
Compression to ventilation ratio, in CPR, 980
Computer, unit-dose medication and, 837
Contaminated material, disposal of, 250–251, 251F
Conditioning exercises, 692–693
Conduction, heat, 434
Cones, 722
Confidentiality, nurse-client relationship and, 9
Conflict
  behavior-needs activity in, 27–28
  reflection of content and, 80
  value, 34
Confusion, self-disclosure and, 39–40
Congruence, 39
Connective tissue
  fibrosis, 705
  ROM exercises and, 705
Consciousness
  airway obstruction removal and, 990F, 991F
  fluid balance and, 489
  swallowing dysfunction and, 518

Consent sheet, 146
Constipation, 606
  enteral feeding and, 533
Container
  calibrated, 493
  in IV therapy, 940F
    changing of, 955
  insulated, food service and, 509F, 510F
Contaminated activity, definition of, 243
Contaminated material, disposal of, 250–251, 251F
Contamination, definition of, 267
Content, reflection of, 79–84
  activities,
    experiencing and using, 83
    ineffective, 82
    reflecting content statements, 81
    simulations, 83
  critical points summary, 84
  effective, 80–81
  empathetic response and, 80
  examples of, 82
  execution, 82–83
  experiencing and using activity, 83
  function of, 79
  ineffective, 81–82
  introduction, 79–80
  negotiations and, 80
  performance checklist, 84
  preparation, 80–82
  review questions, 84
  simulation activity, 83
  student objectives, 79
  validating and, 80
Continuous suture, removal of, 316
Control, time and, 56
Controlled substances
  administration of, 843
  oral administration of, 854
  packaging of, 843, 844F
  sign-out sheet, 845F
Convection, 434
Conversion, heat, 434
Cornstarch bath, 363
Corpse, care of
  chin strap, 427F
  client history and, 426
  collecting valuables, 427
  comforting survivors, 426
  critical points summary, 429
  data base, 426
  death papers, 426
  definition of, 425
  equipment, 426
  execution, 426–429, 427F
  introduction, 425
  learning activities, 429
  performance checklist, 430–431
  physiological changes and, 425–426
  preparation, 425–426
  recorded data and, 426
  recording
    sample narrative, 429
    sample POR, 429
  review questions, 429–430
  shroud packs, 426
  shrouding and transferring, 427–429
  skill sequence, 428
  student objectives, 425
Cotton cloth-backed tape, 299–301F
Cotton flannel bandage, 455
Cotton gauze bandage, 455
Coughing, execution of, 781

Council of State Boards of Nursing, medication errors and, 843
Counseling, cultural variables in, 10
CPR. See Cardiopulmonary resuscitation
Crab lice, 399
Crackles, 775, 776
Cramping, enema and, 613
Cream
  bathing, 366
  topical, 868T
Crust, definition of, 360, 363F
Crutches
  auxillary, 695F
  base of support for, 700F
  four-point gait and, 700F
  gait and, 700–701
  Lofstrand, 695F
  measuring for, 700
  narrative recording sample, 701
  platform, 695F
  POR recording sample, 701
  swing-through gait and, 701F
  swing-to gait and, 701F
  three-point gait and, 700F
  two-point gait and, 699–701, 699F
  types of, 694–695, 695F
  using, 699–700, 699F
Cryotherapy, 434
Culture
  eating and, 481
  eye contact and, 47, 72
  food consumption and, 502
  helping concept and, 10
  nonverbal communication and, 47, 49–50
  personal space and, 63
  self-disclosure and, 36
  touch and, 63
  wound. See Wound culture specimen collection
Culture and sensitivity test, wound infection and, 321
Culture tube, wound specimen collection and, 322F, 323F
Curity thermal system, in wet-to-dry dressing, 346F
Cyanosis, 786
  appearance of, 364
  definition of, 359

Dakin's solution, in wet-to-dry dressing, 345
Damping, in percussion, 174
Dangling, 693
  assisting, 695, 696F
  performance checklist, 702–703
  recording, 700–701
  skill sequence, 696–697
  stages of, 696
  steps for, 696–697
Data base, in record-keeping, 143F
Death, comforting survivors after, 426
Death papers, 426
Debridement, wound repair and, 351
Decay, tooth, 386
Deciduous teeth, 385
Decision making
  alternative solutions in, 102
  assisting with, 101–103, 104
  experiencing activity, 104
  follow-up on, 102–103
  giving advice and, 103

Decision making (cont.)
   problem-solving approach to, 101–102
   providing information for, 102
   referrals and, 102
   self-disclosure and, 102
   simulation activity, 104
Deconditioning, 691
Decubitus ulcer, positioning and, 718.
      See also Sore, pressure
Defecation
   habit pattern of, 590
   isometric exercises and, 692
   Valsalva's maneuver and, 590
Deglutition. See Swallowing
Dehiscence, wound repair and, 295F
Dehydration, hyperosmolar, 533
Deltoid muscle, injection in, 893, 894F
Dennis tube, 570F, 571
Dental caries, 386
Dental pulp, 385
Dentin, 385
Dentist, medication order by, 834
Dentrifice, in oral care, 389
Dentures, care of, 392F
Denture cup, 389
Dependence, enema and, 608
Dependent edema, 488
Depersonalization
   communication skills and, 2
   personal space and, 63
Depression, nonverbal communication and, 48
Dermis, 359
Development, self-concept and, 22
Dextran, IV, 933–934
Dextrose solution, IV, 931–933, 932T
Diabetes insipidus, 866
Diabetic therapy and education sheet, 136–137F, 152, 155F
Diagnostic testing, defecation and, 590
Diarrhea, definition of, 593
Diastolic blood pressure, measurement of, 212
Diet
   assessment of, 113F
   clear liquid, 504
   defecation and, 590
   full liquid, 504
   hospital, 504–505
   liquid, 504
   mechanical soft, 505
   normal, 504–505
   nutritional assessment of, 505–507, 506T
   soft, 505
Diet order, implementation, 509–510
Dietary service, health-care agencies and, 504
Dietitian, 504
Digestion, assessment of, 113F
Dignity, communication skills and, 2
Diluent, injection, 896, 901
Disapproval, reflection of feelings and, 88
Discharge summary, 144
Disclosing solution in oral care, 390
Disclosure, self-. See Self-disclosure
Discomfort, teaching-learning and, 129
Disinfectant, dermal administration of, 867
Disinfection, 271–272, 272T
   boiling water, 272T
   ultraviolet radiation, 272
Disposal
   isolation precautions and, 250–251, 251F
   of used equipment, 275
Distress, interviewing and, 119
Donuts, antidecubitus, 723
Dorsalis pedis pulse, 197, 198F
   measurement of, 203
Dosage, drug
   activities
      of injectable medications, 897–898
      of infusion flow rates, 937–938
         key, 1014
      of IV medication flow rates, 938
         key, 1014–1015
      of oral medications, 850
   calculation of, 828, 831–834
      drops per minute, 937, 938
      factor-label method, 831–833, 850, 897, 937, 938
      in children, 834
      milliliters per hour, 937, 938
      of oral medications, 848–849
      proportion equation method of, 833–834, 850, 897
   definition of, 828
   injection, 896–898
   of injectable medications, 897
   of intravenous fluid flow rates, 937
   of intravenous medication flow rate, 938–939
   oral medication, calculation of, 848–849
   practice problems, 850, 897–898, 937–938
      injectable, 897–898
      intravenous fluids, 937–938
      intravenous medications, 937–938
      oral, 850
Dose, definition of, 828
Double-bag technique, 251F
Douche. See Vagina, irrigation of
Douche kit, 412–413, 413F
Drain
   gravity closed wound drainage system, 329
   Penrose, 329–330, 331–334F
      technique, 336–337
   portable closed wound suction system, 329
   surgical, 329–330
Drainage
   isolation precautions, 258T, 259
   postural, airway resistance and, 779
   serosanguineous, wound repair and, 295
   Trendelenberg position and, 720
   urinary drainage collection bag, 636, 638
      positioning of, 639F
   wound. See Wound drainage and irrigation
Drainage collection bag, 636, 638
   positioning of, 639F
Dram, 830
Drapes, sterile field and, 279
Drawsheet, 760
Dressing technique, isolation and, 252T
Dressing tray, 302
Dressings and wound care, 292–309
   adhesive tape, 222–302, 299F, 300F
   binders and bandages, 302
   burn, 298
   changing techniques, 305–307
   critical points summary, 307–308
   data base for, 297
   delayed healing and, 296–297
   dressing trays, 302
   dry sterile, 346
   duoderm, 299
   equipment for, 298–302
   execution, 302–307
   fibroblastic activity and, 293
   flat, 298
   fluff, 298
   hazards, 299
   hydrophilic, 298
   hydrophobic, 298
   in wound irrigation, 332
   inspection of, 297
   introduction, 292–293
   IV therapy changing of, 956
   learning activities, 308
   medicated, 298
   Montgomery strap 300–301, 301F
   nonadhering, 298
   nonocclusive, 298
   occlusive, 298
   packing strip, 298
   palpation in, 297
   performance checklist, 309
   physical appraisal skills, 297
   preparation, 293–302
   recording
      sample narrative, 307
      sample POR, 307
   review questions, 308
   self-care of, 296–297
   sense of smell in, 297
   skill sequence, 305–307, 306–307
   spray-on, 298–299
   student objectives, 292
   technique, 302–303
   types of, 298–299
   wet sterile. See Wet sterile dressing
   wet-to-dry. See Wet-to-dry dressing
   wound care and, 296
   wound cleansing and, 303–305, 304F
   wound complications, 295–296
   wound healing and, 294–295
   wound repair and, 293–296
Drinking straw, in nasogastric intubation, 573
Drop factor, in infusion flow, 937
Dropper
   eye. See Eye dropper
   oral medication administration via, 853F
   standardization of, 830
Drug
   absorption of, 895
      food and, 848
   cards, 846F
   dispensing unit, 844F
   dosage. See Dosage, drug
   generic, 843, 844
   generic substitution, 853
   knowledge base for, 844–846
   local administration of. See Topical medication
   measurement of, 829
   names for, 843–844
   powdered, injection dosage, 896
   references, nurse-oriented, 844–846
   strength, 848
   swish and swallow, 870
   topical administration of. See Topical medication
Drug use, wound repair and, 294

INDEX **1025**

Dry heat, 437
Dry heat sterilization, 271
Dry kit system, in thermometer cleaning, 186
Dry sterile dressing, 346
Dullness, in percussion, 175*F*
Dumping syndrome, 529
Duoderm dressing, 299
Duval Redi-Vac system, in wound drainage, 331
Dysphagia, 517
Dyspnea, 206–207

Ear
  cleaning of, 361
  inspection, 364
  medication administration in, 872–873, 873*F*
    skill sequence, 873–874
  skin care, 361
  topical medication in, 866
Ear drops, 866
  administration of, 872–874, 873*F*
Earache, intubation and, 564
Earpiece, stethoscope, 178*F*
Eating
  culture and, 481
  facilitation of, 518–522
Eating assistance
  being fed and self-worth, 518
  characteristics of, 516
  critical points summary, 524
  data base, 522
  eating facilitation and, 518–522
  equipment, 522
  execution, 522–523
  feeding clients, 523–524
  introduction, 518
  learning activities, 525
  need determination, 516–517
  neurosensory facilitation techniques, 519–523, 520*F*, 521*F*
  performance checklist, 525–526
  preparation, 516–522
  recording
    sample narrative, 524
    sample POR, 524
  review questions, 525
  self-worth and, 516
  skill sequence, 523–524
  student objectives, 515–516
  swallowing and, 517–518
Eating utensil, isolation and, 252
Ecchymosis, 359
Economic status, food consumption and, 502
Edema
  appearance of, 364
  cast and, 475
  dependent, 488
  fibrosis and, 705
  fluid balance and, 487–488, 488*F*, 492
  interstitial, 487
  nonpitting, 488
  pitting, 487–488, 488*F*
  pulmonary. *See* Pulmonary edema
  thermal application in, 437
Education, self-disclosure and, 36
Effleurage, in massage, 447
Effort arm, 688
Elastic bandage, 456
Elastic foam tape, 300

Elastic stocking, 456, 460–462, 461*F*
  skill sequence, 461–462
Elastin, function of, 359
Elbow
  flexion, 710*F*
  pronation, 710*F*
  restraint, 467, 468*F*
  ROM exercises for, 708, 710*F*
    performance checklist, 716
  supination, 710*F*
Elderly, atelectasis in, 774
Electrical appliance, in hair care, 400
Electrolyte
  assessment of, 113–114*F*
  balance. *See* Electrolyte balance
  fluid balance and, 482
  intubation and, 565
  measurement of, 829
Electrolyte balance
  enemas and, 608
  enteral feeding and, 533
  intubation and, 565
  total parenteral nutrition and, 550
Electrolyte solution, IV, 932*T*, 933
Electronic thermometer, 186–187
  technique, 190*F*
Elimination
  diarrhea and, 593
  fecal problems of, 592
  inducement of, 592–593
  physiological factors in, 589–590
  psychosocial factors in, 589–590
  urinary problems of, 592
Elimination assistance
  abdominal appraisal in, 561
  bedpans, 588–605
  bowel procedures, 605–620
  clinical applications of, 562
  gastrointestinal tube. *See* Gastrointestinal tube
  pressure principles of fluid movement, 561–562
  self-care in, 561
  urinals, 588–605
  urinary incontinence, 620–627
Embolism, IV therapy and, 936
Emergency medical services system, 970
Emergency, technique
  airway obstruction removal, 988–997
  cardiopulmonary resuscitation, 971–987
  types of, 969–970
Emery board, 408
Emesis basin
  in nasogastric intubation, 573
  in nasogastric irrigation, 573
  in oral care, 390
Emollient enema, 608
Emotional status
  assessment of, 112*F*
  caring relationship and, 14–15
  nonverbal communication and, 47
  self-catheterization and, 634
Empathy
  Carkhuff scale of, 13
  definition of, 12
  experiencing activity, 14
  helping relationship and, 12–14
  reflection of content and, 80
Emphysema, tracheostomy and, 801*F*
Employee health, infection control and, 249–250
Enema. *See also* Bowel elimination procedures

  1-2-3, 608
  anthelmintic, 608
  carminative, 608
  cleansing, 607–608
  colon irrigation, 608–609
  contraindications, 608
  definition of, 605
  emollient, 608
  equipment for, 609–611, 610–611*F*
    execution, 612–615, 613–615*F*
  glycerin and water, 608
  Harris flush, 608
  hazards of, 607–608
  large-volume, 607
    execution, 612–614
  Mayo, 608
  medicated, 608
  milk and molasses, 608
  nutritive, 608
  oil-retention, 608
  retention, 608
    execution, 614
  return-flow, 608
  small-volume, 607
    execution, 614
  solution containers, 610
  types of, 607–609
  Valsalva's maneuver and, 597
Enema bag, 610
Energy, client, 129
Enteral feeding set, 535*F*
Enteral formula
  adaptation to, 532–533
  administration sets, 535
  concentration of, 530
  containers, 534–535
  definition of, 527
  temperature of, 532
  types of, 530–531
Enteral nutritional support, 527–546
  adaptation, 532–533
  administration, 532
  administration rate, 532
  administration sets, 535
  aspiration pneumonia and, 533
  auscultation in, 534
  bolus feeding, 539–540
  caloric needs and, 531
  commercial formulas, 530
  constipation and, 533
  continuous, 539
  continuous drip, 529
  critical points summary, 542–543
  data base, 534
  definition of, 527–528
  electrolyte balance and, 533
  equipment, 534–537
  execution, 537–540, 538–539*F*, 540*T*
  feeding methods, 530
  feeding routes, 528–529
  feeding sets, 535
  feeding tubes, 535–536, 536*F*
  fluid balance and, 533
  fluid needs, 531–532
  formula containers, 534–535
  formulas, 530–532
  glucosuria and, 533
  heartburn and, 533
  hydrolyzed formula, 531
  hyperosmolar dehydration and, 533
  inspection in, 534
  intact formula, 530–531
  intermittent, 539–540
  intolerance, 533

Enteral nutritional support (cont.)
  introduction, 527–528
  learning activities, 543
  Levin tubes, 536
  methods of, 529
  monitoring, 540
  nausea and, 533
  noncommercial blenderized, 531
  palpation in, 534
  performance checklist, 543–546
  physical appraisal skills in, 534
  physiological problems, 533
  preparation, 528–530F, 535–537F
  psychosocial adaptation to, 533
  pumps, 535, 537F
  rate of administration, 532
  recording
    sample narrative, 542
    sample POR, 542
  review questions, 543
  routes of, 528–529F
  self-care and, 534
  skill sequence, 540–542
    giving continuous enteral feedings, 540–541
    giving intermittent enteral feedings, 541–542
  skin care and, 538
  specialty formula, 531
  student objectives, 527
  supplemental formula, 531
  temperature and, 532
  time tape, 539F
  tube placement and, 537–538
  tubes, 535–536, 536F
  volume of administration, 532
Envelope-wrapped package, opening of, 276F
Environment
  assessment of, 112F
  food service and, 510
  in teaching-learning, 135
  listening and, 76
  nonverbal communication and, 49
Epidermis, 358–359
Erection
  in perineal care, 373
  urinary catheterization and, 634
Erythema
  appearance of, 364
  definition of, 359
  in breast lesion, 418
Eschar, formation of, 361
Esophagostomy, 528
Ethnic factors, helping concept and, 10
Ethnicity, nonverbal communication and, 49, 50
Ethylene oxide, sterilization and, 270
Eupnea, 206, 207F
Evaluation, definition of, 107
Evaporation, heat, 434–435
Eversion, 705
Evisceration, wound repair and, 295F
Ewald tube, 569F, 570
Exercise
  appetite and, 501
  body temperature and, 183
  chest therapy. See Chest therapy exercise
  conditioning, 692–693
  coughing, 778
    performance checklist, 784
    skill sequence, 782
  deep breathing, 777–778
  defecation and, 590
  diaphragmatic breathing, 778–779
  incentive spirometry, 778, 780F
  isometric, 692
  isotonic, 692–693
  preventive respiratory, 777–778
  pursed lip breathing, 779
  resistive, 692
  restorative respiratory, 778–779
  ROM. See Range of motion, exercises
Exhalation, isometric exercises and, 692
Experience, past, behavior and, 23
Expiration, 774
Exploration, open questions and, 92
Extension, 705
Extracellular fluid, 483
Extremity, supporting and, 707F
Eye
  contact. See Eye contact
  cross-contamination of, 874
  fluid balance and, 489, 492
  inspection of, 869
  irrigation of, 876F
  malnutrition and, 508T
  medication administration to, 874–876
    skill sequence, 875–876
  nonverbal communication and, 47–48
  patching of, 876, 877F
  topical medication in, 866–867
Eye contact, 47
  personal space and, 65
Eye dropper, in topical medication administration, 869
Eye drops, instillation of, 874F
Eye ointment, insertion of, 874F

Face
  fluid balance and, 489
  malnutrition and, 508T
  medication application to, 880
Face sheet, 146
Facial expression, nonverbal communication and, 48
Facial pulse, 197, 198F
Factor-label method
  in dosage calculation, 831–833
  in injection dosage calculation, 897
  in IV flow rate calculation, 937
  in IV medication flow, 938, 939
    rate calculation, 938
  in oral medications, 850
Facts and Comparison, 844
Family, assessment of, 112F
Farenheit temperature, 182–183
Fat, body, 224
Fat emulsion, total parenteral nutrition and, 550
Fatty acid deficiency, TPN and, 550
Feces
  appraisal of, 591–592
  disimpaction of, 615
  impaction of, 606
  incontinence, 607
  isolation and, 252
Feedback
  communication skills and, 4
  reciprocal relatedness of, 18F
Feeding
  assistance with, 515–526
  enteral, 481
  food service and, 499–515
  oral, 481
  parenteral, 481
  supplemental, 481

Feeding device, 522F
Feelings
  behavior and, 18–21
  belittling of, 100
  categories of, 86, 87T
  definition, 7
  disregard for, 88
  identification of, 18–20, 19F
  nonverbal communication and, 47
  reflection of. See Feelings, reflection of
  self-awareness and, 20
  self-expression of, 86
  self-recognition of, 86
  time and, 57
  tones, 47
  values and, 33–34
    interactions activity, 33F
Feelings, reflection of, 85–91
  activities
    experiencing and using, 89–90
    identifying feelings, 86–87
    reflecting feelings, 87–88
    simulations of, 89
  critical points summary, 90
  effective, 86–88
  execution, 89–90
  experiencing and using activity, 89–90
  identifying activity, 86–87
  ineffective, 88–89
    examples of, 88–89
  introduction, 85
  performance checklist, 91
  personalizing and, 85
  preparation, 85–89
  reflecting activity, 87–88
  review questions, 90
  simulations activity, 89
  student objectives, 85
  universalizing and, 85–86
Femoral pulse, 197, 198F
  measurement of, 202
Fenestrated drapes
  sterile field and, 279
  urinary catheterization and, 642
Fever, wound infection and, 320
Fibrillation, atrial, 195
Fibroplasia, retrolental, 787
Filter, in IV therapy, 942
Finger
  abduction, 711F
  flexion, 711F
  opposition, 711F
  ROM exercises for, 708, 711F
  performance checklist, 716
Finger cot, in topical medication administration, 869
Finger probe
  definition of, 989
  in unconscious adult, 992–993, 993F
Fingernail. See Nail
"Five Rights", 828
Flashlight, in nasogastric intubation, 573
Flat dressing, 298
Flatness, in percussion, 175F
Flatulence, 606–607
Flexion, 705
Flossing
  dental, 391F
  in oral care, 389
Flotation devices
  air fluidized bed, 724F
  air suspension bed, 724F

alternating pressure air mattress, 723
antidecubitus, 723–724
silicone gel pads, 723
water beds, 723
Flow rate, in IV infusion, problems with, 954
Flow sheet, 143, 151–153, 161
basic care chart, 153F
diabetic therapy and education, 155F
fluid, 493F
in nursing records, 151–153, 152–153F
in record-keeping, 143F
using activity, 161
Fluency, 49
Fluff dressing, 298
Fluid
balance. See Fluid balance
intake of
defecation and, 590
tracheostomy and, 803
movement of, in elimnation, 561
obligatory loss of, 484
Fluid balance
assessment, 485–489, 487F, 488F, 491T, 494
auscultation and, 492
bedside record cards, 494F
body fluid balance, 483–484, 484T
characteristics of, 482–483
client history, 490–491
consciousness level and, 489
critical points summary, 497
data base, 490–492
deficit, 484, 485T
edema, 487–488, 488F
enemas and, 608
enteral feeding and, 533
equipment, 492–494, 493F, 494F
excess, 485T
execution, 494
eyes and, 489
facial appearance and, 489
flow sheet, 493F
fluid deficit, 484, 485T
fluid excess, 485T
fluid imbalance and, 484–485, 485T
fluid intake changes, 489–490
hypervolemia, 485T
hypovolemia, 485T
inspection, 491–492
intake and output measurement, 485–486
promoting accurate, 495–496
self-care and, 490
intake measurement, 494–495
introduction, 482–483
intubation and, 565
jugular vein filling and, 487, 491–492
laboratory data, 490–491
learning activities, 497
measurement of, 496
mucous membrane and, 489
output measurement, 495
palpation and, 492
performance checklist, 498
peripheral pulse and, 486
peripheral vein filling and, 487
physical appraisal skills, 491–492
preparation, 483–494
recorded data, 490–492
recording, 497
records, intake-output, 493
review questions, 497–498
self-care, 490

sense of smell and, 492
skill sequence, 496
skin and, 489
speech and, 489
stool and, 489
student objectives, 482
thirst and, 489
total parenteral nutrition and, 550
turgor, 488F
urine and, 489
vein filling, 487–488, 488F
water intake and output, 484T
Fluid balance assessment, 481
deficit, 484, 485T
edema, 487–488, 488F
excess, 485T
facial appearance and, 489
guide for, 113F, 491T
intake and output measurement, 485–486
monitoring in, 482–499
mucous membrane and, 489
skin and, 489
stool and, 489
thirst, 489
turgor, 488F
urine and, 489
vein filling, 487–488, 488F
vital signs and, 486
weight and, 486
Fluid container, in IV therapy, 940F
Fluidram, 830
Fluids. See Intravenous infusion; Intravenous medications
Fluoride
in oral care, 390
oral care and, 386
Flush method, of blood pressure measurement, 213
Foam
handwashing and, 242–243
silastic, 299
Foam pads, antidecubitus, 723
Foley catheter, 630
Tamper-Evident Seal, 633
Follow-up, learning, 133
Food
appearance of, 502–503
consumption factors, 501–503
insulated cart, 509F
insulated servers, 510F
intake regulation of, 500–501
oral medication and, 848
service. See Food service
temperature-control mechanisms, 509
transportation devices, 509
urine appraisal and, 591
Food history, 505
Food service. See also Nutritional care
health care agencies and, 503–504
implementing diet order, 509–510
nutritional services, 503–504
Food trays, 508–509
identification, 511
serving, 512
Footboards, 722
Force
body mechanics and, 687
disrupting, 687
restoring, 687
Forceps
dressing change and, 301F
in suture removal, 313
sterile, 274–275
Forearm, IV infusion in, 930, 931F

Foreign object removal. See Obstructed airway removal of
Forms, interviewing, 119
Formula intolerance, 533
Fowler's position
dangling and, 695
in bed, 719, 720F
inspiration and, 717
semi-, 870
eye drop instillation and, 875
Friction
body mechanics and, 687
clinical application of, 687
in handwashing, 245
in massage, 447
shearing force, 719
sliding, 719
Friction rub, 777
Fulcrum, 688
Fungicide, vaginal, 867

Gag reflex, 520, 521F
anticholinergics and, 774
Gait
cane-first, 699
cane-together, 699
crutches and, 700–701
data base, 693
four-point, 693
crutches and, 700F
reciprocal walker and, 699
nonverbal communication and, 48
swing-through, 693
crutches and, 701F
swing-to, 693
crutches and, 701F
three-point, 693
crutches and, 700F
two-point, 699F
two-point alternative, 693
crutches and, 700, 701F
reciprocal walker and, 699
walker and, 699F
Gait belt, 695, 698F
Gargles, 870
Gas sterilization, 270
Gassed-out culture tube, wound specimen
collection and, 322
Gastric lavage, 583–584
Gastrointestinal system
malnutrition and, 508T
oral medication and, 848
positioning and, 717
Gastrointestinal tube, insertion and care of
abdominal appraisal and, 565–568
abdominal distention and, 574
auscultation and, 567, 569
Cantor, 570F, 571
client care, 581–582, 582T
client history and, 568
critical points summary, 584
data base, 568–569
definition of, 563
Dennis, 570F, 571
equipment for, 569–570F, 572–573F
execution, 574–577F
extubation, 582–583
insertion of, 582
equipment, 573
nasogastric, 574–578, 575F, 576F
problems after, 564–565

Gastrointestinal tube (cont.)
  insertion of (cont.)
    problems associated with, 564
    skill sequence, 580–581
  inspection and, 566–567, 568–569
  intestinal tubes, 570–571, 571F
    insertion, 582
    removal, 583
  introduction, 563
  irrigation, 573–574
  learning activities, 584–585
  long, 570–571
  Miller-Abbott, 570F
  nasogastric insertion, 574–578
  nasogastric tubes
    Ewald, 569F, 570
    gastric lavage, 583–584
    insertion of, 574–578, 575F
      performance checklist, 586
      skill sequence, 578–579
    irrigating, 579–580
      skill sequence, 580–581
    Levin, 569F
    neck hyperextension and, 576F
    nursing care for, 582T
    performance checklist, 586, 587
    placement check, 576F
    removal, 582–583
      performance checklist, 587
    Salem Sump tube, 569F, 570
    securing, 577F
    Sengstaken-Blakemore, 569F, 570
    short, 569F
    skill sequence, 578–579
    sump tubes, 569F, 570
  negative pressure and, 563–564
  palpation and, 567–568, 569
  client care, skill sequence, 581–582
  percussion and, 567–568, 569
  performance checklist, 586–587
  physical appraisal, 565–568
  pipeline suctioning of, 571
  post-insertion problems, 564–565
  preparation, 563–574, 566F
  problems associated with, 564–565
  recorded data and, 568
  recording
    sample narrative, 584
    sample POR, 584
  removal, 582–583
    equipment, 574
    skill sequence, 582–583
  review questions, 585
  Sengstaken-Blakemore, 569F, 570
  sense of smell and, 569
  siphon action and, 564
  skill sequence, 578–581, 583
    inserting nasogastric tube, 578–579
    irrigating a gastrointestinal tube, 580–581
    removing nasogastric tube, 583
  student objectives, 562–563
  suction equipment
    pipeline suction, 571
    thermotic pumps, 571–572, 573F
    tubing, 573
  suction of, 563, 571–573, 572–573F
  sump, 569F, 570
  thermotic pump, 571–572, 573F
  usage problems, 564–565
Gastrostomy, 528
Gauze
  in IV infusion, 950F
  in wet-to-dry dressing, 352

injection needle and, 900F
  tracheostomy and, 807F
Gauze bandage, 455
Gauze sponge, 298
Gavage feeding, 527
Gel, topical, 868T
Generativity, basic needs and, 26
Generic drugs, 844
Genuineness, empathy and, 13
Germicidal detergent, isolation and, 260–261
Gestures
  attending behavior and, 72
  nonverbal communication and, 48
Gingiva
  definition of, 384–385
  diseases of, 385
  malnutrition and, 508T
Gingivitis, 385
Gland, malnutrition and, 508T
Glass
  fluid balance assessment and, 493
  in sterile supplies, 274
Glass bottle, in IV therapy, 940F
Glass syringe, 899F
Gloves
  donning and removal of sterile, 263, 291
  for wet sterile dressing, 345
  in topical medication administration, 869
  isolation, 260
  lubricant for, 287
  nitroglycerin administration and, 881
  sterile
    client history and, 287
    critical points summary, 290
    data base, 286–287
    donning, 286, 289F
    donning and removing
      performance checklist, 265
      skill sequence, 263
    equipment, 287
    execution, 287–290
    hazards, 287
    inspection of, 287
    introduction, 286
    learning activities, 290–291
    performance checklist, 291
    physical appraisal skills, 287
    preparation, 286–287
    recorded data and, 287
    removing, 263, 290F, 291
    review questions, 291
    skill sequence, 288, 290
      donning, 288
      removal, 290
      removing, 290
    student objectives, 286
    tracheostomy tube and, 805
    urinary catheterization and, 642
  topical medication and, 880
Glucosuria, enteral feeding and, 533
Gluteal muscle
  injection in, 893F, 894, 895F
  isometric exercises and, 692
Glycerin, in oral care, 389
Glycerin and water enema, 608
Glycerin suppository, 867
Glycosuria, TPN and, 549
Gly-oxide, in oral care, 389
Goals, teaching-learning, 130
Gomco Thermotic pump, in gastrointestinal suction, 571, 573F

Gown
  changing of, IV infusion and, 955
  donning and removing of, 261, 262F
    performance checklist, 264–265
    skill sequence, 261–262
  isolation, 250, 260
  IV infusion and, 955
Graduate, 637
Graduated container, in nasogastric intubation, 573
Grain, 830T
Gram, 829
Granulation tissue, formation of, 351
Graphic sheet, in nursing records, 151–152, 152F
Gratification, of basic needs, 25
Gravity
  center of, 686
  line of, 686
Gravity controller, in IV therapy, 943–944
Gravity flow infusion
  IV administration set, 942
  IV fluid infusion, 937
  IV medication infusion, 937
  TPN and, 551
Grooming
  beard, 402
  hair, 401
Growth and development, self-concept and, 22
Growth needs, 25
Gum. See Gingiva
Gum chewing, body temperature and, 184
Gustatory status, assessment of, 113F
Gynecomastia, 419

Hair
  braiding, 401
  care. See Hair care
  growth of, 398
    disorders of, 398–399
  ingrown, 399
  malnutrition and, 508T
  matted, 401
  structure of, 398
  texture of, 399
Hair care
  bed shampoo, 402, 403–404
  client history and, 399–400
  crab lice, 399
  critical points summary, 404
  data base, 399–400
  definition of, 398
  electrical appliances, 400
  equipment for, 400F
  execution, 401–404
  grooming, 401, 402
  growth disorders, 398–399
  head lice, 399
  inspection in, 400
  introduction, 398
  learning activities, 404
  lice, 399
  palpation in, 400
  pediculosis, 399
  performance checklist, 405
  physical appraisal skills, 400
  preparation, 398–401
  preshave lotion, 400–401
  pubic, 399

recorded data and, 399–400
recording
    sample narrative, 404
    sample POR, 404
review questions, 405
shampooing, 400F, 401–402, 403–404
shaving, 402–403
shaving equipment, 400–401
shower shampoo, 401
sink shampoo, 401–402
skill sequence, 403–404
structure, 398
student objectives, 397
Hand
    IV infusion in, 930, 931F
    position of
        in CPR, 978, 979F
        in percussion, 176F
    positioning, in palpation, 171F, 172F
    washing. See Handwashing
Hand cream, handwashing and, 243
Hand-care agents, handwashing and, 242–243
Handrolls, 722
Handwashing
    critical points summary, 246
    data base for, 243–244
    equipment for, 244
    execution, 244F, 245F
    finger massaging, 245F
    hand care agents and, 242–243
    introduction, 241
    isolation precautions and, 250
    learning activities, 246–247
    paper towels and, 245F
    performance checklist, 247
    physical appraisal skills, 244
    position at sink, 244F
    preparation, 214–244
    review questions, 247
    skill sequence, 245–246
    student objectives, 241
    tracheostomy and, 803
Hangnail, 407–408
Harmony, nurse-client relationship and, 12
Harris flush 608
Head lice, 399
Head tilt, in CPR, 974, 976–977, 977F
Headset, stethoscope, 178F
Healing ridge, 293
Health record, 141–163. See also Nursing record
    activity, 146–147
    characteristics of, 142
    critical points summary, 147
    data base, 143
    discharge summaries, 144
    examination, 146–147
    execution, 146–147
    flow sheets, 143
    formats, 145
    initial plans, 143
    introduction, 142
    isolation and, 252, 258
    legal status of, 145–146
    narrative notes, 143
    nursing records. See Nursing record
    preparation, 142–146
    problem list, 143
    problem-oriented system, 142–144, 143T
        nursing records and, 150–151, 151T
    progress notes, 143–144

review questions, 147–148
student objectives, 141
summaries, 144
traditional systems, 144–145
transfer summaries, 144
Health status
    blood pressure, 210–223
    height and weight, 223–237
    measurement of, 181–237
    pulse, 194–205
    respiration, 205–210
    temperature, 182–194
Health-care agency, nutritional services of, 503–504
Hearing
    in percussion, 174–175
    vs. listening, 75
Heart failure, physiology of, 972
Heartburn, enteral feeding and, 533
Heat
    clinical uses of, 437
    contraindications, 436
    dry, 437
    oral pocket of, 183F
    perception of, 436
    physiological effects of, 435
    systemic effects of, 436
    transfer mechanisms, 434–435
    wet, 437
Heat cradle, in thermal application, 439F
Heat lamp, 439–440, 441
Heating pad, 438–439
Heat-sealed package, opening of, 277, 278F, 279
Heel protectors
    antidecubitus, 723
    shearing force and, 719
Height and weight, 223–237
    appraisal of, 223–237
    body composition and, 224
    body fat and, 224
    body mechanics and, 686
    body water and, 224
    client history, 226
    critical points summary, 235
    data base for, 225–226
    desired, 224T, 225T
    desired weights
        calculation, 234
        for men, 224T
        for women, 225T
    equipment for, 226–228F
    execution, 228
    fluid balance and, 486
    inspection in, 226
    introduction, 223–224
    learning activities, 235
    measurement standards, 225
    nutrition and, 224–225
    overnutrition and, 225
    overweight and, 225
    palpation in, 226
    performance checklist, 235–237
    physical appraisal skills, 226
    preparation, 224–228
    recorded data, 226
    recording of, 234–235
    review questions, 235
    skill sequence, 229
        measuring height-length, 229
        measuring skinfold thickness, 233–234
        measuring weight, 229

        measuring with bedside scale, 230–231
    skinfold measurement and, 231–234, 232F, 233F
    standards, 225
    student objectives, 223
    undernutrition and, 224–225
    weight determination, 229–234
    weight measurement, 229
    wound repair and, 294
Help
    direct physical, 98
        offering, 98–99, 105
    nonverbal communication and, 49
    recipients of, 49
Helper
    awareness skills, 11
    characteristics of, 9
    congruence, 3–9
    distance zone of, 64
    empathy in, 12
Helping, cultural variables in, 10
Helping relationship, the
    acceptance and, 10–11
        activity, in, 11
    activities
        experiencing caring, 14
        experiencing empathy, 14
        experiencing of acceptance, 10
        experiencing trust, 11
    awareness of self in, 7–45
    caring and, 14–15, 15F
        activity in, 14
    characteristics of, 8–10
    critical points summary, 16
    cultural variables in, 10
    desire and, 13
    deterrents to, 10
    empathy and, 14
        activity in, 14
    execution of, 15–16
    genuineness and, 13
    identity level, 15
    introduction, 7, 8
    involvement level, 15
    key components of, 10–15
    nurse-client in, 1, 9–10
    preparation, 8–15
    respect and, 13
    review questions, 16
    self-disclosure and, 13
    student objectives, 8
    superficial level, 15
    trust and, 11–12
        activity in, 11
Hematest, 507
Hematocrit, in nutritional assessment, 506T, 507
Hematologic status, in nutritional assessment, 506T, 507
Hemoglobin, in nutritional assessment, 506T, 507
Hemorrhage, tracheostomy and, 801–802
Hemostat
    dressing change and, 301F, 302
    in nasogastric extubation, 574
    in suture removal, 313
    in wet-to-dry dressing, 345
    tissue clamp, 574
Hemovac system, in wound drainage, 331, 332F
Heparin, injection of, 912–913
Heparin lock

Heparin lock *(cont.)*
 IV piggyback administration, 958*F*
 IV push medication, 959
 IV therapy, 943
Hexachlorophene, handwashing and, 242
Heyer-Schulte system, in wound drainage, 331–332*F*
Hip
 abduction, 712*F*
 ball and socket joint, 706
 circumduction, 713*F*
 flexion, 712*F*
 ROM exercises for, 708, 712*F*, 713*F*
  performance checklist, 716
 rotation, 712*F*
Hirsutism, 398–399
History sheet, medical record, 147
Hoarseness, intubation and, 564
Home furnishings, 49
 IV therapy in, 939
Honesty, nurse-client relationship and, 12
Hormones, topical, 867
Hospital diet, 504–505
Hospital formulary, 844
Hot bath, body temperature and, 183
Hot tub, 440
Household system, of measurement, 830
Hubbard tank, in thermal application, 440
Humidification
 of oxygen, 787–788
 tracheostomy and, 803*F*
Humidifiers
 bubble, 789–790
 heated, 790
 simple, 789
Humidity, skin and, 359–360
Hunger, 500
 food consumption and, 502
Hydrocollator pack
 in thermal application, 439*F*, 441–442, 442*F*
 skill sequence, 442–443
Hydrogen peroxide
 in oral care, 389
 in wet-to-dry dressing, 352
 tracheostomy tubes and, 805
Hydrophilic dressing, 298
Hydrophobic dressing, 298
Hygiene. *See* Personal hygiene
Hyperalimentation. *See* Total parenteral nutrition
Hyercapnia, 786
Hyperemia
 nasal, 866
 stages of, 360–361
Hyperextension, 705
Hyperglycemia, TPN and, 550
Hyperosmolar dehydration, 533
Hyperpigmentation, definition of, 359
Hyperplasia, of gingiva, 385
Hyperpnea, 206, 207*F*
Hypertonic fluid, 931
Hypertonic saline, 933
Hyperventilation, 206, 207*F*
Hypervolemia, 485*T*
Hypodermic syringe, 899*F*
Hypoglycemia, TPN and, 550
Hypopigmentation, 359
Hypotension
 airway suctioning and, 816
 orthostatic. *See* Orthostatic hypotension

Hypotonic fluid, 931
Hypotonic saline, 933
Hypoventilation, 206, 207*F*
 oxygen-induced, 787
Hypovolemia, 484, 485*T*
Hypovolemic shock, Trendelenberg position and, 720
Hypoxemia, 786
Hypoxia, 786

Iatrogenic incontinence, 621
Ideals, values and, activity on, 31–32
Identity, basic needs and, 26
Illness
 fluid needs and, 482
 food consumption and, 503
 needs satisfaction and, 28
I-message
 feedback and, 4
 self-disclosure activity on, 41
 touch and, 64
Immobility
 fibrosis and, 705
 orthostatic hypotension and, 693
Immunosuppression, urinary tract infection and, 633
Inattention, selected, 76
Incentive spirometry, 778, 780*F*, 781
Incision, definition of, 293
Incontinence care, 620–626. *See also* Urinary incontinence care
 fecal, 607
Independence, direct physical help and, 98
Individualization, in interviews, 116–117
Inertia, body mechanics and, 687
Infant
 airway obstruction removal in, 994*F*
 blood pressure measurement in, 213
 CPR in, 981–984, 982*F*, 983*F*
 urinary catheterization in, 632
Infection
 candidiasis, 412
 community-acquired, 239
 cycle of, 240
 intravenous therapy and, 935
 monilial, 412
 nosocomial, 239
 stethoscope and, 179
 TPN and, 549–550
 tracheostomy and, 802
 trichomonal, 412
 urinary tract. *See* Urinary tract infection
 vaginal, 867
 wound, 319–321, 320*T*
  culture of. *See* Wound culture specimen collection
 wound irrigation and, 332
 wound repair and, 295
Infection control, assessment of, 112*F*
Infection control practitioner, 240
 isolation precautions and, 253–254
Infective material, definition of, 250–251
Infiltration, in IV therapy, 935
Inflammation, tracheostomy and, 802
Inflammatory response, 293
Inflation system, of sphygmomanometer, 214*F*, 215*F*
Inflection, 49

Information, providing, decision making and, 102
Information system, purpose of, 142
Infusion, intravenous. *See* Intravenous infusions
Infusion control device, 937
 in IV therapy, 944
 selection of, 946
 volumetric, 944
Infusion pump
 in IV therapy, 944
 total parenteral nutrition and, 551
Ingrown hair, 399
Ingrown nail, 408
Inhalants, volatile, 867
Inhalation, medication, 882*F*
Initial plan, 143
 in record-keeping, 143*F*
Initiative, esteem and, 26
Injectable medication administration
 administering, 908–920, 910*F*, 914–920*F*
 ampules, 900, 901*F*
  opening, 905*F*
  withdrawing medication from, 902, 906*F*, 907, 908
 cartridges, 901, 908
  carpuject, 910*F*
  Tubex, 909*F*
 critical points summary, 921
 data base, 898
 dosage calculation, 897–908
 dosage forms, 896–897
 drug absorption and, 895
 drugs, 890
 equipment, 898–901*F*
 execution, 901–920
 intradermal, 891–892
  administration, 908–912, 909*F*
  drug absorption and, 895
  performance checklist, 924–925
  skill sequence, 911
  use of, 890
 intramuscular
  administration of, 911–912, 917–920, 917–919*F*
  drug absorption and, 895
  injection sites, 892–894
  performance checklist, 926
  skill sequence, 920
  use of, 890
  z-track, 917, 919*F*
 learning activities, 897–898
 mixing medications in syringe, 905–906
 needles. *See also* Needle
  destruction, 901, 902*F*
  selection, 902
  types, 898–900
 performance checklist, 923–928
 practice problems, 897–898
  key, 1013–1014
 preparation, 891–901
 preparing, 901–908, 903–906*F*
  skill sequence, 906–908
 routes for, 890
 side effect minimalization, 896
 site selection, 891
 sites, 891–895*F*
  drug dosage and, 895
  intradermal, 891
  intramuscular, 892–894*F*, 895*F*
  subcutaneous, 892*F*, 893*F*
 skill sequence, 906–920

intradermal, 911
intramuscular, 920
preparation, of injectables, 906–908
subcutaneous, 916
student objectives, 890
subcutaneous, 892F, 893F
  administration, 913–916, 913–915F
  drug absorption and, 895
  heparin, 912–913
  insulin, 913–916
  performance checklist, 925–926
  skill sequence, 916
syringe destruction, 901, 902F
syringes, types, 898–900F
vials, 900, 901F. See also Syringe
  withdrawing medications from, 902–907F
Injection. See Injectable medication administration
Insensible water loss, 483
Inspection, 169–170
  critical points summary, 170
  execution, 170
  in airway obstruction, 989
  in ambulation assistance, 694
  in blood pressure measurement, 214
  in breast examination, 419
  in CPR, 975
  in eating assistance, 522
  in elimination, 594
  in hair care, 400
  in height appraisal, 226
  in incontinence, 623
  in injection, 898
  in intubation, 566–567
  in IV therapy, 940
  in massage, 448
  in mechanical restraint, 466
  in nutritional assessment, 508T
  in oral medication administration, 851
  in oxygen therapy, 788
  in perineal care, 374
  in respiration appraisal, 208
  in self-catheterization, 635
  in skin care, 363–364
  in suture removal, 313
  in thermal application, 438
  in weight appraisal, 226
  in wound culture specimen collection, 322
  introduction, 169
  isolation precautions and, 259–260
  learning activities, 170
  of abdomen, 566–567
  of airway suctioning, 816
  of anal area, 869
  of bandages, 455
  of bindings, 455
  of cast, 477
  of ear, 868
  of enema, 609
  of eye, 869
  of fluid balance, 491–492, 492F
  of mouth, 869
  of nail care, 408
  of nose, 869
  of oral care, 387
  of otic medication, 868
  of pressure points, 364–365
  of respiration, 780
  of ROM, 706
  of skin, 869
  of sterile gloves, 287
  of sterile supplies, 272

of topical medication administration, 868–869
of tracheostomy, 804
of vagina, 869
of vaginal irrigation, 412
of wet sterile dressing, 345
of wet-to-dry dressing, 352
of wound care, 297
of wound drainage, 330
preparation, 170
review questions, 170
student objectives, 169
Inspiration, 774
Instillation, of ear drops, 866
Instruction. See Teaching–learning
Insulation, in wet-to-dry dressing, 346
Insulin, injection, 913–916
Insulin syringe, 899F
Intake-output record, of fluids, 493F
Integrity
  basic needs and, 26
  personal space and, 65
Integumentary system, assessment of, 114F
Intellectual capability, in teaching-learning, 130
Intentions, self-awareness and, 20
Intermittent-reading thermometer, 187
Internalizing, 31
International Council of Nurses, client values and, 30–31
Interpersonal process, 1, 3F
Interpersonal relationship
  learning skills, 3
  nurse-client, 9
Interpretation, self-awareness and, 20
Interpreter, in interviewing, 116
Interrupted suture, removal of, 316
Interruptions, 56–57
Intershift report, 154
Intervention, definition of, 107
Interview
  after the, 120
  analysis of, 120T
  client feelings and, 86
  definition of, 108
  purpose of, 116
  questioning skills in, 91
  summarization of, 117
  termination of, 117
Interviewing
  activities
    analyzing interactions 124
    client interviews, 124
    conducting an assessment interview, 123
    evaluating the interview, 123–124
    experiences with interviewing, 111
  analyzing interactions, 124
  characteristics of, 108–109
  client, 124
  client concerns, 116
  communication skills and, 117
  conducting assessment, 123
  critical points summary, 124
  dealing with distress, 119
  establishing purpose, 116
  evaluation, 123–124
  execution, 121–124
  experiences with activity, 111
  guidelines, 116–117
  individualized, 116–117
  introduction, 108–109
  listening and, 118–119

medical history, 112–114F
performance checklist, 125
post-, 120T
preparation, 110–121
printed forms for, 119–120
process recording, 120–121, 121–123T
  guide, 121T
  sample, 122–123T
review questions, 124
special need and, 115–116
special skills, 118–120
student objectives, 108
summarization, 117
Intestine
  auscultation of, 567
  water loss and, 483
Intimacy, basic needs and, 26
Intonation, 49
Intradermal injection. See Injectable medications, intradermal
Intramuscular injection. See Injectable medications, intramuscular
Intrathoracic pressure, isometric exercises and, 692
Intravenous flow rate
  calculation and timing, 937–939
  practice problems, 937
Intravenous fluid. See Intravenous infusions
Intravenous infusions
  administration, performance checklist, 965–966
  administration set, 955–956
  air embolism and, 936
  ambulation and, 955
  blood administration, 955, 960–961
  blood sample collection, 952–953
    performance checklist, 965
    skill sequence, 953
  circulatory overload and, 936
  client care, 953–955
  client instruction, 939
  complications, 934–937
  container, changing of, 956
  critical points summary, 962–963
  data base, 940
  discontinuing, 956–957
  dressing, changing of, 956
  equipment, 940–945F
  equipment changes, 955–956
  execution, 945–962
  flow rate, calculation and timing, 937–939
    IV fluids, 937–938
    IV medications, 938–939
  flow rate, problems with, 954
  fluid balance assessment and, 495
  fluids, 930–934, 932T
  gown changing and, 955
  home therapy, 939
  infection, 935
  infiltration, 935
  infusion discontinuation, 956–957
  infusion preparation, 945–948
  learning activities, 962–963
  medication administration, 934, 957–960, 958F, 959F
  monitoring, 954
  performance checklist, 965–967
  physicians order, 929
  practice problems, 937–939
    IV fluids, 937–938
    IV medications, 938–939
  preparation, 929–945

Intravenous infusions (cont.)
  preparation of, 947–948
    performance checklist, 965
    skill sequence, 947–948
  psychological reaction to, 929
  recording, 961, 962F
  review questions, 963–964
  skill sequence, 946–948, 951–953
    blood collection, 953
    infusion preparation, 946–948
    venipuncture, 951–952
  speed shock, 936
  starting, 948–952, 949F, 950F
  student objectives, 928
  types of, 928–929, 930–934, 932T
  venipuncture, 944F, 948–953
    performance checklist, 967
    site selection, 929–930, 931F
    skill sequence, 951–952
Intravenous medication
  piggyback, 934, 957
  push, 934, 959–960
    administration of, 960–961F
Intubation
  gastrointestinal. See Gastrointestinal tube
  nasogastric. See Nasogastric tube
Inversion, 705
Iodine, handwashing and, 242
Iodophor, handwashing and, 242
Ionizing radiation sterilization, 271
Irrigating solution, for wounds, 332
Irrigating syringe, in wound drainage, 331–332, 333F
Irrigation
  bladder, 649
  catheter equipment, 637
  colostomy, 675–678, 676–678F
    performance checklist, 682–683
    skill sequence, 678–680
  nasogastric tube, equipment, 573–574
  of colon. See Colon, irrigation of
  of perineum. See Perineum, irrigation of
  of vagina. See Vaginal irrigation
  wound. See Wound drains and irrigation
Irrigation device, in oral care, 388
Irritant
  defecation and, 590
  skin and, 360
  values and, activity on, 34
Isolation
  bed linen and, 252
  blood-body precaution in, 258T, 259
  booties, 250, 260
  caps, 250, 260
  category-specific, 256, 257T
  CDC and, 249
  client history, 259
  contact, 256, 257T
  contaminated items disposal, 250–251, 251F
  critical points summary, 263–264
  data base for, 259–260
  definition of, 249
  disease-specific, 256F, 259
  dishes and eating utensils, 252
  drainage-secretion precaution in, 258T, 259
  dressing techniques, 252
  employee health and infection control and, 249–250
  enteric precaution in, 258T, 259

  equipment, 260
  execution, 261–263
  germicidal detergents and, 260–261
  gloves, 263
  gown, 261, 262F
  handwashing and, 250
  health record, 258
  implementation, 253–254
  inspection in, 259–260
  introduction, 249
  laboratory specimens, 252
  learning activities, 264
  mask, 250, 262, 263F
  needles, 251
  performance checklist, 264–265
  personal effects and, 253
  physical appraisal skills, 259–260
  physical barriers and, 250
  postmortem care and, 253
  precautionary techniques, 250–253, 251F, 252T
    implementing, 253–254
    specifications, 254–259
  preparation, 249–261
  private room and, 250
  protective clothing and, 250
  psychosocial impact of, 254
  recorded data, 259
  recording
    sample narrative, 263
    sample POR, 263
  respiratory, 256, 257T, 259
  review questions, 264
  room cleaning and, 253
  shoe covers, 260
  skill sequence, 261–263
    donning and removing gloves, 263
    donning and removing gown, 261–262
    donning and removing mask, 262
  special procedures, 250–251
  specifications, 254–259, 255–256F, 257–258T
  sphygomomanometers, 251
  stethoscope, 251
  strict, 256, 257T
  student objectives, 248
  syringes, 251
  system A, 256–259, 257–258T
  system B, 259
  terminal cleaning and, 253
  thermometers and, 251–252
  tissues and dressings, 252
  toys, books and magazines and, 253
  transportation and, 252–253
  tuberculosis and, 257T, 259
  urine and feces, 258
  visitors and, 252
Isometric exercises, 692
Isopropyl alcohol, tracheostomy tubes and, 805
Isotonic exercises, 692–693
Isotonic fluid, 931
IV. See Intravenous infusions

Jackson-Pratt drains. See Heyer-Schulte system
Jaundice, 359
  appearance of, 364
  definition of, 359
Jaw thrust, in CPR, 974, 976–977, 977F
Jejunostomy, 528

Johari window, 23
Joint Commission on Accreditation of Hospitals, record-keeping requirements, 142–144
Joints
  ankle, ROM exercises for, 708, 713F
  ball and socket, 706
  condyloid, 706
  diarthrodial, 706
  elbow, ROM exercises for, 708, 710F
  finger, ROM exercises for, 708, 711F
  flexibility of, 705
  hinge, 706
  hip, ROM exercises for, 708, 712F, 713F
  knee, ROM exercises for, 708, 713F
  neck, ROM exercises for, 708F
  pivot, 706
  ROM and, 705
  saddle, 706
  shoulder, ROM exercises for, 708, 709–710F
  toe, ROM exercises for, 708, 714F
  wrist, ROM exercises for, 708, 711F
Judgment, value, questions and, 92
Jugular vein, filling, fluid balance and, 487, 491–492, 492F

Kardex system, 153–154, 156–157F, 161
  portable holder, 156F
  use of, 161
  using activity, 161
Key word listening, 75
Kidney, water loss and, 483
Kinesics, 48
Kneading, in massage, 447
Knee
  flexion, 713F, 719
  ROM exercises for, 708, 713F
    performance checklist, 716
Knot, in mechanical restraint, 469F
Knowing ourselves, 17–24
  activities
    feelings identification, 18
    looking at self-identity, 22
    looking at self-worth, 21–22
    past experiences and behavior, 23
    using the self-awareness wheel, 20–21
  critical points summary, 24
  developing self-awareness, 19–20
  execution, 23–24
  feelings identification and, 18–20, 19F
  introduction, 18
  Johari window and, 23F
  preparation, 18–23
  review questions, 24
  self-awareness and, 18–21
  self-concept and, 21–22
  self-understanding and, 22–23
  student objectives, 17
Korotkoff sounds
  augmentation of, 213
  auscultation of, 211–212
  in blood pressure measurement, 211–212, 212F
Kussmaul respiration, 206

Labia, washing of, 375F, 376
Laboratory report, medical report, 147

INDEX

Laboratory specimen, isolation and, 252
Laboratory study, in nutritional assessment, 505–507, 506*T*
Laceration, definition of, 293
Lactose, in enteral formula, 531
Lactose intolerance, 533
Lamp, in thermal application, 439–440, 441
Language perception, assessment of, 113*F*
Laryngectomy, airway suction and, 815
Laundry, incontinence and, 622
Lateral position
  in bed, 719, 731*F*, 732*F*, 733*F*
  turning to, 732
Law
  mechanical restraint and, 465–466
  medical records and, 145–146
  medication administration and, 843–844
  nursing records and, 154
Learner, involvement of, 132
Learning. *See* Teaching-learning
Legal accountability, nursing records and, 155–158
Leukorrhea, 412
Leveling, communication and, 40
Leveling responses, feedback and, 4, 40
Lever arm, 688
Levers, 688–689
Levin tube, 569*F*
Lice, 399
  crab, 399
  head, 399
Life support, 969–997. *See also* Emergency technique
Lifting, body mechanics of, 689
Limb restraint, 467*F*
  skill sequence, 470–471
Linens, handling, 759
Lip, malnutrition and, 508*T*
Liquid, body temperature and, 184
Listening
  attentive, 74–78, 117*F*
    activities
      experiencing and using, 77
      learning to listen, 76
      listening for meaning, 76
      simulations of, 77
    critical points summary, 78
    effective, 75–76, 77
    execution of, 77–78
    ineffective, 76–77
    introduction, 74–75
    performance checklist, 78
    preparation, 75–77
    review questions, 78
    student objectives, 74
  definition of, 74
  effective behavior for, 75–76
  environmental factors and, 76
  experiencing and using activity, 77
  for meaning, 76
  ineffective behavior for, 76–77
  interviewing and, 117*F*, 118–119
  key word, 75
  learning activity, 76
  oral medication administration and, 857
  personal factors in, 76
  physiologic factors in, 76
  prejudice and, 76–77
  response and, 75
  secondary messages and, 75
  selected inattention and, 76
  silence and, 75–76
  theme, 75
  vs. hearing, 75
Livor mortis, 425–426
Logrolling, 737, 738*F*
Lotion
  in nail care, 408
  topical, 868*T*
Loudness, in percussion, 174
Love, psychological needs and, 25
Lubricant
  enema and, 611
  for sterile gloves, 287
  in nasogastric intubation, 573
  in oxygen administration, 793
Lung, gas exchange in, 775

Macrodrip device, in IV therapy, 942
Malnutrition, 501
  hospital clients and, 481
  physical signs of, 508*T*
  types of, 501
Manometer
  aneroid, 214*F*, 216–217, 217*F*
  mercury-gravity, 214*F*, 215–216, 216*F*
Manual thrust. *See* Obstructed airway, removal of
Mask
  donning and removing, 262, 263*F*
    performance checklist, 265
    skill sequence, 262
  isolation, 250, 260
Maslow growth needs, 25
Massage
  back, 449–451
  circulatory effects of, 446–447
  client history and, 448
  compression, 447
  creative use of, 64
  critical points summary, 451–452
  data base, 448
  definition, 446
  effleurage, 447
  equipment, 448
  execution, 448–451
  friction, 447
  inspection in, 448
  introduction, 446
  kneading, 447
  learning activities, 452
  movements, 447–448
  palpation in, 448
  performance checklist, 452–453
  physical appraisal skills, 448
  physiological effects, 446–447
  preparation, 446–448
  principles of, 449
  recorded data and, 448
  recording
    sample narrative, 451
    sample POR, 451
  review questions, 452
  skeletal effects of, 446
  skill sequence, 450–451
  skin effects of, 446
  stroking, 447
  student objectives, 446
  tapotement, 447–448
Mattress pad, 760
Mayo enema, 608
Mealtime care, 510–512
  skill sequence, 512
Meaning
  communication and, 2, 3
  listening for, 76
Measures and weights, in medication administration, 829–831
Mechanical lifters, 746*F*, 747, 752*F*
Mechanical reaction, to adhesive tape, 301
Mechanical restraint. *See* Restraint, mechanical
Mechanical soft diet, 505
Medical asepsis. *See* Asepsis, medical
Medical history
  airway obstruction and, 989
  airway suctioning and, 816
  bandaging and binding and, 455
  blood pressure measurement and, 213–214
  breast examination and, 419
  CPR and, 974–975
  eating assistance and, 522
  elimination and, 594–595
  enema usage and, 609
  fluid balance and, 490
  food consumption and, 505
  gastrointestinal intubation and, 568
  hair care and, 399–400
  height appraisal and, 225–226
  injection and, 898
  isolation precautions and, 259
  IV therapy and, 939–940
  massage and, 448
  mechanical restraint and, 466
  nail care and, 408
  nutritional assessment and, 507
  oral care and, 386–387
  oxygen therapy and, 788
  perineal care and, 373–374
  pulse measurement and, 199
  respiration appraisal and, 207
  ROM and, 706
  self-catheterization and, 635
  skin care and, 363
  suture removal and, 312–313
  temperature measurement and, 184–185
  thermal application and, 437–438
  topical medications and, 868
  tracheostomy and, 804
  vaginal irrigation and, 412
  weight appraisal and, 225–226
  wound care and, 297
  wound drainage and, 330
Medical information system, purpose of, 142
Medical physician, medication order by, 834, 836*F*
Medical record system. *See* Record
Medicated bath, 363
Medicated dressing, 298
Medicated enema, 608
Medication
  administration
    card, 840, 841
      computer systems and, 838, 839*F*
      dosage calculation and, 831–834. *See also* Injectable medications, dosage calculation, *and* Intravenous infusions, flow rate
    "Five Rights" of, 828
    injectable. *See* Injectable medication administration
    intradermal. *See* Injectable

Medication (cont.)
  intradermal (cont.)
    medication administration, intradermal
  intramuscular. See Injectable medication administration, intramuscular
  intravenous. See Intravenous infusion
  kardex, 840, 841
  knowledge base for, 844–846
  law and, 843–844
  learning, 828–829
  manual systems and, 840–842
  oral. See Oral medication administration
  schedule, 833T, 835
  subcutaneous. See Injectable medication administration, subcutaneous
  topical. See Topical medication administration
  weights and measures in, 829–831
  cart, 838
  constipation and, 590
  delivery systems, 837–838
  errors in, 842–843
  food consumption and, 503
  individual supply of, 838
  injection of. See Injectable medication administration
  intramuscular. See Injectable medication administration, intramuscular
  intravenous. See Intravenous infusions
  kardex, 840, 841
  oral. See Oral medication administration
  order. See Medication order
  otic, 866
  piggyback administration of, 934, 957–958
  preparing, 842
  record. See Medication record
  recording, 842
  stock supply of, 838
  subcutaneous. See Injectable medication administration, subcutaneous
  swallowing of, 856
  topical. See Topical medication administration
  unit-dose system of, 837F, 842
Medication errors, 842–843
Medication order, 834–838
  abbreviations used in, 834F
  initiating the, 834–835
  intravenous, 929
  one-time, 835, 836F
  oral medication, 853
  p.r.n., 835, 836
  standard, 835, 836F
  standing, 835, 836F
  telephone, 835
  terms used in, 834F
  transmission of
    computerized systems in, 838, 839F
    manual systems in, 840–842F
    to nursing staff, 838–842, 839F, 840–842
    to pharmacist, 836–837
  types of, 835–836
  verbal, 835
  written, 836F
Medication record
  computerized systems of, 838, 839F
  manual systems of, 840–842F
Medicine cup, 853F
Medicine spoon, 853F
  standardization of, 830
Medicine tray, 841F
Melena, fecal appraisal of, 592
Mental attitude, blood pressure measurement and, 217
Mental status
  assessment of, 112F
  food consumption and, 502
Menu, food service, 508
Mercury glass thermometer, 185–186
  accuracy of, 186
  cleaning of, 186
  hazards of, 186
Mercury-gravity manometer, 214F, 216, 216F
  cleaning, 216F
Message
  facilitative communication skills and, 69
  feeling aspect reflection, 85
  I-. See I-message
  nonverbal. See Communication, nonverbal
  questions to convey, 92
  secondary, listening for, 75
  validation of, 79
  you-. See You-message
Metabolism, positioning and, 717–718
Metacommunication, 3
Meter, 829
  urine, 636
Metric system, 829
  abbreviations, 829
  weights activity, 829
Miconazole nitrate, 867
Microdrip device, in IV therapy, 942
Microorganism
  in surgical gloves, 286
  medical asepsis and, 239
  resident, definition of, 241
  transfer of, 269
Micturition. See Voiding
Milk and molasses enema, 608
Milliequivalent, definition of, 820
Miller-Abbott tube, 570F
Milligram, 829
Minim pipette, 851
Minimal inhibiting concentration test, wound infection and, 321
Minim, 830T
Misrepresentation, 100
Mistrust vs. trust, 26
Mitt, bathing, 365F
Mitt restraint, 467, 468F
Mobility assistance, 685–778
  assessment of, 113F
  balance and, 686–687
  body mechanics principles and, 686–690
  cast and, 476
  force and, 687
  friction and, 687
  inertia and, 687
  lifting and, 689
  momentum and, 687–688
  motion and, 687
  muscle movements and, 689
  safety concepts, 690
  weight and, 686
  work and, 688–689

Moisturizer, bathing and, 366
Momentum, body mechanics and, 687–688
Monilial infection, of vagina, 412
Monitoring, in IV infusion, 954
Montgomery strap, 300–301, 301F
  in wet-to-dry dressing, 345
Mortar and pestle, 851, 853F
Motion, body mechanics and, 687
Motivation, client, 128–129
Motor system
  assessment of, 113F
  positioning and, 717
Mouth
  care of. See Oral care
  dry, intubation and, 564
  facilitated use of, 520F
  inspection of, 869
  temperature measurement via, 183F, 188
  topical medication in, 866, 869–870
    buccal tablets, 866, 869–870, 870F
    sprays, 866, 870
    sublingual tablets, 866, 869–870, 870F
Mouth prop, 390
Mouth-to-mouth ventilation, 977–978
Mouth-to-nose ventilation, 978
Mouth-to-stoma ventilation, 978
Mouthwash, 389–390, 870
Moving. See Turning, moving and positioning
Mucous membrane
  fluid balance and, 489, 492
  structure of, 361
  topical medication and, 867
  urinary catheterization and, 630–633
Muscle
  contraction of, 692
  injection in. See Injectable medication administration, intramuscular
  massage and, 446
  movement of, 689
  thermal applications to, 435
Musculoskeletal system
  assessment of, 113F
  malnutrition and, 508T
Muslin, in sterile supplies, 273
Muslin bandage, 455

Nail
  biting, 407
  care of. See Nail care clubbing of, 407F
  disorders of, 407
  hemorrhages under, 407
  ingrown, 408
  malnutrition and, 508T
  normal appearance of, 407
  structure and function of, 406–407, 407F
  trauma to, 407–408
Nail care
  client history and, 408
  critical points summary, 409
  cyanosis and, 408
  data base for, 408
  definition of, 406
  emery boards, 408
  equipment for, 408
  execution, 408–409
  inspection in, 408
  introduction, 406

INDEX **1035**

learning activities, 410
nail clippers, 408
nail disorders, 407*F*
orange sticks in, 408
pallor and, 408
palpation in, 408
performance checklist, 410
physical appraisal skills, 408
preparation, 406–408, 408–409
recorded data and, 408
recording
    sample narrative, 409
    sample POR, 409
review questions, 410
skill sequence, 409
structure, 406–407, 407*F*
student objectives, 406
trauma and, 407–408
Narcotic, administration of, 843
Narrative notes, 143, 150, 151
    in record-keeping, 143*F*
    nursing records and, 150–151
Nasal cannula, 790*F*
    oxygen administration via, 794–795
    skill sequence, 795–796
Nasal catheter, 790, 791*F*
    skill sequence, 795–796
Nasal sprays, 866
Nasogastric tube. *See also* Gastrointestinal tube
    client care, 581–582, 582*T*
    data base, 568–569
    definition of, 563
    enteral feeding and, 528
    equipment for, 569–570, 572–573*F*
    Ewald, 569*F*, 570
    execution, 574–584
    gastric lavage, 564, 570
    insertion, 574–578
    irrigation, 579–581
    learning activities, 584–585
    Levin, 569*F*
    nasogastric insertion, 574–578
    performance checklist, 586–587
    pipeline suctioning of, 571
    placement of, 576*F*
    post-insertion problems, 564–565
    recording, 584
    removal, skill sequence, 582–583
    review questions, 585
    Sengstaken-Blakemore, 569*F*, 570
    short, 569–570
    skill sequence, 578–581, 583
        insertion, 578–579
        irrigation, 580–581
        removal, 583
    suctioning of, 571–573, 572–573*F*
    sump, 569*F*, 570
    swallowing dysfunction and, 518
    thermotic pump, 571–572, 573*F*
Nasojejunal tube, enteral feeding and, 528
Nasopharynx, airway suctioning and, 815
National League for Nursing, medication errors and, 843
Nausea, enteral feeding and, 533
Nebulizer, 867
    in topical medication administration, 869
    metered-dose, 881*F*
Neck
    hyperextension of, 856
    oral medication administration and, 856
    ROM exercises for, 708*F*
    performance checklist, 715–716
Neck lift, in CPR, 974, 976–977, 977*F*
Needle
    beveled tip, 900*F*
    butterfly, 942–943, 943*F*
    common sizes, 902*T*
    destruction of, 901, 902*F*
    hub, 900*F*
    in IV therapy, 942–943, 943*F*
    injection, 900*F*
    isolation precautions and, 251
    selection of, 902
    shaft, 900*F*
    winged, 942–943, 943*F*
Needs. *See* Basic needs
Negligence, nursing records and, 154
Negotiation, reflection of content and, 80
Nervous system, malnutrition and, 508*T*
Neurogenic incontinence, 621
Neurologic disorder, eating assistance and, 517
Neuromuscular condition, defecation and, 590
Neurosensory eating facilitation, 519–522
Neurovascular status, cast and, 475
Nitroglycerin ointment
    applicator paper, 881*F*
    transdermal, 880
NITROL Tape Surrounded Appli-Ruler, 881
Nomogram, in skinfold measurement, 233*F*, 234
Nonadhering dressing, 298
Nonblanching hyperemia, 360
Nonocclusive dressing, 298
Nonpitting edema, 488
Nonverbal communication, 45–67, 46*F*
    activities
        interpreting nonverbal behavior, 51
        making and reporting observations, 50
        nonverbal communication, 47
        observing nonverbal behavior, real-life settings, 54
        observing nonverbal behavior, simulated settings, 53
        personal modes, 50
    body language and, 48
    caring and, 15*F*
    client observation, 52–53, 53*T*
    critical points summary, 54
    empathy and, 12
    environment and, 49
    execution, 52–54
    eye communication and, 47–48
    facial expressions and, 48
    interpreting, 49–50, 50–51
    introduction, 46
    modes of, 47–49
    nurse-client relationship and, 49–50
    observation guidelines, 53*T*
    observation skills development, 53–54
    preparation, 46–52
    review questions, 54–55
    simulation activity, 53–54
    student objectives, 46
    touch and, 63
    trust and, 11
    understanding, 49–50
    validating perceptions of, 51–52
    -verbal communication congruence, 51
    voice and, 48–49
Nose
    inspection of, 869
    palpation of, 364
    skin care, 362
    topical medication in, 866
    trauma, intubation and, 564
Nose drops
    insertion, 870–871, 871*F*
    skill sequence, 871–872
Nose sprays, administration of, 871
Nosocomial infection, definition of, 239
Nurse
    competence of, client idea of, 42
    interpersonal skills of, 8
    professional value conflicts, 34
    silence on part of, 57–58
    time-orientation of, 56
Nurse practitioner, medication order by, 834
Nurse-client interaction
    characteristics of, 107–108
    interviewing, 108–126
    space in, 64
    structured, 107–140
    teaching-learning, 126–140
Nurse-client relationship
    caring and, 14
    communication and, 1
    confidential, 9
    deterrents to, 10
    helping relationship and, 7–17
    honesty in, 12
    identity level of, 15
    individualized, 9
    involvement level of, 15–16
    nonverbal communication and, 49–50
    questioning skills in, 91
    reflection of content and, 79
    self-disclosure and, 38–40
    superficial level of, 15
    trust and, 12
Nurse-patient relationship. *See* Nurse-client relationship
Nurse's notes, medical record, 147
Nursing, 845
    communication and, 1–3
    use of space in, 62–63
Nursing audit, 149
Nursing care, distance zone and, 64
Nursing history, 110*F*, 147
    nursing assessment, 111–115
Nursing notes, writing, 159–161
Nursing record, 148–163. *See also* Health record
    abbreviations, 159*T*
    activities, writing nursing notes, 159–161
    characteristics of, 149–150
    critical points summary, 161
    execution, 155–161
    flow sheets, 151–153, 161
    introduction, 149–150
    Kardex system, 153–154, 156–157*F*, 161
    legal acceptability guidelines, 155–158
    narrative notes, 150–151
    POMR system, 150–151
    POR format, 151*T*
    preparation, 150–154
    professional accountability guidelines,

Nursing record (cont.)
  professional accountability guidelines (cont.)
    158–159
  reporting observations, 154
  review questions, 161
  student objectives, 148–149
  traditional source-oriented systems, 151
  writing, 159–161
Nutrition
  oral care and, 386
  tracheostomy and, 803
  weight and, 224–225
Nutritional assessment. *See* Nutritional care
Nutritional care, 481, 500, 505–507, 506T
  after meal care, 512
  anthropometric measures in, 507
  appetite and, 502
  arm muscle circumference and, 507
  characteristics of, 481, 500
  client history and, 507
  consistency modification, 504
  consumption factors, 501–503
  critical points summary, 513
  cultural factors and, 502
  data base, 507
  diagnostic modification, 504
  diet order implementation, 509–510
  dietary service, 504
  eating assistance, 515–526
  economic factors and, 502
  emotional status and, 502
  environmental hygiene and, 510
  equipment, 507–509
  evaluation guide, 506T
  execution, 509–513
  fluid balance assessment, 482–499
  food consumption factors, 501–503
  food history in, 505
  food intake regulation, 500–503
  food itself and, 502–503
  food service, 499–515
  food trays, 508–509
  functional abilities and, 501–502
  health-care agencies, 503–504
  hospital diet, 504
  hunger and, 502
  illness conditions and, 503
  implementing diet order, 509–510
  introduction, 500
  laboratory data in, 505–507
  learning activities, 513–514
  malnutrition, 501, 508T
  mealtime care, 510–512, 511F
    skill sequence, 512
  mental status and, 502
  menu selection, 510
  menus, 508
  normal diet, 504–505
  nutritional assessment, 505–507, 506T
  nutritional services, 503–504
  performance checklist, 514
  personal hygiene and, 510
  physical appraisal skills, 507
  physical strength and, 501–502
  positioning for, 511F
  preparation, 500–509
  recorded data, 507
  recording
    sample narrative, 513
    sample POR, 513
  review questions, 514
  skill sequence, 512
  standard hospital diet, 504–505
  student objectives, 499–500
  temperature-control mechanisms, 509
  texture modification, 504
  therapeutic modification, 504
  transportation devices, 509
  tray identification, 511
  tray serving, 512
Nutritional service, 503–504
  dietary services, 504
  food service, 503–504
Nutritional status, 481
  assessment of, 113F
Nutritional support, 481
  enteral. *See* Enteral nutritional support
  parenteral. *See* Total parenteral nutrition
Nutritive enema, 608
Nuturing activities, touch in, 64

Oatmeal bath, 363
Obesity
  atelectasis and, 774
  dangling and, 695
  definition of, 225
  wound repair and, 294
Objective data, in nursing records, 150
Observation, oral medication administration and, 858
Obstructed airway, removal of
  back blows, 990F
  client history and, 989
  complications, 989
  critical points summary, 995–996
  data base, 989–990
  execution, 990–996
  in conscious adult, 990F, 991F
  in infant, 994F
  in unconscious adult, 992–994, 993F
  inspection in, 985
  introduction, 988
  learning activities, 996
  manual thrusts, 990, 991F
  performance checklist, 996–997
  physical appraisal skills, 989–990
  preparation, 988–990
  recorded data and, 989
  recording, 995
    sample narrative, 996
    sample POR, 996
  review questions, 996
  skill sequence, 992, 993–994, 995
    conscious adult, 992
    in infant, 996
    unconscious adult, 993–994
  student objectives, 988
Occlusive dressing, 298
Occult blood, 507
Occultest, 507
Odor
  in skin care, 365
  in topical medication administration, 869
  in vaginal irrigation, 412
  nonverbal communication and, 49
  of feces, 592
  of urine, 591
  of wet sterile dressing, 345
  of wound, 297

  wound infection and, 321
Offering assistance. *See* Assistance
Oil-retention enema, 608
Ointment, 868T
  bathing, 366
  eye, 874F
Olfactory status, assessment of, 113F
Optometrist, medication order by, 834
Oral care
  agents, 389–390
  appraisal guide, 387, 388T
  assistive agents and devices, 390
  bite block, 390
  bulb syringe in, 390
  client history and, 386–387
  complete assistance, 393–394
  critical points summary, 394–395
  data base, 386–387
  definition of, 383–384
  dental floss, 389
  dentifrices, 389
  denture care, 387, 393F
  denture cups, 389
  devices, 387–389
  disclosing preparations, 390
  emesis basin, 390
  enteral feeding and, 538
  equipment, 387–390
  execution, 390–394
  flossing, 391F
  fluoride supplements, 390
  glycerin, 389
  in unconscious client, 392–393, 393F
  inspection in, 387
  introduction, 383–384
  learning activities, 395
  mouth prop, 390
  mouthwashes, 389–390
  nutrition and, 386–390
  oral cavity, 384–386
  oxygenating agents, 389
  palpation in, 387
  performance checklist, 395–396
  petroleum jelly, 390
  physical appraisal skills, 387
  preparation, 384–390, 388T
  recorded data and, 386–387
  recording
    sample narrative, 394
    sample POR, 394
  review questions, 395
  skill sequence, 393–394
  student objectives, 383
  tongue brushing, 391–392
  tongue depressor, 390
  toothbrushes, 387
  toothbrushing, 391F
  toothette, 387–388
  water irrigation device, 388
Oral cavity
  inspection of, 869
  palate, 385
  saliva, 384
  soft tissue, 384–385
  teeth, 385–386
  tongue, 385
  tonsils, 385
  topical medication in, 866, 869–870
    buccal tablets, 866, 869–870, 870F
    sprays, 866, 870
    sublingual tablets, 866, 869–870, 870F
Oral medications
  administration, 847–864, 856–857

controlled substance, 843–851F, 853–854
critical points summary, 860–861
data base for, 850
dosage calculation, 848–850
dosage forms, 849T
equipment for, 851
execution, 851–860
food and, 848
generic substitution, 853
giving instructions about, 860
individual supply 852–853
introduction, 848
knowledge base for, 851–852
learning activities, 861–862
liquid, 849T
  administering, 856–857
  dosage forms, 849T
  measurement of, 848
nasogastric administration of, 859–860
performance checklist, 862–864
physical appraisal skills, 851
practice problems, 850
  key to, 1013
preparation of, 856F
  safety guidelines for, 852–854
  skill sequence, 854–855
preparation skills, 848–851
preparations of, 848
recording, 860
review questions, 862
skill sequence, 854–855, 858–859
  administering, 858–859
  preparing, 854–855
solid, 849T
stock supply, 852–853
strength of, 848
student objectives, 847
through nasogastric tube, 859–860
types of, 848, 849T
unit-dose, 852
Oral report, 154
Orange stick, in nail care, 408
Orogastric tube, enteral feeding and, 528
Oropharynx, airway suctioning and, 815
Orthopnea, 207
Orthostatic hypotension
  dangling and, 695, 696
  immobility and, 693
  recording, 701
Osmolality
  of serum, 489
  of urine, 489
Osteopathic physician, medication order by, 834
Ostomy care, 658–683
  appliance leakage and, 672
  appliance replacement, 673
  appliances
    disposable, 668, 669F
    permanent, 668, 669F
  auscultation in, 667
  bowel diversions, 659–663
  client history and, 667
  client self-, 666–667
  colostomy, 660–661, 660F, 661F
  colostomy irrigation, 675–678
    skill sequence, 678–680
  common problems in, 665–666
  continent ileostomy, 662–663, 662F
  critical points summary, 680–681
  data base for, 667–668

diarrhea and, 665
equipment, 668–671F
execution, 672–680
flatus and, 665
food block and, 665–666
ileal bladder conduit, 663
ileal conduit, 663, 664F
ileostomy, 662–663
inspection of, 667
introduction, 659
irrigation, 661–662, 675–680F
  equipment, 670–671F
leakage, 665
learning activities, 681
management problems, 665–666
odor in, 665, 667–668
palpation of, 667
performance checklist, 682–683
peristomal skin irritation and, 672
physical appraisal skills in, 667–668
pouch replacement, 672–673
preparation, 659–672
problems, 665–666
psychosocial adjustment to, 666
review questions, 681
self-, 666–667
skill sequence, 673–675, 678–680
  colostomy irrigation, 678–680
  replacing ostomy pouch, 673–675
skin irritation and, 665
skin protection products, 670
stoma cap, 670
student objectives, 658–659
ureterostomy, 663, 664F
urinary diversions, 663–664
urinary tract infections and, 666
vesicostomy, 663, 664F
Outcome criteria, nursing records, 149
Overflow safety device, in pipeline suction, 571
Overhead cradles, antidecubitus, 723
Overnutrition, 501
  definition of, 225
Over-the-needle catheter, 943F
Overweight, definition of, 225
Oxygen
  administration of. See Oxygen therapy
  delivery systems
    high flow, 792
    low flow, 790–792
    preparation of, 794
  humidifiers, 789–790
  portable cylinders of, 789F
  supply systems
    portable, 789F
    wall, 788–789, 789F
  tent, 792
    administration via, 796–797
    skill sequence, 795–796
  toxicity of, 787
Oxygen mask
  nonrebreathing, 792
  partial rebreathing, 791F
  simple, 790–791, 791F
  tent, 792
  Venturi, 792F
Oxygen tension, hypoxemia and, 786
Oxygen therapy, 786–788
  absorption atelectasis and, 787
  administering, 794–795
    body temperature and, 184
    catheter, 794–795
    mask, 795
    nasal catheter, 794–795

  skill sequence, 795–796
  tent, 796–797
auscultation in, 788
blood gases and, 788
client preparation for, 792–793
critical points summary, 797
data base, 788
equipment, 788–793
execution, 793–797
flow meter, 788–789, 789F
hazards of, 787
humidification, 787–788
hypoxemia and, 786
hypoxia and, 786
-induced hypoventilation, 787
inspection in, 788
introduction, 785
learning activities, 797
mask administration, 795
oxygen delivery systems, 790, 793T
  high flow, 792–793
  low flow, 790–792
oxygen supply systems, 788–790
palpation in, 788
performance checklist, 798–799
physical appraisal skills in, 788
portable steel cylinders, 789F
preparation, 785–786
recording, 797
retrolental fibroplasia and, 786
review questions, 797–798
skill sequence, 795–796
student objectives, 785
systems preparation, 794
tent administration, 796–797
toxicity, 787
Oxygenating agent, in oral care, 389

Packaging, of sterile supplies, 274
Pad
  incontinence, 624
  perineal care, 374
Pain, injection, 896
Palate, structure of, 385
Pallor
  appearance of, 364
  definition of, 359
Palpation, 171–173
  critical points summary, 172
  deep, 172F
  execution, 171
  in alternating pulse, 196F
  in ambulation assistance, 694
  in bandaging and binding, 455
  in cast care, 477
  in CPR, 975
  in eating assistance, 522
  in elimination, 595
  in fluid balance, 492
  in hair care, 400
  in injection, 898
  in intubation, 567–568
  in IV therapy, 940
  in massage, 448
  in mechanical restraint, 466
  in nail care, 408
  in nutritional assessment, 508T
  in oral care, 387
  in oxygen therapy, 788
  in pulse measurement, 200
  in respiration appraisal, 208
  in ROM exercises, 706

Palpation (cont.)
  in self-catheterization, 635
  in skin care, 364–365
  in suture removal, 313
  in thermal application, 438
  in topical medication administration, 869
  in weight appraisal, 226
  in wound culture specimen collection, 322
  introduction, 171
  learning activities, 172–173
  light, 171F
  of abdomen, 567–568
  of blood pressure, 213, 214
  of breasts, 419
  of pressure points, 364–365
  of tracheostomy, 804
  of wet sterile dressing, 345
  of wet-to-dry dressing, 352
  of wound, 297
  preparation, 171
  review questions, 173
  student objectives, 171
Pants, incontinence, 624
Paper, sterile, 273
Paper tape, 300
Paper towel, handwashing and, 242
Paraphrasing, 80
Paraplegia
  urinary catheterization and, 629
  urinary tract infection and, 631
Parotitis, intubation and, 564–565
Paste, 868T
Patch, eye, 876, 877F
Patient instruction. See Teaching-learning
PDR. See Physicians' Desk Reference
Pediculosis, 399
Pelvic girdle, "tightening" of, 689
Pelvis, exercises, 622
Penetrating wound, definition of, 293
Penis
  catheterization and, 625
  in perineal care, 373
  washing of, 375–377
Penrose drain, 329–330, 331, 334F
  technique, 336–337
Perception, nonverbal communication, 50
Percussion, 173–177
  critical points summary, 176
  definition of, 779
  dull sound, 175
  execution, 176
  flat sound, 175
  in cast care, 477
  in elimination, 595
  in intubation, 567
  in postural drainage, 779
  in self-catheterization, 635
  introduction, 173–174
  learning activitities, 176–177
  of abdomen, 567
  physical appraisal using, 174–175
  preparation, 174–175
  review questions, 177
  sound perception in, 174
  sound wave characteristics and, 174
  student objectives, 173
Peridontal disease, 385
Peridontal tissue, definition of, 384
Perineal care
  client history and, 373–374

critical points summary, 380
data base, 373–374
definition of, 373
equipment, 374F
execution, 374–379
female, 375
hazards, 379
inspection in, 374
introduction, 373
irrigation, 377–378
  performance checklist, 382
  skill sequence, 377–378
learning activities, 380
male, 375–376
performance checklist, 380–383
physical appraisal skills, 374
positioning, 375F
premoistened pads for, 374
preparation, 373–374
recorded data and, 373–374
recording, 379–380
  sample narrative, 380
  sample POR, 379
review questions, 380
sexual response, 373
sitz bath, 374, 379
  cleaning the, 379
  disposable, 374
  performance checklist, 382–383
  skill sequence, 379
skill sequence
  irrigation, 377–378
  sitz bath, 379
  washing, 376–377
student objectives, 372–373
washing, 375–379
  performance checklist, 380–381
  skill sequence, 376–377
Perineum
  care of. See Perineal care
  irrigation of equipment for, 374
  performance checklist, 382
  skill sequence, 377–378
Periodontitis, 385
Peripheral pulse, 197
  fluid balance and, 486, 492
Peripheral vein, filling of, fluid balance and, 487F, 491
Peristaltic pump, in IV therapy, 944
Personal hygiene
  breast examination, 417–424
  corpse care, 425–431
  definition of, 357
  food service and, 510
  hair care, 397–406
  introduction, 357
  nail care, 406–410
  nonverbal communication and, 47
  nutritional care and, 510
  oral care, 383–397
  perineal care, 372–383
  skin care, 358–372
  vaginal irrigation, 411–417
Personal space. See also Space and touch
  communication activity, 62
  intimate distance, 61
  nursing care and, 64–65
  nursing home use of, 62–63
  nursing use of, 62–63
  personal distance, 61
  public distance, 61
  social distance, 61
  territoriality and, 61–62

Personality, needs satisfaction and, 25
Personalizing, 52
  reflection of feelings and, 85–86
Perspiration
  fluid deficit and, 484
  measurement of, 495
  nonverbal communication and, 47
Petrissage, in massage, 447
Petroleum jelly, in oral care, 390
Pharmacist
  medication order transmission to, 836–837
  medication order by, 834
Pharynx, in swallowing, 517
Phlebitis, IV therapy and, 935–936
Phosphate enema, 607
Physical appraisal skills, 169–180
  auscultation, 177–180
  inspection, 169–170
  palpation, 171–173
  percussion, 173–177
Physical help, providing direct, 98–99
Physician order
  diet, 509–510
  for intravenous therapy, 929
Physicians assistant, 834
Physicians' Desk Reference, 845–846
Physicians order sheet, 146
Physics concepts
  angular movement and, 688
  arc and, 688
  effort arm and, 688
  fulcrum and, 688
  levers and, 688
  resistance arm and, 688
Physiological effect, of mechanical restraint, 465
Physiological needs, 25
Piggyback IV medication, 934, 957–958
Pigmentation, 359
Pillow
  cast, 477
  chest therapy and, 780
Pillowcases, 760, 765F
Pin, in bandaging and binding, 462
Pinch test, in skinfold measurement, 231
Pipe cleaner, tracheostomy tube and, 805
Pitch, in percussion, 174
Pitcher
  fluid balance assessment and, 493
  graduated measuring, 535
Pitting edema, 487–488, 488F
Placation, 40
Plan, in nursing records, 151
Planning, definition of, 107
Plaque, dental, 386
Plasma, 933
  substitutes, 933–934
  volume expander, 933–934
Plaster cast, 474, 475
Plastic, in sterile supplies, 273–274
Plastic container, in IV therapy, 940F, 941
Plastic foam pads, antidecubitus, 723
Plastic tape, 300
Platelet, IV, 933
Platitudes, reassurance and, 100
Pleximeter, percussion, 173
Plexor, in percussion, 173
Pneumonia
  aspiration, 533
  hypoxemia and, 786

Podiatrist, medication order by, 834
Pole, in IV therapy, 944
Popliteal pulse, 197, 198F
  measurement of, 202
Positioning. See Turning, moving and positioning
Postmortem care, isolation and, 253
Postural drainage, airway resistance and, 779
Posture
  attending behavior and, 71
  nonverbal communication and, 48
Povidone-iodine
  in wet-to-dry dressing, 352
  urinary catheterization and, 632
Powder
  bathing, 366
  drug, injection dosage, 896
  for sterile gloves, 287
  topical, 868T
Prefilled syringe, 900
Pregnancy, breasts in, 418
Prejudice
  empathy and, 13–14
  listening and, 76–77
Prescription. See Medication order
Presence, reassurance and, 100
Pressure, elimination and, 561–562
Pressure cuff, blood infusion and, 945
Pressure points, 361F, 364–365
  inspection of, 364–365
  massage of, 449
  palpation of, 364–365
  positioning and, 718
  protective aids, 722–724
Pressure sore, 360F. See also Decubitus ulcer
  positioning and, 718
Primary malnutrition, 501
Priorities, in teaching-learning, 132
Privacy
  bedpan use and, 597
  personal space and, 61
Private room, as isolation precaution, 250
Probe, in electronic thermometer, 187
Problem list, 143
  in record-keeping, 143F
Problem solving, in decision making, 101–102
Problem-oriented medical record system
  nursing records and, 150–151, 151T
  use of, 142–144, 143F
Problem-oriented record, 143–144
Procedural touch, 61
Process criteria, nursing records, 149
Progress notes, 143–144
  in record-keeping, 143F
  medical report, 147
Pronation, 705
Prone position, in bed, 718–719, 735, 736F
  turning to, 735F
Proportion equation method, in injection dosage calculation, 897. See Dosage
  drug
    in dosage calculation, 831–833
    in injection dosage calculation, 897
    in IV flow rate calculation, 937
    in IV medication flow, 938, 939
      rate calculation, 938
    in oral medications, 850
Proprietary drugs, 843
Protective intervention, 433

Protective treatment
  bandage application, 453–464
  binder application, 453–464
  cast care, 473–480
  definition, 433
  entry test, 433
  massage, 446–453
  mechanical restraints, 464–473
  thermal applications, 433–446
Protein
  hair growth and, 398
  in enteral formula, 531
  in nutritional assessment, 506T, 507
Protein-calorie malnutrition, 501
Proxemics, 61
Pruritis
  aging skin and, 362
  topical medication and, 870
Psychiatric client, mechanical restraint in, 470
Psychogenic incontinence, 621
Psychological effect
  of intravenous therapy, 929
  of mechanical restraint, 465
  of urinary catheterization, 633–634
Psychological needs, 25
Psychosocial adaptation, to enteral feeding, 533
Psychosocial impact, of isolation, 254
Psychosocial status, assessment of, 112F
Psychosomatic factors, of defecation, 590
Puberty, touch and, 63
Pull sheet, client moving using, 729
Pull-ups, 692F
Pulmonary arrest, physiology of, 972
Pulmonary edema, 487
  bed rest and, 774
Pulp, dental, 385
Pulse appraisal, 194–204
  alternating, 196F
  apical, 201
  apical-radial, 202
  assessment of, 114F
  auscultation in, 200
  atrial fibrillation and, 195
  bounding, 195–196
  brachial, 202
  carotid, 197, 198F
  characteristics of, 195F, 196F
  client history, 199
  comparisons of, 197–199, 198F
  critical points summary, 204
  data base for 199–200
  deficit, 197, 199
  dorsalis pedis, 202
  equipment for, 200
  execution of, 200–204
  facial, 197, 198F
  femoral, 202
  fluid balance and, 486, 492
  inspection in, 200
  introduction, 194–195
  learning activities, 204
  palpation in, 200
  paradoxical, 196F
  performance checklist, 204
  peripheral, 197
    fluid balance and, 486
    rating scale for, 203T
    stick figure for, 203F
  physical appraisal skills, 200
  popliteal, 202
  posterior tibialis, 202
  preparation, 195–200

  presence of, 197
  quality of, 195
  radial, 200–201
  rate of, 195
  recording of, 203F
  recorded data, 199
  review questions, 204
  rhythm of, 195–196
  sample narrative recording, 204
  sites, 196–197, 198F
  skill sequence, 200–203
    apical pulse, 201
    apical-radial pulse, 202
    brachial pulse, 202
    dorsalis pedis pulse, 203
    femoral pulse, 202
    popliteal pulse, 202
    posterior tibialis pulse, 203
    radial pulse, 200–201
  student objectives, 194
  temporal, 197, 198F
  tibialis, posterior, 202
  weak, 195
Pulse rate, fluid balance and, 486
Pulsus alterans, 196F
Pulsus bigeminus, 195F
Pulsus paradoxus, 196F
Pump
  in enteral feedings, 535F
  in IV therapy, 944
  thermotic, in gastric suction, 571–572, 573F
Puncture wound, 293
Pupil, in CPR, 975
Purulent exudate, wound infection and, 320–321
Pushups, 692

Quadriceps, isometric exercises and, 692
Quadriplegia, urinary catheterization and, 629
Questioning
  activities
    questioning and being questioned, 95–96
    simulations of, 95
    using open and closed questions, 93–94
  critical points summary, 96
  execution, 94–96
  introduction, 91–92
  nonproductive, 95–96
  performance checklist, 97
  preparation, 92–94
  productive, 95, 96
  review questions, 96
  simulation activity, 95
  student objectives, 91
Questions
  closed, 93
    examples of, 93
    using activity 93–94
  definition of, 91
  open, 92
    examples of, 92
    using activity, 93–94
  problems with, 94
  wording of, 95
Quick-stretch, eating facilitation, 519, 520F

Racial factors, helping concept and, 10

Radial pulse, 197, 198F
  measurement of, 200–201
Radiant energy in thermal applications, 437
Rales, 776
Range of motion, 704–716
  anatomic neutral position and, 705
  client history and, 706
  client position and, 706–707
  critical points summary, 715
  data base, 706
  equipment and, 706
  execution, 706–714
  exercises, 708–714
    active assistive, 705
    ankle, 708, 713F
    elbow, 708, 710F
    extremities, 707
    finger, 708, 711F
    free active, 705
    hip, 708, 712F, 713F
    implementing, 707–714
    knee, 708, 713F
    neck, 707, 708F
    passive, 705, 707
    recording, 714
    resistive, 705
    shoulder, 707, 708, 709F, 710F
    skill sequence, 714
    support for, 707F
    toe, 708, 714F
    wrist, 708, 711F
  inspection and, 706
  introduction, 704
  joints and, 705–706
  learning activities, 715
  palpation and, 706
  performance checklist, 715–716
  physical appraisal skills, 706
  positioning, 706–707
  preparation, 704–706
  recorded data and, 706
  recording
    sample narrative, 714
    sample POR, 714
  review questions, 715
  skill sequence, 714
  student objectives, 704
  terms, 705
  types of, 705
Rayon taffeta tape, 300
Reassurance
  experiencing activity, 104
  false, 100–101
  genuine, 99–100
  giving activity, 101
  need for, 99
  providing appropriate, 99–101
  receiving activity, 101
  simulation activity, 104
Rebound phenomenon, in thermal application, 435–436
Record. See also Written communication
  health. See Health record nursing. See Nursing record
Recording
  interviewing and, 120–121, 121–123T
  process, 120–121, 121–123T
Rectal tube
  enema, 611
  insertion of, 614–615
Rectum
  medication administration in, 879F
    skill sequence, 879–880

temperature measurement via, 184F
  technique, 189
  topical medication in, 867
Rectus femoris muscle, injection, 894F
Recycle system, in thermometer cleaning, 186
Red blood cell count, in nutritional assessment, 506T, 507
Red blood cells, packed, 933
Referrals
  decision making and, 102
  reassurance and, 100
Reflection of content. See Content, reflection of
Reflection of feelings. See Feelings, reflection of
Reflex, gag, 520, 521F
Regeneration, in wound repair, 293
Reinforcement, learning and, 133
Relationship, goal of, 9
Religion, helping factors and, 10
Repetition, learning and, 133
Reproductive status, assessment of, 112F
Resident organism, definition of, 241
Resistance arm, 688
Resistive exercises, 692
Resonance, in percussion, 175F
Resource availability, in teaching-learning, 135
Respect
  caring and, 14
  level of, 13
Respiration appraisal, 205–209
  assessment of, 114F
  auscultation in, 208
  breath sounds and, 207
  characteristics of, 206–207, 207F
  Cheyne-Stokes, 206, 207F
  client history, 207
  critical points summary, 209
  data base for, 207–208
  depth of, 206
  execution, 208–209
  fluid balance and, 486
  inspection in, 208
  introduction, 205–206
  intubation and, 565
  Kussmaul, 206
  learning activities, 209
  palpation in, 208
  pattern, 206–207
  performance checklist, 209
  physical appraisal skills, 207–208
  positioning and, 717
  preparation, 206–208
  quality of, 774
  rate of, 206
  recorded data, 213
  recording
    sample narrative, 209
    sample POR, 208
  review questions, 209
  rhythm, 206
  skill sequence, 208
  student objectives, 205
Respiratory care, introduction, 773
Respiratory insufficiency, tracheostomy and, 802
Respiratory isolation, 256, 257T, 259
Respiratory system
  appraisal of, 776–777
  breath sounds, 776–777
    auscultation of, 777F

positioning and, 717
Respiratory therapist, 785
Responsibility, record keeping, 141
Restraints
  chest, 467, 468F
  elbow, 467, 468F
  hard, 465
  limb, 467F, 469, 470–471
  mechanical
    applying, 469–470
    chest, 467, 468F
    client care, 470
    client history and, 466
    combative clients and, 470
    critical points summary, 471–472
    data base, 466
    elbow, 368F, 467
    equipment, 465–467, 467F, 468F
    execution, 468–471
    hard, 465, 467F
    inspection of, 466
    introduction, 465
    knots in, 469F
    learning activities, 472
    legal aspects of, 465–466
    limb, 467F, 470–471
    mitt, 467, 468F
    palpation and, 466
    performance checklist, 472–473
    physical appraisal skills, 466
    physiological effects, 465
    preparation, 465–467
    psychiatric clients and, 470
    psychological effects of, 465
    recorded data and, 466
    recording
      sample narrative, 471
      sample POR, 471
    review questions, 472
    safety belts, 466–467
    skill sequence, 470–471
    soft, 465
    student objectives, 464–465
    types of, 465, 466–467
  mitt, 467, 468F
  soft, 465
Resuscitation
cardiopulmonary. See Cardiopulmonary resuscitation
  mouth-to-mouth, 977–978
  mouth-to-nose, 978
  mouth-to-stoma, 978
Retention suture, 312
Reticulum, function of, 359
Retrolental fibroplasia, 787
Return-flow enema, 608
Reusable glass syringe, 899–900
Rhonchi, 776–777
Rigor mortis, 426
RN, 845
Roller bars, 746–747
Room cleaning, isolation and, 253
Rubber bag, in thermal application, 438
Rubber bands, in nasogastric intubation, 573

Safety, bedpans and, 597
Safety belt, 466–467
Safety pin, in nasogastric intubation, 573
Salicylic acid, in wet-to-dry dressing, 345

Saline
  enema and, 607
  in nasogastric irrigation, 574
  in wet sterile dressing, 345
  in wet-to-dry dressing, 352
  IV solution, 932T, 933
  tracheostomy tubes and, 805
Saliva
  characteristics of, 384
  fluid balance and, 489
Sandbags, 722
Satiety, 501
Scale
  accuracy of, 227–228
  balance-beam, 226F, 227F
  bathroom, 226
  bedside, 227F
    skill sequence, 230–231
  physicians, 226F
Scalp
  IV infusion in, 930
  medication administration to, 880
Scapular area, injection in, 892
Scissors
  dressing change and, 301F, 302
  in cast care, 477
  in suture removal, 313
Scopolamine, transdermal, 881–882
Secondary malnutrition, 501
Secretions
  isolation precautions and, 258T, 259
  respiratory, retention of, 775
Sedative
  administration of, 843
  tracheostomy and, 803
Self
  acceptance of, 18
  ideal self relationship, 21
  inner, 23F
  learning about, 24
  perceived, 21
  private, 23F
  public, 23F
  semipublic, 23F
  therapeutic use of, 10
  value conflicts within, 34
Self-actualization, nurse-client relationship and, 29
Self-awareness
  acceptance and, 11
  definition, 7
  developing, 19–20
  feelings identification and, 18–20, 19F
  of values, 35
  wheel, 19, 20F
  using the, 20–21
Self-care
  elimination and, 561
  feeding and, 481
  fluid balance and, 490
  helping relationship and, 10
Self-catheterization
  intermittent, 634–635
  teaching clients, 651–652
Self-concept
  definition, 7
  knowing ourselves and, 21–22
  needs satisfaction and, 27
Self-determination, helping relationship and, 10
Self-disclosure, 36–42
  activities
    communication patterns, 41
    I-messages, 41

  self-disclosure, 37, 38F
  self-disclosure to others, 42
  you-messages, 41
authenticity of, 35
communication and, 40–41
  patterns activity, 41
confusion and, 35
congruence of, 35
critical points summary, 42
decision making and, 102
definition, 7
empathy and, 13
execution of, 41–42
genuineness of, 35
hindrances to, 40
I-messages activity in, 41
intentional, 37
introduction, 36–37
nurse-client relationship and, 38–40
personal, 37–38
  activity, 37, 38F
preparation, 36–41
reciprocal nature of, 39
review questions, 42
student objectives, 36
to others, activity in, 42
you-messages activity in, 41
Self-esteem, self-concept and, 21. See also Self-worth
Self-identity, looking at activity, 22
Self-sufficiency, direct physical help and, 98
Self-understanding
  definition, 7
  knowing ourselves and, 22–23
Self-worth
  being fed and, 518
  direct physical help and, 98–99
  eating assistance and, 516
  self-catheterization and, 634
  self-concept and, 21
Semi-fowler's position. See Fowler's position
Sengstaken-Blakemore tube, 569F, 570
Sensations, self-awareness and, 20
Sensible water loss, 483
Sensory status, assessment of, 112–113F
Serosanguineous drainage, wound repair and, 295
Serous exudate, wound infection and, 320
Serum, osmolality, 489
Sex
  body water composition and, 483
  self-disclosure and, 36
Sexuality status, assessment of, 112F
  adjustment with ostomy, 666
Shampoo, hair care and, 400
Shampoo tray, 400
Shampooing
  hair, 401–402, 403–404
  bed, 402
  shower, 401
  sink, 401–402
Shaving, 402–403
  equipment, 400–401
Shearing force, 719
Sheepskin pads, antidecubitus, 723
Sheets, 760
Shock
  IV therapy and, 936
  speed, 936
Shoulder
  abduction of, 709–710F

  ball and socket joint, 706
  circumduction of, 709F
  depression of, 710F
  elevation of, 710F
  forward flexion of, 709F
  ROM exercises for, 708, 709F, 710F
  rotation of, 709F
Shower, shampoo in, 401
Shroud, 426, 427F
Sighing, 207
  chest therapy exercises and, 774
Silastic foam, 299
Silence. See Time and silence
Silicone gel pads, antidecubitus, 723–724
Sims position
  in bed, 719
  turning to, 734–736
Sink, shampooing in, 401
Sinus, topical medication in, 866
Siphoning, in gastrointestinal tube, 564
Sitz bath
  equipment for, 374F
  performance checklist, 382–383
  skill sequence, 379
Skin
  assessment of, 114F
  bandaging of, 454–455
  barrier properties, 359–360
  binding of, 454–455
  care of. See Skin care
  color of, 359
  fluid balance and, 489, 492
  inspection of, 869
  malnutrition and, 508T
  massage and, 446
  medication adminstration to, 880
    transdermal, 880–882
  pressure sores, 360–361
  protection of, 454–455
  structure and function of, 358–362, 362F
  water loss and, 483
Skin care
  aging skin and, 362
  bath mitts, 365F
  bathing, 362–363
  bed bath, 367–369
  cast and, 476
  client history and, 363
  creams, 366
  critical points summary, 369–370
  data base, 363–365
  ear, 361
  enteral nutritional support and, 538
  equipment, 365F
  execution, 366–369
  hyperemia, 361
  inspection in, 363–365
  introduction, 358
  learning activities, 370
  moisturizing preparations, 366
  mucous membranes, 361
  nose, 362
  palpation in, 364–365
  performance checklist, 370–371
  physical appraisal skills, 363–365
  powders, 366
  preparation, 358–366
  pressure points, 361F
  pressure sores, 360–361
  recorded data, 363
  recording
    sample narrative, 369

Skin care (cont.)
    sample POR, 369
    review questions, 370
    sense of smell in, 365
    skill sequence, 368–369
    soaps, 366
    sponges, 365
    structure and function in, 358–362, 361*F*
    student objectives, 358
    therapeutic baths, 362–363
    washcloth mitt, 365*F*
    water temperature, 366
Skinfold thickness
    calipers, 231, 233–234
    measurement of, 231, 232*F*, 233*F*
    nomogram, 233*F*, 234
    pinch test, 231
Sleep status, assessment of, 114*F*
Sling, 456, 459–460, 460*F*
Smell
    fluid balance and, 492
    in self-catheterization, 635
    in skin care, 365
    in topical medication administration, 869
    in vaginal irrigation, 412
    nonverbal communication and, 49
    of elimination, 595
    of wet sterile dressing, 345
    of wound, 297
    wound infection and, 321
Smoking
    body temperature and, 184
    wound repair and, 294
Soap
    bathing, 366
    handwashing and, 242
Soap-solution enema, 607
Society, values conflicts in, 34
Sodium bicarbonate
    bath, 363
    in oral care, 389
Soft diet, 505
Sore, pressure, 360*F*, 361*F*. *See also* Decubitus ulcer
Sound, in percussion, 174–175
Source-oriented medical record system, 144–145
Space and touch
    activities
        communication distances and comfort, 62
        personal comfort with touch, 65*F*
        personal patterns, 64
        touching and being touched, 66
    critical points summary, 66–67
    culture and, 63
    definition, 60–61
    execution, 64–65
    eye contact and, 65
    in nursing care, 64–65
    intimate distance, 61, 65
    introduction, 60–61
    message of, 63*F*
    nonprocedural touch, 61
    nursing care and, 64–65
    nursing home use of, 62–63
    nursing use of, 62–63, 63*F*, 64
    personal distance, 61, 65
    personal space, 61–62
    personal comfort level with touch, 65–66
    preparation, 61–63, 63–64
    procedural touch, 61
    proxemics and, 61
    public distance, 61
    review questions, 67
    social distance, 61, 65
    student objectives, 60
    territoriality and, 61–62
Speech, fluid balance and, 489
Speed shock, IV therapy and, 936
Sphygmomanometer, 214–217*F*
    aneroid manometer of, 214*F*, 216–217, 217*F*
    inflation system of, 214*F*, 215*F*
    isolation precautions and, 251
    mercury-gravity manometer of, 214*F*, 215–216, 216*F*
Spirometer, incentive, 780*F*
Spirometry, incentive, 778, 781
Splints, 722
Sponge
    bathing, 365
    gauze, 298
    in topical medication administration, 869
Sponge bath, in thermal application, 441
Spoon, medicine, 851
Spray-on dressing, 298–299
Sprays
    nasal, 866
    topical, 868*T*
Sputum, 775–776
    collection of, 776, 822
        airway suction, 816
Sputum specimen container, 818*F*
Squeeze bottle, in topical medication administration, 869
Stain, on cast, 476
Standing, assisting with, 697*F*
Staple suture, 311
    insertion of, 315*F*, 316
State Board Test Pool Examination, medication errors, 843
Steam sterilization, 270
Steatorrhea, 592
Stereotyping, empathy and, 13
Sterile field
    definition of, 279
    preparation of, 279–281, 280*F*
Sterile gloves. *See* Gloves, sterile
Sterile package. *See* Sterile supplies
Sterile solution, pouring of, 281–282, 282*F*
Sterile supplies, 268–284
    aseptic technique, 275–276, 284
    care of, 275
    client history and, 273
    cloth, 273
    critical points summary, 283
    data base for, 273
    definition of, 269
    disposal of, 275
    dry muslin, 273
    envelope-wrapped package, 276*F*
    equipment for, 273–275
    execution, 275–283
        guidelines for, 275–276
    glass, 274
    heat-sealed, 277–279, 278*F*
    inspection of, 273
    introduction, 269
    learning activities, 283
    methods for, 269–272
    microorganism transfer principles and, 269
    opening, 276*F*, 278*F*
    packaging of, 274
    paper, 273
    performance checklist, 284
    physical appraisal skills, 279
    plastic, 273–274
    pouring sterile solutions, 282
    preparation, 269–275
    recorded data and, 273
    recording, 283
    review questions, 283–284
    skill sequence, 277–283, 278*F*
        adding envelope-wrapped items to sterile field, 281
        adding heat-sealed items to sterile field, 281
        opening envelope-wrapped package, 277
        opening heat-sealed package, 279
        pouring sterile solutions, 282
        preparing sterile field, 279
    solutions, pouring, 281–282, 282*F*
    sterile field preparation, 279–282, 280*F*
    sterilization methods, 269–272
    sterilizing indicators, 272
    storage and handling, 273
    student objectives, 268–269
    transfer forceps, 274–275
    wrappers and containers, 273–274
Sterility
    abridged, 267
    definition of, 267–268
Sterilization
    boiling water disinfection, 271–272, 272*T*
    chemical, 271
    cold, 271
    definition of, 267
    disinfection, 271–272, 272*T*
    dry heat, 271
    gas, 270
    indicators, 272
    ionizing radiation, 271
    liquid chemical, 271
    methods, 269–272
    steam, 270
    ultraviolet radiation disinfection, 272
Steri-Strips, application of, 312*F*
Stertor, 207
Stethoscope
    bell and diaphragm chestpieces, 184*F*
    blood pressure measurement and, 217
    cleaning, 179
    components of, 178–179
    in auscultation, 178*F*
    in nasogastric intubation, 573
    isolation precautions and, 251
    maintenance of, 179
Stimulus, perception of, 2–3, 3*F*
Stockinet, in cast application, 454–475
Stockinet bandage, 456
Stocking
    elastic, 456, 460–462, 461*F*
    skill sequence, 461–462
Stomach
    distension of, in CPR, 974–975
    distension of, 565
    mucosal injury, intubation and, 565
Stool
    abnormal components of, 592
    acholic, 592
    black, 592

color of, 592
consistency of, 592
fluid balance and, 489
normal components of, 591–592
odor of, 592
red, 592
testing of, 593
Strapping tape, 300
Stratum, function of, 359–360
Strength, food consumption and, 501–502
Stress
　ciliary function and, 775
　defecation and, 590
Stress incontinence, 621
Stretch pressure, eating facilitation and, 519, 520F
Stretchers, 746
Stridor, 207
Stroke. See Cerebrovascular accident
Stroking, in massage, 447
Subclavian dressing kit, TPN and, 552
Subcutaneous injection. See Injectable medication administration, subcutaneous
Subjective data, in nursing records, 150
Sucking
　evaluation of, 518
　facilitation of, 521F
Suction
　gastrointestinal tube, 563–564
　pipeline regulator, 571, 572F
Suction system
　closed wound, 329
　portable wound, 331
Suctioning, airway. See Airway suctioning
Summarization, interview, 117
Summary, in record-keeping, 144
Sump tube, 569F, 570
Supination, 705
Supine position
　dangling and, 695
　in bed, 718, 732, 733F
　in breast examination, 420F
　turning to, 733–734, 736
Supportive and protective treatment
　bandage application, 453–464
　binder application, 453–464
　cast care, 473–480
　definition, 433
　massage, 446–453
　mechanical restraints, 464–473
　thermal applications, 433–446
Supportive devices
　cones, 722
　footboards, 722
　handrolls, 722
　sandbags, 722
　splints, 722
　trochanter rolls, 722F
Supportive intervention, 433
Suppository
　rectal, 867
　　administration of, 879F
　　skill sequence, 879–880
　vaginal, 878
Surgery
　defecation and, 590
　food consumption and, 503
　ROM exercises and, 705
　urinary catheterization and, 630
Surgical asepsis. See Asepsis, surgical
Surgivac system

in wound drainage, 331
　technique, 335F
Survival, physiological needs for, 25
Suture
　absorbable, 311
　Butterfly closures, 312, 313F
　catgut, 311
　classification of, 311
　continuous, removal of, 316
　cotton, 311
　definition of, 311–312
　interrupted, removal of, 316
　linen, 311
　monofilament, 311
　nonabsorbable, 311
　removal of. See Suture removal
　retention, 312
　silk, 311
　stainless steel wire, 311
　staple, 311
　　insertion of, 315F, 316
　synthetic, 311
Suture removal
　blanket continuous, 316
　client history and, 312–313
　critical points summary, 317
　data base, 312–313
　dressing forceps, 313
　equipment, 313
　execution, 313–315F
　inspection of, 313
　introduction, 311
　learning activities, 317
　mattress continuous, 316
　mattress interrupted, 316
　palpation in, 313
　performance checklist, 317–318
　physical appraisal skills, 313
　plain continuous, 316
　plain interrupted, 313F, 316
　preparation, 311–313, 312F, 313F
　recorded data and, 312–313
　recording
　　sample narrative, 317
　　sample POR, 317
　review questions, 317
　sets, 313
　skill sequence, 316–317
　skin, 314–315F
　student objectives, 311
　thumb forceps, 313
Swab
　catheterization and, 637
　dressing changing and, 301
　in topical medication administration, 869
　in wound culture specimen collection, 322
　injection and, 901
Swallowing
　anticholinergics and, 774
　dysfunction of, 517–518
　evaluation of, 518
　facilitation of, 520, 521F
　medication, 856
　physiology of, 517
　xylocaine and, 870
Syringe
　air removal from, 905F
　asepto, 331–332, 333F
　in oral care, 390
　bulb, 331–332, 333F
　in oral care, 390
　Carpuject, 908, 910F

common sizes, 902T
destruction of, 901, 902F
glass, 899F
hypodermic, 899F
in nasogastric intubation, 573
in nasogastric irrigation, 574
insulin, 899F
irrigating, 331–332, 333F
isolation precautions and, 251
mixing medication in, 905–906
oral medication administration, 852F
prefilled, 900
reusable glass, 899–900
selection of, 902
structure of, 898F
tuberculin, 899F
Tubex, 908, 909F
types of, 898–899F
Syringe pump, in IV therapy, 944
Systolic blood pressure, measurement of, 211–212

Tachycardia, 195
Tachypnea, 206
Tactile status, assessment of, 113F
Tape
　adhesive, 299–301F
　　in cast care, 477
　cotton cloth-backed, 300
　elastic foam, 300
　in bandaging and binding, 462
　in IV therapy, 944
　in nasogastric intubation, 573
　in wet-to-dry dressing, 352
　IV infusion and, 950F
　paper, 300
　plastic, 300
　rayon taffeta, 300
　strapping, 300
　tracheostomy and, 804
　umbilical, 804
　waterproof, 300
Tapotement, in massage, 447–448
Tapping, eating facilitation and, 519
T-binder, 456, 459
T-connector, airway suctioning and, 818
Teacher, assessment of, 134
Teaching-learning
　activities
　　analyzing client-care situation, 137–138
　　evaluation of, 138
　　examining a learning situation, 131
　　experiences with, 127
　analysis of, 130–131, 131T
　analyzing the teaching-learning task, 130, 131T
　background information in, 127–128
　characteristics of, 126–127
　client capabilities, 129–130
　client motivation, 128–129
　client-care situation and, 137–139
　commitment degree and, 134
　content of, 131–132
　critical points summary, 138
　definition of, 126
　documentation, 135
　evaluation of, 138
　execution, 135–137
　incidental, characteristics of, 127
　instructional methods and activities, 132

1044   INDEX

Teaching–learning (cont.)
  introduction, 126–127
  learner assessment, 127–130
  learner involvement, 132–133
  performance checklist, 139
  planned, 127
  preparation, 127–135, 134–135
  process, 130–134
  readiness for, 128–130
  reinforcement, 133
  review questions, 138
  self-assessment in, 134
  setting goals and objectives, 130
  situation, 134–135
  student objectives, 126
Teeth
  brushing, 391F
  decay, 386
  deciduous, 385
  malnutrition and, 508T
  structure of, 385–386
Temperature
  appraisal of. See Temperature appraisal
  assessment of, 114F
  bath, 362–363, 366
  environmental, 183
  fluid balance and, 486
  fluid deficit and, 485
  food, 509F
  heat pockets, 183F
  maximum, 183
  monitor. See Temperature monitor
  of enteral feedings, 532
  of enteral formula, 532
  of wet sterile dressing, 344
  of wound irrigation solution, 337
  thermal application and, 436
Temperature appraisal, 182–194
  axillary measurement, 189
  chemical probe thermometer for, 190–191, 191F
  client history and, 182–183
  critical points summary, 192
  data base for, 184–185
  electronic thermometer for, 190F
  equipment for, 185–187
  execution of, 187–192
  inspection in, 191
  introduction, 182
  learning activities, 192
  measurement sites, 183–184
  mercury glass thermometer in, 185F
  oral measurement, 188
  palpation in, 191
  performance checklist, 192–193
  physical appraisal skills, 185
  preparation, 182–187
  recorded data and, 182–183
  recording, 191F
  rectal measurement, 189
  review questions, 192
  scales for, 182–183
  skill sequence, 188, 189
    axillary temperature, 189
    oral temperature, 188
    rectal temperature, 189
  student objectives, 182
Temperature monitor, in electronic thermometer, 186–187
Temporal pulse, 197, 198F
Territoriality, personal space and, 61–62
Test-tube brush, tracheostomy tube and, 805

Theme, listening for, 75
Therapeutic manner, helping relationship and, 10
Therapeutic relationship, helping relationship and, 8
Therapeutic touch, 64
Therapeutic use of self, 10
Thermal application
  client history and, 437–438
  clinical uses, 437
  cold vs. hot, 437
  conduction, 434
  consensual response, 435
  contraindications, 436
  convection, 434, 440
  conversion, 434
  critical points summary, 443
  data base, 437–438
  dry vs. wet, 437
  equipment, 438F, 439F
  evaporation, 434–435, 440
  execution, 440–443
  heat lamp, 441
  heat transfer mechanisms, 434–435
  hot vs. cold, 437
  hot water, 440
  hydrocollator packs, 441–448, 448F
    skill sequence, 442–443
  ice bags, 440
  introduction, 434
  learning activities, 443–444
  moist compresses, 440–441
  performance checklist, 444–445
  physiological effects, 435–436
  preparation, 435–440
  rebound phenomenon, 435–436
  recorded data and, 437–438
  recording
    sample narrative, 443
    sample POR, 443
  review questions, 444
  sensation perception and, 436
  skill sequence, 442–443
  sponge bath, 441
  student objectives, 433–434
  systemic effects of, 436
  transfer devices, 440
  wet vs. dry, 437
Thermistor, in electronic thermometer, 186
Thermography, 434
Thermometer
  chemical probe, 187
  cleaning, 186
  electronic, 186–187
  hazards, 186
  intermittent-reading, 187
  isolation precautions and, 251
  maximum temperature, 183
  mercury glass, 185F
  Tempa-DOT, 191
  temperature monitor, 186–187
Thigh
  blood pressure measurement and, 218F, 219
  injection in, 892, 893F
"Things I love to do," values and, 32–33
Thinking, valuing, 31
Thirst, fluid balance and, 489
Thoracic pump, 973F
Throat
  sore, intubation and, 564
  topical medication in, 866, 869–870
Thrombocyte, IV, 933

Thromboembolism, bed rest and, 774
Thrombophlebitis, IV therapy and, 935–936
Through-the-needle catheter, 943F
Thumb
  opposition of, 711F
  saddle joint, 706
Tibialis pulse, 197, 198F
  measurement of, 203
Time and silence
  activities
    experiencing silence, 58
    observing silence in others, 58
    personal use of time, 57
    using silence in interactions, 59
  conveying feelings and, 57
  critical points summary, 59
  execution, 58–59
  interruptions and time, 56–57
  introduction, 56
  personal use activity, 57
  preparation, 56–58
  review questions, 59–60
  student objectives, 55–56
  use of time, 56–57, 58
  use of silence, 57–58, 59
  waiting and time, 56
Time tape
  in enteral feedings, 539F
  in IV therapy, 944
  total parenteral nutrition and, 553
Tissue
  in nasogastric intubation, 573
  isolation and, 252
Toe
  abduction, 714F
  flexion, 714F
  ROM exercises for, 708, 714F
  performance checklist, 716
Toilet adapter pan, in fluid balance assessment, 494
Tone, in percussion, 174
Tongue
  brushing of, 391–392
  displacement of, 856
  facilitated use of, 520, 521F
  function of, 385
  in swallowing, 517
  in topical medication administration, 869
  malnutrition and, 508T
  oral medication and, 856
Tongue blade
  airway suctioning and, 818
  dressing change and, 301
  in nasogastric intubation, 573
Tongue depressor, 390, 870
Tonsil, structure of, 385
Toothbrush, 387
Toothette, 387–388
Topical medication administration, 865–889
  advantages of, 866
  buccal, 866
  buccal tablets, 866
  common forms of, 868T
  critical points summary, 883
  data base for, 867–869
  dermal, 867, 868T, 880
  dermal administration of, 867
  disadvantages of, 866
  ear, 866–867, 872–874
  equipment, 869
  execution, 869–883

eye, 866–867, 874F, 877F
hormones, 867
inhalation of, 881F, 882F
inspection, 868–869
introduction, 865–866
learning activities, 883–884
mouth, 866, 869–870, 870F
nasal, 866, 870–872, 871F
optic, 866–867
otic, 866–867
performance checklist, 884–889
preparation skills, 866–869
psychologic benefit of, 865
purposes for, 866–867
record, 882–883
rectal, 879F
respiratory, 881F, 882F
review questions, 884
routes for, 866–867
skill sequence, 871–876, 878–880
  ear medications, 873–874
  eye medications, 875–876
  nasal drops, 871–872
  rectal suppository, 879–880
  vaginal medications, 878–879
student objectives, 865–889
sublingual, 866
sublingual tablets, 866
throat, 866, 870F
transdermal, 867, 880–882
vaginal, 867, 876–879, 877F, 878F
Total parenteral nutrition (TPN), 546–549
  adhesive tape in, 552–553
  administration method, 549
  administration rate, 549
  adverse reactions to, 549–550
  air embolism in, 550
  care goals, 553
  catheter insertion, 548F
  catheter sites for, 547–548
  client history and, 551
  control device, 551
  critical points summary, 556
  data base, 551
  definition of, 547
  dressing changing in, 553
  electrolyte balance and, 553
  equipment, 551–553, 552F
  execution, 553–554
  fat emulsions, 550
  flow rate maintenance, 553
  glycosuria in, 549, 553
  infection and, 549–550
  infection prevention, 553
  infusion pump for, 551
  inspection and, 551
  introduction, 547
  IV infusion equipment in, 551
  learning activities, 556–557
  malnutrition and, 481
  metabolic complications in, 550
  monitoring, 554T
  performance checklist, 557–558
  physical appraisal skills in, 551
  preparation, 547–550
  recorded data, 551
  recording
    sample narrative, 556
    sample POR, 556
  review questions, 557
  self-care, 551
  skill sequence, 554–556
    dressing change, 555–556

tubing and solution change, 554–555
solutions, 548–549
student objectives, 547
subclavian dressing kits, 552F
tubing, changing in, 553
Valsalva's maneuver and, 553
venous complications in, 550
Touch. See also Space and touch
  nonprocedural, 61
  procedural, 61
  therapeutic, 64
Tourniquet, in IV therapy, 944
Towel
  in nasogastric intubation, 573
  in nasogastric irrigation, 574
  paper
    handwashing and, 242
    sterile, 273
TPN. See Total parenteral nutrition
Tracheal dilator, 805–806
Tracheobronchoalveolar system, air movement in, 776
Tracheoesophageal fistula, tracheostomy and, 802
Tracheostomy
  adverse effects of, 801–802
  airway suctioning and, 815
  auscultation in, 804
  body temperature and, 184
  cleansing in, 809
  client care, 802–804
  complications of, 801–802
  critical points summary, 811–812
  cuff inflation and, 809–810
  data base, 804
  disadvantages of, 801
  dressing preparation, 807F
  emergency airway maintenance, 810
  equipment, 804–806
  execution, 806–811
  gauze dressing, 807F
  inspection in, 804
  introduction, 800
  learning activities, 812
  neck tape preparation, 808F
  palpation in, 804
  performance checklist, 812–814
  permanent tube
    changing a, 810
    cleansing a, 809
    performance checklist, 813–814
    skill sequence, 810
  physical appraisal skills in, 804
  physiological effects of, 803
  preparation, 800–806
  procedure, 800–801
  procedure selection, 812–813
  psychological aspects of, 803–804
  recording, 811
  review questions, 812
  routine care, 808–809
  self-care, 811
  skill sequence, 808–809
    changing permanent tube, 810–811
    routine tracheostomy, 808–809
  student objectives, 799–800
  tube. See Tracheostomy tube
  tube ties changing, 807–808
  wound care, 807
Tracheostomy mask, 803
Tracheostomy tube
  catheter insertion in, 820F
  cuffed, 804, 805F

displacement of, 802F
emphysema and, 801F
expulsion of, 802
metal, 804
obturator, 804, 805F
permanent
  changing a, 810
  performance checklist, 813–814
  skill sequence, 810–811
placement of, 801, 802
teaching suctioning for, 822–823
tie-changing, 807–808
  slit method, 808F
  square-knot method, 808
types of, 804
Tracheotomy, 800
Tranquilizer
  administration of, 843
  tracheostomy and, 803
Transactional system, 142
Transdermal medication, 867
Transderm-Nitro, 881
Transfer activities
  bed and chair
    execution, 747–749, 748F, 749F
    performance checklist, 754–755
    skill sequence, 748–749
  bed and stretcher
    execution, 749, 750F
    performance checklist, 755–756
    skill sequence, 750–752
  capability assessment, 745
  chair positioning, 745
  critical points summary, 753
  data base, 745–746
  equipment, 746–747
  execution, 747–753
  introduction, 742
  learning activities, 753–754
  mechanical lift, execution, 752
  mechanical lifters, 746F, 747
  three-person, 756
  performance checklist, 754–756
  physical appraisal skills, 746
  positioning in chair, 745
  preparation, 744–747
  recording of, 752–753
  review questions, 754
  roller bars, 746–747
  skill sequence, 748–752
    from bed to chair, 748–749
    from bed to stretcher, 750–752
    pull sheet, 750–751
    roller bar, 751
    three-person, 751–752
  stretchers, 746
  student objectives, 744
  wheelchairs, 746F
Transfer forceps, 274–275
Transfer summary, 144
  in record-keeping, 144
Transfusion, blood, 960–961
Trapeze, 692
Trauma
  fibrosis and, 705
  injection and, 896
  nail, 407–408
  of CPR, 974
  ROM exercises and, 705
Tray
  food, 508–509
    identification, 511
    serving, 512
  in IV therapy, 944–945

Tray (cont.)
  medicine, 841F
Trendelenburg position
  hypovolemic shock and, 717
  modified, 720, 721F
  regular, 720F
  reverse, 720, 721F
Triceps skinfold, in nutritional assessment, 507
Trichomonal infection, of vagina, 412
Trimethobenzamide suppository, 867
Trochanter roll, 722F, 734F
Trust
  basic needs and, 26
  definition of, 11
  experience activity, 11
  helping relationship and, 11–12
  vs. mistrust, 26
TSAR, 881
T-tube, wound drainage and, 329, 331, 334F
Tube feeding. *See* Enteral nutritional support
Tube–gauze, 456
Tuberculin syringe, 899F
Tuberculosis, isolation in, 257T, 259
Tubex syringe, 908, 909F
Tubing
  intravenous, 212
  rectal, 611
  stethoscope, 178F
Turbo–inhaler device, 882F
Turgor, fluid balance and, 488F, 492
Turning
  in bandage application
    circular, 456–457, 457F
    figure-of-eight, 458F
    recurrent, 458F
    spica, 458F
    spiral, 457F
    spiral reverse, 457F
Turning devices, 724–725
  Bradford, 724
  Circle beds, 725–726
  CircOlectric, 725
  Stryker frames, 724–725
  wedge turning frame, 725F
Turning, moving, and positioning
  antidecubitus pads, 723
  back strain and, 718
  chair, 745
  circle beds, 725–726
  CircOlectric bed, 725–726, 726F
  clients in bed, 727F, 730–737
    skill sequence, 728, 729
  critical points summary, 738
  data base, 721–722
  data base for, 721–722
  drainage collection bag, 639F
  ear medication and, 873
  equipment, 722–724
  execution, 726–732, 727–738
  eye medication and, 874–875
  flotation devices, 723–724
  Fowler's, 719, 720F
  frequency of, 721
  introduction, 717–718
  lateral, 719, 731F
    skill sequence, 732–734
    turning to, 732–734
  learning activities, 738–739
  logrolling, 737, 738F
  mealtime, 511F
  moving

    performance checklist, 739–741
    skill sequence, 728, 729
    side of bed, 728
    up in bed, 729
  nasal medication and, 871
  nutritional care and, 511F
  oral medication and, 856
  performance checklist, 739–743
  positioning
    performance checklist 741–743
    skill sequence, 732–737
      turning to lateral and supine positions, 732–734
      turning to prone and supine positions, 735–737
  preparation, 718–720, 721F
  pressure points and, 718
  prone, 718–719
    turning to, 734–736
  protective devices, 722–724
  pull sheets for, 729–730
  recording
    sample narrative, 738
    sample POR, 737–738
  rectal medication and, 879
  review questions, 739
  ROM exercises and, 706–707
  Sims, 719, 737F
    turning to, 734–736
  skill sequence, 732–736
    moving to side of bed, 728
    moving up in bed, 729
    turning lateral to supine, 732–734
    turning prone to supine, 736
    turning supine to lateral, 732–733
    turning supine to prone, 735–736
  Stryker frame for, 724–725
  student objectives, 717
  supine, 733F
    skill sequence, 732–734
    turning to, 732–734
  support devices, 722–724
  supportive devices, 722
  tissue anoxia and, 717
  to lateral position, 732–734
  to prone position, 734–736
  to side, 731
  to Sims position, 736–737
  to supine position, 732–734, 733F
  tracheostomy and, 803
  Trendelenburg, 720, 721F
    reverse, 721F
  turning
    performance checklist, 741–743
    skill sequence, 732–736
      lateral to supine, 732–734
      prone to supine, 735–736
      supine to lateral, 732–734
      supine to prone, 735–736
    up or down, 729, 731F
    urinary catheterization and, 641–642, 642F
  vaginal medication and, 876
  wedge turning frame, 725F
  with pullsheet, 729–730
  without pullsheet, 729
Tympany, in percussion, 175F

Ulcer
  definition of, 301F, 360
  formation of, 361
Ultraviolet light, skin and, 360

Ultraviolet radiation, disinfection, 272
Umbilical tape, tracheostomy tube and, 804
Unconditional positive regard. *See* Acceptance
Unconsciousness
  airway obstruction removal and, 992–994, 993F
  oral care in, 392–393, 393F
Undernutrition, 501
  definition of, 224–225
Unit–dose system
  errors and, 842
  of medication administration, 837F
Universalizing, 52
  reflection of feelings and, 85–86
Urge incontinence, 621
Urinal. *See* Bedpans and urinals
Urinary bladder. *See* Bladder
Urinary catheterization
  catheter insertion, 641–642, 642F
    anatomic landmarks for, 643F
    in female, 642F, 643F, 646–648
    in male, 644F, 648–649
    positioning, 641–642, 642F
  changing, 634
  client care, 638–640
  client history and, 635
  critical points summary, 652–653
  data base, 635
  drainage collection bag, 632
  equipment, 635–637, 636F
  execution, 638–652
  female
    insertion, 641–649
    performance checklist, 654–655
    positioning, 641–642, 642F
    skill sequence, 646–648
  in–and–out, 630
  indwelling
    long–term use of, 634
  infection
    drainage collection bag and, 632
    extraluminal route, 631F, 632
    intraluminal route, 631F, 632
    rate and, 630–631
  inspection in, 635
  instillation, 633, 649
    skill sequence, 650
  intermittent, 630
  intermittent self–, 634–635
    teaching clients, 651–652
  introduction, 629–630
  irrigation, 633, 649
  irrigation equipment, 637
    performance checklist, 656–657
    skill sequence, 650
  kits, 637
  learning activities, 653
  long–term, 634
  male
    insertion, 641–649, 644F
    performance checklist, 655–656
    skill sequence, 648–649
  palpation in, 635
  percussion in, 635
  performance checklist, 654–657
  physical appraisal skills, 635
  positioning, 641–642, 642F
  preparation, 630–637
  psychological aspects of, 633–634
  recorded data and, 635
  recording, 652
  reflux prevention and, 639–640

removal of, 651
review questions, 653
self–, intermittent, 634–635
sense of smell in, 635
  size, 630
skill sequence, 646–649
  inserting catheter: female, 646–648
  inserting catheter: male, 648–649
student objectives, 629
  types, 635, 636F
  urinary tract infection and, 630–633, 634
  prevention of, 631–632
urine specimen collection and, 640–641
Urinary incontinence care
  bladder training, 622
  catheterization for, 624–626
  clothing protection, 623
  critical points summary, 627
  data base, 623
  definition of, 620–621
  equipment, 623–624
  execution, 624–626
  external catheters, 622–623, 623–624
    applying, 625–626
    maintenance care, 626
    preparation, 625
  iatrogenic, 621
  inspection in, 623
  introduction, 620
  laundry and, 622
  learning activities, 627
  management of, 622–623
  neurogenic, 621
  odor problems, 622
  pants and pads, 624
  pelvic exercises, 622
  physical appraisal skills, 623
  preparation, 621–624
  problems associated with, 621–622
  protection, 623
  psychogenic, 621
  recording
    sample narrative, 627
    sample POR, 627
  review questions, 627
  sense of smell in, 623
  skill sequence, 626–627
  skin problems of, 622
  sociopsychological problems of, 621–622
  stress, 621
  student objectives, 620
  types of, 621
  urge, 621
Urinary system, positioning and, 717
Urinary tract infection
  catheter insertion and, 631, 632
  catheterization and, 630–633
  drainage collection bag and, 632
  extraluminal route, 631F, 632
  indwelling catheter and, 630–631
  intraluminal route, 631F, 632
  rate and, 630–631
  paraplegia and, 631
  postpartum, 631
  prevention of, 631–633
Urination. See Voiding
Urine
  acid, 632
  appraisal of, 591
  calibrated measuring container, 637
  collection bag, 632

collection procedure, 594
color of, 591
fluid balance and, 489
isolation and, 252
odor of, 591
opacity of, 591
osmolality of, 489
output of, 484
pH, 591
reflux prevention, 632, 639–640
retention of, 593
  with overflow, 593
sediment, 591
specific gravity of, 591
specimen, 640–641, 641F
  collection procedure, 594
  testing, 593–594
volume of, 484
Urine meter, 636

Vagina
  bacterial infection of, 412
  candidiasis of, 412
  environment of, 411–412
  factors affecting health of, 411–412
  infection of, 412, 867
  inspection of, 869
  irrigation of. See Vaginal irrigation
  medication administration in, 876–879, 877F
  monilial infection of, 412
  topical medication in, 867
  trichomonal infection of, 412
Vaginal irrigation, 411–416
  client history and, 412
  critical points summary, 415
  data base, 412
  douche kit, 412, 413F
  execution, 413–415, 414F
  hazards of, 414
  inspection and, 412
  introduction, 411
  irrigating bag, 412
  learning activities, 415
  performance checklist, 416
  physical appraisal skills, 412
  preparation, 411–413
  recorded data and, 412
  recording
    sample narrative, 415
    sample POR, 415
  review questions, 415
  skill sequence, 414–415
  smell and, 412
  solutions for, 413
  student objectives, 411
Vagus nerve, stimulation of, enema and, 608
Validating, reflection of content and, 80
Validation, open questions and, 92
Valsalva's maneuver
  bowel elimination and, 590
  enemas and, 597
  isometric exercises and, 692
  TPN dressing change and, 553
Value judgments, questions and, 94
Values
  actions and, 33
  activities
    "things I love to do", 32F
    values and actions, 33
    values and feelings in interaction, 33F

values and ideals, 31–32
values and irritants, 34
basic needs and, 31
behavior and, 32–33
conflicts, 34
definition of, 7, 30
development of, 31–32
feelings and, 33–34
identification of, 30–36
  critical points summary, 35
  execution, 34–35
  introduction, 30–32
  preparation, 31–34
  review questions, 35
  student objectives, 30
institutions, conflict with, 34
internalizing, 31
needs satisfaction and, 27
personal, 34
professional, 34
self-awareness of, 35
shared, 31
societal, 34
trade-offs in, 34
Valuing, 31
Vascular pressure, positioning and, 718
Vasoconstriction
  nose drops and, 866
  wet sterile dressing and, 344
Vasopressin, 866
Vastus lateralis muscle, injection in, 893, 894F
Vein, filling of, fluid balance and, 487F, 491–492, 492F
Venipuncture
  in IV push medication, 959
  performance checklist, 966–967
  site selection, 929–930
  skill sequence, 951–953
  technique, 948–953
    blood sample collection, 952–953
    starting infusion, 948–952, 949F, 950F
Venipuncture device, 934F, 942–943
Venous pressure, positionng and, 718
Ventilation
  in children, 982
  mechanics of, 974
  mouth-to-mouth, 977–978
  mouth-to-nose, 978
  mouth-to-stoma, 978
Ventrogluteal muscle, injection in, 893F
Venturi mask, 792F
Vesicle
  definition of, 360, 361F
  formation of, 361
Vesicular sounds, 776
Vial
  injection, 900, 901F
  medication removal from, 902–907, 903F, 904F, 905F
Vibration
  definition of, 779
  in postural drainage, 779
  eating facilitation and, 519, 520F
Vision, assessment of, 112–113F
Visitors, isolation and, 252
Vital signs
  blood pressure, 210–223
  fluid balance and, 486
  measurement of, 181–223
  pulse, 194–205
  respiration, 205–210
  temperature, 182–194

Vocabulary, in questioning, 92, 95
Vocal patterns, nonverbal communication and, 49
Voice
 fluency, 49
 inflection, 49
 intonation, 49
 nonverbal communication and, 48–49
 pitch, 48–49
 rate, 48
 volume, 49
Voiding
 difficulty, 592
 frequency of, drug use and, 589–590
 inducement of, 592–593
 physiological factors, 589
 psychosocial factors, 590
Volume-control container, in IV therapy, 941F

Waiting, 56
Walker
 four-point gait and, 699
 reciprocal, 694, 695F
 standard, 694
 tote bag attachment to, 699
 two-point gait and, 699F
Warmer, blood, 945
Washcloth, bathing, 365F
Water
 body composition and, 483
 deficit of, 484, 485T
 enema and, 607
 excess of, 485
 in body, 224
 in nasogastric intubation, 573
 in thermal applications, 437T
 intake and output of, 484T
 loss of, 483–484
 sources of, 483
 tepid, 440
Waterproof tape, 300
Weight, appraisal of. See Height and weight
Weight lifting, 693
Weights and measures
 abbreviations and symbols, 1013
 apothecary system of, 830
 conversion table, 831T
 household system of, 830
 in medication administration, 829–831
 metric system of, 829
 system exchanges, 830–831, 831T
Wet heat, 437
Wet kit system, in thermometer cleaning, 186
Wet sterile dressing
 client history and, 345
 critical points summary, 349
 data base, 345
 definition, 343
 equipment, 345–346
 execution, 346–348
 hazards of, 344–345
 inspection of, 345
 insulating materials, 346
 introduction, 343
 learning activities, 349
 Montgomery straps for, 345
 palpation and, 345
 performance checklist, 350
 physical appraisal skills, 345

preparation, 343–346
 recorded data and, 345
 recording
  sample narrative, 348
  sample POR, 348
 review questions, 349
 sense of smell and, 345
 skill sequence, 347–348
 student objectives, 343
 temperature recommendations, 344
Wet-to-dry dressing
 application of, 353–354
 client history and, 352
 critical points summary, 354
 data base, 352
 definition of, 351
 equipment, 353–354
 hazards, 352–353
 inspection of, 352
 introduction, 351
 learning activities, 354
 palpation and, 352
 performance checklist, 355
 physical appraisal skills, 352
 preparation of, 351–353
 recorded data and, 352
 recording
  sample narrative, 354
  sample POR, 354
 review questions, 354
 skill sequence, 353–354
 student objectives, 351
Wheelchairs, 746F
Wheezes, 775, 776–777
Wheezing, 207
Whirlpool bath, in thermal application, 440
Window, Johari, 23
Winged needle, in IV therapy, 942–943, 943F
Work, body mechanics and, 688–689
Wound
 cleansing of, 303, 304F
  closed, 292
  suction system, 329
 culture specimen collection. See Wound culture specimen collection
 definition of, 292–293
 dehiscence, 295F
 drainage. See Wound drains and irrigation
 dressings. See Dressings and wound care
 evisceration, 295F
 healing. See Wound healing
 irrigation. See Wound drains and irrigation
 open, 292
 penetrating, 293
 perforating, 293
 puncture, 293
 repair
  complications, 295F
  delayed healing, 294–295
  drainage and, 296
  drug use and, 294
  first intention in, 294F
  healing types and, 294F
  process, 293–294
  promoting factors, 296
  second intention in, 294F
  third intention in, 294F
 superficial, 293
Wound culture specimen collection

aerobic, 324–325
 anerobic, 325
 auscultation in, 322
 client history and, 322
 critical points summary, 326
 culture tubes, 322
 data base for, 322
 equipment for, 322F
 execution, 323–326
 infection characteristics and, 320–321
 infection risk, 320T
 infection sources and, 319–320, 320T
 infection treatment and, 321
 inspection in, 322
 introduction, 318–319
 learning activities, 326
 minimal inhibiting concentration test, 321
 palpation in, 322
 performance checklist, 327
 physical appraisal skills, 322
 preparation, 319–323
 recorded data and, 322
 recording
  sample narrative, 226
  sample POR, 226
 review questions, 326–327
 sensitivity, 321
 skill sequence, 224–225
  aerobic culture collection, 224–225
  anaerobic culture collection, 225
 student objectives, 318
 syringes, 322–323
Wound drains and irrigation
 auscultation and, 330–331
 basins for, 332
 client history and, 330
 critical points summary, 339
 data base, 330–331
 definition, 328
 dressings for, 332
 equipment, 331–333, 332F, 333F
 execution, 333–339, 337F, 340F
 gravity closed system of, 329
 hazards, 332–333
 inspection and, 330
 introduction, 228–229
 irrigating syringes, 331–332
 learning activity, 339–340
 open, 338–339
 open wound irrigation, 337–338
 Penrose drain, 331, 335
 performance checklist, 341–342
 physical appraisal skills, 330–331
 portable closed wound suction system, 331
 preparation, 329–338, 330–332
 recorded data and, 330
 recording
  sample narrative, 339
  sample POR, 339
 review questions, 341
 skill sequence, 336–337, 338–339
 open wound irrigation, 338–339
 Penrose drain, 336–337
 Snyder Hemovac evacuator, 332F, 338F
 Snyder Surgivac evacuator, 332F
 solutions, 332
 student objectives, 328
 surgical drains, 329–330
 T-tubes, 331
Wound healing
 complications, 295–296

delayed, 294–295
factors promoting, 296
first intention, 294F
process of, 293–294
second intention, 294F
third intention, 294F
types of, 294
Wrist
adduction, 711F
condyloid joint, 706
flexion, 711F
ROM exercises for, 708, 711F
performance checklist, 716
Written communication, 141–163
characteristics of, 141
health record use, 141–148
nursing records, 148–163

Xerostomia, saliva and, 384

Xylocaine, swallowing and, 870

Y-connector, airway suctioning and, 818, 819
You-message, self-disclosure through, 41

Z-track intramuscular injection, 917–920, 919F